OPTUM360°®

PROFESSIONAL

Current Procedural Coding Expert

CPT® codes with Medicare essentials for enhanced accuracy

2021

optum360coding.com

Notice

The *2021 Current Procedural Coding Expert, Professional Edition,* is designed to be an accurate and authoritative source of information about the CPT® coding system. Every effort has been made to verify the accuracy of the listings, and all information is believed reliable at the time of publication. Absolute accuracy cannot be guaranteed, however. This publication is made available with the understanding that the publisher is not engaged in rendering legal or other services that require a professional license.

American Medical Association Notice

Fee schedules, relative value units, conversion factors and/or related components are not assigned by the AMA, are not part of CPT, and the AMA is not recommending their use. The AMA does not directly or indirectly practice medicine or dispense medical services. The AMA assumes no liability for data contained or not contained herein.

CPT is a registered trademark of the American Medical Association.

Our Commitment to Accuracy

Optum360 is committed to producing accurate and reliable materials.

To report corrections, please email accuracy@optum.com. You can also reach customer service by calling 1.800.464.3649, option 1.

Copyright

Made in the USA

ISBN 978-1-62254-553-7

Acknowledgments

Gregory A. Kemp, MA, *Product Manager*
Stacy Perry, *Manager, Desktop Publishing*
Elizabeth Leibold, RHIT, *Subject Matter Expert*
Anita Schmidt, BS, RHIA, AHIMA-approved ICD-10-CM/PCS Trainer, *Subject Matter Expert*
LaJuana Green, RHIA, CCS, *Subject Matter Expert*
Tracy Betzler, *Senior Desktop Publishing Specialist*
Hope M. Dunn, *Senior Desktop Publishing Specialist*
Katie Russell, *Desktop Publishing Specialist*
Kate Holden, *Editor*

About the Contributors

Elizabeth Leibold, RHIT

Ms. Leibold has more than 25 years of experience in the health care profession. She has served in a variety of roles, ranging from patient registration to billing and collections, and has an extensive background in both physician and hospital outpatient coding and compliance. She has worked for large health care systems and health information management services companies, and has wide-ranging experience in facility and professional component coding, along with CPT expertise in interventional procedures, infusion services, emergency department, observation, and ambulatory surgery coding. Her areas of expertise include chart-to-claim coding audits and providing staff education to both tenured and new coding staff. She is an active member of the American Health Information Management Association (AHIMA) and West Tennessee Health Information Management Association (WTHIMA).

Anita Schmidt, BS, RHIA, AHIMA-approved ICD-10-CM/PCS Trainer

Ms. Schmidt has expertise in ICD-10-CM/PCS, DRG, and CPT with more than 15 years' experience in coding in multiple settings, including inpatient, observation, and same-day surgery. Her experience includes analysis of medical record documentation, assignment of ICD-10-CM and PCS codes, and DRG validation. She has conducted training for ICD-10-CM/PCS and electronic health record. She has also collaborated with clinical documentation specialists to identify documentation needs and potential areas for physician education. Most recently she has been developing content for resource and educational products related to ICD-10-CM, ICD-10-PCS, DRG, and CPT. Ms. Schmidt is an AHIMA-approved ICD-10-CM/PCS trainer and is an active member of the American Health Information Management Association (AHIMA) and the Minnesota Health Information Management Association.

LaJuana Green, RHIA, CCS

Ms. Green is a Registered Health Information Administrator with over 35 years of experience in multiple areas of information management. She has proven expertise in the analysis of medical record documentation, assignment of ICD-10-CM and PCS codes, DRG validation, and CPT code assignment in ambulatory surgery units and the hospital outpatient setting. Her experience includes serving as a director of a health information management department, clinical technical editing, new technology research and writing, medical record management, utilization review activities, quality assurance, tumor registry, medical library services, and chargemaster maintenance. Ms. Green is an active member of the American Health Information Management Association (AHIMA).

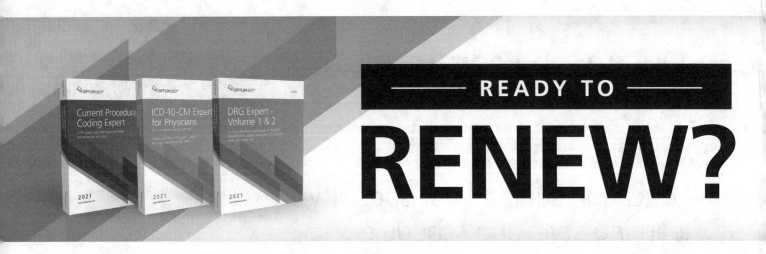

Contents

Introduction

Welcome to Optum360's *Current Procedural Coding Expert, Professional Edition*, an exciting Medicare coding and reimbursement tool and definitive procedure coding source that combines the work of the Centers for Medicare and Medicaid Services, American Medical Association, and Optum360 experts with the technical components you need for proper reimbursement and coding accuracy.

This approach to CPT® Medicare coding utilizes innovative and intuitive ways of communicating the information you need to code claims accurately and efficiently. *Includes* and *Excludes* notes, similar to those found in the ICD-10-CM manual, help determine what services are related to the codes you are reporting. Icons help you crosswalk the code you are reporting to laboratory and radiology procedures necessary for proper reimbursement. CMS-mandated icons and relative value units (RVUs) help you determine which codes are most appropriate for the service you are reporting. Add to that additional information identifying age and sex edits, ambulatory surgery center (ASC) and ambulatory payment classification (APC) indicators, and Medicare coverage and payment rule citations, and *Current Procedural Coding Expert, Professional Edition* provides the best in Medicare procedure reporting.

Current Procedural Coding Expert, Professional Edition includes the information needed to submit claims to federal contractors and most commercial payers, and is correct at the time of printing. However, CMS, federal contractors, and commercial payers may change payment rules at any time throughout the year. *Current Procedural Coding Expert, Professional Edition* includes effective codes that will not be published in the AMA's Current Procedural Terminology (CPT) book until the following year. Commercial payers will announce changes through monthly news or information posted on their websites. CMS will post changes in policy on its website at http://www.cms.gov/transmittals. National and local coverage determinations (NCDs and LCDs) provide universal and individual contractor guidelines for specific services. The existence of a procedure code does not imply coverage under any given insurance plan.

Current Procedural Coding Expert, Professional Edition is based on the AMA's Current Procedural Terminology coding system, which is copyrighted and owned by the physician organization. The CPT codes are the nation's official, Health Information Portability and Accountability Act (HIPAA) compliant code set for procedures and services provided by physicians, ambulatory surgery centers (ASCs), and hospital outpatient services, as well as laboratories, imaging centers, physical therapy clinics, urgent care centers, and others.

Getting Started with *Current Procedural Coding Expert, Professional Edition*

Current Procedural Coding Expert, Professional Edition is an exciting tool combining the most current material at the time of our publication from the AMA's CPT 2021, CMS's online manual system, the Correct Coding initiative, CMS fee schedules, official Medicare guidelines for reimbursement and coverage, the Integrated Outpatient Code Editor (I/OCE), and Optum360's own coding expertise.

These coding rules and guidelines are incorporated into more specific section notes and code notes. Section notes are listed under a range of codes and apply to all codes in that range. Code notes are found under individual codes and apply to the single code.

Material is presented in a logical fashion for those billing Medicare, Medicaid, and many private payers. The format, based on customer comments, better addresses what customers tell us they need in a comprehensive Medicare procedure coding guide.

Designed to be easy to use and full of information, this product is an excellent companion to your AMA CPT manual, and other Optum360 and Medicare resources.

For mid-year code updates, official errata changes, correction notices, and any other changes pertinent to the information in *Current Procedural Coding Expert, Professional Edition*, see our product update page at https://www.optum360coding.com/ProductUpdates/. The password for 2021 is PROCEDURE2021.

Note: The AMA releases code changes quarterly as well as errata or corrections to CPT codes and guidelines and posts them on their web site. Some of these changes may not appear in the AMA's CPT book until the following year. *Current Procedural Coding Expert, Professional Edition* incorporates the most recent errata or release notes found on the AMA's web site at our publication time, including new, revised and deleted codes. *Current Procedural Coding Expert, Professional Edition* identifies these new or revised codes from the AMA website errata or release notes with an icon similar to the AMA's current new ● and revised ▲ icons. For purposes of this publication, new CPT codes and revisions that won't be in the AMA book until the next edition are indicated with a ● and a ▲ icon. For the next year's edition of *Current Procedural Coding Expert, Professional Edition*, these codes will appear with standard black new or revised icons, as appropriate, to correspond with those changes as indicated in the AMA's CPT book. CPT codes that were new for 2020 and appeared in the 2020 *Current Procedural Coding Expert, Professional Edition* but did not appear in the AMA's CPT code book until 2021 are identified in appendix B as "Web Release New and Revised Codes."

General Conventions

Many of the sources of information in this book can be determined by color.

- All CPT codes and descriptions and the Evaluation and Management guidelines from the American Medical Association are in **black text**.
- Includes, Excludes, and other notes appear in **blue text**. The resources used for this information are a variety of Medicare policy manuals, the *National Correct Coding Initiative Policy Manual* (NCCI), AMA resources and guidelines, and specialty association resources and our Optum360 clinical experts.

Resequencing of CPT Codes

The American Medical Association (AMA) uses a numbering methodology of resequencing, which is the practice of displaying codes outside of their numerical order according to the description relationship. According to the AMA, there are instances in which a new code is needed within an existing grouping of codes but an unused code number is not available. In these situations, the AMA will resequence the codes. In other words, it will assign a code that is not in numeric sequence with the related codes. However, the code and description will appear in the CPT manual with the other related codes.

An example of resequencing from *Current Procedural Coding Expert, Professional Edition* follows:

	21555	**Excision, tumor, soft tissue of neck or anterior thorax, subcutaneous; less than 3 cm**
#	**21552**	**3 cm or greater**
	21556	**Excision, tumor, soft tissue of neck or anterior thorax, subfascial (eg, intramuscular); less than 5 cm**
#	**21554**	**5 cm or greater**

In *Current Procedural Coding Expert, Professional Edition* the resequenced codes are listed twice. They appear in their resequenced position as shown above as well as in their original numeric position with a note indicating that the code is out of numerical sequence and where it can be found. (See example below.)

21554 **Resequenced code. See code following 21556.**

This differs from the AMA CPT book, in which the coder is directed to a code range that contains the resequenced code and description, rather than to a specific location.

Resequenced codes will appear in brackets in the headers, section notes, and code ranges. For example:

27327-27339 [27337, 27339] Excision Soft Tissue Tumors Femur/Knee. Codes [27337, 27339] are included in section 27327-27339 in their resequenced positions.

Code also toxoid/vaccine (90476-90749 [90620, 90621, 90625, 90630, 90644, 90672, 90673, 90674, 90750, 90756])

This shows codes 90620, 90621, 90625, 90630, 90644, 90672, 90673, 90674, 90750, and 90756 are resequenced in this range of codes.

Code Ranges for Medicare Billing

Appendix E identifies all resequenced CPT codes. Optum360 will display the resequenced coding as assigned by the AMA in its CPT products so that the user may understand the code description relationships.

Each particular group of CPT codes in *Current Procedural Coding Expert, Professional Edition* is organized in a more intuitive fashion for Medicare billing, being grouped by the Medicare rules and regulations as found in the official CMS online manuals that govern payment of these particular procedures and services, as in this example:

99221-99233 Inpatient Hospital Visits: Initial and Subsequent
CMS: 100-4,11,40.1.3 Independent Attending Physician Services; 100-4,12,100.1.1 Teaching Physicians E/M Services; 100-4,12,30.6.10 Consultation Services; 100-4,12,30.6.15.1 Prolonged Services With Direct Face-to-Face Patient Contact; 100-4,12,30.6.4 Services Furnished Incident to Physician's Service; 100-4,12,30.6.9 Hospital Visit and Critical Care on Same Day

Icons

● **New Codes**
Codes that have been added since the last edition of the AMA CPT book was printed.

▲ **Revised Codes**
Codes that have been revised since the last edition of the AMA CPT book was printed.

● **New Web Release**
Codes that are new for the current year but will not be in the AMA CPT book until 2022.

▲ **Revised Web Release**
Codes that have been revised for the current year, but will not be in the AMA CPT book until 2022.

Resequenced Codes
Codes that are out of numeric order but apply to the appropriate category.

★ **Telemedicine Services**
Codes that may be reported for telemedicine services. Modifier 95 must be appended to code.

❍ **Reinstated Code**
Codes that have been reinstated since the last edition of the book was printed.

Pink Color Bar—Not Covered by Medicare
Services and procedures identified by this color bar are never covered benefits under Medicare. Services and procedures that are not covered may be billed directly to the patient at the time of the service.

Gray Color Bar—Unlisted Procedure
Unlisted CPT codes report procedures that have not been assigned a specific code number. An unlisted code delays payment due to the extra time necessary for review.

Green Color Bar—Resequenced Codes
Resequenced codes are codes that are out of numeric sequence—they are indicated with a green color bar. They are listed twice, in their resequenced position as well as in their original numeric position with a note that the code is out of numerical sequence and where the resequenced code and description can be found.

INCLUDES **Includes notes**
Includes notes identify procedures and services that would be bundled in the procedure code. These are derived from AMA, CMS, NCCI, and Optum360 coding guidelines. This is not meant to be an all-inclusive list.

EXCLUDES **Excludes notes**
Excludes notes may lead the user to other codes. They may identify services that are not bundled and may be separately reported, OR may lead the user to another more appropriate code. These are derived from AMA, CMS, NCCI, and Optum360 coding guidelines. This is not meant to be an all-inclusive list.

Code Also This note identifies an additional code that should be reported with the service and may relate to another CPT code or an appropriate HCPCS code(s) that should be reported along with the CPT code when appropriate.

Code First Found under add-on codes, this note identifies codes for primary procedures that should be reported first, with the add-on code reported as a secondary code.

Laboratory/Pathology Crosswalk
This icon denotes CPT codes in the laboratory and pathology section of CPT that may be reported separately with the primary CPT code.

Radiology Crosswalk
This icon denotes codes in the radiology section that may be used with the primary CPT code being reported.

TC **Technical Component Only**
Codes with this icon represent only the technical component (staff and equipment costs) of a procedure or service. Do not use either modifier 26 (professional component) or TC (technical component) with these codes.

26 **Professional Component**
Only codes with this icon represent the physician's work or professional component of a procedure or service. Do not use either modifier 26 (professional component) or TC (technical component) with these codes.

50 **Bilateral Procedure**
This icon identifies codes that can be reported bilaterally when the same surgeon provides the service for the same patient on the same date. Medicare allows payment for both procedures at 150 percent of the usual amount for one procedure. The modifier does not apply to bilateral procedures inclusive to one code.

80 **Assist-at-Surgery Allowed**
Services noted by this icon are allowed an assistant at surgery with a Medicare payment equal to 16 percent of the allowed amount for the global surgery for that procedure. No documentation is required.

80 **Assist-at-Surgery Allowed with Documentation**
Services noted by this icon are allowed an assistant at surgery with a Medicare payment equal to 16 percent of the allowed amount for the global surgery for that procedure. Documentation is required.

\+ **Add-on Codes**
This icon identifies procedures reported in addition to the primary procedure. The icon "**+**" denotes add-on codes. An add-on code is neither a stand-alone code nor subject to multiple procedure rules since it describes work in addition to the primary procedure.

According to Medicare guidelines, add-on codes may be identified in the following ways:

- The code is found on Change Request (CR) 7501 or successive CRs as a Type I, Type II, or Type III add-on code.

- The add-on code most often has a global period of "ZZZ" in the Medicare Physician Fee Schedule Database.
- The code is found in the CPT book with the icon "+" appended. Add-on code descriptors typically include the phrases "each additional" or "(List separately in addition to primary procedure)."

(50) **Optum Modifier 50 Exempt**
Codes identified by this icon indicate that the procedure should not be reported with modifier 50 (Bilateral procedures).

⊘ **Modifier 51 Exempt**
Codes identified by this icon indicate that the procedure should not be reported with modifier 51 (Multiple procedures).

(51) **Optum Modifier 51 Exempt**
Codes identified by this Optum360 icon Indicate that the procedure should not be reported with modifier 51 (Multiple procedures). Any code with this icon is backed by official AMA guidelines but was not identified by the AMA with their modifier 51 exempt icon.

Correct Coding Initiative (CCI)
Current Procedural Coding Expert, Professional Edition identifies those codes with corresponding CCI edits. The CCI edits define correct coding practices that serve as the basis of the national Medicare policy for paying claims. The code noted is the major service/procedure. The code may represent a column 1 code within the column 1/column 2 correct coding edits table or a code pair that is mutually exclusive of each other.

CLIA Waived Test
This symbol is used to distinguish those laboratory tests that can be performed using test systems that are waived from regulatory oversight established by the Clinical Laboratory Improvement Amendments of 1988 (CLIA). The applicable CPT code for a CLIA waived test may be reported by providers who perform the testing but do not hold a CLIA license.

(63) **Modifier 63 Exempt**
This icon identifies procedures performed on infants that weigh less than 4 kg. Due to the complexity of performing procedures on infants less than 4 kg, modifier 63 may be added to the surgery codes to inform the payers of the special circumstances involved.

A2–Z3 **ASC Payment Indicators**
This icon identifies ASC status payment indicators. They indicate how the ASC payment rate was derived and/or how the procedure, item, or service is treated under the revised ASC payment system. For more information about these indicators and how they affect billing, consult Optum360's *Revenue Cycle Pro*.

A2 Surgical procedure on ASC list in 2007; payment based on OPPS relative payment weight.

B5 Alternative code may be available; no payment made.

Deleted/discontinued code; no payment made.

F4 Corneal tissue acquisition; hepatitis B vaccine; paid at reasonable cost.

G2 Non-office-based surgical procedure added in CY 2008 or later; payment based on OPPS relative payment weight.

H2 Brachytherapy source paid separately when provided integral to a surgical procedure on ASC list; payment based on OPPS rate.

J7 OPPS pass-through device paid separately when provided integral to a surgical procedure on ASC list; payment contractor-priced.

J8 Device-intensive procedure; paid at adjusted rate.

K2 Drugs and biologicals paid separately when provided integral to a surgical procedure on ASC list; payment based on OPPS rate.

K7 Unclassified drugs and biologicals; payment contractor-priced.

L1 Influenza vaccine; pneumococcal vaccine. Packaged item/service; no separate payment made.

L6 New technology intraocular lens (NTIOL); special payment.

N1 Packaged service/item; no separate payment made.

P2 Office-based surgical procedure added to ASC list in CY 2008 or later with MPFS nonfacility practice expense (PE) RVUs; payment based on OPPS relative payment weight.

P3 Office-based surgical procedure added to ASC list in CY 2008 or later with MPFS nonfacility PE RVUs; payment based on MPFS nonfacility PE RVUs.

R2 Office-based surgical procedure added to ASC list in CY 2008 or later without MPFS nonfacility PE RVUs; payment based on OPPS relative payment weight.

Z2 Radiology or diagnostic service paid separately when provided integral to a surgical procedure on ASC list; payment based on OPPS relative payment weight.

Z3 Radiology or diagnostic service paid separately when provided integral to a surgical procedure on ASC list; payment based on MPFS nonfacility PE RVUs.

A **Age Edit**
This icon denotes codes intended for use with a specific age group, such as neonate, newborn, pediatric, and adult. This edit is based on age specifications in the CPT code descriptors, the product/service represented by the code *may* have age restrictions, and/or updates from the Integrated Outpatient Code Editor (I/OCE). Carefully review the code description to ensure the code you report most appropriately reflects the patient's age.

M **Maternity**
This icon identifies procedures that by definition should be used only for maternity patients generally between 9 and 64 years of age based on CMS I/OCE designations.

♀ **Female Only**
This icon identifies procedures designated by CMS for females only based on CMS I/OCE designations.

♂ **Male Only**
This icon identifies procedures designated by CMS for males only based on CMS I/OCE designations.

Facility RVU
This icon precedes the facility RVU from CMS's 2018 physician fee schedule (PFS). It can be found under the code description.

New codes include no RVU information.

Nonfacility RVU
This icon precedes the nonfacility RVU from CMS's 2018 PFS. It can be found under the code description.

New codes include no RVU information.

FUD: Global days are sometimes referred to as "follow-up days" or FUDs. The global period is the time following surgery during which routine care by the physician is considered postoperative and included in the surgical fee. Office visits or other routine care related to the original surgery cannot be separately reported if provided during the global period. The statuses are:

000 No follow-up care included in this procedure

010 Normal postoperative care is included in this procedure for ten days

090 Normal postoperative care is included in the procedure for 90 days

MMM Maternity codes; usual global period does not apply

XXX The global concept does not apply to the code

YYY The carrier is to determine whether the global concept applies and establishes postoperative period, if appropriate, at time of pricing

ZZZ The code is related to another service and is always included in the global period of the other service

CMS: This notation indicates that there is a specific CMS guideline pertaining to this code in the CMS Online Manual System which includes the internet-only manual (IOM) *National Coverage Determinations Manual* (NCD). These CMS sources present the rules for submitting these services to the federal government or its contractors and a link to the IOMs is included in appendix G of this book.

AMA: This indicates discussion of the code in the American Medical Association's *CPT Assistant* newsletter. Use the citation to find the correct issue. This includes citations for the current year and the preceding six years. In the event no citations can be found during this time period, the most recent citations that can be found are used.

⁄ **Drug Not Approved by FDA**
The AMA CPT Editorial Panel is publishing new vaccine product codes prior to Food and Drug Administration approval. This symbol indicates which of these codes are pending FDA approval at press time.

[A]–[Y] **OPPS Status Indicators (OPSI)**
Status indicators identify how individual CPT codes are paid or not paid under the latest available hospital outpatient prospective payment system (OPPS). The same status indicator is assigned to all the codes within an ambulatory payment classification (APC). Consult your payer or other resource to learn which CPT codes fall within various APCs.

[A] Services furnished to a hospital outpatient that are paid under a fee schedule or payment system other than OPPS. For example:
- Ambulance services
- Separately payable clinical diagnostic laboratory services
- Separately payable non-implantable prosthetics and orthotics
- Physical, occupational, and speech therapy
- Diagnostic mammography
- Screening mammography

[B] Codes that are not recognized by OPPS when submitted on an outpatient hospital Part B bill type (12x and 13x)

[C] Inpatient procedures

[D] Discontinued codes

[E] Items, codes, and services:
- Not covered by any Medicare outpatient benefit category
- Statutorily excluded by Medicare
- Not reasonable and necessary

[NC] Items, codes, and services for which pricing information and claims data are not available

[F] Corneal tissue acquisition; certain CRNA services and hepatitis B vaccines

[G] Pass-through drugs and biologicals

[H] Pass-through device categories

[J1] Hospital Part B services paid through a comprehensive APC

[J2] Hospital Part B services that may be paid through a comprehensive APC

[K] Nonpass-through drugs and nonimplantable biologicals, including therapeutic radiopharmaceuticals

[L] Influenza vaccine; pneumococcal pneumonia vaccine

[M] Items and services not billable to the MAC

[N] Items and services packaged into APC rates

[P] Partial hospitalization

[Q1] STV-packaged codes

[Q2] T-packaged codes

[Q3] Codes that may be paid through a composite APC

[Q4] Conditionally packaged laboratory tests

[R] Blood and blood products

[S] Procedure or service, not discounted when multiple

[T] Procedure or service, multiple procedure reduction applies

[U] Brachytherapy sources

[V] Clinic or emergency department visit

[Y] Nonimplantable durable medical equipment

Appendixes

Appendix A: Modifiers—This appendix identifies modifiers. A modifier is a two-position alpha or numeric code that is appended to a CPT or HCPCS code to clarify the services being billed. Modifiers provide a means by which a service can be altered without changing the procedure code. They add more information, such as anatomical site, to the code. In addition, they help eliminate the appearance of duplicate billing and unbundling. Modifiers are used to increase the accuracy in reimbursement and coding consistency, ease editing, and capture payment data.

Appendix B: New, Revised, and Deleted Codes—This is a list of new, revised, and deleted CPT codes for the current year. This appendix also includes a list of web release new and revised codes, which indicate official code changes in *Current Procedural Coding Expert, Professional Edition* that will not be in the CPT code book until the following year.

Appendix C: Evaluation and Management Extended Guidelines—This appendix presents an overview of evaluation and management (E/M) services that augment the official AMA CPT E/M services. It includes tables that distinguish documentation components of each E/M code and the federal documentation guidelines (1995 and 1997) currently in use by the Centers for Medicare and Medicaid Services (CMS).

Appendix D: Crosswalk of Deleted Codes—This appendix is a cross-reference from a deleted CPT code to an active code when one is available. The deleted code cross-reference will also appear under the deleted code description in the tabular section of the book.

Appendix E: Resequenced Codes—This appendix contains a list of codes that are not in numeric order in the book. AMA resequenced some of the code numbers to relocate codes in the same category but not in numeric sequence. In addition to the list of codes, this appendix provides the page number where the resequenced code may be found..

Appendix F: Add-on, Optum Modifier 50 Exempt, Modifier 51 Exempt, Optum Modifier 51 Exempt, Modifier 63 Exempt, and Modifier 95 Telemedicine Services—This list includes add-on codes that cannot be reported alone, codes that are exempt from modifiers 50 and 51, codes that should not be reported with modifier 63, and codes identified by the ★ icon to which modifier 95 may be appended when the service is provided as a synchronous telemedicine service.

Appendix G: Medicare Internet-only Manual (IOMs)—Previously, this appendix contained a verbatim printout of the Medicare Internet-only Manual references pertaining to specific codes. This appendix now contains a link to the IOMs on the Centers for Medicare and Medicaid Services website. The IOM references applicable to specific codes can still be found at the code level. For example:

93784-93790 Ambulatory Blood Pressure Monitoring
CMS: 100-3,20.19 Ambulatory Blood Pressure Monitoring (20.19); 100-4,32,10.1 Ambulatory Blood Pressure Monitoring Billing Requirements

Appendix H: Quality Payment Program (QPP)—Previously, this appendix contained lists of the numerators and denominators applicable to the Medicare PQRS. However, with the implementation of the Quality Payment Program (QPP) mandated by passage of the Medicare Access and Chip Reauthorization Act (MACRA) of 2015, the PQRS system will be obsolete. This appendix now contains information pertinent to that legislation as well as a brief overview of the proposed changes for the following year.

Appendix I: Medically Unlikely Edits—This appendix contains the published medically unlikely edits (MUEs). These edits establish maximum daily allowable units of service. The edits will be applied to the services provided to the same patient, for the same CPT code, on the same date of service when billed by the same provider. Included are the physician and facility edits.

Appendix J: Inpatient-Only Procedures—This appendix identifies services with the status indicator "C." Medicare will not pay an OPPS hospital or ASC when these procedures are performed on a Medicare patient as an outpatient. Physicians should refer to this list when scheduling Medicare patients for surgical procedures. CMS updates this list quarterly.

Appendix K: Place of Service and Type of Service—This appendix contains lists of place-of-service codes that should be used on professional claims and type-of-service codes used by the Medicare Common Working File.

Appendix L: Multianalyte Assays with Algorithmic Analyses —This appendix lists the administrative codes for multianalyte assays with algorithmic analyses. The AMA updates this list three times a year.

Appendix M: Glossary—This appendix contains general terms and definitions as well as those that would apply to or be helpful for billing and reimbursement.

Appendix N: Listing of Sensory, Motor, and Mixed Nerves—This appendix lists a summary of each sensory, motor, and mixed nerve with its appropriate nerve conduction study code.

Note: All data current as of November 12, 2020.

Anatomical Illustrations

Body Planes and Movements

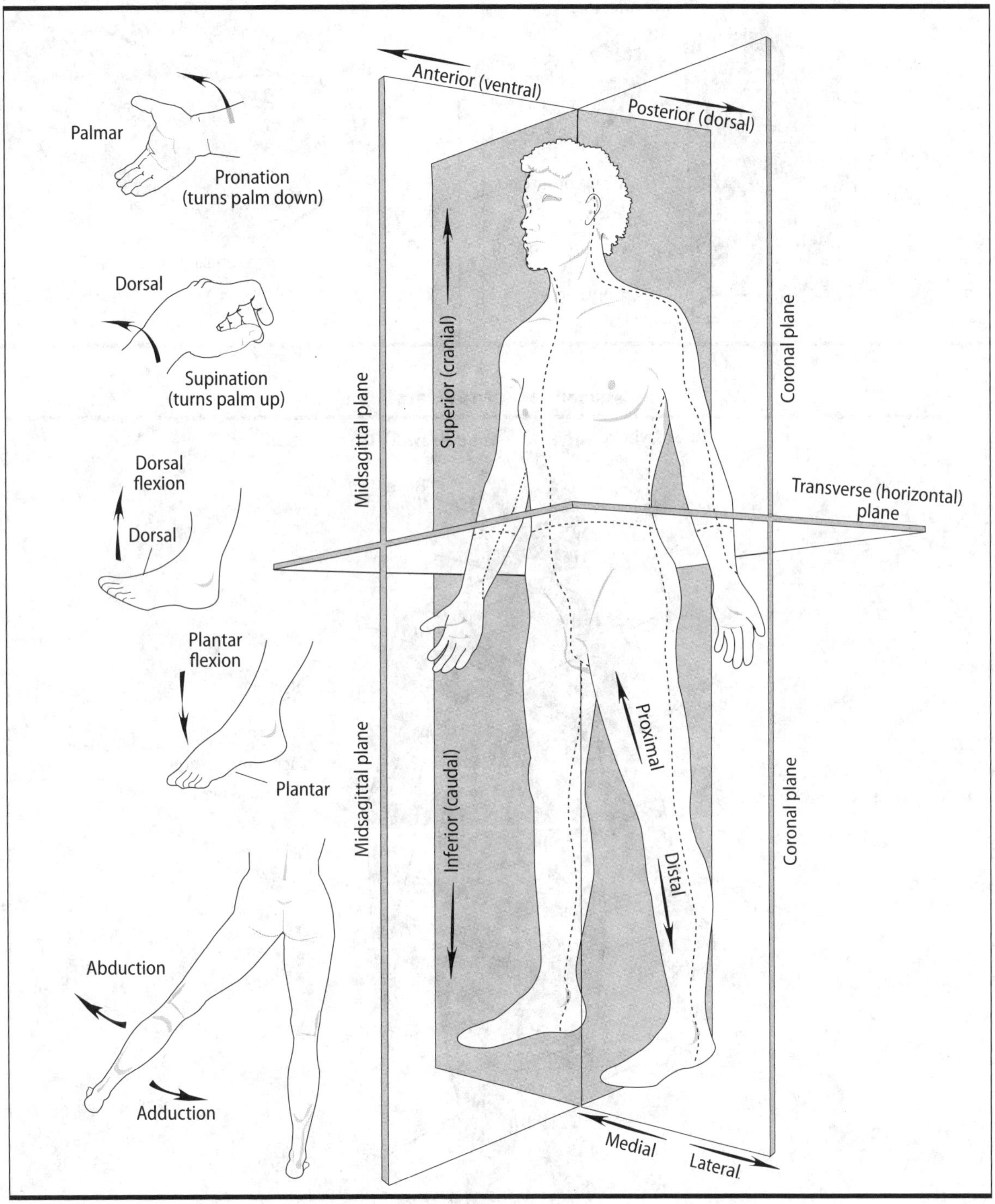

Integumentary System

Skin and Subcutaneous Tissue

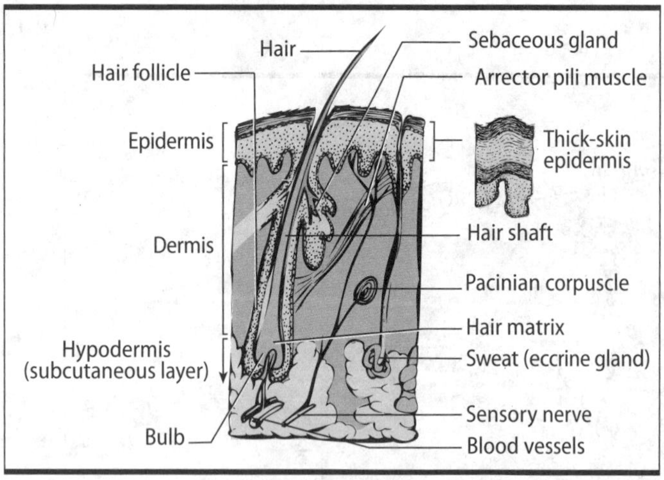

Nail Anatomy

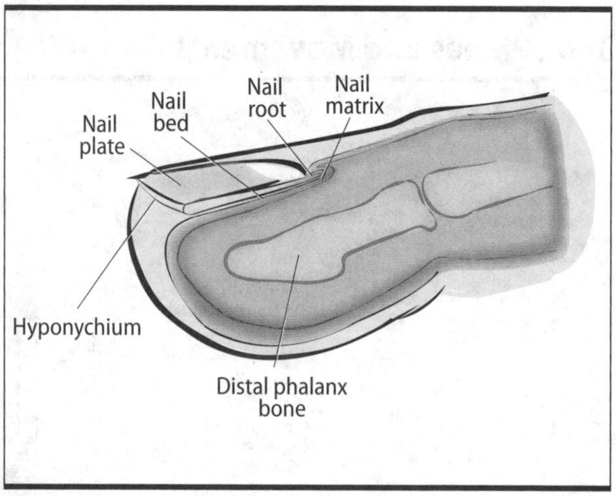

Assessment of Burn Surface Area

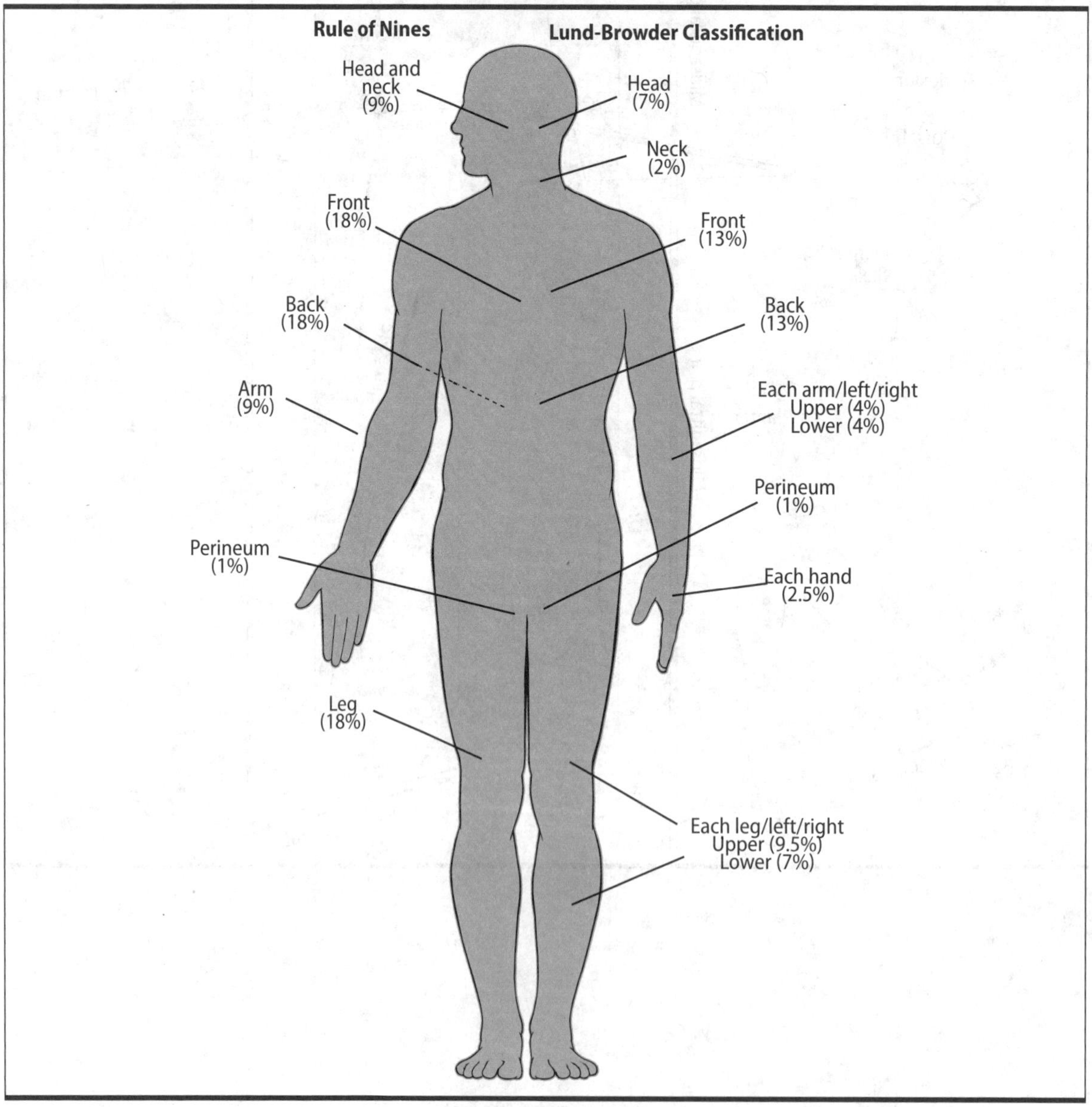

Musculoskeletal System

Bones and Joints

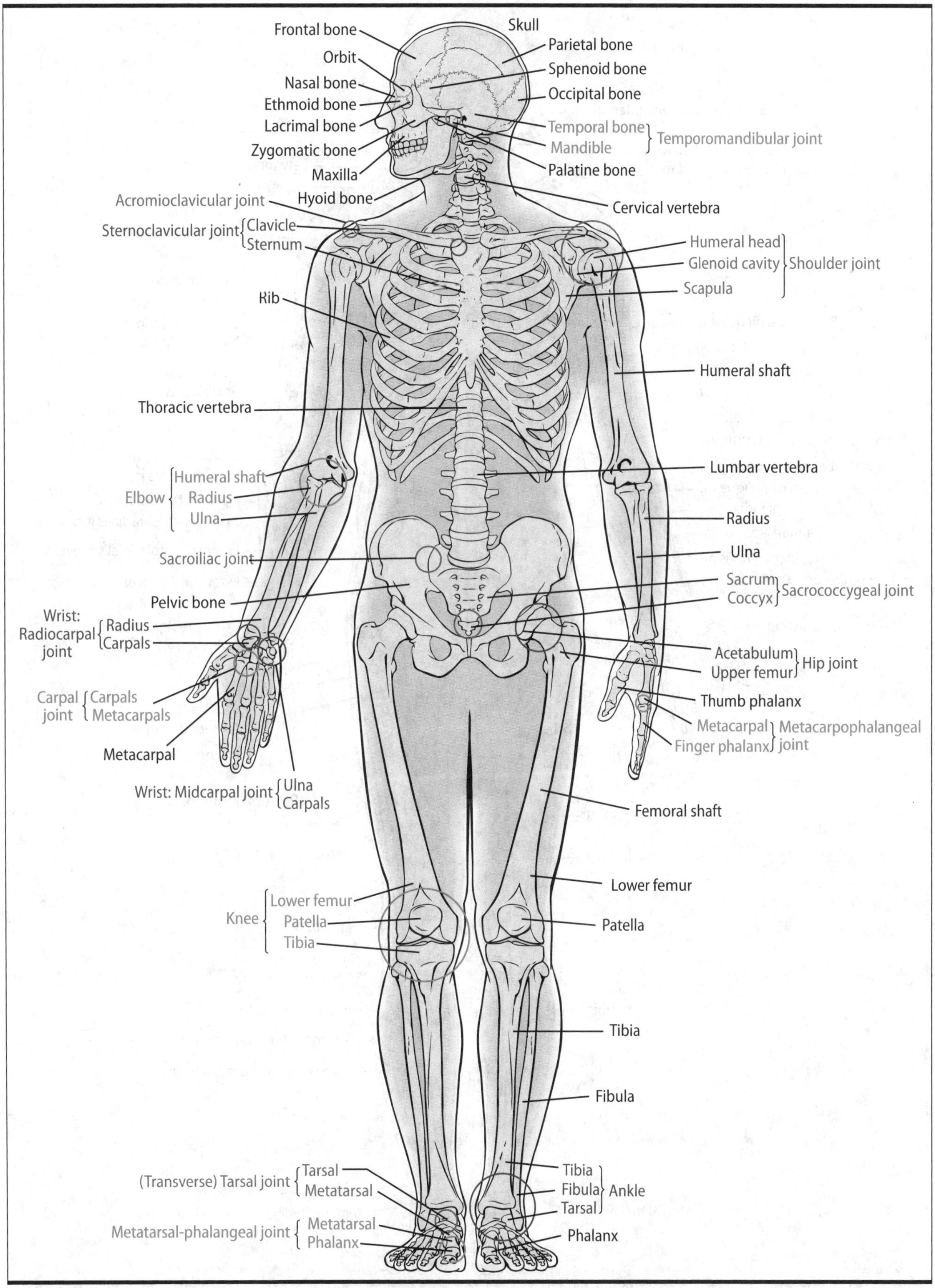
Frontal bone
Skull
Parietal bone
Orbit
Sphenoid bone
Nasal bone
Occipital bone
Ethmoid bone
Lacrimal bone
Temporal bone
Mandible
Temporomandibular joint
Zygomatic bone
Palatine bone
Maxilla
Acromioclavicular joint
Hyoid bone
Cervical vertebra
Sternoclavicular joint
Clavicle
Sternum
Humeral head
Glenoid cavity
Shoulder joint
Scapula
Rib
Humeral shaft
Thoracic vertebra
Lumbar vertebra
Elbow
Humeral shaft
Radius
Ulna
Radius
Ulna
Sacroiliac joint
Sacrum
Coccyx
Sacrococcygeal joint
Pelvic bone
Wrist: Radiocarpal joint
Radius
Carpals
Acetabulum
Upper femur
Hip joint
Thumb phalanx
Carpal joint
Carpals
Metacarpals
Metacarpal
Finger phalanx
Metacarpophalangeal joint
Metacarpal
Wrist: Midcarpal joint
Ulna
Carpals
Femoral shaft
Knee
Lower femur
Patella
Tibia
Lower femur
Patella
Tibia
Fibula
(Transverse) Tarsal joint
Tarsal
Metatarsal
Tibia
Fibula
Tarsal
Ankle
Metatarsal-phalangeal joint
Metatarsal
Phalanx
Phalanx

Muscles

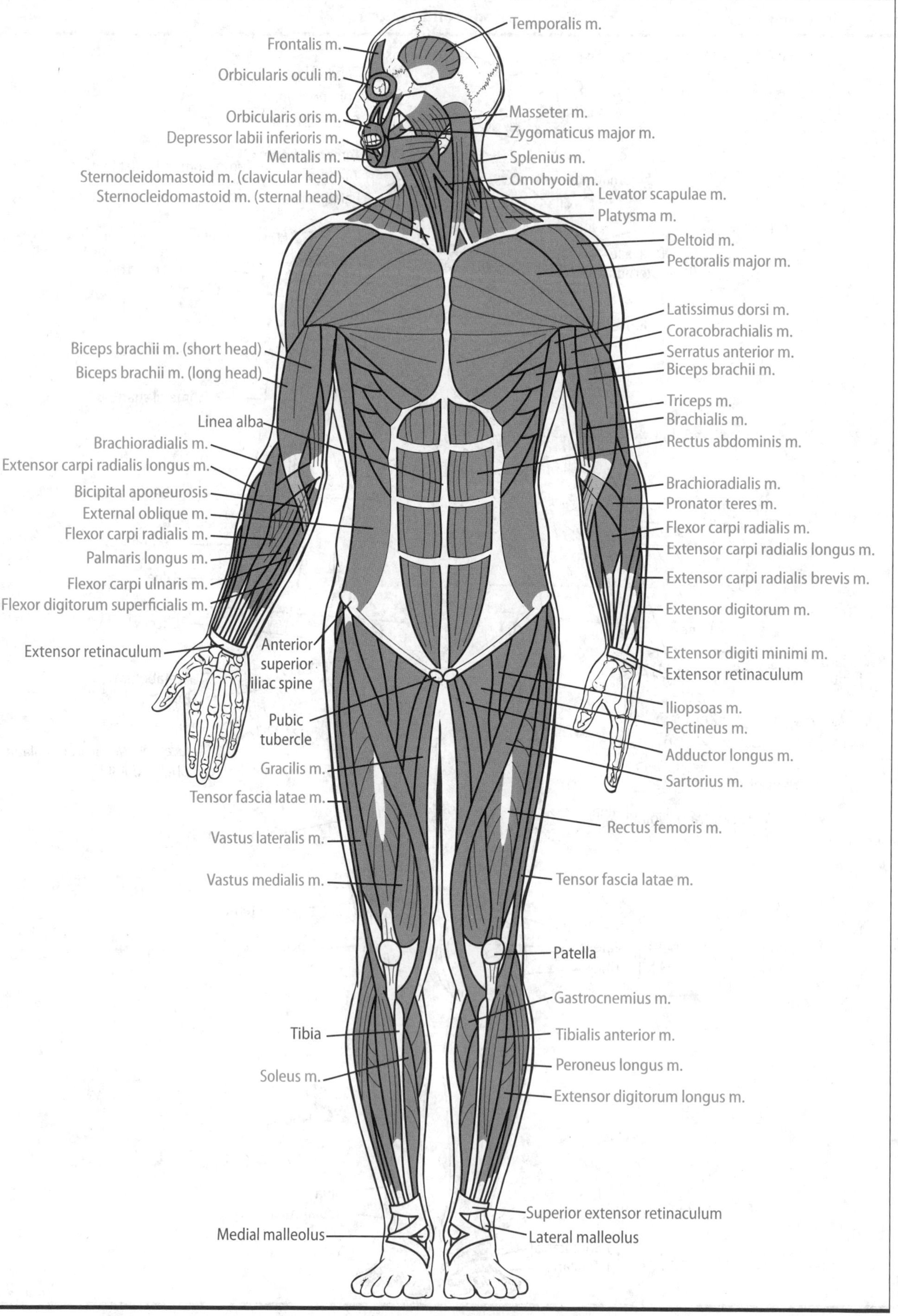
Temporalis m.
Frontalis m.
Orbicularis oculi m.
Orbicularis oris m.
Depressor labii inferioris m.
Mentalis m.
Sternocleidomastoid m. (clavicular head)
Sternocleidomastoid m. (sternal head)
Masseter m.
Zygomaticus major m.
Splenius m.
Omohyoid m.
Levator scapulae m.
Platysma m.
Deltoid m.
Pectoralis major m.
Latissimus dorsi m.
Coracobrachialis m.
Serratus anterior m.
Biceps brachii m.
Biceps brachii m. (short head)
Biceps brachii m. (long head)
Triceps m.
Brachialis m.
Linea alba
Rectus abdominis m.
Brachioradialis m.
Extensor carpi radialis longus m.
Bicipital aponeurosis
External oblique m.
Flexor carpi radialis m.
Palmaris longus m.
Flexor carpi ulnaris m.
Flexor digitorum superficialis m.
Brachioradialis m.
Pronator teres m.
Flexor carpi radialis m.
Extensor carpi radialis longus m.
Extensor carpi radialis brevis m.
Extensor digitorum m.
Extensor retinaculum
Anterior superior iliac spine
Extensor digiti minimi m.
Extensor retinaculum
Iliopsoas m.
Pectineus m.
Pubic tubercle
Adductor longus m.
Gracilis m.
Sartorius m.
Tensor fascia latae m.
Rectus femoris m.
Vastus lateralis m.
Vastus medialis m.
Tensor fascia latae m.
Patella
Gastrocnemius m.
Tibia
Tibialis anterior m.
Peroneus longus m.
Soleus m.
Extensor digitorum longus m.
Superior extensor retinaculum
Medial malleolus
Lateral malleolus

Head and Facial Bones

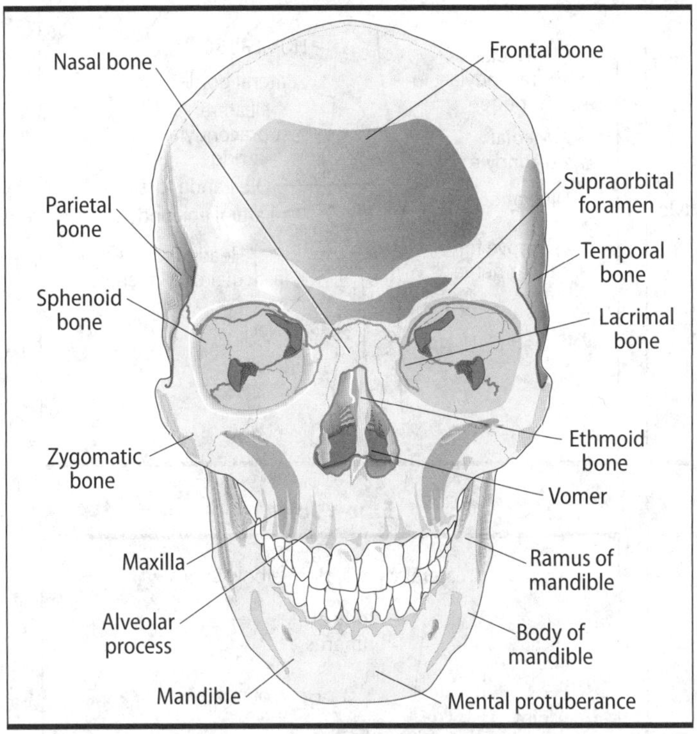
Nasal bone
Frontal bone
Parietal bone
Supraorbital foramen
Temporal bone
Sphenoid bone
Lacrimal bone
Ethmoid bone
Zygomatic bone
Vomer
Maxilla
Ramus of mandible
Alveolar process
Body of mandible
Mandible
Mental protuberance

Nose

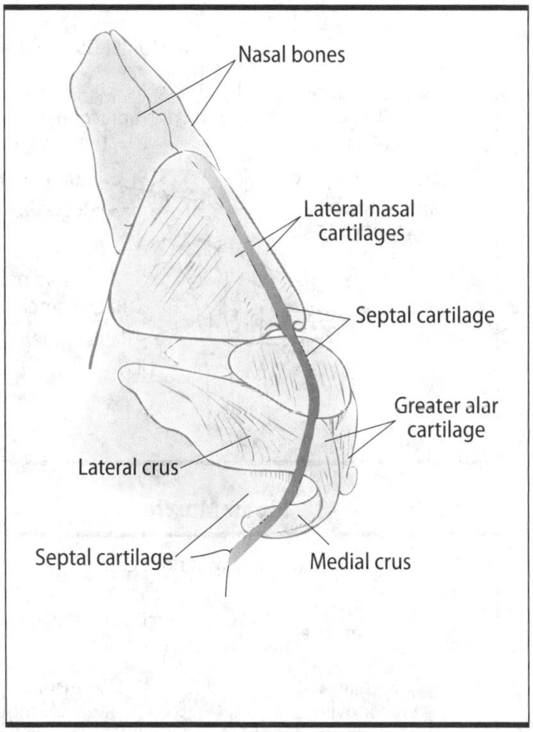
Nasal bones
Lateral nasal cartilages
Septal cartilage
Greater alar cartilage
Lateral crus
Septal cartilage
Medial crus

Shoulder (Anterior View)

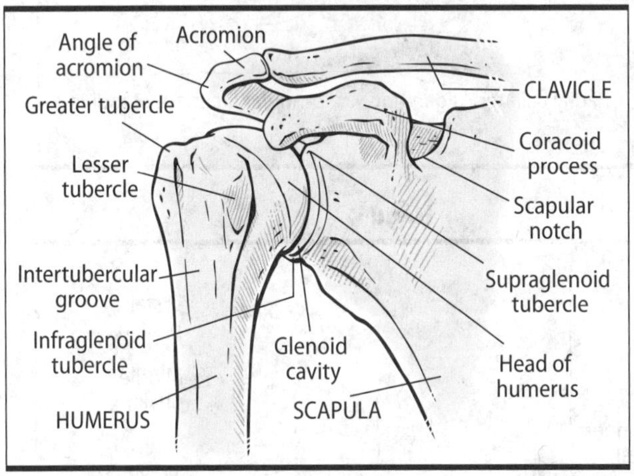
Angle of acromion
Acromion
CLAVICLE
Greater tubercle
Coracoid process
Lesser tubercle
Scapular notch
Intertubercular groove
Supraglenoid tubercle
Infraglenoid tubercle
Glenoid cavity
Head of humerus
HUMERUS
SCAPULA

Shoulder (Posterior View)

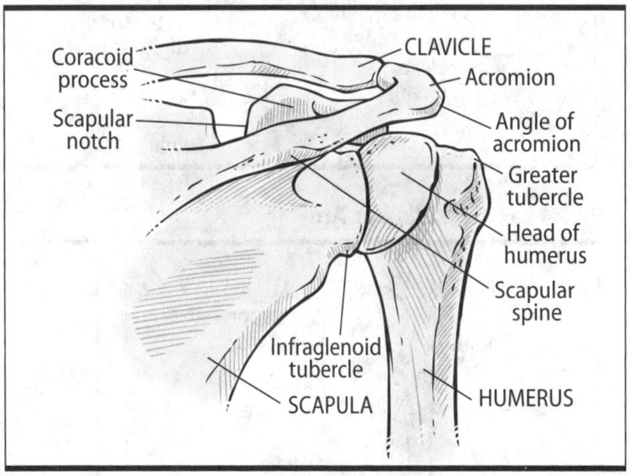
Coracoid process
CLAVICLE
Acromion
Scapular notch
Angle of acromion
Greater tubercle
Head of humerus
Scapular spine
Infraglenoid tubercle
SCAPULA
HUMERUS

Shoulder Muscles

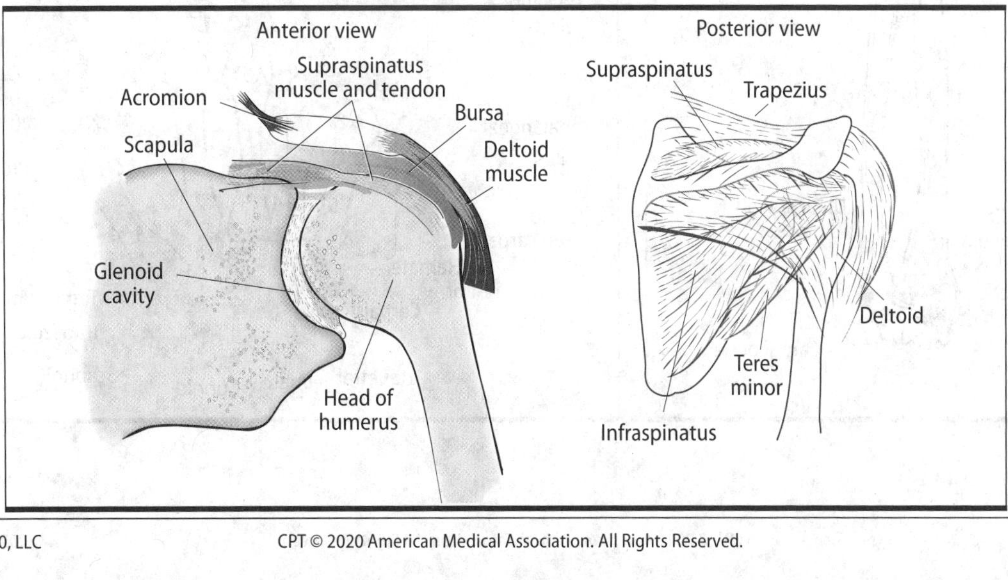
Anterior view
Supraspinatus muscle and tendon
Acromion
Bursa
Scapula
Deltoid muscle
Glenoid cavity
Head of humerus
Posterior view
Supraspinatus
Trapezius
Deltoid
Teres minor
Infraspinatus

Elbow (Anterior View)

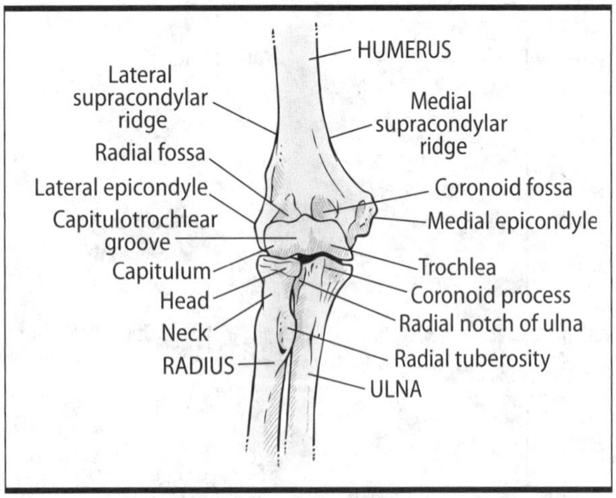

Elbow (Posterior View)

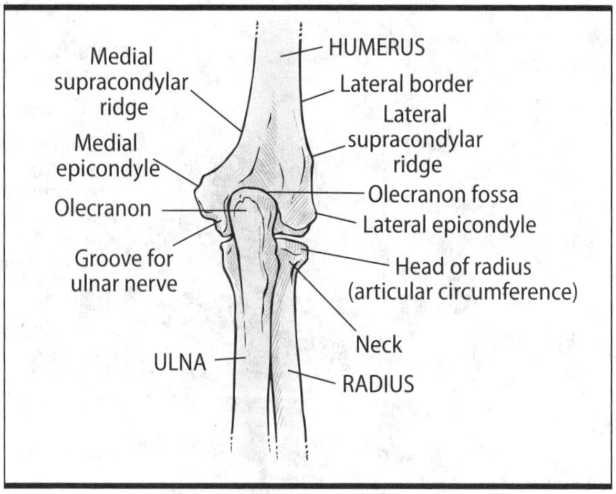

Elbow Muscles

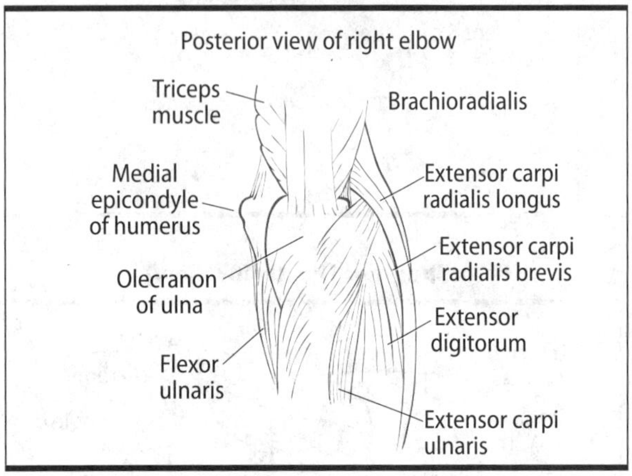

Elbow Joint

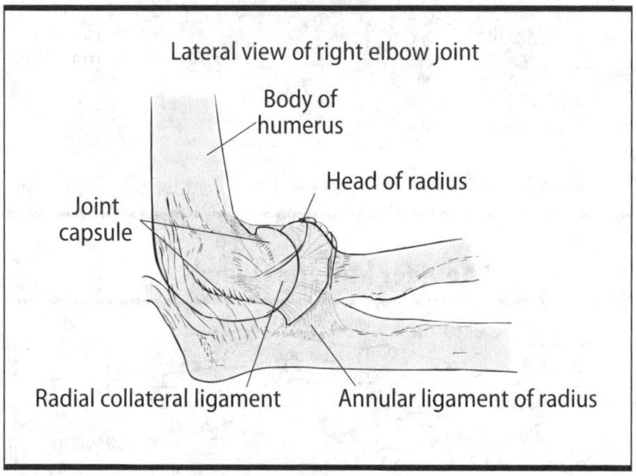

Lower Arm

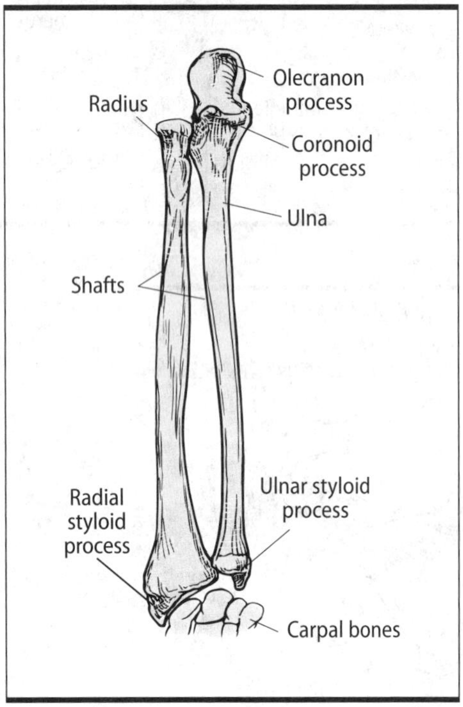

Hand

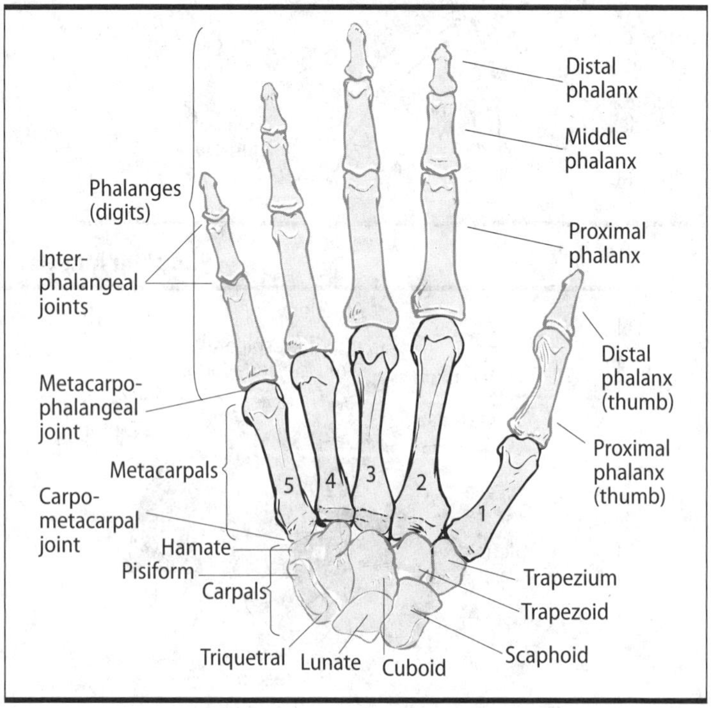

Hip (Anterior View)

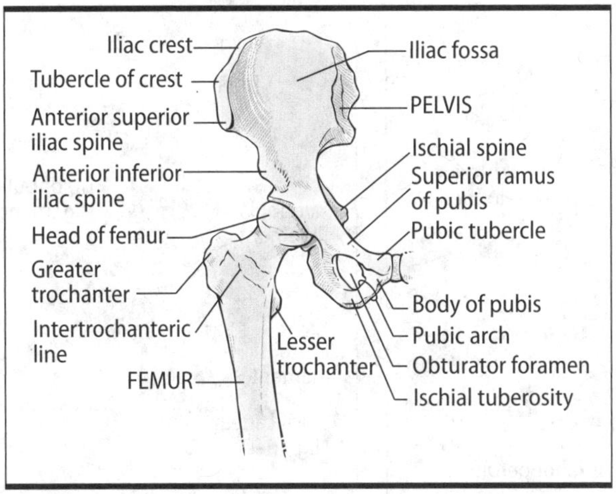
Iliac crest
Tubercle of crest
Anterior superior iliac spine
Anterior inferior iliac spine
Head of femur
Greater trochanter
Intertrochanteric line
FEMUR
Lesser trochanter
Iliac fossa
PELVIS
Ischial spine
Superior ramus of pubis
Pubic tubercle
Body of pubis
Pubic arch
Obturator foramen
Ischial tuberosity

Hip (Posterior View)

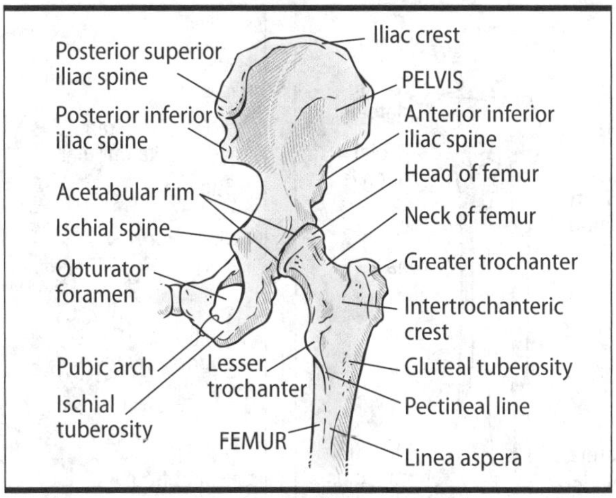
Posterior superior iliac spine
Posterior inferior iliac spine
Acetabular rim
Ischial spine
Obturator foramen
Pubic arch
Ischial tuberosity
Lesser trochanter
FEMUR
Iliac crest
PELVIS
Anterior inferior iliac spine
Head of femur
Neck of femur
Greater trochanter
Intertrochanteric crest
Gluteal tuberosity
Pectineal line
Linea aspera

Knee (Anterior View)

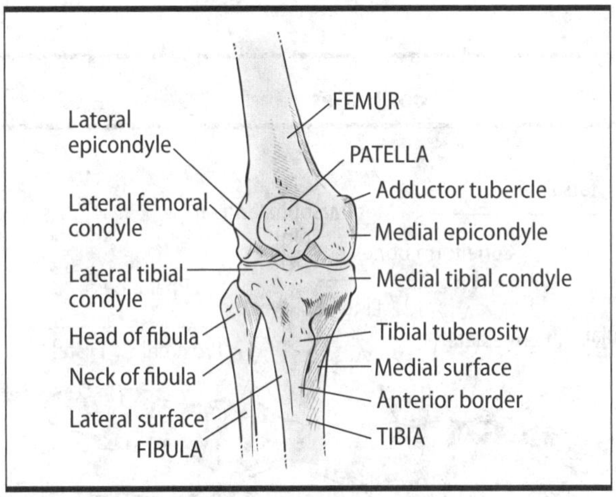
Lateral epicondyle
Lateral femoral condyle
Lateral tibial condyle
Head of fibula
Neck of fibula
Lateral surface
FIBULA
FEMUR
PATELLA
Adductor tubercle
Medial epicondyle
Medial tibial condyle
Tibial tuberosity
Medial surface
Anterior border
TIBIA

Knee (Posterior View)

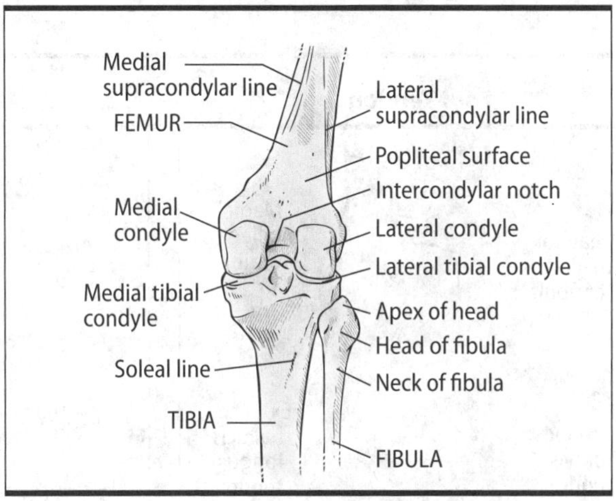
Medial supracondylar line
FEMUR
Medial condyle
Medial tibial condyle
Soleal line
TIBIA
Lateral supracondylar line
Popliteal surface
Intercondylar notch
Lateral condyle
Lateral tibial condyle
Apex of head
Head of fibula
Neck of fibula
FIBULA

Knee Joint (Anterior View)

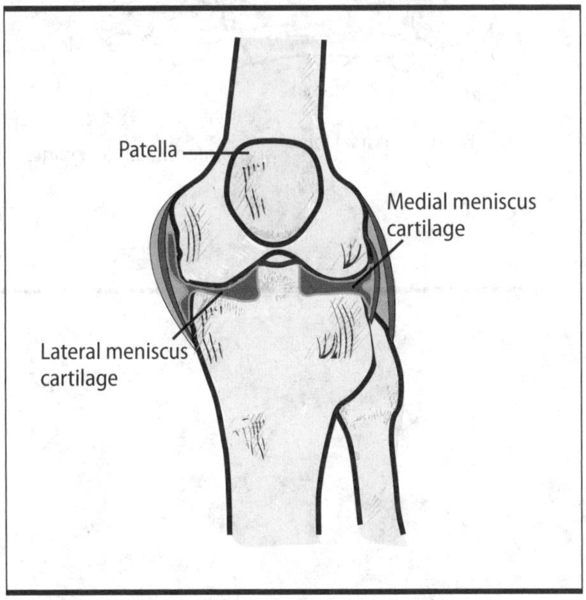
Patella
Medial meniscus cartilage
Lateral meniscus cartilage

Knee Joint (Lateral View)

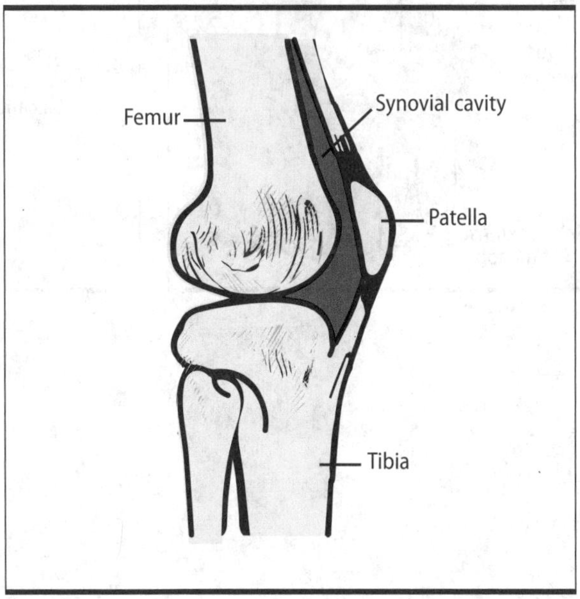
Femur
Synovial cavity
Patella
Tibia

Lower Leg

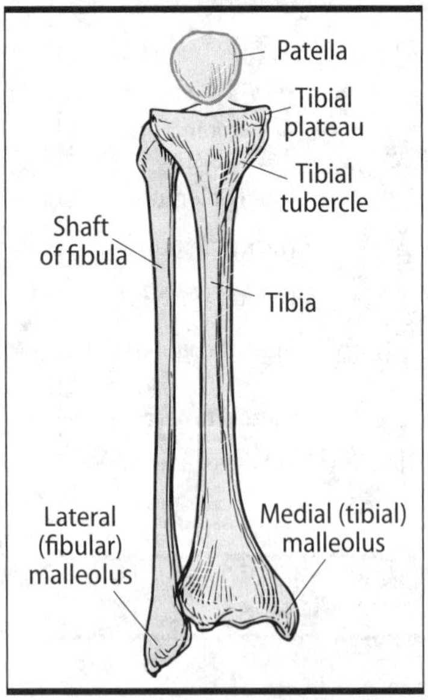
Patella
Tibial plateau
Tibial tubercle
Shaft of fibula
Tibia
Lateral (fibular) malleolus
Medial (tibial) malleolus

Ankle Ligament (Lateral View)

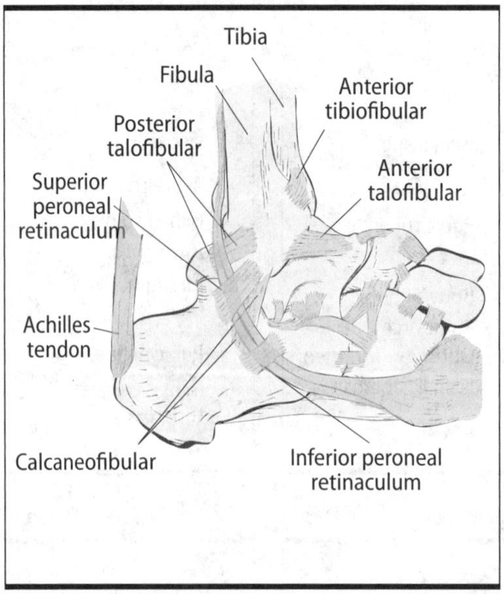
Tibia
Fibula
Anterior tibiofibular
Posterior talofibular
Superior peroneal retinaculum
Anterior talofibular
Achilles tendon
Calcaneofibular
Inferior peroneal retinaculum

Ankle Ligament (Posterior View)

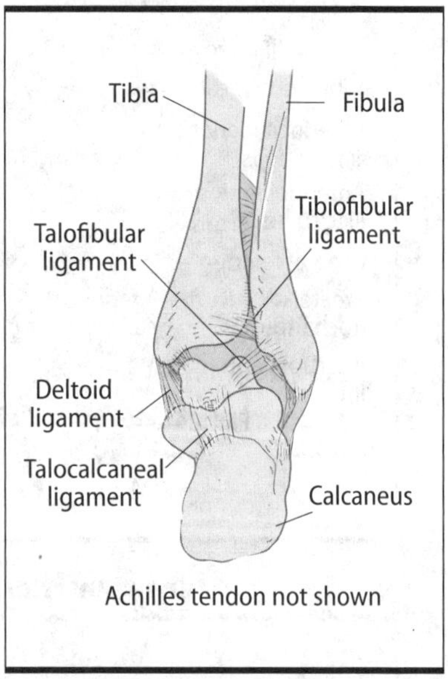
Tibia
Fibula
Tibiofibular ligament
Talofibular ligament
Deltoid ligament
Talocalcaneal ligament
Calcaneus
Achilles tendon not shown

Foot Tendons

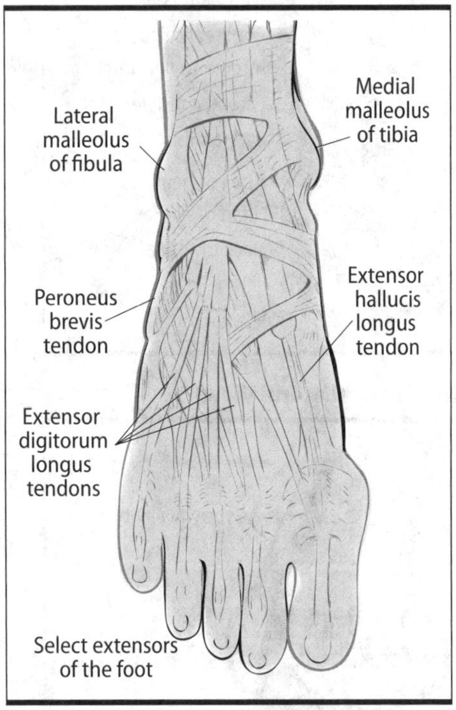
Lateral malleolus of fibula
Medial malleolus of tibia
Peroneus brevis tendon
Extensor hallucis longus tendon
Extensor digitorum longus tendons
Select extensors of the foot

Foot Bones

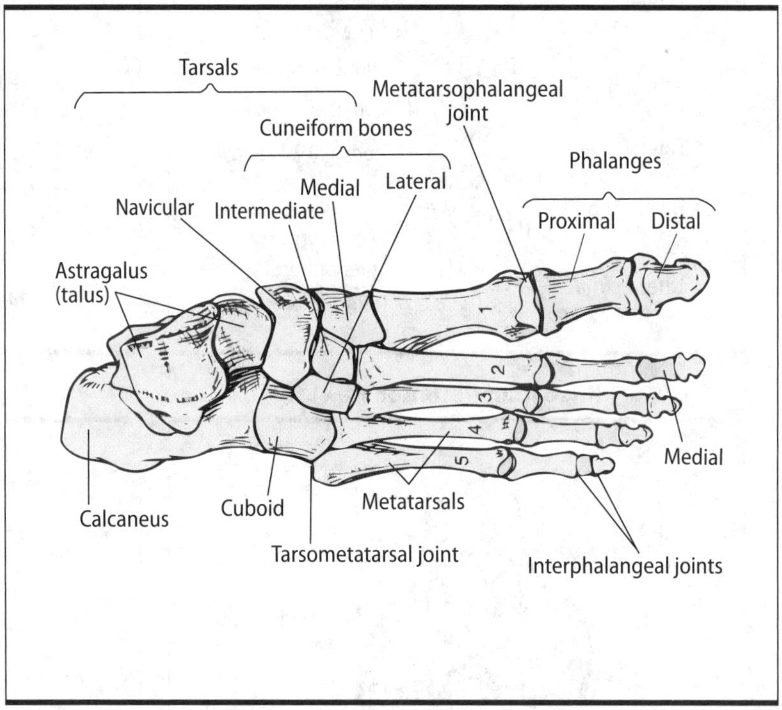
Tarsals
Metatarsophalangeal joint
Cuneiform bones
Phalanges
Medial
Lateral
Navicular
Intermediate
Proximal
Distal
Astragalus (talus)
1
2
3
4
5
Medial
Calcaneus
Cuboid
Metatarsals
Tarsometatarsal joint
Interphalangeal joints

Respiratory System

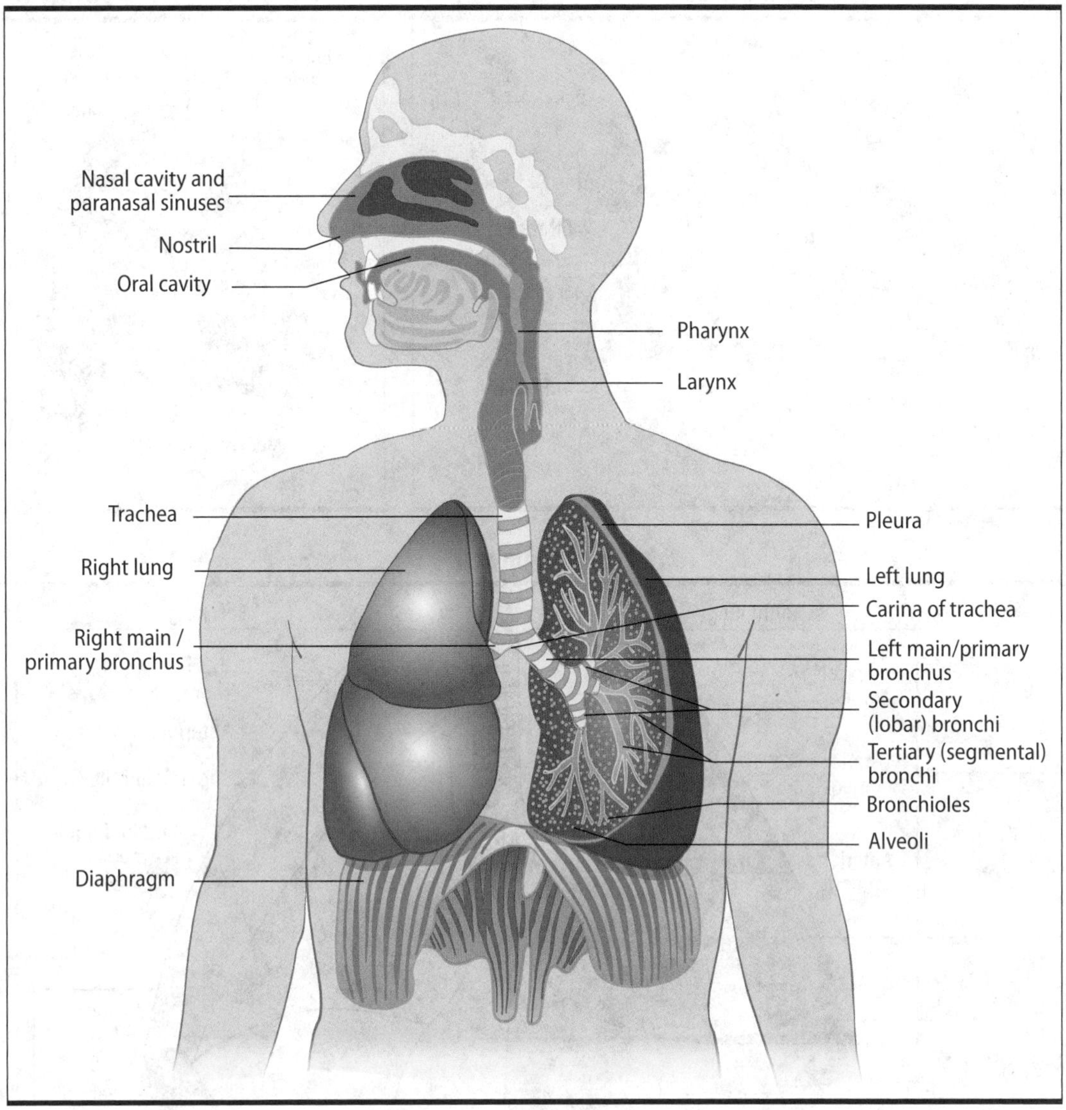
Nasal cavity and paranasal sinuses
Nostril
Oral cavity
Pharynx
Larynx
Trachea
Right lung
Right main / primary bronchus
Pleura
Left lung
Carina of trachea
Left main/primary bronchus
Secondary (lobar) bronchi
Tertiary (segmental) bronchi
Bronchioles
Alveoli
Diaphragm

Upper Respiratory System

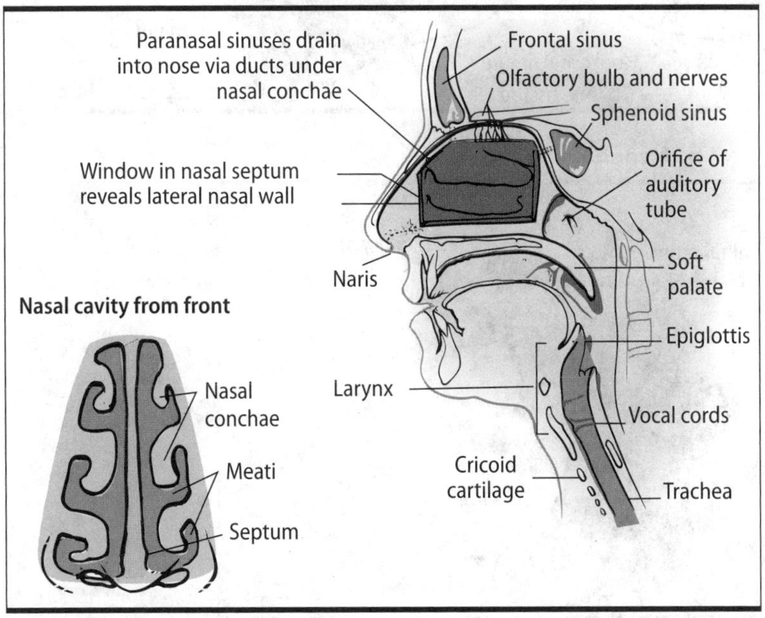
Paranasal sinuses drain into nose via ducts under nasal conchae
Frontal sinus
Olfactory bulb and nerves
Sphenoid sinus
Window in nasal septum reveals lateral nasal wall
Orifice of auditory tube
Naris
Soft palate
Nasal cavity from front
Epiglottis
Nasal conchae
Larynx
Vocal cords
Meati
Cricoid cartilage
Trachea
Septum

Nasal Turbinates

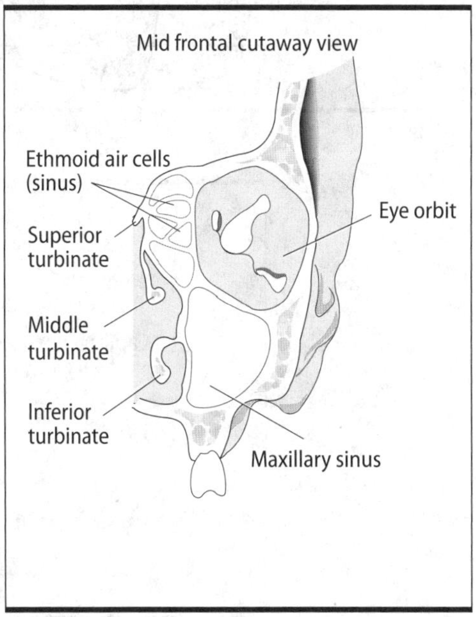
Mid frontal cutaway view
Ethmoid air cells (sinus)
Eye orbit
Superior turbinate
Middle turbinate
Inferior turbinate
Maxillary sinus

Paranasal Sinuses

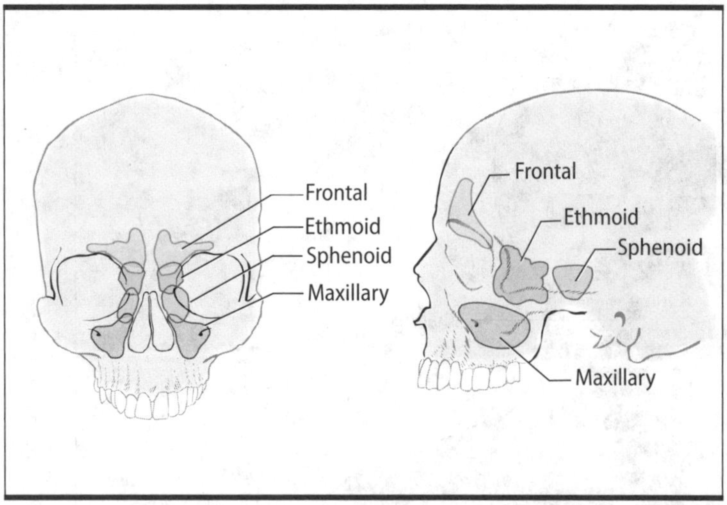
Frontal
Ethmoid
Sphenoid
Maxillary
Frontal
Ethmoid
Sphenoid
Maxillary

Lower Respiratory System

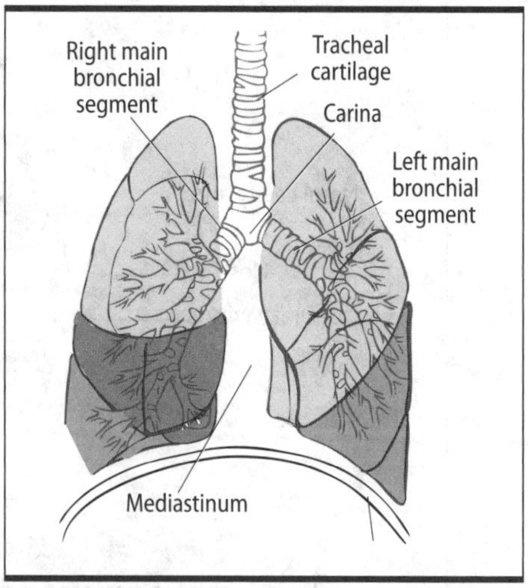
Right main bronchial segment
Tracheal cartilage
Carina
Left main bronchial segment
Mediastinum

Lung Segments

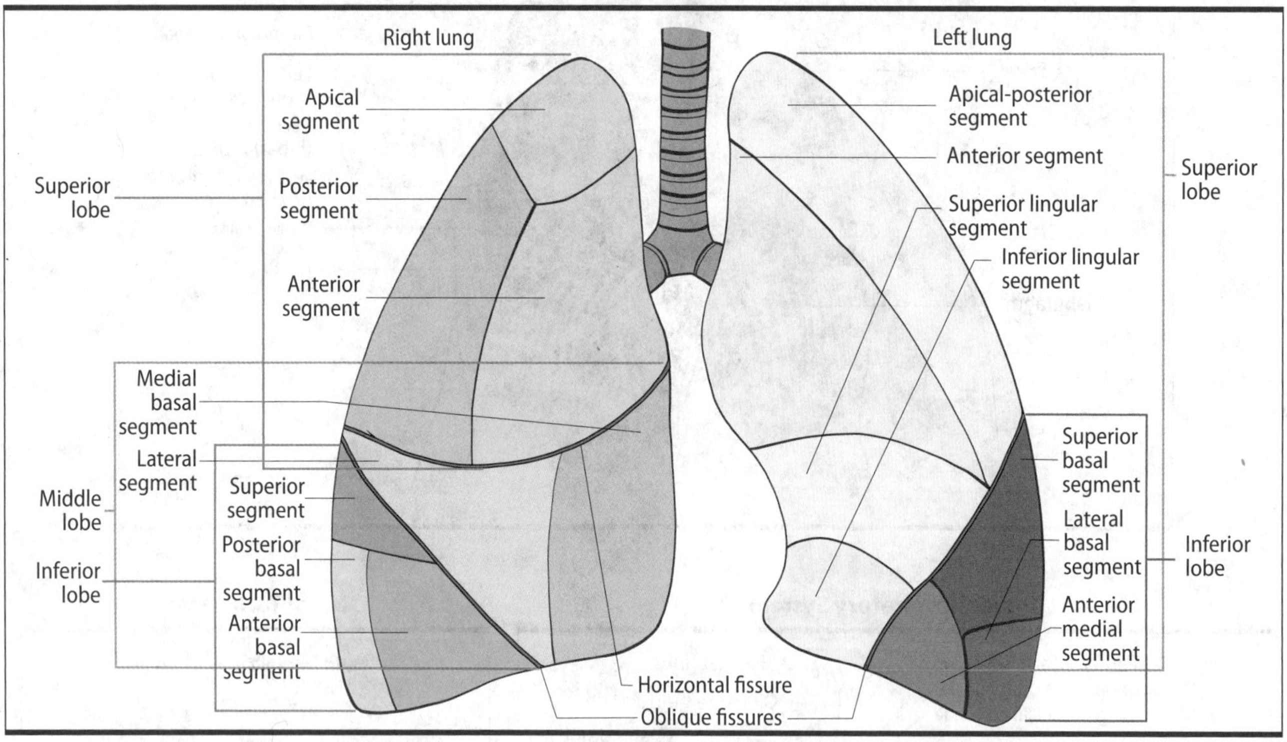
Right lung
Left lung
Apical segment
Superior lobe
Posterior segment
Anterior segment
Medial basal segment
Lateral segment
Middle lobe
Superior segment
Inferior lobe
Posterior basal segment
Anterior basal segment
Apical-posterior segment
Anterior segment
Superior lobe
Superior lingular segment
Inferior lingular segment
Superior basal segment
Lateral basal segment
Inferior lobe
Anterior medial segment
Horizontal fissure
Oblique fissures

Alveoli

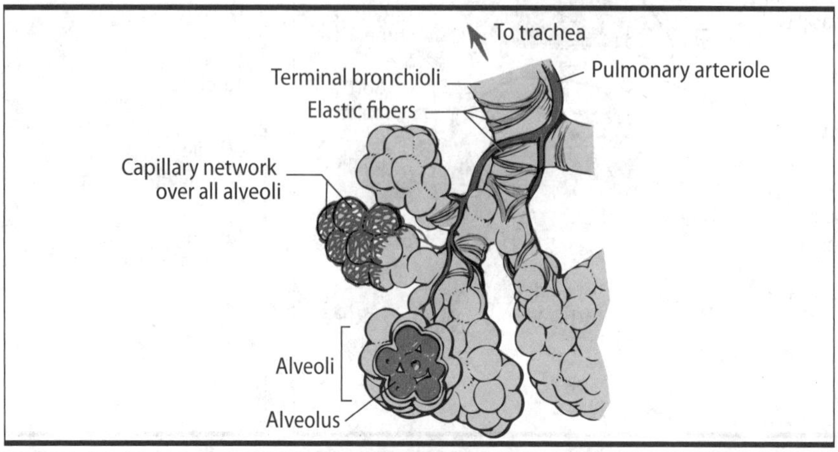
To trachea
Terminal bronchioli
Pulmonary arteriole
Elastic fibers
Capillary network over all alveoli
Alveoli
Alveolus

Arterial System

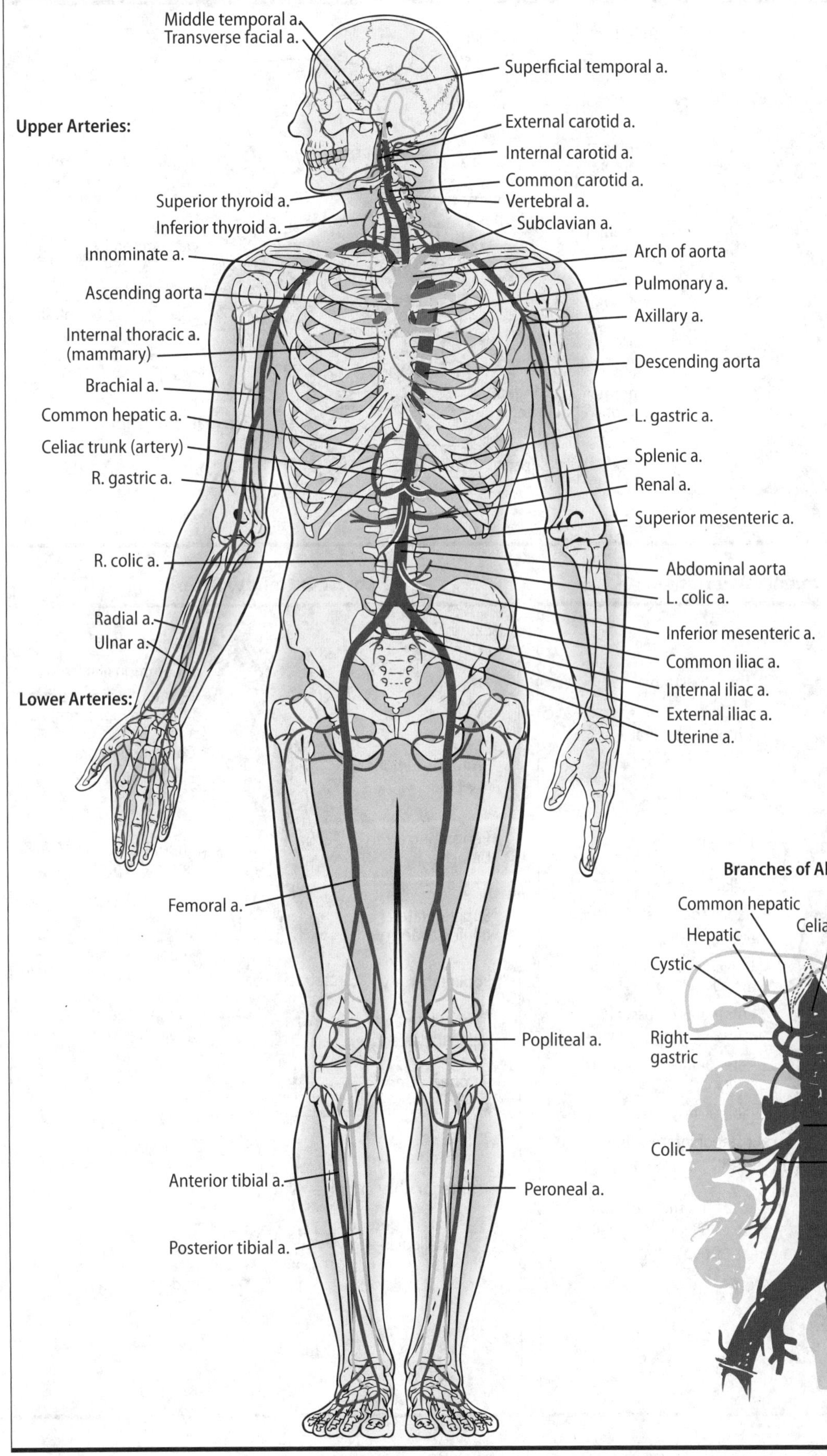
Middle temporal a.
Transverse facial a.
Superficial temporal a.
Upper Arteries:
External carotid a.
Internal carotid a.
Common carotid a.
Superior thyroid a.
Vertebral a.
Inferior thyroid a.
Subclavian a.
Innominate a.
Arch of aorta
Ascending aorta
Pulmonary a.
Axillary a.
Internal thoracic a. (mammary)
Descending aorta
Brachial a.
Common hepatic a.
L. gastric a.
Celiac trunk (artery)
Splenic a.
R. gastric a.
Renal a.
Superior mesenteric a.
R. colic a.
Abdominal aorta
L. colic a.
Radial a.
Inferior mesenteric a.
Ulnar a.
Common iliac a.
Lower Arteries:
Internal iliac a.
External iliac a.
Uterine a.
Femoral a.
Popliteal a.
Anterior tibial a.
Peroneal a.
Posterior tibial a.

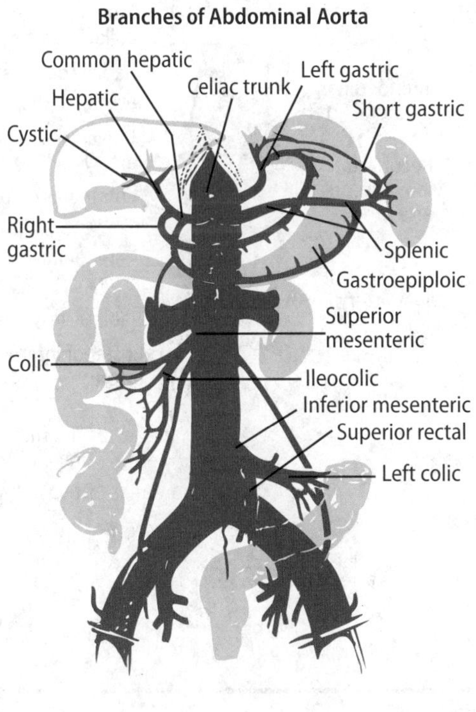
Branches of Abdominal Aorta
Common hepatic
Left gastric
Celiac trunk
Hepatic
Short gastric
Cystic
Right gastric
Splenic
Gastroepiploic
Superior mesenteric
Colic
Ileocolic
Inferior mesenteric
Superior rectal
Left colic

Internal Carotid and Arteries and Branches

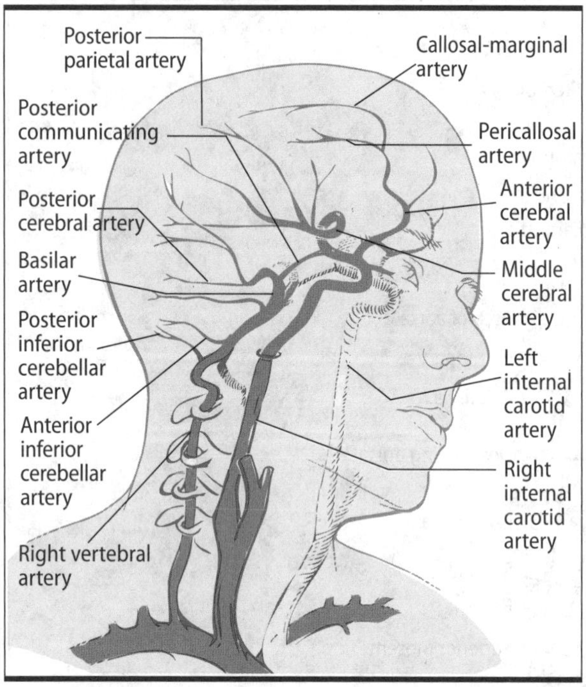
Posterior parietal artery
Callosal-marginal artery
Posterior communicating artery
Pericallosal artery
Posterior cerebral artery
Anterior cerebral artery
Basilar artery
Middle cerebral artery
Posterior inferior cerebellar artery
Left internal carotid artery
Anterior inferior cerebellar artery
Right internal carotid artery
Right vertebral artery

External Carotid Arteries and Branches

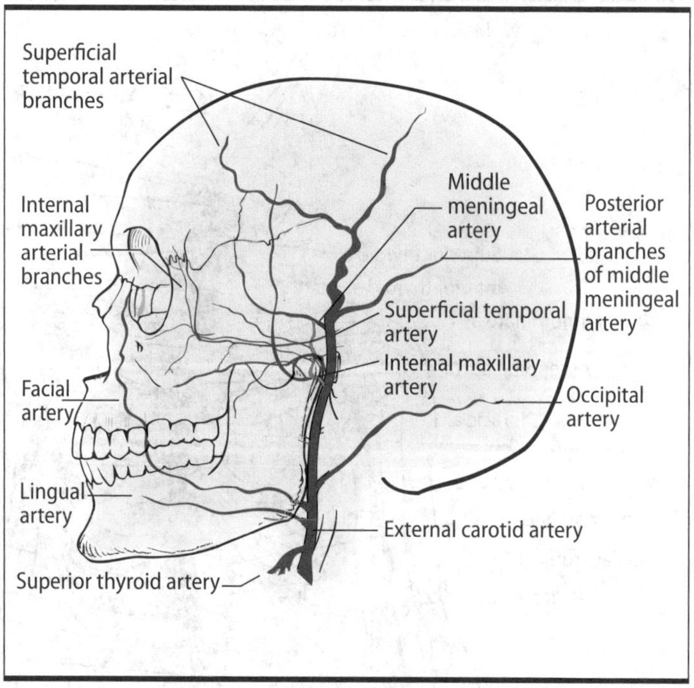
Superficial temporal arterial branches
Middle meningeal artery
Posterior arterial branches of middle meningeal artery
Internal maxillary arterial branches
Superficial temporal artery
Internal maxillary artery
Facial artery
Occipital artery
Lingual artery
External carotid artery
Superior thyroid artery

Upper Extremity Arteries

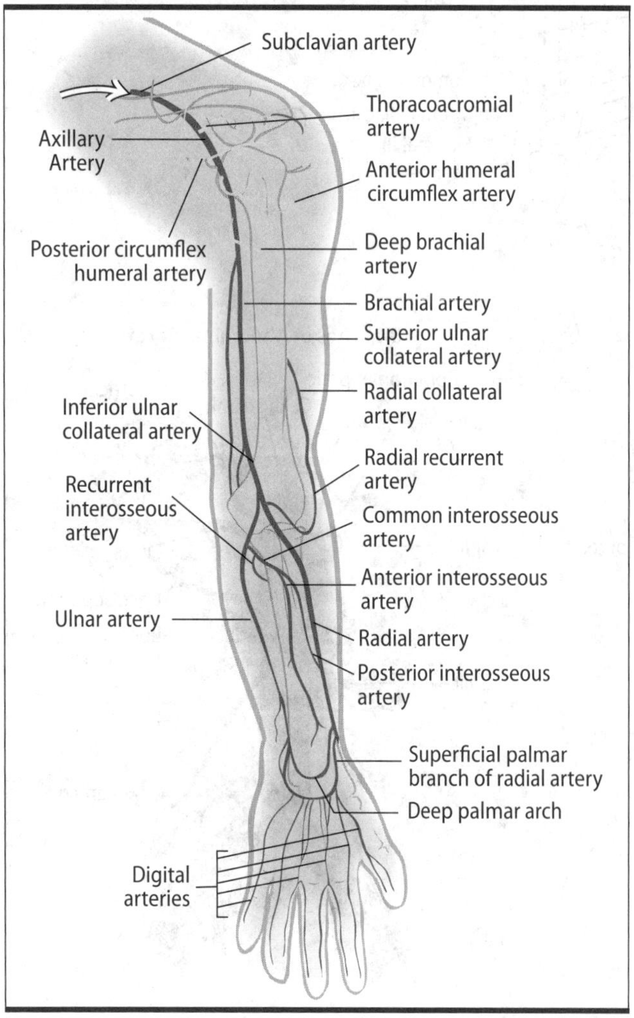
Subclavian artery
Thoracoacromial artery
Axillary Artery
Anterior humeral circumflex artery
Posterior circumflex humeral artery
Deep brachial artery
Brachial artery
Superior ulnar collateral artery
Radial collateral artery
Inferior ulnar collateral artery
Radial recurrent artery
Recurrent interosseous artery
Common interosseous artery
Anterior interosseous artery
Ulnar artery
Radial artery
Posterior interosseous artery
Superficial palmar branch of radial artery
Deep palmar arch
Digital arteries

Lower Extremity Arteries

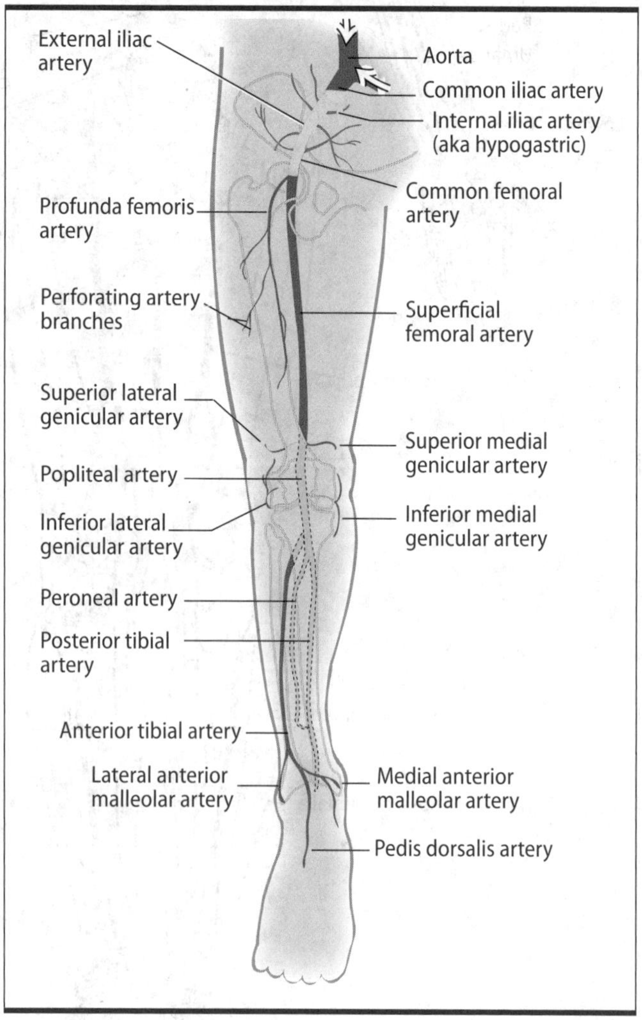
External iliac artery
Aorta
Common iliac artery
Internal iliac artery (aka hypogastric)
Common femoral artery
Profunda femoris artery
Perforating artery branches
Superficial femoral artery
Superior lateral genicular artery
Superior medial genicular artery
Popliteal artery
Inferior lateral genicular artery
Inferior medial genicular artery
Peroneal artery
Posterior tibial artery
Anterior tibial artery
Lateral anterior malleolar artery
Medial anterior malleolar artery
Pedis dorsalis artery

Venous System

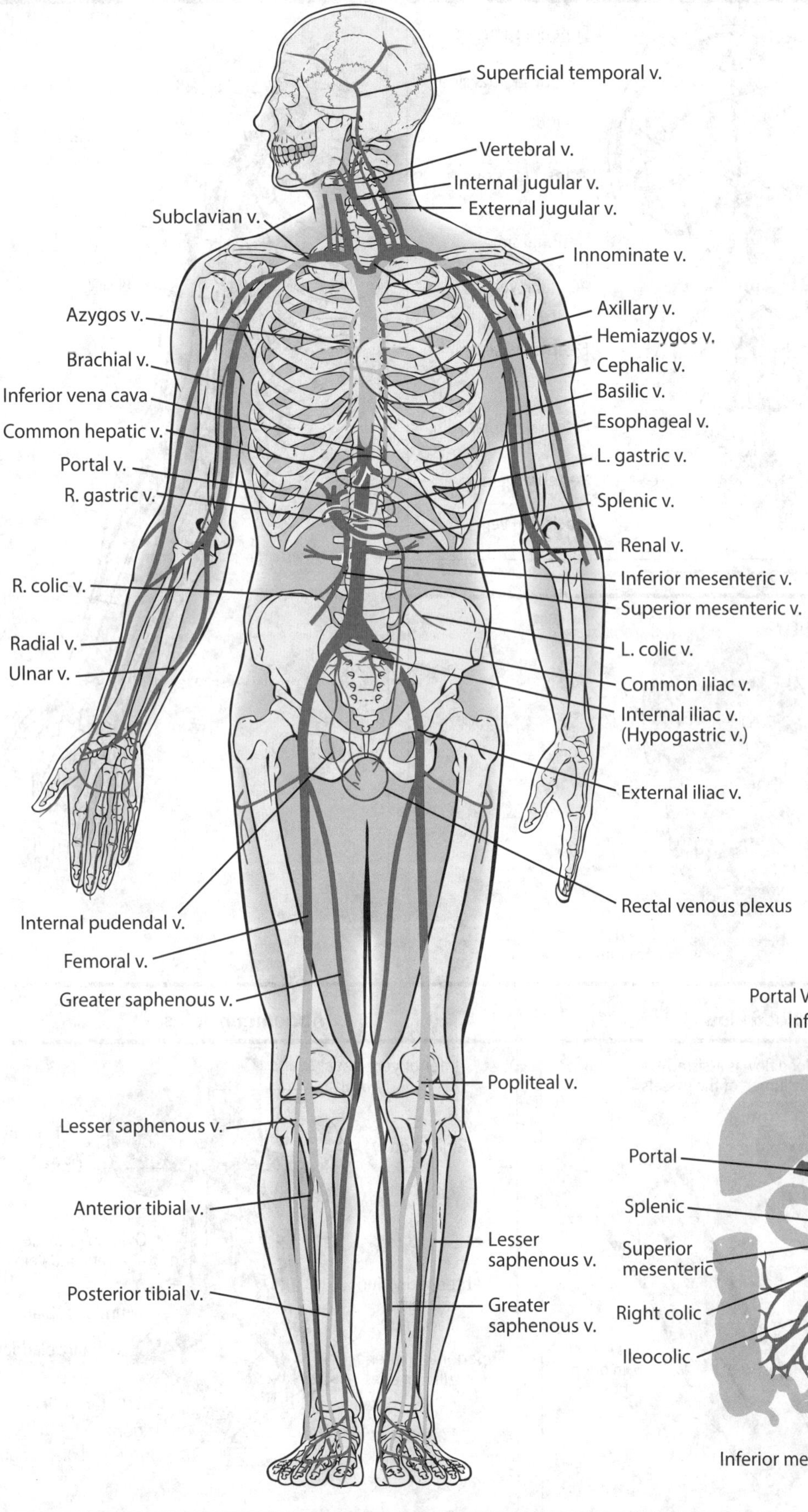
Superficial temporal v.
Vertebral v.
Internal jugular v.
External jugular v.
Subclavian v.
Innominate v.
Azygos v.
Axillary v.
Hemiazygos v.
Brachial v.
Cephalic v.
Inferior vena cava
Basilic v.
Common hepatic v.
Esophageal v.
Portal v.
L. gastric v.
R. gastric v.
Splenic v.
Renal v.
R. colic v.
Inferior mesenteric v.
Superior mesenteric v.
Radial v.
L. colic v.
Ulnar v.
Common iliac v.
Internal iliac v.
(Hypogastric v.)
External iliac v.
Rectal venous plexus
Internal pudendal v.
Femoral v.
Greater saphenous v.
Popliteal v.
Lesser saphenous v.
Anterior tibial v.
Lesser
saphenous v.
Posterior tibial v.
Greater
saphenous v.

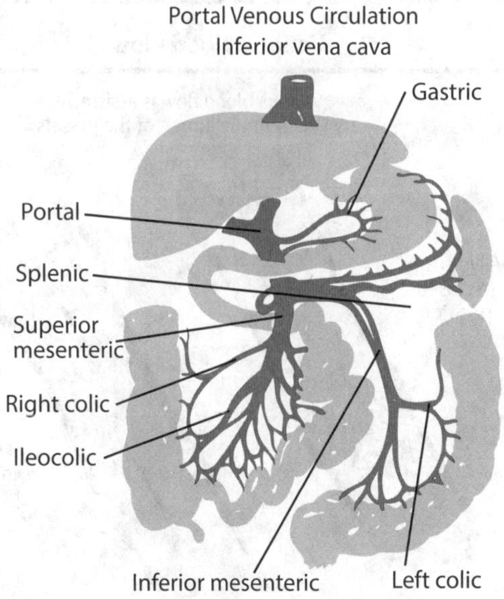
Portal Venous Circulation
Inferior vena cava
Gastric
Portal
Splenic
Superior
mesenteric
Right colic
Ileocolic
Inferior mesenteric
Left colic

Head and Neck Veins

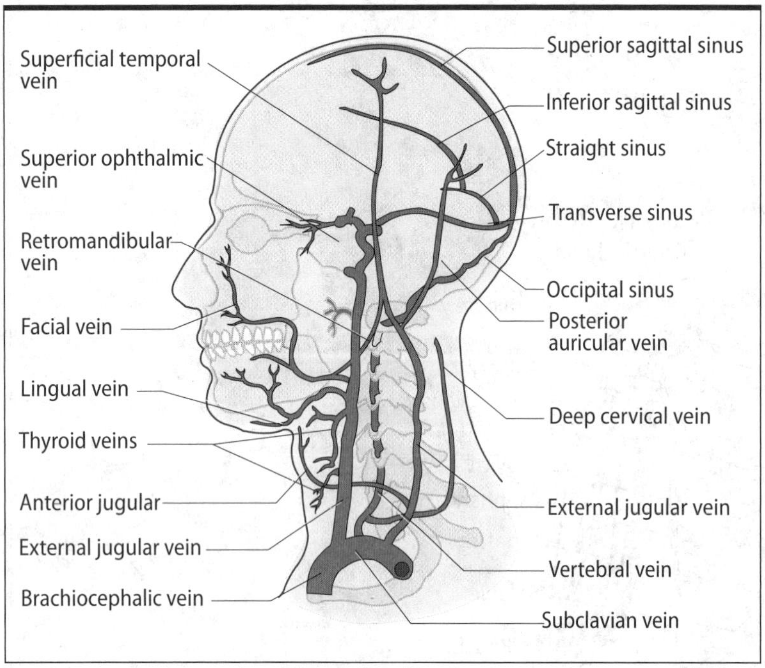
Superficial temporal vein
Superior ophthalmic vein
Retromandibular vein
Facial vein
Lingual vein
Thyroid veins
Anterior jugular
External jugular vein
Brachiocephalic vein
Superior sagittal sinus
Inferior sagittal sinus
Straight sinus
Transverse sinus
Occipital sinus
Posterior auricular vein
Deep cervical vein
External jugular vein
Vertebral vein
Subclavian vein

Upper Extremity Veins

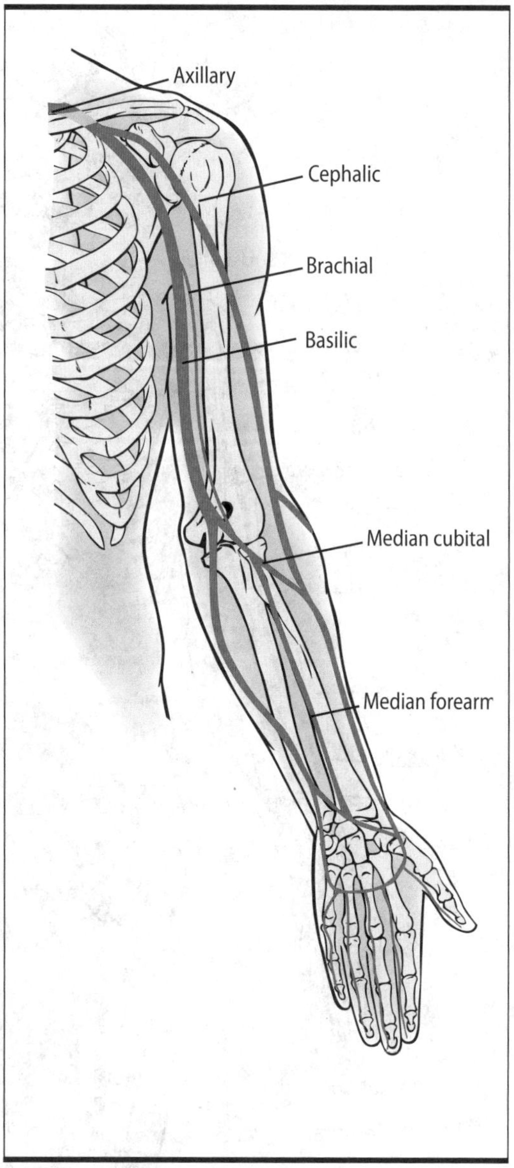
Axillary
Cephalic
Brachial
Basilic
Median cubital
Median forearm

Venae Comitantes

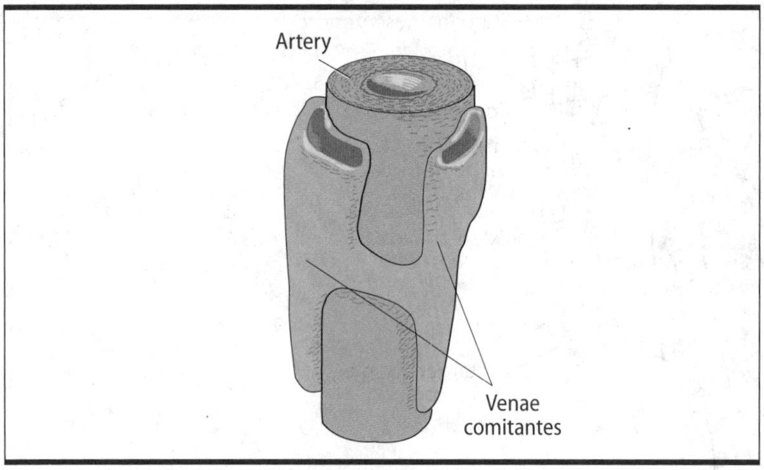
Artery
Venae comitantes

Venous Blood Flow

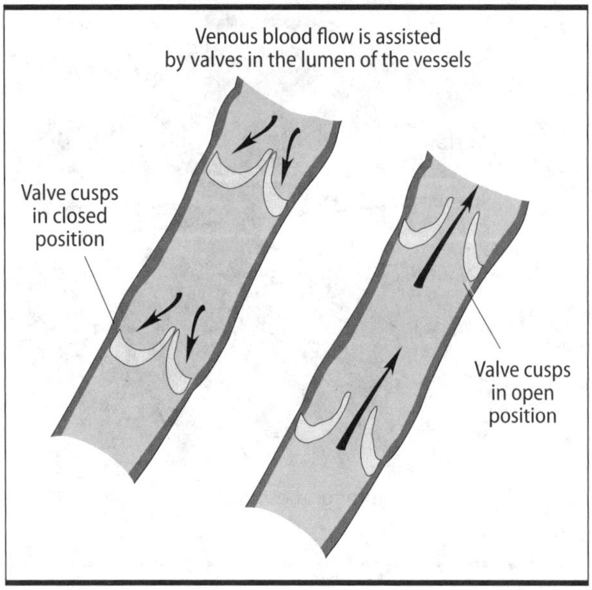
Venous blood flow is assisted by valves in the lumen of the vessels
Valve cusps in closed position
Valve cusps in open position

Abdominal Veins

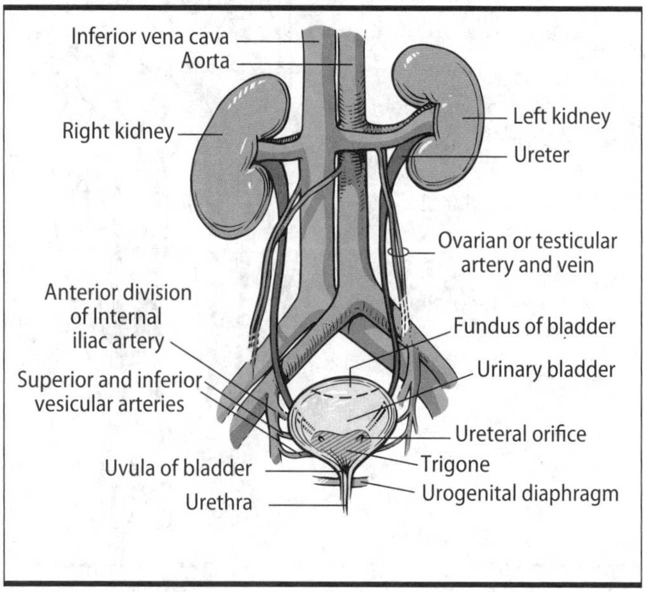
Inferior vena cava
Aorta
Right kidney
Left kidney
Ureter
Ovarian or testicular artery and vein
Anterior division of Internal iliac artery
Fundus of bladder
Urinary bladder
Superior and inferior vesicular arteries
Ureteral orifice
Trigone
Uvula of bladder
Urogenital diaphragm
Urethra

Cardiovascular System

Coronary Veins

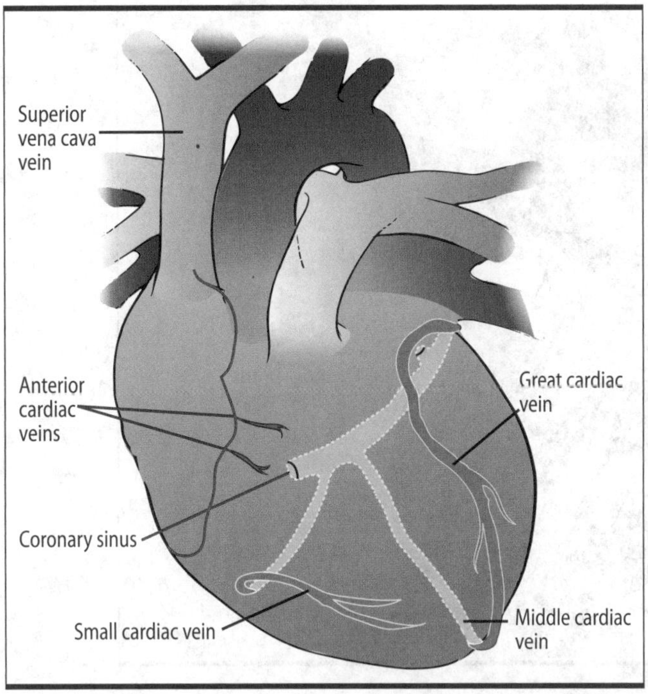

Anatomy of the Heart

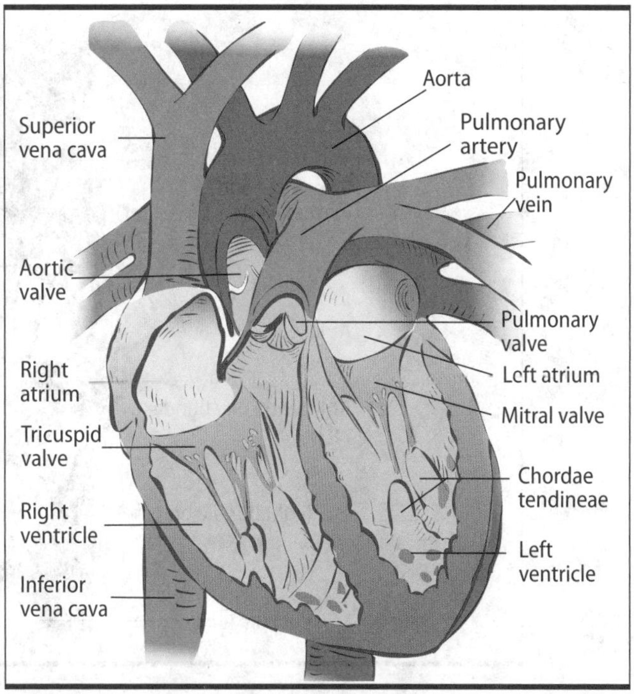

Heart Cross Section

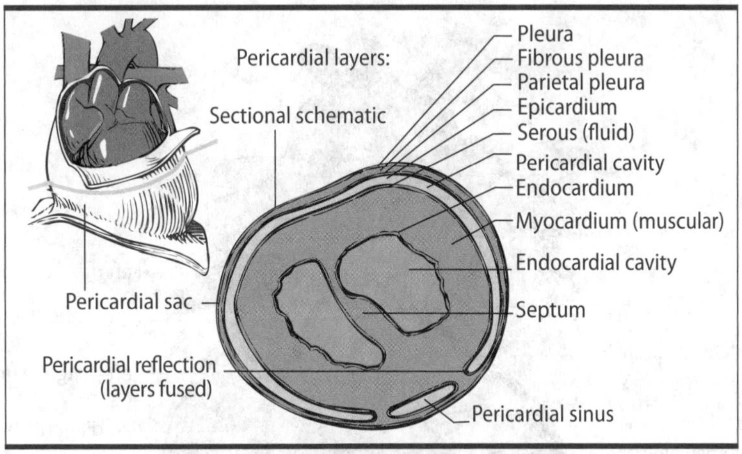

Heart Valves

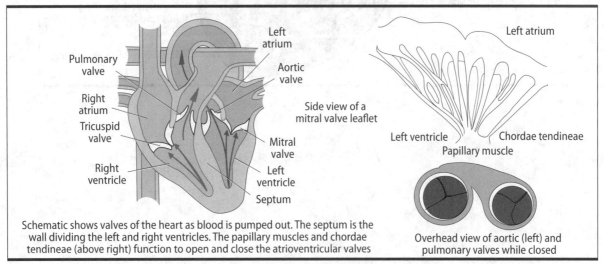

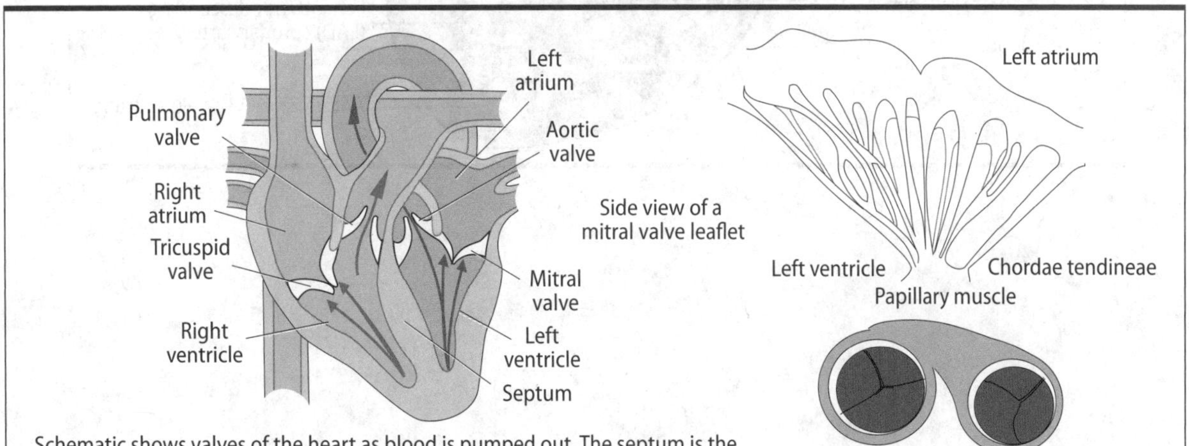

Schematic shows valves of the heart as blood is pumped out. The septum is the wall dividing the left and right ventricles. The papillary muscles and chordae tendineae (above right) function to open and close the atrioventricular valves

Overhead view of aortic (left) and pulmonary valves while closed

Heart Conduction System

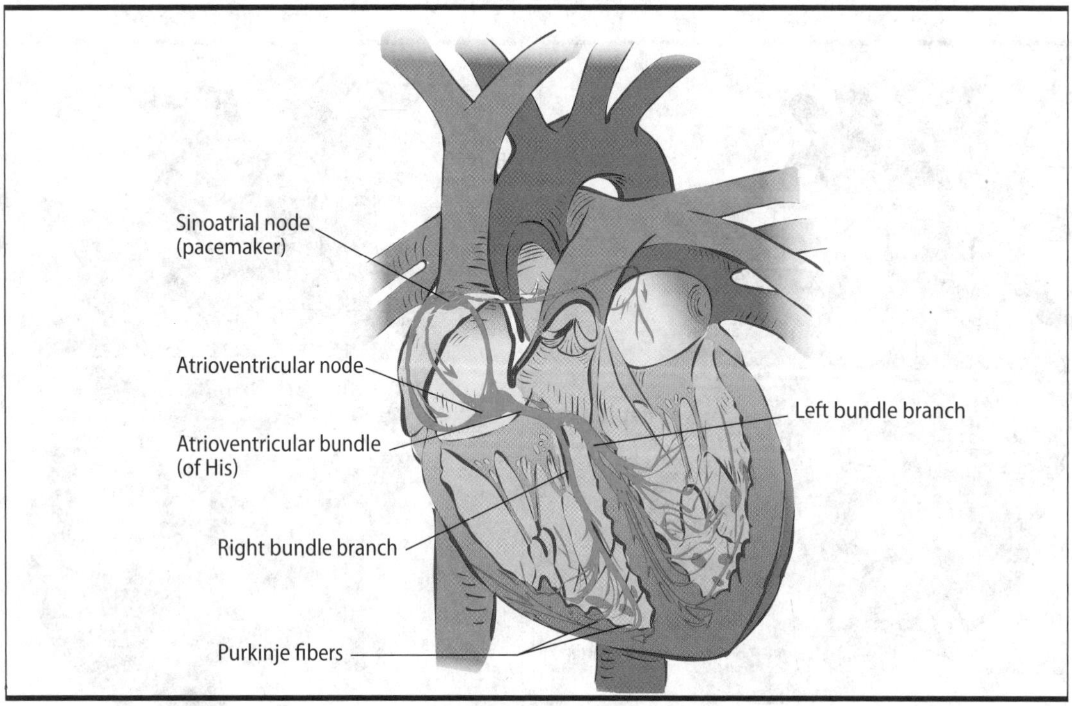
Sinoatrial node
(pacemaker)
Atrioventricular node
Atrioventricular bundle
(of His)
Right bundle branch
Purkinje fibers
Left bundle branch

Coronary Arteries

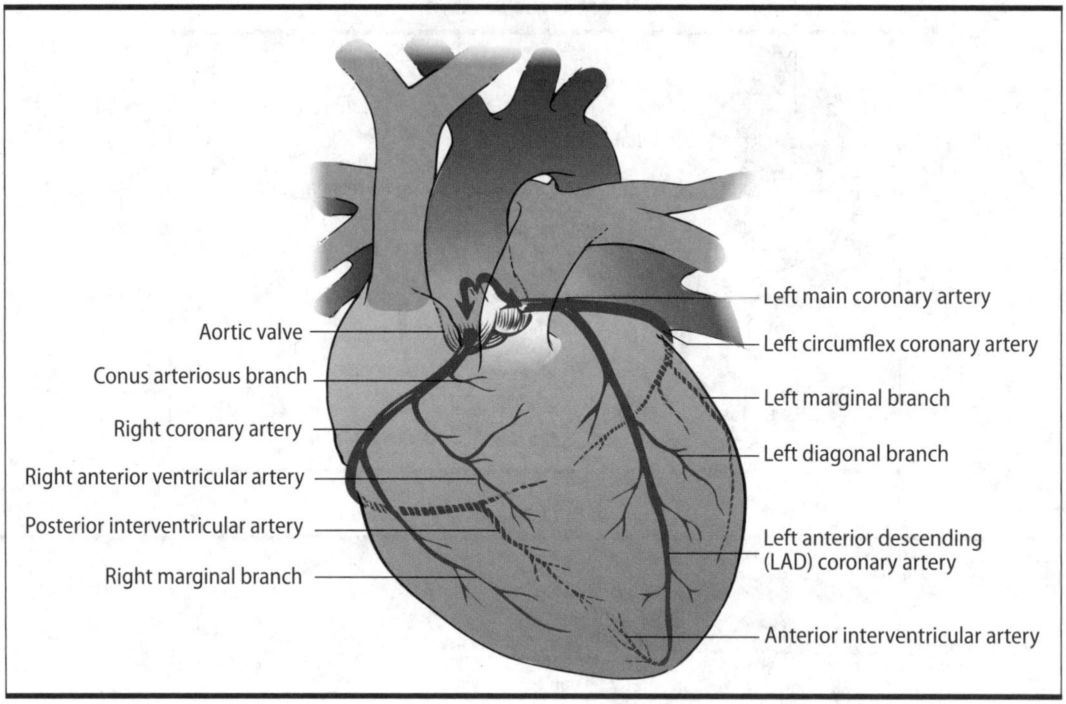
Aortic valve
Conus arteriosus branch
Right coronary artery
Right anterior ventricular artery
Posterior interventricular artery
Right marginal branch
Left main coronary artery
Left circumflex coronary artery
Left marginal branch
Left diagonal branch
Left anterior descending
(LAD) coronary artery
Anterior interventricular artery

Lymphatic System

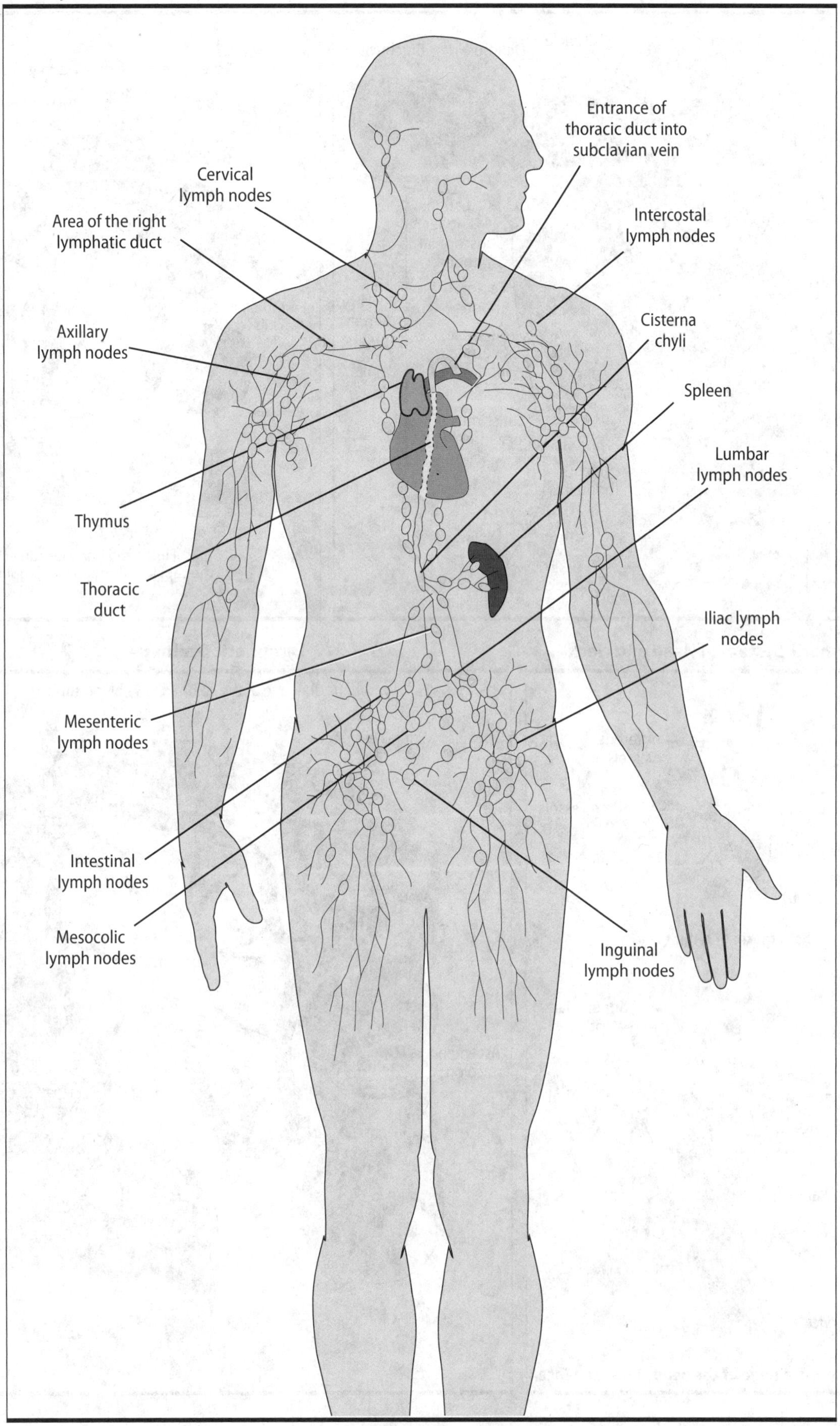
Entrance of thoracic duct into subclavian vein
Cervical lymph nodes
Area of the right lymphatic duct
Intercostal lymph nodes
Axillary lymph nodes
Cisterna chyli
Spleen
Lumbar lymph nodes
Thymus
Thoracic duct
Iliac lymph nodes
Mesenteric lymph nodes
Intestinal lymph nodes
Mesocolic lymph nodes
Inguinal lymph nodes

Axillary Lymph Nodes

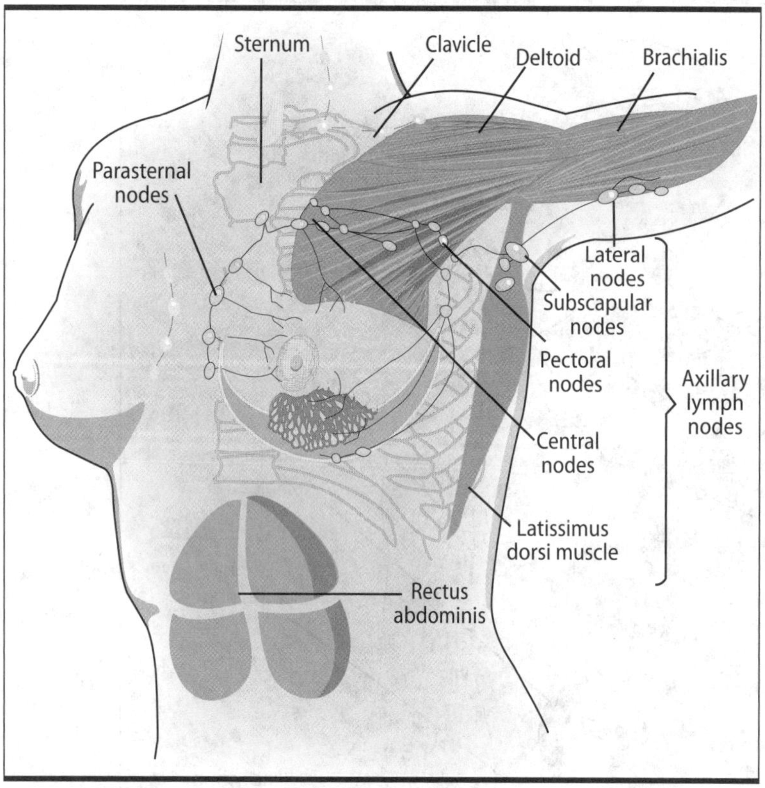

Lymphatic Capillaries

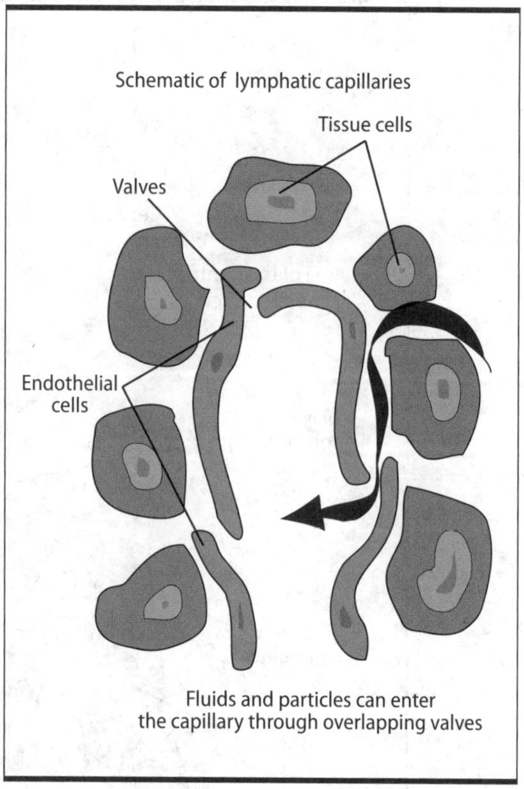

Lymphatic System of Head and Neck

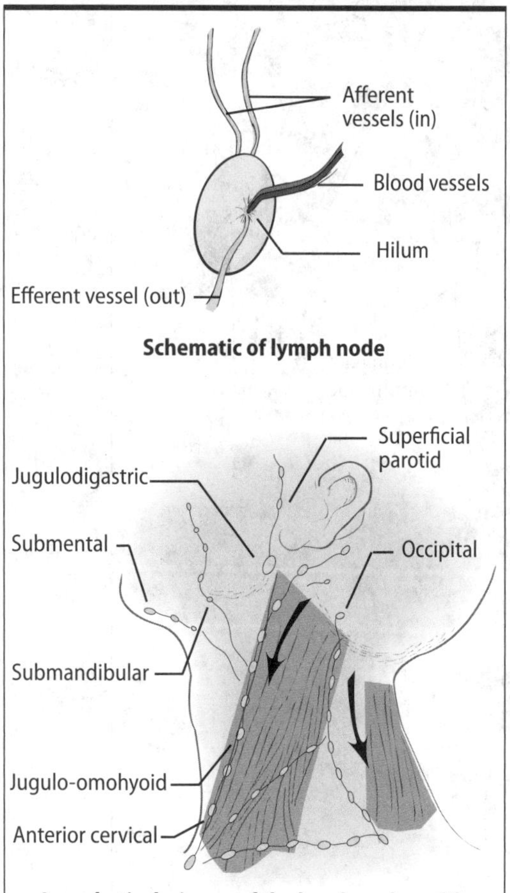

Lymphatic drainage of the head, neck, and face

Lymphatic Drainage

Lymphatic drainage of the colon follows blood supply

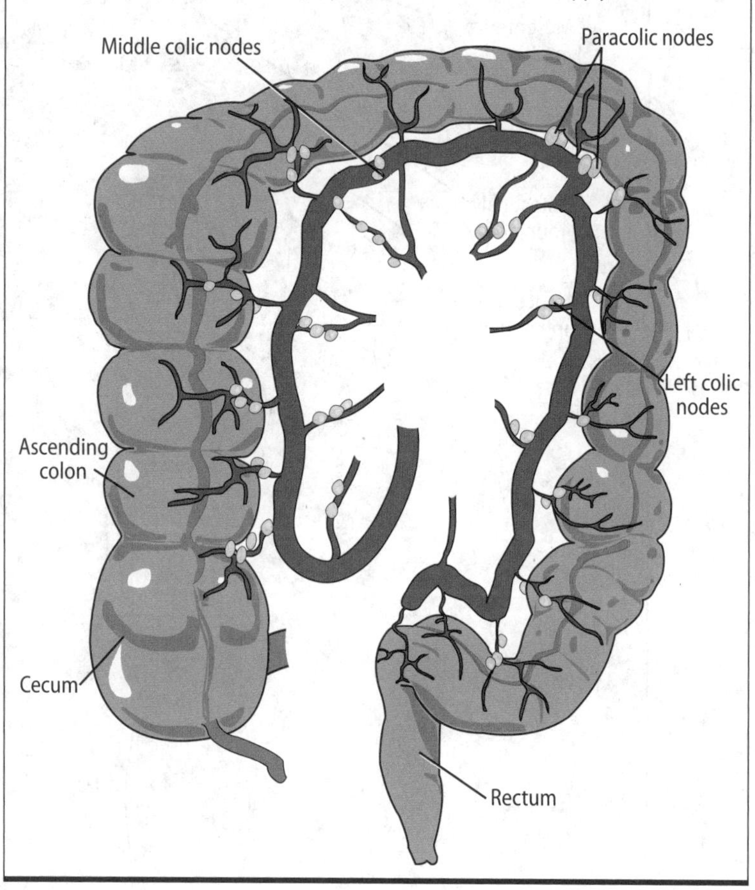

Spleen Internal Structures

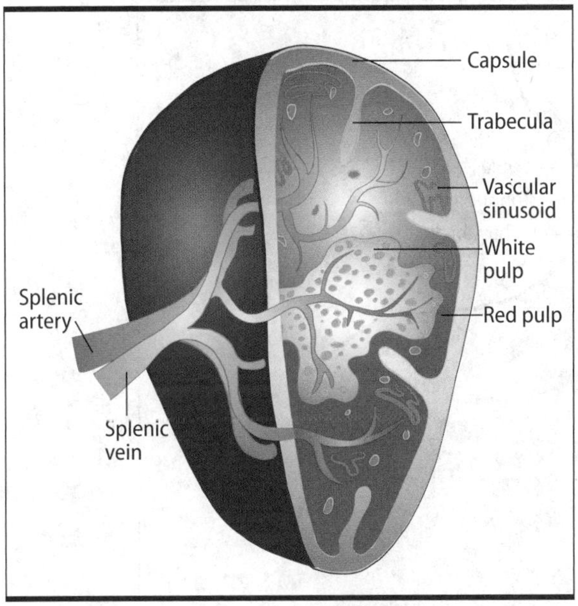

Spleen External Structures

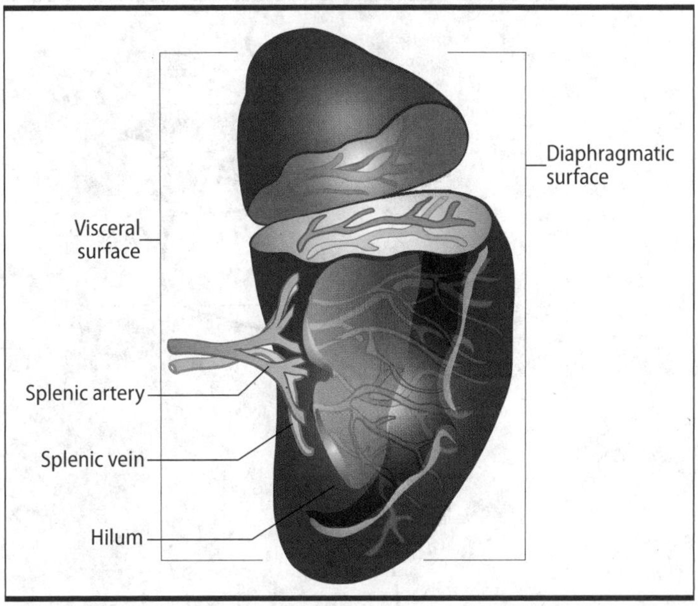

Digestive System

Pharynx
Salivary glands
Parotid
Sublingual
Submandibular
Oral cavity
Uvula
Tongue
Wharton duct
Esophagus
Stomach
Liver
Splenic flexure
Pancreas
Gallbladder
Common bile duct
Hepatic flexure
Duodenum
Jejunum
Ileum
Small intestine
Mesentery
Transverse colon
Ascending colon
Descending colon
Ileocecal valve
Cecum
Appendix
Rectum
Sigmoid colon
Anus

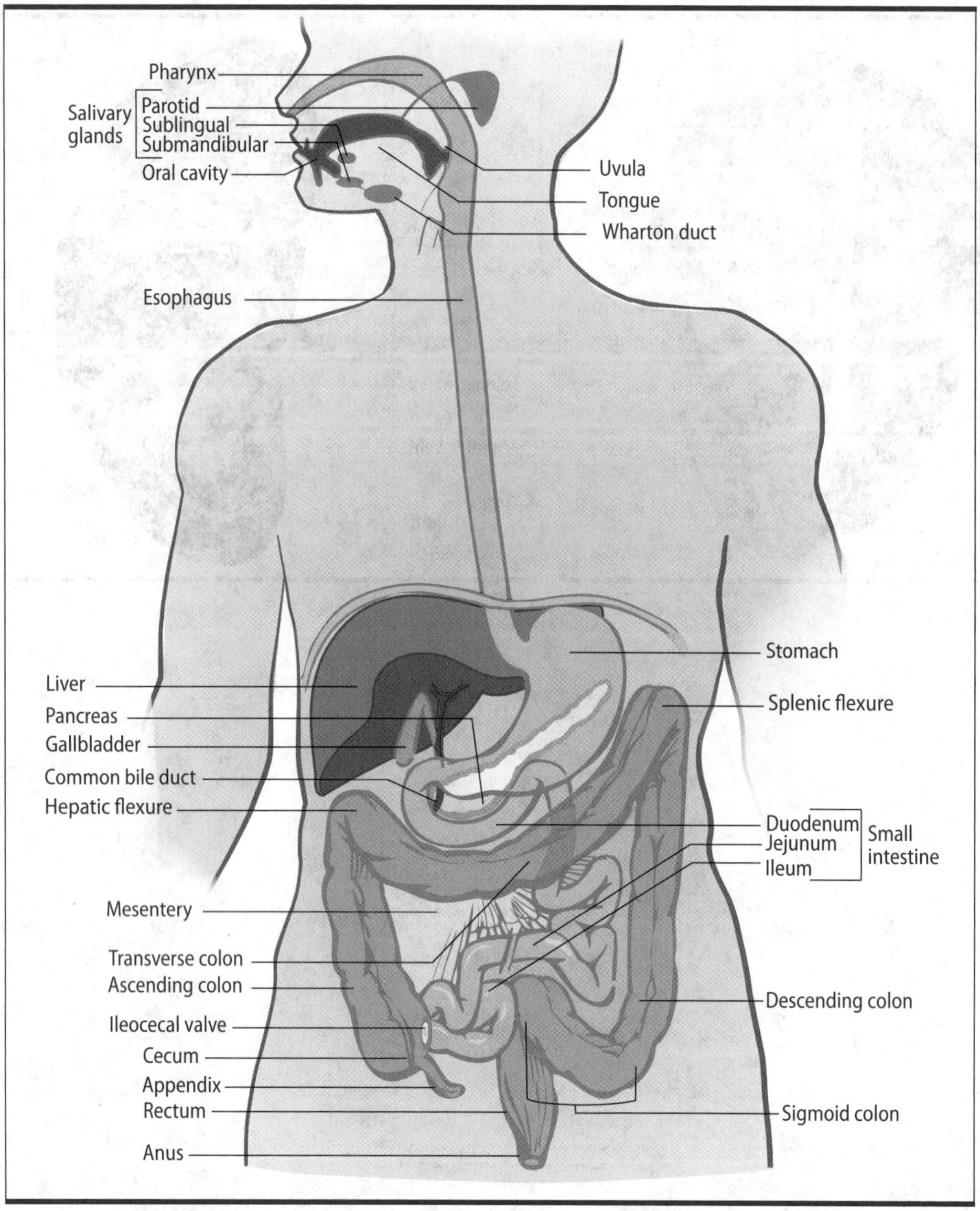

Gallbladder

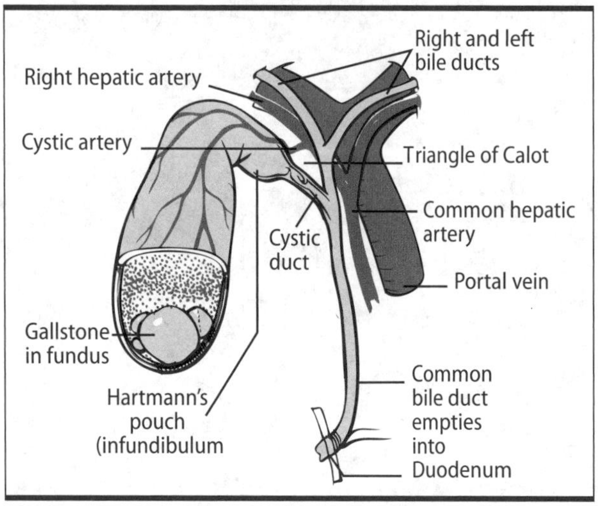

Stomach

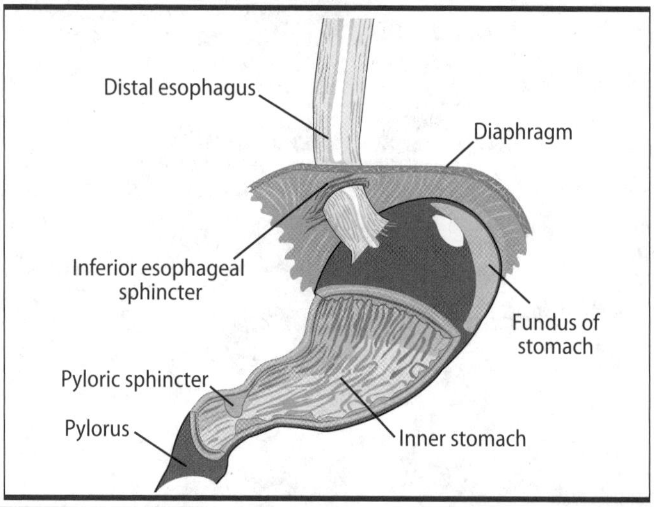

Mouth (Upper)

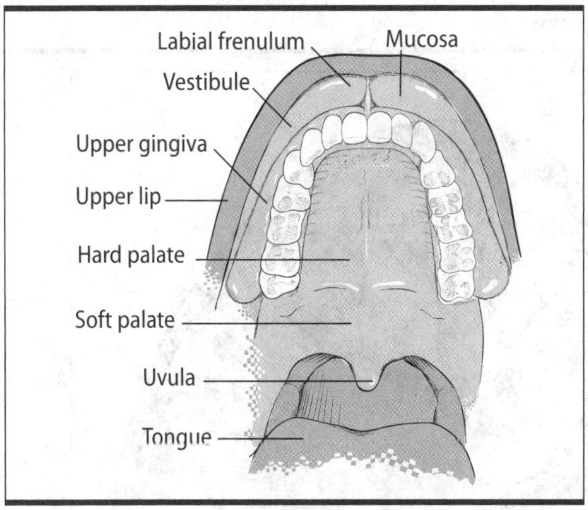

Mouth (Lower)

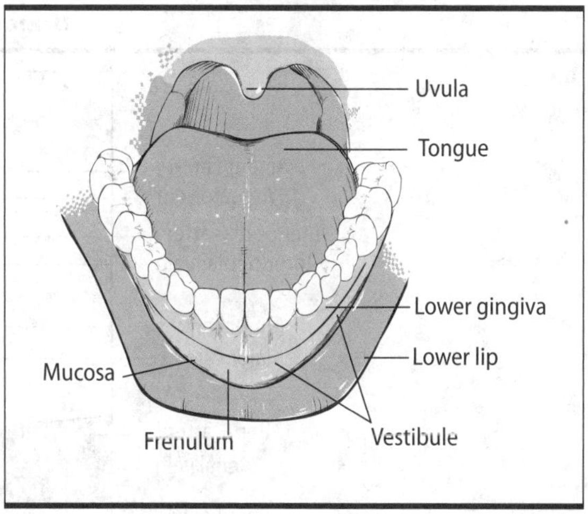

Pancreas

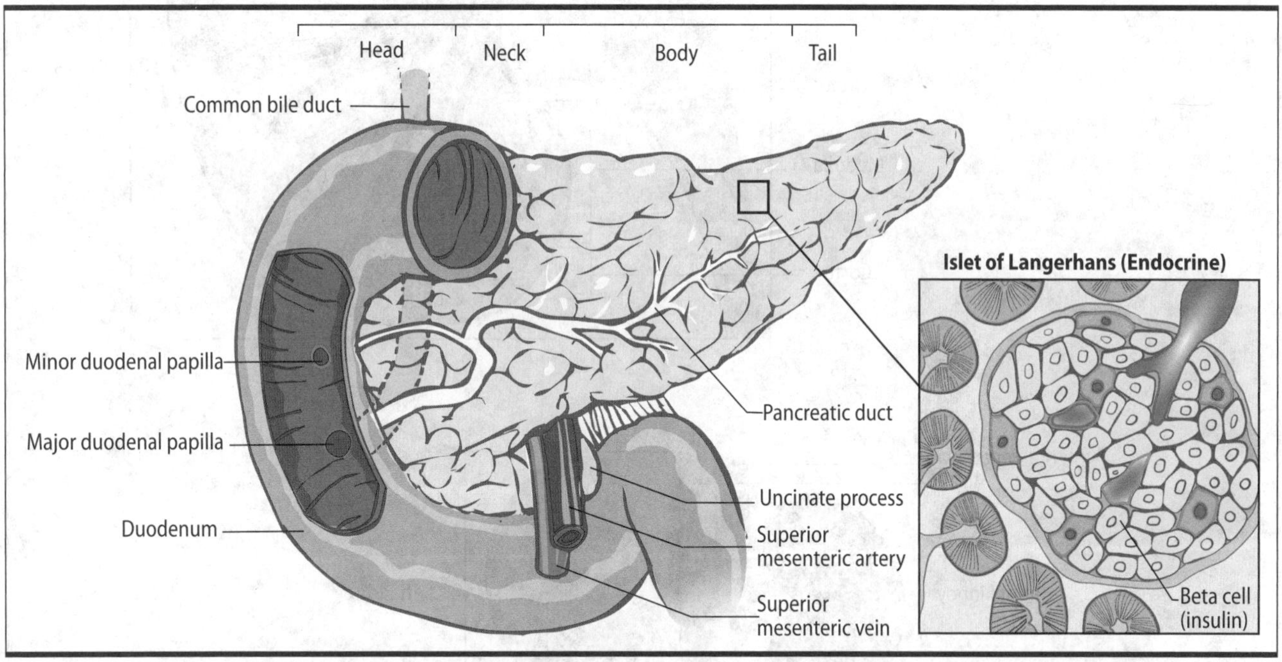

Liver

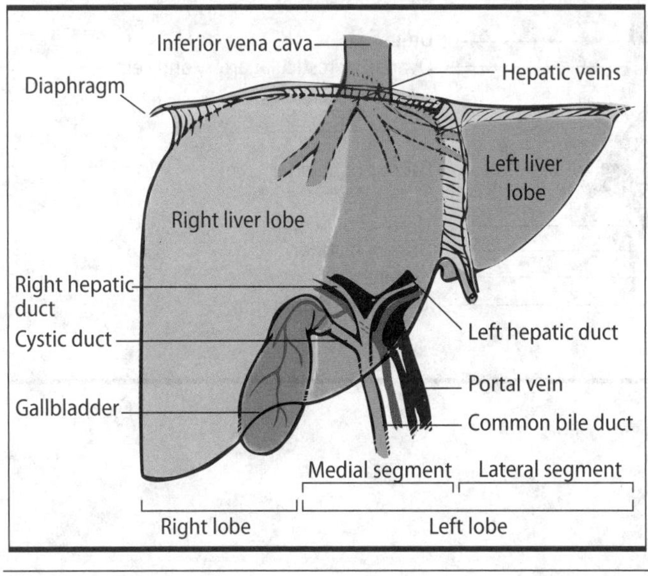

Anus

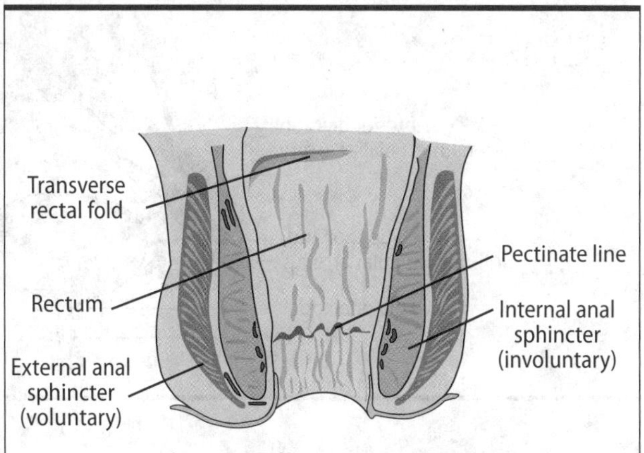

Detail cutaway of lower rectum and anus

Genitourinary System

Urinary System

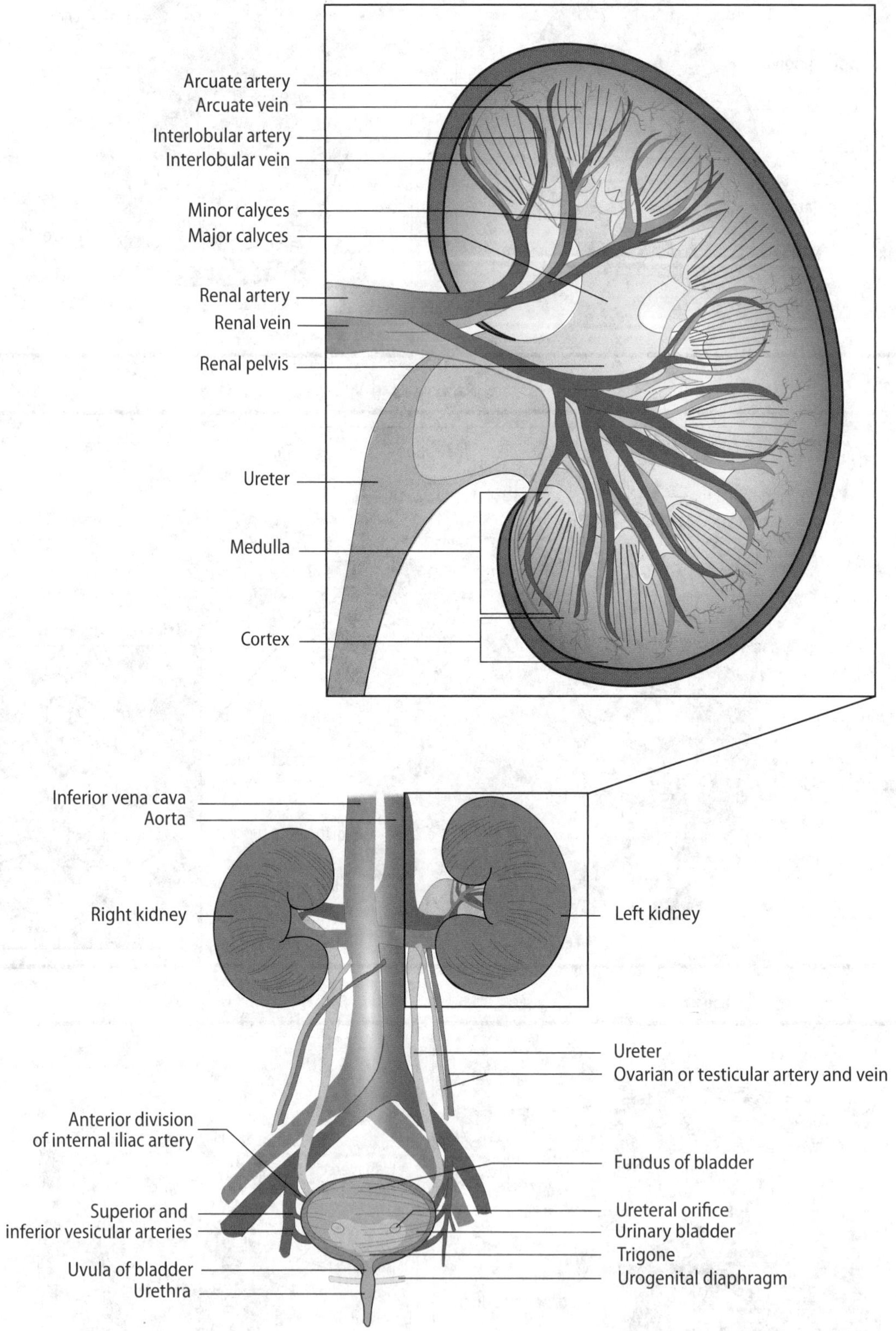
Arcuate artery
Arcuate vein
Interlobular artery
Interlobular vein
Minor calyces
Major calyces
Renal artery
Renal vein
Renal pelvis
Ureter
Medulla
Cortex
Inferior vena cava
Aorta
Right kidney
Left kidney
Ureter
Ovarian or testicular artery and vein
Anterior division of internal iliac artery
Fundus of bladder
Superior and inferior vesicular arteries
Ureteral orifice
Urinary bladder
Trigone
Uvula of bladder
Urogenital diaphragm
Urethra

Nephron

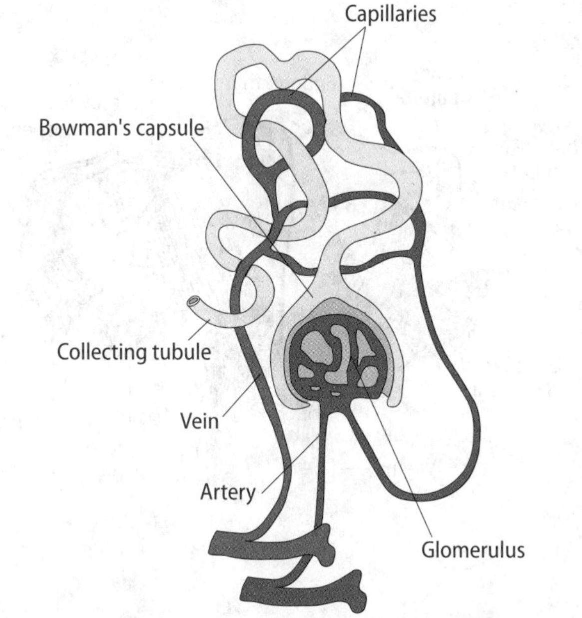

Schematic of nephron, the tiny filtering mechanism of the kidney

Male Genitourinary

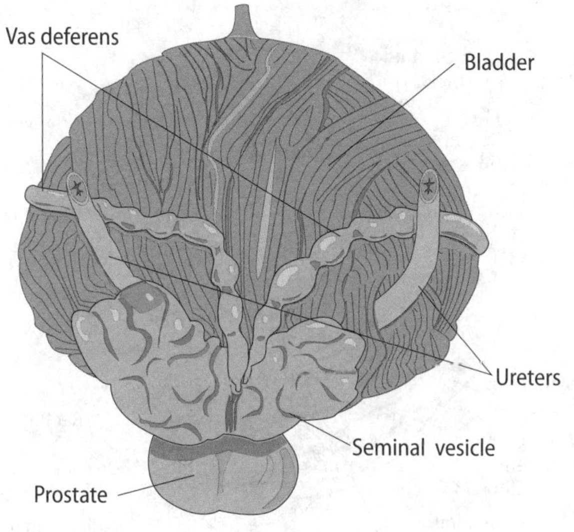

Posterior view of male bladder and prostate

Testis and Associate Structures

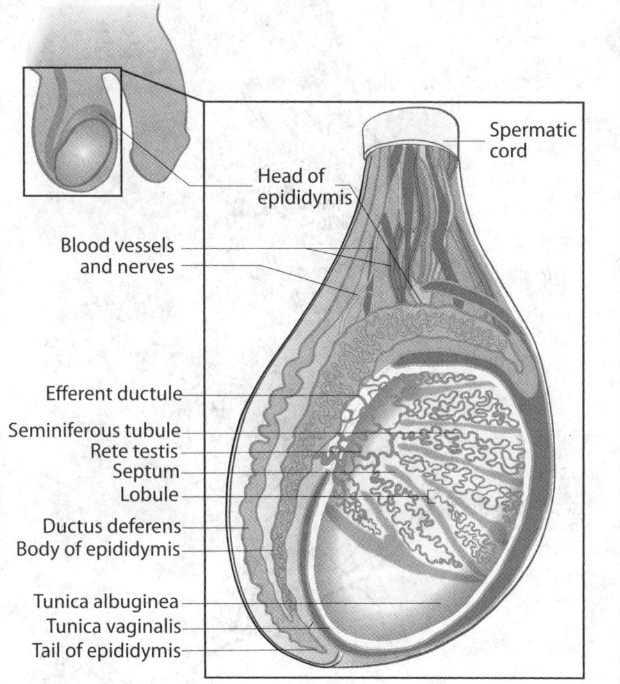

Male Genitourinary System

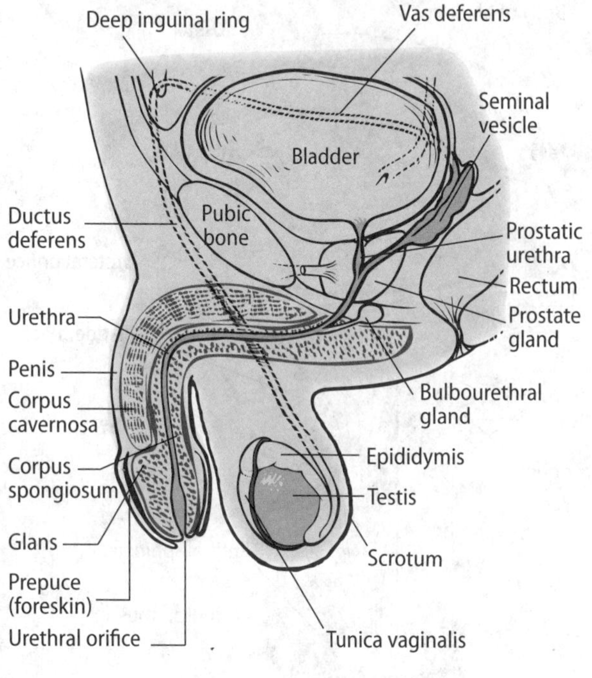

Female Genitourinary

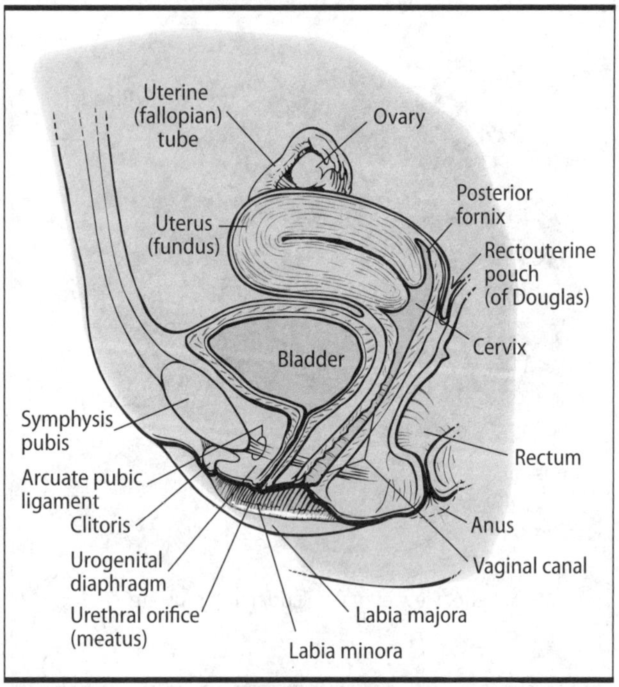

Female Reproductive System

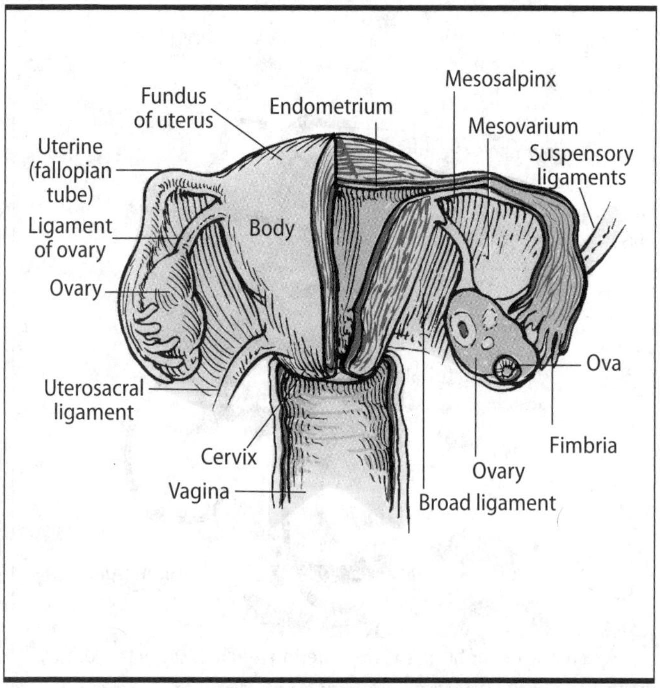

Female Bladder

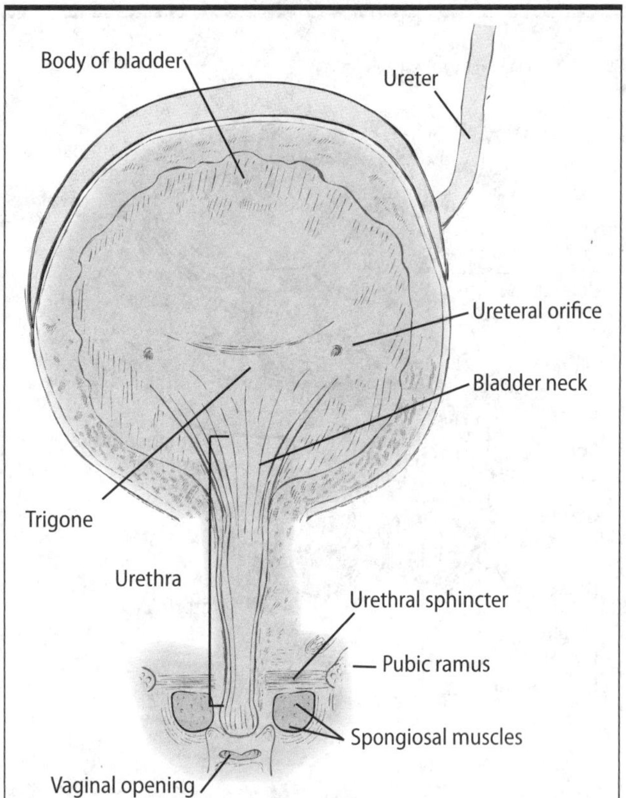

Female Breast

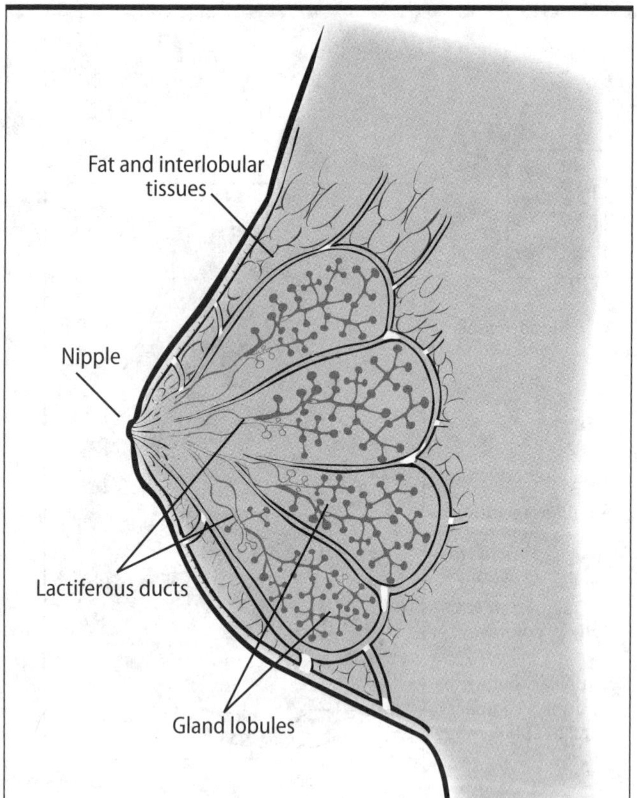

Endocrine System

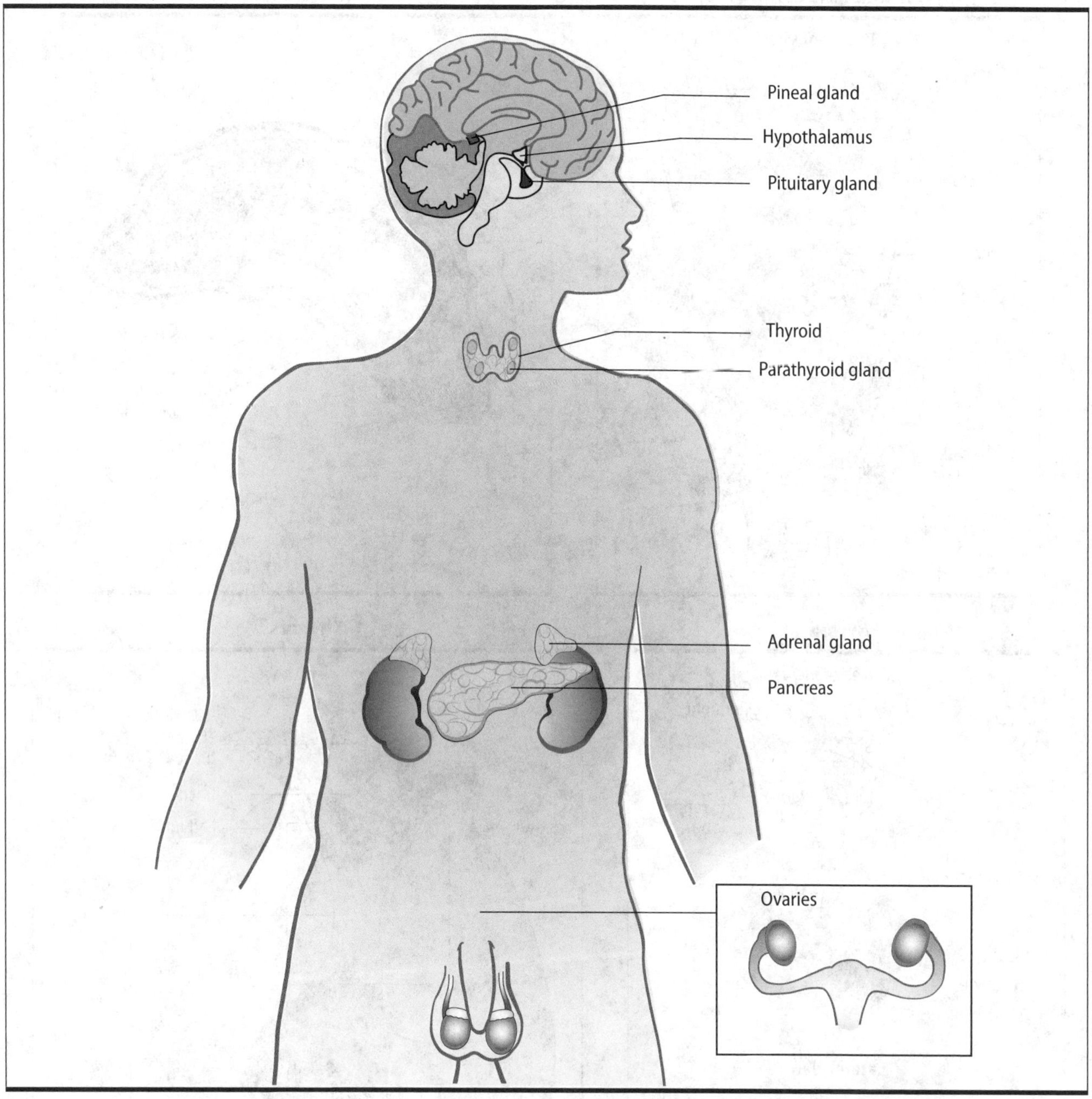

Structure of an Ovary

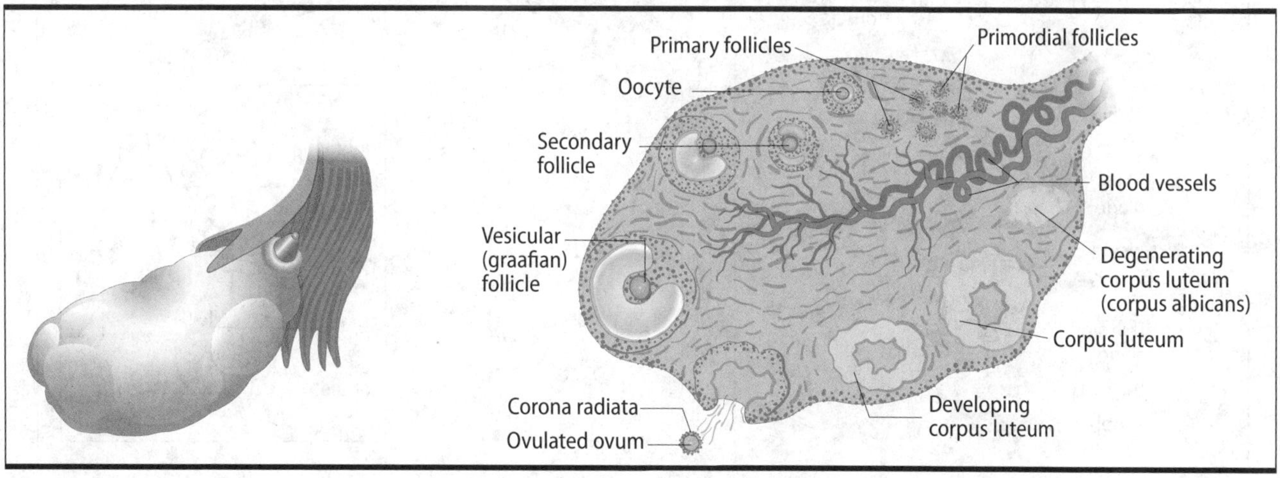

Thyroid and Parathyroid Glands

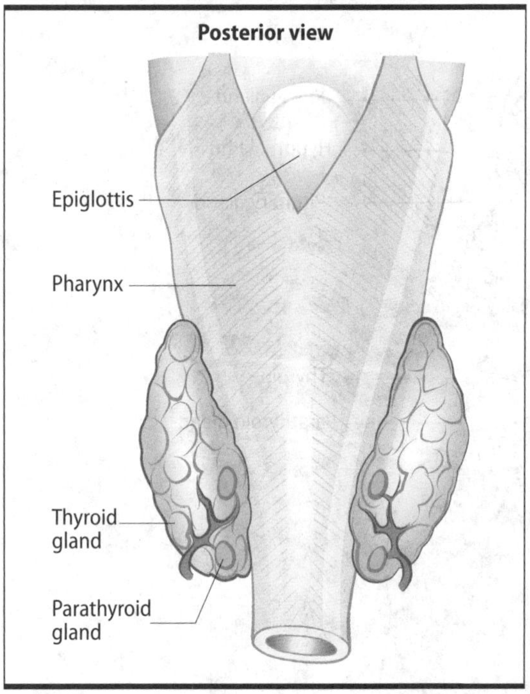

Adrenal Gland

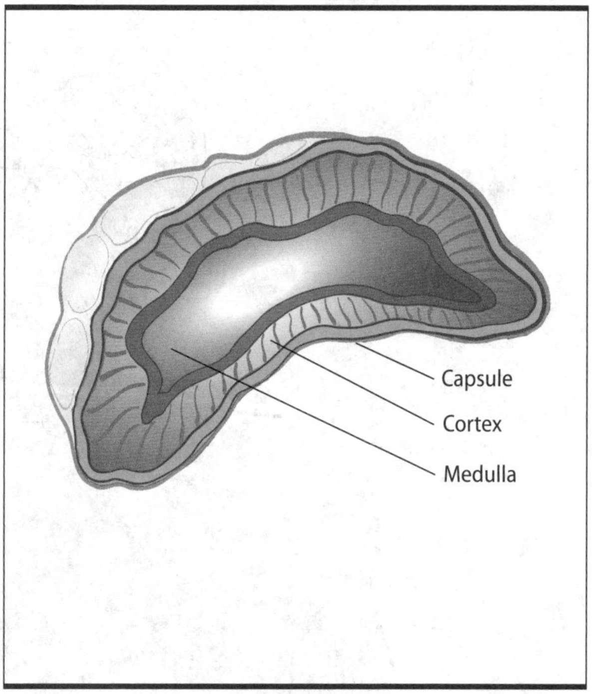

Thyroid

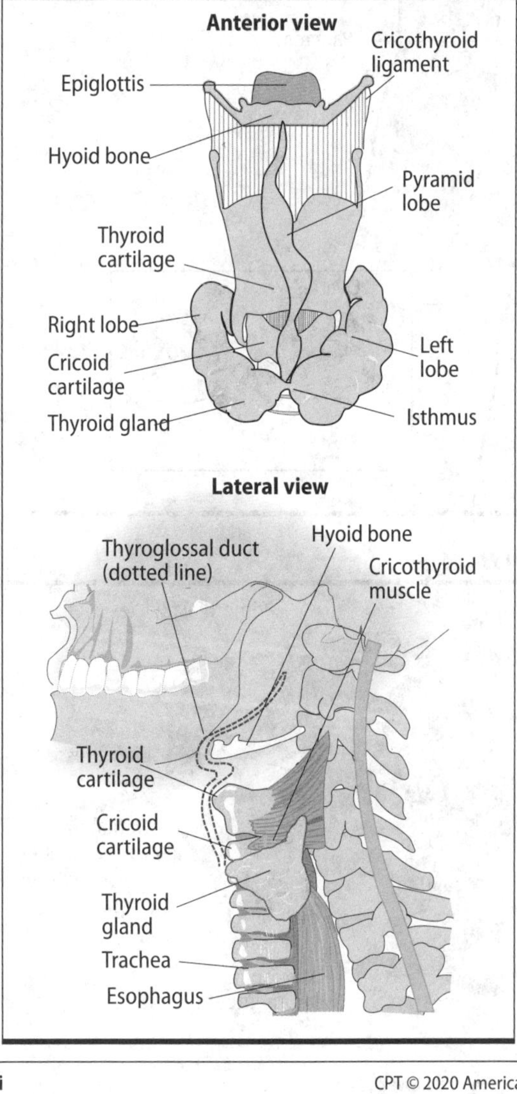

Thymus

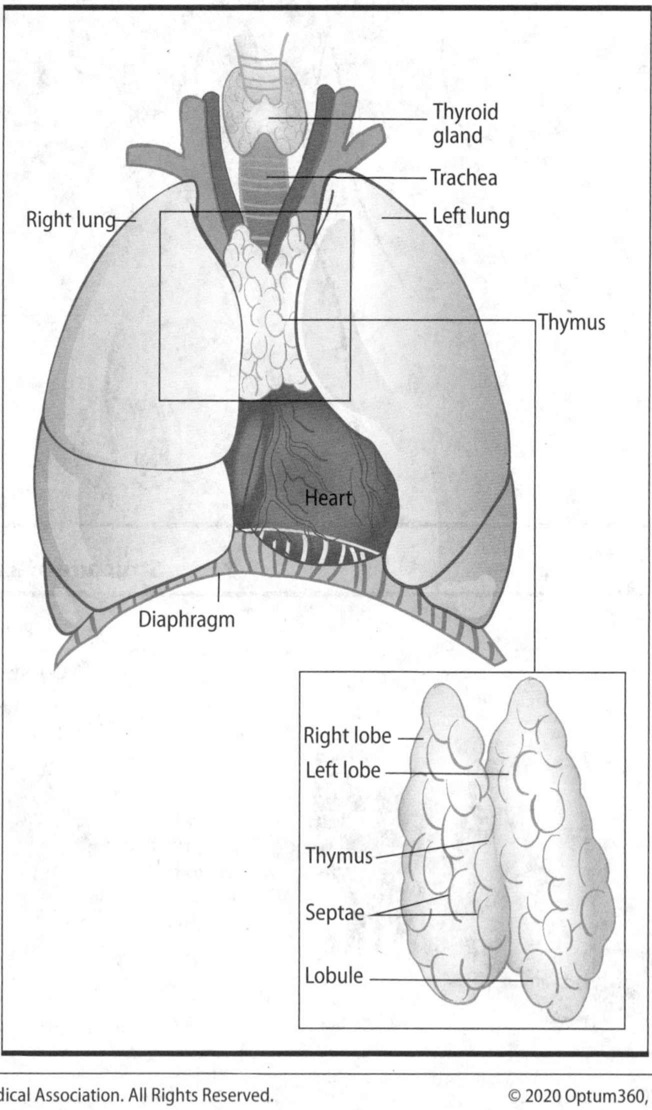

Nervous System

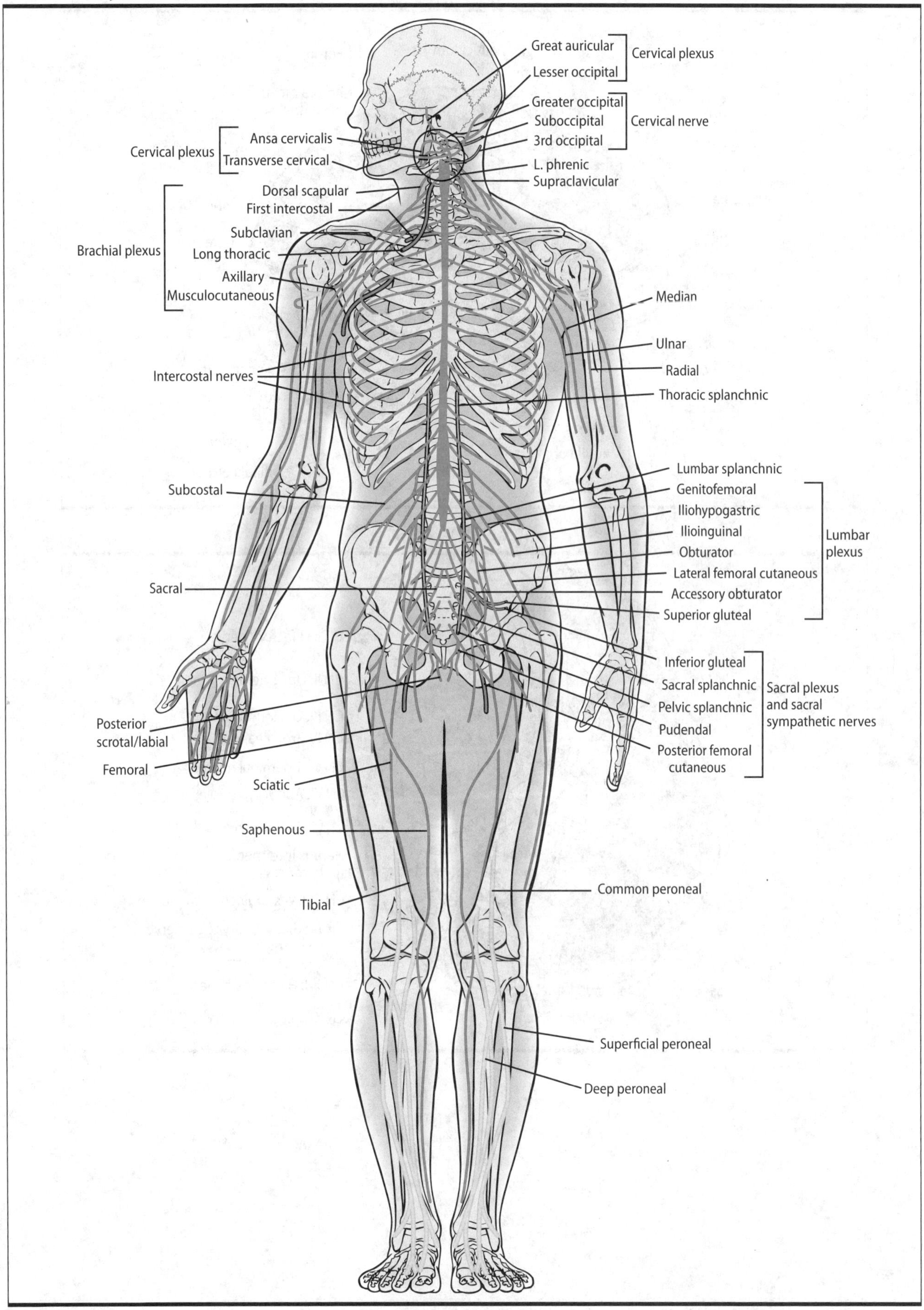
Great auricular
Lesser occipital
Cervical plexus
Greater occipital
Suboccipital
3rd occipital
Cervical nerve
L. phrenic
Supraclavicular
Cervical plexus
Ansa cervicalis
Transverse cervical
Dorsal scapular
First intercostal
Subclavian
Brachial plexus
Long thoracic
Axillary
Musculocutaneous
Median
Ulnar
Radial
Intercostal nerves
Thoracic splanchnic
Lumbar splanchnic
Genitofemoral
Iliohypogastric
Ilioinguinal
Obturator
Lateral femoral cutaneous
Accessory obturator
Superior gluteal
Lumbar plexus
Subcostal
Sacral
Inferior gluteal
Sacral splanchnic
Pelvic splanchnic
Pudendal
Posterior femoral cutaneous
Sacral plexus and sacral sympathetic nerves
Posterior scrotal/labial
Femoral
Sciatic
Saphenous
Common peroneal
Tibial
Superficial peroneal
Deep peroneal

Brain

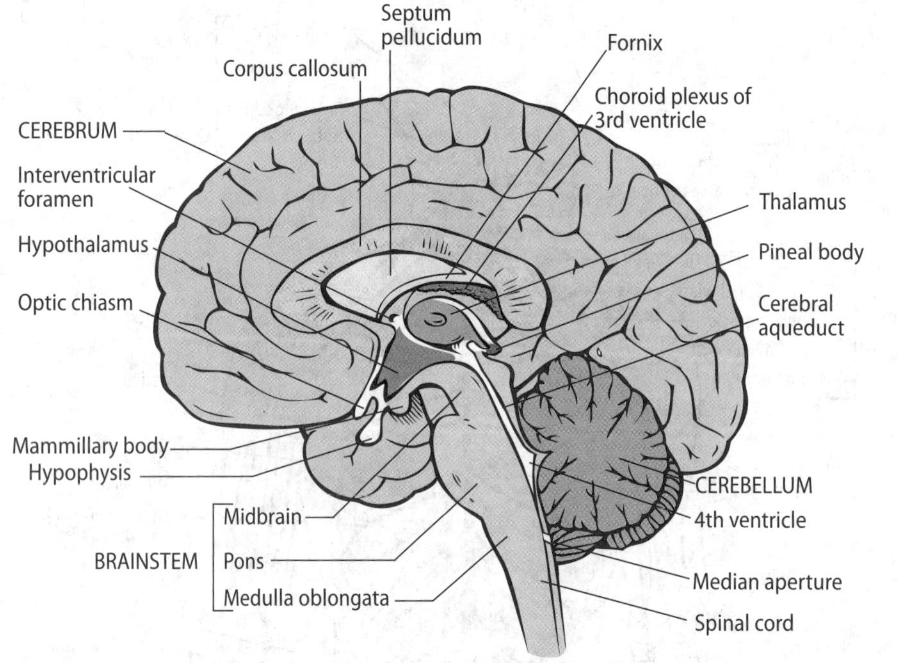
Septum pellucidum
Fornix
Corpus callosum
Choroid plexus of 3rd ventricle
CEREBRUM
Interventricular foramen
Thalamus
Hypothalamus
Pineal body
Optic chiasm
Cerebral aqueduct
Mammillary body
Hypophysis
CEREBELLUM
Midbrain
4th ventricle
BRAINSTEM
Pons
Median aperture
Medulla oblongata
Spinal cord

Cranial Nerves

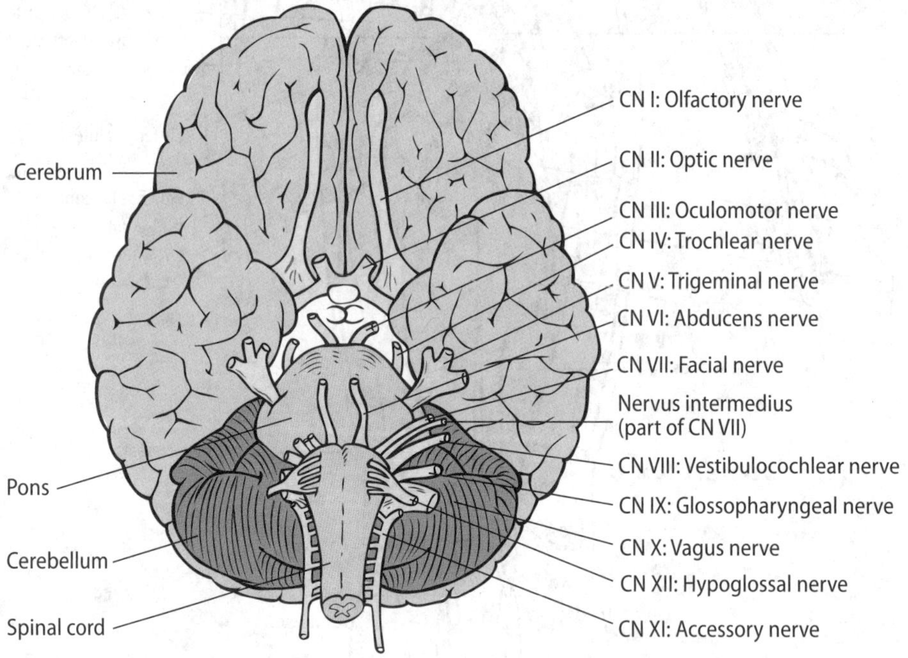
CN I: Olfactory nerve
Cerebrum
CN II: Optic nerve
CN III: Oculomotor nerve
CN IV: Trochlear nerve
CN V: Trigeminal nerve
CN VI: Abducens nerve
CN VII: Facial nerve
Nervus intermedius (part of CN VII)
CN VIII: Vestibulocochlear nerve
Pons
CN IX: Glossopharyngeal nerve
CN X: Vagus nerve
Cerebellum
CN XII: Hypoglossal nerve
Spinal cord
CN XI: Accessory nerve

Spinal Cord and Spinal Nerves

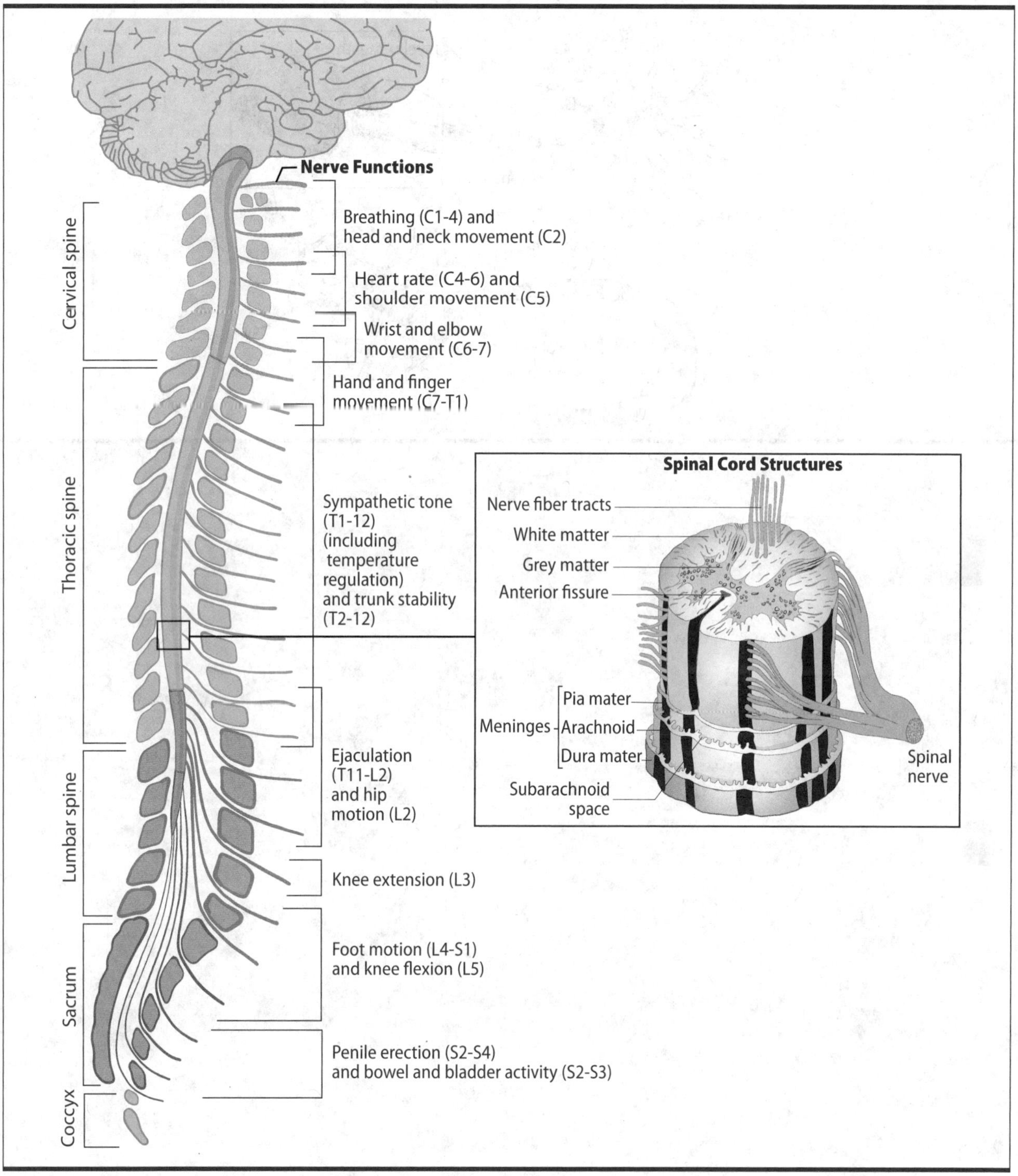
Nerve Functions
Cervical spine
Thoracic spine
Lumbar spine
Sacrum
Coccyx
Breathing (C1-4) and head and neck movement (C2)
Heart rate (C4-6) and shoulder movement (C5)
Wrist and elbow movement (C6-7)
Hand and finger movement (C7-T1)
Sympathetic tone (T1-12) (including temperature regulation) and trunk stability (T2-12)
Ejaculation (T11-L2) and hip motion (L2)
Knee extension (L3)
Foot motion (L4-S1) and knee flexion (L5)
Penile erection (S2-S4) and bowel and bladder activity (S2-S3)
Spinal Cord Structures
Nerve fiber tracts
White matter
Grey matter
Anterior fissure
Meninges
Pia mater
Arachnoid
Dura mater
Subarachnoid space
Spinal nerve

Nerve Cell

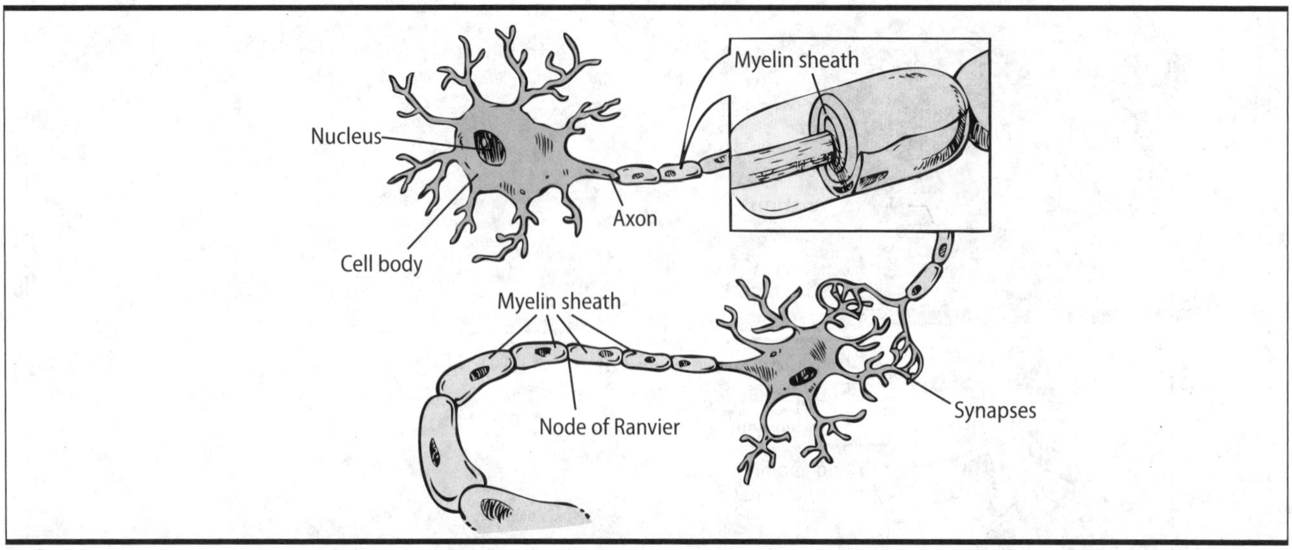
Myelin sheath
Nucleus
Axon
Cell body
Myelin sheath
Synapses
Node of Ranvier

Eye

Eye Structure

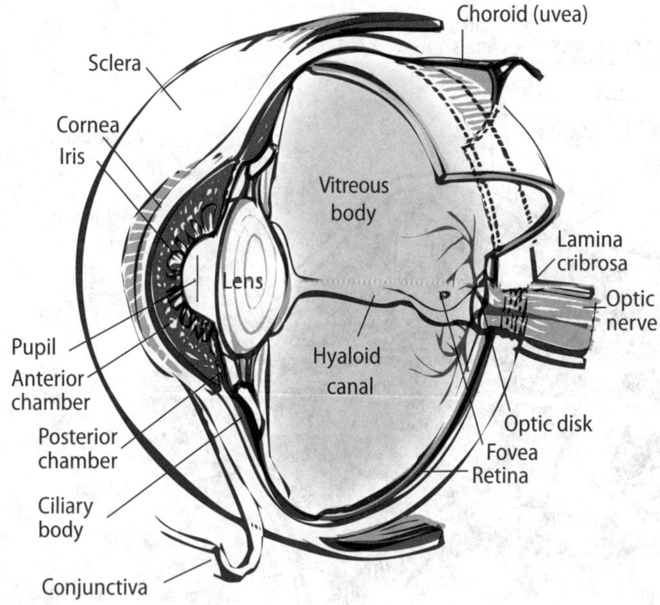

Posterior Pole of Globe/Flow of Aqueous Humor

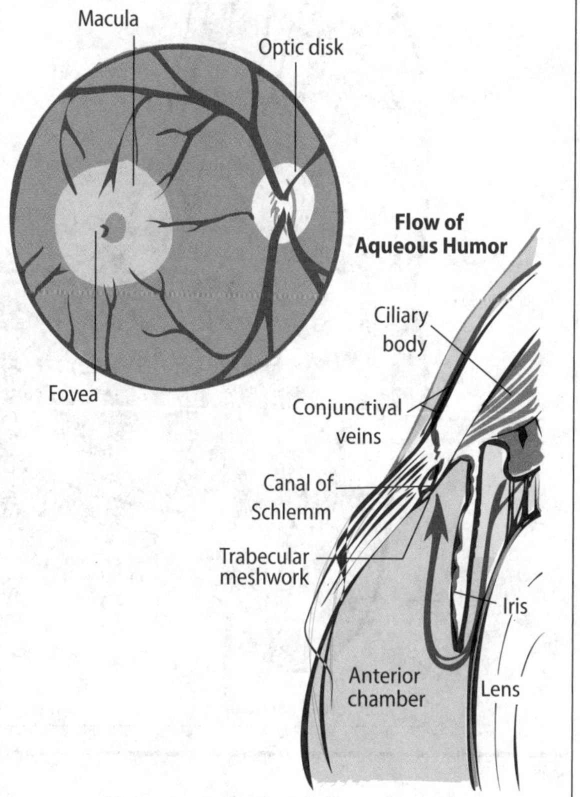

Eye Musculature

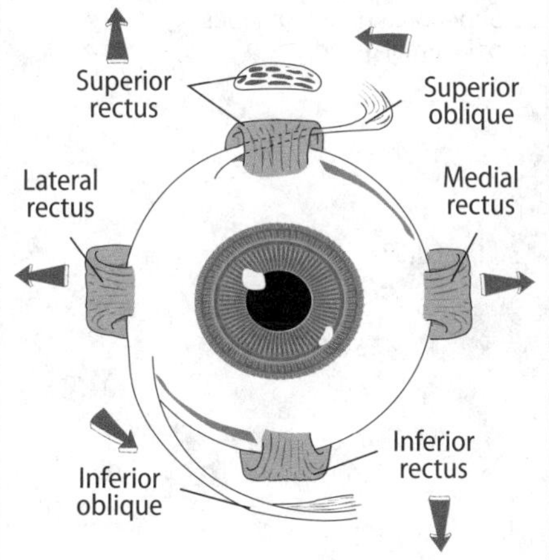

Muscles and actions (right eye)

Eyelid Structures

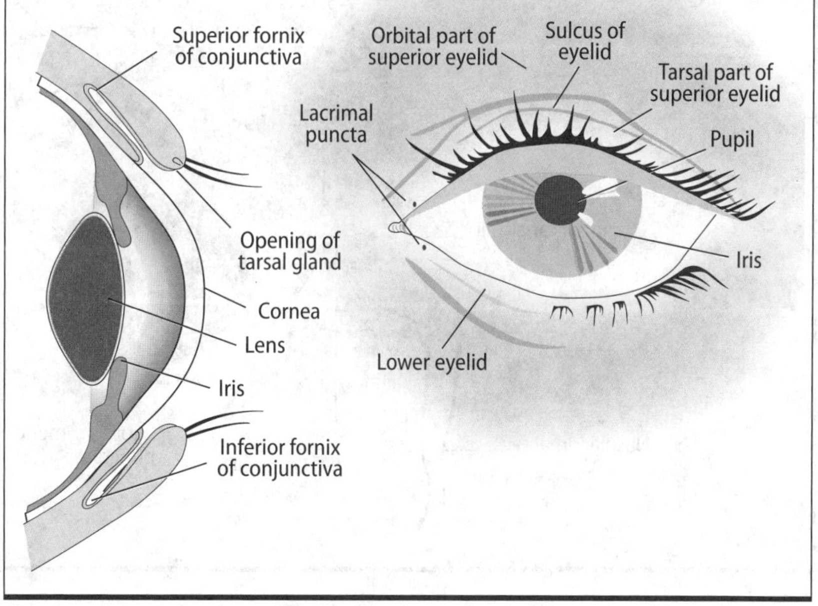

Ear and Lacrimal System

Ear Anatomy

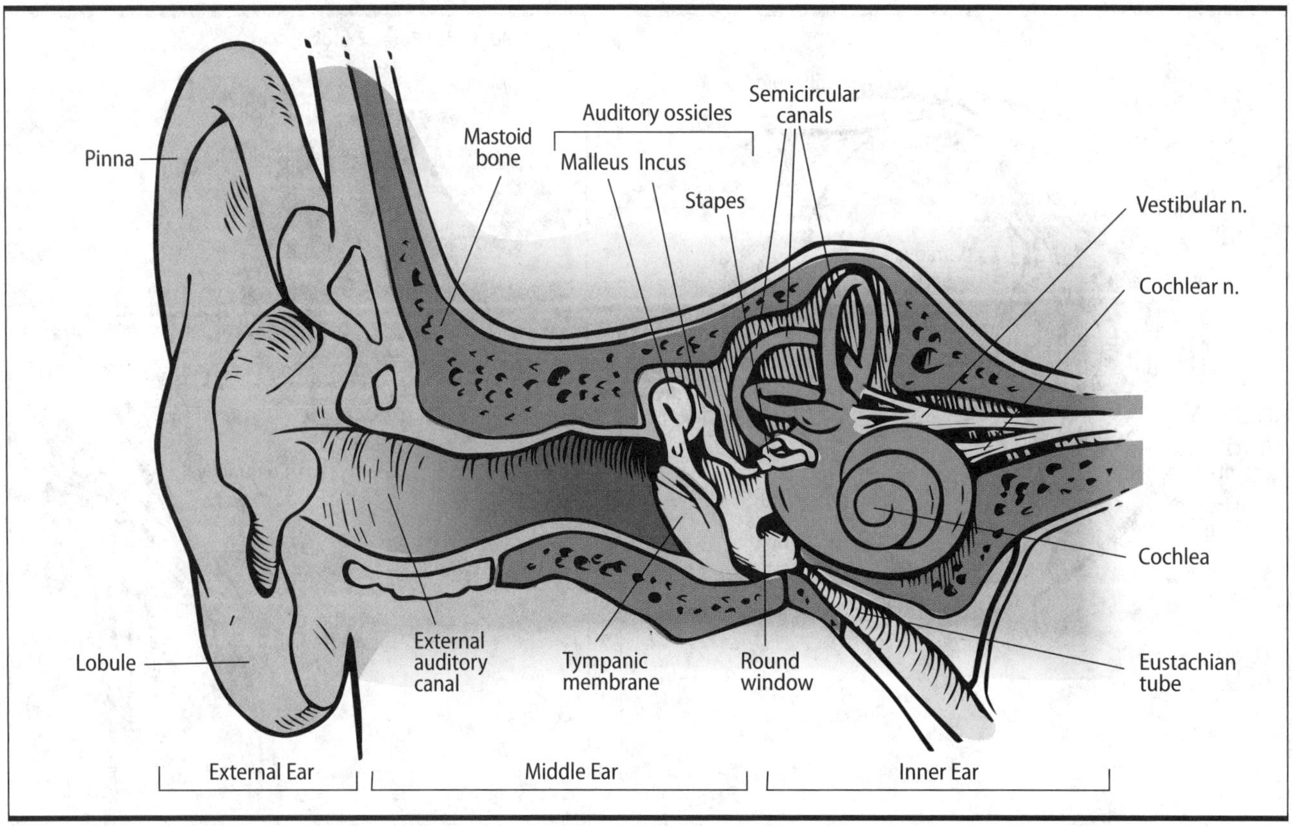

Lacrimal System

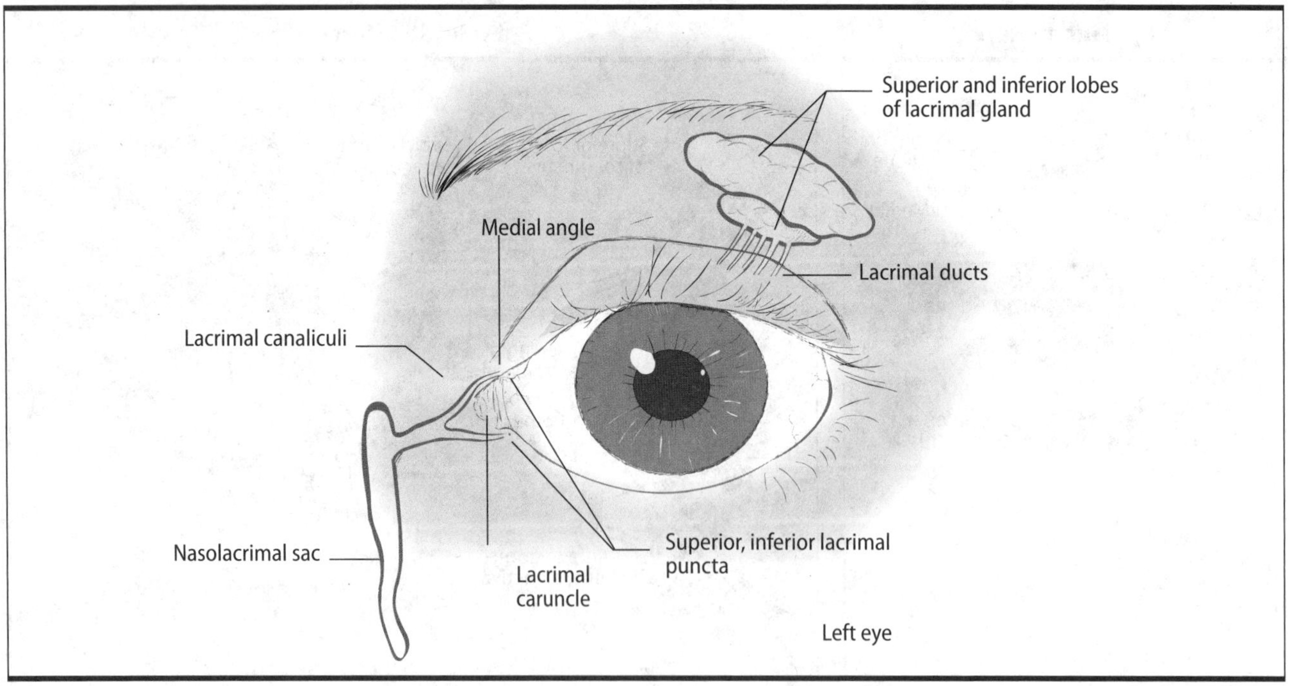

[Resequenced]

 [Resequenced]

 [Resequenced]

 [Resequenced]

C

 [Resequenced]

 [Resequenced]

D

 [Resequenced]

E

 [Resequenced]

 [Resequenced]

F

 [Resequenced]

 [Resequenced]

J

K

L

 [Resequenced]

M

Index
Monitoring — Mycophenolate

 [Resequenced]

 [Resequenced]

 [Resequenced]

S

 [Resequenced]

 [Resequenced]

[Resequenced]

 [Resequenced]

U

 [Resequenced]

 [Resequenced]

X

 [Resequenced]

Y

Z

00100-00126 Anesthesia for Cleft Lip, Ear, ECT, Eyelid, and Salivary Gland Procedures

CMS: 100-04,12,140.1 Qualified Nonphysician Anesthetists; 100-04,12,140.3 Payment for Qualified Nonphysician Anesthetists; 100-04,12,140.3.3 Billing Modifiers; 100-04,12,140.3.4 General Billing Instructions; 100-04,12,140.4.1 Anesthesiologist/Qualified Nonphysican Anesthetist; 100-04,12,140.4.2 Anesthetist and Anesthesiologist in a Single Procedure; 100-04,12,140.4.3 Payment for Medical /Surgical Services by CRNAs; 100-04,12,140.4.4 Conversion Factors for Anesthesia Services; 100-04,12,140.5 Payment for Anesthesia Services Furnished by a Teaching CRNA; 100-04,4,250.3.2 Anesthesia in a Hospital Outpatient Setting

00100 **Anesthesia for procedures on salivary glands, including biopsy**
0.00 0.00 **FUD** XXX N
AMA: 2019,Oct,10; 2018,Jan,8; 2017,Dec,8; 2017,Jan,8; 2016,Jan,13; 2015,Jan,16

00102 **Anesthesia for procedures involving plastic repair of cleft lip**
0.00 0.00 **FUD** XXX N
AMA: 2019,Oct,10; 2018,Jan,8; 2017,Dec,8; 2017,Jan,8; 2016,Jan,13; 2015,Jan,16

00103 **Anesthesia for reconstructive procedures of eyelid (eg, blepharoplasty, ptosis surgery)**
0.00 0.00 **FUD** XXX N
AMA: 2019,Oct,10; 2018,Jan,8; 2017,Dec,8; 2017,Jan,8; 2016,Jan,13; 2015,Jan,16

00104 **Anesthesia for electroconvulsive therapy**
0.00 0.00 **FUD** XXX N
AMA: 2019,Oct,10; 2018,Jan,8; 2017,Dec,8; 2017,Jan,8; 2016,Jan,13; 2015,Jan,16

00120 **Anesthesia for procedures on external, middle, and inner ear including biopsy; not otherwise specified**
0.00 0.00 **FUD** XXX N
AMA: 2019,Oct,10; 2018,Jan,8; 2017,Dec,8; 2017,Jan,8; 2016,Jan,13; 2015,Jan,16

00124 **otoscopy**
0.00 0.00 **FUD** XXX N
AMA: 2019,Oct,10; 2018,Jan,8; 2017,Dec,8; 2017,Jan,8; 2016,Jan,13; 2015,Jan,16

00126 **tympanotomy**
0.00 0.00 **FUD** XXX N
AMA: 2019,Oct,10; 2018,Jan,8; 2017,Dec,8; 2017,Jan,8; 2016,Jan,13; 2015,Jan,16

00140-00148 Anesthesia for Eye Procedures

CMS: 100-04,12,140.1 Qualified Nonphysician Anesthetists; 100-04,12,140.3 Payment for Qualified Nonphysician Anesthetists; 100-04,12,140.3.3 Billing Modifiers; 100-04,12,140.3.4 General Billing Instructions; 100-04,12,140.4.1 Anesthesiologist/Qualified Nonphysican Anesthetist; 100-04,12,140.4.2 Anesthetist and Anesthesiologist in a Single Procedure; 100-04,12,140.4.3 Payment for Medical /Surgical Services by CRNAs; 100-04,12,140.4.4 Conversion Factors for Anesthesia Services; 100-04,12,140.5 Payment for Anesthesia Services Furnished by a Teaching CRNA; 100-04,4,250.3.2 Anesthesia in a Hospital Outpatient Setting

00140 **Anesthesia for procedures on eye; not otherwise specified**
0.00 0.00 **FUD** XXX N
AMA: 2019,Oct,10; 2018,Jan,8; 2017,Dec,8; 2017,Jan,8; 2016,Jan,13; 2015,Jan,16

00142 **lens surgery**
0.00 0.00 **FUD** XXX N
AMA: 2019,Oct,10; 2018,Jan,8; 2017,Dec,8; 2017,Jan,8; 2016,Jan,13; 2015,Jan,16

00144 **corneal transplant**
0.00 0.00 **FUD** XXX N
AMA: 2019,Oct,10; 2018,Jan,8; 2017,Dec,8; 2017,Jan,8; 2016,Jan,13; 2015,Jan,16

00145 **vitreoretinal surgery**
0.00 0.00 **FUD** XXX N
AMA: 2019,Oct,10; 2018,Jan,8; 2017,Dec,8; 2017,Jan,8; 2016,Jan,13; 2015,Jan,16

00147 **iridectomy**
0.00 0.00 **FUD** XXX N
AMA: 2019,Oct,10; 2018,Jan,8; 2017,Dec,8; 2017,Jan,8; 2016,Jan,13; 2015,Jan,16

00148 **ophthalmoscopy**
0.00 0.00 **FUD** XXX N
AMA: 2019,Oct,10; 2018,Jan,8; 2017,Dec,8; 2017,Jan,8; 2016,Jan,13; 2015,Jan,16

00160-00326 Anesthesia for Face and Head Procedures

CMS: 100-04,12,140.1 Qualified Nonphysician Anesthetists; 100-04,12,140.3 Payment for Qualified Nonphysician Anesthetists; 100-04,12,140.3.3 Billing Modifiers; 100-04,12,140.3.4 General Billing Instructions; 100-04,12,140.4.1 Anesthesiologist/Qualified Nonphysican Anesthetist; 100-04,12,140.4.2 Anesthetist and Anesthesiologist in a Single Procedure; 100-04,12,140.4.4 Conversion Factors for Anesthesia Services; 100-04,12,140.5 Payment for Anesthesia Services Furnished by a Teaching CRNA; 100-04,4,250.3.2 Anesthesia in a Hospital Outpatient Setting

00160 **Anesthesia for procedures on nose and accessory sinuses; not otherwise specified**
0.00 0.00 **FUD** XXX N
AMA: 2019,Oct,10; 2018,Jan,8; 2017,Dec,8; 2017,Jan,8; 2016,Jan,13; 2015,Jan,16

00162 **radical surgery**
0.00 0.00 **FUD** XXX N
AMA: 2019,Oct,10; 2018,Jan,8; 2017,Dec,8; 2017,Jan,8; 2016,Jan,13; 2015,Jan,16

00164 **biopsy, soft tissue**
0.00 0.00 **FUD** XXX N
AMA: 2019,Oct,10; 2018,Jan,8; 2017,Dec,8; 2017,Jan,8; 2016,Jan,13; 2015,Jan,16

00170 **Anesthesia for intraoral procedures, including biopsy; not otherwise specified**
0.00 0.00 **FUD** XXX N
AMA: 2019,Oct,10; 2018,Jan,8; 2017,Dec,8; 2017,Jan,8; 2016,Jan,13; 2015,Jan,16

00172 **repair of cleft palate**
0.00 0.00 **FUD** XXX N
AMA: 2019,Oct,10; 2018,Jan,8; 2017,Dec,8; 2017,Jan,8; 2016,Jan,13; 2015,Jan,16

00174 **excision of retropharyngeal tumor**
0.00 0.00 **FUD** XXX N
AMA: 2019,Oct,10; 2018,Jan,8; 2017,Dec,8; 2017,Jan,8; 2016,Jan,13; 2015,Jan,16

00176 **radical surgery**
0.00 0.00 **FUD** XXX C
AMA: 2019,Oct,10; 2018,Jan,8; 2017,Dec,8; 2017,Jan,8; 2016,Jan,13; 2015,Jan,16

00190 **Anesthesia for procedures on facial bones or skull; not otherwise specified**
0.00 0.00 **FUD** XXX N
AMA: 2019,Oct,10; 2018,Jan,8; 2017,Dec,8; 2017,Jan,8; 2016,Jan,13; 2015,Jan,16

00192 **radical surgery (including prognathism)**
0.00 0.00 **FUD** XXX C
AMA: 2019,Oct,10; 2018,Jan,8; 2017,Dec,8; 2017,Jan,8; 2016,Jan,13; 2015,Jan,16

00210 **Anesthesia for intracranial procedures; not otherwise specified**
0.00 0.00 **FUD** XXX N
AMA: 2019,Oct,10; 2018,Jan,8; 2017,Dec,8; 2017,Jan,8; 2016,Jan,13; 2015,Jan,16

00211 **craniotomy or craniectomy for evacuation of hematoma**
0.00 0.00 **FUD** XXX C
AMA: 2019,Oct,10; 2018,Jan,8; 2017,Dec,8; 2017,Jan,8; 2016,Jan,13; 2015,Jan,16

00212 **subdural taps**
0.00 0.00 **FUD** XXX N
AMA: 2019,Oct,10; 2018,Jan,8; 2017,Dec,8; 2017,Jan,8; 2016,Jan,13; 2015,Jan,16

00214 **burr holes, including ventriculography**
0.00 0.00 **FUD** XXX C
AMA: 2019,Oct,10; 2018,Jan,8; 2017,Dec,8; 2017,Jan,8; 2016,Jan,13; 2015,Jan,16

00215 **cranioplasty or elevation of depressed skull fracture, extradural (simple or compound)**
0.00 0.00 FUD XXX C
AMA: 2019,Oct,10; 2018,Jan,8; 2017,Dec,8; 2017,Jan,8; 2016,Jan,13; 2015,Jan,16

00216 **vascular procedures**
0.00 0.00 FUD XXX N
AMA: 2019,Oct,10; 2018,Jan,8; 2017,Dec,8; 2017,Jan,8; 2016,Jan,13; 2015,Jan,16

00218 **procedures in sitting position**
0.00 0.00 FUD XXX N
AMA: 2019,Oct,10; 2018,Jan,8; 2017,Dec,8; 2017,Jan,8; 2016,Jan,13; 2015,Jan,16

00220 **cerebrospinal fluid shunting procedures**
0.00 0.00 FUD XXX N
AMA: 2019,Oct,10; 2018,Jan,8; 2017,Dec,8; 2017,Jan,8; 2016,Jan,13; 2015,Jan,16

00222 **electrocoagulation of intracranial nerve**
0.00 0.00 FUD XXX N
AMA: 2019,Oct,10; 2018,Jan,8; 2017,Dec,8; 2017,Jan,8; 2016,Jan,13; 2015,Jan,16

00300 **Anesthesia for all procedures on the integumentary system, muscles and nerves of head, neck, and posterior trunk, not otherwise specified**
0.00 0.00 FUD XXX N
AMA: 2019,Oct,10; 2018,Jan,8; 2017,Dec,8; 2017,Jan,8; 2016,Jan,13; 2015,Jan,16

00320 **Anesthesia for all procedures on esophagus, thyroid, larynx, trachea and lymphatic system of neck; not otherwise specified, age 1 year or older**
0.00 0.00 FUD XXX N
AMA: 2019,Oct,10; 2018,Jan,8; 2017,Dec,8; 2017,Jan,8; 2016,Jan,13; 2015,Jan,16

00322 **needle biopsy of thyroid**
EXCLUDES *Cervical spine and spinal cord procedures (00600, 00604, 00670)*
0.00 0.00 FUD XXX N
AMA: 2019,Oct,10; 2018,Jan,8; 2017,Dec,8; 2017,Jan,8; 2016,Jan,13; 2015,Jan,16

00326 **Anesthesia for all procedures on the larynx and trachea in children younger than 1 year of age** A
INCLUDES Anesthesia for patient of extreme age, younger than 1 year and older than 70 (99100)
0.00 0.00 FUD XXX N
AMA: 2019,Oct,10; 2018,Jan,8; 2017,Dec,8; 2017,Jan,8; 2016,Jan,13; 2015,Jan,16

00350-00352 Anesthesia for Neck Vessel Procedures

CMS: 100-04,12,140.1 Qualified Nonphysician Anesthetists; 100-04,12,140.3 Payment for Qualified Nonphysician Anesthetists; 100-04,12,140.3.3 Billing Modifiers; 100-04,12,140.3.4 General Billing Instructions; 100-04,12,140.4.1 Anesthesiologist/Qualified Nonphysican Anesthetist; 100-04,12,140.4.2 Anesthetist and Anesthesiologist in a Single Procedure; 100-04,12,140.4.3 Payment for Medical /Surgical Services by CRNAs; 100-04,12,140.4.4 Conversion Factors for Anesthesia Services; 100-04,12,140.5 Payment for Anesthesia Services Furnished by a Teaching CRNA; 100-04,4,250.3.2 Anesthesia in a Hospital Outpatient Setting

EXCLUDES *Arteriography (01916)*

00350 **Anesthesia for procedures on major vessels of neck; not otherwise specified**
0.00 0.00 FUD XXX N
AMA: 2019,Oct,10; 2018,Jan,8; 2017,Dec,8; 2017,Jan,8; 2016,Jan,13; 2015,Jan,16

00352 **simple ligation**
0.00 0.00 FUD XXX N
AMA: 2019,Oct,10; 2018,Jan,8; 2017,Dec,8; 2017,Jan,8; 2016,Jan,13; 2015,Jan,16

00400-00529 Anesthesia for Chest/Pectoral Girdle Procedures

CMS: 100-04,12,140.1 Qualified Nonphysician Anesthetists; 100-04,12,140.3 Payment for Qualified Nonphysician Anesthetists; 100-04,12,140.3.3 Billing Modifiers; 100-04,12,140.3.4 General Billing Instructions; 100-04,12,140.4.1 Anesthesiologist/Qualified Nonphysican Anesthetist; 100-04,12,140.4.2 Anesthetist and Anesthesiologist in a Single Procedure; 100-04,12,140.4.3 Payment for Medical /Surgical Services by CRNAs; 100-04,12,140.4.4 Conversion Factors for Anesthesia Services; 100-04,12,140.5 Payment for Anesthesia Services Furnished by a Teaching CRNA; 100-04,4,250.3.2 Anesthesia in a Hospital Outpatient Setting

00400 **Anesthesia for procedures on the integumentary system on the extremities, anterior trunk and perineum; not otherwise specified**
0.00 0.00 FUD XXX N
AMA: 2019,Oct,10; 2018,Jan,8; 2017,Dec,8; 2017,Jan,8; 2016,Jan,13; 2015,Jan,16

00402 **reconstructive procedures on breast (eg, reduction or augmentation mammoplasty, muscle flaps)**
0.00 0.00 FUD XXX N
AMA: 2019,Oct,10; 2018,Jan,8; 2017,Dec,8; 2017,Jan,8; 2016,Jan,13; 2015,Jan,16

00404 **radical or modified radical procedures on breast**
0.00 0.00 FUD XXX N
AMA: 2019,Oct,10; 2018,Jan,8; 2017,Dec,8; 2017,Jan,8; 2016,Jan,13; 2015,Jan,16

00406 **radical or modified radical procedures on breast with internal mammary node dissection**
0.00 0.00 FUD XXX N
AMA: 2019,Oct,10; 2018,Jan,8; 2017,Dec,8; 2017,Jan,8; 2016,Jan,13; 2015,Jan,16

00410 **electrical conversion of arrhythmias**
0.00 0.00 FUD XXX N
AMA: 2019,Oct,10; 2018,Jan,8; 2017,Dec,8; 2017,Jan,8; 2016,Jan,13; 2015,Jan,16

00450 **Anesthesia for procedures on clavicle and scapula; not otherwise specified**
0.00 0.00 FUD XXX N
AMA: 2019,Oct,10; 2018,Jan,8; 2017,Dec,8; 2017,Jan,8; 2016,Jan,13; 2015,Jan,16

00454 **biopsy of clavicle**
0.00 0.00 FUD XXX N
AMA: 2019,Oct,10; 2018,Jan,8; 2017,Dec,8; 2017,Jan,8; 2016,Jan,13; 2015,Jan,16

00470 **Anesthesia for partial rib resection; not otherwise specified**
0.00 0.00 FUD XXX N
AMA: 2019,Oct,10; 2018,Jan,8; 2017,Dec,8; 2017,Jan,8; 2016,Jan,13; 2015,Jan,16

00472 **thoracoplasty (any type)**
0.00 0.00 FUD XXX N
AMA: 2019,Oct,10; 2018,Jan,8; 2017,Dec,8; 2017,Jan,8; 2016,Jan,13; 2015,Jan,16

00474 **radical procedures (eg, pectus excavatum)**
0.00 0.00 FUD XXX C
AMA: 2019,Oct,10; 2018,Jan,8; 2017,Dec,8; 2017,Jan,8; 2016,Jan,13; 2015,Jan,16

00500 **Anesthesia for all procedures on esophagus**
0.00 0.00 FUD XXX N
AMA: 2019,Oct,10; 2018,Jan,8; 2017,Dec,8; 2017,Jan,8; 2016,Jan,13; 2015,Jan,16

00520 **Anesthesia for closed chest procedures; (including bronchoscopy) not otherwise specified**
0.00 0.00 FUD XXX N
AMA: 2019,Oct,10; 2018,Jan,8; 2017,Dec,8; 2017,Jan,8; 2016,Jan,13; 2015,Jan,16

00522 **needle biopsy of pleura**
0.00 0.00 FUD XXX N
AMA: 2019,Oct,10; 2018,Jan,8; 2017,Dec,8; 2017,Jan,8; 2016,Jan,13; 2015,Jan,16

00524 **pneumocentesis**
0.00 0.00 **FUD** XXX C
AMA: 2019,Oct,10; 2018,Jan,8; 2017,Dec,8; 2017,Jan,8; 2016,Jan,13; 2015,Jan,16

00528 **mediastinoscopy and diagnostic thoracoscopy not utilizing 1 lung ventilation**
EXCLUDES *Tracheobronchial reconstruction (00539)*
0.00 0.00 **FUD** XXX N
AMA: 2019,Oct,10; 2018,Jan,8; 2017,Dec,8; 2017,Jan,8; 2016,Jan,13; 2015,Jan,16

00529 **mediastinoscopy and diagnostic thoracoscopy utilizing 1 lung ventilation**
0.00 0.00 **FUD** XXX N
AMA: 2019,Oct,10; 2018,Jan,8; 2017,Dec,8; 2017,Jan,8; 2016,Jan,13; 2015,Jan,16

00530 Anesthesia for Cardiac Pacemaker Procedure

CMS: 100-03,10.6 Anesthesia in Cardiac Pacemaker Surgery; 100-04,12,140.1 Qualified Nonphysician Anesthetists; 100-04,12,140.3 Payment for Qualified Nonphysician Anesthetists; 100-04,12,140.3.3 Billing Modifiers; 100-04,12,140.3.4 General Billing Instructions; 100-04,12,140.4.1 Anesthesiologist/Qualified Nonphysican Anesthetist; 100-04,12,140.4.2 Anesthetist and Anesthesiologist in a Single Procedure; 100-04,12,140.4.3 Payment for Medical /Surgical Services by CRNAs; 100-04,12,140.4.4 Conversion Factors for Anesthesia Services; 100-04,12,140.5 Payment for Anesthesia Services Furnished by a Teaching CRNA; 100-04,4,250.3.2 Anesthesia in a Hospital Outpatient Setting

00530 **Anesthesia for permanent transvenous pacemaker insertion**
0.00 0.00 **FUD** XXX N
AMA: 2019,Oct,10; 2018,Jan,8; 2017,Dec,8; 2017,Jan,8; 2016,Jan,13; 2015,Jan,16

00532-00550 Anesthesia for Heart and Lung Procedures

CMS: 100-04,12,140.1 Qualified Nonphysician Anesthetists; 100-04,12,140.3 Payment for Qualified Nonphysician Anesthetists; 100-04,12,140.3.3 Billing Modifiers; 100-04,12,140.3.4 General Billing Instructions; 100-04,12,140.4.1 Anesthesiologist/Qualified Nonphysican Anesthetist; 100-04,12,140.4.2 Anesthetist and Anesthesiologist in a Single Procedure; 100-04,12,140.4.3 Payment for Medical /Surgical Services by CRNAs; 100-04,12,140.4.4 Conversion Factors for Anesthesia Services; 100-04,12,140.5 Payment for Anesthesia Services Furnished by a Teaching CRNA; 100-04,4,250.3.2 Anesthesia in a Hospital Outpatient Setting

00532 **Anesthesia for access to central venous circulation**
0.00 0.00 **FUD** XXX N
AMA: 2019,Oct,10; 2018,Jan,8; 2017,Dec,8; 2017,Jan,8; 2016,Jan,13; 2015,Jan,16

00534 **Anesthesia for transvenous insertion or replacement of pacing cardioverter-defibrillator**
EXCLUDES *Transthoracic approach (00560)*
0.00 0.00 **FUD** XXX N
AMA: 2019,Oct,10; 2018,Jan,8; 2017,Dec,8; 2017,Jan,8; 2016,Jan,13; 2015,Jan,16

00537 **Anesthesia for cardiac electrophysiologic procedures including radiofrequency ablation**
0.00 0.00 **FUD** XXX N
AMA: 2019,Oct,10; 2018,Jan,8; 2017,Dec,8; 2017,Jan,8; 2016,Jan,13; 2015,Jan,16

00539 **Anesthesia for tracheobronchial reconstruction**
0.00 0.00 **FUD** XXX N
AMA: 2019,Oct,10; 2018,Jan,8; 2017,Dec,8; 2017,Jan,8; 2016,Jan,13; 2015,Jan,16

00540 **Anesthesia for thoracotomy procedures involving lungs, pleura, diaphragm, and mediastinum (including surgical thoracoscopy); not otherwise specified**
EXCLUDES *Thoracic spine and spinal cord procedures via anterior transthoracic approach (00625-00626)*
0.00 0.00 **FUD** XXX C
AMA: 2019,Oct,10; 2018,Jan,8; 2017,Dec,8; 2017,Jan,8; 2016,Jan,13; 2015,Jan,16

00541 **utilizing 1 lung ventilation**
EXCLUDES *Thoracic spine and spinal cord procedures via anterior transthoracic approach (00625-00626)*
0.00 0.00 **FUD** XXX N
AMA: 2019,Oct,10; 2018,Jan,8; 2017,Dec,8; 2017,Jan,8; 2016,Jan,13; 2015,Jan,16

00542 **decortication**
0.00 0.00 **FUD** XXX C
AMA: 2019,Oct,10; 2018,Jan,8; 2017,Dec,8; 2017,Jan,8; 2016,Jan,13; 2015,Jan,16

00546 **pulmonary resection with thoracoplasty**
0.00 0.00 **FUD** XXX C
AMA: 2019,Oct,10; 2018,Jan,8; 2017,Dec,8; 2017,Jan,8; 2016,Jan,13; 2015,Jan,16

00548 **intrathoracic procedures on the trachea and bronchi**
0.00 0.00 **FUD** XXX N
AMA: 2019,Oct,10; 2018,Jan,8; 2017,Dec,8; 2017,Jan,8; 2016,Jan,13; 2015,Jan,16

00550 **Anesthesia for sternal debridement**
0.00 0.00 **FUD** XXX N
AMA: 2019,Oct,10; 2018,Jan,8; 2017,Dec,8; 2017,Jan,8; 2016,Jan,13; 2015,Jan,16

00560-00580 Anesthesia for Open Heart Procedures

CMS: 100-04,12,140.1 Qualified Nonphysician Anesthetists; 100-04,12,140.3 Payment for Qualified Nonphysician Anesthetists; 100-04,12,140.3.3 Billing Modifiers; 100-04,12,140.3.4 General Billing Instructions; 100-04,12,140.4.1 Anesthesiologist/Qualified Nonphysican Anesthetist; 100-04,12,140.4.2 Anesthetist and Anesthesiologist in a Single Procedure; 100-04,12,140.4.3 Payment for Medical /Surgical Services by CRNAs; 100-04,12,140.4.4 Conversion Factors for Anesthesia Services; 100-04,12,140.5 Payment for Anesthesia Services Furnished by a Teaching CRNA; 100-04,4,250.3.2 Anesthesia in a Hospital Outpatient Setting

00560 **Anesthesia for procedures on heart, pericardial sac, and great vessels of chest; without pump oxygenator**
0.00 0.00 **FUD** XXX C
AMA: 2019,Oct,10; 2018,Jan,8; 2017,Dec,8; 2017,Jan,8; 2016,Jan,13; 2015,Jan,16

00561 **with pump oxygenator, younger than 1 year of age** A
INCLUDES Anesthesia complicated by utilization of controlled hypotension (99135)
Anesthesia complicated by utilization of total body hypothermia (99116)
Anesthesia for patient of extreme age, younger than 1 year and older than 70 (99100)
0.00 0.00 **FUD** XXX C
AMA: 2019,Oct,10; 2018,Jan,8; 2017,Dec,8; 2017,Jan,8; 2016,Jan,13; 2015,Jan,16

00562 **with pump oxygenator, age 1 year or older, for all noncoronary bypass procedures (eg, valve procedures) or for re-operation for coronary bypass more than 1 month after original operation** A
0.00 0.00 **FUD** XXX C
AMA: 2019,Oct,10; 2018,Jan,8; 2017,Dec,8; 2017,Jan,8; 2016,Jan,13; 2015,Jan,16

00563 **with pump oxygenator with hypothermic circulatory arrest**
0.00 0.00 **FUD** XXX N
AMA: 2019,Oct,10; 2018,Jan,8; 2017,Dec,8; 2017,Jan,8; 2016,Jan,13; 2015,Jan,16

00566 **Anesthesia for direct coronary artery bypass grafting; without pump oxygenator**
0.00 0.00 **FUD** XXX N
AMA: 2019,Oct,10; 2018,Jan,8; 2017,Dec,8; 2017,Jan,8; 2016,Jan,13; 2015,Jan,16

00567 **with pump oxygenator**
0.00 0.00 **FUD** XXX C
AMA: 2019,Oct,10; 2018,Jan,8; 2017,Dec,8; 2017,Jan,8; 2016,Jan,13; 2015,Jan,16

00580 **Anesthesia for heart transplant or heart/lung transplant**
0.00 0.00 **FUD** XXX C
AMA: 2019,Oct,10; 2018,Jan,8; 2017,Dec,8; 2017,Jan,8; 2016,Jan,13; 2015,Jan,16

00600-00670 Anesthesia for Spinal Procedures

CMS: 100-04,12,140.1 Qualified Nonphysician Anesthetists; 100-04,12,140.3 Payment for Qualified Nonphysician Anesthetists; 100-04,12,140.3.3 Billing Modifiers; 100-04,12,140.3.4 General Billing Instructions; 100-04,12,140.4.1 Anesthesiologist/Qualified Nonphysican Anesthetist; 100-04,12,140.4.2 Anesthetist and Anesthesiologist in a Single Procedure; 100-04,12,140.4.3 Payment for Medical /Surgical Services by CRNAs; 100-04,12,140.4.4 Conversion Factors for Anesthesia Services; 100-04,12,140.5 Payment for Anesthesia Services Furnished by a Teaching CRNA; 100-04,4,250.3.2 Anesthesia in a Hospital Outpatient Setting

00600 **Anesthesia for procedures on cervical spine and cord; not otherwise specified**

EXCLUDES *Percutaneous image-guided spine and spinal cord anesthesia services (01935-01936)*

0.00 0.00 **FUD** XXX N

AMA: 2019,Oct,10; 2018,Jan,8; 2017,Dec,8; 2017,Jan,8; 2016,Jan,13; 2015,Jan,16

00604 **procedures with patient in the sitting position**

0.00 0.00 **FUD** XXX C

AMA: 2019,Oct,10; 2018,Jan,8; 2017,Dec,8; 2017,Jan,8; 2016,Jan,13; 2015,Jan,16

00620 **Anesthesia for procedures on thoracic spine and cord, not otherwise specified**

0.00 0.00 **FUD** XXX N

AMA: 2019,Oct,10; 2018,Jan,8; 2017,Dec,8; 2017,Jan,8; 2016,Jan,13; 2015,Jan,16

00625 **Anesthesia for procedures on the thoracic spine and cord, via an anterior transthoracic approach; not utilizing 1 lung ventilation**

EXCLUDES *Anesthesia services for thoracotomy procedures other than spine (00540-00541)*

0.00 0.00 **FUD** XXX N

AMA: 2019,Oct,10; 2018,Jan,8; 2017,Dec,8; 2017,Jan,8; 2016,Jan,13; 2015,Jan,16

00626 **utilizing 1 lung ventilation**

EXCLUDES *Anesthesia services for thoracotomy procedures other than spine (00540-00541)*

0.00 0.00 **FUD** XXX N

AMA: 2019,Oct,10; 2018,Jan,8; 2017,Dec,8; 2017,Jan,8; 2016,Jan,13; 2015,Jan,16

00630 **Anesthesia for procedures in lumbar region; not otherwise specified**

0.00 0.00 **FUD** XXX N

AMA: 2019,Oct,10; 2018,Jan,8; 2017,Dec,8; 2017,Jan,8; 2016,Jan,13; 2015,Jan,16

00632 **lumbar sympathectomy**

0.00 0.00 **FUD** XXX C

AMA: 2019,Oct,10; 2018,Jan,8; 2017,Dec,8; 2017,Jan,8; 2016,Jan,13; 2015,Jan,16

00635 **diagnostic or therapeutic lumbar puncture**

0.00 0.00 **FUD** XXX N

AMA: 2019,Oct,10; 2018,Jan,8; 2017,Dec,8; 2017,Jan,8; 2016,Jan,13; 2015,Jan,16

00640 **Anesthesia for manipulation of the spine or for closed procedures on the cervical, thoracic or lumbar spine**

0.00 0.00 **FUD** XXX N

AMA: 2019,Oct,10; 2018,Jan,8; 2017,Dec,8; 2017,Jan,8; 2016,Jan,13; 2015,Jan,16

00670 **Anesthesia for extensive spine and spinal cord procedures (eg, spinal instrumentation or vascular procedures)**

0.00 0.00 **FUD** XXX C

AMA: 2019,Oct,10; 2018,Jan,8; 2017,Dec,8; 2017,Jan,8; 2016,Jan,13; 2015,Jan,16

00700-00882 Anesthesia for Abdominal Procedures

CMS: 100-04,12,140.1 Qualified Nonphysician Anesthetists; 100-04,12,140.3 Payment for Qualified Nonphysician Anesthetists; 100-04,12,140.3.3 Billing Modifiers; 100-04,12,140.3.4 General Billing Instructions; 100-04,12,140.4.1 Anesthesiologist/Qualified Nonphysican Anesthetist; 100-04,12,140.4.2 Anesthetist and Anesthesiologist in a Single Procedure; 100-04,12,140.4.3 Payment for Medical /Surgical Services by CRNAs; 100-04,12,140.4.4 Conversion Factors for Anesthesia Services; 100-04,12,140.5 Payment for Anesthesia Services Furnished by a Teaching CRNA; 100-04,4,250.3.2 Anesthesia in a Hospital Outpatient Setting

00700 **Anesthesia for procedures on upper anterior abdominal wall; not otherwise specified**

0.00 0.00 **FUD** XXX N

AMA: 2019,Oct,10; 2018,Jan,8; 2017,Dec,8; 2017,Jan,8; 2016,Jan,13; 2015,Jan,16

00702 **percutaneous liver biopsy**

0.00 0.00 **FUD** XXX N

AMA: 2019,Oct,10; 2018,Jan,8; 2017,Dec,8; 2017,Jan,8; 2016,Jan,13; 2015,Jan,16

00730 **Anesthesia for procedures on upper posterior abdominal wall**

0.00 0.00 **FUD** XXX N

AMA: 2019,Oct,10; 2018,Jan,8; 2017,Dec,8; 2017,Jan,8; 2016,Jan,13; 2015,Jan,16

00731 **Anesthesia for upper gastrointestinal endoscopic procedures, endoscope introduced proximal to duodenum; not otherwise specified**

EXCLUDES *Combination of upper and lower endoscopic gastrointestinal procedures (00813)*

0.00 0.00 **FUD** XXX N

AMA: 2019,Oct,10; 2018,Jan,8; 2017,Dec,8

00732 **endoscopic retrograde cholangiopancreatography (ERCP)**

EXCLUDES *Combination of upper and lower endoscopic gastrointestinal procedures (00813)*

0.00 0.00 **FUD** XXX N

AMA: 2019,Oct,10; 2018,Jan,8; 2017,Dec,8

00750 **Anesthesia for hernia repairs in upper abdomen; not otherwise specified**

0.00 0.00 **FUD** XXX N

AMA: 2019,Oct,10; 2018,Jan,8; 2017,Dec,8; 2017,Jan,8; 2016,Jan,13; 2015,Jan,16

00752 **lumbar and ventral (incisional) hernias and/or wound dehiscence**

0.00 0.00 **FUD** XXX N

AMA: 2019,Oct,10; 2018,Jan,8; 2017,Dec,8; 2017,Jan,8; 2016,Jan,13; 2015,Jan,16

00754 **omphalocele**

0.00 0.00 **FUD** XXX N

AMA: 2019,Oct,10; 2018,Jan,8; 2017,Dec,8; 2017,Jan,8; 2016,Jan,13; 2015,Jan,16

00756 **transabdominal repair of diaphragmatic hernia**

0.00 0.00 **FUD** XXX N

AMA: 2019,Oct,10; 2018,Jan,8; 2017,Dec,8; 2017,Jan,8; 2016,Jan,13; 2015,Jan,16

00770 **Anesthesia for all procedures on major abdominal blood vessels**

0.00 0.00 **FUD** XXX N

AMA: 2019,Oct,10; 2018,Jan,8; 2017,Dec,8; 2017,Jan,8; 2016,Jan,13; 2015,Jan,16

00790 **Anesthesia for intraperitoneal procedures in upper abdomen including laparoscopy; not otherwise specified**

0.00 0.00 **FUD** XXX N

AMA: 2019,Oct,10; 2018,Jan,8; 2017,Dec,8; 2017,Jan,8; 2016,Jan,13; 2015,Jan,16

00792 **partial hepatectomy or management of liver hemorrhage (excluding liver biopsy)**

0.00 0.00 **FUD** XXX C

AMA: 2019,Oct,10; 2018,Jan,8; 2017,Dec,8; 2017,Jan,8; 2016,Jan,13; 2015,Jan,16

00794 **pancreatectomy, partial or total (eg, Whipple procedure)**
0.00 0.00 **FUD** XXX C
AMA: 2019,Oct,10; 2018,Jan,8; 2017,Dec,8; 2017,Jan,8; 2016,Jan,13; 2015,Jan,16

00796 **liver transplant (recipient)**
EXCLUDES *Physiological support during liver harvest (01990)*
0.00 0.00 **FUD** XXX C
AMA: 2019,Oct,10; 2018,Jan,8; 2017,Dec,8; 2017,Jan,8; 2016,Jan,13; 2015,Jan,16

00797 **gastric restrictive procedure for morbid obesity**
0.00 0.00 **FUD** XXX N
AMA: 2019,Oct,10; 2018,Jan,8; 2017,Dec,8; 2017,Jan,8; 2016,Jan,13; 2015,Jan,16

00800 **Anesthesia for procedures on lower anterior abdominal wall; not otherwise specified**
0.00 0.00 **FUD** XXX N
AMA: 2019,Oct,10, 2018,Jan,8, 2017,Dec,8; 2017,Jan,8; 2016,Jan,13; 2015,Jan,16

00802 **panniculectomy**
0.00 0.00 **FUD** XXX C
AMA: 2019,Oct,10; 2018,Jan,8; 2017,Dec,8; 2017,Jan,8; 2016,Jan,13; 2015,Jan,16

00811 **Anesthesia for lower intestinal endoscopic procedures, endoscope introduced distal to duodenum; not otherwise specified**
0.00 0.00 **FUD** XXX N
AMA: 2019,Oct,10; 2018,Jan,8; 2017,Dec,8

00812 **screening colonoscopy**
INCLUDES Anesthesia services for all screening colonoscopy irrespective of findings
0.00 0.00 **FUD** XXX N
AMA: 2019,Oct,10; 2018,Jan,8; 2017,Dec,8

00813 **Anesthesia for combined upper and lower gastrointestinal endoscopic procedures, endoscope introduced both proximal to and distal to the duodenum**
0.00 0.00 **FUD** XXX N
AMA: 2019,Oct,10; 2018,Jan,8; 2017,Dec,8

00820 **Anesthesia for procedures on lower posterior abdominal wall**
0.00 0.00 **FUD** XXX N
AMA: 2019,Oct,10; 2018,Jan,8; 2017,Dec,8; 2017,Jan,8; 2016,Jan,13; 2015,Jan,16

00830 **Anesthesia for hernia repairs in lower abdomen; not otherwise specified**
EXCLUDES *Anesthesia for hernia repairs on infants one year old or less (00834, 00836)*
0.00 0.00 **FUD** XXX N
AMA: 2019,Oct,10; 2018,Jan,8; 2017,Dec,8; 2017,Jan,8; 2016,Jan,13; 2015,Jan,16

00832 **ventral and incisional hernias**
EXCLUDES *Anesthesia for hernia repairs on infants one year old or less (00834, 00836)*
0.00 0.00 **FUD** XXX N
AMA: 2019,Oct,10; 2018,Jan,8; 2017,Dec,8; 2017,Jan,8; 2016,Jan,13; 2015,Jan,16

00834 **Anesthesia for hernia repairs in the lower abdomen not otherwise specified, younger than 1 year of age** A
INCLUDES Anesthesia for patient of extreme age, younger than 1 year and older than 70 (99100)
0.00 0.00 **FUD** XXX N
AMA: 2019,Oct,10; 2018,Jan,8; 2017,Dec,8; 2017,Jan,8; 2016,Jan,13; 2015,Jan,16

00836 **Anesthesia for hernia repairs in the lower abdomen not otherwise specified, infants younger than 37 weeks gestational age at birth and younger than 50 weeks gestational age at time of surgery** A
INCLUDES Anesthesia for patient of extreme age, younger than 1 year and older than 70 (99100)
0.00 0.00 **FUD** XXX N
AMA: 2019,Oct,10; 2018,Jan,8; 2017,Dec,8; 2017,Jan,8; 2016,Jan,13; 2015,Jan,16

00840 **Anesthesia for intraperitoneal procedures in lower abdomen including laparoscopy; not otherwise specified**
0.00 0.00 **FUD** XXX N
AMA: 2019,Oct,10; 2018,Jan,8; 2017,Dec,8; 2017,Jan,8; 2016,Jan,13; 2015,Jan,16

00842 **amniocentesis** M ♀
0.00 0.00 **FUD** XXX N
AMA: 2019,Oct,10; 2018,Jan,8; 2017,Dec,8; 2017,Jan,8; 2016,Jan,13; 2015,Jan,16

00844 **abdominoperineal resection**
0.00 0.00 **FUD** XXX C
AMA: 2019,Oct,10; 2018,Jan,8; 2017,Dec,8; 2017,Jan,8; 2016,Jan,13; 2015,Jan,16

00846 **radical hysterectomy** ♀
0.00 0.00 **FUD** XXX C
AMA: 2019,Oct,10; 2018,Jan,8; 2017,Dec,8; 2017,Jan,8; 2016,Jan,13; 2015,Jan,16

00848 **pelvic exenteration**
0.00 0.00 **FUD** XXX C
AMA: 2019,Oct,10; 2018,Jan,8; 2017,Dec,8; 2017,Jan,8; 2016,Jan,13; 2015,Jan,16

00851 **tubal ligation/transection** ♀
0.00 0.00 **FUD** XXX N
AMA: 2019,Oct,10; 2018,Jan,8; 2017,Dec,8; 2017,Jan,8; 2016,Jan,13; 2015,Jan,16

00860 **Anesthesia for extraperitoneal procedures in lower abdomen, including urinary tract; not otherwise specified**
0.00 0.00 **FUD** XXX N
AMA: 2019,Oct,10; 2018,Jan,8; 2017,Dec,8; 2017,Jan,8; 2016,Jan,13; 2015,Jan,16

00862 **renal procedures, including upper one-third of ureter, or donor nephrectomy**
0.00 0.00 **FUD** XXX N
AMA: 2019,Oct,10; 2018,Jan,8; 2017,Dec,8; 2017,Jan,8; 2016,Jan,13; 2015,Jan,16

00864 **total cystectomy**
0.00 0.00 **FUD** XXX C
AMA: 2019,Oct,10; 2018,Jan,8; 2017,Dec,8; 2017,Jan,8; 2016,Jan,13; 2015,Jan,16

00865 **radical prostatectomy (suprapubic, retropubic)** ♂
0.00 0.00 **FUD** XXX C
AMA: 2019,Oct,10; 2018,Jan,8; 2017,Dec,8; 2017,Jan,8; 2016,Jan,13; 2015,Jan,16

00866 **adrenalectomy**
0.00 0.00 **FUD** XXX C
AMA: 2019,Oct,10; 2018,Jan,8; 2017,Dec,8; 2017,Jan,8; 2016,Jan,13; 2015,Jan,16

00868 **renal transplant (recipient)**
EXCLUDES *Anesthesia for donor nephrectomy (00862)*
Physiological support during kidney harvest (01990)
0.00 0.00 **FUD** XXX C
AMA: 2019,Oct,10; 2018,Jan,8; 2017,Dec,8; 2017,Jan,8; 2016,Jan,13; 2015,Jan,16

00870 **cystolithotomy**
0.00 0.00 **FUD** XXX N
AMA: 2019,Oct,10; 2018,Jan,8; 2017,Dec,8; 2017,Jan,8; 2016,Jan,13; 2015,Jan,16

00872 **Anesthesia for lithotripsy, extracorporeal shock wave; with water bath**
0.00 0.00 **FUD** XXX N
AMA: 2019,Oct,10; 2018,Jan,8; 2017,Dec,8; 2017,Jan,8; 2016,Jan,13; 2015,Jan,16

00873 **without water bath**
0.00 0.00 **FUD** XXX N
AMA: 2019,Oct,10; 2018,Jan,8; 2017,Dec,8; 2017,Jan,8; 2016,Jan,13; 2015,Jan,16

00880 **Anesthesia for procedures on major lower abdominal vessels; not otherwise specified**
0.00 0.00 **FUD** XXX N
AMA: 2019,Oct,10; 2018,Jan,8; 2017,Dec,8; 2017,Jan,8; 2016,Jan,13; 2015,Jan,16

00882 **inferior vena cava ligation**
0.00 0.00 **FUD** XXX C
AMA: 2019,Oct,10; 2018,Jan,8; 2017,Dec,8; 2017,Jan,8; 2016,Jan,13; 2015,Jan,16

00902-00952 Anesthesia for Genitourinary Procedures

CMS: 100-04,12,140.1 Qualified Nonphysician Anesthetists; 100-04,12,140.3 Payment for Qualified Nonphysician Anesthetists; 100-04,12,140.3.3 Billing Modifiers; 100-04,12,140.3.4 General Billing Instructions; 100-04,12,140.4.1 Anesthesiologist/Qualified Nonphysican Anesthetist; 100-04,12,140.4.2 Anesthetist and Anesthesiologist in a Single Procedure; 100-04,12,140.4.3 Payment for Medical /Surgical Services by CRNAs; 100-04,12,140.4.4 Conversion Factors for Anesthesia Services; 100-04,12,140.5 Payment for Anesthesia Services Furnished by a Teaching CRNA; 100-04,4,250.3.2 Anesthesia in a Hospital Outpatient Setting

EXCLUDES *Procedures on perineal skin, muscles, and nerves (00300, 00400)*

00902 **Anesthesia for; anorectal procedure**
0.00 0.00 **FUD** XXX N
AMA: 2019,Oct,10; 2018,Jan,8; 2017,Dec,8; 2017,Jan,8; 2016,Jan,13; 2015,Jan,16

00904 **radical perineal procedure**
0.00 0.00 **FUD** XXX C
AMA: 2019,Oct,10; 2018,Jan,8; 2017,Dec,8; 2017,Jan,8; 2016,Jan,13; 2015,Jan,16

00906 **vulvectomy** ♀
0.00 0.00 **FUD** XXX N
AMA: 2019,Oct,10; 2018,Jan,8; 2017,Dec,8; 2017,Jan,8; 2016,Jan,13; 2015,Jan,16

00908 **perineal prostatectomy** ♂
0.00 0.00 **FUD** XXX C
AMA: 2019,Oct,10; 2018,Jan,8; 2017,Dec,8; 2017,Jan,8; 2016,Jan,13; 2015,Jan,16

00910 **Anesthesia for transurethral procedures (including urethrocystoscopy); not otherwise specified**
0.00 0.00 **FUD** XXX N
AMA: 2019,Oct,10; 2018,Jan,8; 2017,Dec,8; 2017,Jan,8; 2016,Jan,13; 2015,Jan,16

00912 **transurethral resection of bladder tumor(s)**
0.00 0.00 **FUD** XXX N
AMA: 2019,Oct,10; 2018,Jan,8; 2017,Dec,8; 2017,Jan,8; 2016,Jan,13; 2015,Jan,16

00914 **transurethral resection of prostate** ♂
0.00 0.00 **FUD** XXX N
AMA: 2019,Oct,10; 2018,Jan,8; 2017,Dec,8; 2017,Jan,8; 2016,Jan,13; 2015,Jan,16

00916 **post-transurethral resection bleeding**
0.00 0.00 **FUD** XXX N
AMA: 2019,Oct,10; 2018,Jan,8; 2017,Dec,8; 2017,Jan,8; 2016,Jan,13; 2015,Jan,16

00918 **with fragmentation, manipulation and/or removal of ureteral calculus**
0.00 0.00 **FUD** XXX N
AMA: 2019,Oct,10; 2018,Jan,8; 2017,Dec,8; 2017,Jan,8; 2016,Jan,13; 2015,Jan,16

00920 **Anesthesia for procedures on male genitalia (including open urethral procedures); not otherwise specified** ♂
0.00 0.00 **FUD** XXX N
AMA: 2019,Oct,10; 2018,Jan,8; 2017,Dec,8; 2017,Jan,8; 2016,Jan,13; 2015,Jan,16

00921 **vasectomy, unilateral or bilateral** ♂
0.00 0.00 **FUD** XXX N
AMA: 2019,Oct,10; 2018,Jan,8; 2017,Dec,8; 2017,Jan,8; 2016,Jan,13; 2015,Jan,16

00922 **seminal vesicles** ♂
0.00 0.00 **FUD** XXX N
AMA: 2019,Oct,10; 2018,Jan,8; 2017,Dec,8; 2017,Jan,8; 2016,Jan,13; 2015,Jan,16

00924 **undescended testis, unilateral or bilateral** ♂
0.00 0.00 **FUD** XXX N
AMA: 2019,Oct,10; 2018,Jan,8; 2017,Dec,8; 2017,Jan,8; 2016,Jan,13; 2015,Jan,16

00926 **radical orchiectomy, inguinal** ♂
0.00 0.00 **FUD** XXX N
AMA: 2019,Oct,10; 2018,Jan,8; 2017,Dec,8; 2017,Jan,8; 2016,Jan,13; 2015,Jan,16

00928 **radical orchiectomy, abdominal** ♂
0.00 0.00 **FUD** XXX N
AMA: 2019,Oct,10; 2018,Jan,8; 2017,Dec,8; 2017,Jan,8; 2016,Jan,13; 2015,Jan,16

00930 **orchiopexy, unilateral or bilateral** ♂
0.00 0.00 **FUD** XXX N
AMA: 2019,Oct,10; 2018,Jan,8; 2017,Dec,8; 2017,Jan,8; 2016,Jan,13; 2015,Jan,16

00932 **complete amputation of penis** ♂
0.00 0.00 **FUD** XXX C
AMA: 2019,Oct,10; 2018,Jan,8; 2017,Dec,8; 2017,Jan,8; 2016,Jan,13; 2015,Jan,16

00934 **radical amputation of penis with bilateral inguinal lymphadenectomy** ♂
0.00 0.00 **FUD** XXX C
AMA: 2019,Oct,10; 2018,Jan,8; 2017,Dec,8; 2017,Jan,8; 2016,Jan,13; 2015,Jan,16

00936 **radical amputation of penis with bilateral inguinal and iliac lymphadenectomy** ♂
0.00 0.00 **FUD** XXX C
AMA: 2019,Oct,10; 2018,Jan,8; 2017,Dec,8; 2017,Jan,8; 2016,Jan,13; 2015,Jan,16

00938 **insertion of penile prosthesis (perineal approach)** ♂
0.00 0.00 **FUD** XXX N
AMA: 2019,Oct,10; 2018,Jan,8; 2017,Dec,8; 2017,Jan,8; 2016,Jan,13; 2015,Jan,16

00940 **Anesthesia for vaginal procedures (including biopsy of labia, vagina, cervix or endometrium); not otherwise specified** ♀
0.00 0.00 **FUD** XXX N
AMA: 2019,Oct,10; 2018,Jan,8; 2017,Dec,8; 2017,Jan,8; 2016,Jan,13; 2015,Jan,16

00942 **colpotomy, vaginectomy, colporrhaphy, and open urethral procedures** ♀
0.00 0.00 **FUD** XXX N
AMA: 2019,Oct,10; 2018,Jan,8; 2017,Dec,8; 2017,Jan,8; 2016,Jan,13; 2015,Jan,16

00944 **vaginal hysterectomy** ♀
0.00 0.00 **FUD** XXX C
AMA: 2019,Oct,10; 2018,Jan,8; 2017,Dec,8; 2017,Jan,8; 2016,Jan,13; 2015,Jan,16

00948 **cervical cerclage** ♀
0.00 0.00 **FUD** XXX N
AMA: 2019,Oct,10; 2018,Jan,8; 2017,Dec,8; 2017,Jan,8; 2016,Jan,13; 2015,Jan,16

00950 culdoscopy ♀
0.00 0.00 FUD XXX N
AMA: 2019,Oct,10; 2018,Jan,8; 2017,Dec,8; 2017,Jan,8; 2016,Jan,13; 2015,Jan,16

00952 hysteroscopy and/or hysterosalpingography ♀
0.00 0.00 FUD XXX N
AMA: 2019,Oct,10; 2018,Jan,8; 2017,Dec,8; 2017,Jan,8; 2016,Jan,13; 2015,Jan,16

01112-01522 Anesthesia for Lower Extremity Procedures

CMS: 100-04,12,140.1 Qualified Nonphysician Anesthetists; 100-04,12,140.3 Payment for Qualified Nonphysician Anesthetists; 100-04,12,140.3.3 Billing Modifiers; 100-04,12,140.3.4 General Billing Instructions; 100-04,12,140.4.1 Anesthesiologist/Qualified Nonphysican Anesthetist; 100-04,12,140.4.2 Anesthetist and Anesthesiologist in a Single Procedure; 100-04,12,140.4.3 Payment for Medical /Surgical Services by CRNAs; 100-04,12,140.4.4 Conversion Factors for Anesthesia Services; 100-04,12,140.5 Payment for Anesthesia Services Furnished by a Teaching CRNA; 100-04,4,250.3.2 Anesthesia in a Hospital Outpatient Setting

01112 Anesthesia for bone marrow aspiration and/or biopsy, anterior or posterior iliac crest
0.00 0.00 FUD XXX N
AMA: 2019,Oct,10; 2018,Jan,8; 2017,Dec,8; 2017,Jan,8; 2016,Jan,13; 2015,Jan,16

01120 Anesthesia for procedures on bony pelvis
0.00 0.00 FUD XXX N
AMA: 2019,Oct,10; 2018,Jan,8; 2017,Dec,8; 2017,Jan,8; 2016,Jan,13; 2015,Jan,16

01130 Anesthesia for body cast application or revision
0.00 0.00 FUD XXX N
AMA: 2019,Oct,10; 2018,Jan,8; 2017,Dec,8; 2017,Jan,8; 2016,Jan,13; 2015,Jan,16

01140 Anesthesia for interpelviabdominal (hindquarter) amputation
0.00 0.00 FUD XXX C
AMA: 2019,Oct,10; 2018,Jan,8; 2017,Dec,8; 2017,Jan,8; 2016,Jan,13; 2015,Jan,16

01150 Anesthesia for radical procedures for tumor of pelvis, except hindquarter amputation
0.00 0.00 FUD XXX C
AMA: 2019,Oct,10; 2018,Jan,8; 2017,Dec,8; 2017,Jan,8; 2016,Jan,13; 2015,Jan,16

01160 Anesthesia for closed procedures involving symphysis pubis or sacroiliac joint
0.00 0.00 FUD XXX N
AMA: 2019,Oct,10; 2018,Jan,8; 2017,Dec,8; 2017,Jan,8; 2016,Jan,13; 2015,Jan,16

01170 Anesthesia for open procedures involving symphysis pubis or sacroiliac joint
0.00 0.00 FUD XXX N
AMA: 2019,Oct,10; 2018,Jan,8; 2017,Dec,8; 2017,Jan,8; 2016,Jan,13; 2015,Jan,16

01173 Anesthesia for open repair of fracture disruption of pelvis or column fracture involving acetabulum
0.00 0.00 FUD XXX N
AMA: 2019,Oct,10; 2018,Jan,8; 2017,Dec,8; 2017,Jan,8; 2016,Jan,13; 2015,Jan,16

01200 Anesthesia for all closed procedures involving hip joint
0.00 0.00 FUD XXX N
AMA: 2019,Oct,10; 2018,Jan,8; 2017,Dec,8; 2017,Jan,8; 2016,Jan,13; 2015,Jan,16

01202 Anesthesia for arthroscopic procedures of hip joint
0.00 0.00 FUD XXX N
AMA: 2019,Oct,10; 2018,Jan,8; 2017,Dec,8; 2017,Jan,8; 2016,Jan,13; 2015,Jan,16

01210 Anesthesia for open procedures involving hip joint; not otherwise specified
0.00 0.00 FUD XXX N
AMA: 2019,Oct,10; 2018,Jan,8; 2017,Dec,8; 2017,Jan,8; 2016,Jan,13; 2015,Jan,16

01212 hip disarticulation
0.00 0.00 FUD XXX C
AMA: 2019,Oct,10; 2018,Jan,8; 2017,Dec,8; 2017,Jan,8; 2016,Jan,13; 2015,Jan,16

01214 total hip arthroplasty
0.00 0.00 FUD XXX C
AMA: 2019,Oct,10; 2018,Jan,8; 2017,Dec,8; 2017,Jan,8; 2016,Jan,13; 2015,Jan,16

01215 revision of total hip arthroplasty
0.00 0.00 FUD XXX N
AMA: 2019,Oct,10; 2018,Jan,8; 2017,Dec,8; 2017,Jan,8; 2016,Jan,13; 2015,Jan,16

01220 Anesthesia for all closed procedures involving upper two-thirds of femur
0.00 0.00 FUD XXX N
AMA: 2019,Oct,10; 2018,Jan,8; 2017,Dec,8; 2017,Jan,8; 2016,Jan,13; 2015,Jan,16

01230 Anesthesia for open procedures involving upper two-thirds of femur; not otherwise specified
0.00 0.00 FUD XXX N
AMA: 2019,Oct,10; 2018,Jan,8; 2017,Dec,8; 2017,Jan,8; 2016,Jan,13; 2015,Jan,16

01232 amputation
0.00 0.00 FUD XXX C
AMA: 2019,Oct,10; 2018,Jan,8; 2017,Dec,8; 2017,Jan,8; 2016,Jan,13; 2015,Jan,16

01234 radical resection
0.00 0.00 FUD XXX C
AMA: 2019,Oct,10; 2018,Jan,8; 2017,Dec,8; 2017,Jan,8; 2016,Jan,13; 2015,Jan,16

01250 Anesthesia for all procedures on nerves, muscles, tendons, fascia, and bursae of upper leg
0.00 0.00 FUD XXX N
AMA: 2019,Oct,10; 2018,Jan,8; 2017,Dec,8; 2017,Jan,8; 2016,Jan,13; 2015,Jan,16

01260 Anesthesia for all procedures involving veins of upper leg, including exploration
0.00 0.00 FUD XXX N
AMA: 2019,Oct,10; 2018,Jan,8; 2017,Dec,8; 2017,Jan,8; 2016,Jan,13; 2015,Jan,16

01270 Anesthesia for procedures involving arteries of upper leg, including bypass graft; not otherwise specified
0.00 0.00 FUD XXX N
AMA: 2019,Oct,10; 2018,Jan,8; 2017,Dec,8; 2017,Jan,8; 2016,Jan,13; 2015,Jan,16

01272 femoral artery ligation
0.00 0.00 FUD XXX C
AMA: 2019,Oct,10; 2018,Jan,8; 2017,Dec,8; 2017,Jan,8; 2016,Jan,13; 2015,Jan,16

01274 femoral artery embolectomy
0.00 0.00 FUD XXX C
AMA: 2019,Oct,10; 2018,Jan,8; 2017,Dec,8; 2017,Jan,8; 2016,Jan,13; 2015,Jan,16

01320 Anesthesia for all procedures on nerves, muscles, tendons, fascia, and bursae of knee and/or popliteal area
0.00 0.00 FUD XXX N
AMA: 2019,Oct,10; 2018,Jan,8; 2017,Dec,8; 2017,Jan,8; 2016,Jan,13; 2015,Jan,16

01340 Anesthesia for all closed procedures on lower one-third of femur
0.00 0.00 FUD XXX N
AMA: 2019,Oct,10; 2018,Jan,8; 2017,Dec,8; 2017,Jan,8; 2016,Jan,13; 2015,Jan,16

01360 Anesthesia for all open procedures on lower one-third of femur
0.00 0.00 FUD XXX N
AMA: 2019,Oct,10; 2018,Jan,8; 2017,Dec,8; 2017,Jan,8; 2016,Jan,13; 2015,Jan,16

01380 **Anesthesia for all closed procedures on knee joint**
0.00 0.00 **FUD** XXX N
AMA: 2019,Oct,10; 2018,Jan,8; 2017,Dec,8; 2017,Jan,8; 2016,Jan,13; 2015,Jan,16

01382 **Anesthesia for diagnostic arthroscopic procedures of knee joint**
0.00 0.00 **FUD** XXX N
AMA: 2019,Oct,10; 2018,Jan,8; 2017,Dec,8; 2017,Jan,8; 2016,Jan,13; 2015,Jan,16

01390 **Anesthesia for all closed procedures on upper ends of tibia, fibula, and/or patella**
0.00 0.00 **FUD** XXX N
AMA: 2019,Oct,10; 2018,Jan,8; 2017,Dec,8; 2017,Jan,8; 2016,Jan,13; 2015,Jan,16

01392 **Anesthesia for all open procedures on upper ends of tibia, fibula, and/or patella**
0.00 0.00 **FUD** XXX N
AMA: 2019,Oct,10; 2018,Jan,8; 2017,Dec,8; 2017,Jan,8; 2016,Jan,13; 2015,Jan,16

01400 **Anesthesia for open or surgical arthroscopic procedures on knee joint; not otherwise specified**
0.00 0.00 **FUD** XXX N
AMA: 2019,Oct,10; 2018,Jan,8; 2017,Dec,8; 2017,Jan,8; 2016,Jan,13; 2015,Jan,16

01402 **total knee arthroplasty**
0.00 0.00 **FUD** XXX C
AMA: 2019,Oct,10; 2018,Jan,8; 2017,Dec,8; 2017,Jan,8; 2016,Jan,13; 2015,Jan,16

01404 **disarticulation at knee**
0.00 0.00 **FUD** XXX C
AMA: 2019,Oct,10; 2018,Jan,8; 2017,Dec,8; 2017,Jan,8; 2016,Jan,13; 2015,Jan,16

01420 **Anesthesia for all cast applications, removal, or repair involving knee joint**
0.00 0.00 **FUD** XXX N
AMA: 2019,Oct,10; 2018,Jan,8; 2017,Dec,8; 2017,Jan,8; 2016,Jan,13; 2015,Jan,16

01430 **Anesthesia for procedures on veins of knee and popliteal area; not otherwise specified**
0.00 0.00 **FUD** XXX N
AMA: 2019,Oct,10; 2018,Jan,8; 2017,Dec,8; 2017,Jan,8; 2016,Jan,13; 2015,Jan,16

01432 **arteriovenous fistula**
0.00 0.00 **FUD** XXX N
AMA: 2019,Oct,10; 2018,Jan,8; 2017,Dec,8; 2017,Jan,8; 2016,Jan,13; 2015,Jan,16

01440 **Anesthesia for procedures on arteries of knee and popliteal area; not otherwise specified**
0.00 0.00 **FUD** XXX N
AMA: 2019,Oct,10; 2018,Jan,8; 2017,Dec,8; 2017,Jan,8; 2016,Jan,13; 2015,Jan,16

01442 **popliteal thromboendarterectomy, with or without patch graft**
0.00 0.00 **FUD** XXX C
AMA: 2019,Oct,10; 2018,Jan,8; 2017,Dec,8; 2017,Jan,8; 2016,Jan,13; 2015,Jan,16

01444 **popliteal excision and graft or repair for occlusion or aneurysm**
0.00 0.00 **FUD** XXX C
AMA: 2019,Oct,10; 2018,Jan,8; 2017,Dec,8; 2017,Jan,8; 2016,Jan,13; 2015,Jan,16

01462 **Anesthesia for all closed procedures on lower leg, ankle, and foot**
0.00 0.00 **FUD** XXX N
AMA: 2019,Oct,10; 2018,Jan,8; 2017,Dec,8; 2017,Jan,8; 2016,Jan,13; 2015,Jan,16

01464 **Anesthesia for arthroscopic procedures of ankle and/or foot**
0.00 0.00 **FUD** XXX N
AMA: 2019,Oct,10; 2018,Jan,8; 2017,Dec,8; 2017,Jan,8; 2016,Jan,13; 2015,Jan,16

01470 **Anesthesia for procedures on nerves, muscles, tendons, and fascia of lower leg, ankle, and foot; not otherwise specified**
0.00 0.00 **FUD** XXX N
AMA: 2019,Oct,10; 2018,Jan,8; 2017,Dec,8; 2017,Jan,8; 2016,Jan,13; 2015,Jan,16

01472 **repair of ruptured Achilles tendon, with or without graft**
0.00 0.00 **FUD** XXX N
AMA: 2019,Oct,10; 2018,Jan,8; 2017,Dec,8; 2017,Jan,8; 2016,Jan,13; 2015,Jan,16

01474 **gastrocnemius recession (eg, Strayer procedure)**
0.00 0.00 **FUD** XXX N
AMA: 2019,Oct,10; 2018,Jan,8; 2017,Dec,8; 2017,Jan,8; 2016,Jan,13; 2015,Jan,16

01480 **Anesthesia for open procedures on bones of lower leg, ankle, and foot; not otherwise specified**
0.00 0.00 **FUD** XXX N
AMA: 2019,Oct,10; 2018,Jan,8; 2017,Dec,8; 2017,Jan,8; 2016,Jan,13; 2015,Jan,16

01482 **radical resection (including below knee amputation)**
0.00 0.00 **FUD** XXX N
AMA: 2019,Oct,10; 2018,Jan,8; 2017,Dec,8; 2017,Jan,8; 2016,Jan,13; 2015,Jan,16

01484 **osteotomy or osteoplasty of tibia and/or fibula**
0.00 0.00 **FUD** XXX N
AMA: 2019,Oct,10; 2018,Jan,8; 2017,Dec,8; 2017,Jan,8; 2016,Jan,13; 2015,Jan,16

01486 **total ankle replacement**
0.00 0.00 **FUD** XXX C
AMA: 2019,Oct,10; 2018,Jan,8; 2017,Dec,8; 2017,Jan,8; 2016,Jan,13; 2015,Jan,16

01490 **Anesthesia for lower leg cast application, removal, or repair**
0.00 0.00 **FUD** XXX N
AMA: 2019,Oct,10; 2018,Jan,8; 2017,Dec,8; 2017,Jan,8; 2016,Jan,13; 2015,Jan,16

01500 **Anesthesia for procedures on arteries of lower leg, including bypass graft; not otherwise specified**
0.00 0.00 **FUD** XXX N
AMA: 2019,Oct,10; 2018,Jan,8; 2017,Dec,8; 2017,Jan,8; 2016,Jan,13; 2015,Jan,16

01502 **embolectomy, direct or with catheter**
0.00 0.00 **FUD** XXX C
AMA: 2019,Oct,10; 2018,Jan,8; 2017,Dec,8; 2017,Jan,8; 2016,Jan,13; 2015,Jan,16

01520 **Anesthesia for procedures on veins of lower leg; not otherwise specified**
0.00 0.00 **FUD** XXX N
AMA: 2019,Oct,10; 2018,Jan,8; 2017,Dec,8; 2017,Jan,8; 2016,Jan,13; 2015,Jan,16

01522 **venous thrombectomy, direct or with catheter**
0.00 0.00 **FUD** XXX N
AMA: 2019,Oct,10; 2018,Jan,8; 2017,Dec,8; 2017,Jan,8; 2016,Jan,13; 2015,Jan,16

01610-01680 Anesthesia for Shoulder Procedures

CMS: 100-04,12,140.1 Qualified Nonphysician Anesthetists; 100-04,12,140.3 Payment for Qualified Nonphysician Anesthetists; 100-04,12,140.3.3 Billing Modifiers; 100-04,12,140.3.4 General Billing Instructions; 100-04,12,140.4.1 Anesthesiologist/Qualified Nonphysican Anesthetist; 100-04,12,140.4.2 Anesthetist and Anesthesiologist in a Single Procedure; 100-04,12,140.4.3 Payment for Medical /Surgical Services by CRNAs; 100-04,12,140.4.4 Conversion Factors for Anesthesia Services; 100-04,12,140.5 Payment for Anesthesia Services Furnished by a Teaching CRNA; 100-04,4,250.3.2 Anesthesia in a Hospital Outpatient Setting

INCLUDES Acromioclavicular joint
Humeral head and neck
Shoulder joint
Sternoclavicular joint

01610 Anesthesia for all procedures on nerves, muscles, tendons, fascia, and bursae of shoulder and axilla
0.00 0.00 **FUD** XXX N
AMA: 2019,Oct,10; 2018,Jan,8; 2017,Dec,8; 2017,Jan,8; 2016,Jan,13; 2015,Jan,16

01620 Anesthesia for all closed procedures on humeral head and neck, sternoclavicular joint, acromioclavicular joint, and shoulder joint
0.00 0.00 **FUD** XXX N
AMA: 2019,Oct,10; 2018,Jan,8; 2017,Dec,8; 2017,Jan,8; 2016,Jan,13; 2015,Jan,16

01622 Anesthesia for diagnostic arthroscopic procedures of shoulder joint
0.00 0.00 **FUD** XXX N
AMA: 2019,Oct,10; 2018,Jan,8; 2017,Dec,8; 2017,Jan,8; 2016,Jan,13; 2015,Jan,16

01630 Anesthesia for open or surgical arthroscopic procedures on humeral head and neck, sternoclavicular joint, acromioclavicular joint, and shoulder joint; not otherwise specified
0.00 0.00 **FUD** XXX N
AMA: 2019,Oct,10; 2018,Jan,8; 2017,Dec,8; 2017,Jan,8; 2016,Jan,13; 2015,Jan,16

01634 shoulder disarticulation
0.00 0.00 **FUD** XXX C
AMA: 2019,Oct,10; 2018,Jan,8; 2017,Dec,8; 2017,Jan,8; 2016,Jan,13; 2015,Jan,16

01636 interthoracoscapular (forequarter) amputation
0.00 0.00 **FUD** XXX C
AMA: 2019,Oct,10; 2018,Jan,8; 2017,Dec,8; 2017,Jan,8; 2016,Jan,13; 2015,Jan,16

01638 total shoulder replacement
0.00 0.00 **FUD** XXX C
AMA: 2019,Oct,10; 2018,Jan,8; 2017,Dec,8; 2017,Jan,8; 2016,Jan,13; 2015,Jan,16

01650 Anesthesia for procedures on arteries of shoulder and axilla; not otherwise specified
0.00 0.00 **FUD** XXX N
AMA: 2019,Oct,10; 2018,Jan,8; 2017,Dec,8; 2017,Jan,8; 2016,Jan,13; 2015,Jan,16

01652 axillary-brachial aneurysm
0.00 0.00 **FUD** XXX C
AMA: 2019,Oct,10; 2018,Jan,8; 2017,Dec,8; 2017,Jan,8; 2016,Jan,13; 2015,Jan,16

01654 bypass graft
0.00 0.00 **FUD** XXX C
AMA: 2019,Oct,10; 2018,Jan,8; 2017,Dec,8; 2017,Jan,8; 2016,Jan,13; 2015,Jan,16

01656 axillary-femoral bypass graft
0.00 0.00 **FUD** XXX C
AMA: 2019,Oct,10; 2018,Jan,8; 2017,Dec,8; 2017,Jan,8; 2016,Jan,13; 2015,Jan,16

01670 Anesthesia for all procedures on veins of shoulder and axilla
0.00 0.00 **FUD** XXX N
AMA: 2019,Oct,10; 2018,Jan,8; 2017,Dec,8; 2017,Jan,8; 2016,Jan,13; 2015,Jan,16

01680 Anesthesia for shoulder cast application, removal or repair, not otherwise specified
0.00 0.00 **FUD** XXX N
AMA: 2019,Oct,10; 2018,Jan,8; 2017,Dec,8; 2017,Jan,8; 2016,Jan,13; 2015,Jan,16

01710-01860 Anesthesia for Upper Extremity Procedures

CMS: 100-04,12,140.1 Qualified Nonphysician Anesthetists; 100-04,12,140.3 Payment for Qualified Nonphysician Anesthetists; 100-04,12,140.3.3 Billing Modifiers; 100-04,12,140.3.4 General Billing Instructions; 100-04,12,140.4.1 Anesthesiologist/Qualified Nonphysican Anesthetist; 100-04,12,140.4.2 Anesthetist and Anesthesiologist in a Single Procedure; 100-04,12,140.4.3 Payment for Medical /Surgical Services by CRNAs; 100-04,12,140.4.4 Conversion Factors for Anesthesia Services; 100-04,12,140.5 Payment for Anesthesia Services Furnished by a Teaching CRNA; 100-04,4,250.3.2 Anesthesia in a Hospital Outpatient Setting

01710 Anesthesia for procedures on nerves, muscles, tendons, fascia, and bursae of upper arm and elbow; not otherwise specified
0.00 0.00 **FUD** XXX N
AMA: 2019,Oct,10; 2018,Jan,8; 2017,Dec,8; 2017,Jan,8; 2016,Jan,13; 2015,Jan,16

01712 tenotomy, elbow to shoulder, open
0.00 0.00 **FUD** XXX N
AMA: 2019,Oct,10; 2018,Jan,8; 2017,Dec,8; 2017,Jan,8; 2016,Jan,13; 2015,Jan,16

01714 tenoplasty, elbow to shoulder
0.00 0.00 **FUD** XXX N
AMA: 2019,Oct,10; 2018,Jan,8; 2017,Dec,8; 2017,Jan,8; 2016,Jan,13; 2015,Jan,16

01716 tenodesis, rupture of long tendon of biceps
0.00 0.00 **FUD** XXX N
AMA: 2019,Oct,10; 2018,Jan,8; 2017,Dec,8; 2017,Jan,8; 2016,Jan,13; 2015,Jan,16

01730 Anesthesia for all closed procedures on humerus and elbow
0.00 0.00 **FUD** XXX N
AMA: 2019,Oct,10; 2018,Jan,8; 2017,Dec,8; 2017,Jan,8; 2016,Jan,13; 2015,Jan,16

01732 Anesthesia for diagnostic arthroscopic procedures of elbow joint
0.00 0.00 **FUD** XXX N
AMA: 2019,Oct,10; 2018,Jan,8; 2017,Dec,8; 2017,Jan,8; 2016,Jan,13; 2015,Jan,16

01740 Anesthesia for open or surgical arthroscopic procedures of the elbow; not otherwise specified
0.00 0.00 **FUD** XXX N
AMA: 2019,Oct,10; 2018,Jan,8; 2017,Dec,8; 2017,Jan,8; 2016,Jan,13; 2015,Jan,16

01742 osteotomy of humerus
0.00 0.00 **FUD** XXX N
AMA: 2019,Oct,10; 2018,Jan,8; 2017,Dec,8; 2017,Jan,8; 2016,Jan,13; 2015,Jan,16

01744 repair of nonunion or malunion of humerus
0.00 0.00 **FUD** XXX N
AMA: 2019,Oct,10; 2018,Jan,8; 2017,Dec,8; 2017,Jan,8; 2016,Jan,13; 2015,Jan,16

01756 radical procedures
0.00 0.00 **FUD** XXX C
AMA: 2019,Oct,10; 2018,Jan,8; 2017,Dec,8; 2017,Jan,8; 2016,Jan,13; 2015,Jan,16

01758 excision of cyst or tumor of humerus
0.00 0.00 **FUD** XXX N
AMA: 2019,Oct,10; 2018,Jan,8; 2017,Dec,8; 2017,Jan,8; 2016,Jan,13; 2015,Jan,16

01760 total elbow replacement
0.00 0.00 **FUD** XXX N
AMA: 2019,Oct,10; 2018,Jan,8; 2017,Dec,8; 2017,Jan,8; 2016,Jan,13; 2015,Jan,16

01770 **Anesthesia for procedures on arteries of upper arm and elbow; not otherwise specified**
0.00 0.00 FUD XXX N
AMA: 2019,Oct,10; 2018,Jan,8; 2017,Dec,8; 2017,Jan,8; 2016,Jan,13; 2015,Jan,16

01772 **embolectomy**
0.00 0.00 FUD XXX N
AMA: 2019,Oct,10; 2018,Jan,8; 2017,Dec,8; 2017,Jan,8; 2016,Jan,13; 2015,Jan,16

01780 **Anesthesia for procedures on veins of upper arm and elbow; not otherwise specified**
0.00 0.00 FUD XXX N
AMA: 2019,Oct,10; 2018,Jan,8; 2017,Dec,8; 2017,Jan,8; 2016,Jan,13; 2015,Jan,16

01782 **phleborrhaphy**
0.00 0.00 FUD XXX N
AMA: 2019,Oct,10; 2018,Jan,8; 2017,Dec,8; 2017,Jan,8; 2016,Jan,13; 2015,Jan,16

01810 **Anesthesia for all procedures on nerves, muscles, tendons, fascia, and bursae of forearm, wrist, and hand**
0.00 0.00 FUD XXX N
AMA: 2019,Oct,10; 2018,Jan,8; 2017,Dec,8; 2017,Jan,8; 2016,Jan,13; 2015,Jan,16

01820 **Anesthesia for all closed procedures on radius, ulna, wrist, or hand bones**
0.00 0.00 FUD XXX N
AMA: 2019,Oct,10; 2018,Jan,8; 2017,Dec,8; 2017,Jan,8; 2016,Jan,13; 2015,Jan,16

01829 **Anesthesia for diagnostic arthroscopic procedures on the wrist**
0.00 0.00 FUD XXX N
AMA: 2019,Oct,10; 2018,Jan,8; 2017,Dec,8; 2017,Jan,8; 2016,Jan,13; 2015,Jan,16

01830 **Anesthesia for open or surgical arthroscopic/endoscopic procedures on distal radius, distal ulna, wrist, or hand joints; not otherwise specified**
0.00 0.00 FUD XXX N
AMA: 2019,Oct,10; 2018,Jan,8; 2017,Dec,8; 2017,Jan,8; 2016,Jan,13; 2015,Jan,16

01832 **total wrist replacement**
0.00 0.00 FUD XXX N
AMA: 2019,Oct,10; 2018,Jan,8; 2017,Dec,8; 2017,Jan,8; 2016,Jan,13; 2015,Jan,16

01840 **Anesthesia for procedures on arteries of forearm, wrist, and hand; not otherwise specified**
0.00 0.00 FUD XXX N
AMA: 2019,Oct,10; 2018,Jan,8; 2017,Dec,8; 2017,Jan,8; 2016,Jan,13; 2015,Jan,16

01842 **embolectomy**
0.00 0.00 FUD XXX N
AMA: 2019,Oct,10; 2018,Jan,8; 2017,Dec,8; 2017,Jan,8; 2016,Jan,13; 2015,Jan,16

01844 **Anesthesia for vascular shunt, or shunt revision, any type (eg, dialysis)**
0.00 0.00 FUD XXX N
AMA: 2019,Oct,10; 2018,Jan,8; 2017,Dec,8; 2017,Jan,8; 2016,Jan,13; 2015,Jan,16

01850 **Anesthesia for procedures on veins of forearm, wrist, and hand; not otherwise specified**
0.00 0.00 FUD XXX N
AMA: 2019,Oct,10; 2018,Jan,8; 2017,Dec,8; 2017,Jan,8; 2016,Jan,13; 2015,Jan,16

01852 **phleborrhaphy**
0.00 0.00 FUD XXX N
AMA: 2019,Oct,10; 2018,Jan,8; 2017,Dec,8; 2017,Jan,8; 2016,Jan,13; 2015,Jan,16

01860 **Anesthesia for forearm, wrist, or hand cast application, removal, or repair**
0.00 0.00 FUD XXX N
AMA: 2019,Oct,10; 2018,Jan,8; 2017,Dec,8; 2017,Jan,8; 2016,Jan,13; 2015,Jan,16

01916-01936 Anesthesia for Interventional Radiology Procedures

CMS: 100-04,12,140.1 Qualified Nonphysician Anesthetists; 100-04,12,140.3 Payment for Qualified Nonphysician Anesthetists; 100-04,12,140.3.3 Billing Modifiers; 100-04,12,140.3.4 General Billing Instructions; 100-04,12,140.4.1 Anesthesiologist/Qualified Nonphysican Anesthetist; 100-04,12,140.4.2 Anesthetist and Anesthesiologist in a Single Procedure; 100-04,12,140.4.3 Payment for Medical /Surgical Services by CRNAs; 100-04,12,140.4.4 Conversion Factors for Anesthesia Services; 100-04,12,140.5 Payment for Anesthesia Services Furnished by a Teaching CRNA; 100-04,4,250.3.2 Anesthesia in a Hospital Outpatient Setting

01916 **Anesthesia for diagnostic arteriography/venography**
EXCLUDES *Anesthesia for therapeutic interventional radiological procedures involving the arterial system (01924-01926)*
Anesthesia for therapeutic interventional radiological procedures involving the venous/lymphatic system (01930-01933)
0.00 0.00 FUD XXX N
AMA: 2019,Oct,10; 2018,Jan,8; 2017,Dec,8; 2017,Jan,8; 2016,Jan,13; 2015,Jan,16

01920 **Anesthesia for cardiac catheterization including coronary angiography and ventriculography (not to include Swan-Ganz catheter)**
0.00 0.00 FUD XXX N
AMA: 2019,Oct,10; 2018,Jan,8; 2017,Dec,8; 2017,Jan,8; 2016,Jan,13; 2015,Jan,16

01922 **Anesthesia for non-invasive imaging or radiation therapy**
0.00 0.00 FUD XXX N
AMA: 2019,Oct,10; 2018,Jan,8; 2017,Dec,8; 2017,Jan,8; 2016,Jan,13; 2015,Jan,16

01924 **Anesthesia for therapeutic interventional radiological procedures involving the arterial system; not otherwise specified**
0.00 0.00 FUD XXX N
AMA: 2019,Oct,10; 2018,Jan,8; 2017,Dec,8; 2017,Jan,8; 2016,Jan,13; 2015,Jan,16

01925 **carotid or coronary**
0.00 0.00 FUD XXX N
AMA: 2019,Oct,10; 2018,Jan,8; 2017,Dec,8; 2017,Jan,8; 2016,Jan,13; 2015,Jan,16

01926 **intracranial, intracardiac, or aortic**
0.00 0.00 FUD XXX N
AMA: 2019,Oct,10; 2018,Jan,8; 2017,Dec,8; 2017,Jan,8; 2016,Jan,13; 2015,Jan,16

01930 **Anesthesia for therapeutic interventional radiological procedures involving the venous/lymphatic system (not to include access to the central circulation); not otherwise specified**
0.00 0.00 FUD XXX N
AMA: 2019,Oct,10; 2018,Jan,8; 2017,Dec,8; 2017,Jan,8; 2016,Jan,13; 2015,Jan,16

01931 **intrahepatic or portal circulation (eg, transvenous intrahepatic portosystemic shunt[s] [TIPS])**
0.00 0.00 FUD XXX N
AMA: 2019,Oct,10; 2018,Jan,8; 2017,Dec,8; 2017,Jan,8; 2016,Jan,13; 2015,Jan,16

01932 **intrathoracic or jugular**
0.00 0.00 FUD XXX N
AMA: 2019,Oct,10; 2018,Jan,8; 2017,Dec,8; 2017,Jan,8; 2016,Jan,13; 2015,Jan,16

01933 **intracranial**
0.00 0.00 FUD XXX N
AMA: 2019,Oct,10; 2018,Jan,8; 2017,Dec,8; 2017,Jan,8; 2016,Jan,13; 2015,Jan,16

01935 **Anesthesia for percutaneous image guided procedures on the spine and spinal cord; diagnostic**
0.00 0.00 **FUD** XXX N
AMA: 2019,Oct,10; 2018,Jan,8; 2017,Dec,8; 2017,Jan,8; 2016,Jan,13; 2015,Jan,16

01936 **therapeutic**
0.00 0.00 **FUD** XXX N
AMA: 2019,Oct,10; 2018,Jan,8; 2017,Dec,8; 2017,Jan,8; 2016,Jan,13; 2015,Jan,16

01951-01953 Anesthesia for Burn Procedures

CMS: 100-04,12,140.1 Qualified Nonphysician Anesthetists; 100-04,12,140.3 Payment for Qualified Nonphysician Anesthetists; 100-04,12,140.3.3 Billing Modifiers; 100-04,12,140.3.4 General Billing Instructions; 100-04,12,140.4.1 Anesthesiologist/Qualified Nonphysican Anesthetist; 100-04,12,140.4.2 Anesthetist and Anesthesiologist in a Single Procedure; 100-04,12,140.4.3 Payment for Medical /Surgical Services by CRNAs; 100-04,12,140.4.4 Conversion Factors for Anesthesia Services; 100-04,12,140.5 Payment for Anesthesia Services Furnished by a Teaching CRNA; 100-04,4,250.3.2 Anesthesia in a Hospital Outpatient Setting

01951 **Anesthesia for second and third-degree burn excision or debridement with or without skin grafting, any site, for total body surface area (TBSA) treated during anesthesia and surgery; less than 4% total body surface area**
0.00 0.00 **FUD** XXX N
AMA: 2019,Oct,10; 2018,Jan,8; 2017,Dec,8; 2017,Jan,8; 2016,Jan,13; 2015,Jan,16

01952 **between 4% and 9% of total body surface area**
0.00 0.00 **FUD** XXX N
AMA: 2019,Oct,10; 2018,Jan,8; 2017,Dec,8; 2017,Jan,8; 2016,Jan,13; 2015,Jan,16

\+ **01953** **each additional 9% total body surface area or part thereof (List separately in addition to code for primary procedure)**
Code first (01952)
0.00 0.00 **FUD** XXX N
AMA: 2019,Oct,10; 2018,Jan,8; 2017,Dec,8; 2017,Jan,8; 2016,Jan,13; 2015,Jan,16

01958-01969 Anesthesia for Obstetric Procedures

CMS: 100-04,12,140.1 Qualified Nonphysician Anesthetists; 100-04,12,140.3 Payment for Qualified Nonphysician Anesthetists; 100-04,12,140.3.3 Billing Modifiers; 100-04,12,140.3.4 General Billing Instructions; 100-04,12,140.4.1 Anesthesiologist/Qualified Nonphysican Anesthetist; 100-04,12,140.4.2 Anesthetist and Anesthesiologist in a Single Procedure; 100-04,12,140.4.3 Payment for Medical /Surgical Services by CRNAs; 100-04,12,140.4.4 Conversion Factors for Anesthesia Services; 100-04,12,140.5 Payment for Anesthesia Services Furnished by a Teaching CRNA; 100-04,4,250.3.2 Anesthesia in a Hospital Outpatient Setting

01958 **Anesthesia for external cephalic version procedure** M
0.00 0.00 **FUD** XXX N
AMA: 2019,Oct,10; 2018,Jan,8; 2017,Dec,8; 2017,Jan,8; 2016,Jan,13; 2015,Jan,16

01960 **Anesthesia for vaginal delivery only** M ♀
0.00 0.00 **FUD** XXX N
AMA: 2019,Oct,10; 2018,Jan,8; 2017,Dec,8; 2017,Jan,8; 2016,Jan,13; 2015,Jan,16

01961 **Anesthesia for cesarean delivery only** M ♀
0.00 0.00 **FUD** XXX N
AMA: 2019,Oct,10; 2018,Jan,8; 2017,Dec,8; 2017,Jan,8; 2016,Jan,13; 2015,Jan,16

01962 **Anesthesia for urgent hysterectomy following delivery** M ♀
0.00 0.00 **FUD** XXX N
AMA: 2019,Oct,10; 2018,Jan,8; 2017,Dec,8; 2017,Jan,8; 2016,Jan,13; 2015,Jan,16

01963 **Anesthesia for cesarean hysterectomy without any labor analgesia/anesthesia care** M ♀
0.00 0.00 **FUD** XXX N
AMA: 2019,Oct,10; 2018,Jan,8; 2017,Dec,8; 2017,Jan,8; 2016,Jan,13; 2015,Jan,16

01965 **Anesthesia for incomplete or missed abortion procedures** M ♀
0.00 0.00 **FUD** XXX N
AMA: 2019,Oct,10; 2018,Jan,8; 2017,Dec,8; 2017,Jan,8; 2016,Jan,13; 2015,Jan,16

01966 **Anesthesia for induced abortion procedures** M ♀
0.00 0.00 **FUD** XXX N
AMA: 2019,Oct,10; 2018,Jan,8; 2017,Dec,8; 2017,Jan,8; 2016,Jan,13; 2015,Jan,16

01967 **Neuraxial labor analgesia/anesthesia for planned vaginal delivery (this includes any repeat subarachnoid needle placement and drug injection and/or any necessary replacement of an epidural catheter during labor)** M ♀
0.00 0.00 **FUD** XXX N
AMA: 2019,Oct,10; 2018,Jan,8; 2017,Dec,8; 2017,Jan,8; 2016,Jan,13; 2015,Jan,16

\+ **01968** **Anesthesia for cesarean delivery following neuraxial labor analgesia/anesthesia (List separately in addition to code for primary procedure performed)** M ♀
Code first (01967)
0.00 0.00 **FUD** XXX N
AMA: 2019,Oct,10; 2018,Jan,8; 2017,Dec,8; 2017,Jan,8; 2016,Jan,13; 2015,Jan,16

\+ **01969** **Anesthesia for cesarean hysterectomy following neuraxial labor analgesia/anesthesia (List separately in addition to code for primary procedure performed)** M ♀
Code first (01967)
0.00 0.00 **FUD** XXX N
AMA: 2019,Oct,10; 2018,Jan,8; 2017,Dec,8; 2017,Jan,8; 2016,Jan,13; 2015,Jan,16

01990-01999 Anesthesia Miscellaneous

CMS: 100-04,12,140.1 Qualified Nonphysician Anesthetists; 100-04,12,140.3 Payment for Qualified Nonphysician Anesthetists; 100-04,12,140.3.3 Billing Modifiers; 100-04,12,140.3.4 General Billing Instructions; 100-04,12,140.4.1 Anesthesiologist/Qualified Nonphysican Anesthetist; 100-04,12,140.4.2 Anesthetist and Anesthesiologist in a Single Procedure; 100-04,12,140.4.3 Payment for Medical /Surgical Services by CRNAs; 100-04,12,140.4.4 Conversion Factors for Anesthesia Services; 100-04,12,140.5 Payment for Anesthesia Services Furnished by a Teaching CRNA; 100-04,4,250.3.2 Anesthesia in a Hospital Outpatient Setting

01990 **Physiological support for harvesting of organ(s) from brain-dead patient**
0.00 0.00 **FUD** XXX C
AMA: 2019,Oct,10; 2018,Jan,8; 2017,Dec,8; 2017,Jan,8; 2016,Jan,13; 2015,Jan,16

01991 **Anesthesia for diagnostic or therapeutic nerve blocks and injections (when block or injection is performed by a different physician or other qualified health care professional); other than the prone position**
EXCLUDES *Bier block for pain management (64999)*
Moderate Sedation (99151-99153, 99155-99157)
Pain management via intra-arterial or IV therapy (96373-96374)
Regional or local anesthesia of arms or legs for surgical procedure
0.00 0.00 **FUD** XXX N
AMA: 2019,Oct,10; 2018,Jan,8; 2017,Dec,8; 2017,Jan,8; 2016,Jan,13; 2015,Jan,16

01992 **prone position**
EXCLUDES *Bier block for pain management (64999)*
Moderate sedation (99151-99153, 99155-99157)
Pain management via intra-arterial or IV therapy (96373-96374)
Regional or local anesthesia of arms or legs for surgical procedure
0.00 0.00 **FUD** XXX N
AMA: 2019,Oct,10; 2018,Jan,8; 2017,Dec,8; 2017,Jan,8; 2016,Jan,13; 2015,Jan,16

01996 **Daily hospital management of epidural or subarachnoid continuous drug administration**

INCLUDES Continuous epidural or subarachnoid drug services performed after insertion of an epidural or subarachnoid catheter

0.00 0.00 **FUD** XXX N

AMA: 2019,Oct,10; 2018,Jan,8; 2017,Dec,8; 2017,Sep,6; 2017,Jan,8; 2016,Jan,13; 2015,May,10; 2015,Jan,16

01999 **Unlisted anesthesia procedure(s)**

0.00 0.00 **FUD** XXX N

AMA: 2019,Oct,10; 2018,Jan,8; 2017,Dec,8; 2017,Jan,8; 2016,Jan,13; 2015,May,10; 2015,Jan,16

10004-10012 [10004, 10005, 10006, 10007, 10008, 10009, 10010, 10011, 10012] Fine Needle Aspiration

EXCLUDES *Core needle biopsy, lung or mediastinum (32408)*
Percutaneous localization clip placement during breast biopsy (19081-19086)
Percutaneous needle biopsy:
Abdominal or retroperitoneal mass (49180)
Epididymis (54800)
Kidney (50200)
Liver (47000-47001)
Lymph node (38505)
Muscle (20206)
Nucleus pulposus, paravertebral tissue, intervertebral disc (62267)
Pancreas (48102)
Pleura (32400)
Prostate (55700, 55706)
Salivary gland (42400)
Spinal cord (62269)
Testis (54500)
Thyroid (60100)
Soft tissue percutaneous fluid drainage by catheter using image guidance (10030)
Thyroid cyst (60300)

Code also multiple biopsies on same service date:
FNA biopsies using same imaging guidance: report imaging add-on code for second and successive procedures
FNA biopsies separate lesions, different imaging guidance: append modifier 59 to codes for additional imaging modality used
FNA and core needle biopsy same lesion, same imaging guidance, procedure includes imaging guidance for core needle procedure
FNA and core needle biopsies separate lesions, same or different imaging guidance, append modifier 59 to code for core needle biopsy and imaging guidance

10004 **Resequenced code. See code following 10021.**
10005 **Resequenced code. See code following 10021.**
10006 **Resequenced code. See code following 10021.**
10007 **Resequenced code. See code following 10021.**
10008 **Resequenced code. See code following 10021.**
10009 **Resequenced code. See code following 10021.**
10010 **Resequenced code. See code following 10021.**
10011 **Resequenced code. See code following 10021.**
10012 **Resequenced code. See code following 10021.**

10021 **Fine needle aspiration biopsy, without imaging guidance; first lesion**
(88172-88173, [88177])
1.60 2.80 FUD XXX T P3 80
AMA: 2019,May,10; 2019,Apr,4; 2019,Feb,8; 2018,Jan,8; 2017,Jan,8; 2016,Jan,13; 2015,Jan,16

\+ # 10004 **each additional lesion (List separately in addition to code for primary procedure)**
EXCLUDES *Fine needle biopsy using other imaging methods for same lesion ([10005, 10006, 10007, 10008, 10009, 10010, 10011, 10012])*
Imaging guidance (76942)
(88172-88173, [88177])
Code first (10021)
1.25 1.48 FUD ZZZ N1 80
AMA: 2019,Apr,4; 2019,Feb,8

\# 10005 **Fine needle aspiration biopsy, including ultrasound guidance; first lesion**
INCLUDES Imaging guidance (76942)
(88172-88173, [88177])
2.10 3.59 FUD XXX P3 80
AMA: 2019,May,10; 2019,Feb,8; 2019,Apr,4

\+ # 10006 **each additional lesion (List separately in addition to code for primary procedure)**
INCLUDES Imaging guidance (76942)
(88172-88173, [88177])
Code first ([10005])
1.42 1.70 FUD ZZZ N1 80
AMA: 2019,Apr,4; 2019,Feb,8

\# 10007 **Fine needle aspiration biopsy, including fluoroscopic guidance; first lesion**
INCLUDES Imaging guidance (77002)
(88172-88173, [88177])
2.70 8.09 FUD XXX P3 80
AMA: 2019,Apr,4; 2019,Feb,8

\+ # 10008 **each additional lesion (List separately in addition to code for primary procedure)**
INCLUDES Imaging guidance (77002)
(88172-88173, [88177])
Code first ([10007])
1.76 4.79 FUD ZZZ N1 80
AMA: 2019,Apr,4; 2019,Feb,8

\# 10009 **Fine needle aspiration biopsy, including CT guidance; first lesion**
INCLUDES Imaging guidance (77012)
(88172-88173, [88177])
3.28 13.3 FUD XXX P2 80
AMA: 2019,Apr,4; 2019,Feb,8

\+ # 10010 **each additional lesion (List separately in addition to code for primary procedure)**
INCLUDES Imaging guidance (77012)
(88172-88173, [88177])
Code first ([10009])
2.38 8.02 FUD ZZZ N1 80
AMA: 2019,Apr,4; 2019,Feb,8

\# 10011 **Fine needle aspiration biopsy, including MR guidance; first lesion**
INCLUDES Imaging guidance (77021)
(88172-88173, [88177])
0.00 0.00 FUD XXX R2 80
AMA: 2019,Apr,4; 2019,Feb,8

\+ # 10012 **each additional lesion (List separately in addition to code for primary procedure)**
INCLUDES Imaging guidance (77021)
(88172-88173, [88177])
Code first ([10011])
0.00 0.00 FUD ZZZ N1 80
AMA: 2019,Apr,4; 2019,Feb,8

10030-10180 Treatment of Lesions: Skin and Subcutaneous Tissues

EXCLUDES *Excision benign lesion (11400-11471)*

10030 **Image-guided fluid collection drainage by catheter (eg, abscess, hematoma, seroma, lymphocele, cyst), soft tissue (eg, extremity, abdominal wall, neck), percutaneous**
INCLUDES Radiologic guidance (75989, 76942, 77002-77003, 77012, 77021)
EXCLUDES *Percutaneous drainage with imaging guidance:*
Peritoneal or retroperitoneal collections (49406)
Visceral collections (49405)
Transvaginal or transrectal drainage with imaging guidance peritoneal or retroperitoneal collections (49407)
Code also every instance of fluid collection drained using a separate catheter (10030)
3.98 17.5 FUD 000 T G2 80
AMA: 2019,Apr,4; 2018,Jan,8; 2017,Aug,9; 2017,Jan,8; 2016,Jan,13; 2015,Jan,16

Integumentary System
10004 — 10030

10035 **Placement of soft tissue localization device(s) (eg, clip, metallic pellet, wire/needle, radioactive seeds), percutaneous, including imaging guidance; first lesion**

INCLUDES Radiologic guidance (76942, 77002, 77012, 77021)

EXCLUDES *Sites with more specific code descriptor, such as breast*

Reporting code more than one time per site, regardless number markers used

Code also each additional target on same or opposite side (10036)

2.46 12.8 FUD 000 T N1 80 50

AMA: 2018,Jan,8; 2017,Jan,8; 2016,Jun,3

\+ **10036** **each additional lesion (List separately in addition to code for primary procedure)**

INCLUDES Radiologic guidance (76942, 77002, 77012, 77021)

EXCLUDES *Sites with more specific code descriptor, such as breast*

Reporting code more than one time per site, regardless number markers used

Code first (10035)

1.25 11.7 FUD ZZZ N N1 80

AMA: 2018,Jan,8; 2017,Jan,8; 2016,Jun,3

10040 **Acne surgery (eg, marsupialization, opening or removal of multiple milia, comedones, cysts, pustules)**

1.53 3.11 FUD 010 01 N1

AMA: 2018,Jan,8; 2017,Jan,8; 2016,Jan,13; 2015,Jan,16

10060 **Incision and drainage of abscess (eg, carbuncle, suppurative hidradenitis, cutaneous or subcutaneous abscess, cyst, furuncle, or paronychia); simple or single**

2.87 3.44 FUD 010 T P3

AMA: 2018,Jan,8; 2017,Jan,8; 2016,Jan,13; 2015,Jan,16

10061 **complicated or multiple**

5.16 5.87 FUD 010 T P3

AMA: 2018,Jan,8; 2017,Jan,8; 2016,Jan,13; 2015,Jan,16

10080 **Incision and drainage of pilonidal cyst; simple**

2.95 5.99 FUD 010 T P3

AMA: 2018,Jan,8; 2017,Jan,8; 2016,Jan,13; 2015,Jan,16

10081 **complicated**

EXCLUDES *Excision pilonidal cyst (11770-11772)*

4.93 8.67 FUD 010 T P3

AMA: 2018,Jan,8; 2017,Jan,8; 2016,Jan,13; 2015,Jan,16

10120 **Incision and removal of foreign body, subcutaneous tissues; simple**

2.94 4.31 FUD 010 T P3

AMA: 2018,Jan,8; 2017,Jan,8; 2016,Jan,13; 2015,Jan,16

10121 **complicated**

EXCLUDES *Debridement associated with fracture or dislocation (11010-11012)*

Exploration penetrating wound (20100-20103)

5.33 7.76 FUD 010 J A2

AMA: 2018,Jan,8; 2017,Jan,8; 2016,Jan,13; 2015,Jan,16

10140 **Incision and drainage of hematoma, seroma or fluid collection**

(76942, 77002, 77012, 77021)

3.40 4.77 FUD 010 J P3

AMA: 2018,Jan,8; 2017,Jan,8; 2016,Jan,13; 2015,Jan,16

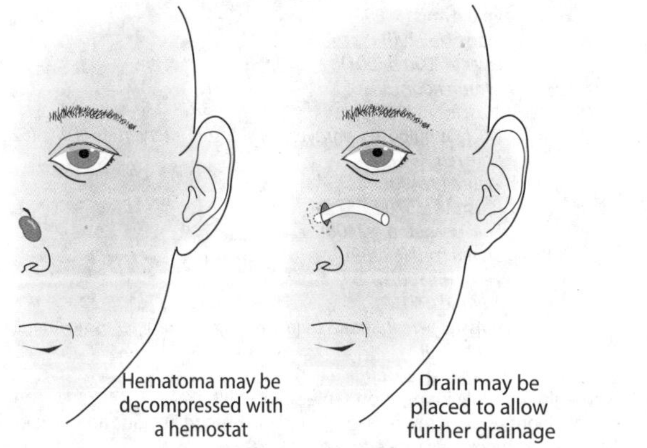
Hematoma may be decompressed with a hemostat
Drain may be placed to allow further drainage

10160 **Puncture aspiration of abscess, hematoma, bulla, or cyst**

(76942, 77002, 77012, 77021)

2.71 3.71 FUD 010 T P3

AMA: 2018,Jan,8; 2017,Aug,9; 2017,Jan,8; 2016,Jan,13; 2015,Jan,16

10180 **Incision and drainage, complex, postoperative wound infection**

EXCLUDES *Wound dehiscence (12020-12021, 13160)*

5.10 7.12 FUD 010 J A2

AMA: 2018,Jan,8; 2017,Jan,8; 2016,Jan,13; 2015,Jan,16

11000-11012 Removal of Foreign Substances and Infected/Devitalized Tissue

EXCLUDES *Debridement:*

Burns (16000-16030)

Deeper tissue (11042-11047 [11045, 11046])

Nails (11720-11721)

Nonelective debridement/active care management (97597-97598)

Wounds (11042-11047 [11045, 11046])

Dermabrasions (15780-15783)

Pressure ulcer excision (15920-15999)

11000 **Debridement of extensive eczematous or infected skin; up to 10% of body surface**

EXCLUDES *Necrotizing soft tissue infection:*

Abdominal wall (11005-11006)

External genitalia and perineum (11004, 11006)

0.82 1.61 FUD 000 T P3

AMA: 2018,Feb,10; 2018,Jan,8; 2017,Jan,8; 2016,Jan,13; 2015,Jan,16

\+ **11001** **each additional 10% of the body surface, or part thereof (List separately in addition to code for primary procedure)**

EXCLUDES *Necrotizing soft tissue infection:*

Abdominal wall (11005-11006)

External genitalia and perineum (11004, 11006)

Code first (11000)

0.41 0.62 FUD ZZZ N N1

AMA: 2018,Feb,10; 2018,Jan,8; 2017,Jan,8; 2016,Jan,13; 2015,Jan,16

11004 **Debridement of skin, subcutaneous tissue, muscle and fascia for necrotizing soft tissue infection; external genitalia and perineum**

Code also skin grafts or flaps, when performed (14000-14350, 15040-15770 [15769], 15771-15776)

16.6 16.6 FUD 000 C

AMA: 2019,Nov,14; 2018,Feb,10; 2018,Jan,8; 2017,Jan,8; 2016,Jan,13; 2015,Jan,16

11005 **abdominal wall, with or without fascial closure**

Code also skin grafts or flaps, when performed (14000-14350, 15040-15770 [15769], 15771-15776)

22.6 22.6 FUD 000 C 80

AMA: 2019,Nov,14; 2018,Feb,10; 2018,Jan,8; 2017,Jan,8; 2016,Jan,13; 2015,Jan,16

11006 **external genitalia, perineum and abdominal wall, with or without fascial closure**

EXCLUDES *Orchiectomy (54520)*
Testicular transplant (54680)

Code also skin grafts or flaps, when performed (14000-14350, 15040-15770 [15769], 15771-15776)

20.4 20.4 FUD 000 C

AMA: 2019,Nov,14; 2018,Jan,8; 2017,Jan,8; 2016,Jan,13; 2015,Jan,16

+ **11008** **Removal of prosthetic material or mesh, abdominal wall for infection (eg, for chronic or recurrent mesh infection or necrotizing soft tissue infection) (List separately in addition to code for primary procedure)**

EXCLUDES *Debridement (11000-11001, 11010-11044 [11045, 11046])*
Insertion mesh (49568)

Code also skin grafts or flaps, when performed (14000-14350, 15040-15770 [15769], 15771-15776)

Code first (10180, 11004-11006)

7.99 7.99 FUD ZZZ C 80

AMA: 2019,Jan,14; 2018,Jan,8; 2017,Jan,8; 2016,Jan,13; 2015,Jan,16

11010 **Debridement including removal of foreign material at the site of an open fracture and/or an open dislocation (eg, excisional debridement); skin and subcutaneous tissues**

7.96 13.5 FUD 010 T A2

AMA: 2018,Jan,8; 2017,Jan,8; 2016,Jan,13; 2015,Jan,16

11011 **skin, subcutaneous tissue, muscle fascia, and muscle**

8.68 15.2 FUD 000 T A2

AMA: 2018,Jan,8; 2017,Jan,8; 2016,Jan,13; 2015,Jan,16

11012 **skin, subcutaneous tissue, muscle fascia, muscle, and bone**

12.0 19.3 FUD 000 J A2

AMA: 2018,Jan,8; 2017,Jan,8; 2016,Jan,13; 2015,Jan,16

11042-11047 [11045, 11046] Removal of Infected/Devitalized Tissue

INCLUDES Debridement reported by size and depth
Debridement reported for multiple wounds by adding total surface area wounds with same depth
Injuries, wounds, chronic ulcers, infections

EXCLUDES *Debridement:*
Burn (16020-16030)
Eczematous or infected skin (11000-11001)
Nails (11720-11721)
Necrotizing soft tissue infection external genitalia, perineum, or abdominal wall (11004-11006)
Non-elective debridement/active care management same wound (97597-97602)
Dermabrasions (15780-15783)
Excision pressure ulcers (15920-15999)

Code also each additional single wound with different depths
Code also modifier 59 for additional wound debridement
Code also multiple wound groups with different depths

11042 **Debridement, subcutaneous tissue (includes epidermis and dermis, if performed); first 20 sq cm or less**

1.75 3.57 FUD 000 T A2

AMA: 2018,Jan,8; 2017,Jan,8; 2016,Oct,3; 2016,Aug,9; 2016,Feb,13; 2016,Jan,13; 2015,Jan,16

+ # **11045** **each additional 20 sq cm, or part thereof (List separately in addition to code for primary procedure)**

Code first (11042)

0.77 1.19 FUD ZZZ N N1 80

AMA: 2018,Jan,8; 2017,Jan,8; 2016,Oct,3; 2016,Aug,9; 2016,Jan,13; 2015,Jan,16

11043 **Debridement, muscle and/or fascia (includes epidermis, dermis, and subcutaneous tissue, if performed); first 20 sq cm or less**

4.47 6.64 FUD 000 T A2

AMA: 2020,Apr,8; 2018,Jan,8; 2017,Jan,8; 2016,Oct,3; 2016,Aug,9; 2016,Jan,13; 2015,Jan,16

+ # **11046** **each additional 20 sq cm, or part thereof (List separately in addition to code for primary procedure)**

Code first (11043)

1.62 2.12 FUD ZZZ N N1 80

AMA: 2018,Jan,8; 2017,Jan,8; 2016,Oct,3; 2016,Aug,9; 2016,Jan,13; 2015,Jan,16

11044 **Debridement, bone (includes epidermis, dermis, subcutaneous tissue, muscle and/or fascia, if performed); first 20 sq cm or less**

6.58 8.93 FUD 000 J A2

AMA: 2018,Jan,8; 2017,Jan,8; 2016,Oct,3; 2016,Aug,9; 2016,Jan,13; 2015,Jan,16

11045 **Resequenced code. See code following 11042.**

11046 **Resequenced code. See code following 11043.**

+ **11047** **each additional 20 sq cm, or part thereof (List separately in addition to code for primary procedure)**

Code first (11044)

2.86 3.53 FUD ZZZ N N1 80

AMA: 2018,Jan,8; 2017,Jan,8; 2016,Oct,3; 2016,Aug,9; 2016,Jan,13; 2015,Jan,16

11055-11057 Excision Benign Hypertrophic Skin Lesions

CMS: 100-04,32,80.8 CSF Edits: Routine Foot Care

EXCLUDES *Destruction benign lesions other than cutaneous vascular proliferative lesions or skin tags (17110-17111)*

11055 **Paring or cutting of benign hyperkeratotic lesion (eg, corn or callus); single lesion**

0.46 1.78 FUD 000 Q1 N1

AMA: 2018,Jan,8; 2017,Jan,8; 2016,Jan,13; 2015,Jan,16

11056 **2 to 4 lesions**

0.65 1.90 FUD 000 Q1 N1

AMA: 2018,Jan,8; 2017,Jan,8; 2016,Jan,13; 2015,Jan,16

11057 **more than 4 lesions**

0.85 2.31 FUD 000 T P3

AMA: 2018,Jan,8; 2017,Jan,8; 2016,Jan,13; 2015,Jan,16

11102-11107 Surgical Biopsy Skin and Mucous Membranes

INCLUDES Attaining tissue for pathologic exam

EXCLUDES *Biopsies performed during related procedures*
Biopsy:
Anterior 2/3 tongue (41100)
Conjunctiva (68100)
Ear (69100)
Eyelid ([67810])
Floor of mouth (41108)
Intranasal (30100)
Lip (40490)
Nail (11755)
Penis (54100)
Perineum/vulva (56605-56606)
Vestibule of mouth (40808)

11102 **Tangential biopsy of skin (eg, shave, scoop, saucerize, curette); single lesion**

1.12 2.84 FUD 000 P3

AMA: 2020,May,13; 2019,Dec,9; 2019,Jan,9

+ **11103** **each separate/additional lesion (List separately in addition to code for primary procedure)**

Code first different biopsy techniques used for additional separate lesions, when performed (11102, 11104, 11106)

0.66 1.51 FUD ZZZ N1

AMA: 2020,May,13; 2019,Dec,9; 2019,Jan,9

11104 **Punch biopsy of skin (including simple closure, when performed); single lesion**

1.40 3.57 FUD 000 P2

AMA: 2019,Dec,9; 2019,Jan,9

+ **11105** **each separate/additional lesion (List separately in addition to code for primary procedure)**
Code first different biopsy techniques used for additional separate lesions, when performed (11104, 11106)
0.76 1.72 **FUD** ZZZ N1
AMA: 2019,Dec,9; 2019,Jan,9

11106 **Incisional biopsy of skin (eg, wedge) (including simple closure, when performed); single lesion**
1.74 4.26 **FUD** 000 P3
AMA: 2019,Dec,9; 2019,Jan,9

+ **11107** **each separate/additional lesion (List separately in addition to code for primary procedure)**
Code first (11106)
0.93 2.04 **FUD** ZZZ N1
AMA: 2019,Dec,9; 2019,Jan,9

11200-11201 Skin Tag Removal - All Techniques

INCLUDES
- Chemical destruction
- Electrocauterization
- Electrosurgical destruction
- Ligature strangulation
- Removal with or without local anesthesia
- Sharp excision or scissoring

11200 **Removal of skin tags, multiple fibrocutaneous tags, any area; up to and including 15 lesions**
2.10 2.52 **FUD** 010 Q1 N1
AMA: 2018,Jan,8; 2017,Jan,8; 2016,Jan,13; 2015,Jan,16

+ **11201** **each additional 10 lesions, or part thereof (List separately in addition to code for primary procedure)**
Code first (11200)
0.48 0.54 **FUD** ZZZ N N1
AMA: 2018,Jan,8; 2017,Jan,8; 2016,Jan,13; 2015,Jan,16

11300-11313 Skin Lesion Removal: Shaving

INCLUDES
- Local anesthesia
- Partial thickness excision by horizontal slicing
- Wound cauterization

11300 **Shaving of epidermal or dermal lesion, single lesion, trunk, arms or legs; lesion diameter 0.5 cm or less**
0.99 2.84 **FUD** 000 Q1 N1 80
AMA: 2019,Jan,9; 2018,Feb,10; 2018,Jan,8; 2017,Dec,14; 2017,Jan,8; 2016,Jan,13; 2015,Jan,16

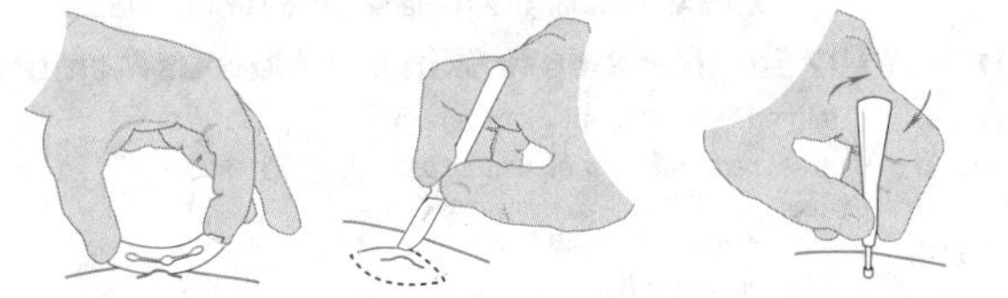

Shave excision of an elevated lesion; technique also used to biopsy

Elliptical excision is often used when tissue removal is larger than 4 mm or when deep pathology is suspected

A punch biopsy cuts a core of tissue as the tool is twisted downward

11301 **lesion diameter 0.6 to 1.0 cm**
1.50 3.45 **FUD** 000 Q1 N1 80
AMA: 2019,Jan,9; 2018,Feb,10; 2018,Jan,8; 2017,Dec,14; 2017,Jan,8; 2016,Jan,13; 2015,Jan,16

11302 **lesion diameter 1.1 to 2.0 cm**
1.76 3.99 **FUD** 000 Q1 N1 80
AMA: 2019,Jan,9; 2018,Feb,10; 2018,Jan,8; 2017,Dec,14; 2017,Jan,8; 2016,Jan,13; 2015,Jan,16

11303 **lesion diameter over 2.0 cm**
2.07 4.39 **FUD** 000 Q1 N1 80
AMA: 2019,Jan,9; 2018,Feb,10; 2018,Jan,8; 2017,Dec,14; 2017,Jan,8; 2016,Jan,13; 2015,Jan,16

11305 **Shaving of epidermal or dermal lesion, single lesion, scalp, neck, hands, feet, genitalia; lesion diameter 0.5 cm or less**
1.12 2.90 **FUD** 000 Q1 N1 80
AMA: 2019,Jan,9; 2018,Feb,10; 2018,Jan,8; 2017,Dec,14; 2017,Jan,8; 2016,Jan,13; 2015,Jan,16

11306 **lesion diameter 0.6 to 1.0 cm**
1.45 3.50 **FUD** 000 Q1 N1 80
AMA: 2019,Jan,9; 2018,Feb,10; 2018,Jan,8; 2017,Dec,14; 2017,Jan,8; 2016,Jan,13; 2015,Jan,16

11307 **lesion diameter 1.1 to 2.0 cm**
1.87 4.09 **FUD** 000 T P2 80
AMA: 2019,Jan,9; 2018,Feb,10; 2018,Jan,8; 2017,Dec,14; 2017,Jan,8; 2016,Jan,13; 2015,Jan,16

11308 **lesion diameter over 2.0 cm**
2.11 4.37 **FUD** 000 Q1 N1 80
AMA: 2019,Jan,9; 2018,Feb,10; 2018,Jan,8; 2017,Dec,14; 2017,Jan,8; 2016,Jan,13; 2015,Jan,16

11310 **Shaving of epidermal or dermal lesion, single lesion, face, ears, eyelids, nose, lips, mucous membrane; lesion diameter 0.5 cm or less**
1.34 3.29 **FUD** 000 T P3 80
AMA: 2019,Jan,9; 2018,Feb,10; 2018,Jan,8; 2017,Dec,14; 2017,Jan,8; 2016,Jan,13; 2015,Jan,16

11311 **lesion diameter 0.6 to 1.0 cm**
1.88 3.86 **FUD** 000 T P2 80
AMA: 2019,Jan,9; 2018,Feb,10; 2018,Jan,8; 2017,Dec,14; 2017,Jan,8; 2016,Jan,13; 2015,Jan,16

11312 **lesion diameter 1.1 to 2.0 cm**
2.17 4.51 **FUD** 000 T P3 80
AMA: 2019,Jan,9; 2018,Feb,10; 2018,Jan,8; 2017,Dec,14; 2017,Jan,8; 2016,Jan,13; 2015,Jan,16

11313 **lesion diameter over 2.0 cm**
2.82 5.27 **FUD** 000 T P3 80
AMA: 2019,Jan,9; 2018,Feb,10; 2018,Jan,8; 2017,Dec,14; 2017,Jan,8; 2016,Jan,13; 2015,Jan,16

11400-11446 Skin Lesion Removal: Benign

INCLUDES
- Biopsy on same lesion
- Cicatricial lesion excision
- Full thickness removal including margins
- Lesion measurement before excision at largest diameter plus margin
- Local anesthesia
- Simple, nonlayered closure

EXCLUDES
- *Adjacent tissue transfer: report only adjacent tissue transfer (14000-14302)*
- *Biopsy eyelid ([67810])*
- *Destruction:*
  - *Benign lesions, any method (17110-17111)*
  - *Cutaneous vascular proliferative lesions (17106-17108)*
  - *Destruction of eyelid lesion (67850)*
  - *Malignant lesions (17260-17286)*
  - *Premalignant lesions (17000, 17003-17004)*
- *Escharotomy (16035-16036)*
- *Excision and reconstruction eyelid (67961-67975)*
- *Excision chalazion (67800-67808)*
- *Eyelid procedures involving more than skin (67800 and subsequent codes)*
- *Laser fenestration for scars (0479T-0480T)*
- *Shave removal (11300-11313)*

Code also complex closure (13100-13153)
Code also each separate lesion
Code also intermediate closure (12031-12057)
Code also modifier 22 when excision complicated or unusual
Code also reconstruction (15002-15261, 15570-15770)

11400 **Excision, benign lesion including margins, except skin tag (unless listed elsewhere), trunk, arms or legs; excised diameter 0.5 cm or less**
2.33 3.57 **FUD** 010 T P3
AMA: 2019,Nov,3; 2018,Sep,7; 2018,Feb,10; 2018,Jan,8; 2017,Jan,8; 2016,Apr,3; 2016,Jan,13; 2015,Jan,16

11401 **excised diameter 0.6 to 1.0 cm**
2.96 4.35 **FUD** 010 T P3
AMA: 2019,Nov,3; 2018,Sep,7; 2018,Feb,10; 2018,Jan,8; 2017,Jan,8; 2016,Apr,3; 2016,Jan,13; 2015,Jan,16

11402 **excised diameter 1.1 to 2.0 cm**
3.29 4.78 **FUD** 010 T P3
AMA: 2019,Nov,3; 2018,Sep,7; 2018,Feb,10; 2018,Jan,8; 2017,Jan,8; 2016,Apr,3; 2016,Jan,13; 2015,Jan,16

11403 **excised diameter 2.1 to 3.0 cm**
4.23 5.58 **FUD** 010 T P3
AMA: 2019,Nov,3; 2018,Sep,7; 2018,Feb,10; 2018,Jan,8; 2017,Jan,8; 2016,Apr,3; 2016,Jan,13; 2015,Jan,16

11404 **excised diameter 3.1 to 4.0 cm**
4.66 6.34 **FUD** 010 J A2
AMA: 2019,Nov,3; 2018,Sep,7; 2018,Feb,10; 2018,Jan,8; 2017,Jan,8; 2016,Apr,3; 2016,Jan,13; 2015,Jan,16

11406 **excised diameter over 4.0 cm**
7.09 9.07 **FUD** 010 J A2
AMA: 2019,Nov,3; 2018,Sep,7; 2018,Feb,10; 2018,Jan,8; 2017,Jan,8; 2016,Apr,3; 2016,Jan,13; 2015,Jan,16

11420 **Excision, benign lesion including margins, except skin tag (unless listed elsewhere), scalp, neck, hands, feet, genitalia; excised diameter 0.5 cm or less**
2.34 3.60 **FUD** 010 J P3
AMA: 2019,Nov,3; 2018,Sep,7; 2018,Feb,10; 2018,Jan,8; 2017,Jan,8; 2016,Apr,3; 2016,Jan,13; 2015,Jan,16

11421 **excised diameter 0.6 to 1.0 cm**
3.15 4.49 **FUD** 010 T P3
AMA: 2019,Nov,3; 2018,Sep,7; 2018,Feb,10; 2018,Jan,8; 2017,Jan,8; 2016,Apr,3; 2016,Jan,13; 2015,Jan,16

11422 **excised diameter 1.1 to 2.0 cm**
3.88 5.11 **FUD** 010 J P3
AMA: 2019,Nov,3; 2018,Sep,7; 2018,Feb,10; 2018,Jan,8; 2017,Jan,8; 2016,Apr,3; 2016,Jan,13; 2015,Jan,16

11423 **excised diameter 2.1 to 3.0 cm**
4.45 5.81 **FUD** 010 J P3
AMA: 2019,Nov,3; 2018,Sep,7; 2018,Feb,10; 2018,Jan,8; 2017,Jan,8; 2016,Apr,3; 2016,Jan,13; 2015,Jan,16

11424 **excised diameter 3.1 to 4.0 cm**
5.11 6.71 **FUD** 010 J A2
AMA: 2019,Nov,3; 2018,Sep,7; 2018,Feb,10; 2018,Jan,8; 2017,Jan,8; 2016,Apr,3; 2016,Jan,13; 2015,Jan,16

11426 **excised diameter over 4.0 cm**
7.89 9.63 **FUD** 010 J A2
AMA: 2019,Nov,3; 2018,Sep,7; 2018,Feb,10; 2018,Jan,8; 2017,Jan,8; 2016,Apr,3; 2016,Jan,13; 2015,Jan,16

11440 **Excision, other benign lesion including margins, except skin tag (unless listed elsewhere), face, ears, eyelids, nose, lips, mucous membrane; excised diameter 0.5 cm or less**
2.96 3.91 **FUD** 010 T P3
AMA: 2019,Nov,3; 2019,Jan,14; 2018,Sep,7; 2018,Feb,10; 2018,Jan,8; 2017,Jan,8; 2016,Apr,3; 2016,Jan,13; 2015,Jan,16

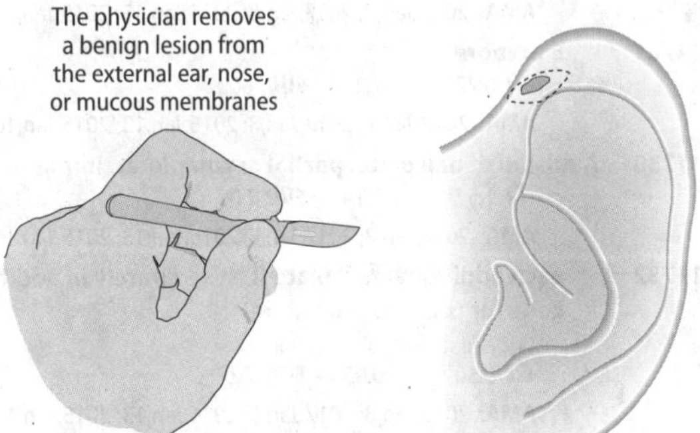

11441 **excised diameter 0.6 to 1.0 cm**
3.73 4.88 **FUD** 010 T P3
AMA: 2019,Nov,3; 2019,Jan,14; 2018,Sep,7; 2018,Feb,10; 2018,Jan,8; 2017,Jan,8; 2016,Apr,3; 2016,Jan,13; 2015,Jan,16

11442 **excised diameter 1.1 to 2.0 cm**
4.14 5.43 **FUD** 010 T P3
AMA: 2019,Nov,3; 2019,Jan,14; 2018,Sep,7; 2018,Feb,10; 2018,Jan,8; 2017,Jan,8; 2016,Apr,3; 2016,Jan,13; 2015,Jan,16

11443 **excised diameter 2.1 to 3.0 cm**
5.08 6.45 **FUD** 010 J P3
AMA: 2019,Nov,3; 2019,Jan,14; 2018,Sep,7; 2018,Feb,10; 2018,Jan,8; 2017,Jan,8; 2016,Apr,3; 2016,Jan,13; 2015,Jan,16

11444 **excised diameter 3.1 to 4.0 cm**
6.49 8.09 **FUD** 010 J A2
AMA: 2019,Nov,3; 2019,Jan,14; 2018,Sep,7; 2018,Feb,10; 2018,Jan,8; 2017,Jan,8; 2016,Apr,3; 2016,Jan,13; 2015,Jan,16

11446 **excised diameter over 4.0 cm**
9.33 11.1 **FUD** 010 J A2
AMA: 2019,Nov,3; 2019,Jan,14; 2018,Sep,7; 2018,Feb,10; 2018,Jan,8; 2017,Jan,8; 2016,Apr,3; 2016,Jan,13; 2015,Jan,16

11450-11471 Treatment of Hidradenitis: Excision and Repair

Code also closure by skin graft or flap (14000-14350, 15040-15770 [15769], 15771-15776)

11450 **Excision of skin and subcutaneous tissue for hidradenitis, axillary; with simple or intermediate repair**
7.36 11.6 **FUD** 090 J A2 50
AMA: 2019,Nov,3; 2018,Sep,7; 2018,Feb,10; 2018,Jan,8; 2017,Jan,8; 2016,Aug,9; 2016,Jan,13; 2015,Jan,16

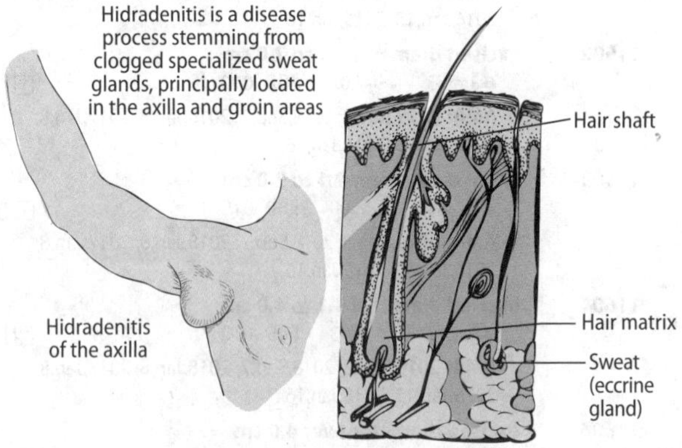

11451 **with complex repair**
9.41 14.5 **FUD** 090 J A2 80 50
AMA: 2019,Nov,3; 2018,Sep,7; 2018,Feb,10; 2018,Jan,8; 2017,Jan,8; 2016,Aug,9; 2016,Jan,13; 2015,Jan,16

11462 **Excision of skin and subcutaneous tissue for hidradenitis, inguinal; with simple or intermediate repair**
7.01 11.3 **FUD** 090 J A2 80 50
AMA: 2019,Nov,3; 2018,Sep,7; 2018,Feb,10; 2018,Jan,8; 2017,Jan,8; 2016,Aug,9; 2016,Jan,13; 2015,Jan,16

11463 **with complex repair**
9.42 14.3 **FUD** 090 J A2 80 50
AMA: 2019,Nov,3; 2018,Sep,7; 2018,Feb,10; 2018,Jan,8; 2017,Jan,8; 2016,Aug,9; 2016,Jan,13; 2015,Jan,16

11470 **Excision of skin and subcutaneous tissue for hidradenitis, perianal, perineal, or umbilical; with simple or intermediate repair**
8.08 12.0 **FUD** 090 J A2
AMA: 2019,Nov,3; 2018,Sep,7; 2018,Feb,10; 2018,Jan,8; 2017,Jan,8; 2016,Aug,9; 2016,Jan,13; 2015,Jan,16

11471 **with complex repair**
10.0 15.0 **FUD** 090 J A2 80
AMA: 2019,Nov,3; 2018,Sep,7; 2018,Feb,10; 2018,Jan,8; 2017,Jan,8; 2016,Aug,9; 2016,Jan,13; 2015,Jan,16

11600-11646 Skin Lesion Removal: Malignant

INCLUDES Biopsy on same lesion
Excision additional margin at same operative session
Full thickness removal including margins
Lesion measurement before excision at largest diameter plus margin
Local anesthesia
Simple, nonlayered closure

EXCLUDES *Adjacent tissue transfer. Report only adjacent tissue transfer (14000-14302)*
Destruction (17260-17286)
Excision additional margin at subsequent operative session (11600-11646)

Code also complex closure (13100-13153)
Code also each separate lesion
Code also intermediate closure (12031-12057)
Code also modifier 58 when re-excision performed during postoperative period
Code also reconstruction (15002-15261, 15570-15770)

11600 Excision, malignant lesion including margins, trunk, arms, or legs; excised diameter 0.5 cm or less
3.46 5.61 FUD 010 T P3
AMA: 2019,Nov,3; 2018,Sep,7; 2018,Jan,8; 2017,Jan,8; 2016,Jan,13; 2015,Jan,16

11601 excised diameter 0.6 to 1.0 cm
4.29 6.52 FUD 010 T P3
AMA: 2019,Nov,3; 2018,Sep,7; 2018,Jan,8; 2017,Jan,8; 2016,Jan,13; 2015,Jan,16

11602 excised diameter 1.1 to 2.0 cm
4.63 7.02 FUD 010 T P2
AMA: 2019,Nov,3; 2018,Sep,7; 2018,Jan,8; 2017,Jan,8; 2016,Jan,13; 2015,Jan,16

11603 excised diameter 2.1 to 3.0 cm
5.54 8.00 FUD 010 T P3
AMA: 2019,Nov,3; 2018,Sep,7; 2018,Jan,8; 2017,Jan,8; 2016,Jan,13; 2015,Jan,16

11604 excised diameter 3.1 to 4.0 cm
6.12 8.93 FUD 010 T A2
AMA: 2019,Nov,3; 2018,Sep,7; 2018,Jan,8; 2017,Jan,8; 2016,Jan,13; 2015,Jan,16

11606 excised diameter over 4.0 cm
9.24 12.8 FUD 010 J A2
AMA: 2019,Nov,3; 2018,Sep,7; 2018,Jan,8; 2017,Jan,8; 2016,Jan,13; 2015,Jan,16

11620 Excision, malignant lesion including margins, scalp, neck, hands, feet, genitalia; excised diameter 0.5 cm or less
3.50 5.64 FUD 010 J P3
AMA: 2019,Nov,3; 2018,Sep,7; 2018,Jan,8; 2017,Jan,8; 2016,Jan,13; 2015,Jan,16

11621 excised diameter 0.6 to 1.0 cm
4.27 6.55 FUD 010 T P3
AMA: 2019,Nov,3; 2018,Sep,7; 2018,Jan,8; 2017,Jan,8; 2016,Jan,13; 2015,Jan,16

11622 excised diameter 1.1 to 2.0 cm
4.93 7.30 FUD 010 T P3
AMA: 2019,Nov,3; 2018,Sep,7; 2018,Jan,8; 2017,Jan,8; 2016,Jan,13; 2015,Jan,16

11623 excised diameter 2.1 to 3.0 cm
6.03 8.52 FUD 010 J P3
AMA: 2019,Nov,3; 2018,Sep,7; 2018,Jan,8; 2017,Jan,8; 2016,Jan,13; 2015,Jan,16

11624 excised diameter 3.1 to 4.0 cm
6.85 9.65 FUD 010 J A2
AMA: 2019,Nov,3; 2018,Sep,7; 2018,Jan,8; 2017,Jan,8; 2016,Jan,13; 2015,Jan,16

11626 excised diameter over 4.0 cm
8.44 11.6 FUD 010 J A2
AMA: 2019,Nov,3; 2018,Sep,7; 2018,Jan,8; 2017,Jan,8; 2016,Jan,13; 2015,Jan,16

11640 Excision, malignant lesion including margins, face, ears, eyelids, nose, lips; excised diameter 0.5 cm or less
EXCLUDES *Eyelid excision involving more than skin (67800-67808, 67840-67850, 67961-67966)*
3.59 5.77 FUD 010 T P3
AMA: 2019,Nov,3; 2018,Sep,7; 2018,Jan,8; 2017,Jan,8; 2016,Jan,13; 2015,Jan,16

11641 excised diameter 0.6 to 1.0 cm
EXCLUDES *Eyelid excision involving more than skin (67800-67808, 67840-67850, 67961-67966)*
4.45 6.78 FUD 010 T P3
AMA: 2019,Nov,3; 2018,Sep,7; 2018,Jan,8; 2017,Jan,8; 2016,Jan,13; 2015,Jan,16

11642 excised diameter 1.1 to 2.0 cm
EXCLUDES *Eyelid excision involving more than skin (67800-67808, 67840-67850, 67961-67966)*
5.30 7.73 FUD 010 T P3
AMA: 2019,Nov,3; 2018,Sep,7; 2018,Jan,8; 2017,Jan,8; 2016,Jan,13; 2015,Jan,16

11643 excised diameter 2.1 to 3.0 cm
EXCLUDES *Eyelid excision involving more than skin (67800-67808, 67840-67850, 67961-67966)*
6.55 9.06 FUD 010 J P3
AMA: 2019,Nov,3; 2018,Sep,7; 2018,Jan,8; 2017,Jan,8; 2016,Jan,13; 2015,Jan,16

11644 excised diameter 3.1 to 4.0 cm
EXCLUDES *Eyelid excision involving more than skin (67800-67808, 67840-67850, 67961-67966)*
8.14 11.1 FUD 010 J A2
AMA: 2019,Nov,3; 2018,Sep,7; 2018,Jan,8; 2017,Jan,8; 2016,Jan,13; 2015,Jan,16

11646 excised diameter over 4.0 cm
EXCLUDES *Eyelid excision involving more than skin (67800-67808, 67840-67850, 67961-67966)*
11.2 14.5 FUD 010 J A2
AMA: 2019,Nov,3; 2018,Sep,7; 2018,Jan,8; 2017,Jan,8; 2016,Jan,13; 2015,Jan,16

11719-11765 Nails and Supporting Structures

CMS: 100-02,15,290 Foot Care
EXCLUDES *Drainage paronychia or onychia (10060-10061)*

11719 Trimming of nondystrophic nails, any number
0.22 0.41 FUD 000 Q1 N1
AMA: 2018,Jan,8; 2017,Jan,8; 2016,Jan,13; 2015,Jan,16

11720 Debridement of nail(s) by any method(s); 1 to 5
0.42 0.93 FUD 000 Q1 N1
AMA: 2018,Jan,8; 2017,Jan,8; 2016,Jan,13; 2015,Jan,16

11721 6 or more
0.72 1.29 FUD 000 Q1 N1
AMA: 2018,Jan,8; 2017,Jan,8; 2016,Jan,13; 2015,Jan,16

11730 Avulsion of nail plate, partial or complete, simple; single
1.57 3.14 FUD 000 Q1 N1
AMA: 2018,Jan,8; 2017,Jan,8; 2016,Jan,13; 2015,Jan,16

+ **11732 each additional nail plate (List separately in addition to code for primary procedure)**
Code first (11730)
0.50 0.95 FUD ZZZ N N1
AMA: 2018,Jan,8; 2017,Jan,8; 2016,Jan,13; 2015,Jan,16

11740 Evacuation of subungual hematoma
0.90 1.52 FUD 000 Q1 N1
AMA: 2018,Jan,8; 2017,Jan,8; 2016,Jan,13; 2015,Jan,16

11750 Excision of nail and nail matrix, partial or complete (eg, ingrown or deformed nail), for permanent removal;
EXCLUDES *Pinch graft (15050)*
2.92 4.41 FUD 010 T P3
AMA: 2018,Jan,8; 2017,Jan,8; 2016,Jan,13; 2015,Jan,16

11755 **Biopsy of nail unit (eg, plate, bed, matrix, hyponychium, proximal and lateral nail folds) (separate procedure)**
1.79 3.47 FUD 000 T P3 80
AMA: 2019,Jan,9; 2018,Jan,8; 2017,Jan,8; 2016,Jan,13; 2015,Jan,16

11760 **Repair of nail bed**
3.27 5.46 FUD 010 T G2
AMA: 2018,Jan,8; 2017,Jan,8; 2016,Jan,13; 2015,Jan,16

11762 **Reconstruction of nail bed with graft**
5.33 8.15 FUD 010 T P3
AMA: 2018,Jan,8; 2017,Jan,8; 2016,Jan,13; 2015,Jan,16

11765 **Wedge excision of skin of nail fold (eg, for ingrown toenail)**
INCLUDES Cotting's operation
2.64 4.80 FUD 010 Q1 N1
AMA: 2018,Jan,8; 2017,Jan,8; 2016,Jan,13; 2015,Jan,16

11770-11772 Treatment Pilonidal Cyst: Excision

EXCLUDES *Incision of pilonidal cyst (10080-10081)*

11770 **Excision of pilonidal cyst or sinus; simple**
5.34 8.92 FUD 010 J A2

11771 **extensive**
12.7 17.2 FUD 090 J A2

11772 **complicated**
16.6 20.9 FUD 090 J A2
AMA: 2018,Jan,8; 2017,Jan,8; 2016,Jan,13; 2015,Sep,12

11900-11901 Treatment of Lesions: Injection

EXCLUDES *Injection local anesthesia performed preoperatively*
Injection veins (36470-36471)
Intralesional chemotherapy (96405-96406)

11900 **Injection, intralesional; up to and including 7 lesions**
0.90 1.54 FUD 000 Q1 N1
AMA: 2018,Jan,8; 2017,Jan,8; 2016,Jan,13; 2015,Jan,16

11901 **more than 7 lesions**
1.36 1.97 FUD 000 Q1 N1
AMA: 2018,Jan,8; 2017,Jan,8; 2016,Jan,13; 2015,Jan,16

11920-11971 Tattoos, Tissue Expanders, and Dermal Fillers

CMS: 100-02,16,10 Exclusions from Coverage; 100-02,16,120 Cosmetic Procedures; 100-02,16,180 Services Related to Noncovered Procedures

11920 **Tattooing, intradermal introduction of insoluble opaque pigments to correct color defects of skin, including micropigmentation; 6.0 sq cm or less**
3.23 5.33 FUD 000 T P3 80
AMA: 2018,Jan,8; 2017,Jan,8; 2016,Aug,9

11921 **6.1 to 20.0 sq cm**
3.81 6.08 FUD 000 T P3 80
AMA: 2018,Jan,8; 2017,Jan,8; 2016,Aug,9

\+ 11922 **each additional 20.0 sq cm, or part thereof (List separately in addition to code for primary procedure)**
Code first (11921)
0.86 1.71 FUD ZZZ N N1 80

11950 **Subcutaneous injection of filling material (eg, collagen); 1 cc or less**
1.51 2.26 FUD 000 T P3 80
AMA: 2019,Aug,10; 2018,Jan,8; 2017,Jan,8; 2016,Jan,13; 2015,Jan,16

11951 **1.1 to 5.0 cc**
1.98 2.80 FUD 000 T P3 80
AMA: 2019,Aug,10; 2018,Jan,8; 2017,Jan,8; 2016,Jan,13; 2015,Jan,16

11952 **5.1 to 10.0 cc**
3.03 4.13 FUD 000 T P3 80
AMA: 2019,Aug,10; 2018,Jan,8; 2017,Jan,8; 2016,Jan,13; 2015,Jan,16

11954 **over 10.0 cc**
3.21 4.41 FUD 000 T P3 80
AMA: 2019,Aug,10; 2018,Jan,8; 2017,Jan,8; 2016,Jan,13; 2015,Jan,16

11960 **Insertion of tissue expander(s) for other than breast, including subsequent expansion**
EXCLUDES *Breast reconstruction with tissue expander(s) (19357)*
Decompression, nerve (64722-64726)
Endoscopic release transverse carpal ligament (29848)
Neuroplasty (64702-64721)
Removal tissue expander without implant insertion (11971)
Secondary closure, surgical wound or dehiscence (13160)
28.1 28.1 FUD 090 T A2
AMA: 1991,Win,1

▲ 11970 **Replacement of tissue expander with permanent implant**
17.6 17.6 FUD 090 J A2 50
AMA: 2018,Jan,8; 2017,Jan,8; 2016,Jan,13; 2015,Jan,16

▲ 11971 **Removal of tissue expander without insertion of implant**
EXCLUDES *Insertion/replacement tissue expander (11960, 11970)*
9.31 13.7 FUD 090 Q2 A2 80 50
AMA: 2018,Jan,8; 2017,Jan,8; 2016,Jan,13; 2015,Jan,16

11976-11983 Drug Implantation

11976 **Removal, implantable contraceptive capsules** ♀
2.73 4.15 FUD 000 Q2 P3 80
AMA: 1992,Win,1; 1991,Win,1

11980 **Subcutaneous hormone pellet implantation (implantation of estradiol and/or testosterone pellets beneath the skin)**
1.61 2.69 FUD 000 Q1 N1
AMA: 2018,Jan,8; 2017,Jan,8; 2016,Jan,13; 2015,Jan,16

11981 **Insertion, non-biodegradable drug delivery implant**
EXCLUDES *Insertion deep drug-delivery device:*
Intra-articular (20704)
Intramedullary (20702)
Subfascial (20700)
1.86 2.96 FUD 000 Q1 N1 80
AMA: 2018,Jan,8; 2017,Jan,8; 2016,Jan,13; 2015,Jan,16

11982 **Removal, non-biodegradable drug delivery implant**
EXCLUDES *Removal deep drug-delivery device:*
Intra-articular (20705)
Intramedullary (20703)
Subfascial (20701)
2.87 4.49 FUD XXX Q1 N1 80

11983 **Removal with reinsertion, non-biodegradable drug delivery implant**
3.01 4.15 FUD 000 Q1 N1 80

12001-12021 Suturing of Superficial Wounds

INCLUDES Administration local anesthesia
Cauterization without closure
Simple:
Exploration nerves, blood vessels, tendons
Vessel ligation, in wound
Simple repair that involves:
Routine debridement and decontamination
Simple one layer closure
Superficial tissues
Sutures, staples, tissue adhesives
Total length several repairs in same code category

EXCLUDES *Adhesive strips only, see appropriate E/M service*
Complex repair nerves, blood vessels, tendons (see appropriate anatomical section)
Debridement requiring:
Comprehensive cleaning
Removal significant tissue
Removal soft tissue and/or bone, no fracture/dislocation, performed separately (11042-11047 [11045, 11046])
Removal soft tissue and/or bone with open fracture/dislocation (11010-11012)
Deep tissue repair (12031-13153)
Major exploration (20100-20103)
Repair nerves, blood vessels, tendons (See appropriate anatomical section. These repairs include simple and intermediate closure. Report complex closure with modifier 59.)
Secondary closure/dehiscence (13160)

Code also modifier 59 added to less complicated procedure code when reporting more than one wound repair classification

12001 **Simple repair of superficial wounds of scalp, neck, axillae, external genitalia, trunk and/or extremities (including hands and feet); 2.5 cm or less**
1.30 2.58 **FUD** 000 Q1 N1
AMA: 2018,Sep,7; 2018,Jan,8; 2017,Dec,14; 2017,Jan,8; 2016,Jan,13; 2015,Jan,16

12002 **2.6 cm to 7.5 cm**
1.67 3.08 **FUD** 000 Q1 N1
AMA: 2018,Sep,7; 2018,Jan,8; 2017,Jan,8; 2016,Jan,13; 2015,Jan,16

12004 **7.6 cm to 12.5 cm**
2.15 3.69 **FUD** 000 Q1 N1
AMA: 2018,Sep,7; 2018,Jan,8; 2017,Jan,8; 2016,Jan,13; 2015,Jan,16

12005 **12.6 cm to 20.0 cm**
2.71 4.69 **FUD** 000 Q1 A2
AMA: 2018,Sep,7; 2018,Jan,8; 2017,Jan,8; 2016,Jan,13; 2015,Jan,16

12006 **20.1 cm to 30.0 cm**
3.43 5.76 **FUD** 000 Q2 A2
AMA: 2018,Sep,7; 2018,Jan,8; 2017,Jan,8; 2016,Jan,13; 2015,Jan,16

12007 **over 30.0 cm**
4.23 6.58 **FUD** 000 T A2
AMA: 2018,Sep,7; 2018,Jan,8; 2017,Jan,8; 2016,Jan,13; 2015,Jan,16

12011 **Simple repair of superficial wounds of face, ears, eyelids, nose, lips and/or mucous membranes; 2.5 cm or less**
1.57 3.09 **FUD** 000 Q1 N1
AMA: 2018,Sep,7; 2018,Jan,8; 2017,Jan,8; 2016,Nov,7; 2016,Jan,13; 2015,Jan,16

12013 **2.6 cm to 5.0 cm**
1.72 3.29 **FUD** 000 Q1 N1
AMA: 2018,Sep,7; 2018,Jan,8; 2017,Jan,8; 2016,Jan,13; 2015,Jan,16

12014 **5.1 cm to 7.5 cm**
2.20 4.00 **FUD** 000 Q1 N1
AMA: 2018,Sep,7; 2018,Jan,8; 2017,Jan,8; 2016,Jan,13; 2015,Jan,16

12015 **7.6 cm to 12.5 cm**
2.78 4.84 **FUD** 000 Q1 G2
AMA: 2018,Sep,7; 2018,Jan,8; 2017,Jan,8; 2016,Jan,13; 2015,Jan,16

12016 **12.6 cm to 20.0 cm**
3.77 6.16 **FUD** 000 Q1 A2
AMA: 2018,Sep,7; 2018,Jan,8; 2017,Jan,8; 2016,Jan,13; 2015,Jan,16

12017 **20.1 cm to 30.0 cm**
4.48 4.48 **FUD** 000 Q1 A2 80
AMA: 2018,Sep,7; 2018,Jan,8; 2017,Jan,8; 2016,Jan,13; 2015,Jan,16

12018 **over 30.0 cm**
5.08 5.08 **FUD** 000 Q1 A2 80
AMA: 2018,Sep,7; 2018,Jan,8; 2017,Jan,8; 2016,Jan,13; 2015,Jan,16

12020 **Treatment of superficial wound dehiscence; simple closure**
EXCLUDES *Secondary closure major/complex wound or dehiscence (13160)*
5.43 8.41 **FUD** 010 T A2
AMA: 2019,Nov,3; 2018,Jan,8; 2017,Jan,8; 2016,Jan,13; 2015,Jan,16

12021 **with packing**
EXCLUDES *Secondary closure major/complex wound or dehiscence (13160)*
4.01 4.90 **FUD** 010 T A2
AMA: 2019,Nov,3; 2018,Jan,8; 2017,Jan,8; 2016,Jan,13; 2015,Jan,16

12031-12057 Suturing of Intermediate Wounds

INCLUDES Administration local anesthesia
Repair that involves:
Closure contaminated single layer wound
Layered closure (e.g., subcutaneous tissue, superficial fascia)
Limited undermining
Removal foreign material (e.g., gravel, glass)
Routine debridement and decontamination
Simple:
Exploration nerves, blood vessels, tendons in wound
Vessel ligation, in wound
Total length several repairs in same code category

EXCLUDES *Debridement requiring:*
Removal soft tissue and/or bone, no fracture/dislocation, performed separately (11042-11047 [11045, 11046])
Removal soft tissue/bone due to open fracture/dislocation (11010-11012)
Major exploration (20100-20103)
Repair nerves, blood vessels, tendons (See appropriate anatomical section. These repairs include simple and intermediate closure. Report complex closure with modifier 59.)
Secondary closure major/complex wound or dehiscence (13160)
Wound repair involving more than layered closure

Code also modifier 59 added to less complicated procedure code when reporting more than one wound repair classification

12031 **Repair, intermediate, wounds of scalp, axillae, trunk and/or extremities (excluding hands and feet); 2.5 cm or less**
4.36 7.17 **FUD** 010 T P2
AMA: 2019,Nov,3; 2018,Sep,7; 2018,Jan,8; 2017,Jan,8; 2016,Jan,13; 2015,Jan,16

12032 **2.6 cm to 7.5 cm**
5.46 8.59 **FUD** 010 T P2
AMA: 2019,Nov,3; 2018,Sep,7; 2018,Jan,8; 2017,Jan,8; 2016,Jan,13; 2015,Jan,16

12034 **7.6 cm to 12.5 cm**
5.96 9.07 **FUD** 010 T A2
AMA: 2019,Nov,3; 2018,Sep,7; 2018,Jan,8; 2017,Jan,8; 2016,Jan,13; 2015,Jan,16

12035 **12.6 cm to 20.0 cm**
6.94 11.0 **FUD** 010 T A2
AMA: 2019,Nov,3; 2018,Sep,7; 2018,Jan,8; 2017,Jan,8; 2016,Jan,13; 2015,Jan,16

12036 **20.1 cm to 30.0 cm**
8.15 12.3 **FUD** 010 T A2
AMA: 2019,Nov,3; 2018,Sep,7; 2018,Jan,8; 2017,Jan,8; 2016,Jan,13; 2015,Jan,16

12037 **over 30.0 cm**
9.53 | 14.0 | **FUD** 010 | T A2 80
AMA: 2019,Nov,3; 2018,Sep,7; 2018,Jan,8; 2017,Jan,8; 2016,Jan,13; 2015,Jan,16

12041 **Repair, intermediate, wounds of neck, hands, feet and/or external genitalia; 2.5 cm or less**
4.22 | 7.19 | **FUD** 010 | Q2 P2
AMA: 2019,Nov,3; 2018,Sep,7; 2018,Jan,8; 2017,Jan,8; 2016,Jan,13; 2015,Jan,16

12042 **2.6 cm to 7.5 cm**
5.75 | 8.41 | **FUD** 010 | T P2
AMA: 2019,Nov,3; 2018,Sep,7; 2018,Jan,8; 2017,Jan,8; 2016,Jan,13; 2015,Jan,16

12044 **7.6 cm to 12.5 cm**
6.16 | 10.6 | **FUD** 010 | T A2
AMA: 2019,Nov,3; 2018,Sep,7; 2018,Jan,8; 2017,Jan,8; 2016,Jan,13; 2015,Jan,16

12045 **12.6 cm to 20.0 cm**
7.71 | 11.4 | **FUD** 010 | T A2
AMA: 2019,Nov,3; 2018,Sep,7; 2018,Jan,8; 2017,Jan,8; 2016,Jan,13; 2015,Jan,16

12046 **20.1 cm to 30.0 cm**
9.01 | 13.8 | **FUD** 010 | T A2 80
AMA: 2019,Nov,3; 2018,Sep,7; 2018,Jan,8; 2017,Jan,8; 2016,Jan,13; 2015,Jan,16

12047 **over 30.0 cm**
10.1 | 15.4 | **FUD** 010 | T A2 80
AMA: 2019,Nov,3; 2018,Sep,7; 2018,Jan,8; 2017,Jan,8; 2016,Jan,13; 2015,Jan,16

12051 **Repair, intermediate, wounds of face, ears, eyelids, nose, lips and/or mucous membranes; 2.5 cm or less**
4.85 | 7.73 | **FUD** 010 | T P2
AMA: 2019,Nov,3; 2018,Sep,7; 2018,Jan,8; 2017,Jan,8; 2016,Jan,13; 2015,Jan,16

12052 **2.6 cm to 5.0 cm**
5.74 | 8.67 | **FUD** 010 | T P2
AMA: 2019,Nov,3; 2018,Sep,7; 2018,Jan,8; 2017,Jan,8; 2016,Jan,13; 2015,Jan,16

12053 **5.1 cm to 7.5 cm**
6.20 | 10.1 | **FUD** 010 | T P2
AMA: 2019,Nov,3; 2018,Sep,7; 2018,Jan,8; 2017,Jan,8; 2016,Jan,13; 2015,Jan,16

12054 **7.6 cm to 12.5 cm**
6.35 | 10.7 | **FUD** 010 | Q2 A2
AMA: 2019,Nov,3; 2018,Sep,7; 2018,Jan,8; 2017,Jan,8; 2016,Jan,13; 2015,Jan,16

12055 **12.6 cm to 20.0 cm**
8.66 | 13.9 | **FUD** 010 | T A2
AMA: 2019,Nov,3; 2018,Sep,7; 2018,Jan,8; 2017,Jan,8; 2016,Jan,13; 2015,Jan,16

12056 **20.1 cm to 30.0 cm**
11.0 | 15.9 | **FUD** 010 | Q2 A2 80
AMA: 2019,Nov,3; 2018,Sep,7; 2018,Jan,8; 2017,Jan,8; 2016,Jan,13; 2015,Jan,16

12057 **over 30.0 cm**
12.2 | 16.9 | **FUD** 010 | T A2 80
AMA: 2019,Nov,3; 2018,Sep,7; 2018,Jan,8; 2017,Jan,8; 2016,Jan,13; 2015,Jan,16

13100-13160 Suturing of Complicated Wounds

INCLUDES Creation limited defect for repair
Debridement complicated wounds/avulsions
Repair with layered closure that involves at least one of the following:
- Debridement wound edges
- Exposure underlying structures, such as bone, cartilage, tendon, or named neovascular structure
- Extensive undermining
- Free margin involvement helical or nostril rim or vermillion border
- Retention suture placement

Simple:
- Exploration nerves, vessels, tendons in wound
- Vessel ligation in wound

Total length several repairs in same code category

EXCLUDES *Excision:*
- *Benign lesions (11400-11446)*
- *Extensive debridement open fracture/dislocation (11010-11012)*
- *Extensive debridement penetrating or blunt trauma not associated with open fracture/dislocation (11042-11047 [11045, 11046])*
- *Malignant lesions (11600-11646)*
- *Surgical preparation wound bed (15002-15005)*

Extensive exploration (20100-20103)
Repair nerves, blood vessel, tendons (See appropriate anatomical section. These repairs include simple and intermediate closure. Report complex closure with modifier 59.)

Code also modifier 59 added to less complicated procedure code when reporting more than one wound repair classification

13100 **Repair, complex, trunk; 1.1 cm to 2.5 cm**
EXCLUDES *Complex repair 1.0 cm or less (12001, 12031)*
5.81 | 9.72 | **FUD** 010 | T A2
AMA: 2019,Nov,14; 2019,Nov,3; 2018,Sep,7; 2018,Jan,8; 2017,Apr,9; 2017,Jan,8; 2016,Jan,13; 2015,Jan,16

13101 **2.6 cm to 7.5 cm**
7.14 | 11.4 | **FUD** 010 | T A2
AMA: 2019,Dec,14; 2019,Nov,3; 2018,Sep,7; 2018,Jan,8; 2017,Apr,9; 2017,Jan,8; 2016,Jan,13; 2015,Jan,16

\+ 13102 **each additional 5 cm or less (List separately in addition to code for primary procedure)**
Code first (13101)
2.14 | 3.46 | **FUD** ZZZ | N N1
AMA: 2019,Nov,14; 2019,Nov,3; 2018,Sep,7; 2018,Jan,8; 2017,Apr,9; 2017,Jan,8; 2016,Jan,13; 2015,Jan,16

13120 **Repair, complex, scalp, arms, and/or legs; 1.1 cm to 2.5 cm**
EXCLUDES *Complex repair 1.0 cm or less (12001, 12031)*
6.68 | 10.1 | **FUD** 010 | T A2
AMA: 2019,Nov,3; 2018,Sep,7; 2018,Jan,8; 2017,Jan,8; 2016,Jan,13; 2015,Jan,16

13121 **2.6 cm to 7.5 cm**
7.67 | 12.2 | **FUD** 010 | T A2
AMA: 2019,Nov,3; 2018,Sep,7; 2018,Jan,8; 2017,Jan,8; 2016,Jan,13; 2015,Jan,16

\+ 13122 **each additional 5 cm or less (List separately in addition to code for primary procedure)**
Code first (13121)
2.42 | 3.74 | **FUD** ZZZ | N N1
AMA: 2019,Nov,3; 2018,Sep,7; 2018,Jan,8; 2017,Jan,8; 2016,Jan,13; 2015,Jan,16

13131 **Repair, complex, forehead, cheeks, chin, mouth, neck, axillae, genitalia, hands and/or feet; 1.1 cm to 2.5 cm**
EXCLUDES *Complex repair 1.0 cm or less (12001, 12011, 12031, 12041, 12051)*
7.04 | 11.1 | **FUD** 010 | T A2
AMA: 2019,Nov,3; 2018,Sep,7; 2018,Jan,8; 2017,Apr,9; 2017,Jan,8; 2016,Jan,13; 2015,Jan,16

13132 **2.6 cm to 7.5 cm**
8.81 | 13.5 | **FUD** 010 | T A2
AMA: 2019,Nov,3; 2018,Sep,7; 2018,Jan,8; 2017,Apr,9; 2017,Jan,8; 2016,Jan,13; 2015,Jan,16

+ **13133** **each additional 5 cm or less (List separately in addition to code for primary procedure)**

Code first (13132)

3.69 4.98 **FUD** ZZZ N N1

AMA: 2019,Nov,3; 2018,Sep,7; 2018,Jan,8; 2017,Apr,9; 2017,Jan,8; 2016,Jan,13; 2015,Jan,16

13151 **Repair, complex, eyelids, nose, ears and/or lips; 1.1 cm to 2.5 cm**

EXCLUDES *Complex repair 1.0 cm or less (12011, 12051)*

8.25 12.1 **FUD** 010 T A2

AMA: 2019,Nov,3; 2018,Sep,7; 2018,Jan,8; 2017,Jan,8; 2016,Jan,13; 2015,Jan,16

13152 **2.6 cm to 7.5 cm**

9.74 14.3 **FUD** 010 T A2

AMA: 2019,Nov,3; 2018,Sep,7; 2018,Jan,8; 2017,Jan,8; 2016,Jan,13; 2015,Jan,16

+ **13153** **each additional 5 cm or less (List separately in addition to code for primary procedure)**

Code first (13152)

4.02 5.45 **FUD** ZZZ N N1

AMA: 2019,Nov,3; 2018,Sep,7; 2018,Jan,8; 2017,Jan,8; 2016,Jan,13; 2015,Jan,16

13160 **Secondary closure of surgical wound or dehiscence, extensive or complicated**

EXCLUDES *Insertion tissue expander, other than breast (11960)*
Packing or simple secondary wound closure (12020-12021)

22.9 22.9 **FUD** 090 T A2

AMA: 2019,Nov,3; 2018,Jan,8; 2017,Jan,8; 2016,Jan,13; 2015,Jan,16

14000-14350 Reposition Contiguous Tissue

INCLUDES Excision (with or without lesion) with repair by adjacent tissue transfer or tissue rearrangement
Size includes primary (due to excision) and secondary (due to flap design)
Z-plasty, W-plasty, VY-plasty, rotation flap, advancement flap, double pedicle flap, random island flap

EXCLUDES *Closure wounds by undermining surrounding tissue without additional incisions (13100-13160)*
Full thickness closure:
Eyelid (67930-67935, 67961-67975)
Lip (40650-40654)

Code also skin graft necessary to repair secondary defect (15040-15731)

14000 **Adjacent tissue transfer or rearrangement, trunk; defect 10 sq cm or less**

INCLUDES Burrow's operation

EXCLUDES *Excision lesion with repair by adjacent tissue transfer or tissue rearrangement (11400-11446, 11600-11646)*

14.3 17.8 **FUD** 090 T A2

AMA: 2018,Jan,8; 2017,Oct,9; 2017,Jan,8; 2016,Jan,13; 2015,Sep,12; 2015,Feb,10; 2015,Jan,16

Example of common Z-plasty. Lesion is removed with oval-shaped incision

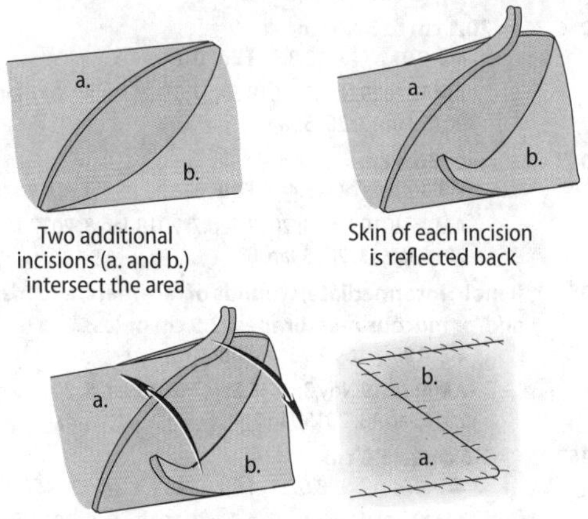
a.
b.
Two additional incisions (a. and b.) intersect the area
Skin of each incision is reflected back

The flaps are then transposed and the repair is closed

An adjacent flap, or other rearrangement flap, is performed to repair a defect

14001 **defect 10.1 sq cm to 30.0 sq cm**

EXCLUDES *Excision lesion with repair by adjacent tissue transfer or tissue rearrangement (11400-11446, 11600-11646)*

18.7 22.8 **FUD** 090 T A2

AMA: 2018,Jan,8; 2017,Oct,9; 2017,Jan,8; 2016,Jan,13; 2015,Feb,10; 2015,Jan,16

14020 **Adjacent tissue transfer or rearrangement, scalp, arms and/or legs; defect 10 sq cm or less**

EXCLUDES *Excision lesion with repair by adjacent tissue transfer or tissue rearrangement (11400-11446, 11600-11646)*

16.0 19.8 **FUD** 090 T A2

AMA: 2018,Jan,8; 2017,Jan,8; 2016,Jan,13; 2015,Jan,16

14021 **defect 10.1 sq cm to 30.0 sq cm**

EXCLUDES *Excision lesion with repair by adjacent tissue transfer or tissue rearrangement (11400-11446, 11600-11646)*

20.5 24.7 **FUD** 090 T A2

AMA: 2018,Jan,8; 2017,Jan,8; 2016,Jan,13; 2015,Jan,16

14040 Adjacent tissue transfer or rearrangement, forehead, cheeks, chin, mouth, neck, axillae, genitalia, hands and/or feet; defect 10 sq cm or less

INCLUDES Krimer's palatoplasty

EXCLUDES *Excision lesion with repair by adjacent tissue transfer or tissue rearrangement (11400-11446, 11600-11646)*

18.1 21.7 FUD 090 T A2

AMA: 2018,Jan,8; 2017,Nov,6; 2017,Jan,8; 2016,Jan,13; 2015,Jan,16

14041 defect 10.1 sq cm to 30.0 sq cm

EXCLUDES *Excision lesion with repair by adjacent tissue transfer or tissue rearrangement (11400-11446, 11600-11646)*

22.3 26.7 FUD 090 T A2

AMA: 2018,Jan,8; 2017,Nov,6; 2017,Jan,8; 2016,Jan,13; 2015,Jan,16

14060 Adjacent tissue transfer or rearrangement, eyelids, nose, ears and/or lips; defect 10 sq cm or less

INCLUDES Denonvillier's operation

EXCLUDES *Excision lesion with repair by adjacent tissue transfer or tissue rearrangement (11400-11446, 11600-11646)*

Eyelid, full thickness (67961-67966)

19.0 21.9 FUD 090 T A2

AMA: 2018,Jan,8; 2017,Nov,6; 2017,Jan,8; 2016,Jan,13; 2015,Jan,16

14061 defect 10.1 sq cm to 30.0 sq cm

EXCLUDES *Excision lesion with repair by adjacent tissue transfer or tissue rearrangement (11400-11446, 11600-11646)*

Eyelid, full thickness (67961 and subsequent codes)

23.4 28.3 FUD 090 T A2

AMA: 2018,Jan,8; 2017,Nov,6; 2017,Jan,8; 2016,Jan,13; 2015,Jan,16

14301 Adjacent tissue transfer or rearrangement, any area; defect 30.1 sq cm to 60.0 sq cm

EXCLUDES *Excision lesion with repair by adjacent tissue transfer or tissue rearrangement (11400-11446, 11600-11646)*

25.0 30.8 FUD 090 T G2 80

AMA: 2018,Jan,8; 2017,Nov,6; 2017,Apr,9; 2017,Jan,8; 2016,Jan,13; 2015,Jan,16

+ **14302 each additional 30.0 sq cm, or part thereof (List separately in addition to code for primary procedure)**

EXCLUDES *Excision lesion with repair by adjacent tissue transfer or tissue rearrangement (11400-11446, 11600-11646)*

Code first (14301)

6.31 6.31 FUD ZZZ N N1 80

AMA: 2018,Jan,8; 2017,Nov,6; 2017,Jan,8; 2016,Jan,13; 2015,Jan,16

14350 Filleted finger or toe flap, including preparation of recipient site

19.7 19.7 FUD 090 T A2 80

AMA: 2018,Jan,8; 2017,Jan,8; 2016,Jan,13; 2015,Jan,16

15002-15005 Development of Base for Tissue Grafting

INCLUDES Add together surface area multiple wounds in same anatomical locations as indicated in code descriptor groups, such as face and scalp. Do not add together multiple wounds at different anatomical site groups such as trunk and face

Ankle or wrist when code description describes leg or arm

Cleaning and preparing viable wound surface for grafting or negative pressure wound therapy used to heal wound primarily

Code selection based on defect size and location

Percentage applies to children younger than age 10

Removal nonviable tissue in nonchronic wounds for primary healing

Square centimeters applies to children and adults age 10 or older

EXCLUDES *Chronic wound management on wounds left to heal by secondary intention (11042-11047 [11045, 11046], 97597-97598)*

Necrotizing soft tissue infections for specific anatomical locations (11004-11008)

15002 Surgical preparation or creation of recipient site by excision of open wounds, burn eschar, or scar (including subcutaneous tissues), or incisional release of scar contracture, trunk, arms, legs; first 100 sq cm or 1% of body area of infants and children

EXCLUDES *Linear scar revision (13100-13153)*

6.45 10.0 FUD 000 T A2 80

AMA: 2019,Nov,3; 2018,Jan,8; 2017,Jan,8; 2016,Jan,13; 2015,Jan,16

+ **15003 each additional 100 sq cm, or part thereof, or each additional 1% of body area of infants and children (List separately in addition to code for primary procedure)**

Code first (15002)

1.32 2.11 FUD ZZZ N N1 80

AMA: 2019,Nov,3; 2018,Jan,8; 2017,Jan,8; 2016,Jan,13; 2015,Jan,16

15004 Surgical preparation or creation of recipient site by excision of open wounds, burn eschar, or scar (including subcutaneous tissues), or incisional release of scar contracture, face, scalp, eyelids, mouth, neck, ears, orbits, genitalia, hands, feet and/or multiple digits; first 100 sq cm or 1% of body area of infants and children

7.65 11.4 FUD 000 T A2 80

AMA: 2019,Nov,3; 2018,Jan,8; 2017,Jan,8; 2016,Jan,13; 2015,Jan,16

+ **15005 each additional 100 sq cm, or part thereof, or each additional 1% of body area of infants and children (List separately in addition to code for primary procedure)**

Code first (15004)

2.66 3.50 FUD ZZZ N N1 80

AMA: 2019,Nov,3; 2018,Jan,8; 2017,Jan,8; 2016,Jan,13; 2015,Jan,16

15040 Obtain Autograft

INCLUDES Ankle or wrist when code description describes leg or arm

Percentage applies to children younger than age 10

Square centimeters applies to children and adults age 10 or older

15040 Harvest of skin for tissue cultured skin autograft, 100 sq cm or less

3.60 7.47 FUD 000 T A2

AMA: 2018,Jan,8; 2017,Jan,8; 2016,Jan,13; 2015,Jan,16

15050 Pinch Graft

INCLUDES Autologous skin graft harvest and application

Current graft removal

Fixation and anchoring skin graft

Simple cleaning

EXCLUDES *Removal devitalized tissue from wound(s), non-selective debridement, without anesthesia (97602)*

Code also graft or flap necessary to repair donor site

15050 Pinch graft, single or multiple, to cover small ulcer, tip of digit, or other minimal open area (except on face), up to defect size 2 cm diameter

13.0 16.7 FUD 090 T A2

AMA: 2018,Jan,8; 2017,Jan,8; 2016,Jun,8; 2016,Jan,13; 2015,Jan,16

Integumentary System

14040 — 15050

15100-15261 Skin Grafts and Replacements

INCLUDES Add together surface area multiple wounds in same anatomical locations as indicated in code descriptor groups, such as face and scalp. Do not add together multiple wounds at different anatomical site groups such as trunk and face
Ankle or wrist when code description describes leg or arm
Autologous skin graft harvest and application
Code selection based on recipient site location and graft size and type
Current graft removal
Fixation and anchoring skin graft
Percentage applies to children younger than age 10
Simple cleaning
Simple tissue debridement
Square centimeters applies to children and adults age 10 or older

EXCLUDES *Debridement without immediate primary closure, when wound grossly contaminated and extensive cleaning needed, or when necrotic or contaminated tissue removed (11042-11047 [11045, 11046], 97597-97598)*
Removal devitalized tissue from wound(s), non-selective debridement, without anesthesia (97602)

Code also graft or flap necessary to repair donor site
Code also primary procedure requiring skin graft for definitive closure

15100 Split-thickness autograft, trunk, arms, legs; first 100 sq cm or less, or 1% of body area of infants and children (except 15050)
20.5 24.5 FUD 090 T A2
AMA: 2018,Jan,8; 2017,Jan,8; 2016,Jun,8; 2016,Jan,13; 2015,Jan,16

\+ **15101 each additional 100 sq cm, or each additional 1% of body area of infants and children, or part thereof (List separately in addition to code for primary procedure)**
Code first (15100)
3.24 5.40 FUD ZZZ N N1
AMA: 2018,Jan,8; 2017,Jan,8; 2016,Jun,8; 2016,Jan,13; 2015,Jan,16

15110 Epidermal autograft, trunk, arms, legs; first 100 sq cm or less, or 1% of body area of infants and children
19.9 23.1 FUD 090 T A2
AMA: 2018,Jan,8; 2017,Jan,8; 2016,Jan,13; 2015,Jan,16

\+ **15111 each additional 100 sq cm, or each additional 1% of body area of infants and children, or part thereof (List separately in addition to code for primary procedure)**
Code first (15110)
3.02 3.33 FUD ZZZ N N1
AMA: 2018,Jan,8; 2017,Jan,8; 2016,Jan,13; 2015,Jan,16

15115 Epidermal autograft, face, scalp, eyelids, mouth, neck, ears, orbits, genitalia, hands, feet, and/or multiple digits; first 100 sq cm or less, or 1% of body area of infants and children
19.6 22.8 FUD 090 T A2
AMA: 2018,Jan,8; 2017,Jan,8; 2016,Jan,13; 2015,Jan,16

\+ **15116 each additional 100 sq cm, or each additional 1% of body area of infants and children, or part thereof (List separately in addition to code for primary procedure)**
Code first (15115)
4.39 4.81 FUD ZZZ N N1
AMA: 2018,Jan,8; 2017,Jan,8; 2016,Jan,13; 2015,Jan,16

15120 Split-thickness autograft, face, scalp, eyelids, mouth, neck, ears, orbits, genitalia, hands, feet, and/or multiple digits; first 100 sq cm or less, or 1% of body area of infants and children (except 15050)
EXCLUDES *Other eyelid repair (67961-67975)*
19.9 24.3 FUD 090 T A2
AMA: 2018,Jan,8; 2017,Jan,8; 2016,Jun,8; 2016,Jan,13; 2015,Jan,16

\+ **15121 each additional 100 sq cm, or each additional 1% of body area of infants and children, or part thereof (List separately in addition to code for primary procedure)**
EXCLUDES *Other eyelid repair (67961-67975)*
Code first (15120)
3.86 5.95 FUD ZZZ N N1
AMA: 2018,Jan,8; 2017,Jan,8; 2016,Jun,8; 2016,Jan,13; 2015,Jan,16

15130 Dermal autograft, trunk, arms, legs; first 100 sq cm or less, or 1% of body area of infants and children
17.1 20.6 FUD 090 T A2
AMA: 2018,Jan,8; 2017,Jan,8; 2016,Jan,13; 2015,Jan,16

\+ **15131 each additional 100 sq cm, or each additional 1% of body area of infants and children, or part thereof (List separately in addition to code for primary procedure)**
Code first (15130)
2.65 2.86 FUD ZZZ N N1
AMA: 2018,Jan,8; 2017,Jan,8; 2016,Jan,13; 2015,Jan,16

15135 Dermal autograft, face, scalp, eyelids, mouth, neck, ears, orbits, genitalia, hands, feet, and/or multiple digits; first 100 sq cm or less, or 1% of body area of infants and children
21.4 24.5 FUD 090 T A2
AMA: 2018,Jan,8; 2017,Jan,8; 2016,Jan,13; 2015,Jan,16

\+ **15136 each additional 100 sq cm, or each additional 1% of body area of infants and children, or part thereof (List separately in addition to code for primary procedure)**
Code first (15135)
2.65 2.83 FUD ZZZ N N1
AMA: 2018,Jan,8; 2017,Jan,8; 2016,Jan,13; 2015,Jan,16

15150 Tissue cultured skin autograft, trunk, arms, legs; first 25 sq cm or less
18.4 20.3 FUD 090 T A2
AMA: 2018,Jan,8; 2017,Jan,8; 2016,Jan,13; 2015,Jan,16

\+ **15151 additional 1 sq cm to 75 sq cm (List separately in addition to code for primary procedure)**
EXCLUDES *Grafts over 75 sq cm (15152)*
Reporting code more than one time per session
Code first (15150)
3.19 3.45 FUD ZZZ N N1
AMA: 2018,Jan,8; 2017,Jan,8; 2016,Jan,13; 2015,Jan,16

\+ **15152 each additional 100 sq cm, or each additional 1% of body area of infants and children, or part thereof (List separately in addition to code for primary procedure)**
Code first (15151)
4.22 4.47 FUD ZZZ N N1
AMA: 2018,Jan,8; 2017,Jan,8; 2016,Jan,13; 2015,Jan,16

15155 Tissue cultured skin autograft, face, scalp, eyelids, mouth, neck, ears, orbits, genitalia, hands, feet, and/or multiple digits; first 25 sq cm or less
21.1 23.0 FUD 090 T A2
AMA: 2018,Jan,8; 2017,Jan,8; 2016,Jan,13; 2015,Jan,16

\+ **15156 additional 1 sq cm to 75 sq cm (List separately in addition to code for primary procedure)**
EXCLUDES *Grafts over 75 sq cm (15157)*
Reporting code more than one time per session
Code first (15155)
4.39 4.64 FUD ZZZ N N1
AMA: 2018,Jan,8; 2017,Jan,8; 2016,Jan,13; 2015,Jan,16

\+ **15157 each additional 100 sq cm, or each additional 1% of body area of infants and children, or part thereof (List separately in addition to code for primary procedure)**
Code first (15156)
4.78 5.17 FUD ZZZ N N1
AMA: 2018,Jan,8; 2017,Jan,8; 2016,Jan,13; 2015,Jan,16

15200 **Full thickness graft, free, including direct closure of donor site, trunk; 20 sq cm or less**
19.2 23.9 FUD 090 T A2
AMA: 2018,Jan,8; 2017,Jan,8; 2016,Jun,8; 2016,Jan,13; 2015,Jan,16

+ 15201 **each additional 20 sq cm, or part thereof (List separately in addition to code for primary procedure)**
Code first (15200)
2.26 4.20 FUD ZZZ N N1
AMA: 2018,Jan,8; 2017,Jan,8; 2016,Jun,8; 2016,Jan,13; 2015,Jan,16

15220 **Full thickness graft, free, including direct closure of donor site, scalp, arms, and/or legs; 20 sq cm or less**
17.4 21.9 FUD 090 T A2
AMA: 2018,Jan,8; 2017,Jan,8; 2016,Jun,8; 2016,Jan,13; 2015,Jan,16

+ 15221 **each additional 20 sq cm, or part thereof (List separately in addition to code for primary procedure)**
Code first (15220)
2.03 3.86 FUD ZZZ N N1
AMA: 2018,Jan,8; 2017,Jan,8; 2016,Jun,8; 2016,Jan,13; 2015,Jan,16

15240 **Full thickness graft, free, including direct closure of donor site, forehead, cheeks, chin, mouth, neck, axillae, genitalia, hands, and/or feet; 20 sq cm or less**
EXCLUDES *Fingertip graft (15050)*
Syndactyly repair fingers (26560-26562)
23.0 26.6 FUD 090 T A2
AMA: 2018,Jan,8; 2017,Jan,8; 2016,Jun,8; 2016,Jan,13; 2015,Jan,16

+ 15241 **each additional 20 sq cm, or part thereof (List separately in addition to code for primary procedure)**
Code first (15240)
3.18 5.22 FUD ZZZ N N1
AMA: 2018,Jan,8; 2017,Jan,8; 2016,Jun,8; 2016,Jan,13; 2015,Jan,16

15260 **Full thickness graft, free, including direct closure of donor site, nose, ears, eyelids, and/or lips; 20 sq cm or less**
EXCLUDES *Other eyelid repair (67961-67975)*
24.1 28.5 FUD 090 T A2
AMA: 2018,Jan,8; 2017,Jan,8; 2016,Jun,8; 2016,Jan,13; 2015,Jan,16

+ 15261 **each additional 20 sq cm, or part thereof (List separately in addition to code for primary procedure)**
EXCLUDES *Other eyelid repair (67961-67975)*
Code first (15260)
3.96 5.99 FUD ZZZ N N1
AMA: 2018,Jan,8; 2017,Jan,8; 2016,Jun,8; 2016,Jan,13; 2015,Jan,16

15271-15278 Skin Substitute Graft Application

INCLUDES Add together surface area multiple wounds in same anatomical locations as indicated in code descriptor groups, such as face and scalp. Do not add together multiple wounds at different anatomical site groups such as trunk and face
Ankle or wrist when code description describes leg or arm
Code selection based on defect site location and size
Fixation and anchoring skin graft
Graft types include:
- Biological material used for tissue engineering (e.g., scaffold) for growing skin
- Nonautologous human skin such as:
  - Acellular
  - Allograft
  - Cellular
  - Dermal
  - Epidermal
  - Homograft
- Nonhuman grafts

Percentage applies to children younger than age 10
Removing current graft
Simple cleaning
Simple tissue debridement
Square centimeters applies to children and adults age 10 or older

EXCLUDES *Application nongraft dressing*
Injected skin substitutes
Removal devitalized tissue from wound(s), non-selective debridement, without anesthesia (97602)
Skin application procedures, low cost (C5271-C5278)

Code also biologic implant for soft tissue reinforcement (15777)
Code also primary procedure requiring skin graft for definitive closure
Code also supply high-cost skin substitute product (C1849, C9363, Q4101, Q4103-Q4110, Q4116, Q4121-Q4123, Q4126-Q4128, Q4132-Q4133, Q4137-Q4138, Q4140-Q4141, Q4143, Q4146-Q4148, Q4150-Q4161, Q4163-Q4164, Q4169, Q4173, Q4175, Q4176, Q4178, Q4179, Q4180, Q4181, Q4183, Q4184, Q4186-Q4187, Q4194, Q4195, Q4196, Q4197, Q4203, Q4205, Q4208, Q4226, Q4234)

15271 **Application of skin substitute graft to trunk, arms, legs, total wound surface area up to 100 sq cm; first 25 sq cm or less wound surface area**
EXCLUDES *Total wound area greater than or equal to 100 sq cm (15273-15274)*
2.42 4.14 FUD 000 T G2
AMA: 2018,Jan,8; 2017,Oct,9; 2017,Jan,8; 2016,Jan,13; 2015,Jan,16

+ 15272 **each additional 25 sq cm wound surface area, or part thereof (List separately in addition to code for primary procedure)**
EXCLUDES *Total wound area greater than or equal to 100 sq cm (15273-15274)*
Code first (15271)
0.50 0.76 FUD ZZZ N N1
AMA: 2018,Jan,8; 2017,Jan,8; 2016,Jan,13; 2015,Jan,16

15273 **Application of skin substitute graft to trunk, arms, legs, total wound surface area greater than or equal to 100 sq cm; first 100 sq cm wound surface area, or 1% of body area of infants and children**
EXCLUDES *Total wound surface area up to 100 cm (15271-15272)*
5.84 8.73 FUD 000 T G2
AMA: 2018,Jan,8; 2017,Jan,8; 2016,Jan,13; 2015,Jan,16

+ 15274 **each additional 100 sq cm wound surface area, or part thereof, or each additional 1% of body area of infants and children, or part thereof (List separately in addition to code for primary procedure)**
EXCLUDES *Total wound surface area up to 100 cm (15271-15272)*
Code first (15273)
1.33 2.15 FUD ZZZ N N1
AMA: 2018,Jan,8; 2017,Jan,8; 2016,Jan,13; 2015,Jan,16

15275 **Application of skin substitute graft to face, scalp, eyelids, mouth, neck, ears, orbits, genitalia, hands, feet, and/or multiple digits, total wound surface area up to 100 sq cm; first 25 sq cm or less wound surface area**

EXCLUDES *Total wound area greater than or equal to 100 sq cm (15277-15278)*

2.74 4.37 **FUD** 000 T G2

AMA: 2018,Jan,8; 2017,Jan,8; 2016,Jan,13; 2015,Jan,16

\+ **15276** **each additional 25 sq cm wound surface area, or part thereof (List separately in addition to code for primary procedure)**

EXCLUDES *Total wound area greater than or equal to 100 sq cm (15277-15278)*

Code first (15275)

0.73 0.98 **FUD** ZZZ N N1

AMA: 2018,Jan,8; 2017,Jan,8; 2016,Jan,13; 2015,Jan,16

15277 **Application of skin substitute graft to face, scalp, eyelids, mouth, neck, ears, orbits, genitalia, hands, feet, and/or multiple digits, total wound surface area greater than or equal to 100 sq cm; first 100 sq cm wound surface area, or 1% of body area of infants and children**

EXCLUDES *Total surface area up to 100 sq cm (15275-15276)*

6.60 9.55 **FUD** 000 T G2

AMA: 2018,Jan,8; 2017,Jan,8; 2016,Jan,13; 2015,Jan,16

\+ **15278** **each additional 100 sq cm wound surface area, or part thereof, or each additional 1% of body area of infants and children, or part thereof (List separately in addition to code for primary procedure)**

EXCLUDES *Total surface area up to 100 sq cm (15275-15276)*

Code first (15277)

1.66 2.54 **FUD** ZZZ N N1

AMA: 2018,Jan,8; 2017,Jan,8; 2016,Jan,13; 2015,Jan,16

15570-15731 Wound Reconstruction: Skin Flaps

INCLUDES Ankle or wrist when code description describes leg or arm
Code selection based on recipient site when flap attached in transfer or to final site and based on donor site when tube created for transfer later or when flap delayed prior to transfer
Fixation and anchoring skin graft
Simple tissue debridement
Tube formation for later transfer

EXCLUDES *Contiguous tissue transfer flaps (14040-14041, 14060-14061, 14301-14302)*
Debridement without immediate primary closure (11042-11047 [11045, 11046], 97597-97598)
Excision:
Benign lesion (11400-11471)
Burn eschar or scar (15002-15005)
Malignant lesion (11600-11646)
Microvascular repair (15756-15758)
Primary procedure--see appropriate anatomical site

Code also application extensive immobilization apparatus
Code also repair donor site with skin grafts or flaps

15570 **Formation of direct or tubed pedicle, with or without transfer; trunk**

INCLUDES Flaps without vascular pedicle

21.1 26.2 **FUD** 090 T A2

AMA: 2018,Jan,8; 2017,Jan,8; 2016,Jan,13; 2015,Jan,16

Pedicle flap

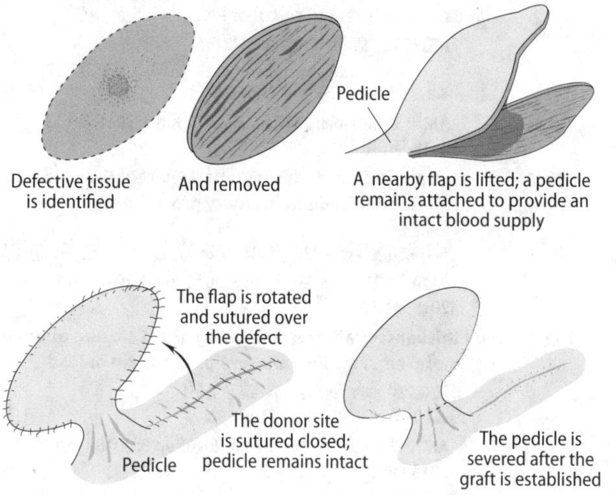
Defective tissue is identified
And removed
Pedicle
A nearby flap is lifted; a pedicle remains attached to provide an intact blood supply
The flap is rotated and sutured over the defect
The donor site is sutured closed; pedicle remains intact
Pedicle
The pedicle is severed after the graft is established

15572 **scalp, arms, or legs**

INCLUDES Flaps without vascular pedicle

21.2 25.3 **FUD** 090 T A2

AMA: 2018,Jan,8; 2017,Jan,8; 2016,Jan,13; 2015,Jan,16

15574 **forehead, cheeks, chin, mouth, neck, axillae, genitalia, hands or feet**

INCLUDES Flaps without vascular pedicle

21.6 25.7 **FUD** 090 T A2

AMA: 2018,Jan,8; 2017,Jan,8; 2016,Jan,13; 2015,Jan,16

15576 **eyelids, nose, ears, lips, or intraoral**

INCLUDES Flaps without vascular pedicle

19.1 22.9 **FUD** 090 T A2

AMA: 2018,Jan,8; 2017,Jan,8; 2016,Jan,13; 2015,Jan,16

15600 **Delay of flap or sectioning of flap (division and inset); at trunk**

5.96 9.47 **FUD** 090 T A2 80

AMA: 2019,Jun,14; 2018,Jan,8; 2017,Jan,8; 2016,Jan,13; 2015,Jan,16

15610 **at scalp, arms, or legs**

6.89 10.2 **FUD** 090 T A2 80

AMA: 2018,Jan,8; 2017,Jan,8; 2016,Jan,13; 2015,Jan,16

15620 **at forehead, cheeks, chin, neck, axillae, genitalia, hands, or feet**
9.26 12.6 FUD 090 T A2
AMA: 2018,Jan,8; 2017,Jan,8; 2016,Jan,13; 2015,Jan,16

15630 **at eyelids, nose, ears, or lips**
9.77 13.0 FUD 090 T A2
AMA: 2018,Jan,8; 2017,Jan,8; 2016,Jan,13; 2015,Jan,16

15650 **Transfer, intermediate, of any pedicle flap (eg, abdomen to wrist, Walking tube), any location**
EXCLUDES *Defatting, revision, or rearranging transferred pedicle flap or skin graft (13100-14302)*
Eyelids, ears, lips, and nose - refer to anatomical area
11.0 14.5 FUD 090 T A2 80
AMA: 2018,Jan,8; 2017,Jan,8; 2016,Jan,13; 2015,Jan,16

15730 **Midface flap (ie, zygomaticofacial flap) with preservation of vascular pedicle(s)**
26.3 42.9 FUD 090 T G2
AMA: 2018,Apr,10; 2018,Jan,8; 2017,Nov,6

15731 **Forehead flap with preservation of vascular pedicle (eg, axial pattern flap, paramedian forehead flap)**
EXCLUDES *Muscle, myocutaneous, or fasciocutaneous flap head or neck (15733)*
28.6 32.0 FUD 090 T A2 80
AMA: 2018,Jan,8; 2017,Nov,6; 2017,Jan,8; 2016,Jan,13; 2015,Jan,16

15733-15738 Wound Reconstruction: Muscle Flaps

INCLUDES Code based on donor site
EXCLUDES *Contiguous tissue transfer flaps (14040-14041, 14060-14061, 14301-14302)*
Microvascular repair (15756-15758)
Code also application extensive immobilization apparatus
Code also repair donor site with skin grafts or flaps

15733 **Muscle, myocutaneous, or fasciocutaneous flap; head and neck with named vascular pedicle (ie, buccinators, genioglossus, temporalis, masseter, sternocleidomastoid, levator scapulae)**
INCLUDES Repair extracranial defect by anterior pericranial flap on vascular pedicle (15731)
29.9 29.9 FUD 090 T A2
AMA: 2018,Apr,10; 2018,Jan,8; 2017,Nov,6

15734 **trunk**
43.6 43.6 FUD 090 T A2 80
AMA: 2018,Aug,10; 2018,Jan,8; 2017,Nov,6; 2017,Jan,8; 2016,Jan,13; 2015,Jan,16

15736 **upper extremity**
35.3 35.3 FUD 090 T A2
AMA: 2018,Jan,8; 2017,Nov,6; 2017,Jan,8; 2016,Jan,13; 2015,Jan,16

15738 **lower extremity**
37.4 37.4 FUD 090 T A2 80
AMA: 2018,Jan,8; 2017,Nov,6; 2017,Jan,8; 2016,Jan,13; 2015,Jan,16

15740-15758 Wound Reconstruction: Other

INCLUDES Fixation and anchoring skin graft
Routine dressing
Simple tissue debridement
EXCLUDES *Adjacent tissue transfer (14000-14302)*
Excision:
Benign lesion (11400-11471)
Burn eschar or scar (15002-15005)
Malignant lesion (11600-11646)
Flaps without vascular pedicle addition (15570-15576)
Primary procedure--see appropriate anatomical section
Skin graft for repair donor site (15050-15278)
Code also repair donor site with skin grafts or flaps (14000-14350, 15050-15278)

15740 **Flap; island pedicle requiring identification and dissection of an anatomically named axial vessel**
EXCLUDES *V-Y subcutaneous flaps, random island flaps, and other flaps from adjacent areas (14000-14302)*
24.2 28.8 FUD 090 T A2
AMA: 2018,Jan,8; 2017,Dec,14; 2017,Jan,8; 2016,Jan,13; 2015,Jan,16

15750 **neurovascular pedicle**
EXCLUDES *V-Y subcutaneous flaps, random island flaps, and other flaps from adjacent areas (14000-14302)*
26.4 26.4 FUD 090 T A2 80
AMA: 2018,Jan,8; 2017,Dec,14

15756 **Free muscle or myocutaneous flap with microvascular anastomosis**
INCLUDES Operating microscope (69990)
66.0 66.0 FUD 090 C 80
AMA: 2019,Dec,5; 2018,Jan,8; 2017,Jan,8; 2016,Feb,12; 2016,Jan,13; 2015,Jan,16

15757 **Free skin flap with microvascular anastomosis**
INCLUDES Operating microscope (69990)
65.5 65.5 FUD 090 C 80
AMA: 2019,Dec,5; 2018,Jan,8; 2017,Jan,8; 2016,Apr,8; 2016,Feb,12; 2016,Jan,13; 2015,Jan,16

15758 **Free fascial flap with microvascular anastomosis**
INCLUDES Operating microscope (69990)
66.0 66.0 FUD 090 C 80
AMA: 2019,Dec,5; 2018,Jan,8; 2017,Jan,8; 2016,Feb,12; 2016,Jan,13; 2015,Jan,16

15760-15774 [15769] Other Grafts

EXCLUDES *Adjacent tissue transfer (14000-14302)*
Excision:
Benign lesion (11400-11471)
Burn eschar or scar (15002-15005)
Malignant lesion (11600-11646)
Flaps without vascular pedicle addition (15570-15576)
Microvascular repair (15756-15758)
Primary procedure (see appropriate anatomical site)
Repair donor site with skin grafts or flaps (14000-14350, 15050-15278)

15760 **Graft; composite (eg, full thickness of external ear or nasal ala), including primary closure, donor area**
INCLUDES Fixation and anchoring skin graft
Routine dressing
Simple tissue debridement
20.2 24.2 FUD 090 T A2
AMA: 2018,Jan,8; 2017,Jan,8; 2016,Jan,13; 2015,Jan,16

15769 **Resequenced code. See code following 15770.**

15770 **derma-fat-fascia**
INCLUDES Fixation and anchoring skin graft
Routine dressing
Simple tissue debridement
19.0 19.0 FUD 090 T A2 80
AMA: 2019,Oct,5; 2018,Jan,8; 2017,Jan,8; 2016,Jan,13; 2015,Jan,16

\# **15769** **Grafting of autologous soft tissue, other, harvested by direct excision (eg, fat, dermis, fascia)**

INCLUDES Excisional graft harvest and recipient site placement

EXCLUDES *Autologous grafts specific tissue types, such as skin, bone, nerve, tendon, fascia lata, or vessels*
Autologous white blood cell concentrate injection (0481T)
Harvesting adipose tissue for adipose-derived regenerative cell therapy (0489T-0490T)
Platelet-rich plasma injection (0232T)
Suction assisted lipectomy (15876-15879)

13.8 13.8 **FUD** 090 G2

15771 **Grafting of autologous fat harvested by liposuction technique to trunk, breasts, scalp, arms, and/or legs; 50 cc or less injectate**

INCLUDES Add together injectate volume harvested from each anatomical area indicated in code description, such as face and neck, to report total volume. Do not add together injectate harvested from different anatomical site groups, such as trunk and face
Code based on recipient site

EXCLUDES *Autologous white blood cell concentrate injection (0481T)*
Liposuction not for grafting purposes (15876-15879)
Obtaining tissue for adipose-derived regenerative cell therapy (0489T-0490T)
Platelet-rich plasma injection (0232T)
Subcutaneous injection filling material, at same anatomical site (11950-11954)
Reporting code more than one time per session

13.7 16.5 **FUD** 090 G2

AMA: 2020,Apr,10

\+ **15772** **each additional 50 cc injectate, or part thereof (List separately in addition to code for primary procedure)**

Code first (15771)

4.07 5.22 **FUD** ZZZ

AMA: 2020,Apr,10

15773 **Grafting of autologous fat harvested by liposuction technique to face, eyelids, mouth, neck, ears, orbits, genitalia, hands, and/or feet; 25 cc or less injectate**

INCLUDES Add together injectate volume harvested from each anatomical area indicated in code description, such as face and neck, to report total volume. Do not add together injectate harvested from different anatomical site groups, such as trunk and face
Code based on recipient site

EXCLUDES *Autologous white blood cell concentrate injection (0481T)*
Liposuction not for grafting purposes (15876-15879)
Obtaining tissue for adipose-derived regenerative cell therapy (0489T-0490T)
Platelet-rich plasma injection (0232T)
Subcutaneous injection filling material, at same anatomical site (11950-11954)
Reporting code more than one time per session

13.9 16.7 **FUD** 090 G2

\+ **15774** **each additional 25 cc injectate, or part thereof (List separately in addition to code for primary procedure)**

Code first (15773)

3.91 5.06 **FUD** ZZZ

15775-15839 Plastic, Reconstructive, and Aesthetic Surgery

CMS: 100-02,16,10 Exclusions from Coverage; 100-02,16,120 Cosmetic Procedures; 100-02,16,180 Services Related to Noncovered Procedures

15775 **Punch graft for hair transplant; 1 to 15 punch grafts**

EXCLUDES *Strip transplant (15220)*

6.42 8.74 **FUD** 000 T A2 80

AMA: 2018,Jan,8; 2017,Jan,8; 2016,Jan,13; 2015,Jan,16

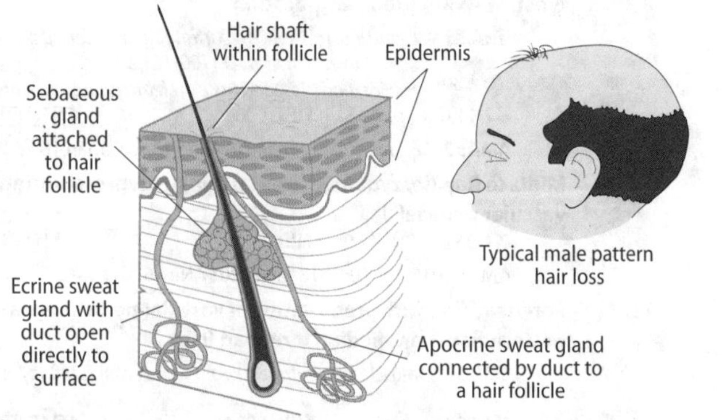

15776 **more than 15 punch grafts**

EXCLUDES *Strip transplant (15220)*

10.2 14.5 **FUD** 000 T A2 80

AMA: 2018,Jan,8; 2017,Jan,8; 2016,Jan,13; 2015,Jan,16

\+ **15777** **Implantation of biologic implant (eg, acellular dermal matrix) for soft tissue reinforcement (ie, breast, trunk) (List separately in addition to code for primary procedure)**

EXCLUDES *Application high cost skin substitute to external wound (15271-15278)*
Application low cost skin substitute to external wound (C5271-C5278)
Mesh implantation for:
Open repair ventral or incisional hernia (49560-49566) and (49568)
Repair devitalized soft tissue infection (11004-11006) and (49568)
Repair pelvic floor (57267)
Repair anorectal fistula with plug (46707)
Soft tissue reinforcement with biologic implants other than in the breast or trunk (17999)
Reporting modifier 50 for bilateral breast procedure. Report once for each side when performed bilaterally

Code also supply biologic implant
Code also synthetic or non-biological implant to reinforce abdominal wall (0437T)
Code first primary procedure

6.25 6.25 **FUD** ZZZ N N1 50

AMA: 2019,Nov,14; 2019,Jan,14; 2018,Jan,8; 2017,Jan,8; 2016,Jan,13; 2015,Jan,16

15780 **Dermabrasion; total face (eg, for acne scarring, fine wrinkling, rhytids, general keratosis)**

19.3 25.2 **FUD** 090 J P3 80

AMA: 2018,Jan,8; 2017,Jan,8; 2016,Jan,13; 2015,Jan,16

15781 **segmental, face**

12.3 15.6 **FUD** 090 T P2

AMA: 1997,Nov,1

15782 **regional, other than face**

11.2 15.3 **FUD** 090 J P3 80

AMA: 1997,Nov,1

15783 **superficial, any site (eg, tattoo removal)**

10.6 13.6 **FUD** 090 T P2 80

AMA: 2018,Jan,8; 2017,Jan,8; 2016,Jan,13; 2015,Jan,16

15786 **Abrasion; single lesion (eg, keratosis, scar)**

3.85 6.87 **FUD** 010 01 N1

AMA: 1997,Nov,1

\+ **15787** **each additional 4 lesions or less (List separately in addition to code for primary procedure)**
Code first (15786)
0.50 | 1.27 | **FUD** ZZZ | N N1
AMA: 1997,Nov,1

15788 **Chemical peel, facial; epidermal**
6.55 | 12.2 | **FUD** 090 | Q1 N1
AMA: 1997,Nov,1; 1993,Win,1

15789 **dermal**
11.6 | 15.3 | **FUD** 090 | T P2
AMA: 1997,Nov,1; 1993,Win,1

15792 **Chemical peel, nonfacial; epidermal**
6.61 | 10.9 | **FUD** 090 | Q1 N1 80
AMA: 1997,Nov,1; 1993,Win,1

15793 **dermal**
10.0 | 13.6 | **FUD** 090 | Q1 N1 80
AMA: 1997,Nov,1; 1993,Win,1

15819 **Cervicoplasty**
22.7 | 22.7 | **FUD** 090 | T G2 80
AMA: 1997,Nov,1

15820 **Blepharoplasty, lower eyelid;**
14.5 | 16.2 | **FUD** 090 | T A2 80 50
AMA: 2018,Jan,8; 2017,Jan,8; 2016,Jan,13; 2015,Jan,16

15821 **with extensive herniated fat pad**
15.5 | 17.4 | **FUD** 090 | T A2 80 50
AMA: 2018,Jan,8; 2017,Jan,8; 2016,Jan,13; 2015,Jan,16

15822 **Blepharoplasty, upper eyelid;**
11.2 | 12.9 | **FUD** 090 | T A2 50
AMA: 2018,Jan,8; 2017,Jan,8; 2016,Jan,13; 2015,Jan,16

15823 **with excessive skin weighting down lid**
15.5 | 17.4 | **FUD** 090 | T A2 50
AMA: 2018,Jan,8; 2017,Jan,8; 2016,Jan,13; 2015,Jan,16

15824 **Rhytidectomy; forehead**
EXCLUDES *Repair brow ptosis (67900)*
0.00 | 0.00 | **FUD** 000 | T A2 80 50
AMA: 2018,Jan,8; 2017,Apr,9

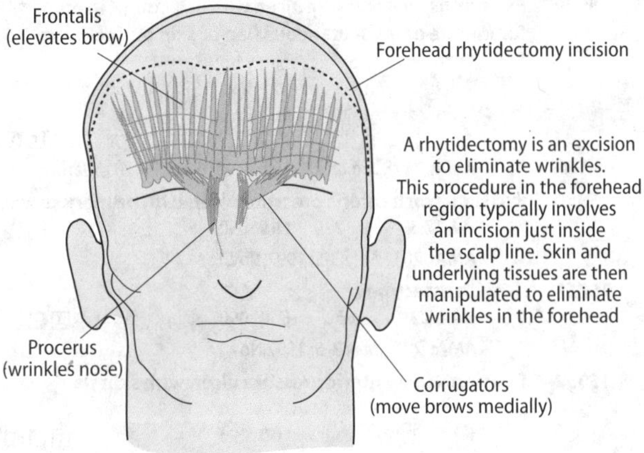

A rhytidectomy is an excision to eliminate wrinkles. This procedure in the forehead region typically involves an incision just inside the scalp line. Skin and underlying tissues are then manipulated to eliminate wrinkles in the forehead

15825 **neck with platysmal tightening (platysmal flap, P-flap)**
0.00 | 0.00 | **FUD** 000 | T A2 80 50
AMA: 2018,Jan,8; 2017,Apr,9

15826 **glabellar frown lines**
0.00 | 0.00 | **FUD** 000 | T A2 80 50
AMA: 1997,Nov,1

15828 **cheek, chin, and neck**
0.00 | 0.00 | **FUD** 000 | T A2 80 50
AMA: 1997,Nov,1

15829 **superficial musculoaponeurotic system (SMAS) flap**
0.00 | 0.00 | **FUD** 000 | T A2 80 50
AMA: 1997,Nov,1

15830 **Excision, excessive skin and subcutaneous tissue (includes lipectomy); abdomen, infraumbilical panniculectomy**
EXCLUDES *For same wound:*
Adjacent tissue transfer, trunk (14000-14001, 14302)
Complex wound repair, trunk (13100-13102)
Intermediate wound repair, trunk (12031-12032, 12034-12037)
Other abdominoplasty (17999)
Code also, when performed (15847)
33.9 | 33.9 | **FUD** 090 | J A2 80

15832 **thigh**
26.5 | 26.5 | **FUD** 090 | J A2 80 50
AMA: 1997,Nov,1

15833 **leg**
25.2 | 25.2 | **FUD** 090 | J A2 80 50
AMA: 1997,Nov,1

15834 **hip**
25.7 | 25.7 | **FUD** 090 | J A2 80 50
AMA: 1997,Nov,1

15835 **buttock**
26.9 | 26.9 | **FUD** 090 | J A2 80
AMA: 1997,Nov,1

15836 **arm**
22.6 | 22.6 | **FUD** 090 | J A2 80 50
AMA: 1997,Nov,1

15837 **forearm or hand**
20.6 | 24.7 | **FUD** 090 | J G2 80
AMA: 1997,Nov,1

15838 **submental fat pad**
18.5 | 18.5 | **FUD** 090 | J G2 80
AMA: 1998,Feb,1; 1997,Nov,1

15839 **other area**
21.2 | 25.4 | **FUD** 090 | J A2 80
AMA: 1997,Nov,1

15840-15845 Reanimation of the Paralyzed Face

INCLUDES Routine dressing and supplies
EXCLUDES *Intravenous fluorescein evaluation blood flow in graft or flap (15860)*
Nerve:
Decompression (69720, 69725, 69955)
Pedicle transfer (64905, 64907)
Suture (64831-64876, 69740, 69745)
Code also repair donor site with skin grafts or flaps

15840 **Graft for facial nerve paralysis; free fascia graft (including obtaining fascia)**
28.9 | 28.9 | **FUD** 090 | T A2
AMA: 1997,Nov,1

15841 **free muscle graft (including obtaining graft)**
51.2 | 51.2 | **FUD** 090 | T A2 80
AMA: 1997,Nov,1

15842 **free muscle flap by microsurgical technique**
INCLUDES Operating microscope (69990)
78.5 | 78.5 | **FUD** 090 | T G2 80
AMA: 2016,Feb,12

15845 **regional muscle transfer**
28.8 | 28.8 | **FUD** 090 | T A2 80
AMA: 1998,Feb,1; 1997,Nov,1

15847 Removal of Excess Abdominal Tissue Add-on

CMS: 100-02,16,10 Exclusions from Coverage; 100-02,16,120 Cosmetic Procedures; 100-02,16,180 Services Related to Noncovered Procedures

\+ **15847** **Excision, excessive skin and subcutaneous tissue (includes lipectomy), abdomen (eg, abdominoplasty) (includes umbilical transposition and fascial plication) (List separately in addition to code for primary procedure)**
EXCLUDES *Abdominal wall hernia repair (49491-49587)*
Other abdominoplasty (17999)
Code first (15830)
0.00 | 0.00 | **FUD** YYY | N N1 80

15850-15852 Suture Removal/Dressing Change: Anesthesia Required

15850 **Removal of sutures under anesthesia (other than local), same surgeon**
1.14 2.57 FUD XXX T G2
AMA: 2018,Jan,8; 2017,Jan,8; 2016,Jan,13; 2015,Jan,16

15851 **Removal of sutures under anesthesia (other than local), other surgeon**
1.31 2.85 FUD 000 T P3
AMA: 2018,Jan,8; 2017,Jan,8; 2016,Jan,13; 2015,Jan,16

15852 **Dressing change (for other than burns) under anesthesia (other than local)**
EXCLUDES *Dressing change for burns (16020-16030)*
1.34 1.34 FUD 000 Q1 N1
AMA: 1997,Nov,1

15860 Injection for Vascular Flow Determination

15860 **Intravenous injection of agent (eg, fluorescein) to test vascular flow in flap or graft**
3.13 3.13 FUD 000 Q1 N1 80
AMA: 2002,May,7; 1997,Nov,1

15876-15879 Liposuction

CMS: 100-02,16,10 Exclusions from Coverage; 100-02,16,120 Cosmetic Procedures; 100-02,16,180 Services Related to Noncovered Procedures

EXCLUDES *Liposuction for autologous fat grafting (15771-15774)*
Obtaining tissue for adipose-derived regenerative cell therapy (0489T-0490T)

15876 **Suction assisted lipectomy; head and neck**
0.00 0.00 FUD 000 T A2 80
AMA: 2019,Oct,5; 2019,Aug,10; 2018,Sep,12

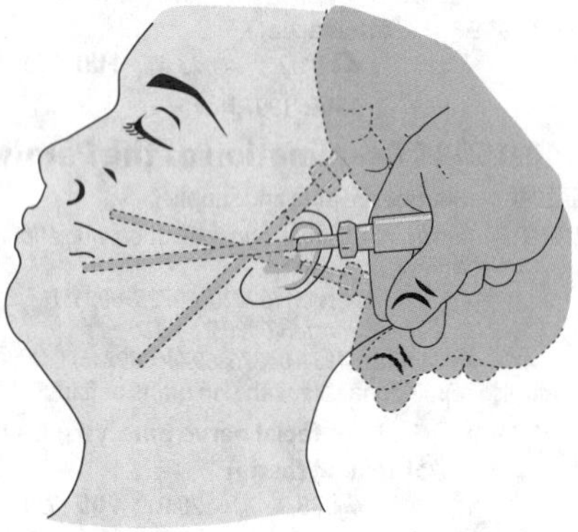

Cannula typically inserted through incision in front of ear

15877 **trunk**
0.00 0.00 FUD 000 T A2 80
AMA: 2019,Oct,5; 2019,Aug,10; 2018,Sep,12; 2018,Jan,8; 2017,Jan,8; 2016,Jan,13; 2015,Jan,16

15878 **upper extremity**
0.00 0.00 FUD 000 T A2 80 50
AMA: 2019,Oct,5; 2019,Aug,10; 2018,Sep,12

15879 **lower extremity**
0.00 0.00 FUD 000 T A2 80 50
AMA: 2019,Oct,5; 2019,Aug,10; 2018,Sep,12

15920-15999 Treatment of Decubitus Ulcers

Code also free skin graft to repair ulcer or donor site

15920 **Excision, coccygeal pressure ulcer, with coccygectomy; with primary suture**
17.8 17.8 FUD 090 J A2 80
AMA: 2011,May,3-5; 1997,Nov,1

15922 **with flap closure**
22.8 22.8 FUD 090 T A2 80
AMA: 2011,May,3-5; 1997,Nov,1

15931 **Excision, sacral pressure ulcer, with primary suture;**
20.1 20.1 FUD 090 J A2
AMA: 2011,May,3-5; 1997,Nov,1

15933 **with ostectomy**
24.5 24.5 FUD 090 J A2 80
AMA: 2011,May,3-5; 1997,Nov,1

15934 **Excision, sacral pressure ulcer, with skin flap closure;**
27.3 27.3 FUD 090 T A2
AMA: 2011,May,3-5; 1997,Nov,1

15935 **with ostectomy**
31.6 31.6 FUD 090 T A2 80
AMA: 2011,May,3-5; 1997,Nov,1

15936 **Excision, sacral pressure ulcer, in preparation for muscle or myocutaneous flap or skin graft closure;**
Code also any defect repair with:
Muscle or myocutaneous flap (15734, 15738)
Split skin graft (15100-15101)
26.0 26.0 FUD 090 T A2
AMA: 2011,May,3-5; 1998,Nov,1

15937 **with ostectomy**
Code also any defect repair with:
Muscle or myocutaneous flap (15734, 15738)
Split skin graft (15100-15101)
30.1 30.1 FUD 090 T A2
AMA: 2011,May,3-5; 1998,Nov,1

15940 **Excision, ischial pressure ulcer, with primary suture;**
20.1 20.1 FUD 090 J A2
AMA: 2011,May,3-5; 1997,Nov,1

15941 **with ostectomy (ischiectomy)**
26.4 26.4 FUD 090 J A2 80
AMA: 2011,May,3-5; 1997,Nov,1

15944 **Excision, ischial pressure ulcer, with skin flap closure;**
26.2 26.2 FUD 090 T A2 80
AMA: 2011,May,3-5; 1997,Nov,1

15945 **with ostectomy**
29.3 29.3 FUD 090 T A2 80
AMA: 2011,May,3-5; 1997,Nov,1

15946 **Excision, ischial pressure ulcer, with ostectomy, in preparation for muscle or myocutaneous flap or skin graft closure**
Code also any defect repair with:
Muscle or myocutaneous flap (15734, 15738)
Split skin graft (15100-15101)
47.0 47.0 FUD 090 T A2
AMA: 2018,Jan,8; 2017,Jan,8; 2016,Jan,13; 2015,Jan,16

15950 **Excision, trochanteric pressure ulcer, with primary suture;**
17.6 17.6 FUD 090 J A2
AMA: 2011,May,3-5; 1997,Nov,1

15951 **with ostectomy**
25.2 25.2 FUD 090 J A2 80
AMA: 2011,May,3-5; 1997,Nov,1

15952 **Excision, trochanteric pressure ulcer, with skin flap closure;**
26.3 26.3 FUD 090 T A2 80
AMA: 2011,May,3-5; 1997,Nov,1

15953 **with ostectomy**
28.9 28.9 FUD 090 T A2
AMA: 2011,May,3-5; 1997,Nov,1

15956 **Excision, trochanteric pressure ulcer, in preparation for muscle or myocutaneous flap or skin graft closure;**
Code also any defect repair with:
Muscle or myocutaneous flap (15734, 15738)
Split skin graft (15100-15101)
33.3 33.3 FUD 090 T A2
AMA: 2011,May,3-5; 1998,Nov,1

15958 **with ostectomy**
Code also any defect repair with:
Muscle or myocutaneous flap (15734-15738)
Split skin graft (15100-15101)
34.0 34.0 **FUD** 090 T A2
AMA: 2011,May,3-5; 1998,Nov,1

15999 **Unlisted procedure, excision pressure ulcer**
0.00 0.00 **FUD** YYY T 80
AMA: 2011,May,3-5; 1997,Nov,1

16000-16036 Burn Care

INCLUDES Local care burn surface only
EXCLUDES *Application skin grafts and flaps including all services described in:(15100-15777)*
E/M services
Laser fenestration for scars (0479T-0480T)

16000 **Initial treatment, first degree burn, when no more than local treatment is required**
1.33 2.09 **FUD** 000 Q1 N1
AMA: 2018,Jan,8; 2017,Jan,8; 2016,Jan,13; 2015,Jan,16

16020 **Dressings and/or debridement of partial-thickness burns, initial or subsequent; small (less than 5% total body surface area)**
INCLUDES Wound coverage other than skin graft
1.56 2.35 **FUD** 000 Q1 N1
AMA: 2018,Jan,8; 2017,Jan,8; 2016,Jan,13; 2015,Jan,16

16025 **medium (eg, whole face or whole extremity, or 5% to 10% total body surface area)**
INCLUDES Wound coverage other than skin graft
3.16 4.26 **FUD** 000 T A2
AMA: 2018,Jan,8; 2017,Jan,8; 2016,Jan,13; 2015,Jan,16

16030 **large (eg, more than 1 extremity, or greater than 10% total body surface area)**
INCLUDES Wound coverage other than skin graft
3.84 5.54 **FUD** 000 T A2
AMA: 2018,Jan,8; 2017,Jan,8; 2016,Jan,13; 2015,Jan,16

16035 **Escharotomy; initial incision**
EXCLUDES *Debridement scraping of burn (16020-16030)*
5.71 5.71 **FUD** 000 T G2
AMA: 2018,Jan,8; 2017,Jan,8; 2016,Jan,13; 2015,Jan,16

+ 16036 **each additional incision (List separately in addition to code for primary procedure)**
EXCLUDES *Debridement or scraping burn (16020-16030)*
Code first (16035)
2.37 2.37 **FUD** ZZZ C
AMA: 2018,Jan,8; 2017,Jan,8; 2016,Jan,13; 2015,Jan,16

17000-17004 Destruction Any Method: Premalignant Lesion

CMS: 100-03,140.5 Laser Procedures
EXCLUDES *Cryotherapy acne (17340)*
Destruction, skin:
Benign lesions other than cutaneous vascular proliferative lesions (17110-17111)
Cutaneous vascular proliferative lesions (17106-17108)
Malignant lesions (17260-17286)
Destruction lesion:
Anus (46900-46917, 46924)
Conjunctiva (68135)
Eyelid (67850)
Penis (54050-54057, 54065)
Vagina (57061, 57065)
Vestibule of mouth (40820)
Vulva (56501, 56515)
Destruction or excision skin tags (11200-11201)
Escharotomy (16035-16036)
Excision benign lesion (11400-11446)
Laser fenestration for scars (0479T-0480T)
Localized chemotherapy treatment see appropriate office visit service code
Paring or excision benign hyperkeratotic lesion (11055-11057)
Shaving skin lesions (11300-11313)
Treatment inflammatory skin disease via laser (96920-96922)

17000 **Destruction (eg, laser surgery, electrosurgery, cryosurgery, chemosurgery, surgical curettement), premalignant lesions (eg, actinic keratoses); first lesion**
1.53 1.85 **FUD** 010 Q1 N1
AMA: 2018,Jan,8; 2017,Dec,14; 2017,Jan,8; 2016,Apr,3; 2016,Jan,13; 2015,Jan,16

+ 17003 **second through 14 lesions, each (List separately in addition to code for first lesion)**
Code first (17000)
0.06 0.17 **FUD** ZZZ N N1
AMA: 2018,Jan,8; 2017,Dec,14; 2017,Jan,8; 2016,Apr,3; 2016,Jan,13; 2015,Jan,16

17004 **Destruction (eg, laser surgery, electrosurgery, cryosurgery, chemosurgery, surgical curettement), premalignant lesions (eg, actinic keratoses), 15 or more lesions**
EXCLUDES *Reporting code for destruction less than 15 lesions (17000-17003)*
2.79 4.48 **FUD** 010 T P3
AMA: 2018,Jan,8; 2017,Dec,14; 2017,Jan,8; 2016,Apr,3; 2016,Jan,13; 2015,Jan,16

17106-17250 Destruction Any Method: Vascular Proliferative Lesion

CMS: 100-02,16,10 Exclusions from Coverage; 100-02,16,120 Cosmetic Procedures
EXCLUDES *Cryotherapy acne (17340)*
Destruction, skin:
Malignant lesions (17260-17286)
Premalignant lesions (17000-17004)
Destruction lesion:
Anus (46900-46917, 46924)
Conjunctiva (68135)
Eyelid (67850)
Penis (54050-54057, 54065)
Vagina (57061, 57065)
Vestibule of mouth (40820)
Vulva (56501, 56515)
Destruction or excision skin tags (11200-11201)
Escharotomy (16035-16036)
Excision benign lesion (11400-11446)
Laser fenestration for scars (0479T-0480T)
Localized chemotherapy treatment see appropriate office visit service code
Paring or excision benign hyperkeratotic lesion (11055-11057)
Shaving skin lesions (11300-11313)
Treatment inflammatory skin disease via laser (96920-96922)

17106 **Destruction of cutaneous vascular proliferative lesions (eg, laser technique); less than 10 sq cm**
7.84 9.72 **FUD** 090 T P2
AMA: 2019,Sep,10; 2018,Jan,8; 2017,Dec,14; 2017,Jan,8; 2016,Apr,3; 2016,Jan,13; 2015,Jan,16

17107 **10.0 to 50.0 sq cm**

10.1 12.7 **FUD** 090 T P2

AMA: 2018,Jan,8; 2017,Dec,14; 2017,Jan,8; 2016,Apr,3; 2016,Jan,13; 2015,Jan,16

17108 **over 50.0 sq cm**

15.0 18.1 **FUD** 090 T P3 80

AMA: 2018,Jan,8; 2017,Dec,14; 2017,Jan,8; 2016,Apr,3; 2016,Jan,13; 2015,Jan,16

17110 **Destruction (eg, laser surgery, electrosurgery, cryosurgery, chemosurgery, surgical curettement), of benign lesions other than skin tags or cutaneous vascular proliferative lesions; up to 14 lesions**

1.91 3.17 **FUD** 010 Q1 N1

AMA: 2020,Apr,10; 2018,Jan,8; 2017,Dec,14; 2017,Jan,8; 2016,Apr,3; 2016,Jan,13; 2015,Jan,16

17111 **15 or more lesions**

EXCLUDES *Destruction neurofibromas, 50-100 lesions (0419T-0420T)*

2.34 3.72 **FUD** 010 Q1 N1

AMA: 2018,Jan,8; 2017,Dec,14; 2017,Jan,8; 2016,Apr,3; 2016,Jan,13; 2015,Jan,16

17250 **Chemical cauterization of granulation tissue (ie, proud flesh)**

EXCLUDES *Excision/removal codes for same lesion*
Chemical cauterization when applied for wound hemostasis
Wound care management (97597-97598, 97602)

1.05 2.31 **FUD** 000 Q1 N1

AMA: 2018,Jan,8; 2017,Dec,14; 2017,Jan,8; 2016,Jan,13; 2015,Jan,16

17260-17286 Destruction, Any Method: Malignant Lesion

CMS: 100-03,140.5 Laser Procedures

EXCLUDES *Cryotherapy acne (17340)*
Destruction, skin:
Benign lesions other than cutaneous vascular proliferative lesions (17110-17111)
Cutaneous vascular proliferative lesions (17106-17108)
Premalignant lesions (17000-17004)
Destruction lesion:
Anus (46900-46917, 46924)
Conjunctiva (68135)
Eyelid (67850)
Penis (54050-54057, 54065)
Vestibule of mouth (40820)
Vulva (56501-56515)
Destruction or excision skin tags (11200-11201)
Escharotomy (16035-16036)
Excision benign lesion (11400-11446)
Laser fenestration for scars (0479T-0480T)
Localized chemotherapy treatment see appropriate office visit service code
Paring or excision benign hyperkeratotic lesion (11055-11057)
Shaving skin lesion (11300-11313)
Treatment inflammatory skin disease via laser (96920-96922)

17260 **Destruction, malignant lesion (eg, laser surgery, electrosurgery, cryosurgery, chemosurgery, surgical curettement), trunk, arms or legs; lesion diameter 0.5 cm or less**

2.03 2.71 **FUD** 010 Q1 N1

AMA: 2018,Jan,8; 2017,Dec,14; 2017,Jan,8; 2016,Jan,13; 2015,Jan,16

17261 **lesion diameter 0.6 to 1.0 cm**

2.58 4.11 **FUD** 010 Q1 N1

AMA: 2018,Jan,8; 2017,Dec,14; 2017,Jan,8; 2016,Jan,13; 2015,Jan,16

17262 **lesion diameter 1.1 to 2.0 cm**

3.30 5.01 **FUD** 010 Q1 N1

AMA: 2018,Jan,8; 2017,Dec,14; 2017,Jan,8; 2016,Jan,13; 2015,Jan,16

17263 **lesion diameter 2.1 to 3.0 cm**

3.55 5.45 **FUD** 010 Q1 N1

AMA: 2018,Jan,8; 2017,Dec,14; 2017,Jan,8; 2016,Jan,13; 2015,Jan,16

17264 **lesion diameter 3.1 to 4.0 cm**

3.79 5.84 **FUD** 010 T P3

AMA: 2018,Jan,8; 2017,Dec,14; 2017,Jan,8; 2016,Jan,13; 2015,Jan,16

17266 **lesion diameter over 4.0 cm**

4.47 6.66 **FUD** 010 T P3

AMA: 2018,Jan,8; 2017,Dec,14; 2017,Jan,8; 2016,Jan,13; 2015,Jan,16

17270 **Destruction, malignant lesion (eg, laser surgery, electrosurgery, cryosurgery, chemosurgery, surgical curettement), scalp, neck, hands, feet, genitalia; lesion diameter 0.5 cm or less**

2.74 4.22 **FUD** 010 T P2

AMA: 2018,Jan,8; 2017,Dec,14; 2017,Jan,8; 2016,Jan,13; 2015,Jan,16

17271 **lesion diameter 0.6 to 1.0 cm**

3.14 4.67 **FUD** 010 T P2

AMA: 2018,Jan,8; 2017,Dec,14; 2017,Jan,8; 2016,Jan,13; 2015,Jan,16

17272 **lesion diameter 1.1 to 2.0 cm**

3.52 5.32 **FUD** 010 Q1 N1

AMA: 2018,Jan,8; 2017,Dec,14; 2017,Jan,8; 2016,Jan,13; 2015,Jan,16

17273 **lesion diameter 2.1 to 3.0 cm**

4.11 5.94 **FUD** 010 T P3

AMA: 2018,Jan,8; 2017,Dec,14; 2017,Jan,8; 2016,Jan,13; 2015,Jan,16

17274 **lesion diameter 3.1 to 4.0 cm**

4.88 6.97 **FUD** 010 T P3

AMA: 2018,Jan,8; 2017,Dec,14; 2017,Jan,8; 2016,Jan,13; 2015,Jan,16

17276 **lesion diameter over 4.0 cm**

5.86 8.07 **FUD** 010 T P2

AMA: 2018,Jan,8; 2017,Dec,14; 2017,Jan,8; 2016,Jan,13; 2015,Jan,16

17280 **Destruction, malignant lesion (eg, laser surgery, electrosurgery, cryosurgery, chemosurgery, surgical curettement), face, ears, eyelids, nose, lips, mucous membrane; lesion diameter 0.5 cm or less**

2.48 3.94 **FUD** 010 Q1 N1

AMA: 2018,Jan,8; 2017,Dec,14; 2017,Jan,8; 2016,Jan,13; 2015,Jan,16

17281 **lesion diameter 0.6 to 1.0 cm**

3.54 5.09 **FUD** 010 T P3

AMA: 2018,Jan,8; 2017,Dec,14; 2017,Jan,8; 2016,Jan,13; 2015,Jan,16

17282 **lesion diameter 1.1 to 2.0 cm**

3.97 5.82 **FUD** 010 T P3

AMA: 2018,Jan,8; 2017,Dec,14; 2017,Jan,8; 2016,Jan,13; 2015,Jan,16

17283 **lesion diameter 2.1 to 3.0 cm**

4.97 6.94 **FUD** 010 T P3

AMA: 2018,Jan,8; 2017,Dec,14; 2017,Jan,8; 2016,Jan,13; 2015,Jan,16

17284 **lesion diameter 3.1 to 4.0 cm**

5.80 7.90 **FUD** 010 T P3

AMA: 2018,Jan,8; 2017,Dec,14; 2017,Jan,8; 2016,Jan,13; 2015,Jan,16

17286 **lesion diameter over 4.0 cm**

7.86 10.1 **FUD** 010 T P3

AMA: 2018,Jan,8; 2017,Dec,14; 2017,Jan,8; 2016,Jan,13; 2015,Jan,16

17311-17315 Mohs Surgery

INCLUDES Surgical/pathology services performed by same physician or other qualified health care provider:
Evaluation skin margins by surgeon
Pathology exam on Mohs surgery specimen (by Mohs surgeon) (88302-88309)
Routine frozen section stain (88314)
Tumor removal, mapping, preparation, and examination lesion

EXCLUDES *Frozen section if no prior diagnosis determination has been performed (88331)*

Code also any special histochemical stain on frozen section, nonroutine (with modifier 59) (88311-88314, 88342)
Code also biopsy (with modifier 59) when no prior diagnosis determination has been performed, biopsy indeterminate, or performed more than 90 days preoperatively (11102, 11104, 11106)
Code also complex repair (13100-13160)
Code also flaps or grafts (14000-14350, 15050-15770)
Code also intermediate repair (12031-12057)
Code also simple repair (12001-12021)

17311 Mohs micrographic technique, including removal of all gross tumor, surgical excision of tissue specimens, mapping, color coding of specimens, microscopic examination of specimens by the surgeon, and histopathologic preparation including routine stain(s) (eg, hematoxylin and eosin, toluidine blue), head, neck, hands, feet, genitalia, or any location with surgery directly involving muscle, cartilage, bone, tendon, major nerves, or vessels; first stage, up to 5 tissue blocks
10.4 18.8 FUD 000 T P2
AMA: 2018,Jan,8; 2017,Jan,8; 2016,Jan,13; 2015,Jan,16

\+ **17312 each additional stage after the first stage, up to 5 tissue blocks (List separately in addition to code for primary procedure)**
Code first (17311)
5.76 11.2 FUD ZZZ N N1
AMA: 2018,Jan,8; 2017,Jan,8; 2016,Jan,13; 2015,Jan,16

17313 Mohs micrographic technique, including removal of all gross tumor, surgical excision of tissue specimens, mapping, color coding of specimens, microscopic examination of specimens by the surgeon, and histopathologic preparation including routine stain(s) (eg, hematoxylin and eosin, toluidine blue), of the trunk, arms, or legs; first stage, up to 5 tissue blocks
9.34 17.6 FUD 000 T P2
AMA: 2018,Jan,8; 2017,Jan,8; 2016,Jan,13; 2015,Jan,16

\+ **17314 each additional stage after the first stage, up to 5 tissue blocks (List separately in addition to code for primary procedure)**
Code first (17313)
5.14 10.8 FUD ZZZ N N1
AMA: 2018,Jan,8; 2017,Jan,8; 2016,Jan,13; 2015,Jan,16

\+ **17315 Mohs micrographic technique, including removal of all gross tumor, surgical excision of tissue specimens, mapping, color coding of specimens, microscopic examination of specimens by the surgeon, and histopathologic preparation including routine stain(s) (eg, hematoxylin and eosin, toluidine blue), each additional block after the first 5 tissue blocks, any stage (List separately in addition to code for primary procedure)**
Code first (17311-17314)
1.47 2.22 FUD ZZZ N N1
AMA: 2018,Jan,8; 2017,Jan,8; 2016,Jan,13; 2015,Jan,16

17340-17999 Treatment for Active Acne and Permanent Hair Removal

CMS: 100-02,16,10 Exclusions from Coverage; 100-02,16,120 Cosmetic Procedures

17340 Cryotherapy (CO2 slush, liquid N2) for acne
1.40 1.49 FUD 010 Q1 N1
AMA: 2018,Jan,8; 2017,Jan,8; 2016,Jan,13; 2015,Jan,16

17360 Chemical exfoliation for acne (eg, acne paste, acid)
2.77 3.61 FUD 010 Q1 N1
AMA: 2018,Jan,8; 2017,Jan,8; 2016,Jan,13; 2015,Jan,16

17380 Electrolysis epilation, each 30 minutes
EXCLUDES *Actinotherapy (96900)*
0.00 0.00 FUD 000 T R2 80
AMA: 2018,Jan,8; 2017,Jan,8; 2016,Jan,13; 2015,Jan,16

17999 Unlisted procedure, skin, mucous membrane and subcutaneous tissue
0.00 0.00 FUD YYY Q1 80
AMA: 2019,Sep,10; 2019,Mar,10; 2019,Jan,14; 2018,Jan,8; 2017,Dec,13; 2017,Jan,8; 2016,May,13; 2016,Jan,13; 2015,Jan,16

19000-19030 Treatment of Breast Abscess and Cyst with Injection, Aspiration, Incision

19000 Puncture aspiration of cyst of breast;
(76942, 77021)
1.26 3.11 FUD 000 T P3
AMA: 2018,Jan,8; 2017,Jan,8; 2016,Jan,13; 2015,Jan,16

\+ **19001 each additional cyst (List separately in addition to code for primary procedure)**
Code first (19000)
(76942, 77021)
0.62 0.77 FUD ZZZ N N1
AMA: 2018,Jan,8; 2017,Jan,8; 2016,Jan,13; 2015,Jan,16

19020 Mastotomy with exploration or drainage of abscess, deep
8.93 13.5 FUD 090 J A2 50
AMA: 2018,Jan,8; 2017,Jan,8; 2016,Jan,13; 2015,Jan,16

19030 Injection procedure only for mammary ductogram or galactogram
(77053-77054)
2.23 4.74 FUD 000 N N1 50
AMA: 2018,Jan,8; 2017,Jan,8; 2016,Jan,13; 2015,Jan,16

19081-19086 Breast Biopsy with Imaging Guidance

CMS: 100-03,220.13 Percutaneous Image-guided Breast Biopsy; 100-04,12,40.7 Bilateral Procedures; 100-04,13,80.1 Physician Presence; 100-04,13,80.2 S&I Multiple Procedure Reduction

INCLUDES Breast biopsy with placement localization devices
Fluoroscopic guidance for needle placement (77002)
Magnetic resonance guidance for needle placement (77021)
Radiological examination, surgical specimen (76098)
Ultrasonic guidance for needle placement (76942)

EXCLUDES *Biopsy breast without imaging guidance (19100-19101)*
Lesion removal without concentration on surgical margins (19110-19126)
Open biopsy after placement localization device (19101)
Partial mastectomy (19301-19302)
Placement localization devices only (19281-19288)
Total mastectomy (19303-19307)

Code also additional biopsies performed with different imaging modalities

19081 Biopsy, breast, with placement of breast localization device(s) (eg, clip, metallic pellet), when performed, and imaging of the biopsy specimen, when performed, percutaneous; first lesion, including stereotactic guidance
4.82 17.3 FUD 000 J G2 80 50
AMA: 2019,Apr,4; 2018,Jan,8; 2017,Jan,8; 2016,Jun,3; 2016,Jan,13; 2015,May,8; 2015,Mar,5; 2015,Jan,16

\+ **19082 each additional lesion, including stereotactic guidance (List separately in addition to code for primary procedure)**
Code first (19081)
2.42 13.9 FUD ZZZ N N1 80
AMA: 2019,Apr,4; 2018,Jan,8; 2017,Jan,8; 2016,Jun,3; 2016,Jan,13; 2015,May,8; 2015,Mar,5; 2015,Jan,16

19083 Biopsy, breast, with placement of breast localization device(s) (eg, clip, metallic pellet), when performed, and imaging of the biopsy specimen, when performed, percutaneous; first lesion, including ultrasound guidance
4.56 17.1 FUD 000 J G2 80 50
AMA: 2019,Apr,4; 2018,Jan,8; 2017,Jan,8; 2016,Jun,3; 2016,Jan,13; 2015,May,8; 2015,Mar,5; 2015,Jan,16

\+ 19084 **each additional lesion, including ultrasound guidance (List separately in addition to code for primary procedure)**

Code first (19083)

2.25 13.6 **FUD** ZZZ N N1 80

AMA: 2019,Apr,4; 2018,Jan,8; 2017,Jan,8; 2016,Jun,3; 2016,Jan,13; 2015,May,8; 2015,Mar,5; 2015,Jan,16

19085 **Biopsy, breast, with placement of breast localization device(s) (eg, clip, metallic pellet), when performed, and imaging of the biopsy specimen, when performed, percutaneous; first lesion, including magnetic resonance guidance**

5.28 26.1 **FUD** 000 J G2 80 50

AMA: 2019,Apr,4; 2018,Jan,8; 2017,Jan,8; 2016,Jun,3; 2016,Jan,13; 2015,May,8; 2015,Mar,5; 2015,Jan,16

\+ 19086 **each additional lesion, including magnetic resonance guidance (List separately in addition to code for primary procedure)**

Code first (19085)

2.65 21.9 **FUD** ZZZ N N1 80

AMA: 2019,Apr,4; 2018,Jan,8; 2017,Jan,8; 2016,Jun,3; 2016,Jan,13; 2015,May,8; 2015,Mar,5; 2015,Jan,16

19100-19101 Breast Biopsy Without Imaging Guidance

EXCLUDES *Biopsy breast with imaging guidance (19081-19086)*
Lesion removal without concentration on surgical margins (19110-19126)
Partial mastectomy (19301-19302)
Total mastectomy (19303-19307)

19100 **Biopsy of breast; percutaneous, needle core, not using imaging guidance (separate procedure)**

EXCLUDES *Fine needle aspiration:*
With imaging guidance ([10005, 10006, 10007, 10008, 10009, 10010, 10011, 10012])
Without imaging guidance (10021, [10004])

2.03 4.32 **FUD** 000 J A2 50

AMA: 2018,Jan,8; 2017,Jan,8; 2016,Jan,13; 2015,Jan,16

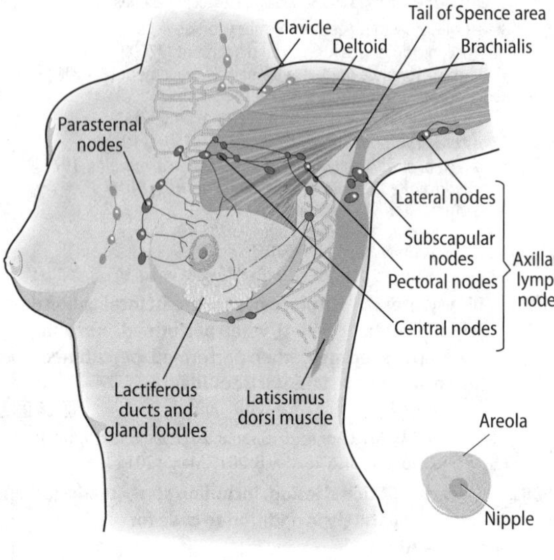

19101 **open, incisional**

Code also placement localization device with imaging guidance (19281-19288)

6.45 9.62 **FUD** 010 J A2 50

AMA: 2018,Jan,8; 2017,Jan,8; 2016,Jan,13; 2015,Jan,16

19105 Treatment of Fibroadenoma: Cryoablation

CMS: 100-04,13,80.1 Physician Presence; 100-04,13,80.2 S&I Multiple Procedure Reduction

INCLUDES Adjacent lesions treated with one cryoprobe
Ultrasound guidance (76940, 76942)

EXCLUDES *Cryoablation malignant breast tumors (0581T)*

19105 **Ablation, cryosurgical, of fibroadenoma, including ultrasound guidance, each fibroadenoma**

6.14 77.6 **FUD** 000 J G2 50

AMA: 2007,Mar,7-8

19110-19126 Excisional Procedures: Breast

INCLUDES Open removal breast mass without concentration on surgical margins

Code also placement localization device with imaging guidance (19281-19288)

19110 **Nipple exploration, with or without excision of a solitary lactiferous duct or a papilloma lactiferous duct**

9.94 13.9 **FUD** 090 J A2 50

AMA: 2018,Jan,8; 2017,Jan,8; 2016,Jan,13; 2015,Jan,16

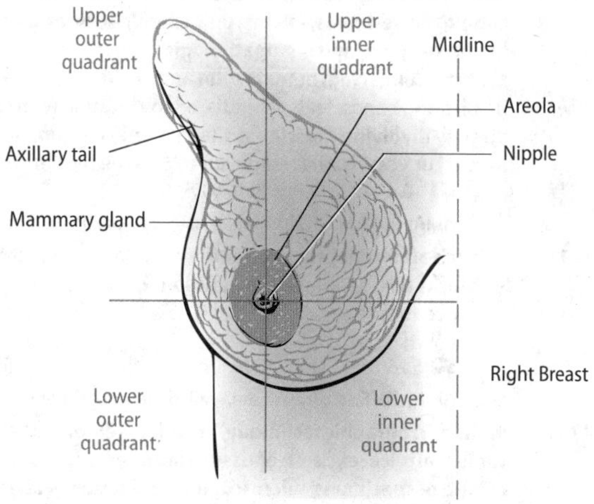

19112 **Excision of lactiferous duct fistula**

9.12 13.2 **FUD** 090 J A2 80 50

AMA: 2018,Jan,8; 2017,Jan,8; 2016,Jan,13; 2015,Jan,16

19120 **Excision of cyst, fibroadenoma, or other benign or malignant tumor, aberrant breast tissue, duct lesion, nipple or areolar lesion (except 19300), open, male or female, 1 or more lesions**

12.0 14.5 **FUD** 090 J A2 50

AMA: 2018,Jan,8; 2017,Jan,8; 2016,Jan,13; 2015,Mar,5; 2015,Jan,16

19125 **Excision of breast lesion identified by preoperative placement of radiological marker, open; single lesion**

INCLUDES Intraoperative clip placement

13.2 15.8 **FUD** 090 J A2 50

AMA: 2018,Jan,8; 2017,Jan,8; 2016,Jan,13; 2015,Mar,5; 2015,Jan,16

\+ 19126 **each additional lesion separately identified by a preoperative radiological marker (List separately in addition to code for primary procedure)**

INCLUDES Intraoperative clip placement

Code first (19125)

4.68 4.68 **FUD** ZZZ N N1

AMA: 2018,Jan,8; 2017,Jan,8; 2016,Jan,13; 2015,Jan,16

19281-19288 Placement of Localization Markers

INCLUDES Placement localization devices only

EXCLUDES *Biopsy breast without imaging guidance (19100-19101)*
When performed on same lesion:
Fluoroscopic guidance for needle placement (77002)
Localization device placement with biopsy breast (19081-19086)
Magnetic resonance guidance for needle placement (77021)
Ultrasonic guidance for needle placement (76942)

Code also open excision of breast lesion when performed after localization device placement (19110-19126)

Code also open incisional breast biopsy when performed after localization device placement (19101)

Code also radiography surgical specimen (76098)

19281 Placement of breast localization device(s) (eg, clip, metallic pellet, wire/needle, radioactive seeds), percutaneous; first lesion, including mammographic guidance
2.91 6.90 FUD 000 Q1 N1 80 50
AMA: 2018,Jan,8; 2017,Jan,8; 2016,Jun,3; 2016,Jan,13; 2015,May,8; 2015,Jan,16

+ **19282 each additional lesion, including mammographic guidance (List separately in addition to code for primary procedure)**
Code first (19281)
1.46 4.92 FUD ZZZ N N1 80
AMA: 2018,Jan,8; 2017,Jan,8; 2016,Jun,3; 2016,Jan,13; 2015,May,8; 2015,Jan,16

19283 Placement of breast localization device(s) (eg, clip, metallic pellet, wire/needle, radioactive seeds), percutaneous; first lesion, including stereotactic guidance
2.93 7.74 FUD 000 Q1 N1 80 50
AMA: 2018,Jan,8; 2017,Jan,8; 2016,Jun,3; 2016,May,13; 2016,Jan,13; 2015,May,8; 2015,Jan,16

+ **19284 each additional lesion, including stereotactic guidance (List separately in addition to code for primary procedure)**
Code first (19283)
1.49 5.90 FUD ZZZ N N1 80
AMA: 2018,Jan,8; 2017,Jan,8; 2016,Jun,3; 2016,May,13; 2016,Jan,13; 2015,May,8; 2015,Jan,16

19285 Placement of breast localization device(s) (eg, clip, metallic pellet, wire/needle, radioactive seeds), percutaneous; first lesion, including ultrasound guidance
2.49 12.9 FUD 000 Q1 N1 80 50
AMA: 2018,Jan,8; 2017,Jan,8; 2016,Jun,3; 2016,May,13; 2016,Jan,13; 2015,May,8; 2015,Jan,16

+ **19286 each additional lesion, including ultrasound guidance (List separately in addition to code for primary procedure)**
Code first (19285)
1.25 11.9 FUD ZZZ N N1 80
AMA: 2018,Jan,8; 2017,Jan,8; 2016,Jun,3; 2016,May,13; 2016,Jan,13; 2015,May,8; 2015,Jan,16

19287 Placement of breast localization device(s) (eg clip, metallic pellet, wire/needle, radioactive seeds), percutaneous; first lesion, including magnetic resonance guidance
3.72 22.1 FUD 000 Q1 N1 80 50
AMA: 2018,Jan,8; 2017,Jan,8; 2016,Jun,3; 2016,May,13; 2016,Jan,13; 2015,Jan,16

+ **19288 each additional lesion, including magnetic resonance guidance (List separately in addition to code for primary procedure)**
Code first (19287)
1.87 18.6 FUD ZZZ N N1 80
AMA: 2018,Jan,8; 2017,Jan,8; 2016,Jun,3; 2016,May,13; 2016,Jan,13; 2015,Jan,16

19294-19298 Radioelement Application

+ **19294 Preparation of tumor cavity, with placement of a radiation therapy applicator for intraoperative radiation therapy (IORT) concurrent with partial mastectomy (List separately in addition to code for primary procedure)**
Code first (19301-19302)
4.71 4.71 FUD ZZZ N N1 80
AMA: 2020,May,9

19296 Placement of radiotherapy afterloading expandable catheter (single or multichannel) into the breast for interstitial radioelement application following partial mastectomy, includes imaging guidance; on date separate from partial mastectomy
6.11 114. FUD 000 J J8 80 50
AMA: 2020,May,9; 2018,Jan,8; 2017,Jan,8; 2016,Jan,13; 2015,Jan,16

+ **19297 concurrent with partial mastectomy (List separately in addition to code for primary procedure)**
Code first (19301-19302)
2.75 2.75 FUD ZZZ N N1 80
AMA: 2020,May,9; 2019,Apr,10; 2018,Jan,8; 2017,Jan,8; 2016,Jan,13; 2015,Jan,16

19298 Placement of radiotherapy after loading brachytherapy catheters (multiple tube and button type) into the breast for interstitial radioelement application following (at the time of or subsequent to) partial mastectomy, includes imaging guidance
9.22 28.4 FUD 000 J G2 80 50
AMA: 2020,May,9; 2018,Jan,8; 2017,Jan,8; 2016,Jan,13; 2015,Jan,16

19300-19307 Mastectomies: Partial, Simple, Radical

CMS: 100-04,12,40.7 Bilateral Procedures

INCLUDES Intraoperative clip placement

EXCLUDES *Insertion prosthesis (19340, 19342)*

19300 Mastectomy for gynecomastia ♂
EXCLUDES *Removal breast tissue for:*
Other than gynecomastia (19318)
Treatment or prevention breast cancer (19301-19307)
12.1 15.8 FUD 090 J A2 50
AMA: 2020,May,9; 2018,Jan,8; 2017,Jan,8; 2016,Jan,13; 2015,Jan,16

19301 Mastectomy, partial (eg, lumpectomy, tylectomy, quadrantectomy, segmentectomy);
EXCLUDES *Insertion radiotherapy afterloading balloon during separate encounter (19296)*
Code also intraoperative radiofrequency spectroscopy margin assessment and report (0546T)
Code also insertion radiotherapy afterloading balloon catheter, when performed at same time (19297)
Code also insertion radiotherapy afterloading brachytherapy catheter, when performed at same time (19298)
Code also tumor cavity preparation with intraoperative radiation therapy applicator, when performed (19294)
19.0 19.0 FUD 090 J A2 80 50
AMA: 2020,May,9; 2018,Jan,8; 2017,Oct,9; 2017,Jan,8; 2016,Jan,13; 2015,Mar,5; 2015,Jan,16

19302 with axillary lymphadenectomy
EXCLUDES *Insertion radiotherapy afterloading balloon during separate encounter (19296)*
Code also intraoperative radiofrequency spectroscopy margin assessment and report (0546T)
Code also insertion radiotherapy afterloading balloon catheter, when performed at same time (19297)
Code also insertion radiotherapy afterloading brachytherapy catheter, when performed at same time (19298)
Code also tumor cavity preparation with intraoperative radiation therapy applicator, when performed (19294)
25.9 25.9 FUD 090 J A2 80 50
AMA: 2020,May,9; 2019,Feb,8; 2018,Jan,8; 2017,Jan,8; 2016,Jan,13; 2015,Mar,5; 2015,Jan,16

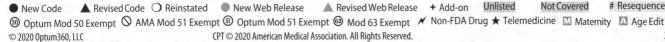

19303 Mastectomy, simple, complete

EXCLUDES *Excision pectoral muscles and axillary or internal mammary lymph nodes*
Removal breast tissue for:
Gynecomastia (19300)
Other than gynecomastia (19318)

Facility RVU 27.6 Non-Facility RVU 27.6 FUD 090 J A2 80 50

AMA: 2020,May,9; 2019,Dec,4; 2018,Jan,8; 2017,Jan,8; 2016,Jan,13; 2015,Mar,5; 2015,Jan,16

19305 Mastectomy, radical, including pectoral muscles, axillary lymph nodes

Facility RVU 33.0 Non-Facility RVU 33.0 FUD 090 C 80 50

AMA: 2020,May,9; 2018,Jan,8; 2017,Jan,8; 2016,Jan,13; 2015,Jan,16

19306 Mastectomy, radical, including pectoral muscles, axillary and internal mammary lymph nodes (Urban type operation)

Facility RVU 34.7 Non-Facility RVU 34.7 FUD 090 C 80 50

AMA: 2020,May,9; 2018,Jan,8; 2017,Jan,8; 2016,Jan,13; 2015,Jan,16

19307 Mastectomy, modified radical, including axillary lymph nodes, with or without pectoralis minor muscle, but excluding pectoralis major muscle

Facility RVU 34.6 Non-Facility RVU 34.6 FUD 090 J 80 50

AMA: 2020,May,9; 2019,Feb,8; 2018,Jan,8; 2017,Jan,8; 2016,Jan,13; 2015,Mar,5; 2015,Jan,16

19316-19499 Plastic, Reconstructive, and Aesthetic Breast Procedures

CMS: 100-03,140.2 Breast Reconstruction Following Mastectomy; 100-04,12,40.7 Bilateral Procedures

Code also biologic implant for tissue reinforcement (15777)

19316 Mastopexy

Facility RVU 22.3 Non-Facility RVU 22.3 FUD 090 J A2 80 50

AMA: 2018,Jan,8; 2017,Jan,8; 2016,Jan,13; 2015,Jan,16

▲ **19318 Breast reduction**

INCLUDES Aries-Pitanguy mammaplasty
Biesenberger mammaplasty

Facility RVU 31.5 Non-Facility RVU 31.5 FUD 090 J A2 80 50

AMA: 2020,May,9; 2018,Jan,8; 2017,Jan,8; 2016,Jan,13; 2015,Jan,16

~~**19324 Mammaplasty, augmentation; without prosthetic implant**~~

To report, see (15771-15772)

▲ **19325 Breast augmentation with implant**

EXCLUDES *Flap or graft (15100-15650)*

Code also fat grafting, when performed (15771-15772)

Facility RVU 18.6 Non-Facility RVU 18.6 FUD 090 J G2 80 50

AMA: 2018,Jan,8; 2017,Jan,8; 2016,Jan,13; 2015,Jan,16

▲ **19328 Removal of intact breast implant**

EXCLUDES *Removal tissue expander (11970-11971)*
Revision peri-implant capsule, breast (19370)

Facility RVU 14.4 Non-Facility RVU 14.4 FUD 090 Q2 A2 50

AMA: 2018,Jan,8; 2017,Jan,8; 2016,Jan,13; 2015,Jan,16

▲ **19330 Removal of ruptured breast implant, including implant contents (eg, saline, silicone gel)**

EXCLUDES *Insertion new breast implant during same operative session (19342)*
Removal ruptured tissue expander (11970-11971)

Facility RVU 18.3 Non-Facility RVU 18.3 FUD 090 Q2 A2 50

AMA: 2018,Jan,8; 2017,Jan,8; 2016,Jan,13; 2015,Jan,16

▲ **19340 Insertion of breast implant on same day of mastectomy (ie, immediate)**

EXCLUDES *Preparation moulage for custom breast implant (19396)*
Supply prosthetic implant (99070, C1789, L8600)

Facility RVU 28.6 Non-Facility RVU 28.6 FUD 090 J A2 50

AMA: 2020,May,9; 2018,Jan,8; 2017,Jan,8; 2016,Jan,13; 2015,Dec,18; 2015,Jan,16

▲ **19342 Insertion or replacement of breast implant on separate day from mastectomy**

EXCLUDES *Preparation moulage for custom breast implant (19396)*
Removal intact breast implant (19328)
Removal tissue expander with insertion breast implant (11970)
Supply prosthetic implant (99070, C1789, L8600)

Facility RVU 26.7 Non-Facility RVU 26.7 FUD 090 J A2 80 50

AMA: 2020,May,9; 2018,Jan,8; 2017,Jan,8; 2016,Jan,13; 2015,Nov,10; 2015,Jan,16

19350 Nipple/areola reconstruction

INCLUDES Adjacent tissue transfer, trunk (14000-14001)
Full-thickness graft, trunk (15200-15201)
Split-thickness autograft, trunk, arms, legs (15100)
Tattooing to correct skin color defects (11920-11922)

Facility RVU 19.4 Non-Facility RVU 23.8 FUD 090 J A2 50

AMA: 2018,Jan,8; 2017,Jan,8; 2016,Aug,9; 2016,Jan,13; 2015,Jan,16

19355 Correction of inverted nipples

Facility RVU 17.8 Non-Facility RVU 21.7 FUD 090 J A2 80 50

AMA: 2018,Jan,8; 2017,Jan,8; 2016,Jan,13; 2015,Jan,16

▲ **19357 Tissue expander placement in breast reconstruction, including subsequent expansion(s)**

Facility RVU 43.1 Non-Facility RVU 43.1 FUD 090 J J8 80 50

AMA: 2018,Jan,8; 2017,Jan,8; 2016,Jan,13; 2015,Feb,10; 2015,Jan,16

▲ **19361 Breast reconstruction; with latissimus dorsi flap**

INCLUDES Closure donor site
Harvesting skin graft
Inset shaping flap into breast

EXCLUDES *Implant prosthesis with latissimus dorsi implant:*
performed different day than mastectomy (19342)
performed same day as mastectomy (19340)
Insertion tissue expander with latissimus dorsi flap (19357)

Facility RVU 45.4 Non-Facility RVU 45.4 FUD 090 C 80 50

AMA: 2019,Nov,14; 2018,Jan,8; 2017,Jan,8; 2016,Jan,13; 2015,Feb,10; 2015,Jan,16

▲ **19364 with free flap (eg, fTRAM, DIEP, SIEA, GAP flap)**

INCLUDES Closure donor site
Harvesting skin graft
Inset shaping flap into breast
Microvascular repair
Operating microscope (69990)

Facility RVU 79.7 Non-Facility RVU 79.7 FUD 090 C 80 50

AMA: 2019,Nov,14; 2018,Jan,8; 2017,Jan,8; 2016,Feb,12; 2016,Jan,13; 2015,Feb,10; 2015,Jan,16

~~**19366 Breast reconstruction with other technique**~~

▲ **19367 with single-pedicled transverse rectus abdominis myocutaneous (TRAM) flap**

INCLUDES Closure donor site
Harvesting skin graft
Inset shaping flap into breast

Facility RVU 51.5 Non-Facility RVU 51.5 FUD 090 C 80 50

AMA: 2019,Nov,14; 2018,Jan,8; 2017,Jan,8; 2016,Jan,13; 2015,Feb,10; 2015,Jan,16

▲ **19368 with single-pedicled transverse rectus abdominis myocutaneous (TRAM) flap, requiring separate microvascular anastomosis (supercharging)**

INCLUDES Closure donor site
Harvesting skin graft
Inset shaping flap into breast
Operating microscope (69990)

Facility RVU 63.2 Non-Facility RVU 63.2 FUD 090 C 80 50

AMA: 2019,Nov,14; 2018,Jan,8; 2017,Jan,8; 2016,Feb,12; 2016,Jan,13; 2015,Feb,10; 2015,Jan,16

▲ **19369 with bipedicled transverse rectus abdominis myocutaneous (TRAM) flap**

INCLUDES Closure donor site
Harvesting skin graft
Inset shaping flap into breast

59.0 59.0 FUD 090 C 80 50

AMA: 2019,Nov,14; 2018,Jan,8; 2017,Jan,8; 2016,Jan,13; 2015,Feb,10; 2015,Jan,16

▲ **19370 Revision of peri-implant capsule, breast, including capsulotomy, capsulorrhaphy, and/or partial capsulectomy**

EXCLUDES *Removal and replacement with new implant (19342)*
Removal intact breast implant (19328)

19.9 19.9 FUD 090 J A2 50

AMA: 2018,Jan,8; 2017,Jan,8; 2016,Jan,13; 2015,Dec,18; 2015,Jan,16

▲ **19371 Peri-implant capsulectomy, breast, complete, including removal of all intracapsular contents**

EXCLUDES *Removal and replacement with new implant (19342)*
Removal intact breast implant (19328)
Removal ruptured breast implant (19330)
Revision peri-implant capsule on same breast (19370)

22.5 22.5 FUD 090 J A2 50

AMA: 2018,Jan,8; 2017,Jan,8; 2016,Jan,13; 2015,Jan,16

▲ **19380 Revision of reconstructed breast (eg, significant removal of tissue, re-advancement and/or re-inset of flaps in autologous reconstruction or significant capsular revision combined with soft tissue excision in implant-based reconstruction)**

INCLUDES Removal portion or reshaping flap
Revision flap position on chest wall
Revision scar(s)
When performed on same breast:
Breast reduction (19318)
Mastopexy (19316)
Repair complex, trunk (13100-13102)
Repair intermediate, trunk (12031-12037)
Revision peri-implant capsule, breast (19370)
Suction assisted lipectomy; trunk (15877)

EXCLUDES *Autologuous fat graft (15771-15772)*
Implant replacement (19342)

22.4 22.4 FUD 090 J A2 50

AMA: 2019,Nov,14; 2018,Jan,8; 2017,Dec,13; 2017,Jan,8; 2016,Jan,13; 2015,Dec,18; 2015,Jan,16

19396 Preparation of moulage for custom breast implant

4.17 8.23 FUD 000 J G2 80 50

AMA: 2018,Jan,8; 2017,Jan,8; 2016,Jan,13; 2015,Jan,16

19499 Unlisted procedure, breast

0.00 0.00 FUD YYY J 80 50

AMA: 2019,Aug,10; 2019,Apr,10; 2018,Jan,8; 2017,Jan,8; 2016,Dec,16; 2016,Jan,13; 2015,Mar,5; 2015,Jan,16

20100-20103 Exploratory Surgery of Traumatic Wound

INCLUDES Debridement
Expanded dissection wound for exploration
Extraction foreign material
Open examination
Tying or coagulation small vessels

EXCLUDES *Cutaneous/subcutaneous incision and drainage procedures (10060-10061)*
Laparotomy (49000-49010)
Repair major vessels:
Abdomen (35221, 35251, 35281)
Chest (35211, 35216, 35241, 35246, 35271, 35276)
Extremity (35206-35207, 35226, 35236, 35256, 35266, 35286)
Neck (35201, 35231, 35261)
Thoracotomy (32100-32160)

20100 Exploration of penetrating wound (separate procedure); neck
17.4 17.4 **FUD** 010 T 80 50
AMA: 2018,Jan,8; 2017,Jan,8; 2016,Jan,13; 2015,Jan,16

20101 chest
6.10 13.7 **FUD** 010 T
AMA: 2018,Jan,8; 2017,Jan,8; 2016,Jan,13; 2015,Jan,16

20102 abdomen/flank/back
7.39 14.0 **FUD** 010 T
AMA: 2020,Jan,6; 2018,Jan,8; 2017,Jan,8; 2016,Jan,13; 2015,Jan,16

20103 extremity
10.0 16.5 **FUD** 010 T G2 80
AMA: 2018,Jan,8; 2017,Jan,8; 2016,Jan,13; 2015,Jan,16

20150 Epiphyseal Bar Resection

20150 Excision of epiphyseal bar, with or without autogenous soft tissue graft obtained through same fascial incision
29.0 29.0 **FUD** 090 J G2 80 50
AMA: 1996,Nov,1

20200-20206 Muscle Biopsy

EXCLUDES *Removal of muscle tumor (see appropriate anatomic section)*

20200 Biopsy, muscle; superficial
2.73 6.07 **FUD** 000 J A2

20205 deep
4.44 8.47 **FUD** 000 J A2

20206 Biopsy, muscle, percutaneous needle
EXCLUDES *Fine needle aspiration (10021, [10004, 10005, 10006, 10007, 10008, 10009, 10010, 10011, 10012])*
(76942, 77002, 77012, 77021)
(88172-88173)
1.67 6.76 **FUD** 000 J A2
AMA: 2019,Apr,4

20220-20225 Percutaneous Bone Biopsy

EXCLUDES *Bone marrow aspiration(s) or biopsy(ies) (38220-38222)*

20220 Biopsy, bone, trocar, or needle; superficial (eg, ilium, sternum, spinous process, ribs)
(77002, 77012, 77021)
2.55 7.04 **FUD** 000 J A2
AMA: 2018,Jan,8; 2017,Jan,8; 2016,Jan,13; 2015,Jan,16

20225 deep (eg, vertebral body, femur)
EXCLUDES *When performed at same level:*
Percutaneous vertebroplasty (22510-22515)
Percutaneous sacral augmentation (sacroplasty) (0200T-0201T)
(77002, 77012, 77021)
3.07 14.7 **FUD** 000 J A2
AMA: 2018,Jan,8; 2017,Jan,8; 2016,Jan,13; 2015,Jan,8; 2015,Jan,16

20240-20251 Open Bone Biopsy

EXCLUDES *Sequestrectomy or incision and drainage of bone abscess of:*
Calcaneus (28120)
Carpal bone (25145)
Clavicle (23170)
Humeral head (23174)
Humerus (24134)
Olecranon process (24138)
Radius (24136, 25145)
Scapula (23172)
Skull (61501)
Talus (28120)
Ulna (24138, 24145)

20240 Biopsy, bone, open; superficial (eg, sternum, spinous process, rib, patella, olecranon process, calcaneus, tarsal, metatarsal, carpal, metacarpal, phalanx)
4.21 4.21 **FUD** 000 J A2
AMA: 2018,Jan,8; 2017,Jan,8; 2016,Jan,13; 2015,Jan,16

20245 deep (eg, humeral shaft, ischium, femoral shaft)
10.1 10.1 **FUD** 000 J A2
AMA: 2018,Jan,8; 2017,Jan,8; 2016,Jan,13; 2015,Jan,16

20250 Biopsy, vertebral body, open; thoracic
11.3 11.3 **FUD** 010 J A2
AMA: 2018,Jan,8; 2017,Jan,8; 2016,Jan,13; 2015,Jan,16

20251 lumbar or cervical
12.4 12.4 **FUD** 010 J A2 80
AMA: 2018,Jan,8; 2017,Jan,8; 2016,Jan,13; 2015,Jan,16

20500-20501 Injection Fistula/Sinus Tract

EXCLUDES *Arthrography injection of:*
Ankle (27648)
Elbow (24220)
Hip (27093, 27095)
Sacroiliac joint (27096)
Shoulder (23350)
Temporomandibular joint (TMJ) (21116)
Wrist (25246)
Autologous adipose-derived regenerative cells injection (0489T-0490T)

20500 Injection of sinus tract; therapeutic (separate procedure)
(76080)
2.49 3.25 **FUD** 010 T P3

20501 diagnostic (sinogram)
EXCLUDES *Contrast injection or injections for radiological evaluation existing gastrostomy, duodenostomy, jejunostomy, gastro-jejunostomy, or cecostomy (or other colonic) tube from percutaneous approach (49465)*
(76080)
1.09 3.62 **FUD** 000 N N1

20520-20525 Foreign Body Removal

20520 Removal of foreign body in muscle or tendon sheath; simple
4.22 6.03 **FUD** 010 J P3

20525 deep or complicated
7.11 13.6 **FUD** 010 J A2

20526-20561 [20560, 20561] Therapeutic Injections: Tendons, Trigger Points

20526 Injection, therapeutic (eg, local anesthetic, corticosteroid), carpal tunnel
1.66 2.20 **FUD** 000 T P3 50
AMA: 2018,Jan,8; 2017,Jan,8; 2016,Jan,13; 2015,Jan,16

20527 Injection, enzyme (eg, collagenase), palmar fascial cord (ie, Dupuytren's contracture)
EXCLUDES *Post injection palmar fascial cord manipulation (26341)*
1.90 2.39 **FUD** 000 T P3 50
AMA: 2018,Jan,8; 2017,Jan,8; 2016,Jan,13; 2015,Jan,16

20550 **Injection(s); single tendon sheath, or ligament, aponeurosis (eg, plantar "fascia")**

EXCLUDES *Autologous WBC injection (0481T)*
Morton's neuroma (64455, 64632)
Platelet rich plasma injection (0232T)

(76942, 77002, 77021)

1.13 1.51 FUD 000 T P3 50

AMA: 2018,Jan,8; 2017,Jan,8; 2016,Jan,13; 2015,Jan,16

20551 **single tendon origin/insertion**

EXCLUDES *Autologous WBC injection (0481T)*
Platelet rich plasma injection (0232T)

(76942, 77002, 77021)

1.15 1.60 FUD 000 T P3

AMA: 2018,Jan,8; 2017,Dec,13; 2017,Jan,8; 2016,Jan,13; 2015,Jan,16

20552 **Injection(s); single or multiple trigger point(s), 1 or 2 muscle(s)**

EXCLUDES *Autologous WBC injection (0481T)*
Needle insertion(s) without injection(s) for same muscle(s) ([20560, 20561])
Platelet rich plasma injection (0232T)

(76942, 77002, 77021)

1.11 1.59 FUD 000 T P3

AMA: 2020,Feb,9; 2018,Jan,8; 2017,Dec,13; 2017,Jun,10; 2017,Jan,8; 2016,Jan,13; 2015,Jan,16

20553 **single or multiple trigger point(s), 3 or more muscles**

EXCLUDES *Needle insertion(s) without injection(s) for same muscle(s) ([20560, 20561])*

(76942, 77002, 77021)

1.25 1.82 FUD 000 T P3

AMA: 2020,Feb,9; 2018,Dec,8; 2018,Dec,8; 2018,Jan,8; 2017,Jun,10; 2017,Jan,8; 2016,Jan,13; 2015,Jan,16

\# **20560** **Needle insertion(s) without injection(s); 1 or 2 muscle(s)**

INCLUDES Dry needling and trigger-point acupuncture

0.47 0.74 FUD XXX

AMA: 2020,Feb,9

\# **20561** **3 or more muscles**

INCLUDES Dry needling and trigger-point acupuncture

0.71 1.10 FUD XXX

AMA: 2020,Feb,9

20555-20561 [20560, 20561] Placement of Catheters/Needles for Brachytherapy

Code also interstitial radioelement application (77770-77772, 77778)

20555 **Placement of needles or catheters into muscle and/or soft tissue for subsequent interstitial radioelement application (at the time of or subsequent to the procedure)**

EXCLUDES *Interstitial radioelement:*
Devices placed into breast (19296-19298)
Placement needle, catheters, or devices into muscle or soft tissue head and neck (41019)
Placement needles or catheters into pelvic organs or genitalia (55920)
Placement needles or catheters into prostate (55875)

(76942, 77002, 77012, 77021)

9.49 9.49 FUD 000 J A2 80

AMA: 2018,Jan,8; 2017,Jan,8; 2016,Jan,13; 2015,Jan,16

20560 **Resequenced code. See code following 20553.**

20561 **Resequenced code. See code before 20555.**

20600-20611 Aspiration and/or Injection of Joint

CMS: 100-03,150.7 Prolotherapy, Joint Sclerotherapy, and Ligamentous Injections with Sclerosing Agents

20600 **Arthrocentesis, aspiration and/or injection, small joint or bursa (eg, fingers, toes); without ultrasound guidance**

EXCLUDES *Autologous adipose-derived regenerative cells injection (0489T-0490T)*
Platelet rich plasma (PRP) injections (0232T)
Ultrasound guidance (76942)

(77002, 77012, 77021)

1.04 1.44 FUD 000 T P3 50

AMA: 2018,Sep,12; 2018,Jan,8; 2017,Aug,9; 2017,Jan,8; 2016,Jan,13; 2015,Nov,10; 2015,Feb,6; 2015,Jan,16

20604 **with ultrasound guidance, with permanent recording and reporting**

INCLUDES Ultrasound guidance (76942)

EXCLUDES *Autologous adipose-derived regenerative cells injection (0489T-0490T)*
Platelet rich plasma (PRP) injections (0232T)

(77002, 77012, 77021)

1.32 2.17 FUD 000 T P3 50

AMA: 2018,Sep,12; 2018,Jan,8; 2017,Jan,8; 2016,Jan,13; 2015,Jul,10; 2015,Feb,6

20605 **Arthrocentesis, aspiration and/or injection, intermediate joint or bursa (eg, temporomandibular, acromioclavicular, wrist, elbow or ankle, olecranon bursa); without ultrasound guidance**

EXCLUDES *Ultrasound guidance (76942)*

(77002, 77012, 77021)

1.08 1.49 FUD 000 T P3 50

AMA: 2018,Jan,8; 2017,Aug,9; 2017,Jan,8; 2016,Jan,13; 2015,Nov,10; 2015,Feb,6; 2015,Jan,16

20606 **with ultrasound guidance, with permanent recording and reporting**

INCLUDES Ultrasound guidance (76942)

EXCLUDES *Platelet rich plasma (PRP) injections (0232T)*

(77002, 77012, 77021)

1.53 2.32 FUD 000 T P3 50

AMA: 2018,Jan,8; 2017,Jan,8; 2016,Jan,13; 2015,Jul,10; 2015,Feb,6

20610 **Arthrocentesis, aspiration and/or injection, major joint or bursa (eg, shoulder, hip, knee, subacromial bursa); without ultrasound guidance**

EXCLUDES *Injection contrast for knee arthrography (27369)*
Platelet rich plasma (PRP) injections (0232T)
Ultrasound guidance (76942)

(77002, 77012, 77021)

1.32 1.77 FUD 000 T P3 50

AMA: 2019,Aug,7; 2018,Jan,8; 2017,Apr,9; 2017,Jan,8; 2016,Jan,13; 2015,Nov,10; 2015,Aug,6; 2015,Feb,6; 2015,Jan,16

20611 **with ultrasound guidance, with permanent recording and reporting**

INCLUDES Ultrasound guidance (76942)

EXCLUDES *Injection contrast for knee arthrography (27369)*
Platelet rich plasma (PRP) injections (0232T)

(77002, 77012, 77021)

1.75 2.61 FUD 000 T P3 50

AMA: 2019,Aug,7; 2018,Jan,8; 2017,Jan,8; 2016,Jan,13; 2015,Nov,10; 2015,Aug,6; 2015,Jul,10; 2015,Feb,6

20612-20615 Aspiration and/or Injection of Cyst

20612 **Aspiration and/or injection of ganglion cyst(s) any location**

Code also modifier 59 for multiple ganglion aspirations or injections

1.19 1.76 FUD 000 T P3

20615 **Aspiration and injection for treatment of bone cyst**

4.60 7.10 FUD 010 T P3

20650-20697 Procedures Related to Bony Fixation

20650 Insertion of wire or pin with application of skeletal traction, including removal (separate procedure)
4.54 6.08 FUD 010 J A2

20660 Application of cranial tongs, caliper, or stereotactic frame, including removal (separate procedure)
7.00 7.00 FUD 000 Q2
AMA: 2018,Jan,8; 2017,Jan,8; 2016,Jan,13; 2015,Jan,16

20661 Application of halo, including removal; cranial
14.4 14.4 FUD 090 C
AMA: 2018,Jan,8; 2017,Jan,8; 2016,Jan,13; 2015,Jan,16

20662 pelvic
14.8 14.8 FUD 090 J R2 80

20663 femoral
13.6 13.6 FUD 090 J R2 80 50

20664 Application of halo, including removal, cranial, 6 or more pins placed, for thin skull osteology (eg, pediatric patients, hydrocephalus, osteogenesis imperfecta)
25.0 25.0 FUD 090 C
AMA: 2018,Jan,8; 2017,Jan,8; 2016,Jan,13; 2015,Jan,16

20665 Removal of tongs or halo applied by another individual
2.65 3.13 FUD 010 Q1 G2 80
AMA: 2018,Jan,8; 2017,Jan,8; 2016,Jan,13; 2015,Jan,16

20670 Removal of implant; superficial (eg, buried wire, pin or rod) (separate procedure)
4.18 10.5 FUD 010 Q2 A2
AMA: 2018,Jan,3; 2018,Jan,8; 2017,Jan,8; 2016,Jan,13; 2015,Jan,16

20680 deep (eg, buried wire, pin, screw, metal band, nail, rod or plate)
EXCLUDES *Removal and reinsertion sinus tarsi implant ([0511T])*
Removal sinus tarsi implant ([0510T])
12.1 17.6 FUD 090 Q2 A2 80
AMA: 2018,Jan,3; 2018,Jan,8; 2017,Jan,8; 2016,Nov,9; 2016,Jan,13; 2015,Nov,10; 2015,Jan,16

20690 Application of a uniplane (pins or wires in 1 plane), unilateral, external fixation system
17.2 17.2 FUD 090 J J8
AMA: 2018,Jan,3; 2018,Jan,8; 2017,Jan,8; 2016,Jan,13; 2015,Jan,16

20692 Application of a multiplane (pins or wires in more than 1 plane), unilateral, external fixation system (eg, Ilizarov, Monticelli type)
32.2 32.2 FUD 090 J J8 80
AMA: 2019,May,10; 2018,Jan,8; 2018,Jan,3; 2017,Jan,8; 2016,Jan,13; 2015,Jan,16

20693 Adjustment or revision of external fixation system requiring anesthesia (eg, new pin[s] or wire[s] and/or new ring[s] or bar[s])
12.7 12.7 FUD 090 J A2
AMA: 2018,Jan,3; 2018,Jan,8; 2017,Jan,8; 2016,Jan,13; 2015,Jan,16

20694 Removal, under anesthesia, of external fixation system
9.72 12.2 FUD 090 Q2 A2
AMA: 2018,Jan,3; 2018,Jan,8; 2017,Jan,8; 2016,Jan,13; 2015,Jan,16

20696 Application of multiplane (pins or wires in more than 1 plane), unilateral, external fixation with stereotactic computer-assisted adjustment (eg, spatial frame), including imaging; initial and subsequent alignment(s), assessment(s), and computation(s) of adjustment schedule(s)
EXCLUDES *Application multiplane external fixation system (20692)*
Osteotomy with insertion intramedullary lengthening device, humerus (0594T)
Removal and replacement each strut (20697)
34.4 34.4 FUD 090 J J8 80
AMA: 2018,Jan,3; 2018,Jan,8; 2017,Jan,8; 2016,Jan,13; 2015,Jan,16

20697 exchange (ie, removal and replacement) of strut, each
EXCLUDES *Application multiplane external fixation system (20692)*
Exchange strut for multiplane external fixation system (20697)
58.9 58.9 FUD 000 ⊘ J P2 80 TC
AMA: 2018,Jan,3; 2018,Jan,8; 2017,Jan,8; 2016,Jan,13; 2015,Jan,16

20700-20705 Drug Delivery Device

\+ **20700 Manual preparation and insertion of drug-delivery device(s), deep (eg, subfascial) (List separately in addition to code for primary procedure)**
INCLUDES Combining therapeutic agents, including antibiotics, with carrier substance during operative episode
Forming resulting mixture into drug delivery devices (beads, nails, spacers)
Insertion therapeutic device/agent once per anatomic location
EXCLUDES *Insertion drug delivery implant, non-biodegradable (11981)*
Insertion prefabricated drug device
Code first (11010-11012, 11043, [11046], 11044, 11047, 20240-20251, 21010, 21025-21026, 21501-21510, 21627-21630, 22010-22015, 23030-23044, 23170-23184, 23334-23335, 23930-24000, 24134-24140, 24147, 24160, 25031-25040, 25145-25151, 26070, 26230-26236, 26990-26992, 27030, 27070-27071, 27090, 27301-27303, 27310, 27360, 27603-27604, 27610, 27640-27641, 28001-28003, 28020, 28120-28122)
2.44 2.44 FUD ZZZ 80

\+ **20701 Removal of drug-delivery device(s), deep (eg, subfascial) (List separately in addition to code for primary procedure)**
INCLUDES Removal therapeutic device/agent once per anatomic location from subfascial tissues
EXCLUDES *Removal drug delivery device, performed alone (20680)*
Removal drug delivery implant, non-biodegradable (11982)
Code first (11010-11012, 11043, [11046], 11044, 11047, 20240-20251, 21010, 21025-21026, 21501-21510, 21627-21630, 22010-22015, 23030-23044, 23170-23184, 23334-23335, 23930-24000, 24134-24140, 24147, 24160, 25031-25040, 25145-25151, 26070, 26230-26236, 26990-26992, 27030, 27070-27071, 27090, 27301-27303, 27310, 27360, 27603-27604, 27610, 27640-27641, 28001-28003, 28020, 28120-28122)
1.82 1.82 FUD ZZZ 80

Musculoskeletal System

20650 — 20701

\+ **20702** **Manual preparation and insertion of drug-delivery device(s), intramedullary (List separately in addition to code for primary procedure)**

INCLUDES Combining therapeutic agents, including antibiotics, with carrier substance during operative episode
Forming resulting mixture into drug delivery devices (beads, nails, spacers)
Insertion therapeutic device/agent once per anatomic location into intramedullary spaces

EXCLUDES *Insertion drug delivery implant, non-biodegradable (11981)*
Insertion prefabricated drug device

Code first (20680-20692, 20694, 20802-20805, 20838, 21510, 23035, 23170, 23180, 23184, 23515, 23615, 23935, 24134, 24138-24140, 24147, 24430, 24516, 25035, 25145-25151, 25400, 25515, 25525-25526, 25545, 25574-25575, 27245, 27259, 27360, 27470, 27506, 27640, 27720)

4.06 4.06 **FUD** ZZZ 80

\+ **20703** **Removal of drug-delivery device(s), intramedullary (List separately in addition to code for primary procedure)**

INCLUDES Removal therapeutic device/agent once per anatomic location from intramedullary spaces

EXCLUDES *Removal drug delivery device, performed alone (20680)*
Removal drug delivery implant, non-biodegradable (11982)

Code first (20690-20692, 20694, 20802-20805, 20838, 21510, 23035, 23170, 23180, 23184, 23515, 23615, 23935, 24134, 24138-24140, 24147, 24430, 24516, 25035, 25145-25151, 25400, 25515, 25525-25526, 25545, 25574-25575, 27245, 27259, 27360, 27470, 27506, 27640, 27720)

2.91 2.91 **FUD** ZZZ 80

\+ **20704** **Manual preparation and insertion of drug-delivery device(s), intra-articular (List separately in addition to code for primary procedure)**

INCLUDES Combining therapeutic agents, including antibiotics, with carrier substance during operative episode
Forming resulting mixture into drug delivery devices (beads, nails, spacers)
Insertion therapeutic device/agent once per anatomic location into intra-articular spaces

EXCLUDES *Insertion drug delivery implant, non-biodegradable (11981)*
Insertion prefabricated drug device
Removal hip prosthesis (27091)
Removal knee prosthesis (27488)

Code first (22864-22865, 23040-23044, 23334, 24000, 24160, 25040, 25250-25251, 26070-26080, 26990, 27030, 27090, 27301, 27310, 27603, 27610, 28020)

4.23 4.23 **FUD** ZZZ 80

\+ **20705** **Removal of drug-delivery device(s), intra-articular (List separately in addition to code for primary procedure)**

INCLUDES Removal therapeutic device/agent once per anatomic location from intra-articular space(s)

EXCLUDES *Open treatment femoral neck fracture/internal fixation or prosthetic replacement (27236)*
Partial knee replacement (27446)
Partial or total hip replacement (27125-27130)
Patella arthroplasty with prosthesis (27438)
Removal drug delivery device, performed alone (20680)
Removal drug delivery implant, non-biodegradable (11982)
Removal hip prosthesis (27091)
Removal knee prosthesis (27488)
Removal shoulder prosthesis (23335)
Revision hip arthroplasty (27134-27138)
Revision knee arthroplasty (27486-27487)

Code first (22864-22865, 23040-23044, 23334, 24000, 24160, 25040, 25250-25251, 26070-26080, 26990, 27030, 27090, 27301, 27310, 27603, 27610, 28020)

3.48 3.48 **FUD** ZZZ 80

20802-20838 Reimplantation Procedures

EXCLUDES *Repair incomplete amputation (see individual repair codes for bone(s), ligament(s), tendon(s), nerve(s), or blood vessel(s) and append modifier 52)*

20802 **Replantation, arm (includes surgical neck of humerus through elbow joint), complete amputation**

79.5 79.5 **FUD** 090 C 80 50

AMA: 1997,Apr,4

20805 **Replantation, forearm (includes radius and ulna to radial carpal joint), complete amputation**

94.7 94.7 **FUD** 090 C 80 50

AMA: 1997,Apr,4

20808 **Replantation, hand (includes hand through metacarpophalangeal joints), complete amputation**

114. 114. **FUD** 090 C 80 50

AMA: 1997,Apr,4

20816 **Replantation, digit, excluding thumb (includes metacarpophalangeal joint to insertion of flexor sublimis tendon), complete amputation**

59.5 59.5 **FUD** 090 C 80

AMA: 2018,Jan,8; 2017,Jan,8; 2016,Jan,13; 2015,Jan,16

20822 **Replantation, digit, excluding thumb (includes distal tip to sublimis tendon insertion), complete amputation**

51.2 51.2 **FUD** 090 J G2 80

AMA: 1997,Apr,4

20824 **Replantation, thumb (includes carpometacarpal joint to MP joint), complete amputation**

59.7 59.7 **FUD** 090 C 80 50

AMA: 1997,Apr,4

20827 **Replantation, thumb (includes distal tip to MP joint), complete amputation**

52.6 52.6 **FUD** 090 C 80 50

AMA: 1997,Apr,4

20838 **Replantation, foot, complete amputation**

80.6 80.6 **FUD** 090 C 80 50

AMA: 1997,Apr,4

20900-20924 Bone and Tissue Autografts

EXCLUDES *Acquisition autogenous bone, bone marrow, cartilage, tendon, fascia lata or other grafts through distinct incision unless included in code description*
Autologous fat graft obtained by liposuction (15771-15774)
Bone graft procedures on spine (20930-20938)
Other autologous soft tissue grafts (fat, dermis, fascia) harvested by direct excision ([15769])

20900 **Bone graft, any donor area; minor or small (eg, dowel or button)**

5.33 11.6 **FUD** 000 J A2 80

AMA: 2020,May,13; 2018,Jul,14; 2018,Jan,8; 2017,Jan,8; 2016,Jan,13; 2015,Jan,16

20902 **major or large**

8.20 8.20 **FUD** 000 J A2 80

AMA: 2020,May,13; 2018,Jul,14; 2018,Jan,8; 2017,Jan,8; 2016,Jan,13; 2015,Jan,16

20910 **Cartilage graft; costochondral**

EXCLUDES *Graft with ear cartilage (21235)*

13.5 13.5 **FUD** 090 T A2 80

AMA: 2020,May,13; 2018,Jul,14; 2018,Jan,8; 2017,Jan,8; 2016,Jan,13; 2015,Jan,16

20912 **nasal septum**

EXCLUDES *Graft with ear cartilage (21235)*

13.6 13.6 **FUD** 090 T A2 80

AMA: 2020,May,13; 2018,Jul,14

20920 **Fascia lata graft; by stripper**

11.3 11.3 **FUD** 090 T A2

AMA: 2020,May,13; 2018,Jul,14; 2018,Jan,8; 2017,Jan,8; 2016,Jan,13; 2015,Jan,16

20922 **by incision and area exposure, complex or sheet**
13.9 17.0 FUD 090 T A2 80
AMA: 2020,May,13; 2018,Jul,14; 2018,Jan,8; 2017,Jan,8; 2016,Jan,13; 2015,Jan,16

20924 **Tendon graft, from a distance (eg, palmaris, toe extensor, plantaris)**
14.6 14.6 FUD 090 J A2 80
AMA: 2020,May,13; 2018,Jul,14

20930-20939 Bone Allograft and Autograft of Spine

EXCLUDES *Acquisition autogenous bone, bone marrow, cartilage, tendon, fascia lata, or other grafts through distinct incision unless included in code description*
Autologous fat graft obtained by liposuction (15771-15774)
Other autologous soft tissue grafts (fat, dermis, fascia) harvested by direct excision ([15769])

\+ 20930 **Allograft, morselized, or placement of osteopromotive material, for spine surgery only (List separately in addition to code for primary procedure)**
Code first (22319, 22532-22533, 22548-22558, 22590-22612, 22630, 22633-22634, 22800-22812)
0.00 0.00 FUD XXX N N1
AMA: 2020,May,13; 2019,May,7; 2018,Jul,14; 2018,Jan,8; 2017,Mar,7; 2017,Jan,8; 2016,Jan,13; 2015,Jan,16

\+ 20931 **Allograft, structural, for spine surgery only (List separately in addition to code for primary procedure)**
Code first (22319, 22532-22533, 22548-22558, 22590-22612, 22630, 22633-22634, 22800-22812)
3.26 3.26 FUD ZZZ N N1
AMA: 2020,May,13; 2019,May,7; 2018,Jul,14; 2018,Jan,8; 2017,Mar,7; 2017,Jan,8; 2016,Jan,13; 2015,Jan,16

\+ 20932 **Allograft, includes templating, cutting, placement and internal fixation, when performed; osteoarticular, including articular surface and contiguous bone (List separately in addition to code for primary procedure)**
EXCLUDES *Allograft, intercalary (20933-20934)*
Injection contrast for ankle arthrography (27648)
Osteotomy, femur (27448)
Radical resection tumor:
Clavicle (23200)
Fibula (27646)
Ischial tuberosity/greater trochanter femur (27078)
Radial head or neck (24152)
Talus or calcaneus (27647)
Removal hip prosthesis (27090-27091)
Code also insertion joint prosthesis
Code first (23210, 23220, 24150, 25170, 27075-27077, 27365, 27645, 27704)
20.6 20.6 FUD ZZZ N1 80
AMA: 2020,May,13; 2019,May,7

\+ 20933 **hemicortical intercalary, partial (ie, hemicylindrical) (List separately in addition to code for primary procedure)**
EXCLUDES *Allograft, intercalary, complete (20934)*
Allograft, osteoarticular (20932)
Arthroplasty procedures, hip (27130, 27132, 27134, 27138)
Bone graft (20955-20957, 20962)
Excision cyst with allograft (23146, 23156, 24116, 24126, 25126, 25136, 27356, 27638, 28103, 28107)
Injection contrast for ankle arthrography (27648)
Open treatment femoral fractures (27236, 27244)
Osteotomy, femur (27448)
Radical resection tumor:
Clavicle (23200)
Fibula (27646)
Ischial tuberosity/greater trochanter femur (27078)
Radial head or neck (24152)
Talus or calcaneus (27647)
Removal hip prosthesis (27090-27091)
Code also insertion joint prosthesis
Code first (23210, 23220, 24150, 25170, 27075-27077, 27365, 27645, 27704)
18.9 18.9 FUD ZZZ N1 80
AMA: 2020,May,13; 2019,May,7

\+ 20934 **intercalary, complete (ie, cylindrical) (List separately in addition to code for primary procedure)**
Allograft, intercalary, partial (20933)
Allograft, osteoarticular (20932)
Excision cyst with allograft (23146, 23156)
Injection contrast for ankle arthrography (27648)
Osteotomy, femur (27448)
Radical resection tumor:
Clavicle (23200)
Fibula (27646)
Ischial tuberosity/greater trochanter femur (27078)
Radial head or neck (24152)
Talus or calcaneus (27647)
Removal hip prosthesis (27090-27091)
Code also insertion joint prosthesis
Code first (23210, 23220, 24150, 25170, 27075-27077, 27365, 27645, 27704)
20.6 20.6 FUD ZZZ N1 80
AMA: 2020,May,13; 2019,May,7

\+ 20936 **Autograft for spine surgery only (includes harvesting the graft); local (eg, ribs, spinous process, or laminar fragments) obtained from same incision (List separately in addition to code for primary procedure)**
Code first (22319, 22532-22533, 22548-22558, 22590-22612, 22630, 22633-22634, 22800-22812)
0.00 0.00 FUD XXX N N1
AMA: 2020,May,13; 2018,Jul,14; 2018,Jan,8; 2017,Mar,7; 2017,Jan,8; 2016,Jan,13; 2015,Jan,16

\+ 20937 **morselized (through separate skin or fascial incision) (List separately in addition to code for primary procedure)**
Code first (22319, 22532-22533, 22548-22558, 22590-22612, 22630, 22633-22634, 22800-22812)
4.85 4.85 FUD ZZZ N N1 80
AMA: 2020,May,13; 2018,Jul,14; 2018,Jan,8; 2017,Mar,7; 2017,Jan,8; 2016,Jan,13; 2015,Jan,16

\+ 20938 **structural, bicortical or tricortical (through separate skin or fascial incision) (List separately in addition to code for primary procedure)**
EXCLUDES *Bone marrow for bone grafting in spinal surgery (20939)*
Code first (22319, 22532-22533, 22548-22558, 22590-22612, 22630, 22633-22634, 22800-22812)
5.34 5.34 FUD ZZZ N N1 80
AMA: 2020,May,13; 2018,Jul,14; 2018,Jan,8; 2017,Mar,7; 2017,Jan,8; 2016,Jan,13; 2015,Jan,16

+ **20939 Bone marrow aspiration for bone grafting, spine surgery only, through separate skin or fascial incision (List separately in addition to code for primary procedure)**

EXCLUDES *Bone marrow aspiration for other than bone grafting in spinal surgery (20999)*
Diagnostic bone marrow aspiration (38220, 38222)
Platelet rich plasma injection (0232T)
Reporting with modifier 50. Report once for each side when performed bilaterally

Code first (22319, 22532-22534, 22548, 22551-22552, 22554, 22556, 22558, 22590, 22595, 22600, 22610, 22612, 22630, 22633-22634, 22800, 22802, 22804, 22808, 22810, 22812)

2.03 | 2.03 | **FUD** ZZZ | N N1 80 50

AMA: 2018,May,3

20950 Measurement of Intracompartmental Pressure

20950 Monitoring of interstitial fluid pressure (includes insertion of device, eg, wick catheter technique, needle manometer technique) in detection of muscle compartment syndrome

2.56 | 7.43 | **FUD** 000 | T G2 80

AMA: 2018,Jan,8; 2017,Jan,8; 2016,Jan,13; 2015,Jan,16

20955-20973 Bone and Osteocutaneous Grafts

INCLUDES Operating microscope (69990)

20955 Bone graft with microvascular anastomosis; fibula

70.9 | 70.9 | **FUD** 090 | C 80

AMA: 2019,Dec,5; 2019,May,7; 2018,Jan,8; 2017,Jan,8; 2016,Feb,12; 2016,Jan,13; 2015,Jan,16

20956 iliac crest

76.6 | 76.6 | **FUD** 090 | C 80

AMA: 2019,Dec,5; 2019,May,7; 2018,Jan,8; 2017,Jan,8; 2016,Feb,12; 2016,Jan,13; 2015,Jan,16

20957 metatarsal

79.6 | 79.6 | **FUD** 090 | C 80

AMA: 2019,Dec,5; 2019,May,7; 2018,Jan,8; 2017,Jan,8; 2016,Feb,12; 2016,Jan,13; 2015,Jan,16

20962 other than fibula, iliac crest, or metatarsal

76.9 | 76.9 | **FUD** 090 | C 80

AMA: 2019,Dec,5; 2019,May,7; 2016,Feb,12

20969 Free osteocutaneous flap with microvascular anastomosis; other than iliac crest, metatarsal, or great toe

78.6 | 78.6 | **FUD** 090 | C 80

AMA: 2019,Dec,5; 2019,Oct,10; 2018,Jan,8; 2017,Jan,8; 2016,Feb,12; 2016,Jan,13; 2015,Jan,16

20970 iliac crest

82.6 | 82.6 | **FUD** 090 | C 80

AMA: 2019,Dec,5; 2018,Jan,8; 2017,Jan,8; 2016,Feb,12; 2016,Jan,13; 2015,Jan,16

20972 metatarsal

82.4 | 82.4 | **FUD** 090 | J G2 80

AMA: 2019,Dec,5; 2018,Jan,8; 2017,Jan,8; 2016,Feb,12; 2016,Jan,13; 2015,Jan,16

20973 great toe with web space

EXCLUDES *Great toe wrap-around with bone graft (26551)*

87.0 | 87.0 | **FUD** 090 | J R2 80 50

AMA: 2019,Dec,5; 2018,Jan,8; 2017,Jan,8; 2016,Feb,12; 2016,Jan,13; 2015,Jan,16

20974-20979 Osteogenic Stimulation

CMS: 100-03,150.2 Osteogenic Stimulation

20974 Electrical stimulation to aid bone healing; noninvasive (nonoperative)

1.45 | 2.26 | **FUD** 000 | ⊘ A

AMA: 2018,Jan,8; 2017,Jan,8; 2016,Jan,13; 2015,Jan,16

20975 invasive (operative)

5.18 | 5.18 | **FUD** 000 | ⊘ N N1 80

AMA: 2002,Apr,13; 2000,Nov,8

20979 Low intensity ultrasound stimulation to aid bone healing, noninvasive (nonoperative)

0.93 | 1.53 | **FUD** 000 | Q1 N1

AMA: 2018,Jan,8; 2017,Jan,8; 2016,Jan,13; 2015,Jan,16

20982-20999 General Musculoskeletal Procedures

20982 Ablation therapy for reduction or eradication of 1 or more bone tumors (eg, metastasis) including adjacent soft tissue when involved by tumor extension, percutaneous, including imaging guidance when performed; radiofrequency

EXCLUDES *Radiologic guidance (76940, 77002, 77013, 77022)*

10.5 | 110. | **FUD** 000 | J G2 50

AMA: 2018,Jan,8; 2017,Jan,8; 2016,Jan,13; 2015,Sep,12; 2015,Jul,8

20983 cryoablation

EXCLUDES *Radiologic guidance (76940, 77002, 77013, 77022)*

10.1 | 163. | **FUD** 000 | J J8 50

AMA: 2018,Jan,8; 2017,Jan,8; 2016,Jan,13; 2015,Jul,8

+ **20985 Computer-assisted surgical navigational procedure for musculoskeletal procedures, image-less (List separately in addition to code for primary procedure)**

EXCLUDES *Image guidance derived from intraoperative and preoperative obtained images (0054T-0055T)*
Stereotactic computer-assisted navigational procedure; cranial or intradural (61781-61783)

Code first primary procedure

4.24 | 4.24 | **FUD** ZZZ | N N1 80

AMA: 2018,Jan,8; 2017,Jan,8; 2016,Jan,13; 2015,Jan,16

20999 Unlisted procedure, musculoskeletal system, general

0.00 | 0.00 | **FUD** YYY | T 80

AMA: 2018,May,3; 2018,Jan,8; 2017,Jan,8; 2016,Jan,13; 2015,Jul,8; 2015,Jan,16

21010 Temporomandibular Joint Arthrotomy

21010 Arthrotomy, temporomandibular joint

EXCLUDES *Cutaneous/subcutaneous abscess and hematoma drainage (10060-10061)*
Excision foreign body from dentoalveolar site (41805-41806)

22.0 | 22.0 | **FUD** 090 | J A2 80 50

AMA: 2002,Apr,13

21011-21016 Excision Soft Tissue Tumors Face and Scalp

INCLUDES Any necessary elevation tissue planes or dissection
Measurement tumor and necessary margin at greatest diameter prior to excision
Simple and intermediate repairs
Excision types:
- Fascial or subfascial soft tissue tumors: simple and marginal resection tumors found either in or below deep fascia, not including bone or excision substantial amount normal tissue; primarily benign and intramuscular tumors
- Radical resection soft tissue tumor: wide resection tumor involving substantial margins normal tissue and may include tissue removal from one or more layers; most often malignant or aggressive benign
- Subcutaneous: simple and marginal resection tumors in subcutaneous tissue above deep fascia; most often benign

EXCLUDES *Complex repair*
Excision benign cutaneous lesions (eg, sebaceous cyst) (11420-11426)
Radical resection cutaneous tumors (eg, melanoma) (11620-11646)
Significant vessel exploration or neuroplasty

21011 Excision, tumor, soft tissue of face or scalp, subcutaneous; less than 2 cm

7.38 | 10.3 | **FUD** 090 | J P3 80

AMA: 2018,Sep,7; 2018,Jan,8; 2017,Jan,8; 2016,Jan,13; 2015,Jan,16

21012 2 cm or greater

9.72 | 9.72 | **FUD** 090 | J R2 80

AMA: 2018,Sep,7; 2018,Jan,8; 2017,Jan,8; 2016,Jan,13; 2015,Jan,16

21013 **Excision, tumor, soft tissue of face and scalp, subfascial (eg, subgaleal, intramuscular); less than 2 cm**
11.5 15.1 FUD 090 J P3 80
AMA: 2018,Sep,7; 2018,Jan,8; 2017,Jan,8; 2016,Jan,13; 2015,Jan,16

21014 **2 cm or greater**
15.0 15.0 FUD 090 J R2 80
AMA: 2018,Sep,7; 2018,Jan,8; 2017,Jan,8; 2016,Jan,13; 2015,Jan,16

21015 **Radical resection of tumor (eg, sarcoma), soft tissue of face or scalp; less than 2 cm**
EXCLUDES *Removal of cranial tumor for osteomyelitis (61501)*
20.3 20.3 FUD 090 J G2
AMA: 2018,Sep,7; 2018,Jan,8; 2017,Jan,8; 2016,Jan,13; 2015,Jan,16

21016 **2 cm or greater**
29.0 29.0 FUD 090 J G2 80
AMA: 2018,Sep,7; 2018,Jan,8; 2017,Jan,8; 2016,Jan,13; 2015,Jan,16

21025-21070 Procedures of Cranial and Facial Bones

INCLUDES Any necessary elevation tissue planes or dissection
Measurement tumor and necessary margins prior to excision
Radical resection bone tumor involves resection tumor (may include entire bone) and wide margins normal tissue primarily for malignant or aggressive benign tumors
Simple and intermediate repairs

EXCLUDES *Complex repair*
Excision soft tissue tumors, face and scalp (21011-21016)
Radical resection cutaneous tumors (e.g., melanoma) (11620-11646)
Significant vessel exploration, neuroplasty, reconstruction, or complex bone repair

21025 **Excision of bone (eg, for osteomyelitis or bone abscess); mandible**
19.9 23.6 FUD 090 J A2
AMA: 2018,Sep,7; 2018,Jan,8; 2017,Jan,8; 2016,Jan,13; 2015,Jan,16

21026 **facial bone(s)**
12.9 16.0 FUD 090 J A2
AMA: 2018,Sep,7

21029 **Removal by contouring of benign tumor of facial bone (eg, fibrous dysplasia)**
17.9 21.8 FUD 090 J A2 80
AMA: 2018,Sep,7

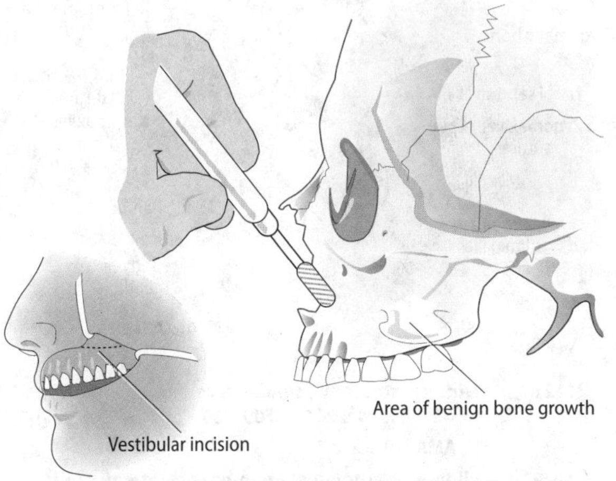

21030 **Excision of benign tumor or cyst of maxilla or zygoma by enucleation and curettage**
11.1 14.0 FUD 090 J P3 50
AMA: 2018,Sep,7; 2018,Jan,8; 2017,Jan,8; 2016,Jan,13; 2015,Jan,16

21031 **Excision of torus mandibularis**
8.03 11.1 FUD 090 J P3 50
AMA: 2018,Sep,7

21032 **Excision of maxillary torus palatinus**
8.21 11.3 FUD 090 J P3
AMA: 2018,Sep,7

21034 **Excision of malignant tumor of maxilla or zygoma**
33.0 37.5 FUD 090 J A2 80
AMA: 2018,Sep,7; 2018,Jan,8; 2017,Jan,8; 2016,Jan,13; 2015,Jan,16

21040 **Excision of benign tumor or cyst of mandible, by enucleation and/or curettage**
INCLUDES Removal benign tumor or cyst without osteotomy
EXCLUDES *Removal benign tumor or cyst with osteotomy (21046-21047)*
11.1 14.1 FUD 090 J A2
AMA: 2018,Sep,7; 2018,Jan,8; 2017,Jan,8; 2016,Jan,13; 2015,Jan,16

21044 **Excision of malignant tumor of mandible;**
25.0 25.0 FUD 090 J A2 80
AMA: 2018,Sep,7

21045 **radical resection**
Code also bone graft procedure (21215)
34.6 34.6 FUD 090 C 80
AMA: 2018,Sep,7

21046 **Excision of benign tumor or cyst of mandible; requiring intra-oral osteotomy (eg, locally aggressive or destructive lesion[s])**
30.0 30.0 FUD 090 J A2 80
AMA: 2018,Sep,7; 2018,Jan,8; 2017,Jan,8; 2016,Jan,13; 2015,Jan,16

21047 **requiring extra-oral osteotomy and partial mandibulectomy (eg, locally aggressive or destructive lesion[s])**
36.7 36.7 FUD 090 J A2 80
AMA: 2018,Sep,7; 2018,Jan,8; 2017,Jan,8; 2016,Jan,13; 2015,Jan,16

21048 **Excision of benign tumor or cyst of maxilla; requiring intra-oral osteotomy (eg, locally aggressive or destructive lesion[s])**
30.5 30.5 FUD 090 J R2 80
AMA: 2018,Sep,7; 2018,Jan,8; 2017,Jan,8; 2016,Jan,13; 2015,Jan,16

21049 **requiring extra-oral osteotomy and partial maxillectomy (eg, locally aggressive or destructive lesion[s])**
34.6 34.6 FUD 090 J 80
AMA: 2018,Sep,7; 2018,Jan,8; 2017,Jan,8; 2016,Jan,13; 2015,Jan,16

21050 **Condylectomy, temporomandibular joint (separate procedure)**
25.2 25.2 FUD 090 J A2 80 50
AMA: 2018,Sep,7

21060 **Meniscectomy, partial or complete, temporomandibular joint (separate procedure)**
22.9 22.9 FUD 090 J A2 80 50
AMA: 2018,Sep,7

21070 **Coronoidectomy (separate procedure)**
18.3 18.3 FUD 090 J A2 80 50
AMA: 2018,Sep,7

21073 Temporomandibular Joint Manipulation with Anesthesia

21073 **Manipulation of temporomandibular joint(s) (TMJ), therapeutic, requiring an anesthesia service (ie, general or monitored anesthesia care)**

EXCLUDES *Closed treatment TMJ dislocation (21480, 21485)*
Manipulation TMJ without general or MAC anesthesia (97140, 98925-98929, 98943)

7.19 10.9 **FUD** 090 T P3 80 50

AMA: 2018,Sep,7; 2018,Jan,8; 2018,Jan,3; 2017,Jan,8; 2016,Jan,13; 2015,Jan,16

21076-21089 Medical Impressions for Fabrication Maxillofacial Prosthesis

INCLUDES Design, preparation, and professional services rendered by physician or other qualified health care professional

EXCLUDES *Application or removal caliper or tongs (20660, 20665)*
Professional services rendered for outside laboratory designed and prepared prosthesis

21076 **Impression and custom preparation; surgical obturator prosthesis**
23.1 27.6 **FUD** 010 T P3 80
AMA: 2018,Sep,7; 2018,Jan,8; 2017,Jan,8; 2016,Jan,13; 2015,Jan,16

21077 **orbital prosthesis**
53.4 64.0 **FUD** 090 J P3 80 50
AMA: 2018,Sep,7; 2018,Jan,8; 2017,Jan,8; 2016,Jan,13; 2015,Jan,16

21079 **interim obturator prosthesis**
35.8 43.5 **FUD** 090 J P3
AMA: 2018,Sep,7; 2018,Jan,8; 2017,Jan,8; 2016,Jan,13; 2015,Jan,16

21080 **definitive obturator prosthesis**
40.4 49.8 **FUD** 090 J P3
AMA: 2018,Sep,7; 2018,Jan,8; 2017,Jan,8; 2016,Jan,13; 2015,Jan,16

21081 **mandibular resection prosthesis**
37.0 45.7 **FUD** 090 J P3 80
AMA: 2018,Sep,7; 2018,Jan,8; 2017,Jan,8; 2016,Jan,13; 2015,Jan,16

21082 **palatal augmentation prosthesis**
34.0 42.4 **FUD** 090 J P3 80
AMA: 2018,Sep,7; 2018,Jan,8; 2017,Jan,8; 2016,Jan,13; 2015,Jan,16

21083 **palatal lift prosthesis**
31.6 40.4 **FUD** 090 J P3 80
AMA: 2018,Sep,7; 2018,Jan,8; 2017,Jan,8; 2016,Jan,13; 2015,Jan,16

21084 **speech aid prosthesis**
36.5 46.2 **FUD** 090 J P3 80
AMA: 2018,Sep,7; 2018,Jan,8; 2017,Jan,8; 2016,Jan,13; 2015,Jan,16

21085 **oral surgical splint**
15.7 21.0 **FUD** 010 T P2 80
AMA: 2018,Sep,7; 2018,Jan,8; 2017,Sep,14; 2017,Jan,8; 2016,Jan,13; 2015,Jan,16

21086 **auricular prosthesis**
39.4 47.6 **FUD** 090 J P3 80 50
AMA: 2018,Sep,7; 2018,Jan,8; 2017,Jan,8; 2016,Jan,13; 2015,Jan,16

21087 **nasal prosthesis**
42.7 51.1 **FUD** 090 J P3 80
AMA: 2018,Sep,7; 2018,Jan,8; 2017,Jan,8; 2016,Jan,13; 2015,Jan,16

21088 **facial prosthesis**
0.00 0.00 **FUD** 090 J R2 80
AMA: 2018,Sep,7; 2018,Jan,8; 2017,Jan,8; 2016,Jan,13; 2015,Jan,16

21089 **Unlisted maxillofacial prosthetic procedure**
0.00 0.00 **FUD** YYY T
AMA: 2018,Sep,7; 2018,Jan,8; 2017,Jan,8; 2016,Jan,13; 2015,Jan,16

21100-21110 Application Fixation Device

21100 **Application of halo type appliance for maxillofacial fixation, includes removal (separate procedure)**
10.6 18.9 **FUD** 090 J A2 80
AMA: 2018,Sep,7

21110 **Application of interdental fixation device for conditions other than fracture or dislocation, includes removal**

EXCLUDES *Interdental fixation device removal by different provider (20670-20680)*

19.5 23.3 **FUD** 090 02 P2
AMA: 2018,Sep,7; 2018,Jan,8; 2017,Jan,8; 2016,Jan,13; 2015,Jan,16

21116 Injection for TMJ Arthrogram

CMS: 100-02,15,150.1 Treatment of Temporomandibular Joint (TMJ) Syndrome; 100-04,13,80.1 Physician Presence; 100-04,13,80.2 S&I Multiple Procedure Reduction

21116 **Injection procedure for temporomandibular joint arthrography**
(70332)
1.34 5.62 **FUD** 000 N N1 50
AMA: 2018,Sep,7; 2018,Jan,8; 2017,Jan,8; 2016,May,13; 2016,Jan,13; 2015,Aug,6

21120-21299 Repair/Reconstruction Craniofacial Bones

EXCLUDES *Cranioplasty (21179-21180, 62120, 62140-62147)*

21120 **Genioplasty; augmentation (autograft, allograft, prosthetic material)**
15.0 19.2 **FUD** 090 J G2
AMA: 2018,Sep,7

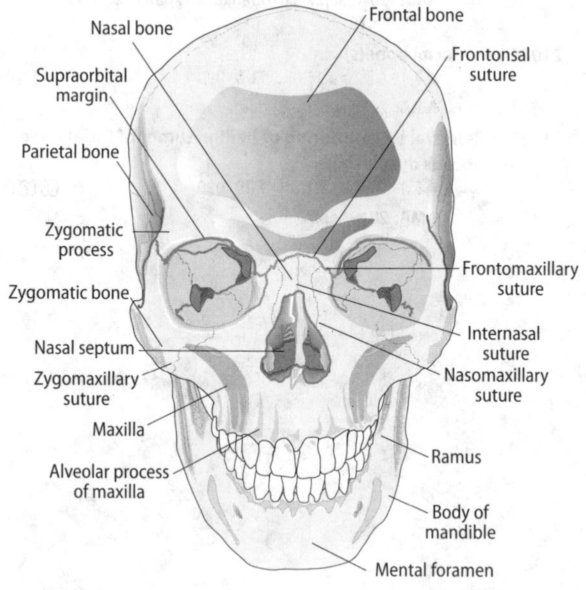

21121 **sliding osteotomy, single piece**
17.8 20.9 **FUD** 090 J A2 80
AMA: 2018,Sep,7

21122 **sliding osteotomies, 2 or more osteotomies (eg, wedge excision or bone wedge reversal for asymmetrical chin)**
22.1 22.1 **FUD** 090 J A2 80
AMA: 2018,Sep,7

21123 **sliding, augmentation with interpositional bone grafts (includes obtaining autografts)**
26.1 26.1 **FUD** 090 J A2 80
AMA: 2018,Sep,7

21125 Augmentation, mandibular body or angle; prosthetic material
19.8 80.8 FUD 090 J A2 80
AMA: 2018,Sep,7

21127 with bone graft, onlay or interpositional (includes obtaining autograft)
24.6 112. FUD 090 J A2 80
AMA: 2018,Sep,7

21137 Reduction forehead; contouring only
21.7 21.7 FUD 090 J G2 80
AMA: 2018,Sep,7

21138 contouring and application of prosthetic material or bone graft (includes obtaining autograft)
26.5 26.5 FUD 090 J G2 80
AMA: 2018,Sep,7

21139 contouring and setback of anterior frontal sinus wall
32.0 32.0 FUD 090 J G2 80
AMA: 2018,Sep,7

21141 Reconstruction midface, LeFort I; single piece, segment movement in any direction (eg, for Long Face Syndrome), without bone graft
39.4 39.4 FUD 090 C 80
AMA: 2018,Sep,7

21142 2 pieces, segment movement in any direction, without bone graft
40.5 40.5 FUD 090 C 80
AMA: 2018,Sep,7

21143 3 or more pieces, segment movement in any direction, without bone graft
41.0 41.0 FUD 090 C 80
AMA: 2018,Sep,7

21145 single piece, segment movement in any direction, requiring bone grafts (includes obtaining autografts)
46.2 46.2 FUD 090 C 80
AMA: 2018,Sep,7

21146 2 pieces, segment movement in any direction, requiring bone grafts (includes obtaining autografts) (eg, ungrafted unilateral alveolar cleft)
46.8 46.8 FUD 090 C 80
AMA: 2018,Sep,7

21147 3 or more pieces, segment movement in any direction, requiring bone grafts (includes obtaining autografts) (eg, ungrafted bilateral alveolar cleft or multiple osteotomies)
50.8 50.8 FUD 090 C 80
AMA: 2018,Sep,7

21150 Reconstruction midface, LeFort II; anterior intrusion (eg, Treacher-Collins Syndrome)
47.3 47.3 FUD 090 J G2 80
AMA: 2018,Sep,7

21151 any direction, requiring bone grafts (includes obtaining autografts)
52.0 52.0 FUD 090 C 80
AMA: 2018,Sep,7

21154 Reconstruction midface, LeFort III (extracranial), any type, requiring bone grafts (includes obtaining autografts); without LeFort I
56.0 56.0 FUD 090 C 80
AMA: 2018,Sep,7

21155 with LeFort I
62.2 62.2 FUD 090 C 80
AMA: 2018,Sep,7

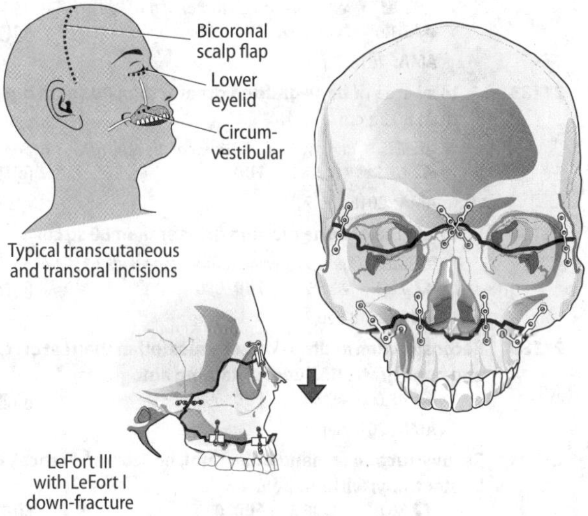

21159 Reconstruction midface, LeFort III (extra and intracranial) with forehead advancement (eg, mono bloc), requiring bone grafts (includes obtaining autografts); without LeFort I
74.5 74.5 FUD 090 C 80
AMA: 2018,Sep,7

21160 with LeFort I
81.4 81.4 FUD 090 C 80
AMA: 2018,Sep,7

21172 Reconstruction superior-lateral orbital rim and lower forehead, advancement or alteration, with or without grafts (includes obtaining autografts)
EXCLUDES *Frontal or parietal craniotomy for craniosynostosis (61556)*
60.2 60.2 FUD 090 J 80
AMA: 2018,Sep,7

21175 Reconstruction, bifrontal, superior-lateral orbital rims and lower forehead, advancement or alteration (eg, plagiocephaly, trigonocephaly, brachycephaly), with or without grafts (includes obtaining autografts)
EXCLUDES *Bifrontal craniotomy for craniosynostosis (61557)*
64.3 64.3 FUD 090 J 80
AMA: 2018,Sep,7

21179 Reconstruction, entire or majority of forehead and/or supraorbital rims; with grafts (allograft or prosthetic material)
EXCLUDES *Extensive craniotomy for numerous suture craniosynostosis (61558-61559)*
44.2 44.2 FUD 090 C 80
AMA: 2018,Sep,7

21180 with autograft (includes obtaining grafts)
EXCLUDES *Extensive craniotomy for numerous suture craniosynostosis (61558-61559)*
49.4 49.4 FUD 090 C 80
AMA: 2018,Sep,7

21181 Reconstruction by contouring of benign tumor of cranial bones (eg, fibrous dysplasia), extracranial
21.4 21.4 FUD 090 J A2 80
AMA: 2018,Sep,7

21182 **Reconstruction of orbital walls, rims, forehead, nasoethmoid complex following intra- and extracranial excision of benign tumor of cranial bone (eg, fibrous dysplasia), with multiple autografts (includes obtaining grafts); total area of bone grafting less than 40 sq cm**
EXCLUDES *Removal obenign tumor of the skull (61563-61564)*
61.6 61.6 **FUD** 090 C 80
AMA: 2018,Sep,7

21183 **total area of bone grafting greater than 40 sq cm but less than 80 sq cm**
EXCLUDES *Removal benign tumor of the skull (61563-61564)*
67.1 67.1 **FUD** 090 C 80
AMA: 2018,Sep,7

21184 **total area of bone grafting greater than 80 sq cm**
EXCLUDES *Removal benign tumor of the skull (61563-61564)*
72.3 72.3 **FUD** 090 C 80
AMA: 2018,Sep,7

21188 **Reconstruction midface, osteotomies (other than LeFort type) and bone grafts (includes obtaining autografts)**
48.0 48.0 **FUD** 090 C 80
AMA: 2018,Sep,7

21193 **Reconstruction of mandibular rami, horizontal, vertical, C, or L osteotomy; without bone graft**
36.8 36.8 **FUD** 090 J 80
AMA: 2018,Sep,7; 2018,Jan,8; 2017,Jan,8; 2016,Jan,13; 2015,Jan,16

21194 **with bone graft (includes obtaining graft)**
41.2 41.2 **FUD** 090 C 80
AMA: 2018,Sep,7; 2018,Jan,8; 2017,Jan,8; 2016,Jan,13; 2015,Jan,16

21195 **Reconstruction of mandibular rami and/or body, sagittal split; without internal rigid fixation**
39.5 39.5 **FUD** 090 J 80
AMA: 2018,Sep,7; 2018,Jan,8; 2017,Jan,8; 2016,Jan,13; 2015,Jan,16

21196 **with internal rigid fixation**
40.9 40.9 **FUD** 090 C 80
AMA: 2018,Sep,7; 2018,Jan,8; 2017,Jan,8; 2016,Jan,13; 2015,Jan,16

21198 **Osteotomy, mandible, segmental;**
EXCLUDES *Total maxillary osteotomy (21141-21160)*
33.0 33.0 **FUD** 090 J G2 80
AMA: 2018,Sep,7; 2018,Jan,8; 2017,Jan,8; 2016,Jan,13; 2015,Jan,16

21199 **with genioglossus advancement**
EXCLUDES *Total maxillary osteotomy (21141-21160)*
31.0 31.0 **FUD** 090 J G2 80
AMA: 2018,Sep,7; 2018,Jan,8; 2017,Jan,8; 2016,Jan,13; 2015,Jan,16

21206 **Osteotomy, maxilla, segmental (eg, Wassmund or Schuchard)**
34.1 34.1 **FUD** 090 J A2 80
AMA: 2018,Sep,7

21208 **Osteoplasty, facial bones; augmentation (autograft, allograft, or prosthetic implant)**
23.2 49.9 **FUD** 090 J J8 80
AMA: 2018,Sep,7

21209 **reduction**
17.4 22.9 **FUD** 090 J A2 80
AMA: 2018,Sep,7

21210 **Graft, bone; nasal, maxillary or malar areas (includes obtaining graft)**
EXCLUDES *Cleft palate procedures (42200-42225)*
22.3 56.5 **FUD** 090 J A2
AMA: 2018,Sep,7

21215 **mandible (includes obtaining graft)**
24.9 114. **FUD** 090 J A2
AMA: 2018,Sep,7

21230 **Graft; rib cartilage, autogenous, to face, chin, nose or ear (includes obtaining graft)**
EXCLUDES *Augmentation facial bones (21208)*
21.3 21.3 **FUD** 090 J A2 80
AMA: 2018,Sep,7

21235 **ear cartilage, autogenous, to nose or ear (includes obtaining graft)**
EXCLUDES *Augmentation facial bones (21208)*
16.2 20.7 **FUD** 090 J A2
AMA: 2018,Sep,7; 2018,Jan,8; 2017,Jan,8; 2016,Jan,13; 2015,Jan,16

21240 **Arthroplasty, temporomandibular joint, with or without autograft (includes obtaining graft)**
30.8 30.8 **FUD** 090 J A2 80 50
AMA: 2018,Sep,7

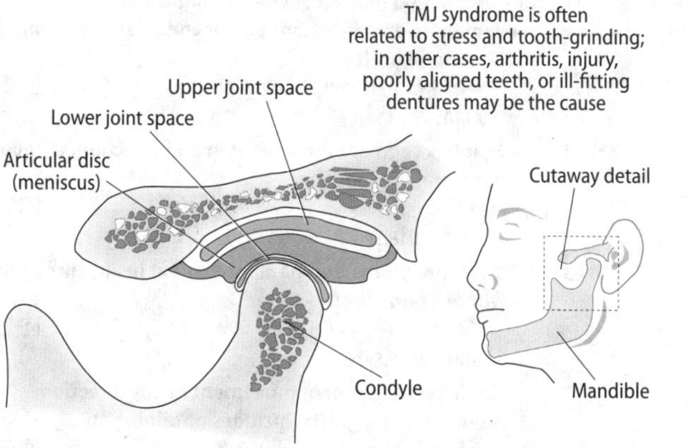

Cutaway view of temporomandibular joint (TMJ)

Symptoms include facial pain and chewing problems; TMJ syndrome occurs more frequently in women

21242 **Arthroplasty, temporomandibular joint, with allograft**
29.2 29.2 **FUD** 090 J A2 80 50
AMA: 2018,Sep,7

21243 **Arthroplasty, temporomandibular joint, with prosthetic joint replacement**
48.9 48.9 **FUD** 090 J J8 80 50
AMA: 2018,Sep,7

21244 **Reconstruction of mandible, extraoral, with transosteal bone plate (eg, mandibular staple bone plate)**
29.3 29.3 **FUD** 090 J G2 80
AMA: 2018,Sep,7

21245 **Reconstruction of mandible or maxilla, subperiosteal implant; partial**
26.8 34.5 **FUD** 090 J A2 80
AMA: 2018,Sep,7

21246 **complete**
25.4 25.4 **FUD** 090 J A2 80
AMA: 2018,Sep,7

21247 **Reconstruction of mandibular condyle with bone and cartilage autografts (includes obtaining grafts) (eg, for hemifacial microsomia)**
45.9 45.9 **FUD** 090 C 80 50
AMA: 2018,Sep,7

21248 **Reconstruction of mandible or maxilla, endosteal implant (eg, blade, cylinder); partial**
EXCLUDES *Midface reconstruction (21141-21160)*
25.3 31.1 **FUD** 090 J A2
AMA: 2018,Sep,7

21249 **complete**

EXCLUDES *Midface reconstruction (21141-21160)*

33.4 40.1 **FUD** 090 J A2 80

AMA: 2018,Sep,7

21255 **Reconstruction of zygomatic arch and glenoid fossa with bone and cartilage (includes obtaining autografts)**

40.6 40.6 **FUD** 090 C 80 50

AMA: 2018,Sep,7

21256 **Reconstruction of orbit with osteotomies (extracranial) and with bone grafts (includes obtaining autografts) (eg, micro-ophthalmia)**

35.9 35.9 **FUD** 090 J 80 50

AMA: 2018,Sep,7

21260 **Periorbital osteotomies for orbital hypertelorism, with bone grafts; extracranial approach**

40.1 40.1 **FUD** 090 J G2 80

AMA: 2018,Sep,7

21261 **combined intra- and extracranial approach**

71.1 71.1 **FUD** 090 J 80

AMA: 2018,Sep,7

21263 **with forehead advancement**

65.7 65.7 **FUD** 090 J 80

AMA: 2018,Sep,7

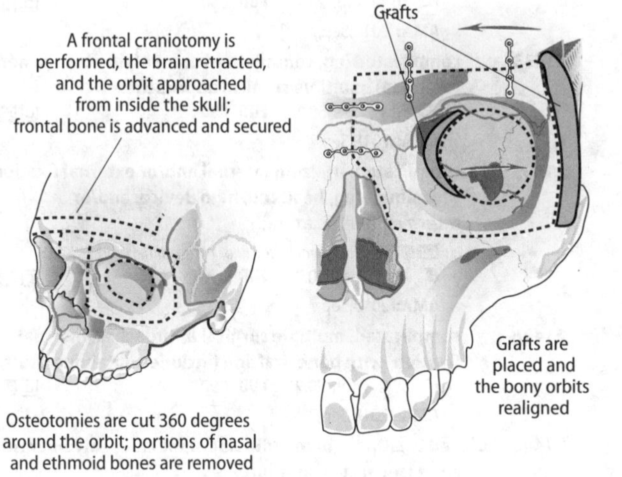

21267 **Orbital repositioning, periorbital osteotomies, unilateral, with bone grafts; extracranial approach**

46.8 46.8 **FUD** 090 J A2 80 50

AMA: 2018,Sep,7

21268 **combined intra- and extracranial approach**

58.8 58.8 **FUD** 090 C 80 50

AMA: 2018,Sep,7

21270 **Malar augmentation, prosthetic material**

EXCLUDES *Augmentation procedure with bone graft (21210)*

21.7 29.1 **FUD** 090 J A2 80 50

AMA: 2018,Sep,7

21275 **Secondary revision of orbitocraniofacial reconstruction**

24.1 24.1 **FUD** 090 J G2 80

AMA: 2018,Sep,7

21280 **Medial canthopexy (separate procedure)**

EXCLUDES *Reconstruction canthus (67950)*

16.4 16.4 **FUD** 090 J A2 80 50

AMA: 2018,Sep,7

21282 **Lateral canthopexy**

11.0 11.0 **FUD** 090 J A2 50

AMA: 2018,Sep,7

21295 **Reduction of masseter muscle and bone (eg, for treatment of benign masseteric hypertrophy); extraoral approach**

5.39 5.39 **FUD** 090 T A2 80 50

AMA: 2018,Sep,7

21296 **intraoral approach**

11.7 11.7 **FUD** 090 J A2 80 50

AMA: 2018,Sep,7

21299 **Unlisted craniofacial and maxillofacial procedure**

0.00 0.00 **FUD** YYY T 80

AMA: 2018,Sep,7

21310-21499 Care of Fractures/Dislocations of the Cranial and Facial Bones

EXCLUDES *Closed treatment skull fracture, report with appropriate E/M service*
Open treatment skull fracture (62000-62010)

21310 **Closed treatment of nasal bone fracture without manipulation**

0.78 3.76 **FUD** 000 T A2

AMA: 2019,Nov,12; 2019,Sep,3; 2018,Sep,7; 2018,Jan,3

21315 **Closed treatment of nasal bone fracture; without stabilization**

4.31 7.80 **FUD** 010 T A2

AMA: 2019,Nov,12; 2019,Sep,3; 2018,Sep,7; 2018,Jan,3

21320 **with stabilization**

3.83 7.23 **FUD** 010 J A2

AMA: 2019,Sep,3; 2018,Sep,7

21325 **Open treatment of nasal fracture; uncomplicated**

12.4 12.4 **FUD** 090 J A2 80

AMA: 2018,Sep,7

21330 **complicated, with internal and/or external skeletal fixation**

16.0 16.0 **FUD** 090 J A2 80

AMA: 2018,Sep,7

21335 **with concomitant open treatment of fractured septum**

20.3 20.3 **FUD** 090 J A2

AMA: 2018,Sep,7

21336 **Open treatment of nasal septal fracture, with or without stabilization**

18.2 18.2 **FUD** 090 J A2 80

AMA: 2018,Sep,7

21337 **Closed treatment of nasal septal fracture, with or without stabilization**

8.41 11.7 **FUD** 090 J A2 80

AMA: 2019,Sep,3; 2018,Sep,7

21338 **Open treatment of nasoethmoid fracture; without external fixation**

18.8 18.8 **FUD** 090 J J8 80

AMA: 2018,Sep,7

21339 **with external fixation**

21.3 21.3 **FUD** 090 J A2 80

AMA: 2018,Sep,7

21340 **Percutaneous treatment of nasoethmoid complex fracture, with splint, wire or headcap fixation, including repair of canthal ligaments and/or the nasolacrimal apparatus**

21.3 21.3 **FUD** 090 J A2 80

AMA: 2018,Sep,7

21343 **Open treatment of depressed frontal sinus fracture**

30.7 30.7 **FUD** 090 C 80

AMA: 2018,Sep,7

21344 **Open treatment of complicated (eg, comminuted or involving posterior wall) frontal sinus fracture, via coronal or multiple approaches**

39.7 39.7 **FUD** 090 C 80

AMA: 2018,Sep,7

21345 **Closed treatment of nasomaxillary complex fracture (LeFort II type), with interdental wire fixation or fixation of denture or splint**
17.9 22.2 FUD 090 T A2 80
AMA: 2018,Sep,7

21346 **Open treatment of nasomaxillary complex fracture (LeFort II type); with wiring and/or local fixation**
27.4 27.4 FUD 090 J
AMA: 2018,Sep,7

21347 **requiring multiple open approaches**
29.0 29.0 FUD 090 C 80
AMA: 2018,Sep,7

21348 **with bone grafting (includes obtaining graft)**
31.0 31.0 FUD 090 C 80
AMA: 2018,Sep,7

21355 **Percutaneous treatment of fracture of malar area, including zygomatic arch and malar tripod, with manipulation**
9.18 12.2 FUD 010 J A2 80 50
AMA: 2018,Sep,7

21356 **Open treatment of depressed zygomatic arch fracture (eg, Gillies approach)**
10.7 14.2 FUD 010 J A2 80 50
AMA: 2018,Sep,7

21360 **Open treatment of depressed malar fracture, including zygomatic arch and malar tripod**
14.6 14.6 FUD 090 J G2 80 50
AMA: 2018,Sep,7

21365 **Open treatment of complicated (eg, comminuted or involving cranial nerve foramina) fracture(s) of malar area, including zygomatic arch and malar tripod; with internal fixation and multiple surgical approaches**
31.6 31.6 FUD 090 J 80 50
AMA: 2018,Sep,7

21366 **with bone grafting (includes obtaining graft)**
36.5 36.5 FUD 090 C 80 50
AMA: 2018,Sep,7

21385 **Open treatment of orbital floor blowout fracture; transantral approach (Caldwell-Luc type operation)**
21.5 21.5 FUD 090 J 80 50
AMA: 2018,Sep,7

21386 **periorbital approach**
18.7 18.7 FUD 090 J 80 50
AMA: 2018,Sep,7

21387 **combined approach**
22.5 22.5 FUD 090 J 80 50
AMA: 2018,Sep,7

21390 **periorbital approach, with alloplastic or other implant**
22.9 22.9 FUD 090 J G2 80 50
AMA: 2018,Sep,7

21395 **periorbital approach with bone graft (includes obtaining graft)**
29.0 29.0 FUD 090 J 80 50
AMA: 2018,Sep,7

21400 **Closed treatment of fracture of orbit, except blowout; without manipulation**
4.59 5.77 FUD 090 T A2 80 50
AMA: 2018,Sep,7

21401 **with manipulation**
9.23 14.7 FUD 090 T A2 80 50
AMA: 2018,Sep,7

21406 **Open treatment of fracture of orbit, except blowout; without implant**
16.7 16.7 FUD 090 J G2 80 50
AMA: 2018,Sep,7

21407 **with implant**
18.4 18.4 FUD 090 J G2 80 50
AMA: 2018,Sep,7

21408 **with bone grafting (includes obtaining graft)**
26.1 26.1 FUD 090 J 80 50
AMA: 2018,Sep,7

21421 **Closed treatment of palatal or maxillary fracture (LeFort I type), with interdental wire fixation or fixation of denture or splint**
17.2 20.3 FUD 090 J A2 80
AMA: 2018,Sep,7

21422 **Open treatment of palatal or maxillary fracture (LeFort I type);**
18.4 18.4 FUD 090 C 80
AMA: 2018,Sep,7

21423 **complicated (comminuted or involving cranial nerve foramina), multiple approaches**
22.0 22.0 FUD 090 C 80
AMA: 2018,Sep,7

21431 **Closed treatment of craniofacial separation (LeFort III type) using interdental wire fixation of denture or splint**
19.9 19.9 FUD 090 C 80
AMA: 2018,Sep,7

21432 **Open treatment of craniofacial separation (LeFort III type); with wiring and/or internal fixation**
20.7 20.7 FUD 090 C 80
AMA: 2018,Sep,7

21433 **complicated (eg, comminuted or involving cranial nerve foramina), multiple surgical approaches**
50.1 50.1 FUD 090 C 80
AMA: 2018,Sep,7

21435 **complicated, utilizing internal and/or external fixation techniques (eg, head cap, halo device, and/or intermaxillary fixation)**
EXCLUDES *Removal internal or external fixation (20670)*
40.7 40.7 FUD 090 C 80
AMA: 2018,Sep,7

21436 **complicated, multiple surgical approaches, internal fixation, with bone grafting (includes obtaining graft)**
59.2 59.2 FUD 090 C 80
AMA: 2018,Sep,7

21440 **Closed treatment of mandibular or maxillary alveolar ridge fracture (separate procedure)**
14.0 17.3 FUD 090 J P3 80
AMA: 2018,Sep,7

21445 **Open treatment of mandibular or maxillary alveolar ridge fracture (separate procedure)**
17.9 22.2 FUD 090 J A2 80
AMA: 2018,Sep,7

21450 **Closed treatment of mandibular fracture; without manipulation**
13.4 16.4 FUD 090 T A2 80
AMA: 2018,Sep,7

21451 **with manipulation**
18.0 21.5 FUD 090 T A2 80
AMA: 2018,Sep,7

26/TC PC/TC Only | A2-Z3 ASC Payment | 50 Bilateral | ♂ Male Only | ♀ Female Only | Facility RVU | Non-Facility RVU | CCI | CLIA
FUD Follow-up Days | CMS: IOM | AMA: CPT Asst | A-Y OPPSI | 80/80 Surg Assist Allowed / w/Doc | Lab Crosswalk | Radiology Crosswalk

21452 **Percutaneous treatment of mandibular fracture, with external fixation**
12.0 20.1 **FUD** 090 J A2 80
AMA: 2018,Sep,7

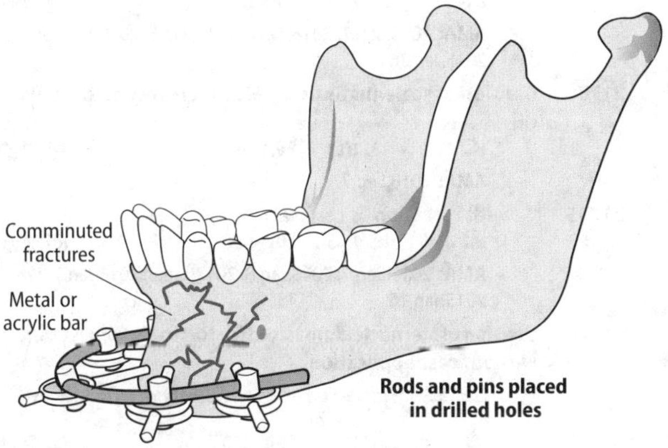

21453 **Closed treatment of mandibular fracture with interdental fixation**
23.6 27.6 **FUD** 090 J A2 80
AMA: 2018,Sep,7; 2018,Jan,8; 2017,Jan,8; 2016,Jan,13; 2015,Jan,16

21454 **Open treatment of mandibular fracture with external fixation**
15.6 15.6 **FUD** 090 J A2 80
AMA: 2018,Sep,7

21461 **Open treatment of mandibular fracture; without interdental fixation**
28.8 57.4 **FUD** 090 J J8
AMA: 2018,Sep,7

21462 **with interdental fixation**
31.9 61.4 **FUD** 090 J J8 80
AMA: 2018,Sep,7

21465 **Open treatment of mandibular condylar fracture**
24.1 24.1 **FUD** 090 J A2 80 50
AMA: 2018,Sep,7

21470 **Open treatment of complicated mandibular fracture by multiple surgical approaches including internal fixation, interdental fixation, and/or wiring of dentures or splints**
34.5 34.5 **FUD** 090 J 80
AMA: 2018,Sep,7; 2018,Jan,8; 2017,Jan,8; 2016,Jan,13; 2015,Jan,16

21480 **Closed treatment of temporomandibular dislocation; initial or subsequent**
0.91 3.07 **FUD** 000 T A2 50
AMA: 2018,Sep,7

21485 **complicated (eg, recurrent requiring intermaxillary fixation or splinting), initial or subsequent**
20.6 25.2 **FUD** 090 T A2 80 50
AMA: 2018,Sep,7

21490 **Open treatment of temporomandibular dislocation**
EXCLUDES *Closed treatment larynx fracture, report with appropriate E/M service*
Interdental wiring (21497)
23.7 23.7 **FUD** 090 J A2 80 50
AMA: 2018,Sep,7

21497 **Interdental wiring, for condition other than fracture**
16.4 19.6 **FUD** 090 T A2 80
AMA: 2018,Sep,7; 2018,Jan,8; 2017,Jan,8; 2016,Jan,13; 2015,Jan,16

21499 **Unlisted musculoskeletal procedure, head**
EXCLUDES *Unlisted procedures craniofacial or maxillofacial areas (21299)*
0.00 0.00 **FUD** YYY T 80
AMA: 2018,Sep,7

21501-21510 Surgical Incision for Drainage: Chest and Soft Tissues of Neck

EXCLUDES *Biopsy flank or back (21920-21925)*
Simple incision and drainage abscess or hematoma (10060, 10140)
Tumor removal flank or back (21930-21936)

21501 **Incision and drainage, deep abscess or hematoma, soft tissues of neck or thorax;**
EXCLUDES *Deep incision and drainage posterior spine (22010-22015)*
9.37 13.4 **FUD** 090 J A2
AMA: 2018,Sep,7; 2018,Jan,8; 2017,Jan,8; 2016,Jan,13; 2015,Jan,16

21502 **with partial rib ostectomy**
14.5 14.5 **FUD** 090 J A2 80
AMA: 2018,Sep,7

21510 **Incision, deep, with opening of bone cortex (eg, for osteomyelitis or bone abscess), thorax**
12.9 12.9 **FUD** 090 C 80
AMA: 2018,Sep,7

21550 Soft Tissue Biopsy of Chest or Neck

EXCLUDES *Biopsy bone (20220-20251)*
Soft tissue needle biopsy (20206)

21550 **Biopsy, soft tissue of neck or thorax**
4.47 7.50 **FUD** 010 J G2
AMA: 2018,Sep,7

21552-21558 [21552, 21554] Excision Soft Tissue Tumors Chest and Neck

INCLUDES Any necessary elevation tissue planes or dissection
Measurement tumor and necessary margin at greatest diameter prior to excision
Resection without removal significant normal tissue
Simple and intermediate repairs
Excision types:
Fascial or subfascial soft tissue tumors: simple and marginal resection tumors found either in or below deep fascia, not involving bone or excision substantial amount normal tissue; primarily benign and intramuscular tumors
Radical resection soft tissue tumor: wide resection tumor, involving substantial margins normal tissue and may involve tissue removal from one or more layers; most often malignant or aggressive benign
Subcutaneous: simple and marginal resection tumors in subcutaneous tissue above deep fascia; most often benign

EXCLUDES *Complex repair*
Excision benign cutaneous lesions (eg, sebaceous cyst) (11400-11426)
Radical resection cutaneous tumors (eg, melanoma) (11600-11626)
Significant vessel exploration or neuroplasty

21552 **Resequenced code. See code following 21555.**

21554 **Resequenced code. See code following 21556.**

21555 **Excision, tumor, soft tissue of neck or anterior thorax, subcutaneous; less than 3 cm**
8.79 12.2 **FUD** 090 J G2
AMA: 2018,Sep,7; 2018,Jan,8; 2017,Jan,8; 2016,Jan,13; 2015,Jan,16

21552 **3 cm or greater**
12.8 12.8 **FUD** 090 J G2 80
AMA: 2018,Sep,7

21556 **Excision, tumor, soft tissue of neck or anterior thorax, subfascial (eg, intramuscular); less than 5 cm**
15.2 15.2 **FUD** 090 J G2
AMA: 2018,Sep,7

21554 **5 cm or greater**
21.0 21.0 **FUD** 090 J G2 80
AMA: 2018,Sep,7

21557 **Radical resection of tumor (eg, sarcoma), soft tissue of neck or anterior thorax; less than 5 cm**
27.5 27.5 **FUD** 090 J G2 80
AMA: 2020,Apr,10; 2018,Sep,7; 2018,Jan,8; 2017,Jan,8; 2016,Jan,13; 2015,Jan,16

21558 **5 cm or greater**
38.8 38.8 **FUD** 090 J G2 80
AMA: 2020,Apr,10; 2018,Sep,7

21600-21632 Bony Resection Chest and Neck

21600 **Excision of rib, partial**
EXCLUDES *Extensive debridement (11044, 11047)*
Radical resection, chest wall/rib cage for tumor (21601)
15.9 15.9 **FUD** 090 J A2 80
AMA: 2018,Sep,7; 2018,Jan,8; 2017,Jan,8; 2016,Jan,13; 2015,Jan,16

21601 **Excision of chest wall tumor including rib(s)**
EXCLUDES *Exploratory thoracotomy (32100)*
Resection apical lung tumor (32503-32504)
Thoracentesis (32554-32555)
Tube thoracostomy (32551)
34.1 34.1 **FUD** 090 80
AMA: 2019,Dec,4

21602 **Excision of chest wall tumor involving rib(s), with plastic reconstruction; without mediastinal lymphadenectomy**
EXCLUDES *Exploratory thoracotomy (32100)*
Resection apical lung tumor (32503-32504)
Thoracentesis (32554-32555)
Tube thoracostomy (32551)
45.8 45.8 **FUD** 090 80
AMA: 2019,Dec,4

21603 **with mediastinal lymphadenectomy**
EXCLUDES *Exploratory thoracotomy (32100)*
Resection apical lung tumor (32503-32504)
Thoracentesis (32554-32555)
Tube thoracostomy (32551)
50.7 50.7 **FUD** 090 80
AMA: 2019,Dec,4

21610 **Costotransversectomy (separate procedure)**
34.5 34.5 **FUD** 090 J A2 80
AMA: 2018,Sep,7

21615 **Excision first and/or cervical rib;**
17.8 17.8 **FUD** 090 C 80 50
AMA: 2018,Sep,7; 2018,Jan,8; 2017,Jan,8; 2016,Jan,13; 2015,Jan,16

21616 **with sympathectomy**
20.7 20.7 **FUD** 090 C 80 50
AMA: 2018,Sep,7

21620 **Ostectomy of sternum, partial**
14.6 14.6 **FUD** 090 C 80
AMA: 2018,Sep,7

21627 **Sternal debridement**
EXCLUDES *Debridement with sternotomy closure (21750)*
15.5 15.5 **FUD** 090 C 80
AMA: 2018,Sep,7; 2018,Jan,8; 2017,Jan,8; 2016,Jan,13; 2015,Jan,16

21630 **Radical resection of sternum;**
35.1 35.1 **FUD** 090 C 80
AMA: 2018,Sep,7

21632 **with mediastinal lymphadenectomy**
34.9 34.9 **FUD** 090 C 80
AMA: 2018,Sep,7

21685-21750 Repair/Reconstruction Chest and Soft Tissues Neck

EXCLUDES *Repair simple wounds (12001-12007)*

21685 **Hyoid myotomy and suspension**
28.2 28.2 **FUD** 090 J G2 80
AMA: 2018,Sep,7; 2018,Jan,8; 2017,Jan,8; 2016,Jan,13; 2015,Jan,16

21700 **Division of scalenus anticus; without resection of cervical rib**
10.3 10.3 **FUD** 090 J A2 80 50
AMA: 2018,Sep,7

21705 **with resection of cervical rib**
15.5 15.5 **FUD** 090 C 80 50
AMA: 2018,Sep,7; 2018,Jan,8; 2017,Jan,8; 2016,Jan,13; 2015,Jan,16

21720 **Division of sternocleidomastoid for torticollis, open operation; without cast application**
EXCLUDES *Transection spinal accessory and cervical nerves (63191, 64722)*
15.0 15.0 **FUD** 090 J A2 80
AMA: 2018,Sep,7

21725 **with cast application**
EXCLUDES *Transection spinal accessory and cervical nerves (63191, 64722)*
15.5 15.5 **FUD** 090 T A2 80
AMA: 2018,Sep,7

21740 **Reconstructive repair of pectus excavatum or carinatum; open**
29.7 29.7 **FUD** 090 C 80
AMA: 2018,Sep,7

21742 **minimally invasive approach (Nuss procedure), without thoracoscopy**
0.00 0.00 **FUD** 090 J 80
AMA: 2018,Sep,7

21743 **minimally invasive approach (Nuss procedure), with thoracoscopy**
0.00 0.00 **FUD** 090 J 80
AMA: 2019,Nov,14; 2018,Sep,7

21750 **Closure of median sternotomy separation with or without debridement (separate procedure)**
19.7 19.7 **FUD** 090 C 80
AMA: 2018,Sep,7; 2018,Jan,8; 2017,Jan,8; 2016,Jan,13; 2015,Jan,16

21811-21825 Fracture Care: Ribs and Sternum

EXCLUDES *Closed treatment uncomplicated rib fractures, report appropriate E/M services*

21811 **Open treatment of rib fracture(s) with internal fixation, includes thoracoscopic visualization when performed, unilateral; 1-3 ribs**
17.2 17.2 **FUD** 000 J 80 50
AMA: 2018,Sep,7; 2018,Jan,8; 2017,Jan,8; 2016,Jan,13; 2015,Aug,3

21812 **4-6 ribs**
21.0 21.0 **FUD** 000 J 80 50
AMA: 2018,Sep,7; 2018,Jan,8; 2017,Jan,8; 2016,Jan,13; 2015,Aug,3

21813 **7 or more ribs**
28.7 28.7 **FUD** 000 J 80 50
AMA: 2018,Sep,7; 2018,Jan,8; 2017,Jan,8; 2016,Jan,13; 2015,Aug,3

21820 **Closed treatment of sternum fracture**
4.15 4.18 **FUD** 090 T A2
AMA: 2018,Sep,7

21825 **Open treatment of sternum fracture with or without skeletal fixation**
EXCLUDES *Treatment sternoclavicular dislocation (23520-23532)*
15.6 15.6 FUD 090 C 80
AMA: 2018,Sep,7

21899 Unlisted Procedures of Chest or Neck

CMS: 100-04,4,180.3 Unlisted Service or Procedure

21899 **Unlisted procedure, neck or thorax**
0.00 0.00 FUD YYY T 80
AMA: 2018,Sep,7; 2018,Jan,8; 2017,Jan,8; 2016,Jan,13; 2015,Aug,3

21920-21925 Biopsy Soft Tissue of Back and Flank

EXCLUDES *Soft tissue needle biopsy (20206)*

21920 **Biopsy, soft tissue of back or flank; superficial**
4.55 7.30 FUD 010 J P3
AMA: 2018,Sep,7

21925 **deep**
10.4 13.4 FUD 090 J A2
AMA: 2018,Sep,7

21930-21936 Excision Soft Tissue Tumors Back or Flank

INCLUDES Any necessary elevation tissue planes or dissection
Measurement tumor and necessary margin at greatest diameter prior to excision
Simple and intermediate repairs
Excision types:
Fascial or subfascial soft tissue tumors: simple and marginal resection tumors found either in or below deep fascia, not involving bone or excision substantial amount normal tissue; most often benign and intramuscular tumors
Radical resection soft tissue tumor: wide resection of tumor, involving substantial margins normal tissue and may include tissue removal from one or more layers; most often malignant or aggressive benign
Subcutaneous: simple and marginal resection tumors in subcutaneous tissue above deep fascia; most often benign

EXCLUDES *Complex repair*
Excision benign cutaneous lesions (eg, sebaceous cyst) (11400-11406)
Radical resection cutaneous tumors (eg, melanoma) (11600-11606)
Significant vessel exploration or neuroplasty

21930 **Excision, tumor, soft tissue of back or flank, subcutaneous; less than 3 cm**
10.4 14.1 FUD 090 J G2
AMA: 2018,Sep,7; 2018,Jan,8; 2017,Jan,8; 2016,Jan,13; 2015,Jan,16

21931 **3 cm or greater**
13.6 13.6 FUD 090 J G2 80
AMA: 2018,Sep,7

21932 **Excision, tumor, soft tissue of back or flank, subfascial (eg, intramuscular); less than 5 cm**
19.0 19.0 FUD 090 J G2 80
AMA: 2018,Sep,7

21933 **5 cm or greater**
21.3 21.3 FUD 090 J G2 80
AMA: 2018,Sep,7

21935 **Radical resection of tumor (eg, sarcoma), soft tissue of back or flank; less than 5 cm**
29.7 29.7 FUD 090 J G2
AMA: 2018,Sep,7

21936 **5 cm or greater**
40.9 40.9 FUD 090 J G2 80
AMA: 2018,Sep,7

22010-22015 Incision for Drainage of Deep Spinal Abscess

EXCLUDES *Incision and drainage hematoma (10060, 10140)*
Injection:
Chemonucleolysis (62292)
Discography (62290-62291)
Facet joint (64490-64495, [64633, 64634, 64635, 64636])
Myelography (62284)
Needle/trocar biopsy (20220-20225)

22010 **Incision and drainage, open, of deep abscess (subfascial), posterior spine; cervical, thoracic, or cervicothoracic**
27.7 27.7 FUD 090 C 80
AMA: 2018,Sep,7

22015 **lumbar, sacral, or lumbosacral**
EXCLUDES *Incision and drainage, complex, postoperative wound infection (10180)*
Incision and drainage, open, deep abscess (subfascial), posterior spine; cervical, thoracic, or cervicothoracic (22010)
Removal posterior nonsegmental instrumentation (eg, Harrington rod) (22850)
Removal posterior segmental instrumentation (22852)
27.2 27.2 FUD 090 C
AMA: 2018,Sep,7

22100-22103 Partial Resection Vertebral Component

EXCLUDES *Back or flank biopsy (21920-21925)*
Bone biopsy (20220-20251)
Bone grafting procedures (20930-20938)
Harvest bone graft (20931, 20938)
Injection:
Chemonucleolysis (62292)
Discography (62290-62291)
Facet joint (64490-64495, [64633, 64634, 64635, 64636])
Myelography (62284)
Osteotomy (22210-22226)
Reconstruction after vertebral body resection (22585, 63082, 63086, 63088, 63091)
Removal tumor flank or back (21930)
Soft tissue needle biopsy (20206)
Spinal reconstruction with bone graft or vertebral body prosthesis:
Cervical (20931, 20938, 22554, 63081)
Lumbar (20931, 20938, 22558, 63087, 63090)
Thoracic (20931, 20938, 22556, 63085, 63087)
Vertebral corpectomy (63081-63091)

22100 **Partial excision of posterior vertebral component (eg, spinous process, lamina or facet) for intrinsic bony lesion, single vertebral segment; cervical**
24.8 24.8 FUD 090 J 80
AMA: 2018,Sep,7; 2018,Jan,8; 2017,Mar,7; 2017,Jan,8; 2016,Jan,13; 2015,Jan,16

22101 **thoracic**
25.1 25.1 FUD 090 J 80
AMA: 2018,Sep,7; 2018,Jan,8; 2017,Mar,7; 2017,Jan,8; 2016,Jan,13; 2015,Jan,16

22102 **lumbar**
Code also posterior spinous process distraction device insertion, when applicable (22867-22870)
23.6 23.6 FUD 090 J G2 80
AMA: 2018,Sep,7; 2018,Jan,8; 2017,Mar,7; 2017,Jan,8; 2016,Jan,13; 2015,Jan,16

+ **22103** **each additional segment (List separately in addition to code for primary procedure)**
Code first (22100-22102)
4.09 4.09 FUD ZZZ N N1 80
AMA: 2018,Sep,7

22110-22116 Partial Resection Vertebral Component without Decompression

EXCLUDES *Back or flank biopsy (21920-21925)*
Bone biopsy (20220-20251)
Bone grafting procedures (20930-20938)
Harvest bone graft (20931, 20938)
Injection:
Chemonucleolysis (62292)
Discography (62290-62291)
Facet joint (64490-64495, [64633, 64634, 64635, 64636])
Myelography (62284)
Osteotomy (22210-22226)
Reconstruction after vertebral body resection (22585, 63082, 63086, 63088, 63091)
Removal tumor flank or back (21930)
Soft tissue needle biopsy (20206)
Spinal reconstruction with bone graft or vertebral body prosthesis:
Cervical (20931, 20938, 22554, 22853-22854 [22859], 63081)
Lumbar (20931, 20938, 22558, 22853-22854 [22859], 63087, 63090)
Thoracic (20931, 20938, 22556, 22853-22854 [22859], 63085, 63087)
Vertebral corpectomy (63081-63091)

22110 Partial excision of vertebral body, for intrinsic bony lesion, without decompression of spinal cord or nerve root(s), single vertebral segment; cervical
30.1 30.1 **FUD** 090 C 80
AMA: 2018,Sep,7; 2018,Jan,8; 2017,Mar,7; 2017,Jan,8; 2016,Jan,13; 2015,Jan,16

22112 thoracic
32.7 32.7 **FUD** 090 C 80
AMA: 2018,Sep,7; 2018,Jan,8; 2017,Mar,7; 2017,Jan,8; 2016,Jan,13; 2015,Jan,16

22114 lumbar
32.4 32.4 **FUD** 090 C 80
AMA: 2018,Sep,7; 2018,Jan,8; 2017,Mar,7; 2017,Jan,8; 2016,Jan,13; 2015,Jan,16

+ **22116 each additional vertebral segment (List separately in addition to code for primary procedure)**
Code first (22110-22114)
4.12 4.12 **FUD** ZZZ C 80
AMA: 2018,Sep,7

22206-22216 Spinal Osteotomy: Posterior/Posterolateral Approach

EXCLUDES *Decompression spinal cord and/or nerve roots (63001-63308)*
Injection:
Chemonucleolysis (62292)
Discography (62290-62292)
Facet joint (64490-64495, [64633, 64634, 64635, 64636])
Myelography (62284)
Vertebral corpectomy (63081-63091)
Code also arthrodesis (22590-22632)
Code also bone grafting procedures (20930-20938)
Code also spinal instrumentation (22840-22855 [22859])

22206 Osteotomy of spine, posterior or posterolateral approach, 3 columns, 1 vertebral segment (eg, pedicle/vertebral body subtraction); thoracic
EXCLUDES *Osteotomy spine, posterior or posterolateral approach, lumbar (22207)*
Procedures performed at same level (22210-22226, 22830, 63001-63048, 63055-63066, 63075-63091, 63101-63103)
71.3 71.3 **FUD** 090 C 80
AMA: 2018,Sep,7; 2018,Jan,8; 2017,Mar,7; 2017,Jan,8; 2016,Jan,13; 2015,Jan,16

22207 lumbar
EXCLUDES *Osteotomy spine, posterior or posterolateral approach, thoracic (22206)*
Procedures performed at same level (22210-22226, 22830, 63001-63048, 63055-63066, 63075-63091, 63101-63103)
69.8 69.8 **FUD** 090 C 80
AMA: 2018,Sep,7; 2018,Jan,8; 2017,Mar,7; 2017,Jan,8; 2016,Jan,13; 2015,Jan,16

+ **22208 each additional vertebral segment (List separately in addition to code for primary procedure)**
EXCLUDES *Procedures performed at same level (22210-22226, 22830, 63001-63048, 63055-63066, 63075-63091, 63101-63103)*
Code first (22206, 22207)
17.1 17.1 **FUD** ZZZ C 80
AMA: 2018,Sep,7; 2018,Jan,8; 2017,Jan,8; 2016,Jan,13; 2015,Jan,16

22210 Osteotomy of spine, posterior or posterolateral approach, 1 vertebral segment; cervical
51.7 51.7 **FUD** 090 C 80
AMA: 2018,Sep,7; 2018,Jan,8; 2017,Mar,7; 2017,Jan,8; 2016,Jan,13; 2015,Jan,16

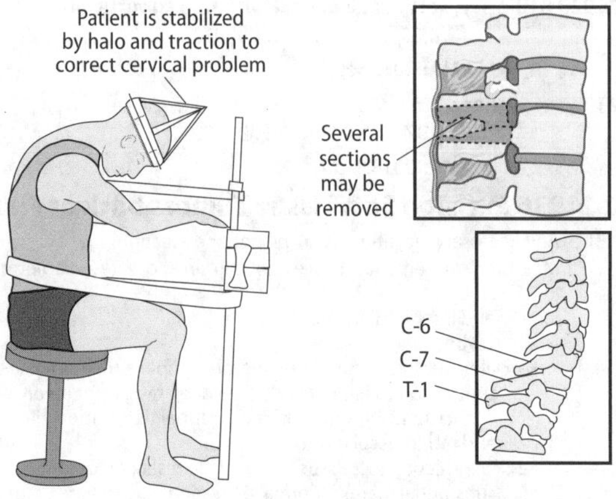

Patient is stabilized by halo and traction to correct cervical problem
Several sections may be removed
C-6
C-7
T-1

Physician removes spinous processes, lamina

22212 thoracic
43.2 43.2 **FUD** 090 C 80
AMA: 2018,Sep,7; 2018,Jan,8; 2017,Mar,7; 2017,Jan,8; 2016,Jan,13; 2015,Jan,16

22214 lumbar
43.4 43.4 **FUD** 090 C 80
AMA: 2018,Sep,7; 2018,Jan,8; 2017,Mar,7; 2017,Jan,8; 2016,Jan,13; 2015,Jan,16

+ **22216 each additional vertebral segment (List separately in addition to primary procedure)**
Code first (22210-22214)
10.5 10.5 **FUD** ZZZ C 80
AMA: 2018,Sep,7; 2018,Jan,8; 2017,Jan,8; 2016,Jan,13; 2015,Jan,16

22220-22226 Spinal Osteotomy: Anterior Approach

EXCLUDES *Decompression spinal cord and/or nerve roots (63001-63308)*
Injection:
Chemonucleolysis (62292)
Discography (62290-62291)
Facet joint (64490-64495, [64633, 64634, 64635, 64636])
Myelography (62284)
Needle/trocar biopsy (20220-20225)
Verterbral corpectomy (63081-63091)
Code also arthrodesis (22590-22632)
Code also bone grafting procedures (20930-20938)
Code also spinal instrumentation (22840-22855 [22859])

22220 Osteotomy of spine, including discectomy, anterior approach, single vertebral segment; cervical
47.0 47.0 **FUD** 090 C 80
AMA: 2018,Sep,7; 2018,Jan,8; 2017,Mar,7; 2017,Jan,8; 2016,Jan,13; 2015,Jan,16

22222 thoracic
51.1 51.1 **FUD** 090 C 80
AMA: 2018,Sep,7; 2018,Jan,8; 2017,Jan,8; 2017,Jan,8; 2016,Jan,13; 2015,Jan,16

22224 **lumbar**
46.1 46.1 **FUD** 090 C 80
AMA: 2018,Sep,7; 2018,Jan,8; 2017,Mar,7; 2017,Jan,8; 2016,Jan,13; 2015,Jan,16

+ 22226 **each additional vertebral segment (List separately in addition to code for primary procedure)**
Code first (22220-22224)
10.5 10.5 **FUD** ZZZ C 80
AMA: 2018,Sep,7

22310-22315 Closed Treatment Vertebral Fractures

EXCLUDES *Injection:*
Chemonucleolysis (62292)
Discography (62290-62291)
Facet joint (64490-64495, [64633, 64634, 64635, 64636])
Myelography (62284)
Percutaneous vertebroplasty at same level (22510-22515)
Code also arthrodesis (22590-22632)
Code also bone grafting procedures (20930-20938)
Code also spinal instrumentation (22840-22855 [22859])

22310 **Closed treatment of vertebral body fracture(s), without manipulation, requiring and including casting or bracing**
8.38 8.70 **FUD** 090 T A2
AMA: 2018,Sep,7; 2018,Jan,8; 2017,Mar,7; 2017,Jan,8; 2016,Jan,13; 2015,Jan,16; 2015,Jan,8

22315 **Closed treatment of vertebral fracture(s) and/or dislocation(s) requiring casting or bracing, with and including casting and/or bracing by manipulation or traction**
EXCLUDES *Spinal manipulation (97140)*
22.2 25.3 **FUD** 090 J A2
AMA: 2018,Sep,7; 2018,Jan,8; 2017,Mar,7; 2017,Jan,8; 2016,Jan,13; 2015,Jan,8; 2015,Jan,16

22318-22319 Open Treatment Odontoid Fracture: Anterior Approach

EXCLUDES *Injection:*
Chemonucleolysis (62292)
Discography (62290-62291)
Facet joint (64490-64495, [64633, 64634, 64635, 64636])
Myelography (62284)
Needle/trocar biopsy (20220-20225)
Code also arthrodesis (22590-22632)
Code also bone grafting procedures (20930-20938)
Code also spinal instrumentation (22840-22855 [22859])

22318 **Open treatment and/or reduction of odontoid fracture(s) and or dislocation(s) (including os odontoideum), anterior approach, including placement of internal fixation; without grafting**
47.6 47.6 **FUD** 090 C 80
AMA: 2018,Sep,7; 2018,Jan,8; 2017,Mar,7; 2017,Jan,8; 2016,Jan,13; 2015,Jan,16

22319 **with grafting**
53.6 53.6 **FUD** 090 C 80
AMA: 2018,Sep,7; 2018,May,3; 2018,Jan,8; 2017,Mar,7; 2017,Jan,8; 2016,Jan,13; 2015,Jan,16

22325-22328 Open Treatment Vertebral Fractures: Posterior Approach

EXCLUDES *Injection:*
Chemonucleolysis (62292)
Discography (62290-62291)
Facet joint (64490-64495, [64633, 64634, 64635, 64636])
Myelography (62284)
Needle/trocar biopsy (20220-20225)
Spine decompression (63001-63091)
Vertebral corpectomy (63081-63091)
Vertebral fracture care by arthrodesis (22548-22632)
Code also arthrodesis (22548-22632)
Code also bone grafting procedures (20930-20938)
Code also spinal instrumentation (22840-22855 [22859])

22325 **Open treatment and/or reduction of vertebral fracture(s) and/or dislocation(s), posterior approach, 1 fractured vertebra or dislocated segment; lumbar**
EXCLUDES *Percutaneous vertebral augmentation performed at same level (22514-22515)*
Percutaneous vertebroplasty performed at same level (22511-22512)
41.9 41.9 **FUD** 090 C 80
AMA: 2018,Sep,7; 2018,Jan,8; 2017,Aug,9; 2017,Mar,7; 2017,Jan,8; 2016,Jan,13; 2015,Jan,16; 2015,Jan,8

22326 **cervical**
EXCLUDES *Percutaneous vertebroplasty performed at same level (22510, 22512)*
43.4 43.4 **FUD** 090 C 80
AMA: 2018,Sep,7; 2018,Jan,8; 2017,Mar,7; 2017,Jan,8; 2016,Jan,13; 2015,Jan,16

22327 **thoracic**
EXCLUDES *Percutaneous vertebral augmentation performed at same level (22515)*
Percutaneous vertebroplasty performed at same level (22510, 22512-22513)
43.7 43.7 **FUD** 090 C 80
AMA: 2018,Sep,7; 2018,Jan,8; 2017,Mar,7; 2017,Jan,8; 2016,Jan,13; 2015,Jan,8; 2015,Jan,16

+ 22328 **each additional fractured vertebra or dislocated segment (List separately in addition to code for primary procedure)**
Code first (22325-22327)
8.25 8.25 **FUD** ZZZ C 80
AMA: 2018,Sep,7

22505 Spinal Manipulation with Anesthesia

EXCLUDES *Manipulation not requiring anesthesia (97140)*

22505 **Manipulation of spine requiring anesthesia, any region**
3.76 3.76 **FUD** 010 J A2
AMA: 2018,Sep,7; 2018,Jan,8; 2017,Jan,8; 2016,Jan,13; 2015,Jan,16

22510-22515 Percutaneous Vertebroplasty/Kyphoplasty

INCLUDES Radiological guidance
When performed at same level:
Bone biopsy (20225)
Closed treatment vertebral fractures (22310, 22315)
Open treatment/reduction vertebral fractures (22325, 22327)
EXCLUDES *Sacroplasty/augmentation (0200T-0201T)*

22510 **Percutaneous vertebroplasty (bone biopsy included when performed), 1 vertebral body, unilateral or bilateral injection, inclusive of all imaging guidance; cervicothoracic**
12.5 49.8 **FUD** 010 J G2
AMA: 2018,Sep,7; 2018,Jan,8; 2017,Jan,8; 2016,Jan,13; 2015,Jan,8

22511 **lumbosacral**
11.7 49.3 **FUD** 010 J G2
AMA: 2018,Sep,7; 2018,Jan,8; 2017,Jan,8; 2016,Jan,13; 2015,Apr,8; 2015,Jan,8

\+ **22512** **each additional cervicothoracic or lumbosacral vertebral body (List separately in addition to code for primary procedure)**

Code first (22510-22511)

5.96 24.4 **FUD** ZZZ N N1

AMA: 2018,Sep,7; 2018,Jan,8; 2017,Jan,8; 2016,Jan,13; 2015,Jan,8

22513 **Percutaneous vertebral augmentation, including cavity creation (fracture reduction and bone biopsy included when performed) using mechanical device (eg, kyphoplasty), 1 vertebral body, unilateral or bilateral cannulation, inclusive of all imaging guidance; thoracic**

14.9 195. **FUD** 010 J G2

AMA: 2018,Sep,7; 2018,Jan,8; 2017,Jan,8; 2016,Jan,13; 2015,Jan,8

22514 **lumbar**

13.9 194. **FUD** 010 J G2

AMA: 2018,Sep,7; 2018,Jan,8; 2017,Jan,8; 2016,Jan,13; 2015,Jan,8

\+ **22515** **each additional thoracic or lumbar vertebral body (List separately in addition to code for primary procedure)**

Code first (22513-22514)

6.39 105. **FUD** ZZZ N N1

AMA: 2018,Sep,7; 2018,Jan,8; 2017,Jan,8; 2016,Jan,13; 2015,Jan,8

22526-22527 Percutaneous Annuloplasty

CMS: 100-04,32,220.1 Thermal Intradiscal Procedures (TIPS)

INCLUDES Fluoroscopic guidance (77002, 77003)

EXCLUDES *Needle/trocar biopsy (20220-20225)*
Injection:
Chemonucleolysis (62292)
Discography (62290-62291)
Facet joint (64490-64495, [64633, 64634, 64635, 64636])
Myelography (62284)
Procedure performed by other methods (22899)

22526 **Percutaneous intradiscal electrothermal annuloplasty, unilateral or bilateral including fluoroscopic guidance; single level**

9.76 65.0 **FUD** 010 E

AMA: 2018,Sep,7; 2018,Jan,8; 2017,Jan,8; 2016,Jan,13; 2015,Jan,8; 2015,Jan,16

\+ **22527** **1 or more additional levels (List separately in addition to code for primary procedure)**

Code first (22526)

4.44 53.1 **FUD** ZZZ E

AMA: 2018,Sep,7; 2018,Jan,8; 2017,Jan,8; 2016,Jan,13; 2015,Jan,8; 2015,Jan,16

22532-22534 Spinal Fusion: Lateral Extracavitary Approach

EXCLUDES *Corpectomy (63101-63103)*
Exploration spinal fusion (22830)
Fracture care (22310-22328)
Injection:
Chemonucleolysis (62292)
Discography (62290-62291)
Facet joint (64490-64495, [64633, 64634, 64635, 64636])
Myelography (62284)
Laminectomy (63001-63017)
Needle/trocar biopsy (20220-20225)
Osteotomy (22206-22226)

Code also bone grafting procedures (20930-20938)
Code also spinal instrumentation (22840-22855 [22859])

22532 **Arthrodesis, lateral extracavitary technique, including minimal discectomy to prepare interspace (other than for decompression); thoracic**

52.1 52.1 **FUD** 090 C 80

AMA: 2020,May,13; 2018,Sep,7; 2018,May,3; 2018,Jan,8; 2017,Mar,7; 2017,Feb,9; 2017,Jan,8; 2016,Jan,13; 2015,Jan,16

22533 **lumbar**

48.0 48.0 **FUD** 090 C 80

AMA: 2020,May,13; 2018,Sep,7; 2018,May,3; 2018,Jan,8; 2017,Mar,7; 2017,Feb,9; 2017,Jan,8; 2016,Jan,13; 2015,Jan,16

\+ **22534** **thoracic or lumbar, each additional vertebral segment (List separately in addition to code for primary procedure)**

Code first (22532-22533)

10.5 10.5 **FUD** ZZZ C 80

AMA: 2020,May,13; 2018,Sep,7; 2018,May,3; 2017,Feb,9

22548-22634 Spinal Fusion: Anterior and Posterior Approach

EXCLUDES *Corpectomy (63081-63091)*
Exploration spinal fusion (22830)
Fracture care (22310-22328)
Injection:
Chemonucleolysis (62292)
Discography (62290-62291)
Facet joint (64490-64495, [64633, 64634, 64635, 64636])
Myelography (62284)
Laminectomy (63001-63017)
Needle/trocar biopsy (20220-20225)
Osteotomy (22206-22226)

Code also bone grafting procedures (20930-20938)
Code also spinal instrumentation (22840-22855 [22859])

22548 **Arthrodesis, anterior transoral or extraoral technique, clivus-C1-C2 (atlas-axis), with or without excision of odontoid process**

EXCLUDES *Laminectomy or laminotomy with disc removal (63020-63042)*

56.4 56.4 **FUD** 090 C 80

AMA: 2020,May,13; 2018,Sep,7; 2018,May,3; 2018,Jan,8; 2017,Mar,7; 2017,Jan,8; 2016,Jan,13; 2015,Jan,16

22551 **Arthrodesis, anterior interbody, including disc space preparation, discectomy, osteophytectomy and decompression of spinal cord and/or nerve roots; cervical below C2**

INCLUDES Operating microscope (69990)

49.3 49.3 **FUD** 090 J J8 80

AMA: 2020,May,13; 2018,Sep,7; 2018,Aug,10; 2018,May,3; 2018,Jan,8; 2017,Mar,7; 2017,Jan,8; 2016,May,13; 2016,Feb,12; 2016,Jan,13; 2015,Jan,16; 2015,Jan,13

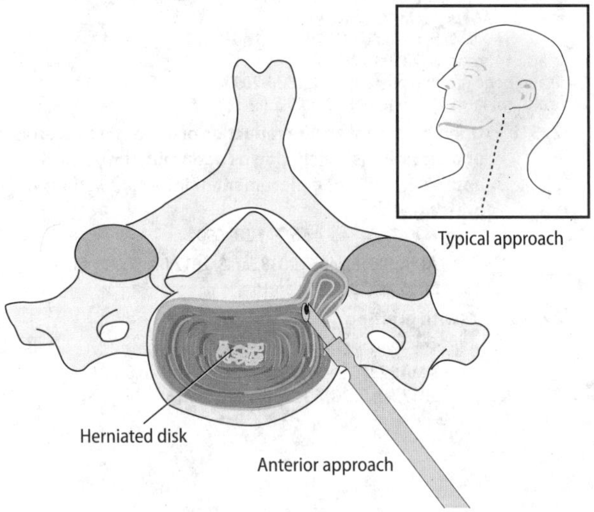

\+ **22552** **cervical below C2, each additional interspace (List separately in addition to code for separate procedure)**

INCLUDES Operating microscope (69990)

Code first (22551)

11.6 11.6 **FUD** ZZZ N N1 80

AMA: 2020,May,13; 2018,Sep,7; 2018,Aug,10; 2018,May,3; 2018,Jan,8; 2017,Mar,7; 2017,Jan,8; 2016,Feb,12; 2016,Jan,13; 2015,Jan,16

22554 Arthrodesis, anterior interbody technique, including minimal discectomy to prepare interspace (other than for decompression); cervical below C2

EXCLUDES *Anterior discectomy and interbody fusion during same operative session (regardless if performed by multiple surgeons) (22551)*

Discectomy, anterior, with decompression spinal cord and/or nerve root(s), cervical (even by separate individual) (63075-63076)

36.3 36.3 **FUD** 090 J J8 80

AMA: 2020,May,13; 2018,Sep,7; 2018,May,3; 2018,Jan,8; 2017,Mar,7; 2017,Jan,8; 2016,Jan,13; 2015,Apr,7; 2015,Jan,16

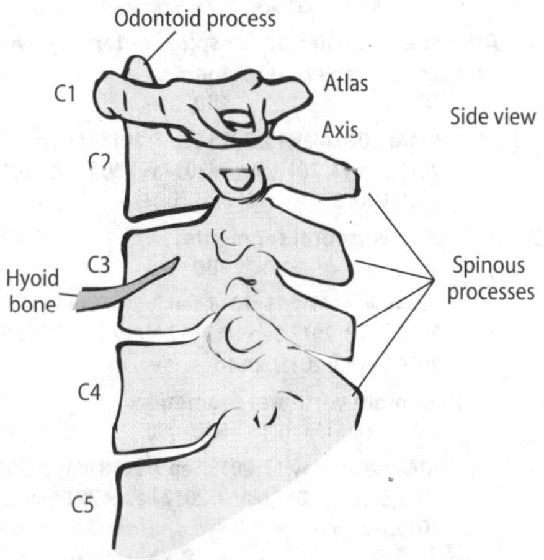

22556 thoracic

48.1 48.1 **FUD** 090 C 80

AMA: 2020,May,13; 2018,Sep,7; 2018,May,3; 2018,Jan,8; 2017,Mar,7; 2017,Jan,8; 2016,Jan,13; 2015,Jan,16

22558 lumbar

EXCLUDES *Arthrodesis using pre-sacral interbody technique (22586)*

44.3 44.3 **FUD** 090 C 80

AMA: 2020,May,13; 2018,Sep,7; 2018,May,3; 2018,Jan,8; 2017,Mar,7; 2017,Feb,9; 2017,Jan,8; 2016,Jan,13; 2015,Mar,9; 2015,Jan,16

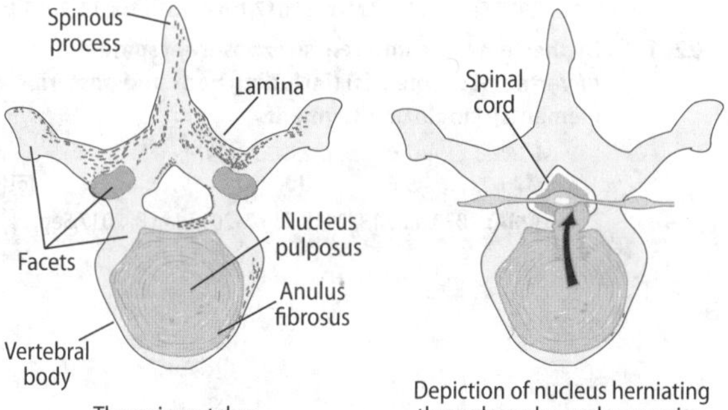

Thoracic vertebra (superior views)

Depiction of nucleus herniating through anulus and pressuring spinal nerve

\+ **22585 each additional interspace (List separately in addition to code for primary procedure)**

EXCLUDES *Anterior discectomy and interbody fusion during same operative session (regardless if performed by multiple surgeons) (22552)*

Discectomy, anterior, with decompression spinal cord and/or nerve root(s), cervical (even by separate individual) (63075)

Code first (22554-22558)

9.51 9.51 **FUD** ZZZ N N1 80

AMA: 2020,May,13; 2018,Sep,7; 2018,Jan,8; 2017,Jan,8; 2016,Jan,13; 2015,Jan,16

22586 Arthrodesis, pre-sacral interbody technique, including disc space preparation, discectomy, with posterior instrumentation, with image guidance, includes bone graft when performed, L5-S1 interspace

INCLUDES Radiologic guidance (77002-77003, 77011-77012)

EXCLUDES *Allograft and autograft spinal bone (20930-20938)*

Epidurography, radiological supervision and interpretation (72275)

Pelvic fixation, other than sacrum (22848)

Posterior non-segmental instrumentation (22840)

59.6 59.6 **FUD** 090 C 80

AMA: 2020,May,13; 2018,Sep,7

22590 Arthrodesis, posterior technique, craniocervical (occiput-C2)

EXCLUDES *Posterior intrafacet implant insertion (0219T-0222T)*

45.6 45.6 **FUD** 090 C 80

AMA: 2020,May,13; 2018,Sep,7; 2018,May,3; 2018,Jan,8; 2017,Mar,7; 2017,Jan,8; 2016,Jan,13; 2015,Jan,16

Skull and cervical vertebrae; posterior view

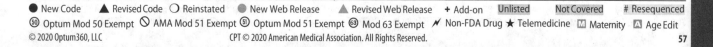

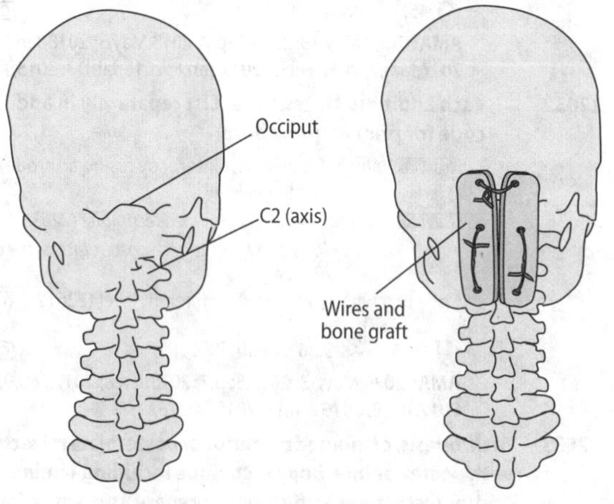

The physician fuses skull to C2 (axis) to stabilize cervical vertebrae; anchor holes are drilled in the occiput of the skull

22595 Arthrodesis, posterior technique, atlas-axis (C1-C2)

EXCLUDES *Posterior intrafacet implant insertion (0219T-0222T)*

43.8 43.8 **FUD** 090 C 80

AMA: 2020,May,13; 2018,Sep,7; 2018,May,3; 2018,Jan,8; 2017,Mar,7; 2017,Jan,8; 2016,Jan,13; 2015,Jan,16

22600 Arthrodesis, posterior or posterolateral technique, single level; cervical below C2 segment

EXCLUDES *Posterior intrafacet implant insertion (0219T-0222T)*

37.4 37.4 **FUD** 090 C 80

AMA: 2020,May,13; 2018,Sep,7; 2018,May,3; 2018,Jan,8; 2017,Mar,7; 2017,Jan,8; 2016,Jan,13; 2015,Jan,16

22610 thoracic (with lateral transverse technique, when performed)

EXCLUDES *Posterior intrafacet implant insertion (0219T-0222T)*

36.7 36.7 **FUD** 090 C 80

AMA: 2020,May,13; 2018,Sep,7; 2018,May,3; 2018,Jan,8; 2017,Mar,7; 2017,Jan,8; 2016,Jan,13; 2015,Jan,16

22612 lumbar (with lateral transverse technique, when performed)

EXCLUDES *Arthrodesis performed at same interspace and segment (22630)*

Combined technique at same interspace and segment (22633)

Posterior intrafacet implant insertion (0219T-0222T)

46.0 46.0 **FUD** 090 J J8 80

AMA: 2020,May,13; 2018,Sep,7; 2018,May,3; 2018,Jan,8; 2017,Mar,7; 2017,Feb,9; 2017,Jan,8; 2016,Jan,13; 2015,Jan,16

\+ **22614** **each additional vertebral segment (List separately in addition to code for primary procedure)**

INCLUDES Additional level fusion arthrodesis posterior or posterolateral interbody

EXCLUDES *Additional level interbody arthrodesis combined posterolateral or posterior with posterior interbody arthrodesis (22634)*
Additional level posterior interbody arthrodesis (22632)
Posterior intrafacet implant insertion (0219T-0222T)

Code first when performed at different level (22600, 22610, 22612, 22630, 22633)

Facility RVU 11.4 Non-Facility RVU 11.4 **FUD** ZZZ N N1 80

AMA: 2020,May,13; 2018,Sep,7; 2018,Jan,8; 2017,Feb,9; 2017,Jan,8; 2016,Jan,13; 2015,Jan,16

22630 **Arthrodesis, posterior interbody technique, including laminectomy and/or discectomy to prepare interspace (other than for decompression), single interspace; lumbar**

EXCLUDES *Arthrodesis performed at same interspace and segment (22612)*
Combined technique (22612 and 22630) for same interspace and segment (22633)

Facility RVU 45.5 Non-Facility RVU 45.5 **FUD** 090 C 80

AMA: 2020,May,13; 2018,Sep,7; 2018,May,3; 2018,Jan,8; 2017,Mar,7; 2017,Feb,9; 2017,Jan,8; 2016,Jan,13; 2015,Jan,16

\+ **22632** **each additional interspace (List separately in addition to code for primary procedure)**

INCLUDES Includes posterior interbody fusion arthrodesis, additional level

EXCLUDES *Additional level combined technique (22634)*
Additional level posterior or posterolateral fusion (22614)

Code first when performed at different level (22612, 22630, 22633)

Facility RVU 9.36 Non-Facility RVU 9.36 **FUD** ZZZ C 80

AMA: 2020,May,13; 2018,Sep,7; 2018,Jan,8; 2017,Feb,9; 2017,Jan,8; 2016,Jan,13; 2015,Jan,16

22633 **Arthrodesis, combined posterior or posterolateral technique with posterior interbody technique including laminectomy and/or discectomy sufficient to prepare interspace (other than for decompression), single interspace and segment; lumbar**

EXCLUDES *Arthrodesis performed at same interspace and segment (22612, 22630)*

Facility RVU 53.8 Non-Facility RVU 53.8 **FUD** 090 C 80

AMA: 2020,May,13; 2018,Sep,7; 2018,Jul,14; 2018,May,9; 2018,May,3; 2018,Jan,8; 2017,Mar,7; 2017,Feb,9; 2017,Jan,8; 2016,Oct,11; 2016,Jan,13; 2015,Jan,16

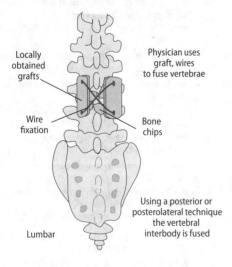

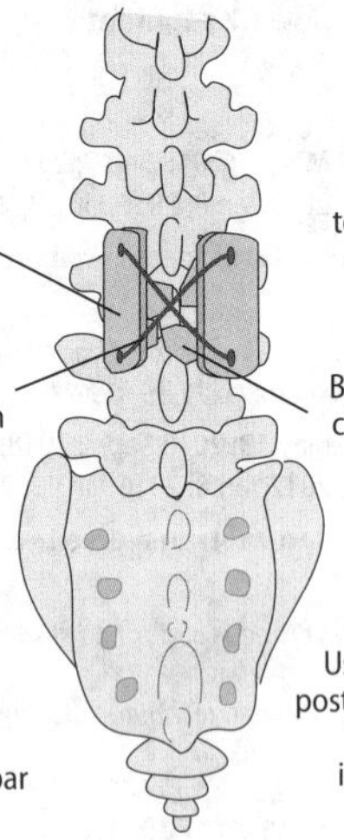
Locally obtained grafts
Physician uses graft, wires to fuse vertebrae
Wire fixation
Bone chips
Using a posterior or posterolateral technique the vertebral interbody is fused
Lumbar

\+ **22634** **each additional interspace and segment (List separately in addition to code for primary procedure)**

Code first (22633)

Facility RVU 14.4 Non-Facility RVU 14.4 **FUD** ZZZ C 80

AMA: 2020,May,13; 2018,Sep,7; 2018,Jul,14; 2018,May,3; 2018,Jan,8; 2017,Mar,7; 2017,Feb,9; 2017,Jan,8; 2016,Jan,13; 2015,Jan,16

22800-22819 Procedures to Correct Anomalous Spinal Vertebrae

CMS: 100-03,150.2 Osteogenic Stimulation

EXCLUDES *Facet injection (64490-64495, [64633, 64634, 64635, 64636])*

Code also bone grafting procedures (20930-20938)
Code also spinal instrumentation (22840-22855 [22859])

22800 **Arthrodesis, posterior, for spinal deformity, with or without cast; up to 6 vertebral segments**

Facility RVU 39.3 Non-Facility RVU 39.3 **FUD** 090 C 80

AMA: 2020,May,13; 2018,Sep,7; 2018,May,3; 2018,Jan,8; 2017,Sep,14; 2017,Mar,7; 2017,Feb,9; 2017,Jan,8; 2016,Jan,13; 2015,Jan,16

22802 **7 to 12 vertebral segments**

Facility RVU 61.0 Non-Facility RVU 61.0 **FUD** 090 C 80

AMA: 2020,May,13; 2018,Sep,7; 2018,Jul,14; 2018,May,3; 2018,Jan,8; 2017,Sep,14; 2017,Mar,7; 2017,Feb,9; 2017,Jan,8; 2016,Jan,13; 2015,Jan,16

22804 **13 or more vertebral segments**

Facility RVU 70.3 Non-Facility RVU 70.3 **FUD** 090 C 80

AMA: 2020,May,13; 2018,Sep,7; 2018,May,3; 2018,Jan,8; 2017,Sep,14; 2017,Mar,7; 2017,Feb,9; 2017,Jan,8; 2016,Jan,13; 2015,Jan,16

22808 **Arthrodesis, anterior, for spinal deformity, with or without cast; 2 to 3 vertebral segments**

INCLUDES Smith-Robinson arthrodesis

Facility RVU 53.1 Non-Facility RVU 53.1 **FUD** 090 C 80

AMA: 2020,May,13; 2018,Sep,7; 2018,May,3; 2018,Jan,8; 2017,Sep,14; 2017,Mar,7; 2017,Jan,8; 2016,Jan,13; 2015,Jan,16

22810 **4 to 7 vertebral segments**

Facility RVU 60.2 Non-Facility RVU 60.2 **FUD** 090 C 80

AMA: 2020,May,13; 2018,Sep,7; 2018,May,3; 2018,Jan,8; 2017,Sep,14; 2017,Mar,7; 2017,Jan,8; 2016,Jan,13; 2015,Jan,16

22812 **8 or more vertebral segments**

Facility RVU 63.9 Non-Facility RVU 63.9 **FUD** 090 C 80

AMA: 2020,May,13; 2018,Sep,7; 2018,May,3; 2018,Jan,8; 2017,Sep,14; 2017,Mar,7; 2017,Jan,8; 2016,Jan,13; 2015,Jan,16

22818 **Kyphectomy, circumferential exposure of spine and resection of vertebral segment(s) (including body and posterior elements); single or 2 segments**

EXCLUDES *Arthrodesis (22800-22804)*

Facility RVU 62.6 Non-Facility RVU 62.6 **FUD** 090 C 80

AMA: 2020,May,13; 2018,Sep,7; 2018,Jan,8; 2017,Sep,14

22819 **3 or more segments**

EXCLUDES *Arthrodesis (22800-22804)*

72.2 72.2 **FUD** 090 C 80

AMA: 2020,May,13; 2018,Sep,7; 2018,Jan,8; 2017,Sep,14

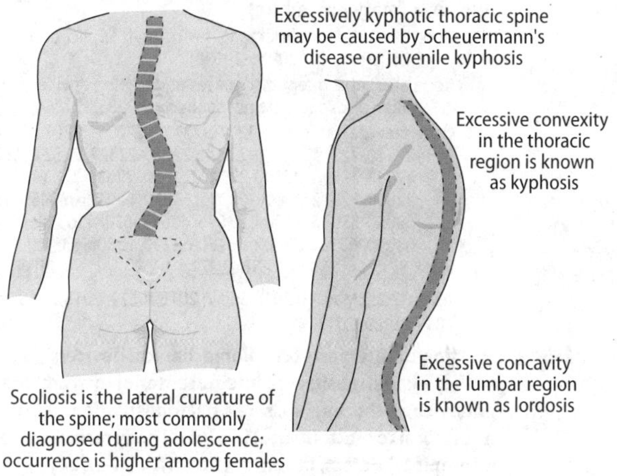

22830 Surgical Exploration Previous Spinal Fusion

CMS: 100-03,150.2 Osteogenic Stimulation

EXCLUDES *Arthrodesis (22532-22819)*
Bone grafting procedures (20930-20938)
Instrumentation removal (22850, 22852, 22855)
Spinal decompression (63001-63103)

Code also spinal instrumentation (22840-22855 [22859])

22830 **Exploration of spinal fusion**

23.6 23.6 **FUD** 090 C 80

AMA: 2018,Sep,7; 2018,Jan,8; 2017,Jan,8; 2016,Jan,13; 2015,Jan,16

22840-22848 Posterior, Anterior, Pelvic Spinal Instrumentation

INCLUDES Removal or revision previously placed spinal instrumentation during same session as insertion new instrumentation at levels including all or part of previously instrumented segments (22849, 22850, 22852, 22855)

EXCLUDES *Arthrodesis (22532-22534, 22548-22812)*
Bone grafting procedures (20930-20938)
Exploration spinal fusion (22830)
Fracture treatment (22325-22328)
Reporting more than one instrumentation code per incision

\+ **22840** **Posterior non-segmental instrumentation (eg, Harrington rod technique, pedicle fixation across 1 interspace, atlantoaxial transarticular screw fixation, sublaminar wiring at C1, facet screw fixation) (List separately in addition to code for primary procedure)**

Code first (22100-22102, 22110-22114, 22206-22207, 22210-22214, 22220-22224, 22310-22327, 22532-22533, 22548-22558, 22590-22612, 22630, 22633-22634, 22800-22812, 63001-63030, 63040-63042, 63045-63047, 63050-63056, 63064, 63075, 63077, 63081, 63085, 63087, 63090, 63101-63102, 63170-63290, 63300-63307)

22.2 22.2 **FUD** ZZZ N N1 80

AMA: 2020,May,13; 2018,Sep,7; 2018,Jan,8; 2017,Jun,10; 2017,Feb,9; 2017,Jan,8; 2016,Jan,13; 2015,Jan,16

\+ **22841** **Internal spinal fixation by wiring of spinous processes (List separately in addition to code for primary procedure)**

Code first (22100-22102, 22110-22114, 22206-22207, 22210-22214, 22220-22224, 22310-22327, 22532-22533, 22548-22558, 22590-22612, 22630, 22633-22634, 22800-22812, 63001-63030, 63040-63042, 63045-63047, 63050-63056, 63064, 63075, 63077, 63081, 63085, 63087, 63090, 63101-63102, 63170-63290, 63300-63307)

0.00 0.00 **FUD** XXX C

AMA: 2020,May,13; 2018,Sep,7; 2018,Jan,8; 2017,Feb,9; 2017,Jan,8; 2016,Jan,13; 2015,Jan,16

\+ **22842** **Posterior segmental instrumentation (eg, pedicle fixation, dual rods with multiple hooks and sublaminar wires); 3 to 6 vertebral segments (List separately in addition to code for primary procedure)**

Code first (22100-22102, 22110-22114, 22206-22207, 22210-22214, 22220-22224, 22310-22327, 22532-22533, 22548-22558, 22590-22612, 22630, 22633-22634, 22800-22812, 63001-63030, 63040-63042, 63045-63047, 63050-63056, 63064, 63075, 63077, 63081, 63085, 63087, 63090, 63101-63102, 63170-63290, 63300-63307)

22.1 22.1 **FUD** ZZZ N N1 80

AMA: 2020,May,13; 2018,Sep,7; 2018,Jan,8; 2017,Feb,9; 2017,Jan,8; 2016,Jan,13; 2015,Jan,16

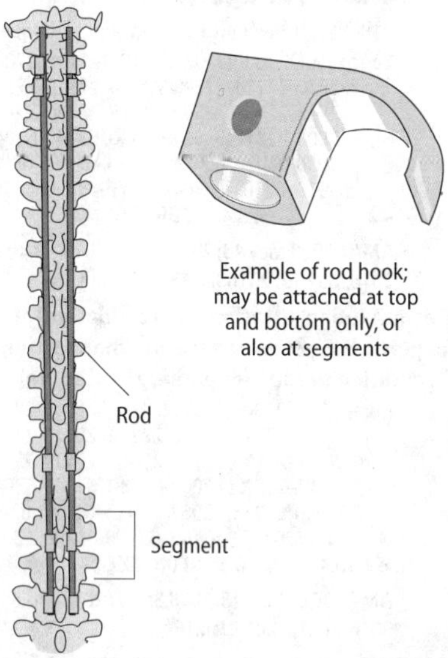

\+ **22843** **7 to 12 vertebral segments (List separately in addition to code for primary procedure)**

Code first (22100-22102, 22110-22114, 22206-22207, 22210-22214, 22220-22224, 22310-22327, 22532-22533, 22548-22558, 22590-22612, 22630, 22633-22634, 22800-22812, 63001-63030, 63040-63042, 63045-63047, 63050-63056, 63064, 63075, 63077, 63081, 63085, 63087, 63090, 63101-63102, 63170-63290, 63300-63307)

23.8 23.8 **FUD** ZZZ C 80

AMA: 2020,May,13; 2018,Sep,7; 2018,Jul,14; 2018,Jan,8; 2017,Jan,8; 2016,Jan,13; 2015,Jan,16

\+ **22844** **13 or more vertebral segments (List separately in addition to code for primary procedure)**

Code first (22100-22102, 22110-22114, 22206-22207, 22210-22214, 22220-22224, 22310-22327, 22532-22533, 22548-22558, 22590-22612, 22630, 22633-22634, 22800-22812, 63001-63030, 63040-63042, 63045-63047, 63050-63056, 63064, 63075, 63077, 63081, 63085, 63087, 63090, 63101-63102, 63170-63290, 63300-63307)

28.6 28.6 **FUD** ZZZ C 80

AMA: 2020,May,13; 2018,Sep,7; 2018,Jan,8; 2017,Jan,8; 2016,Jan,13; 2015,Jan,16

\+ **22845** **Anterior instrumentation; 2 to 3 vertebral segments (List separately in addition to code for primary procedure)**

INCLUDES Dwyer instrumentation technique

Code first (22100-22102, 22110-22114, 22206-22207, 22210-22214, 22220-22224, 22310-22327, 22532-22533, 22548-22558, 22590-22612, 22630, 22633-22634, 22800-22812, 63001-63030, 63040-63042, 63045-63047, 63050-63056, 63064, 63075, 63077, 63081, 63085, 63087, 63090, 63101-63102, 63170-63290, 63300-63307)

21.1 21.1 **FUD** ZZZ N N1 80

AMA: 2020,May,13; 2018,Sep,7; 2018,Jan,8; 2017,Mar,7; 2017,Jan,8; 2016,May,13; 2016,Jan,13; 2015,Apr,7; 2015,Mar,9; 2015,Jan,13; 2015,Jan,16

+ **22846** **4 to 7 vertebral segments (List separately in addition to code for primary procedure)**

INCLUDES Dwyer instrumentation technique

Code first (22100-22102, 22110-22114, 22206-22207, 22210-22214, 22220-22224, 22310-22327, 22532-22533, 22548-22558, 22590-22612, 22630, 22633-22634, 22800-22812, 63001-63030, 63040-63042, 63045-63047, 63050-63056, 63064, 63075, 63077, 63081, 63085, 63087, 63090, 63101-63102, 63170-63290, 63300-63307)

22.0 22.0 **FUD** ZZZ C 80

AMA: 2020,May,13; 2018,Sep,7; 2018,Jan,8; 2017,Jan,8; 2016,May,13; 2016,Jan,13; 2015,Jan,16

+ **22847** **8 or more vertebral segments (List separately in addition to code for primary procedure)**

INCLUDES Dwyer instrumentation technique

Code first (22100-22102, 22110-22114, 22206-22207, 22210-22214, 22220-22224, 22310-22327, 22532-22533, 22548-22558, 22590-22612, 22630, 22633-22634, 22800-22812, 63001-63030, 63040-63042, 63045-63047, 63050-63056, 63064, 63075, 63077, 63081, 63085, 63087, 63090, 63101-63102, 63170-63290, 63300-63307)

23.4 23.4 **FUD** ZZZ C 80

AMA: 2020,May,13; 2018,Sep,7; 2018,Jan,8; 2017,Jan,8; 2016,May,13; 2016,Jan,13; 2015,Jan,16

+ **22848** **Pelvic fixation (attachment of caudal end of instrumentation to pelvic bony structures) other than sacrum (List separately in addition to code for primary procedure)**

Code first (22100-22102, 22110-22114, 22206-22207, 22210-22214, 22220-22224, 22310-22327, 22532-22533, 22548-22558, 22590-22612, 22630, 22633-22634, 22800-22812, 63001-63030, 63040-63042, 63045-63047, 63050-63056, 63064, 63075, 63077, 63081, 63085, 63087, 63090, 63101-63102, 63170-63290, 63300-63307)

10.4 10.4 **FUD** ZZZ C 80

AMA: 2020,May,13; 2018,Sep,7; 2018,Jan,8; 2017,Jan,8; 2016,Jan,13; 2015,Jan,16

22849-22855 [22859] Miscellaneous Spinal Instrumentation

EXCLUDES *Arthrodesis (22532-22534, 22548-22812)*
Bone grafting procedures (20930-20938)
Exploration spinal fusion (22830)
Facet injection (64490-64495, [64633, 64634, 64635, 64636])
Fracture treatment (22325-22328)

22849 **Reinsertion of spinal fixation device**

INCLUDES Removal of instrumentation at the same level (22850, 22852, 22855)

37.7 37.7 **FUD** 090 C 80

AMA: 2020,May,13; 2018,Sep,7; 2018,Jan,8; 2017,Jun,10; 2017,Jan,8; 2016,May,13; 2016,Jan,13; 2015,Jan,16

22850 **Removal of posterior nonsegmental instrumentation (eg, Harrington rod)**

21.0 21.0 **FUD** 090 C 80

AMA: 2020,May,13; 2018,Sep,7; 2018,Jan,8; 2017,Jun,10; 2017,Jan,8; 2016,May,13; 2016,Jan,13; 2015,Jan,16

22852 **Removal of posterior segmental instrumentation**

20.2 20.2 **FUD** 090 C 80

AMA: 2020,May,13; 2018,Sep,7; 2018,Jan,8; 2017,Jun,10; 2017,Jan,8; 2016,Jan,13; 2015,Jan,16

+ **22853** **Insertion of interbody biomechanical device(s) (eg, synthetic cage, mesh) with integral anterior instrumentation for device anchoring (eg, screws, flanges), when performed, to intervertebral disc space in conjunction with interbody arthrodesis, each interspace (List separately in addition to code for primary procedure)**

Code also intervertebral bone device/graft application (20930-20931, 20936-20938)

Code also subsequent disc spaces undergoing device insertion when disc spaces are not connected (22853-22854, [22859])

Code first (22100-22102, 22110-22114, 22206-22207, 22210-22214, 22220-22224, 22310-22327, 22532-22533, 22548-22558, 22590-22612, 22630, 22633-22634, 22800-22812, 63001-63030, 63040, 63042, 63045-63047, 63050-63056, 63064, 63075, 63077, 63081, 63085, 63087, 63090, 63101-63102, 63170-63290, 63300-63307)

7.52 7.52 **FUD** ZZZ N N1 80

AMA: 2020,May,13; 2018,Sep,7; 2018,Jul,14; 2018,Jan,8; 2017,Aug,9; 2017,Mar,7

+ **22854** **Insertion of intervertebral biomechanical device(s) (eg, synthetic cage, mesh) with integral anterior instrumentation for device anchoring (eg, screws, flanges), when performed, to vertebral corpectomy(ies) (vertebral body resection, partial or complete) defect, in conjunction with interbody arthrodesis, each contiguous defect (List separately in addition to code for primary procedure)**

Code also intervertebral bone device/graft application (20930-20931, 20936-20938)

Code also subsequent disc spaces undergoing device insertion when disc spaces are not connected (22853-22854, [22859])

Code first (22100-22102, 22110-22114, 22206-22207, 22210-22214, 22220-22224, 22310-22327, 22532-22533, 22548-22558, 22590-22612, 22630, 22633-22634, 22800-22812, 63001-63030, 63040, 63042, 63045-63047, 63050-63056, 63064, 63075, 63077, 63081, 63085, 63087, 63090, 63101-63102, 63170-63290, 63300-63307)

9.74 9.74 **FUD** ZZZ N N1 80

AMA: 2020,May,13; 2018,Sep,7; 2018,Jan,8; 2017,Mar,7

+ # **22859** **Insertion of intervertebral biomechanical device(s) (eg, synthetic cage, mesh, methylmethacrylate) to intervertebral disc space or vertebral body defect without interbody arthrodesis, each contiguous defect (List separately in addition to code for primary procedure)**

Code also intervertebral bone device/graft application (20930-20931, 20936-20938)

Code also subsequent disc spaces undergoing device insertion when disc spaces are not connected (22853-22854, 22854)

Code first (22100-22102, 22110-22114, 22206-22207, 22210-22214, 22220-22224, 22310-22327, 22532-22533, 22548-22558, 22590-22612, 22630, 22633-22634, 22800-22812, 63001-63030, 63040-63042, 63045-63047, 63050-63056, 63064, 63075, 63077, 63081, 63085, 63087, 63090, 63101-63102, 63170-63290, 63300-63307)

9.74 9.74 **FUD** ZZZ N N1 80

AMA: 2020,May,13; 2018,Sep,7; 2018,Jan,8; 2017,Mar,7

22855 **Removal of anterior instrumentation**

32.1 32.1 **FUD** 090 C 80

AMA: 2020,May,13; 2018,Sep,7; 2018,Jan,8; 2017,Jun,10; 2017,Jan,8; 2016,Jan,13; 2015,Jan,16

22856-22865 [22858, 22859] Artificial Disc Replacement

EXCLUDES *Fluoroscopy*
Spinal decompression (63001-63048)

22856 Total disc arthroplasty (artificial disc), anterior approach, including discectomy with end plate preparation (includes osteophytectomy for nerve root or spinal cord decompression and microdissection); single interspace, cervical

INCLUDES Operating microscope (69990)
EXCLUDES *Application intervertebral biomechanical device(s) at same level (22853-22854, [22859])*
Arthrodesis at same level (22554)
Discectomy at same level (63075)
Insertion instrumentation at same level (22845)
Code also arthroplasty more than one interspace, when performed ([22858])
47.3 47.3 FUD 090 J J8 80
AMA: 2020,May,13; 2018,Sep,7; 2018,Jan,8; 2017,Jan,8; 2016,Feb,12; 2016,Jan,13; 2015,Apr,7

\+ # **22858 second level, cervical (List separately in addition to code for primary procedure)**

Code first (22856)
14.8 14.8 FUD ZZZ N N1 80
AMA: 2020,May,13; 2018,Sep,7; 2018,Jan,8; 2017,Jan,8; 2016,Feb,12; 2016,Jan,13; 2015,Apr,7

22857 Total disc arthroplasty (artificial disc), anterior approach, including discectomy to prepare interspace (other than for decompression), single interspace, lumbar

INCLUDES Operating microscope (69990)
EXCLUDES *Application intervertebral biomechanical device(s) at same level (22853-22854, [22859])*
Arthrodesis at same level (22558)
Insertion instrumentation at same level (22845)
Retroperitoneal exploration (49010)
Code also arthroplasty more than one interspace, when performed (0163T)
50.8 50.8 FUD 090 C 80
AMA: 2020,May,13; 2018,Sep,7; 2016,Feb,12

22858 **Resequenced code. See code following 22856.**

22859 **Resequenced code. See code following 22854.**

22861 Revision including replacement of total disc arthroplasty (artificial disc), anterior approach, single interspace; cervical

INCLUDES Operating microscope (69990)
EXCLUDES *Procedures performed at same level (22845, 22853-22854, [22859], 22864, 63075)*
Revision additional cervical arthroplasty (0098T)
66.9 66.9 FUD 090 C 80
AMA: 2020,May,13; 2018,Sep,7; 2016,Feb,12

22862 lumbar

EXCLUDES *Arthroplasty revision more than one interspace (0165T)*
Procedures performed at same level (22558, 22845, 22853-22854, [22859], 22865, 49010)
66.8 66.8 FUD 090 C 80
AMA: 2020,May,13; 2018,Sep,7; 2018,Jan,8; 2017,Jan,8; 2016,Jan,13; 2015,Jan,16

22864 Removal of total disc arthroplasty (artificial disc), anterior approach, single interspace; cervical

INCLUDES Operating microscope (69990)
EXCLUDES *Cervical total disc arthroplasty with additional interspace removal (0095T)*
Revision total disc arthroplasty (22861)
59.7 59.7 FUD 090 C 80
AMA: 2020,May,13; 2018,Sep,7

22865 lumbar

EXCLUDES *Arthroplasty more than one level (0164T)*
Exploration, retroperitoneal area with or without biopsy(s) (49010)
65.1 65.1 FUD 090 C 80
AMA: 2020,May,13; 2018,Sep,7; 2018,Jan,8; 2017,Jan,8; 2016,Jan,13; 2015,Jan,16

22867-22899 Spinal Distraction/Stabilization Device

22867 Insertion of interlaminar/interspinous process stabilization/distraction device, without fusion, including image guidance when performed, with open decompression, lumbar; single level

EXCLUDES *Interlaminar/interspinous stabilization/distraction device insertion (22869, 22870)*
Procedures at same level (22532-22534, 22558, 22612, 22614, 22630, 22632-22634, 22800, 22802, 22804, 22840-22842, 22869-22870, 63005, 63012, 63017, 63030, 63035, 63042, 63044, 63047-63048, 77003)
28.2 20.2 FUD 090 J J8 80
AMA: 2020,May,13; 2018,Sep,7; 2018,Jan,8; 2017,Feb,9

\+ **22868 second level (List separately in addition to code for primary procedure)**

EXCLUDES *Interlaminar/interspinous stabilization/distraction device insertion (22869-22870)*
Procedures at same level (22532-22534, 22558, 22612, 22614, 22630, 22632-22634, 22800, 22802, 22804, 22840-22842, 22869-22870, 63005, 63012, 63017, 63030, 63035, 63042, 63044, 63047-63048, 77003)
Code first (22867)
7.08 7.08 FUD ZZZ N N1 80
AMA: 2020,May,13; 2018,Sep,7; 2018,Jan,8; 2017,Feb,9

22869 Insertion of interlaminar/interspinous process stabilization/distraction device, without open decompression or fusion, including image guidance when performed, lumbar; single level

EXCLUDES *Procedures at the same level (22532-22534, 22558, 22612, 22614, 22630, 22632-22634, 22800, 22802, 22804, 22840-22842, 63005, 63012, 63017, 63030, 63035, 63042, 63044, 63047-63048, 77003)*
12.8 12.8 FUD 090 J J8 80
AMA: 2020,May,13; 2018,Sep,7; 2018,Jan,8; 2017,Feb,9

\+ **22870 second level (List separately in addition to code for primary procedure)**

EXCLUDES *Procedures at the same level (22532-22534, 22558, 22612, 22614, 22630, 22632-22634, 22800, 22802, 22804, 22840-22842, 63005, 63012, 63017, 63030, 63035, 63042, 63044, 63047-63048, 77003)*
Code first (22869)
3.96 3.96 FUD ZZZ N N1 80
AMA: 2020,May,13; 2018,Sep,7; 2018,Jan,8; 2017,Feb,9

22899 Unlisted procedure, spine

0.00 0.00 FUD YYY T 80
AMA: 2020,Jun,14; 2018,Sep,7; 2018,May,10; 2018,Jan,8; 2017,Feb,9; 2017,Jan,8; 2016,Jan,13; 2015,Jan,8; 2015,Jan,16

22900-22999 Musculoskeletal Procedures of Abdomen

INCLUDES Any necessary elevation tissue planes or dissection
Measurement tumor and necessary margin at greatest diameter prior to excision
Simple and intermediate repairs
Excision types:
Fascial or subfascial soft tissue tumors: simple and marginal resection tumors found either in or below deep fascia, not involving bone or excision substantial amount normal tissue; primarily benign and intramuscular tumors
Radical resection soft tissue tumor: wide resection tumor involving substantial margins normal tissue and may include tissue removal from one or more layers; most often malignant or aggressive benign
Subcutaneous: simple and marginal resection tumors in subcutaneous tissue above deep fascia; most often benign

EXCLUDES *Complex repair*
Excision benign cutaneous lesions (eg, sebaceous cyst) (11400-11406)
Radical resection cutaneous tumors (eg, melanoma) (11600-11606)
Significant vessel exploration or neuroplasty

22900 **Excision, tumor, soft tissue of abdominal wall, subfascial (eg, intramuscular); less than 5 cm**
16.3 16.3 FUD 090 J G2 80
AMA: 2018,Sep,7

22901 **5 cm or greater**
19.3 19.3 FUD 090 J G2 80
AMA: 2018,Sep,7

22902 **Excision, tumor, soft tissue of abdominal wall, subcutaneous; less than 3 cm**
9.57 13.1 FUD 090 J G2 80
AMA: 2018,Sep,7

22903 **3 cm or greater**
12.6 12.6 FUD 090 J G2 80
AMA: 2018,Sep,7

22904 **Radical resection of tumor (eg, sarcoma), soft tissue of abdominal wall; less than 5 cm**
30.5 30.5 FUD 090 J G2 80
AMA: 2018,Sep,7

22905 **5 cm or greater**
38.5 38.5 FUD 090 J G2 80
AMA: 2018,Sep,7

22999 **Unlisted procedure, abdomen, musculoskeletal system**
0.00 0.00 FUD YYY T 80
AMA: 2018,Sep,7

23000-23044 Surgical Incision Shoulder: Drainage, Foreign Body Removal, Contracture Release

23000 **Removal of subdeltoid calcareous deposits, open**
EXCLUDES *Arthroscopic removal calcium deposits bursa (29999)*
10.5 16.4 FUD 090 J A2 80 50
AMA: 2018,Sep,7

23020 **Capsular contracture release (eg, Sever type procedure)**
EXCLUDES *Simple incision and drainage (10040-10160)*
19.9 19.9 FUD 090 J A2 80 50
AMA: 2018,Sep,7

23030 **Incision and drainage, shoulder area; deep abscess or hematoma**
7.20 12.4 FUD 010 J A2
AMA: 2018,Sep,7

23031 **infected bursa**
6.01 11.5 FUD 010 J A2 50
AMA: 2018,Sep,7

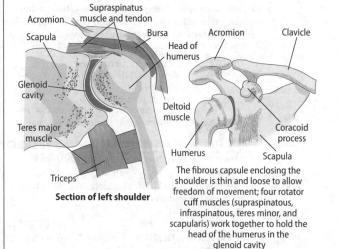

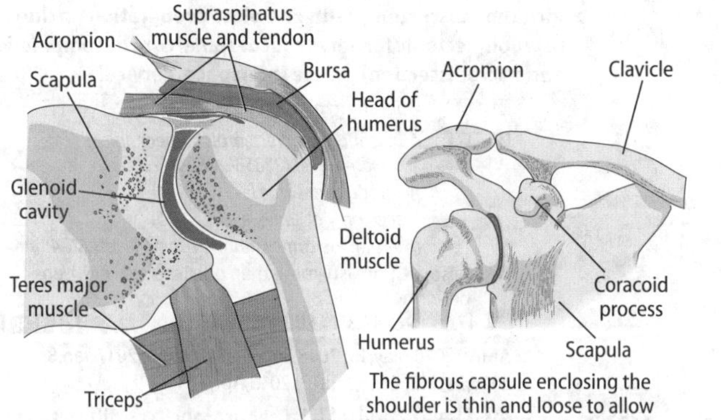

Section of left shoulder

The fibrous capsule enclosing the shoulder is thin and loose to allow freedom of movement; four rotator cuff muscles (supraspinatous, infraspinatous, teres minor, and scapularis) work together to hold the head of the humerus in the glenoid cavity

23035 **Incision, bone cortex (eg, osteomyelitis or bone abscess), shoulder area**
19.6 19.6 FUD 090 J A2 80 50
AMA: 2018,Sep,7

23040 **Arthrotomy, glenohumeral joint, including exploration, drainage, or removal of foreign body**
20.7 20.7 FUD 090 J A2 80 50
AMA: 2018,Sep,7

23044 **Arthrotomy, acromioclavicular, sternoclavicular joint, including exploration, drainage, or removal of foreign body**
16.3 16.3 FUD 090 J A2 50
AMA: 2018,Sep,7

23065-23066 Shoulder Biopsy

EXCLUDES *Soft tissue needle biopsy (20206)*

23065 **Biopsy, soft tissue of shoulder area; superficial**
4.81 6.34 FUD 010 J P3 50
AMA: 2018,Sep,7

23066 **deep**
10.4 16.2 FUD 090 J A2 50
AMA: 2018,Sep,7

23071-23078 [23071, 23073] Excision Soft Tissue Tumors of Shoulder

INCLUDES Any necessary elevation tissue planes or dissection
Measurement tumor and necessary margin at greatest diameter prior to excision
Simple and intermediate repairs
Excision types:
Fascial or subfascial soft tissue tumors: simple and marginal resection tumors found either in or below deep fascia, not involving bone or excision substantial amount normal tissue; primarily benign and intramuscular tumors
Radical resection soft tissue tumor: wide resection tumor, involving substantial margins normal tissue and may involve tissue removal from one or more layers; most often malignant or aggressive benign
Subcutaneous: simple and marginal resection tumors in subcutaneous tissue above deep fascia; most often benign

EXCLUDES *Complex repair*
Excision benign cutaneous lesions (eg, sebaceous cyst) (11400-11406)
Radical resection cutaneous tumors (eg, melanoma) (11600-11606)
Significant vessel exploration or neuroplasty

23071 **Resequenced code. See code following 23075.**

23073 **Resequenced code. See code following 23076.**

23075 **Excision, tumor, soft tissue of shoulder area, subcutaneous; less than 3 cm**
9.44 14.3 FUD 090 J G2 50
AMA: 2018,Sep,7; 2018,Jan,8; 2017,Jan,8; 2016,Jan,13; 2015,Jan,16

23071 **3 cm or greater**
12.1 12.1 FUD 090 J G2 80 50
AMA: 2018,Sep,7

23076 **Excision, tumor, soft tissue of shoulder area, subfascial (eg, intramuscular); less than 5 cm**
15.6 15.6 FUD 090 J G2 50
AMA: 2018,Sep,7; 2018,Jan,8; 2017,Jan,8; 2016,Jan,13; 2015,Jan,16

23073 **5 cm or greater**
20.1 20.1 FUD 090 J G2 80 50
AMA: 2018,Sep,7

23077 **Radical resection of tumor (eg, sarcoma), soft tissue of shoulder area; less than 5 cm**
32.7 32.7 FUD 090 J G2 80 50
AMA: 2018,Sep,7

23078 **5 cm or greater**
41.4 41.4 FUD 090 J G2 80 50
AMA: 2018,Sep,7

23100-23195 Bone and Joint Procedures of Shoulder

INCLUDES Acromioclavicular joint
Clavicle
Head and neck of humerus
Scapula
Shoulder joint
Sternoclavicular joint

23100 **Arthrotomy, glenohumeral joint, including biopsy**
14.5 14.5 FUD 090 J A2 80 50
AMA: 2018,Sep,7

23101 **Arthrotomy, acromioclavicular joint or sternoclavicular joint, including biopsy and/or excision of torn cartilage**
13.1 13.1 FUD 090 J A2 50
AMA: 2018,Sep,7

23105 **Arthrotomy; glenohumeral joint, with synovectomy, with or without biopsy**
18.3 18.3 FUD 090 J A2 80 50
AMA: 2018,Sep,7

23106 **sternoclavicular joint, with synovectomy, with or without biopsy**
14.3 14.3 FUD 090 J A2 50
AMA: 2018,Sep,7

23107 **Arthrotomy, glenohumeral joint, with joint exploration, with or without removal of loose or foreign body**
19.0 19.0 FUD 090 J A2 80 50
AMA: 2018,Sep,7

23120 **Claviculectomy; partial**
INCLUDES Mumford operation
EXCLUDES *Arthroscopic claviculectomy (29824)*
16.8 16.8 FUD 090 J A2 80 50
AMA: 2018,Sep,7; 2018,Jan,8; 2017,Jan,8; 2016,Jan,13; 2015,Jan,16

23125 **total**
20.4 20.4 FUD 090 J A2 80 50
AMA: 2018,Sep,7

23130 **Acromioplasty or acromionectomy, partial, with or without coracoacromial ligament release**
17.6 17.6 FUD 090 J A2 50
AMA: 2018,Sep,7; 2018,Jan,8; 2017,Jan,8; 2016,Jan,13; 2015,Mar,7; 2015,Feb,10; 2015,Jan,16

23140 **Excision or curettage of bone cyst or benign tumor of clavicle or scapula;**
15.9 15.9 FUD 090 J A2 50
AMA: 2018,Sep,7

23145 **with autograft (includes obtaining graft)**
20.0 20.0 FUD 090 J A2 80 50
AMA: 2018,Sep,7

23146 **with allograft**
17.9 17.9 FUD 090 J A2 80 50
AMA: 2019,May,7; 2018,Sep,7

23150 **Excision or curettage of bone cyst or benign tumor of proximal humerus;**
19.2 19.2 FUD 090 J A2 80 50
AMA: 2018,Sep,7

23155 **with autograft (includes obtaining graft)**
22.9 22.9 FUD 090 J A2 80 50
AMA: 2018,Sep,7

23156 **with allograft**
19.4 19.4 FUD 090 J J8 80 50
AMA: 2019,May,7; 2018,Sep,7

23170 **Sequestrectomy (eg, for osteomyelitis or bone abscess), clavicle**
16.2 16.2 FUD 090 J A2 50
AMA: 2018,Sep,7

23172 **Sequestrectomy (eg, for osteomyelitis or bone abscess), scapula**
16.3 16.3 FUD 090 J A2 80 50
AMA: 2018,Sep,7

23174 **Sequestrectomy (eg, for osteomyelitis or bone abscess), humeral head to surgical neck**
21.9 21.9 FUD 090 J A2 80 50
AMA: 2018,Sep,7

23180 **Partial excision (craterization, saucerization, or diaphysectomy) bone (eg, osteomyelitis), clavicle**
19.1 19.1 FUD 090 J A2 50
AMA: 2018,Sep,7

23182 **Partial excision (craterization, saucerization, or diaphysectomy) bone (eg, osteomyelitis), scapula**
19.0 19.0 FUD 090 J A2 80 50
AMA: 2018,Sep,7

23184 **Partial excision (craterization, saucerization, or diaphysectomy) bone (eg, osteomyelitis), proximal humerus**
21.1 21.1 FUD 090 J A2 80 50
AMA: 2018,Sep,7

23190 **Ostectomy of scapula, partial (eg, superior medial angle)**
16.5 16.5 FUD 090 J A2 80 50
AMA: 2018,Sep,7

23195 **Resection, humeral head**
EXCLUDES *Arthroplasty with replacement with implant (23470)*
21.5 21.5 FUD 090 J A2 80 50
AMA: 2018,Sep,7

23200-23220 Radical Resection of Bone Tumors of Shoulder

INCLUDES Any necessary elevation tissue planes or dissection
Excision adjacent soft tissue during bone tumor resection (23071-23078 [23071, 23073])
Measurement tumor and necessary margin at greatest diameter prior to excision
Radical resection cutaneous tumors (e.g., melanoma)
Resection tumor (may include entire bone) and wide margins normal tissues primarily for malignant or aggressive benign tumors
Simple and intermediate repairs
EXCLUDES *Complex repair*
Significant vessel exploration, neuroplasty, reconstruction, or complex bone repair

23200 **Radical resection of tumor; clavicle**
43.6 43.6 FUD 090 C 80 50
AMA: 2019,May,7; 2018,Sep,7

23210 **scapula**
51.2 51.2 FUD 090 C 80 50
AMA: 2019,May,7; 2018,Sep,7

23220 **Radical resection of tumor, proximal humerus**
56.3 56.3 FUD 090 C 80 50
AMA: 2019,May,7; 2018,Sep,7

23330-23335 Removal Implant/Foreign Body from Shoulder

EXCLUDES *Bursal arthrocentesis or needling (20610)*
K-wire or pin insertion (20650)
K-wire or pin removal (20670, 20680)

23330 **Removal of foreign body, shoulder; subcutaneous**
4.79 8.03 FUD 010 T A2 80 50
AMA: 2018,Sep,7; 2018,Jan,8; 2017,Jan,8; 2016,Jan,13; 2015,Jan,16

23333 **deep (subfascial or intramuscular)**
13.2 13.2 FUD 090 J G2 80 50
AMA: 2018,Sep,7; 2018,Jan,8; 2017,Jan,8; 2016,Jan,13; 2015,Jan,16

23334 **Removal of prosthesis, includes debridement and synovectomy when performed; humeral or glenoid component**
EXCLUDES *Foreign body removal (23330, 23333)*
Prosthesis removal and replacement in same shoulder (eg, glenoid and/or humeral components) (23473-23474)
30.8 30.8 FUD 090 J G2 50
AMA: 2018,Sep,7; 2018,Jan,8; 2017,Jan,8; 2016,Jan,13; 2015,Jan,16

23335 **humeral and glenoid components (eg, total shoulder)**
EXCLUDES *Foreign body removal (23330, 23333)*
Prosthesis removal and replacement in same shoulder (eg, glenoid and/or humeral components) (23473-23474)
36.7 36.7 FUD 090 C 50
AMA: 2018,Sep,7; 2018,Jan,8; 2017,Jan,8; 2016,Jan,13; 2015,Jan,16

23350 Injection for Shoulder Arthrogram

23350 **Injection procedure for shoulder arthrography or enhanced CT/MRI shoulder arthrography**
EXCLUDES *Shoulder biopsy (29805-29826)*
(73040, 73201-73202, 73222-73223, 77002)
1.47 3.97 FUD 000 N N1 50
AMA: 2018,Sep,7; 2018,Jan,8; 2017,Jan,8; 2016,May,13; 2016,Jan,13; 2015,Aug,6; 2015,Jan,16

23395-23491 Repair/Reconstruction of Shoulder

23395 **Muscle transfer, any type, shoulder or upper arm; single**
37.0 37.0 FUD 090 J A2 80
AMA: 2018,Sep,7

23397 **multiple**
32.9 32.9 FUD 090 J A2 80
AMA: 2018,Sep,7

23400 **Scapulopexy (eg, Sprengels deformity or for paralysis)**
28.0 28.0 FUD 090 J A2 80 50
AMA: 2018,Sep,7

23405 **Tenotomy, shoulder area; single tendon**
17.8 17.8 FUD 090 J A2 80
AMA: 2018,Sep,7

23406 **multiple tendons through same incision**
22.2 22.2 FUD 090 J J8 80
AMA: 2018,Sep,7

23410 **Repair of ruptured musculotendinous cuff (eg, rotator cuff) open; acute**
EXCLUDES *Arthroscopic repair (29827)*
23.6 23.6 FUD 090 J A2 80 50
AMA: 2018,Sep,7; 2018,Jan,8; 2017,Jan,8; 2016,Jan,13; 2015,Jan,16

23412 **chronic**
EXCLUDES *Arthroscopic repair (29827)*
24.5 24.5 FUD 090 J A2 80 50
AMA: 2018,Sep,7; 2018,Jan,8; 2017,Jan,8; 2016,Jan,13; 2015,Jun,10; 2015,Feb,10; 2015,Jan,16

23415 **Coracoacromial ligament release, with or without acromioplasty**
EXCLUDES *Arthroscopic repair (29826)*
20.1 20.1 FUD 090 J A2 50
AMA: 2018,Sep,7; 2018,Jan,8; 2017,Jan,8; 2016,Jan,13; 2015,Mar,7

23420 **Reconstruction of complete shoulder (rotator) cuff avulsion, chronic (includes acromioplasty)**
28.0 28.0 FUD 090 J A2 80 50
AMA: 2018,Sep,7; 2018,Jan,8; 2017,Jan,8; 2016,Jan,13; 2015,Jan,16

23430 **Tenodesis of long tendon of biceps**
EXCLUDES *Arthroscopic biceps tenodesis (29828)*
21.4 21.4 FUD 090 J A2 80 50
AMA: 2018,Sep,7

23440 **Resection or transplantation of long tendon of biceps**
21.7 21.7 FUD 090 J A2 80 50
AMA: 2018,Sep,7

23450 **Capsulorrhaphy, anterior; Putti-Platt procedure or Magnuson type operation**
EXCLUDES *Arthroscopic thermal capsulorrhaphy (29999)*
27.3 27.3 FUD 090 J A2 80 50
AMA: 2018,Sep,7

23455 **with labral repair (eg, Bankart procedure)**
EXCLUDES *Arthroscopic repair (29806)*
28.7 28.7 FUD 090 J A2 80 50
AMA: 2018,Sep,7

23460 **Capsulorrhaphy, anterior, any type; with bone block**
INCLUDES Bristow procedure
31.4 31.4 FUD 090 J A2 80 50
AMA: 2018,Sep,7

23462 **with coracoid process transfer**
EXCLUDES *Open thermal capsulorrhaphy (23929)*
30.9 30.9 FUD 090 J A2 80 50
AMA: 2018,Sep,7

23465 **Capsulorrhaphy, glenohumeral joint, posterior, with or without bone block**
EXCLUDES *Sternoclavicular and acromioclavicular joint repair (23530, 23550)*
32.3 32.3 FUD 090 J G2 80 50
AMA: 2018,Sep,7

23466 **Capsulorrhaphy, glenohumeral joint, any type multi-directional instability**
32.0 32.0 FUD 090 J A2 80 50
AMA: 2018,Sep,7

23470 **Arthroplasty, glenohumeral joint; hemiarthroplasty**
34.7 34.7 FUD 090 J 80 50
AMA: 2018,Sep,7; 2018,Jan,8; 2017,Jan,8; 2016,Jan,13; 2015,Jan,16

23472 **total shoulder (glenoid and proximal humeral replacement (eg, total shoulder))**
EXCLUDES *Proximal humerus osteotomy (24400)*
Removal total shoulder components (23334-23335)
41.9 41.9 FUD 090 C 80 50
AMA: 2018,Sep,7; 2018,Jan,8; 2017,Jan,8; 2016,Jan,13; 2015,Jan,16

23473 **Revision of total shoulder arthroplasty, including allograft when performed; humeral or glenoid component**

EXCLUDES *Removal prosthesis only (glenoid and/or humeral component) same shoulder/same operative sessions (23334-23335)*

46.7 46.7 FUD 090 J 80 50

AMA: 2018,Sep,7; 2018,Jan,8; 2017,Jan,8; 2016,Jan,13; 2015,Jan,16

23474 **humeral and glenoid component**

EXCLUDES *Removal prosthesis only (glenoid and/or humeral component) same shoulder/same operative sessions (23334-23335)*

50.5 50.5 FUD 090 C 80 50

AMA: 2018,Sep,7; 2018,Jan,8; 2017,Jan,8; 2016,Jan,13; 2015,Jan,16

23480 **Osteotomy, clavicle, with or without internal fixation;**

23.7 23.7 FUD 090 J A2 50

AMA: 2018,Sep,7

23485 **with bone graft for nonunion or malunion (includes obtaining graft and/or necessary fixation)**

27.6 27.6 FUD 090 J J8 80 50

AMA: 2018,Sep,7

23490 **Prophylactic treatment (nailing, pinning, plating or wiring) with or without methylmethacrylate; clavicle**

24.6 24.6 FUD 090 J A2 80 50

AMA: 2018,Sep,7

23491 **proximal humerus**

29.3 29.3 FUD 090 J J8 80 50

AMA: 2018,Sep,7

23500-23680 Treatment of Shoulder Fracture/Dislocation

23500 **Closed treatment of clavicular fracture; without manipulation**

6.37 6.24 FUD 090 T A2 50

AMA: 2018,Sep,7

23505 **with manipulation**

9.61 10.2 FUD 090 J A2 50

AMA: 2018,Sep,7

23515 **Open treatment of clavicular fracture, includes internal fixation, when performed**

20.7 20.7 FUD 090 J J8 80 50

AMA: 2018,Sep,7; 2018,Jan,8; 2017,Jan,8; 2016,Jan,13; 2015,Jan,16

23520 **Closed treatment of sternoclavicular dislocation; without manipulation**

6.73 6.72 FUD 090 J A2 80 50

AMA: 2018,Sep,7

23525 **with manipulation**

10.2 11.1 FUD 090 T A2 80 50

AMA: 2018,Sep,7

23530 **Open treatment of sternoclavicular dislocation, acute or chronic;**

16.5 16.5 FUD 090 J A2 80 50

AMA: 2018,Sep,7

23532 **with fascial graft (includes obtaining graft)**

18.0 18.0 FUD 090 J A2 80 50

AMA: 2018,Sep,7

23540 **Closed treatment of acromioclavicular dislocation; without manipulation**

6.64 6.67 FUD 090 T A2 50

AMA: 2018,Sep,7

23545 **with manipulation**

8.93 9.91 FUD 090 T A2 80 50

AMA: 2018,Sep,7

23550 **Open treatment of acromioclavicular dislocation, acute or chronic;**

16.3 16.3 FUD 090 J A2 80 50

AMA: 2018,Sep,7

23552 **with fascial graft (includes obtaining graft)**

18.8 18.8 FUD 090 J J8 80 50

AMA: 2019,Nov,14; 2018,Sep,7

23570 **Closed treatment of scapular fracture; without manipulation**

6.89 6.69 FUD 090 T A2 50

AMA: 2018,Sep,7

23575 **with manipulation, with or without skeletal traction (with or without shoulder joint involvement)**

10.8 11.6 FUD 090 J A2 80 50

AMA: 2018,Sep,7

23585 **Open treatment of scapular fracture (body, glenoid or acromion) includes internal fixation, when performed**

28.2 28.2 FUD 090 J A2 80 50

AMA: 2018,Sep,7; 2018,Jan,8; 2017,Jan,8; 2016,Jan,13; 2015,Jan,16

23600 **Closed treatment of proximal humeral (surgical or anatomical neck) fracture; without manipulation**

8.92 9.45 FUD 090 T P2 50

AMA: 2018,Sep,7

23605 **with manipulation, with or without skeletal traction**

12.2 13.4 FUD 090 J A2 50

AMA: 2018,Sep,7

23615 **Open treatment of proximal humeral (surgical or anatomical neck) fracture, includes internal fixation, when performed, includes repair of tuberosity(s), when performed;**

25.5 25.5 FUD 090 J J8 80 50

AMA: 2018,Sep,7; 2018,Jan,8; 2017,Jan,8; 2016,Jan,13; 2015,Jan,16

23616 **with proximal humeral prosthetic replacement**

35.7 35.7 FUD 090 J J8 80 50

AMA: 2018,Sep,7

23620 **Closed treatment of greater humeral tuberosity fracture; without manipulation**

7.32 7.65 FUD 090 T P2 50

AMA: 2018,Sep,7

23625 **with manipulation**

10.1 10.9 FUD 090 J A2 50

AMA: 2018,Sep,7

23630 **Open treatment of greater humeral tuberosity fracture, includes internal fixation, when performed**

22.4 22.4 FUD 090 J J8 80 50

AMA: 2018,Sep,7

23650 **Closed treatment of shoulder dislocation, with manipulation; without anesthesia**

8.36 9.18 FUD 090 T A2 50

AMA: 2018,Sep,7

23655 **requiring anesthesia**

11.5 11.5 FUD 090 J A2 50

AMA: 2018,Sep,7

23660 **Open treatment of acute shoulder dislocation**

EXCLUDES *Chronic dislocation repair (23450-23466)*

16.8 16.8 FUD 090 J A2 80 50

AMA: 2018,Sep,7; 2018,Jan,8; 2017,Jan,8; 2016,Jan,13; 2015,Jan,16

23665 **Closed treatment of shoulder dislocation, with fracture of greater humeral tuberosity, with manipulation**

11.4 12.3 FUD 090 J A2 50

AMA: 2019,Feb,10; 2018,Sep,7

23670 **Open treatment of shoulder dislocation, with fracture of greater humeral tuberosity, includes internal fixation, when performed**

25.2 25.2 FUD 090 J A2 80 50

AMA: 2018,Sep,7

23675 **Closed treatment of shoulder dislocation, with surgical or anatomical neck fracture, with manipulation**
14.4 15.9 FUD 090 J A2 50
AMA: 2018,Sep,7

23680 **Open treatment of shoulder dislocation, with surgical or anatomical neck fracture, includes internal fixation, when performed**
26.8 26.8 FUD 090 J J8 80 50
AMA: 2018,Sep,7

23700-23929 Other/Unlisted Shoulder Procedures

23700 **Manipulation under anesthesia, shoulder joint, including application of fixation apparatus (dislocation excluded)**
5.63 5.63 FUD 010 J A2 50
AMA: 2018,Sep,7; 2018,Jan,8; 2017,Jan,8; 2016,Jan,13; 2015,Jun,10; 2015,Jan,16

23800 **Arthrodesis, glenohumeral joint;**
29.6 29.6 FUD 090 J G2 80 50
AMA: 2020,May,13; 2018,Sep,7

23802 **with autogenous graft (includes obtaining graft)**
37.0 37.0 FUD 090 J G2 80 50
AMA: 2020,May,13; 2018,Sep,7

23900 **Interthoracoscapular amputation (forequarter)**
40.0 40.0 FUD 090 C 80
AMA: 2018,Sep,7

23920 **Disarticulation of shoulder;**
32.4 32.4 FUD 090 C 80 50
AMA: 2018,Sep,7

23921 **secondary closure or scar revision**
13.5 13.5 FUD 090 T A2 50
AMA: 2018,Sep,7

23929 **Unlisted procedure, shoulder**
0.00 0.00 FUD YYY T 80
AMA: 2018,Sep,7

23930-24006 Surgical Incision Elbow/Upper Arm

EXCLUDES *Simple incision and drainage procedures (10040-10160)*

23930 **Incision and drainage, upper arm or elbow area; deep abscess or hematoma**
6.12 10.2 FUD 010 J A2 50
AMA: 2018,Sep,7

23931 **bursa**
4.48 8.19 FUD 010 J A2 50
AMA: 2018,Sep,7

23935 **Incision, deep, with opening of bone cortex (eg, for osteomyelitis or bone abscess), humerus or elbow**
14.7 14.7 FUD 090 J A2 80 50
AMA: 2018,Sep,7

24000 **Arthrotomy, elbow, including exploration, drainage, or removal of foreign body**
13.7 13.7 FUD 090 J A2 80 50
AMA: 2018,Sep,7

24006 **Arthrotomy of the elbow, with capsular excision for capsular release (separate procedure)**
20.5 20.5 FUD 090 J A2 80 50
AMA: 2018,Sep,7

24065-24066 Biopsy of Elbow/Upper Arm

EXCLUDES *Soft tissue needle biopsy (20206)*

24065 **Biopsy, soft tissue of upper arm or elbow area; superficial**
4.71 7.41 FUD 010 J P3 50
AMA: 2018,Sep,7

24066 **deep (subfascial or intramuscular)**
12.0 18.0 FUD 090 J A2 50
AMA: 2018,Sep,7

24071-24079 [24071, 24073] Excision Soft Tissue Tumors Elbow/Upper Arm

INCLUDES Any necessary elevation tissue planes or dissection
Measurement tumor and necessary margin at greatest diameter prior to excision
Excision types:
- Fascial or subfascial soft tissue tumors: simple and marginal resection tumors found either in or below deep fascia, not involving bone or excision substantial amount normal tissue; primarily benign and intramuscular tumors
- Radical resection soft tissue tumor: wide resection tumor involving substantial margins normal tissue and may involve tissue removal from one or more layers; most often malignant or aggressive benign
- Subcutaneous: simple and marginal resection tumors found in subcutaneous tissue above deep fascia; most often benign

EXCLUDES *Complex repair*
Excision benign cutaneous lesion (eg, sebaceous cyst) (11400-11406)
Radical resection cutaneous tumors (eg, melanoma) (11600-11606)
Significant vessel exploration or neuroplasty

24071 **Resequenced code. See code following 24075.**

24073 **Resequenced code. See code following 24076.**

24075 **Excision, tumor, soft tissue of upper arm or elbow area, subcutaneous; less than 3 cm**
9.47 14.8 FUD 090 J G2 50
AMA: 2018,Sep,7

\# **24071** **3 cm or greater**
11.7 11.7 FUD 090 J G2 80 50
AMA: 2018,Sep,7

24076 **Excision, tumor, soft tissue of upper arm or elbow area, subfascial (eg, intramuscular); less than 5 cm**
15.6 15.6 FUD 090 J G2 50
AMA: 2018,Sep,7

\# **24073** **5 cm or greater**
19.9 19.9 FUD 090 J G2 80 50
AMA: 2018,Sep,7

24077 **Radical resection of tumor (eg, sarcoma), soft tissue of upper arm or elbow area; less than 5 cm**
29.9 29.9 FUD 090 J G2 50
AMA: 2018,Sep,7

24079 **5 cm or greater**
38.3 38.3 FUD 090 J G2 80 50
AMA: 2018,Sep,7

24100-24149 Bone/Joint Procedures Upper Arm/Elbow

24100 **Arthrotomy, elbow; with synovial biopsy only**
12.0 12.0 FUD 090 J A2 80 50
AMA: 2018,Sep,7

24101 **with joint exploration, with or without biopsy, with or without removal of loose or foreign body**
14.4 14.4 FUD 090 J A2 80 50
AMA: 2018,Sep,7

24102 **with synovectomy**
17.7 17.7 FUD 090 J A2 80 50
AMA: 2018,Sep,7

24105 **Excision, olecranon bursa**
10.1 10.1 FUD 090 J A2 50
AMA: 2018,Sep,7

24110 **Excision or curettage of bone cyst or benign tumor, humerus;**
16.8 16.8 FUD 090 J A2 50
AMA: 2018,Sep,7

24115 **with autograft (includes obtaining graft)**
21.2 21.2 FUD 090 J A2 80 50
AMA: 2018,Sep,7

24116 **with allograft**
24.8 24.8 FUD 090 J A2 80 50
AMA: 2019,May,7; 2018,Sep,7

24120 **Excision or curettage of bone cyst or benign tumor of head or neck of radius or olecranon process;**
15.3 15.3 FUD 090 J A2 80 50
AMA: 2018,Sep,7

24125 **with autograft (includes obtaining graft)**
17.9 17.9 FUD 090 J A2 80 50
AMA: 2018,Sep,7

24126 **with allograft**
18.7 18.7 FUD 090 J J8 80 50
AMA: 2019,May,7; 2018,Sep,7

24130 **Excision, radial head**
EXCLUDES *Radial head arthroplasty with implant (24366)*
14.6 14.6 FUD 090 J A2 50
AMA: 2018,Sep,7

24134 **Sequestrectomy (eg, for osteomyelitis or bone abscess), shaft or distal humerus**
21.4 21.4 FUD 090 J A2 80 50
AMA: 2018,Sep,7

24136 **Sequestrectomy (eg, for osteomyelitis or bone abscess), radial head or neck**
18.2 18.2 FUD 090 J A2 50
AMA: 2018,Sep,7

24138 **Sequestrectomy (eg, for osteomyelitis or bone abscess), olecranon process**
19.6 19.6 FUD 090 J A2 80 50
AMA: 2018,Sep,7

24140 **Partial excision (craterization, saucerization, or diaphysectomy) bone (eg, osteomyelitis), humerus**
20.2 20.2 FUD 090 J A2 80 50
AMA: 2018,Sep,7

24145 **Partial excision (craterization, saucerization, or diaphysectomy) bone (eg, osteomyelitis), radial head or neck**
17.1 17.1 FUD 090 J A2 50
AMA: 2018,Sep,7

24147 **Partial excision (craterization, saucerization, or diaphysectomy) bone (eg, osteomyelitis), olecranon process**
17.9 17.9 FUD 090 J A2 50
AMA: 2018,Sep,7

24149 **Radical resection of capsule, soft tissue, and heterotopic bone, elbow, with contracture release (separate procedure)**
EXCLUDES *Capsular and soft tissue release (24006)*
33.8 33.8 FUD 090 J G2 80 50
AMA: 2018,Sep,7

24150-24152 Radical Resection Bone Tumor Upper Arm

INCLUDES Any necessary elevation tissue planes or dissection
Excision adjacent soft tissue during bone tumor resection (24071-24079 [24071, 24073])
Measurement tumor and necessary margin at greatest diameter prior to excision
Resection tumor (may include entire bone) and wide margins normal tissue primarily for malignant or aggressive benign tumors
Simple and intermediate repairs

EXCLUDES *Complex repair*
Significant vessel exploration, neuroplasty, reconstruction, or complex bone repair

24150 **Radical resection of tumor, shaft or distal humerus**
44.9 44.9 FUD 090 J 80 50
AMA: 2019,May,7; 2018,Sep,7

24152 **Radical resection of tumor, radial head or neck**
38.9 38.9 FUD 090 J G2 80 50
AMA: 2019,May,7; 2018,Sep,7

24155 Elbow Arthrectomy

24155 **Resection of elbow joint (arthrectomy)**
24.6 24.6 FUD 090 J A2 80 50
AMA: 2018,Sep,7

24160-24201 Removal Implant/Foreign Body from Elbow/Upper Arm

EXCLUDES *Bursal or joint arthrocentesis or needling (20605)*
K-wire or pin insertion (20650)
K-wire or pin removal (20670, 20680)

24160 **Removal of prosthesis, includes debridement and synovectomy when performed; humeral and ulnar components**
INCLUDES Prosthesis removal and replacement in same elbow (eg, humeral and/or ulnar component(s)) (24370-24371)
EXCLUDES *Foreign body removal (24200-24201)*
Hardware removal other than prosthesis (20680)
36.3 36.3 FUD 090 Q2 A2 50
AMA: 2018,Sep,7; 2018,Jan,8; 2017,Jan,8; 2016,Jan,13; 2015,Jan,16

24164 **radial head**
EXCLUDES *Foreign body removal (24200-24201)*
Hardware removal other than prosthesis (20680)
20.8 20.8 FUD 090 Q2 A2 50
AMA: 2018,Sep,7; 2018,Jan,8; 2017,Jan,8; 2016,Jan,13; 2015,Jan,16

24200 **Removal of foreign body, upper arm or elbow area; subcutaneous**
4.05 6.20 FUD 010 J P3 80 50
AMA: 2018,Sep,7; 2018,Jan,8; 2017,Jan,8; 2016,Jan,13; 2015,Jan,16

24201 **deep (subfascial or intramuscular)**
10.4 15.7 FUD 090 J A2 50
AMA: 2018,Sep,7; 2018,Jan,8; 2017,Jan,8; 2016,Jan,13; 2015,Jan,16

24220 Injection for Elbow Arthrogram

24220 **Injection procedure for elbow arthrography**
EXCLUDES *Injection tennis elbow (20550)*
(73085)
1.95 4.71 FUD 000 N N1 80 50
AMA: 2018,Sep,7; 2018,Jan,8; 2017,Jan,8; 2016,May,13; 2016,Jan,13; 2015,Aug,6

24300-24498 Repair/Reconstruction of Elbow/Upper Arm

24300 **Manipulation, elbow, under anesthesia**
EXCLUDES *External fixation (20690, 20692)*
12.2 12.2 FUD 090 J G2 50
AMA: 2018,Sep,7

24301 **Muscle or tendon transfer, any type, upper arm or elbow, single (excluding 24320-24331)**
21.6 21.6 FUD 090 J A2 80
AMA: 2018,Sep,7

24305 **Tendon lengthening, upper arm or elbow, each tendon**
16.7 16.7 FUD 090 J A2 80
AMA: 2018,Sep,7

24310 **Tenotomy, open, elbow to shoulder, each tendon**
13.5 13.5 FUD 090 J A2 80
AMA: 2018,Sep,7

24320 **Tenoplasty, with muscle transfer, with or without free graft, elbow to shoulder, single (Seddon-Brookes type procedure)**
22.5 22.5 FUD 090 J A2 80
AMA: 2018,Sep,7

24330 **Flexor-plasty, elbow (eg, Steindler type advancement);**
20.6 20.6 FUD 090 J A2 80 50
AMA: 2018,Sep,7

24331 **with extensor advancement**
22.7 22.7 FUD 090 J A2 80 50
AMA: 2018,Sep,7

24332 Tenolysis, triceps
Facility RVU 17.6 Non-Facility RVU 17.6 FUD 090 J G2 50 CCI
AMA: 2018,Sep,7

24340 Tenodesis of biceps tendon at elbow (separate procedure)
Facility RVU 17.7 Non-Facility RVU 17.7 FUD 090 J A2 80 50 CCI
AMA: 2018,Sep,7

24341 Repair, tendon or muscle, upper arm or elbow, each tendon or muscle, primary or secondary (excludes rotator cuff)
Facility RVU 21.4 Non-Facility RVU 21.4 FUD 090 J A2 80 50 CCI
AMA: 2018,Sep,7

24342 Reinsertion of ruptured biceps or triceps tendon, distal, with or without tendon graft
Facility RVU 22.3 Non-Facility RVU 22.3 FUD 090 J A2 80 50 CCI
AMA: 2018,Sep,7; 2018,Jan,8; 2017,Apr,9

24343 Repair lateral collateral ligament, elbow, with local tissue
Facility RVU 20.4 Non-Facility RVU 20.4 FUD 090 J G2 80 50 CCI
AMA: 2018,Sep,7

24344 Reconstruction lateral collateral ligament, elbow, with tendon graft (includes harvesting of graft)
Facility RVU 31.5 Non-Facility RVU 31.5 FUD 090 J G2 80 50 CCI
AMA: 2018,Sep,7

24345 Repair medial collateral ligament, elbow, with local tissue
Facility RVU 20.2 Non-Facility RVU 20.2 FUD 090 J A2 80 50 CCI
AMA: 2018,Sep,7

24346 Reconstruction medial collateral ligament, elbow, with tendon graft (includes harvesting of graft)
Facility RVU 31.7 Non-Facility RVU 31.7 FUD 090 J G2 80 50 CCI
AMA: 2018,Sep,7

24357 Tenotomy, elbow, lateral or medial (eg, epicondylitis, tennis elbow, golfer's elbow); percutaneous
EXCLUDES *Arthroscopy, elbow, surgical; debridement (29837-29838)*
Facility RVU 11.9 Non-Facility RVU 11.9 FUD 090 J G2 80 50 CCI
AMA: 2018,Sep,7; 2018,Jan,8; 2017,Jan,8; 2016,Jan,13; 2015,Jan,16

24358 debridement, soft tissue and/or bone, open
EXCLUDES *Arthroscopy, elbow, surgical; debridement (29837-29838)*
Facility RVU 15.1 Non-Facility RVU 15.1 FUD 090 J G2 80 50 CCI
AMA: 2018,Sep,7; 2018,Jan,8; 2017,Jan,8; 2016,Jan,13; 2015,Jan,16

24359 debridement, soft tissue and/or bone, open with tendon repair or reattachment
EXCLUDES *Arthroscopy, elbow, surgical; debridement (29837-29838)*
Facility RVU 19.0 Non-Facility RVU 19.0 FUD 090 J G2 80 50 CCI
AMA: 2018,Sep,7; 2018,Jan,8; 2017,Jan,8; 2016,Jan,13; 2015,Jan,16

24360 Arthroplasty, elbow; with membrane (eg, fascial)
Facility RVU 26.0 Non-Facility RVU 26.0 FUD 090 J A2 80 50 CCI
AMA: 2018,Sep,7

24361 with distal humeral prosthetic replacement
Facility RVU 29.0 Non-Facility RVU 29.0 FUD 090 J J8 80 50 CCI
AMA: 2018,Sep,7

24362 with implant and fascia lata ligament reconstruction
Facility RVU 30.6 Non-Facility RVU 30.6 FUD 090 J A2 80 50 CCI
AMA: 2018,Sep,7

24363 with distal humerus and proximal ulnar prosthetic replacement (eg, total elbow)
EXCLUDES *Total elbow implant revision (24370-24371)*
Facility RVU 41.9 Non-Facility RVU 41.9 FUD 090 J J8 80 50 CCI
AMA: 2018,Sep,7; 2018,Jan,8; 2017,Jan,8; 2016,Jan,13; 2015,Jan,16

24365 Arthroplasty, radial head;
Facility RVU 18.4 Non-Facility RVU 18.4 FUD 090 J J8 80 50 CCI
AMA: 2018,Sep,7

24366 with implant
Facility RVU 19.7 Non-Facility RVU 19.7 FUD 090 J J8 80 50 CCI
AMA: 2018,Sep,7

24370 Revision of total elbow arthroplasty, including allograft when performed; humeral or ulnar component
EXCLUDES *Prosthesis removal without replacement in same elbow (eg, humeral and/or ulnar component/s) (24160)*
Facility RVU 44.7 Non-Facility RVU 44.7 FUD 090 J J8 80 50 CCI
AMA: 2018,Sep,7; 2018,Jan,8; 2017,Jan,8; 2016,Jan,13; 2015,Jan,16

24371 humeral and ulnar component
EXCLUDES *Prosthesis removal without replacement in same elbow (eg, humeral and/or ulnar component/s) (24160)*
Facility RVU 51.3 Non-Facility RVU 51.3 FUD 090 J J8 80 50 CCI
AMA: 2018,Sep,7; 2018,Jan,8; 2017,Jan,8; 2016,Jan,13; 2015,Jan,16

24400 Osteotomy, humerus, with or without internal fixation
EXCLUDES *Osteotomy with insertion intramedullary lengthening device, humerus (0594T)*
Facility RVU 23.7 Non-Facility RVU 23.7 FUD 090 J A2 80 50 CCI
AMA: 2018,Sep,7; 2018,Jan,8; 2017,Jan,8; 2016,Jan,13; 2015,Jan,16

24410 Multiple osteotomies with realignment on intramedullary rod, humeral shaft (Sofield type procedure)
EXCLUDES *Osteotomy with insertion intramedullary lengthening device, humerus (0594T)*
Facility RVU 30.5 Non-Facility RVU 30.5 FUD 090 J G2 80 50 CCI
AMA: 2018,Sep,7

24420 Osteoplasty, humerus (eg, shortening or lengthening) (excluding 64876)
EXCLUDES *Osteotomy with insertion intramedullary lengthening device, humerus (0594T)*
Facility RVU 29.5 Non-Facility RVU 29.5 FUD 090 J A2 80 50 CCI
AMA: 2018,Sep,7

24430 Repair of nonunion or malunion, humerus; without graft (eg, compression technique)
EXCLUDES *Repair proximal radius and/or ulna (25400-25420)*
Facility RVU 30.5 Non-Facility RVU 30.5 FUD 090 J J8 80 50 CCI
AMA: 2018,Sep,7

24435 with iliac or other autograft (includes obtaining graft)
EXCLUDES *Repair proximal radius and/or ulna (25400-25420)*
Facility RVU 31.0 Non-Facility RVU 31.0 FUD 090 J J8 80 50 CCI
AMA: 2018,Sep,7

24470 Hemiepiphyseal arrest (eg, cubitus varus or valgus, distal humerus)
Facility RVU 19.3 Non-Facility RVU 19.3 FUD 090 J A2 80 50 CCI
AMA: 2018,Sep,7

24495 Decompression fasciotomy, forearm, with brachial artery exploration
Facility RVU 23.4 Non-Facility RVU 23.4 FUD 090 J A2 80 50 CCI
AMA: 2018,Sep,7

24498 Prophylactic treatment (nailing, pinning, plating or wiring), with or without methylmethacrylate, humeral shaft
Facility RVU 24.9 Non-Facility RVU 24.9 FUD 090 J J8 80 50 CCI
AMA: 2018,Sep,7

24500-24685 Treatment of Fracture/Dislocation of Elbow/Upper Arm

INCLUDES Treatment for either closed or open fractures or dislocations

24500 Closed treatment of humeral shaft fracture; without manipulation
Facility RVU 9.46 Non-Facility RVU 10.2 FUD 090 T A2 50 CCI
AMA: 2018,Sep,7

24505 with manipulation, with or without skeletal traction
Facility RVU 12.9 Non-Facility RVU 14.3 FUD 090 J A2 50 CCI
AMA: 2018,Sep,7

24515 **Open treatment of humeral shaft fracture with plate/screws, with or without cerclage**
25.3 25.3 FUD 090 J J8 80 50
AMA: 2018,Sep,7

24516 **Treatment of humeral shaft fracture, with insertion of intramedullary implant, with or without cerclage and/or locking screws**
EXCLUDES *Osteotomy with insertion intramedullary lengthening device, humerus (0594T)*
24.7 24.7 FUD 090 J J8 80 50
AMA: 2018,Sep,7; 2018,Jan,8; 2018,Jan,3; 2017,Jan,8; 2016,Jan,13; 2015,Jan,16

24530 **Closed treatment of supracondylar or transcondylar humeral fracture, with or without intercondylar extension; without manipulation**
9.96 10.9 FUD 090 T A2 50
AMA: 2018,Sep,7

24535 **with manipulation, with or without skin or skeletal traction**
16.3 17.7 FUD 090 J A2 50
AMA: 2018,Sep,7

24538 **Percutaneous skeletal fixation of supracondylar or transcondylar humeral fracture, with or without intercondylar extension**
21.5 21.5 FUD 090 J A2 50
AMA: 2018,Sep,7; 2018,Jan,8; 2017,Jan,8; 2016,Jan,13; 2015,Jan,16

24545 **Open treatment of humeral supracondylar or transcondylar fracture, includes internal fixation, when performed; without intercondylar extension**
26.8 26.8 FUD 090 J J8 80 50
AMA: 2018,Sep,7

24546 **with intercondylar extension**
29.9 29.9 FUD 090 J J8 80 50
AMA: 2018,Sep,7

24560 **Closed treatment of humeral epicondylar fracture, medial or lateral; without manipulation**
8.41 9.43 FUD 090 T A2 50
AMA: 2018,Sep,7

24565 **with manipulation**
14.1 15.3 FUD 090 J A2 50
AMA: 2018,Sep,7

24566 **Percutaneous skeletal fixation of humeral epicondylar fracture, medial or lateral, with manipulation**
20.6 20.6 FUD 090 J A2 50
AMA: 2018,Sep,7

24575 **Open treatment of humeral epicondylar fracture, medial or lateral, includes internal fixation, when performed**
21.0 21.0 FUD 090 J J8 80 50
AMA: 2018,Sep,7

24576 **Closed treatment of humeral condylar fracture, medial or lateral; without manipulation**
8.75 9.80 FUD 090 T A2 50
AMA: 2018,Sep,7

24577 **with manipulation**
14.4 15.8 FUD 090 J A2 50
AMA: 2018,Sep,7

24579 **Open treatment of humeral condylar fracture, medial or lateral, includes internal fixation, when performed**
EXCLUDES *Closed treatment without manipulation (24530, 24560, 24576, 24650, 24670)*
Repair with manipulation (24535, 24565, 24577, 24675)
24.0 24.0 FUD 090 J J8 80 50
AMA: 2018,Sep,7

24582 **Percutaneous skeletal fixation of humeral condylar fracture, medial or lateral, with manipulation**
23.3 23.3 FUD 090 J A2 50
AMA: 2018,Sep,7

24586 **Open treatment of periarticular fracture and/or dislocation of the elbow (fracture distal humerus and proximal ulna and/or proximal radius);**
31.2 31.2 FUD 090 J G2 80 50
AMA: 2018,Sep,7

24587 **with implant arthroplasty**
EXCLUDES *Distal humerus arthroplasty with implant (24361)*
31.4 31.4 FUD 090 J J8 80 50
AMA: 2018,Sep,7

24600 **Treatment of closed elbow dislocation; without anesthesia**
9.71 10.6 FUD 090 T A2 50
AMA: 2018,Sep,7

24605 **requiring anesthesia**
13.6 13.6 FUD 090 J A2 50
AMA: 2018,Sep,7

24615 **Open treatment of acute or chronic elbow dislocation**
20.6 20.6 FUD 090 J A2 80 50
AMA: 2018,Sep,7

24620 **Closed treatment of Monteggia type of fracture dislocation at elbow (fracture proximal end of ulna with dislocation of radial head), with manipulation**
15.8 15.8 FUD 090 J A2 80 50
AMA: 2018,Sep,7

24635 **Open treatment of Monteggia type of fracture dislocation at elbow (fracture proximal end of ulna with dislocation of radial head), includes internal fixation, when performed**
19.3 19.3 FUD 090 J J8 80 50
AMA: 2018,Sep,7

24640 **Closed treatment of radial head subluxation in child, nursemaid elbow, with manipulation** A
2.26 2.89 FUD 010 T P3 80 50
AMA: 2018,Sep,7

24650 **Closed treatment of radial head or neck fracture; without manipulation**
6.96 7.51 FUD 090 T P2 50
AMA: 2018,Sep,7

24655 **with manipulation**
11.4 12.6 FUD 090 J A2 50
AMA: 2018,Sep,7

24665 **Open treatment of radial head or neck fracture, includes internal fixation or radial head excision, when performed;**
18.8 18.8 FUD 090 J A2 80 50
AMA: 2018,Sep,7

24666 **with radial head prosthetic replacement**
21.1 21.1 FUD 090 J J8 80 50
AMA: 2018,Sep,7

24670 **Closed treatment of ulnar fracture, proximal end (eg, olecranon or coronoid process[es]); without manipulation**
7.53 8.28 FUD 090 T A2 50
AMA: 2018,Sep,7

24675 **with manipulation**
11.9 13.1 FUD 090 J A2 50
AMA: 2018,Sep,7

24685 **Open treatment of ulnar fracture, proximal end (eg, olecranon or coronoid process[es]), includes internal fixation, when performed**
EXCLUDES *Arthrotomy, elbow (24100-24102)*
18.8 18.8 FUD 090 J J8 80 50
AMA: 2018,Sep,7; 2018,Jan,3

24800-24999 Other/Unlisted Elbow/Upper Arm Procedures

24800 **Arthrodesis, elbow joint; local**
23.9 23.9 FUD 090 J A2 80 50
AMA: 2020,May,13; 2018,Sep,7

24802 **with autogenous graft (includes obtaining graft)**
28.9 28.9 FUD 090 J G2 80 50
AMA: 2020,May,13; 2018,Sep,7

24900 **Amputation, arm through humerus; with primary closure**
21.3 21.3 FUD 090 C 80 50
AMA: 2018,Sep,7

24920 **open, circular (guillotine)**
21.1 21.1 FUD 090 C 80 50
AMA: 2018,Sep,7

24925 **secondary closure or scar revision**
16.3 16.3 FUD 090 J A2 80 50
AMA: 2018,Sep,7

24930 **re-amputation**
22.3 22.3 FUD 090 C 80 50
AMA: 2018,Sep,7

24931 **with implant**
26.9 26.9 FUD 090 C 80 50
AMA: 2018,Sep,7

24935 **Stump elongation, upper extremity**
33.6 33.6 FUD 090 J 80 50
AMA: 2018,Sep,7

24940 **Cineplasty, upper extremity, complete procedure**
0.00 0.00 FUD 090 C 80 50
AMA: 2018,Sep,7

24999 **Unlisted procedure, humerus or elbow**
0.00 0.00 FUD YYY T 80 50
AMA: 2018,Sep,7

25000-25001 Incision Tendon Sheath of Wrist

25000 **Incision, extensor tendon sheath, wrist (eg, deQuervains disease)**
EXCLUDES *Carpal tunnel release (64721)*
9.70 9.70 FUD 090 J A2 50
AMA: 2018,Sep,7

25001 **Incision, flexor tendon sheath, wrist (eg, flexor carpi radialis)**
9.88 9.88 FUD 090 J G2 50
AMA: 2018,Sep,7

25020-25025 Decompression Fasciotomy Forearm/Wrist

25020 **Decompression fasciotomy, forearm and/or wrist, flexor OR extensor compartment; without debridement of nonviable muscle and/or nerve**
EXCLUDES *Brachial artery exploration (24495)*
Superficial incision and drainage (10060-10160)
16.4 16.4 FUD 090 J A2 50
AMA: 2018,Sep,7

25023 **with debridement of nonviable muscle and/or nerve**
EXCLUDES *Debridement (11000-11044 [11045, 11046])*
Decompression fasciotomy with exploration brachial artery exploration (24495)
Superficial incision and drainage (10060-10160)
34.4 34.4 FUD 090 J A2 80 50
AMA: 2018,Sep,7

25024 **Decompression fasciotomy, forearm and/or wrist, flexor AND extensor compartment; without debridement of nonviable muscle and/or nerve**
22.5 22.5 FUD 090 J A2 50
AMA: 2018,Sep,7

25025 **with debridement of nonviable muscle and/or nerve**
34.8 34.8 FUD 090 J A2 80 50
AMA: 2018,Sep,7

25028-25040 Incision for Drainage/Foreign Body Removal

25028 **Incision and drainage, forearm and/or wrist; deep abscess or hematoma**
17.0 17.0 FUD 090 J A2 50
AMA: 2018,Sep,7

25031 **bursa**
10.0 10.0 FUD 090 J A2 80 50
AMA: 2018,Sep,7

25035 **Incision, deep, bone cortex, forearm and/or wrist (eg, osteomyelitis or bone abscess)**
16.8 16.8 FUD 090 J A2 80 50
AMA: 2018,Sep,7

25040 **Arthrotomy, radiocarpal or midcarpal joint, with exploration, drainage, or removal of foreign body**
16.1 16.1 FUD 090 J A2 80 50
AMA: 2018,Sep,7

25065-25066 Biopsy Forearm/Wrist

EXCLUDES *Soft tissue needle biopsy (20206)*

25065 **Biopsy, soft tissue of forearm and/or wrist; superficial**
4.59 7.37 FUD 010 J P3 50
AMA: 2018,Sep,7

25066 **deep (subfascial or intramuscular)**
10.3 10.3 FUD 090 J A2 50
AMA: 2018,Sep,7

25071-25078 [25071, 25073] Excision Soft Tissue Tumors Forearm/Wrist

INCLUDES Any necessary elevation tissue planes or dissection
Measurement tumor and necessary margin at greatest diameter prior to excision
Simple and intermediate repairs
Excision types:
Fascial or subfascial soft tissue tumors: simple and marginal resection tumors found either in or below deep fascia, not involving bone or excision substantial amount normal tissue; primarily benign and intramuscular tumors
Radical resection soft tissue tumor: wide resection tumor involving substantial margins normal tissue and may include tissue removal from one or more layers; most often malignant or aggressive benign
Subcutaneous: simple and marginal resection tumors in subcutaneous tissue above deep fascia; most often benign

EXCLUDES *Complex repair*
Excision benign cutaneous lesions (eg, sebaceous cyst) (11400-11406)
Radical resection cutaneous tumors (eg, melanoma) (11600-11606)
Significant vessel exploration or neuroplasty

25071 **Resequenced code. See code following 25075.**

25073 **Resequenced code. See code following 25076.**

25075 **Excision, tumor, soft tissue of forearm and/or wrist area, subcutaneous; less than 3 cm**
9.09 14.5 FUD 090 J G2 50
AMA: 2018,Sep,7

\# **25071** **3 cm or greater**
12.2 12.2 FUD 090 J G2 80 50
AMA: 2018,Sep,7

25076 **Excision, tumor, soft tissue of forearm and/or wrist area, subfascial (eg, intramuscular); less than 3 cm**
14.9 14.9 FUD 090 J G2 50
AMA: 2018,Sep,7

\# **25073** **3 cm or greater**
15.4 15.4 FUD 090 J G2 80 50
AMA: 2018,Sep,7

25077 **Radical resection of tumor (eg, sarcoma), soft tissue of forearm and/or wrist area; less than 3 cm**
25.6 25.6 FUD 090 J G2 50
AMA: 2018,Sep,7

25078 **3 cm or greater**
33.6 33.6 FUD 090 J G2 80 50
AMA: 2018,Sep,7

25085-25240 Procedures of Bones/Joints Lower Arm/Wrist

25085 Capsulotomy, wrist (eg, contracture)
12.9 12.9 FUD 090 J A2 80 50
AMA: 2018,Sep,7

25100 Arthrotomy, wrist joint; with biopsy
10.0 10.0 FUD 090 J A2 80 50
AMA: 2018,Sep,7

25101 with joint exploration, with or without biopsy, with or without removal of loose or foreign body
11.6 11.6 FUD 090 J A2 80 50
AMA: 2018,Sep,7

25105 with synovectomy
13.9 13.9 FUD 090 J A2 80 50
AMA: 2018,Sep,7

25107 Arthrotomy, distal radioulnar joint including repair of triangular cartilage, complex
17.7 17.7 FUD 090 J A2 80 50
AMA: 2018,Sep,7

25109 Excision of tendon, forearm and/or wrist, flexor or extensor, each
15.4 15.4 FUD 090 J G2 50
AMA: 2018,Sep,7

25110 Excision, lesion of tendon sheath, forearm and/or wrist
9.84 9.84 FUD 090 J A2 50
AMA: 2018,Sep,7

25111 Excision of ganglion, wrist (dorsal or volar); primary
EXCLUDES *Excision ganglion hand or finger (26160)*
9.24 9.24 FUD 090 J A2 50
AMA: 2018,Sep,7

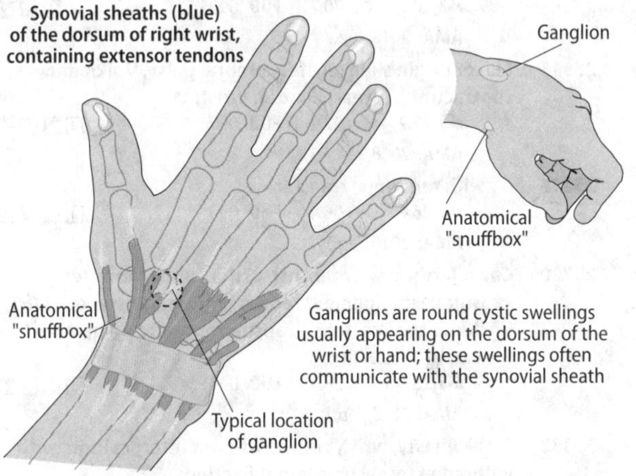

25112 recurrent
EXCLUDES *Excision ganglion hand or finger (26160)*
11.1 11.1 FUD 090 J A2 50
AMA: 2018,Sep,7

25115 Radical excision of bursa, synovia of wrist, or forearm tendon sheaths (eg, tenosynovitis, fungus, Tbc, or other granulomas, rheumatoid arthritis); flexors
EXCLUDES *Finger synovectomy (26145)*
21.8 21.8 FUD 090 J A2 50
AMA: 2018,Sep,7; 2018,Jan,8; 2017,Jan,8; 2016,Jan,13; 2015,Jan,16

25116 extensors, with or without transposition of dorsal retinaculum
EXCLUDES *Finger synovectomy (26145)*
17.3 17.3 FUD 090 J A2 80 50
AMA: 2018,Sep,7

25118 Synovectomy, extensor tendon sheath, wrist, single compartment;
EXCLUDES *Finger synovectomy (26145)*
10.9 10.9 FUD 090 J A2 50
AMA: 2018,Sep,7; 2018,Jan,8; 2017,Jan,8; 2016,Jan,13; 2015,Jun,10; 2015,Jan,16

25119 with resection of distal ulna
EXCLUDES *Finger synovectomy (26145)*
14.2 14.2 FUD 090 J A2 80 50
AMA: 2018,Sep,7

25120 Excision or curettage of bone cyst or benign tumor of radius or ulna (excluding head or neck of radius and olecranon process);
EXCLUDES *Removal bone cyst or tumor radial head, neck, or olecranon process (24120-24126)*
14.4 14.4 FUD 090 J A2 80 50
AMA: 2018,Sep,7

25125 with autograft (includes obtaining graft)
17.0 17.0 FUD 090 J A2 80 50
AMA: 2018,Sep,7

25126 with allograft
17.2 17.2 FUD 090 J A2 80 50
AMA: 2019,May,7; 2018,Sep,7

25130 Excision or curettage of bone cyst or benign tumor of carpal bones;
12.9 12.9 FUD 090 J A2 80 50
AMA: 2018,Sep,7

25135 with autograft (includes obtaining graft)
16.0 16.0 FUD 090 J A2 80 50
AMA: 2018,Sep,7

25136 with allograft
14.0 14.0 FUD 090 J J8 80 50
AMA: 2019,May,7; 2018,Sep,7

25145 Sequestrectomy (eg, for osteomyelitis or bone abscess), forearm and/or wrist
14.9 14.9 FUD 090 J A2 80 50
AMA: 2018,Sep,7

25150 Partial excision (craterization, saucerization, or diaphysectomy) of bone (eg, for osteomyelitis); ulna
16.2 16.2 FUD 090 J A2 50
AMA: 2018,Sep,7

25151 radius
EXCLUDES *Partial removal radial head, neck, or olecranon process (24145, 24147)*
16.8 16.8 FUD 090 J A2 80 50
AMA: 2018,Sep,7

25170 Radical resection of tumor, radius or ulna
INCLUDES Any necessary elevation tissue planes or dissection
Excision adjacent soft tissue during bone tumor resection (25071-25078 [25071, 25073])
Measurement tumor and necessary margin at greatest diameter prior to excision
Resection tumor (may include entire bone) and wide margins normal tissues primarily for malignant or aggressive benign tumors
Resection without removal significant normal tissue
Simple and intermediate repairs
EXCLUDES *Complex repair*
Radical resection cutaneous tumors (e.g., melanoma) (11600-11646)
Significant vessel exploration, neuroplasty, reconstruction, or complex bone repair
42.5 42.5 FUD 090 J 80 50
AMA: 2019,May,7; 2018,Sep,7

25210 Carpectomy; 1 bone
EXCLUDES *Carpectomy with insertion implant (25441-25445)*
14.0 14.0 FUD 090 J A2 80
AMA: 2018,Sep,7

25215 all bones of proximal row
17.8 17.8 **FUD** 090 J A2 80 50
AMA: 2019,Dec,14; 2019,Feb,10; 2018,Sep,7

25230 Radial styloidectomy (separate procedure)
12.4 12.4 **FUD** 090 J A2 50
AMA: 2018,Sep,7

25240 Excision distal ulna partial or complete (eg, Darrach type or matched resection)
EXCLUDES *Acquisition fascia for interposition (20920, 20922)*
Implant replacement (25442)
12.3 12.3 **FUD** 090 J A2 80 50
AMA: 2018,Sep,7

25246 Injection for Wrist Arthrogram

25246 Injection procedure for wrist arthrography
EXCLUDES *Excision superficial foreign body (20520)*
(73115)
2.14 5.25 **FUD** 000 N N1 50
AMA: 2018,Sep,7; 2018,Jan,8; 2017,Jan,8; 2016,Jan,13; 2015,Aug,6

25248-25251 Removal Foreign Body of Wrist

EXCLUDES *Excision superficial foreign body (20520)*
K-wire, pin, or rod insertion (20650)
K-wire, pin, or rod removal (20670, 20680)

25248 Exploration with removal of deep foreign body, forearm or wrist
11.8 11.8 **FUD** 090 J A2 50
AMA: 2018,Sep,7

25250 Removal of wrist prosthesis; (separate procedure)
15.3 15.3 **FUD** 090 Q2 A2 80 50
AMA: 2018,Sep,7

25251 complicated, including total wrist
20.7 20.7 **FUD** 090 Q2 A2 80 50
AMA: 2018,Sep,7

25259 Manipulation of Wrist with Anesthesia

25259 Manipulation, wrist, under anesthesia
EXCLUDES *Application external fixation (20690, 20692)*
12.1 12.1 **FUD** 090 J G2 50
AMA: 2018,Sep,7; 2018,Jan,8; 2017,Jan,8; 2016,Jan,13; 2015,Jan,16

25260-25492 Repair/Reconstruction of Forearm/Wrist

25260 Repair, tendon or muscle, flexor, forearm and/or wrist; primary, single, each tendon or muscle
18.1 18.1 **FUD** 090 J A2
AMA: 2018,Sep,7

25263 secondary, single, each tendon or muscle
18.1 18.1 **FUD** 090 J A2 80
AMA: 2018,Sep,7

25265 secondary, with free graft (includes obtaining graft), each tendon or muscle
21.4 21.4 **FUD** 090 J A2 80
AMA: 2018,Sep,7

25270 Repair, tendon or muscle, extensor, forearm and/or wrist; primary, single, each tendon or muscle
14.1 14.1 **FUD** 090 J A2 80
AMA: 2018,Sep,7

25272 secondary, single, each tendon or muscle
15.9 15.9 **FUD** 090 J A2 80
AMA: 2018,Sep,7

25274 secondary, with free graft (includes obtaining graft), each tendon or muscle
19.1 19.1 **FUD** 090 J A2 80
AMA: 2018,Sep,7

25275 Repair, tendon sheath, extensor, forearm and/or wrist, with free graft (includes obtaining graft) (eg, for extensor carpi ulnaris subluxation)
19.3 19.3 **FUD** 090 J A2 80 50
AMA: 2018,Sep,7

25280 Lengthening or shortening of flexor or extensor tendon, forearm and/or wrist, single, each tendon
16.3 16.3 **FUD** 090 J A2 80
AMA: 2018,Sep,7

25290 Tenotomy, open, flexor or extensor tendon, forearm and/or wrist, single, each tendon
12.5 12.5 **FUD** 090 J A2
AMA: 2018,Sep,7

25295 Tenolysis, flexor or extensor tendon, forearm and/or wrist, single, each tendon
15.1 15.1 **FUD** 090 J A2
AMA: 2018,Sep,7; 2018,Jan,8; 2017,Jan,8; 2016,Jan,13; 2015,Jan,16

25300 Tenodesis at wrist; flexors of fingers
19.5 19.5 **FUD** 090 J A2 80 50
AMA: 2018,Sep,7

25301 extensors of fingers
18.5 18.5 **FUD** 090 J A2 80 50
AMA: 2018,Sep,7

25310 Tendon transplantation or transfer, flexor or extensor, forearm and/or wrist, single; each tendon
17.8 17.8 **FUD** 090 J A2 80
AMA: 2018,Sep,7; 2018,Jan,8; 2017,Jan,8; 2016,Jan,13; 2015,Jan,16

25312 with tendon graft(s) (includes obtaining graft), each tendon
20.7 20.7 **FUD** 090 J A2 80
AMA: 2018,Sep,7

25315 Flexor origin slide (eg, for cerebral palsy, Volkmann contracture), forearm and/or wrist;
22.2 22.2 **FUD** 090 J A2 80 50
AMA: 2018,Sep,7

25316 with tendon(s) transfer
26.4 26.4 **FUD** 090 J A2 80 50
AMA: 2018,Sep,7

25320 Capsulorrhaphy or reconstruction, wrist, open (eg, capsulodesis, ligament repair, tendon transfer or graft) (includes synovectomy, capsulotomy and open reduction) for carpal instability
28.3 28.3 **FUD** 090 J A2 80 50
AMA: 2018,Sep,7

25332 Arthroplasty, wrist, with or without interposition, with or without external or internal fixation
EXCLUDES *Acquiring fascia for interposition (20920, 20922)*
Arthroplasty with prosthesis (25441-25446)
24.2 24.2 **FUD** 090 J A2 80 50
AMA: 2019,Feb,10; 2018,Sep,7; 2018,Jan,8; 2017,Jan,8; 2016,Jan,13; 2015,Jan,16

25335 Centralization of wrist on ulna (eg, radial club hand)
27.2 27.2 **FUD** 090 J A2 80 50
AMA: 2018,Sep,7; 2018,May,10

25337 Reconstruction for stabilization of unstable distal ulna or distal radioulnar joint, secondary by soft tissue stabilization (eg, tendon transfer, tendon graft or weave, or tenodesis) with or without open reduction of distal radioulnar joint
EXCLUDES *Acquiring fascia lata graft (20920, 20922)*
25.5 25.5 **FUD** 090 J A2 50
AMA: 2018,Sep,7

25350 Osteotomy, radius; distal third
19.4 19.4 **FUD** 090 J J8 80 50
AMA: 2018,Sep,7

25355 **middle or proximal third**
22.0 22.0 **FUD** 090 J A2 80 50
AMA: 2018,Sep,7

25360 **Osteotomy; ulna**
18.8 18.8 **FUD** 090 J A2 80 50
AMA: 2018,Sep,7

25365 **radius AND ulna**
26.4 26.4 **FUD** 090 J A2 80 50
AMA: 2018,Sep,7

25370 **Multiple osteotomies, with realignment on intramedullary rod (Sofield type procedure); radius OR ulna**
29.0 29.0 **FUD** 090 J A2 80 50
AMA: 2018,Sep,7

25375 **radius AND ulna**
27.5 27.5 **FUD** 090 J A2 80 50
AMA: 2018,Sep,7

25390 **Osteoplasty, radius OR ulna; shortening**
22.1 22.1 **FUD** 090 J J8 80 50
AMA: 2018,Sep,7

25391 **lengthening with autograft**
28.7 28.7 **FUD** 090 J J8 80 50
AMA: 2018,Sep,7

25392 **Osteoplasty, radius AND ulna; shortening (excluding 64876)**
29.3 29.3 **FUD** 090 J A2 80 50
AMA: 2018,Sep,7

25393 **lengthening with autograft**
32.6 32.6 **FUD** 090 J A2 80 50
AMA: 2018,Sep,7

25394 **Osteoplasty, carpal bone, shortening**
22.6 22.6 **FUD** 090 J G2 80 50
AMA: 2018,Sep,7

25400 **Repair of nonunion or malunion, radius OR ulna; without graft (eg, compression technique)**
23.1 23.1 **FUD** 090 J J8 80 50
AMA: 2018,Sep,7

25405 **with autograft (includes obtaining graft)**
29.9 29.9 **FUD** 090 J J8 80 50
AMA: 2018,Sep,7

25415 **Repair of nonunion or malunion, radius AND ulna; without graft (eg, compression technique)**
27.8 27.8 **FUD** 090 J J8 80 50
AMA: 2018,Sep,7

25420 **with autograft (includes obtaining graft)**
33.5 33.5 **FUD** 090 J G2 80 50
AMA: 2018,Sep,7

25425 **Repair of defect with autograft; radius OR ulna**
27.6 27.6 **FUD** 090 J A2 80 50
AMA: 2018,Sep,7

25426 **radius AND ulna**
32.4 32.4 **FUD** 090 J G2 80 50
AMA: 2018,Sep,7

25430 **Insertion of vascular pedicle into carpal bone (eg, Hori procedure)**
21.0 21.0 **FUD** 090 J G2 50
AMA: 2018,Sep,7

25431 **Repair of nonunion of carpal bone (excluding carpal scaphoid (navicular)) (includes obtaining graft and necessary fixation), each bone**
22.7 22.7 **FUD** 090 J G2 80 50
AMA: 2018,Sep,7

25440 **Repair of nonunion, scaphoid carpal (navicular) bone, with or without radial styloidectomy (includes obtaining graft and necessary fixation)**
22.1 22.1 **FUD** 090 J A2 80 50
AMA: 2018,Sep,7

25441 **Arthroplasty with prosthetic replacement; distal radius**
27.0 27.0 **FUD** 090 J J8 80 50
AMA: 2018,Sep,7; 2018,Jan,8; 2017,Aug,9; 2017,Jan,8; 2016,Jan,13; 2015,Jan,16

25442 **distal ulna**
23.2 23.2 **FUD** 090 J J8 80 50
AMA: 2018,Sep,7; 2018,Jan,8; 2017,Aug,9; 2017,Jan,8; 2016,Jan,13; 2015,Jan,16

25443 **scaphoid carpal (navicular)**
22.6 22.6 **FUD** 090 J J8 80 50
AMA: 2018,Sep,7; 2018,Jan,8; 2017,Jan,8; 2016,Jan,13; 2015,Jan,16

25444 **lunate**
23.7 23.7 **FUD** 090 J J8 80 50
AMA: 2018,Sep,7; 2018,Jan,8; 2017,Jan,8; 2016,Jan,13; 2015,Jan,16

25445 **trapezium**
20.8 20.8 **FUD** 090 J J8 50
AMA: 2018,Sep,7; 2018,Jan,8; 2017,Jan,8; 2016,Jan,13; 2015,Jan,16

25446 **distal radius and partial or entire carpus (total wrist)**
33.8 33.8 **FUD** 090 J J8 80 50
AMA: 2018,Sep,7; 2018,Jan,8; 2017,Jan,8; 2016,Jan,13; 2015,Jan,16

25447 **Arthroplasty, interposition, intercarpal or carpometacarpal joints**
EXCLUDES *Wrist arthroplasty (25332)*
23.8 23.8 **FUD** 090 J A2 80 50
AMA: 2018,Sep,7; 2018,Jan,8; 2017,Jan,8; 2016,Jan,13; 2015,Jan,16

25449 **Revision of arthroplasty, including removal of implant, wrist joint**
29.8 29.8 **FUD** 090 J A2 80 50
AMA: 2018,Sep,7

25450 **Epiphyseal arrest by epiphysiodesis or stapling; distal radius OR ulna**
17.7 17.7 **FUD** 090 J A2 50
AMA: 2018,Sep,7

25455 **distal radius AND ulna**
21.0 21.0 **FUD** 090 J A2 50
AMA: 2018,Sep,7

25490 **Prophylactic treatment (nailing, pinning, plating or wiring) with or without methylmethacrylate; radius**
20.7 20.7 **FUD** 090 J A2 80 50
AMA: 2018,Sep,7

25491 **ulna**
21.3 21.3 **FUD** 090 J A2 80 50
AMA: 2018,Sep,7

25492 **radius AND ulna**
26.1 26.1 **FUD** 090 J A2 80 50
AMA: 2018,Sep,7

25500-25695 Treatment of Fracture/Dislocation of Forearm/Wrist

Code also external fixation, when performed (20690, 20692)

25500 **Closed treatment of radial shaft fracture; without manipulation**
7.25 7.98 **FUD** 090 T P2 50
AMA: 2018,Sep,7

25505 **with manipulation**
13.2 14.4 **FUD** 090 J A2 50
AMA: 2018,Sep,7

25515 **Open treatment of radial shaft fracture, includes internal fixation, when performed**
19.2 19.2 **FUD** 090 J J8 80 50
AMA: 2018,Sep,7

25520 Closed treatment of radial shaft fracture and closed treatment of dislocation of distal radioulnar joint (Galeazzi fracture/dislocation)
15.5 16.4 **FUD** 090 J A2 50
AMA: 2018,Sep,7

25525 Open treatment of radial shaft fracture, includes internal fixation, when performed, and closed treatment of distal radioulnar joint dislocation (Galeazzi fracture/ dislocation), includes percutaneous skeletal fixation, when performed
22.6 22.6 **FUD** 090 J A2 80 50
AMA: 2018,Sep,7

25526 Open treatment of radial shaft fracture, includes internal fixation, when performed, and open treatment of distal radioulnar joint dislocation (Galeazzi fracture/ dislocation), includes internal fixation, when performed, includes repair of triangular fibrocartilage complex
27.5 27.5 **FUD** 090 J J8 80 50
AMA: 2018,Sep,7

25530 Closed treatment of ulnar shaft fracture; without manipulation
6.88 7.52 **FUD** 090 T P2 50
AMA: 2018,Sep,7

25535 with manipulation
13.0 14.0 **FUD** 090 T A2 50
AMA: 2018,Sep,7

25545 Open treatment of ulnar shaft fracture, includes internal fixation, when performed
17.9 17.9 **FUD** 090 J J8 80 50
AMA: 2018,Sep,7; 2018,Jan,8; 2017,Jan,8; 2016,Jan,13; 2015,Jan,16

25560 Closed treatment of radial and ulnar shaft fractures; without manipulation
7.31 8.15 **FUD** 090 T P2 50
AMA: 2018,Sep,7

25565 with manipulation
13.2 14.7 **FUD** 090 J A2 50
AMA: 2018,Sep,7

25574 Open treatment of radial AND ulnar shaft fractures, with internal fixation, when performed; of radius OR ulna
19.4 19.4 **FUD** 090 J J8 80 50
AMA: 2018,Sep,7; 2018,Jan,8; 2017,Jan,8; 2016,Jan,13; 2015,Jan,16

25575 of radius AND ulna
25.9 25.9 **FUD** 090 J J8 80 50
AMA: 2018,Sep,7

25600 Closed treatment of distal radial fracture (eg, Colles or Smith type) or epiphyseal separation, includes closed treatment of fracture of ulnar styloid, when performed; without manipulation
INCLUDES Closed treatment ulnar styloid fracture (25650)
9.06 9.51 **FUD** 090 T P2 50
AMA: 2018,Sep,7; 2018,Jan,8; 2017,Jan,8; 2016,Jan,13; 2015,Jan,16

25605 with manipulation
INCLUDES Closed treatment ulnar styloid fracture (25650)
14.7 15.5 **FUD** 090 J A2 50
AMA: 2018,Sep,7; 2018,Jan,8; 2017,Jan,8; 2016,Jan,13; 2015,Jan,16

25606 Percutaneous skeletal fixation of distal radial fracture or epiphyseal separation
EXCLUDES *Closed treatment ulnar styloid fracture (25650)*
Open repair ulnar styloid fracture (25652)
Percutaneous repair ulnar styloid fracture (25651)
19.1 19.1 **FUD** 090 J A2 50
AMA: 2018,Sep,7

25607 Open treatment of distal radial extra-articular fracture or epiphyseal separation, with internal fixation
EXCLUDES *Closed treatment ulnar styloid fracture (25650)*
Open repair ulnar styloid fracture (25652)
Percutaneous repair ulnar styloid fracture (25651)
21.1 21.1 **FUD** 090 J J8 80 50
AMA: 2018,Sep,7; 2018,Jan,8; 2017,Jan,8; 2016,Jan,13; 2015,Jan,16

25608 Open treatment of distal radial intra-articular fracture or epiphyseal separation; with internal fixation of 2 fragments
EXCLUDES *Closed treatment ulnar styloid fracture (25650)*
Open repair ulnar styloid fracture (25652)
Open treatment distal radial intra-articular fracture or epiphyseal separation; with internal fixation of 3 or more fragments (25609)
Percutaneous repair ulnar styloid fracture (25651)
23.7 23.7 **FUD** 090 J J8 80 50
AMA: 2018,Sep,7; 2018,Jan,8; 2017,Jan,8; 2016,Jan,13; 2015,Jan,16

25609 with internal fixation of 3 or more fragments
EXCLUDES *Closed treatment ulnar styloid fracture (25650)*
Open repair ulnar styloid fracture (25652)
Percutaneous repair ulnar styloid fracture (25651)
30.2 30.2 **FUD** 090 J J8 80 50
AMA: 2018,Sep,7; 2018,Jan,8; 2017,Jan,8; 2016,Jan,13; 2015,Jan,16

25622 Closed treatment of carpal scaphoid (navicular) fracture; without manipulation
8.07 8.76 **FUD** 090 T P2 50
AMA: 2018,Sep,7

25624 with manipulation
12.6 13.8 **FUD** 090 J A2 80 50
AMA: 2018,Sep,7

25628 Open treatment of carpal scaphoid (navicular) fracture, includes internal fixation, when performed
20.7 20.7 **FUD** 090 J A2 80 50
AMA: 2018,Sep,7

25630 Closed treatment of carpal bone fracture (excluding carpal scaphoid [navicular]); without manipulation, each bone
8.13 8.77 **FUD** 090 T P2 50
AMA: 2018,Sep,7

25635 with manipulation, each bone
11.9 13.1 **FUD** 090 J A2 80 50
AMA: 2018,Sep,7

25645 Open treatment of carpal bone fracture (other than carpal scaphoid [navicular]), each bone
16.4 16.4 **FUD** 090 J A2 80 50
AMA: 2018,Sep,7

25650 Closed treatment of ulnar styloid fracture
EXCLUDES *Closed treatment distal radial fracture (25600, 25605)*
Open treatment distal radial extra-articular fracture or epiphyseal separation, with internal fixation (25607-25609)
8.70 9.35 **FUD** 090 T P2 50
AMA: 2018,Sep,7; 2018,Jan,8; 2017,Jan,8; 2016,Jan,13; 2015,Jan,16

25651 Percutaneous skeletal fixation of ulnar styloid fracture
14.0 14.0 **FUD** 090 J G2 80 50
AMA: 2018,Sep,7

25652 Open treatment of ulnar styloid fracture
17.9 17.9 **FUD** 090 J G2 50
AMA: 2018,Sep,7; 2018,Jan,8; 2017,Jan,8; 2016,Jan,13; 2015,Jan,16

25660 Closed treatment of radiocarpal or intercarpal dislocation, 1 or more bones, with manipulation
11.9 11.9 **FUD** 090 T A2 80 50
AMA: 2018,Sep,7

25670 **Open treatment of radiocarpal or intercarpal dislocation, 1 or more bones**
17.5 17.5 FUD 090 J A2 80 50
AMA: 2018,Sep,7

25671 **Percutaneous skeletal fixation of distal radioulnar dislocation**
15.3 15.3 FUD 090 J A2 50
AMA: 2018,Sep,7

25675 **Closed treatment of distal radioulnar dislocation with manipulation**
11.2 12.4 FUD 090 T A2 80 50
AMA: 2018,Sep,7

25676 **Open treatment of distal radioulnar dislocation, acute or chronic**
18.0 18.0 FUD 090 J A2 80 50
AMA: 2018,Sep,7

25680 **Closed treatment of trans-scaphoperilunar type of fracture dislocation, with manipulation**
15.1 15.1 FUD 090 T A2 80 50
AMA: 2018,Sep,7

25685 **Open treatment of trans-scaphoperilunar type of fracture dislocation**
21.2 21.2 FUD 090 J A2 80 50
AMA: 2018,Sep,7

25690 **Closed treatment of lunate dislocation, with manipulation**
14.0 14.0 FUD 090 J A2 80 50
AMA: 2018,Sep,7

25695 **Open treatment of lunate dislocation**
18.2 18.2 FUD 090 J A2 80 50
AMA: 2018,Sep,7

25800-25830 Wrist Fusion

25800 **Arthrodesis, wrist; complete, without bone graft (includes radiocarpal and/or intercarpal and/or carpometacarpal joints)**
21.0 21.0 FUD 090 J J8 80 50
AMA: 2020,May,13; 2018,Sep,7

25805 **with sliding graft**
24.4 24.4 FUD 090 J J8 80 50
AMA: 2020,May,13; 2018,Sep,7

25810 **with iliac or other autograft (includes obtaining graft)**
24.9 24.9 FUD 090 J J8 80 50
AMA: 2020,May,13; 2018,Sep,7

25820 **Arthrodesis, wrist; limited, without bone graft (eg, intercarpal or radiocarpal)**
18.1 18.1 FUD 090 J J8 80 50
AMA: 2020,May,13; 2018,Sep,7

25825 **with autograft (includes obtaining graft)**
22.3 22.3 FUD 090 J J8 80 50
AMA: 2020,May,13; 2018,Sep,7; 2018,Jan,8; 2017,Jan,8; 2016,Jan,13; 2015,Jan,16

25830 **Arthrodesis, distal radioulnar joint with segmental resection of ulna, with or without bone graft (eg, Sauve-Kapandji procedure)**
27.0 27.0 FUD 090 J J8 80 50
AMA: 2020,May,13; 2018,Sep,7

25900-25999 Amputation Through Forearm/Wrist

25900 **Amputation, forearm, through radius and ulna;**
20.5 20.5 FUD 090 C 80 50
AMA: 2018,Sep,7

25905 **open, circular (guillotine)**
20.2 20.2 FUD 090 C 80 50
AMA: 2018,Sep,7

25907 **secondary closure or scar revision**
17.6 17.6 FUD 090 J A2 80 50
AMA: 2018,Sep,7

25909 **re-amputation**
19.7 19.7 FUD 090 J 80 50
AMA: 2018,Sep,7

25915 **Krukenberg procedure**
33.7 33.7 FUD 090 C 80 50
AMA: 2018,Sep,7

25920 **Disarticulation through wrist;**
20.5 20.5 FUD 090 C 80 50
AMA: 2018,Sep,7

25922 **secondary closure or scar revision**
17.7 17.7 FUD 090 J A2 80 50
AMA: 2018,Sep,7

25924 **re-amputation**
20.0 20.0 FUD 090 C 80 50
AMA: 2018,Sep,7

25927 **Transmetacarpal amputation;**
24.0 24.0 FUD 090 C 80 50
AMA: 2018,Sep,7

25929 **secondary closure or scar revision**
17.2 17.2 FUD 090 T A2 80 50
AMA: 2018,Sep,7

25931 **re-amputation**
22.1 22.1 FUD 090 J G2 50
AMA: 2018,Sep,7

25999 **Unlisted procedure, forearm or wrist**
0.00 0.00 FUD YYY T 80 50
AMA: 2019,Feb,10; 2018,Sep,7

26010-26037 Incision Hand/Fingers

26010 **Drainage of finger abscess; simple**
3.97 8.62 FUD 010 T P2
AMA: 2018,Sep,7

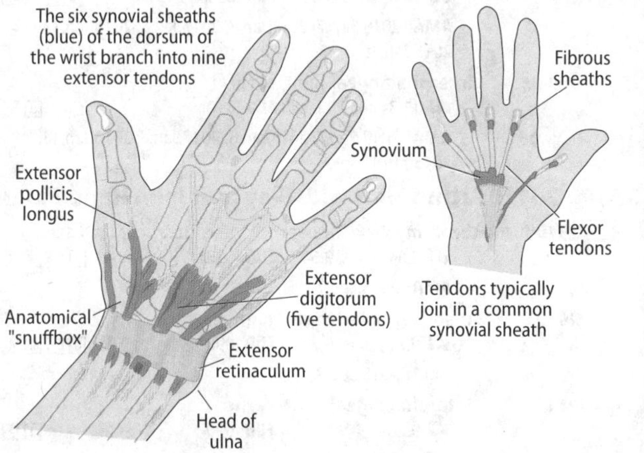

26011 **complicated (eg, felon)**
5.32 12.4 FUD 010 J A2
AMA: 2018,Sep,7

26020 **Drainage of tendon sheath, digit and/or palm, each**
15.9 15.9 FUD 090 J A2
AMA: 2018,Sep,7

26025 **Drainage of palmar bursa; single, bursa**
12.1 12.1 FUD 090 J A2 80 50
AMA: 2018,Sep,7

26030 **multiple bursa**
14.0 14.0 FUD 090 J A2 80 50
AMA: 2018,Sep,7

26034 **Incision, bone cortex, hand or finger (eg, osteomyelitis or bone abscess)**
15.7 15.7 FUD 090 J A2
AMA: 2018,Sep,7

26035 Decompression fingers and/or hand, injection injury (eg, grease gun)

    🖫 24.7   24.7   **FUD** 090   J G2 80 ▣

    AMA: 2018,Sep,7

26037 Decompressive fasciotomy, hand (excludes 26035)

    EXCLUDES   *Injection injury (26035)*

    🖫 16.3   16.3   **FUD** 090   J G2 80 50 ▣

    AMA: 2018,Sep,7

26040-26045 Incision Palmar Fascia

EXCLUDES   *Enzyme injection fasciotomy (20527, 26341)*
          Fasciectomy (26121, 26123, 26125)

26040 Fasciotomy, palmar (eg, Dupuytren's contracture); percutaneous

    🖫 9.00   9.00   **FUD** 090   J A2 50 ▣

    AMA: 2018,Sep,7; 2018,Jan,8; 2017,Jan,8; 2016,Jan,13; 2015,Jan,16

26045 open, partial

    🖫 13.5   13.5   **FUD** 090   J A2 50 ▣

    AMA: 2018,Sep,7; 2018,Jan,8; 2017,Jan,8; 2016,Jan,13; 2015,Jan,16

26055-26080 Incision Tendon/Joint of Fingers/Hand

26055 Tendon sheath incision (eg, for trigger finger)

    🖫 8.91   16.1   **FUD** 090   J A2 ▣

    AMA: 2018,Sep,7

26060 Tenotomy, percutaneous, single, each digit

    🖫 7.41   7.41   **FUD** 090   J A2 80 ▣

    AMA: 2018,Sep,7

26070 Arthrotomy, with exploration, drainage, or removal of loose or foreign body; carpometacarpal joint

    🖫 9.23   9.23   **FUD** 090   J A2 50 ▣

    AMA: 2018,Sep,7

26075 metacarpophalangeal joint, each

    🖫 9.64   9.64   **FUD** 090   J A2 50 ▣

    AMA: 2018,Sep,7; 2018,Jan,8; 2017,Jan,8; 2016,Jan,13; 2015,Jan,16

26080 interphalangeal joint, each

    🖫 11.3   11.3   **FUD** 090   J A2 ▣

    AMA: 2018,Sep,7; 2018,Jan,8; 2017,Jan,8; 2016,Jan,13; 2015,Jan,16

26100-26110 Arthrotomy with Biopsy of Joint Hand/Fingers

26100 Arthrotomy with biopsy; carpometacarpal joint, each

    🖫 9.64   9.64   **FUD** 090   J A2 80 50 ▣

    AMA: 2018,Sep,7

26105 metacarpophalangeal joint, each

    🖫 9.71   9.71   **FUD** 090   J A2 80 50 ▣

    AMA: 2018,Sep,7

26110 interphalangeal joint, each

    🖫 9.28   9.28   **FUD** 090   J A2 ▣

    AMA: 2018,Sep,7

26111-26118 [26111, 26113] Excision Soft Tissue Tumors Fingers and Hand

INCLUDES   Any necessary elevation tissue planes or dissection
Measurement tumor and necessary margin at greatest diameter prior to excision
Simple and intermediate repairs
Excision types:
    Fascial or subfascial soft tissue tumors: simple and marginal resection tumors found either in or below deep fascia, not involving bone or excision substantial amount normal tissue; primarily benign and intramuscular tumors
    Tumors fingers and toes involving joint capsules, tendons and tendon sheaths
    Radical resection soft tissue tumor: wide resection tumor, involving substantial margins normal tissue and may include tissue removal from one or more layers; most often malignant or aggressive benign
    Tumors fingers and toes adjacent to joints, tendons and tendon sheaths
    Subcutaneous: simple and marginal resection tumors found in subcutaneous tissue above deep fascia; most often benign

EXCLUDES   *Complex repair*
    Excision benign cutaneous lesions (eg, sebaceous cyst) (11420-11426)
    Radical resection cutaneous tumors (eg, melanoma) (11620-11626)
    Significant vessel exploration or neuroplasty

26111 Resequenced code. See code following 26115.

26113 Resequenced code. See code following 26116.

26115 Excision, tumor or vascular malformation, soft tissue of hand or finger, subcutaneous; less than 1.5 cm

    🖫 9.51   15.2   **FUD** 090   J G2 ▣

    AMA: 2018,Sep,7

\# **26111** 1.5 cm or greater

    🖫 11.9   11.9   **FUD** 090   J G2 80 ▣

    AMA: 2018,Sep,7

26116 Excision, tumor, soft tissue, or vascular malformation, of hand or finger, subfascial (eg, intramuscular); less than 1.5 cm

    🖫 15.1   15.1   **FUD** 090   J G2 ▣

    AMA: 2018,Sep,7; 2018,Jan,8; 2017,Jan,8; 2016,Jan,13; 2015,Jan,16

\# **26113** 1.5 cm or greater

    🖫 15.7   15.7   **FUD** 090   J G2 80 ▣

    AMA: 2018,Sep,7

26117 Radical resection of tumor (eg, sarcoma), soft tissue of hand or finger; less than 3 cm

    🖫 21.4   21.4   **FUD** 090   J G2 ▣

    AMA: 2018,Sep,7

26118 3 cm or greater

    🖫 30.3   30.3   **FUD** 090   J G2 80 ▣

    AMA: 2018,Sep,7

26121-26236 Procedures of Bones, Fascia, Joints and Tendons Hands and Fingers

26121 Fasciectomy, palm only, with or without Z-plasty, other local tissue rearrangement, or skin grafting (includes obtaining graft)

    EXCLUDES   *Enzyme injection fasciotomy (20527, 26341)*
              Fasciotomy (26040, 26045)

    🖫 17.2   17.2   **FUD** 090   J A2 50 ▣

    AMA: 2018,Sep,7; 2018,Jan,8; 2017,Jan,8; 2016,Jan,13; 2015,Jan,16

26123 Fasciectomy, partial palmar with release of single digit including proximal interphalangeal joint, with or without Z-plasty, other local tissue rearrangement, or skin grafting (includes obtaining graft);

    EXCLUDES   *Enzyme injection fasciotomy (20527, 26341)*
              Fasciotomy (26040, 26045)

    🖫 24.0   24.0   **FUD** 090   J A2 50 ▣

    AMA: 2018,Sep,7; 2018,Jan,8; 2017,Jan,8; 2016,Jan,13; 2015,Jan,16

+ **26125** **each additional digit (List separately in addition to code for primary procedure)**
EXCLUDES *Enzyme injection fasciotomy (20527, 26341)*
Fasciotomy (26040, 26045)
Code first (26123)
7.87 7.87 **FUD** ZZZ N N1
AMA: 2018,Sep,7; 2018,Jan,8; 2017,Jan,8; 2016,Jan,13; 2015,Jan,16

26130 **Synovectomy, carpometacarpal joint**
13.4 13.4 **FUD** 090 J A2 50
AMA: 2018,Sep,7

26135 **Synovectomy, metacarpophalangeal joint including intrinsic release and extensor hood reconstruction, each digit**
15.9 15.9 **FUD** 090 J A2 80
AMA: 2018,Sep,7

26140 **Synovectomy, proximal interphalangeal joint, including extensor reconstruction, each interphalangeal joint**
14.5 14.5 **FUD** 090 J A2
AMA: 2018,Sep,7

26145 **Synovectomy, tendon sheath, radical (tenosynovectomy), flexor tendon, palm and/or finger, each tendon**
EXCLUDES *Wrist synovectomy (25115-25116)*
14.7 14.7 **FUD** 090 J A2
AMA: 2018,Sep,7

26160 **Excision of lesion of tendon sheath or joint capsule (eg, cyst, mucous cyst, or ganglion), hand or finger**
EXCLUDES *Trigger finger (26055)*
Wrist ganglion removal (25111-25112)
9.04 16.3 **FUD** 090 J A2
AMA: 2019,Jul,10; 2018,Sep,7

26170 **Excision of tendon, palm, flexor or extensor, single, each tendon**
EXCLUDES *Excision extensor tendon, with implantation synthetic rod for delayed tendon graft, hand or finger, each rod (26415)*
Excision flexor tendon, with implantation synthetic rod for delayed tendon graft, hand or finger, each rod (26390)
11.7 11.7 **FUD** 090 J A2 80
AMA: 2018,Sep,7; 2018,Jan,8; 2017,Jan,8; 2016,Jan,13; 2015,Jan,16

26180 **Excision of tendon, finger, flexor or extensor, each tendon**
EXCLUDES *Excision extensor tendon, with implantation synthetic rod for delayed tendon graft, hand or finger, each rod (26415)*
Excision flexor tendon, with implantation synthetic rod for delayed tendon graft, hand or finger, each rod (26390)
12.8 12.8 **FUD** 090 J A2 80
AMA: 2018,Sep,7

26185 **Sesamoidectomy, thumb or finger (separate procedure)**
15.8 15.8 **FUD** 090 J A2 80 50
AMA: 2018,Sep,7

26200 **Excision or curettage of bone cyst or benign tumor of metacarpal;**
13.0 13.0 **FUD** 090 J A2 80
AMA: 2018,Sep,7

26205 **with autograft (includes obtaining graft)**
17.3 17.3 **FUD** 090 J A2
AMA: 2018,Sep,7

26210 **Excision or curettage of bone cyst or benign tumor of proximal, middle, or distal phalanx of finger;**
12.7 12.7 **FUD** 090 J A2
AMA: 2018,Sep,7

26215 **with autograft (includes obtaining graft)**
16.2 16.2 **FUD** 090 J A2
AMA: 2018,Sep,7

26230 **Partial excision (craterization, saucerization, or diaphysectomy) bone (eg, osteomyelitis); metacarpal**
14.4 14.4 **FUD** 090 J A2 80
AMA: 2018,Sep,7

26235 **proximal or middle phalanx of finger**
14.1 14.1 **FUD** 090 J A2 80
AMA: 2019,Jul,10; 2018,Sep,7

26236 **distal phalanx of finger**
12.6 12.6 **FUD** 090 J A2
AMA: 2019,Jul,10; 2018,Sep,7

26250-26262 Radical Resection Bone Tumor of Hand/Finger

INCLUDES Any necessary elevation tissue planes or dissection
Excision adjacent soft tissue during bone tumor resection (26111-26118 [26111, 26113])
Measurement tumor and necessary margin at greatest diameter prior to excision
Resection tumor (may include entire bone) and wide margins normal tissue primarily for malignant or aggressive benign tumors
Simple and intermediate repairs
EXCLUDES *Complex repair*
Significant vessel exploration, neuroplasty, reconstruction, or complex bone repair

26250 **Radical resection of tumor, metacarpal**
30.8 30.8 **FUD** 090 J A2 80
AMA: 2018,Sep,7

26260 **Radical resection of tumor, proximal or middle phalanx of finger**
23.0 23.0 **FUD** 090 J A2 80
AMA: 2018,Sep,7

26262 **Radical resection of tumor, distal phalanx of finger**
18.1 18.1 **FUD** 090 J A2 80
AMA: 2018,Sep,7

26320 Implant Removal Hand/Finger

26320 **Removal of implant from finger or hand**
EXCLUDES *Excision foreign body (20520, 20525)*
9.98 9.98 **FUD** 090 Q2 A2
AMA: 2018,Sep,7

26340-26548 Repair/Reconstruction of Fingers and Hand

26340 **Manipulation, finger joint, under anesthesia, each joint**
EXCLUDES *Application external fixation (20690, 20692)*
9.67 9.67 **FUD** 090 J G2 50
AMA: 2018,Sep,7; 2018,Jan,8; 2017,Jan,8; 2016,Jan,13; 2015,Jan,16

26341 **Manipulation, palmar fascial cord (ie, Dupuytren's cord), post enzyme injection (eg, collagenase), single cord**
EXCLUDES *Enzyme injection fasciotomy (20527)*
Code also custom orthotic fabrication and/or fitting
2.17 2.90 **FUD** 010 T P3 50
AMA: 2018,Sep,7; 2018,Jan,8; 2017,Jan,8; 2016,Jan,13; 2015,Jan,16

26350 **Repair or advancement, flexor tendon, not in zone 2 digital flexor tendon sheath (eg, no man's land); primary or secondary without free graft, each tendon**
20.8 20.8 **FUD** 090 J A2
AMA: 2018,Sep,7

26352 **secondary with free graft (includes obtaining graft), each tendon**
23.3 23.3 **FUD** 090 J A2 80
AMA: 2018,Sep,7

26356 **Repair or advancement, flexor tendon, in zone 2 digital flexor tendon sheath (eg, no man's land); primary, without free graft, each tendon**
22.8 22.8 **FUD** 090 J A2
AMA: 2018,Sep,7; 2018,Jan,8; 2017,Dec,14; 2017,Jan,8; 2016,Jan,13; 2015,Jan,16

26357 **secondary, without free graft, each tendon**
Facility RVU 25.6 Non-Facility RVU 25.6 FUD 090 J A2 80 CCI
AMA: 2018,Sep,7

26358 **secondary, with free graft (includes obtaining graft), each tendon**
Facility RVU 28.3 Non-Facility RVU 28.3 FUD 090 J A2 80 CCI
AMA: 2018,Sep,7

26370 **Repair or advancement of profundus tendon, with intact superficialis tendon; primary, each tendon**
Facility RVU 21.9 Non-Facility RVU 21.9 FUD 090 J A2 80 CCI
AMA: 2018,Sep,7; 2018,Jan,8; 2017,Jan,8; 2016,Jan,13; 2015,Jan,16

26372 **secondary with free graft (includes obtaining graft), each tendon**
Facility RVU 25.7 Non-Facility RVU 25.7 FUD 090 J A2 80 CCI
AMA: 2018,Sep,7

26373 **secondary without free graft, each tendon**
Facility RVU 24.7 Non-Facility RVU 24.7 FUD 090 J A2 80 CCI
AMA: 2018,Sep,7

26390 **Excision flexor tendon, with implantation of synthetic rod for delayed tendon graft, hand or finger, each rod**
Facility RVU 23.6 Non-Facility RVU 23.6 FUD 090 J J8 80 CCI
AMA: 2018,Sep,7

26392 **Removal of synthetic rod and insertion of flexor tendon graft, hand or finger (includes obtaining graft), each rod**
Facility RVU 27.4 Non-Facility RVU 27.4 FUD 090 J A2 80 CCI
AMA: 2018,Sep,7

26410 **Repair, extensor tendon, hand, primary or secondary; without free graft, each tendon**
Facility RVU 16.5 Non-Facility RVU 16.5 FUD 090 J A2 CCI
AMA: 2018,Sep,7

26412 **with free graft (includes obtaining graft), each tendon**
Facility RVU 19.7 Non-Facility RVU 19.7 FUD 090 J A2 80 CCI
AMA: 2018,Sep,7

26415 **Excision of extensor tendon, with implantation of synthetic rod for delayed tendon graft, hand or finger, each rod**
Facility RVU 23.7 Non-Facility RVU 23.7 FUD 090 J A2 80 CCI
AMA: 2018,Sep,7

26416 **Removal of synthetic rod and insertion of extensor tendon graft (includes obtaining graft), hand or finger, each rod**
Facility RVU 25.7 Non-Facility RVU 25.7 FUD 090 J A2 CCI
AMA: 2018,Sep,7; 2018,Jan,8; 2017,Jan,8; 2016,Jan,13; 2015,Jan,16

26418 **Repair, extensor tendon, finger, primary or secondary; without free graft, each tendon**
Facility RVU 16.2 Non-Facility RVU 16.2 FUD 090 J A2 CCI
AMA: 2018,Sep,7; 2018,Jan,8; 2017,Jan,8; 2016,Jan,13; 2015,Jan,16

26420 **with free graft (includes obtaining graft) each tendon**
Facility RVU 20.6 Non-Facility RVU 20.6 FUD 090 J A2 80 CCI
AMA: 2018,Sep,7

26426 **Repair of extensor tendon, central slip, secondary (eg, boutonniere deformity); using local tissue(s), including lateral band(s), each finger**
Facility RVU 14.4 Non-Facility RVU 14.4 FUD 090 J A2 CCI
AMA: 2018,Sep,7

26428 **with free graft (includes obtaining graft), each finger**
Facility RVU 21.3 Non-Facility RVU 21.3 FUD 090 J A2 80 CCI
AMA: 2018,Sep,7

26432 **Closed treatment of distal extensor tendon insertion, with or without percutaneous pinning (eg, mallet finger)**
Facility RVU 13.9 Non-Facility RVU 13.9 FUD 090 J A2 CCI
AMA: 2018,Sep,7

26433 **Repair of extensor tendon, distal insertion, primary or secondary; without graft (eg, mallet finger)**
EXCLUDES *Trigger finger (26055)*
Facility RVU 15.6 Non-Facility RVU 15.6 FUD 090 J A2 CCI
AMA: 2018,Sep,7

26434 **with free graft (includes obtaining graft)**
EXCLUDES *Trigger finger (26055)*
Facility RVU 18.2 Non-Facility RVU 18.2 FUD 090 J A2 80 CCI
AMA: 2018,Sep,7

26437 **Realignment of extensor tendon, hand, each tendon**
Facility RVU 17.5 Non-Facility RVU 17.5 FUD 090 J A2 CCI
AMA: 2018,Sep,7

26440 **Tenolysis, flexor tendon; palm OR finger, each tendon**
Facility RVU 18.0 Non-Facility RVU 18.0 FUD 090 J A2 CCI
AMA: 2018,Sep,7; 2018,Jan,8; 2017,Jan,8; 2016,Jan,13; 2015,Jun,10; 2015,Jan,16

26442 **palm AND finger, each tendon**
Facility RVU 27.1 Non-Facility RVU 27.1 FUD 090 J A2 CCI
AMA: 2018,Sep,7

26445 **Tenolysis, extensor tendon, hand OR finger, each tendon**
Facility RVU 16.8 Non-Facility RVU 16.8 FUD 090 J A2 CCI
AMA: 2018,Sep,7; 2018,Jan,8; 2017,Jan,8; 2016,Jan,13; 2015,Jan,16

26449 **Tenolysis, complex, extensor tendon, finger, including forearm, each tendon**
Facility RVU 19.9 Non-Facility RVU 19.9 FUD 090 J A2 80 CCI
AMA: 2018,Sep,7

26450 **Tenotomy, flexor, palm, open, each tendon**
Facility RVU 11.4 Non-Facility RVU 11.4 FUD 090 J A2 80 CCI
AMA: 2018,Sep,7

26455 **Tenotomy, flexor, finger, open, each tendon**
Facility RVU 12.1 Non-Facility RVU 12.1 FUD 090 J A2 80 CCI
AMA: 2018,Sep,7

26460 **Tenotomy, extensor, hand or finger, open, each tendon**
Facility RVU 11.8 Non-Facility RVU 11.8 FUD 090 J A2 CCI
AMA: 2018,Sep,7

26471 **Tenodesis; of proximal interphalangeal joint, each joint**
Facility RVU 18.0 Non-Facility RVU 18.0 FUD 090 J A2 80 CCI
AMA: 2018,Sep,7

26474 **of distal joint, each joint**
Facility RVU 17.7 Non-Facility RVU 17.7 FUD 090 J A2 80 CCI
AMA: 2018,Sep,7

26476 **Lengthening of tendon, extensor, hand or finger, each tendon**
Facility RVU 17.5 Non-Facility RVU 17.5 FUD 090 J A2 CCI
AMA: 2018,Sep,7

26477 **Shortening of tendon, extensor, hand or finger, each tendon**
Facility RVU 16.3 Non-Facility RVU 16.3 FUD 090 J A2 CCI
AMA: 2018,Sep,7

26478 **Lengthening of tendon, flexor, hand or finger, each tendon**
Facility RVU 18.2 Non-Facility RVU 18.2 FUD 090 J A2 80 CCI
AMA: 2018,Sep,7; 2018,Jan,8; 2017,Jan,8; 2016,Jan,13; 2015,Jan,16

26479 **Shortening of tendon, flexor, hand or finger, each tendon**
Facility RVU 17.6 Non-Facility RVU 17.6 FUD 090 J A2 80 CCI
AMA: 2018,Sep,7

26480 **Transfer or transplant of tendon, carpometacarpal area or dorsum of hand; without free graft, each tendon**
Facility RVU 21.1 Non-Facility RVU 21.1 FUD 090 J A2 80 CCI
AMA: 2018,Sep,7; 2018,Jan,8; 2017,Jan,8; 2016,Jan,13; 2015,Jan,16

26/TC PC/TC Only A2-Z3 ASC Payment 50 Bilateral ♂ Male Only ♀ Female Only Facility RVU Non-Facility RVU CCI X CLIA
FUD Follow-up Days CMS: IOM AMA: CPT Asst A-Y OPPSI 80/80 Surg Assist Allowed / w/Doc Lab Crosswalk Radiology Crosswalk

26483 with free tendon graft (includes obtaining graft), each tendon

24.4 24.4 FUD 090 J A2 80

AMA: 2018,Sep,7

26485 Transfer or transplant of tendon, palmar; without free tendon graft, each tendon

22.7 22.7 FUD 090 J A2 80

AMA: 2018,Sep,7

26489 with free tendon graft (includes obtaining graft), each tendon

27.1 27.1 FUD 090 J A2 80

AMA: 2018,Sep,7

26490 Opponensplasty; superficialis tendon transfer type, each tendon

EXCLUDES *Thumb fusion (26820)*

22.5 22.5 FUD 090 J A2 80

AMA: 2018,Sep,7

26492 tendon transfer with graft (includes obtaining graft), each tendon

EXCLUDES *Thumb fusion (26820)*

25.0 25.0 FUD 090 J A2 80

AMA: 2018,Sep,7

26494 hypothenar muscle transfer

EXCLUDES *Thumb fusion (26820)*

23.3 23.3 FUD 090 J A2 80

AMA: 2018,Sep,7

26496 other methods

EXCLUDES *Thumb fusion (26820)*

24.9 24.9 FUD 090 J A2 80

AMA: 2018,Sep,7

26497 Transfer of tendon to restore intrinsic function; ring and small finger

25.2 25.2 FUD 090 J A2 80

AMA: 2018,Sep,7

26498 all 4 fingers

33.2 33.2 FUD 090 J A2 80

AMA: 2018,Sep,7

26499 Correction claw finger, other methods

24.2 24.2 FUD 090 J A2 80

AMA: 2018,Sep,7

26500 Reconstruction of tendon pulley, each tendon; with local tissues (separate procedure)

18.2 18.2 FUD 090 J A2 80

AMA: 2018,Sep,7

26502 with tendon or fascial graft (includes obtaining graft) (separate procedure)

20.8 20.8 FUD 090 J A2 80

AMA: 2018,Sep,7

26508 Release of thenar muscle(s) (eg, thumb contracture)

18.6 18.6 FUD 090 J A2 80 50

AMA: 2018,Sep,7

26510 Cross intrinsic transfer, each tendon

17.6 17.6 FUD 090 J A2 80

AMA: 2018,Sep,7

26516 Capsulodesis, metacarpophalangeal joint; single digit

20.5 20.5 FUD 090 J A2 80 50

AMA: 2018,Sep,7

26517 2 digits

24.1 24.1 FUD 090 J A2 80 50

AMA: 2018,Sep,7

26518 3 or 4 digits

24.4 24.4 FUD 090 J A2 80 50

AMA: 2018,Sep,7

26520 Capsulectomy or capsulotomy; metacarpophalangeal joint, each joint

EXCLUDES *Carpometacarpal joint arthroplasty (25447)*

18.2 18.2 FUD 090 J A2

AMA: 2018,Sep,7

26525 interphalangeal joint, each joint

EXCLUDES *Carpometacarpal joint arthroplasty (25447)*

18.9 18.9 FUD 090 J A2

AMA: 2018,Sep,7; 2018,Jan,8; 2017,Jan,8; 2016,Jan,13; 2015,Jun,10; 2015,Jan,16

26530 Arthroplasty, metacarpophalangeal joint; each joint

EXCLUDES *Carpometacarpal joint arthroplasty (25447)*

15.4 15.4 FUD 090 J A2 80

AMA: 2018,Sep,7

26531 with prosthetic implant, each joint

EXCLUDES *Carpometacarpal joint arthroplasty (25447)*

18.0 18.0 FUD 090 J J8 80

AMA: 2018,Sep,7; 2018,Jan,8; 2017,Jan,8; 2016,Jan,13; 2015,Jan,16

26535 Arthroplasty, interphalangeal joint; each joint

EXCLUDES *Carpometacarpal joint arthroplasty (25447)*

12.3 12.3 FUD 090 J A2

AMA: 2018,Sep,7

26536 with prosthetic implant, each joint

EXCLUDES *Carpometacarpal joint arthroplasty (25447)*

20.8 20.8 FUD 090 J J8 80

AMA: 2018,Sep,7

26540 Repair of collateral ligament, metacarpophalangeal or interphalangeal joint

19.3 19.3 FUD 090 J A2 80

AMA: 2018,Sep,7

26541 Reconstruction, collateral ligament, metacarpophalangeal joint, single; with tendon or fascial graft (includes obtaining graft)

22.5 22.5 FUD 090 J A2 80

AMA: 2018,Sep,7; 2018,Jan,8; 2017,Jan,8; 2016,Jan,13; 2015,Jan,16

26542 with local tissue (eg, adductor advancement)

19.9 19.9 FUD 090 J A2 80

AMA: 2018,Sep,7; 2018,Jan,8; 2017,Jan,8; 2016,Jan,13; 2015,Jan,16

26545 Reconstruction, collateral ligament, interphalangeal joint, single, including graft, each joint

20.7 20.7 FUD 090 J A2 80

AMA: 2018,Sep,7

26546 Repair non-union, metacarpal or phalanx (includes obtaining bone graft with or without external or internal fixation)

28.9 28.9 FUD 090 J A2 80 50

AMA: 2018,Sep,7

26548 Repair and reconstruction, finger, volar plate, interphalangeal joint

22.2 22.2 FUD 090 J A2 80

AMA: 2018,Sep,7

26550-26556 Reconstruction Procedures with Finger and Toe Transplants

26550 Pollicization of a digit

46.8 46.8 FUD 090 J A2 80 50

AMA: 2018,Sep,7

26551 Transfer, toe-to-hand with microvascular anastomosis; great toe wrap-around with bone graft

INCLUDES Operating microscope (69990)

EXCLUDES *Big toe with web space (20973)*

95.1 95.1 FUD 090 C 80 50

AMA: 2018,Sep,7; 2018,Jan,8; 2017,Jan,8; 2016,Feb,12; 2016,Jan,13; 2015,Jan,16

26553 **other than great toe, single**
INCLUDES Operating microscope (69990)
Facility RVU 94.5 Non-Facility RVU 94.5 FUD 090 C 80 50
AMA: 2018,Sep,7; 2018,Jan,8; 2017,Jan,8; 2016,Feb,12; 2016,Jan,13; 2015,Jan,16

26554 **other than great toe, double**
INCLUDES Operating microscope (69990)
Facility RVU 109. Non-Facility RVU 109. FUD 090 C 80 50
AMA: 2018,Sep,7; 2018,Jan,8; 2017,Jan,8; 2016,Feb,12; 2016,Jan,13; 2015,Jan,16

26555 **Transfer, finger to another position without microvascular anastomosis**
Facility RVU 39.6 Non-Facility RVU 39.6 FUD 090 J A2 80
AMA: 2018,Sep,7

26556 **Transfer, free toe joint, with microvascular anastomosis**
INCLUDES Operating microscope (69990)
EXCLUDES *Big toe to hand transfer (20973)*
Facility RVU 98.2 Non-Facility RVU 98.2 FUD 090 C 80
AMA: 2018,Sep,7; 2018,Jan,8; 2017,Jan,8; 2016,Feb,12; 2016,Jan,13; 2015,Jan,16

26560-26596 Repair of Other Deformities of the Fingers/Hand

26560 **Repair of syndactyly (web finger) each web space; with skin flaps**
Facility RVU 16.5 Non-Facility RVU 16.5 FUD 090 J A2 80
AMA: 2018,Sep,7

26561 **with skin flaps and grafts**
Facility RVU 27.5 Non-Facility RVU 27.5 FUD 090 J A2 80
AMA: 2018,Sep,7

26562 **complex (eg, involving bone, nails)**
Facility RVU 38.8 Non-Facility RVU 38.8 FUD 090 J A2 80
AMA: 2018,Sep,7

26565 **Osteotomy; metacarpal, each**
Facility RVU 19.0 Non-Facility RVU 19.0 FUD 090 J A2 80
AMA: 2018,Sep,7

26567 **phalanx of finger, each**
Facility RVU 19.9 Non-Facility RVU 19.9 FUD 090 J A2 80
AMA: 2018,Sep,7; 2018,Jan,8; 2017,Jan,8; 2016,Jan,13; 2015,Jan,16

26568 **Osteoplasty, lengthening, metacarpal or phalanx**
Facility RVU 26.1 Non-Facility RVU 26.1 FUD 090 J A2 80
AMA: 2018,Sep,7

26580 **Repair cleft hand**
INCLUDES Barsky's procedure
Facility RVU 43.7 Non-Facility RVU 43.7 FUD 090 J A2 80 50
AMA: 2018,Sep,7

26587 **Reconstruction of polydactylous digit, soft tissue and bone**
EXCLUDES *Soft tissue removal only (11200)*
Facility RVU 30.0 Non-Facility RVU 30.0 FUD 090 J A2 80
AMA: 2018,Sep,7; 2018,Jan,8; 2017,Jan,8; 2016,Jan,13; 2015,Jan,16

26590 **Repair macrodactylia, each digit**
Facility RVU 40.7 Non-Facility RVU 40.7 FUD 090 J A2 80
AMA: 2018,Sep,7; 2018,Jan,8; 2017,Jan,8; 2016,Jan,13; 2015,Jan,16

26591 **Repair, intrinsic muscles of hand, each muscle**
Facility RVU 13.0 Non-Facility RVU 13.0 FUD 090 J A2 80
AMA: 2018,Sep,7; 2018,Jan,8; 2017,Jan,8; 2016,Jan,13; 2015,Jan,16

26593 **Release, intrinsic muscles of hand, each muscle**
Facility RVU 17.6 Non-Facility RVU 17.6 FUD 090 J A2
AMA: 2018,Sep,7

26596 **Excision of constricting ring of finger, with multiple Z-plasties**
EXCLUDES *Graft repair or scar contracture release (11042, 14040-14041, 15120, 15240)*
Facility RVU 22.5 Non-Facility RVU 22.5 FUD 090 J A2 80
AMA: 2018,Sep,7

26600-26785 Treatment of Fracture/Dislocation of Fingers and Hand

INCLUDES Closed, percutaneous, and open treatment fractures or dislocations

26600 **Closed treatment of metacarpal fracture, single; without manipulation, each bone**
Facility RVU 8.06 Non-Facility RVU 8.50 FUD 090 T P2
AMA: 2018,Sep,7

26605 **with manipulation, each bone**
Facility RVU 8.45 Non-Facility RVU 9.33 FUD 090 T A2
AMA: 2018,Sep,7

26607 **Closed treatment of metacarpal fracture, with manipulation, with external fixation, each bone**
Facility RVU 13.9 Non-Facility RVU 13.9 FUD 090 J A2 80
AMA: 2018,Sep,7

26608 **Percutaneous skeletal fixation of metacarpal fracture, each bone**
Facility RVU 13.7 Non-Facility RVU 13.7 FUD 090 J A2 80
AMA: 2018,Sep,7

26615 **Open treatment of metacarpal fracture, single, includes internal fixation, when performed, each bone**
Facility RVU 16.5 Non-Facility RVU 16.5 FUD 090 J A2
AMA: 2018,Sep,7

26641 **Closed treatment of carpometacarpal dislocation, thumb, with manipulation**
Facility RVU 9.97 Non-Facility RVU 11.0 FUD 090 T P2 80 50
AMA: 2018,Sep,7

26645 **Closed treatment of carpometacarpal fracture dislocation, thumb (Bennett fracture), with manipulation**
Facility RVU 11.3 Non-Facility RVU 12.3 FUD 090 J A2 80 50
AMA: 2018,Sep,7

26650 **Percutaneous skeletal fixation of carpometacarpal fracture dislocation, thumb (Bennett fracture), with manipulation**
Facility RVU 13.7 Non-Facility RVU 13.7 FUD 090 J A2 50
AMA: 2018,Sep,7

26665 **Open treatment of carpometacarpal fracture dislocation, thumb (Bennett fracture), includes internal fixation, when performed**
Facility RVU 18.0 Non-Facility RVU 18.0 FUD 090 J A2 50
AMA: 2018,Sep,7

26670 **Closed treatment of carpometacarpal dislocation, other than thumb, with manipulation, each joint; without anesthesia**
Facility RVU 8.87 Non-Facility RVU 9.86 FUD 090 T P2 80
AMA: 2018,Sep,7

26675 **requiring anesthesia**
Facility RVU 12.0 Non-Facility RVU 13.1 FUD 090 J A2 80
AMA: 2018,Sep,7

26676 **Percutaneous skeletal fixation of carpometacarpal dislocation, other than thumb, with manipulation, each joint**
Facility RVU 14.5 Non-Facility RVU 14.5 FUD 090 J A2
AMA: 2018,Sep,7

26685 **Open treatment of carpometacarpal dislocation, other than thumb; includes internal fixation, when performed, each joint**
Facility RVU 16.5 Non-Facility RVU 16.5 FUD 090 J A2
AMA: 2018,Sep,7

26686 **complex, multiple, or delayed reduction**
Facility RVU 18.0 Non-Facility RVU 18.0 FUD 090 J A2 80
AMA: 2018,Sep,7

26700 **Closed treatment of metacarpophalangeal dislocation, single, with manipulation; without anesthesia**
8.73 9.38 FUD 090 T P2
AMA: 2018,Sep,7

26705 **requiring anesthesia**
10.9 11.9 FUD 090 J A2 80
AMA: 2018,Sep,7

26706 **Percutaneous skeletal fixation of metacarpophalangeal dislocation, single, with manipulation**
12.6 12.6 FUD 090 J A2
AMA: 2018,Sep,7

26715 **Open treatment of metacarpophalangeal dislocation, single, includes internal fixation, when performed**
16.4 16.4 FUD 090 J A2 80
AMA: 2018,Sep,7

26720 **Closed treatment of phalangeal shaft fracture, proximal or middle phalanx, finger or thumb; without manipulation, each**
5.26 5.62 FUD 090 T P2
AMA: 2018,Sep,7

26725 **with manipulation, with or without skin or skeletal traction, each**
8.73 9.75 FUD 090 T P2
AMA: 2018,Sep,7

26727 **Percutaneous skeletal fixation of unstable phalangeal shaft fracture, proximal or middle phalanx, finger or thumb, with manipulation, each**
13.5 13.5 FUD 090 J A2
AMA: 2018,Sep,7

26735 **Open treatment of phalangeal shaft fracture, proximal or middle phalanx, finger or thumb, includes internal fixation, when performed, each**
17.1 17.1 FUD 090 J A2
AMA: 2018,Sep,7

26740 **Closed treatment of articular fracture, involving metacarpophalangeal or interphalangeal joint; without manipulation, each**
6.25 6.60 FUD 090 T P2
AMA: 2018,Sep,7

26742 **with manipulation, each**
9.64 10.6 FUD 090 J A2
AMA: 2018,Sep,7

26746 **Open treatment of articular fracture, involving metacarpophalangeal or interphalangeal joint, includes internal fixation, when performed, each**
21.3 21.3 FUD 090 J A2
AMA: 2018,Sep,7

26750 **Closed treatment of distal phalangeal fracture, finger or thumb; without manipulation, each**
5.35 5.32 FUD 090 T P2
AMA: 2018,Sep,7

26755 **with manipulation, each**
7.77 8.99 FUD 090 T G2
AMA: 2018,Sep,7

26756 **Percutaneous skeletal fixation of distal phalangeal fracture, finger or thumb, each**
12.1 12.1 FUD 090 J A2 80
AMA: 2018,Sep,7

26765 **Open treatment of distal phalangeal fracture, finger or thumb, includes internal fixation, when performed, each**
14.3 14.3 FUD 090 J A2
AMA: 2018,Sep,7

26770 **Closed treatment of interphalangeal joint dislocation, single, with manipulation; without anesthesia**
7.41 8.08 FUD 090 T G2
AMA: 2018,Sep,7

26775 **requiring anesthesia**
9.96 11.0 FUD 090 T P2
AMA: 2018,Sep,7

26776 **Percutaneous skeletal fixation of interphalangeal joint dislocation, single, with manipulation**
12.8 12.8 FUD 090 J A2
AMA: 2018,Sep,7

26785 **Open treatment of interphalangeal joint dislocation, includes internal fixation, when performed, single**
15.7 15.7 FUD 090 J A2
AMA: 2018,Sep,7

26820-26863 Fusion of Joint(s) of Fingers or Hand

26820 **Fusion in opposition, thumb, with autogenous graft (includes obtaining graft)**
22.2 22.2 FUD 090 J J8 80 50
AMA: 2020,May,13; 2018,Sep,7

26841 **Arthrodesis, carpometacarpal joint, thumb, with or without internal fixation;**
21.2 21.2 FUD 090 J A2 80 50
AMA: 2020,May,13; 2018,Sep,7

26842 **with autograft (includes obtaining graft)**
22.8 22.8 FUD 090 J A2 80 50
AMA: 2020,May,13; 2018,Sep,7

26843 **Arthrodesis, carpometacarpal joint, digit, other than thumb, each;**
21.6 21.6 FUD 090 J A2 80
AMA: 2020,May,13; 2018,Sep,7; 2018,Jan,8; 2017,Jan,8; 2016,Jan,13; 2015,Jan,16

26844 **with autograft (includes obtaining graft)**
23.9 23.9 FUD 090 J A2 80
AMA: 2020,May,13; 2018,Sep,7

26850 **Arthrodesis, metacarpophalangeal joint, with or without internal fixation;**
20.2 20.2 FUD 090 J A2 80
AMA: 2020,May,13; 2018,Sep,7

26852 **with autograft (includes obtaining graft)**
23.2 23.2 FUD 090 J A2 80
AMA: 2020,May,13; 2018,Sep,7

26860 **Arthrodesis, interphalangeal joint, with or without internal fixation;**
15.9 15.9 FUD 090 J A2
AMA: 2020,May,13; 2018,Sep,7; 2018,Jan,8; 2017,Jan,8; 2016,Jan,13; 2015,Jan,16

\+ **26861** **each additional interphalangeal joint (List separately in addition to code for primary procedure)**
Code first (26860)
2.98 2.98 FUD ZZZ N N1
AMA: 2020,May,13; 2018,Sep,7; 2018,Jan,8; 2017,Jan,8; 2016,Jan,13; 2015,Jan,16

26862 **with autograft (includes obtaining graft)**
21.1 21.1 FUD 090 J A2 80
AMA: 2020,May,13; 2018,Sep,7

\+ **26863** **with autograft (includes obtaining graft), each additional joint (List separately in addition to code for primary procedure)**
Code first (26862)
6.62 6.62 FUD ZZZ N N1 80
AMA: 2020,May,13; 2018,Sep,7

26910-26989 Amputations and Unlisted Procedures Finger/Hand

26910 **Amputation, metacarpal, with finger or thumb (ray amputation), single, with or without interosseous transfer**
EXCLUDES *Repositioning (26550, 26555)*
Transmetacarpal amputation hand (25927)
20.4 20.4 FUD 090 J A2
AMA: 2018,Sep,7

26951 **Amputation, finger or thumb, primary or secondary, any joint or phalanx, single, including neurectomies; with direct closure**

EXCLUDES *Repair necessitating flaps or grafts (15050-15758)*
Transmetacarpal amputation hand (25927)

Facility RVU 19.1 Non-Facility RVU 19.1 **FUD** 090 J A2 CCI

AMA: 2018,Sep,7

26952 **with local advancement flaps (V-Y, hood)**

EXCLUDES *Repair necessitating flaps or grafts (15050-15758)*
Transmetacarpal amputation hand (25927)

Facility RVU 18.9 Non-Facility RVU 18.9 **FUD** 090 J A2 CCI

AMA: 2018,Sep,7

26989 **Unlisted procedure, hands or fingers**

Facility RVU 0.00 Non-Facility RVU 0.00 **FUD** YYY T CCI

AMA: 2018,Sep,7

26990-26992 Incision for Drainage of Pelvis or Hip

EXCLUDES *Simple incision and drainage procedures (10040-10160)*

26990 **Incision and drainage, pelvis or hip joint area; deep abscess or hematoma**

Facility RVU 18.8 Non-Facility RVU 18.8 **FUD** 090 J A2 CCI

AMA: 2018,Sep,7

26991 **infected bursa**

Facility RVU 15.1 Non-Facility RVU 20.4 **FUD** 090 J A2 80 CCI

AMA: 2018,Sep,7

26992 **Incision, bone cortex, pelvis and/or hip joint (eg, osteomyelitis or bone abscess)**

Facility RVU 28.5 Non-Facility RVU 28.5 **FUD** 090 C 80 CCI

AMA: 2018,Sep,7; 2018,Jan,8; 2017,Jan,8; 2016,Jan,13; 2015,Jan,16

27000-27006 Tenotomy Procedures of Hip

27000 **Tenotomy, adductor of hip, percutaneous (separate procedure)**

Facility RVU 11.6 Non-Facility RVU 11.6 **FUD** 090 J A2 50 CCI

AMA: 2018,Sep,7

27001 **Tenotomy, adductor of hip, open**

Facility RVU 15.6 Non-Facility RVU 15.6 **FUD** 090 J A2 80 50 CCI

AMA: 2018,Sep,7

27003 **Tenotomy, adductor, subcutaneous, open, with obturator neurectomy**

Facility RVU 17.1 Non-Facility RVU 17.1 **FUD** 090 J A2 80 50 CCI

AMA: 2018,Sep,7

27005 **Tenotomy, hip flexor(s), open (separate procedure)**

Facility RVU 20.8 Non-Facility RVU 20.8 **FUD** 090 C 80 50 CCI

AMA: 2018,Sep,7

27006 **Tenotomy, abductors and/or extensor(s) of hip, open (separate procedure)**

Facility RVU 20.7 Non-Facility RVU 20.7 **FUD** 090 J 80 50 CCI

AMA: 2018,Sep,7

27025-27036 Surgical Incision of Hip

27025 **Fasciotomy, hip or thigh, any type**

Facility RVU 26.5 Non-Facility RVU 26.5 **FUD** 090 C 80 50 CCI

AMA: 2018,Sep,7

27027 **Decompression fasciotomy(ies), pelvic (buttock) compartment(s) (eg, gluteus medius-minimus, gluteus maximus, iliopsoas, and/or tensor fascia lata muscle), unilateral**

Facility RVU 25.8 Non-Facility RVU 25.8 **FUD** 090 J 80 50 CCI

AMA: 2018,Sep,7

27030 **Arthrotomy, hip, with drainage (eg, infection)**

Facility RVU 27.1 Non-Facility RVU 27.1 **FUD** 090 C 80 50 CCI

AMA: 2018,Sep,7

27033 **Arthrotomy, hip, including exploration or removal of loose or foreign body**

Facility RVU 28.1 Non-Facility RVU 28.1 **FUD** 090 J A2 80 50 CCI

AMA: 2018,Sep,7; 2018,Jan,8; 2017,Jan,8; 2016,Jan,13; 2015,Jan,16

27035 **Denervation, hip joint, intrapelvic or extrapelvic intra-articular branches of sciatic, femoral, or obturator nerves**

EXCLUDES *Transection obturator nerve (64763, 64766)*

Facility RVU 32.8 Non-Facility RVU 32.8 **FUD** 090 J A2 80 50 CCI

AMA: 2018,Sep,7; 2018,Jan,8; 2017,Jan,8; 2016,Jan,13; 2015,Jan,16

27036 **Capsulectomy or capsulotomy, hip, with or without excision of heterotopic bone, with release of hip flexor muscles (ie, gluteus medius, gluteus minimus, tensor fascia latae, rectus femoris, sartorius, iliopsoas)**

Facility RVU 29.1 Non-Facility RVU 29.1 **FUD** 090 C 80 50 CCI

AMA: 2018,Sep,7

27040-27041 Biopsy of Hip/Pelvis

EXCLUDES *Soft tissue needle biopsy (20206)*

27040 **Biopsy, soft tissue of pelvis and hip area; superficial**

Facility RVU 5.70 Non-Facility RVU 9.83 **FUD** 010 J A2 50 CCI

AMA: 2018,Sep,7

27041 **deep, subfascial or intramuscular**

Facility RVU 20.1 Non-Facility RVU 20.1 **FUD** 090 J A2 50 CCI

AMA: 2018,Sep,7

27043-27059 [27043, 27045, 27059] Excision Soft Tissue Tumors Hip/ Pelvis

INCLUDES Any necessary elevation tissue planes or dissection
Measurement tumor and necessary margin at greatest diameter prior to excision
Simple and intermediate repairs
Excision types:
- Fascial or subfascial soft tissue tumors: simple and marginal resection tumors found either in or below deep fascia, not involving bone or excision substantial amount normal tissue; primarily benign and intramuscular tumors
- Radical resection soft tissue tumor: wide resection tumor involving substantial margins normal tissue and may involve tissue removal from one or more layers; mostly malignant or aggressive benign
- Subcutaneous: simple and marginal resection tumors found in subcutaneous tissue above deep fascia; most often benign

EXCLUDES *Complex repair*
Excision benign cutaneous lesions (eg, sebaceous cyst) (11400-11406)
Radical resection cutaneous tumors (eg, melanoma) (11600-11606)
Significant vessel exploration, neuroplasty, reconstruction, or complex bone repair

27043 **Resequenced code. See code following 27047.**

27045 **Resequenced code. See code following 27048.**

27047 **Excision, tumor, soft tissue of pelvis and hip area, subcutaneous; less than 3 cm**

Facility RVU 10.4 Non-Facility RVU 13.6 **FUD** 090 J G2 50 CCI

AMA: 2018,Sep,7

\# **27043** **3 cm or greater**

Facility RVU 13.5 Non-Facility RVU 13.5 **FUD** 090 J G2 50 CCI

AMA: 2018,Sep,7

27048 **Excision, tumor, soft tissue of pelvis and hip area, subfascial (eg, intramuscular); less than 5 cm**

Facility RVU 17.6 Non-Facility RVU 17.6 **FUD** 090 J G2 80 50 CCI

AMA: 2018,Sep,7

\# **27045** **5 cm or greater**

Facility RVU 21.3 Non-Facility RVU 21.3 **FUD** 090 J G2 80 50 CCI

AMA: 2018,Sep,7

27049 **Radical resection of tumor (eg, sarcoma), soft tissue of pelvis and hip area; less than 5 cm**

Facility RVU 38.6 Non-Facility RVU 38.6 **FUD** 090 J G2 80 50 CCI

AMA: 2018,Sep,7

\# **27059** **5 cm or greater**
52.6 52.6 **FUD** 090 J G2 80 50
AMA: 2018,Sep,7

27050-27071 [27059] Procedures of Bones and Joints of Hip and Pelvis

27050 **Arthrotomy, with biopsy; sacroiliac joint**
11.5 11.5 **FUD** 090 J A2 80 50
AMA: 2018,Sep,7

27052 **hip joint**
16.6 16.6 **FUD** 090 J A2 80 50
AMA: 2018,Sep,7

27054 **Arthrotomy with synovectomy, hip joint**
19.8 19.8 **FUD** 090 C 80 50
AMA: 2018,Sep,7

27057 **Decompression fasciotomy(ies), pelvic (buttock) compartment(s) (eg, gluteus medius-minimus, gluteus maximus, iliopsoas, and/or tensor fascia lata muscle) with debridement of nonviable muscle, unilateral**
29.2 29.2 **FUD** 090 J 80 50
AMA: 2018,Sep,7

27059 **Resequenced code. See code following 27049.**

27060 **Excision; ischial bursa**
13.4 13.4 **FUD** 090 J A2 50
AMA: 2018,Sep,7

27062 **trochanteric bursa or calcification**
EXCLUDES *Arthrocentesis (20610)*
13.1 13.1 **FUD** 090 J A2 50
AMA: 2018,Sep,7

27065 **Excision of bone cyst or benign tumor, wing of ilium, symphysis pubis, or greater trochanter of femur; superficial, includes autograft, when performed**
15.0 15.0 **FUD** 090 J A2 80 50
AMA: 2018,Sep,7

27066 **deep (subfascial), includes autograft, when performed**
23.1 23.1 **FUD** 090 J A2 80 50
AMA: 2018,Sep,7

27067 **with autograft requiring separate incision**
29.8 29.8 **FUD** 090 J A2 80 50
AMA: 2018,Sep,7

27070 **Partial excision, wing of ilium, symphysis pubis, or greater trochanter of femur, (craterization, saucerization) (eg, osteomyelitis or bone abscess); superficial**
25.3 25.3 **FUD** 090 C 80 50
AMA: 2018,Sep,7

27071 **deep (subfascial or intramuscular)**
27.2 27.2 **FUD** 090 C 80 50
AMA: 2018,Sep,7

27075-27078 Radical Resection Bone Tumor of Hip/Pelvis

INCLUDES Any necessary elevation tissue planes or dissection
Excision adjacent soft tissue during bone tumor resection (27043-27049 [27043, 27045, 27059])
Measurement tumor and necessary margin at greatest diameter prior to excision
Resection tumor (may include entire bone) and wide margins normal tissue primarily for malignant or aggressive benign tumors
Simple and intermediate repairs

EXCLUDES *Complex repair*
Significant vessel exploration, neuroplasty, reconstruction, or complex bone repair

27075 **Radical resection of tumor; wing of ilium, 1 pubic or ischial ramus or symphysis pubis**
60.5 60.5 **FUD** 090 C 80
AMA: 2019,May,7; 2018,Sep,7

27076 **ilium, including acetabulum, both pubic rami, or ischium and acetabulum**
73.5 73.5 **FUD** 090 C 80
AMA: 2019,May,7; 2018,Sep,7

27077 **innominate bone, total**
81.8 81.8 **FUD** 090 C 80
AMA: 2019,May,7; 2018,Sep,7

27078 **ischial tuberosity and greater trochanter of femur**
59.6 59.6 **FUD** 090 C 80 50
AMA: 2019,May,7; 2018,Sep,7

27080 Excision of Coccyx

EXCLUDES *Surgical excision decubitus ulcers (15920, 15922, 15931-15958)*

27080 **Coccygectomy, primary**
14.7 14.7 **FUD** 090 J A2 80
AMA: 2018,Sep,7

27086-27091 Removal Foreign Body or Hip Prosthesis

27086 **Removal of foreign body, pelvis or hip; subcutaneous tissue**
4.82 8.78 **FUD** 010 J A2 80 50
AMA: 2018,Sep,7; 2018,Jan,8; 2017,Jan,8; 2016,Jan,13; 2015,Jan,16

27087 **deep (subfascial or intramuscular)**
17.7 17.7 **FUD** 090 J A2 80 50
AMA: 2018,Sep,7

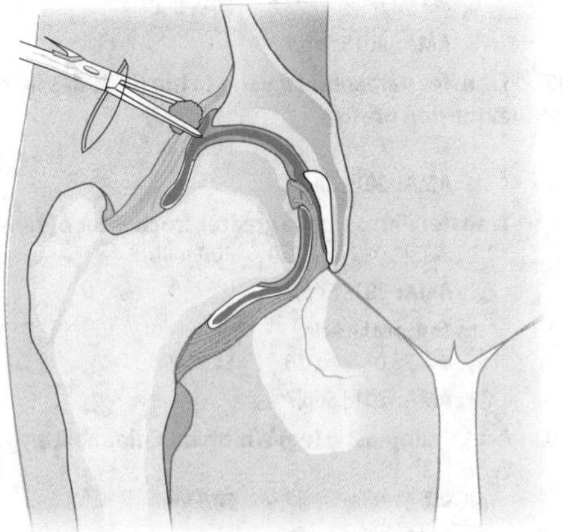

A foreign body is removed from the pelvis or hip

27090 **Removal of hip prosthesis; (separate procedure)**
24.0 24.0 **FUD** 090 C 80 50
AMA: 2019,May,7; 2018,Sep,7

27091 **complicated, including total hip prosthesis, methylmethacrylate with or without insertion of spacer**
46.0 46.0 **FUD** 090 C 80 50
AMA: 2019,May,7; 2018,Sep,7; 2018,Jan,8; 2017,Jan,8; 2016,Jan,13; 2015,Jan,16

27093-27096 Injection for Arthrogram Hip/Sacroiliac Joint

27093 **Injection procedure for hip arthrography; without anesthesia**
(73525)
2.01 5.72 **FUD** 000 N N1 50
AMA: 2018,Sep,7; 2018,Jan,8; 2017,Jan,8; 2016,Jan,13; 2015,Aug,6; 2015,Jan,16

27095 **with anesthesia**
(73525)
2.43 8.36 **FUD** 000 N N1 50
AMA: 2018,Sep,7; 2018,Jan,8; 2017,Jan,8; 2016,Jan,13; 2016,Jan,11; 2015,Aug,6; 2015,Jan,16

27096 **Injection procedure for sacroiliac joint, anesthetic/steroid, with image guidance (fluoroscopy or CT) including arthrography when performed**

INCLUDES Confirmation intra-articular needle placement with CT or fluoroscopy

Fluoroscopic guidance (77002-77003)

EXCLUDES *Procedure performed without fluoroscopy or CT guidance (20552)*

2.39 | 4.61 | **FUD** 000 | B 50

AMA: 2018,Sep,7; 2018,Jan,8; 2017,Jan,8; 2016,Jan,13; 2015,Aug,6; 2015,Jan,16

27097-27187 Revision/Reconstruction Hip and Pelvis

INCLUDES Closed, open and percutaneous treatment fractures and dislocations

27097 **Release or recession, hamstring, proximal**

19.7 | 19.7 | **FUD** 090 | J A2 80 50

AMA: 2018,Sep,7

27098 **Transfer, adductor to ischium**

20.0 | 20.0 | **FUD** 090 | J A2 80 50

AMA: 2018,Sep,7

27100 **Transfer external oblique muscle to greater trochanter including fascial or tendon extension (graft)**

INCLUDES Eggers procedure

23.6 | 23.6 | **FUD** 090 | J A2 80 50

AMA: 2018,Sep,7

27105 **Transfer paraspinal muscle to hip (includes fascial or tendon extension graft)**

25.0 | 25.0 | **FUD** 090 | J A2 80 50

AMA: 2018,Sep,7

27110 **Transfer iliopsoas; to greater trochanter of femur**

28.0 | 28.0 | **FUD** 090 | J A2 80 50

AMA: 2018,Sep,7

27111 **to femoral neck**

26.0 | 26.0 | **FUD** 090 | J A2 80 50

AMA: 2018,Sep,7

27120 **Acetabuloplasty; (eg, Whitman, Colonna, Haygroves, or cup type)**

37.5 | 37.5 | **FUD** 090 | C 80 50

AMA: 2018,Sep,7

27122 **resection, femoral head (eg, Girdlestone procedure)**

31.7 | 31.7 | **FUD** 090 | C 80 50

AMA: 2018,Sep,7

27125 **Hemiarthroplasty, hip, partial (eg, femoral stem prosthesis, bipolar arthroplasty)**

EXCLUDES *Hip replacement following hip fracture (27236)*

32.7 | 32.7 | **FUD** 090 | C 80 50

AMA: 2018,Sep,7; 2018,Jan,8; 2017,Jan,8; 2016,Jan,13; 2015,Jan,16

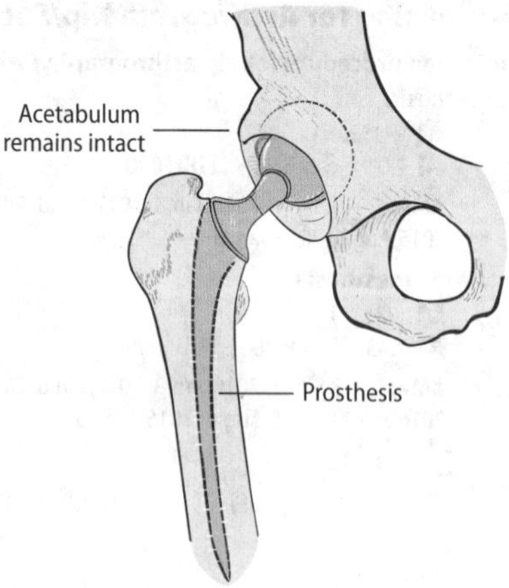

27130 **Arthroplasty, acetabular and proximal femoral prosthetic replacement (total hip arthroplasty), with or without autograft or allograft**

39.2 | 39.2 | **FUD** 090 | C 80 50

AMA: 2019,May,7; 2018,Sep,7; 2018,Jan,8; 2017,Jan,8; 2016,Jan,13; 2015,Jan,16

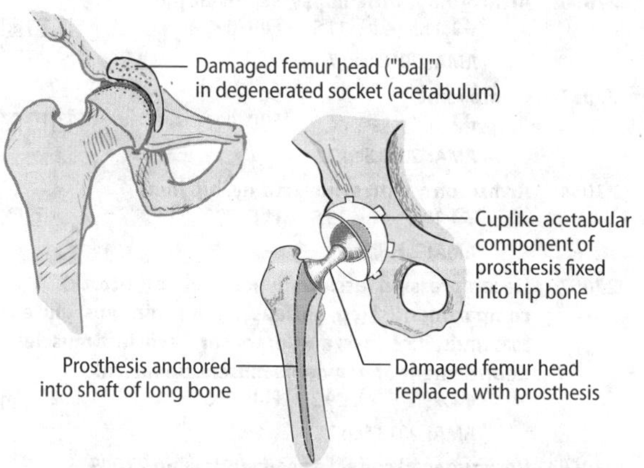

27132 **Conversion of previous hip surgery to total hip arthroplasty, with or without autograft or allograft**

48.3 | 48.3 | **FUD** 090 | C 80 50

AMA: 2019,May,7; 2018,Sep,7; 2018,Jan,8; 2017,Sep,14; 2017,Jan,8; 2016,Jan,13; 2015,Jan,16

27134 **Revision of total hip arthroplasty; both components, with or without autograft or allograft**

55.3 | 55.3 | **FUD** 090 | C 80 50

AMA: 2019,May,7; 2018,Sep,7; 2018,Jan,8; 2017,Jan,8; 2016,Jan,13; 2015,Jan,16

27137 **acetabular component only, with or without autograft or allograft**

42.5 | 42.5 | **FUD** 090 | C 80 50

AMA: 2018,Sep,7; 2018,Jan,8; 2017,Jan,8; 2016,Jan,13; 2015,Jan,16

27138 **femoral component only, with or without allograft**

44.1 | 44.1 | **FUD** 090 | C 80 50

AMA: 2019,May,7; 2018,Sep,7; 2018,Jan,8; 2017,Jan,8; 2016,Jan,13; 2015,Jan,16

27140 **Osteotomy and transfer of greater trochanter of femur (separate procedure)**

25.8 | 25.8 | **FUD** 090 | C 80 50

AMA: 2018,Sep,7

27146 **Osteotomy, iliac, acetabular or innominate bone;**

INCLUDES Salter osteotomy

36.9 | 36.9 | **FUD** 090 | C 80 50

AMA: 2018,Sep,7; 2018,Jan,8; 2017,Jan,8; 2016,Jan,13; 2015,Jan,16

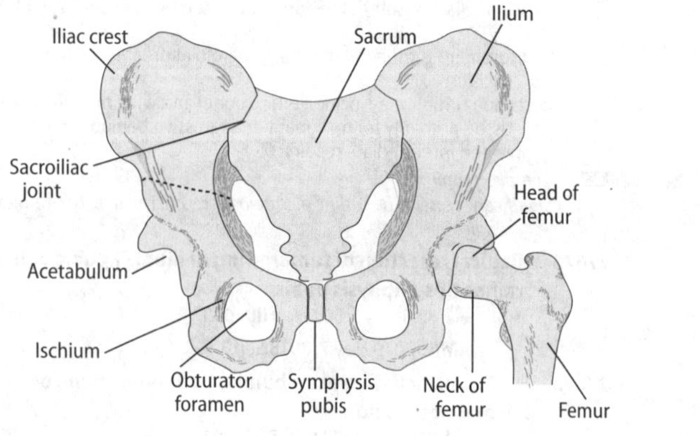

27147 **with open reduction of hip**

INCLUDES Pemberton osteotomy

42.4 42.4 **FUD** 090 C 80 50

AMA: 2018,Sep,7

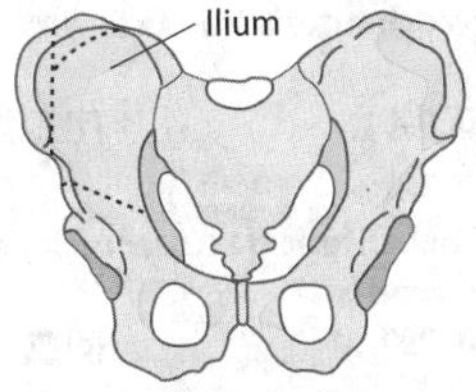

Example of innominate osteotomy

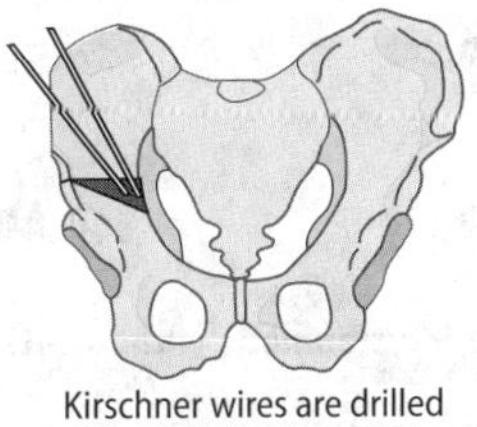

Kirschner wires are drilled through the ilium and into lower fragment

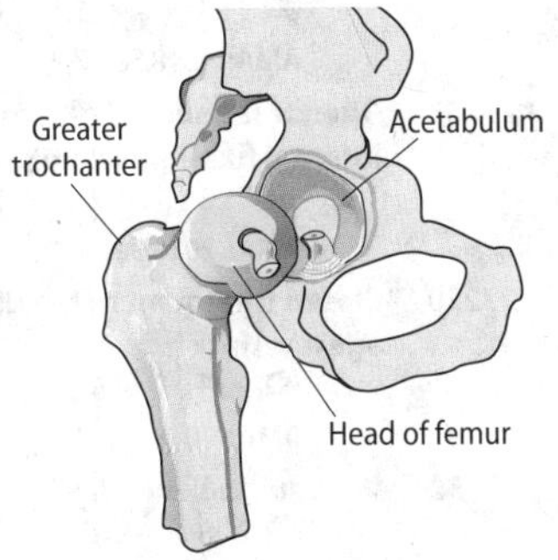

Femoral head is reduced into the acetabulum

27151 **with femoral osteotomy**

45.9 45.9 **FUD** 090 C 80 50

AMA: 2018,Sep,7

27156 **with femoral osteotomy and with open reduction of hip**

INCLUDES Chiari osteotomy

49.5 49.5 **FUD** 090 C 80 50

AMA: 2018,Sep,7

27158 **Osteotomy, pelvis, bilateral (eg, congenital malformation)**

40.5 40.5 **FUD** 090 C 80

AMA: 2018,Sep,7

27161 **Osteotomy, femoral neck (separate procedure)**

35.2 35.2 **FUD** 090 C 80 50

AMA: 2018,Sep,7

27165 **Osteotomy, intertrochanteric or subtrochanteric including internal or external fixation and/or cast**

39.6 39.6 **FUD** 090 C 80 50

AMA: 2018,Sep,7; 2018,Jan,8; 2017,Jan,8; 2016,Jan,13; 2015,Jan,16

27170 **Bone graft, femoral head, neck, intertrochanteric or subtrochanteric area (includes obtaining bone graft)**

33.9 33.9 **FUD** 090 C 80 50

AMA: 2018,Sep,7; 2018,Jan,8; 2017,Jan,8; 2016,Jan,13; 2015,Jan,16

27175 **Treatment of slipped femoral epiphysis; by traction, without reduction**

19.2 19.2 **FUD** 090 C 80 50

AMA: 2018,Sep,7

27176 **by single or multiple pinning, in situ**

26.5 26.5 **FUD** 090 C 80 50

AMA: 2018,Sep,7

27177 **Open treatment of slipped femoral epiphysis; single or multiple pinning or bone graft (includes obtaining graft)**

32.1 32.1 **FUD** 090 C 80 50

AMA: 2018,Sep,7

27178 **closed manipulation with single or multiple pinning**

26.5 26.5 **FUD** 090 C 80 50

AMA: 2018,Sep,7

27179 **osteoplasty of femoral neck (Heyman type procedure)**

28.2 28.2 **FUD** 090 J 80 50

AMA: 2018,Sep,7

27181 **osteotomy and internal fixation**

32.3 32.3 **FUD** 090 C 80 50

AMA: 2018,Sep,7

27185 **Epiphyseal arrest by epiphysiodesis or stapling, greater trochanter of femur**

20.7 20.7 **FUD** 090 C 50

AMA: 2018,Sep,7

27187 **Prophylactic treatment (nailing, pinning, plating or wiring) with or without methylmethacrylate, femoral neck and proximal femur**

28.7 28.7 **FUD** 090 C 80 50

AMA: 2018,Sep,7; 2018,Jan,8; 2017,Jan,8; 2016,Jan,13; 2015,Jan,16

27197-27269 Treatment of Fracture/Dislocation Hip/Pelvis

27197 **Closed treatment of posterior pelvic ring fracture(s), dislocation(s), diastasis or subluxation of the ilium, sacroiliac joint, and/or sacrum, with or without anterior pelvic ring fracture(s) and/or dislocation(s) of the pubic symphysis and/or superior/inferior rami, unilateral or bilateral; without manipulation**

3.68 3.68 **FUD** 000 T G2

AMA: 2018,Sep,7; 2018,Jan,8; 2017,Jun,9

27198 **with manipulation, requiring more than local anesthesia (ie, general anesthesia, moderate sedation, spinal/epidural)**

EXCLUDES *Closed treatment anterior pelvic ring, pubic symphysis, inferior rami fracture/dislocation--see appropriate E/M codes*

8.84 8.84 **FUD** 000 T G2 80

AMA: 2018,Sep,7; 2018,Jan,3; 2018,Jan,8; 2017,Jun,9

27200 **Closed treatment of coccygeal fracture**

5.40 5.32 **FUD** 090 T P2

AMA: 2018,Sep,7

27202 **Open treatment of coccygeal fracture**

15.2 15.2 **FUD** 090 J A2 80

AMA: 2018,Sep,7

27215 **Open treatment of iliac spine(s), tuberosity avulsion, or iliac wing fracture(s), unilateral, for pelvic bone fracture patterns that do not disrupt the pelvic ring, includes internal fixation, when performed**

17.4 17.4 **FUD** 090 E

AMA: 2018,Sep,7

27216 **Percutaneous skeletal fixation of posterior pelvic bone fracture and/or dislocation, for fracture patterns that disrupt the pelvic ring, unilateral (includes ipsilateral ilium, sacroiliac joint and/or sacrum)**

EXCLUDES *Sacroiliac joint arthrodesis without fracture and/or dislocation, percutaneous or minimally invasive (27279)*

26.7 26.7 **FUD** 090 E

AMA: 2018,Sep,7; 2018,Jan,8; 2017,Jan,8; 2016,Jan,13; 2015,Jan,16

27217 **Open treatment of anterior pelvic bone fracture and/or dislocation for fracture patterns that disrupt the pelvic ring, unilateral, includes internal fixation, when performed (includes pubic symphysis and/or ipsilateral superior/inferior rami)**

25.0 25.0 **FUD** 090 E

AMA: 2018,Sep,7

27218 **Open treatment of posterior pelvic bone fracture and/or dislocation, for fracture patterns that disrupt the pelvic ring, unilateral, includes internal fixation, when performed (includes ipsilateral ilium, sacroiliac joint and/or sacrum)**
EXCLUDES *Sacroiliac joint arthrodesis without fracture and/or dislocation, percutaneous or minimally invasive (27279)*
34.6 34.6 **FUD** 090 E
AMA: 2018,Sep,7; 2018,Jan,8; 2017,Jan,8; 2016,Jan,13; 2015,Jan,16

27220 **Closed treatment of acetabulum (hip socket) fracture(s); without manipulation**
12.2 12.4 **FUD** 090 T G2 50
AMA: 2018,Sep,7

27222 **with manipulation, with or without skeletal traction**
28.1 28.1 **FUD** 090 C 50
AMA: 2018,Sep,7

27226 **Open treatment of posterior or anterior acetabular wall fracture, with internal fixation**
30.4 30.4 **FUD** 090 C 80 50
AMA: 2018,Sep,7

27227 **Open treatment of acetabular fracture(s) involving anterior or posterior (one) column, or a fracture running transversely across the acetabulum, with internal fixation**
47.9 47.9 **FUD** 090 C 80 50
AMA: 2018,Sep,7

27228 **Open treatment of acetabular fracture(s) involving anterior and posterior (two) columns, includes T-fracture and both column fracture with complete articular detachment, or single column or transverse fracture with associated acetabular wall fracture, with internal fixation**
54.3 54.3 **FUD** 090 C 80 50
AMA: 2018,Sep,7

27230 **Closed treatment of femoral fracture, proximal end, neck; without manipulation**
13.6 13.8 **FUD** 090 T A2 50
AMA: 2018,Sep,7

27232 **with manipulation, with or without skeletal traction**
21.6 21.6 **FUD** 090 C 50
AMA: 2018,Sep,7

27235 **Percutaneous skeletal fixation of femoral fracture, proximal end, neck**
26.2 26.2 **FUD** 090 J 50
AMA: 2018,Sep,7; 2018,Jan,8; 2017,Jan,8; 2016,Jan,13; 2015,Jan,16

27236 **Open treatment of femoral fracture, proximal end, neck, internal fixation or prosthetic replacement**
34.4 34.4 **FUD** 090 C 80 50
AMA: 2019,May,7; 2018,Sep,7; 2018,Jan,8; 2017,Jan,8; 2016,Nov,9; 2016,Jan,13; 2015,Jan,16

27238 **Closed treatment of intertrochanteric, peritrochanteric, or subtrochanteric femoral fracture; without manipulation**
13.3 13.3 **FUD** 090 J A2 50
AMA: 2018,Sep,7; 2018,Jan,8; 2017,Jan,8; 2016,Jan,13; 2015,Jan,16

27240 **with manipulation, with or without skin or skeletal traction**
27.5 27.5 **FUD** 090 C 50
AMA: 2018,Sep,7; 2018,Jan,8; 2017,Jan,8; 2016,Jan,13; 2015,Jan,16

27244 **Treatment of intertrochanteric, peritrochanteric, or subtrochanteric femoral fracture; with plate/screw type implant, with or without cerclage**
35.5 35.5 **FUD** 090 C 80 50
AMA: 2019,May,7; 2018,Sep,7; 2018,Jan,8; 2017,Jan,8; 2016,Jan,13; 2015,Jan,16

27245 **with intramedullary implant, with or without interlocking screws and/or cerclage**
35.5 35.5 **FUD** 090 C 80 50
AMA: 2018,Sep,7; 2018,Jan,8; 2017,Jan,8; 2016,Jan,13; 2015,Jan,16

27246 **Closed treatment of greater trochanteric fracture, without manipulation**
11.1 11.1 **FUD** 090 T A2 50
AMA: 2018,Sep,7

27248 **Open treatment of greater trochanteric fracture, includes internal fixation, when performed**
21.5 21.5 **FUD** 090 C 80 50
AMA: 2018,Sep,7

27250 **Closed treatment of hip dislocation, traumatic; without anesthesia**
5.33 5.33 **FUD** 000 T A2 50
AMA: 2018,Sep,7

27252 **requiring anesthesia**
21.8 21.8 **FUD** 090 J A2 50
AMA: 2018,Sep,7

27253 **Open treatment of hip dislocation, traumatic, without internal fixation**
27.2 27.2 **FUD** 090 C 80 50
AMA: 2018,Sep,7

27254 **Open treatment of hip dislocation, traumatic, with acetabular wall and femoral head fracture, with or without internal or external fixation**
EXCLUDES *Acetabular fracture treatment (27226-27227)*
36.4 36.4 **FUD** 090 C 80 50
AMA: 2018,Sep,7

27256 **Treatment of spontaneous hip dislocation (developmental, including congenital or pathological), by abduction, splint or traction; without anesthesia, without manipulation**
6.78 8.73 **FUD** 010 T G2 80 50
AMA: 2018,Sep,7

27257 **with manipulation, requiring anesthesia**
10.4 10.4 **FUD** 010 J A2 80 50
AMA: 2018,Sep,7

27258 **Open treatment of spontaneous hip dislocation (developmental, including congenital or pathological), replacement of femoral head in acetabulum (including tenotomy, etc);**
INCLUDES Lorenz's operation
32.1 32.1 **FUD** 090 C 80 50
AMA: 2018,Sep,7

27259 **with femoral shaft shortening**
44.7 44.7 **FUD** 090 C 80 50
AMA: 2018,Sep,7

27265 **Closed treatment of post hip arthroplasty dislocation; without anesthesia**
11.6 11.6 **FUD** 090 T A2 50
AMA: 2018,Sep,7

27266 **requiring regional or general anesthesia**
16.8 16.8 **FUD** 090 J A2 50
AMA: 2018,Sep,7

27267 **Closed treatment of femoral fracture, proximal end, head; without manipulation**
12.5 12.5 **FUD** 090 J G2 80 50
AMA: 2018,Sep,7; 2018,Jan,8; 2017,Jan,8; 2016,Jan,13; 2015,Jan,16

27268 **with manipulation**
15.6 15.6 **FUD** 090 C 80 50
AMA: 2018,Sep,7; 2018,Jan,8; 2017,Jan,8; 2016,Jan,13; 2015,Jan,16

27269 **Open treatment of femoral fracture, proximal end, head, includes internal fixation, when performed**

EXCLUDES *Arthrotomy, hip (27033)*
Open treatment hip dislocation, traumatic, without internal fixation (27253)

35.9 35.9 FUD 090 C 80 50

AMA: 2018,Sep,7; 2018,Jan,8; 2017,Jan,8; 2016,Jan,13; 2015,Jan,16

27275 Hip Manipulation with Anesthesia

27275 **Manipulation, hip joint, requiring general anesthesia**

5.26 5.26 FUD 010 J A2

AMA: 2018,Sep,7; 2018,Jan,8; 2017,Jan,8; 2016,May,13; 2016,Jan,11; 2016,Jan,13; 2015,Jan,16

27279-27286 Arthrodesis of Hip and Pelvis

27279 **Arthrodesis, sacroiliac joint, percutaneous or minimally invasive (indirect visualization), with image guidance, includes obtaining bone graft when performed, and placement of transfixing device**

25.3 25.3 FUD 090 J J8 80 50

AMA: 2020,May,13; 2018,Sep,7

27280 **Arthrodesis, open, sacroiliac joint, including obtaining bone graft, including instrumentation, when performed**

EXCLUDES *Sacroiliac joint arthrodesis without fracture and/or dislocation, percutaneous or minimally invasive (27279)*

39.2 39.2 FUD 090 C 80 50

AMA: 2020,May,13; 2018,Sep,7; 2018,Jan,8; 2017,Jan,8; 2016,Jan,13; 2015,Jan,16

27282 **Arthrodesis, symphysis pubis (including obtaining graft)**

24.7 24.7 FUD 090 C 80

AMA: 2020,May,13; 2018,Sep,7

27284 **Arthrodesis, hip joint (including obtaining graft);**

46.6 46.6 FUD 090 C 80 50

AMA: 2020,May,13; 2018,Sep,7

27286 **with subtrochanteric osteotomy**

47.6 47.6 FUD 090 C 80 50

AMA: 2020,May,13; 2018,Sep,7; 2018,Jan,8; 2017,Jan,8; 2016,Jan,13; 2015,Jan,16

27290-27299 Amputations and Unlisted Procedures of Hip and Pelvis

27290 **Interpelviabdominal amputation (hindquarter amputation)**

46.9 46.9 FUD 090 C 80

AMA: 2018,Sep,7; 2018,Jan,8; 2017,Jan,8; 2016,Jan,13; 2015,Jan,16

27295 **Disarticulation of hip**

36.4 36.4 FUD 090 C 80 50

AMA: 2018,Sep,7; 2018,Jan,8; 2017,Jan,8; 2016,Jan,13; 2015,Jan,16

27299 **Unlisted procedure, pelvis or hip joint**

0.00 0.00 FUD YYY T 80 50

AMA: 2018,Sep,7; 2018,Jan,8; 2017,Jan,8; 2016,Jun,8; 2016,Jan,13; 2015,Jan,16

27301-27310 Incisional Procedures Femur or Knee

EXCLUDES *Superficial incision and drainage (10040-10160)*

27301 **Incision and drainage, deep abscess, bursa, or hematoma, thigh or knee region**

14.5 19.4 FUD 090 J A2 50

AMA: 2018,Sep,7; 2018,Jan,8; 2017,Jan,8; 2016,Jan,13; 2015,Jan,16

27303 **Incision, deep, with opening of bone cortex, femur or knee (eg, osteomyelitis or bone abscess)**

18.5 18.5 FUD 090 C 80 50

AMA: 2018,Sep,7

27305 **Fasciotomy, iliotibial (tenotomy), open**

EXCLUDES *Ober-Yount (gluteal-iliotibial) fasciotomy (27025)*

13.8 13.8 FUD 090 J A2 80 50

AMA: 2018,Sep,7

27306 **Tenotomy, percutaneous, adductor or hamstring; single tendon (separate procedure)**

9.89 9.89 FUD 090 J A2 80 50

AMA: 2018,Sep,7; 2018,Jan,8; 2017,Aug,9

27307 **multiple tendons**

13.8 13.8 FUD 090 J A2 80 50

AMA: 2018,Sep,7; 2018,Jan,8; 2017,Aug,9

27310 **Arthrotomy, knee, with exploration, drainage, or removal of foreign body (eg, infection)**

21.1 21.1 FUD 090 J A2 80 50

AMA: 2018,Sep,7; 2018,Jan,8; 2017,Jan,8; 2016,Jan,13; 2015,Jan,16

27323-27324 Biopsy Femur or Knee

EXCLUDES *Soft tissue needle biopsy (20206)*

27323 **Biopsy, soft tissue of thigh or knee area; superficial**

5.08 7.91 FUD 010 J A2 50

AMA: 2018,Sep,7; 2018,Jan,8; 2017,Jan,8; 2016,Jan,13; 2015,Jan,16

27324 **deep (subfascial or intramuscular)**

11.6 11.6 FUD 090 J A2 50

AMA: 2018,Sep,7; 2018,Jan,8; 2017,Jan,8; 2016,Jan,13; 2015,Jan,16

27325-27326 Neurectomy

27325 **Neurectomy, hamstring muscle**

16.1 16.1 FUD 090 J A2 80 50

AMA: 2018,Sep,7

27326 **Neurectomy, popliteal (gastrocnemius)**

14.9 14.9 FUD 090 J A2 80 50

AMA: 2018,Sep,7

27327-27339 [27329, 27337, 27339] Excision Soft Tissue Tumors Femur/ Knee

INCLUDES Any necessary elevation tissue planes or dissection
Measurement tumor and necessary margin at greatest diameter prior to excision
Simple and intermediate repairs
Excision types:
Fascial or subfascial soft tissue tumors: simple and marginal resection tumors found either in or below deep fascia, not including bone or excision substantial amount normal tissue; primarily benign and intramuscular tumors
Radical resection soft tissue tumor: wide resection tumor involving substantial margins normal tissue and may involve tissue removal from one or more layers; most often malignant or aggressive benign
Subcutaneous: simple and marginal resection tumors in subcutaneous tissue above deep fascia; most often benign

EXCLUDES *Complex repair*
Excision benign cutaneous lesions (eg, sebaceous cyst) (11400-11406)
Radical resection cutaneous tumors (eg, melanoma) (11600-11606)
Significant vessel exploration or neuroplasty

27327 **Excision, tumor, soft tissue of thigh or knee area, subcutaneous; less than 3 cm**

9.00 13.5 FUD 090 J G2 50

AMA: 2018,Sep,7

\# **27337** **3 cm or greater**

12.1 12.1 FUD 090 J G2 80 50

AMA: 2018,Sep,7

27328 **Excision, tumor, soft tissue of thigh or knee area, subfascial (eg, intramuscular); less than 5 cm**

18.0 18.0 FUD 090 J G2 50

AMA: 2018,Sep,7; 2018,Jan,8; 2017,Jan,8; 2016,Nov,9

27329 **Resequenced code. See code following 27360.**

\# **27339** **5 cm or greater**

21.7 21.7 FUD 090 J G2 80 50

AMA: 2018,Sep,7

27330-27360 [27337, 27339] Resection Procedures Thigh/Knee

27330 Arthrotomy, knee; with synovial biopsy only
🔪 11.9 ⚕ 11.9 **FUD** 090 J A2 50 ▣
AMA: 2018,Sep,7; 2018,Jan,8; 2017,Jan,8; 2016,Jan,13; 2015,Jan,16

27331 including joint exploration, biopsy, or removal of loose or foreign bodies
🔪 13.6 ⚕ 13.6 **FUD** 090 J A2 80 50 ▣
AMA: 2018,Sep,7; 2018,Jan,8; 2017,Jan,8; 2016,Jan,13; 2015,Jan,16

27332 Arthrotomy, with excision of semilunar cartilage (meniscectomy) knee; medial OR lateral
🔪 18.5 ⚕ 18.5 **FUD** 090 J A2 80 50 ▣
AMA: 2018,Sep,7

Lateral meniscus
Posterior cruciate ligament
Medial meniscus
Anterior horns
Posterior horns
Patellar ligament
Anterior cruciate ligament

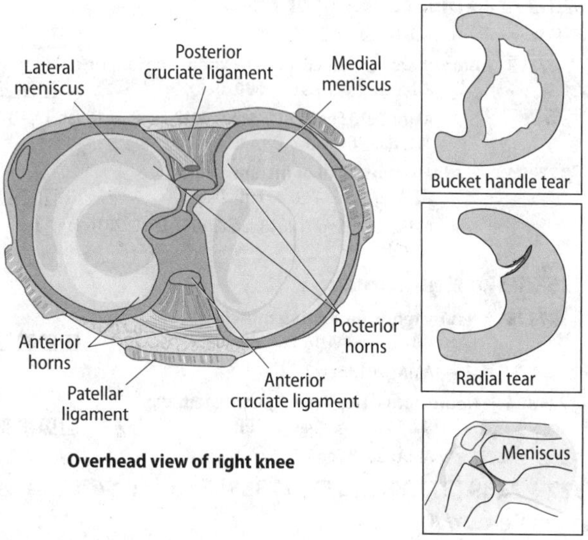

Overhead view of right knee

Bucket handle tear

Radial tear

Meniscus

27333 medial AND lateral
🔪 16.9 ⚕ 16.9 **FUD** 090 J A2 80 50 ▣
AMA: 2018,Sep,7; 2018,Jan,8; 2017,Jan,8; 2016,Jan,13; 2015,Jan,16

27334 Arthrotomy, with synovectomy, knee; anterior OR posterior
🔪 19.7 ⚕ 19.7 **FUD** 090 J A2 80 50 ▣
AMA: 2018,Sep,7

27335 anterior AND posterior including popliteal area
🔪 22.0 ⚕ 22.0 **FUD** 090 J A2 80 50 ▣
AMA: 2018,Sep,7

27337 Resequenced code. See code following 27327.

27339 Resequenced code. See code before 27330.

27340 Excision, prepatellar bursa
🔪 10.6 ⚕ 10.6 **FUD** 090 J A2 50 ▣
AMA: 2018,Sep,7

27345 Excision of synovial cyst of popliteal space (eg, Baker's cyst)
🔪 13.9 ⚕ 13.9 **FUD** 090 J A2 80 50 ▣
AMA: 2018,Sep,7

27347 Excision of lesion of meniscus or capsule (eg, cyst, ganglion), knee
🔪 15.1 ⚕ 15.1 **FUD** 090 J A2 80 50 ▣
AMA: 2018,Sep,7

27350 Patellectomy or hemipatellectomy
🔪 18.8 ⚕ 18.8 **FUD** 090 J A2 80 50 ▣
AMA: 2018,Sep,7

27355 Excision or curettage of bone cyst or benign tumor of femur;
🔪 17.4 ⚕ 17.4 **FUD** 090 J A2 80 50 ▣
AMA: 2018,Sep,7

27356 with allograft
🔪 21.3 ⚕ 21.3 **FUD** 090 J G2 80 50 ▣
AMA: 2019,May,7; 2018,Sep,7

27357 with autograft (includes obtaining graft)
🔪 23.5 ⚕ 23.5 **FUD** 090 J A2 80 50 ▣
AMA: 2018,Sep,7; 2018,Jan,8; 2017,Jan,8; 2016,Jan,13; 2015,Jan,16

+ 27358 with internal fixation (List in addition to code for primary procedure)
Code first (27355-27357)
🔪 8.03 ⚕ 8.03 **FUD** ZZZ N N1 80 ▣
AMA: 2018,Sep,7

27360 Partial excision (craterization, saucerization, or diaphysectomy) bone, femur, proximal tibia and/or fibula (eg, osteomyelitis or bone abscess)
🔪 24.7 ⚕ 24.7 **FUD** 090 J A2 80 50 ▣
AMA: 2018,Sep,7

27329-27365 [27329] Radical Resection Tumor Knee/Thigh

INCLUDES Any necessary elevation tissue planes or dissection
Excision adjacent soft tissue during bone tumor resection
Measurement tumor and necessary margin at greatest diameter prior to excision
Radical resection bone tumor: resection tumor (may include entire bone) and wide margins normal tissue primarily for malignant or aggressive benign tumors
Radical resection soft tissue tumor: wide resection tumor involving substantial margins normal tissue that may include tissue removal from one or more layers; most often malignant or aggressive benign
Simple and intermediate repairs

EXCLUDES Complex repair
Radical resection cutaneous tumors (eg, melanoma) (11600-11606)
Significant vessel exploration, neuroplasty, reconstruction, or complex bone repair

 # 27329 Radical resection of tumor (eg, sarcoma), soft tissue of thigh or knee area; less than 5 cm
🔪 30.1 ⚕ 30.1 **FUD** 090 J G2 80 50 ▣
AMA: 2018,Sep,7

27364 5 cm or greater
🔪 45.2 ⚕ 45.2 **FUD** 090 J G2 80 50 ▣
AMA: 2018,Sep,7

27365 Radical resection of tumor, femur or knee
EXCLUDES Soft tissue tumor excision thigh or knee area (27329, 27364)
🔪 59.6 ⚕ 59.6 **FUD** 090 C 80 50 ▣
AMA: 2019,May,7; 2018,Sep,7

27369 Injection for Arthrogram of Knee

EXCLUDES Arthrocentesis, aspiration and/or injection, knee (20610-20611)
Arthroscopy, knee (29871)

27369 Injection procedure for contrast knee arthrography or contrast enhanced CT/MRI knee arthrography
Code also fluoroscopic guidance, when performed for CT/MRI arthrography (73701-73702, 73722-73723, 77002)
📷 (73580, 73701-73702, 73722-73723)
🔪 1.17 ⚕ 4.06 **FUD** 000 N1 50 ▣
AMA: 2019,Aug,7

27372 Foreign Body Removal Femur or Knee

EXCLUDES Arthroscopic procedures (29870-29887)
Removal knee prosthesis (27488)

27372 Removal of foreign body, deep, thigh region or knee area
🔪 11.4 ⚕ 17.0 **FUD** 090 J A2 80 50 ▣
AMA: 2018,Sep,7

27380-27499 Repair/Reconstruction of Femur or Knee

27380 Suture of infrapatellar tendon; primary
🔪 17.5 ⚕ 17.5 **FUD** 090 J A2 80 50 ▣
AMA: 2018,Sep,7

27381 **secondary reconstruction, including fascial or tendon graft**
23.0 23.0 FUD 090 J A2 80 50
AMA: 2018,Sep,7

27385 **Suture of quadriceps or hamstring muscle rupture; primary**
16.9 16.9 FUD 090 J A2 80 50
AMA: 2018,Sep,7; 2018,Jan,8; 2017,Aug,9

27386 **secondary reconstruction, including fascial or tendon graft**
24.3 24.3 FUD 090 J A2 80 50
AMA: 2020,Apr,10; 2018,Sep,7

27390 **Tenotomy, open, hamstring, knee to hip; single tendon**
12.9 12.9 FUD 090 J A2 80 50
AMA: 2018,Sep,7

27391 **multiple tendons, 1 leg**
16.2 16.2 FUD 090 J A2 80
AMA: 2018,Sep,7

27392 **multiple tendons, bilateral**
20.4 20.4 FUD 090 J A2 80
AMA: 2018,Sep,7

27393 **Lengthening of hamstring tendon; single tendon**
14.6 14.6 FUD 090 J A2 80 50
AMA: 2018,Sep,7

27394 **multiple tendons, 1 leg**
18.8 18.8 FUD 090 J A2 80
AMA: 2018,Sep,7

27395 **multiple tendons, bilateral**
25.4 25.4 FUD 090 J A2 80
AMA: 2018,Sep,7

27396 **Transplant or transfer (with muscle redirection or rerouting), thigh (eg, extensor to flexor); single tendon**
17.7 17.7 FUD 090 J A2 80 50
AMA: 2018,Sep,7

27397 **multiple tendons**
26.3 26.3 FUD 090 J G2 80 50
AMA: 2018,Sep,7

27400 **Transfer, tendon or muscle, hamstrings to femur (eg, Egger's type procedure)**
20.0 20.0 FUD 090 J A2 80 50
AMA: 2018,Sep,7

27403 **Arthrotomy with meniscus repair, knee**
EXCLUDES *Arthroscopic treatment (29882)*
18.5 18.5 FUD 090 J J8 80 50
AMA: 2019,May,10; 2018,Sep,7

27405 **Repair, primary, torn ligament and/or capsule, knee; collateral**
19.5 19.5 FUD 090 J A2 80 50
AMA: 2018,Sep,7; 2018,Jan,8; 2017,Jan,8; 2016,Jan,13; 2015,Jan,16

27407 **cruciate**
EXCLUDES *Reconstruction (27427)*
22.9 22.9 FUD 090 J A2 80 50
AMA: 2018,Sep,7

27409 **collateral and cruciate ligaments**
EXCLUDES *Reconstruction (27427-27429)*
27.9 27.9 FUD 090 J A2 80 50
AMA: 2018,Sep,7

27412 **Autologous chondrocyte implantation, knee**
EXCLUDES *Arthrotomy, knee (27331)*
Autologous fat graft obtained by liposuction (15771-15774)
Manipulation knee joint under general anesthesia (27570)
Obtaining chondrocytes (29870)
Other autologous soft tissue grafts (fat, dermis, fascia) harvested by direct excision ([15769])
47.1 47.1 FUD 090 J 80 50
AMA: 2018,Sep,7

27415 **Osteochondral allograft, knee, open**
EXCLUDES *Arthroscopic procedure (29867)*
Osteochondral autograft knee (27416)
39.6 39.6 FUD 090 J J8 80 50
AMA: 2019,Apr,10; 2018,Sep,7; 2018,Jan,8; 2017,Jan,8; 2016,Jan,13; 2015,Jan,16

27416 **Osteochondral autograft(s), knee, open (eg, mosaicplasty) (includes harvesting of autograft[s])**
EXCLUDES *Procedures in same compartment (29874, 29877, 29879, 29885-29887)*
Procedures performed at same surgical session (27415, 29870-29871, 29875, 29884)
Surgical arthroscopy knee with osteochondral autograft(s) (29866)
28.3 28.3 FUD 090 J G2 80 50
AMA: 2018,Sep,7; 2018,Jan,8; 2017,Jan,8; 2016,Jan,13; 2015,Jan,16

27418 **Anterior tibial tubercleplasty (eg, Maquet type procedure)**
23.8 23.8 FUD 090 J A2 80 50
AMA: 2018,Sep,7; 2018,Jan,8; 2017,Jan,8; 2016,Jan,13; 2015,Jan,16

27420 **Reconstruction of dislocating patella; (eg, Hauser type procedure)**
21.4 21.4 FUD 090 J A2 80 50
AMA: 2018,Sep,7; 2018,Jan,8; 2017,Jan,8; 2016,Jan,13; 2015,Jan,16

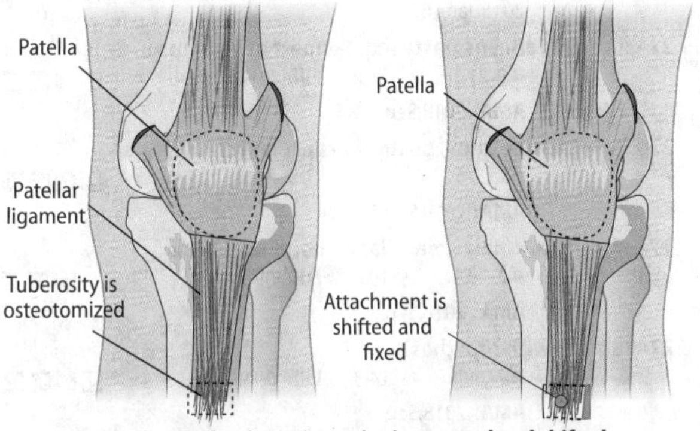

Patellar tendon insertion point is resected and shifted

27422 **with extensor realignment and/or muscle advancement or release (eg, Campbell, Goldwaite type procedure)**
21.4 21.4 FUD 090 J A2 80 50
AMA: 2018,Sep,7; 2018,Jan,8; 2017,Jan,8; 2016,Jan,13; 2015,Jan,16

27424 **with patellectomy**
21.5 21.5 FUD 090 J A2 80 50
AMA: 2018,Sep,7

27425 **Lateral retinacular release, open**

EXCLUDES *Arthroscopic release (29873)*

12.9 — 12.9 **FUD** 090 J A2 50

AMA: 2018,Sep,7; 2018,Jan,8; 2017,Jan,8; 2016,Jan,13; 2015,Nov,7; 2015,Jan,16

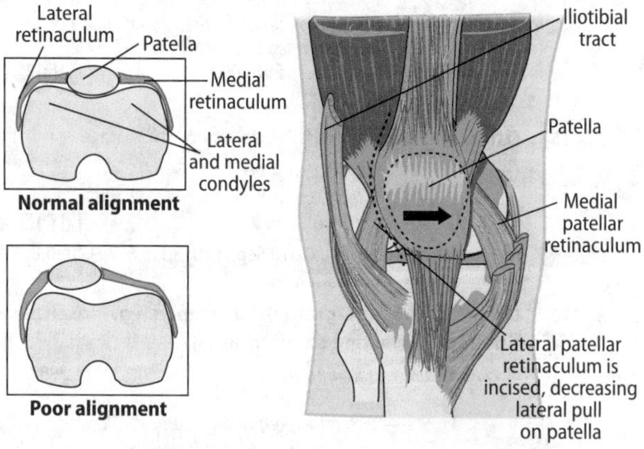

27427 **Ligamentous reconstruction (augmentation), knee; extra-articular**

EXCLUDES *Primary repair ligament(s) (27405, 27407, 27409)*

20.5 — 20.5 **FUD** 090 J J8 80 50

AMA: 2018,Sep,7; 2018,Jan,8; 2017,Jan,8; 2016,Jan,13; 2015,Jan,16

27428 **intra-articular (open)**

EXCLUDES *Primary repair ligament(s) (27405, 27407, 27409)*

32.2 — 32.2 **FUD** 090 J J8 80 50

AMA: 2018,Sep,7; 2018,Jan,8; 2017,Jan,8; 2016,Jan,13; 2015,Jan,16

27429 **intra-articular (open) and extra-articular**

EXCLUDES *Primary repair ligament(s) (27405, 27407, 27409)*

36.2 — 36.2 **FUD** 090 J J8 80 50

AMA: 2018,Sep,7; 2018,Jan,8; 2017,Jan,8; 2016,Jan,13; 2015,Jan,16

27430 **Quadricepsplasty (eg, Bennett or Thompson type)**

21.2 — 21.2 **FUD** 090 J A2 80 50

AMA: 2018,Sep,7

27435 **Capsulotomy, posterior capsular release, knee**

23.2 — 23.2 **FUD** 090 J A2 80 50

AMA: 2018,Sep,7

27437 **Arthroplasty, patella; without prosthesis**

19.0 — 19.0 **FUD** 090 J A2 50

AMA: 2018,Sep,7

27438 **with prosthesis**

24.3 — 24.3 **FUD** 090 J J8 80 50

AMA: 2018,Sep,7

27440 **Arthroplasty, knee, tibial plateau;**

23.0 — 23.0 **FUD** 090 J J8 80 50

AMA: 2018,Sep,7

27441 **with debridement and partial synovectomy**

23.8 — 23.8 **FUD** 090 J G2 80 50

AMA: 2018,Sep,7

27442 **Arthroplasty, femoral condyles or tibial plateau(s), knee;**

25.2 — 25.2 **FUD** 090 J J8 80 50

AMA: 2018,Sep,7; 2018,Jan,8; 2017,Jan,8; 2016,Jun,8

27443 **with debridement and partial synovectomy**

23.4 — 23.4 **FUD** 090 J J8 80 50

AMA: 2018,Sep,7

27445 **Arthroplasty, knee, hinge prosthesis (eg, Walldius type)**

EXCLUDES *Removal knee prosthesis (27488)*
Revision knee arthroplasty (27487)

36.1 — 36.1 **FUD** 090 C 80 50

AMA: 2018,Sep,7

27446 **Arthroplasty, knee, condyle and plateau; medial OR lateral compartment**

EXCLUDES *Removal knee prosthesis (27488)*
Revision knee arthroplasty (27487)

33.4 — 33.4 **FUD** 090 J J8 80 50

AMA: 2018,Sep,7; 2018,Jan,8; 2017,Dec,13

27447 **medial AND lateral compartments with or without patella resurfacing (total knee arthroplasty)**

EXCLUDES *Removal knee prosthesis (27488)*
Revision knee arthroplasty (27487)

39.0 — 39.0 **FUD** 090 J J8 80 50

AMA: 2018,Sep,7; 2018,Jan,8; 2017,Jan,8; 2016,Jan,13; 2015,Jan,16

27448 **Osteotomy, femur, shaft or supracondylar; without fixation**

23.7 — 23.7 **FUD** 090 C 80 50

AMA: 2019,May,7; 2018,Sep,7

27450 **with fixation**

29.3 — 29.3 **FUD** 090 C 80 50

AMA: 2018,Sep,7

27454 **Osteotomy, multiple, with realignment on intramedullary rod, femoral shaft (eg, Sofield type procedure)**

37.4 — 37.4 **FUD** 090 C 80 50

AMA: 2018,Sep,7

27455 **Osteotomy, proximal tibia, including fibular excision or osteotomy (includes correction of genu varus [bowleg] or genu valgus [knock-knee]); before epiphyseal closure**

27.5 — 27.5 **FUD** 090 C 80 50

AMA: 2018,Sep,7

27457 **after epiphyseal closure**

27.8 — 27.8 **FUD** 090 C 80 50

AMA: 2018,Sep,7

27465 **Osteoplasty, femur; shortening (excluding 64876)**

36.1 — 36.1 **FUD** 090 C 80 50

AMA: 2018,Sep,7

27466 **lengthening**

34.0 — 34.0 **FUD** 090 C 80 50

AMA: 2018,Sep,7

27468 **combined, lengthening and shortening with femoral segment transfer**

38.8 — 38.8 **FUD** 090 C 80 50

AMA: 2018,Sep,7

27470 **Repair, nonunion or malunion, femur, distal to head and neck; without graft (eg, compression technique)**

34.0 — 34.0 **FUD** 090 C 80 50

AMA: 2018,Sep,7

27472 **with iliac or other autogenous bone graft (includes obtaining graft)**

36.5 — 36.5 **FUD** 090 C 80 50

AMA: 2018,Sep,7

27475 **Arrest, epiphyseal, any method (eg, epiphysiodesis); distal femur**

19.1 — 19.1 **FUD** 090 J G2 50

AMA: 2018,Sep,7

27477 **tibia and fibula, proximal**

21.1 — 21.1 **FUD** 090 J 50

AMA: 2018,Sep,7

27479 **combined distal femur, proximal tibia and fibula**

26.5 — 26.5 **FUD** 090 J G2 80 50

AMA: 2018,Sep,7

27485 **Arrest, hemiepiphyseal, distal femur or proximal tibia or fibula (eg, genu varus or valgus)**
19.3 19.3 FUD 090 J 50
AMA: 2018,Sep,7

27486 **Revision of total knee arthroplasty, with or without allograft; 1 component**
40.6 40.6 FUD 090 C 80 50
AMA: 2018,Sep,7; 2018,Apr,10; 2018,Jan,8; 2017,Jan,8; 2016,Jan,13; 2015,Jul,10; 2015,Jan,16

27487 **femoral and entire tibial component**
50.8 50.8 FUD 090 C 80 50
AMA: 2018,Sep,7; 2018,Jan,8; 2017,Jan,8; 2016,Jan,13; 2015,Jan,16

27488 **Removal of prosthesis, including total knee prosthesis, methylmethacrylate with or without insertion of spacer, knee**
34.7 34.7 FUD 090 C 80 50
AMA: 2018,Sep,7; 2018,Jan,8; 2017,Jan,8; 2016,Jan,13; 2015,Jan,16

27495 **Prophylactic treatment (nailing, pinning, plating, or wiring) with or without methylmethacrylate, femur**
32.5 32.5 FUD 090 C 80 50
AMA: 2018,Sep,7

27496 **Decompression fasciotomy, thigh and/or knee, 1 compartment (flexor or extensor or adductor);**
15.7 15.7 FUD 090 J A2 50
AMA: 2018,Sep,7

27497 **with debridement of nonviable muscle and/or nerve**
16.7 16.7 FUD 090 J A2 80 50
AMA: 2018,Sep,7

27498 **Decompression fasciotomy, thigh and/or knee, multiple compartments;**
18.8 18.8 FUD 090 J A2 80 50
AMA: 2018,Sep,7

27499 **with debridement of nonviable muscle and/or nerve**
20.2 20.2 FUD 090 J A2 80 50
AMA: 2018,Sep,7

27500-27566 Treatment of Fracture/Dislocation of Femur/Knee

INCLUDES Closed, percutaneous, and open treatment fractures and dislocations

27500 **Closed treatment of femoral shaft fracture, without manipulation**
13.8 15.0 FUD 090 T A2 50
AMA: 2018,Sep,7

27501 **Closed treatment of supracondylar or transcondylar femoral fracture with or without intercondylar extension, without manipulation**
14.3 14.5 FUD 090 T A2 80 50
AMA: 2018,Sep,7

27502 **Closed treatment of femoral shaft fracture, with manipulation, with or without skin or skeletal traction**
21.9 21.9 FUD 090 J A2 50
AMA: 2018,Sep,7; 2018,Jan,8; 2017,Jan,8; 2016,Jan,13; 2015,Jan,16

27503 **Closed treatment of supracondylar or transcondylar femoral fracture with or without intercondylar extension, with manipulation, with or without skin or skeletal traction**
23.1 23.1 FUD 090 J A2 80 50
AMA: 2018,Sep,7

27506 **Open treatment of femoral shaft fracture, with or without external fixation, with insertion of intramedullary implant, with or without cerclage and/or locking screws**
38.6 38.6 FUD 090 C 80 50
AMA: 2018,Sep,7; 2018,Jan,8; 2017,Jan,8; 2016,Jan,13; 2015,Jan,16

27507 **Open treatment of femoral shaft fracture with plate/screws, with or without cerclage**
28.0 28.0 FUD 090 C 80 50
AMA: 2018,Sep,7

27508 **Closed treatment of femoral fracture, distal end, medial or lateral condyle, without manipulation**
14.3 15.0 FUD 090 T A2 50
AMA: 2018,Sep,7

27509 **Percutaneous skeletal fixation of femoral fracture, distal end, medial or lateral condyle, or supracondylar or transcondylar, with or without intercondylar extension, or distal femoral epiphyseal separation**
18.6 18.6 FUD 090 J A2 80 50
AMA: 2018,Dec,10; 2018,Dec,10; 2018,Sep,7

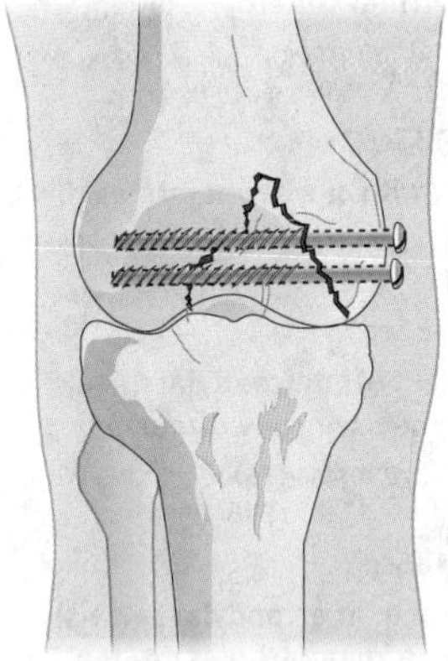

27510 **Closed treatment of femoral fracture, distal end, medial or lateral condyle, with manipulation**
19.6 19.6 FUD 090 J A2 50
AMA: 2018,Sep,7

27511 **Open treatment of femoral supracondylar or transcondylar fracture without intercondylar extension, includes internal fixation, when performed**
28.8 28.8 FUD 090 C 80 50
AMA: 2018,Sep,7

27513 **Open treatment of femoral supracondylar or transcondylar fracture with intercondylar extension, includes internal fixation, when performed**
35.9 35.9 FUD 090 C 80 50
AMA: 2018,Sep,7

27514 **Open treatment of femoral fracture, distal end, medial or lateral condyle, includes internal fixation, when performed**
27.9 27.9 FUD 090 C 80 50
AMA: 2018,Sep,7

27516 **Closed treatment of distal femoral epiphyseal separation; without manipulation**
13.8 14.7 FUD 090 T A2 50
AMA: 2018,Sep,7

27517 **with manipulation, with or without skin or skeletal traction**
19.6 19.6 FUD 090 J A2 80 50
AMA: 2018,Sep,7

27519 **Open treatment of distal femoral epiphyseal separation, includes internal fixation, when performed**
25.7 25.7 FUD 090 C 80 50
AMA: 2018,Sep,7

27520 **Closed treatment of patellar fracture, without manipulation**
8.54 9.25 FUD 090 T A2 50
AMA: 2018,Sep,7

27524 **Open treatment of patellar fracture, with internal fixation and/or partial or complete patellectomy and soft tissue repair**
21.7 21.7 FUD 090 J G2 80 50
AMA: 2018,Sep,7

27530 **Closed treatment of tibial fracture, proximal (plateau); without manipulation**
EXCLUDES *Arthroscopic repair (29855-29856)*
8.05 8.63 FUD 090 T A2 50
AMA: 2018,Sep,7

27532 **with or without manipulation, with skeletal traction**
EXCLUDES *Arthroscopic repair (29855-29856)*
16.5 17.7 FUD 090 J A2 50
AMA: 2018,Sep,7

27535 **Open treatment of tibial fracture, proximal (plateau); unicondylar, includes internal fixation, when performed**
EXCLUDES *Arthroscopic repair (29855-29856)*
25.9 25.9 FUD 090 C 80 50
AMA: 2018,Sep,7

27536 **bicondylar, with or without internal fixation**
EXCLUDES *Arthroscopic repair (29855-29856)*
34.3 34.3 FUD 090 C 80 50
AMA: 2018,Sep,7

27538 **Closed treatment of intercondylar spine(s) and/or tuberosity fracture(s) of knee, with or without manipulation**
EXCLUDES *Arthroscopic repair (29850-29851)*
12.7 13.6 FUD 090 T A2 80 50
AMA: 2018,Sep,7

27540 **Open treatment of intercondylar spine(s) and/or tuberosity fracture(s) of the knee, includes internal fixation, when performed**
23.4 23.4 FUD 090 C 80 50
AMA: 2018,Sep,7

27550 **Closed treatment of knee dislocation; without anesthesia**
13.8 14.9 FUD 090 T A2 80 50
AMA: 2018,Sep,7

27552 **requiring anesthesia**
18.0 18.0 FUD 090 J A2 80 50
AMA: 2018,Sep,7

27556 **Open treatment of knee dislocation, includes internal fixation, when performed; without primary ligamentous repair or augmentation/reconstruction**
25.3 25.3 FUD 090 C 80 50
AMA: 2018,Sep,7

27557 **with primary ligamentous repair**
30.2 30.2 FUD 090 C 80 50
AMA: 2018,Sep,7

27558 **with primary ligamentous repair, with augmentation/reconstruction**
34.5 34.5 FUD 090 C 80 50
AMA: 2018,Sep,7

27560 **Closed treatment of patellar dislocation; without anesthesia**
EXCLUDES *Recurrent dislocation (27420-27424)*
9.66 10.5 FUD 090 T A2 50
AMA: 2018,Sep,7

27562 **requiring anesthesia**
EXCLUDES *Recurrent dislocation (27420-27424)*
13.9 13.9 FUD 090 T A2 80 50
AMA: 2018,Sep,7

27566 **Open treatment of patellar dislocation, with or without partial or total patellectomy**
EXCLUDES *Recurrent dislocation (27420-27424)*
25.8 25.8 FUD 090 J A2 80 50
AMA: 2018,Sep,7

27570 Knee Manipulation with Anesthesia

27570 **Manipulation of knee joint under general anesthesia (includes application of traction or other fixation devices)**
4.34 4.34 FUD 010 J A2 50
AMA: 2018,Sep,7; 2018,Jan,8; 2017,Jan,8; 2016,Jan,13; 2015,Jan,16

27580 Knee Arthrodesis

27580 **Arthrodesis, knee, any technique**
42.1 42.1 FUD 090 C 80 50
AMA: 2020,May,13; 2018,Sep,7

27590-27599 Amputations and Unlisted Procedures at Femur or Knee

27590 **Amputation, thigh, through femur, any level;**
23.0 23.0 FUD 090 C 80 50
AMA: 2018,Sep,7; 2018,Jan,8; 2017,Dec,13

27591 **immediate fitting technique including first cast**
27.9 27.9 FUD 090 C 80 50
AMA: 2018,Sep,7

27592 **open, circular (guillotine)**
19.5 19.5 FUD 090 C 80 50
AMA: 2018,Sep,7

27594 **secondary closure or scar revision**
14.6 14.6 FUD 090 J A2 50
AMA: 2018,Sep,7

27596 **re-amputation**
20.6 20.6 FUD 090 C 50
AMA: 2018,Sep,7

27598 **Disarticulation at knee**
INCLUDES Batch-Spittler-McFaddin operation
Callander knee disarticulation
Gritti amputation
20.6 20.6 FUD 090 C 80 50
AMA: 2018,Sep,7

27599 **Unlisted procedure, femur or knee**
0.00 0.00 FUD YYY T 80 50
AMA: 2019,Apr,10; 2018,Dec,10; 2018,Dec,10; 2018,Sep,7; 2018,Apr,10; 2018,Jan,8; 2017,Aug,9; 2017,Mar,10; 2017,Jan,8; 2016,Nov,9; 2016,Jun,8; 2016,Jan,13; 2015,Jan,13; 2015,Jan,16

27600-27602 Decompression Fasciotomy of Leg

EXCLUDES *Fasciotomy with debridement (27892-27894)*
Simple incision and drainage (10140-10160)

27600 **Decompression fasciotomy, leg; anterior and/or lateral compartments only**
11.7 11.7 FUD 090 J A2 50
AMA: 2018,Sep,7

27601 **posterior compartment(s) only**
12.8 12.8 FUD 090 J A2 50
AMA: 2018,Sep,7

27602 **anterior and/or lateral, and posterior compartment(s)**
14.0 14.0 FUD 090 J A2 80 50
AMA: 2018,Sep,7

27603-27612 Incisional Procedures Lower Leg and Ankle

27603 **Incision and drainage, leg or ankle; deep abscess or hematoma**
11.1 15.2 FUD 090 J A2 50
AMA: 2018,Sep,7

27604 **infected bursa**
9.61 13.6 FUD 090 J A2 80 50
AMA: 2018,Sep,7

27605 **Tenotomy, percutaneous, Achilles tendon (separate procedure); local anesthesia**
5.34 9.83 FUD 010 J A2 80 50
AMA: 2018,Sep,14; 2018,Sep,7

27606 general anesthesia
7.99 | 7.99 | FUD 010 | J A2 50
AMA: 2018,Sep,7; 2018,Sep,14

27607 Incision (eg, osteomyelitis or bone abscess), leg or ankle
17.5 | 17.5 | FUD 090 | J A2 50
AMA: 2018,Sep,7

27610 Arthrotomy, ankle, including exploration, drainage, or removal of foreign body
18.7 | 18.7 | FUD 090 | J A2 50
AMA: 2018,Sep,7

27612 Arthrotomy, posterior capsular release, ankle, with or without Achilles tendon lengthening
EXCLUDES *Lengthening or shortening tendon (27685)*
16.0 | 16.0 | FUD 090 | J A2 80 50
AMA: 2018,Sep,7

27613-27614 Biopsy Lower Leg and Ankle

EXCLUDES *Needle biopsy (20206)*

27613 Biopsy, soft tissue of leg or ankle area; superficial
4.60 | 7.22 | FUD 010 | J P3 50
AMA: 2018,Sep,7

27614 deep (subfascial or intramuscular)
11.7 | 16.6 | FUD 090 | J A2 50
AMA: 2018,Sep,7

27615-27634 [27632, 27634] Excision Soft Tissue Tumors Lower Leg/Ankle

INCLUDES Any necessary elevation tissue planes or dissection
Measurement tumor and necessary margin at greatest diameter prior to excision
Resection without removal significant normal tissue
Simple and intermediate repairs
Excision types:
Fascial or subfascial soft tissue tumors: simple and marginal resection most often benign and intramuscular tumors found either in or below deep fascia, not involving bone
Resection tumor (may include entire bone) and wide margins normal tissue primarily for malignant or aggressive benign tumors
Subcutaneous: simple and marginal resection most often benign tumors found in subcutaneous tissue above deep fascia

EXCLUDES *Complex repair*
Excision benign cutaneous lesions (eg, sebaceous cyst) (11400-11406)
Radical resection cutaneous tumors (eg, melanoma) (11600-11606)
Significant vessel exploration or neuroplasty

27615 Radical resection of tumor (eg, sarcoma), soft tissue of leg or ankle area; less than 5 cm
29.6 | 29.6 | FUD 090 | J G2 80 50
AMA: 2018,Sep,7

27616 5 cm or greater
36.6 | 36.6 | FUD 090 | J G2 80 50
AMA: 2018,Sep,7

27618 Excision, tumor, soft tissue of leg or ankle area, subcutaneous; less than 3 cm
8.83 | 13.2 | FUD 090 | J G2 50
AMA: 2018,Sep,7; 2018,Jan,8; 2017,Jan,8; 2016,Jan,13; 2015,Jan,16

\# **27632** 3 cm or greater
11.9 | 11.9 | FUD 090 | J G2 80 50
AMA: 2018,Sep,7

27619 Excision, tumor, soft tissue of leg or ankle area, subfascial (eg, intramuscular); less than 5 cm
13.3 | 13.3 | FUD 090 | J G2 50
AMA: 2018,Sep,7

\# **27634** 5 cm or greater
19.7 | 19.7 | FUD 090 | J G2 80 50
AMA: 2018,Sep,7

27620-27641 [27632, 27634] Bone and Joint Procedures Ankle/Leg

27620 Arthrotomy, ankle, with joint exploration, with or without biopsy, with or without removal of loose or foreign body
12.9 | 12.9 | FUD 090 | J A2 80 50
AMA: 2018,Sep,7

27625 Arthrotomy, with synovectomy, ankle;
16.4 | 16.4 | FUD 090 | J A2 80 50
AMA: 2018,Sep,7

27626 including tenosynovectomy
17.4 | 17.4 | FUD 090 | J A2 80 50
AMA: 2018,Sep,7

27630 Excision of lesion of tendon sheath or capsule (eg, cyst or ganglion), leg and/or ankle
10.4 | 15.9 | FUD 090 | J A2 50
AMA: 2018,Sep,7

27632 Resequenced code. See code following 27618.

27634 Resequenced code. See code following 27619.

27635 Excision or curettage of bone cyst or benign tumor, tibia or fibula;
16.7 | 16.7 | FUD 090 | J A2 50
AMA: 2018,Sep,7; 2018,Jan,8; 2017,Jan,8; 2016,Jan,13; 2015,Jan,16

27637 with autograft (includes obtaining graft)
21.5 | 21.5 | FUD 090 | J A2 80 50
AMA: 2018,Sep,7

27638 with allograft
22.0 | 22.0 | FUD 090 | J A2 80 50
AMA: 2019,May,7; 2018,Sep,7

27640 Partial excision (craterization, saucerization, or diaphysectomy), bone (eg, osteomyelitis); tibia
EXCLUDES *Excision exostosis (27635)*
23.9 | 23.9 | FUD 090 | J A2 50
AMA: 2018,Sep,7; 2018,Jan,8; 2017,Jan,8; 2016,Jan,13; 2015,Jan,16

27641 fibula
EXCLUDES *Excision exostosis (27635)*
19.0 | 19.0 | FUD 090 | J A2 50
AMA: 2018,Sep,7

27645-27647 Radical Resection Bone Tumor Ankle/Leg

INCLUDES Any necessary elevation tissue planes or dissection
Excision adjacent soft tissue during bone tumor resection (27615-27619 [27632, 27634])
Measurement tumor and necessary margin at greatest diameter prior to excision
Resection tumor (may include entire bone) and wide margins normal tissue primarily for malignant or aggressive benign tumors
Simple and intermediate repairs

EXCLUDES *Complex repair*
Significant vessel exploration, neuroplasty, reconstruction, or complex bone repair

27645 Radical resection of tumor; tibia
51.2 | 51.2 | FUD 090 | C 80 50
AMA: 2019,May,7; 2018,Sep,7

27646 fibula
44.5 | 44.5 | FUD 090 | C 80 50
AMA: 2019,May,7; 2018,Sep,7

27647 talus or calcaneus
29.3 | 29.3 | FUD 090 | J A2 80 50
AMA: 2019,May,7; 2018,Sep,7

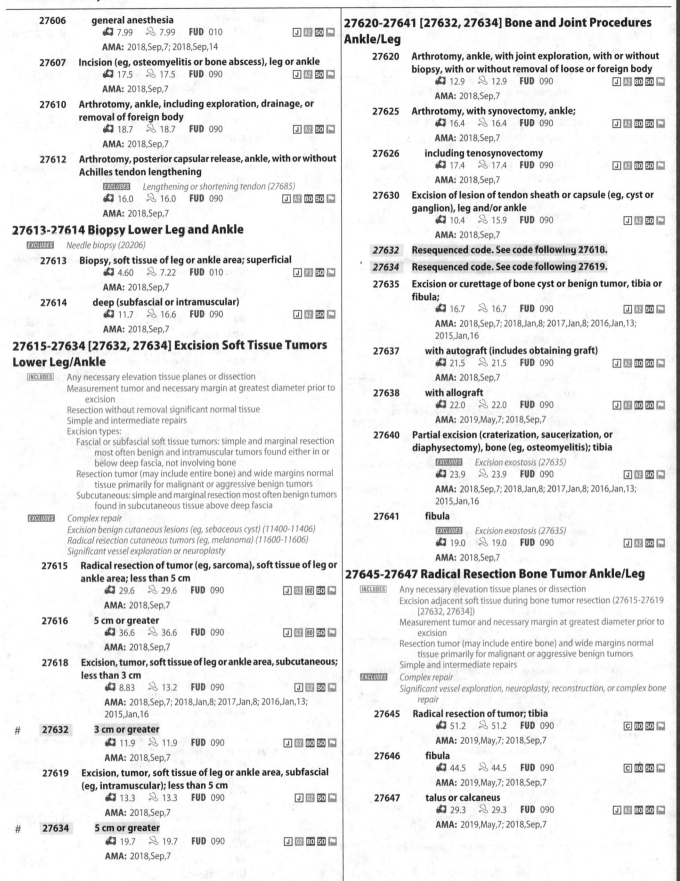

27648 Injection for Ankle Arthrogram

EXCLUDES *Arthroscopy (29894-29898)*

27648 Injection procedure for ankle arthrography
(73615)
🔧 1.52 ⚕ 5.22 **FUD** 000 N N1 80 50 ▪

AMA: 2019,May,7; 2018,Sep,7; 2018,Jan,8; 2017,Jan,8; 2016,Jan,13; 2015,Aug,6

27650-27745 Repair/Reconstruction Lower Leg/Ankle

27650 Repair, primary, open or percutaneous, ruptured Achilles tendon;
🔧 18.9 ⚕ 18.9 **FUD** 090 J A2 80 50 ▪

AMA: 2020,Jun,14; 2018,Sep,7; 2018,Jan,8; 2017,Jan,8; 2016,Jan,13; 2015,Jan,16

27652 with graft (includes obtaining graft)
🔧 19.1 ⚕ 19.1 **FUD** 090 J A2 50 ▪

AMA: 2018,Sep,7; 2018,Jan,8; 2017,Jan,8; 2016,Jan,13; 2015,Jan,16

27654 Repair, secondary, Achilles tendon, with or without graft
🔧 20.4 ⚕ 20.4 **FUD** 090 J A2 80 50 ▪

AMA: 2020,Jun,14; 2020,Apr,8; 2018,Sep,7; 2018,Jan,8; 2017,Jan,8; 2016,Dec,16; 2016,Jan,13; 2015,Jan,16

27656 Repair, fascial defect of leg
🔧 11.4 ⚕ 18.2 **FUD** 090 J A2 80 50 ▪

AMA: 2018,Sep,7

27658 Repair, flexor tendon, leg; primary, without graft, each tendon
🔧 10.6 ⚕ 10.6 **FUD** 090 J A2 80 ▪

AMA: 2018,Sep,7

27659 secondary, with or without graft, each tendon
🔧 13.5 ⚕ 13.5 **FUD** 090 J A2 80 ▪

AMA: 2018,Sep,7; 2018,Jan,8; 2017,Jan,8; 2016,Jan,13; 2015,Jan,13

27664 Repair, extensor tendon, leg; primary, without graft, each tendon
🔧 10.3 ⚕ 10.3 **FUD** 090 J A2 80 ▪

AMA: 2018,Sep,7; 2018,Jan,8; 2017,Jan,8; 2016,Jan,13; 2015,Jan,13

27665 secondary, with or without graft, each tendon
🔧 11.9 ⚕ 11.9 **FUD** 090 J A2 80 ▪

AMA: 2018,Sep,7

27675 Repair, dislocating peroneal tendons; without fibular osteotomy
🔧 14.1 ⚕ 14.1 **FUD** 090 J A2 80 50 ▪

AMA: 2018,Sep,7

27676 with fibular osteotomy
🔧 17.2 ⚕ 17.2 **FUD** 090 J A2 80 50 ▪

AMA: 2018,Sep,7

27680 Tenolysis, flexor or extensor tendon, leg and/or ankle; single, each tendon
🔧 12.2 ⚕ 12.2 **FUD** 090 J A2 ▪

AMA: 2018,Sep,7; 2018,Jan,8; 2017,Jan,8; 2016,Jan,13; 2015,Jan,16

27681 multiple tendons (through separate incision[s])
🔧 15.7 ⚕ 15.7 **FUD** 090 J A2 50 ▪

AMA: 2018,Sep,7

27685 Lengthening or shortening of tendon, leg or ankle; single tendon (separate procedure)
🔧 13.3 ⚕ 19.0 **FUD** 090 J A2 80 50 ▪

AMA: 2018,Sep,7; 2018,Sep,14; 2018,Jan,8; 2017,Jan,8; 2016,Jan,13; 2015,Jan,16

27686 multiple tendons (through same incision), each
🔧 15.6 ⚕ 15.6 **FUD** 090 J A2 50 ▪

AMA: 2018,Sep,7; 2018,Jan,8; 2017,Jan,8; 2016,Jan,13; 2015,Jan,16

27687 Gastrocnemius recession (eg, Strayer procedure)
🔧 13.0 ⚕ 13.0 **FUD** 090 J A2 80 50 ▪

AMA: 2018,Sep,7

27690 Transfer or transplant of single tendon (with muscle redirection or rerouting); superficial (eg, anterior tibial extensors into midfoot)
INCLUDES Toe extensors considered single tendon with transplant into midfoot
🔧 18.3 ⚕ 18.3 **FUD** 090 J A2 80 50 ▪

AMA: 2018,Sep,7

27691 deep (eg, anterior tibial or posterior tibial through interosseous space, flexor digitorum longus, flexor hallucis longus, or peroneal tendon to midfoot or hindfoot)
INCLUDES Barr procedure
Toe extensors considered single tendon with transplant into midfoot
🔧 21.4 ⚕ 21.4 **FUD** 090 J A2 80 50 ▪

AMA: 2018,Sep,7

+ **27692** each additional tendon (List separately in addition to code for primary procedure)
INCLUDES Toe extensors considered single tendon with transplant into midfoot
Code first (27690-27691)
🔧 3.01 ⚕ 3.01 **FUD** ZZZ N N1 80 ▪

AMA: 2018,Sep,7

27695 Repair, primary, disrupted ligament, ankle; collateral
🔧 13.6 ⚕ 13.6 **FUD** 090 J A2 50 ▪

AMA: 2018,Nov,11; 2018,Sep,7; 2018,Jan,8; 2017,Jan,8; 2016,Jan,13; 2015,Jan,16

Fibula
Tibia
Lateral view of right ankle showing components of the collateral ligament
Posterior talofibular
Anterior talofibular
Calcaneus
Calcaneofibular

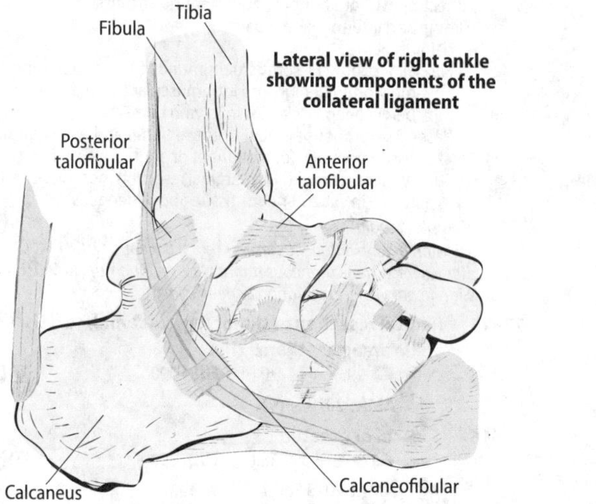

27696 both collateral ligaments
🔧 16.0 ⚕ 16.0 **FUD** 090 J A2 50 ▪

AMA: 2018,Nov,11; 2018,Sep,7; 2018,Jan,8; 2017,Jan,8; 2016,Jan,13; 2015,Jan,16

27698 Repair, secondary, disrupted ligament, ankle, collateral (eg, Watson-Jones procedure)
🔧 18.3 ⚕ 18.3 **FUD** 090 J A2 80 50 ▪

AMA: 2018,Sep,7; 2018,Jan,8; 2017,Jan,8; 2016,Jan,13; 2015,Jan,16

27700 Arthroplasty, ankle;
🔧 17.6 ⚕ 17.6 **FUD** 090 J A2 80 50 ▪

AMA: 2018,Sep,7

27702 with implant (total ankle)
🔧 27.7 ⚕ 27.7 **FUD** 090 C 80 50 ▪

AMA: 2018,Sep,7

27703 revision, total ankle
🔧 32.2 ⚕ 32.2 **FUD** 090 C 80 50 ▪

AMA: 2018,Sep,7

27704 **Removal of ankle implant**
16.5 16.5 FUD 090 Q2 A2 50
AMA: 2019,May,7; 2018,Sep,7

27705 **Osteotomy; tibia**
EXCLUDES *Genu varus or genu valgus repair (27455-27457)*
21.8 21.8 FUD 090 J J8 80 50
AMA: 2018,Sep,7

27707 **fibula**
EXCLUDES *Genu varus or genu valgus repair (27455-27457)*
11.4 11.4 FUD 090 J A2 50
AMA: 2018,Sep,7

27709 **tibia and fibula**
EXCLUDES *Genu varus or genu valgus repair (27455-27457)*
33.6 33.6 FUD 090 J A2 80 50
AMA: 2018,Sep,7

27712 **multiple, with realignment on intramedullary rod (eg, Sofield type procedure)**
EXCLUDES *Genu varus or genu valgus repair (27455-27457)*
31.8 31.8 FUD 090 C 80 50
AMA: 2018,Sep,7

27715 **Osteoplasty, tibia and fibula, lengthening or shortening**
INCLUDES Anderson tibial lengthening
30.9 30.9 FUD 090 C 80 50
AMA: 2018,Sep,7

27720 **Repair of nonunion or malunion, tibia; without graft, (eg, compression technique)**
25.1 25.1 FUD 090 J J8 80 50
AMA: 2018,Sep,7

27722 **with sliding graft**
25.7 25.7 FUD 090 J 80 50
AMA: 2018,Sep,7

27724 **with iliac or other autograft (includes obtaining graft)**
36.4 36.4 FUD 090 C 80 50
AMA: 2018,Sep,7; 2018,Jan,8; 2017,Jan,8; 2016,Jan,13; 2015,Jan,16

27725 **by synostosis, with fibula, any method**
35.1 35.1 FUD 090 C 80 50
AMA: 2018,Sep,7

27726 **Repair of fibula nonunion and/or malunion with internal fixation**
INCLUDES Osteotomy; fibula (27707)
27.6 27.6 FUD 090 J J8 50
AMA: 2018,Sep,7; 2018,Jan,8; 2017,Jan,8; 2016,Jan,13; 2015,Jan,16

27727 **Repair of congenital pseudarthrosis, tibia**
29.9 29.9 FUD 090 C 80 50
AMA: 2018,Sep,7

27730 **Arrest, epiphyseal (epiphysiodesis), open; distal tibia**
16.9 16.9 FUD 090 J A2 50
AMA: 2018,Sep,7

27732 **distal fibula**
12.9 12.9 FUD 090 J A2 50
AMA: 2018,Sep,7

27734 **distal tibia and fibula**
18.9 18.9 FUD 090 J A2 50
AMA: 2018,Sep,7

27740 **Arrest, epiphyseal (epiphysiodesis), any method, combined, proximal and distal tibia and fibula;**
EXCLUDES *Epiphyseal arrest proximal tibia and fibula (27477)*
20.4 20.4 FUD 090 J G2 80 50
AMA: 2018,Sep,7

27742 **and distal femur**
EXCLUDES *Epiphyseal arrest proximal tibia and fibula (27477)*
22.4 22.4 FUD 090 J A2 80 50
AMA: 2018,Sep,7

27745 **Prophylactic treatment (nailing, pinning, plating or wiring) with or without methylmethacrylate, tibia**
21.7 21.7 FUD 090 J J8 80 50
AMA: 2018,Sep,7

27750-27848 Treatment of Fracture/Dislocation Lower Leg/Ankle

INCLUDES Treatment open or closed fracture or dislocation

27750 **Closed treatment of tibial shaft fracture (with or without fibular fracture); without manipulation**
9.18 9.91 FUD 090 T A2 50
AMA: 2018,Sep,7; 2018,Jan,8; 2017,Jan,8; 2016,Jan,13; 2015,Jan,16

27752 **with manipulation, with or without skeletal traction**
14.1 15.4 FUD 090 J A2 50
AMA: 2018,Sep,7; 2018,Jan,8; 2018,Jan,3; 2017,Jan,8; 2016,Jan,13; 2015,Jan,16

27756 **Percutaneous skeletal fixation of tibial shaft fracture (with or without fibular fracture) (eg, pins or screws)**
16.6 16.6 FUD 090 J J8 80 50
AMA: 2018,Sep,7; 2018,Jan,8; 2017,Jan,8; 2016,Jan,13; 2015,Jan,16

27758 **Open treatment of tibial shaft fracture (with or without fibular fracture), with plate/screws, with or without cerclage**
25.8 25.8 FUD 090 J J8 80 50
AMA: 2018,Sep,7; 2018,Jan,8; 2017,Jan,8; 2016,Jan,13; 2015,Jan,16

27759 **Treatment of tibial shaft fracture (with or without fibular fracture) by intramedullary implant, with or without interlocking screws and/or cerclage**
28.8 28.8 FUD 090 J J8 80 50
AMA: 2018,Sep,7; 2018,Jan,8; 2017,Jan,8; 2016,Jan,13; 2015,Jan,16

27760 **Closed treatment of medial malleolus fracture; without manipulation**
8.81 9.56 FUD 090 T A2 50
AMA: 2018,Sep,7

27762 **with manipulation, with or without skin or skeletal traction**
12.4 13.7 FUD 090 J A2 50
AMA: 2018,Sep,7

27766 **Open treatment of medial malleolus fracture, includes internal fixation, when performed**
17.4 17.4 FUD 090 J A2 50
AMA: 2018,Sep,7

27767 **Closed treatment of posterior malleolus fracture; without manipulation**
EXCLUDES *Treatment bimalleolar ankle fracture (27808-27814)*
Treatment trimalleolar ankle fracture (27816-27823)
8.20 8.24 FUD 090 T P2 50
AMA: 2018,Sep,7

27768 **with manipulation**
EXCLUDES *Treatment bimalleolar ankle fracture (27808-27814)*
Treatment trimalleolar ankle fracture (27816-27823)
12.7 12.7 FUD 090 J G2 50
AMA: 2018,Sep,7

27769 **Open treatment of posterior malleolus fracture, includes internal fixation, when performed**
EXCLUDES *Treatment bimalleolar ankle fracture (27808-27814)*
Treatment trimalleolar ankle fracture (27816-27823)
21.0 21.0 FUD 090 J G2 50
AMA: 2018,Sep,7

27780 **Closed treatment of proximal fibula or shaft fracture; without manipulation**
8.08 8.80 FUD 090 T A2 50
AMA: 2018,Sep,7; 2018,Jan,8; 2017,Jan,8; 2016,Jan,13; 2015,Jan,16

Musculoskeletal System

27704 — 27780

27781 with manipulation
11.3 12.3 FUD 090 J A2 50
AMA: 2018,Sep,7

27784 Open treatment of proximal fibula or shaft fracture, includes internal fixation, when performed
20.6 20.6 FUD 090 J A2 50
AMA: 2018,Sep,7; 2018,Jan,8; 2017,Jan,8; 2016,Jan,13; 2015,Jan,16

27786 Closed treatment of distal fibular fracture (lateral malleolus); without manipulation
8.25 9.01 FUD 090 T A2 50
AMA: 2018,Sep,7

27788 with manipulation
11.1 12.2 FUD 090 T A2 50
AMA: 2018,Sep,7

27792 Open treatment of distal fibular fracture (lateral malleolus), includes internal fixation, when performed
EXCLUDES *Repair tibia and fibula shaft fracture (27750-27759)*
18.6 18.6 FUD 090 J J8 50
AMA: 2018,Sep,7; 2018,Jan,8; 2017,Jan,8; 2016,Jan,13; 2015,Jan,16

27808 Closed treatment of bimalleolar ankle fracture (eg, lateral and medial malleoli, or lateral and posterior malleoli or medial and posterior malleoli); without manipulation
8.70 9.57 FUD 090 T A2 50
AMA: 2018,Sep,7

27810 with manipulation
12.1 13.3 FUD 090 J A2 50
AMA: 2018,Sep,7

27814 Open treatment of bimalleolar ankle fracture (eg, lateral and medial malleoli, or lateral and posterior malleoli, or medial and posterior malleoli), includes internal fixation, when performed
22.1 22.1 FUD 090 J J8 80 50
AMA: 2018,Sep,7; 2018,Jan,8; 2017,Jan,8; 2016,Feb,13

27816 Closed treatment of trimalleolar ankle fracture; without manipulation
8.36 9.36 FUD 090 T A2 50
AMA: 2018,Sep,7

27818 with manipulation
12.4 13.9 FUD 090 J A2 50
AMA: 2018,Sep,7

27822 Open treatment of trimalleolar ankle fracture, includes internal fixation, when performed, medial and/or lateral malleolus; without fixation of posterior lip
24.9 24.9 FUD 090 J J8 80 50
AMA: 2018,Sep,7

27823 with fixation of posterior lip
28.0 28.0 FUD 090 J J8 80 50
AMA: 2018,Sep,7

27824 Closed treatment of fracture of weight bearing articular portion of distal tibia (eg, pilon or tibial plafond), with or without anesthesia; without manipulation
8.71 9.02 FUD 090 T A2 50
AMA: 2018,Sep,7

27825 with skeletal traction and/or requiring manipulation
14.2 15.7 FUD 090 J A2 80 50
AMA: 2018,Sep,7

27826 Open treatment of fracture of weight bearing articular surface/portion of distal tibia (eg, pilon or tibial plafond), with internal fixation, when performed; of fibula only
24.2 24.2 FUD 090 J J8 80 50
AMA: 2018,Sep,7

27827 of tibia only
32.0 32.0 FUD 090 J J8 80 50
AMA: 2018,Sep,7

27828 of both tibia and fibula
38.1 38.1 FUD 090 J J8 80 50
AMA: 2018,Sep,7; 2018,Jan,8; 2017,Jan,8; 2016,Jan,13; 2015,Jan,16

27829 Open treatment of distal tibiofibular joint (syndesmosis) disruption, includes internal fixation, when performed
20.0 20.0 FUD 090 J A2 80 50
AMA: 2018,Sep,7; 2018,Jan,8; 2017,Jan,8; 2016,Feb,13; 2016,Jan,13; 2015,Jan,16

27830 Closed treatment of proximal tibiofibular joint dislocation; without anesthesia
10.2 11.1 FUD 090 T A2 80 50
AMA: 2018,Sep,7

27831 requiring anesthesia
11.6 11.6 FUD 090 J A2 80 50
AMA: 2018,Sep,7

27832 Open treatment of proximal tibiofibular joint dislocation, includes internal fixation, when performed, or with excision of proximal fibula
21.8 21.8 FUD 090 J A2 80 50
AMA: 2018,Sep,7

27840 Closed treatment of ankle dislocation; without anesthesia
10.7 10.7 FUD 090 T A2 50
AMA: 2018,Sep,7

27842 requiring anesthesia, with or without percutaneous skeletal fixation
14.2 14.2 FUD 090 J A2 50
AMA: 2018,Sep,7

27846 Open treatment of ankle dislocation, with or without percutaneous skeletal fixation; without repair or internal fixation
EXCLUDES *Arthroscopy (29894-29898)*
20.6 20.6 FUD 090 J A2 80 50
AMA: 2018,Sep,7

27848 with repair or internal or external fixation
EXCLUDES *Arthroscopy (29894-29898)*
23.0 23.0 FUD 090 J J8 80 50
AMA: 2018,Sep,7

27860 Ankle Manipulation with Anesthesia

27860 Manipulation of ankle under general anesthesia (includes application of traction or other fixation apparatus)
4.91 4.91 FUD 010 J A2 80 50
AMA: 2018,Sep,7

27870-27871 Arthrodesis Lower Leg/Ankle

27870 Arthrodesis, ankle, open
EXCLUDES *Arthroscopic arthrodesis ankle (29899)*
29.5 29.5 FUD 090 J J8 80 50
AMA: 2020,May,13; 2018,Sep,7

27871 Arthrodesis, tibiofibular joint, proximal or distal
19.8 19.8 FUD 090 J J8 80 50
AMA: 2020,May,13; 2018,Sep,7

27880-27889 Amputations of Lower Leg/Ankle

27880 Amputation, leg, through tibia and fibula;
INCLUDES Burgess amputation
26.3 26.3 FUD 090 C 80 50
AMA: 2018,Sep,7

27881 with immediate fitting technique including application of first cast
24.8 24.8 FUD 090 C 80 50
AMA: 2018,Sep,7

27882 open, circular (guillotine)
17.3 17.3 FUD 090 C 80 50
AMA: 2018,Sep,7

27884 secondary closure or scar revision
16.5 16.5 FUD 090 J A2 50
AMA: 2018,Sep,7

27886 re-amputation
18.9 18.9 FUD 090 C 50
AMA: 2018,Sep,7

27888 Amputation, ankle, through malleoli of tibia and fibula (eg, Syme, Pirogoff type procedures), with plastic closure and resection of nerves
18.9 18.9 FUD 090 C 80 50
AMA: 2018,Sep,7

27889 Ankle disarticulation
18.6 18.6 FUD 090 J A2 50
AMA: 2018,Sep,7

27892-27899 Decompression Fasciotomy Lower Leg

EXCLUDES *Decompression fasciotomy without debridement (27600-27602)*

27892 Decompression fasciotomy, leg; anterior and/or lateral compartments only, with debridement of nonviable muscle and/or nerve
15.8 15.8 FUD 090 J A2 80 50
AMA: 2018,Sep,7

27893 posterior compartment(s) only, with debridement of nonviable muscle and/or nerve
17.5 17.5 FUD 090 J A2 80 50
AMA: 2018,Sep,7

27894 anterior and/or lateral, and posterior compartment(s), with debridement of nonviable muscle and/or nerve
24.3 24.3 FUD 090 J A2 80 50
AMA: 2018,Sep,7

27899 Unlisted procedure, leg or ankle
0.00 0.00 FUD YYY T 80 50
AMA: 2020,Apr,8; 2018,Sep,7; 2018,Jan,8; 2017,Jan,8; 2016,Dec,16; 2016,Jan,13; 2015,Jan,16

28001-28008 Surgical Incision Foot/Toe

EXCLUDES *Simple incision and drainage (10060-10160)*

28001 Incision and drainage, bursa, foot
4.90 8.03 FUD 010 J P3
AMA: 2018,Sep,7

28002 Incision and drainage below fascia, with or without tendon sheath involvement, foot; single bursal space
9.20 12.7 FUD 010 J A2
AMA: 2018,Sep,7

28003 multiple areas
16.0 20.1 FUD 090 J A2
AMA: 2018,Sep,7

28005 Incision, bone cortex (eg, osteomyelitis or bone abscess), foot
16.6 16.6 FUD 090 J A2
AMA: 2018,Sep,7

28008 Fasciotomy, foot and/or toe
EXCLUDES *Plantar fascia division (28250)*
Plantar fasciectomy (28060, 28062)
8.46 12.5 FUD 090 J A2 50
AMA: 2018,Sep,7

28010-28011 Tenotomy/Toe

EXCLUDES *Open tenotomy (28230-28234)*
Simple incision and drainage (10140-10160)

28010 Tenotomy, percutaneous, toe; single tendon
5.99 6.69 FUD 090 J P3
AMA: 2018,Sep,7

28011 multiple tendons
8.10 9.09 FUD 090 J A2
AMA: 2018,Sep,7

28020-28024 Arthrotomy Foot/Toe

EXCLUDES *Simple incision and drainage (10140-10160)*

28020 Arthrotomy, including exploration, drainage, or removal of loose or foreign body; intertarsal or tarsometatarsal joint
10.3 15.5 FUD 090 J A2
AMA: 2018,Sep,7

28022 metatarsophalangeal joint
9.36 14.0 FUD 090 J A2
AMA: 2018,Sep,7

28024 interphalangeal joint
8.71 13.1 FUD 090 J A2
AMA: 2018,Sep,7

28035 Tarsal Tunnel Release

EXCLUDES *Other nerve decompression (64722)*
Other neuroplasty (64704)

28035 Release, tarsal tunnel (posterior tibial nerve decompression)
10.2 15.2 FUD 090 J A2 50
AMA: 2018,Sep,7

28039-28047 [28039, 28041] Excision Soft Tissue Tumors Foot/Toe

INCLUDES Any necessary elevation tissue planes or dissection
Measurement tumor and necessary margin at greatest diameter prior to excision
Simple and intermediate repairs
Excision types:
Fascial or subfascial soft tissue tumors: simple and marginal resection tumors found either in or below deep fascia, not involving bone or excision substantial amount normal tissue; primarily benign and intramuscular tumors
Tumors fingers and toes involving joint capsules, tendons and tendon sheaths
Radical resection soft tissue tumor: wide resection tumor, involving substantial margins normal tissue and may involve tissue removal from one or more layers; most often malignant or aggressive benign
Tumors fingers and toes adjacent to joints, tendons and tendon sheaths
Subcutaneous: simple and marginal resection tumors in subcutaneous tissue above deep fascia; most often benign

EXCLUDES *Complex repair*
Excision benign cutaneous lesions (eg, sebaceous cyst) (11420-11426)
Radical resection cutaneous tumors (eg, melanoma) (11620-11626)
Significant vessel exploration, neuroplasty, or reconstruction

28039 Resequenced code. See code following 28043.

28041 Resequenced code. See code following 28045.

28043 Excision, tumor, soft tissue of foot or toe, subcutaneous; less than 1.5 cm
7.52 11.3 FUD 090 J G2 50
AMA: 2018,Sep,7

\# 28039 1.5 cm or greater
9.94 14.3 FUD 090 J G2 80 50
AMA: 2018,Sep,7

28045 Excision, tumor, soft tissue of foot or toe, subfascial (eg, intramuscular); less than 1.5 cm
9.97 14.0 FUD 090 J G2 80 50
AMA: 2018,Sep,7

\# 28041 1.5 cm or greater
13.0 13.0 FUD 090 J G2 80 50
AMA: 2018,Sep,7

28046 Radical resection of tumor (eg, sarcoma), soft tissue of foot or toe; less than 3 cm
20.6 20.6 FUD 090 J G2 50
AMA: 2018,Sep,7

28047 3 cm or greater
30.1 30.1 FUD 090 J G2 80 50
AMA: 2018,Sep,7

28050-28160 Resection Procedures Foot/Toes

28050 **Arthrotomy with biopsy; intertarsal or tarsometatarsal joint**
8.03 12.1 **FUD** 090 J A2 50
AMA: 2002,Apr,13; 1998,Nov,1

28052 **metatarsophalangeal joint**
8.15 12.8 **FUD** 090 J A2 50
AMA: 2002,Apr,13

28054 **interphalangeal joint**
6.77 10.8 **FUD** 090 J A2 80 50
AMA: 2002,Apr,13

28055 **Neurectomy, intrinsic musculature of foot**
11.1 11.1 **FUD** 090 J A2 80 50

28060 **Fasciectomy, plantar fascia; partial (separate procedure)**
EXCLUDES *Plantar fasciotomy (28008, 28250)*
10.3 15.0 **FUD** 090 J A2 50
AMA: 2018,Jan,8; 2017,Jan,8; 2016,Jan,13; 2015,Jan,16

28062 **radical (separate procedure)**
EXCLUDES *Plantar fasciotomy (28008, 28250)*
11.7 16.7 **FUD** 090 J A2 50
AMA: 2002,Apr,13

28070 **Synovectomy; intertarsal or tarsometatarsal joint, each**
10.1 15.2 **FUD** 090 J A2
AMA: 2002,Apr,13

28072 **metatarsophalangeal joint, each**
9.23 14.0 **FUD** 090 J A2
AMA: 2002,Apr,13

28080 **Excision, interdigital (Morton) neuroma, single, each**
10.6 15.1 **FUD** 090 J A2 80
AMA: 2018,Jan,8; 2017,Jan,8; 2016,Jan,13; 2015,Jan,16

Plantar view of right foot showing common location of Morton neuroma

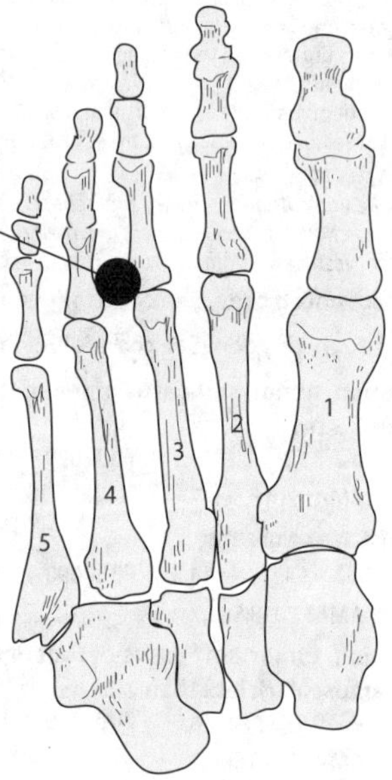

Morton neuroma is a chronic inflammation or irritation of the nerves in the web space between the heads of the metatarsals and phalanges

28086 **Synovectomy, tendon sheath, foot; flexor**
10.2 15.4 **FUD** 090 J A2 80 50
AMA: 2002,Apr,13

28088 **extensor**
7.92 12.5 **FUD** 090 J A2 80 50
AMA: 2002,Apr,13

28090 **Excision of lesion, tendon, tendon sheath, or capsule (including synovectomy) (eg, cyst or ganglion); foot**
8.86 13.5 **FUD** 090 J A2 50
AMA: 2002,Apr,13; 1998,Nov,1

28092 **toe(s), each**
7.75 12.2 **FUD** 090 J A2
AMA: 2002,Apr,13; 1998,Nov,1

28100 **Excision or curettage of bone cyst or benign tumor, talus or calcaneus;**
11.9 17.6 **FUD** 090 J A2 80 50
AMA: 2002,Apr,13

28102 **with iliac or other autograft (includes obtaining graft)**
17.5 17.5 **FUD** 090 J A2 80 50
AMA: 2002,Apr,13

28103 **with allograft**
11.2 11.2 **FUD** 090 J A2 80 50
AMA: 2019,May,7

28104 **Excision or curettage of bone cyst or benign tumor, tarsal or metatarsal, except talus or calcaneus;**
10.2 15.2 **FUD** 090 J A2 80
AMA: 2002,May,7; 2002,Apr,13

28106 **with iliac or other autograft (includes obtaining graft)**
12.3 12.3 **FUD** 090 J A2 80
AMA: 2002,May,7; 2002,Apr,13

28107 **with allograft**
10.0 14.7 **FUD** 090 J A2 80
AMA: 2019,May,7

28108 **Excision or curettage of bone cyst or benign tumor, phalanges of foot**
EXCLUDES *Partial excision bone, toe (28124)*
8.30 12.7 **FUD** 090 J A2
AMA: 2002,Apr,13

28110 **Ostectomy, partial excision, fifth metatarsal head (bunionette) (separate procedure)**
8.35 13.3 **FUD** 090 J A2 50
AMA: 2018,Jan,8; 2017,Jan,8; 2016,Jan,13; 2015,Jan,16

28111 **Ostectomy, complete excision; first metatarsal head**
9.33 14.0 **FUD** 090 J A2 50
AMA: 2002,Apr,13

28112 **other metatarsal head (second, third or fourth)**
9.00 14.0 **FUD** 090 J A2 50
AMA: 2002,Apr,13

28113 **fifth metatarsal head**
12.1 16.9 **FUD** 090 J A2 80 50
AMA: 2002,Apr,13

28114 **all metatarsal heads, with partial proximal phalangectomy, excluding first metatarsal (eg, Clayton type procedure)**
23.9 30.7 **FUD** 090 J A2 80 50
AMA: 2002,Apr,13; 1998,Nov,1

28116 **Ostectomy, excision of tarsal coalition**
16.6 22.0 **FUD** 090 J A2 50
AMA: 2002,Apr,13

28118 **Ostectomy, calcaneus;**
11.9 17.2 **FUD** 090 J A2 80 50
AMA: 2018,Jan,8; 2017,Jan,8; 2016,Jan,13; 2015,Jan,13; 2015,Jan,16

28119 **for spur, with or without plantar fascial release**
10.3 15.1 **FUD** 090 J A2 50
AMA: 2018,Jan,8; 2017,Jan,8; 2016,Jan,13; 2015,Jan,16

28120 **Partial excision (craterization, saucerization, sequestrectomy, or diaphysectomy) bone (eg, osteomyelitis or bossing); talus or calcaneus**
INCLUDES Barker operation
14.3 19.5 **FUD** 090 J A2 50
AMA: 2018,Jan,8; 2017,Jan,8; 2016,Jan,13; 2015,Jan,16

28122 **tarsal or metatarsal bone, except talus or calcaneus**

EXCLUDES *Hallux rigidus cheilectomy (28289)*
Partial removal talus or calcaneus (28120)

12.6 17.2 FUD 090 J A2 80 50

AMA: 2020,Aug,14

28124 **phalanx of toe**

9.55 13.8 FUD 090 J P3 50

AMA: 2002,Apr,13

28126 **Resection, partial or complete, phalangeal base, each toe**

7.11 11.3 FUD 090 J A2

AMA: 2018,Jan,8; 2017,Jan,8; 2016,Jan,13; 2015,Mar,9

28130 **Talectomy (astragalectomy)**

INCLUDES Whitman astragalectomy

EXCLUDES *Calcanectomy (28118)*

18.2 18.2 FUD 090 J J8 80 50

AMA: 2002,Apr,13

28140 **Metatarsectomy**

12.5 16.9 FUD 090 J A2

AMA: 2002,Apr,13

28150 **Phalangectomy, toe, each toe**

8.04 12.2 FUD 090 J A2

AMA: 2002,Apr,13; 1998,Nov,1

28153 **Resection, condyle(s), distal end of phalanx, each toe**

7.63 11.9 FUD 090 J A2

AMA: 2018,Jan,8; 2017,Jan,8; 2016,Jan,13; 2015,Jan,16

28160 **Hemiphalangectomy or interphalangeal joint excision, toe, proximal end of phalanx, each**

7.69 11.9 FUD 090 J A2

AMA: 2002,Apr,13; 1998,Nov,1

28171-28175 Radical Resection Bone Tumor Foot/Toes

INCLUDES Any necessary elevation tissue planes or dissection
Excision adjacent soft tissue during bone tumor resection (28039-28047 [28039, 28041])
Measurement tumor and necessary margin at greatest diameter prior to excision
Resection tumor (may include entire bone) and wide margins normal tissue primarily for malignant or aggressive benign tumors
Simple and intermediate repairs

EXCLUDES *Complex repair*
Radical tumor resection calcaneus or talus (27647)
Significant vessel exploration, neuroplasty, reconstruction, or complex bone repair

28171 **Radical resection of tumor; tarsal (except talus or calcaneus)**

32.1 32.1 FUD 090 J A2 80

AMA: 2002,Apr,13; 1994,Win,1

28173 **metatarsal**

21.3 21.3 FUD 090 J A2

AMA: 2002,Apr,13; 1994,Win,1

28175 **phalanx of toe**

13.6 13.6 FUD 090 J A2

AMA: 2002,Apr,13

28190-28193 Foreign Body Removal: Foot

28190 **Removal of foreign body, foot; subcutaneous**

3.85 7.35 FUD 010 T P3 50

AMA: 2018,Jan,8; 2017,Jan,8; 2016,Jan,13; 2015,Jan,16

28192 **deep**

9.01 13.5 FUD 090 J A2 50

AMA: 2018,Jan,8; 2017,Jan,8; 2016,Jan,13; 2015,Jan,16

28193 **complicated**

10.6 15.2 FUD 090 J A2 50

AMA: 2002,Apr,13

28200-28360 [28295] Repair/Reconstruction of Foot/Toe

INCLUDES Closed, open, and percutaneous treatment fractures and dislocations

28200 **Repair, tendon, flexor, foot; primary or secondary, without free graft, each tendon**

9.33 14.2 FUD 090 J A2

AMA: 2018,Jan,8; 2017,Jan,8; 2016,Feb,15; 2016,Jan,13; 2015,Jan,16

28202 **secondary with free graft, each tendon (includes obtaining graft)**

12.4 17.4 FUD 090 J A2 80

AMA: 2002,Apr,13

28208 **Repair, tendon, extensor, foot; primary or secondary, each tendon**

9.11 13.9 FUD 090 J A2

AMA: 2002,Apr,13; 1998,Nov,1

28210 **secondary with free graft, each tendon (includes obtaining graft)**

12.0 16.9 FUD 090 J A2 80

AMA: 2002,Apr,13

28220 **Tenolysis, flexor, foot; single tendon**

8.72 13.0 FUD 090 J P3 50

AMA: 2002,Apr,13; 1998,Nov,1

28222 **multiple tendons**

10.2 14.9 FUD 090 J A2 50

AMA: 2002,Apr,13; 1998,Nov,1

28225 **Tenolysis, extensor, foot; single tendon**

7.59 12.0 FUD 090 J A2 50

AMA: 2002,Apr,13; 1998,Nov,1

28226 **multiple tendons**

11.3 17.6 FUD 090 J A2 50

AMA: 2002,Apr,13; 1998,Nov,1

28230 **Tenotomy, open, tendon flexor; foot, single or multiple tendon(s) (separate procedure)**

8.16 12.5 FUD 090 J P3 50

AMA: 2002,Apr,13; 1998,Nov,1

28232 **toe, single tendon (separate procedure)**

6.95 11.1 FUD 090 J P3

AMA: 2020,Apr,10; 2018,Jan,8; 2017,Jan,8; 2016,Jan,13; 2015,Mar,9

28234 **Tenotomy, open, extensor, foot or toe, each tendon**

EXCLUDES *Tendon transfer (27690-27691)*

7.59 11.8 FUD 090 J A2

AMA: 2018,Jan,8; 2017,Jan,8; 2016,Jan,13; 2015,Jan,16

28238 **Reconstruction (advancement), posterior tibial tendon with excision of accessory tarsal navicular bone (eg, Kidner type procedure)**

EXCLUDES *Extensor hallucis longus transfer with big toe fusion (Jones procedure) (28760)*
Subcutaneous tenotomy (28010-28011)
Transfer or transplant tendon with muscle redirection or rerouting (27690-27692)

13.9 19.2 FUD 090 J A2 80 50

AMA: 2002,Apr,13; 2002,May,7

28240 **Tenotomy, lengthening, or release, abductor hallucis muscle**

8.46 12.9 FUD 090 J A2 50

AMA: 2002,Apr,13

28250 **Division of plantar fascia and muscle (eg, Steindler stripping) (separate procedure)**

11.6 16.7 FUD 090 J A2 80 50

AMA: 2002,Apr,13; 1998,Nov,1

28260 **Capsulotomy, midfoot; medial release only (separate procedure)**

14.9 20.2 FUD 090 J A2 80 50

AMA: 2002,Apr,13

28261 **with tendon lengthening**
27.0 34.6 **FUD** 090 J A2 80 50
AMA: 2002,Apr,13

28262 **extensive, including posterior talotibial capsulotomy and tendon(s) lengthening (eg, resistant clubfoot deformity)**
32.5 40.4 **FUD** 090 J J8 80 50
AMA: 2002,Apr,13; 1998,Nov,1

28264 **Capsulotomy, midtarsal (eg, Heyman type procedure)**
22.2 29.1 **FUD** 090 J A2 80 50
AMA: 2002,Apr,13; 1998,Nov,1

28270 **Capsulotomy; metatarsophalangeal joint, with or without tenorrhaphy, each joint (separate procedure)**
9.64 14.2 **FUD** 090 J A2 50
AMA: 2018,Jan,8; 2017,Jan,8; 2016,Jan,13; 2015,Jan,16

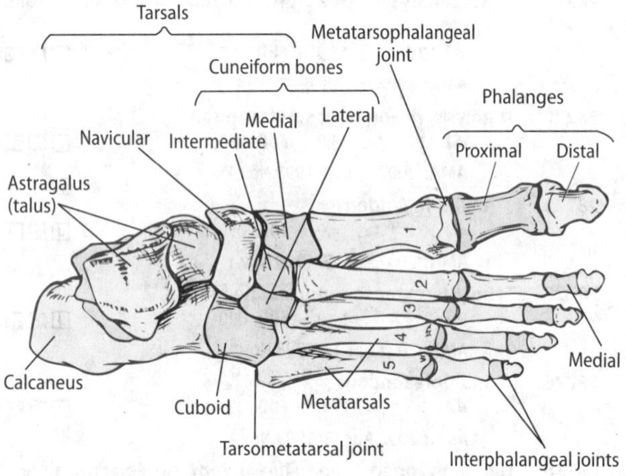

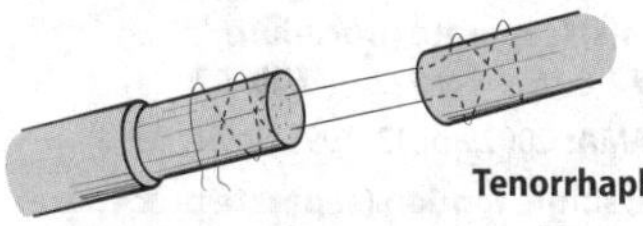

28272 **interphalangeal joint, each joint (separate procedure)**
7.27 11.3 **FUD** 090 J P3 50
AMA: 2018,Jan,8; 2017,Jan,8; 2016,Jan,13; 2015,Jan,16

28280 **Syndactylization, toes (eg, webbing or Kelikian type procedure)**
10.0 14.8 **FUD** 090 J A2 80 50
AMA: 2002,Apr,13; 1998,Nov,1

28285 **Correction, hammertoe (eg, interphalangeal fusion, partial or total phalangectomy)**
10.9 15.5 **FUD** 090 J A2 50
AMA: 2018,Jan,8; 2017,Jan,8; 2016,Jun,8; 2016,Jan,13; 2015,Mar,9; 2015,Jan,16

28286 **Correction, cock-up fifth toe, with plastic skin closure (eg, Ruiz-Mora type procedure)**
8.56 12.8 **FUD** 090 J A2 50
AMA: 2002,Apr,13; 1998,Nov,1

28288 **Ostectomy, partial, exostectomy or condylectomy, metatarsal head, each metatarsal head**
12.4 17.5 **FUD** 090 J A2
AMA: 2002,Apr,13; 1998,Nov,1

28289 **Hallux rigidus correction with cheilectomy, debridement and capsular release of the first metatarsophalangeal joint; without implant**
13.2 20.5 **FUD** 090 J A2 80 50
AMA: 2020,Aug,14; 2020,Jul,13; 2018,Jan,8; 2017,Jan,8; 2016,Dec,3; 2016,Jan,13; 2015,Sep,12; 2015,Jan,16

28291 **with implant**
14.1 21.0 **FUD** 090 J J8 80 50
AMA: 2020,Aug,14; 2018,Jan,8; 2017,Nov,10; 2017,Jan,8; 2016,Dec,3

28292 **Correction, hallux valgus (bunionectomy), with sesamoidectomy, when performed; with resection of proximal phalanx base, when performed, any method**
13.9 21.3 **FUD** 090 J A2 80 50
AMA: 2018,Jan,8; 2017,Jan,8; 2016,Dec,3; 2016,Jan,13; 2015,Jan,16

28295 **Resequenced code. See code following 28296.**

28296 **with distal metatarsal osteotomy, any method**
14.8 26.3 **FUD** 090 J A2 80 50
AMA: 2020,Jul,13; 2018,Sep,14; 2018,Jan,8; 2017,Jan,8; 2016,Dec,3; 2016,Jan,13; 2015,Jan,16

28295 **with proximal metatarsal osteotomy, any method**
16.1 28.5 **FUD** 090 J G2 80 50
AMA: 2018,Jan,8; 2017,Jan,8; 2016,Dec,3

28297 **with first metatarsal and medial cuneiform joint arthrodesis, any method**
17.4 30.2 **FUD** 090 J J8 80 50
AMA: 2018,Jan,8; 2017,Jan,8; 2016,Dec,3; 2016,Jan,13; 2015,Jan,16

28298 **with proximal phalanx osteotomy, any method**
INCLUDES Akin procedure
14.3 24.3 **FUD** 090 J A2 80 50
AMA: 2018,Jan,8; 2017,Jan,8; 2016,Dec,3; 2016,Jan,13; 2015,Jan,16

28299 **with double osteotomy, any method**
16.8 29.1 **FUD** 090 J A2 80 50
AMA: 2018,Jan,8; 2017,Jan,8; 2016,Dec,3; 2016,Apr,8; 2016,Jan,13; 2015,Jan,16

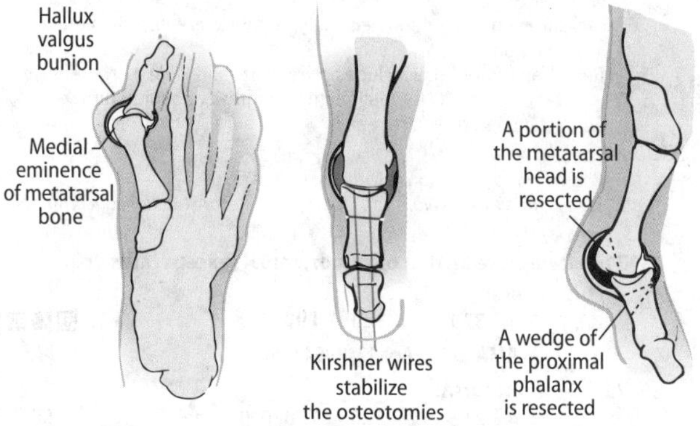

28300 **Osteotomy; calcaneus (eg, Dwyer or Chambers type procedure), with or without internal fixation**
18.7 18.7 **FUD** 090 J J8 80 50
AMA: 2002,Apr,13; 1998,Nov,1

28302 **talus**
20.6 20.6 **FUD** 090 J A2 80 50
AMA: 2002,Apr,13

28304 **Osteotomy, tarsal bones, other than calcaneus or talus;**
17.3 23.6 **FUD** 090 J A2 80 50
AMA: 2002,Apr,13; 1998,Nov,1

28305 **with autograft (includes obtaining graft) (eg, Fowler type)**
19.3 19.3 **FUD** 090 J J8 80 50
AMA: 2002,Apr,13; 1998,Nov,1

28306 **Osteotomy, with or without lengthening, shortening or angular correction, metatarsal; first metatarsal**
11.6 17.6 **FUD** 090 J A2 80 50
AMA: 2018,Jan,8; 2017,Jan,8; 2016,Jan,13; 2015,Jan,16

28307 first metatarsal with autograft (other than first toe)
11.9 17.9 FUD 090 J A2 80 50
AMA: 2002,Apr,13; 1998,Nov,1

28308 other than first metatarsal, each
10.9 16.4 FUD 090 J A2 80 50
AMA: 2002,Apr,13; 1998,Nov,1

28309 multiple (eg, Swanson type cavus foot procedure)
25.5 25.5 FUD 090 J A2 80 50
AMA: 2018,Jan,8; 2017,Jan,8; 2016,Jan,13; 2015,Jan,16

28310 Osteotomy, shortening, angular or rotational correction; proximal phalanx, first toe (separate procedure)
10.3 15.7 FUD 090 J A2 50
AMA: 2018,Jan,8; 2017,Jan,8; 2016,Jan,13; 2015,Jan,16

28312 other phalanges, any toe
9.12 14.4 FUD 090 J A2
AMA: 2002,Apr,13

28313 Reconstruction, angular deformity of toe, soft tissue procedures only (eg, overlapping second toe, fifth toe, curly toes)
10.2 15.1 FUD 090 J A2
AMA: 2002,Apr,13; 1998,Nov,1

28315 Sesamoidectomy, first toe (separate procedure)
9.38 13.9 FUD 090 J A2 50
AMA: 2002,Apr,13

28320 Repair, nonunion or malunion; tarsal bones
17.5 17.5 FUD 090 J J8 80 50
AMA: 2002,Apr,13; 1998,Nov,1

28322 metatarsal, with or without bone graft (includes obtaining graft)
16.5 22.5 FUD 090 J J8 80
AMA: 2002,Apr,13

28340 Reconstruction, toe, macrodactyly; soft tissue resection
11.8 16.5 FUD 090 J A2
AMA: 2002,Apr,13

28341 requiring bone resection
14.1 19.3 FUD 090 J A2
AMA: 2002,Apr,13

28344 Reconstruction, toe(s); polydactyly
8.04 12.2 FUD 090 J A2 50
AMA: 2002,Apr,13

28345 syndactyly, with or without skin graft(s), each web
10.5 14.9 FUD 090 J A2 80
AMA: 2002,Apr,13

28360 Reconstruction, cleft foot
31.4 31.4 FUD 090 J 80 50
AMA: 2002,Apr,13

28400-28675 Treatment of Fracture/Dislocation of Foot/Toe

28400 Closed treatment of calcaneal fracture; without manipulation
6.55 7.09 FUD 090 T A2 50
AMA: 2002,Apr,13

28405 with manipulation
INCLUDES Bohler reduction
10.0 11.1 FUD 090 T A2 80 50
AMA: 2002,Apr,13

28406 Percutaneous skeletal fixation of calcaneal fracture, with manipulation
15.1 15.1 FUD 090 J A2 80 50
AMA: 2002,Apr,13

28415 Open treatment of calcaneal fracture, includes internal fixation, when performed;
32.2 32.2 FUD 090 J J8 80 50
AMA: 2002,Apr,13

28420 with primary iliac or other autogenous bone graft (includes obtaining graft)
37.1 37.1 FUD 090 J J8 80 50
AMA: 2002,Apr,13

28430 Closed treatment of talus fracture; without manipulation
6.03 6.85 FUD 090 T P2 50
AMA: 2002,Apr,13

28435 with manipulation
9.31 10.4 FUD 090 J A2 80 50
AMA: 2002,Apr,13

28436 Percutaneous skeletal fixation of talus fracture, with manipulation
12.9 12.9 FUD 090 J G2 50
AMA: 2002,Apr,13

28445 Open treatment of talus fracture, includes internal fixation, when performed
29.9 29.9 FUD 090 J J8 80 50
AMA: 2002,Apr,13

28446 Open osteochondral autograft, talus (includes obtaining graft[s])
INCLUDES Osteotomy; fibula (27707)
Osteotomy; tibia (27705)
EXCLUDES *Arthroscopically aided osteochondral talus graft (29892)*
Open osteochondral allograft or repairs with industrial grafts (28899)
35.3 35.3 FUD 090 J G2 80 50
AMA: 2018,Jan,8; 2017,Jan,8; 2016,Jan,13; 2015,Jan,16

28450 Treatment of tarsal bone fracture (except talus and calcaneus); without manipulation, each
5.47 6.07 FUD 090 T P2
AMA: 2018,Jan,8; 2017,Jan,8; 2016,Jan,13; 2015,Jan,16

28455 with manipulation, each
7.40 8.27 FUD 090 J P3 80
AMA: 2002,Apr,13

28456 Percutaneous skeletal fixation of tarsal bone fracture (except talus and calcaneus), with manipulation, each
9.74 9.74 FUD 090 J A2
AMA: 2002,Apr,13

28465 Open treatment of tarsal bone fracture (except talus and calcaneus), includes internal fixation, when performed, each
18.1 18.1 FUD 090 J J8
AMA: 2019,Aug,10

28470 Closed treatment of metatarsal fracture; without manipulation, each
5.85 6.26 FUD 090 T P2
AMA: 2002,Apr,13

28475 with manipulation, each
6.52 7.37 FUD 090 T P2
AMA: 2002,Apr,13

28476 Percutaneous skeletal fixation of metatarsal fracture, with manipulation, each
10.5 10.5 FUD 090 J A2 80
AMA: 2002,Apr,13

28485 Open treatment of metatarsal fracture, includes internal fixation, when performed, each
15.8 15.8 FUD 090 J J8
AMA: 2019,Aug,10

28490 Closed treatment of fracture great toe, phalanx or phalanges; without manipulation
3.57 4.12 FUD 090 T P3 50
AMA: 2002,Apr,13

28495 with manipulation
4.25 5.10 FUD 090 T P2 50
AMA: 2002,Apr,13

28496 **Percutaneous skeletal fixation of fracture great toe, phalanx or phalanges, with manipulation**
6.93 12.9 **FUD** 090 J A2 50
AMA: 2002,Apr,13

28505 **Open treatment of fracture, great toe, phalanx or phalanges, includes internal fixation, when performed**
14.3 19.1 **FUD** 090 J A2 50
AMA: 2002,Apr,13

28510 **Closed treatment of fracture, phalanx or phalanges, other than great toe; without manipulation, each**
3.41 3.47 **FUD** 090 T P3
AMA: 2002,Apr,13

28515 **with manipulation, each**
4.08 4.67 **FUD** 090 T P3
AMA: 2002,Apr,13

28525 **Open treatment of fracture, phalanx or phalanges, other than great toe, includes internal fixation, when performed, each**
11.6 16.5 **FUD** 090 J A2 80
AMA: 2002,Apr,13

28530 **Closed treatment of sesamoid fracture**
2.88 3.30 **FUD** 090 T P3 80 50
AMA: 2002,Apr,13

28531 **Open treatment of sesamoid fracture, with or without internal fixation**
5.22 9.73 **FUD** 090 J A2 50
AMA: 2002,Apr,13

28540 **Closed treatment of tarsal bone dislocation, other than talotarsal; without anesthesia**
5.01 5.57 **FUD** 090 T P2 80 50
AMA: 2002,Apr,13

28545 **requiring anesthesia**
7.62 8.67 **FUD** 090 J G2 80 50
AMA: 2002,Apr,13

28546 **Percutaneous skeletal fixation of tarsal bone dislocation, other than talotarsal, with manipulation**
9.85 16.7 **FUD** 090 J A2 80 50
AMA: 2002,Apr,13

28555 **Open treatment of tarsal bone dislocation, includes internal fixation, when performed**
18.7 24.6 **FUD** 090 J A2 80 50
AMA: 2002,Apr,13

28570 **Closed treatment of talotarsal joint dislocation; without anesthesia**
5.52 6.57 **FUD** 090 T P2 80 50
AMA: 2002,Apr,13

28575 **requiring anesthesia**
9.57 10.6 **FUD** 090 J A2 80 50
AMA: 2002,Apr,13

28576 **Percutaneous skeletal fixation of talotarsal joint dislocation, with manipulation**
11.1 11.1 **FUD** 090 J A2 80 50
AMA: 2002,Apr,13

28585 **Open treatment of talotarsal joint dislocation, includes internal fixation, when performed**
19.6 25.0 **FUD** 090 J J8 80 50
AMA: 2018,Jan,8; 2017,Jan,8; 2016,Jan,13; 2015,Jan,16

28600 **Closed treatment of tarsometatarsal joint dislocation; without anesthesia**
5.35 6.26 **FUD** 090 T P2 80
AMA: 2002,Apr,13

28605 **requiring anesthesia**
8.57 9.58 **FUD** 090 T A2 80
AMA: 2002,Apr,13

28606 **Percutaneous skeletal fixation of tarsometatarsal joint dislocation, with manipulation**
11.1 11.1 **FUD** 090 J A2
AMA: 2002,Apr,13

28615 **Open treatment of tarsometatarsal joint dislocation, includes internal fixation, when performed**
23.4 23.4 **FUD** 090 J J8 80
AMA: 2002,Apr,13

28630 **Closed treatment of metatarsophalangeal joint dislocation; without anesthesia**
3.15 4.49 **FUD** 010 T P3 80
AMA: 2002,Apr,13

28635 **requiring anesthesia**
3.81 5.04 **FUD** 010 J A2 80
AMA: 2002,Apr,13

28636 **Percutaneous skeletal fixation of metatarsophalangeal joint dislocation, with manipulation**
5.74 8.98 **FUD** 010 J A2
AMA: 2002,Apr,13

28645 **Open treatment of metatarsophalangeal joint dislocation, includes internal fixation, when performed**
14.0 18.9 **FUD** 090 J A2
AMA: 2018,Jan,8; 2017,Jan,8; 2016,Jan,13; 2015,Jan,16

28660 **Closed treatment of interphalangeal joint dislocation; without anesthesia**
2.56 3.38 **FUD** 010 T P3
AMA: 2002,Apr,13

28665 **requiring anesthesia**
3.72 4.41 **FUD** 010 T A2 80
AMA: 2002,Apr,13

28666 **Percutaneous skeletal fixation of interphalangeal joint dislocation, with manipulation**
4.79 4.79 **FUD** 010 J A2
AMA: 2002,Apr,13

28675 **Open treatment of interphalangeal joint dislocation, includes internal fixation, when performed**
11.6 16.4 **FUD** 090 J A2
AMA: 2002,Apr,13

28705-28760 Arthrodesis of Foot/Toe

28705 **Arthrodesis; pantalar**
35.4 35.4 **FUD** 090 J J8 80 50
AMA: 2020,May,13

28715 **triple**
27.1 27.1 **FUD** 090 J J8 80 50
AMA: 2020,May,13

28725 **subtalar**
INCLUDES Dunn arthrodesis
Grice arthrodesis
22.4 22.4 **FUD** 090 J J8 80 50
AMA: 2020,May,13; 2018,Jan,8; 2017,Jan,8; 2016,Jan,13; 2015,Jan,16

28730 **Arthrodesis, midtarsal or tarsometatarsal, multiple or transverse;**
INCLUDES Lambrinudi arthrodesis
21.2 21.2 **FUD** 090 J J8 80 50
AMA: 2020,May,13

28735 **with osteotomy (eg, flatfoot correction)**
22.4 22.4 **FUD** 090 J J8 80 50
AMA: 2020,May,13; 2019,May,10

28737 **Arthrodesis, with tendon lengthening and advancement, midtarsal, tarsal navicular-cuneiform (eg, Miller type procedure)**
19.8 19.8 **FUD** 090 J J8 80 50
AMA: 2020,May,13

28740 **Arthrodesis, midtarsal or tarsometatarsal, single joint**
17.9 24.3 FUD 090 J J8 80 50
AMA: 2020,May,13; 2018,Jan,8; 2017,Jan,8; 2016,Jan,13; 2015,Jan,16

28750 **Arthrodesis, great toe; metatarsophalangeal joint**
16.8 22.9 FUD 090 J J8 80 50
AMA: 2020,May,13; 2018,Jan,8; 2017,Jan,8; 2016,Dec,3; 2016,Jan,13; 2015,Jan,16

28755 **interphalangeal joint**
9.56 14.7 FUD 090 J A2 50
AMA: 2020,May,13

28760 **Arthrodesis, with extensor hallucis longus transfer to first metatarsal neck, great toe, interphalangeal joint (eg, Jones type procedure)**
INCLUDES Jones procedure
EXCLUDES *Hammer toe repair or interphalangeal fusion (28285)*
16.6 22.5 FUD 090 J A2 80 50
AMA: 2020,May,13

28800-28825 Amputation Foot/Toe

28800 **Amputation, foot; midtarsal (eg, Chopart type procedure)**
15.4 15.4 FUD 090 C 80 50
AMA: 2002,Apr,13; 1998,Nov,1

28805 **transmetatarsal**
20.9 20.9 FUD 090 J 80 50
AMA: 2002,Apr,13; 1997,May,4

28810 **Amputation, metatarsal, with toe, single**
12.3 12.3 FUD 090 J A2 80
AMA: 2002,Apr,13

28820 **Amputation, toe; metatarsophalangeal joint**
11.3 16.1 FUD 090 J A2
AMA: 2002,Apr,13; 1997,May,4

28825 **interphalangeal joint**
10.6 15.4 FUD 090 J A2
AMA: 2002,Apr,13

28890-28899 Other/Unlisted Procedures Foot/Toe

28890 **Extracorporeal shock wave, high energy, performed by a physician or other qualified health care professional, requiring anesthesia other than local, including ultrasound guidance, involving the plantar fascia**
EXCLUDES *Extracorporeal shock wave therapy integumentary system not otherwise specified, when performed on same treatment area ([0512T, 0513T])*
Extracorporeal shock wave therapy musculoskeletal system not otherwise specified (0101T-0102T)
6.38 9.18 FUD 090 J P3 50
AMA: 2018,Dec,5; 2018,Dec,5; 2018,Jan,8; 2017,Jan,8; 2016,Jan,13; 2015,Jan,16

28899 **Unlisted procedure, foot or toes**
0.00 0.00 FUD YYY T 80
AMA: 2018,Oct,11; 2018,Jan,8; 2017,Nov,10; 2017,Sep,14; 2017,Jan,8; 2016,Dec,3; 2016,Jun,8; 2016,Jan,13; 2015,Nov,10; 2015,Jan,16

29000-29086 Casting: Arm/Shoulder/Torso

INCLUDES Application cast or strapping when provided as:
Initial service to stabilize fracture or injury without restorative treatment
Replacement procedure
Removal cast
EXCLUDES *Cast or splint material*
E/M services provided as initial service when restorative treatment not provided
Orthotic supervision and training (97760-97763)

29000 **Application of halo type body cast (see 20661-20663 for insertion)**
5.57 9.69 FUD 000 T G2 80
AMA: 2018,Jan,8; 2018,Jan,3; 2017,Jan,8; 2016,Jan,13; 2015,Jan,16

29010 **Application of Risser jacket, localizer, body; only**
4.58 7.63 FUD 000 T P2 80
AMA: 2018,Jan,8; 2018,Jan,3; 2017,Jan,8; 2016,Jan,13; 2015,Jan,16

29015 **including head**
5.18 8.22 FUD 000 T P2 80
AMA: 2018,Jan,8; 2018,Jan,3; 2017,Jan,8; 2016,Jan,13; 2015,Jan,16

29035 **Application of body cast, shoulder to hips;**
4.08 7.13 FUD 000 T P2 80
AMA: 2018,Jan,8; 2018,Jan,3; 2017,Jan,8; 2016,Jan,13; 2015,Jan,16

29040 **including head, Minerva type**
4.95 8.17 FUD 000 T G2 80
AMA: 2018,Jan,8; 2018,Jan,3; 2017,Jan,8; 2016,Jan,13; 2015,Jan,16

29044 **including 1 thigh**
4.78 8.01 FUD 000 T P2 80
AMA: 2018,Jan,8; 2018,Jan,3; 2017,Jan,8; 2016,Jan,13; 2015,Jan,16

29046 **including both thighs**
5.37 8.78 FUD 000 T G2 80
AMA: 2018,Jan,8; 2018,Jan,3; 2017,Jan,8; 2016,Jan,13; 2015,Jan,16

29049 **Application, cast; figure-of-eight**
2.00 2.79 FUD 000 T P3 80
AMA: 2018,Jan,3; 2018,Jan,8; 2017,Jan,8; 2016,Jan,13; 2015,Jan,16

29055 **shoulder spica**
3.93 6.22 FUD 000 T P2 80
AMA: 2018,Jan,8; 2018,Jan,3; 2017,Jan,8; 2016,Jan,13; 2015,Jan,16

29058 **plaster Velpeau**
2.71 3.51 FUD 000 T P3 80
AMA: 2018,Jan,8; 2018,Jan,3; 2017,Jan,8; 2016,Jan,13; 2015,Jan,16

29065 **shoulder to hand (long arm)**
1.95 2.70 FUD 000 T P3 50
AMA: 2018,Jan,8; 2018,Jan,3; 2017,Jan,8; 2016,Jan,13; 2015,Jan,16

29075 **elbow to finger (short arm)**
1.76 2.43 FUD 000 T P3 50
AMA: 2018,Jan,8; 2018,Jan,3; 2017,Jan,8; 2016,Jan,13; 2015,Jan,16

29085 **hand and lower forearm (gauntlet)**
1.92 2.68 FUD 000 T P3 50
AMA: 2018,Jan,3; 2018,Jan,8; 2017,Jan,8; 2016,Jan,13; 2015,Jan,16

29086 **finger (eg, contracture)**
1.47 2.22 FUD 000 T P3 50
AMA: 2018,Jan,8; 2018,Jan,3; 2017,Jan,8; 2016,Jan,13; 2015,Jan,16

29105-29280 Splinting and Strapping: Torso/Upper Extremities

INCLUDES Application splint or strapping when provided as:
Initial service to stabilize fracture or dislocation
Replacement procedure
EXCLUDES *E/M services provided as initial service when restorative treatment not provided*
Orthotic supervision and training (97760-97763)
Splinting and strapping material

29105 **Application of long arm splint (shoulder to hand)**
1.38 2.33 FUD 000 T P3 50
AMA: 2018,Jan,3; 2018,Jan,8; 2017,Jan,8; 2016,Jan,13; 2015,Jan,16

29125 **Application of short arm splint (forearm to hand); static**
1.13 1.82 FUD 000 Q1 N1 50
AMA: 2018,Jan,8; 2018,Jan,3; 2017,Jan,8; 2016,Jan,13; 2015,Jan,16

29126 **dynamic**
1.40 2.18 **FUD** 000 Q1 N1 50
AMA: 2018,Jan,8; 2018,Jan,3; 2017,Jan,8; 2016,Jan,13; 2015,Jan,16

29130 **Application of finger splint; static**
0.85 1.18 **FUD** 000 Q1 N1 50
AMA: 2018,Jan,8; 2018,Jan,3; 2017,Jan,8; 2016,Jan,13; 2015,Jan,16

29131 **dynamic**
0.98 1.48 **FUD** 000 Q1 N1 50
AMA: 2018,Jan,8; 2018,Jan,3; 2017,Jan,8; 2016,Jan,13; 2015,Jan,16

29200 **Strapping; thorax**
EXCLUDES *Strapping of low back (29799)*
0.54 0.93 **FUD** 000 T P3
AMA: 2018,Jan,8; 2018,Jan,3; 2017,Jan,8; 2016,Jan,13; 2015,Jan,16

29240 **shoulder (eg, Velpeau)**
0.54 0.87 **FUD** 000 Q1 N1 50
AMA: 2018,Jan,3; 2018,Jan,8; 2017,Jan,8; 2016,Jan,13; 2015,Jan,16

29260 **elbow or wrist**
0.56 0.86 **FUD** 000 Q1 N1 50
AMA: 2018,Jan,8; 2018,Jan,3; 2017,Jan,8; 2016,Jan,13; 2015,Jan,16

29280 **hand or finger**
0.60 0.88 **FUD** 000 Q1 N1 50
AMA: 2018,Jan,8; 2018,Jan,3; 2017,Jan,8; 2016,Jan,13; 2015,Jan,16

29305-29450 Casting: Legs

INCLUDES Application cast when provided as:
Initial service to stabilize fracture or injury without restorative treatment
Replacement procedure
Removal cast

EXCLUDES *Cast or splint materials*
E/M services provided as part initial service when restorative treatment is not provided
Orthotic supervision and training (97760-97763)

29305 **Application of hip spica cast; 1 leg**
EXCLUDES *Hip spica cast thighs only (29046)*
4.57 7.02 **FUD** 000 T P2 80
AMA: 2018,Jan,8; 2018,Jan,3; 2017,Jan,8; 2016,Jan,13; 2015,Jan,16

29325 **1 and one-half spica or both legs**
EXCLUDES *Hip spica cast thighs only (29046)*
5.11 7.75 **FUD** 000 T P2 80
AMA: 2018,Jan,8; 2018,Jan,3; 2017,Jan,8; 2016,Jan,13; 2015,Jan,16

29345 **Application of long leg cast (thigh to toes);**
2.87 3.85 **FUD** 000 T P3 50
AMA: 2018,Jan,3; 2018,Jan,8; 2017,Jan,8; 2016,Jan,13; 2015,Jan,16

29355 **walker or ambulatory type**
3.07 4.03 **FUD** 000 T P3 50
AMA: 2018,Jan,3; 2018,Jan,8; 2017,Jan,8; 2016,Jan,13; 2015,Jan,16

29358 **Application of long leg cast brace**
2.96 4.51 **FUD** 000 T P3 50
AMA: 2018,Jan,3; 2018,Jan,8; 2017,Jan,8; 2016,Jan,13; 2015,Jan,16

29365 **Application of cylinder cast (thigh to ankle)**
2.51 3.49 **FUD** 000 T P3 50
AMA: 2018,Jan,3; 2018,Jan,8; 2017,Jan,8; 2016,Jan,13; 2015,Jan,16

29405 **Application of short leg cast (below knee to toes);**
1.69 2.26 **FUD** 000 T P3 50
AMA: 2018,Jan,3; 2018,Jan,8; 2017,Jan,8; 2016,Jan,13; 2015,Jan,16

29425 **walking or ambulatory type**
1.59 2.17 **FUD** 000 T P3 50
AMA: 2018,Jan,8; 2018,Jan,3; 2018,Jan,8; 2017,Jan,8; 2016,Jan,13; 2015,Jan,16

29435 **Application of patellar tendon bearing (PTB) cast**
2.35 3.25 **FUD** 000 T P3 50
AMA: 2018,Jan,3; 2018,Jan,8; 2017,Jan,8; 2016,Jan,13; 2015,Jan,16

29440 **Adding walker to previously applied cast**
0.83 1.23 **FUD** 000 T P3 50
AMA: 2018,Jan,8; 2018,Jan,3; 2017,Jan,8; 2016,Jan,13; 2015,Jan,16

29445 **Application of rigid total contact leg cast**
2.94 3.73 **FUD** 000 T P3 50
AMA: 2018,Jan,3; 2018,Jan,8; 2017,Jan,8; 2016,Jan,13; 2015,Jan,16

29450 **Application of clubfoot cast with molding or manipulation, long or short leg**
3.26 4.11 **FUD** 000 T P3 50
AMA: 2018,Jan,8; 2018,Jan,3; 2017,Jan,8; 2016,Jan,13; 2015,Jan,16

29505-29584 Splinting and Strapping Ankle/Foot/Leg/Toes

INCLUDES Application splinting and strapping when provided as:
Initial service to stabilize fracture or injury without restorative treatment
Replacement procedure

EXCLUDES *E/M services provided as part initial service when restorative treatment not provided*
Orthotic supervision and training (97760-97763)

29505 **Application of long leg splint (thigh to ankle or toes)**
1.45 2.41 **FUD** 000 T P3 50
AMA: 2018,Jan,3; 2018,Jan,8; 2017,Jan,8; 2016,Jan,13; 2015,Jan,16

29515 **Application of short leg splint (calf to foot)**
1.42 2.01 **FUD** 000 T P3 50
AMA: 2019,Oct,10; 2018,Jan,8; 2018,Jan,3; 2017,Jan,8; 2016,Jan,13; 2015,Jan,16

29520 **Strapping; hip**
EXCLUDES *For treatment in same extremity:*
Endovenous ablation therapy incompetent vein (36473-36479, [36482], [36483])
Sclerosal injection for incompetent vein(s) ([36465], [36466], 36468-36471)
0.55 1.00 **FUD** 000 Q1 N1 80 50
AMA: 2018,Jan,8; 2018,Jan,3; 2017,Jan,8; 2016,Jan,13; 2015,Jan,16

29530 **knee**
EXCLUDES *For treatment in same extremity:*
Endovenous ablation therapy incompetent vein (36473-36479, [36482], [36483])
Sclerosal injection for incompetent vein(s) ([36465], [36466], 36468-36471)
0.54 0.87 **FUD** 000 Q1 N1 50
AMA: 2018,Jan,3; 2018,Jan,8; 2017,Jan,8; 2016,Jan,13; 2015,Jan,16

29540 **ankle and/or foot**
EXCLUDES *For treatment in same extremity:*
Endovenous ablation therapy incompetent vein (36473-36479, [36482, 36483])
Multi-layer compression system (29581)
Sclerosal injection for incompetent vein(s) ([36465], [36466], 36468-36471)
Unna boot (29580)
0.51 0.81 **FUD** 000 T P3 50
AMA: 2018,Jan,3; 2018,Jan,8; 2017,Jan,8; 2016,Aug,3; 2016,Jan,13; 2015,Jan,16

29550 **toes**

EXCLUDES *For treatment in same extremity:*
Endovenous ablation therapy incompetent vein (36473-36479, [36482, 36483])
Sclerosal injection for incompetent vein(s) ([36465], [36466], 36468-36471)

0.33 0.54 FUD 000 Q1 N1 50

AMA: 2018,Jan,8; 2018,Jan,3; 2017,Jan,8; 2016,Jan,13; 2015,Jan,16

29580 **Unna boot**

EXCLUDES *Application multilayer compression system (29581)*
For treatment in same extremity:
Endovenous ablation therapy incompetent vein (36473-36479, [36482, 36483])
Sclerosal injection for incompetent vein(s) ([36465], [36466], 36468-36471)
Strapping ankle or foot (29540)

0.79 1.80 FUD 000 T P3 50

AMA: 2018,Jan,3; 2018,Jan,8; 2017,Jan,8; 2016,Aug,3; 2016,Jan,13; 2015,Jan,16

29581 **Application of multi-layer compression system; leg (below knee), including ankle and foot**

EXCLUDES *For treatment in same extremity:*
Endovenous ablation therapy incompetent vein (36473-36479, [36482, 36483])
Sclerosal injection for incompetent vein(s) ([36465], [36466], 36468-36471)
Strapping (29540, 29580)

0.80 2.47 FUD 000 T P2 80 50

AMA: 2018,Mar,3; 2018,Jan,8; 2018,Jan,3; 2017,Jan,8; 2016,Nov,3; 2016,Aug,3; 2016,Jan,13; 2015,Mar,9; 2015,Jan,16

29584 **upper arm, forearm, hand, and fingers**

EXCLUDES *For treatment in same extremity:*
Endovenous ablation therapy incompetent vein (36473-36479, [36482], [36483])
Sclerosal injection for incompetent vein(s) ([36465], [36466], 36468-36471)

0.47 2.29 FUD 000 T P2 80 50

AMA: 2018,Jan,3; 2018,Jan,8; 2017,Jan,8; 2016,Aug,3; 2016,Jan,13; 2015,Mar,9

29700-29799 Casting Services Other Than Application

INCLUDES Casts applied by treating individual
Removal casts applied by treating individual

29700 **Removal or bivalving; gauntlet, boot or body cast**

0.96 1.78 FUD 000 T P3

AMA: 2018,Jan,3; 2018,Jan,8; 2017,Jan,8; 2016,Jan,13; 2015,Jan,16

29705 **full arm or full leg cast**

1.31 1.82 FUD 000 T P3 50

AMA: 2018,Jan,3; 2018,Jan,8; 2017,Jan,8; 2016,Jan,13; 2015,Jan,16

29710 **shoulder or hip spica, Minerva, or Risser jacket, etc.**

2.41 3.48 FUD 000 T P3 80 50

AMA: 2018,Jan,3; 2018,Jan,8; 2017,Jan,8; 2016,Jan,13; 2015,Jan,16

29720 **Repair of spica, body cast or jacket**

1.26 2.38 FUD 000 T P3

AMA: 2018,Jan,3; 2018,Jan,8; 2017,Jan,8; 2016,Jan,13; 2015,Jan,16

29730 **Windowing of cast**

1.25 1.76 FUD 000 T P3

AMA: 2018,Jan,3; 2018,Jan,8; 2017,Jan,8; 2016,Jan,13; 2015,Jan,16

29740 **Wedging of cast (except clubfoot casts)**

2.02 2.82 FUD 000 T P3

AMA: 2018,Jan,3; 2018,Jan,8; 2017,Jan,8; 2016,Jan,13; 2015,Jan,16

29750 **Wedging of clubfoot cast**

2.26 3.07 FUD 000 T P3 80 50

AMA: 2018,Jan,3; 2018,Jan,8; 2017,Jan,8; 2016,Jan,13; 2015,Jan,16

29799 **Unlisted procedure, casting or strapping**

0.00 0.00 FUD YYY T 80

AMA: 2018,Jan,3; 2018,Jan,8; 2017,Jan,8; 2016,Aug,3; 2016,Jan,13; 2015,Jan,16

29800-29999 [29914, 29915, 29916] Arthroscopic Procedures

INCLUDES Diagnostic arthroscopy with surgical arthroscopy
EXCLUDES *Reporting removal foreign or loose body(ies) smaller than arthroscopic cannula diameter utilized for procedure*
Code also modifier 51 when arthroscopy performed with arthrotomy

29800 **Arthroscopy, temporomandibular joint, diagnostic, with or without synovial biopsy (separate procedure)**

15.2 15.2 FUD 090 J A2 80 50

AMA: 2018,Jan,8; 2017,Jan,8; 2016,Jan,13; 2015,Jan,16

29804 **Arthroscopy, temporomandibular joint, surgical**

EXCLUDES *Open surgery (21010)*

17.7 17.7 FUD 090 J A2 80 50

AMA: 2018,Jan,8; 2017,Jan,8; 2016,Jan,13; 2015,Jan,16

29805 **Arthroscopy, shoulder, diagnostic, with or without synovial biopsy (separate procedure)**

EXCLUDES *Open surgery (23065-23066, 23100-23101)*

13.5 13.5 FUD 090 J A2 50

AMA: 2018,Jan,8; 2017,Jan,8; 2016,Jan,13; 2015,Jun,10; 2015,Jan,16

29806 **Arthroscopy, shoulder, surgical; capsulorrhaphy**

EXCLUDES *Open surgery (23450-23466)*
Thermal capsulorrhaphy (29999)

30.5 30.5 FUD 090 J A2 50

AMA: 2018,Jun,11; 2018,Jan,8; 2017,Jan,8; 2016,Jan,13; 2015,Jul,10; 2015,Mar,7; 2015,Jan,16

29807 **repair of SLAP lesion**

29.8 29.8 FUD 090 J A2 50

AMA: 2018,Jan,8; 2017,Jan,8; 2016,Jan,13; 2015,Mar,7; 2015,Jan,16

29819 **with removal of loose body or foreign body**

EXCLUDES *Open surgery (23040-23044, 23107)*

16.9 16.9 FUD 090 J A2 50

AMA: 2018,Jun,11; 2018,Jan,8; 2017,Jan,8; 2016,Jan,13; 2015,Mar,7; 2015,Jan,16

29820 **synovectomy, partial**

EXCLUDES *Open surgery (23105)*

15.3 15.3 FUD 090 J A2 80 50

AMA: 2018,Jan,8; 2017,Jan,8; 2016,Jan,13; 2015,Mar,7; 2015,Jan,16

29821 **synovectomy, complete**

EXCLUDES *Open surgery (23105)*

17.1 17.1 FUD 090 J A2 80 50

AMA: 2018,Jan,8; 2017,Jan,8; 2016,Jan,13; 2015,Mar,7; 2015,Jan,16

▲ **29822** **debridement, limited, 1 or 2 discrete structures (eg, humeral bone, humeral articular cartilage, glenoid bone, glenoid articular cartilage, biceps tendon, biceps anchor complex, labrum, articular capsule, articular side of the rotator cuff, bursal side of the rotator cuff, subacromial bursa, foreign body[ies])**

EXCLUDES *Open surgery (see specific shoulder section)*

16.6 16.6 FUD 090 J A2 80 50

AMA: 2018,Jan,7; 2018,Jan,8; 2017,Jan,8; 2016,Jan,13; 2015,Mar,7; 2015,Jan,16

▲ **29823** **debridement, extensive, 3 or more discrete structures (eg, humeral bone, humeral articular cartilage, glenoid bone, glenoid articular cartilage, biceps tendon, biceps anchor complex, labrum, articular capsule, articular side of the rotator cuff, bursal side of the rotator cuff, subacromial bursa, foreign body[ies])**

EXCLUDES *Open surgery (see specific shoulder section)*

18.1 18.1 FUD 090 J A2 80 50

AMA: 2018,Jan,7; 2018,Jan,8; 2017,Jan,8; 2016,Dec,16; 2016,Jan,13; 2015,Mar,7; 2015,Jan,16

29824 **distal claviculectomy including distal articular surface (Mumford procedure)**

EXCLUDES *Open surgery (23120)*

19.1 19.1 FUD 090 J A2 80 50

AMA: 2018,Jan,8; 2017,Jan,8; 2016,Jan,13; 2015,Mar,7; 2015,Jan,16

29825 **with lysis and resection of adhesions, with or without manipulation**

EXCLUDES *Open surgery (see specific shoulder section)*

16.9 16.9 FUD 090 J A2 80 50

AMA: 2018,Jan,8; 2017,Jan,8; 2016,Jan,13; 2015,Mar,7; 2015,Jan,16

+ **29826** **decompression of subacromial space with partial acromioplasty, with coracoacromial ligament (ie, arch) release, when performed (List separately in addition to code for primary procedure)**

EXCLUDES *Open surgery (23130, 23415)*

Code first (29806-29825, 29827-29828)

5.07 5.07 FUD ZZZ N N1 80 50

AMA: 2018,Jan,8; 2017,Jan,8; 2016,Jan,13; 2015,Mar,7; 2015,Jan,16

29827 **with rotator cuff repair**

EXCLUDES *Distal clavicle excision (29824)*
Open surgery or mini open repair (23412)
Subacromial decompression (29826)

30.9 30.9 FUD 090 J A2 80 50

AMA: 2018,Jan,8; 2017,Jan,8; 2016,Jul,8; 2016,Jan,13; 2015,Mar,7; 2015,Jan,16

29828 **biceps tenodesis**

EXCLUDES *Arthroscopy, shoulder, diagnostic, with or without synovial biopsy (29805)*
Arthroscopy, shoulder, surgical; debridement, limited (29822)
Arthroscopy, shoulder, surgical; synovectomy, partial (29820)
Tenodesis long tendon biceps (23430)

26.5 26.5 FUD 090 J G2 80 50

AMA: 2018,Jan,8; 2017,Jan,8; 2016,Jul,8; 2016,Jan,13; 2015,Mar,7; 2015,Jan,16

29830 **Arthroscopy, elbow, diagnostic, with or without synovial biopsy (separate procedure)**

13.1 13.1 FUD 090 J A2 50

AMA: 2018,Jan,8; 2017,Jan,8; 2016,Jan,13; 2015,Jan,16

29834 **Arthroscopy, elbow, surgical; with removal of loose body or foreign body**

13.9 13.9 FUD 090 J A2 80 50

AMA: 2018,Jan,8; 2017,Jan,8; 2016,Jan,13; 2015,Jan,16

29835 **synovectomy, partial**

14.4 14.4 FUD 090 J A2 80 50

AMA: 2018,Jan,8; 2017,Jan,8; 2016,Jan,13; 2015,Jan,16

29836 **synovectomy, complete**

16.8 16.8 FUD 090 J A2 80 50

AMA: 2018,Jan,8; 2017,Jan,8; 2016,Jan,13; 2015,Jan,16

29837 **debridement, limited**

15.2 15.2 FUD 090 J A2 80 50

AMA: 2018,Jan,8; 2017,Jan,8; 2016,Jan,13; 2015,Jan,16

29838 **debridement, extensive**

17.0 17.0 FUD 090 J A2 80 50

AMA: 2018,Jan,8; 2017,Jan,8; 2016,Jan,13; 2015,Jan,16

29840 **Arthroscopy, wrist, diagnostic, with or without synovial biopsy (separate procedure)**

12.9 12.9 FUD 090 J A2 80 50

AMA: 2018,Jan,8; 2017,Jan,8; 2016,Jan,13; 2015,Jan,16

29843 **Arthroscopy, wrist, surgical; for infection, lavage and drainage**

14.0 14.0 FUD 090 J A2 80 50

AMA: 2018,Jan,8; 2017,Jan,8; 2016,Jan,13; 2015,Jan,16

29844 **synovectomy, partial**

14.2 14.2 FUD 090 J A2 80 50

AMA: 2018,Jan,8; 2017,Jan,8; 2016,Jan,13; 2015,Jan,16

29845 **synovectomy, complete**

16.8 16.8 FUD 090 J A2 80 50

AMA: 2018,Jan,8; 2017,Jan,8; 2016,Jan,13; 2015,Jan,16

29846 **excision and/or repair of triangular fibrocartilage and/or joint debridement**

15.0 15.0 FUD 090 J A2 80 50

AMA: 2018,Jan,8; 2017,Jan,8; 2016,Jan,13; 2015,Jan,16

29847 **internal fixation for fracture or instability**

15.6 15.6 FUD 090 J A2 80 50

AMA: 2018,Jan,8; 2017,Jan,8; 2016,Jan,13; 2015,Jan,16

29848 **Endoscopy, wrist, surgical, with release of transverse carpal ligament**

EXCLUDES *Open surgery (64721)*
Tissue expander, other than breast (11960)

14.7 14.7 FUD 090 J A2 50

AMA: 2018,Apr,10; 2018,Jan,8; 2017,Jan,8; 2017,Jan,6; 2016,Jan,13; 2015,Jul,10; 2015,Jan,16

29850 **Arthroscopically aided treatment of intercondylar spine(s) and/or tuberosity fracture(s) of the knee, with or without manipulation; without internal or external fixation (includes arthroscopy)**

17.9 17.9 FUD 090 J A2 80 50

AMA: 2018,Jan,8; 2017,Jan,8; 2016,Jan,13; 2015,Jan,16

29851 **with internal or external fixation (includes arthroscopy)**

EXCLUDES *Bone graft (20900, 20902)*

26.8 26.8 FUD 090 J A2 80 50

AMA: 2018,Jan,8; 2017,Jan,8; 2016,Jan,13; 2015,Jan,16

29855 **Arthroscopically aided treatment of tibial fracture, proximal (plateau); unicondylar, includes internal fixation, when performed (includes arthroscopy)**

EXCLUDES *Bone graft (20900, 20902)*

22.5 22.5 FUD 090 J J8 80 50

AMA: 2019,Nov,13; 2018,Sep,14; 2018,Jan,8; 2017,Jan,8; 2016,Jan,13; 2015,Jan,16

29856 **bicondylar, includes internal fixation, when performed (includes arthroscopy)**

EXCLUDES *Bone graft (20900, 20902)*

28.6 28.6 FUD 090 J J8 80 50

AMA: 2018,Jan,8; 2017,Jan,8; 2016,Jan,13; 2015,Jan,16

29860 **Arthroscopy, hip, diagnostic with or without synovial biopsy (separate procedure)**

19.2 19.2 FUD 090 J A2 80 50

AMA: 2018,Jan,8; 2017,Jan,8; 2016,Jan,13; 2015,Jan,16

29861 **Arthroscopy, hip, surgical; with removal of loose body or foreign body**

20.8 20.8 FUD 090 J A2 80 50

AMA: 2018,Jan,8; 2017,Jan,8; 2016,Jan,13; 2015,Jan,16

29862 **with debridement/shaving of articular cartilage (chondroplasty), abrasion arthroplasty, and/or resection of labrum**

23.4 23.4 FUD 090 J A2 80 50

AMA: 2018,Jan,8; 2017,Jan,8; 2016,Jan,13; 2015,Jan,16

29863 **with synovectomy**
23.2 23.2 FUD 090 J A2 80 50
AMA: 2018,Jan,8; 2017,Jan,8; 2016,Jan,13; 2015,Jan,16

29914 **with femoroplasty (ie, treatment of cam lesion)**
INCLUDES Chondroplasty (29862)
Synovectomy (29863)
28.7 28.7 FUD 090 J G2 80 50
AMA: 2018,Jan,8; 2017,Jan,8; 2016,Jan,13; 2015,Jan,16

29915 **with acetabuloplasty (ie, treatment of pincer lesion)**
INCLUDES Chondroplasty (29862)
Synovectomy (29863)
29.5 29.5 FUD 090 J G2 80 50
AMA: 2018,Jan,8; 2017,Jan,8; 2016,Jan,13; 2015,Jan,16

29916 **with labral repair**
INCLUDES Acetabuloplasty ([29915])
Chondroplasty (29862)
Synovectomy (29863)
29.5 29.5 FUD 090 J G2 80 50
AMA: 2018,Jan,8; 2017,Jan,8; 2016,Jan,13; 2015,Jan,16

29866 **Arthroscopy, knee, surgical; osteochondral autograft(s) (eg, mosaicplasty) (includes harvesting of the autograft[s])**
EXCLUDES *Open osteochondral autograft knee (27416)*
Procedures performed at same surgical session (29870-29871, 29875, 29884)
Procedures performed in same compartment (29874, 29877, 29879, 29885-29887)
30.3 30.3 FUD 090 J G2 80 50
AMA: 2018,Jan,8; 2017,Jan,8; 2016,Jan,13; 2015,Jan,16

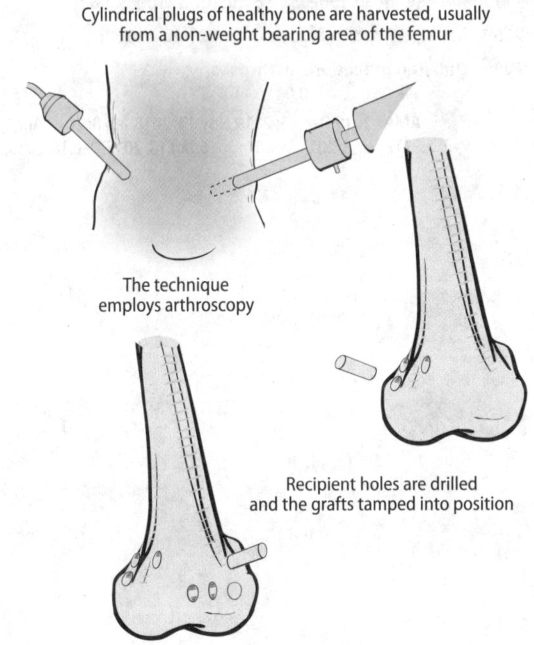

Cylindrical plugs of healthy bone are harvested, usually from a non-weight bearing area of the femur
The technique employs arthroscopy
Recipient holes are drilled and the grafts tamped into position

29867 **osteochondral allograft (eg, mosaicplasty)**
EXCLUDES *Procedures performed at same surgical session (27415, 27570, 29870-29871, 29875, 29884)*
Procedures performed in same compartment (29874, 29877, 29879, 29885-29887)
36.9 36.9 FUD 090 J J8 80 50
AMA: 2018,Jan,8; 2017,Jan,8; 2016,Jan,13; 2015,Jan,16

29868 **meniscal transplantation (includes arthrotomy for meniscal insertion), medial or lateral**
EXCLUDES *Procedures performed at same surgical session (29870-29871, 29875, 29880, 29883-29884)*
Procedures performed in same compartment (29874, 29877, 29881-29882)
48.4 48.4 FUD 090 J 80 50
AMA: 2018,Jan,8; 2017,Jan,8; 2016,Jan,13; 2015,Jan,16

29870 **Arthroscopy, knee, diagnostic, with or without synovial biopsy (separate procedure)**
EXCLUDES *Open procedure (27412)*
11.7 16.4 FUD 090 J A2 50
AMA: 2019,Nov,14; 2018,Jan,8; 2017,Jan,8; 2016,Jan,13; 2015,Jan,16

29871 **Arthroscopy, knee, surgical; for infection, lavage and drainage**
EXCLUDES *Injection contrast for knee arthrography (27369)*
Osteochondral graft (27412, 27415, 29866-29867)
14.8 14.8 FUD 090 J A2 50
AMA: 2019,Aug,7; 2018,Jan,8; 2017,Jan,8; 2016,Jan,13; 2015,Aug,6; 2015,Jan,16

29873 **with lateral release**
EXCLUDES *Open procedure (27425)*
15.2 15.2 FUD 090 J A2 50
AMA: 2018,Jan,8; 2017,Jan,8; 2016,Jan,13; 2015,Nov,7; 2015,Jan,16

29874 **for removal of loose body or foreign body (eg, osteochondritis dissecans fragmentation, chondral fragmentation)**
15.5 15.5 FUD 090 J A2 80 50
AMA: 2018,Jan,8; 2017,Jan,8; 2016,Jan,13; 2015,Jan,16

29875 **synovectomy, limited (eg, plica or shelf resection) (separate procedure)**
14.3 14.3 FUD 090 J A2 80 50
AMA: 2018,Jan,8; 2017,Jan,8; 2016,Jan,13; 2016,Jan,11; 2015,Jan,16

29876 **synovectomy, major, 2 or more compartments (eg, medial or lateral)**
18.8 18.8 FUD 090 J A2 50
AMA: 2018,Jan,8; 2017,Jan,8; 2016,Jan,13; 2015,Jan,16

29877 **debridement/shaving of articular cartilage (chondroplasty)**
EXCLUDES *Arthroscopy, knee, surgical; with meniscectomy (29880-29881)*
17.9 17.9 FUD 090 J A2 80 50
AMA: 2020,May,13; 2018,Jan,8; 2017,Jan,8; 2016,Jan,13; 2015,Jan,16

29879 **abrasion arthroplasty (includes chondroplasty where necessary) or multiple drilling or microfracture**
19.0 19.0 FUD 090 J A2 80 50
AMA: 2018,Jan,8; 2017,Jan,8; 2016,Jan,13; 2015,Jan,16

29880 **with meniscectomy (medial AND lateral, including any meniscal shaving) including debridement/shaving of articular cartilage (chondroplasty), same or separate compartment(s), when performed**
16.1 16.1 FUD 090 J A2 80 50
AMA: 2018,Jan,8; 2017,Jan,8; 2016,Jan,13; 2015,Jan,16

29881 **with meniscectomy (medial OR lateral, including any meniscal shaving) including debridement/shaving of articular cartilage (chondroplasty), same or separate compartment(s), when performed**
15.5 15.5 FUD 090 J A2 80 50
AMA: 2020,Sep,14; 2020,May,13; 2019,Nov,14; 2018,Jan,8; 2017,Jan,8; 2016,Jan,13; 2016,Jan,11; 2015,Jan,16

29882 with meniscus repair (medial OR lateral)

EXCLUDES *Meniscus transplant (29868)*

🏥 19.9 👤 19.9 **FUD** 090 〔J〕〔A2〕〔50〕▢

AMA: 2019,May,10; 2018,Jan,8; 2017,Jan,8; 2016,Jan,13; 2015,Jan,16

29883 with meniscus repair (medial AND lateral)

EXCLUDES *Meniscus transplant (29868)*

🏥 24.2 👤 24.2 **FUD** 090 〔J〕〔A2〕〔80〕〔50〕▢

AMA: 2018,Jan,8; 2017,Jan,8; 2016,Jan,13; 2015,Jan,16

29884 with lysis of adhesions, with or without manipulation (separate procedure)

🏥 17.8 👤 17.8 **FUD** 090 〔J〕〔A2〕〔80〕〔50〕▢

AMA: 2018,Jan,8; 2017,Jan,8; 2016,Jan,13; 2015,Jan,16

29885 drilling for osteochondritis dissecans with bone grafting, with or without internal fixation (including debridement of base of lesion)

🏥 21.7 👤 21.7 **FUD** 090 〔J〕〔A2〕〔80〕〔50〕▢

AMA: 2018,Jan,8; 2017,Jan,8; 2016,Jan,13; 2015,Jan,16

29886 drilling for intact osteochondritis dissecans lesion

🏥 18.3 👤 18.3 **FUD** 090 〔J〕〔A2〕〔50〕▢

AMA: 2018,Jan,8; 2017,Jan,8; 2016,Jan,13; 2015,Jan,16

29887 drilling for intact osteochondritis dissecans lesion with internal fixation

🏥 21.5 👤 21.5 **FUD** 090 〔J〕〔A2〕〔80〕〔50〕▢

AMA: 2018,Jan,8; 2017,Jan,8; 2016,Jan,13; 2015,Jan,16

29888 Arthroscopically aided anterior cruciate ligament repair/augmentation or reconstruction

🏥 28.3 👤 28.3 **FUD** 090 〔J〕〔J8〕〔80〕〔50〕▢

AMA: 2018,Jan,8; 2017,Jan,8; 2016,Nov,9; 2016,Jan,13; 2015,Jan,16

29889 Arthroscopically aided posterior cruciate ligament repair/augmentation or reconstruction

🏥 35.3 👤 35.3 **FUD** 090 〔J〕〔J8〕〔80〕〔50〕▢

AMA: 2018,Jan,8; 2017,Jan,8; 2016,Jan,13; 2015,Jan,16

29891 Arthroscopy, ankle, surgical, excision of osteochondral defect of talus and/or tibia, including drilling of the defect

🏥 19.3 👤 19.3 **FUD** 090 〔J〕〔A2〕〔80〕〔50〕▢

AMA: 2018,Jan,8; 2017,Jan,8; 2016,Jan,13; 2015,Jan,16

29892 Arthroscopically aided repair of large osteochondritis dissecans lesion, talar dome fracture, or tibial plafond fracture, with or without internal fixation (includes arthroscopy)

🏥 18.7 👤 18.7 **FUD** 090 〔J〕〔A2〕〔80〕〔50〕▢

AMA: 2018,Jan,8; 2017,Jan,8; 2016,Jan,13; 2015,Jan,16

29893 Endoscopic plantar fasciotomy

🏥 12.3 👤 17.8 **FUD** 090 〔J〕〔A2〕〔50〕▢

AMA: 2018,Jan,8; 2017,Jan,8; 2016,Jan,13; 2015,Jan,16

29894 Arthroscopy, ankle (tibiotalar and fibulotalar joints), surgical; with removal of loose body or foreign body

🏥 14.2 👤 14.2 **FUD** 090 〔J〕〔A2〕〔80〕〔50〕▢

AMA: 2018,Jan,8; 2017,Jan,8; 2016,Jan,13; 2015,Jan,16

29895 synovectomy, partial

🏥 13.4 👤 13.4 **FUD** 090 〔J〕〔A2〕〔80〕〔50〕▢

AMA: 2018,Jan,8; 2017,Jan,8; 2016,Jan,13; 2015,Jan,16

29897 debridement, limited

🏥 14.4 👤 14.4 **FUD** 090 〔J〕〔A2〕〔80〕〔50〕▢

AMA: 2018,Jan,8; 2017,Jan,8; 2016,Jan,13; 2015,Jan,16

29898 debridement, extensive

🏥 16.1 👤 16.1 **FUD** 090 〔J〕〔A2〕〔80〕〔50〕▢

AMA: 2018,Jan,8; 2017,Jan,8; 2016,Jan,13; 2015,Jan,16

29899 with ankle arthrodesis

EXCLUDES *Open procedure (27870)*

🏥 29.7 👤 29.7 **FUD** 090 〔J〕〔J8〕〔80〕〔50〕▢

AMA: 2018,Jan,8; 2017,Jan,8; 2016,Jan,13; 2015,Jan,16

29900 Arthroscopy, metacarpophalangeal joint, diagnostic, includes synovial biopsy

EXCLUDES *Arthroscopy, metacarpophalangeal joint, surgical (29901-29902)*

🏥 14.3 👤 14.3 **FUD** 090 〔J〕〔A2〕〔80〕〔50〕▢

AMA: 2018,Jan,8; 2017,Jan,8; 2016,Jan,13; 2015,Jan,16

29901 Arthroscopy, metacarpophalangeal joint, surgical; with debridement

🏥 15.4 👤 15.4 **FUD** 090 〔J〕〔A2〕〔80〕〔50〕▢

AMA: 2018,Jan,8; 2017,Jan,8; 2016,Jan,13; 2015,Jan,16

29902 with reduction of displaced ulnar collateral ligament (eg, Stenar lesion)

🏥 16.4 👤 16.4 **FUD** 090 〔J〕〔A2〕〔80〕〔50〕▢

AMA: 2018,Jan,8; 2017,Jan,8; 2016,Jan,13; 2015,Jan,16

29904 Arthroscopy, subtalar joint, surgical; with removal of loose body or foreign body

🏥 18.3 👤 18.3 **FUD** 090 〔J〕〔02〕〔80〕〔50〕▢

AMA: 2018,Jan,8; 2017,Jan,8; 2016,Jan,13; 2015,Jan,16

29905 with synovectomy

🏥 14.9 👤 14.9 **FUD** 090 〔J〕〔02〕〔80〕〔50〕▢

AMA: 2018,Jan,8; 2017,Jan,8; 2016,Jan,13; 2015,Jan,16

29906 with debridement

🏥 19.5 👤 19.5 **FUD** 090 〔J〕〔02〕〔80〕〔50〕▢

AMA: 2018,Jan,8; 2017,Jan,8; 2016,Jan,13; 2015,Jan,16

29907 with subtalar arthrodesis

🏥 25.3 👤 25.3 **FUD** 090 〔J〕〔J8〕〔80〕〔50〕▢

AMA: 2018,Jan,8; 2017,Jan,8; 2016,Jan,13; 2015,Jan,16

29914 Resequenced code. See code following 29863.

29915 Resequenced code. See code following 29863.

29916 Resequenced code. See code before 29866.

29999 Unlisted procedure, arthroscopy

🏥 0.00 👤 0.00 **FUD** YYY 〔T〕〔80〕〔50〕▢

AMA: 2019,Dec,12; 2019,Nov,13; 2018,Jan,8; 2017,Apr,9; 2017,Jan,8; 2016,Dec,16; 2016,Jan,13; 2015,Dec,16; 2015,Jan,16

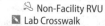

30000-30115 I&D, Biopsy, Excision Procedures of the Nose

30000 Drainage abscess or hematoma, nasal, internal approach

EXCLUDES *Incision and drainage (10060, 10140)*

3.38 | 7.18 | FUD 010 | T P2 80

AMA: 2005,May,13-14; 1994,Spr,24

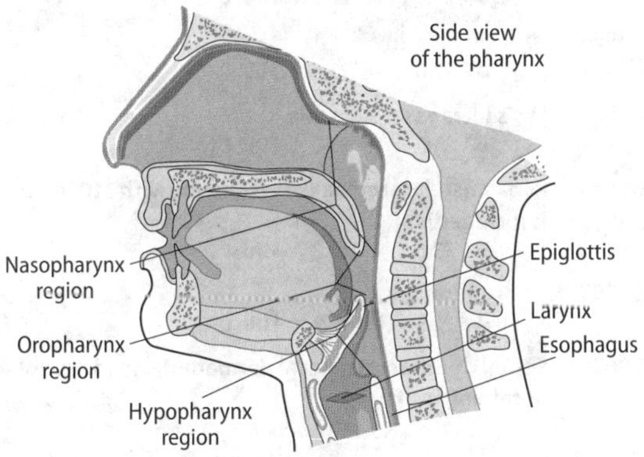

Side view of the pharynx
Nasopharynx region
Oropharynx region
Hypopharynx region
Epiglottis
Larynx
Esophagus

The nasopharynx is the membranous passage above the level of the soft palate; the oropharynx is the region between the soft palate and the upper edge of the epiglottis; the hypopharynx is the region of the epiglottis to the juncture of the larynx and esophagus; the three regions are collectively known as the pharynx

30020 Drainage abscess or hematoma, nasal septum

EXCLUDES *Lateral rhinotomy incision (30118, 30320)*

3.37 | 6.90 | FUD 010 | T P3

30100 Biopsy, intranasal

EXCLUDES *Superficial biopsy nose (11102-11107)*

1.91 | 4.03 | FUD 000 | T P3

AMA: 2019,Jan,9

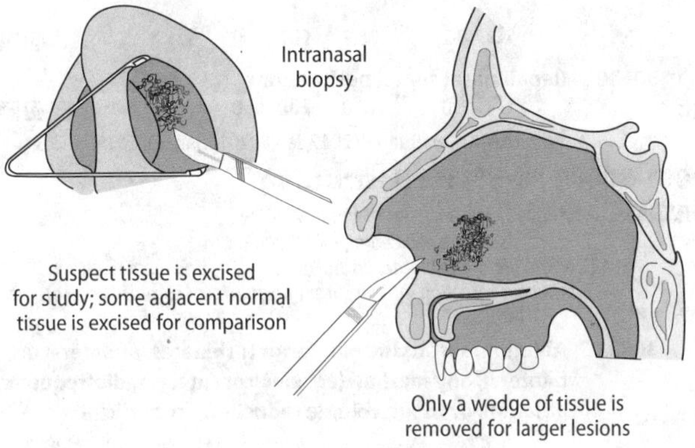

Intranasal biopsy
Suspect tissue is excised for study; some adjacent normal tissue is excised for comparison
Only a wedge of tissue is removed for larger lesions

30110 Excision, nasal polyp(s), simple

3.70 | 6.82 | FUD 010 | T P3 50

30115 Excision, nasal polyp(s), extensive

12.7 | 12.7 | FUD 090 | J A2 50

30117-30118 Destruction Procedures Nose

CMS: 100-03,140.5 Laser Procedures

30117 Excision or destruction (eg, laser), intranasal lesion; internal approach

9.47 | 26.4 | FUD 090 | J A2

AMA: 2020,Sep,14; 2019,Nov,14; 2019,Jul,10

30118 external approach (lateral rhinotomy)

22.0 | 22.0 | FUD 090 | J A2

30120-30140 Excision Procedures Nose, Turbinate

30120 Excision or surgical planing of skin of nose for rhinophyma

12.3 | 14.6 | FUD 090 | J A2

AMA: 2018,Jan,8; 2017,Jan,8; 2016,Jan,13; 2015,Jan,16

30124 Excision dermoid cyst, nose; simple, skin, subcutaneous

8.33 | 8.33 | FUD 090 | T R2

30125 complex, under bone or cartilage

17.5 | 17.5 | FUD 090 | J A2 80

30130 Excision inferior turbinate, partial or complete, any method

EXCLUDES *Ablation, soft tissue inferior turbinates, unilateral or bilateral, any method (30801-30802)*
Excision middle/superior turbinate(s) (30999)
Fracture nasal inferior turbinate(s), therapeutic (30930)

11.2 | 11.2 | FUD 090 | J A2 50

AMA: 2018,Jan,8; 2017,Jan,8; 2016,Jan,13; 2015,Jan,16

30140 Submucous resection inferior turbinate, partial or complete, any method

EXCLUDES *Ablation, soft tissue inferior turbinates, unilateral or bilateral, any method (30801-30802)*
Endoscopic resection concha bullosa middle turbinate (31240)
Fracture nasal inferior turbinate(s), therapeutic (30930)
Submucous resection:
Nasal septum (30520)
Superior or middle turbinate (30999)

5.12 | 7.92 | FUD 000 | J A2 50

AMA: 2020,Jan,12; 2018,Jan,8; 2017,Jan,8; 2016,Jan,13; 2015,Jan,16

30150-30160 Surgical Removal: Nose

EXCLUDES *Reconstruction and/or closure (primary or delayed primary intention) (13151-13160, 14060-14302, 15120-15121, 15260-15261, 15760, 20900-20912)*

30150 Rhinectomy; partial

22.4 | 22.4 | FUD 090 | J A2

30160 total

22.6 | 22.6 | FUD 090 | J A2 80

30200-30320 Turbinate Injection, Removal Foreign Substance in the Nose

30200 Injection into turbinate(s), therapeutic

1.66 | 3.18 | FUD 000 | T P3

AMA: 2018,Jan,8; 2017,Jan,8; 2016,Jan,13; 2015,Jan,16

30210 Displacement therapy (Proetz type)

2.82 | 4.24 | FUD 010 | T P3

AMA: 2018,Jan,8; 2017,Jan,8; 2016,Jan,13; 2015,Jan,16

30220 Insertion, nasal septal prosthesis (button)

3.57 | 8.70 | FUD 010 | T A2

30300 Removal foreign body, intranasal; office type procedure

3.23 | 5.40 | FUD 010 | Q1 N1

AMA: 2018,Jan,8; 2017,Jan,8; 2016,Jan,13; 2015,Jan,16

30310 requiring general anesthesia

5.80 | 5.80 | FUD 010 | J A2 80

30320 by lateral rhinotomy

13.2 | 13.2 | FUD 090 | T A2 80

30400-30630 Reconstruction or Repair of Nose

EXCLUDES *Harvesting bone/tissue/fat grafts ([15769], 15773-15774, 20900-20924, 21210)*
Liposuction for autologous fat grafting (15773-15774)

30400 Rhinoplasty, primary; lateral and alar cartilages and/or elevation of nasal tip

INCLUDES Carpue's operation

EXCLUDES *Reconstruction columella (13151-13153)*

34.3 | 34.3 | FUD 090 | J A2 80

30410 complete, external parts including bony pyramid, lateral and alar cartilages, and/or elevation of nasal tip

39.8 | 39.8 | FUD 090 | J A2 80

30420 **including major septal repair**
40.3 40.3 **FUD** 090 J A2
AMA: 2018,Jan,8; 2017,Nov,11; 2017,Jan,8; 2016,Jul,8

30430 **Rhinoplasty, secondary; minor revision (small amount of nasal tip work)**
29.7 29.7 **FUD** 090 J A2 80

30435 **intermediate revision (bony work with osteotomies)**
37.6 37.6 **FUD** 090 J A2 80

30450 **major revision (nasal tip work and osteotomies)**
49.8 49.8 **FUD** 090 J A2 80

30460 **Rhinoplasty for nasal deformity secondary to congenital cleft lip and/or palate, including columellar lengthening; tip only**
23.5 23.5 **FUD** 090 J A2 80
AMA: 2018,Jan,8; 2017,Jan,8; 2016,Jan,13; 2015,Jan,16

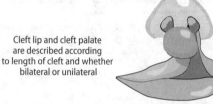

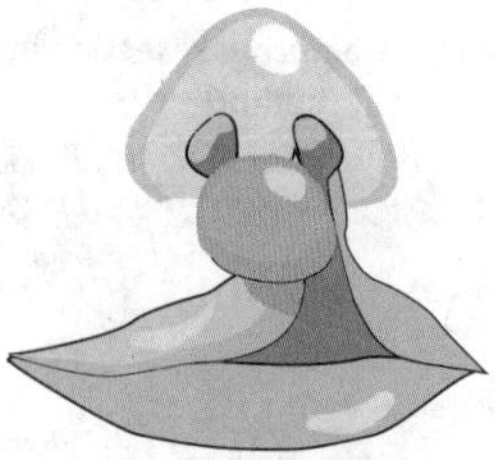
Cleft lip and cleft palate are described according to length of cleft and whether bilateral or unilateral

Complete unilateral cleft lip

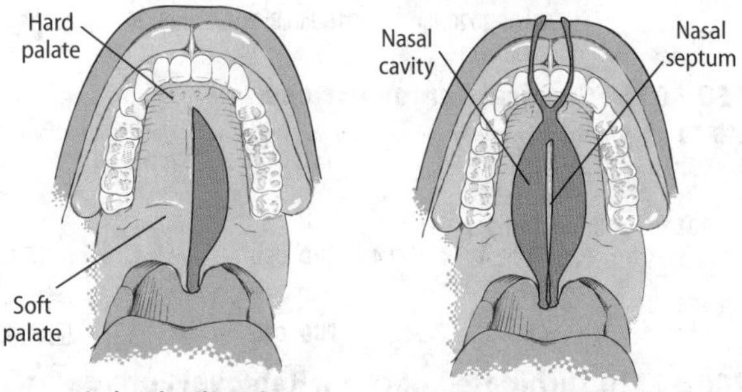
Hard palate
Soft palate
Nasal cavity
Nasal septum

Isolated unilateral complete cleft of palate

Bilateral complete cleft of lip and palate

30462 **tip, septum, osteotomies**
45.1 45.1 **FUD** 090 J A2 80
AMA: 2018,Jan,8; 2017,Jan,8; 2016,Jan,13; 2015,Jan,16

30465 **Repair of nasal vestibular stenosis (eg, spreader grafting, lateral nasal wall reconstruction)**
INCLUDES Bilateral procedure
EXCLUDES *Harvesting ear cartilage graft, autogenous (21235)*
Repair nasal valve or vestibular lateral wall collapse with implants same side during same operative session (30468)
Repair nasal vestibular stenosis without graft, implant, or reconstruction lateral wall (30999)
Code also modifier 52 for unilateral procedure
28.5 28.5 **FUD** 090 J A2 80
AMA: 2020,Sep,14

● **30468** **Repair of nasal valve collapse with subcutaneous/submucosal lateral wall implant(s)**
INCLUDES Bilateral procedure
EXCLUDES *Repair nasal vestibular stenosis same side during same operative session (30465)*
Repair nasal vestibular stenosis without graft, implant, or reconstruction lateral wall (30999)
Code also modifier 52 for unilateral procedure

30520 **Septoplasty or submucous resection, with or without cartilage scoring, contouring or replacement with graft**
EXCLUDES *Turbinate resection (30140)*
18.0 18.0 **FUD** 090 J A2
AMA: 2019,Jul,10; 2018,Jan,8; 2017,Jan,8; 2016,Jan,13; 2015,Jul,10; 2015,Jan,16

30540 **Repair choanal atresia; intranasal**
20.2 20.2 **FUD** 090 63 J A2 80

30545 **transpalatine**
27.6 27.6 **FUD** 090 63 J A2 80

30560 **Lysis intranasal synechia**
3.95 7.96 **FUD** 010 T A2

30580 **Repair fistula; oromaxillary (combine with 31030 if antrotomy is included)**
13.6 17.8 **FUD** 090 J A2

30600 **oronasal**
12.3 16.8 **FUD** 090 J A2 80

30620 **Septal or other intranasal dermatoplasty (does not include obtaining graft)**

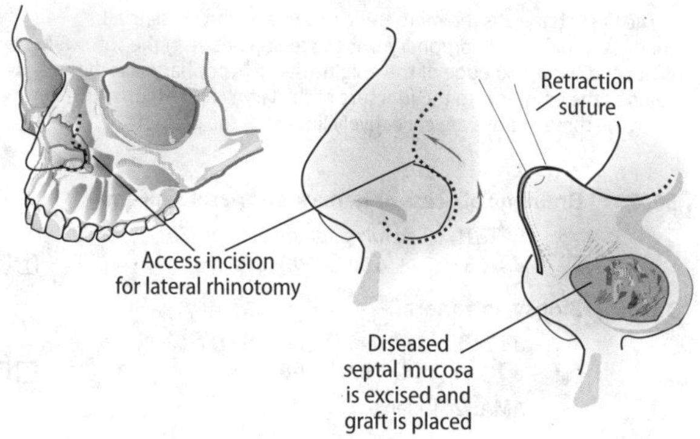
Retraction suture
Access incision for lateral rhinotomy
Diseased septal mucosa is excised and graft is placed

18.2 18.2 **FUD** 090 J A2

30630 **Repair nasal septal perforations**
18.0 18.0 **FUD** 090 J A2 80
AMA: 2018,Jan,8; 2017,Jan,8; 2016,Jan,13; 2015,Jan,16

30801-30802 Turbinate Destruction

EXCLUDES *Ablation middle/superior turbinates (30999)*
Cautery to stop nasal bleeding (30901-30906)
Excision inferior turbinate, partial or complete, any method (30130)
Submucous resection inferior turbinate, partial or complete, any method (30140)

30801 **Ablation, soft tissue of inferior turbinates, unilateral or bilateral, any method (eg, electrocautery, radiofrequency ablation, or tissue volume reduction); superficial**
EXCLUDES *Submucosal ablation inferior turbinates (30802)*
4.10 6.18 **FUD** 010 T A2
AMA: 2019,Jul,10

30802 **intramural (ie, submucosal)**
EXCLUDES *Superficial ablation inferior turbinates (30801)*
5.58 7.86 **FUD** 010 T A2
AMA: 2019,Jul,10; 2018,Jan,8; 2017,Jan,8; 2016,Jan,13; 2015,Jan,16

30901-30920 Control Nose Bleed

30901 **Control nasal hemorrhage, anterior, simple (limited cautery and/or packing) any method**
1.64 4.09 **FUD** 000 Q1 N1 50
AMA: 2020,Jul,13

30903 **Control nasal hemorrhage, anterior, complex (extensive cautery and/or packing) any method**
2.28 6.49 **FUD** 000 T A2 50
AMA: 1990,Win,4

30905 **Control nasal hemorrhage, posterior, with posterior nasal packs and/or cautery, any method; initial**
3.07 9.64 FUD 000 T A2
AMA: 2018,Jan,8; 2017,Jan,8; 2016,Jan,13; 2015,Jan,16

30906 **subsequent**
3.92 10.0 FUD 000 T A2
AMA: 2002,May,7

30915 **Ligation arteries; ethmoidal**
EXCLUDES *External carotid artery (37600)*
16.7 16.7 FUD 090 T A2

30920 **internal maxillary artery, transantral**
EXCLUDES *External carotid artery (37600)*
24.3 24.3 FUD 090 T A2

30930-30999 Other and Unlisted Procedures of Nose

30930 **Fracture nasal inferior turbinate(s), therapeutic**
EXCLUDES *Excision inferior turbinate, partial or complete, any method (30130)*
Fracture superior or middle turbinate(s) (30999)
Submucous resection inferior turbinate, partial or complete, any method (30140)
3.43 3.43 FUD 010 J A2
AMA: 2018,Jan,8; 2017,Nov,11; 2017,Jan,8; 2016,Jul,8; 2016,Jan,13; 2015,Jan,16

30999 **Unlisted procedure, nose**
0.00 0.00 FUD YYY T 80
AMA: 2020,Sep,14; 2019,Nov,14; 2018,Jan,8; 2017,Jan,8; 2016,Jan,13; 2015,Jan,16

31000-31230 Opening Sinuses

31000 **Lavage by cannulation; maxillary sinus (antrum puncture or natural ostium)**
3.02 5.17 FUD 010 T P2 50
AMA: 2018,Jan,8; 2017,Jan,8; 2016,Jan,13; 2015,Jan,16

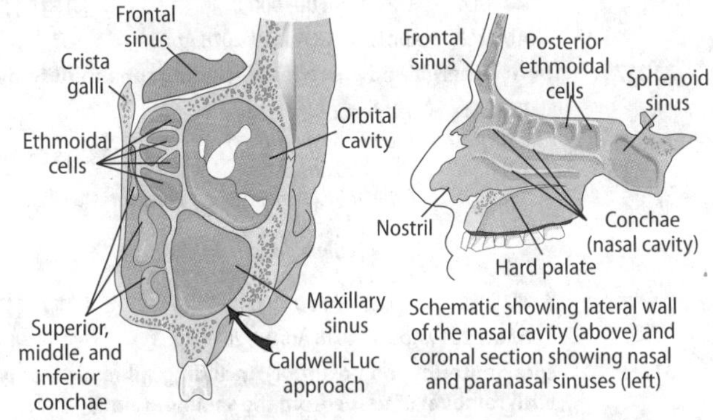

Schematic showing lateral wall of the nasal cavity (above) and coronal section showing nasal and paranasal sinuses (left)

31002 **sphenoid sinus**
5.39 5.39 FUD 010 T R2 80 50

31020 **Sinusotomy, maxillary (antrotomy); intranasal**
10.4 13.6 FUD 090 J A2 50

31030 **radical (Caldwell-Luc) without removal of antrochoanal polyps**
14.7 18.4 FUD 090 J A2 50

31032 **radical (Caldwell-Luc) with removal of antrochoanal polyps**
16.5 16.5 FUD 090 J A2 50

31040 **Pterygomaxillary fossa surgery, any approach**
EXCLUDES *Transantral ligation internal maxillary artery (30920)*
22.0 22.0 FUD 090 J R2 50

31050 **Sinusotomy, sphenoid, with or without biopsy;**
14.1 14.1 FUD 090 J A2 50

31051 **with mucosal stripping or removal of polyp(s)**
19.0 19.0 FUD 090 J A2 50

31070 **Sinusotomy frontal; external, simple (trephine operation)**
INCLUDES Killian operation
EXCLUDES *Intranasal frontal sinusotomy (31276)*
12.9 12.9 FUD 090 J A2 50

31075 **transorbital, unilateral (for mucocele or osteoma, Lynch type)**
22.8 22.8 FUD 090 J A2 80 50

31080 **obliterative without osteoplastic flap, brow incision (includes ablation)**
INCLUDES Ridell sinusotomy
30.0 30.0 FUD 090 J A2 80 50

31081 **obliterative, without osteoplastic flap, coronal incision (includes ablation)**
32.3 32.3 FUD 090 J A2 80 50

31084 **obliterative, with osteoplastic flap, brow incision**
33.5 33.5 FUD 090 J A2 80 50

31085 **obliterative, with osteoplastic flap, coronal incision**
34.6 34.6 FUD 090 J A2 80 50

31086 **nonobliterative, with osteoplastic flap, brow incision**
32.6 32.6 FUD 090 J A2 80 50

31087 **nonobliterative, with osteoplastic flap, coronal incision**
31.2 31.2 FUD 090 J A2 80 50

31090 **Sinusotomy, unilateral, 3 or more paranasal sinuses (frontal, maxillary, ethmoid, sphenoid)**
30.3 30.3 FUD 090 J A2 50
AMA: 1998,Nov,1; 1997,Nov,1

31200 **Ethmoidectomy; intranasal, anterior**
16.7 16.7 FUD 090 J A2 50
AMA: 2018,Jan,8; 2017,Jan,8; 2016,Feb,10

31201 **intranasal, total**
21.9 21.9 FUD 090 J A2 50
AMA: 2018,Jan,8; 2017,Jan,8; 2016,Feb,10

31205 **extranasal, total**
26.3 26.3 FUD 090 J A2 80 50
AMA: 2018,Jan,8; 2017,Jan,8; 2016,Feb,10

31225 **Maxillectomy; without orbital exenteration**
52.1 52.1 FUD 090 C 80 50

31230 **with orbital exenteration (en bloc)**
EXCLUDES *Orbital exenteration without maxillectomy (65110-65114)*
Skin grafts (15120-15121)
58.3 58.3 FUD 090 C 80 50

31231-31235 Nasal Endoscopy, Diagnostic

INCLUDES Complete sinus exam (e.g., nasal cavity, turbinates, sphenoethmoidal recess)
Code also stereotactic navigation, when performed (61782)

31231 **Nasal endoscopy, diagnostic, unilateral or bilateral (separate procedure)**
1.82 5.48 FUD 000 T P2
AMA: 2018,Apr,3; 2018,Jan,8; 2017,Jul,7; 2017,Jan,8; 2017,Jan,6; 2016,Dec,13; 2016,Feb,10; 2016,Jan,13; 2015,Jan,16

31233 **Nasal/sinus endoscopy, diagnostic; with maxillary sinusoscopy (via inferior meatus or canine fossa puncture)**
EXCLUDES *When performed on same side:*
Dilation of maxillary sinus ostium (31295)
Maxillary antrostomy (31256, 31267)
3.87 7.41 FUD 000 T A2 80 50
AMA: 2018,Apr,3; 2018,Jan,8; 2017,Jan,8; 2016,Jan,13; 2015,Jan,16

31235 **with sphenoid sinusoscopy (via puncture of sphenoidal face or cannulation of ostium)**

EXCLUDES *Insertion drug-eluting implant performed with biopsy, debridement, or polypectomy (31237)*
Insertion drug-eluting implant without other nasal/sinus endoscopic procedure (31299)
When performed on same side:
Sinus dilation (31297-31298)
Sphenoidotomy (31287-31288)
Total ethmoidectomy with sphenoidotomy ([31257, 31259])

4.54   8.49   **FUD** 000   J A2 80 50

AMA: 2018,Apr,3; 2018,Jan,8; 2017,Jan,8; 2016,Jan,13; 2015,Jan,16

31237-31253 [31253] Nasal Endoscopy, Surgical

INCLUDES Diagnostic nasal/sinus endoscopy
Code also stereotactic navigation, when performed (61782)

31237 **Nasal/sinus endoscopy, surgical; with biopsy, polypectomy or debridement (separate procedure)**

EXCLUDES *When performed on same side:*
Frontal sinus exploration (31276)
Maxillary antrostomy (31256, 31267)
Nasal hemorrhage control (31238)
Optic nerve decompression (31294)
Orbital wall decompression, medial and/or inferior (31292-31293)
Other total ethmoidectomy procedures ([31253], 31255, [31257], [31259])
Partial ethmoidectomy (31254)
Repair CSF leak (31290-31291)
Sphenoidotomy (31287-31288)

4.54   7.21   **FUD** 000   J A2 50

AMA: 2020,Jan,12; 2019,Jul,7; 2019,Apr,10; 2018,Apr,3; 2018,Jan,8; 2017,Jan,8; 2016,Feb,10; 2016,Jan,13; 2015,Jan,16; 2015,Jan,13

31238 **with control of nasal hemorrhage**

EXCLUDES *When performed on same side:*
Biopsy, polypectomy, or debridement (31237)
Sphenopalatine artery ligation (31241)

4.80   7.17   **FUD** 000   J A2 80 50

AMA: 2018,Apr,3; 2018,Jan,8; 2017,Jan,8; 2016,Jan,13; 2015,Jan,16

31239 **with dacryocystorhinostomy**

17.4   17.4   **FUD** 010   J A2 80 50

AMA: 2018,Apr,3; 2018,Jan,8; 2017,Jan,8; 2016,Jan,13; 2015,Jan,16

31240 **with concha bullosa resection**

4.52   4.52   **FUD** 000   J A2 80 50

AMA: 2018,Apr,3; 2018,Jan,8; 2017,Jan,8; 2016,Feb,10; 2016,Jan,13; 2015,Jan,16

31241 **with ligation of sphenopalatine artery**

EXCLUDES *When performed on same side:*
Nasal hemorrhage control (31238)

12.7   12.7   **FUD** 000   C 80 50

AMA: 2018,Apr,3

31253 **Resequenced code. See code following 31255.**

31254-31259 [31253, 31257, 31259] Nasal Endoscopy with Ethmoid Removal

INCLUDES Diagnostic nasal/sinus endoscopy
Sinusotomy, when applicable
EXCLUDES *When performed on same side:*
Biopsy, polypectomy, or debridement (31237)
Optic nerve decompression (31294)
Orbital wall decompression, medial, and/or inferior (31292-31293)
Repair CSF leak (31290-31291)
Code also stereotactic navigation, when performed (61782)

31254 **Nasal/sinus endoscopy, surgical with ethmoidectomy; partial (anterior)**

EXCLUDES *When performed on same side:*
Other total ethmoidectomy procedures (31253, 31255, [31257], [31259])

7.01   11.7   **FUD** 000   J A2 50

AMA: 2019,Apr,10; 2018,Apr,3; 2018,Jan,8; 2017,Jan,8; 2016,Feb,10; 2016,Jan,13; 2015,Jan,16

31255 **with ethmoidectomy, total (anterior and posterior)**

EXCLUDES *When performed on same side:*
Frontal sinus exploration (31276)
Other total ethmoidectomy procedures (31253, [31257], [31259])
Partial ethmoidectomy (31254)
Sphenoidotomy (31287-31288)

9.31   9.31   **FUD** 000   J A2 50

AMA: 2019,Apr,10; 2018,Apr,3; 2018,Apr,10; 2018,Jan,8; 2017,Jan,8; 2016,Feb,10; 2016,Jan,13; 2015,Jan,16

31253 **total (anterior and posterior), including frontal sinus exploration, with removal of tissue from frontal sinus, when performed**

EXCLUDES *When performed on same side:*
Dilation sinus (31296, 31298)
Frontal sinus exploration (31276)
Partial ethmoidectomy (31254)
Total ethmoidectomy (31255)

14.4   14.4   **FUD** 000   J G2 50

AMA: 2019,Apr,10; 2018,Apr,10; 2018,Apr,3

31257 **total (anterior and posterior), including sphenoidotomy**

EXCLUDES *When performed on same side:*
Diagnostic sphenoid sinusoscopy (31235)
Dilation sinus (31297-31298)
Other total ethmoidectomy procedures (31255, [31259])
Partial ethmoidectomy (31254)
Sphenoidotomy (31287-31288)

12.8   12.8   **FUD** 000   J G2 50

AMA: 2019,Apr,10; 2018,Apr,10; 2018,Apr,3

31259 **total (anterior and posterior), including sphenoidotomy, with removal of tissue from the sphenoid sinus**

EXCLUDES *When performed on same side:*
Diagnostic sphenoid sinusoscopy (31235)
Dilation sinus (31297-31298)
Other total ethmoidectomy procedures (31255, [31257])
Partial ethmoidectomy (31254)
Sphenoidotomy (31287-31288)

13.6   13.6   **FUD** 000   J G2 50

AMA: 2019,Apr,10; 2018,Apr,3

31256-31267 [31257, 31259] Nasal Endoscopy with Maxillary Procedures

INCLUDES Diagnostic nasal/sinus endoscopy
Sinusotomy, when applicable

EXCLUDES *When performed on same side:*
Biopsy, polypectomy, or debridement (31237)
Dilation maxillary sinus ostium (31295)
Maxillary sinusoscopy (31233)

Code also stereotactic navigation, when performed (61782)

31256 **Nasal/sinus endoscopy, surgical, with maxillary antrostomy;**

EXCLUDES *When performed on the same side:*
Maxillary antrostomy with removal of tissue from maxillary sinus (31267)

5.19 5.19 **FUD** 000 J A2 50

AMA: 2019,Apr,10; 2018,Apr,3; 2018,Apr,10; 2018,Jan,8; 2017,Jan,8; 2016,Jan,13; 2015,Jan,16

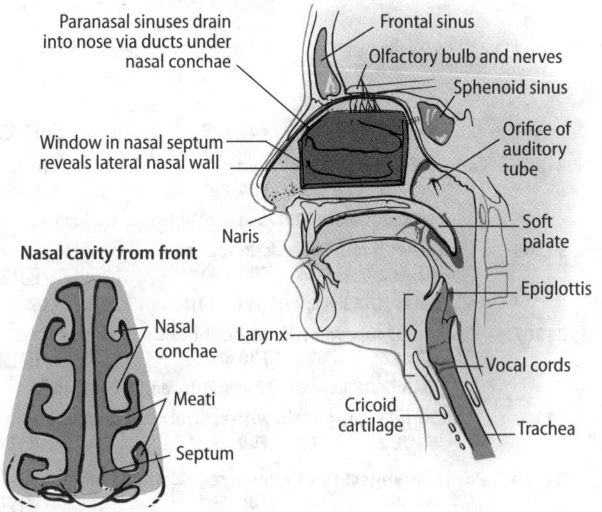

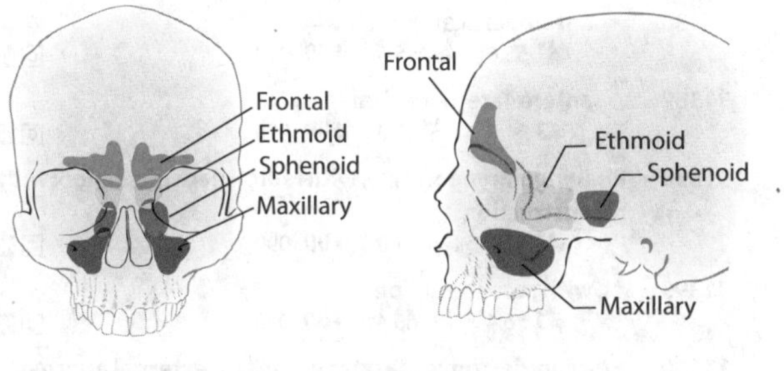

31257 **Resequenced code. See code following 31255.**

31259 **Resequenced code. See code following 31255.**

31267 **with removal of tissue from maxillary sinus**

EXCLUDES *When performed on same side:*
Maxillary antrostomy without removal tissue (31256)

7.61 7.61 **FUD** 000 J A2 50

AMA: 2019,Apr,10; 2018,Apr,3; 2018,Jan,8; 2017,Jan,8; 2016,Jan,13; 2015,Jan,16

31276 Nasal Endoscopy with Frontal Sinus Examination

INCLUDES Diagnostic nasal/sinus endoscopy
Sinusotomy, when applicable

EXCLUDES *When performed on same side:*
Biopsy, polypectomy, or debridement (31237)
Dilation frontal or frontal and sphenoid sinus (31296, 31298)
Other total ethmoidectomy procedures (31253, 31255)

Code also stereotactic navigation, when performed (61782)

31276 **Nasal/sinus endoscopy, surgical, with frontal sinus exploration, including removal of tissue from frontal sinus, when performed**

10.9 10.9 **FUD** 000 J A2 50

AMA: 2019,Apr,10; 2018,Apr,3; 2018,Apr,10; 2018,Jan,8; 2017,Jan,8; 2016,Jan,13; 2015,Jan,16

31287-31288 Nasal Endoscopy with Sphenoid Procedures

EXCLUDES *Sinus dilation (31297-31298)*
When performed on same side:
Biopsy, polypectomy, or debridement (31237)
Diagnostic sphenoid sinusoscopy (31235)
Optic nerve decompression (31294)
Other total ethmoidectomy procedures (31255, [31257], [31259])
Repair CSF leak (31291)

Code also stereotactic navigation, when performed (61782)

31287 **Nasal/sinus endoscopy, surgical, with sphenoidotomy;**

EXCLUDES *When performed on same side:*
Sphenoidotomy with removal tissue (31288)

5.78 5.78 **FUD** 000 J A2 80 50

AMA: 2019,Apr,10; 2018,Apr,3; 2018,Jan,8; 2017,Jan,8; 2016,Jan,13; 2015,Jan,16

31288 **with removal of tissue from the sphenoid sinus**

EXCLUDES *When performed on same side:*
Sphenoidotomy without removal tissue (31287)

6.71 6.71 **FUD** 000 J A2 80 50

AMA: 2019,Apr,10; 2018,Apr,3; 2018,Jan,8; 2017,Jan,8; 2016,Feb,10; 2016,Jan,13; 2015,Jan,16

31290-31294 Nasal Endoscopy with Repair and Decompression

INCLUDES Diagnostic nasal/sinus endoscopy
Sinusotomy, when applicable

EXCLUDES *When performed on same side:*
Biopsy, polypectomy, or debridement (31237)
Other total ethmoidectomy procedures ([31253], 31255, [31257], [31259])
Partial ethmoidectomy (31254)

Code also stereotactic navigation, when performed (61782)

31290 **Nasal/sinus endoscopy, surgical, with repair of cerebrospinal fluid leak; ethmoid region**

32.7 32.7 **FUD** 010 C 80 50

AMA: 2018,Apr,3; 2018,Jan,8; 2017,Jan,8; 2016,Feb,10; 2016,Jan,13; 2015,Jan,16

31291 **sphenoid region**

EXCLUDES *When performed on same side:*
Sphenoidotomy (31287-31288)

34.9 34.9 **FUD** 010 C 80 50

AMA: 2018,Apr,3; 2018,Jan,8; 2017,Jan,8; 2016,Jan,13; 2015,Jan,16

31292 **Nasal/sinus endoscopy, surgical, with orbital decompression; medial or inferior wall**

EXCLUDES *When performed on same side:*
Dilation frontal sinus only (31296)
Orbital wall decompression, medial and inferior (31293)

28.4 28.4 **FUD** 010 J 80 50

AMA: 2018,Apr,3; 2018,Jan,8; 2017,Jan,8; 2016,Jan,13; 2015,Jan,16

31293 **medial and inferior wall**

EXCLUDES *When performed on same side:*
Orbital wall decompression, medial or inferior (31292)

30.7 30.7 **FUD** 010 J 80 50

AMA: 2018,Apr,3; 2018,Jan,8; 2017,Jan,8; 2016,Jan,13; 2015,Jan,16

31294 Nasal/sinus endoscopy, surgical, with optic nerve decompression

EXCLUDES *When performed on same side:*
Sphenoidotomy (31287-31288)

35.2 35.2 FUD 010 J 80 50

AMA: 2018,Apr,3; 2018,Jan,8; 2017,Jan,8; 2016,Jan,13; 2015,Jan,16

31295-31298 Nasal Endoscopy with Sinus Ostia Dilation

INCLUDES Any method tissue displacement
Fluoroscopy, when performed

Code also stereotactic navigation, when performed (61782)

31295 Nasal/sinus endoscopy, surgical, with dilation (eg, balloon dilation); maxillary sinus ostium, transnasal or via canine fossa

EXCLUDES *When performed on same side:*
Maxillary antrostomy (31256-31267)
Maxillary sinusoscopy (31233)

4.55 55.6 FUD 000 J P3 80 50

AMA: 2020,Jun,14; 2018,Apr,3; 2018,Jan,8; 2017,Jan,8; 2016,Jan,13; 2015,Jan,16

31296 frontal sinus ostium

EXCLUDES *When performed on same side:*
Frontal sinus exploration (31276)
Dilation frontal and sphenoid sinus (31298)
Dilation sphenoid sinus only (31297)
Total ethmoidectomy (31253)

5.15 54.2 FUD 000 J P3 80 50

AMA: 2020,Jun,14; 2018,Apr,3; 2018,Jan,8; 2017,Jan,8; 2016,Jan,13; 2015,Jan,16

31297 sphenoid sinus ostium

EXCLUDES *When performed on same side:*
Diagnostic sphenoid sinusoscopy (31235)
Dilation frontal and sphenoid sinus (31298)
Dilation frontal sinus only (31296)
Sphenoidotomy (31287-31288)
Total ethmoidectomy procedures ([31257], [31259])

4.12 53.1 FUD 000 J P3 80 50

AMA: 2020,Jun,14; 2018,Apr,3; 2018,Jan,8; 2017,Jan,8; 2016,Jan,13; 2015,Jan,16

31298 frontal and sphenoid sinus ostia

EXCLUDES *When performed on same side:*
Diagnostic sphenoid sinusoscopy (31235)
Dilation frontal sinus only (31296)
Dilation sphenoid sinus only (31297)
Frontal sinus exploration (31276)
Other total ethmoidectomy procedures (31253, [31257], [31259])
Sphenoidotomy (31287-31288)

7.34 102. FUD 000 J P2 80 50

AMA: 2020,Jun,14; 2018,Apr,3

31299 Unlisted Procedures of Accessory Sinuses

CMS: 100-04,4,180.3 Unlisted Service or Procedure

EXCLUDES *Hypophysectomy (61546, 61548)*

31299 Unlisted procedure, accessory sinuses

0.00 0.00 FUD YYY T 80

AMA: 2019,Jul,7; 2019,Apr,10; 2018,Jan,8; 2017,Nov,11; 2017,Jan,8; 2016,Feb,10; 2016,Jan,13; 2015,Jul,10; 2015,Jan,16

31300-31502 Procedures of the Larynx

31300 Laryngotomy (thyrotomy, laryngofissure), with removal of tumor or laryngocele, cordectomy

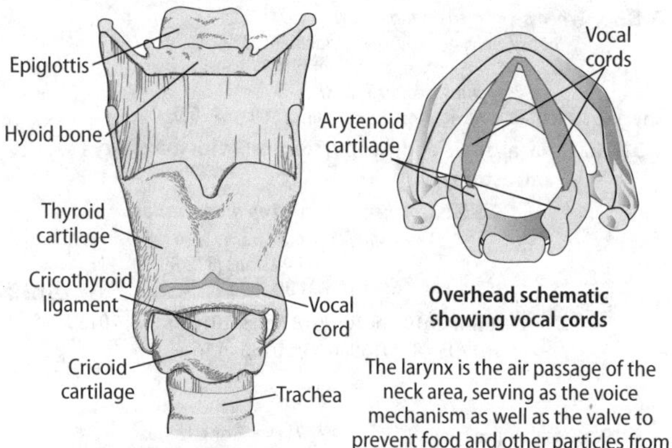

Frontal view of the major structures of the larynx

Overhead schematic showing vocal cords

The larynx is the air passage of the neck area, serving as the voice mechanism as well as the valve to prevent food and other particles from entering the respiratory tract

36.6 36.6 FUD 090 J A2 80

31360 Laryngectomy; total, without radical neck dissection

59.2 59.2 FUD 090 C 80

AMA: 2018,Jan,8; 2017,Jan,8; 2016,Jan,13; 2015,Jan,16

31365 total, with radical neck dissection

73.2 73.2 FUD 090 C 80

AMA: 2018,Jan,8; 2017,Jan,8; 2016,Jan,13; 2015,Jan,16

31367 subtotal supraglottic, without radical neck dissection

62.6 62.6 FUD 090 C 80

AMA: 2018,Jan,8; 2017,Jan,8; 2016,Jan,13; 2015,Jan,16

31368 subtotal supraglottic, with radical neck dissection

70.2 70.2 FUD 090 C 80

31370 Partial laryngectomy (hemilaryngectomy); horizontal

59.4 59.4 FUD 090 C 80

31375 laterovertical

55.8 55.8 FUD 090 C 80

31380 anterovertical

55.6 55.6 FUD 090 C 80

31382 antero-latero-vertical

61.0 61.0 FUD 090 C 80

31390 Pharyngolaryngectomy, with radical neck dissection; without reconstruction

81.0 81.0 FUD 090 C 80

31395 with reconstruction

86.4 86.4 FUD 090 C 80

31400 Arytenoidectomy or arytenoidopexy, external approach

EXCLUDES *Endoscopic arytenoidectomy (31560)*

28.0 28.0 FUD 090 J A2 80

31420 Epiglottidectomy

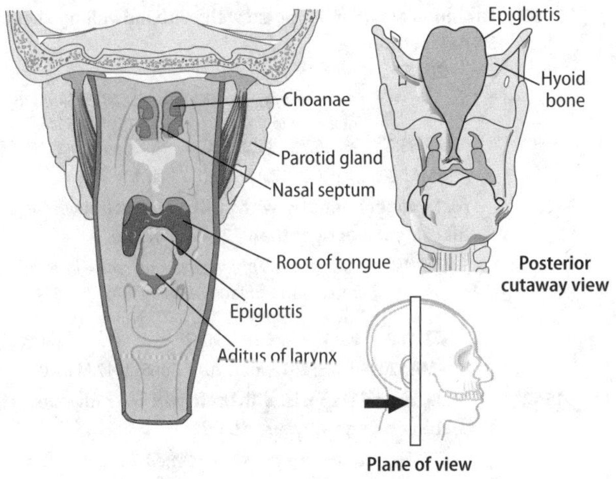

23.4 23.4 FUD 090 J A2 80

31500 Intubation, endotracheal, emergency procedure

EXCLUDES *Chest x-ray performed to confirm endotracheal tube position*

4.14 4.14 FUD 000 T G2

AMA: 2018,Jan,8; 2017,Jan,8; 2016,Oct,8; 2016,May,3; 2016,Jan,13; 2015,Jan,16

31502 Tracheotomy tube change prior to establishment of fistula tract

1.01 1.01 FUD 000 T G2

AMA: 1990,Win,4

31505-31541 Endoscopy of the Larynx

31505 Laryngoscopy, indirect; diagnostic (separate procedure)

1.39 2.48 FUD 000 T P3

AMA: 2018,Jan,8; 2017,Jan,8; 2016,Jan,13; 2015,Jan,16

31510 with biopsy

3.46 6.01 FUD 000 J A2 80

AMA: 2018,Jan,8; 2017,Jan,8; 2016,Jan,13; 2015,Jan,16

31511 with removal of foreign body

3.79 6.04 FUD 000 T A2

AMA: 2018,Jan,8; 2017,Jan,8; 2016,Jan,13; 2015,Jan,16

31512 with removal of lesion

3.70 5.92 FUD 000 J A2 80

AMA: 2018,Jan,8; 2017,Jan,8; 2016,Jan,13; 2015,Jan,16

31513 with vocal cord injection

3.76 3.76 FUD 000 T A2 80

AMA: 2018,Jan,8; 2017,Jan,8; 2016,Jan,13; 2015,Jan,16

31515 Laryngoscopy direct, with or without tracheoscopy; for aspiration

3.12 5.79 FUD 000 T A2

AMA: 1998,Nov,1; 1997,Nov,1

31520 diagnostic, newborn A

4.48 4.48 FUD 000 63 T G2 80

AMA: 1998,Nov,1; 1997,Nov,1

31525 diagnostic, except newborn

4.56 7.15 FUD 000 J A2

AMA: 2018,Jan,8; 2017,Jan,8; 2016,Jan,13; 2015,Jan,16

31526 diagnostic, with operating microscope or telescope

INCLUDES Operating microscope (69990)

4.49 4.49 FUD 000 J A2

AMA: 2018,Jan,8; 2017,Jun,10; 2016,Feb,12

31527 with insertion of obturator

5.55 5.55 FUD 000 J A2 80

AMA: 1998,Nov,1; 1997,Nov,1

31528 with dilation, initial

4.09 4.09 FUD 000 J A2 80

AMA: 2002,May,7; 1998,Nov,1

31529 with dilation, subsequent

4.59 4.59 FUD 000 J A2 80

AMA: 2002,May,7; 1998,Nov,1

31530 Laryngoscopy, direct, operative, with foreign body removal;

5.70 5.70 FUD 000 J A2

AMA: 1998,Nov,1; 1997,Nov,1

31531 with operating microscope or telescope

INCLUDES Operating microscope (69990)

6.08 6.08 FUD 000 J A2 80

AMA: 2018,Jan,8; 2017,Jun,10; 2016,Feb,12

31535 Laryngoscopy, direct, operative, with biopsy;

5.39 5.39 FUD 000 J A2

AMA: 1998,Nov,1; 1997,Nov,1

31536 with operating microscope or telescope

INCLUDES Operating microscope (69990)

6.00 6.00 FUD 000 J A2

AMA: 2018,Jan,8; 2017,Jun,10; 2016,Feb,12

31540 Laryngoscopy, direct, operative, with excision of tumor and/or stripping of vocal cords or epiglottis;

6.89 6.89 FUD 000 J A2

AMA: 1998,Nov,1; 1997,Nov,1

31541 with operating microscope or telescope

INCLUDES Operating microscope (69990)

7.52 7.52 FUD 000 J A2

AMA: 2019,Sep,10; 2019,Jul,10; 2018,Jan,8; 2017,Jun,10; 2016,Feb,12

31545-31554 [31551, 31552, 31553, 31554] Endoscopy of Larynx with Reconstruction

INCLUDES Operating microscope (69990)

EXCLUDES *Laryngoscopy, direct, operative, with excision tumor and/or vocal cord or epiglottis stripping (31540-31541)*
Vocal cord reconstruction with allograft (31599)

31545 Laryngoscopy, direct, operative, with operating microscope or telescope, with submucosal removal of non-neoplastic lesion(s) of vocal cord; reconstruction with local tissue flap(s)

10.3 10.3 FUD 000 J A2 50

AMA: 2016,Feb,12

31546 reconstruction with graft(s) (includes obtaining autograft)

EXCLUDES *Autologous fat graft obtained by liposuction (15771-15774)*
Autologous soft tissue grafts obtained by direct excision ([15769])

15.7 15.7 FUD 000 J A2 50

AMA: 2018,Jan,8; 2017,Jan,8; 2016,Feb,12; 2016,Jan,13; 2015,Jan,16

31551 **Resequenced code. See code following 31580.**

31552 **Resequenced code. See code following 31580.**

31553 **Resequenced code. See code following 31580.**

31554 **Resequenced code. See code following 31580.**

31560-31571 Endoscopy of Larynx with Arytenoid Removal, Vocal Cord Injection

31560 Laryngoscopy, direct, operative, with arytenoidectomy;

8.97 8.97 FUD 000 J A2 80

AMA: 1998,Nov,1; 1997,Nov,1

31561 with operating microscope or telescope

INCLUDES Operating microscope (69990)

9.82 9.82 FUD 000 J A2 80

AMA: 2018,Jan,8; 2017,Jun,10; 2016,Feb,12

31570 **Laryngoscopy, direct, with injection into vocal cord(s), therapeutic;**
6.53 9.68 FUD 000 J A2
AMA: 2018,Jan,8; 2017,Jan,8; 2017,Jan,6; 2016,Jan,13; 2015,Jan,16

31571 **with operating microscope or telescope**
INCLUDES *Operating microscope (69990)*
7.14 7.14 FUD 000 J A2
AMA: 2018,Jan,8; 2017,Jun,10; 2017,Jan,8; 2017,Jan,6; 2016,Feb,12; 2016,Jan,13; 2015,Jan,16

31572-31579 [31572, 31573, 31574] Endoscopy of Larynx, Flexible Fiberoptic

EXCLUDES *Evaluation by flexible fiberoptic endoscope:*
Sensory assessment (92614-92615)
Swallowing (92612-92613)
Swallowing and sensory assessment (92616-92617)
Flexible fiberoptic endoscopic examination/testing by cine or video recording (92612-92617)

31572 **Resequenced code. See code following 31578.**

31573 **Resequenced code. See code following 31578.**

31574 **Resequenced code. See code following 31578.**

31575 **Laryngoscopy, flexible; diagnostic**
EXCLUDES *Diagnostic nasal endoscopy not through additional endoscope (31231)*
Procedures during same session (31572-31574, 31576-31578, 43197-43198, 92511, 92612, 92614, 92616)
1.90 3.49 FUD 000 T P2
AMA: 2018,Jan,8; 2017,Jul,7; 2017,Apr,8; 2017,Jan,8; 2016,Dec,13

31576 **with biopsy(ies)**
EXCLUDES *Destruction or excision lesion (31572, 31578)*
3.38 7.63 FUD 000 J A2
AMA: 2018,Jan,8; 2017,Jul,7; 2017,Apr,8; 2017,Jan,8; 2016,Dec,13

31577 **with removal of foreign body(s)**
3.82 7.93 FUD 000 T A2 80
AMA: 2018,Jan,8; 2017,Jul,7; 2017,Apr,8; 2017,Jan,8; 2016,Dec,13

31578 **with removal of lesion(s), non-laser**
4.27 8.59 FUD 000 J A2 80
AMA: 2018,Jan,8; 2017,Jul,7; 2017,Apr,8; 2017,Jan,8; 2016,Dec,13

\# **31572** **with ablation or destruction of lesion(s) with laser, unilateral**
EXCLUDES *Biopsy or excision lesion (31576, 31578)*
5.15 14.7 FUD 000 J G2 80 50
AMA: 2019,Sep,10; 2018,Jan,8; 2017,Jul,7; 2017,Apr,8; 2017,Jan,8; 2016,Dec,13

\# **31573** **with therapeutic injection(s) (eg, chemodenervation agent or corticosteroid, injected percutaneous, transoral, or via endoscope channel), unilateral**
4.27 7.61 FUD 000 J P3 80 50
AMA: 2018,May,7; 2018,Jan,8; 2017,Jul,7; 2017,Apr,8; 2017,Jan,8; 2016,Dec,13

\# **31574** **with injection(s) for augmentation (eg, percutaneous, transoral), unilateral**
4.27 28.7 FUD 000 J G2 80 50
AMA: 2018,May,7; 2018,Jan,8; 2017,Jul,7; 2017,Apr,8; 2017,Jan,8; 2016,Dec,13

31579 **Laryngoscopy, flexible or rigid telescopic, with stroboscopy**
3.41 5.46 FUD 000 T P3
AMA: 2018,Jan,8; 2017,Jul,7; 2017,Apr,8; 2017,Jan,8; 2016,Dec,13

31580-31599 [31551, 31552, 31553, 31554] Larynx Reconstruction

31580 **Laryngoplasty; for laryngeal web, with indwelling keel or stent insertion**
EXCLUDES *Keel or stent removal (31599)*
Tracheostomy (31600-31601, 31603, 31605, 31610)
Treatment laryngeal stenosis (31551-31554)
35.7 35.7 FUD 090 J A2 80
AMA: 2018,Jan,8; 2017,Apr,5; 2017,Mar,10

\# **31551** **for laryngeal stenosis, with graft, without indwelling stent placement, younger than 12 years of age** A
EXCLUDES *Cartilage graft obtained through same incision*
Procedure during same session (31552-31554, 31580)
Tracheostomy (31600-31601, 31603, 31605, 31610)
41.2 41.2 FUD 090 J G2 80
AMA: 2018,Jan,8; 2017,Jul,7; 2017,Apr,5; 2017,Mar,10

\# **31552** **for laryngeal stenosis, with graft, without indwelling stent placement, age 12 years or older** A
EXCLUDES *Cartilage graft obtained through same incision*
Procedure during same session (31551, 31553-31554, 31580)
Tracheostomy (31600-31601, 31603, 31605, 31610)
42.0 42.0 FUD 090 J G2 80
AMA: 2018,Jan,8; 2017,Jul,7; 2017,Apr,5; 2017,Mar,10

\# **31553** **for laryngeal stenosis, with graft, with indwelling stent placement, younger than 12 years of age** A
EXCLUDES *Cartilage graft obtained through same incision*
Procedure during same session (31551-31552, 31554, 31580)
Stent removal (31599)
Tracheostomy (31600-31601, 31603, 31605, 31610)
47.8 47.8 FUD 090 J G2 80
AMA: 2018,Jan,8; 2017,Jul,7; 2017,Apr,5; 2017,Mar,10

\# **31554** **for laryngeal stenosis, with graft, with indwelling stent placement, age 12 years or older** A
EXCLUDES *Cartilage graft obtained through same incision*
Procedure during same session (31551-31553, 31580)
Stent removal (31599)
Tracheostomy (31600-31601, 31603, 31605, 31610)
47.8 47.8 FUD 090 J G2 80
AMA: 2018,Jan,8; 2017,Jul,7; 2017,Apr,5; 2017,Mar,10

31584 **with open reduction and fixation of (eg, plating) fracture, includes tracheostomy, if performed**
EXCLUDES *Cartilage graft obtained through same incision*
39.6 39.6 FUD 090 J 80
AMA: 2018,Jan,8; 2017,Apr,5; 2017,Mar,10

31587 **Laryngoplasty, cricoid split, without graft placement**
EXCLUDES *Tracheostomy (31600-31601, 31603, 31605, 31610)*
33.2 33.2 FUD 090 J 80
AMA: 2018,Jan,8; 2017,Apr,5; 2017,Mar,10

31590 **Laryngeal reinnervation by neuromuscular pedicle**
24.9 24.9 FUD 090 J A2 80
AMA: 2018,Jan,8; 2017,Mar,10

31591 **Laryngoplasty, medialization, unilateral**
30.7 30.7 FUD 090 J G2 80
AMA: 2018,Jan,8; 2017,Jul,7; 2017,Apr,5; 2017,Mar,10

31592 **Cricotracheal resection**
EXCLUDES *Advancement or rotational flaps performed not requiring additional incision*
Cartilage graft obtained through same incision
Tracheal stenosis excision/anastomosis (31780-31781)
Tracheostomy (31600-31601, 31603, 31605, 31610)
49.2 49.2 FUD 090 J G2 80
AMA: 2018,Jan,8; 2017,Jul,7; 2017,Apr,5; 2017,Mar,10; 2017,Feb,14

31599 **Unlisted procedure, larynx**
0.00 | 0.00 | FUD YYY | T 80
AMA: 2018,Jan,8; 2017,Apr,5; 2017,Mar,10; 2017,Jan,8; 2017,Jan,6; 2016,Dec,13; 2016,Jan,13; 2015,Jan,16

31600-31610 Stoma Creation: Trachea

EXCLUDES *Aspiration trachea, direct vision (31515)*
Endotracheal intubation (31500)

31600 **Tracheostomy, planned (separate procedure);**
8.91 | 8.91 | FUD 000 | J
AMA: 2019,Sep,10; 2017,Apr,5

31601 **younger than 2 years** A
12.9 | 12.9 | FUD 000 | J 80
AMA: 2017,Apr,5

31603 **Tracheostomy, emergency procedure; transtracheal**
9.30 | 9.30 | FUD 000 | T A2
AMA: 2017,Apr,5

31605 **cricothyroid membrane**
9.70 | 9.70 | FUD 000 | T G2
AMA: 2017,Apr,5

31610 **Tracheostomy, fenestration procedure with skin flaps**
27.2 | 27.2 | FUD 090 | J
AMA: 2017,Apr,5

31611-31614 Procedures of the Trachea

31611 **Construction of tracheoesophageal fistula and subsequent insertion of an alaryngeal speech prosthesis (eg, voice button, Blom-Singer prosthesis)**
15.1 | 15.1 | FUD 090 | J A2 80

31612 **Tracheal puncture, percutaneous with transtracheal aspiration and/or injection**
EXCLUDES *Tracheal aspiration under direct vision (31515)*
1.37 | 2.46 | FUD 000 | J A2 80
AMA: 1994,Win,1

31613 **Tracheostoma revision; simple, without flap rotation**
12.6 | 12.6 | FUD 090 | J A2

31614 **complex, with flap rotation**
20.7 | 20.7 | FUD 090 | J A2

31615 Endoscopy Through Tracheostomy

INCLUDES Diagnostic bronchoscopy
EXCLUDES *Endobronchial ultrasound [EBUS] guided biopsies mediastinal or hilar lymph nodes (31652-31653)*
Tracheoscopy (31515-31578)
Code also endobronchial ultrasound [EBUS] during diagnostic/therapeutic peripheral lesion intervention (31654)

31615 **Tracheobronchoscopy through established tracheostomy incision**
3.29 | 4.83 | FUD 000 | T A2
AMA: 2018,Jan,8; 2017,Jan,8; 2016,Jan,13; 2015,Jan,16

31622-31654 [31651] Endoscopy of Lung

INCLUDES Diagnostic bronchoscopy with surgical bronchoscopy procedures
Fluoroscopic imaging guidance, when performed

31622 **Bronchoscopy, rigid or flexible, including fluoroscopic guidance, when performed; diagnostic, with cell washing, when performed (separate procedure)**
3.78 | 6.84 | FUD 000 | J A2
AMA: 2018,Jan,8; 2017,Jan,8; 2016,Apr,5; 2016,Jan,13; 2015,Jan,16

31623 **with brushing or protected brushings**
3.82 | 7.66 | FUD 000 | J A2
AMA: 2018,Jan,8; 2017,Jan,8; 2016,Apr,5; 2016,Jan,13; 2015,Jan,16

31624 **with bronchial alveolar lavage**
3.87 | 7.16 | FUD 000 | J A2
AMA: 2018,Jan,8; 2017,Jun,10; 2017,Jan,8; 2016,Apr,5; 2016,Jan,13; 2015,Jan,16

31625 **with bronchial or endobronchial biopsy(s), single or multiple sites**
4.50 | 9.80 | FUD 000 | J A2
AMA: 2018,Jan,8; 2017,Jan,8; 2016,Apr,5; 2016,Jan,13; 2015,Jan,16

31626 **with placement of fiducial markers, single or multiple**
Code also device
5.72 | 23.9 | FUD 000 | J G2 80
AMA: 2018,Jan,8; 2017,Jun,10; 2017,Jan,8; 2016,Apr,5; 2016,Jan,13; 2015,Jun,6; 2015,Jan,16

+ **31627** **with computer-assisted, image-guided navigation (List separately in addition to code for primary procedure[s])**
INCLUDES 3D reconstruction (76376-76377)
Code first (31615, 31622-31626, 31628-31631, 31635-31636, 31638-31643)
2.78 | 36.3 | FUD ZZZ | N N1 80
AMA: 2018,Jan,8; 2017,Jan,8; 2016,Jan,13; 2015,Jan,16

31628 **with transbronchial lung biopsy(s), single lobe**
INCLUDES All biopsies taken from lobe
EXCLUDES *Transbronchial biopsies by needle aspiration (31629, 31633)*
Code also transbronchial biopsies additional lobe(s) (31632)
5.06 | 10.4 | FUD 000 | J A2
AMA: 2018,Jan,8; 2017,Jun,10; 2017,Jan,8; 2016,Apr,5; 2016,Jan,13; 2015,Jan,16

31629 **with transbronchial needle aspiration biopsy(s), trachea, main stem and/or lobar bronchus(i)**
INCLUDES All biopsies from same lobe or upper airway
EXCLUDES *Transbronchial biopsies lung (31628, 31632)*
Code also transbronchial needle biopsies additional lobe(s) (31633)
5.37 | 12.8 | FUD 000 | J A2
AMA: 2018,Jan,8; 2017,Jan,8; 2016,Apr,5; 2016,Jan,13; 2015,Jan,16

31630 **with tracheal/bronchial dilation or closed reduction of fracture**
5.72 | 5.72 | FUD 000 | J A2
AMA: 2018,Jan,8; 2017,Jan,8; 2016,Jan,13; 2015,Jan,16

31631 **with placement of tracheal stent(s) (includes tracheal/bronchial dilation as required)**
EXCLUDES *Bronchial stent placement (31636-31637)*
Revision bronchial or tracheal stent (31638)
6.58 | 6.58 | FUD 000 | J A2
AMA: 2018,Jan,8; 2017,Jan,8; 2016,Jan,13; 2015,Jan,16

+ **31632** **with transbronchial lung biopsy(s), each additional lobe (List separately in addition to code for primary procedure)**
INCLUDES All biopsies taken from additional lobe lung
Code first (31628)
1.43 | 1.82 | FUD ZZZ | N N1
AMA: 2018,Jan,8; 2017,Jan,8; 2016,Jan,13; 2015,Jan,16

+ **31633** **with transbronchial needle aspiration biopsy(s), each additional lobe (List separately in addition to code for primary procedure)**
INCLUDES All needle biopsies from another lobe or from trachea
Code first (31629)
1.82 | 2.26 | FUD ZZZ | N N1
AMA: 2018,Jan,8; 2017,Jan,8; 2016,Jan,13; 2015,Jan,16

31634 **with balloon occlusion, with assessment of air leak, with administration of occlusive substance (eg, fibrin glue), if performed**
EXCLUDES *When performed during same operative session:*
Bronchoscopy, rigid or flexible, including fluoroscopic guidance; with balloon occlusio, assessment air leak, airway sizing, and insertion bronchial valve(s), initial lobe (31647, [31651])
5.53 | 49.4 | FUD 000 | J G2 80
AMA: 2018,Jan,8; 2017,Jan,8; 2016,Jan,13; 2015,Jan,16

31635 **with removal of foreign body**
EXCLUDES *Removal implanted bronchial valves (31648-31649)*
5.06 8.03 FUD 000 J A2
AMA: 2018,Jan,8; 2017,Jan,8; 2016,Jan,13; 2015,Jan,16

31636 **with placement of bronchial stent(s) (includes tracheal/bronchial dilation as required), initial bronchus**
6.33 6.33 FUD 000 J J8
AMA: 2018,Jan,8; 2017,Jan,8; 2016,Jan,13; 2015,Jan,16

+ **31637** **each additional major bronchus stented (List separately in addition to code for primary procedure)**
Code first (31636)
2.22 2.22 FUD ZZZ N N1
AMA: 2018,Jan,8; 2017,Jan,8; 2016,Jan,13; 2015,Jan,16

31638 **with revision of tracheal or bronchial stent inserted at previous session (includes tracheal/bronchial dilation as required)**
7.21 7.21 FUD 000 J A2
AMA: 2018,Jan,8; 2017,Jan,8; 2016,Jan,13; 2015,Jan,16

31640 **with excision of tumor**
7.21 7.21 FUD 000 J A2
AMA: 2018,Jan,8; 2017,Jan,8; 2016,Apr,5; 2016,Jan,13; 2015,Jan,16

31641 **with destruction of tumor or relief of stenosis by any method other than excision (eg, laser therapy, cryotherapy)**
Code also any photodynamic therapy via bronchoscopy (96570-96571)
7.39 7.39 FUD 000 J A2
AMA: 2018,Jan,8; 2017,Jan,8; 2016,Jan,13; 2015,Jan,16

31643 **with placement of catheter(s) for intracavitary radioelement application**
Code also when appropriate (77761-77763, 77770-77772)
5.04 5.04 FUD 000 J A2
AMA: 2018,Jan,8; 2017,Jan,8; 2016,Apr,5; 2016,Jan,13; 2015,Jan,16

31645 **with therapeutic aspiration of tracheobronchial tree, initial (eg, drainage of lung abscess)**
EXCLUDES *Bedside aspiration trachea, bronchi (31725)*
4.21 7.42 FUD 000 J A2
AMA: 2018,Jan,8; 2017,Jan,8; 2016,Apr,5; 2016,Jan,13; 2015,Jan,16

31646 **with therapeutic aspiration of tracheobronchial tree, subsequent**
EXCLUDES *Bedside aspiration trachea, bronchi (31725)*
4.08 4.08 FUD 000 T A2
AMA: 2018,Sep,3; 2018,Jan,8; 2017,Jan,8; 2016,Apr,5; 2016,Jan,13; 2015,Jan,16

31647 **with balloon occlusion, when performed, assessment of air leak, airway sizing, and insertion of bronchial valve(s), initial lobe**
6.10 6.10 FUD 000 J J8
AMA: 2018,Sep,3; 2018,Jan,8; 2017,Jan,8; 2016,Jan,13; 2015,Jan,16

+ # **31651** **with balloon occlusion, when performed, assessment of air leak, airway sizing, and insertion of bronchial valve(s), each additional lobe (List separately in addition to code for primary procedure[s])**
Code first (31647)
2.13 2.13 FUD ZZZ N N1
AMA: 2018,Sep,3; 2018,Jan,8; 2017,Jan,8; 2016,Jan,13; 2015,Jan,16

31648 **with removal of bronchial valve(s), initial lobe**
EXCLUDES *Removal with reinsertion bronchial valve during same session (31647 and 31648) and ([31651])*
5.80 5.80 FUD 000 J G2
AMA: 2018,Sep,3; 2018,Jan,8; 2017,Jan,8; 2016,Jan,13; 2015,Jan,16

+ **31649** **with removal of bronchial valve(s), each additional lobe (List separately in addition to code for primary procedure)**
Code first (31648)
1.94 1.94 FUD ZZZ Q2 G2
AMA: 2018,Sep,3; 2018,Jan,8; 2017,Jan,8; 2016,Jan,13; 2015,Jan,16

31651 **Resequenced code. See code following 31647.**

31652 **with endobronchial ultrasound (EBUS) guided transtracheal and/or transbronchial sampling (eg, aspiration[s]/biopsy[ies]), one or two mediastinal and/or hilar lymph node stations or structures**
EXCLUDES *Procedures performed more than one time per session*
6.38 31.2 FUD 000 J G2
AMA: 2018,Jan,8; 2017,Jan,8; 2016,Apr,5

31653 **with endobronchial ultrasound (EBUS) guided transtracheal and/or transbronchial sampling (eg, aspiration[s]/biopsy[ies]), 3 or more mediastinal and/or hilar lymph node stations or structures**
EXCLUDES *Procedures performed more than one time per session*
7.08 28.7 FUD 000 J G2
AMA: 2018,Jan,8; 2017,Jan,8; 2016,Apr,5

+ **31654** **with transendoscopic endobronchial ultrasound (EBUS) during bronchoscopic diagnostic or therapeutic intervention(s) for peripheral lesion(s) (List separately in addition to code for primary procedure[s])**
EXCLUDES *Endobronchial ultrasound [EBUS] for mediastinal/hilar lymph node station/adjacent structure access (31652-31653)*
Procedures performed more than one time per session
Code first (31622-31626, 31628-31629, 31640, 31643-31646)
1.94 3.48 FUD ZZZ N N1
AMA: 2018,Jan,8; 2017,Jan,8; 2016,Apr,5

31660-31661 Bronchial Thermoplasty

INCLUDES Fluoroscopic imaging guidance, when performed

31660 **Bronchoscopy, rigid or flexible, including fluoroscopic guidance, when performed; with bronchial thermoplasty, 1 lobe**
5.62 5.62 FUD 000 J
AMA: 2018,Jan,8; 2017,Jan,8; 2016,Jan,13; 2015,Jan,16

31661 **with bronchial thermoplasty, 2 or more lobes**
5.93 5.93 FUD 000 J
AMA: 2018,Jan,8; 2017,Jan,8; 2016,Jan,13; 2015,Jan,16

31717-31899 Respiratory Procedures

EXCLUDES *Endotracheal intubation (31500)*
Tracheal aspiration under direct vision (31515)

31717 **Catheterization with bronchial brush biopsy**
3.18 7.98 FUD 000 T A2
AMA: 2018,Jan,8; 2017,Jan,8; 2016,Jan,13; 2015,Jan,16

31720 **Catheter aspiration (separate procedure); nasotracheal**
1.59 1.59 FUD 000 Q1 N1
AMA: 1994,Win,1

31725 **tracheobronchial with fiberscope, bedside**
2.27 2.27 FUD 000 C

31730 **Transtracheal (percutaneous) introduction of needle wire dilator/stent or indwelling tube for oxygen therapy**
4.33 33.8 FUD 000 J A2
AMA: 1992,Win,1

31750 **Tracheoplasty; cervical**
39.1 39.1 FUD 090 J A2 80

31755 **tracheopharyngeal fistulization, each stage**
49.1 49.1 FUD 090 J A2 80

31760 **intrathoracic**
39.6 39.6 FUD 090 C 80

31766 **Carinal reconstruction**
51.3 51.3 FUD 090 C 80

31770 **Bronchoplasty; graft repair**

EXCLUDES *Bronchoplasty done with lobectomy (32501)*

38.4 38.4 **FUD** 090 C 80

31775 **excision stenosis and anastomosis**

EXCLUDES *Bronchoplasty done with lobectomy (32501)*

40.4 40.4 **FUD** 090 C 80

31780 **Excision tracheal stenosis and anastomosis; cervical**

34.2 34.2 **FUD** 090 C 80

AMA: 2018,Jan,8; 2017,Apr,5; 2017,Feb,14

31781 **cervicothoracic**

39.8 39.8 **FUD** 090 C 80

AMA: 2018,Jan,8; 2017,Apr,5; 2017,Feb,14

31785 **Excision of tracheal tumor or carcinoma; cervical**

30.8 30.8 **FUD** 090 J 80

AMA: 2003,Jan,1

31786 **thoracic**

41.6 41.6 **FUD** 090 C 80

31800 **Suture of tracheal wound or injury; cervical**

20.3 20.3 **FUD** 090 C 80

AMA: 1994,Win,1

31805 **intrathoracic**

23.5 23.5 **FUD** 090 C 80

31820 **Surgical closure tracheostomy or fistula; without plastic repair**

EXCLUDES *Tracheoesophageal fistula repair (43305, 43312)*

9.35 12.3 **FUD** 090 J A2 80

31825 **with plastic repair**

EXCLUDES *Tracheoesophageal fistula repair (43305, 43312)*

13.6 17.1 **FUD** 090 J A2 80

31830 **Revision of tracheostomy scar**

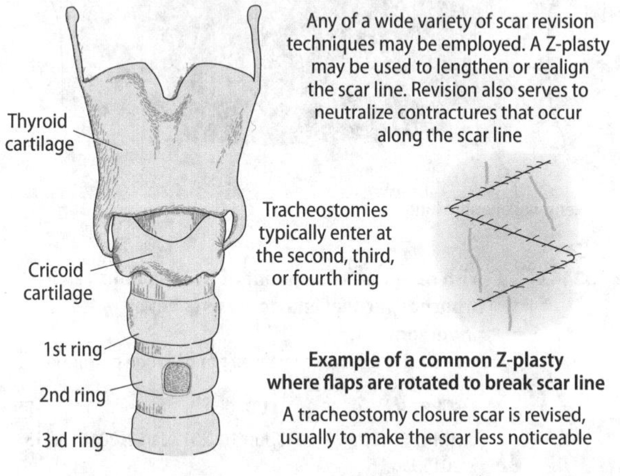

10.0 13.2 **FUD** 090 J A2 80

31899 **Unlisted procedure, trachea, bronchi**

0.00 0.00 **FUD** YYY T 80

AMA: 2018,Jan,8; 2017,Jan,8; 2016,Jan,13; 2015,Jan,16

32035-32036 Procedures for Empyema

EXCLUDES *Wound exploration without thoracotomy for penetrating chest wound (20101)*

32035 **Thoracostomy; with rib resection for empyema**

21.0 21.0 **FUD** 090 C 80 50

32036 **with open flap drainage for empyema**

22.3 22.3 **FUD** 090 C 80 50

32096-32098 Open Biopsy of Chest and Pleura

INCLUDES Varying amounts of lung tissue excised for analysis
Wedge technique with tissue obtained without precise consideration of margins

EXCLUDES *Core needle biopsy, lung or mediastinum (32408)*
Percutaneous needle biopsy pleura (32400)
Thoracoscopy:
with biopsy (32607-32609)
with diagnostic wedge resection resulting in anatomic lung resection (32668)
with diagnostic wedge resection resulting in anatomic lung resection (32507)

32096 **Thoracotomy, with diagnostic biopsy(ies) of lung infiltrate(s) (eg, wedge, incisional), unilateral**

EXCLUDES *Procedure performed more than one time per lung*
Removal lung (32440-32445, 32488)

Code also appropriate add-on code for the more extensive procedure at the same location if diagnostic wedge resection results in the need for further surgery (32507, 32668)

23.2 23.2 **FUD** 090 C 80

AMA: 2018,Jan,8; 2017,Jan,8; 2016,Jan,13; 2015,Jan,16

32097 **Thoracotomy, with diagnostic biopsy(ies) of lung nodule(s) or mass(es) (eg, wedge, incisional), unilateral**

EXCLUDES *Procedure performed more than one time per lung*
Removal lung (32440-32445, 32488)

Code also appropriate add-on code for the more extensive procedure in the same location if diagnostic wedge resection results in the need for further surgery (32507, 32668)

23.1 23.1 **FUD** 090 C 80

AMA: 2018,Jan,8; 2017,Jan,8; 2016,Jan,13; 2015,Jan,16

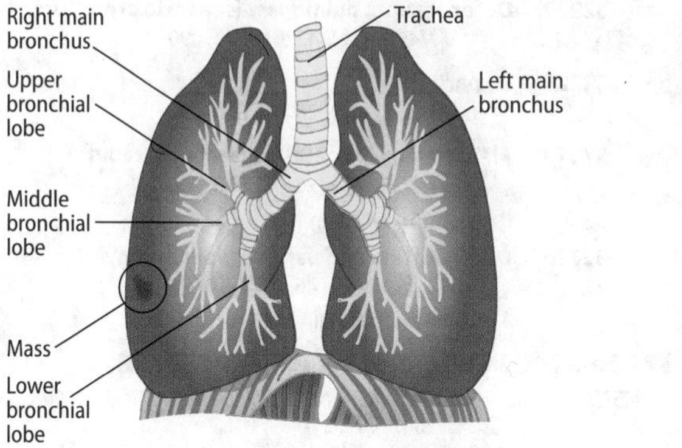

32098 **Thoracotomy, with biopsy(ies) of pleura**

21.9 21.9 **FUD** 090 C 80

AMA: 2018,Jan,8; 2017,Jan,8; 2016,Jan,13; 2015,Jan,16

32100-32160 Open Procedures: Chest

INCLUDES Exploration penetrating chest wound

EXCLUDES *Lung resection (32480-32504)*
Wound exploration without thoracotomy for penetrating chest wound (20101)

32100 **Thoracotomy; with exploration**

EXCLUDES *Excision chest wall tumor, when performed (21601-21603)*
Extracorporeal membrane oxygenation (ECMO)/extracorporeal life support (ECLS) (33955-33957, [33963, 33964])
Resection apical lung tumor (32503-32504)

23.3 23.3 **FUD** 090 C 80

AMA: 2019,Dec,5; 2019,Dec,4; 2018,Jan,8; 2017,Jan,8; 2016,Jan,13; 2015,Jul,3; 2015,Jan,16

32110 **with control of traumatic hemorrhage and/or repair of lung tear**

42.4 42.4 **FUD** 090 C 80

AMA: 2018,Jan,8; 2017,Jan,8; 2016,Jan,13; 2015,Jan,16

32120 **for postoperative complications**

25.2 25.2 **FUD** 090 C 80

32124 **with open intrapleural pneumonolysis**
26.7 26.7 FUD 090 C 80
AMA: 2018,Jan,8; 2017,Jan,8; 2016,Jan,13; 2015,Jan,16

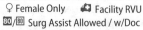

32140 **with cyst(s) removal, includes pleural procedure when performed**
28.5 28.5 FUD 090 C 80
AMA: 2018,Jan,8; 2017,Jan,8; 2016,Jan,13; 2015,Jan,16

32141 **with resection-plication of bullae, includes any pleural procedure when performed**
EXCLUDES *Lung volume reduction (32491)*
44.0 44.0 FUD 090 C 80
AMA: 2018,Jan,8; 2017,Jan,8; 2016,Jan,13; 2015,Jan,16

32150 **with removal of intrapleural foreign body or fibrin deposit**
28.9 28.9 FUD 090 C 80
AMA: 2018,Jan,8; 2017,Jan,8; 2016,Jan,13; 2015,Jan,16

32151 **with removal of intrapulmonary foreign body**
29.0 29.0 FUD 090 C 80

32160 **with cardiac massage**
22.9 22.9 FUD 090 C 80

32200-32320 Open Procedures: Lung

32200 **Pneumonostomy, with open drainage of abscess or cyst**
EXCLUDES *Image-guided, percutaneous drainage (eg, abscess, cyst) of lungs/mediastinum via catheter (49405)*
(75989)
32.7 32.7 FUD 090 C 80
AMA: 2013,Nov,9; 1997,Nov,1

32215 **Pleural scarification for repeat pneumothorax**
23.0 23.0 FUD 090 C 80 50

32220 **Decortication, pulmonary (separate procedure); total**
45.9 45.9 FUD 090 C 80 50

32225 **partial**
28.7 28.7 FUD 090 C 80 50

32310 **Pleurectomy, parietal (separate procedure)**
26.3 26.3 FUD 090 C 80
AMA: 1994,Win,1

32320 **Decortication and parietal pleurectomy**
46.1 46.1 FUD 090 C 80
AMA: 1994,Fall,1

32400-32408 Lung Biopsy

EXCLUDES *Fine needle aspiration ([10004, 10005, 10006, 10007, 10008, 10009, 10010, 10011, 10012], 10021)*
Open lung biopsy (32096-32097)
Open mediastinal biopsy (39000-39010)
Thoracoscopic (VATS) biopsy lung, pericardium, pleural, or mediastinal space (32604-32609)

32400 **Biopsy, pleura, percutaneous needle**
(76942, 77002, 77012, 77021)
2.48 4.56 FUD 000 J A2
AMA: 2019,Apr,4; 2018,Jan,8; 2017,Jan,8; 2016,Jan,13; 2015,Jan,16

~~**32405** **Biopsy, lung or mediastinum, percutaneous needle**~~
To report, see ([32408])

● **32408** **Core needle biopsy, lung or mediastinum, percutaneous, including imaging guidance, when performed**
INCLUDES Imaging guidance performed during tsame session on same lesion (76942, 77002, 77012, 77021)
Code also core needle biopsy performed during same operative session:
other anatomical site; report both codes and append modifier 59 on second code
same anatomical site, different lesion; report 32408 for each lesion biopsied and append modifier 59 on second code
Code also FNA biopsy and core needle biopsy performed during same operative session:
different lesion, utilizing same or different imaging guidance; report both codes and append modifier 59 on either code
same lesion, utilizing different imaging guidance; report both image-guided biopsy codes and append modifier 59 on either code
same lesion, utilizing same imaging guidance; report both codes and append modifier 52 on either code

32440-32501 Lung Resection

32440 **Removal of lung, pneumonectomy;**
Code also excision chest wall tumor, when performed (21601-21603)
45.1 45.1 FUD 090 C 80
AMA: 2018,Jan,8; 2017,Jan,8; 2016,Jan,13; 2015,Jan,16

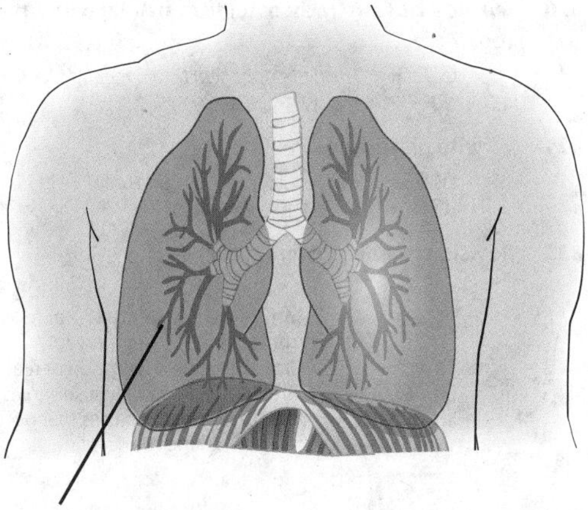

32442 **with resection of segment of trachea followed by broncho-tracheal anastomosis (sleeve pneumonectomy)**
Code also excision chest wall tumor, when performed (21601-21603)
88.9 88.9 FUD 090 C 80
AMA: 2018,Jan,8; 2017,Jun,10; 2017,Jan,8; 2016,Jan,13; 2015,Jan,16

32445 **extrapleural**
Code also empyemectomy with extrapleural pneumonectomy (32540)
Code also excision chest wall tumor, when performed (21601-21603)
102. 102. FUD 090 C 80
AMA: 2018,Jan,8; 2017,Jan,8; 2016,Jan,13; 2015,Jan,16

32480 **Removal of lung, other than pneumonectomy; single lobe (lobectomy)**
EXCLUDES *Lung removal with bronchoplasty (32501)*
Code also decortication (32320)
Code also excision chest wall tumor, when performed (21601-21603)
42.6 42.6 FUD 090 C 80
AMA: 2018,Jan,8; 2017,Jan,8; 2016,Jan,13; 2015,Jan,16

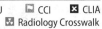

32482 **2 lobes (bilobectomy)**

EXCLUDES *Lung removal with bronchoplasty (32501)*

Code also decortication (32320)

Code also excision chest wall tumor, when performed (21601-21603)

45.8 45.8 **FUD** 090 C 80

AMA: 2018,Jan,8; 2017,Jan,8; 2016,Jan,13; 2015,Jan,16

32484 **single segment (segmentectomy)**

EXCLUDES *Lung removal with bronchoplasty (32501)*

Code also decortication (32320)

Code also excision chest wall tumor, when performed (21601-21603)

41.3 41.3 **FUD** 090 C 80

AMA: 2018,Jan,8; 2017,Jan,8; 2016,Jan,13; 2015,Jan,16

32486 **with circumferential resection of segment of bronchus followed by broncho-bronchial anastomosis (sleeve lobectomy)**

Code also decortication (32320)

Code also excision chest wall tumor, when performed (21601-21603)

68.1 68.1 **FUD** 090 C 80

AMA: 2018,Jan,8; 2017,Jun,10; 2017,Jan,8; 2016,Jan,13; 2015,Jan,16

32488 **with all remaining lung following previous removal of a portion of lung (completion pneumonectomy)**

Code also decortication (32320)

Code also excision chest wall tumor, when performed (21601-21603)

69.1 69.1 **FUD** 090 C 80

AMA: 2018,Jan,8; 2017,Jan,8; 2016,Jan,13; 2015,Jan,16

32491 **with resection-plication of emphysematous lung(s) (bullous or non-bullous) for lung volume reduction, sternal split or transthoracic approach, includes any pleural procedure, when performed**

Code also decortication (32320)

Code also excision chest wall tumor, when performed (21601-21603)

42.4 42.4 **FUD** 090 C 80 50

AMA: 2018,Jan,8; 2017,Jan,8; 2016,Jan,13; 2015,Jan,16

\+ **32501** **Resection and repair of portion of bronchus (bronchoplasty) when performed at time of lobectomy or segmentectomy (List separately in addition to code for primary procedure)**

INCLUDES Plastic closure bronchus, not closure resected bronchus

Code first (32480-32484)

7.04 7.04 **FUD** ZZZ C 80

AMA: 1995,Win,1

32503-32504 Excision of Lung Neoplasm

EXCLUDES *Excision chest wall tumor (21601-21603)*
Thoracentesis, needle or catheter, aspiration pleural space (32554-32555)
Thoracotomy; with exploration (32100)
Tube thoracostomy (32551)

32503 **Resection of apical lung tumor (eg, Pancoast tumor), including chest wall resection, rib(s) resection(s), neurovascular dissection, when performed; without chest wall reconstruction(s)**

51.9 51.9 **FUD** 090 C 80

AMA: 2019,Dec,4

32504 **with chest wall reconstruction**

59.1 59.1 **FUD** 090 C 80

AMA: 2019,Dec,4

32505-32507 Thoracotomy with Wedge Resection

INCLUDES Wedge technique with tissue obtained with precise consideration margins and complete resection

Code also resection chest wall tumor with lung resection, when performed (21601-21603)

32505 **Thoracotomy; with therapeutic wedge resection (eg, mass, nodule), initial**

EXCLUDES *Removal lung (32440, 32442, 32445, 32488)*

Code also more extensive procedure lung when performed on contralateral lung or different lobe with modifier 59 despite intraoperative pathology consultation

26.8 26.8 **FUD** 090 C 80

AMA: 2018,Jan,8; 2017,Jan,8; 2016,Jan,13; 2015,Jan,16

\+ **32506** **with therapeutic wedge resection (eg, mass or nodule), each additional resection, ipsilateral (List separately in addition to code for primary procedure)**

Code also more extensive procedure lung when performed on contralateral lung or different lobe with modifier 59 despite intraoperative pathology consultation

Code first (32505)

4.53 4.53 **FUD** ZZZ C 80

AMA: 2018,Jan,8; 2017,Jan,8; 2016,Jan,13; 2015,Jan,16

\+ **32507** **with diagnostic wedge resection followed by anatomic lung resection (List separately in addition to code for primary procedure)**

INCLUDES Classification as diagnostic wedge resection when intraoperative pathology consultation dictates more extensive resection in same anatomical area

EXCLUDES *Diagnostic wedge resection by thoracoscopy (32668)*
Therapeutic wedge resection (32505-32506, 32666-32667)

Code first (32440, 32442, 32445, 32480-32488, 32503-32504)

4.52 4.52 **FUD** ZZZ C 80

AMA: 2018,Jan,8; 2017,Jan,8; 2016,Jan,13; 2015,Jan,16

32540 Removal of Empyema

32540 **Extrapleural enucleation of empyema (empyemectomy)**

Code also appropriate removal lung code when done with lobectomy (32480-32488)

50.1 50.1 **FUD** 090 C 80

AMA: 1994,Fall,1

32550-32552 Chest Tube/Catheter

32550 **Insertion of indwelling tunneled pleural catheter with cuff**

EXCLUDES *Procedures performed on same side chest with (32554-32557)*

(75989)

5.98 21.2 **FUD** 000 J G2

AMA: 2018,Jan,8; 2017,Jan,8; 2016,Jan,13; 2015,Jan,16

32551 **Tube thoracostomy, includes connection to drainage system (eg, water seal), when performed, open (separate procedure)**

EXCLUDES *Procedures performed on same side chest with (33020, 33025)*

4.56 4.56 **FUD** 000 T 50

AMA: 2019,Dec,4; 2018,Jul,7; 2018,Jan,8; 2017,Jun,10; 2017,Jan,8; 2016,Jan,13; 2015,Jan,16

32552 **Removal of indwelling tunneled pleural catheter with cuff**

4.55 5.28 **FUD** 010 Q2 G2 80

AMA: 2018,Jan,8; 2017,Jan,8; 2016,Jan,13; 2015,Jan,16

32553 Intrathoracic Placement Radiation Therapy Devices

EXCLUDES *Percutaneous placement interstitial device(s) for radiation therapy guidance: intra-abdominal, intrapelvic, and/or retroperitoneal (49411)*

Code also device

32553 **Placement of interstitial device(s) for radiation therapy guidance (eg, fiducial markers, dosimeter), percutaneous, intra-thoracic, single or multiple**
(76942, 77002, 77012, 77021)
5.17 15.1 **FUD** 000 S G2 80
AMA: 2018,Jan,8; 2017,Jan,8; 2016,Jun,3; 2016,Jan,13; 2015,Jun,6; 2015,Jan,16

32554-32557 Pleural Aspiration and Drainage

EXCLUDES *Chest x-ray performed to confirm chest tube position, complications, procedure adequacy*
Open tube thoracostomy (32551)
Placement indwelling tunneled pleural drainage catheter (cuffed) (32550)

32554 **Thoracentesis, needle or catheter, aspiration of the pleural space; without imaging guidance**
EXCLUDES *Radiologic guidance (75989, 76942, 77002, 77012, 77021)*
2.58 6.01 **FUD** 000 T G2 50
AMA: 2019,Dec,4; 2018,Jan,8; 2017,Jan,8; 2016,Jan,13; 2015,Jan,16

32555 **with imaging guidance**
INCLUDES Radiologic guidance (75989, 76942, 77002, 77012, 77021)
3.22 8.51 **FUD** 000 T G2 50
AMA: 2019,Dec,4; 2018,Jan,8; 2017,Jan,8; 2016,Jan,13; 2015,Jan,16

32556 **Pleural drainage, percutaneous, with insertion of indwelling catheter; without imaging guidance**
EXCLUDES *Radiologic guidance (75989, 76942, 77002, 77012, 77021)*
3.55 17.4 **FUD** 000 J G2 50
AMA: 2018,Jan,8; 2017,Jan,8; 2016,Jan,13; 2015,Jan,16

32557 **with imaging guidance**
INCLUDES Radiologic guidance (75989, 76942, 77002, 77012, 77021)
4.39 16.0 **FUD** 000 T G2 50
AMA: 2018,Jan,8; 2017,Jan,8; 2016,Jan,13; 2015,Jan,16

32560-32562 Instillation Drug/Chemical by Chest Tube

EXCLUDES *Insertion chest tube (32551)*

32560 **Instillation, via chest tube/catheter, agent for pleurodesis (eg, talc for recurrent or persistent pneumothorax)**
2.25 7.38 **FUD** 000 T
AMA: 2018,Jan,8; 2017,Jan,8; 2016,Jan,13; 2015,Jan,16

32561 **Instillation(s), via chest tube/catheter, agent for fibrinolysis (eg, fibrinolytic agent for break up of multiloculated effusion); initial day**
EXCLUDES *Reporting code more than one time on initial treatment date*
1.95 2.66 **FUD** 000 T 80
AMA: 2018,Jan,8; 2017,Jan,8; 2016,Jan,13; 2015,Jan,16

32562 **subsequent day**
EXCLUDES *Reporting code more than one time on each day subsequent treatment*
1.75 2.40 **FUD** 000 T 80
AMA: 2018,Jan,8; 2017,Jan,8; 2016,Jan,13; 2015,Jan,16

32601-32674 Thoracic Surgery: Video-Assisted (VATS)

INCLUDES Diagnostic thoracoscopy in surgical thoracoscopy

32601 **Thoracoscopy, diagnostic (separate procedure); lungs, pericardial sac, mediastinal or pleural space, without biopsy**
8.90 8.90 **FUD** 000 J 80
AMA: 2018,Jan,8; 2017,Jan,8; 2016,Jan,13; 2015,Jan,16

32604 **pericardial sac, with biopsy**
EXCLUDES *Open biopsy pericardium (39010)*
13.8 13.8 **FUD** 000 J 80
AMA: 2018,Jan,8; 2017,Jan,8; 2016,Jan,13; 2015,Jan,16

32606 **mediastinal space, with biopsy**
13.3 13.3 **FUD** 000 J 80
AMA: 2018,Jan,8; 2017,Jan,8; 2016,Jan,13; 2015,Jan,16

32607 **Thoracoscopy; with diagnostic biopsy(ies) of lung infiltrate(s) (eg, wedge, incisional), unilateral**
EXCLUDES *Removal lung (32440-32445, 32488)*
Thoracoscopy, surgical; with removal lung (32671)
Reporting code more than one time per lung
8.89 8.89 **FUD** 000 J 80
AMA: 2018,Jan,8; 2017,Jan,8; 2016,Jan,13; 2015,Jan,16

32608 **with diagnostic biopsy(ies) of lung nodule(s) or mass(es) (eg, wedge, incisional), unilateral**
EXCLUDES *Removal lung (32440-32445, 32488)*
Thoracoscopy, surgical; with removal lung (32671)
Reporting code more than one time per lung
10.9 10.9 **FUD** 000 J 80
AMA: 2018,Jan,8; 2017,Jan,8; 2016,Jan,13; 2015,Jan,16

32609 **with biopsy(ies) of pleura**
7.45 7.45 **FUD** 000 J 80
AMA: 2018,Jan,8; 2017,Jan,8; 2016,Jan,13; 2015,Jan,16

32650 **Thoracoscopy, surgical; with pleurodesis (eg, mechanical or chemical)**
19.1 19.1 **FUD** 090 C 80 50
AMA: 2018,Jan,8; 2017,Jan,8; 2016,Jan,13; 2015,Jan,16

32651 **with partial pulmonary decortication**
31.6 31.6 **FUD** 090 C 80 50
AMA: 2018,Jan,8; 2017,Jan,8; 2016,Jan,13; 2015,Jan,16

32652 **with total pulmonary decortication, including intrapleural pneumonolysis**
47.9 47.9 **FUD** 090 C 80 50
AMA: 2018,Jan,8; 2017,Jan,8; 2016,Jan,13; 2015,Jan,16

32653 **with removal of intrapleural foreign body or fibrin deposit**
30.6 30.6 **FUD** 090 C 80
AMA: 2018,Jan,8; 2017,Jan,8; 2016,Jan,13; 2015,Jan,16

32654 **with control of traumatic hemorrhage**
33.5 33.5 **FUD** 090 C 80 50
AMA: 2018,Jan,8; 2017,Jan,8; 2016,Jan,13; 2015,Jan,16

32655 **with resection-plication of bullae, includes any pleural procedure when performed**
EXCLUDES *Thoracoscopic lung volume reduction surgery (32672)*
27.5 27.5 **FUD** 090 C 80 50
AMA: 2018,Jan,8; 2017,Jan,8; 2016,Jan,13; 2015,Jan,16

32656 **with parietal pleurectomy**
23.0 23.0 **FUD** 090 C 80 50
AMA: 2018,Jan,8; 2017,Jan,8; 2016,Jan,13; 2015,Jan,16

32658 **with removal of clot or foreign body from pericardial sac**
20.6 20.6 **FUD** 090 C 80
AMA: 2018,Jan,8; 2017,Jan,8; 2016,Jan,13; 2015,Jan,16

32659 **with creation of pericardial window or partial resection of pericardial sac for drainage**
21.1 21.1 **FUD** 090 C 80
AMA: 2018,Jan,8; 2017,Jan,8; 2016,Jan,13; 2015,Jan,16

32661 **with excision of pericardial cyst, tumor, or mass**
23.0 23.0 **FUD** 090 C 80
AMA: 2018,Jan,8; 2017,Jan,8; 2016,Jan,13; 2015,Jan,16

32662 **with excision of mediastinal cyst, tumor, or mass**
25.7 25.7 **FUD** 090 C 80
AMA: 2018,Jan,8; 2017,Jan,8; 2016,Jan,13; 2015,Jan,16

32663 with lobectomy (single lobe)

EXCLUDES *Thoracoscopic segmentectomy (32669)*

40.4 40.4 FUD 090 C 80

AMA: 2018,Jan,8; 2017,Jan,8; 2016,Jan,13; 2015,Jan,16

32664 with thoracic sympathectomy

24.4 24.4 FUD 090 C 80 50

AMA: 2018,Jan,8; 2017,Jan,8; 2016,Jan,13; 2015,Dec,16; 2015,Jan,16

32665 with esophagomyotomy (Heller type)

EXCLUDES *Exploratory thoracoscopy with and without biopsy (32601-32609)*

35.6 35.6 FUD 090 C 80

AMA: 2018,Jan,8; 2017,Jan,8; 2016,Jan,13; 2015,Jan,16

32666 with therapeutic wedge resection (eg, mass, nodule), initial unilateral

EXCLUDES *Removal lung (32440-32445, 32488)*
Thoracoscopy, surgical; with removal lung (32671)

Code also more extensive procedure lung when performed on contralateral lung or different lobe with modifier 59 despite pathology consultation

25.1 25.1 FUD 090 C 80 50

AMA: 2018,Jan,8; 2017,Jan,8; 2016,Jan,13; 2015,Jan,16

+ **32667 with therapeutic wedge resection (eg, mass or nodule), each additional resection, ipsilateral (List separately in addition to code for primary procedure)**

EXCLUDES *Removal lung (32440-32445, 32488)*
Thoracoscopy, surgical; with removal lung (32671)

Code also more extensive procedure lung when performed on contralateral lung or different lobe with modifier 59 despite intraoperative pathology consultation

Code first (32666)

4.54 4.54 FUD ZZZ C 80

AMA: 2018,Jan,8; 2017,Jan,8; 2016,Jan,13; 2015,Jan,16

+ **32668 with diagnostic wedge resection followed by anatomic lung resection (List separately in addition to code for primary procedure)**

INCLUDES Classification as diagnostic wedge resection when intraoperative pathology consultation dictates more extensive resection in same anatomical area

Code first (32440-32488, 32503-32504, 32663, 32669-32671)

4.54 4.54 FUD ZZZ C 80

AMA: 2018,Jan,8; 2017,Jan,8; 2016,Jan,13; 2015,Jan,16

32669 with removal of a single lung segment (segmentectomy)

38.7 38.7 FUD 090 C 80

AMA: 2018,Jan,8; 2017,Jan,8; 2016,Jan,13; 2015,Jan,16

32670 with removal of two lobes (bilobectomy)

46.2 46.2 FUD 090 C 80

AMA: 2018,Jan,8; 2017,Jan,8; 2016,Jan,13; 2015,Jan,16

32671 with removal of lung (pneumonectomy)

51.5 51.5 FUD 090 C 80

AMA: 2018,Jan,8; 2017,Jan,8; 2016,Jan,13; 2015,Jan,16

32672 with resection-plication for emphysematous lung (bullous or non-bullous) for lung volume reduction (LVRS), unilateral includes any pleural procedure, when performed

44.0 44.0 FUD 090 C 80

AMA: 2018,Jan,8; 2017,Jan,8; 2016,Jan,13; 2015,Jan,16

32673 with resection of thymus, unilateral or bilateral

EXCLUDES *Exploratory thoracoscopy with and without biopsy (32601-32609)*
Open excision mediastinal cyst (39200)
Open excision mediastinal tumor (39220)
Open thymectomy (60520-60522)

35.0 35.0 FUD 090 C 80

AMA: 2018,Jan,8; 2017,Jan,8; 2016,Jan,13; 2015,Jan,16

+ **32674 with mediastinal and regional lymphadenectomy (List separately in addition to code for primary procedure)**

INCLUDES Mediastinal lymph nodes:
- Left side:
  - Aortopulmonary window
  - Inferior pulmonary ligament
  - Paraesophageal
  - Subcarinal
- Right side:
  - Inferior pulmonary ligament
  - Paraesophageal
  - Paratracheal
  - Subcarinal

EXCLUDES *Mediastinal and regional lymphadenectomy by thoracotomy (38746)*

Code first (21601, 31760, 31766, 31786, 32096-32200, 32220-32320, 32440-32491, 32503-32505, 32601-32663, 32666, 32669-32673, 32815, 33025, 33030, 33050-33130, 39200-39220, 39560-39561, 43101, 43112, 43117-43118, 43122-43123, 43287-43288, 43351, 60270, 60505)

6.24 6.24 FUD ZZZ C 80

AMA: 2018,Jan,8; 2017,Jan,8; 2016,Jan,13; 2015,Jan,16

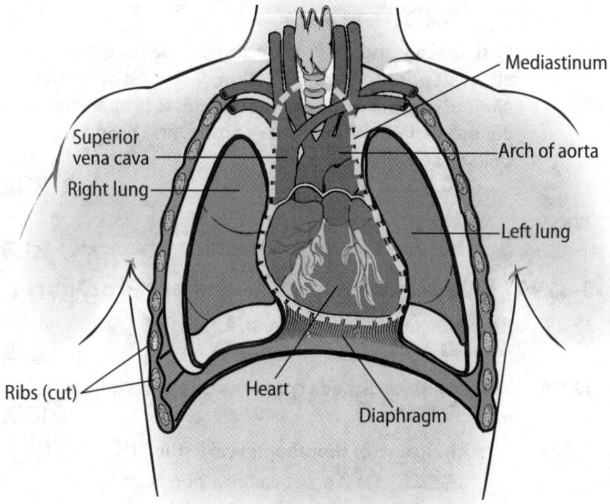

32701 Target Delineation for Stereotactic Radiation Therapy

INCLUDES Collaboration between radiation oncologist and surgeon
Correlation tumor and contiguous body structures
Determination borders and volume of tumor
Identification fiducial markers
Verification target when fiducial markers not used

EXCLUDES *Fiducial marker insertion (31626, 32553)*
Procedure performed by same physician as radiation treatment management (77427-77499)
Radiation oncology services (77295, 77331, 77370, 77373, 77435)
Therapeutic radiology (77261-77799 [77295, 77385, 77386, 77387, 77424, 77425])

32701 Thoracic target(s) delineation for stereotactic body radiation therapy (SRS/SBRT), (photon or particle beam), entire course of treatment

6.21 6.21 FUD XXX B 80 26

AMA: 2018,Jan,8; 2017,Jan,8; 2016,Jan,13; 2015,Jun,6

32800-32820 Chest Repair and Reconstruction Procedures

32800 Repair lung hernia through chest wall

27.0 27.0 FUD 090 C 80

32810 Closure of chest wall following open flap drainage for empyema (Clagett type procedure)

26.0 26.0 FUD 090 C 80

32815 Open closure of major bronchial fistula

81.0 81.0 FUD 090 C 80

32820 Major reconstruction, chest wall (posttraumatic)

38.3 38.3 FUD 090 C 80

32850-32856 Lung Transplant Procedures

INCLUDES Harvesting donor lung(s), cold preservation, preparation donor lung(s), transplantation into recipient

EXCLUDES *Assessment marginal cadaver donor lungs (0494T-0496T)*
Repairs or resection donor lung(s) (32491, 32505-32507, 35216, 35276)

32850 Donor pneumonectomy(s) (including cold preservation), from cadaver donor
0.00 0.00 FUD XXX C
AMA: 1993,Win,1

32851 Lung transplant, single; without cardiopulmonary bypass
94.8 94.8 FUD 090 C 80
AMA: 1993,Win,1

32852 with cardiopulmonary bypass
103. 103. FUD 090 C 80
AMA: 2017,Dec,3

32853 Lung transplant, double (bilateral sequential or en bloc); without cardiopulmonary bypass
133. 133. FUD 090 C 80
AMA: 1993,Win,1

32854 with cardiopulmonary bypass
141. 141. FUD 090 C 80
AMA: 2017,Dec,3

32855 Backbench standard preparation of cadaver donor lung allograft prior to transplantation, including dissection of allograft from surrounding soft tissues to prepare pulmonary venous/atrial cuff, pulmonary artery, and bronchus; unilateral
0.00 0.00 FUD XXX C 80

32856 bilateral
0.00 0.00 FUD XXX C 80

32900-32997 [32994] Chest and Respiratory Procedures

32900 Resection of ribs, extrapleural, all stages
41.0 41.0 FUD 090 C 80

32905 Thoracoplasty, Schede type or extrapleural (all stages);
38.5 38.5 FUD 090 C 80

32906 with closure of bronchopleural fistula
EXCLUDES *Open closure bronchial fistula (32815)*
Resection first rib for thoracic compression (21615-21616)
47.6 47.6 FUD 090 C 80

32940 Pneumonolysis, extraperiosteal, including filling or packing procedures
35.7 35.7 FUD 090 C 80

32960 Pneumothorax, therapeutic, intrapleural injection of air
2.62 3.61 FUD 000 T G2

***32994* Resequenced code. See code following 32998.**

32997 Total lung lavage (unilateral)
EXCLUDES *Broncho-alveolar lavage by bronchoscopy (31624)*
9.84 9.84 FUD 000 C 50
AMA: 2018,Jan,8; 2017,Jan,8; 2016,Jan,13; 2015,Jan,16

32998-32999 [32994] Destruction of Lung Neoplasm

32998 Ablation therapy for reduction or eradication of 1 or more pulmonary tumor(s) including pleura or chest wall when involved by tumor extension, percutaneous, including imaging guidance when performed, unilateral; radiofrequency
12.7 99.5 FUD 000 J G2 80 50
AMA: 2018,Jan,8; 2017,Nov,8

\# **32994 cryoablation**
12.8 155. FUD 000 J G2 80 50
AMA: 2018,Jan,8; 2017,Nov,8

32999 Unlisted procedure, lungs and pleura
0.00 0.00 FUD YYY T
AMA: 2018,Jan,8; 2017,Jan,8; 2016,Jan,13; 2015,Dec,16; 2015,Jun,6; 2015,Jan,16

33016-33050 Procedures of the Pericardial Sac

EXCLUDES *Surgical thoracoscopy (video-assisted thoracic surgery [VATS]) procedures pericardium (32601, 32604, 32658-32659, 32661)*

33016 Pericardiocentesis, including imaging guidance, when performed

INCLUDES Imaging guidance for needle placement:
Computed tomography (77012)
Fluoroscopy (77002)
Magnetic resonance (77021)
Ultrasound (76942)

EXCLUDES *Echocardiography for pericardiocentesis guidance (93303-93325)*

6.85 6.85 **FUD** 000

AMA: 2020,Jan,7

33017 Pericardial drainage with insertion of indwelling catheter, percutaneous, including fluoroscopy and/or ultrasound guidance, when performed; 6 years and older without congenital cardiac anomaly

INCLUDES Catheters that remain in patient at procedure conclusion
Imaging guidance for needle placement:
Fluoroscopy (77002)
Magnetic resonance (77021)
Ultrasound (76942)

EXCLUDES *CT guided pericardial drainage (33019)*
Echocardiography for pericardiocentesis guidance (93303-93325)
Pericardial drainage for patients:
Any age with congenital cardiac anomaly (33018)
Younger than 6 years of age (33018)
Radiologically guided catheter placement for percutaneous drainage (75989)

7.10 7.10 **FUD** 000

AMA: 2020,Jan,7

33018 birth through 5 years of age or any age with congenital cardiac anomaly

INCLUDES Catheters that remain in patient at procedure conclusion
Imaging guidance for needle placement:
Fluoroscopy (77002)
Magnetic resonance (77021)
Ultrasound (76942)
Patient age birth to 5 years without congenital cardiac anomaly
Patient any age with congenital cardiac anomaly, such as heterotaxy, dextrocardia, mesocardia, or single ventricle anomaly, or 90 days following repair congenital cardiac anomaly

EXCLUDES *CT guided pericardial drainage (33019)*
Echocardiography for pericardiocentesis guidance (93303-93325)
Radiologically guided catheter placement for percutaneous drainage (75989)

8.09 8.09 **FUD** 000

AMA: 2020,Jan,7

33019 Pericardial drainage with insertion of indwelling catheter, percutaneous, including CT guidance

INCLUDES Catheters that remain in patient at procedure conclusion
Imaging guidance for needle placement:
Computed tomography (77012)
Fluoroscopy (77002)
Magnetic resonance (77021)
Ultrasound (76942)

EXCLUDES *Radiologically guided catheter placement for percutaneous drainage (75989)*

6.57 6.57 **FUD** 000

AMA: 2020,Jan,7

33020 Pericardiotomy for removal of clot or foreign body (primary procedure)

INCLUDES Tube thoracostomy when chest tube or pleural drain placed on same side (32551)

23.8 23.8 **FUD** 090 C 80

AMA: 1997,Nov,1

33025 Creation of pericardial window or partial resection for drainage

INCLUDES Tube thoracostomy when chest tube or pleural drain placed on same side (32551)

EXCLUDES *Surgical thoracoscopy (video-assisted thoracic surgery [VATS]) creation of pericardial window (32659)*

22.2 22.2 **FUD** 090 C 80

AMA: 1997,Nov,1

33030 Pericardiectomy, subtotal or complete; without cardiopulmonary bypass

INCLUDES Delorme pericardiectomy

57.8 57.8 **FUD** 090 C 80

AMA: 1997,Nov,1; 1994,Win,1

33031 with cardiopulmonary bypass

71.7 71.7 **FUD** 090 C 80

AMA: 2017,Dec,3

33050 Resection of pericardial cyst or tumor

EXCLUDES *Open biopsy pericardium (39010)*
Surgical thoracoscopy (video-assisted thoracic surgery [VATS]) resection of cyst, mass, or tumor pericardium (32661)

28.9 28.9 **FUD** 090 C 80

AMA: 1997,Nov,1

33120-33130 Neoplasms of Heart

Code also removal thrombus through separate heart incision, when performed (33310-33315); append modifier 59 to (33315)

33120 Excision of intracardiac tumor, resection with cardiopulmonary bypass

60.6 60.6 **FUD** 090 C 80

AMA: 2018,Jan,8; 2017,Dec,3; 2017,Jan,8; 2016,Jan,13; 2015,Jan,16

33130 Resection of external cardiac tumor

39.5 39.5 **FUD** 090 C 80

AMA: 2018,Jan,8; 2017,Jan,8; 2016,Jan,13; 2015,Jan,16

33140-33141 Transmyocardial Revascularization

33140 Transmyocardial laser revascularization, by thoracotomy; (separate procedure)

45.5 45.5 **FUD** 090 C 80

AMA: 2018,Jan,8; 2017,Jan,8; 2016,Jan,13; 2015,Jan,16

\+ **33141 performed at the time of other open cardiac procedure(s) (List separately in addition to code for primary procedure)**

Code first (33390-33391, 33404-33496, 33510-33536, 33542)

3.80 3.80 **FUD** ZZZ C 80

AMA: 2018,Jan,8; 2017,Jan,8; 2016,Jan,13; 2015,Jan,16

33202-33203 Placement Epicardial Leads

INCLUDES Imaging guidance:
- Fluoroscopy (76000)
- Ultrasound (76942, 76998, 93318)

Temporary pacemaker (33210-33211)

Code also insertion pulse generator when performed by same physician/same surgical session (33212-33213, [33221], 33230-33231, 33240)

33202 Insertion of epicardial electrode(s); open incision (eg, thoracotomy, median sternotomy, subxiphoid approach)

22.3 22.3 **FUD** 090 C

AMA: 2019,Mar,6; 2018,Jan,8; 2017,Jan,8; 2016,Aug,5; 2016,May,5; 2016,Jan,13; 2015,May,3; 2015,Jan,16

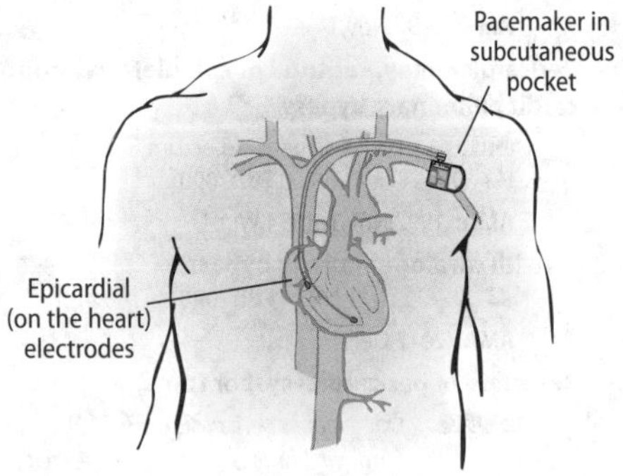

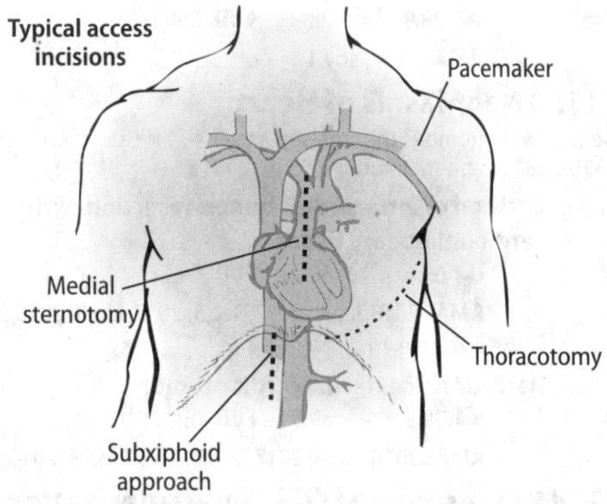

33203 endoscopic approach (eg, thoracoscopy, pericardioscopy)

23.3 23.3 **FUD** 090 C

AMA: 2019,Mar,6; 2018,Jan,8; 2017,Jan,8; 2016,Aug,5; 2016,May,5; 2016,Jan,13; 2015,May,3; 2015,Jan,16

33206-33214 [33221] Pacemakers

INCLUDES Device evaluation (93279-93298 [93260, 93261])

Dual lead: device that paces and senses in two heart chambers

Imaging guidance:
- Fluoroscopy (76000)
- Ultrasound (76942, 76998, 93318)

Multiple lead: device that paces and senses in three or more heart chambers

Radiological supervision and interpretation for pacemaker procedure

Single lead: device that paces and senses in one heart chamber

Skin pocket revision, when performed

Temporary pacemaker (33210-33211)

EXCLUDES *Electrode repositioning:*
- *Left ventricle (33226)*
- *Pacemaker (33215)*

Insertion lead for left ventricular (biventricular) pacing (33224-33225)

Leadless pacemaker systems ([33274, 33275])

Code also wound infection or hematoma incision/drainage, when performed (10140, 10180, 11042-11047 [11045, 11046])

33206 Insertion of new or replacement of permanent pacemaker with transvenous electrode(s); atrial

INCLUDES Pulse generator insertion/single transvenous electrode placement

EXCLUDES *Insertion transvenous electrode only (33216-33217)*

Removal with immediate replacement pacemaker pulse generator only, single lead system ([33227])

Code also removal old pacemaker pulse generator and electrode, when replacement entire system performed:
- Electrode (33234)
- Pulse generator (33233)

13.1 13.1 **FUD** 090 J J8

AMA: 2019,Oct,3; 2019,Mar,6; 2018,Jan,8; 2017,Jan,8; 2016,Aug,5; 2016,May,5; 2016,Jan,13; 2015,May,3; 2015,Jan,16

33207 ventricular

INCLUDES Pulse generator insertion/single transvenous electrode placement

EXCLUDES *Insertion transvenous electrode only (33216-33217)*

Removal with immediate replacement pacemaker pulse generator only, single lead system ([33227])

Code also removal old pacemaker pulse generator and electrode, when replacement entire system performed:
- Electrode (33234)
- Pulse generator (33233)

13.9 13.9 **FUD** 090 J J8

AMA: 2019,Oct,3; 2019,Mar,6; 2018,Jan,8; 2017,Jan,8; 2016,Aug,5; 2016,May,5; 2016,Jan,13; 2015,May,3; 2015,Jan,16

33208 atrial and ventricular

INCLUDES Pulse generator insertion/dual transvenous electrode placement

EXCLUDES *Insertion transvenous electrode(s) only (33216-33217)*

Removal with immediate replacement pacemaker pulse generator only, dual or multiple lead system ([33228, 33229])

Code also removal old pacemaker pulse generator and electrode, when replacement entire system performed:
- Electrodes (33235)
- Pulse generator (33233)

15.1 15.1 **FUD** 090 J J8

AMA: 2019,Oct,3; 2019,Mar,6; 2018,Jan,8; 2017,Jan,8; 2016,Aug,5; 2016,May,5; 2016,Jan,13; 2015,May,3; 2015,Jan,16

33210 Insertion or replacement of temporary transvenous single chamber cardiac electrode or pacemaker catheter (separate procedure)

4.74 4.74 **FUD** 000 J G2

AMA: 2019,Oct,3; 2019,Mar,6; 2018,Jan,8; 2017,Jan,8; 2016,Aug,5; 2016,May,5; 2016,Jan,13; 2015,May,3; 2015,Jan,16

33211 Insertion or replacement of temporary transvenous dual chamber pacing electrodes (separate procedure)

4.90 4.90 **FUD** 000 J J8

AMA: 2019,Oct,3; 2019,Mar,6; 2018,Jan,8; 2017,Jan,8; 2016,Aug,5; 2016,May,5; 2016,Jan,13; 2015,May,3; 2015,Jan,16

33212 **Insertion of pacemaker pulse generator only; with existing single lead**

EXCLUDES *Insertion for replacement single lead pacemaker pulse generator ([33227])*
Insertion transvenous electrode(s) (33216-33217)
Removal permanent pacemaker pulse generator only (33233)

Code also placement epicardial leads by same physician/same surgical session (33202-33203)

9.31 9.31 **FUD** 090 J J8

AMA: 2019,Oct,3; 2019,Mar,6; 2018,Jan,8; 2017,Jan,8; 2016,Aug,5; 2016,May,5; 2016,Jan,13; 2015,May,3; 2015,Jan,16

33213 **with existing dual leads**

EXCLUDES *Insertion for replacement dual lead pacemaker pulse generator ([33228])*
Insertion transvenous electrode(s) (33216-33217)
Removal permanent pacemaker pulse generator only (33233)

Code also placement epicardial leads by same physician/same surgical session (33202-33203)

9.73 9.73 **FUD** 090 J J8

AMA: 2019,Oct,3; 2019,Mar,6; 2018,Jan,8; 2017,Jan,8; 2016,Aug,5; 2016,May,5; 2016,Jan,13; 2015,May,3; 2015,Jan,16

33221 **with existing multiple leads**

EXCLUDES *Insertion for replacement multiple lead pacemaker pulse generator ([33229])*
Insertion transvenous electrode(s) (33216-33217)
Removal permanent pacemaker pulse generator only (33233)

Code also placement epicardial leads by same physician/same surgical session (33202-33203)

10.4 10.4 **FUD** 090 J J8

AMA: 2019,Oct,3; 2019,Mar,6; 2018,Jan,8; 2017,Jan,8; 2016,Aug,5; 2016,May,5; 2016,Jan,13; 2015,May,3; 2015,Jan,16

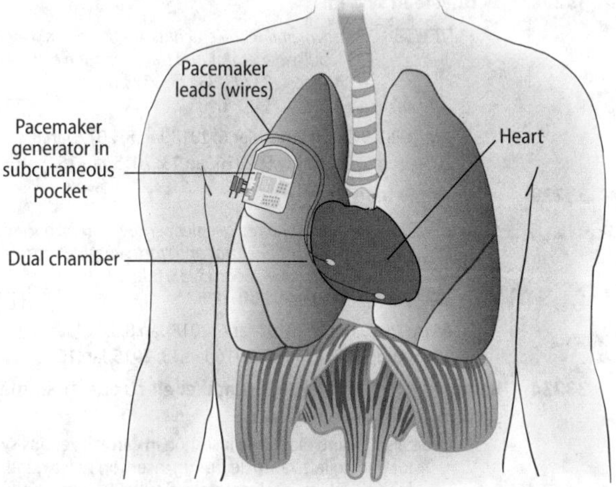

33214 **Upgrade of implanted pacemaker system, conversion of single chamber system to dual chamber system (includes removal of previously placed pulse generator, testing of existing lead, insertion of new lead, insertion of new pulse generator)**

EXCLUDES *Insertion transvenous electrode(s) (33216-33217)*
Removal and replacement pacemaker pulse generator (33227-33229)

13.8 13.8 **FUD** 090 J J8 80

AMA: 2019,Oct,3; 2019,Mar,6; 2018,Jan,8; 2017,Jan,8; 2016,Aug,5; 2016,May,5; 2016,Jan,13; 2015,May,3; 2015,Jan,16

33215-33249 [33221, 33227, 33228, 33229, 33230, 33231, 33262, 33263, 33264] Pacemakers/Implantable Defibrillator/Electrode Insertion/Replacement/Revision/Repair

INCLUDES Device evaluation (93279-93298 [93260, 93261])
Dual lead: device that paces and senses in two heart chambers
Imaging guidance:
Fluoroscopy (76000)
Ultrasound (76942, 76998, 93318)
Multiple lead: device that paces and senses in three or more heart chambers
Radiological supervision and interpretation for pacemaker or pacing cardioverter-defibrillator procedure
Single lead: device that paces and senses in one heart chamber
Skin pocket revision, when performed
Temporary pacemaker (33210-33211)

EXCLUDES *Electrode repositioning:*
Left ventricle (33226)
Pacemaker or implantable defibrillator (33215)
Insertion lead for left ventricular (biventricular) pacing (33224-33225)
Removal leadless pacemaker system ([33275])
Removal subcutaneous implantable defibrillator electrode ([33272])
Testing defibrillator threshold (DFT) during follow-up evaluation (93642-93644)
Testing defibrillator threshold (DFT) during insertion/replacement (93640-93641)

Code also wound infection or hematoma incision/drainage, when performed (10140, 10180, 11042-11047 [11045, 11046])

33215 **Repositioning of previously implanted transvenous pacemaker or implantable defibrillator (right atrial or right ventricular) electrode**

9.01 9.01 **FUD** 090 T G2

AMA: 2019,Oct,3; 2019,Mar,6; 2018,Jan,8; 2017,Jan,8; 2016,Aug,5; 2016,May,5; 2016,Jan,13; 2015,May,3; 2015,Jan,16

33216 **Insertion of a single transvenous electrode, permanent pacemaker or implantable defibrillator**

EXCLUDES *Insertion or replacement lead for cardiac venous system (33224-33225)*
Insertion or replacement permanent implantable defibrillator generator or system (33249)
Removal and replacement permanent pacemaker or implantable defibrillator (33206-33208, 33212-33213, [33221], 33227-33229, 33230-33231, 33240, [33262, 33263, 33264])

10.7 10.7 **FUD** 090 J J8

AMA: 2019,Oct,3; 2019,Mar,6; 2018,Jan,8; 2017,Jan,8; 2016,Aug,5; 2016,May,5; 2016,Jan,13; 2015,May,3; 2015,Jan,16

33217 **Insertion of 2 transvenous electrodes, permanent pacemaker or implantable defibrillator**

EXCLUDES *Insertion or replacement lead for cardiac venous system (33224-33225)*
Insertion or replacement permanent implantable defibrillator generator or system (33249)
Removal and replacement permanent pacemaker or implantable defibrillator (33206-33208, 33212-33213, [33221], 33227-33229, 33230-33231, 33240, [33262, 33263, 33264])

10.6 10.6 **FUD** 090 J J8

AMA: 2019,Oct,3; 2019,Mar,6; 2018,Jan,8; 2017,Jan,8; 2016,Aug,5; 2016,May,5; 2016,Jan,13; 2015,May,3; 2015,Jan,16

33218 **Repair of single transvenous electrode, permanent pacemaker or implantable defibrillator**

Code also removal old generator with insertion new generator replacement, when performed:
Implantable defibrillator ([33262, 33263, 33264])
Pacemaker ([33227, 33228, 33229])

11.2 11.2 **FUD** 090 T G2

AMA: 2019,Oct,3; 2019,Mar,6; 2018,Jan,8; 2017,Jan,8; 2016,Aug,5; 2016,May,5; 2016,Jan,13; 2015,May,3; 2015,Jan,16

33220 Repair of 2 transvenous electrodes for permanent pacemaker or implantable defibrillator

Code also modifier 52 Reduced services, when one electrode in two-chamber system repaired

Code also removal old generator with insertion new generator replacement, when performed:

Implantable defibrillator ([33263, 33264])

Pacemaker ([33228, 33229])

10.9 10.9 **FUD** 090 T J8

AMA: 2019,Oct,3; 2019,Mar,6; 2018,Jan,8; 2017,Jan,8; 2016,Aug,5; 2016,May,5; 2016,Jan,13; 2015,May,3; 2015,Jan,16

***33221* Resequenced code. See code following 33213.**

33222 Relocation of skin pocket for pacemaker

INCLUDES Formation new pocket

Procedures related to existing pocket:

Accessing pocket

Incision/drainage abscess or hematoma (10140, 10180)

Pocket closure (13100-13102)

EXCLUDES *Debridement, subcutaneous tissue (11042-11047 [11045, 11046])*

Code also removal and replacement existing generator

9.84 9.84 **FUD** 090 T A2

AMA: 2019,Oct,3; 2019,Mar,6; 2018,Jan,8; 2017,Jan,8; 2016,Aug,5; 2016,May,5; 2016,Jan,13; 2015,May,3; 2015,Jan,16

33223 Relocation of skin pocket for implantable defibrillator

INCLUDES Formation new pocket

Procedures related to existing pocket:

Accessing pocket

Incision/drainage abscess or hematoma (10140, 10180)

Pocket closure (13100-13102)

EXCLUDES *Debridement, subcutaneous tissue (11042-11047 [11045, 11046])*

Code also removal and replacement existing generator

11.8 11.8 **FUD** 090 T A2 80

AMA: 2019,Oct,3; 2019,Mar,6; 2018,Jan,8; 2017,Jan,8; 2016,Aug,5; 2016,Jan,13; 2015,Jan,16

33224 Insertion of pacing electrode, cardiac venous system, for left ventricular pacing, with attachment to previously placed pacemaker or implantable defibrillator pulse generator (including revision of pocket, removal, insertion, and/or replacement of existing generator)

Code also placement epicardial electrode when appropriate (33202-33203)

14.9 14.9 **FUD** 000 J J8

AMA: 2019,Oct,3; 2019,Mar,6; 2018,Jan,8; 2017,Jan,8; 2016,Aug,5; 2016,May,5; 2016,Jan,13; 2015,May,3; 2015,Jan,16

+ **33225 Insertion of pacing electrode, cardiac venous system, for left ventricular pacing, at time of insertion of implantable defibrillator or pacemaker pulse generator (eg, for upgrade to dual chamber system) (List separately in addition to code for primary procedure)**

Code also placement epicardial electrode when appropriate (33202-33203)

Code first (33206-33208, 33212-33213, [33221], 33214, 33216-33217, 33223, 33228-33229, 33230-33231, 33233, 33234-33235, 33240, [33263, 33264], 33249)

Code first (33223) for relocation pocket for implantable defibrillator

Code first (33222) for relocation pocket for pacemaker pulse generator

13.6 13.6 **FUD** ZZZ N N1

AMA: 2019,Oct,3; 2019,Mar,6; 2018,Jan,8; 2017,Jan,8; 2016,Aug,5; 2016,May,5; 2016,Jan,13; 2015,May,3; 2015,Jan,16

33226 Repositioning of previously implanted cardiac venous system (left ventricular) electrode (including removal, insertion and/or replacement of existing generator)

14.4 14.4 **FUD** 000 T G2

AMA: 2019,Oct,3; 2019,Mar,6; 2018,Jan,8; 2017,Jan,8; 2016,Aug,5; 2016,May,5; 2016,Jan,13; 2015,May,3; 2015,Jan,16

***33227* Resequenced code. See code following 33233.**

***33228* Resequenced code. See code following 33233.**

***33229* Resequenced code. See code before 33234.**

***33230* Resequenced code. See code following 33240.**

***33231* Resequenced code. See code before 33241.**

33233 Removal of permanent pacemaker pulse generator only

EXCLUDES *Removal with immediate replacement pacemaker pulse generator, without replacement electrode(s):*

Dual lead system ([33228])

Multiple lead system ([33229])

Single lead system ([33227])

Code also insertion replacement pacemaker pulse generator with transvenous electrode(s) (total system), when performed:

Pacemaker and dual leads (33208)

Pacemaker and single atrial lead (33206)

Pacemaker and single ventricular lead (33207)

Code also removal electrode(s), when removal total system without replacement performed:

Dual leads (atrial and ventricular) (33235)

Single lead (atrial or ventricular) (33234)

6.68 6.68 **FUD** 090 Q2 J8

AMA: 2019,Oct,3; 2019,Mar,6; 2018,Jan,8; 2017,Jan,8; 2016,Aug,5; 2016,May,5; 2016,Jan,13; 2015,Jan,16

33227 Removal of permanent pacemaker pulse generator with replacement of pacemaker pulse generator; single lead system

EXCLUDES *Removal and replacement entire system, pacemaker pulse generator and transvenous electrode, report (33206-33207, 33233, 33234)*

Removal and replacement for conversion from single chamber to dual chamber system (33214)

9.82 9.82 **FUD** 090 J J8

AMA: 2019,Oct,3; 2019,Mar,6; 2018,Jan,8; 2017,Jan,8; 2016,Aug,5; 2016,May,5; 2016,Jan,13; 2015,Jan,16

33228 dual lead system

EXCLUDES *Removal and replacement entire system, pacemaker pulse generator and transvenous electrode(s), report (33208, 33233, 33235)*

10.2 10.2 **FUD** 090 J J8

AMA: 2019,Oct,3; 2019,Mar,6; 2018,Jan,8; 2017,Jan,8; 2016,Aug,5; 2016,May,5; 2016,Jan,13; 2015,Jan,16

33229 multiple lead system

EXCLUDES *Removal and replacement entire system, pacemaker pulse generator and transvenous electrode(s), report (33208, 33233, 33235)*

10.8 10.8 **FUD** 090 J J8

AMA: 2019,Oct,3; 2019,Mar,6; 2018,Jan,8; 2017,Jan,8; 2016,Aug,5; 2016,May,5; 2016,Jan,13; 2015,Jan,16

33234 Removal of transvenous pacemaker electrode(s); single lead system, atrial or ventricular

Code also pacing electrode insertion in cardiac venous system for pacing left ventricle during insertion pulse generator (pacemaker or implantable defibrillator) when performed (33225)

Code also removal old pacemaker pulse generator and insertion replacement pacemaker pulse generator with transvenous electrode (total system), when performed:

Insertion pacemaker and atrial lead (33206) OR

Insertion pacemaker and ventricular lead (33207) AND

Removal generator (33233)

Code also thoracotomy to remove electrode, when performed, for unsuccessful transvenous removal (33238)

14.0 14.0 **FUD** 090 Q2 G2

AMA: 2019,Oct,3; 2019,Mar,6; 2018,Jan,8; 2017,Jan,8; 2016,Aug,5; 2016,May,5; 2016,Jan,13; 2015,Jan,16

33235 dual lead system

Code also pacing electrode insertion in cardiac venous system for pacing left ventricle during insertion pulse generator (pacemaker or implantable defibrillator) when performed (33225)

Code also removal old pacemaker pulse generator and insertion replacement pacemaker pulse generator with transvenous electrodes (total system), when performed:

Insertion generator and dual leads (33208) AND

Insertion pacemaker and atrial lead (33206) OR

Insertion pacemaker and ventricular lead (33207) AND

Removal generator (33233)

Code also thoracotomy to remove electrode, when performed, for unsuccessful transvenous removal (33238)

18.5 18.5 **FUD** 090 Q2 J8

AMA: 2019,Oct,3; 2019,Mar,6; 2018,Jan,8; 2017,Jan,8; 2016,Aug,5; 2016,May,5; 2016,Jan,13; 2015,Jan,16

33236 Removal of permanent epicardial pacemaker and electrodes by thoracotomy; single lead system, atrial or ventricular

EXCLUDES *Removal implantable defibrillator electrode(s) by thoracotomy (33243)*

Removal transvenous electrodes by thoracotomy (33238)

Removal transvenous pacemaker electrodes, single or dual lead system; without thoracotomy (33234, 33235)

22.5 22.5 **FUD** 090 C 80

AMA: 2019,Oct,3; 2019,Mar,6; 2018,Jan,8; 2017,Jan,8; 2016,Aug,5; 2016,May,5; 2016,Jan,13; 2015,Jan,16

33237 dual lead system

EXCLUDES *Removal implantable defibrillator electrode(s) by thoracotomy (33243)*

Removal transvenous electrodes by thoracotomy (33238)

Removal transvenous pacemaker electrodes, single or dual lead system; without thoracotomy (33234, 33235)

24.1 24.1 **FUD** 090 C 80

AMA: 2019,Oct,3; 2019,Mar,6; 2018,Jan,8; 2017,Jan,8; 2016,Aug,5; 2016,May,5; 2016,Jan,13; 2015,Jan,16

33238 Removal of permanent transvenous electrode(s) by thoracotomy

EXCLUDES *Removal implantable defibrillator electrode(s) by thoracotomy (33243)*

Removal transvenous pacemaker electrodes, single or dual lead system; without thoracotomy (33234, 33235)

27.0 27.0 **FUD** 090 C 80

AMA: 2019,Oct,3; 2018,Jan,8; 2017,Jan,8; 2016,Aug,5; 2016,May,5; 2016,Jan,13; 2015,Jan,16

33240 Insertion of implantable defibrillator pulse generator only; with existing single lead

EXCLUDES *Insertion electrode(s) (33216-33217, [33271])*

Removal and replacement implantable defibrillator pulse generator only ([33262, 33263, 33264])

Code also placement epicardial leads by same physician/same surgical session as generator insertion (33202-33203)

10.5 10.5 **FUD** 090 J J8

AMA: 2019,Oct,3; 2018,Jan,8; 2017,Jan,8; 2016,Aug,5; 2016,Jan,13; 2015,Jan,16

\# **33230 with existing dual leads**

EXCLUDES *Insertion single transvenous electrode, permanent pacemaker or implantable defibrillator (33216-33217)*

Removal and replacement implantable defibrillator pulse generator only ([33262, 33263, 33264])

Code also placement epicardial leads by same physician/same surgical session as generator insertion (33202-33203)

11.0 11.0 **FUD** 090 J J8

AMA: 2019,Oct,3; 2019,Mar,6; 2018,Jan,8; 2017,Jan,8; 2016,Aug,5; 2016,Jan,13; 2015,Jan,16

\# **33231 with existing multiple leads**

EXCLUDES *Insertion single transvenous electrode, permanent pacemaker or implantable defibrillator (33216-33217)*

Removal and replacement implantable defibrillator pulse generator only ([33262, 33263, 33264])

Code also placement epicardial leads by same physician/same surgical session as generator placement (33202-33203)

11.6 11.6 **FUD** 090 J J8

AMA: 2019,Oct,3; 2019,Mar,6; 2018,Jan,8; 2017,Jan,8; 2016,Aug,5; 2016,Jan,13; 2015,Jan,16

33241 Removal of implantable defibrillator pulse generator only

EXCLUDES *Removal substernal implantable defibrillator pulse generator only (0580T)*

Removal with immediate replacement implantable defibrillator pulse generator only ([33262, 33263, 33264])

Code also removal electrode(s) and insertion replacement defibrillator with electrode(s) (total system), when performed:

Removal electrode(s) (33243-33244) AND

Insertion defibrillator system, single or dual (33249) OR

Removal subcutaneous electrode ([33272]) AND

Insertion subcutaneous defibrillator system ([33270])

Code also removal electrode(s), when total system removed without replacement:

Subcutaneous electrode ([33272])

Transvenous electrode(s) (33243)

6.20 6.20 **FUD** 090 Q2 G2

AMA: 2019,Oct,3; 2018,Jan,8; 2017,Jan,8; 2016,Aug,5; 2016,Jan,13; 2015,Jan,16

\# **33262 Removal of implantable defibrillator pulse generator with replacement of implantable defibrillator pulse generator; single lead system**

EXCLUDES *Insertion electrode(s) (33216-33217, [33271])*

Removal and replacement implantable defibrillator pulse generator and electrode(s) (total system) (33241, 33243-33244, 33249)

Removal and replacement subcutaneous defibrillator pulse generator and electrode(s) (total system) (33241, [33270], [33272])

Removal and replacement substernal implantable defibrillator pulse generator ([0614T])

Removal implantable defibrillator pulse generator only (33241)

Repair implantable defibrillator pulse generator and/or leads (33218, 33220)

Code also electrode(s) removal by thoracotomy (33243)

Code also subcutaneous electrode removal ([33272])

Code also transvenous removal of electrode(s) (33244)

10.8 10.8 **FUD** 090 J J8

AMA: 2019,Oct,3; 2018,Jan,8; 2017,Jan,8; 2016,Aug,5; 2016,Jan,13; 2015,Jan,16

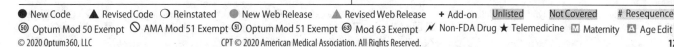

33263 **dual lead system**

EXCLUDES *Insertion single transvenous electrode, permanent pacemaker or implantable defibrillator (33216-33217)*
Removal and replacement implantable defibrillator pulse generator and electrode(s) (total system) (33241, 33243-33244, 33249)
Removal and replacement subcutaneous defibrillator pulse generator and electrode (total system) (33241, [33270], [33272])
Removal implantable defibrillator pulse generator only (33241)
Repair implantable defibrillator pulse generator and/or leads (33218, 33220)

Code also removal electrodes by thoracotomy (33243)
Code also transvenous removal electrodes (33244)

11.2 11.2 **FUD** 090 J J8

AMA: 2019,Oct,3; 2018,Jan,8; 2017,Jan,8; 2016,Aug,5; 2016,Jan,13; 2015,Jan,16

33264 **multiple lead system**

EXCLUDES *Insertion single transvenous electrode, permanent pacemaker or implantable defibrillator (33216-33217)*
Removal and replacement implantable defibrillator pulse generator and electrode(s) (total system) (33241, 33243-33244, 33249)
Removal and replacement subcutaneous defibrillator pulse generator and electrode(s) (total system) (33241, [33270], [33272])
Removal implantable defibrillator pulse generator only (33241)
Repair implantable defibrillator pulse generator and/or leads (33218, 33220)

Code also removal electrodes by thoracotomy (33243)
Code also transvenous removal electrodes (33244)

11.7 11.7 **FUD** 090 J J8

AMA: 2019,Oct,3; 2018,Jan,8; 2017,Jan,8; 2016,Aug,5; 2016,Jan,13; 2015,Jan,16

33243 **Removal of single or dual chamber implantable defibrillator electrode(s); by thoracotomy**

EXCLUDES *Transvenous removal defibrillator electrode(s) (33244)*

Code also removal implantable defibrillator pulse generator and insertion replacement defibrillator with electrodes (total system), when entire system replaced:
Insertion defibrillator system, single or dual (33249)
Removal generator (33241)
Code also removal implantable defibrillator pulse generator, when entire system removed without replacement (33241)
Code also replacement implantable defibrillator pulse generator, when performed:
Dual lead system ([33263])
Multiple lead system ([33264])
Single lead system ([33262])

39.6 39.6 **FUD** 090 C 80

AMA: 2019,Oct,3; 2018,Jan,8; 2017,Jan,8; 2016,Aug,5; 2016,Jan,13; 2015,Jan,16

33244 **by transvenous extraction**

Code also removal implantable defibrillator pulse generator and insertion replacement defibrillator with electrodes (total system), when entire system replaced:
Insertion defibrillator system, single or dual (33249)
Removal generator (33241)
Code also removal implantable defibrillator pulse generator, when entire system removed without replacement (33241)
Code also replacement implantable defibrillator pulse generator, when performed:
Dual lead system ([33263])
Multiple lead system ([33264])
Single lead system ([33262])
Code also thoracotomy to remove electrode, when performed, if transvenous removal unsuccessful (33238, 33243)

25.1 25.1 **FUD** 090 Q2

AMA: 2019,Oct,3; 2018,Jan,8; 2017,Jan,8; 2016,Aug,5; 2016,Jan,13; 2015,Jan,16

33249 **Insertion or replacement of permanent implantable defibrillator system, with transvenous lead(s), single or dual chamber**

EXCLUDES *Insertion single transvenous electrode, permanent pacemaker or implantable defibrillator (33216-33217)*

Code also removal defibrillator generator when upgrading from single to dual-chamber system (33241)
Code also removal implantable defibrillator pulse generator and removal electrode(s), when entire system replaced:
Removal electrode(s) (33243-33244)
Removal generator (33241)

26.6 26.6 **FUD** 090 J J8

AMA: 2019,Oct,3; 2018,Jan,8; 2017,Jan,8; 2016,Aug,5; 2016,Jan,13; 2015,Jan,16

33270-33275 [33270, 33271, 33272, 33273, 33274, 33275] Subcutaneous Implantable Defibrillator

INCLUDES Programming and interrogation of:
Leadless pacemaker (93279, 93286, 93288, 93294, 93296)
Subcutaneous implantable defibrillator ([93260, 93261])

33270 **Insertion or replacement of permanent subcutaneous implantable defibrillator system, with subcutaneous electrode, including defibrillation threshold evaluation, induction of arrhythmia, evaluation of sensing for arrhythmia termination, and programming or reprogramming of sensing or therapeutic parameters, when performed**

INCLUDES Electrophysiologic evaluation at initial insertion (93644)

EXCLUDES *Insertion subcutaneous implantable defibrillator electrode only ([33271])*
Insertion/replacement permanent implantable defibrillator system with substernal electrode (0571T)

Code also electrophysiologic evaluation following replacement subcutaneous implantable defibrillator, when performed (93644)
Code also removal subcutaneous implantable defibrillator and removal subcutaneous electrode, when entire system is being replaced:
Defibrillator (33241)
Electrode ([33272])

16.4 16.4 **FUD** 090 J J8

AMA: 2019,Oct,3; 2018,Jan,8; 2017,Jan,8; 2016,Aug,5; 2016,Jan,13; 2015,Jan,16

33271 **Insertion of subcutaneous implantable defibrillator electrode**

EXCLUDES *Insertion implantable defibrillator pulse generator only, other than subcutaneous:*
Initial insertion (33240)
Removal/replacement ([33262])
Insertion subcutaneous implantable defibrillator and electrode (total system) ([33270])
Insertion substernal defibrillator electrode (0572T)

13.1 13.1 **FUD** 090 J J8

AMA: 2019,Oct,3; 2018,Jan,8; 2017,Jan,8; 2016,Aug,5; 2016,Jan,13; 2015,Jan,16

33272 **Removal of subcutaneous implantable defibrillator electrode**

EXCLUDES *Removal substernal defibrillator electrode (0573T)*

Code also removal implantable defibrillator, when performed:
Removal with replacement ([33262])
Removal without replacement (33241)
Code also removal subcutaneous implantable defibrillator and insertion replacement implantable subcutaneous defibrillator with electrode (total system), when entire system is being replaced:
Insertion total system ([33270])
Removal defibrillator (33241)

10.0 10.0 **FUD** 090 Q2

AMA: 2019,Oct,3; 2018,Jan,8; 2017,Jan,8; 2016,Aug,5; 2016,Jan,13; 2015,Jan,16

33273 **Repositioning of previously implanted subcutaneous implantable defibrillator electrode**

EXCLUDES *Repositioning substernal defibrillator electrode (0574T)*

11.5 11.5 FUD 090 T G2

AMA: 2019,Oct,3; 2018,Jan,8; 2017,Jan,8; 2016,Aug,5; 2016,Jan,13; 2015,Jan,16

33274 **Transcatheter insertion or replacement of permanent leadless pacemaker, right ventricular, including imaging guidance (eg, fluoroscopy, venous ultrasound, ventriculography, femoral venography) and device evaluation (eg, interrogation or programming), when performed**

INCLUDES Cardiac catheterization for insertion leadless pacemaker (93451, 93453, 93456-93457, 93460-93461, 93530-93533)
Femoral venography (75820)
Imaging guidance (76000, 76937, 77002)
Right ventriculography (93566)

EXCLUDES *Removal permanent leadless pacemaker ([33275])*
Services for pacemakers with leads (33202-33203, 33206-33208, 33212-33214 [33221], 33215-33218, 33220, 33233-33237 [33227, 33228, 33229])

14.2 14.2 FUD 090 J8

AMA: 2019,Mar,6

33275 **Transcatheter removal of permanent leadless pacemaker, right ventricular, including imaging guidance (eg, fluoroscopy, venous ultrasound, ventriculography, femoral venography), when performed**

INCLUDES Cardiac catheterization for insertion leadless pacemaker (93451, 93453, 93456-93457, 93460-93461, 93530-93533)
Femoral venography (75820)
Imaging guidance (76000, 76937, 77002)
Right ventriculography (93566)

EXCLUDES *Insertion/replacement leadless pacemaker ([33274])*
Services for pacemakers with leads (33202-33203, 33206-33208, 33212-33214 [33221], 33215-33218, 33220, 33233-33237 [33227, 33228, 33229])

15.4 15.4 FUD 090 G2

AMA: 2019,Mar,6

33250-33251 Surgical Ablation Arrhythmogenic Foci, Supraventricular

INCLUDES Procedures using cryotherapy, laser, microwave, radiofrequency, and ultrasound

33250 **Operative ablation of supraventricular arrhythmogenic focus or pathway (eg, Wolff-Parkinson-White, atrioventricular node re-entry), tract(s) and/or focus (foci); without cardiopulmonary bypass**

EXCLUDES *Pacing and mapping during surgery by other provider (93631)*

41.7 41.7 FUD 090 C 80

AMA: 2018,Jan,8; 2017,Jan,8; 2016,Jan,13; 2015,Jan,16

33251 **with cardiopulmonary bypass**

47.0 47.0 FUD 090 C 80

AMA: 2018,Jan,8; 2017,Dec,3; 2017,Jan,8; 2016,Jan,13; 2015,Jan,16

33254-33256 Surgical Ablation Arrhythmogenic Foci, Atrial (e.g., Maze)

INCLUDES Excision or isolation left atrial appendage
Procedures using cryotherapy, laser, microwave, radiofrequency, and ultrasound

EXCLUDES *Any procedure involving median sternotomy or cardiopulmonary bypass*
Aortic valve procedures (33390-33391, 33404-33415)
Aortoplasty (33417)
Ascending aorta graft (33858-33859, 33863-33864)
Coronary artery bypass (33510-33516, 33517-33523, 33533-33536)
Excision intracardiac tumor, resection (33120)
Mitral valve procedures (33418-33430)
Outflow tract augmentation (33478)
Prosthetic valve repair (33496)
Pulmonary artery embolectomy (33910-33920)
Pulmonary valve procedures (33470-33477)
Repair aberrant coronary artery anatomy (33500-33507)
Repair aberrant heart anatomy (33600-33853)
Resection external cardiac tumor (33130)
Temporary pacemaker (33210-33211)
Thoracotomy; with exploration (32100)
Tricuspid valve procedures (33460-33468)
Tube thoracostomy, includes connection to drainage system (32551)
Ventricular reconstruction (33542-33548)
Ventriculomyotomy (33416)

33254 **Operative tissue ablation and reconstruction of atria, limited (eg, modified maze procedure)**

39.0 39.0 FUD 090 C 80

AMA: 2018,Jan,8; 2017,Jan,8; 2016,Jan,13; 2015,Jan,16

33255 **Operative tissue ablation and reconstruction of atria, extensive (eg, maze procedure); without cardiopulmonary bypass**

47.4 47.4 FUD 090 C 80

AMA: 2018,Jan,8; 2017,Jan,8; 2016,Jan,13; 2015,Jan,16

33256 **with cardiopulmonary bypass**

56.1 56.1 FUD 090 C 80

AMA: 2018,Jan,8; 2017,Dec,3; 2017,Jan,8; 2016,Jan,13; 2015,Jan,16

33257-33259 Surgical Ablation Arrhythmogenic Foci, Atrial, with Other Heart Procedure(s)

EXCLUDES *Operative tissue ablation and reconstruction atria (without other cardiac procedure), limited or extensive:*
Endoscopic (33265-33266)
Open (33254-33256)
Temporary pacemaker (33210-33211)
Tube thoracostomy, includes connection to drainage system (32551)

+ 33257 **Operative tissue ablation and reconstruction of atria, performed at the time of other cardiac procedure(s), limited (eg, modified maze procedure) (List separately in addition to code for primary procedure)**

Code first (33120-33130, 33250-33251, 33261, 33300-33335, 33365, 33390-33391, 33404-33417 [33440], 33420-33430, 33460-33476, 33478, 33496, 33500-33507, 33510-33516, 33533-33548, 33600-33619, 33641-33697, 33702-33732, 33735-33767, 33770-33877, 33910-33922, 33925-33926, 33975-33983)

16.8 16.8 FUD ZZZ C 80

+ 33258 **Operative tissue ablation and reconstruction of atria, performed at the time of other cardiac procedure(s), extensive (eg, maze procedure), without cardiopulmonary bypass (List separately in addition to code for primary procedure)**

Code first, when performed without cardiopulmonary bypass (33130, 33250, 33300, 33310, 33320-33321, 33330, 33365, 33420, 33470-33471, 33501-33503, 33510-33516, 33533-33536, 33690, 33735, 33737, 33750-33766, 33800-33813, 33820-33824, 33840-33852, 33875, 33877, 33915, 33925, 33981, 33982)

18.7 18.7 FUD ZZZ C 80

\+ **33259** **Operative tissue ablation and reconstruction of atria, performed at the time of other cardiac procedure(s), extensive (eg, maze procedure), with cardiopulmonary bypass (List separately in addition to code for primary procedure)**

Code first, when performed with cardiopulmonary bypass (33120, 33251, 33261, 33305, 33315, 33322, 33335, 33390-33391, 33404-33410, 33411-33417, 33422-33430, 33460-33468, 33474-33478, 33496, 33500, 33504-33507, 33510-33516, 33533-33548, 33600-33688, 33692-33726, 33730, 33732, 33736, 33767, 33770, 33783, 33786-33788, 33814, 33853, 33858-33877, 33910, 33916-33922, 33926, 33975-33980, 33983)

24.3 24.3 **FUD** ZZZ C 80

AMA: 2017,Dec,3

33261-33264 [33262, 33263, 33264] Surgical Ablation Arrhythmogenic Foci, Ventricular

33261 **Operative ablation of ventricular arrhythmogenic focus with cardiopulmonary bypass**

47.0 47.0 **FUD** 090 C 80

AMA: 2018,Jan,8; 2017,Dec,3; 2017,Jan,8; 2016,Jan,13; 2015,Jan,16

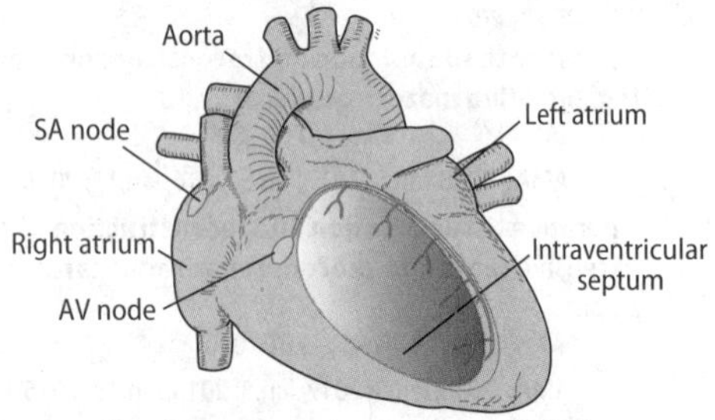

Impulse centers that are causing arrhythmia are treated with ablation

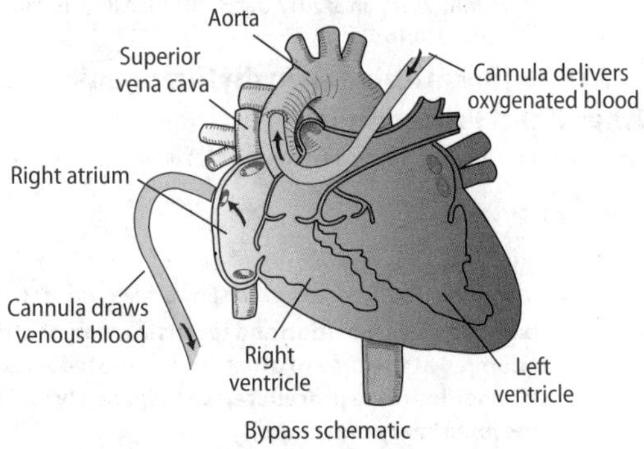

Bypass schematic

33262 **Resequenced code. See code following 33241.**

33263 **Resequenced code. See code following 33241.**

33264 **Resequenced code. See code before 33243.**

33265-33275 [33270, 33271, 33272, 33273, 33274, 33275] Surgical Ablation Arrhythmogenic Foci, Endoscopic

EXCLUDES *Insertion or replacement temporary transvenous single chamber cardiac electrode or pacemaker catheter (separate procedure) (33210-33211)*
Tube thoracostomy, includes connection to drainage system (32551)

33265 **Endoscopy, surgical; operative tissue ablation and reconstruction of atria, limited (eg, modified maze procedure), without cardiopulmonary bypass**

39.3 39.3 **FUD** 090 C 80

AMA: 2018,Jan,8; 2017,Jan,8; 2016,Jan,13; 2015,Jan,16

33266 **operative tissue ablation and reconstruction of atria, extensive (eg, maze procedure), without cardiopulmonary bypass**

53.4 53.4 **FUD** 090 C 80

AMA: 2018,Jan,8; 2017,Jan,8; 2016,Jan,13; 2015,Jan,16

33270 **Resequenced code. See code following 33249.**

33271 **Resequenced code. See code following 33249.**

33272 **Resequenced code. See code following 33249.**

33273 **Resequenced code. See code following 33249.**

33274 **Resequenced code. See code following 33249.**

33275 **Resequenced code. See code following 33249.**

33285-33289 Cardiac Rhythm Monitor System

33285 **Insertion, subcutaneous cardiac rhythm monitor, including programming**

INCLUDES Implantation device into subcutaneous prepectoral pocket
Initial programming

EXCLUDES *Successive analysis and/or reprogramming (93285, 93291, 93298)*

2.57 142. **FUD** 000 J8

AMA: 2019,Oct,3; 2019,Apr,3

33286 **Removal, subcutaneous cardiac rhythm monitor**

2.54 3.80 **FUD** 000 G2

AMA: 2019,Apr,3

33289 **Transcatheter implantation of wireless pulmonary artery pressure sensor for long-term hemodynamic monitoring, including deployment and calibration of the sensor, right heart catheterization, selective pulmonary catheterization, radiological supervision and interpretation, and pulmonary artery angiography, when performed**

INCLUDES Device implantation into subcutaneous pocket
Fluoroscopy (76000)
Pulmonary artery angiography/injection (75741, 75743, 75746, 93568)
Pulmonary artery catheterization (36013-36015)
Radiologic supervision and interpretation
Remote monitoring (93264)
Right heart catheterization (93451, 93453, 93456-93457, 93460-93461, 93530-93533)
Sensor deployment and calibration

9.55 9.55 **FUD** 000 80

AMA: 2019,Jun,3

33300-33315 Procedures for Injury of the Heart

INCLUDES Procedures with and without cardiopulmonary bypass

Code also transvascular ventricular support, when performed:
Balloon pump (33967, 33968, 33970-33974)
Extracorporeal membrane oxygenation (ECMO)/extracorporeal life support (ECLS) (33946-33949)
Ventricular assist device (33975-33983, [33995], 33990-33993 [33997])

33300 **Repair of cardiac wound; without bypass**

71.0 71.0 **FUD** 090 C 80

AMA: 1997,Nov,1

33305 **with cardiopulmonary bypass**

118. 118. **FUD** 090 C 80

AMA: 2017,Dec,3

33310 **Cardiotomy, exploratory (includes removal of foreign body, atrial or ventricular thrombus); without bypass**

EXCLUDES *Other cardiac procedures unless separate incision into heart necessary to remove thrombus*

33.7 33.7 **FUD** 090 C 80

AMA: 1997,Nov,1

33315 **with cardiopulmonary bypass**

EXCLUDES *Other cardiac procedures unless separate incision into heart necessary to remove thrombus*

Code also excision thrombus with cardiopulmonary bypass and append modifier 59 when separate incision required with (33120, 33130, 33420-33430, 33460-33468, 33496, 33542, 33545, 33641-33647, 33670, 33681, 33975-33980)

55.3 55.3 **FUD** 090 C 80

AMA: 2018,Jan,8; 2017,Dec,3; 2017,Jan,8; 2016,Jan,13; 2015,Jan,16

33320-33335 Procedures for Injury of the Aorta/Great Vessels

Code also transvascular ventricular support, when performed:
Balloon pump (33967, 33968, 33970-33974)
Extracorporeal membrane oxygenation (ECMO)/extracorporeal life support (ECLS) (33946-33949)
Ventricular assist device (33975-33983, [33995], 33990-33993 [33997])

33320 Suture repair of aorta or great vessels; without shunt or cardiopulmonary bypass
30.5 30.5 **FUD** 090 C 80
AMA: 2018,Jun,11; 2018,Jan,8; 2017,Jan,8; 2016,Jan,13; 2015,Jan,16

33321 with shunt bypass
34.3 34.3 **FUD** 090 C 80
AMA: 2018,Jun,11

33322 with cardiopulmonary bypass
40.2 40.2 **FUD** 090 C 80
AMA: 2018,Jun,11; 2018,Jan,8; 2017,Dec,3; 2017,Jan,8; 2016,Jan,13; 2015,Jan,16

33330 Insertion of graft, aorta or great vessels; without shunt, or cardiopulmonary bypass
41.2 41.2 **FUD** 090 C 80
AMA: 2018,Jun,11

33335 with cardiopulmonary bypass
54.6 54.6 **FUD** 090 C 80
AMA: 2018,Jun,11; 2017,Dec,3

33340 Closure Left Atrial Appendage

EXCLUDES *Cardiac catheterization except for reasons other than closure left atrial appendage (93451-93453, 93456, 93458-93461, 93462, 93530-93533)*
Code also transvascular ventricular support, when performed:
Balloon pump (33967, 33968, 33970-33974)
Extracorporeal membrane oxygenation (ECMO)/extracorporeal life support (ECLS) (33946-33949)
Ventricular assist device (33975-33983, [33995], 33990-33993 [33997])

33340 Percutaneous transcatheter closure of the left atrial appendage with endocardial implant, including fluoroscopy, transseptal puncture, catheter placement(s), left atrial angiography, left atrial appendage angiography, when performed, and radiological supervision and interpretation
22.9 22.9 **FUD** 000 C 80
AMA: 2018,Jan,8; 2017,Jul,3

33361-33369 Transcatheter Aortic Valve Replacement

CMS: 100-03,20.32 Transcatheter Aortic Valve Replacement (TAVR); 100-04,32,290.3 Claims Processing TAVR Inpatient; 100-04,32,290.4 Payment of TAVR for MA Plan Participants

INCLUDES Access and implantation aortic valve (33361-33366)
Access sheath placement
Advancement valve delivery system
Arteriotomy closure
Balloon aortic valvuloplasty
Cardiac or open arterial approach
Deployment of valve
Percutaneous access
Radiology procedures:
Angiography during and after procedure
Assessment access site for closure
Documentation intervention completion
Guidance for valve placement
Supervision and interpretation
Temporary pacemaker
Valve repositioning when necessary

EXCLUDES *Cardiac catheterization procedures included in TAVR/TAVI service (93452 93453, 93458-93461, 93567)*
Percutaneous coronary interventional procedures

Code also cardiac catheterization services for purposes other than TAVR/TAVI
Code also diagnostic coronary angiography at different session from interventional procedure
Code also diagnostic coronary angiography same time as TAVR/TAVI when:
Previous study available, but documentation states patient's condition has changed since previous study, visualization anatomy/pathology inadequate, or change occurs during procedure warranting additional evaluation outside current target area
No previous catheter-based coronary angiography study available, and full diagnostic study performed, with decision to perform intervention based on that study
Code also modifier 59 when diagnostic coronary angiography procedures performed as separate and distinct procedural services on same day or session as TAVR/TAVI
Code also modifier 62 as all TAVI/TAVR procedures require work two physicians
Code also transvascular ventricular support, when performed:
Balloon pump (33967, 33970, 33973)
Ventricular assist device (33975-33976, [33995], 33990-33993 [33997])

33361 Transcatheter aortic valve replacement (TAVR/TAVI) with prosthetic valve; percutaneous femoral artery approach
Code also cardiopulmonary bypass when performed (33367-33369)
39.4 39.4 **FUD** 000 C 80
AMA: 2018,Jan,8; 2017,Jan,8; 2016,Jan,13; 2015,Mar,9; 2015,Jan,16

33362 open femoral artery approach
Code also cardiopulmonary bypass when performed (33367-33369)
43.1 43.1 **FUD** 000 C 80
AMA: 2018,Jan,8; 2017,Dec,3; 2017,Jan,8; 2016,Jan,13; 2015,Mar,9; 2015,Jan,16

33363 open axillary artery approach
Code also cardiopulmonary bypass when performed (33367-33369)
44.6 44.6 **FUD** 000 C 80
AMA: 2018,Jan,8; 2017,Dec,3; 2017,Jan,8; 2016,Jan,13; 2015,Mar,9; 2015,Jan,16

33364 open iliac artery approach
Code also cardiopulmonary bypass when performed (33367-33369)
46.1 46.1 **FUD** 000 C 80
AMA: 2018,Jan,8; 2017,Dec,3; 2017,Jan,8; 2016,Jan,13; 2015,Mar,9; 2015,Jan,16

33365 transaortic approach (eg, median sternotomy, mediastinotomy)
Code also cardiopulmonary bypass when performed (33367-33369)
51.8 51.8 **FUD** 000 C 80
AMA: 2018,Jan,8; 2017,Jan,8; 2016,Jan,13; 2015,Mar,9; 2015,Jan,16

33366 **transapical exposure (eg, left thoracotomy)**

Code also cardiopulmonary bypass when performed (33367-33369)

45.7 45.7 FUD 000 C 80

AMA: 2018,Jan,8; 2017,Jan,8; 2016,Jan,13; 2015,Mar,9; 2015,Jan,16

+ **33367** **cardiopulmonary bypass support with percutaneous peripheral arterial and venous cannulation (eg, femoral vessels) (List separately in addition to code for primary procedure)**

EXCLUDES *Cardiopulmonary bypass support with open or central arterial and venous cannulation (33368-33369)*

Code first (33361-33366, 33418, 33477, 0483T-0484T, 0544T, 0545T, 0569T-0570T)

18.2 18.2 FUD ZZZ C 80

AMA: 2018,Jan,8; 2017,Jan,8; 2016,Mar,5; 2016,Jan,13; 2015,Sep,3; 2015,Jan,16

+ **33368** **cardiopulmonary bypass support with open peripheral arterial and venous cannulation (eg, femoral, iliac, axillary vessels) (List separately in addition to code for primary procedure)**

EXCLUDES *Cardiopulmonary bypass support with percutaneous or central arterial and venous cannulation (33367, 33369)*

Code first (33361-33366, 33418, 33477, 0483T-0484T, 0544T, 0545T, 0569T-0570T)

21.7 21.7 FUD ZZZ C 80

AMA: 2018,Jan,8; 2017,Jan,8; 2016,Mar,5; 2016,Jan,13; 2015,Sep,3; 2015,Jan,16

+ **33369** **cardiopulmonary bypass support with central arterial and venous cannulation (eg, aorta, right atrium, pulmonary artery) (List separately in addition to code for primary procedure)**

EXCLUDES *Cardiopulmonary bypass support with percutaneous or open arterial and venous cannulation (33367-33368)*

Code first (33361-33366, 33418, 33477, 0483T-0484T, 0544T, 0545T, 0569T-0570T)

28.6 28.6 FUD ZZZ C 80

AMA: 2018,Jan,8; 2017,Jan,8; 2016,Mar,5; 2016,Jan,13; 2015,Sep,3; 2015,Jan,16

33390-33415 [33440] Aortic Valve Procedures

Code also transvascular ventricular support, when performed:

Balloon pump (33967, 33968, 33970-33974)

Extracorporeal membrane oxygenation (ECMO)/extracorporeal life support (ECLS) (33946-33949)

Ventricular assist device (33975-33983, [33995], 33990-33993 [33997])

33390 **Valvuloplasty, aortic valve, open, with cardiopulmonary bypass; simple (ie, valvotomy, debridement, debulking, and/or simple commissural resuspension)**

54.9 54.9 FUD 090 C 80

AMA: 2018,Jan,8; 2017,Dec,3

33391 **complex (eg, leaflet extension, leaflet resection, leaflet reconstruction, or annuloplasty)**

INCLUDES Simple aortic valvuloplasty (33390)

66.4 66.4 FUD 090 C 80

AMA: 2018,Jan,8; 2017,Dec,3

33404 **Construction of apical-aortic conduit**

50.6 50.6 FUD 090 C 80

AMA: 2018,Jan,8; 2017,Dec,3; 2017,Jan,8; 2016,Jan,13; 2015,Jan,16

33405 **Replacement, aortic valve, open, with cardiopulmonary bypass; with prosthetic valve other than homograft or stentless valve**

65.7 65.7 FUD 090 C 80

AMA: 2019,Nov,9; 2019,Apr,6; 2018,Jan,8; 2017,Dec,3; 2017,Jan,8; 2016,Jan,13; 2015,Jan,16

33406 **with allograft valve (freehand)**

83.4 83.4 FUD 090 C 80

AMA: 2019,Nov,9; 2019,Apr,6; 2018,Jan,8; 2017,Dec,3; 2017,Jan,8; 2016,Jan,13; 2015,Jan,16

33410 **with stentless tissue valve**

73.6 73.6 FUD 090 C 80

AMA: 2019,Nov,9; 2019,Apr,6; 2018,Jan,8; 2017,Dec,3; 2017,Jan,8; 2016,Jan,13; 2015,Jan,16

33440 **Replacement, aortic valve; by translocation of autologous pulmonary valve and transventricular aortic annulus enlargement of the left ventricular outflow tract with valved conduit replacement of pulmonary valve (Ross-Konno procedure)**

INCLUDES Open replacement aortic valve with aortic annulus enlargement (33411-33412)

Open replacement aortic valve with translocation pulmonary valve (33413)

EXCLUDES *Aortoplasty for supravalvular stenosis (33417)*

Open replacement aortic valve (33405-33406, 33410)

Repair complex cardiac anomaly (except pulmonary atresia) (33608)

Repair left ventricular outlet obstruction (33414)

Repair pulmonary atresia (33920)

Replacement pulmonary valve (33475)

Resection/incision subvalvular tissue for aortic stenosis (33416)

98.1 98.1 FUD 090 80

AMA: 2019,Apr,6

33411 **with aortic annulus enlargement, noncoronary sinus**

97.4 97.4 FUD 090 C 80

AMA: 2019,Nov,9; 2019,Apr,6; 2018,Jan,8; 2017,Dec,3; 2017,Jan,8; 2016,Jan,13; 2015,Jan,16

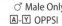

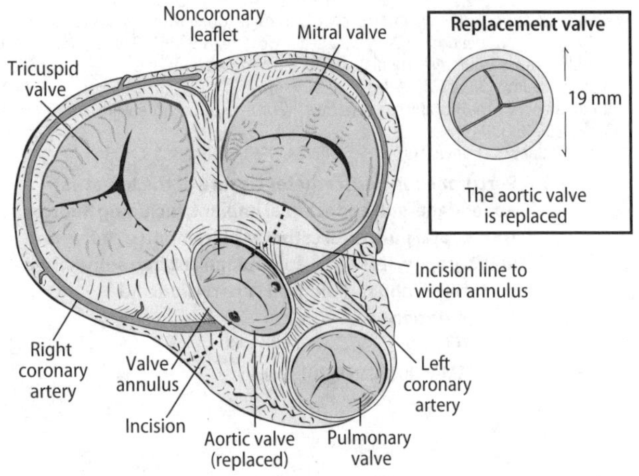

Overhead schematic of major heart valves

33412 **with transventricular aortic annulus enlargement (Konno procedure)**

EXCLUDES *Replacement aortic valve by translocation pulmonary valve, aortic annulus enlargement, valved conduit pulmonary valve replacement ([33440])*

Replacement aortic valve with translocation pulmonary valve (33413)

91.4 91.4 FUD 090 C 80

AMA: 2019,Nov,9; 2019,Apr,6; 2018,Jan,8; 2017,Dec,3; 2017,Jan,8; 2016,Jan,13; 2015,Jan,16

33413 **by translocation of autologous pulmonary valve with allograft replacement of pulmonary valve (Ross procedure)**

EXCLUDES *Replacement aortic valve by translocation pulmonary valve, aortic annulus enlargement, valved conduit pulmonary valve replacement ([33440])*

Replacement aortic valve with transventricular aortic annulus enlargement (33412)

94.3 94.3 FUD 090 C 80

AMA: 2019,Nov,9; 2019,Apr,6; 2018,Jan,8; 2017,Dec,3; 2017,Jan,8; 2016,Jan,13; 2015,Jan,16

33414 **Repair of left ventricular outflow tract obstruction by patch enlargement of the outflow tract**
62.2 62.2 FUD 090 C 80
AMA: 2019,Apr,6; 2018,Jan,8; 2017,Dec,3; 2017,Jan,8; 2016,Jan,13; 2015,Jan,16

33415 **Resection or incision of subvalvular tissue for discrete subvalvular aortic stenosis**
58.7 58.7 FUD 090 C 80
AMA: 2018,Jan,8; 2017,Dec,3; 2017,Jan,8; 2016,Jan,13; 2015,Jan,16

33416 Ventriculectomy

CMS: 100-03,20.26 Partial Ventriculectomy

EXCLUDES *Percutaneous transcatheter septal reduction therapy (93583)*

Code also transvascular ventricular support, when performed:
Balloon pump (33967, 33968, 33970-33974)
Extracorporeal membrane oxygenation (ECMO)/extracorporeal life support (ECLS) (33946-33949)
Ventricular assist device (33975-33983, [33995], 33990-33993 [33997])

33416 **Ventriculomyotomy (-myectomy) for idiopathic hypertrophic subaortic stenosis (eg, asymmetric septal hypertrophy)**
58.5 58.5 FUD 090 C 80
AMA: 2019,Apr,6; 2018,Jan,8; 2017,Dec,3; 2017,Jan,8; 2016,Jan,13; 2015,Jan,16

33417 Repair of Supravalvular Stenosis by Aortoplasty

Code also transvascular ventricular support, when performed:
Balloon pump (33967, 33968, 33970-33974)
Extracorporeal membrane oxygenation (ECMO)/extracorporeal life support (ECLS) (33946-33949)
Ventricular assist device (33975-33983, [33995], 33990-33993 [33997])

33417 **Aortoplasty (gusset) for supravalvular stenosis**
48.2 48.2 FUD 090 C 80
AMA: 2019,Apr,6; 2018,Jan,8; 2017,Dec,3; 2017,Jan,8; 2016,Jan,13; 2015,Jan,16

33418-33419 Transcatheter Mitral Valve Procedures

INCLUDES Access sheath placement
Advancement valve delivery system
Deployment valve
Radiology procedures:
Angiography during and after procedure
Documentation intervention completion
Guidance for valve placement
Supervision and interpretation
Valve repositioning when necessary

EXCLUDES *Cardiac catheterization services for purposes other than TMVR*
Diagnostic angiography different session from interventional procedure
Percutaneous approach through the coronary sinus for TMVR (0345T)
Percutaneous coronary interventional procedures
Transcatheter mitral valve annulus reconstruction (0544T)
Transcatheter TMVI by percutaneous or transthoracic approach (0483T-0484T)

Code also cardiopulmonary bypass:
Central (33369)
Open peripheral (33368)
Percutaneous peripheral (33367)
Code also diagnostic coronary angiography and cardiac catheterization procedures when:
No previous study available and full diagnostic study performed
Previous study inadequate or patient's clinical indication for study changed prior to or during procedure
Report modifier 59 with cardiac catheterization procedures when on same day or same session as TMVR
Code also transvascular ventricular support, when performed:
Balloon pump (33967, 33970, 33973)
Ventricular assist device ([33995], 33990-33993 [33997])

33418 **Transcatheter mitral valve repair, percutaneous approach, including transseptal puncture when performed; initial prosthesis**
Code also left heart catheterization when performed by transapical puncture (93462)
52.1 52.1 FUD 090 C 80
AMA: 2018,Jan,8; 2017,Jan,8; 2016,Jan,13; 2015,Sep,3

\+ 33419 **additional prosthesis(es) during same session (List separately in addition to code for primary procedure)**
EXCLUDES *Procedures performed more than one time per session*
Code first (33418)
12.3 12.3 FUD ZZZ N 80
AMA: 2018,Jan,8; 2017,Jan,8; 2016,Jan,13; 2015,Sep,3

33420-33440 [33440] Mitral Valve Procedures

Code also thrombus removal through separate heart incision, when performed (33310-33315); append modifier 59 to (33315)
Code also transvascular ventricular support, when performed:
Balloon pump (33967, 33968, 33970-33974)
Extracorporeal membrane oxygenation (ECMO)/extracorporeal life support (ECLS) (33946-33949)
Ventricular assist device (33975-33983, [33995], 33990-33993 [33997])

33420 **Valvotomy, mitral valve; closed heart**
42.3 42.3 FUD 090 C
AMA: 2018,Jan,8; 2017,Jan,8; 2016,Jan,13; 2015,Sep,3; 2015,Jan,16

33422 **open heart, with cardiopulmonary bypass**
48.1 48.1 FUD 090 C 80
AMA: 2018,Jan,8; 2017,Dec,3; 2017,Jan,8; 2016,Jan,13; 2015,Sep,3; 2015,Jan,16

33425 **Valvuloplasty, mitral valve, with cardiopulmonary bypass;**
79.1 79.1 FUD 090 C 80
AMA: 2018,Jan,8; 2017,Dec,3; 2017,Jan,8; 2016,Jan,13; 2015,Sep,3; 2015,Jan,16

33426 **with prosthetic ring**
69.0 69.0 FUD 090 C 80
AMA: 2018,Jan,8; 2017,Dec,3; 2017,Jan,8; 2016,Jan,13; 2015,Sep,3; 2015,Jan,16

33427 **radical reconstruction, with or without ring**
70.7 70.7 FUD 090 C 80
AMA: 2018,Jan,8; 2017,Dec,3; 2017,Jan,8; 2016,Jan,13; 2015,Sep,3; 2015,Jan,16

33430 **Replacement, mitral valve, with cardiopulmonary bypass**
81.1 81.1 FUD 090 C 80
AMA: 2018,Jan,8; 2017,Dec,3; 2017,Jan,8; 2016,Jan,13; 2015,Sep,3; 2015,Jan,16

33440 **Resequenced code. See code following 33410.**

33460-33468 Tricuspid Valve Procedures

EXCLUDES *Transcatheter tricuspid valve annulus reconstruction (0545T)*
Transcatheter tricuspid valve repair (0569T-0570T)

Code also thrombus removal through separate heart incision, when performed (33310-33315); append modifier 59 to (33315)
Code also transvascular ventricular support, when performed:
Balloon pump (33967, 33968, 33970-33974)
Extracorporeal membrane oxygenation (ECMO)/extracorporeal life support (ECLS) (33946-33949)
Ventricular assist device (33975-33983, [33995], 33990-33993 [33997])

33460 **Valvectomy, tricuspid valve, with cardiopulmonary bypass**
69.6 69.6 FUD 090 C 80
AMA: 2018,Jan,8; 2017,Dec,3; 2017,Jan,8; 2016,Jan,13; 2015,Jan,16

33463 **Valvuloplasty, tricuspid valve; without ring insertion**
89.5 89.5 FUD 090 C 80
AMA: 2018,Jan,8; 2017,Dec,3; 2017,Jan,8; 2016,Jan,13; 2015,Jan,16

33464 **with ring insertion**
70.7 70.7 FUD 090 C 80
AMA: 2018,Jan,8; 2017,Dec,3; 2017,Jan,8; 2016,Jan,13; 2015,Jan,16

33465 **Replacement, tricuspid valve, with cardiopulmonary bypass**
79.9 79.9 FUD 090 C 80
AMA: 2018,Jan,8; 2017,Dec,3; 2017,Jan,8; 2016,Jan,13; 2015,Jan,16

33468 **Tricuspid valve repositioning and plication for Ebstein anomaly**
71.0 71.0 FUD 090 C 80
AMA: 2018,Jan,8; 2017,Dec,3; 2017,Jan,8; 2016,Jan,13; 2015,Jan,16

33470-33474 Pulmonary Valvotomy

INCLUDES Brock's operation
Code also concurrent systemic-to-pulmonary artery shunt ligation/takedown (33924)
Code also transvascular ventricular support, when performed:
Balloon pump (33967, 33968, 33970-33974)
Extracorporeal membrane oxygenation (ECMO)/extracorporeal life support (ECLS) (33946-33949)
Ventricular assist device (33975-33983, [33995], 33990-33993 [33997])

33470 **Valvotomy, pulmonary valve, closed heart; transventricular**
35.8 35.8 FUD 090 63 C 80
AMA: 2018,Jan,8; 2017,Jan,8; 2016,Jan,13; 2015,Jan,16

33471 **via pulmonary artery**
EXCLUDES *Percutaneous valvuloplasty pulmonary valve (92990)*
38.3 38.3 FUD 090 C 80
AMA: 2018,Jan,8; 2017,Jan,8; 2016,Jan,13; 2015,Jan,16

33474 **Valvotomy, pulmonary valve, open heart, with cardiopulmonary bypass**
63.0 63.0 FUD 090 C 80
AMA: 2017,Dec,3

33475-33476 Other Procedures Pulmonary Valve

Code also concurrent systemic-to-pulmonary artery shunt ligation/takedown (33924)
Code also transvascular ventricular support, when performed:
Balloon pump (33967, 33968, 33970-33974)
Extracorporeal membrane oxygenation (ECMO)/extracorporeal life support (ECLS) (33946-33949)
Ventricular assist device (33975-33983, [33995], 33990-33993 [33997])

33475 **Replacement, pulmonary valve**
67.5 67.5 FUD 090 C 80
AMA: 2019,Apr,6; 2018,Jan,8; 2017,Dec,3; 2017,Jan,8; 2016,Jan,13; 2015,Jan,16

33476 **Right ventricular resection for infundibular stenosis, with or without commissurotomy**
INCLUDES Brock's operation
44.0 44.0 FUD 090 C 80
AMA: 2018,Jan,8; 2017,Dec,3; 2017,Jan,8; 2016,Jan,13; 2015,Jan,16

33477 Transcatheter Pulmonary Valve Implantation

INCLUDES Cardiac catheterization, contrast injection, angiography, fluoroscopic guidance and supervision and interpretation for device placement
Percutaneous balloon angioplasty within treatment area
Pre-, intra-, and postoperative hemodynamic measurements
Valvuloplasty or stent insertion in pulmonary valve conduit (37236-37237, 92997-92998)
EXCLUDES *Fluoroscopy (76000)*
Injection procedure during cardiac catheterization (93563, 93566-93568)
Percutaneous cardiac intervention procedures, when performed
Procedures performed more than one time per session
Right heart catheterization (93451, 93453-93461, 93530-93533)
Code also concurrent systemic-to-pulmonary artery shunt ligation/takedown (33924)
Code also transvascular ventricular support, when performed:
Balloon pump (33967, 33970, 33973)
Extracorporeal membrane oxygenation (ECMO)/extracorporeal life support (ECLS) (33946-33959, [33962], [33963], [33964], [33965], [33966], [33969], [33984], [33985], [33986], [33987], [33988], [33989])
Ventricular assist device ([33995], 33990-33993 [33997])

33477 **Transcatheter pulmonary valve implantation, percutaneous approach, including pre-stenting of the valve delivery site, when performed**
39.4 39.4 FUD 000 C 80
AMA: 2018,Jan,8; 2017,Jan,8; 2016,Aug,9; 2016,Mar,5

33478 Outflow Tract Augmentation

Code also for cavopulmonary anastomosis to second superior vena cava (33768)
Code also concurrent ligation/takedown systemic-to-pulmonary artery shunt (33924)
Code also transvascular ventricular support, when performed:
Balloon pump (33967, 33968, 33970-33974)
Extracorporeal membrane oxygenation (ECMO)/extracorporeal life support (ECLS) (33946-33949)
Ventricular assist device (33975-33983, [33995], 33990-33993 [33997])

33478 **Outflow tract augmentation (gusset), with or without commissurotomy or infundibular resection**
45.4 45.4 FUD 090 C 80
AMA: 2018,Jan,8; 2017,Dec,3; 2017,Jan,8; 2016,Jan,13; 2015,Jan,16

33496 Prosthetic Valve Repair

Code also thrombus removal through separate heart incision, when performed (33310-33315); append modifier 59 to (33315)
Code also reoperation if performed (33530)

33496 **Repair of non-structural prosthetic valve dysfunction with cardiopulmonary bypass (separate procedure)**
48.5 48.5 FUD 090 C 80
AMA: 2018,Jan,8; 2017,Dec,3; 2017,Jan,8; 2016,Jan,13; 2015,Jan,16

33500-33507 Repair Aberrant Coronary Artery Anatomy

INCLUDES Angioplasty and/or endarterectomy

33500 **Repair of coronary arteriovenous or arteriocardiac chamber fistula; with cardiopulmonary bypass**
45.5 45.5 FUD 090 C 80
AMA: 2017,Dec,3

33501 **without cardiopulmonary bypass**
32.2 32.2 FUD 090 C 80
AMA: 2007,Mar,1-3; 1997,Nov,1

33502 **Repair of anomalous coronary artery from pulmonary artery origin; by ligation**
36.9 36.9 FUD 090 63 C 80
AMA: 2017,Dec,3

33503 **by graft, without cardiopulmonary bypass**
38.3 38.3 FUD 090 63 C 80
AMA: 2007,Mar,1-3; 1997,Nov,1

33504 **by graft, with cardiopulmonary bypass**
42.3 42.3 FUD 090 C 80
AMA: 2017,Dec,3

33505 **with construction of intrapulmonary artery tunnel (Takeuchi procedure)**
59.8 59.8 FUD 090 63 C 80
AMA: 2017,Dec,3

33506 **by translocation from pulmonary artery to aorta**
59.7 59.7 FUD 090 63 C 80
AMA: 2017,Dec,3

33507 **Repair of anomalous (eg, intramural) aortic origin of coronary artery by unroofing or translocation**
49.8 49.8 FUD 090 C 80
AMA: 2018,Jan,8; 2017,Dec,3; 2017,Jan,8; 2016,Jan,13; 2015,Jan,16

33508 Endoscopic Harvesting of Venous Graft

INCLUDES Diagnostic endoscopy
EXCLUDES *Harvesting vein upper extremity (35500)*
Code first (33510-33523)

\+ **33508** **Endoscopy, surgical, including video-assisted harvest of vein(s) for coronary artery bypass procedure (List separately in addition to code for primary procedure)**
0.48 0.48 FUD ZZZ N N1 80
AMA: 1997,Nov,1

33510-33516 Coronary Artery Bypass: Venous Grafts

INCLUDES Obtaining saphenous vein grafts
Venous bypass grafting only

EXCLUDES *Arterial bypass (33533-33536)*
Combined arterial-venous bypass (33517-33523, 33533-33536)
Obtaining vein graft:
Femoropopliteal vein (35572)
Upper extremity vein (35500)
Percutaneous ventricular assist devices ([33995], 33990-33993 [33997])

Code also modifier 80 when assistant at surgery obtains grafts

33510 Coronary artery bypass, vein only; single coronary venous graft
56.0 56.0 **FUD** 090 C 80
AMA: 2018,Jan,8; 2017,Dec,3; 2017,Jan,8; 2016,Jan,13; 2015,Jan,16

33511 2 coronary venous grafts
61.4 61.4 **FUD** 090 C 80
AMA: 2018,Jan,8; 2017,Dec,3; 2017,Jan,8; 2016,Jan,13; 2015,Jan,16

33512 3 coronary venous grafts
70.0 70.0 **FUD** 090 C 80
AMA: 2018,Jan,8; 2017,Dec,3; 2017,Jan,8; 2016,Jan,13; 2015,Jan,16

33513 4 coronary venous grafts
71.9 71.9 **FUD** 090 C 80
AMA: 2018,Jan,8; 2017,Dec,3; 2017,Jan,8; 2016,Jan,13; 2015,Jan,16

33514 5 coronary venous grafts
75.6 75.6 **FUD** 090 C 80
AMA: 2018,Jan,8; 2017,Dec,3; 2017,Jan,8; 2016,Jan,13; 2015,Jan,16

33516 6 or more coronary venous grafts
78.1 78.1 **FUD** 090 C 80
AMA: 2018,Jan,8; 2017,Dec,3; 2017,Jan,8; 2016,Jan,13; 2015,Jan,16

33517-33523 Coronary Artery Bypass: Venous AND Arterial Grafts

INCLUDES Obtaining saphenous vein grafts

EXCLUDES *Obtaining arterial graft:*
Upper extremity (35600)
Obtaining vein graft:
Femoropopliteal vein graft (35572)
Upper extremity (35500)
Percutaneous ventricular assist devices ([33995], 33990-33993 [33997])

Code also modifier 80 when assistant at surgery obtains grafts
Code first (33533-33536)

\+ **33517 Coronary artery bypass, using venous graft(s) and arterial graft(s); single vein graft (List separately in addition to code for primary procedure)**
5.44 5.44 **FUD** ZZZ C 80
AMA: 2018,Jan,8; 2017,Jan,8; 2016,Jan,13; 2015,Jan,16

\+ **33518 2 venous grafts (List separately in addition to code for primary procedure)**
11.9 11.9 **FUD** ZZZ C 80
AMA: 2018,Jan,8; 2017,Jan,8; 2016,Jan,13; 2015,Jan,16

\+ **33519 3 venous grafts (List separately in addition to code for primary procedure)**
15.8 15.8 **FUD** ZZZ C 80
AMA: 2018,Jan,8; 2017,Jan,8; 2016,Jan,13; 2015,Jan,16

\+ **33521 4 venous grafts (List separately in addition to code for primary procedure)**
18.9 18.9 **FUD** ZZZ C 80
AMA: 2018,Jan,8; 2017,Jan,8; 2016,Jan,13; 2015,Jan,16

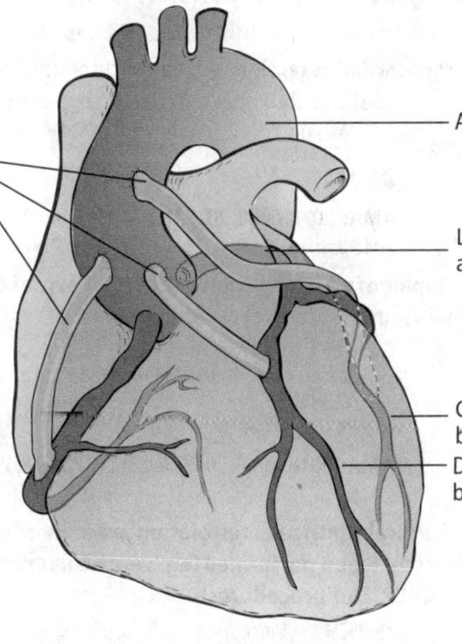

\+ **33522 5 venous grafts (List separately in addition to code for primary procedure)**
21.2 21.2 **FUD** ZZZ C 80
AMA: 2018,Jan,8; 2017,Jan,8; 2016,Jan,13; 2015,Jan,16

\+ **33523 6 or more venous grafts (List separately in addition to code for primary procedure)**
24.0 24.0 **FUD** ZZZ C 80
AMA: 2018,Jan,8; 2017,Jan,8; 2016,Jan,13; 2015,Jan,16

33530 Reoperative Coronary Artery Bypass Graft or Valve Procedure

EXCLUDES *Percutaneous ventricular assist devices (33990-33993)*

Code first (33390-33391, 33404-33496, 33510-33536, 33863)

\+ **33530 Reoperation, coronary artery bypass procedure or valve procedure, more than 1 month after original operation (List separately in addition to code for primary procedure)**
15.2 15.2 **FUD** ZZZ C 80
AMA: 2018,Jan,8; 2017,Jan,8; 2016,Jan,13; 2015,Jan,16

33533-33536 Coronary Artery Bypass: Arterial Grafts

INCLUDES Obtaining arterial graft (eg, epigastric, internal mammary, gastroepiploic and others)

EXCLUDES *Obtaining arterial graft:*
Upper extremity (35600)
Obtaining venous graft:
Femoropopliteal vein (35572)
Upper extremity (35500)
Percutaneous ventricular assist devices ([33995], 33990-33993 [33997])
Venous bypass (33510-33516)

Code also for combined arterial venous grafts (33517-33523)
Code also modifier 80 when assistant at surgery obtains grafts

33533 Coronary artery bypass, using arterial graft(s); single arterial graft
54.1 54.1 **FUD** 090 C 80
AMA: 2018,Jan,8; 2017,Dec,3; 2017,Jan,8; 2016,Jan,13; 2015,Jan,16

33534 2 coronary arterial grafts
63.6 63.6 **FUD** 090 C 80
AMA: 2018,Jan,8; 2017,Dec,3; 2017,Jan,8; 2016,Jan,13; 2015,Jan,16

33535 3 coronary arterial grafts
70.9 70.9 **FUD** 090 C 80
AMA: 2018,Jan,8; 2017,Dec,3; 2017,Jan,8; 2016,Jan,13; 2015,Jan,16

33536 **4 or more coronary arterial grafts**
76.1 76.1 **FUD** 090 C 80
AMA: 2018,Jan,8; 2017,Dec,3; 2017,Jan,8; 2016,Jan,13; 2015,Jan,16

33542-33548 Ventricular Reconstruction

EXCLUDES *Percutaneous ventricular assist devices ([33995], 33990-33993 [33997])*

33542 **Myocardial resection (eg, ventricular aneurysmectomy)**
Code also thrombus removal through separate heart incision, when performed (33310-33315); append modifier 59 to (33315)
76.1 76.1 **FUD** 090 C 80
AMA: 2018,Jan,8; 2017,Dec,3; 2017,Jan,8; 2016,Jan,13; 2015,Jan,16

33545 **Repair of postinfarction ventricular septal defect, with or without myocardial resection**
Code also thrombus removal through separate heart incision, when performed (33310-33315); append modifier 59 to (33315)
89.0 89.0 **FUD** 090 C 80
AMA: 2018,Jan,8; 2017,Dec,3; 2017,Jan,8; 2016,Jan,13; 2015,Jan,16

33548 **Surgical ventricular restoration procedure, includes prosthetic patch, when performed (eg, ventricular remodeling, SVR, SAVER, Dor procedures)**
EXCLUDES *Batista procedure or pachopexy (33999)*
Cardiotomy, exploratory (33310, 33315)
Temporary pacemaker (33210-33211)
Tube thoracostomy (32551)
85.8 85.8 **FUD** 090 C 80
AMA: 2018,Jan,8; 2017,Dec,3; 2017,Jan,8; 2016,Jan,13; 2015,Jan,16

33572 Endarterectomy with CABG (LAD, RCA, Cx)

Code first (33510-33516, 33533-33536)

\+ 33572 **Coronary endarterectomy, open, any method, of left anterior descending, circumflex, or right coronary artery performed in conjunction with coronary artery bypass graft procedure, each vessel (List separately in addition to primary procedure)**
6.67 6.67 **FUD** ZZZ C 80
AMA: 1997,Nov,1; 1994,Win,1

33600-33622 Repair Aberrant Heart Anatomy

33600 **Closure of atrioventricular valve (mitral or tricuspid) by suture or patch**
49.7 49.7 **FUD** 090 C 80
AMA: 2018,Jan,8; 2017,Dec,3; 2017,Jan,8; 2016,Jan,13; 2015,Jan,16

33602 **Closure of semilunar valve (aortic or pulmonary) by suture or patch**
Code also concurrent systemic-to-pulmonary artery shunt ligation/takedown (33924)
48.2 48.2 **FUD** 090 C 80
AMA: 2017,Dec,3

33606 **Anastomosis of pulmonary artery to aorta (Damus-Kaye-Stansel procedure)**
Code also concurrent systemic-to-pulmonary artery shunt ligation/takedown (33924)
51.4 51.4 **FUD** 090 C 80
AMA: 2017,Dec,3

33608 **Repair of complex cardiac anomaly other than pulmonary atresia with ventricular septal defect by construction or replacement of conduit from right or left ventricle to pulmonary artery**
EXCLUDES *Unifocalization arborization anomalies pulmonary artery (33925, 33926)*
Code also concurrent systemic-to-pulmonary artery shunt ligation/takedown (33924)
52.2 52.2 **FUD** 090 C 80
AMA: 2019,Apr,6; 2017,Dec,3

33610 **Repair of complex cardiac anomalies (eg, single ventricle with subaortic obstruction) by surgical enlargement of ventricular septal defect**
Code also concurrent systemic-to-pulmonary artery shunt ligation/takedown (33924)
51.5 51.5 **FUD** 090 63 C 80
AMA: 2017,Dec,3

33611 **Repair of double outlet right ventricle with intraventricular tunnel repair;**
Code also concurrent systemic-to-pulmonary artery shunt ligation/takedown (33924)
56.5 56.5 **FUD** 090 63 C 80
AMA: 2017,Dec,3

33612 **with repair of right ventricular outflow tract obstruction**
Code also concurrent systemic-to-pulmonary artery shunt ligation/takedown (33924)
58.2 58.2 **FUD** 090 C 80
AMA: 2017,Dec,3

33615 **Repair of complex cardiac anomalies (eg, tricuspid atresia) by closure of atrial septal defect and anastomosis of atria or vena cava to pulmonary artery (simple Fontan procedure)**
Code also concurrent systemic-to-pulmonary artery shunt ligation/takedown (33924)
58.0 58.0 **FUD** 090 C 80
AMA: 2017,Dec,3

33617 **Repair of complex cardiac anomalies (eg, single ventricle) by modified Fontan procedure**
Code also cavopulmonary anastomosis to second superior vena cava (33768)
Code also concurrent systemic-to-pulmonary artery shunt ligation/takedown (33924)
62.6 62.6 **FUD** 090 C 80
AMA: 2017,Dec,3

33619 **Repair of single ventricle with aortic outflow obstruction and aortic arch hypoplasia (hypoplastic left heart syndrome) (eg, Norwood procedure)**
79.2 79.2 **FUD** 090 63 C 80
AMA: 2018,Jan,8; 2017,Dec,3; 2017,Jan,8; 2016,Jul,3; 2016,Jan,13; 2015,Jan,16

33620 **Application of right and left pulmonary artery bands (eg, hybrid approach stage 1)**
EXCLUDES *Banding main pulmonary artery related to septal defect (33690)*
Code also transthoracic insertion catheter for stent placement with catheter removal and closure when performed during same session (33621)
47.7 47.7 **FUD** 090 C 80
AMA: 2018,Jan,8; 2017,Dec,3; 2017,Jan,8; 2016,Jul,3; 2016,Jan,13; 2015,Jan,16

33621 **Transthoracic insertion of catheter for stent placement with catheter removal and closure (eg, hybrid approach stage 1)**
Code also application right and left pulmonary artery bands when performed during same session (33620)
Code also stent placement (37236)
26.9 26.9 **FUD** 090 C 80
AMA: 2018,Jan,8; 2017,Dec,3; 2017,Jan,8; 2016,Jul,3; 2016,Jan,13; 2015,Jan,16

33622 **Reconstruction of complex cardiac anomaly (eg, single ventricle or hypoplastic left heart) with palliation of single ventricle with aortic outflow obstruction and aortic arch hypoplasia, creation of cavopulmonary anastomosis, and removal of right and left pulmonary bands (eg, hybrid approach stage 2, Norwood, bidirectional Glenn, pulmonary artery debanding)**

EXCLUDES *Excision coarctation aorta (33840, 33845, 33851)*
Repair hypoplastic or interrupted aortic arch (33853)
Repair patent ductus arteriosus (33822)
Repair pulmonary artery stenosis by reconstruction with patch or graft (33917)
Repair single ventricle with aortic outflow obstruction and aortic arch hypoplasia (33619)
Shunt; superior vena cava to pulmonary artery for flow to both lungs (33767)

Code also anastomosis, cavopulmonary, second superior vena cava for bilateral bidirectional Glenn procedure (33768)
Code also concurrent systemic-to-pulmonary artery shunt ligation/takedown (33924)

100. 100. **FUD** 090 C 80

AMA: 2018,Jan,8; 2017,Dec,3; 2017,Jan,8; 2016,Jul,3; 2016,Jan,13; 2015,Jan,16

33641-33645 Closure of Defect: Atrium

Code also thrombus removal through separate heart incision, when performed (33310-33315); append modifier 59 to (33315)

33641 **Repair atrial septal defect, secundum, with cardiopulmonary bypass, with or without patch**

47.3 47.3 **FUD** 090 C 80

AMA: 2018,Jan,8; 2017,Dec,3; 2017,Jan,8; 2016,Jan,13; 2015,Jan,16

33645 **Direct or patch closure, sinus venosus, with or without anomalous pulmonary venous drainage**

EXCLUDES *Repair isolated partial anomalous pulmonary venous return (33724)*
Repair pulmonary venous stenosis (33726)

50.2 50.2 **FUD** 090 C 80

AMA: 2017,Dec,3

33647 Closure of Septal Defect: Atrium AND Ventricle

EXCLUDES *Tricuspid atresia repair procedures (33615)*

Code also thrombus removal through separate heart incision, when performed (33310-33315); append modifier 59 to (33315)

33647 **Repair of atrial septal defect and ventricular septal defect, with direct or patch closure**

52.6 52.6 **FUD** 090 63 C 80

AMA: 2017,Dec,3

33660-33670 Closure of Defect: Atrioventricular Canal

33660 **Repair of incomplete or partial atrioventricular canal (ostium primum atrial septal defect), with or without atrioventricular valve repair**

50.8 50.8 **FUD** 090 C 80

AMA: 2017,Dec,3

33665 **Repair of intermediate or transitional atrioventricular canal, with or without atrioventricular valve repair**

55.6 55.6 **FUD** 090 C 80

AMA: 2017,Dec,3

33670 **Repair of complete atrioventricular canal, with or without prosthetic valve**

Code also thrombus removal through separate heart incision, when performed (33310-33315); append modifier 59 to (33315)

57.1 57.1 **FUD** 090 63 C 80

AMA: 2017,Dec,3

33675-33677 Closure of Multiple Septal Defects: Ventricle

EXCLUDES *Closure single ventricular septal defect (33681, 33684, 33688)*
Insertion or replacement temporary transvenous single chamber cardiac electrode or pacemaker catheter (33210)
Percutaneous closure (93581)
Thoracentesis (32554-32555)
Thoracotomy (32100)
Tube thoracostomy (32551)

33675 **Closure of multiple ventricular septal defects;**

57.1 57.1 **FUD** 090 C 80

AMA: 2018,Jan,8; 2017,Dec,3; 2017,Jan,8; 2016,Jan,13; 2015,Jan,16

33676 **with pulmonary valvotomy or infundibular resection (acyanotic)**

58.6 58.6 **FUD** 090 C 80

AMA: 2018,Jan,8; 2017,Dec,3; 2017,Jan,8; 2016,Jan,13; 2015,Jan,16

33677 **with removal of pulmonary artery band, with or without gusset**

60.9 60.9 **FUD** 090 C 80

AMA: 2018,Jan,8; 2017,Dec,3; 2017,Jan,8; 2016,Jan,13; 2015,Jan,16

33681-33688 Closure of Septal Defect: Ventricle

EXCLUDES *Repair pulmonary vein that requires creating an atrial septal defect (33724)*

33681 **Closure of single ventricular septal defect, with or without patch;**

Code also thrombus removal through separate heart incision, when performed (33310-33315); append modifier 59 to (33315)

53.2 53.2 **FUD** 090 C 80

AMA: 2018,Jan,8; 2017,Dec,3; 2017,Jan,8; 2016,Jan,13; 2015,Jan,16

33684 **with pulmonary valvotomy or infundibular resection (acyanotic)**

Code also concurrent systemic-to-pulmonary artery shunt ligation/takedown, if performed (33924)

54.7 54.7 **FUD** 090 C 80

AMA: 2017,Dec,3

33688 **with removal of pulmonary artery band, with or without gusset**

Code also concurrent systemic-to-pulmonary artery shunt ligation/takedown, if performed (33924)

54.8 54.8 **FUD** 090 C 80

AMA: 2017,Dec,3

33690 Reduce Pulmonary Overcirculation in Septal Defects

EXCLUDES *Left and right pulmonary artery banding in single ventricle (33620)*

33690 **Banding of pulmonary artery**

34.7 34.7 **FUD** 090 63 C 80

AMA: 2018,Jan,8; 2017,Jan,8; 2016,Jan,13; 2015,Jan,16

33692-33697 Repair of Defects of Tetralogy of Fallot

Code also concurrent systemic-to-pulmonary artery shunt ligation/takedown, when performed (33924)

33692 **Complete repair tetralogy of Fallot without pulmonary atresia;**

56.6 56.6 **FUD** 090 C 80

AMA: 2017,Dec,3

33694 **with transannular patch**

56.5 56.5 **FUD** 090 63 C 80

AMA: 2017,Dec,3

33697 **Complete repair tetralogy of Fallot with pulmonary atresia including construction of conduit from right ventricle to pulmonary artery and closure of ventricular septal defect**

59.5 59.5 **FUD** 090 C 80

AMA: 2018,Jan,8; 2017,Dec,3; 2017,Jan,8; 2016,Jan,13; 2015,Jan,16

33702-33722 Repair Anomalies Sinus of Valsalva

33702 Repair sinus of Valsalva fistula, with cardiopulmonary bypass;

44.2 44.2 **FUD** 090 C 80

AMA: 2018,Jan,8; 2017,Dec,3; 2017,Jan,8; 2016,Jan,13; 2015,Jan,16

33710 with repair of ventricular septal defect

59.4 59.4 **FUD** 090 C 80

AMA: 2017,Dec,3

33720 Repair sinus of Valsalva aneurysm, with cardiopulmonary bypass

44.7 44.7 **FUD** 090 C 80

AMA: 2017,Dec,3

33722 Closure of aortico-left ventricular tunnel

47.1 47.1 **FUD** 090 C 80

AMA: 2018,Jan,8; 2017,Dec,3; 2017,Jan,8; 2016,Jan,13; 2015,Jan,16

33724-33732 Repair Aberrant Pulmonary Venous Connection

33724 Repair of isolated partial anomalous pulmonary venous return (eg, Scimitar Syndrome)

EXCLUDES *Temporary pacemaker (33210-33211)*
Tube thoracostomy (32551)

44.2 44.2 **FUD** 090 C 80

AMA: 2018,Jan,8; 2017,Dec,3; 2017,Jan,8; 2016,Jan,13; 2015,Jan,16

33726 Repair of pulmonary venous stenosis

EXCLUDES *Temporary pacemaker (33210-33211)*
Tube thoracostomy (32551)

58.8 58.8 **FUD** 090 C 80

AMA: 2018,Jan,8; 2017,Dec,3; 2017,Jan,8; 2016,Jan,13; 2015,Jan,16

33730 Complete repair of anomalous pulmonary venous return (supracardiac, intracardiac, or infracardiac types)

EXCLUDES *Partial anomalous pulmonary venous return (33724)*
Repair pulmonary venous stenosis (33726)

58.0 58.0 **FUD** 090 63 C 80

AMA: 2018,Jan,8; 2017,Dec,3; 2017,Jan,8; 2016,Jan,13; 2015,Jan,16

33732 Repair of cor triatriatum or supravalvular mitral ring by resection of left atrial membrane

47.6 47.6 **FUD** 090 63 C 80

AMA: 2018,Jan,8; 2017,Dec,3; 2017,Jan,8; 2016,Jan,13; 2015,Jan,16

33735-33737 Creation of Atrial Septal Defect

Code also concurrent systemic-to-pulmonary artery shunt ligation/takedown, when performed (33924)

33735 Atrial septectomy or septostomy; closed heart (Blalock-Hanlon type operation)

37.4 37.4 **FUD** 090 63 C 80

AMA: 2018,Jan,8; 2017,Jan,8; 2016,Jan,13; 2015,Jan,16

33736 open heart with cardiopulmonary bypass

39.6 39.6 **FUD** 090 63 C 80

AMA: 2017,Dec,3

33737 open heart, with inflow occlusion

37.6 37.6 **FUD** 090 C 80

AMA: 2007,Mar,1-3; 1997,Nov,1

33741-33746 Transcatheter Procedures

● **33741 Transcatheter atrial septostomy (TAS) for congenital cardiac anomalies to create effective atrial flow, including all imaging guidance by the proceduralist, when performed, any method (eg, Rashkind, Sang-Park, balloon, cutting balloon, blade)**

INCLUDES Angiography to carry out procedure
Fluoroscopic and ultrasound guidance for access and intervention
Percutaneous access, access sheath placement, advancement transcatheter delivery system, creation effective intracardiac blood flow

EXCLUDES *Left heart catheterization via transseptal puncture (93462)*
Septostomy performed for noncongenital indications (93799)

Code also diagnostic congenital cardiac catheterization procedures when patient's condition (clinical indication) changed since intervention or prior study, no available prior catheter-based diagnostic study in treatment zone, or prior study not adequate, and append modifier 59 (93530-93533)

Code also diagnostic cardiac catheterization, when performed distinctly separate from shunt creation (93451-93453, 93456, 93458, 93460, 93530-93533)

Code also injection, diagnostic angiography, when performed separate from shunt creation and append modifier 59 (93563, 93565-93568)

0.00 0.00 **FUD** 000 63

● **33745 Transcatheter intracardiac shunt (TIS) creation by stent placement for congenital cardiac anomalies to establish effective intracardiac flow, including all imaging guidance by the proceduralist, when performed, left and right heart diagnostic cardiac catherization for congenital cardiac anomalies, and target zone angioplasty, when performed (eg, atrial septum, Fontan fenestration, right ventricular outflow tract, Mustard/Senning/Warden baffles); initial intracardiac shunt**

INCLUDES Angiography to carry out procedure
Balloon angioplasty(ies) and dilation(s) performed in target lesion
Fluoroscopic and ultrasound guidance for access and intervention
Intracardiac stent(s), including angioplasty before and after placement
Percutaneous access, access sheath placement, advancement transcatheter delivery system, creation effective intracardiac blood flow

EXCLUDES *Right heart catheterization for congenital cardiac anomalies (93530-93533)*

Code also diagnostic cardiac catheterization, when performed distinctly separate from shunt creation (93451-93453, 93456, 93458, 93460, 93530-93533)

Code also injection, diagnostic angiography, when performed separate from shunt creation and append modifier 59 (93563, 93565-93568)

● + **33746 each additional intracardiac shunt location (List separately in addition to code for primary procedure)**

INCLUDES Balloon angioplasty(ies) and dilation(s) performed in target lesion
Intracardiac stent(s), including angioplasty before and after placement

EXCLUDES *Right heart catheterization for congenital cardiac anomalies (93530-93533)*

Code also angioplasty performed in distinctly separate cardiac lesion

Code first (33745)

0.00 0.00 **FUD** 000

33750-33767 Systemic Vessel to Pulmonary Artery Shunts

Code also concurrent systemic-to-pulmonary artery shunt ligation/takedown, when performed (33924)

33750 Shunt; subclavian to pulmonary artery (Blalock-Taussig type operation)

36.5 36.5 **FUD** 090 63 C 80

AMA: 2017,Dec,3

33755 **ascending aorta to pulmonary artery (Waterston type operation)**
38.0 38.0 FUD 090 ⑥③ C 80
AMA: 2017,Dec,3

33762 **descending aorta to pulmonary artery (Potts-Smith type operation)**
37.1 37.1 FUD 090 ⑥③ C 80
AMA: 2017,Dec,3

33764 **central, with prosthetic graft**
38.0 38.0 FUD 090 C 80
AMA: 2017,Dec,3

33766 **superior vena cava to pulmonary artery for flow to 1 lung (classical Glenn procedure)**
38.6 38.6 FUD 090 C 80
AMA: 2017,Dec,3

33767 **superior vena cava to pulmonary artery for flow to both lungs (bidirectional Glenn procedure)**
41.1 41.1 FUD 090 C 80
AMA: 2018,Jan,8; 2017,Dec,3; 2017,Jan,8; 2016,Jul,3

33768 Cavopulmonary Anastomosis to Decrease Volume Load

EXCLUDES *Temporary pacemaker (33210-33211)*
Tube thoracostomy (32551)
Code first (33478, 33617, 33622, 33767)

\+ **33768** **Anastomosis, cavopulmonary, second superior vena cava (List separately in addition to primary procedure)**
12.0 12.0 FUD ZZZ C 80
AMA: 2018,Jan,8; 2017,Jan,8; 2016,Jul,3; 2016,Jan,13; 2015,Jan,16

33770-33783 Repair Aberrant Anatomy: Transposition Great Vessels

Code also concurrent systemic-to-pulmonary artery shunt ligation/takedown, when performed (33924)

33770 **Repair of transposition of the great arteries with ventricular septal defect and subpulmonary stenosis; without surgical enlargement of ventricular septal defect**
61.3 61.3 FUD 090 C 80
AMA: 2018,Jan,8; 2017,Dec,3; 2017,Jan,8; 2016,Jan,13; 2015,Jan,16

33771 **with surgical enlargement of ventricular septal defect**
63.1 63.1 FUD 090 C 80
AMA: 2017,Dec,3

33774 **Repair of transposition of the great arteries, atrial baffle procedure (eg, Mustard or Senning type) with cardiopulmonary bypass;**
52.0 52.0 FUD 090 C 80
AMA: 2017,Dec,3

33775 **with removal of pulmonary band**
53.6 53.6 FUD 090 C 80
AMA: 2017,Dec,3

33776 **with closure of ventricular septal defect**
56.7 56.7 FUD 090 C 80
AMA: 2017,Dec,3

33777 **with repair of subpulmonic obstruction**
54.9 54.9 FUD 090 C 80
AMA: 2017,Dec,3

33778 **Repair of transposition of the great arteries, aortic pulmonary artery reconstruction (eg, Jatene type);**
68.0 68.0 FUD 090 ⑥③ C 80
AMA: 2017,Dec,3

33779 **with removal of pulmonary band**
67.4 67.4 FUD 090 C 80
AMA: 2017,Dec,3

33780 **with closure of ventricular septal defect**
68.6 68.6 FUD 090 C 80
AMA: 2017,Dec,3

33781 **with repair of subpulmonic obstruction**
67.0 67.0 FUD 090 C 80
AMA: 2018,Jan,8; 2017,Dec,3; 2017,Jan,8; 2016,Jan,13; 2015,Jan,16

33782 **Aortic root translocation with ventricular septal defect and pulmonary stenosis repair (ie, Nikaidoh procedure); without coronary ostium reimplantation**
EXCLUDES *Closure single ventricular septal defect (33681)*
Repair complex cardiac anomaly other than pulmonary atresia (33608)
Repair pulmonary atresia with ventricular septal defect (33920)
Repair transposition great arteries (33770-33771, 33778, 33780)
Replacement, aortic valve (33412-33413)
93.6 93.6 FUD 090 C 80
AMA: 2017,Dec,3

33783 **with reimplantation of 1 or both coronary ostia**
101. 101. FUD 090 C 80
AMA: 2017,Dec,3

33786-33788 Repair Aberrant Anatomy: Truncus Arteriosus

33786 **Total repair, truncus arteriosus (Rastelli type operation)**
Code also concurrent systemic-to-pulmonary artery shunt ligation/takedown, when performed (33924)
66.0 66.0 FUD 090 ⑥③ C 80
AMA: 2018,Jan,8; 2017,Dec,3; 2017,Jan,8; 2016,Jan,13; 2015,Jan,16

33788 **Reimplantation of an anomalous pulmonary artery**
EXCLUDES *Pulmonary artery banding (33690)*
44.3 44.3 FUD 090 C 80
AMA: 2018,Jan,8; 2017,Dec,3; 2017,Jan,8; 2016,Jan,13; 2015,Jan,16

33800-33853 Repair Aberrant Anatomy: Aorta

33800 **Aortic suspension (aortopexy) for tracheal decompression (eg, for tracheomalacia) (separate procedure)**
28.5 28.5 FUD 090 C 80
AMA: 2018,Jan,8; 2017,Jan,8; 2016,Jan,13; 2015,Jan,16

33802 **Division of aberrant vessel (vascular ring);**
31.3 31.3 FUD 090 C 80
AMA: 2017,Dec,3

33803 **with reanastomosis**
33.4 33.4 FUD 090 C 80
AMA: 2017,Dec,3

33813 **Obliteration of aortopulmonary septal defect; without cardiopulmonary bypass**
35.8 35.8 FUD 090 C 80
AMA: 2007,Mar,1-3; 1997,Nov,1

33814 **with cardiopulmonary bypass**
44.1 44.1 FUD 090 C 80
AMA: 2017,Dec,3

33820 **Repair of patent ductus arteriosus; by ligation**
EXCLUDES *Percutaneous transcatheter closure patent ductus arteriosus (93582)*
27.9 27.9 FUD 090 C 80
AMA: 2018,Jan,8; 2017,Dec,3; 2017,Jan,8; 2016,Jan,13; 2015,Jan,16

33822 **by division, younger than 18 years** A
EXCLUDES *Percutaneous transcatheter closure patent ductus arteriosus (93582)*
29.6 29.6 FUD 090 C 80
AMA: 2018,Jan,8; 2017,Dec,3; 2017,Jan,8; 2016,Jul,3; 2016,Jan,13; 2015,Jan,16

33824 **by division, 18 years and older**
EXCLUDES *Percutaneous closure patent ductus arteriosus (93582)*
34.2 34.2 FUD 090 C 80
AMA: 2017,Dec,3

33840 **Excision of coarctation of aorta, with or without associated patent ductus arteriosus; with direct anastomosis**

35.8 35.8 **FUD** 090 C 80

AMA: 2018,Jan,8; 2017,Dec,3; 2017,Jan,8; 2016,Jul,3

33845 **with graft**

37.9 37.9 **FUD** 090 C 80

AMA: 2018,Jan,8; 2017,Dec,3; 2017,Jan,8; 2016,Jul,3

33851 **repair using either left subclavian artery or prosthetic material as gusset for enlargement**

36.8 36.8 **FUD** 090 C 80

AMA: 2018,Jan,8; 2017,Dec,3; 2017,Jan,8; 2016,Jul,3

33852 **Repair of hypoplastic or interrupted aortic arch using autogenous or prosthetic material; without cardiopulmonary bypass**

EXCLUDES *Hypoplastic left heart syndrome repair by excision coarctation of aorta (33619)*

40.5 40.5 **FUD** 090 C 80

AMA: 2007,Mar,1-3; 1997,Nov,1

33853 **with cardiopulmonary bypass**

EXCLUDES *Hypoplastic left heart syndrome repair by excision coarctation of aorta (33619)*

53.0 53.0 **FUD** 090 C 80

AMA: 2018,Jan,8; 2017,Dec,3; 2017,Jan,8; 2016,Jul,3; 2016,Jan,13; 2015,Jan,16

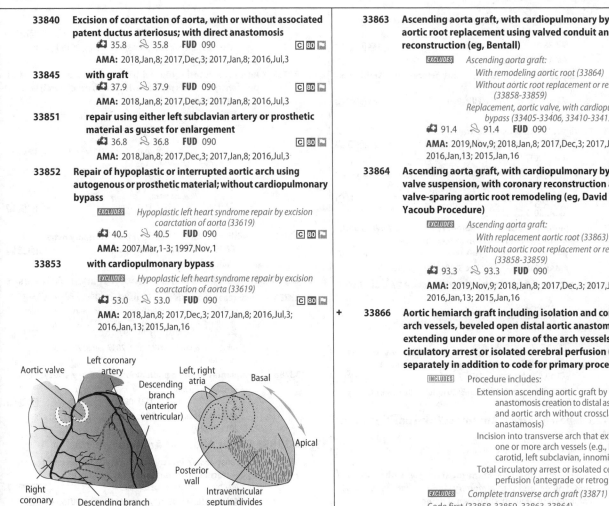

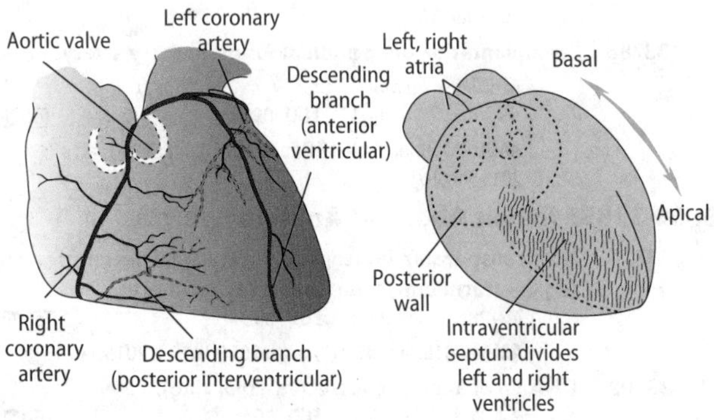

33858-33877 Aortic Graft Procedures

33858 **Ascending aorta graft, with cardiopulmonary bypass, includes valve suspension, when performed; for aortic dissection**

INCLUDES Treatment for aortic dissection

EXCLUDES *Ascending aorta graft:*
- *Treatment other aortic disease(s), such as aneurysm (33859)*
- *With remodeling aortic root (33864)*
- *With replacement aortic root (33863)*

98.5 98.5 **FUD** 090 80

33859 **for aortic disease other than dissection (eg, aneurysm)**

INCLUDES Treatment of aortic disease(s) other than dissection, such as aneurysm

EXCLUDES *Ascending aorta graft:*
- *Treatment other aortic dissection (33858)*
- *With remodeling aortic root (33864)*
- *With replacement aortic root (33863)*

70.7 70.7 **FUD** 090 80

33863 **Ascending aorta graft, with cardiopulmonary bypass, with aortic root replacement using valved conduit and coronary reconstruction (eg, Bentall)**

EXCLUDES *Ascending aorta graft:*
- *With remodeling aortic root (33864)*
- *Without aortic root replacement or remodeling (33858-33859)*

Replacement, aortic valve, with cardiopulmonary bypass (33405-33406, 33410-33413)

91.4 91.4 **FUD** 090 C 80

AMA: 2019,Nov,9; 2018,Jan,8; 2017,Dec,3; 2017,Jan,8; 2016,Jan,13; 2015,Jan,16

33864 **Ascending aorta graft, with cardiopulmonary bypass with valve suspension, with coronary reconstruction and valve-sparing aortic root remodeling (eg, David Procedure, Yacoub Procedure)**

EXCLUDES *Ascending aorta graft:*
- *With replacement aortic root (33863)*
- *Without aortic root replacement or remodeling (33858-33859)*

93.3 93.3 **FUD** 090 C 80

AMA: 2019,Nov,9; 2018,Jan,8; 2017,Dec,3; 2017,Jan,8; 2016,Jan,13; 2015,Jan,16

\+ **33866** **Aortic hemiarch graft including isolation and control of the arch vessels, beveled open distal aortic anastomosis extending under one or more of the arch vessels, and total circulatory arrest or isolated cerebral perfusion (List separately in addition to code for primary procedure)**

INCLUDES Procedure includes:
- Extension ascending aortic graft by beveled anastomosis creation to distal ascending aorta and aortic arch without crossclamp (open anastamosis)
- Incision into transverse arch that extends under one or more arch vessels (e.g., left common carotid, left subclavian, innominate artery)
- Total circulatory arrest or isolated cerebral perfusion (antegrade or retrograde)

EXCLUDES *Complete transverse arch graft (33871)*

Code first (33858-33859, 33863-33864)

26.7 26.7 **FUD** ZZZ N1 80

AMA: 2019,Nov,9

33871 **Transverse aortic arch graft, with cardiopulmonary bypass, with profound hypothermia, total circulatory arrest and isolated cerebral perfusion with reimplantation of arch vessel(s) (eg, island pedicle or individual arch vessel reimplantation)**

EXCLUDES *Ascending aortic graft (33858-33859, 33863-33864)*

Hemiarch aortic graft performed in addition to ascending aortta graft (33866)

94.7 94.7 **FUD** 090 80

33875 **Descending thoracic aorta graft, with or without bypass**

79.5 79.5 **FUD** 090 C 80

AMA: 2017,Dec,3

33877 **Repair of thoracoabdominal aortic aneurysm with graft, with or without cardiopulmonary bypass**
105. 105. FUD 090
AMA: 2017,Dec,3

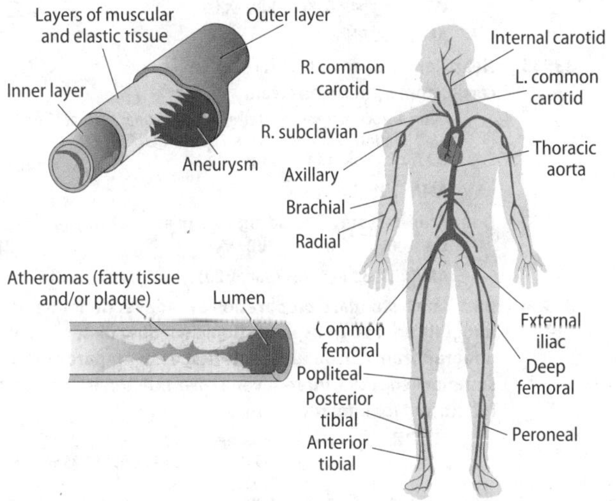

33880-33891 Endovascular Repair Aortic Aneurysm: Thoracic

INCLUDES Balloon angioplasty
Introduction, manipulation, placement, and device deployment
Stent deployment

EXCLUDES *Additional interventional procedures provided during endovascular repair*
Carotid-carotid bypass (33891)
Guidewire and catheter insertion (36140, 36200-36218)
Open exposure artery/subsequent closure ([34812], 34714-34716 [34820, 34833, 34834])
Subclavian to carotid artery transposition (33889)
Substantial artery repair/replacement (35226, 35286)

33880 **Endovascular repair of descending thoracic aorta (eg, aneurysm, pseudoaneurysm, dissection, penetrating ulcer, intramural hematoma, or traumatic disruption); involving coverage of left subclavian artery origin, initial endoprosthesis plus descending thoracic aortic extension(s), if required, to level of celiac artery origin**
INCLUDES Placement distal extensions in distal thoracic aorta
EXCLUDES *Proximal extensions*
(75956)
52.0 52.0 FUD 090
AMA: 2018,Jan,8; 2017,Dec,3; 2017,Jan,8; 2016,Jan,13; 2015,Jan,16

33881 **not involving coverage of left subclavian artery origin, initial endoprosthesis plus descending thoracic aortic extension(s), if required, to level of celiac artery origin**
INCLUDES Placement distal extensions in distal thoracic aorta
EXCLUDES *Procedure where extension placement includes coverage left subclavian artery origin (33880)*
Proximal extensions
(75957)
44.6 44.6 FUD 090
AMA: 2018,Jan,8; 2017,Dec,3; 2017,Jan,8; 2016,Jan,13; 2015,Jan,16

33883 **Placement of proximal extension prosthesis for endovascular repair of descending thoracic aorta (eg, aneurysm, pseudoaneurysm, dissection, penetrating ulcer, intramural hematoma, or traumatic disruption); initial extension**
EXCLUDES *Procedure where extension placement includes coverage left subclavian artery origin (33880)*
(75958)
32.3 32.3 FUD 090
AMA: 2018,Jan,8; 2017,Dec,3; 2017,Jan,8; 2016,Jan,13; 2015,Jan,16

\+ **33884** **each additional proximal extension (List separately in addition to code for primary procedure)**
Code first (33883)
(75958)
11.5 11.5 FUD ZZZ
AMA: 2018,Jan,8; 2017,Dec,3; 2017,Jan,8; 2016,Jan,13; 2015,Jan,16

33886 **Placement of distal extension prosthesis(s) delayed after endovascular repair of descending thoracic aorta**
INCLUDES All modules deployed
EXCLUDES *Endovascular repair descending thoracic aorta (33880, 33881)*
(75959)
27.7 27.7 FUD 090
AMA: 2018,Jan,8; 2017,Dec,3; 2017,Jan,8; 2016,Jan,13; 2015,Jan,16

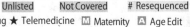

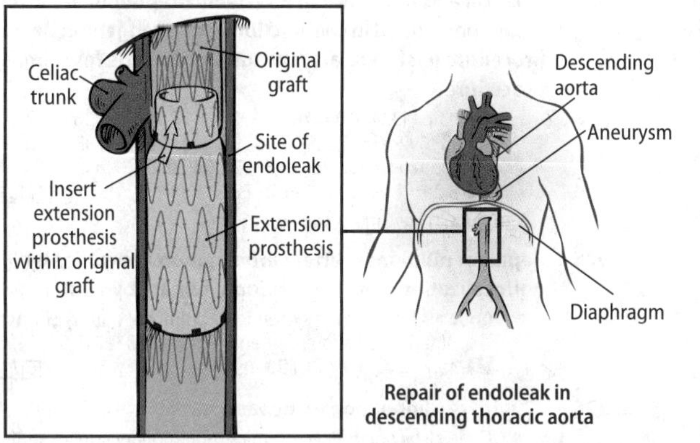

Repair of endoleak in descending thoracic aorta

33889 **Open subclavian to carotid artery transposition performed in conjunction with endovascular repair of descending thoracic aorta, by neck incision, unilateral**
EXCLUDES *Transposition and/or reimplantation; subclavian to carotid artery (35694)*
22.9 22.9 FUD 000
AMA: 2018,Jan,8; 2017,Jan,8; 2016,Jan,13; 2015,Jan,16

33891 **Bypass graft, with other than vein, transcervical retropharyngeal carotid-carotid, performed in conjunction with endovascular repair of descending thoracic aorta, by neck incision**
EXCLUDES *Bypass graft (35509, 35601)*
28.0 28.0 FUD 000
AMA: 2018,Jan,8; 2017,Jan,8; 2016,Jan,13; 2015,Jan,16

33910-33926 Surgical Procedures of Pulmonary Artery

33910 **Pulmonary artery embolectomy; with cardiopulmonary bypass**
77.1 77.1 FUD 090
AMA: 2018,Jan,8; 2017,Dec,3; 2017,Jan,8; 2016,Jan,13; 2015,Jan,16

33915 **without cardiopulmonary bypass**
39.8 39.8 FUD 090
AMA: 2018,Jan,8; 2017,Jan,8; 2016,Jan,13; 2015,Jan,16

33916 **Pulmonary endarterectomy, with or without embolectomy, with cardiopulmonary bypass**
123. 123. FUD 090
AMA: 2018,Jan,8; 2017,Dec,3; 2017,Jan,8; 2016,Jan,13; 2015,Jan,16

33917 **Repair of pulmonary artery stenosis by reconstruction with patch or graft**
Code also concurrent systemic-to-pulmonary artery shunt ligation/takedown, when performed (33924)
42.1 42.1 FUD 090
AMA: 2018,Jan,8; 2017,Dec,3; 2017,Jan,8; 2016,Jul,3; 2016,Jan,13; 2015,Jan,16

Cardiovascular, Hemic, and Lymphatic
33877 — 33917

33920 Repair of pulmonary atresia with ventricular septal defect, by construction or replacement of conduit from right or left ventricle to pulmonary artery

EXCLUDES *Repair complicated cardiac anomalies by creating/replacing conduit from ventricle to pulmonary artery (33608)*

Code also concurrent systemic-to-pulmonary artery shunt ligation/takedown, when performed (33924)

52.4 52.4 **FUD** 090 C 80

AMA: 2019,Apr,6; 2018,Jan,8; 2017,Dec,3; 2017,Jan,8; 2016,Jan,13; 2015,Jan,16

33922 Transection of pulmonary artery with cardiopulmonary bypass

Code also concurrent systemic-to-pulmonary artery shunt ligation/takedown, when performed (33924)

40.1 40.1 **FUD** 090 63 C 80

AMA: 2017,Dec,3

+ **33924 Ligation and takedown of a systemic-to-pulmonary artery shunt, performed in conjunction with a congenital heart procedure (List separately in addition to code for primary procedure)**

Code first (33470-33478, 33600-33617, 33622, 33684-33688, 33692-33697, 33735-33767, 33770-33783, 33786, 33917, 33920-33922, 33925-33926, 33935, 33945)

8.29 8.29 **FUD** ZZZ C 80

AMA: 1997,Nov,1; 1995,Win,1

33925 Repair of pulmonary artery arborization anomalies by unifocalization; without cardiopulmonary bypass

Code also concurrent systemic-to-pulmonary artery shunt ligation/takedown, when performed (33924)

49.7 49.7 **FUD** 090 C 80

33926 with cardiopulmonary bypass

Code also concurrent systemic-to-pulmonary artery shunt ligation/takedown, when performed (33924)

70.3 70.3 **FUD** 090 C 80

AMA: 2017,Dec,3

33927-33945 Heart and Heart-Lung Transplants

INCLUDES Backbench work to prepare donor heart and/or lungs for transplantation (33933, 33944)
Harvesting donor organs with cold preservation (33930, 33940)
Transplantation heart and/or lungs into recipient (33935, 33945)

33927 Implantation of a total replacement heart system (artificial heart) with recipient cardiectomy

EXCLUDES *Implantation ventricular assist device:*
Extracorporeal (33975-33976)
Intracorporeal (33979)
Percutaneous ([33995], 33990-33991)

74.2 74.2 **FUD** XXX C 80

AMA: 2018,Jun,3

33928 Removal and replacement of total replacement heart system (artificial heart)

EXCLUDES *Replacement or revision elements artificial heart (33999)*

0.00 0.00 **FUD** XXX C 80

AMA: 2018,Jun,3

+ **33929 Removal of a total replacement heart system (artificial heart) for heart transplantation (List separately in addition to code for primary procedure)**

Code first (33945)

0.00 0.00 **FUD** ZZZ C 80

AMA: 2018,Jun,3

33930 Donor cardiectomy-pneumonectomy (including cold preservation)

0.00 0.00 **FUD** XXX C

AMA: 1997,Nov,1

33933 Backbench standard preparation of cadaver donor heart/lung allograft prior to transplantation, including dissection of allograft from surrounding soft tissues to prepare aorta, superior vena cava, inferior vena cava, and trachea for implantation

0.00 0.00 **FUD** XXX C 80

AMA: 1997,Nov,1

33935 Heart-lung transplant with recipient cardiectomy-pneumonectomy

Code also concurrent systemic-to-pulmonary artery shunt ligation/takedown, when performed (33924)

143. 143. **FUD** 090 C 80

AMA: 2017,Dec,3

33940 Donor cardiectomy (including cold preservation)

0.00 0.00 **FUD** XXX C

AMA: 2018,Jan,8; 2017,Jan,8; 2016,Jan,13; 2015,Jan,16

33944 Backbench standard preparation of cadaver donor heart allograft prior to transplantation, including dissection of allograft from surrounding soft tissues to prepare aorta, superior vena cava, inferior vena cava, pulmonary artery, and left atrium for implantation

EXCLUDES *Procedures performed on donor heart (33300, 33310, 33320, 33390, 33463-33464, 33510, 33641, 35216, 35276, 35685)*

0.00 0.00 **FUD** XXX C 80

AMA: 1997,Nov,1

33945 Heart transplant, with or without recipient cardiectomy

Code also concurrent systemic-to-pulmonary artery shunt ligation/takedown, when performed (33924)

141. 141. **FUD** 090 C 80

AMA: 2018,Jun,3; 2017,Dec,3

33946-33989 [33962, 33963, 33964, 33965, 33966, 33969, 33984, 33985, 33986, 33987, 33988, 33989] Extracorporeal Circulatory and Respiratory Support

INCLUDES Cannula repositioning and cannula insertion performed during same procedure
Multiple physician and nonphysician team collaboration
Veno-arterial ECMO/ECLS for heart and lung support
Veno-venous ECMO/ECLS for lung support

Code also extensive arterial repair/replacement (35266, 35286, 35371, 35665)
Code also overall daily management services needed to manage patient; report appropriate observation, hospital inpatient, or critical care E/M codes

33946 Extracorporeal membrane oxygenation (ECMO)/extracorporeal life support (ECLS) provided by physician; initiation, veno-venous

EXCLUDES *Daily ECMO/ECLS veno-venous management initial service date (33948)*
Repositioning ECMO/ECLS cannula initial service date (33957-33959 [33962, 33963, 33964])

Code also cannula insertion (33951-33956)

8.95 8.95 **FUD** XXX 63 C

AMA: 2018,Jan,8; 2017,Jan,8; 2016,Mar,5; 2016,Jan,13; 2015,Jul,3

33947 initiation, veno-arterial

EXCLUDES *Daily ECMO/ECLS veno-venous management initial service date (33948)*
Repositioning ECMO/ECLS cannula initial service date (33957-33959 [33962, 33963, 33964])

Code also cannula insertion (33951-33956)

9.97 9.97 **FUD** XXX 63 C

AMA: 2018,Jan,8; 2017,Jan,8; 2016,Mar,5; 2016,Jan,13; 2015,Jul,3

33948 daily management, each day, veno-venous

EXCLUDES *ECMO/ECLS initiation, veno-venous (33946)*

6.91 6.91 **FUD** XXX 63 C

AMA: 2018,Jan,8; 2017,Jan,8; 2016,Mar,5; 2016,Jan,13; 2015,Jul,3

33949 daily management, each day, veno-arterial

EXCLUDES *ECMO/ECLS initiation, veno-arterial (33947)*

6.73 6.73 **FUD** XXX 63 C

AMA: 2018,Jan,8; 2017,Jan,8; 2016,Mar,5; 2016,Jan,13; 2015,Jul,3

33951 **insertion of peripheral (arterial and/or venous) cannula(e), percutaneous, birth through 5 years of age (includes fluoroscopic guidance, when performed)** A

INCLUDES Cannula replacement same vessel
Cannula repositioning during same episode care

Code also cannula removal when new cannula inserted in different vessel with ([33965, 33966, 33969, 33984, 33985, 33986])

Code also ECMO/ECLS initiation or daily management (33946-33947, 33948-33949)

12.3 12.3 **FUD** 000 C 80

AMA: 2018,Jan,8; 2017,Jan,8; 2016,Mar,5; 2016,Jan,13; 2015,Jul,3

33952 **insertion of peripheral (arterial and/or venous) cannula(e), percutaneous, 6 years and older (includes fluoroscopic guidance, when performed)** A

INCLUDES Cannula replacement same vessel
Cannula repositioning during same episode care

Code also cannula removal when new cannula inserted in different vessel with ([33965, 33966, 33969, 33984, 33985, 33986])

Code also ECMO/ECLS initiation or daily management (33946-33947, 33948-33949)

12.4 12.4 **FUD** 000 C 80

AMA: 2018,Jan,8; 2017,Jan,8; 2016,Mar,5; 2016,Jan,13; 2015,Jul,3

33953 **insertion of peripheral (arterial and/or venous) cannula(e), open, birth through 5 years of age** A

INCLUDES Cannula replacement same vessel
Cannula repositioning during same episode care

EXCLUDES *Open artery exposure for delivery/deployment endovascular prosthesis ([34812], 34714-34716 [34820, 34833, 34834], [34820])*

Code also cannula removal when new cannula inserted in different vessel with ([33965, 33966, 33969, 33984, 33985, 33986])

Code also ECMO/ECLS initiation or daily management (33496-33947, 33948-33949)

13.8 13.8 **FUD** 000 C 80

AMA: 2018,Jan,8; 2017,Dec,3; 2017,Jan,8; 2016,Mar,5; 2016,Jan,13; 2015,Jul,3

33954 **insertion of peripheral (arterial and/or venous) cannula(e), open, 6 years and older** A

INCLUDES Cannula replacement same vessel
Cannula repositioning during same episode care

EXCLUDES *Open artery exposure for delivery/deployment endovascular prosthesis ([34812], 34714-34716 [34820, 34833, 34834])*

Code also cannula removal when new cannula inserted in different vessel with ([33965, 33966, 33969, 33984, 33985, 33986])

Code also ECMO/ECLS initiation or daily management (33946-33947, 33948-33949)

13.8 13.8 **FUD** 000 C 80

AMA: 2018,Jan,8; 2017,Dec,3; 2017,Jan,8; 2016,Mar,5; 2016,Jan,13; 2015,Jul,3

33955 **insertion of central cannula(e) by sternotomy or thoracotomy, birth through 5 years of age** A

INCLUDES Cannula replacement same vessel
Cannula repositioning during same episode care

EXCLUDES *Mediastinotomy (39010)*
Thoracotomy (32100)

Code also cannula removal when new cannula inserted in different vessel with ([33965, 33966, 33969, 33984, 33985, 33986])

Code also ECMO/ECLS initiation or daily management (33946-33947, 33948-33949)

24.0 24.0 **FUD** 000 C 80

AMA: 2018,Jan,8; 2017,Jan,8; 2016,Mar,5; 2016,Jan,13; 2015,Jul,3

33956 **insertion of central cannula(e) by sternotomy or thoracotomy, 6 years and older** A

INCLUDES Cannula replacement same vessel
Cannula repositioning during same episode care

EXCLUDES *Mediastinotomy (39010)*
Thoracotomy (32100)

Code also cannula removal when new cannula inserted in different vessel with ([33965, 33966, 33969, 33984, 33985, 33986])

Code also ECMO/ECLS initiation or daily management (33946-33947, 33948-33949)

24.2 24.2 **FUD** 000 C 80

AMA: 2018,Jan,8; 2017,Jan,8; 2016,Mar,5; 2016,Jan,13; 2015,Jul,3

33957 **reposition peripheral (arterial and/or venous) cannula(e), percutaneous, birth through 5 years of age (includes fluoroscopic guidance, when performed)** A

INCLUDES Fluoroscopic guidance

EXCLUDES *ECMO/ECLS initiation, veno-arterial (33947)*
ECMO/ECLS initiation, veno-venous (33946)
ECMO/ECLS insertion cannula (33951-33956)
Percutaneous access and closure femoral artery for endograft delivery (34713)

5.36 5.36 **FUD** 000 C 80

AMA: 2018,Jan,8; 2017,Jan,8; 2016,Mar,5; 2016,Jan,13; 2015,Jul,3

33958 **reposition peripheral (arterial and/or venous) cannula(e), percutaneous, 6 years and older (includes fluoroscopic guidance, when performed)** A

INCLUDES Fluoroscopic guidance

EXCLUDES *ECMO/ECLS initiation, veno-arterial (33947)*
ECMO/ECLS initiation, veno-venous (33946)
ECMO/ECLS insertion of cannula (33951-33956)
Percutaneous access and closure femoral artery for endograft delivery (34713)

5.36 5.36 **FUD** 000 C 80

AMA: 2018,Jan,8; 2017,Jan,8; 2016,Mar,5; 2016,Jan,13; 2015,Jul,3

33959 **reposition peripheral (arterial and/or venous) cannula(e), open, birth through 5 years of age (includes fluoroscopic guidance, when performed)** A

INCLUDES Fluoroscopic guidance

EXCLUDES *ECMO/ECLS initiation, veno-arterial (33947)*
ECMO/ECLS initiation, veno-venous (33946)
ECMO/ECLS insertion of cannula (33951-33956)
Open artery exposure for delivery/deployment endovascular prosthesis ([34812], 34714-34716 [34820, 34833, 34834])

6.84 6.84 **FUD** 000 C 80

AMA: 2018,Jan,8; 2017,Dec,3; 2017,Jan,8; 2016,Mar,5; 2016,Jan,13; 2015,Jul,3

\# **33962** **reposition peripheral (arterial and/or venous) cannula(e), open, 6 years and older (includes fluoroscopic guidance, when performed)** A

INCLUDES Fluoroscopic guidance

EXCLUDES *ECMO/ECLS initiation, veno-arterial (33947)*
ECMO/ECLS initiation, veno-venous (33946)
ECMO/ECLS insertion of cannula (33951-33956)
Open artery exposure for delivery/deployment endovascular prosthesis ([34812], 34714-34716 [34820, 34833, 34834])

6.79 6.79 **FUD** 000 C 80

AMA: 2018,Jan,8; 2017,Dec,3; 2017,Jan,8; 2016,Mar,5; 2016,Jan,13; 2015,Jul,3

 # 33963 reposition of central cannula(e) by sternotomy or thoracotomy, birth through 5 years of age (includes fluoroscopic guidance, when performed) A

INCLUDES Fluoroscopic guidance

EXCLUDES *ECMO/ECLS initiation, veno-arterial (33947)*
ECMO/ECLS initiation, veno-venous (33946)
ECMO/ECLS insertion of cannula (33951-33956)
Open artery exposure for delivery/deployment endovascular prosthesis ([34812], 34714-34716 [34820, 34833, 34834])

Facility RVU 13.5 Non-Facility RVU 13.5 FUD 000 C 80

AMA: 2018,Jan,8; 2017,Jan,8; 2016,Mar,5; 2016,Jan,13; 2015,Jul,3

 # 33964 reposition central cannula(e) by sternotomy or thoracotomy, 6 years and older (includes fluoroscopic guidance, when performed) A

INCLUDES Fluoroscopic guidance

EXCLUDES *ECMO/ECLS initiation, veno-arterial (33947)*
ECMO/ECLS initiation, veno-venous (33946)
ECMO/ECLS insertion cannula (33951-33956)
Mediastinotomy (39010)
Thoracotomy (32100)

Facility RVU 14.3 Non-Facility RVU 14.3 FUD 000 C 80

AMA: 2018,Jan,8; 2017,Jan,8; 2016,Mar,5; 2016,Jan,13; 2015,Jul,3

 # 33965 removal of peripheral (arterial and/or venous) cannula(e), percutaneous, birth through 5 years of age A

Code also extensive arterial repair/replacement, when performed (35266, 35286, 35371, 35665)

Code also new cannula insertion into different vessel (33951-33956)

Facility RVU 5.36 Non-Facility RVU 5.36 FUD 000 C 80

AMA: 2018,Jan,8; 2017,Jan,8; 2016,Mar,5; 2016,Jan,13; 2015,Jul,3

 # 33966 removal of peripheral (arterial and/or venous) cannula(e), percutaneous, 6 years and older A

Code also extensive arterial repair/replacement, when performed (35266, 35286, 35371, 35665)

Code also new cannula insertion into different vessel (33951, 33956)

Facility RVU 6.87 Non-Facility RVU 6.87 FUD 000 C 80

AMA: 2018,Jan,8; 2017,Jan,8; 2016,Mar,5; 2016,Jan,13; 2015,Jul,3

 # 33969 removal of peripheral (arterial and/or venous) cannula(e), open, birth through 5 years of age A

EXCLUDES *Open artery exposure for delivery/deployment endovascular prosthesis ([34812], 34714-34716 [34820, 34833, 34834])*
Repair blood vessel (35201, 35206, 35211, 35216, 35226)

Code also extensive arterial repair/replacement, when performed (35266, 35286, 35371, 35665)

Code also new cannula insertion into different vessel (33951-33956)

Facility RVU 7.98 Non-Facility RVU 7.98 FUD 000 C 80

AMA: 2018,Jan,8; 2017,Dec,3; 2017,Jan,8; 2016,Mar,5; 2016,Jan,13; 2015,Jul,3

 # 33984 removal of peripheral (arterial and/or venous) cannula(e), open, 6 years and older A

EXCLUDES *Open artery exposure for delivery/deployment endovascular prosthesis ([34812], 34714-34716 [34820, 34833, 34834])*
Repair blood vessel (35201, 35206, 35211, 35216, 35226)

Facility RVU 8.25 Non-Facility RVU 8.25 FUD 000 C 80

AMA: 2018,Jan,8; 2017,Dec,3; 2017,Jan,8; 2016,Mar,5; 2016,Jan,13; 2015,Jul,3

 # 33985 removal of central cannula(e) by sternotomy or thoracotomy, birth through 5 years of age A

EXCLUDES *Repair blood vessel (35201, 35206, 35211, 35216, 35226)*

Code also extensive arterial repair/replacement, when performed (35266, 35286, 35371, 35665)

Code also new cannula insertion into different vessel (33951-33956)

Facility RVU 14.9 Non-Facility RVU 14.9 FUD 000 C 80

AMA: 2018,Jan,8; 2017,Jan,8; 2016,Mar,5; 2016,Jan,13; 2015,Jul,3

 # 33986 removal of central cannula(e) by sternotomy or thoracotomy, 6 years and older A

EXCLUDES *Repair blood vessel (35201, 35206, 35211, 35216, 35226)*

Code also extensive arterial repair/replacement, when performed (35266, 35286, 35371, 35665)

Code also new cannula insertion into different vessel (33951-33956)

Facility RVU 15.1 Non-Facility RVU 15.1 FUD 000 C 80

AMA: 2018,Jan,8; 2017,Jan,8; 2016,Mar,5; 2016,Jan,13; 2015,Jul,3

+ # 33987 Arterial exposure with creation of graft conduit (eg, chimney graft) to facilitate arterial perfusion for ECMO/ECLS (List separately in addition to code for primary procedure)

EXCLUDES *Open artery exposure for delivery/deployment endovascular prosthesis ([34812], 34714-34716 [34820, 34833, 34834])*

Code first (33953-33956)

Facility RVU 6.09 Non-Facility RVU 6.09 FUD ZZZ C 80

AMA: 2018,Jan,8; 2017,Dec,3; 2017,Jan,8; 2016,Mar,5; 2016,Jan,13; 2015,Jul,3

 # 33988 Insertion of left heart vent by thoracic incision (eg, sternotomy, thoracotomy) for ECMO/ECLS

Facility RVU 22.5 Non-Facility RVU 22.5 FUD 000 C 80

AMA: 2018,Jan,8; 2017,Jan,8; 2016,Mar,5; 2016,Jan,13; 2015,Jul,3

 # 33989 Removal of left heart vent by thoracic incision (eg, sternotomy, thoracotomy) for ECMO/ECLS

Facility RVU 14.3 Non-Facility RVU 14.3 FUD 000 C 80

AMA: 2018,Jan,8; 2017,Jan,8; 2016,Mar,5; 2016,Jan,13; 2015,Jul,3

33962-33999 [33962, 33963, 33964, 33965, 33966, 33969, 33984, 33985, 33986, 33987, 33988, 33989, 33995, 33997] Mechanical Circulatory Support

33962 **Resequenced code. See code following 33959.**

33963 **Resequenced code. See code following 33959.**

33964 **Resequenced code. See code following 33959.**

33965 **Resequenced code. See code following 33959.**

33966 **Resequenced code. See code following 33959.**

33967 Insertion of intra-aortic balloon assist device, percutaneous

Facility RVU 7.51 Non-Facility RVU 7.51 FUD 000 C 80

AMA: 2018,Jan,8; 2017,Jan,8; 2016,Mar,5; 2016,Jan,13; 2015,Sep,3; 2015,Jul,3; 2015,Jan,16

33968 Removal of intra-aortic balloon assist device, percutaneous

EXCLUDES *Removal implantable aortic counterpulsation ventricular assist system (0455T-0458T)*

Facility RVU 0.98 Non-Facility RVU 0.98 FUD 000 C

AMA: 2018,Jan,8; 2017,Jan,8; 2016,Mar,5; 2016,Jan,13; 2015,Jul,3; 2015,Jan,16

33969 **Resequenced code. See code following 33959.**

33970 Insertion of intra-aortic balloon assist device through the femoral artery, open approach

EXCLUDES *Insertion/replacement implantable aortic counterpulsation ventricular assist system (0451T-0454T)*
Percutaneous insertion intra-aortic balloon assist device (33967)

Facility RVU 10.2 Non-Facility RVU 10.2 FUD 000 C 80

AMA: 2018,Jan,8; 2017,Jan,8; 2016,Mar,5; 2016,Jan,13; 2015,Sep,3; 2015,Jul,3; 2015,Jan,16

33971 Removal of intra-aortic balloon assist device including repair of femoral artery, with or without graft

EXCLUDES *Removal implantable aortic counterpulsation ventricular assist system (0455T-0458T)*

Facility RVU 20.3 Non-Facility RVU 20.3 FUD 090 C

AMA: 2018,Jan,8; 2017,Jan,8; 2016,Mar,5; 2016,Jan,13; 2015,Jul,3; 2015,Jan,16

33973 Insertion of intra-aortic balloon assist device through the ascending aorta

EXCLUDES *Insertion/replacement implantable aortic counterpulsation ventricular assist system (0451T-0454T)*

14.8 14.8 FUD 000 C 80

AMA: 2018,Jan,8; 2017,Jan,8; 2016,Mar,5; 2016,Jan,13; 2015,Sep,3; 2015,Jul,3; 2015,Jan,16

33974 Removal of intra-aortic balloon assist device from the ascending aorta, including repair of the ascending aorta, with or without graft

EXCLUDES *Removal implantable aortic counterpulsation ventricular assist system (0455T-0458T)*

25.7 25.7 FUD 090 C

AMA: 2018,Jan,8; 2017,Jan,8; 2016,Mar,5; 2016,Jan,13; 2015,Jul,3; 2015,Jan,16

33975 Insertion of ventricular assist device; extracorporeal, single ventricle

INCLUDES Insertion new pump with de-airing, connection, and initiation
Removal old pump with replacement entire ventricular assist device system, including pump(s) and cannulas
Transthoracic approach

EXCLUDES *Percutaneous approach ([33995], 33990-33991)*

Code also removal thrombus through separate heart incision, when performed (33310-33315); append modifier 59 to (33315)

37.8 37.8 FUD XXX C 80

AMA: 2018,Jun,3; 2018,Jan,8; 2017,Dec,3; 2017,Jan,8; 2016,Mar,5; 2016,Jan,13; 2015,Jul,3; 2015,Jan,16

33976 extracorporeal, biventricular

INCLUDES Insertion new pump with de-airing, connection, and initiation
Removal with replacement entire ventricular assist device system, including pump(s) and cannulas
Transthoracic approach

EXCLUDES *Percutaneous approach ([33995], 33990-33991)*

Code also removal thrombus through separate heart incision, when performed (33310-33315); append modifier 59 to (33315)

46.0 46.0 FUD XXX C 80

AMA: 2018,Jun,3; 2018,Jan,8; 2017,Dec,3; 2017,Jan,8; 2016,Mar,5; 2016,Jan,13; 2015,Jul,3; 2015,Jan,16

33977 Removal of ventricular assist device; extracorporeal, single ventricle

INCLUDES Removal entire device and cannulas

EXCLUDES *Removal ventricular assist device when performed same time as new device insertion*

Code also thrombus removal through separate heart incision, when performed (33310-33315); append modifier 59 to (33315)

32.6 32.6 FUD XXX C 80

AMA: 2018,Jan,8; 2017,Dec,3; 2017,Jan,8; 2016,Mar,5; 2016,Jan,13; 2015,Jul,3; 2015,Jan,16

33978 extracorporeal, biventricular

INCLUDES Removal entire device and cannulas

EXCLUDES *Removal ventricular assist device when performed same time as new device insertion*

Code also thrombus removal through separate heart incision, when performed (33310-33315); append modifier 59 to (33315)

38.5 38.5 FUD XXX C 80

AMA: 2018,Jan,8; 2017,Dec,3; 2017,Jan,8; 2016,Mar,5; 2016,Jan,13; 2015,Jul,3; 2015,Jan,16

33979 Insertion of ventricular assist device, implantable intracorporeal, single ventricle

INCLUDES New pump insertion with connection, de-airing, and initiation
Removal with replacement entire ventricular assist device system, including pump(s) and cannulas
Transthoracic approach

EXCLUDES *Insertion/replacement implantable aortic counterpulsation ventricular assist system (0451T-0454T)*
Percutaneous approach ([33995], 33990-33991)

Code also thrombus removal through separate heart incision, when performed (33310-33315); append modifier 59 to (33315)

56.5 56.5 FUD XXX C 80

AMA: 2018,Jun,3; 2018,Jan,8; 2017,Dec,3; 2017,Jan,8; 2016,Mar,5; 2016,Jan,13; 2015,Jul,3; 2015,Jan,16

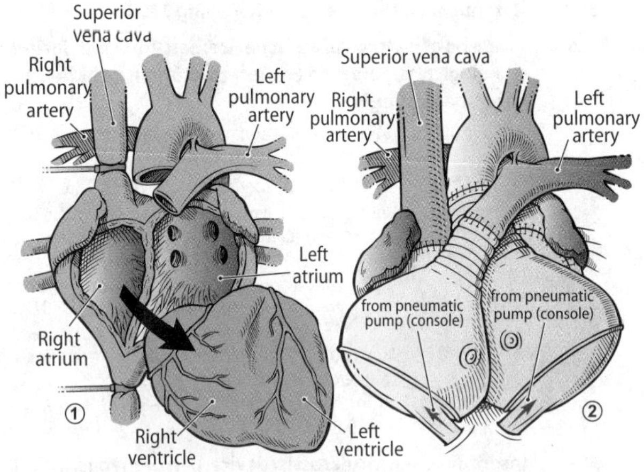

33980 Removal of ventricular assist device, implantable intracorporeal, single ventricle

INCLUDES Removal entire device and cannulas

EXCLUDES *Removal implantable aortic counterpulsation ventricular assist system (0455T-0458T)*
Removal ventricular assist device when performed same time as new device insertion

Code also thrombus removal through separate heart incision, when performed (33310-33315); append modifier 59 to (33315)

51.5 51.5 FUD XXX C 80

AMA: 2018,Jan,8; 2017,Dec,3; 2017,Jan,8; 2016,Mar,5; 2016,Jan,13; 2015,Jul,3; 2015,Jan,16

33981 Replacement of extracorporeal ventricular assist device, single or biventricular, pump(s), single or each pump

INCLUDES New pump insertion with de-airing, connection, and initiation
Removal old pump

24.3 24.3 FUD XXX C 80

AMA: 2018,Jan,8; 2017,Jan,8; 2016,Mar,5; 2016,Jan,13; 2015,Jul,3; 2015,Jan,16

33982 Replacement of ventricular assist device pump(s); implantable intracorporeal, single ventricle, without cardiopulmonary bypass

INCLUDES New pump insertion with connection, de-airing, and initiation
Removal old pump

57.1 57.1 FUD XXX C 80

AMA: 2018,Jan,8; 2017,Jan,8; 2016,Mar,5; 2016,Jan,13; 2015,Jul,3; 2015,Jan,16

33983 **implantable intracorporeal, single ventricle, with cardiopulmonary bypass**

INCLUDES Removal old pump

EXCLUDES *Insertion/replacement implantable aortic counterpulsation ventricular assist system (0451T-0454T)*

Percutaneous transseptal approach (33999)

67.0 67.0 **FUD** XXX C 80

AMA: 2018,Jan,8; 2017,Dec,3; 2017,Jan,8; 2016,Mar,5; 2016,Jan,13; 2015,Jul,3; 2015,Jan,16

33984 **Resequenced code. See code following 33959.**

33985 **Resequenced code. See code following 33959.**

33986 **Resequenced code. See code following 33959.**

33987 **Resequenced code. See code following 33959.**

33988 **Resequenced code. See code following 33959.**

33989 **Resequenced code. See code following 33959.**

● # 33995 **Insertion of ventricular assist device, percutaneous, including radiological supervision and interpretation; right heart, venous access only**

INCLUDES Initial insertion and replacement percutaneous ventricular assist device

EXCLUDES *Extensive artery repair/replacement (35226, 35286)*

Insertion/replacement implantable aortic counterpulsation ventricular assist system (0451T-0454T)

Open arterial approach to aid insertion percutaneous ventricular assist device, when used ([34812], 34714-34716 [34820, 34833, 34834])

Removal percutaneous ventricular assist device with entire system replacement (33992)

Transthoracic approach (33975-33976, 33979)

0.00 0.00 **FUD** 000

▲ 33990 **Insertion of ventricular assist device, percutaneous, including radiological supervision and interpretation; left heart, arterial access only**

INCLUDES Initial insertion and replacement percutaneous ventricular assist device

EXCLUDES *Extensive artery repair/replacement (35226, 35286)*

Insertion/replacement implantable aortic counterpulsation ventricular assist system (0451T-0454T)

Open arterial approach to aid insertion percutaneous ventricular assist device, when used ([34812], 34714-34716 [34820, 34833, 34834])

Removal percutaneous ventricular assist device with entire system replacement (33992)

Transthoracic approach (33975-33976, 33979)

12.4 12.4 **FUD** XXX C 80

AMA: 2018,Jun,3; 2018,Jan,8; 2017,Dec,3; 2017,Jan,8; 2016,Mar,5; 2016,Jan,13; 2015,Sep,3; 2015,Jan,16

▲ 33991 **left heart, both arterial and venous access, with transseptal puncture**

INCLUDES Initial insertion and replacement percutaneous ventricular assist device

EXCLUDES *Extensive artery repair/replacement (35226, 35286)*

Insertion/replacement implantable aortic counterpulsation ventricular assist system (0451T-0454T)

Open arterial approach to aid with insertion percutaneous ventricular assist device, when performed ([34812], 34714-34716 [34820, 34833, 34834])

Removal percutaneous ventricular assist device with entire system replacement (33992)

Transthoracic approach (33975-33976, 33979)

18.1 18.1 **FUD** XXX C 80

AMA: 2018,Jun,3; 2018,Jan,8; 2017,Dec,3; 2017,Jan,8; 2016,Mar,5; 2016,Jan,13; 2015,Sep,3; 2015,Jan,16

▲ 33992 **Removal of percutaneous left heart ventricular assist device, arterial or arterial and venous cannula(s), at separate and distinct session from insertion**

INCLUDES Removal device and cannulas

EXCLUDES *Removal implantable aortic counterpulsation ventricular assist system (0455T-0458T)*

Code also modifier 59 when percutaneous ventricular assist device removed on same day as insertion, but different session

5.80 5.80 **FUD** XXX C 80

AMA: 2018,Jan,8; 2017,Jan,8; 2016,Mar,5; 2016,Jan,13; 2015,Sep,3; 2015,Jan,16

● # 33997 **Removal of percutaneous right heart ventricular assist device, venous cannula, at separate and distinct session from insertion**

EXCLUDES *Removal ventricular assist device, open approach, report appropriate vessel repair code(s)*

0.00 0.00 **FUD** 000

▲ 33993 **Repositioning of percutaneous right or left heart ventricular assist device with imaging guidance at separate and distinct session from insertion**

EXCLUDES *Repositioning percutaneous ventricular assist device without image guidance*

Repositioning device/electrode (0460T-0461T)

Repositioning percutaneous ventricular assist device same session as insertion (33990-33991)

Skin pocket relocation with replacement implantable aortic counterpulsation ventricular assist device and electrodes (0459T)

Code also modifier 59 when percutaneous ventricular assist device repositioned using imaging guidance on same day as insertion, but different session

5.09 5.09 **FUD** XXX C 80

AMA: 2018,Jan,8; 2017,Jan,8; 2016,Mar,5; 2016,Jan,13; 2015,Sep,3; 2015,Jan,16

33995 **Resequenced code. See code following 33983.**

33997 **Resequenced code. See code following 33992.**

33999 **Unlisted procedure, cardiac surgery**

0.00 0.00 **FUD** YYY T 80

AMA: 2019,Apr,10; 2019,Jan,14; 2018,Jun,3; 2018,Jan,8; 2017,Jan,8; 2016,May,5; 2016,Jan,13; 2015,Jan,16

34001-34530 Surgical Revascularization: Veins and Arteries

INCLUDES Repair blood vessel

Surgeon's component operative arteriogram

34001 **Embolectomy or thrombectomy, with or without catheter; carotid, subclavian or innominate artery, by neck incision**

27.8 27.8 **FUD** 090 C 80 50

AMA: 1997,Nov,1

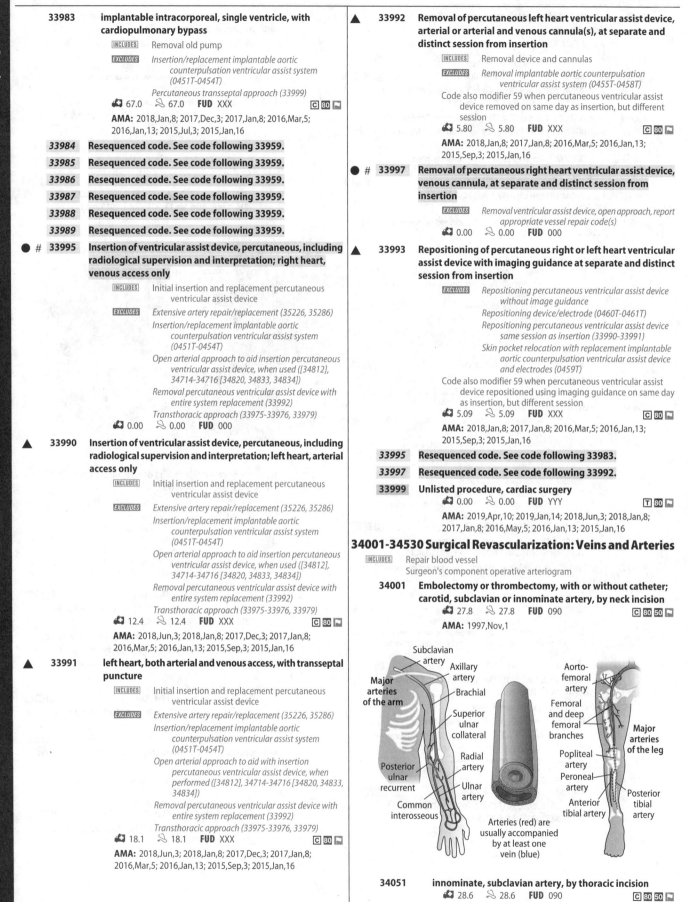

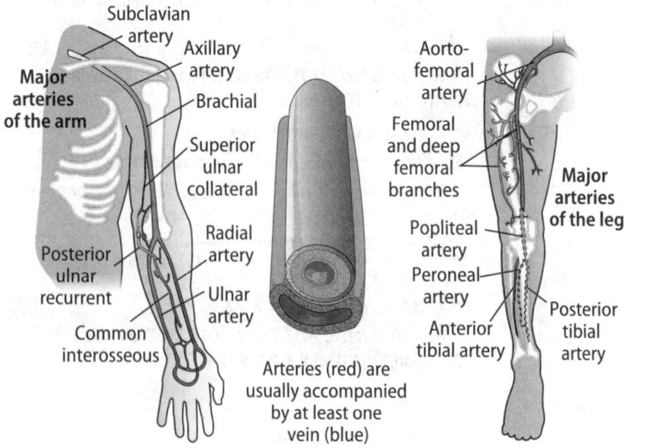

34051 **innominate, subclavian artery, by thoracic incision**

28.6 28.6 **FUD** 090 C 80 50

AMA: 1997,Nov,1

34101 **axillary, brachial, innominate, subclavian artery, by arm incision**
17.3 17.3 **FUD** 090 T 80 50
AMA: 1997,Nov,1

34111 **radial or ulnar artery, by arm incision**
17.3 17.3 **FUD** 090 T 80 50
AMA: 1997,Nov,1

34151 **renal, celiac, mesentery, aortoiliac artery, by abdominal incision**
40.4 40.4 **FUD** 090 C 80 50
AMA: 1997,Nov,1

34201 **femoropopliteal, aortoiliac artery, by leg incision**
29.8 29.8 **FUD** 090 T 80 50
AMA: 2018,Jan,8; 2017,Jan,8; 2016,Jan,13; 2015,Jan,16

34203 **popliteal-tibio-peroneal artery, by leg incision**
27.6 27.6 **FUD** 090 T 80 50
AMA: 1997,Nov,1

34401 **Thrombectomy, direct or with catheter; vena cava, iliac vein, by abdominal incision**
42.4 42.4 **FUD** 090 C 80 50
AMA: 1997,Nov,1

34421 **vena cava, iliac, femoropopliteal vein, by leg incision**
21.5 21.5 **FUD** 090 T 80 50
AMA: 2018,Jan,8; 2017,Jan,8; 2016,Jan,13; 2015,Jan,16

34451 **vena cava, iliac, femoropopliteal vein, by abdominal and leg incision**
41.7 41.7 **FUD** 090 C 80 50
AMA: 1997,Nov,1

34471 **subclavian vein, by neck incision**
31.1 31.1 **FUD** 090 T 50
AMA: 1997,Nov,1

34490 **axillary and subclavian vein, by arm incision**
18.5 18.5 **FUD** 090 T 62 50
AMA: 1997,Nov,1

34501 **Valvuloplasty, femoral vein**
25.8 25.8 **FUD** 090 T 80 50
AMA: 1997,Nov,1

34502 **Reconstruction of vena cava, any method**
44.7 44.7 **FUD** 090 C 80
AMA: 1997,Nov,1

34510 **Venous valve transposition, any vein donor**
29.6 29.6 **FUD** 090 T 80 50
AMA: 1997,Nov,1

34520 **Cross-over vein graft to venous system**
28.7 28.7 **FUD** 090 T 80 50
AMA: 1997,Nov,1

34530 **Saphenopopliteal vein anastomosis**
27.2 27.2 **FUD** 090 T 80 50
AMA: 1997,Nov,1

34701-34713 [34717, 34718] Abdominal Aorta and Iliac Artery Repairs

INCLUDES Closure artery after endograft delivery using sheath size less than 12 French
Treatment with covered stent for:
- Aneurysm
- Aortic dissection
- Arteriovenous malformation
- Pseudoaneurysm
- Trauma

Treatment zones (vessel(s) in which endograft deployed):
- Iliac artery(ies) (34707-34708, [34717], [34718])
- Infrarenal aorta (34701-34702)
- Infrarenal aorta and both common iliac arteries (34705-34706)
- Infrarenal aorta and ipsilateral common iliac artery (34703-34704)

EXCLUDES *Treatment atherosclerotic occlusive disease with covered stent:*
- *Aorta (37236-37237)*
- *Iliac artery(ies) (37221, 37223)*

Code also open arterial exposure, when appropriate ([34812], 34714 [34820, 34833, 34834], 34715-34716)
Code also percutaneous closure artery when endograft delivered through sheath 12 French or larger (34713)
Code also selective catheterization arteries outside target treatment zone

34701 **Endovascular repair of infrarenal aorta by deployment of an aorto-aortic tube endograft including pre-procedure sizing and device selection, all nonselective catheterization(s), all associated radiological supervision and interpretation, all endograft extension(s) placed in the aorta from the level of the renal arteries to the aortic bifurcation, and all angioplasty/stenting performed from the level of the renal arteries to the aortic bifurcation; for other than rupture (eg, for aneurysm, pseudoaneurysm, dissection, penetrating ulcer)**
INCLUDES Nonselective catheterization
Code also intravascular ultrasound when performed (37252-37253)
36.1 36.1 **FUD** 090 C 80
AMA: 2019,Nov,6; 2018,Jan,8; 2017,Dec,3

34702 **for rupture including temporary aortic and/or iliac balloon occlusion, when performed (eg, for aneurysm, pseudoaneurysm, dissection, penetrating ulcer, traumatic disruption)**
INCLUDES Nonselective catheterization
Code also decompressive laparotomy for treatment abdominal compartment syndrome (49000)
Code also intravascular ultrasound when performed (37252-37253)
53.9 53.9 **FUD** 090 C 80
AMA: 2019,Nov,6; 2018,Jan,8; 2017,Dec,3

34703 **Endovascular repair of infrarenal aorta and/or iliac artery(ies) by deployment of an aorto-uni-iliac endograft including pre-procedure sizing and device selection, all nonselective catheterization(s), all associated radiological supervision and interpretation, all endograft extension(s) placed in the aorta from the level of the renal arteries to the iliac bifurcation, and all angioplasty/stenting performed from the level of the renal arteries to the iliac bifurcation; for other than rupture (eg, for aneurysm, pseudoaneurysm, dissection, penetrating ulcer)**
INCLUDES Endograft extensions ending in common iliac arteries
Nonselective catheterization
Code also intravascular ultrasound when performed (37252-37253)
39.8 39.8 **FUD** 090 C 80
AMA: 2019,Nov,6; 2018,Jan,8; 2017,Dec,3

34704 **for rupture including temporary aortic and/or iliac balloon occlusion, when performed (eg, for aneurysm, pseudoaneurysm, dissection, penetrating ulcer, traumatic disruption)**

INCLUDES Endograft extensions ending in common iliac arteries
Nonselective catheterization

Code also decompressive laparotomy for treatment abdominal compartment syndrome (49000)

Code also intravascular ultrasound when performed (37252-37253)

66.4 66.4 **FUD** 090 C 80

AMA: 2019,Nov,6; 2018,Jan,8; 2017,Dec,3

34705 **Endovascular repair of infrarenal aorta and/or iliac artery(ies) by deployment of an aorto-bi-iliac endograft including pre-procedure sizing and device selection, all nonselective catheterization(s), all associated radiological supervision and interpretation, all endograft extension(s) placed in the aorta from the level of the renal arteries to the iliac bifurcation, and all angioplasty/stenting performed from the level of the renal arteries to the iliac bifurcation; for other than rupture (eg, for aneurysm, pseudoaneurysm, dissection, penetrating ulcer)**

INCLUDES Endograft extensions ending in common iliac arteries
Nonselective catheterization

Code also intravascular ultrasound when performed (37252-37253)

44.5 44.5 **FUD** 090 C 80

AMA: 2019,Nov,6; 2018,Jan,8; 2017,Dec,3

34706 **for rupture including temporary aortic and/or iliac balloon occlusion, when performed (eg, for aneurysm, pseudoaneurysm, dissection, penetrating ulcer, traumatic disruption)**

INCLUDES Endograft extensions ending in common iliac arteries
Nonselective catheterization

Code also decompressive laparotomy for treatment abdominal compartment syndrome (49000)

Code also intravascular ultrasound when performed (37252-37253)

67.1 67.1 **FUD** 090 C 80

AMA: 2019,Nov,6; 2018,Jan,8; 2017,Dec,3

34707 **Endovascular repair of iliac artery by deployment of an ilio-iliac tube endograft including pre-procedure sizing and device selection, all nonselective catheterization(s), all associated radiological supervision and interpretation, and all endograft extension(s) proximally to the aortic bifurcation and distally to the iliac bifurcation, and treatment zone angioplasty/stenting, when performed, unilateral; for other than rupture (eg, for aneurysm, pseudoaneurysm, dissection, arteriovenous malformation)**

INCLUDES Endograft extensions ending in common iliac arteries
Nonselective catheterization

EXCLUDES *Deployment iliac branched endograft:*
At same time as aorto-iliac graft placement ([34717])
Delayed/separate from aorto-iliac endograft deployment ([34718])

Code also intravascular ultrasound when performed (37252-37253)

33.7 33.7 **FUD** 090 C 80 50

AMA: 2019,Nov,6; 2018,Jan,8; 2017,Dec,3

34708 **for rupture including temporary aortic and/or iliac balloon occlusion, when performed (eg, for aneurysm, pseudoaneurysm, dissection, arteriovenous malformation, traumatic disruption)**

INCLUDES Endograft extensions ending in common iliac arteries
Nonselective catheterization

EXCLUDES *Deployment iliac branched endograft:*
At same time as aorto-iliac graft placement ([34717])
Delayed/separate from aorto-iliac endograft deployment ([34718])

Code also decompressive laparotomy for treatment abdominal compartment syndrome (49000)

Code also intravascular ultrasound when performed (37252-37253)

53.8 53.8 **FUD** 090 C 80 50

AMA: 2019,Nov,6; 2018,Jan,8; 2017,Dec,3

+ # **34717** **Endovascular repair of iliac artery at the time of aorto-iliac artery endograft placement by deployment of an iliac branched endograft including pre-procedure sizing and device selection, all ipsilateral selective iliac artery catheterization(s), all associated radiological supervision and interpretation, and all endograft extension(s) proximally to the aortic bifurcation and distally in the internal iliac, external iliac, and common femoral artery(ies), and treatment zone angioplasty/stenting, when performed, for rupture or other than rupture (eg, for aneurysm, pseudoaneurysm, dissection, arteriovenous malformation, penetrating ulcer, traumatic disruption), unilateral (List separately in addition to code for primary procedure)**

INCLUDES Endograft extensions into internal and external iliac, and/or common femoral arteries

EXCLUDES *Delayed deployment branched iliac endograft, separate from aorto-iliac endograft placement ([34718])*
Placement prosthesis extensions on same side (34709, 34710-34711)
Reporting with modifier 50. Report once for each side when performed bilaterally

Code first (34703-34706)

12.9 12.9 **FUD** ZZZ 80

+ **34709** **Placement of extension prosthesis(es) distal to the common iliac artery(ies) or proximal to the renal artery(ies) for endovascular repair of infrarenal abdominal aortic or iliac aneurysm, false aneurysm, dissection, penetrating ulcer, including pre-procedure sizing and device selection, all nonselective catheterization(s), all associated radiological supervision and interpretation, and treatment zone angioplasty/stenting, when performed, per vessel treated (List separately in addition to code for primary procedure)**

EXCLUDES *Placement covered stent (37236-37237)*
Placement iliac branched endograft ([34717], [34718])
Reporting code more than one time for each vessel treated

Code first (34701-34708, 34845-34848)

9.42 9.42 **FUD** ZZZ C 80

AMA: 2019,Nov,6; 2018,Jan,8; 2017,Dec,3

34718 **Endovascular repair of iliac artery, not associated with placement of an aorto-iliac artery endograft at the same session, by deployment of an iliac branched endograft, including pre-procedure sizing and device selection, all ipsilateral selective iliac artery catheterization(s), all associated radiological supervision and interpretation, and all endograft extension(s) proximally to the aortic bifurcation and distally in the internal iliac, external iliac, and common femoral artery(ies), and treatment zone angioplasty/stenting, when performed, for other than rupture (eg, for aneurysm, pseudoaneurysm, dissection, arteriovenous malformation, penetrating ulcer), unilateral**

INCLUDES Endograft extensions into internal and external iliac, and/or common femoral arteries

EXCLUDES *Branched iliac endograft deployed same session as aorto-iliac endograft placement (34703-34706, [34717])*

Placement isolated iliac branched endograft, for rupture (37799)

Placement prosthesis extensions on same side (34709, 34710-34711)

36.0 36.0 **FUD** 090 80

34710 **Delayed placement of distal or proximal extension prosthesis for endovascular repair of infrarenal abdominal aortic or iliac aneurysm, false aneurysm, dissection, endoleak, or endograft migration, including pre-procedure sizing and device selection, all nonselective catheterization(s), all associated radiological supervision and interpretation, and treatment zone angioplasty/stenting, when performed; initial vessel treated**

EXCLUDES *Fenestrated endograft repair (34841-34848)*

Initial endovascular repair by endograft (34701-34709)

Reporting code more than one time per procedure

Code also decompressive laparotomy for treatment abdominal compartment syndrome (49000)

23.3 23.3 **FUD** 090 C 80

AMA: 2019,Nov,6; 2018,Jan,8; 2017,Dec,3

\+ **34711** **each additional vessel treated (List separately in addition to code for primary procedure)**

EXCLUDES *Fenestrated endograft repair (34841-34848)*

Initial endovascular repair by endograft (34701-34709)

Reporting code more than one time per procedure

Code first (34710)

8.68 8.68 **FUD** ZZZ C 80

AMA: 2019,Nov,6; 2018,Jan,8; 2017,Dec,3

34712 **Transcatheter delivery of enhanced fixation device(s) to the endograft (eg, anchor, screw, tack) and all associated radiological supervision and interpretation**

EXCLUDES *Reporting code more than one time per procedure*

19.2 19.2 **FUD** 090 C 80

AMA: 2018,Jan,8; 2017,Dec,3

\+ **34713** **Percutaneous access and closure of femoral artery for delivery of endograft through a large sheath (12 French or larger), including ultrasound guidance, when performed, unilateral (List separately in addition to code for primary procedure)**

INCLUDES Ultrasound imaging guidance

Unilateral procedure through large sheath 12 French or larger

EXCLUDES *Reporting with modifier 50. Report once for each side when performed bilaterally*

Code first (33880-33881, 33883-33884, 33886, 34701-34708, [34718], 34710, 34712, 34841-34848)

3.63 3.63 **FUD** ZZZ N N1 80 50

AMA: 2018,Jan,8; 2017,Dec,3

34812-34834 [34717, 34718, 34812, 34820, 34833, 34834] Open Exposure for Endovascular Prosthesis Delivery

INCLUDES Balloon angioplasty/stent deployment within target treatment zone

Introduction, manipulation, placement, and device deployment

Open exposure femoral or iliac artery/subsequent closure

Thromboendarterectomy at site of aneurysm

EXCLUDES *Additional interventional procedures outside target treatment zone*

Guidewire and catheter insertion (36140, 36200, 36245-36248)

Substantial artery repair/replacement (35226, 35286)

\+ # **34812** **Open femoral artery exposure for delivery of endovascular prosthesis, by groin incision, unilateral (List separately in addition to code for primary procedure)**

EXCLUDES *ECMO/ECLS insertion, removal or repositioning (33953-33954, 33959, [33962], [33969], [33984], [33987])*

Extensive repair femoral artery (35226, 35286, 35371)

Reporting with modifier 50. Report once for each side when performed bilaterally

Code first (33880-33881, 33883-33884, 33886, 33990-33991, 34701-34708, [34718], 34710, 34712, 34841-34848)

6.01 6.01 **FUD** ZZZ C 80 50

AMA: 2018,Jan,8; 2017,Dec,3; 2017,Jan,8; 2016,Jan,13; 2015,Jul,3; 2015,Jan,16

\+ **34714** **Open femoral artery exposure with creation of conduit for delivery of endovascular prosthesis or for establishment of cardiopulmonary bypass, by groin incision, unilateral (List separately in addition to code for primary procedure)**

EXCLUDES *Delivery endovascular prosthesis via open femoral artery ([34812])*

ECMO/ECLS insertion, removal or repositioning on same side (33953-33954, 33959, [33962], [33969], [33984])

Reporting with modifier 50. Report once for each side when performed bilaterally

Transcatheter aortic valve replacement via open axillary artery (33362)

Code first (32852, 32854, 33031, 33120, 33251, 33256, 33259, 33261, 33305, 33315, 33322, 33335, 33390-33391, 33404-33406, 33410, [33440], 33411-33417, 33422, 33425-33427, 33430, 33460, 33463-33465, 33468, 33474-33476, 33478, 33496, 33500, 33502, 33504-33507, 33510-33516, 33533-33536, 33542, 33545, 33548, 33600-33688, 33692, 33694, 33697, 33702, 33710, 33720, 33722, 33724, 33726, 33730, 33732, 33736, 33750, 33755, 33762, 33764, 33766-33767, 33770-33783, 33786, 33788, 33802-33803, 33814, 33820, 33822, 33824, 33840, 33845, 33851, 33853, 33858-33859, 33863-33864, 33871, 33875, 33877, 33880-33881, 33883-33884, 33886, 33910, 33916-33917, 33920, 33922, 33926, 33935, 33945, 33975-33980, 33983, 33990-33991, 34701-34708, [34718], 34710, 34712, 34841-34848)

7.87 7.87 **FUD** ZZZ N N1 80 50

AMA: 2018,Jan,8; 2017,Dec,3

\+ # **34820** **Open iliac artery exposure for delivery of endovascular prosthesis or iliac occlusion during endovascular therapy, by abdominal or retroperitoneal incision, unilateral (List separately in addition to code for primary procedure)**

EXCLUDES *ECMO/ECLS insertion, removal or repositioning (33953-33954, 33959, [33962], [33969], [33984])*

Reporting with modifier 50. Report once for each side when performed bilaterally

Code first (33880-33881, 33883-33884, 33886, 33990-33991, 34701-34708, [34718], 34710, 34712, 34841-34848)

10.1 10.1 **FUD** ZZZ C 80 50

AMA: 2018,Jan,8; 2017,Dec,3; 2017,Jan,8; 2016,Jan,13; 2015,Jul,3; 2015,Jan,16

+ # 34833 Open iliac artery exposure with creation of conduit for delivery of endovascular prosthesis or for establishment of cardiopulmonary bypass, by abdominal or retroperitoneal incision, unilateral (List separately in addition to code for primary procedure)

EXCLUDES *Delivery endovascular prosthesis via open iliac artery ([34820])*
ECMO/ECLS insertion, removal or repositioning on same side (33953-33954, 33959, [33962], [33969], [33984])
Reporting with modifier 50. Report once for each side when performed bilaterally
Transcatheter aortic valve replacement via open iliac artery (33364)

Code first (32852, 32854, 33031, 33256, 33259, 33261, 33305, 33315, 33322, 33335, 33390-33391, 33404-33406, 33410, [33440], 33411-33417, 33422, 33425-33427, 33430, 33460, 33463-33465, 33468, 33474-33476, 33478, 33496, 33500, 33502, 33504-33514, 33516, 33533-33536, 33542, 33545, 33548, 33600-33688, 33692, 33694, 33697, 33702, 33710, 33720, 33722, 33724, 33726, 33730, 33732, 33736, 33750, 33755, 33762, 33764, 33766-33767, 33770-33783, 33786, 33788, 33802-33803, 33814, 33820, 33822, 33824, 33840, 33845, 33851, 33853, 33858-33859, 33863-33864, 33871, 33875, 33877, 33880-33881, 33883-33884, 33886, 33910, 33916-33917, 33920, 33922, 33926, 33935, 33945, 33975-33980, 33983, 33990-33991, 34701-34708, [34718], 34710, 34712, 34841-34848)

11.7 11.7 **FUD** ZZZ C 80 50

AMA: 2018,Jan,8; 2017,Dec,3; 2017,Jan,8; 2016,Jan,13; 2015,Jul,3; 2015,Jan,16

+ # 34834 Open brachial artery exposure for delivery of endovascular prosthesis, unilateral (List separately in addition to code for primary procedure)

EXCLUDES *ECMO/ECLS insertion, removal or repositioning (33953-33954, 33959, [33962], [33969], [33984])*
Reporting with modifier 50. Report once for each side when performed bilaterally

Code first (33880-33881, 33883-33884, 33886, 33990-33991, 34701-34708, [34718], 34710, 34712, 34841-34848)

3.75 3.75 **FUD** ZZZ C 80 50

AMA: 2018,Jan,8; 2017,Dec,3; 2017,Jan,8; 2016,Jan,13; 2015,Jul,3; 2015,Jan,16

+ 34715 Open axillary/subclavian artery exposure for delivery of endovascular prosthesis by infraclavicular or supraclavicular incision, unilateral (List separately in addition to code for primary procedure)

EXCLUDES *ECMO/ECLS insertion, removal or repositioning on same side (33953-33954, 33959, [33962], [33969], [33984])*
Implantation or replacement aortic counterpulsation ventricular assist system (0451T-0452T, 0455T-0456T)
Reporting with modifier 50. Report once for each side when performed bilaterally
Transcatheter aortic valve replacement via open axillary artery (33363)

Code first (33880-33881, 33883-33884, 33886, 33990-33991, 34701-34708, [34718], 34710, 34712, 34841-34848)

8.72 8.72 **FUD** ZZZ N N1 80 50

AMA: 2018,Jan,8; 2017,Dec,3

+ 34716 Open axillary/subclavian artery exposure with creation of conduit for delivery of endovascular prosthesis or for establishment of cardiopulmonary bypass, by infraclavicular or supraclavicular incision, unilateral (List separately in addition to code for primary procedure)

EXCLUDES *ECMO/ECLS insertion, removal or repositioning on same side (33953-33954, 33959, [33962], [33969], [33984])*
Implantation or replacement aortic counterpulsation ventricular assist system (0451T-0452T, 0455T-0456T)
Reporting with modifier 50. Report once for each side when performed bilaterally

Code first (32852, 32854, 33031, 33120, 33251, 33256, 33259, 33261, 33305, 33315, 33322, 33335, 33390-33391, 33404-33406, 33410, [33440], 33411-33417, 33422, 33425-33427, 33430, 33460, 33463-33465, 33468, 33474-33476, 33478, 33496, 33500, 33502, 33504-33514, 33516, 33533-33536, 33542, 33545, 33548, 33600-33688, 33692, 33694, 33697, 33702-33722, 33724, 33726, 33730, 33732, 33736, 33750, 33755, 33762, 33764, 33766-33767, 33770-33783, 33786, 33788, 33802-33803, 33814, 33820, 33822, 33824, 33840, 33845, 33851, 33853, 33858-33859, 33863-33864, 33871, 33875, 33877, 33880-33881, 33883-33884, 33886, 33910, 33916-33917, 33920, 33922, 33926, 33935, 33945, 33975-33980, 33983, 33990-33991, 34701-34708, [34718], 34710, 34712, 34841-34848)

10.8 10.8 **FUD** ZZZ N N1 80 50

AMA: 2018,Jan,8; 2017,Dec,3

34717 **Resequenced code. See code following 34708.**

34718 **Resequenced code. See code following 34709.**

+ 34808 Endovascular placement of iliac artery occlusion device (List separately in addition to code for primary procedure)

Code first (34701-34704, 34707-34708, 34709, 34710, 34813, 34841-34844)

5.81 5.81 **FUD** ZZZ C 80

AMA: 2018,Jan,8; 2017,Jan,8; 2016,Jan,13; 2015,Jan,16

34812 **Resequenced code. See code following 34713.**

+ 34813 Placement of femoral-femoral prosthetic graft during endovascular aortic aneurysm repair (List separately in addition to code for primary procedure)

EXCLUDES *Grafting femoral artery (35521, 35533, 35539, 35540, 35556, 35558, 35566, 35621, 35646, 35654-35661, 35666, 35700)*

Code first ([34812])

6.90 6.90 **FUD** ZZZ C 80

AMA: 2018,Jan,8; 2017,Jan,8; 2016,Jan,13; 2015,Jan,16

34820 **Resequenced code. See code following 34714.**

34830 Open repair of infrarenal aortic aneurysm or dissection, plus repair of associated arterial trauma, following unsuccessful endovascular repair; tube prosthesis

51.2 51.2 **FUD** 090 C 80

AMA: 2018,Jan,8; 2017,Jan,8; 2016,Jan,13; 2015,Jan,16

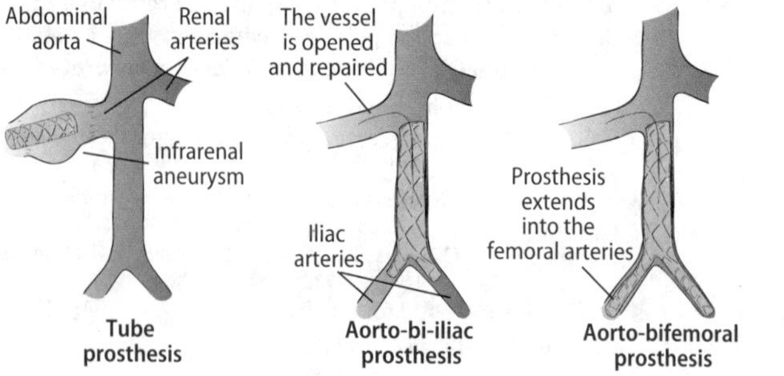

A tube prosthesis is placed and any associated arterial trauma is repaired

34831 aorto-bi-iliac prosthesis

56.0 56.0 **FUD** 090 C 80

AMA: 2018,Jan,8; 2017,Jan,8; 2016,Jan,13; 2015,Jan,16

34832 **aorto-bifemoral prosthesis**
55.0 55.0 **FUD** 090 C 80
AMA: 2018,Jan,8; 2017,Jan,8; 2016,Jan,13; 2015,Jan,16

34833 **Resequenced code. See code following 34714.**

34834 **Resequenced code. See code following 34714.**

34839-34848 Repair Visceral Aorta with Fenestrated Endovascular Grafts

INCLUDES Angiography
Balloon angioplasty before and after graft deployment
Fluoroscopic guidance
Guidewire and catheter insertion vessels in target treatment zone
Radiologic supervision and interpretation
Visceral aorta (34841-34844)
Visceral aorta and associated infrarenal abdominal aorta (34845-34848)

EXCLUDES *Catheterization:*
Arterial families outside treatment zone
Hypogastric arteries
Distal extension prosthesis terminating in common femoral, external iliac, or internal iliac artery (34709-34711 [34718])
Insertion bare metal or covered intravascular stents in visceral branches in target treatment zone (37236-37237)
Interventional procedures outside treatment zone
Open exposure access vessels (34713-34716 [34812, 34820, 34833, 34834])
Placement distal extension prosthesis into internal/external iliac or common femoral artery (34709, [34718], 34710-34711)
Repair abdominal aortic aneurysm without fenestrated graft (34701-34708)
Substantial artery repair (35226, 35286)

Code also associated endovascular repair descending thoracic aorta (33880-33886, 75956-75959)

34839 **Physician planning of a patient-specific fenestrated visceral aortic endograft requiring a minimum of 90 minutes of physician time**
EXCLUDES *3D rendering with interpretation and image reporting (76376-76377)*
Endovascular repair procedure on day of or day after planning (34701-34706, 34841-34848)
Planning on day of or day before endovascular repair procedure
Total planning time less than 90 minutes
0.00 0.00 **FUD** YYY B 80

34841 **Endovascular repair of visceral aorta (eg, aneurysm, pseudoaneurysm, dissection, penetrating ulcer, intramural hematoma, or traumatic disruption) by deployment of a fenestrated visceral aortic endograft and all associated radiological supervision and interpretation, including target zone angioplasty, when performed; including one visceral artery endoprosthesis (superior mesenteric, celiac or renal artery)**
EXCLUDES *Endovascular repair aorta (34701-34706, 34845-34848)*
Physician planning patient-specific fenestrated visceral aortic endograft (34839)
0.00 0.00 **FUD** YYY C 80
AMA: 2018,Jan,8; 2017,Dec,3; 2017,Jul,3; 2017,Jan,8; 2016,Jan,13; 2015,Jan,16

34842 **including two visceral artery endoprostheses (superior mesenteric, celiac and/or renal artery[s])**
INCLUDES Repairs extending from visceral aorta to one or more four visceral artery origins to infrarenal aorta level
EXCLUDES *Endovascular repair aorta (34701-34706, 34845-34848)*
Physician planning patient-specific fenestrated visceral aortic endograft (34839)
0.00 0.00 **FUD** YYY C 80
AMA: 2018,Jan,8; 2017,Dec,3; 2017,Jul,3; 2017,Jan,8; 2016,Jan,13; 2015,Jan,16

34843 **including three visceral artery endoprostheses (superior mesenteric, celiac and/or renal artery[s])**
INCLUDES Repairs extending from visceral aorta to one or more four visceral artery origins to infrarenal aorta level
EXCLUDES *Endovascular repair aorta (34701-34706, 34845-34848)*
Physician planning patient-specific fenestrated visceral aortic endograft (34839)
0.00 0.00 **FUD** YYY C 80
AMA: 2018,Jan,8; 2017,Dec,3; 2017,Jul,3; 2017,Jan,8; 2016,Jan,13; 2015,Jan,16

34844 **including four or more visceral artery endoprostheses (superior mesenteric, celiac and/or renal artery[s])**
INCLUDES Repairs extending from visceral aorta to one or more four visceral artery origins to infrarenal aorta level
EXCLUDES *Endovascular repair aorta (34701-34706, 34845-34848)*
Physician planning patient-specific fenestrated visceral aortic endograft (34839)
0.00 0.00 **FUD** YYY C 80
AMA: 2018,Jan,8; 2017,Dec,3; 2017,Jul,3; 2017,Jan,8; 2016,Jan,13; 2015,Jan,16

34845 **Endovascular repair of visceral aorta and infrarenal abdominal aorta (eg, aneurysm, pseudoaneurysm, dissection, penetrating ulcer, intramural hematoma, or traumatic disruption) with a fenestrated visceral aortic endograft and concomitant unibody or modular infrarenal aortic endograft and all associated radiological supervision and interpretation, including target zone angioplasty, when performed; including one visceral artery endoprosthesis (superior mesenteric, celiac or renal artery)**
INCLUDES Placement device and extensions into common iliac arteries
Repairs extending from visceral aorta to one or more four visceral artery origins to infrarenal aorta level
EXCLUDES *Direct repair aneurysm (35081, 35102)*
Endovascular repair aorta (34701-34706, 34845-34848)
Physician planning patient-specific fenestrated visceral aortic endograft (34839)
Code also iliac artery revascularization when performed outside target treatment zone (37220-37223)
0.00 0.00 **FUD** YYY C 80
AMA: 2018,Jan,8; 2017,Dec,3; 2017,Jul,3; 2017,Jan,8; 2016,Jan,13; 2015,Jan,16

34846 **including two visceral artery endoprostheses (superior mesenteric, celiac and/or renal artery[s])**
INCLUDES Placement device and extensions into common iliac arteries
Repairs extending from visceral aorta to one or more four visceral artery origins to infrarenal aorta level
EXCLUDES *Direct repair aneurysm (35081, 35102)*
Endovascular repair aorta (34701-34706, 34841-34844)
Physician planning patient-specific fenestrated visceral aortic endograft (34839)
Code also iliac artery revascularization when performed outside target treatment zone (37220-37223)
0.00 0.00 **FUD** YYY C 80
AMA: 2018,Jan,8; 2017,Dec,3; 2017,Jul,3; 2017,Jan,8; 2016,Jan,13; 2015,Jan,16

34847 **including three visceral artery endoprostheses (superior mesenteric, celiac and/or renal artery[s])**

INCLUDES Placement device and extensions into common iliac arteries
Repairs extending from visceral aorta to one or more four visceral artery origins to infrarenal aorta level

EXCLUDES *Direct repair aneurysm (35081, 35102)*
Endovascular repair aorta (34701-34706, 34841-34844)
Physician planning patient-specific fenestrated visceral aortic endograft (34839)

Code also iliac artery revascularization when performed outside target treatment zone (37220-37223)

0.00 0.00 **FUD** YYY C 80

AMA: 2018,Jan,8; 2017,Dec,3; 2017,Jul,3; 2017,Jan,8; 2016,Jan,13; 2015,Jan,16

34848 **including four or more visceral artery endoprostheses (superior mesenteric, celiac and/or renal artery[s])**

INCLUDES Placement device and extensions into common iliac arteries
Repairs extending from visceral aorta to one or more four visceral artery origins to infrarenal aorta level

EXCLUDES *Direct repair aneurysm (35081, 35102)*
Endovascular repair aorta (34701-34706, 34841-34844)
Physician planning patient-specific fenestrated visceral aortic endograft (34839)

Code also iliac artery revascularization when performed outside target treatment zone (37220-37223)

0.00 0.00 **FUD** YYY C 80

AMA: 2018,Jan,8; 2017,Dec,3; 2017,Aug,9; 2017,Jul,3; 2017,Jan,8; 2016,Jul,6; 2016,Jan,13; 2015,Jan,16

35001-35152 Repair Aneurysm, False Aneurysm, Related Arterial Disease

INCLUDES Endarterectomy procedures

EXCLUDES *Endovascular repairs:*
Abdominal aortic aneurysm (34701-34716 [34717, 34718, 34812, 34820, 34833, 34834])
Thoracic aortic aneurysm (33858-33859, 33863-33875)
Intracranial aneurysms (61697-61710)
Repairs related to occlusive disease only (35201-35286)

35001 **Direct repair of aneurysm, pseudoaneurysm, or excision (partial or total) and graft insertion, with or without patch graft; for aneurysm and associated occlusive disease, carotid, subclavian artery, by neck incision**

32.6 32.6 **FUD** 090 C 80 50

AMA: 2002,May,7; 2000,Dec,1

35002 **for ruptured aneurysm, carotid, subclavian artery, by neck incision**

33.0 33.0 **FUD** 090 C 80 50

AMA: 2002,May,7; 1997,Nov,1

35005 **for aneurysm, pseudoaneurysm, and associated occlusive disease, vertebral artery**

28.6 28.6 **FUD** 090 C 80 50

AMA: 2002,May,7; 1997,Nov,1

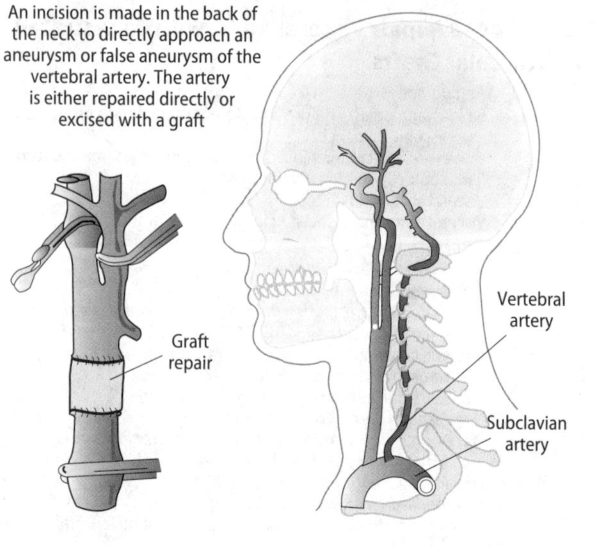
An incision is made in the back of the neck to directly approach an aneurysm or false aneurysm of the vertebral artery. The artery is either repaired directly or excised with a graft
Graft repair
Vertebral artery
Subclavian artery

35011 **for aneurysm and associated occlusive disease, axillary-brachial artery, by arm incision**

29.0 29.0 **FUD** 090 T 80 50

AMA: 2002,May,7; 1997,Nov,1

35013 **for ruptured aneurysm, axillary-brachial artery, by arm incision**

36.6 36.6 **FUD** 090 C 80 50

AMA: 2002,May,7; 1997,Nov,1

35021 **for aneurysm, pseudoaneurysm, and associated occlusive disease, innominate, subclavian artery, by thoracic incision**

36.4 36.4 **FUD** 090 C 80 50

AMA: 2002,May,7; 1997,Nov,1

35022 **for ruptured aneurysm, innominate, subclavian artery, by thoracic incision**

40.6 40.6 **FUD** 090 C 80 50

AMA: 2002,May,7; 1997,Nov,1

35045 **for aneurysm, pseudoaneurysm, and associated occlusive disease, radial or ulnar artery**

28.4 28.4 **FUD** 090 T 80 50

AMA: 2002,May,7; 1997,Nov,1

35081 **for aneurysm, pseudoaneurysm, and associated occlusive disease, abdominal aorta**

50.3 50.3 **FUD** 090 C 80

AMA: 2018,Jan,8; 2017,Jan,8; 2016,Jan,13; 2015,Jan,16

35082 **for ruptured aneurysm, abdominal aorta**

63.4 63.4 **FUD** 090 C 80

AMA: 2002,May,7; 1997,Nov,1

35091 **for aneurysm, pseudoaneurysm, and associated occlusive disease, abdominal aorta involving visceral vessels (mesenteric, celiac, renal)**

52.0 52.0 **FUD** 090 C 80 50

AMA: 2018,Jan,8; 2017,Jan,8; 2016,Jan,13; 2015,Jan,16

35092 **for ruptured aneurysm, abdominal aorta involving visceral vessels (mesenteric, celiac, renal)**

75.7 75.7 **FUD** 090 C 80 50

AMA: 2002,May,7; 1997,Nov,1

35102 **for aneurysm, pseudoaneurysm, and associated occlusive disease, abdominal aorta involving iliac vessels (common, hypogastric, external)**
54.6 54.6 FUD 090 C 80 50
AMA: 2018,Jan,8; 2017,Jan,8; 2016,Jan,13; 2015,Jan,16

35103 **for ruptured aneurysm, abdominal aorta involving iliac vessels (common, hypogastric, external)**
65.0 65.0 FUD 090 C 80 50
AMA: 2002,May,7; 1997,Nov,1

35111 **for aneurysm, pseudoaneurysm, and associated occlusive disease, splenic artery**
38.5 38.5 FUD 090 C 80 50
AMA: 2002,May,7; 1997,Nov,1

35112 **for ruptured aneurysm, splenic artery**
47.4 47.4 FUD 090 C 80 50
AMA: 2002,May,7; 1997,Nov,1

35121 **for aneurysm, pseudoaneurysm, and associated occlusive disease, hepatic, celiac, renal, or mesenteric artery**
45.9 45.9 FUD 090 C 80 50
AMA: 2002,May,7; 1997,Nov,1

35122 **for ruptured aneurysm, hepatic, celiac, renal, or mesenteric artery**
54.9 54.9 FUD 090 C 80 50
AMA: 2002,May,7; 1997,Nov,1

35131 **for aneurysm, pseudoaneurysm, and associated occlusive disease, iliac artery (common, hypogastric, external)**
40.0 40.0 FUD 090 C 80 50
AMA: 2018,Jan,8; 2017,Jan,8; 2016,Jan,13; 2015,Jan,16

35132 **for ruptured aneurysm, iliac artery (common, hypogastric, external)**
47.4 47.4 FUD 090 C 80 50
AMA: 2002,May,7; 1997,Nov,1

35141 **for aneurysm, pseudoaneurysm, and associated occlusive disease, common femoral artery (profunda femoris, superficial femoral)**
32.0 32.0 FUD 090 C 80 50
AMA: 2002,May,7; 1997,Nov,1

35142 **for ruptured aneurysm, common femoral artery (profunda femoris, superficial femoral)**
38.6 38.6 FUD 090 C 80 50
AMA: 2002,May,7; 1997,Nov,1

35151 **for aneurysm, pseudoaneurysm, and associated occlusive disease, popliteal artery**
35.9 35.9 FUD 090 C 80 50
AMA: 2002,May,7; 1997,Nov,1

35152 **for ruptured aneurysm, popliteal artery**
40.5 40.5 FUD 090 C 80 50
AMA: 2002,May,7; 1997,Nov,1

35180-35190 Surgical Repair Arteriovenous Fistula

35180 **Repair, congenital arteriovenous fistula; head and neck**
25.4 25.4 FUD 090 T 80
AMA: 2018,Jan,8; 2017,Jan,8; 2016,Jan,13; 2015,Jan,16

35182 **thorax and abdomen**
51.9 51.9 FUD 090 C 80
AMA: 2018,Jan,8; 2017,Jan,8; 2016,Jan,13; 2015,Jan,16

35184 **extremities**
27.9 27.9 FUD 090 T 80
AMA: 2018,Jan,8; 2017,Jan,8; 2016,Jan,13; 2015,Jan,16

35188 **Repair, acquired or traumatic arteriovenous fistula; head and neck**
36.9 36.9 FUD 090 T A2 80
AMA: 2018,Jan,8; 2017,Jan,8; 2016,Jan,13; 2015,Jan,16

35189 **thorax and abdomen**
43.8 43.8 FUD 090 C 80
AMA: 2018,Jan,8; 2017,Jan,8; 2016,Jan,13; 2015,Jan,16

35190 **extremities**
22.0 22.0 FUD 090 T 80
AMA: 2018,Jan,8; 2017,Jan,8; 2016,Jan,13; 2015,Jan,16

35201-35286 Surgical Repair Artery or Vein

EXCLUDES *Arteriovenous fistula repair (35180-35190)*
Primary open vascular procedures

35201 **Repair blood vessel, direct; neck**
EXCLUDES *Removal ECMO/ECLS cannula ([33969, 33984, 33985, 33986])*
27.3 27.3 FUD 090 T 80 50
AMA: 2019,Dec,5; 2018,Jan,8; 2017,Jan,8; 2016,Jan,13; 2015,Jul,3; 2015,Jan,16

35206 **upper extremity**
EXCLUDES *Removal ECMO/ECLS cannula ([33969, 33984, 33985, 33986])*
22.6 22.6 FUD 090 T 80 50
AMA: 2019,Dec,5; 2018,Jan,8; 2017,Jan,8; 2016,Jan,13; 2015,Jul,3; 2015,Jan,16

35207 **hand, finger**
21.7 21.7 FUD 090 T A2 50
AMA: 2019,Dec,5

35211 **intrathoracic, with bypass**
EXCLUDES *Removal ECMO/ECLS cannula ([33969, 33984, 33985, 33986])*
40.0 40.0 FUD 090 C 80 50
AMA: 2015,Jul,3

35216 **intrathoracic, without bypass**
EXCLUDES *Removal ECMO/ECLS cannula ([33969, 33984, 33985, 33986])*
60.0 60.0 FUD 090 C 80 50
AMA: 2018,Jan,8; 2017,Jan,8; 2016,Jan,13; 2015,Jan,16

35221 **intra-abdominal**
42.4 42.4 FUD 090 C 80 50
AMA: 2012,Apr,3-9; 2003,Feb,1

35226 **lower extremity**
EXCLUDES *Removal ECMO/ECLS cannula ([33969, 33984, 33985, 33986])*
24.1 24.1 FUD 090 T 80 50
AMA: 2019,Jul,10; 2018,Jan,8; 2017,Aug,10; 2017,Jul,3; 2017,Jan,8; 2016,Jul,6; 2016,Jan,13; 2015,Jul,3; 2015,Jan,16

35231 **Repair blood vessel with vein graft; neck**
36.3 36.3 FUD 090 T 80 50
AMA: 2019,Dec,5

35236 **upper extremity**
29.1 29.1 FUD 090 T 80 50
AMA: 2019,Dec,5; 2018,Jan,8; 2017,Jan,8; 2016,Jan,13; 2015,Jan,16

35241 **intrathoracic, with bypass**
41.5 41.5 FUD 090 C 80 50
AMA: 2012,Apr,3-9; 2003,Feb,1

35246 **intrathoracic, without bypass**
45.2 45.2 FUD 090 C 80 50
AMA: 2012,Apr,3-9; 2003,Feb,1

35251 **intra-abdominal**
50.7 50.7 FUD 090 C 80 50
AMA: 2012,Apr,3-9; 2003,Feb,1

35256 **lower extremity**
29.7 29.7 FUD 090 T 80 50
AMA: 2019,Dec,5

35261 **Repair blood vessel with graft other than vein; neck**
28.4 28.4 FUD 090 T 80 50
AMA: 2019,Dec,5

35266 **upper extremity**
25.1 25.1 FUD 090 T 80 50
AMA: 2019,Dec,5; 2018,Jan,8; 2017,Jan,8; 2016,Jan,13; 2015,Jan,16

35271 **intrathoracic, with bypass**
39.9 39.9 **FUD** 090 C 80 50
AMA: 2012,Apr,3-9; 2003,Feb,1

35276 **intrathoracic, without bypass**
42.1 42.1 **FUD** 090 C 80 50
AMA: 2012,Apr,3-9; 2003,Feb,1

35281 **intra-abdominal**
47.3 47.3 **FUD** 090 C 80 50
AMA: 2012,Apr,3-9; 2003,Feb,1

35286 **lower extremity**
27.1 27.1 **FUD** 090 T 80 50
AMA: 2019,Dec,5; 2019,Jul,10; 2018,Jan,8; 2017,Aug,10; 2017,Jul,3; 2017,Jan,8; 2016,Jul,6; 2016,Jan,13; 2015,Jan,16

35301-35372 Surgical Thromboendarterectomy Peripheral and Visceral Arteries

INCLUDES Obtaining saphenous or arm vein for graft
Thrombectomy/embolectomy

EXCLUDES *Coronary artery bypass procedures (33510-33536, 33572)*
Thromboendarterectomy for vascular occlusion on different vessel during same session

35301 **Thromboendarterectomy, including patch graft, if performed; carotid, vertebral, subclavian, by neck incision**
32.7 32.7 **FUD** 090 C 80 50
AMA: 2018,Jan,8; 2017,Jan,8; 2016,Jan,13; 2015,Jan,16

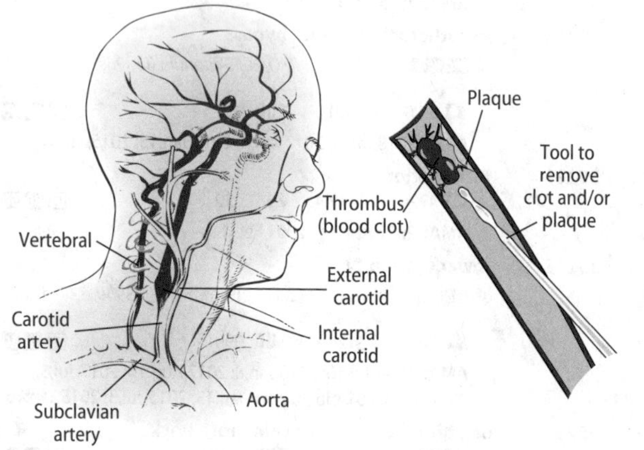

35302 **superficial femoral artery**
EXCLUDES *Revascularization, endovascular, open or percutaneous, femoral, popliteal artery(s) (37225, 37227)*
32.6 32.6 **FUD** 090 C 80 50
AMA: 2018,Jan,8; 2017,Jan,8; 2016,Jan,13; 2015,Jan,16

35303 **popliteal artery**
EXCLUDES *Revascularization, endovascular, open or percutaneous, femoral, popliteal artery(s) (37225, 37227)*
36.0 36.0 **FUD** 090 C 80 50
AMA: 2018,Jan,8; 2017,Jan,8; 2016,Jan,13; 2015,Jan,16

35304 **tibioperoneal trunk artery**
EXCLUDES *Revascularization, endovascular, open or percutaneous, tibial/peroneal artery (37229, 37231, 37233, 37235)*
37.0 37.0 **FUD** 090 C 80 50
AMA: 2018,Jan,8; 2017,Jan,8; 2016,Jan,13; 2015,Jan,16

35305 **tibial or peroneal artery, initial vessel**
EXCLUDES *Revascularization, endovascular, open or percutaneous, tibial/peroneal artery (37229, 37231, 37233, 37235)*
35.6 35.6 **FUD** 090 C 80 50
AMA: 2018,Jan,8; 2017,Jan,8; 2016,Jan,13; 2015,Jan,16

\+ **35306** **each additional tibial or peroneal artery (List separately in addition to code for primary procedure)**
EXCLUDES *Revascularization, endovascular, open or percutaneous, tibial/peroneal artery (37229, 37231, 37233, 37235)*
Code first (35305)
12.9 12.9 **FUD** ZZZ C 80
AMA: 2018,Jan,8; 2017,Jan,8; 2016,Jan,13; 2015,Jan,16

35311 **subclavian, innominate, by thoracic incision**
45.1 45.1 **FUD** 090 C 80 50
AMA: 1997,Nov,1

35321 **axillary-brachial**
25.9 25.9 **FUD** 090 T 80 50
AMA: 1997,Nov,1

35331 **abdominal aorta**
42.3 42.3 **FUD** 090 C 80 50
AMA: 1997,Nov,1

35341 **mesenteric, celiac, or renal**
39.9 39.9 **FUD** 090 C 80 50
AMA: 1997,Nov,1

35351 **iliac**
37.3 37.3 **FUD** 090 C 80 50
AMA: 1997,Nov,1

35355 **iliofemoral**
29.9 29.9 **FUD** 090 C 80 50
AMA: 1997,Nov,1

35361 **combined aortoiliac**
44.2 44.2 **FUD** 090 C 80 50
AMA: 1997,Nov,1

35363 **combined aortoiliofemoral**
47.1 47.1 **FUD** 090 C 80 50
AMA: 1997,Nov,1

35371 **common femoral**
23.7 23.7 **FUD** 090 C 80 50
AMA: 2018,Jan,8; 2017,Aug,10; 2017,Jul,3; 2017,Jan,8; 2016,Jan,13; 2015,Jan,16

35372 **deep (profunda) femoral**
28.4 28.4 **FUD** 090 C 80 50
AMA: 2018,Jan,8; 2017,Jan,8; 2016,Jan,13; 2015,Jan,16

35390 Surgical Thromboendarterectomy: Carotid Reoperation

Code first (35301)

\+ **35390** **Reoperation, carotid, thromboendarterectomy, more than 1 month after original operation (List separately in addition to code for primary procedure)**
4.65 4.65 **FUD** ZZZ C 80
AMA: 1997,Nov,1; 1993,Win,1

35400 Endoscopic Visualization of Vessels

Code first therapeutic intervention

\+ **35400** **Angioscopy (noncoronary vessels or grafts) during therapeutic intervention (List separately in addition to code for primary procedure)**
4.32 4.32 **FUD** ZZZ C 80
AMA: 1997,Dec,1; 1997,Nov,1

35500 Obtain Arm Vein for Graft

EXCLUDES *Endoscopic harvest (33508)*
Harvesting multiple vein segments (35682, 35683)

Code first (33510-33536, 35556, 35566, 35570-35571, 35583-35587)

\+ **35500** **Harvest of upper extremity vein, 1 segment, for lower extremity or coronary artery bypass procedure (List separately in addition to code for primary procedure)**
9.29 9.29 **FUD** ZZZ N 80
AMA: 2018,Jan,8; 2017,Jan,8; 2016,Jan,13; 2015,Jan,16

35501-35571 Arterial Bypass Using Vein Grafts

INCLUDES Obtaining saphenous vein grafts

EXCLUDES *Obtaining multiple vein segments (35682, 35683)*
Obtaining vein grafts, upper extremity or femoropopliteal (35500, 35572)
Treatment different sites with different bypass procedures during same operative session

35501 **Bypass graft, with vein; common carotid-ipsilateral internal carotid**
42.4 42.4 **FUD** 090 C 80 50
AMA: 2018,Jan,8; 2017,Jan,8; 2016,Jan,13; 2015,Jan,16

35506 **carotid-subclavian or subclavian-carotid**
37.0 37.0 **FUD** 090 C 80 50
AMA: 2018,Jan,8; 2017,Jan,8; 2016,Jan,13; 2015,Jan,16

35508 **carotid-vertebral**
INCLUDES Endoscopic procedure
38.5 38.5 **FUD** 090 C 80 50
AMA: 1999,Mar,6; 1999,Apr,11

35509 **carotid-contralateral carotid**
40.8 40.8 **FUD** 090 C 80 50
AMA: 2018,Jan,8; 2017,Jan,8; 2016,Jan,13; 2015,Jan,16

35510 **carotid-brachial**
35.7 35.7 **FUD** 090 C 80 50
AMA: 2018,Jan,8; 2017,Jan,8; 2016,Jan,13; 2015,Jan,16

35511 **subclavian-subclavian**
32.5 32.5 **FUD** 090 C 80 50
AMA: 2018,Jan,8; 2017,Jan,8; 2016,Jan,13; 2015,Jan,16

35512 **subclavian-brachial**
35.0 35.0 **FUD** 090 C 80 50
AMA: 2018,Jan,8; 2017,Jan,8; 2016,Jan,13; 2015,Jan,16

35515 **subclavian-vertebral**
38.5 38.5 **FUD** 090 C 80 50
AMA: 1999,Mar,6; 1999,Apr,11

35516 **subclavian-axillary**
35.4 35.4 **FUD** 090 C 80 50
AMA: 1999,Mar,6; 1999,Apr,11

35518 **axillary-axillary**
33.1 33.1 **FUD** 090 C 80 50
AMA: 2018,Jan,8; 2017,Jan,8; 2016,Jan,13; 2015,Jan,16

35521 **axillary-femoral**
EXCLUDES *Synthetic graft (35621)*
35.6 35.6 **FUD** 090 C 80 50
AMA: 2018,Jan,8; 2017,Jan,8; 2016,Jan,13; 2015,Jan,16

35522 **axillary-brachial**
35.3 35.3 **FUD** 090 C 80 50
AMA: 2018,Jan,8; 2017,Jan,8; 2016,Jan,13; 2015,Jan,16

35523 **brachial-ulnar or -radial**
EXCLUDES *Bypass graft using synthetic conduit (37799)*
Bypass graft, with vein; brachial-brachial (35525)
Distal revascularization and interval ligation (DRIL), upper extremity hemodialysis access (steal syndrome) (36838)
Harvest upper extremity vein, 1 segment, for lower extremity or coronary artery bypass procedure (35500)
Repair blood vessel, direct; upper extremity (35206)
37.1 37.1 **FUD** 090 C 80 50

35525 **brachial-brachial**
33.0 33.0 **FUD** 090 C 80 50
AMA: 2018,Jan,8; 2017,Jan,8; 2016,Jan,13; 2015,Jan,16

35526 **aortosubclavian, aortoinnominate, or aortocarotid**
EXCLUDES *Synthetic graft (35626)*
50.1 50.1 **FUD** 090 C 80 50
AMA: 1999,Mar,6; 1999,Apr,11

35531 **aortoceliac or aortomesenteric**
56.6 56.6 **FUD** 090 C 80 50
AMA: 1999,Mar,6; 1999,Apr,11

35533 **axillary-femoral-femoral**
EXCLUDES *Synthetic graft (35654)*
43.7 43.7 **FUD** 090 C 80 50
AMA: 2012,Apr,3-9; 1999,Mar,6

35535 **hepatorenal**
EXCLUDES *Bypass graft (35536, 35560, 35631, 35636)*
Harvest upper extremity vein, 1 segment, for lower extremity or coronary artery bypass procedure (35500)
Repair blood vessel (35221, 35251, 35281)
55.3 55.3 **FUD** 090 C 80 50

35536 **splenorenal**
49.1 49.1 **FUD** 090 C 80 50
AMA: 2018,Jan,8; 2017,Jan,8; 2016,Jan,13; 2015,Jan,16

35537 **aortoiliac**
EXCLUDES *Bypass graft, with vein; aortobi-iliac (35538)*
Synthetic graft (35637)
60.6 60.6 **FUD** 090 C 80
AMA: 2018,Jan,8; 2017,Jan,8; 2016,Jan,13; 2015,Jan,16

35538 **aortobi-iliac**
EXCLUDES *Bypass graft, with vein; aortoiliac (35537)*
Synthetic graft (35638)
67.9 67.9 **FUD** 090 C 80
AMA: 2018,Jan,8; 2017,Jan,8; 2016,Jan,13; 2015,Jan,16

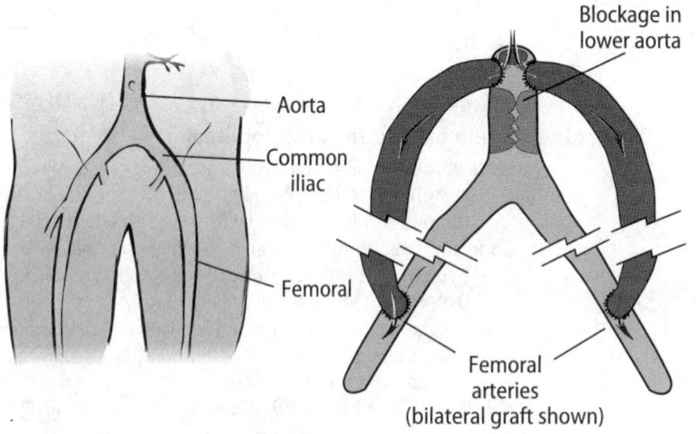

35539 **aortofemoral**
EXCLUDES *Bypass graft, with vein; aortobifemoral (35540)*
Synthetic graft (35647)
63.7 63.7 **FUD** 090 C 80 50
AMA: 2018,Jan,8; 2017,Jan,8; 2016,Jan,13; 2015,Jan,16

35540 **aortobifemoral**
EXCLUDES *Bypass graft, with vein; aortofemoral (35539)*
Synthetic graft (35646)
70.6 70.6 **FUD** 090 C 50
AMA: 2018,Jan,8; 2017,Jan,8; 2016,Jan,13; 2015,Jan,16

35556 **femoral-popliteal**
40.7 40.7 **FUD** 090 C 80 50
AMA: 2018,Jan,8; 2017,Jan,8; 2016,Jan,13; 2015,Jan,16

35558 **femoral-femoral**
35.7 35.7 **FUD** 090 C 80 50
AMA: 2012,Apr,3-9; 1999,Mar,6

35560 **aortorenal**
49.2 49.2 **FUD** 090 C 80 50
AMA: 2018,Jan,8; 2017,Jan,8; 2016,Jan,13; 2015,Jan,16

35563 **ilioiliac**
38.4 38.4 **FUD** 090 C 80 50
AMA: 1999,Mar,6; 1999,Apr,11

35565 **iliofemoral**
38.1 38.1 **FUD** 090 C 80 50
AMA: 2012,Apr,3-9; 2004,Oct,6

35566 **femoral-anterior tibial, posterior tibial, peroneal artery or other distal vessels**
48.6 48.6 **FUD** 090 C 80 50
AMA: 2018,Jan,8; 2017,Jan,8; 2016,Jan,13; 2015,Jan,16

35570 **tibial-tibial, peroneal-tibial, or tibial/peroneal trunk-tibial**
EXCLUDES *Repair blood vessel with graft (35256, 35286)*
42.8 42.8 **FUD** 090 C 80 50
AMA: 2018,Jan,8; 2017,Jan,8; 2016,Jan,13; 2015,Jan,16

35571 **popliteal-tibial, -peroneal artery or other distal vessels**
38.5 38.5 **FUD** 090 C 80 50
AMA: 2018,Jan,8; 2017,Jan,8; 2016,Jan,13; 2015,Jan,16

35572 Obtain Femoropopliteal Vein for Graft

EXCLUDES *Reporting with modifier 50. Report once for each side when performed bilaterally*
Code first (33510-33523, 33533-33536, 34502, 34520, 35001-35002, 35011-35022, 35102-35103, 35121-35152, 35231-35256, 35501-35587, 35879-35907)

\+ **35572** **Harvest of femoropopliteal vein, 1 segment, for vascular reconstruction procedure (eg, aortic, vena caval, coronary, peripheral artery) (List separately in addition to code for primary procedure)**
10.0 10.0 **FUD** ZZZ N N1 80
AMA: 2018,Jan,8; 2017,Jan,8; 2016,Jan,13; 2015,Jan,16

35583-35587 Lower Extremity Revascularization: In-situ Vein Bypass

INCLUDES Obtaining saphenous vein grafts
EXCLUDES *Obtaining multiple vein segments (35682, 35683)*
Obtaining vein graft, upper extremity or femoropopliteal (35500, 35572)

35583 **In-situ vein bypass; femoral-popliteal**
Code also aortobifemoral bypass graft other than vein for aortobifemoral bypass using synthetic conduit and femoral-popliteal bypass with vein conduit in situ (35646)
Code also concurrent aortofemoral bypass for aortofemoral bypass graft with synthetic conduit and femoral-popliteal bypass with vein conduit in-situ (35647)
Code also concurrent aortofemoral bypass (vein) for aortofemoral bypass using vein conduit or femoral-popliteal bypass with vein conduit in-situ (35539)
41.8 41.8 **FUD** 090 C 80 50
AMA: 2018,Jan,8; 2017,Jan,8; 2016,Jan,13; 2015,Jan,16

35585 **femoral-anterior tibial, posterior tibial, or peroneal artery**
48.6 48.6 **FUD** 090 C 80 50
AMA: 2018,Jan,8; 2017,Jan,8; 2016,Jan,13; 2015,Jan,16

35587 **popliteal-tibial, peroneal**
39.6 39.6 **FUD** 090 C 80 50
AMA: 2018,Jan,8; 2017,Jan,8; 2016,Jan,13; 2015,Jan,16

35600 Obtain Arm Artery for Coronary Bypass

EXCLUDES *Transposition and/or reimplantation arteries (35691-35695)*
Code first (33533-33536)

\+ **35600** **Harvest of upper extremity artery, 1 segment, for coronary artery bypass procedure (List separately in addition to code for primary procedure)**
7.43 7.43 **FUD** ZZZ C 80
AMA: 2018,Jan,8; 2017,Jan,8; 2016,Jan,13; 2015,Jan,16

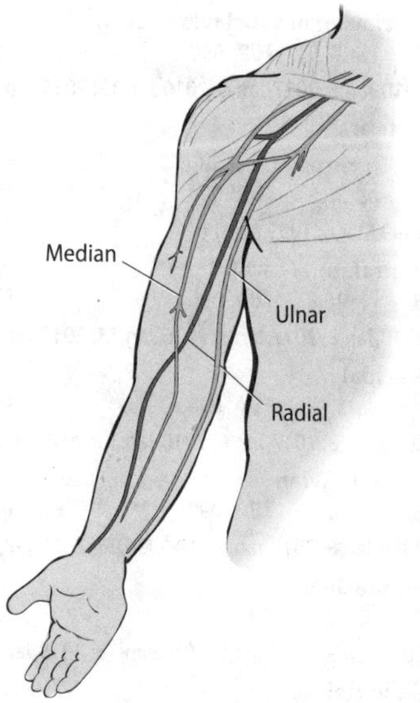

An upper extremity artery or segment is harvested for a coronary artery bypass procedure

35601-35671 Arterial Bypass: Grafts Other Than Veins

EXCLUDES *Transposition and/or reimplantation arteries (35691-35695)*

35601 **Bypass graft, with other than vein; common carotid-ipsilateral internal carotid**
EXCLUDES *Open transcervical common carotid-common carotid bypass with endovascular repair descending thoracic aorta (33891)*
40.4 40.4 **FUD** 090 C 80 50
AMA: 2018,Jan,8; 2017,Jan,8; 2016,Jan,13; 2015,Jan,16

35606 **carotid-subclavian**
EXCLUDES *Open subclavian to carotid artery transposition performed with endovascular thoracic aneurysm repair via neck incision (33889)*
34.0 34.0 **FUD** 090 C 80 50
AMA: 1997,Nov,1

35612 **subclavian-subclavian**
30.3 30.3 **FUD** 090 C 80 50
AMA: 1997,Nov,1

35616 **subclavian-axillary**
32.0 32.0 **FUD** 090 C 80 50
AMA: 1997,Nov,1

35621 **axillary-femoral**
31.8 31.8 **FUD** 090 C 80 50
AMA: 2018,Jan,8; 2017,Jan,8; 2016,Jan,13; 2015,Jan,16

35623 **axillary-popliteal or -tibial**
38.1 38.1 **FUD** 090 C 80 50
AMA: 2012,Apr,3-9; 1997,Nov,1

35626 **aortosubclavian, aortoinnominate, or aortocarotid**
46.1 46.1 **FUD** 090 C 80 50
AMA: 1997,Nov,1

35631 aortoceliac, aortomesenteric, aortorenal
53.8 53.8 FUD 090 C 80 50
AMA: 1997,Nov,1

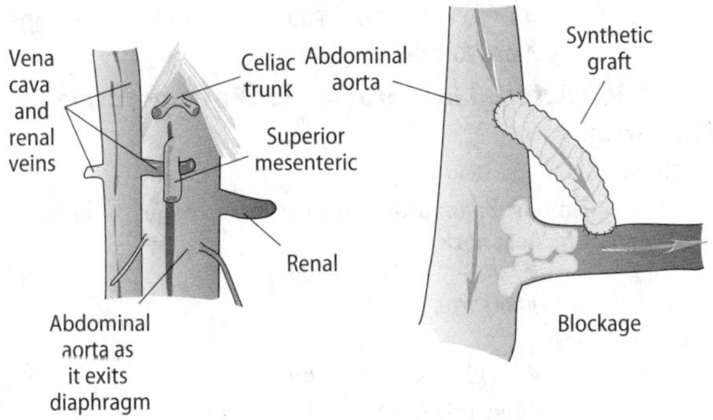

35632 ilio-celiac
EXCLUDES *Bypass graft (35531, 35631)*
Repair blood vessel (35221, 35251, 35281)
52.5 52.5 FUD 090 C 80 50

35633 ilio-mesenteric
EXCLUDES *Bypass graft (35531, 35631)*
Repair blood vessel (35221, 35251, 35281)
57.6 57.6 FUD 090 C 80 50

35634 iliorenal
EXCLUDES *Bypass graft (35536, 35560, 35631)*
Repair blood vessel (35221, 35251, 35281)
51.4 51.4 FUD 090 C 80 50

35636 splenorenal (splenic to renal arterial anastomosis)
46.0 46.0 FUD 090 C 80 50
AMA: 1997,Nov,1; 1994,Win,1

35637 aortoiliac
EXCLUDES *Bypass graft (35638, 35646)*
47.9 47.9 FUD 090 C 80
AMA: 2018,Jan,8; 2017,Jan,8; 2016,Jan,13; 2015,Jan,16

35638 aortobi-iliac
EXCLUDES *Bypass graft (35637, 35646)*
Open placement aorto-bi-iliac prosthesis after failed endovascular repair (34831)
50.7 50.7 FUD 090 C 80
AMA: 2018,Jan,8; 2017,Jan,8; 2016,Jan,13; 2015,Jan,16

35642 carotid-vertebral
28.6 28.6 FUD 090 C 80 50
AMA: 1997,Nov,1

35645 subclavian-vertebral
27.4 27.4 FUD 090 C 80 50
AMA: 1997,Nov,1

35646 aortobifemoral
EXCLUDES *Bypass graft using vein graft (35540)*
Open placement aorto-bi-iliac prosthesis after failed endovascular repair (34831)
49.7 49.7 FUD 090 C 80
AMA: 2018,Jan,8; 2017,Jan,8; 2016,Jan,13; 2015,Jan,16

35647 aortofemoral
EXCLUDES *Bypass graft using vein graft (35539)*
44.9 44.9 FUD 090 C 80 50
AMA: 2018,Jan,8; 2017,Jan,8; 2016,Jan,13; 2015,Jan,16

35650 axillary-axillary
29.6 29.6 FUD 090 C 80 50
AMA: 1997,Nov,1

35654 axillary-femoral-femoral
39.8 39.8 FUD 090 C 80
AMA: 2018,Jan,8; 2017,Jan,8; 2016,Jan,13; 2015,Jan,16

35656 femoral-popliteal
31.4 31.4 FUD 090 C 80 50
AMA: 2018,Jan,8; 2017,Jan,8; 2016,Jan,13; 2015,Jan,16

35661 femoral-femoral
31.5 31.5 FUD 090 C 80 50
AMA: 2018,Jan,8; 2017,Jan,8; 2016,Jan,13; 2015,Jan,16

35663 ilioiliac
35.3 35.3 FUD 090 C 80 50
AMA: 1997,Nov,1

35665 iliofemoral
34.1 34.1 FUD 090 C 80 50
AMA: 2018,Jan,8; 2017,Jan,8; 2016,Jan,13; 2015,Jan,16

35666 femoral-anterior tibial, posterior tibial, or peroneal artery
37.0 37.0 FUD 090 C 80 50
AMA: 2018,Jan,8; 2017,Jan,8; 2016,Jan,13; 2015,Jan,16

35671 popliteal-tibial or peroneal artery
32.6 32.6 FUD 090 C 80 50
AMA: 2012,Apr,3-9; 1997,Nov,1

35681-35683 Arterial Bypass Using Combination Synthetic and Donor Graft

INCLUDES Acquiring multiple vein segments from sites other than extremity for which arterial bypass performed
Anastomosis vein segments to create bypass graft conduits

\+ **35681 Bypass graft; composite, prosthetic and vein (List separately in addition to code for primary procedure)**
EXCLUDES *Bypass graft (35682, 35683)*
Code first primary procedure
2.36 2.36 FUD ZZZ C 80
AMA: 2018,Jan,8; 2017,Jan,8; 2016,Jan,13; 2015,Jan,16

\+ **35682 autogenous composite, 2 segments of veins from 2 locations (List separately in addition to code for primary procedure)**
EXCLUDES *Bypass graft (35681, 35683)*
Code first (35556, 35566, 35570-35571, 35583-35587)
10.2 10.2 FUD ZZZ C 80
AMA: 2018,Jan,8; 2017,Jan,8; 2016,Jan,13; 2015,Jan,16

\+ **35683 autogenous composite, 3 or more segments of vein from 2 or more locations (List separately in addition to code for primary procedure)**
EXCLUDES *Bypass graft (35681-35682)*
Code first (35556, 35566, 35570-35571, 35583-35587)
11.8 11.8 FUD ZZZ C 80
AMA: 2018,Jan,8; 2017,Jan,8; 2016,Jan,13; 2015,Jan,16

35685-35686 Supplemental Procedures

INCLUDES Additional procedures needed with bypass graft to increase graft patency
EXCLUDES *Composite grafts (35681-35683)*

\+ **35685 Placement of vein patch or cuff at distal anastomosis of bypass graft, synthetic conduit (List separately in addition to code for primary procedure)**
INCLUDES Connection vein segment (cuff or patch) between distal portion synthetic graft and native artery
Code first (35656, 35666, 35671)
5.78 5.78 FUD ZZZ N 80
AMA: 2018,Jan,8; 2017,Jan,8; 2016,Jan,13; 2015,Jan,16

\+ **35686 Creation of distal arteriovenous fistula during lower extremity bypass surgery (non-hemodialysis) (List separately in addition to code for primary procedure)**
INCLUDES Creation fistula between peroneal or tibial artery and vein at or past distal anastomosis site
Code first (35556, 35566, 35570-35571, 35583-35587, 35623, 35656, 35666, 35671)
4.68 4.68 FUD ZZZ N 80
AMA: 2018,Jan,8; 2017,Jan,8; 2016,Jan,13; 2015,Jan,16

35691-35697 Arterial Translocation

CMS: 100-03,160.8 Electroencephalographic Monitoring During Cerebral Vasculature Surgery

35691 **Transposition and/or reimplantation; vertebral to carotid artery**

Facility RVU 27.2 Non-Facility RVU 27.2 **FUD** 090 C 80 50

AMA: 1997,Nov,1; 1993,Win,1

35693 **vertebral to subclavian artery**

Facility RVU 24.0 Non-Facility RVU 24.0 **FUD** 090 C 80 50

AMA: 1997,Nov,1; 1994,Sum,29

35694 **subclavian to carotid artery**

EXCLUDES *Subclavian to carotid artery transposition procedure (open) with concurrent repair descending thoracic aorta (endovascular) (33889)*

Facility RVU 28.5 Non-Facility RVU 28.5 **FUD** 090 C 80 50

AMA: 1997,Nov,1; 1993,Win,1

35695 **carotid to subclavian artery**

Facility RVU 29.7 Non-Facility RVU 29.7 **FUD** 090 C 80 50

AMA: 1997,Nov,1; 1993,Win,1

\+ **35697** **Reimplantation, visceral artery to infrarenal aortic prosthesis, each artery (List separately in addition to code for primary procedure)**

EXCLUDES *Repair thoracoabdominal aortic aneurysm with graft (33877)*

Code first primary procedure

Facility RVU 4.29 Non-Facility RVU 4.29 **FUD** ZZZ C 80

AMA: 1997,Nov,1

35700 Reoperative Bypass Lower Extremities

Code first (35556, 35566, 35570-35571, 35583, 35585, 35587, 35656, 35666, 35671)

\+ **35700** **Reoperation, femoral-popliteal or femoral (popliteal)-anterior tibial, posterior tibial, peroneal artery, or other distal vessels, more than 1 month after original operation (List separately in addition to code for primary procedure)**

Facility RVU 4.44 Non-Facility RVU 4.44 **FUD** ZZZ C 80

AMA: 2018,Jan,8; 2017,Jan,8; 2016,Jan,13; 2015,Jan,16

35701-35703 Arterial Exploration without Repair

EXCLUDES *Exploration to identify recipient artery for microvascular free graft/flap anastomosis:*
Bone (20955-20962)
Jejunum (43496)
Muscle, skin or fascia (15756-15758)
Omentum (49906)
Osteocutaneous (20969-20973)
Exploration without surgical repair:
Abdominal artery (49000)
Chest artery (32100)
Other arteries not in neck, upper or lower extremities, chest, abdomen, or retroperitoneum (37799)
Retroperitoneal artery (49010)

Code also nonvascular surgical procedures performed in addition to exploration when exploration through separate incision

35701 **Exploration not followed by surgical repair, artery; neck (eg, carotid, subclavian)**

EXCLUDES *Exploration for postoperative hemorrhage, thrombosis or infection (35800)*
Repair blood vessel on same side neck (35201, 35231, 35261)

Facility RVU 12.6 Non-Facility RVU 12.6 **FUD** 090 C 80 50

AMA: 2019,Dec,5

35702 **upper extremity (eg, axillary, brachial, radial, ulnar)**

EXCLUDES *Exploration for postoperative hemorrhage, thrombosis or infection in same extremity (35860)*
Repair blood vessel in same extremity (35206-35207, 35236, 35266)

Facility RVU 11.9 Non-Facility RVU 11.9 **FUD** 090 80 50

AMA: 2019,Dec,5

35703 **lower extremity (eg, common femoral, deep femoral, superficial femoral, popliteal, tibial, peroneal)**

EXCLUDES *Exploration for postoperative hemorrhage, thrombosis or infection in same extremity (35860)*
Repair blood vessel in same extremity (35256, 35286)

Facility RVU 12.0 Non-Facility RVU 12.0 **FUD** 090 80 50

AMA: 2019,Dec,5

35800-35860 Arterial Exploration for Postoperative Complication

INCLUDES Return to operating room for postoperative hemorrhage

35800 **Exploration for postoperative hemorrhage, thrombosis or infection; neck**

Facility RVU 20.8 Non-Facility RVU 20.8 **FUD** 090 C 80

AMA: 2019,Dec,5

35820 **chest**

Facility RVU 58.2 Non-Facility RVU 58.2 **FUD** 090 C 80

AMA: 1997,Nov,1

35840 **abdomen**

Facility RVU 34.8 Non-Facility RVU 34.8 **FUD** 090 C 80

AMA: 1997,May,4; 1997,Nov,1

35860 **extremity**

Facility RVU 24.2 Non-Facility RVU 24.2 **FUD** 090 T 80

AMA: 2019,Dec,5; 2018,Jan,8; 2017,Jan,8; 2016,Jan,13; 2015,Jan,16

35870 Repair Secondary Aortoenteric Fistula

35870 **Repair of graft-enteric fistula**

Facility RVU 36.1 Non-Facility RVU 36.1 **FUD** 090 C 80

AMA: 1997,Nov,1

35875-35876 Removal of Thrombus from Graft

EXCLUDES *Thrombectomy dialysis fistula or graft (36831, 36833)*
Thrombectomy with blood vessel repair, lower extremity, vein graft (35256)
Thrombectomy with blood vessel repair, lower extremity, with/without patch angioplasty (35226)

35875 **Thrombectomy of arterial or venous graft (other than hemodialysis graft or fistula);**

Facility RVU 17.3 Non-Facility RVU 17.3 **FUD** 090 T A2

AMA: 2018,Jan,8; 2017,Jan,8; 2016,Jan,13; 2015,Jan,16

35876 **with revision of arterial or venous graft**

Facility RVU 27.5 Non-Facility RVU 27.5 **FUD** 090 T A2 80

AMA: 1999,Mar,6; 1999,Nov,1

35879-35884 Revision Lower Extremity Bypass Graft

EXCLUDES *Removal infected graft (35901-35907)*
Revascularization following removal infected graft(s)
Thrombectomy dialysis fistula or graft (36831, 36833)
Thrombectomy with blood vessel repair, lower extremity, vein graft (35256)
Thrombectomy with blood vessel repair, lower extremity, with/without patch angioplasty (35226)
Thrombectomy with graft revision (35876)

35879 **Revision, lower extremity arterial bypass, without thrombectomy, open; with vein patch angioplasty**

Facility RVU 26.8 Non-Facility RVU 26.8 **FUD** 090 T 80 50

AMA: 2018,Jan,8; 2017,Jan,8; 2016,Jan,13; 2015,Jan,16

35881 **with segmental vein interposition**

EXCLUDES *Revision femoral anastomosis synthetic arterial bypass graft (35883-35884)*

Facility RVU 29.6 Non-Facility RVU 29.6 **FUD** 090 T 80 50

AMA: 2018,Jan,8; 2017,Jan,8; 2016,Jan,13; 2015,Jan,16

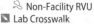

35883 **Revision, femoral anastomosis of synthetic arterial bypass graft in groin, open; with nonautogenous patch graft (eg, Dacron, ePTFE, bovine pericardium)**

EXCLUDES *Reoperation, femoral-popliteal or femoral (popliteal)-anterior tibial, posterior tibial, peroneal artery, or other distal vessels (35700)*
Revision, femoral anastomosis synthetic arterial bypass graft in groin, open; with autogenous vein patch graft (35884)
Thrombectomy arterial or venous graft (35875)

34.8 34.8 **FUD** 090 T 80 50

AMA: 2018,Jan,8; 2017,Jan,8; 2016,Jan,13; 2015,Jan,16

35884 **with autogenous vein patch graft**

EXCLUDES *Reoperation, femoral-popliteal or femoral (popliteal)-anterior tibial, posterior tibial, peroneal artery, or other distal vessels (35700)*
Revision, femoral anastomosis synthetic arterial bypass graft in groin, open; with autogenous vein patch graft (35883)
Thrombectomy arterial or venous graft (35875-35876)

36.0 36.0 **FUD** 090 T 80 50

AMA: 2018,Jan,8; 2017,Jan,8; 2016,Jan,13; 2015,Jan,16

35901-35907 Removal of Infected Graft

35901 **Excision of infected graft; neck**

13.6 13.6 **FUD** 090 C 80

AMA: 1997,Nov,1; 1993,Win,1

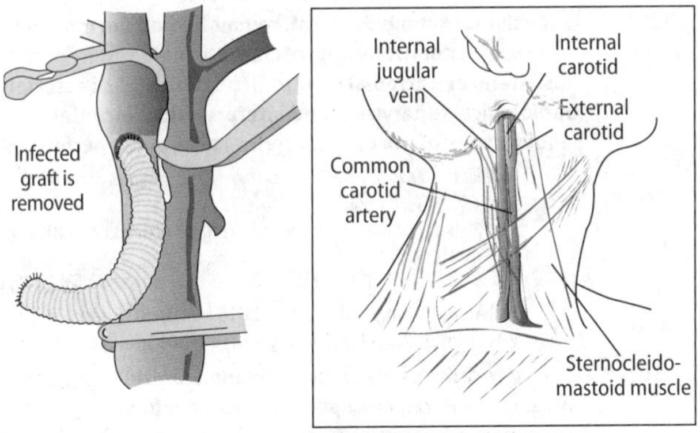

The physician removes an infected graft from the neck and repairs the blood vessel. If a new graft is placed, report the appropriate revascularization code

35903 **extremity**

16.4 16.4 **FUD** 090 T 80

AMA: 2018,Aug,10

35905 **thorax**

51.4 51.4 **FUD** 090 C 80

AMA: 1997,Nov,1; 1993,Win,1

35907 **abdomen**

55.3 55.3 **FUD** 090 C 80

AMA: 1997,Nov,1; 1993,Win,1

36000 Intravenous Access Established

INCLUDES Venous access for phlebotomy, prophylactic intravenous access, infusion therapy, chemotherapy, hydration, transfusion, drug administration, etc., included in primary procedure work value

36000 **Introduction of needle or intracatheter, vein**

0.26 0.79 **FUD** XXX N N1

AMA: 2019,Aug,8; 2018,Mar,3; 2018,Jan,8; 2017,Jan,8; 2016,Nov,3; 2016,Jan,13; 2015,Jan,16

36002 Injection Treatment of Pseudoaneurysm

INCLUDES Insertion needle or catheter, local anesthesia, contrast injection, power injections, and all pre- and postinjection care provided

EXCLUDES *Arteriotomy site sealant*
Compression repair pseudoaneurysm, ultrasound guided (76936)
Medications, contrast material, catheters

36002 **Injection procedures (eg, thrombin) for percutaneous treatment of extremity pseudoaneurysm**

(76942, 77002, 77012, 77021)

3.04 4.43 **FUD** 000 T 62 50

AMA: 2018,Mar,3; 2018,Jan,8; 2017,Jan,8; 2016,Nov,3; 2016,Jan,13; 2015,Jan,16

36005-36015 Insertion Needle or Intracatheter: Venous

INCLUDES Insertion needle or catheter, local anesthesia, contrast injection, power injections, and all pre- and postinjection care provided

EXCLUDES *Medications, contrast materials, catheters*

Code also catheterization second order vessels (or higher) supplied by same first order branch, same vascular family (36012)

Code also each vascular family (e.g., bilateral procedures are separate vascular families)

36005 **Injection procedure for extremity venography (including introduction of needle or intracatheter)**

(75820, 75822)

1.38 8.44 **FUD** 000 N N1 80 50

AMA: 2018,Mar,3; 2018,Jan,8; 2017,Jan,8; 2016,Nov,3; 2016,Jul,6; 2016,Jan,13; 2015,Jan,16

36010 **Introduction of catheter, superior or inferior vena cava**

3.19 15.0 **FUD** XXX N N1 50

AMA: 2018,Jan,8; 2017,Feb,14; 2017,Jan,8; 2016,Jul,6; 2016,Jan,13; 2015,Jan,16

36011 **Selective catheter placement, venous system; first order branch (eg, renal vein, jugular vein)**

4.54 24.0 **FUD** XXX N N1 50

AMA: 2018,Jan,8; 2017,Jan,8; 2016,Jul,6; 2016,Jan,13; 2015,Jan,16

36012 **second order, or more selective, branch (eg, left adrenal vein, petrosal sinus)**

5.04 25.0 **FUD** XXX N N1 50

AMA: 2018,Oct,3; 2018,Jan,8; 2017,Jan,8; 2016,Jul,6; 2016,Jan,13; 2015,Jan,16

36013 **Introduction of catheter, right heart or main pulmonary artery**

3.53 22.7 **FUD** XXX N N1

AMA: 2019,Jun,3; 2018,Jan,8; 2017,Jan,8; 2016,Jul,6; 2016,Jan,13; 2015,Jan,16

36014 **Selective catheter placement, left or right pulmonary artery**

4.38 23.0 **FUD** XXX N N1 50

AMA: 2019,Jun,3; 2018,Jan,8; 2017,Jan,8; 2016,Jul,6; 2016,Jan,13; 2015,Jan,16

36015 **Selective catheter placement, segmental or subsegmental pulmonary artery**

EXCLUDES *Placement Swan Ganz/other flow directed catheter for monitoring (93503)*
Selective blood sampling, specific organs (36500)

5.00 25.7 **FUD** XXX N N1 50

AMA: 2019,Jun,3; 2018,Jan,8; 2017,Jan,8; 2016,Jul,6; 2016,Jan,13; 2015,Jan,16

36100-36218 Insertion Needle or Intracatheter: Arterial

INCLUDES Introduction catheter and catheterization all lesser order vessels used for approach
Local anesthesia, placement catheter/needle, contrast injection, power injections, all pre- and postinjection care

EXCLUDES *Angiography (36222-36228, 75600-75774)*
Angioplasty ([37246, 37247])
Chemotherapy injections (96401-96549)
Injection procedures for cardiac catheterizations (93455, 93457, 93459, 93461, 93530-93533, 93564)
Internal mammary artery angiography without left heart catheterization (36216, 36217)
Medications, contrast, catheters
Transcatheter interventions (37200, 37211, 37213-37214, 37241-37244, 61624, 61626)

Code also additional first order or higher catheterization for vascular families when vascular family supplied by first order vessel different from one already coded

Code also catheterization second and third order vessels supplied by same first order branch, same vascular family (36218, 36248)

36100 Introduction of needle or intracatheter, carotid or vertebral artery
4.54 14.8 **FUD** XXX N N1 50
AMA: 2000,Oct,4; 1998,Apr,1

36140 Introduction of needle or intracatheter, upper or lower extremity artery
EXCLUDES *Arteriovenous cannula insertion (36810-36821)*
2.60 13.6 **FUD** XXX N N1
AMA: 2018,Jan,8; 2017,Jan,8; 2016,Jan,13; 2015,Jan,16

36160 Introduction of needle or intracatheter, aortic, translumbar
3.59 14.6 **FUD** XXX N N1
AMA: 2018,Jan,8; 2017,Jan,8; 2016,Jan,13; 2015,Jan,16

36200 Introduction of catheter, aorta
EXCLUDES *Nonselective angiography extracranial carotid and/or cerebral vessels and cervicocerebral arch (36221)*
4.06 16.8 **FUD** 000 N N1 50
AMA: 2018,Jan,8; 2017,Mar,3; 2017,Jan,8; 2016,Jul,6; 2016,Jan,13; 2015,Jan,16

36215 Selective catheter placement, arterial system; each first order thoracic or brachiocephalic branch, within a vascular family
INCLUDES Introduction catheter into aorta (36200)
EXCLUDES *Placement catheter for coronary angiography (93454-93461)*
6.13 30.7 **FUD** 000 N N1
AMA: 2018,Jan,8; 2017,Mar,3; 2017,Jan,8; 2016,Jul,6; 2016,Jan,13; 2015,Jan,16

36216 initial second order thoracic or brachiocephalic branch, within a vascular family
7.90 32.5 **FUD** 000 N N1
AMA: 2018,Jan,8; 2017,Jan,8; 2016,Jul,6; 2016,Jan,13; 2015,Jan,16

36217 initial third order or more selective thoracic or brachiocephalic branch, within a vascular family
9.52 53.9 **FUD** 000 N N1
AMA: 2018,Jan,8; 2017,Jan,8; 2016,Jul,6; 2016,Jan,13; 2015,Jan,16

+ **36218 additional second order, third order, and beyond, thoracic or brachiocephalic branch, within a vascular family (List in addition to code for initial second or third order vessel as appropriate)**
Code also transcatheter therapy procedures (37200, 37211, 37213-37214, 37236-37239, 37241-37244, 61624, 61626)
Code first (36216-36217, 36225-36226)
1.51 6.89 **FUD** ZZZ N N1
AMA: 2018,Oct,3; 2018,Jan,8; 2017,Jan,8; 2016,Jul,6; 2016,Jan,13; 2015,Jan,16

36221-36228 Diagnostic Studies: Aortic Arch/Carotid/Vertebral Arteries

INCLUDES Accessing vessel
Arterial contrast injection including arterial, capillary, and venous phase imaging, when performed
Arteriotomy closure (pressure or closure device)
Catheter placement
Radiologic supervision and interpretation
Reporting selective catheter placement based on service intensity in following hierarchy:
36226>36225
36224>36223>36222

EXCLUDES *3D rendering when performed (76376-76377)*
Interventional procedures
Ultrasound guidance (76937)

Code also diagnostic angiography upper extremities/other vascular beds during same session, when performed (75774)

36221 Non-selective catheter placement, thoracic aorta, with angiography of the extracranial carotid, vertebral, and/or intracranial vessels, unilateral or bilateral, and all associated radiological supervision and interpretation, includes angiography of the cervicocerebral arch, when performed
EXCLUDES *Selective catheter placement, common carotid or innominate artery (36222-36226)*
Transcatheter intravascular stent placement common carotid or innominate artery on same side (37217)
5.80 29.3 **FUD** 000 02 N1
AMA: 2018,Jan,8; 2017,Jan,8; 2016,Mar,3; 2016,Jan,13; 2015,Nov,3; 2015,May,7; 2015,Jan,16

36222 Selective catheter placement, common carotid or innominate artery, unilateral, any approach, with angiography of the ipsilateral extracranial carotid circulation and all associated radiological supervision and interpretation, includes angiography of the cervicocerebral arch, when performed
EXCLUDES *Transcatheter placement intravascular stent(s) (37215-37218)*
Code also modifier 59 when different territories on both sides body studied
8.22 34.7 **FUD** 000 02 N1 50
AMA: 2018,Jan,8; 2017,Jan,8; 2016,Mar,3; 2016,Jan,13; 2015,Nov,3; 2015,Nov,10; 2015,May,7; 2015,Jan,16

36223 Selective catheter placement, common carotid or innominate artery, unilateral, any approach, with angiography of the ipsilateral intracranial carotid circulation and all associated radiological supervision and interpretation, includes angiography of the extracranial carotid and cervicocerebral arch, when performed
EXCLUDES *Transcatheter placement intravascular stent(s) (37215-37218)*
Code also modifier 59 when different territories on both sides body studied
9.18 43.9 **FUD** 000 02 N1 50
AMA: 2018,Jan,8; 2017,Jan,8; 2016,Mar,3; 2016,Jan,13; 2015,Nov,3; 2015,Jan,16

36224 Selective catheter placement, internal carotid artery, unilateral, with angiography of the ipsilateral intracranial carotid circulation and all associated radiological supervision and interpretation, includes angiography of the extracranial carotid and cervicocerebral arch, when performed
EXCLUDES *Transcatheter placement intravascular stent(s) (37215-37218)*
Code also modifier 59 when different territories on both sides body studied
10.4 56.8 **FUD** 000 02 N1 50
AMA: 2018,Jan,8; 2017,Jan,8; 2016,Mar,3; 2016,Jan,13; 2015,Nov,3; 2015,Jan,16

36225 **Selective catheter placement, subclavian or innominate artery, unilateral, with angiography of the ipsilateral vertebral circulation and all associated radiological supervision and interpretation, includes angiography of the cervicocerebral arch, when performed**

EXCLUDES *Transcatheter placement intravascular stent(s) (37217)*

9.16 42.3 FUD 000 Q2 N1 50

AMA: 2018,Jan,8; 2017,Jan,8; 2016,Mar,3; 2016,Jan,13; 2015,Nov,3; 2015,Jan,16

36226 **Selective catheter placement, vertebral artery, unilateral, with angiography of the ipsilateral vertebral circulation and all associated radiological supervision and interpretation, includes angiography of the cervicocerebral arch, when performed**

EXCLUDES *Transcatheter placement intravascular stent(s) (37217)*

10.3 53.7 FUD 000 Q2 N1 50

AMA: 2018,Jan,8; 2017,Jan,8; 2016,Mar,3; 2016,Jan,13; 2015,Nov,3; 2015,Jan,16

+ **36227** **Selective catheter placement, external carotid artery, unilateral, with angiography of the ipsilateral external carotid circulation and all associated radiological supervision and interpretation (List separately in addition to code for primary procedure)**

EXCLUDES *Reporting with modifier 50. Report once for each side when performed bilaterally*
Transcatheter placement intravascular stent(s) (37217)

Code first (36222-36224)

3.41 7.23 FUD ZZZ N N1 50

AMA: 2018,Jan,8; 2017,Jan,8; 2016,Jan,13; 2015,Nov,10; 2015,Jan,16

+ **36228** **Selective catheter placement, each intracranial branch of the internal carotid or vertebral arteries, unilateral, with angiography of the selected vessel circulation and all associated radiological supervision and interpretation (eg, middle cerebral artery, posterior inferior cerebellar artery) (List separately in addition to code for primary procedure)**

EXCLUDES *Procedure performed more than two times per side*
Reporting with modifier 50. Report once for each side when performed bilaterally

Code first (36223-36226)

7.03 37.6 FUD ZZZ N N1 50

AMA: 2018,Jan,8; 2017,Jan,8; 2016,Jan,13; 2015,Nov,3; 2015,Jan,16

36245-36254 Catheter Placement: Arteries of the Lower Body

INCLUDES Introduction catheter and catheterization all lesser order vessels used for approach
Local anesthesia, placement catheter/needle, contrast injection, power injections

EXCLUDES *Angiography (36222-36228, 75600-75774)*
Chemotherapy injections (96401-96549)
Injection procedures for cardiac catheterizations (93455, 93457, 93459, 93461, 93530-93533, 93564)
Internal mammary artery angiography without left heart catheterization (36216-36217)
Medications, contrast, catheters
Transcatheter procedures (37200, 37211, 37213-37214, 37236-37239, 37241-37244, 61624, 61626)

Code also additional first order or higher catheterization for vascular families when vascular family supplied by first order vessel different from vessel already coded

Code also catheterization second and third order vessels supplied by same first order branch, same vascular family (36218, 36248)

(75600-75774)

36245 **Selective catheter placement, arterial system; each first order abdominal, pelvic, or lower extremity artery branch, within a vascular family**

6.89 38.1 FUD XXX N N1 50

AMA: 2018,Jan,8; 2017,Jan,8; 2016,Jul,6; 2016,Jan,13; 2015,Jan,16

36246 **initial second order abdominal, pelvic, or lower extremity artery branch, within a vascular family**

7.35 24.5 FUD 000 N N1 50

AMA: 2018,Jan,8; 2017,Jan,8; 2016,Jul,6; 2016,Jan,13; 2015,Jan,16

36247 **initial third order or more selective abdominal, pelvic, or lower extremity artery branch, within a vascular family**

8.75 43.2 FUD 000 N N1 50

AMA: 2020,Sep,14; 2018,Jan,8; 2017,Jan,8; 2016,Jul,6; 2016,Jan,13; 2015,Jan,16

+ **36248** **additional second order, third order, and beyond, abdominal, pelvic, or lower extremity artery branch, within a vascular family (List in addition to code for initial second or third order vessel as appropriate)**

Code first (36246, 36247)

1.41 3.92 FUD ZZZ N N1

AMA: 2018,Oct,3; 2018,Jan,8; 2017,Jan,8; 2016,Jul,6; 2016,Jan,13; 2015,Jan,16

36251 **Selective catheter placement (first-order), main renal artery and any accessory renal artery(s) for renal angiography, including arterial puncture and catheter placement(s), fluoroscopy, contrast injection(s), image postprocessing, permanent recording of images, and radiological supervision and interpretation, including pressure gradient measurements when performed, and flush aortogram when performed; unilateral**

INCLUDES Closure device placement at vascular access site

EXCLUDES *Transcatheter renal sympathetic denervation, percutaneous approach (0338T-0339T)*

7.55 39.2 FUD 000 Q2 N1

AMA: 2018,Jan,8; 2017,Jan,8; 2016,Jan,13; 2015,Jan,16

36252 **bilateral**

INCLUDES Closure device placement at vascular access site

EXCLUDES *Transcatheter renal sympathetic denervation, percutaneous approach (0338T-0339T)*

10.4 42.4 FUD 000 Q2 N1

AMA: 2018,Jan,8; 2017,Jan,8; 2016,Jan,13; 2015,Jan,16

36253 **Superselective catheter placement (one or more second order or higher renal artery branches) renal artery and any accessory renal artery(s) for renal angiography, including arterial puncture, catheterization, fluoroscopy, contrast injection(s), image postprocessing, permanent recording of images, and radiological supervision and interpretation, including pressure gradient measurements when performed, and flush aortogram when performed; unilateral**

INCLUDES Closure device placement at vascular access site

EXCLUDES *Procedure performed on same kidney with (36251)*
Transcatheter renal sympathetic denervation, percutaneous approach (0338T-0339T)

10.3 62.6 FUD 000 Q2 N1

AMA: 2018,Jan,8; 2017,Jan,8; 2016,Jan,13; 2015,Jan,16

36254 **bilateral**

INCLUDES Closure device placement at vascular access site

EXCLUDES *Selective catheter placement (first-order), main renal artery and any accessory renal artery(s) for renal angiography (36252)*
Transcatheter renal sympathetic denervation, percutaneous approach (0338T-0339T)

12.1 60.8 FUD 000 Q2 N1

AMA: 2018,Jan,8; 2017,Jan,8; 2016,Jan,13; 2015,Jan,16

36260-36299 Implanted Infusion Pumps: Intra-arterial

36260 **Insertion of implantable intra-arterial infusion pump (eg, for chemotherapy of liver)**

18.8 18.8 FUD 090 T A2

AMA: 2018,Jan,8; 2017,Jan,8; 2016,Jan,13; 2015,Jan,16

36261 **Revision of implanted intra-arterial infusion pump**

11.7 11.7 FUD 090 T J8 80

AMA: 2000,Oct,4; 1997,Nov,1

36262 **Removal of implanted intra-arterial infusion pump**
8.96 8.96 FUD 090 Q2 G2
AMA: 2000,Oct,4; 1997,Nov,1

36299 **Unlisted procedure, vascular injection**
0.00 0.00 FUD YYY N 80
AMA: 2000,Oct,4; 1997,Nov,1

36400-36425 Specimen Collection: Phlebotomy

EXCLUDES *Specimen collection from:*
Completely implantable device (36591)
Established catheter (36592)

36400 **Venipuncture, younger than age 3 years, necessitating the skill of a physician or other qualified health care professional, not to be used for routine venipuncture; femoral or jugular vein** A
0.53 0.75 FUD XXX N N1
AMA: 2018,Jan,8; 2017,Jan,8; 2016,Jan,13; 2015,Jan,16

36405 **scalp vein** A
0.44 0.66 FUD XXX N N1
AMA: 2018,Jan,8; 2017,Jan,8; 2016,Jan,13; 2015,Jan,16

36406 **other vein** A
0.25 0.47 FUD XXX N N1
AMA: 2018,Jan,8; 2017,Jan,8; 2016,Jan,13; 2015,Jan,16

36410 **Venipuncture, age 3 years or older, necessitating the skill of a physician or other qualified health care professional (separate procedure), for diagnostic or therapeutic purposes (not to be used for routine venipuncture)** A
0.27 0.49 FUD XXX N N1
AMA: 2019,Aug,8; 2018,Mar,3; 2018,Jan,8; 2017,Jan,8; 2016,Nov,3; 2016,Jan,13; 2015,Jan,16

36415 **Collection of venous blood by venipuncture**
0.00 0.00 FUD XXX 63 Q
AMA: 2019,Aug,8; 2018,Jan,8; 2017,Jan,8; 2016,Jan,13; 2015,Jan,16

36416 **Collection of capillary blood specimen (eg, finger, heel, ear stick)**
0.00 0.00 FUD XXX N N1
AMA: 2008,Apr,-9; 2003,Feb,7

36420 **Venipuncture, cutdown; younger than age 1 year** A
1.35 1.35 FUD XXX 63 Q1 N1 80
AMA: 2018,Jan,8; 2017,Jan,8; 2016,Jan,13; 2015,Jan,16

36425 **age 1 or over** A
EXCLUDES *Endovenous ablation therapy incompetent vein, extremity (36475-36476, 36478-36479)*
1.15 1.15 FUD XXX Q1 N1
AMA: 2018,Mar,3; 2018,Jan,8; 2017,Jan,8; 2016,Nov,3; 2016,Jan,13; 2015,Jan,16

36430-36460 Transfusions

CMS: 100-01,3,20.5 Blood Deductibles; 100-03,110.16 Transfusion in Kidney Transplants; 100-03,110.7 Blood Transfusions; 100-03,110.8 Blood Platelet Transfusions

36430 **Transfusion, blood or blood components**
EXCLUDES *Infant partial exchange transfusion (36456)*
0.99 0.99 FUD XXX S P3
AMA: 2020,Jun,14; 2019,Jun,5; 2018,Jan,8; 2017,Jul,3; 2017,Jan,8; 2016,Jan,13; 2015,Jan,16

36440 **Push transfusion, blood, 2 years or younger** A
EXCLUDES *Infant partial exchange transfusion (36456)*
1.47 1.47 FUD XXX S R2 80
AMA: 2018,Jan,8; 2017,Jul,3; 2017,Jan,8; 2016,Jan,13; 2015,Jan,16

36450 **Exchange transfusion, blood; newborn** A
EXCLUDES *Automated red cell exchange (36512)*
Infant partial exchange transfusion (36456)
4.93 4.93 FUD XXX 63 S R2 80
AMA: 2018,Jan,8; 2017,Jul,3

36455 **other than newborn** A
EXCLUDES *Automated red cell exchange (36512)*
3.68 3.68 FUD XXX S G2
AMA: 2003,Apr,7; 1997,Nov,1

36456 **Partial exchange transfusion, blood, plasma or crystalloid necessitating the skill of a physician or other qualified health care professional, newborn** A
EXCLUDES *Automated red cell exchange (36512)*
Transfusions other types (36430-36450)
2.93 2.93 FUD XXX 63 S 80
AMA: 2018,Jan,8; 2017,Jul,3

36460 **Transfusion, intrauterine, fetal** A ♀
(76941)
10.1 10.1 FUD XXX 63 S 80
AMA: 2003,Apr,7; 1997,Nov,1

36465-36466 [36465, 36466] Destruction Spider Veins

INCLUDES All supplies, equipment, compression stockings or bandages when performed in physician office
EXCLUDES *Multi-layer compression system applied to leg (29581, 29584)*
Strapping leg: ankle, foot, hip, knee, toes same extremity (29520, 29530, 29540, 29550)
Unna boot (29580)
Reporting code more than one time for each extremity treated
Vascular embolization and occlusion (37241-37244)
Vascular embolization vein in same operative field (37241)

36465 **Resequenced code. See code following 36471.**

36466 **Resequenced code. See code following 36471.**

36468 **Injection(s) of sclerosant for spider veins (telangiectasia), limb or trunk**
(76942)
0.00 0.00 FUD 000 Q1 N1 80
AMA: 2018,Mar,3; 2018,Jan,8; 2017,Jan,8; 2016,Nov,3; 2016,Jan,13; 2015,Apr,10; 2015,Jan,16

36470 **Injection of sclerosant; single incompetent vein (other than telangiectasia)**
EXCLUDES *Injection foam sclerosant with ultrasound guidance for compression maneuvers (36465-36466)*
(76942)
1.10 3.10 FUD 000 T P3 50
AMA: 2018,Dec,10; 2018,Dec,10; 2018,Mar,3; 2018,Jan,8; 2017,Jan,8; 2016,Nov,3; 2016,Jan,13; 2015,Nov,10; 2015,Apr,10; 2015,Jan,16

36471 **multiple incompetent veins (other than telangiectasia), same leg**
EXCLUDES *Injection foam sclerosant with ultrasound guidance for compression maneuvers (36465-36466)*
(76942)
2.21 5.47 FUD 000 T P3 50
AMA: 2018,Dec,10; 2018,Dec,10; 2018,Mar,3; 2018,Jan,8; 2017,Jan,8; 2016,Nov,3; 2016,Jan,13; 2015,Nov,10; 2015,Aug,8; 2015,Apr,10; 2015,Jan,16

36465 **Injection of non-compounded foam sclerosant with ultrasound compression maneuvers to guide dispersion of the injectate, inclusive of all imaging guidance and monitoring; single incompetent extremity truncal vein (eg, great saphenous vein, accessory saphenous vein)**
EXCLUDES *Ablation vein using chemical adhesive ([36482, 36483])*
Injection foam sclerosant with ultrasound guidance for compression maneuvers (36465-36466)
3.48 42.9 FUD 000 T P2 50
AMA: 2019,Feb,9; 2018,Dec,10; 2018,Dec,10; 2018,Mar,3

36466 **multiple incompetent truncal veins (eg, great saphenous vein, accessory saphenous vein), same leg**
EXCLUDES *Ablation vein using chemical adhesive ([36482, 36483])*
Injection foam sclerosant with ultrasound guidance for compression maneuvers (36465-36466)
4.46 47.6 FUD 000 T P2 50
AMA: 2019,Feb,9; 2018,Dec,10; 2018,Dec,10; 2018,Mar,3

36473-36483 [36482, 36483] Vein Ablation

INCLUDES Multi-layer compression system applied to leg (29581, 29584)
Patient monitoring
Radiological guidance (76000, 76937, 76942, 76998, 77002)
Venous access/injections (36000-36005, 36410, 36425)

EXCLUDES *Duplex scans (93970-93971)*
Strapping leg: ankle, foot, hip, knee, toes same extremity (29520, 29530, 29540, 29550)
Transcatheter embolization (75894)
Unna boot (29580)
Vascular embolization vein in same operative field (37241)

36473 Endovenous ablation therapy of incompetent vein, extremity, inclusive of all imaging guidance and monitoring, percutaneous, mechanochemical; first vein treated
INCLUDES Local anesthesia
EXCLUDES *Laser ablation incompetent vein (36478-36479)*
Radiofrequency ablation incompetent vein (36475-36476)
5.18 | 40.4 | FUD 000 | T P3 50
AMA: 2019,Feb,9; 2018,Mar,3; 2018,Jan,8; 2017,Jan,8; 2016,Nov,3

+ **36474 subsequent vein(s) treated in a single extremity, each through separate access sites (List separately in addition to code for primary procedure)**
INCLUDES Local anesthesia
EXCLUDES *Laser ablation incompetent vein (36478-36479)*
Radiofrequency ablation incompetent vein (36475-36476)
Reporting code more than one time per extremity
Code first (36473)
2.60 | 8.23 | FUD ZZZ | N N1 50
AMA: 2019,Feb,9; 2018,Mar,3; 2018,Jan,8; 2017,Jan,8; 2016,Nov,3

36475 Endovenous ablation therapy of incompetent vein, extremity, inclusive of all imaging guidance and monitoring, percutaneous, radiofrequency; first vein treated
INCLUDES Tumescent anesthesia
EXCLUDES *Ablation vein using chemical adhesive ([36482, 36483])*
Endovenous ablation therapy incompetent vein (36478-36479)
8.09 | 38.9 | FUD 000 | T A2 50
AMA: 2018,Mar,3; 2018,Jan,8; 2017,Jan,8; 2016,Nov,3; 2016,Aug,3; 2016,Jan,13; 2015,Apr,10; 2015,Jan,16

+ **36476 subsequent vein(s) treated in a single extremity, each through separate access sites (List separately in addition to code for primary procedure)**
INCLUDES Tumescent anesthesia
EXCLUDES *Ablation vein using chemical adhesive ([36482, 36483])*
Endovenous ablation therapy incompetent vein (36478-36479)
Reporting code more than one time per extremity
Vascular embolization or occlusion (37242-37244)
Code first (36475)
3.92 | 8.81 | FUD ZZZ | N N1 50
AMA: 2018,Mar,3; 2018,Jan,8; 2017,Jan,8; 2016,Nov,3; 2016,Aug,3; 2016,Jan,13; 2015,Apr,10; 2015,Jan,16

36478 Endovenous ablation therapy of incompetent vein, extremity, inclusive of all imaging guidance and monitoring, percutaneous, laser; first vein treated
INCLUDES Tumescent anesthesia
EXCLUDES *Ablation vein using chemical adhesive ([36482, 36483])*
Endovenous ablation therapy incompetent vein (36478-36479)
8.06 | 30.2 | FUD 000 | T A2 50
AMA: 2020,May,13; 2018,Mar,3; 2018,Jan,8; 2017,Jan,8; 2016,Nov,3; 2016,Aug,3; 2016,Jan,13; 2015,Apr,10; 2015,Jan,16

+ **36479 subsequent vein(s) treated in a single extremity, each through separate access sites (List separately in addition to code for primary procedure)**
INCLUDES Tumescent anesthesia
EXCLUDES *Ablation vein using chemical adhesive ([36482, 36483])*
Endovenous ablation therapy incompetent vein (36478-36479)
Vascular embolization or occlusion (37241)
Code first (36478)
3.96 | 9.28 | FUD ZZZ | N N1 50
AMA: 2020,May,13; 2018,Mar,3; 2018,Jan,8; 2017,Jan,8; 2016,Nov,3; 2016,Aug,3; 2016,Jan,13; 2015,Apr,10; 2015,Jan,16

36482 Endovenous ablation therapy of incompetent vein, extremity, by transcatheter delivery of a chemical adhesive (eg, cyanoacrylate) remote from the access site, inclusive of all imaging guidance and monitoring, percutaneous; first vein treated
INCLUDES Local anesthesia
EXCLUDES *Laser ablation incompetent vein (36478-36479)*
Radiofrequency ablation incompetent vein (36475-36476)
5.20 | 54.0 | FUD 000 | T P3 50
AMA: 2019,Feb,9; 2018,Mar,3

+ # **36483 subsequent vein(s) treated in a single extremity, each through separate access sites (List separately in addition to code for primary procedure)**
INCLUDES Local anesthesia
EXCLUDES *Laser ablation incompetent vein (36478-36479)*
Radiofrequency ablation incompetent vein (36475-36476)
Reporting code more than one time per extremity
Code first ([36482])
2.61 | 4.45 | FUD ZZZ | N N1 50
AMA: 2019,Feb,9; 2018,Mar,3

36481-36510 [36482, 36483] Other Venous Catheterization Procedures

EXCLUDES *Specimen collection from:*
Completely implantable device (36591)
Established catheter (36592)

36481 Percutaneous portal vein catheterization by any method
(75885, 75887)
9.56 | 54.6 | FUD 000 | N N1
AMA: 2018,Jan,8; 2017,Jan,8; 2016,Jan,13; 2015,Jan,16

36482 **Resequenced code. See code following 36479.**

36483 **Resequenced code. See code following 36479.**

36500 Venous catheterization for selective organ blood sampling
EXCLUDES *Inferior or superior vena cava catheterization (36010)*
(75893)
5.30 | 5.30 | FUD 000 | N N1
AMA: 2014,Jan,11; 1997,Nov,1

36510 Catheterization of umbilical vein for diagnosis or therapy, newborn A
EXCLUDES *Specimen collection from:*
Capillary blood (36416)
Venipuncture (36415)
1.55 | 2.36 | FUD 000 | 63 N N1 80
AMA: 2018,Jan,8; 2017,Jan,8; 2016,May,3; 2016,Jan,13; 2015,Jan,16

36511-36516 Apheresis

CMS: 100-03,110.14 Apheresis (Therapeutic Pheresis); 100-04,4,231.9 Billing for Pheresis and Apheresis Services

EXCLUDES *Specimen collection for therapeutic treatment from:*
Completely implantable device (36591)
Established catheter (36592)

36511 Therapeutic apheresis; for white blood cells
3.15 | 3.15 | FUD 000 | S G2
AMA: 2018,Jan,8; 2017,Jan,8; 2016,Jan,13; 2015,Jan,16

36512 **for red blood cells**

EXCLUDES *Manual red cell exchange (36450, 36455, 36456)*

3.12 3.12 **FUD** 000 S G2

AMA: 2018,Jan,8; 2017,Jan,8; 2016,Jan,13; 2015,Jan,16

36513 **for platelets**

EXCLUDES *Collection platelets from donors*

3.15 3.15 **FUD** 000 S R2

AMA: 2018,Jan,8; 2017,Jan,8; 2016,Jan,13; 2015,Jan,16

36514 **for plasma pheresis**

2.75 19.1 **FUD** 000 S G2

AMA: 2018,May,10; 2018,Jan,8; 2017,Jan,8; 2016,Jan,13; 2015,Jan,16

36516 **with extracorporeal immunoadsorption, selective adsorption or selective filtration and plasma reinfusion**

Code also modifier 26 for professional evaluation

2.44 55.4 **FUD** 000 S P2

AMA: 2018,Jan,8; 2017,Jan,8; 2016,Jan,13; 2015,Jan,16

36522 Extracorporeal Photopheresis

CMS: 100-03,110.4 Extracorporeal Photopheresis; 100-04,32,190 Billing for Extracorporeal Photopheresis; 100-04,32,190.2 Extracorporeal Photopheresis; 100-04,32,190.3 Medicare Denial Codes; 100-04,4,231.9 Billing for Pheresis and Apheresis Services

36522 **Photopheresis, extracorporeal**

2.79 61.2 **FUD** 000 S G2

AMA: 2018,May,10; 2018,Jan,8; 2017,Jan,8; 2016,Jan,13; 2015,Jan,16

36555-36573 [36572, 36573] Placement of Implantable Venous Access Device

INCLUDES Devices accessed by exposed catheter, or subcutaneous port or pump
Devices inserted via cutdown or percutaneous access:
- Centrally (eg, femoral, jugular, subclavian veins, or inferior vena cava)
- Peripherally (e.g., basilic, cephalic, saphenous vein)

Devices terminating in brachiocephalic (innominate), iliac, subclavian veins, vena cava, or right atrium

EXCLUDES *Insertion midline catheter (36400, 36406, 36410)*
Maintenance/refilling implantable pump/reservoir (96522)

Code also removal central venous access device (if code available) when new device placed through separate venous access

36555 **Insertion of non-tunneled centrally inserted central venous catheter; younger than 5 years of age** A

EXCLUDES *Peripheral insertion (36568)*

(76937, 77001)

2.44 5.35 **FUD** 000 T A2

AMA: 2019,May,3; 2018,Jan,8; 2017,Jan,8; 2016,Jan,13; 2015,Jan,16

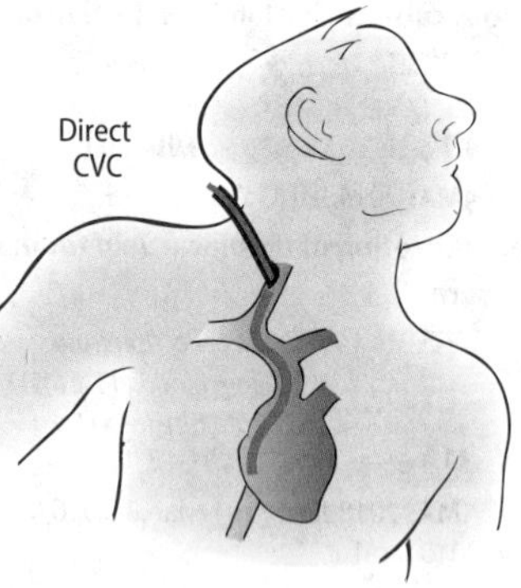

A non-tunneled centrally inserted CVC is inserted

36556 **age 5 years or older** A

EXCLUDES *Peripheral insertion (36569)*

(76937, 77001)

2.46 6.08 **FUD** 000 T A2

AMA: 2019,May,3; 2018,Nov,11; 2018,Jan,8; 2017,Jan,8; 2016,Jan,13; 2015,Jan,16

36557 **Insertion of tunneled centrally inserted central venous catheter, without subcutaneous port or pump; younger than 5 years of age** A

(76937, 77001)

9.25 31.3 **FUD** 010 T A2 80 50

AMA: 2018,Jan,8; 2017,Jan,8; 2016,Jan,13; 2015,Jan,16

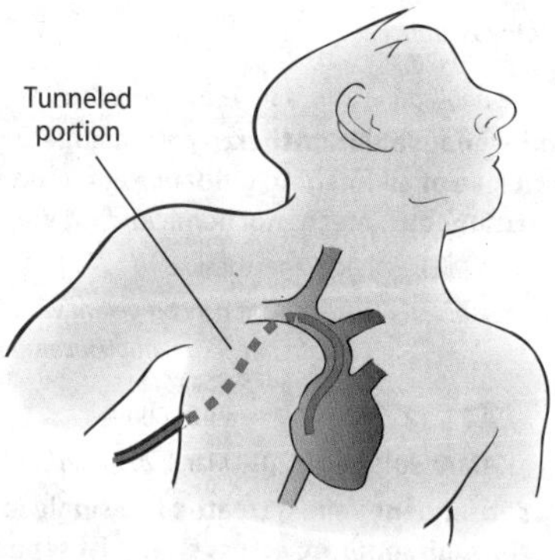

A tunneled centrally inserted CVC is inserted

36558 **age 5 years or older** A

EXCLUDES *Peripheral insertion (36571)*

(76937, 77001)

7.55 23.1 **FUD** 010 T A2 80 50

AMA: 2018,Jan,8; 2017,Jan,8; 2016,Jan,13; 2015,Jan,16; 2015,Jan,13

36560 **Insertion of tunneled centrally inserted central venous access device, with subcutaneous port; younger than 5 years of age** A

EXCLUDES *Peripheral insertion (36570)*

(76937, 77001)

11.0 37.4 **FUD** 010 T G2 80 50

AMA: 2018,Jan,8; 2017,Jan,8; 2016,Jan,13; 2015,Jan,16

36561 **age 5 years or older** A

EXCLUDES *Peripheral insertion (36571)*

(76937, 77001)

9.74 30.6 **FUD** 010 T A2 80 50

AMA: 2018,Jan,8; 2017,Jan,8; 2016,Jan,13; 2015,Jan,16

36563 **Insertion of tunneled centrally inserted central venous access device with subcutaneous pump**

(76937, 77001)

10.6 33.9 **FUD** 010 T A2 80

AMA: 2018,Jan,8; 2017,Jan,8; 2016,Jan,13; 2015,Jan,16

36565 **Insertion of tunneled centrally inserted central venous access device, requiring 2 catheters via 2 separate venous access sites; without subcutaneous port or pump (eg, Tesio type catheter)**

(76937, 77001)

9.71 25.0 **FUD** 010 T A2 80 50

AMA: 2018,Jan,8; 2017,Jan,8; 2016,Jan,13; 2015,Jan,16

36566 **with subcutaneous port(s)**

(76937, 77001)

10.4 132. **FUD** 010 T A2 80 50

AMA: 2018,Jan,8; 2017,Jan,8; 2016,Jan,13; 2015,Jan,16

36568 Insertion of peripherally inserted central venous catheter (PICC), without subcutaneous port or pump, without imaging guidance; younger than 5 years of age　Ⓐ

> EXCLUDES　Centrally inserted placement (36555)
> Imaging guidance (76937, 77001)
> Peripherally inserted ([36572])
> PICC line removal with codes for removal tunneled central venous catheters; report appropriate E/M code

> 🔲 2.65　⚕ 2.65　**FUD** 000　Ⓣ A2 🔲

> **AMA:** 2019,May,3; 2018,Jan,8; 2017,Jan,8; 2016,Jan,13; 2015,Jan,16

36569 age 5 years or older　Ⓐ

> EXCLUDES　Centrally inserted placement (36556)
> Imaging guidance (76937, 77001)
> Peripherally inserted ([36573])
> PICC line removal with codes for removal tunneled central venous catheters; report appropriate E/M code

> 🔲 2.73　⚕ 2.73　**FUD** 000　Ⓣ A2 🔲

> **AMA:** 2019,May,3; 2018,Jan,8; 2017,Jan,8; 2016,Jan,13; 2015,Jan,16

#　36572 Insertion of peripherally inserted central venous catheter (PICC), without subcutaneous port or pump, including all imaging guidance, image documentation, and all associated radiological supervision and interpretation required to perform the insertion; younger than 5 years of age　Ⓐ

> INCLUDES　Verification site catheter tip (71045-71048)

> EXCLUDES　Centrally inserted placement (36555)
> Imaging guidance (76937, 77001)
> Peripherally inserted without imaging guidance (36568)

> 🔲 2.62　⚕ 12.3　**FUD** 000　G2 🔲

> **AMA:** 2019,May,3; 2019,Mar,10

#　36573 age 5 years or older　Ⓐ

> INCLUDES　Verification site catheter tip (71045-71048)

> EXCLUDES　Centrally inserted placement (36556)
> Imaging guidance (76937, 77001)
> Peripherally inserted without imaging guidance (36569)

> 🔲 2.45　⚕ 11.3　**FUD** 000　G2 🔲

> **AMA:** 2019,May,3; 2019,Mar,10

36570 Insertion of peripherally inserted central venous access device, with subcutaneous port; younger than 5 years of age　Ⓐ

> EXCLUDES　Centrally inserted placement (36560)

> 🔲 9.61　⚕ 42.3　**FUD** 010　Ⓣ A2 80 50 🔲

> **AMA:** 2018,Jan,8; 2017,Jan,8; 2016,Jan,13; 2015,Jan,16

36571 age 5 years or older　Ⓐ

> EXCLUDES　Centrally inserted placement (36561)

> 🔲 9.03　⚕ 37.0　**FUD** 010　Ⓣ A2 80 50 🔲

> **AMA:** 2018,Jan,8; 2017,Jan,8; 2016,Jan,13; 2015,Jan,16

36572 Resequenced code. See code following 36569.

36573 Resequenced code. See code following 36569.

36575-36590 Repair, Removal, and Replacement Implantable Venous Access Device

> EXCLUDES　Mechanical removal obstructive material, pericatheter/intraluminal (36595, 36596)
> Code also frequency of two for procedures involving both catheters from multicatheter device

36575 Repair of tunneled or non-tunneled central venous access catheter, without subcutaneous port or pump, central or peripheral insertion site

> INCLUDES　Repair device without replacing any parts
> 🔲 1.01　⚕ 4.57　**FUD** 000　Ⓣ A2 80 🔲

> **AMA:** 2018,Jan,8; 2017,Jan,8; 2016,Jan,13; 2015,Jan,16

36576 Repair of central venous access device, with subcutaneous port or pump, central or peripheral insertion site

> INCLUDES　Repair device without replacing any parts
> 🔲 5.33　⚕ 9.31　**FUD** 010　Ⓣ A2 80 🔲

> **AMA:** 2018,Jan,8; 2017,Jan,8; 2016,Jan,13; 2015,Jan,16

36578 Replacement, catheter only, of central venous access device, with subcutaneous port or pump, central or peripheral insertion site

> INCLUDES　Partial replacement (catheter only)

> EXCLUDES　Total replacement entire device using same venous access sites (36582-36583)

> 🔲 5.89　⚕ 13.4　**FUD** 010　Ⓣ A2 80 🔲

> **AMA:** 2018,Jan,8; 2017,Jan,8; 2016,Jan,13; 2015,Jan,16

36580 Replacement, complete, of a non-tunneled centrally inserted central venous catheter, without subcutaneous port or pump, through same venous access

> INCLUDES　Complete replacement (replace all components/same access site)

> 🔲 1.91　⚕ 6.22　**FUD** 000　Ⓣ A2 🔲

> **AMA:** 2018,Jan,8; 2017,Jan,8; 2016,Jan,13; 2015,Jan,16

36581 Replacement, complete, of a tunneled centrally inserted central venous catheter, without subcutaneous port or pump, through same venous access

> INCLUDES　Complete replacement (replace all components/same access site)

> EXCLUDES　Removal old device and insertion new device using separate venous access site

> 🔲 5.30　⚕ 22.9　**FUD** 010　Ⓣ A2 80 🔲

> **AMA:** 2018,Jan,8; 2017,Jan,8; 2016,Jan,13; 2015,Jan,16

36582 Replacement, complete, of a tunneled centrally inserted central venous access device, with subcutaneous port, through same venous access

> INCLUDES　Complete replacement (replace all components/same access site)

> EXCLUDES　Removal old device and insertion new device using separate venous access site

> 🔲 8.40　⚕ 28.2　**FUD** 010　Ⓣ A2 80 🔲

> **AMA:** 2018,Jan,8; 2017,Jan,8; 2016,Jan,13; 2015,Jan,16

36583 Replacement, complete, of a tunneled centrally inserted central venous access device, with subcutaneous pump, through same venous access

> INCLUDES　Complete replacement (replace all components/same access site)

> EXCLUDES　Removal old device and insertion new device using separate venous access site

> 🔲 9.44　⚕ 35.9　**FUD** 010　Ⓣ J8 80 🔲

> **AMA:** 2018,Jan,8; 2017,Jan,8; 2016,Jan,13; 2015,Jan,16

36584 Replacement, complete, of a peripherally inserted central venous catheter (PICC), without subcutaneous port or pump, through same venous access, including all imaging guidance, image documentation, and all associated radiological supervision and interpretation required to perform the replacement

> INCLUDES　Complete replacement (replace all components/same access site)
> Imaging guidance (76937, 77001)
> Verification site catheter tip (71045-71048)

> EXCLUDES　Replacement PICC line without imaging guidance (37799)

> 🔲 1.73　⚕ 9.92　**FUD** 000　Ⓣ A2 🔲

> **AMA:** 2019,May,3; 2019,Mar,10; 2018,Jan,8; 2017,Jan,8; 2016,Jan,13; 2015,Jan,16

36585 Replacement, complete, of a peripherally inserted central venous access device, with subcutaneous port, through same venous access

> INCLUDES　Complete replacement (replace all components/same access site)

> 🔲 7.86　⚕ 31.4　**FUD** 010　Ⓣ A2 80 🔲

> **AMA:** 2018,Jan,8; 2017,Jan,8; 2016,Jan,13; 2015,Jan,16

36589 **Removal of tunneled central venous catheter, without subcutaneous port or pump**

INCLUDES Complete removal/all components

EXCLUDES *Non-tunneled central venous catheter removal; report appropriate E/M code*

3.97 4.76 FUD 010 Q2 A2 80

AMA: 2018,Jan,8; 2017,Jan,8; 2016,Jan,13; 2015,Nov,10; 2015,Jan,16

36590 **Removal of tunneled central venous access device, with subcutaneous port or pump, central or peripheral insertion**

INCLUDES Complete removal/all components

EXCLUDES *Non-tunneled central venous catheter removal; report appropriate E/M code*

5.51 6.40 FUD 010 Q2 A2 80

AMA: 2018,Jan,8; 2017,Jan,8; 2016,Jan,13; 2015,Jan,16

36591-36592 Obtain Blood Specimen from Implanted Device or Catheter

EXCLUDES *Use of code with any other service except laboratory services*

36591 **Collection of blood specimen from a completely implantable venous access device**

EXCLUDES *Collection:*
Capillary blood specimen (36416)
Venous blood specimen by venipuncture (36415)

0.70 0.70 FUD XXX Q1 N1 80 TC

AMA: 2019,Aug,8; 2018,Jan,8; 2017,Jan,8; 2016,Jan,13; 2015,Jan,16

36592 **Collection of blood specimen using established central or peripheral catheter, venous, not otherwise specified**

EXCLUDES *Collection blood from established arterial catheter (37799)*

0.77 0.77 FUD XXX Q1 N1 80 TC

AMA: 2018,Jan,8; 2017,Jan,8; 2016,Jan,13; 2015,Jan,16

36593-36596 Restore Patency of Occluded Catheter or Device

EXCLUDES *Venous catheterization (36010-36012)*

36593 **Declotting by thrombolytic agent of implanted vascular access device or catheter**

0.89 0.89 FUD XXX T P3 80 TC

AMA: 2018,Jan,8; 2017,Jan,8; 2016,Jan,13; 2015,Jan,16

36595 **Mechanical removal of pericatheter obstructive material (eg, fibrin sheath) from central venous device via separate venous access**

EXCLUDES *Declotting by thrombolytic agent (36593)*

(75901)

5.30 17.3 FUD 000 T G2

AMA: 2018,Jan,8; 2017,Jan,8; 2016,Jan,13; 2015,Jan,16

36596 **Mechanical removal of intraluminal (intracatheter) obstructive material from central venous device through device lumen**

EXCLUDES *Declotting by thrombolytic agent (36593)*

(75902)

1.26 3.47 FUD 000 T G2

AMA: 2018,Jan,8; 2017,Jan,8; 2016,Jan,13; 2015,Jan,16

36597-36598 Repositioning or Assessment of In Situ Venous Access Device

36597 **Repositioning of previously placed central venous catheter under fluoroscopic guidance**

(76000)

1.75 3.79 FUD 000 T G2

AMA: 2018,Jan,8; 2017,Jan,8; 2016,Jan,13; 2015,Jan,16

36598 **Contrast injection(s) for radiologic evaluation of existing central venous access device, including fluoroscopy, image documentation and report**

EXCLUDES *Complete venography studies (75820, 75825, 75827)*
Fluoroscopy (76000)
Mechanical removal pericatheter obstructive material (36595-36596)

1.07 3.44 FUD 000 T P2 80 50

AMA: 2014,Jan,11

36600-36660 Insertion Needle or Catheter: Artery

36600 **Arterial puncture, withdrawal of blood for diagnosis**

EXCLUDES *Critical care services*

0.45 0.86 FUD XXX Q1 N1

AMA: 2019,Aug,8; 2018,Jan,8; 2017,Jan,8; 2016,Jan,13; 2015,Jan,16

36620 **Arterial catheterization or cannulation for sampling, monitoring or transfusion (separate procedure); percutaneous**

1.28 1.28 FUD 000 N N1

AMA: 2018,Jan,8; 2017,Jan,8; 2016,Jan,13; 2015,Jan,16

36625 **cutdown**

3.06 3.06 FUD 000 N N1

AMA: 2018,Jan,8; 2017,Jan,8; 2016,Jan,13; 2015,Jan,16

36640 **Arterial catheterization for prolonged infusion therapy (chemotherapy), cutdown**

EXCLUDES *Intra-arterial chemotherapy (96420-96425)*
Transcatheter embolization (75894)

3.31 3.31 FUD 000 T A2

AMA: 2018,Jan,8; 2017,Jan,8; 2016,Jan,13; 2015,Jan,16

36660 **Catheterization, umbilical artery, newborn, for diagnosis or therapy** A

1.97 1.97 FUD 000 63 C 80

AMA: 2018,Jan,8; 2017,Jan,8; 2016,Jan,13; 2015,Jan,16

36680 Percutaneous Placement of Catheter/Needle into Bone Marrow Cavity

36680 **Placement of needle for intraosseous infusion**

1.74 1.74 FUD 000 Q1 N1 80

AMA: 2018,Jan,8; 2017,Jan,8; 2016,Jan,13; 2015,Jan,16

36800-36821 Vascular Access for Hemodialysis

36800 **Insertion of cannula for hemodialysis, other purpose (separate procedure); vein to vein**

3.55 3.55 FUD 000 T G2

AMA: 2018,Jan,8; 2017,Jan,8; 2016,Jan,13; 2015,Jan,16

36810 **arteriovenous, external (Scribner type)**

6.11 6.11 FUD 000 T A2

AMA: 2018,Jan,8; 2017,Jan,8; 2016,Jan,13; 2015,Jan,16

36815 **arteriovenous, external revision, or closure**

3.92 3.92 FUD 000 T A2

AMA: 2018,Jan,8; 2017,Jan,8; 2016,Jan,13; 2015,Jan,16

36818 **Arteriovenous anastomosis, open; by upper arm cephalic vein transposition**

INCLUDES Two incisions in upper arm: medial incision over brachial artery and lateral incision for exposure to portion of cephalic vein

EXCLUDES *When performed unilaterally with:*
Arteriovenous anastomosis, open (36819-36820)
Creation arteriovenous fistula by other than direct arteriovenous anastomosis (36830)

Code also modifier 50 or 59, as appropriate, for bilateral procedure

20.1 20.1 FUD 090 T A2 80

AMA: 2018,Jan,8; 2017,Mar,3; 2017,Jan,8; 2016,Mar,10; 2016,Jan,13; 2015,Jan,16

36819 **by upper arm basilic vein transposition**

EXCLUDES *When performed unilaterally with:*
Arteriovenous anastomosis, open (36818, 36820-36821)
Creation arteriovenous fistula by other than direct arteriovenous anastomosis (36830)

Code also modifier 50 or 59, as appropriate, for bilateral procedure

21.2 21.2 **FUD** 090 T A2 80

AMA: 2018,Jan,8; 2017,Mar,3; 2017,Jan,8; 2016,Jan,13; 2015,Jan,16

36820 **by forearm vein transposition**

21.2 21.2 **FUD** 090 T A2 80 50

AMA: 2018,Jan,8; 2017,Mar,3; 2017,Jan,8; 2016,Jan,13; 2015,Jan,16

36821 **direct, any site (eg, Cimino type) (separate procedure)**

19.3 19.3 **FUD** 090 T A2 80

AMA: 2018,Jan,8; 2017,Mar,3; 2017,Jan,8, 2016,Jan,13; 2015,Aug,8; 2015,Jan,16

36823 Vascular Access for Extracorporeal Circulation

INCLUDES Chemotherapy perfusion

EXCLUDES *Chemotherapy administration (96409-96425)*
Maintenance for extracorporeal circulation (33946-33949)

36823 **Insertion of arterial and venous cannula(s) for isolated extracorporeal circulation including regional chemotherapy perfusion to an extremity, with or without hyperthermia, with removal of cannula(s) and repair of arteriotomy and venotomy sites**

40.7 40.7 **FUD** 090 C

AMA: 2018,Jan,8; 2017,Mar,3

36825-36835 Permanent Vascular Access Procedures

36825 **Creation of arteriovenous fistula by other than direct arteriovenous anastomosis (separate procedure); autogenous graft**

EXCLUDES *Direct arteriovenous (AV) anastomosis (36821)*

23.0 23.0 **FUD** 090 T A2 80

AMA: 2018,Jan,8; 2017,Mar,3; 2017,Jan,8; 2016,Jan,13; 2015,Jan,16

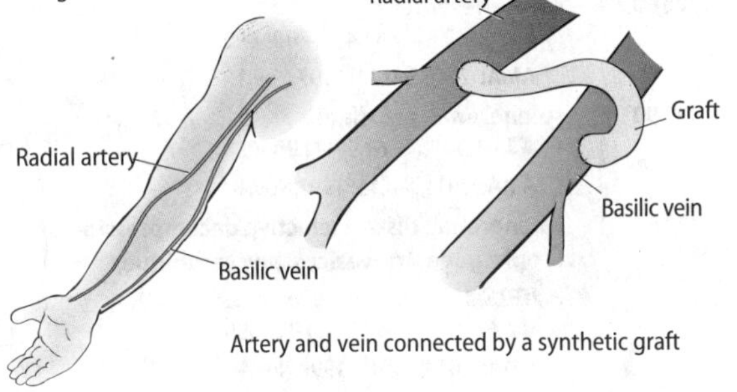

Artery and vein connected by a vein graft in an end-to-side manner, creating an arteriovenous fistula
Radial artery
Graft
Radial artery
Basilic vein
Basilic vein
Artery and vein connected by a synthetic graft

36830 **nonautogenous graft (eg, biological collagen, thermoplastic graft)**

EXCLUDES *Direct arteriovenous (AV) anastomosis (36821)*

19.4 19.4 **FUD** 090 T A2 80

AMA: 2018,Jan,8; 2017,Mar,3; 2017,Jan,8; 2016,Jan,13; 2015,Jan,16; 2015,Jan,13

36831 **Thrombectomy, open, arteriovenous fistula without revision, autogenous or nonautogenous dialysis graft (separate procedure)**

17.9 17.9 **FUD** 090 T A2 80

AMA: 2018,Jan,8; 2017,Mar,3; 2017,Jan,8; 2016,Jan,13; 2015,Jan,16

36832 **Revision, open, arteriovenous fistula; without thrombectomy, autogenous or nonautogenous dialysis graft (separate procedure)**

INCLUDES Revision arteriovenous access fistula or graft

21.9 21.9 **FUD** 090 T A2 80

AMA: 2018,Jan,8; 2017,Mar,3; 2017,Jan,8; 2016,Jan,13; 2015,Jan,16

36833 **with thrombectomy, autogenous or nonautogenous dialysis graft (separate procedure)**

EXCLUDES *Hemodialysis circuit procedures (36901-36906)*

23.5 23.5 **FUD** 090 T A2 80

AMA: 2018,Jan,8; 2017,Mar,3; 2017,Jan,8; 2016,Jan,13; 2015,Jan,16

36835 **Insertion of Thomas shunt (separate procedure)**

13.8 13.8 **FUD** 090 T J8

AMA: 2014,Jan,11; 1997,Nov,1

36838 DRIL Procedure for Ischemic Steal Syndrome

EXCLUDES *Bypass graft, with vein (35512, 35522-35523)*
Ligation (37607, 37618)
Revision, open, arteriovenous fistula (36832)

36838 **Distal revascularization and interval ligation (DRIL), upper extremity hemodialysis access (steal syndrome)**

33.3 33.3 **FUD** 090 T 80 50

AMA: 2014,Jan,11; 1997,Nov,1

36860-36861 Restore Patency of Occluded Cannula or Arteriovenous Fistula

36860 **External cannula declotting (separate procedure); without balloon catheter**

(76000)

3.23 7.05 **FUD** 000 T A2

AMA: 2018,Jan,8; 2017,Jan,8; 2016,Jan,13; 2015,Jan,16

36861 **with balloon catheter**

(76000)

4.05 4.05 **FUD** 000 T A2

AMA: 2018,Jan,8; 2017,Jan,8; 2016,Jan,13; 2015,Jan,16

36901-36909 Hemodialysis Circuit Procedures

EXCLUDES *Arteriography to assess inflow to hemodialysis circuit when performed (76937)*

36901 **Introduction of needle(s) and/or catheter(s), dialysis circuit, with diagnostic angiography of the dialysis circuit, including all direct puncture(s) and catheter placement(s), injection(s) of contrast, all necessary imaging from the arterial anastomosis and adjacent artery through entire venous outflow including the inferior or superior vena cava, fluoroscopic guidance, radiological supervision and interpretation and image documentation and report;**

INCLUDES Access
Catheter advancement (e.g., imaging of accessory veins, assess all circuit sections)
Contrast injection

EXCLUDES *Balloon angioplasty peripheral segment (36902)*
Open revision with thrombectomy arteriovenous fistula (36833)
Percutaneous transluminal procedures peripheral segment (36904-36906)
Stent placement in peripheral segment (36903)
Reporting code more than one time per procedure

4.90 16.9 **FUD** 000 T P3

AMA: 2018,Jan,8; 2017,Mar,3

36902 **with transluminal balloon angioplasty, peripheral dialysis segment, including all imaging and radiological supervision and interpretation necessary to perform the angioplasty**

EXCLUDES *Open revision with thrombectomy arteriovenous fistula (36833)*
Percutaneous transluminal procedures peripheral segment (36904-36906)
Stent placement in peripheral segment (36903)
Reporting code more than one time per procedure

6.94 36.9 FUD 000 J G2

AMA: 2018,Jan,8; 2017,Jul,3; 2017,Mar,3

36903 **with transcatheter placement of intravascular stent(s), peripheral dialysis segment, including all imaging and radiological supervision and interpretation necessary to perform the stenting, and all angioplasty within the peripheral dialysis segment**

INCLUDES Balloon angioplasty peripheral segment (36902)

EXCLUDES *Central hemodialysis circuit procedures (36907-36908)*
Open revision with thrombectomy arteriovenous fistula (36833)
Percutaneous transluminal procedures peripheral segment (36904-36906)
Reporting code more than one time per procedure

9.20 146. FUD 000 J J8

AMA: 2018,Jan,8; 2017,Jul,3; 2017,Mar,3

36904 **Percutaneous transluminal mechanical thrombectomy and/or infusion for thrombolysis, dialysis circuit, any method, including all imaging and radiological supervision and interpretation, diagnostic angiography, fluoroscopic guidance, catheter placement(s), and intraprocedural pharmacological thrombolytic injection(s);**

EXCLUDES *Open thrombectomy arteriovenous fistula with/without revision (36831, 36833)*
Reporting code more than one time per procedure

10.7 54.7 FUD 000 J J8

AMA: 2018,Jan,8; 2017,Jul,3; 2017,Mar,3

36905 **with transluminal balloon angioplasty, peripheral dialysis segment, including all imaging and radiological supervision and interpretation necessary to perform the angioplasty**

INCLUDES Percutaneous mechanical thrombectomy (36904)

EXCLUDES *Reporting code more than one time per procedure*

12.8 68.7 FUD 000 J G2

AMA: 2018,Jan,8; 2017,Jul,3; 2017,Mar,3

36906 **with transcatheter placement of intravascular stent(s), peripheral dialysis segment, including all imaging and radiological supervision and interpretation necessary to perform the stenting, and all angioplasty within the peripheral dialysis circuit**

INCLUDES Percutaneous transluminal balloon angioplasty (36905)
Percutaneous transluminal thrombectomy (36904)

EXCLUDES *Hemodialysis circuit procedures provided by catheter or needle access (36901-36903)*
Reporting code more than one time per procedure

Code also balloon angioplasty central veins, when performed (36907)

Code also stent placement in central veins, when performed (36908)

14.9 193. FUD 000 J J8

AMA: 2018,Jan,8; 2017,Jul,3; 2017,Mar,3

\+ **36907** **Transluminal balloon angioplasty, central dialysis segment, performed through dialysis circuit, including all imaging and radiological supervision and interpretation required to perform the angioplasty (List separately in addition to code for primary procedure)**

INCLUDES All central hemodialysis segment angiography

EXCLUDES *Angiography with stent placement (36908)*

Code first (36818-36833, 36901-36906)

4.25 19.6 FUD ZZZ N N1

AMA: 2018,Jan,8; 2017,Jul,3; 2017,Mar,3

\+ **36908** **Transcatheter placement of intravascular stent(s), central dialysis segment, performed through dialysis circuit, including all imaging and radiological supervision and interpretation required to perform the stenting, and all angioplasty in the central dialysis segment (List separately in addition to code for primary procedure)**

INCLUDES All central hemodialysis segment stent(s) placed
Balloon angioplasty central dialysis segment (36907)

Code first when performed (36818-36833, 36901-36906)

6.02 59.6 FUD ZZZ N N1

AMA: 2018,Jan,8; 2017,Jul,3; 2017,Mar,3

\+ **36909** **Dialysis circuit permanent vascular embolization or occlusion (including main circuit or any accessory veins), endovascular, including all imaging and radiological supervision and interpretation necessary to complete the intervention (List separately in addition to code for primary procedure)**

INCLUDES All embolization/occlusion procedures performed in hemodialysis circuit

EXCLUDES *Banding/ligation arteriovenous fistula (37607)*
Reporting code more than one time per day

Code first (36901-36906)

5.83 56.8 FUD ZZZ N N1

AMA: 2018,Jan,8; 2017,Mar,3

37140-37181 Open Decompression of Portal Circulation

EXCLUDES *Peritoneal-venous shunt (49425)*

37140 **Venous anastomosis, open; portocaval**

67.7 67.7 FUD 090 C

AMA: 2014,Jan,11; 1997,Nov,1

37145 **renoportal**

62.7 62.7 FUD 090 C 80

AMA: 2014,Jan,11; 1997,Nov,1

37160 **caval-mesenteric**

64.4 64.4 FUD 090 C 80

AMA: 2014,Jan,11; 1997,Nov,1

37180 **splenorenal, proximal**

61.9 61.9 FUD 090 C 80

AMA: 2014,Jan,11; 1997,Nov,1

37181 **splenorenal, distal (selective decompression of esophagogastric varices, any technique)**

EXCLUDES *Percutaneous procedure (37182)*

67.7 67.7 FUD 090 C 80

AMA: 2014,Jan,11; 1997,Nov,1

37182-37183 Transvenous Decompression of Portal Circulation

INCLUDES Percutaneous transhepatic portography (75885, 75887)

37182 **Insertion of transvenous intrahepatic portosystemic shunt(s) (TIPS) (includes venous access, hepatic and portal vein catheterization, portography with hemodynamic evaluation, intrahepatic tract formation/dilatation, stent placement and all associated imaging guidance and documentation)**

EXCLUDES *Open procedure (37140)*

23.7 23.7 FUD 000 C 80

AMA: 2018,Jan,8; 2017,Jan,8; 2016,Jan,13; 2015,Jan,16

37183 **Revision of transvenous intrahepatic portosystemic shunt(s) (TIPS) (includes venous access, hepatic and portal vein catheterization, portography with hemodynamic evaluation, intrahepatic tract recanulization/dilatation, stent placement and all associated imaging guidance and documentation)**

EXCLUDES *Arteriovenous (AV) aneurysm repair (36832)*

10.8 176. FUD 000 J 80

AMA: 2018,Jan,8; 2017,Jan,8; 2016,Jan,13; 2015,Jan,16

37184-37188 Removal of Thrombus from Vessel: Percutaneous

INCLUDES Fluoroscopic guidance (76000)
Injection(s) thrombolytics during procedure
Postprocedure evaluation
Pretreatment planning

EXCLUDES *Catheter placement*
Continuous infusion thrombolytics prior to and after procedure (37211-37214)
Diagnostic studies
Intracranial arterial mechanical thrombectomy or infusion (61645)
Mechanical thrombectomy, coronary (92973)
Other interventions performed percutaneously (e.g., balloon angioplasty)
Radiological supervision/interpretation

37184 **Primary percutaneous transluminal mechanical thrombectomy, noncoronary, non-intracranial, arterial or arterial bypass graft, including fluoroscopic guidance and intraprocedural pharmacological thrombolytic injection(s); initial vessel**

EXCLUDES *Intracranial arterial mechanical thrombectomy (61645)*
Mechanical thrombectomy another vascular family/separate access site, append modifier 59 to primary service
Mechanical thrombectomy for embolus/thrombus complicating another percutaneous interventional procedure (37186)
Therapeutic, prophylactic, or diagnostic injection (96374)

12.9 60.2 FUD 000 J J8 50

AMA: 2019,Sep,5; 2018,Jan,8; 2017,Jan,8; 2016,Jul,6; 2016,Mar,3; 2016,Jan,13; 2015,Nov,3; 2015,Apr,10; 2015,Jan,16

\+ 37185 **second and all subsequent vessel(s) within the same vascular family (List separately in addition to code for primary mechanical thrombectomy procedure)**

INCLUDES Treatment second and all succeeding vessel(s) in same vascular family

EXCLUDES *Intravenous drug injections administered subsequent to initial service*
Mechanical thrombectomy another vascular family/separate access site, append modifier 59 to primary service
Therapeutic, prophylactic, or diagnostic injection (96375)

Code first (37184)

4.77 16.9 FUD ZZZ N N1

AMA: 2019,Sep,5; 2018,Jan,8; 2017,Jan,8; 2016,Jul,6; 2016,Jan,13; 2015,Nov,3; 2015,Apr,10; 2015,Jan,16

\+ 37186 **Secondary percutaneous transluminal thrombectomy (eg, nonprimary mechanical, snare basket, suction technique), noncoronary, non-intracranial, arterial or arterial bypass graft, including fluoroscopic guidance and intraprocedural pharmacological thrombolytic injections, provided in conjunction with another percutaneous intervention other than primary mechanical thrombectomy (List separately in addition to code for primary procedure)**

INCLUDES Removal small emboli/thrombi prior to or after another percutaneous procedure

EXCLUDES *Primary percutaneous transluminal mechanical thrombectomy, noncoronary, non-intracranial (37184-37185)*
Therapeutic, prophylactic, or diagnostic injection (96375)

Code first primary procedure

7.10 37.4 FUD ZZZ N N1

AMA: 2019,Sep,5; 2018,Jan,8; 2017,Jan,8; 2016,Jul,6; 2016,Jan,13; 2015,Nov,3; 2015,Jan,16

37187 **Percutaneous transluminal mechanical thrombectomy, vein(s), including intraprocedural pharmacological thrombolytic injections and fluoroscopic guidance**

INCLUDES Secondary or subsequent intravenous injection after another initial service

EXCLUDES *Therapeutic, prophylactic, or diagnostic injection (96375)*

11.4 55.0 FUD 000 J J8 50

AMA: 2018,Jan,8; 2017,Jan,8; 2016,Jul,6; 2016,Mar,3; 2016,Jan,13; 2015,Nov,3; 2015,Jan,16

37188 **Percutaneous transluminal mechanical thrombectomy, vein(s), including intraprocedural pharmacological thrombolytic injections and fluoroscopic guidance, repeat treatment on subsequent day during course of thrombolytic therapy**

EXCLUDES *Therapeutic, prophylactic, or diagnostic injection (96375)*

8.10 46.3 FUD 000 T G2 50

AMA: 2018,Jan,8; 2017,Jan,8; 2016,Jul,6; 2016,Mar,3; 2016,Jan,13; 2015,Nov,3; 2015,Jan,16

37191-37193 Vena Cava Filters

37191 **Insertion of intravascular vena cava filter, endovascular approach including vascular access, vessel selection, and radiological supervision and interpretation, intraprocedural roadmapping, and imaging guidance (ultrasound and fluoroscopy), when performed**

EXCLUDES *Open ligation inferior vena cava via laparotomy or retroperitoneal approach (37619)*

6.49 69.9 FUD 000 T

AMA: 2018,Jan,8; 2017,Feb,14; 2017,Jan,8; 2016,May,11; 2016,Jan,13; 2015,Jan,16

37192 **Repositioning of intravascular vena cava filter, endovascular approach including vascular access, vessel selection, and radiological supervision and interpretation, intraprocedural roadmapping, and imaging guidance (ultrasound and fluoroscopy), when performed**

EXCLUDES *Insertion intravascular vena cava filter (37191)*

9.98 37.4 FUD 000 T

AMA: 2018,Jan,8; 2017,Jan,8; 2016,May,11; 2016,Jan,13; 2015,Jan,16

37193 **Retrieval (removal) of intravascular vena cava filter, endovascular approach including vascular access, vessel selection, and radiological supervision and interpretation, intraprocedural roadmapping, and imaging guidance (ultrasound and fluoroscopy), when performed**

EXCLUDES *Transcatheter retrieval intravascular foreign body, percutaneous (37197)*

10.1 44.0 FUD 000 T

AMA: 2018,Jan,8; 2017,Jan,8; 2016,May,11; 2016,Jan,13; 2015,Jan,16

37195 Intravenous Cerebral Thrombolysis

37195 **Thrombolysis, cerebral, by intravenous infusion**

0.00 0.00 FUD XXX T 80

AMA: 2020,Jan,12

37197-37214 Transcatheter Procedures: Infusions, Biopsy, Foreign Body Removal

37197 **Transcatheter retrieval, percutaneous, of intravascular foreign body (eg, fractured venous or arterial catheter), includes radiological supervision and interpretation, and imaging guidance (ultrasound or fluoroscopy), when performed**

EXCLUDES *Percutaneous vena cava filter retrieval (37193)*
Removal leadless pacemaker system ([33275])

8.78 43.4 FUD 000 T G2

AMA: 2018,Jan,8; 2017,Feb,14; 2017,Jan,8; 2016,May,11; 2016,Jan,13; 2015,Jan,16

37200 Transcatheter biopsy

(75970)

Facility RVU 6.30 Non-Facility RVU 6.30 **FUD** 000 T G2 CCI

AMA: 2014,Jan,11; 1998,Nov,1

37211 Transcatheter therapy, arterial infusion for thrombolysis other than coronary or intracranial, any method, including radiological supervision and interpretation, initial treatment day

INCLUDES Catheter change or position change
E/M services on day of and related to thrombolysis
First day transcatheter thrombolytic infusion
Fluoroscopic guidance
Follow-up arteriography or venography
Radiologic supervision and interpretation

EXCLUDES *Angiography through existing catheter for follow-up study for transcatheter therapy, embolization, or infusion, other than for thrombolysis (75898)*
Catheter placement
Declotting implanted catheter or vascular access device by thrombolytic agent (36593)
Diagnostic studies
Intracranial arterial mechanical thrombectomy or infusion (61645)
Percutaneous interventions
Procedure performed more than one time per date of service
Ultrasound guidance (76937)

Code also significant, separately identifiable E/M service on day of thrombolysis using modifier 25

Facility RVU 11.2 Non-Facility RVU 11.2 **FUD** 000 T G2 50 CCI

AMA: 2019,Sep,6; 2018,Jan,8; 2017,Jan,8; 2016,Jul,6; 2016,Mar,3; 2016,Jan,13; 2015,Nov,3; 2015,Jan,16

37212 Transcatheter therapy, venous infusion for thrombolysis, any method, including radiological supervision and interpretation, initial treatment day

INCLUDES Catheter change or position change
E/M services on day of and related to thrombolysis

EXCLUDES *Angiography through existing catheter for follow-up study for transcatheter therapy, embolization, or infusion, other than for thrombolysis (75898)*
Catheter placement
First day transcatheter thrombolytic infusion
Declotting implanted catheter or vascular access device by thrombolytic agent (36593)
Fluoroscopic guidance
Follow-up arteriography or venography
Diagnostic studies
Initiation and completion thrombolysis on same date of service
Percutaneous interventions
Radiologic supervision and interpretation
Procedure performed more than one time per date of service
Ultrasound guidance (76937)

Code also significant, separately identifiable E/M service on day of thrombolysis using modifier 25

Facility RVU 9.81 Non-Facility RVU 9.81 **FUD** 000 T G2 50 CCI

AMA: 2019,Sep,6; 2018,Jan,8; 2017,Jan,8; 2016,Jul,6; 2016,Mar,3; 2016,Jan,13; 2015,Nov,3; 2015,Jan,16

37213 Transcatheter therapy, arterial or venous infusion for thrombolysis other than coronary, any method, including radiological supervision and interpretation, continued treatment on subsequent day during course of thrombolytic therapy, including follow-up catheter contrast injection, position change, or exchange, when performed;

INCLUDES Continued thrombolytic infusions on subsequent days besides initial and last days of treatment
E/M services on day of and related to thrombolysis
Fluoroscopic guidance
Radiologic supervision and interpretation

EXCLUDES *Angiography through existing catheter for follow-up study for transcatheter therapy, embolization, or infusion, other than for thrombolysis (75898)*
Catheter placement
Declotting implanted catheter or vascular access device by thrombolytic agent (36593)
Diagnostic studies
Percutaneous interventions
Procedure performed more than one time per date of service
Ultrasound guidance (76937)

Code also significant, separately identifiable E/M service on day of thrombolysis using modifier 25

Facility RVU 6.76 Non-Facility RVU 6.76 **FUD** 000 T CCI

AMA: 2019,Sep,6; 2018,Jan,8; 2017,Jan,8; 2016,Jul,6; 2016,Mar,3; 2016,Jan,13; 2015,Nov,3; 2015,Jan,16

37214 cessation of thrombolysis including removal of catheter and vessel closure by any method

INCLUDES E/M services on day of and related to thrombolysis
Fluoroscopic guidance
Last day transcatheter thrombolytic infusions
Radiologic supervision and interpretation

EXCLUDES *Angiography through existing catheter for follow-up study for transcatheter therapy, embolization, or infusion, other than for thrombolysis (75898)*
Catheter placement
Declotting implanted catheter or vascular access device by thrombolytic agent (36593)
Diagnostic studies
Percutaneous interventions
Procedure performed more than one time per date of service
Ultrasound guidance (76937)

Code also significant, separately identifiable E/M service on day of thrombolysis using modifier 25

Facility RVU 3.57 Non-Facility RVU 3.57 **FUD** 000 T CCI

AMA: 2019,Sep,6; 2018,Jan,8; 2017,Jan,8; 2016,Jul,6; 2016,Mar,3; 2016,Jan,13; 2015,Nov,3; 2015,Jan,16

37215-37216 Stenting of Cervical Carotid Artery with/without Insertion Distal Embolic Protection Device

INCLUDES Carotid stenting, if required
Ipsilateral cerebral and cervical carotid diagnostic imaging/supervision and interpretation
Ipsilateral selective carotid catheterization

EXCLUDES *Carotid catheterization and imaging, if carotid stenting not required*
Selective catheter placement, common carotid or innominate artery (36222-36224)
Transcatheter placement extracranial vertebral artery stents, open or percutaneous (0075T, 0076T)

37215 Transcatheter placement of intravascular stent(s), cervical carotid artery, open or percutaneous, including angioplasty, when performed, and radiological supervision and interpretation; with distal embolic protection

29.2 29.2 **FUD** 090 C 80 50

AMA: 2018,Jan,8; 2017,Jul,3; 2017,Jan,8; 2016,Jan,13; 2015,Jan,16

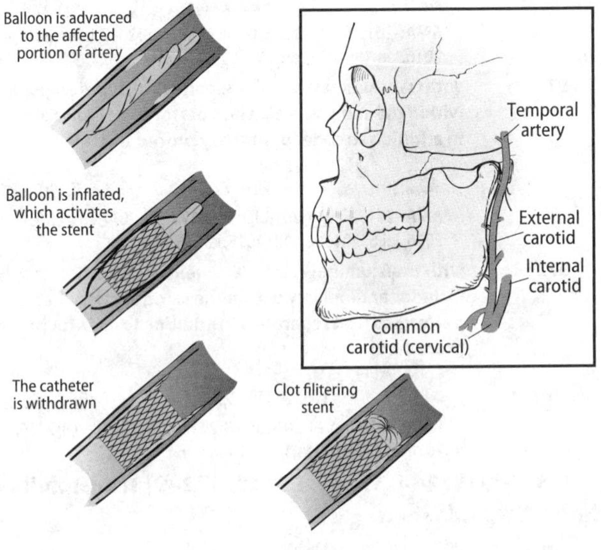
Balloon is advanced to the affected portion of artery
Balloon is inflated, which activates the stent
The catheter is withdrawn
Temporal artery
External carotid
Internal carotid
Common carotid (cervical)
Clot filtering stent

37216 without distal embolic protection

28.2 28.2 **FUD** 090 E

AMA: 2018,Jan,8; 2017,Jul,3; 2017,Jan,8; 2016,Jan,13; 2015,Jan,16

37217-37218 Stenting of Intrathoracic Carotid Artery/Innominate Artery

INCLUDES Access to vessel (open)
Arteriotomy closure by suture
Catheterization vessel (selective) (36222-36227)
Imaging during and after procedure
Radiological supervision and interpretation

EXCLUDES *Carotid artery revascularization procedures when performed during same session*
Transcatheter insertion extracranial vertebral artery stents, open or percutaneous (0075T-0076T)
Transcatheter insertion intracranial stents (61635)
Transcatheter insertion intravascular cervical carotid artery stents, open or percutaneous (37215-37216)

37217 Transcatheter placement of intravascular stent(s), intrathoracic common carotid artery or innominate artery by retrograde treatment, open ipsilateral cervical carotid artery exposure, including angioplasty, when performed, and radiological supervision and interpretation

INCLUDES When performed on same side:
Direct repair blood vessel, neck (35201)
Nonselective catheterization, thoracic aorta (36221)
Transluminal balloon angioplasty (37246-37247 [37246, 37247])

31.3 31.3 **FUD** 090 C 80 50

AMA: 2018,Jan,8; 2017,Jul,3; 2017,Jan,8; 2016,Jan,13; 2015,May,7; 2015,Jan,16

37218 Transcatheter placement of intravascular stent(s), intrathoracic common carotid artery or innominate artery, open or percutaneous antegrade approach, including angioplasty, when performed, and radiological supervision and interpretation

EXCLUDES *Selective catheter placement, common carotid or innominate artery (36222-36224)*

23.7 23.7 **FUD** 090 C 80 50

AMA: 2018,Jan,8; 2017,Jul,3; 2017,Jan,8; 2016,Jan,13; 2015,May,7

37220-37235 Endovascular Revascularization Lower Extremities

INCLUDES Percutaneous and open interventional and associated procedures for lower extremity occlusive disease; unilateral
Accessing vessel
Arteriotomy closure by suturing puncture or pressure with arterial closure device application
Atherectomy (e.g., directional, laser, rotational)
Balloon angioplasty (e.g., cryoplasty, cutting balloon, low-profile)
Catheterization vessel (selective)
Embolic protection
Imaging once procedure complete
Radiological supervision and interpretation
Stenting (e.g., bare metal, balloon-expandable, covered, drug-eluting, self-expanding)
Traversing lesion
Reporting most comprehensive treatment in given vessel according to following hierarchy:
1. Stent and atherectomy
2. Atherectomy
3. Stent
4. PTA
Revascularization procedures for three arterial vascular territories:
Femoral/popliteal vascular territory including common, deep, and superficial femoral arteries, and popliteal artery (one extremity = a single vessel) (37224-37227)
Iliac vascular territory: common iliac, external iliac, internal iliac (37220-37223)
Tibial/peroneal territory: includes anterior tibial, peroneal artery, posterior tibial (37228-37235)

EXCLUDES *Assignment more than one code from this family for each lower extremity vessel treated*
Assignment more than one code when multiple vessels are treated in femoral/popliteal territory (report most complex service for more than one lesion in territory); when contiguous lesion that spans from one territory to another can be opened with single procedure; or when more than one stent deployed in same vessel
Extensive repair or replacement artery (35226, 35286)
Mechanical thrombectomy and/or thrombolysis

Code also add-on codes for different vessels, but not different lesions in same vessel; and for multiple territories in same leg
Code also modifier 59 if same territory(ies) both legs are treated during same surgical session
Code first one primary code for initial service in each leg

37220 Revascularization, endovascular, open or percutaneous, iliac artery, unilateral, initial vessel; with transluminal angioplasty

Code also only when transluminal angioplasty performed outside treatment target zone of (34701-34708, 34709, [34718], 34710-34711, 34845-34848)

11.6 83.7 **FUD** 000 J 62 50

AMA: 2019,Jun,14; 2018,Jan,8; 2017,Jul,3; 2017,Jan,8; 2016,Jul,8; 2016,Jan,13; 2015,Jan,16

37221 with transluminal stent placement(s), includes angioplasty within the same vessel, when performed

Code also only when transluminal angioplasty performed outside treatment target zone of (34701-34708, 34709, [34718], 34710-34711, 34845-34848)

14.3 111. **FUD** 000 J J8 80 50

AMA: 2019,Jun,14; 2018,Jan,8; 2017,Dec,3; 2017,Jul,3; 2017,Jan,8; 2016,Jul,6; 2016,Jul,8; 2016,Jan,13; 2015,Jan,13; 2015,Jan,16

\+ **37222** **Revascularization, endovascular, open or percutaneous, iliac artery, each additional ipsilateral iliac vessel; with transluminal angioplasty (List separately in addition to code for primary procedure)**

Code also only when transluminal angioplasty performed outside treatment target zone of (34701-34708, 34709, [34718], 34710-34711, 34845-34848)

Code first (37220-37221)

5.42 21.2 **FUD** ZZZ N N1 80 50

AMA: 2019,Jun,14; 2018,Jan,8; 2017,Jul,3; 2017,Jan,8; 2016,Jul,8; 2016,Jan,13; 2015,Jan,16

\+ **37223** **with transluminal stent placement(s), includes angioplasty within the same vessel, when performed (List separately in addition to code for primary procedure)**

Code also only when transluminal angioplasty performed outside treatment target zone of (34701-34708, 34709, [34718], 34710-34711, 34845-34848)

Code first (37221)

6.20 62.6 **FUD** ZZZ N N1 80 50

AMA: 2019,Jun,14; 2018,Jan,8; 2017,Dec,3; 2017,Jul,3; 2017,Jan,8; 2016,Jul,8; 2016,Jul,6; 2016,Jan,13; 2015,Jan,16

37224 **Revascularization, endovascular, open or percutaneous, femoral, popliteal artery(s), unilateral; with transluminal angioplasty**

EXCLUDES *Revascularization with intravascular stent grafts in femoral-popliteal segment (0505T)*

12.9 97.6 **FUD** 000 J J8 80 50

AMA: 2019,Jun,14; 2018,Jan,8; 2017,Jul,3; 2017,Jan,8; 2016,Jul,8; 2016,Jan,13; 2015,Jan,16

37225 **with atherectomy, includes angioplasty within the same vessel, when performed**

EXCLUDES *Revascularization with intravascular stent grafts in femoral-popliteal segment (0505T)*

17.5 320. **FUD** 000 J J8 80 50

AMA: 2019,Jun,14; 2018,Jan,8; 2017,Jul,3; 2017,Jan,8; 2016,Jul,8; 2016,Jan,13; 2015,Jan,16

37226 **with transluminal stent placement(s), includes angioplasty within the same vessel, when performed**

EXCLUDES *Revascularization with intravascular stent grafts in femoral-popliteal segment (0505T)*

15.1 285. **FUD** 000 J J8 80 50

AMA: 2019,Jun,14; 2018,Jan,8; 2017,Jul,3; 2017,Jan,8; 2016,Jul,6; 2016,Jul,8; 2016,Jan,13; 2015,Jan,16

37227 **with transluminal stent placement(s) and atherectomy, includes angioplasty within the same vessel, when performed**

EXCLUDES *Revascularization with intravascular stent grafts in femoral-popliteal segment (0505T)*

21.1 444. **FUD** 000 J J8 80 50

AMA: 2019,Jun,14; 2018,Jan,8; 2017,Jul,3; 2017,Jan,8; 2016,Jul,6; 2016,Jul,8; 2016,Jan,13; 2015,Jan,16

37228 **Revascularization, endovascular, open or percutaneous, tibial, peroneal artery, unilateral, initial vessel; with transluminal angioplasty**

15.7 140. **FUD** 000 J J8 80 50

AMA: 2019,Jun,14; 2018,Jan,8; 2017,Jul,3; 2017,Jan,8; 2016,Jul,8; 2016,Jan,13; 2015,Jan,16

37229 **with atherectomy, includes angioplasty within the same vessel, when performed**

20.4 322. **FUD** 000 J J8 80 50

AMA: 2019,Jun,14; 2018,Jan,8; 2017,Jul,3; 2017,Jan,8; 2016,Jul,8; 2016,Jan,13; 2015,Jan,16

37230 **with transluminal stent placement(s), includes angioplasty within the same vessel, when performed**

20.3 289. **FUD** 000 J J8 80 50

AMA: 2020,Jul,13; 2019,Jun,14; 2018,Jan,8; 2017,Jul,3; 2017,Jan,8; 2016,Jul,6; 2016,Jul,8; 2016,Jan,13; 2015,Jan,16

37231 **with transluminal stent placement(s) and atherectomy, includes angioplasty within the same vessel, when performed**

22.0 401. **FUD** 000 J J8 80 50

AMA: 2019,Jun,14; 2018,Jan,8; 2017,Jul,3; 2017,Jan,8; 2016,Jul,8; 2016,Jul,6; 2016,Jan,13; 2015,Jan,16

\+ **37232** **Revascularization, endovascular, open or percutaneous, tibial/peroneal artery, unilateral, each additional vessel; with transluminal angioplasty (List separately in addition to code for primary procedure)**

Code first (37228-37231)

5.83 29.0 **FUD** ZZZ N N1 80 50

AMA: 2019,Jun,14; 2018,Jan,8; 2017,Jul,3; 2017,Jan,8; 2016,Jul,8; 2016,Jan,13; 2015,Jan,16

\+ **37233** **with atherectomy, includes angioplasty within the same vessel, when performed (List separately in addition to code for primary procedure)**

Code first (37229, 37231)

9.48 35.7 **FUD** ZZZ N N1 80 50

AMA: 2019,Jun,14; 2018,Jan,8; 2017,Jul,3; 2017,Jan,8; 2016,Jul,8; 2016,Jan,13; 2015,Jan,16

\+ **37234** **with transluminal stent placement(s), includes angioplasty within the same vessel, when performed (List separately in addition to code for primary procedure)**

Code first (37229-37231)

8.30 110. **FUD** ZZZ N N1 80 50

AMA: 2019,Jun,14; 2018,Jan,8; 2017,Jul,3; 2017,Jan,8; 2016,Jul,8; 2016,Jul,6; 2016,Jan,13; 2015,Jan,16

\+ **37235** **with transluminal stent placement(s) and atherectomy, includes angioplasty within the same vessel, when performed (List separately in addition to code for primary procedure)**

Code first (37231)

11.7 116. **FUD** ZZZ N N1 80 50

AMA: 2019,Jun,14; 2018,Jan,8; 2017,Jul,3; 2017,Jan,8; 2016,Jul,6; 2016,Jul,8; 2016,Jan,13; 2015,Jan,16

37246-37249 [37246, 37247, 37248, 37249] Transluminal Balloon Angioplasty

INCLUDES Open and percutaneous balloon angioplasty
Radiological supervision and interpretation (37220-37235)

EXCLUDES *Angioplasty other vessels:*
Aortic/visceral arteries (with endovascular repair) (34841-34848)
Coronary artery (92920-92944)
Intracranial artery (61630, 61635)
Performed in hemodialysis circuit (36901-36909)
Infusion thrombolytics (37211-37214)
Mechanical thrombectomy (37184-37188)
Pulmonary artery (92997-92998)
Reporting codes more than one time for all services performed in single vessel or treatable with one angioplasty procedure

Code also angioplasty different vessel, when performed ([37247], [37249])
Code also extensive artery repair or replacement, when performed (35226, 35286)
Code also intravascular ultrasound, when performed (37252-37253)

\# **37246** **Transluminal balloon angioplasty (except lower extremity artery(ies) for occlusive disease, intracranial, coronary, pulmonary, or dialysis circuit), open or percutaneous, including all imaging and radiological supervision and interpretation necessary to perform the angioplasty within the same artery; initial artery**

EXCLUDES *Intravascular stent placement except lower extremities (37236-37237)*
Revascularization lower extremities (37220-37235)
Stent placement:
Cervical carotid artery (37215-37216)
Intrathoracic carotid or innominate artery (37217-37218)

Code first (37239)

10.1 58.3 **FUD** 000 J G2 50

AMA: 2018,Jan,8; 2017,Aug,10; 2017,Jul,3

+ # **37247** **each additional artery (List separately in addition to code for primary procedure)**

EXCLUDES *Intravascular stent placement except lower extremities (37236-37237)*
Revascularization lower extremities (37220-37235)
Stent placement:
Cervical carotid artery (37215-37216)
Intrathoracic carotid or innominate artery (37217-37218)

Code first ([37246])

4.97 20.5 **FUD** ZZZ N N1 50

AMA: 2018,Jan,8; 2017,Aug,10; 2017,Jul,3

37248 **Transluminal balloon angioplasty (except dialysis circuit), open or percutaneous, including all imaging and radiological supervision and interpretation necessary to perform the angioplasty within the same vein; initial vein**

EXCLUDES *Endovascular venous arterialization with intravascular stent graft(s) in tibial-peroneal segment (0620T)*
Placement intravascular (venous) stent in same vein, same session as (37238-37239)
Revascularization with intravascular stent grafts in femoral-popliteal segment (0505T)

8.64 42.9 **FUD** 000 J G2 50

AMA: 2018,Jan,8; 2017,Aug,10; 2017,Jul,3; 2017,Mar,3

+ # **37249** **each additional vein (List separately in addition to code for primary procedure)**

EXCLUDES *Endovascular venous arterialization with intravascular stent graft(s) in tibial-peroneal segment (0620T)*
Placement intravascular (venous) stent in same vein, same session as (37238-37239)
Revascularization with intravascular stent grafts in femoral-popliteal segment (0505T)

Code first (37239)

4.24 15.6 **FUD** ZZZ N N1 50

AMA: 2018,Jan,8; 2017,Aug,10; 2017,Jul,3; 2017,Mar,3

37236-37239 Endovascular Revascularization Excluding Lower Extremities

INCLUDES Arteriotomy closure by suturing puncture, pressure, or arterial closure device application
Balloon angioplasty
Post-dilation after stent deployment
Predilation performed as primary or secondary angioplasty
Treatment lesion inside same vessel but outside stented portion
Treatment using different-sized balloons to accomplish procedure
Endovascular revascularization arteries and veins other than carotid, coronary, extracranial, intracranial, lower extremities
Imaging once procedure complete
Radiological supervision and interpretation
Stent placement provided as only treatment

EXCLUDES *Angioplasty in unrelated vessel*
Extensive repair or replacement artery (35226, 35286)
Insertion multiple stents in single vessel using more than one code
Intravascular ultrasound (37252-37253)
Mechanical thrombectomy (37184-37188)
Selective and nonselective catheterization (36005, 36010-36015, 36200, 36215-36218, 36245-36248)
Stent placement in:
Cervical carotid artery (37215-37216)
Extracranial vertebral (0075T-0076T)
Hemodialysis circuit (36903, 36905, 36908)
Intracoronary (92928-92929, 92933-92934, 92937-92938, 92941, 92943-92944)
Intracranial (61635)
Intrathoracic common carotid or innominate artery, retrograde or antegrade approach (37218)
Lower extremity arteries for occlusive disease (37221, 37223, 37226-37227, 37230-37231, 37234-37235)
Visceral arteries with fenestrated aortic repair (34841-34848)
Thrombolytic therapy (37211-37214)
Ultrasound guidance (76937)

Code also add-on codes for different vessels treated during same operative session

37236 **Transcatheter placement of an intravascular stent(s) (except lower extremity artery(s) for occlusive disease, cervical carotid, extracranial vertebral or intrathoracic carotid, intracranial, or coronary), open or percutaneous, including radiological supervision and interpretation and including all angioplasty within the same vessel, when performed; initial artery**

EXCLUDES *Procedures in same target treatment zone with (34841-34848)*

12.9 101. **FUD** 000 J J8 80 50

AMA: 2018,Jan,8; 2017,Dec,3; 2017,Jul,3; 2017,Jan,8; 2016,Jul,3; 2016,Jul,6; 2016,Mar,5; 2016,Jan,13; 2015,May,7; 2015,Jan,16

+ **37237** **each additional artery (List separately in addition to code for primary procedure)**

EXCLUDES *Procedures in same target treatment zone with (34841-34848)*

Code first (37236)

6.18 53.2 **FUD** ZZZ N N1 80 50

AMA: 2018,Jan,8; 2017,Dec,3; 2017,Jul,3; 2017,Jan,8; 2016,Jul,6; 2016,Mar,5; 2016,Jan,13; 2015,Jan,16

37238 **Transcatheter placement of an intravascular stent(s), open or percutaneous, including radiological supervision and interpretation and including angioplasty within the same vessel, when performed; initial vein**

EXCLUDES *Endovascular venous arterialization with intravascular stent graft(s) in tibial-peroneal segment (0620T)*
Revascularization with intravascular stent grafts in femoral-popliteal segment (0505T)

8.88 90.3 **FUD** 000 J J8 80 50

AMA: 2018,Jan,8; 2017,Jul,3; 2017,Mar,3; 2017,Jan,8; 2016,Jul,6; 2016,Jun,8

\+ 37239 **each additional vein (List separately in addition to code for primary procedure)**

EXCLUDES *Endovascular venous arterialization with intravascular stent graft(s) in tibial-peroneal segment (0620T)*
Revascularization with intravascular stent grafts in femoral-popliteal segment (0505T)

Code first (37238)

4.43 41.8 FUD ZZZ N N1 80 50

AMA: 2018,Jan,8; 2017,Jul,3; 2017,Mar,3; 2017,Jan,8; 2016,Jul,6

37241-37249 [37246, 37247, 37248, 37249] Therapeutic Vascular Embolization/Occlusion

INCLUDES Embolization or occlusion arteries, lymphatics, and veins except for head/neck and central nervous system
Imaging once procedure complete
Intraprocedural guidance
Radiological supervision and interpretation
Roadmapping
Stent placement provided as support for embolization

EXCLUDES *Embolization code assigned more than once per operative field*
Head, neck, or central nervous system embolization (61624, 61626, 61710)
Multiple codes for indications that overlap, code only indication needing most immediate attention
Stent deployment as primary aneurysm management, pseudoaneurysm, or vascular extravasation
Vein destruction with sclerosing solution (36468-36471)

Code also additional embolization procedure(s) and appropriate modifiers (e.g., modifier 59) when embolization procedures performed in multiple operative fields

Code also diagnostic angiography and catheter placement using modifier 59 when appropriate

37241 **Vascular embolization or occlusion, inclusive of all radiological supervision and interpretation, intraprocedural roadmapping, and imaging guidance necessary to complete the intervention; venous, other than hemorrhage (eg, congenital or acquired venous malformations, venous and capillary hemangiomas, varices, varicoceles)**

EXCLUDES *Embolization side branch(es) outflow vein from hemodialysis access (36909)*
Procedure in same operative field with:
Endovenous ablation therapy incompetent vein (36475-36479)
Injection sclerosing solution; single vein (36470-36471)
Transcatheter embolization procedures (75894, 75898)
Vein destruction (36468-36479 [36465, 36466])

12.7 140. FUD 000 J P2

AMA: 2019,Sep,6; 2018,Mar,3; 2018,Jan,8; 2017,Mar,3; 2017,Jan,8; 2016,Nov,3; 2016,Jan,13; 2015,Nov,3; 2015,Aug,8; 2015,Apr,10; 2015,Jan,16

37242 **arterial, other than hemorrhage or tumor (eg, congenital or acquired arterial malformations, arteriovenous malformations, arteriovenous fistulas, aneurysms, pseudoaneurysms)**

EXCLUDES *Percutaneous treatment pseudoaneurysm extremity (36002)*

13.8 211. FUD 000 J J8

AMA: 2019,Sep,6; 2018,Jul,14; 2018,Mar,3; 2018,Jan,8; 2017,Jan,8; 2016,Jan,13; 2015,Nov,3; 2015,Jan,16

37243 **for tumors, organ ischemia, or infarction**

INCLUDES Embolization uterine fibroids (37244)

EXCLUDES *Procedure in same operative field:*
Angiography (75898)
Transcatheter embolization in same operative field (75894)

Code also chemotherapy when provided with embolization procedure (96420-96425)

Code also injection radioisotopes when provided with embolization procedure (79445)

16.3 273. FUD 000 J G2

AMA: 2019,Sep,6; 2018,Mar,3; 2018,Jan,8; 2017,Jan,8; 2016,Jan,13; 2015,Nov,3; 2015,Jan,16

37244 **for arterial or venous hemorrhage or lymphatic extravasation**

INCLUDES Embolization uterine arteries for hemorrhage

19.3 200. FUD 000 J

AMA: 2019,Sep,6; 2018,Jul,14; 2018,Mar,3; 2018,Jan,8; 2017,Oct,9; 2017,Jan,8; 2016,Jan,13; 2015,Nov,3; 2015,Jan,16

37246 **Resequenced code. See code following 37235.**

37247 **Resequenced code. See code following 37235.**

37248 **Resequenced code. See code following 37235.**

37249 **Resequenced code. See code following 37235.**

37252-37253 Intravascular Ultrasound: Noncoronary

INCLUDES Manipulation and repositioning transducer prior to and after therapeutic interventional procedures

EXCLUDES *Selective or non-selective catheter placement for access (36005-36248)*
Transcatheter procedures (37200, 37236-37239, 37241-37244, 61624, 61626)
Vena cava filter procedures (37191-37193, 37197)

Code first (33361-33369, 33477, 33880-33886, 34701-34708, 34709, [34718], 34710-34711, 34712, 34841-34848, 36010-36015, 36100-36218, 36221-36228, 36245-36248, 36251-36254, 36481, 36555-36571 [36572, 36573], 36578, 36580-36585, 36595, 36901-36909, 37184-37188, 37200, 37211-37218, 37220-37239 [37246, 37247, 37248, 37249], 37241-37244, 61623, 75600-75635, 75705-75774, 75805, 75807, 75810, 75820-75833, 75860-75872, 75885-75898, 75901-75902, 75956-75959, 75970, 76000, 77001, 0075T-0076T, 0234T-0238T, 0338T)

\+ 37252 **Intravascular ultrasound (noncoronary vessel) during diagnostic evaluation and/or therapeutic intervention, including radiological supervision and interpretation; initial noncoronary vessel (List separately in addition to code for primary procedure)**

Code first primary procedure

2.63 33.2 FUD ZZZ N N1 80

AMA: 2019,Nov,6; 2018,Jan,8; 2017,Dec,3; 2017,Aug,10; 2017,Mar,3; 2017,Jan,8; 2016,Jul,6; 2016,May,11

\+ 37253 **each additional noncoronary vessel (List separately in addition to code for primary procedure)**

Code first (37252)

2.11 5.38 FUD ZZZ N N1 80

AMA: 2019,Nov,6; 2018,Jan,8; 2017,Dec,3; 2017,Aug,10; 2017,Mar,3; 2017,Jan,8; 2016,Jul,6; 2016,May,11

37500-37501 Vascular Endoscopic Procedures

INCLUDES Diagnostic endoscopy

EXCLUDES *Open procedure (37760)*

37500 **Vascular endoscopy, surgical, with ligation of perforator veins, subfascial (SEPS)**

18.3 18.3 FUD 090 T A2 50

AMA: 2018,Jan,8; 2017,Jan,8; 2016,Jan,13; 2015,Jan,16

37501 **Unlisted vascular endoscopy procedure**

0.00 0.00 FUD YYY T 50

AMA: 2014,Jan,11; 1997,Nov,1

37565-37606 Ligation Procedures: Jugular Vein, Carotid Arteries

CMS: 100-03,160.8 Electroencephalographic Monitoring During Cerebral Vasculature Surgery

EXCLUDES *Arterial balloon occlusion, endovascular, temporary (61623)*
Suture arteries and veins (35201-35286)
Transcatheter arterial embolization/occlusion, permanent (61624-61626)
Treatment intracranial aneurysm (61703)

37565 **Ligation, internal jugular vein**

20.7 20.7 FUD 090 T 80 50

AMA: 2014,Jan,11; 1997,Nov,1

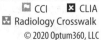

37600 **Ligation; external carotid artery**
21.2 21.2 **FUD** 090 T 80
AMA: 2014,Jan,11; 1997,Nov,1

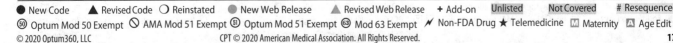

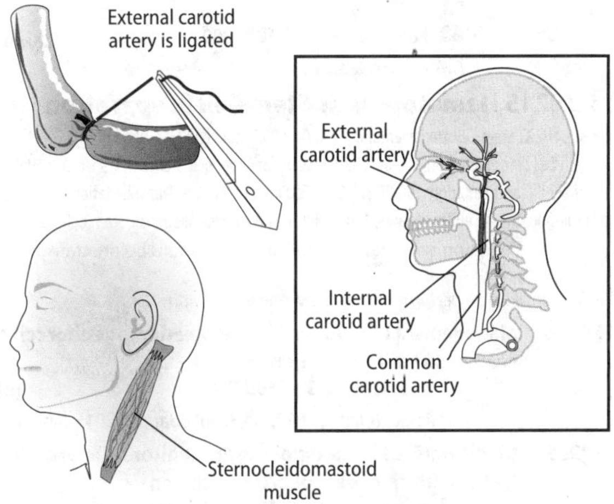

37605 **internal or common carotid artery**
21.4 21.4 **FUD** 090 T 80
AMA: 2014,Jan,11; 1997,Nov,1

37606 **internal or common carotid artery, with gradual occlusion, as with Selverstone or Crutchfield clamp**
20.7 20.7 **FUD** 090 T 80
AMA: 2014,Jan,11; 1997,Nov,1

37607-37609 Ligation Hemodialysis Angioaccess or Temporal Artery

EXCLUDES *Suture arteries and veins (35201-35286)*

37607 **Ligation or banding of angioaccess arteriovenous fistula**
10.8 10.8 **FUD** 090 T A2
AMA: 2014,Jan,11; 1997,Nov,1

37609 **Ligation or biopsy, temporal artery**
5.94 8.94 **FUD** 010 J A2 50
AMA: 2014,Jan,11; 1997,Nov,1

37615-37618 Arterial Ligation, Major Vessel, for Injury/Rupture

EXCLUDES *Suture arteries and veins (35201-35286)*

37615 **Ligation, major artery (eg, post-traumatic, rupture); neck**
INCLUDES Touroff ligation
15.3 15.3 **FUD** 090 T 80
AMA: 2014,Jan,11; 1997,Nov,1

37616 **chest**
INCLUDES Bardenheurer operation
32.0 32.0 **FUD** 090 C 80
AMA: 2014,Jan,11; 1997,Nov,1

37617 **abdomen**
38.6 38.6 **FUD** 090 C 80
AMA: 2018,Jan,8; 2017,Jan,8; 2016,Jan,13; 2015,Jan,16

37618 **extremity**
11.2 11.2 **FUD** 090 C 80
AMA: 2014,Jan,11; 1997,Nov,1

37619 Ligation Inferior Vena Cava

EXCLUDES *Suture arteries and veins (35201-35286)*
Endovascular delivery inferior vena cava filter (37191)

37619 **Ligation of inferior vena cava**
50.1 50.1 **FUD** 090 T 80
AMA: 2018,Jan,8; 2017,Jan,8; 2016,Jan,13; 2015,Jan,16

37650-37660 Venous Ligation, Femoral and Common Iliac

EXCLUDES *Suture arteries and veins (35201-35286)*

37650 **Ligation of femoral vein**
13.2 13.2 **FUD** 090 T A2 50
AMA: 2014,Jan,11; 1997,Nov,1

37660 **Ligation of common iliac vein**
38.3 38.3 **FUD** 090 C 80 50
AMA: 2014,Jan,11; 1997,Nov,1

37700-37785 Treatment of Varicose Veins of Legs

EXCLUDES *Suture arteries and veins (35201-35286)*

37700 **Ligation and division of long saphenous vein at saphenofemoral junction, or distal interruptions**
INCLUDES Babcock operation
EXCLUDES *Ligation, division, and stripping vein (37718, 37722)*
7.08 7.08 **FUD** 090 T A2 50
AMA: 2018,Mar,3; 2018,Jan,8; 2017,Jan,8; 2016,Jan,13; 2015,Jan,16

37718 **Ligation, division, and stripping, short saphenous vein**
EXCLUDES *Ligation, division, and stripping vein (37700, 37735, 37780)*
12.2 12.2 **FUD** 090 T A2 50
AMA: 2018,Mar,3; 2018,Jan,8; 2017,Jan,8

37722 **Ligation, division, and stripping, long (greater) saphenous veins from saphenofemoral junction to knee or below**
EXCLUDES *Ligation, division, and stripping vein (37700, 37718, 37735)*
13.6 13.6 **FUD** 090 T A2 50
AMA: 2018,Mar,3; 2018,Jan,8; 2017,Jan,8

37735 **Ligation and division and complete stripping of long or short saphenous veins with radical excision of ulcer and skin graft and/or interruption of communicating veins of lower leg, with excision of deep fascia**
EXCLUDES *Ligation, division, and stripping vein (37700, 37718, 37722, 37780)*
16.8 16.8 **FUD** 090 T A2 50
AMA: 2018,Mar,3; 2018,Jan,8; 2017,Jan,8; 2016,Jan,13; 2015,Jan,16

37760 **Ligation of perforator veins, subfascial, radical (Linton type), including skin graft, when performed, open,1 leg**
EXCLUDES *Duplex scan extremity veins (93971)*
Ligation subfascial perforator veins, endoscopic (37500)
Ultrasonic guidance (76937, 76942, 76998)
18.0 18.0 **FUD** 090 T A2 50
AMA: 2018,Mar,3; 2018,Jan,8; 2017,Jan,8; 2016,Jan,13; 2015,Jan,16

37761 **Ligation of perforator vein(s), subfascial, open, including ultrasound guidance, when performed, 1 leg**
INCLUDES Ultrasonic guidance (76937, 76942, 76998)
EXCLUDES *Duplex scan extremity veins (93971)*
Ligation subfascial perforator veins, endoscopic (37500)
15.7 15.7 **FUD** 090 T R2 80 50
AMA: 2018,Mar,3; 2018,Jan,8; 2017,Jan,8; 2016,Jan,13; 2015,Jan,16

37765 **Stab phlebectomy of varicose veins, 1 extremity; 10-20 stab incisions**
EXCLUDES *Fewer than 10 incisions (37799)*
More than 20 incisions (37766)
7.88 12.6 **FUD** 010 T P3 50
AMA: 2018,Mar,3; 2018,Jan,8; 2017,Jan,8; 2016,Nov,3; 2016,Jan,13; 2015,Jan,16

37766 **more than 20 incisions**
EXCLUDES *Fewer than 10 incisions (37799)*
10-20 incisions (37765)
15.8 22.0 **FUD** 090 T P3 50
AMA: 2018,Mar,3; 2018,Jan,8; 2017,Jan,8; 2016,Nov,3; 2016,Jan,13; 2015,Jan,16

37780 **Ligation and division of short saphenous vein at saphenopopliteal junction (separate procedure)**
6.75 6.75 FUD 090 T A2 50
AMA: 2018,Jan,8; 2017,Jan,8; 2016,Jan,13; 2015,Jan,16

37785 **Ligation, division, and/or excision of varicose vein cluster(s), 1 leg**
7.45 10.0 FUD 090 T A2 50
AMA: 2018,Jan,8; 2017,Jan,8; 2016,Jan,13; 2015,Jan,16

37788-37790 Treatment of Vascular Disease of the Penis

37788 **Penile revascularization, artery, with or without vein graft** ♂
36.5 36.5 FUD 090 C 80
AMA: 2014,Jan,11; 1997,Nov,1

37790 **Penile venous occlusive procedure**
14.0 14.0 FUD 090 J A2 80
AMA: 2014,Jan,11; 1997,Nov,1

37799 Unlisted Vascular Surgery Procedures

CMS: 100-04,32,161 Intracranial Percutaneous Transluminal Angioplasty (PTA) With Stenting; 100-04,4,180.3 Unlisted Service or Procedure

37799 **Unlisted procedure, vascular surgery**
0.00 0.00 FUD YYY T 80
AMA: 2019,Dec,5; 2019,Nov,6; 2018,Nov,11; 2018,Jan,8; 2017,Jan,8; 2016,Nov,3; 2016,Jan,13; 2015,Apr,10; 2015,Jan,16

38100-38200 Splenic Procedures

38100 **Splenectomy; total (separate procedure)**
33.5 33.5 FUD 090 C 80
AMA: 2018,Jan,8; 2017,Jan,8; 2016,Jan,13; 2015,Jan,16

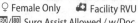

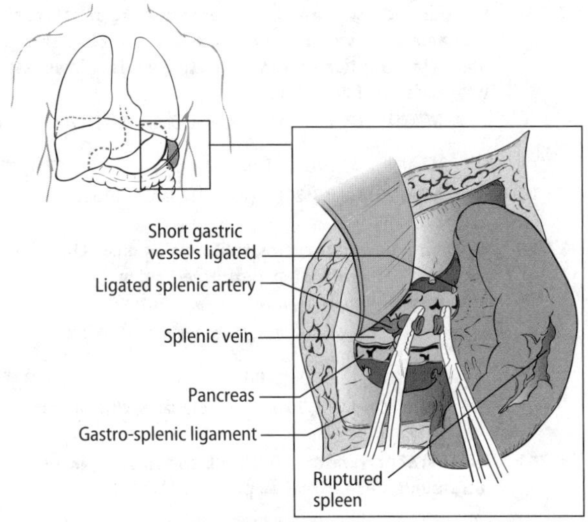

38101 **partial (separate procedure)**
33.5 33.5 FUD 090 C 80
AMA: 2018,Jan,8; 2017,Jan,8; 2016,Jan,13; 2015,Jan,16

+ **38102** **total, en bloc for extensive disease, in conjunction with other procedure (List in addition to code for primary procedure)**
Code first primary procedure
7.63 7.63 FUD ZZZ C 80
AMA: 2018,Jan,8; 2017,Jan,8; 2016,Jan,13; 2015,Jan,16

38115 **Repair of ruptured spleen (splenorrhaphy) with or without partial splenectomy**
37.1 37.1 FUD 090 C 80
AMA: 2018,Jan,8; 2017,Jan,8; 2016,Jan,13; 2015,Jan,16

38120 **Laparoscopy, surgical, splenectomy**
INCLUDES Diagnostic laparoscopy (49320)
30.6 30.6 FUD 090 J 80
AMA: 2018,Jan,8; 2017,Jan,8; 2016,Jan,13; 2015,Jan,16

38129 **Unlisted laparoscopy procedure, spleen**
0.00 0.00 FUD YYY J 80
AMA: 2018,Jan,8; 2017,Jan,8; 2016,Jan,13; 2015,Jan,16

38200 **Injection procedure for splenoportography**
(75810)
3.85 3.85 FUD 000 N N1 80
AMA: 2014,Jan,11

38204-38215 Hematopoietic Stem Cell Preparation

CMS: 100-03,110.23 Stem Cell Transplantation; 100-04,3,90.3 Stem Cell Transplantation; 100-04,3,90.3.1 Allogeneic Stem Cell Transplantation; 100-04,3,90.3.3 Billing for Allogeneic Stem Cell Transplants; 100-04,32,90 Billing for Stem Cell Transplantation; 100-04,32,90.2.1 Coding for Stem Cell Transplantation; 100-04,4,231.10 Billing for Autologous Stem Cell Transplants; 100-04,4,231.11 Billing for Allogeneic Stem Cell Transplants

INCLUDES Preservation, preparation, purification stem cells before transplant or reinfusion

EXCLUDES *Procedure performed more than one time per day*

38204 **Management of recipient hematopoietic progenitor cell donor search and cell acquisition**
3.03 3.03 FUD XXX N N1
AMA: 2018,Jan,8; 2017,Jan,8; 2016,Jan,13; 2015,Jan,16

38205 **Blood-derived hematopoietic progenitor cell harvesting for transplantation, per collection; allogeneic**
2.44 2.44 FUD 000 B 80
AMA: 2018,May,3; 2018,Jan,8; 2017,Jan,8; 2016,Jan,13; 2015,Jan,16

38206 **autologous**
2.39 2.39 FUD 000 S G2 80
AMA: 2018,May,3; 2018,Jan,8; 2017,Jan,8; 2016,Jan,13; 2015,Jan,16

38207 **Transplant preparation of hematopoietic progenitor cells; cryopreservation and storage**
EXCLUDES *Flow cytometry (88182, 88184-88189)*
(88240)
1.31 1.31 FUD XXX S
AMA: 2018,Jan,8; 2017,Jan,8; 2016,Jan,13; 2015,Jan,16

38208 **thawing of previously frozen harvest, without washing, per donor**
EXCLUDES *Flow cytometry (88182, 88184-88189)*
(88241)
0.83 0.83 FUD XXX S
AMA: 2018,Jan,8; 2017,Jan,8; 2016,Jan,13; 2015,Jan,16

38209 **thawing of previously frozen harvest, with washing, per donor**
EXCLUDES *Flow cytometry (88182, 88184-88189)*
0.35 0.35 FUD XXX S
AMA: 2018,Jan,8; 2017,Jan,8; 2016,Jan,13; 2015,Jan,16

38210 **specific cell depletion within harvest, T-cell depletion**
EXCLUDES *Flow cytometry (88182, 88184-88189)*
2.29 2.29 FUD XXX S
AMA: 2018,Jan,8; 2017,Jan,8; 2016,Jan,13; 2015,Jan,16

38211 **tumor cell depletion**
EXCLUDES *Flow cytometry (88182, 88184-88189)*
2.08 2.08 FUD XXX S
AMA: 2018,Jan,8; 2017,Jan,8; 2016,Jan,13; 2015,Jan,16

38212 **red blood cell removal**
EXCLUDES *Flow cytometry (88182, 88184-88189)*
1.39 1.39 FUD XXX S
AMA: 2018,Jan,8; 2017,Jan,8; 2016,Jan,13; 2015,Jan,16

38213 **platelet depletion**
EXCLUDES *Flow cytometry (88182, 88184-88189)*
0.35 0.35 FUD XXX S
AMA: 2018,Jan,8; 2017,Jan,8; 2016,Jan,13; 2015,Jan,16

38214 **plasma (volume) depletion**
EXCLUDES *Flow cytometry (88182, 88184-88189)*
1.23 1.23 FUD XXX S
AMA: 2018,Jan,8; 2017,Jan,8; 2016,Jan,13; 2015,Jan,16

38215 **cell concentration in plasma, mononuclear, or buffy coat layer**

EXCLUDES *Flow cytometry (88182, 88184-88189)*

1.39 1.39 FUD XXX S

AMA: 2018,Jan,8; 2017,Jan,8; 2016,Jan,13; 2015,Jan,16

38220-38232 Bone Marrow Procedures

CMS: 100-03,110.23 Stem Cell Transplantation; 100-04,3,90.3 Stem Cell Transplantation; 100-04,32,90 Billing for Stem Cell Transplantation; 100-04,4,231.11 Billing for Allogeneic Stem Cell Transplants

38220 **Diagnostic bone marrow; aspiration(s)**

EXCLUDES *Aspiration bone marrow for spinal graft (20939)*
Bone marrow biopsy (38221)
Bone marrow for platelet rich stem cell injection (0232T)

Code also biopsy bone marrow during same session (38222)

1.99 4.71 FUD XXX J P3 80 50

AMA: 2018,May,3; 2018,Jan,8; 2017,Jan,8; 2016,Jan,13; 2015,Mar,9; 2015,Jan,16

38221 **biopsy(ies)**

EXCLUDES *Aspiration and biopsy during same session (38222)*
Aspiration bone marrow (38220)

(88305)

2.00 4.47 FUD XXX J P3 80 50

AMA: 2018,May,3; 2018,Jan,8; 2017,Jan,8; 2016,Jan,13; 2015,Mar,9

38222 **biopsy(ies) and aspiration(s)**

EXCLUDES *Aspiration bone marrow only (38221)*
Biopsy bone marrow only (38220)

(88305)

2.24 4.94 FUD XXX J G2 80 50

AMA: 2018,May,3

38230 **Bone marrow harvesting for transplantation; allogeneic**

EXCLUDES *Aspiration bone marrow for platelet rich stem cell injection (0232T)*
Harvesting blood-derived hematopoietic progenitor cells for transplant (allogeneic) (38205)

5.92 5.92 FUD 000 S G2 80

AMA: 2018,Jan,8; 2017,Jan,8; 2016,Jan,13; 2015,Jan,16

38232 **autologous**

EXCLUDES *Aspiration bone marrow (38220, 38222)*
Aspiration bone marrow for platelet rich stem cell injection (0232T)
Aspiration bone marrow for spinal graft (20939)
Harvesting blood-derived peripheral stem cells for transplant (allogenic/autologous) (38205-38206)

5.75 5.75 FUD 000 S G2 80

AMA: 2018,Jan,8; 2017,Jan,8; 2016,Jan,13; 2015,Jan,16

38240-38243 [38243] Hematopoietic Progenitor Cell Transplantation

CMS: 100-03,110.23 Stem Cell Transplantation; 100-04,3,90.3 Stem Cell Transplantation; 100-04,3,90.3.1 Allogeneic Stem Cell Transplantation; 100-04,3,90.3.2 Autologous Stem Cell Transplantation (AuSCT); 100-04,3,90.3.3 Billing for Allogeneic Stem Cell Transplants; 100-04,32,90 Billing for Stem Cell Transplantation; 100-04,32,90.2 Allogeneic Stem Cell Transplantation; 100-04,32,90.2.1 Coding for Stem Cell Transplantation; 100-04,32,90.3 Autologous Stem Cell Transplantation; 100-04,32,90.4 Edits Stem Cell Transplant; 100-04,32,90.6 Clinical Trials for Stem Cell Transplant for Myelodysplastic Syndrome (; 100-04,4,231.10 Billing for Autologous Stem Cell Transplants; 100-04,4,231.11 Billing for Allogeneic Stem Cell Transplants

INCLUDES Evaluation patient prior to, during, and after infusion
Management uncomplicated adverse reactions such as hives or nausea
Monitoring physiological parameters
Physician presence during infusion
Supervision clinical staff

EXCLUDES *Administration fluids for transplant or incidental hydration separately*
Concurrent administration medications with infusion for transplant
Cryopreservation, freezing, and storage hematopoietic progenitor cells for transplant (38207)
Human leukocyte antigen (HLA) testing (81379-81383, 86812-86821)
Modification, treatment, processing hematopoietic progenitor cell specimens for transplant (38210-38215)
Thawing and expansion hematopoietic progenitor cells for transplant (38208-38209)

Code also administration medications and/or fluids not related to transplant with modifier 59

Code also E/M service for treatment more complicated adverse reactions after infusion, as appropriate

Code also separately identifiable E/M service on same date, appending modifier 25 as appropriate (99211-99215, 99217-99220, [99224, 99225, 99226], 99221-99223, 99231-99239, 99471-99472, 99475-99476)

38240 **Hematopoietic progenitor cell (HPC); allogeneic transplantation per donor**

EXCLUDES *Allogeneic lymphocyte infusions on same date of service with (38242)*
Hematopoietic progenitor cell (HPC); HPC boost on same date of service with ([38243])

6.78 6.78 FUD XXX J 80

AMA: 2018,Jan,8; 2017,Jan,8; 2016,Jan,13; 2015,Jan,16

38241 **autologous transplantation**

5.02 5.02 FUD XXX S G2 80

AMA: 2018,Jan,8; 2017,Jan,8; 2016,Jan,13; 2015,Jan,16

\# **38243** **HPC boost**

EXCLUDES *Allogeneic lymphocyte infusions on same date of service with (38242)*
Hematopoietic progenitor cell (HPC); allogeneic transplantation per donor on same date of service with (38240)

3.47 3.47 FUD 000 S R2 80

AMA: 2018,Jan,8; 2017,Jan,8; 2016,Jan,13; 2015,Feb,10; 2015,Jan,16

38242 **Allogeneic lymphocyte infusions**

EXCLUDES *Aspiration bone marrow (38220, 38222)*
Aspiration bone marrow for platelet rich stem cell injection (0232T)
Aspiration bone marrow for spinal graft (20939)
Hematopoietic progenitor cell (HPC); allogeneic transplantation per donor on same date of service with (38240)
Hematopoietic progenitor cell (HPC); HPC boost on same service date with ([38243])

(81379-81383, 86812-86813, 86816-86817, 86821)

3.63 3.63 FUD 000 S R2 80

AMA: 2018,Jan,8; 2017,Jan,8; 2016,Jan,13; 2015,Jan,16

38243 **Resequenced code. See code following 38241.**

38300-38382 Incision Lymphatic Vessels

38300 **Drainage of lymph node abscess or lymphadenitis; simple**

5.91 9.40 FUD 010 J A2

AMA: 2014,Jan,11

38305 **extensive**

14.1 14.1 FUD 090 J A2

AMA: 2014,Jan,11

38308 **Lymphangiotomy or other operations on lymphatic channels**
13.0 13.0 FUD 090 J A2 80
AMA: 2014,Jan,11

38380 **Suture and/or ligation of thoracic duct; cervical approach**
16.3 16.3 FUD 090 C 80
AMA: 2014,Jan,11

38381 **thoracic approach**
23.2 23.2 FUD 090 C 80
AMA: 2014,Jan,11

38382 **abdominal approach**
19.4 19.4 FUD 090 C 80
AMA: 2014,Jan,11

38500-38555 Biopsy/Excision Lymphatic Vessels

EXCLUDES *Injection for sentinel node identification (38792)*
Percutaneous needle biopsy retroperitoneal mass (49180)

38500 **Biopsy or excision of lymph node(s); open, superficial**
EXCLUDES *Lymphadenectomy (38700-38780)*
7.38 9.68 FUD 010 J A2 50
AMA: 2019,Feb,8; 2018,Jan,8; 2017,Jan,8; 2016,Jan,13; 2015,Jan,16

38505 **by needle, superficial (eg, cervical, inguinal, axillary)**
EXCLUDES *Fine needle aspiration (10004-10012, 10021)*
(88172-88173)
(76942, 77002, 77012, 77021)
2.02 3.55 FUD 000 J A2 50
AMA: 2019,Feb,8; 2018,Jan,8; 2017,Jan,8; 2016,Jan,13; 2015,Jan,16

38510 **open, deep cervical node(s)**
12.0 15.1 FUD 010 J A2 50
AMA: 2019,Feb,8; 2018,Jan,8; 2017,Jan,8; 2016,Jan,13; 2015,Jan,16

38520 **open, deep cervical node(s) with excision scalene fat pad**
13.4 13.4 FUD 090 J A2 50
AMA: 2019,Feb,8; 2018,Jan,8; 2017,Jan,8; 2016,Jan,13; 2015,Jan,16

38525 **open, deep axillary node(s)**
12.6 12.6 FUD 090 J A2 50
AMA: 2019,Feb,8; 2018,Jan,8; 2017,Jan,8; 2016,Jan,13; 2015,Mar,5; 2015,Jan,16

38530 **open, internal mammary node(s)**
EXCLUDES *Fine needle aspiration (10005-10012)*
Lymphadenectomy (38720-38746)
16.3 16.3 FUD 090 J A2 80 50
AMA: 2019,Feb,8; 2018,Jan,8; 2017,Jan,8; 2016,Jan,13; 2015,Jan,16

38531 **open, inguinofemoral node(s)**
12.5 12.5 FUD 090 80 50
AMA: 2019,Feb,8

38542 **Dissection, deep jugular node(s)**
EXCLUDES *Complete cervical lymphadenectomy (38720)*
14.8 14.8 FUD 090 J A2 80 50
AMA: 2019,Feb,8; 2018,Jan,8; 2017,Jan,8; 2016,Jan,13; 2015,Jan,16

38550 **Excision of cystic hygroma, axillary or cervical; without deep neurovascular dissection**
14.9 14.9 FUD 090 J A2 80
AMA: 2014,Jan,11; 1994,Win,1

38555 **with deep neurovascular dissection**
29.5 29.5 FUD 090 J A2 80
AMA: 2014,Jan,11; 1994,Win,1

38562-38564 Limited Lymphadenectomy: Staging

38562 **Limited lymphadenectomy for staging (separate procedure); pelvic and para-aortic**
EXCLUDES *Prostatectomy (55812, 55842)*
Radioactive substance inserted into prostate (55862)
20.4 20.4 FUD 090 C 80
AMA: 2019,Feb,8; 2018,Jan,8; 2017,Jan,8; 2016,Jan,13; 2015,Jan,16

38564 **retroperitoneal (aortic and/or splenic)**
20.4 20.4 FUD 090 C 80
AMA: 2019,Feb,8

38570-38589 Laparoscopic Lymph Node Procedures

INCLUDES Diagnostic laparoscopy (49320)
EXCLUDES *Laparoscopy with draining lymphocele to peritoneal cavity (49323)*
Limited lymphadenectomy:
Pelvic (38562)
Retroperitoneal (38564)

38570 **Laparoscopy, surgical; with retroperitoneal lymph node sampling (biopsy), single or multiple**
14.7 14.7 FUD 010 J A2 80
AMA: 2019,Feb,8; 2018,Jan,8; 2017,Jan,8; 2016,Jan,13; 2015,Jan,16

38571 **with bilateral total pelvic lymphadenectomy**
19.1 19.1 FUD 010 J A2 80
AMA: 2019,Feb,8; 2018,Jan,8; 2017,Jan,8; 2016,Jan,13; 2015,Jan,16

38572 **with bilateral total pelvic lymphadenectomy and peri-aortic lymph node sampling (biopsy), single or multiple**
EXCLUDES *Lymphocele drainage into peritoneal cavity (49323)*
26.3 26.3 FUD 010 J A2 80
AMA: 2019,Feb,8; 2018,Jan,8; 2017,Jan,8; 2016,Jan,13; 2015,Jan,13; 2015,Jan,16

38573 **with bilateral total pelvic lymphadenectomy and peri-aortic lymph node sampling, peritoneal washings, peritoneal biopsy(ies), omentectomy, and diaphragmatic washings, including diaphragmatic and other serosal biopsy(ies), when performed**
EXCLUDES *Laparoscopic hysterectomy procedures (58541-58554)*
Laparoscopic omentopexy (separate procedure) (49326)
Laparoscopy abdomen, diagnostic (separate procedure)(49320)
Laparoscopy unlisted (38589)
Laparoscopy without omentectomy (38570-38572)
Lymphadenectomy for staging (38562-38564)
Omentectomy (separate procedure) (49255)
Pelvic lymphadenectomy external iliac, hypogastric, and obturator nodes (38770)
Retroperitoneal lymphadenectomy aortic, pelvic, and renal nodes (separate procedure) (38780)
33.5 33.5 FUD 010 J G2 80
AMA: 2019,Mar,5; 2018,Apr,10

38589 **Unlisted laparoscopy procedure, lymphatic system**
0.00 0.00 FUD YYY J 80 50
AMA: 2018,Apr,10; 2018,Jan,8; 2017,Jan,8; 2016,Jan,13; 2015,Jan,16

38700-38780 Lymphadenectomy Procedures

INCLUDES Lymph node biopsy/excision (38500)
EXCLUDES *Excision lymphedematous skin and subcutaneous tissue (15004-15005)*
Limited lymphadenectomy
Pelvic (38562)
Retroperitoneal (38564)
Repair lymphedematous skin and tissue (15570-15650)

38700 **Suprahyoid lymphadenectomy**
23.1 23.1 FUD 090 J G2 80 50
AMA: 2019,Feb,8; 2018,Jan,8; 2017,Jan,8; 2016,Jan,13; 2015,Jan,16

38720 Cervical lymphadenectomy (complete)
38.5 38.5 **FUD** 090 J 80 50
AMA: 2020,Apr,10; 2019,Feb,8; 2018,Jan,8; 2017,Jan,8; 2016,Jan,13; 2015,Jan,16

38724 Cervical lymphadenectomy (modified radical neck dissection)
41.5 41.5 **FUD** 090 C 80 50
AMA: 2019,Mar,10; 2019,Feb,8; 2018,Jan,8; 2017,Jan,8; 2016,Jan,13; 2015,Jan,16

38740 Axillary lymphadenectomy; superficial
20.2 20.2 **FUD** 090 J A2 80 50
AMA: 2019,Feb,8; 2018,Jan,8; 2017,Jan,8; 2016,Jan,13; 2015,Jan,16

38745 complete
25.4 25.4 **FUD** 090 J A2 80 50
AMA: 2019,Feb,8

\+ **38746 Thoracic lymphadenectomy by thoracotomy, mediastinal and regional lymphadenectomy (List separately in addition to code for primary procedure)**

INCLUDES Left side
- Aortopulmonary window
- Inferior pulmonary ligament
- Paraesophageal
- Subcarinal

Right side
- Inferior pulmonary ligament
- Paraesophageal
- Paratracheal
- Subcarinal

EXCLUDES *Thoracoscopic mediastinal and regional lymphadenectomy (32674)*

Code first (21601, 31760, 31766, 31786, 32096-32200, 32220-32320, 32440-32491, 32503-32505, 33025, 33030, 33050-33130, 39200-39220, 39560-39561, 43101, 43112, 43117-43118, 43122-43123, 43351, 60270, 60505)
6.22 6.22 **FUD** ZZZ C 80
AMA: 2019,Feb,8; 2018,Jan,8; 2017,Jan,8; 2016,Jan,13; 2015,Jan,16

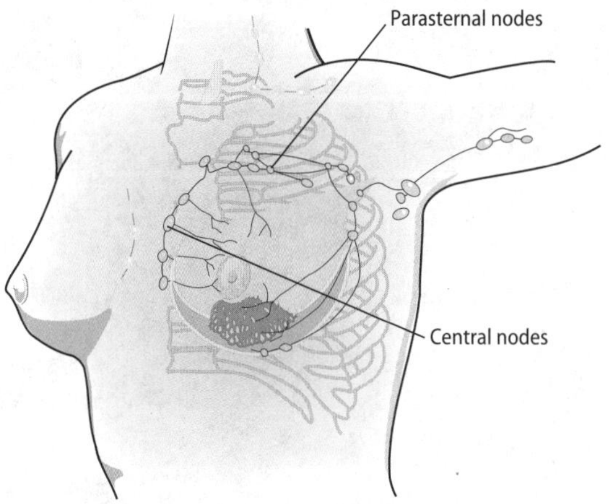

\+ **38747 Abdominal lymphadenectomy, regional, including celiac, gastric, portal, peripancreatic, with or without para-aortic and vena caval nodes (List separately in addition to code for primary procedure)**
Code first primary procedure
7.77 7.77 **FUD** ZZZ C 80
AMA: 2020,Apr,10; 2019,Feb,8

38760 Inguinofemoral lymphadenectomy, superficial, including Cloquet's node (separate procedure)
24.2 24.2 **FUD** 090 J A2 80 50
AMA: 2019,Feb,8; 2018,Jan,8; 2017,Jan,8; 2016,Jan,13; 2015,Jan,16

38765 Inguinofemoral lymphadenectomy, superficial, in continuity with pelvic lymphadenectomy, including external iliac, hypogastric, and obturator nodes (separate procedure)
37.7 37.7 **FUD** 090 C 80 50
AMA: 2019,Feb,8; 2018,Jan,8; 2017,Jan,8; 2016,Jan,13; 2015,Jan,16

38770 Pelvic lymphadenectomy, including external iliac, hypogastric, and obturator nodes (separate procedure)
23.2 23.2 **FUD** 090 C 80 50
AMA: 2019,Feb,8

38780 Retroperitoneal transabdominal lymphadenectomy, extensive, including pelvic, aortic, and renal nodes (separate procedure)
29.9 29.9 **FUD** 090 C 80
AMA: 2019,Feb,8

38790-38999 Cannulation/Injection/Other Procedures

38790 Injection procedure; lymphangiography
(75801-75807)
2.36 2.36 **FUD** 000 N N1 50
AMA: 2014,Jan,11; 1999,Jul,6

38792 radioactive tracer for identification of sentinel node
EXCLUDES *Sentinel node excision (38500-38542)*
Sentinel node(s) identification (mapping) intraoperative with nonradioactive dye injection (38900)
(78195)
0.97 2.37 **FUD** 000 Q1 N1 50
AMA: 2019,Feb,8; 2018,Jan,8; 2017,Jan,8; 2016,Jan,13; 2015,Mar,5; 2015,Jan,16

38794 Cannulation, thoracic duct
8.52 8.52 **FUD** 090 N N1 80
AMA: 2014,Jan,11

\+ **38900 Intraoperative identification (eg, mapping) of sentinel lymph node(s) includes injection of non-radioactive dye, when performed (List separately in addition to code for primary procedure)**
EXCLUDES *Injection tracer for sentinel node identification (38792)*
Code first (19302, 19307, 38500, 38510, 38520, 38525, 38530-38531, 38542, 38562-38564, 38570-38572, 38740, 38745, 38760, 38765, 38770, 38780, 56630-56634, 56637, 56640)
4.03 4.03 **FUD** ZZZ N N1 80 50
AMA: 2019,Feb,8; 2018,Jan,8; 2017,Jan,8; 2016,Jan,13; 2015,Mar,5

38999 Unlisted procedure, hemic or lymphatic system
0.00 0.00 **FUD** YYY S 80
AMA: 2018,Jan,8; 2017,Jan,8; 2016,Jan,13; 2015,Jan,16

39000-39499 Surgical Procedures: Mediastinum

39000 Mediastinotomy with exploration, drainage, removal of foreign body, or biopsy; cervical approach
14.3 14.3 **FUD** 090 C 80
AMA: 2014,Jan,11; 1994,Win,1

39010 transthoracic approach, including either transthoracic or median sternotomy
EXCLUDES *ECMO/ECLS insertion or reposition cannula (33955-33956, [33963, 33964])*
Video-assisted thoracic surgery (VATS) pericardial biopsy (32604)
22.7 22.7 **FUD** 090 C 80
AMA: 2018,Jan,8; 2017,Jan,8; 2016,Jan,13; 2015,Jul,3; 2015,Jan,16

39200 Resection of mediastinal cyst
25.2 25.2 **FUD** 090 C 80
AMA: 2014,Jan,11; 2012,Oct,9-11

39220 Resection of mediastinal tumor

EXCLUDES *Thymectomy (60520)*
Thyroidectomy, substernal (60270)
Video-assisted thoracic surgery (VATS) resection cyst, mass, or tumor of mediastinum (32662)

32.7 32.7 FUD 090 C 80

AMA: 2014,Jan,11; 2012,Oct,9-11

39401 Mediastinoscopy; includes biopsy(ies) of mediastinal mass (eg, lymphoma), when performed

8.93 8.93 FUD 000 J

AMA: 2018,Jan,8; 2017,Jan,8; 2016,Jun,4

39402 with lymph node biopsy(ies) (eg, lung cancer staging)

11.7 11.7 FUD 000 J

AMA: 2018,Jan,8; 2017,Jan,8; 2016,Jun,4

39499 Unlisted procedure, mediastinum

0.00 0.00 FUD YYY C 80

AMA: 2014,Jan,11

39501-39599 Surgical Procedures: Diaphragm

EXCLUDES *Esophagogastric fundoplasty, with fundic patch (43325)*
Repair diaphragmatic (esophageal) hernias:
Laparoscopic with fundoplication (43280-43282)
Laparotomy (43332-43333)
Thoracoabdominal (43336-43337)
Thoracotomy (43334-43335)

39501 Repair, laceration of diaphragm, any approach

24.6 24.6 FUD 090 C 80

AMA: 2018,Jan,8; 2017,Jan,8; 2016,Jan,13; 2015,Jan,16

39503 Repair, neonatal diaphragmatic hernia, with or without chest tube insertion and with or without creation of ventral hernia A

173. 173. FUD 090 63 C 80

AMA: 2018,Jan,8; 2017,Jan,8; 2016,Jan,13; 2015,Jan,16

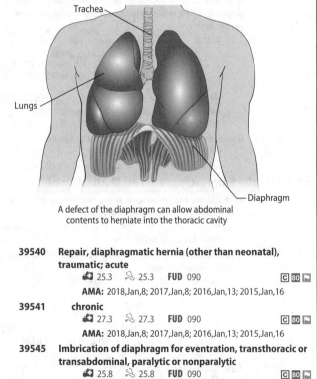

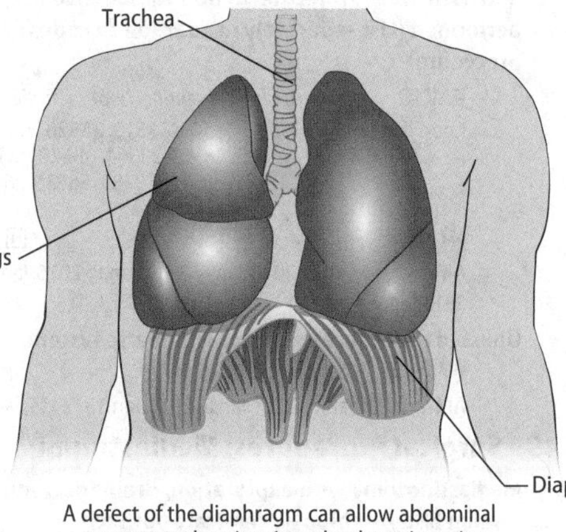

A defect of the diaphragm can allow abdominal contents to herniate into the thoracic cavity

39540 Repair, diaphragmatic hernia (other than neonatal), traumatic; acute

25.3 25.3 FUD 090 C 80

AMA: 2018,Jan,8; 2017,Jan,8; 2016,Jan,13; 2015,Jan,16

39541 chronic

27.3 27.3 FUD 090 C 80

AMA: 2018,Jan,8; 2017,Jan,8; 2016,Jan,13; 2015,Jan,16

39545 Imbrication of diaphragm for eventration, transthoracic or transabdominal, paralytic or nonparalytic

25.8 25.8 FUD 090 C 80

AMA: 2018,Jan,8; 2017,Jan,8; 2016,Jan,13; 2015,Jan,16

39560 Resection, diaphragm; with simple repair (eg, primary suture)

23.1 23.1 FUD 090 C 80

AMA: 2018,Jan,8; 2017,Jan,8; 2016,Jan,13; 2015,Jan,16

39561 with complex repair (eg, prosthetic material, local muscle flap)

35.9 35.9 FUD 090 C 80

AMA: 2018,Jan,8; 2017,Jan,8; 2016,Jan,13; 2015,Jan,16

39599 Unlisted procedure, diaphragm

0.00 0.00 FUD YYY C 80

AMA: 2014,Jan,11

40490-40799 Resection and Repair Procedures of the Lips

EXCLUDES *Procedures on skin of lips — see integumentary section codes*

40490 Biopsy of lip
2.03 3.55 FUD 000 T P3
AMA: 2019,Jan,9

40500 Vermilionectomy (lip shave), with mucosal advancement
10.4 14.7 FUD 090 J A2
AMA: 2014,Jan,11; 2000,Sep,11

40510 Excision of lip; transverse wedge excision with primary closure
EXCLUDES *Excision mucous lesions (40810-40816)*
10.0 13.9 FUD 090 J A2
AMA: 2014,Jan,11

40520 V-excision with primary direct linear closure
EXCLUDES *Excision mucous lesions (40810-40816)*
10.2 14.2 FUD 090 J A2
AMA: 2014,Jan,11; 2000,Sep,11

40525 full thickness, reconstruction with local flap (eg, Estlander or fan)
15.8 15.8 FUD 090 J A2
AMA: 2014,Jan,11

40527 full thickness, reconstruction with cross lip flap (Abbe-Estlander)
INCLUDES Cleft lip repair with cross lip pedicle flap (Abbe-Estlander type), without pedicle sectioning and insertion
EXCLUDES *Cleft lip repair with cross lip pedicle flap (Abbe-Estlander type), with pedicle sectioning and insertion (40761)*
17.7 17.7 FUD 090 J A2 80
AMA: 2014,Jan,11

40530 Resection of lip, more than one-fourth, without reconstruction
EXCLUDES *Reconstruction (13131-13153)*
11.4 15.6 FUD 090 J A2
AMA: 2014,Jan,11

40650 Repair lip, full thickness; vermilion only
8.79 13.2 FUD 090 T A2 80
AMA: 2018,Jan,8; 2017,Jan,8; 2016,Nov,7; 2016,Jan,13; 2015,Jan,16

40652 up to half vertical height
10.2 14.5 FUD 090 T A2 80
AMA: 2018,Jan,8; 2017,Jan,8; 2016,Nov,7; 2016,Jan,13; 2015,Jan,16

40654 over one-half vertical height, or complex
12.1 16.5 FUD 090 T A2
AMA: 2018,Jan,8; 2017,Jan,8; 2016,Nov,7

40700 Plastic repair of cleft lip/nasal deformity; primary, partial or complete, unilateral
EXCLUDES *Cleft lip repair with cross lip pedicle flap (Abbe-Estlander type):*
With pedicle sectioning and insertion (40761)
Without pedicle sectioning and insertion (40527)
Rhinoplasty for nasal deformity secondary to congenital cleft lip (30460, 30462)
29.2 29.2 FUD 090 J A2 80
AMA: 2018,Jan,8; 2017,Jan,8; 2016,Jan,13; 2015,Jan,16

40701 primary bilateral, 1-stage procedure
EXCLUDES *Cleft lip repair with cross lip pedicle flap (Abbe-Estlander type):*
With pedicle sectioning and insertion (40761)
Without pedicle sectioning and insertion (40527)
Rhinoplasty for nasal deformity secondary to congenital cleft lip (30460, 30462)
34.6 34.6 FUD 090 J A2 80
AMA: 2018,Jan,8; 2017,Jan,8; 2016,Jan,13; 2015,Jan,16

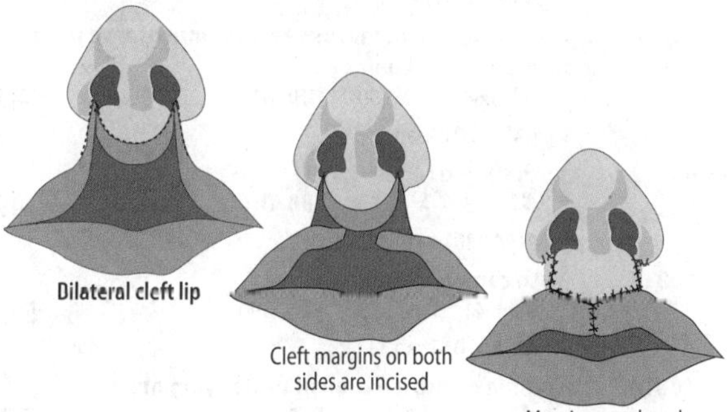
Dilateral cleft lip
Cleft margins on both sides are incised
Margins are closed, correcting cleft

40702 primary bilateral, 1 of 2 stages
EXCLUDES *Cleft lip repair with cross lip pedicle flap (Abbe-Estlander type):*
With pedicle sectioning and insertion (40761)
Without pedicle sectioning and insertion (40527)
Rhinoplasty for nasal deformity secondary to congenital cleft lip (30460, 30462)
29.0 29.0 FUD 090 J R2 80
AMA: 2018,Jan,8; 2017,Jan,8; 2016,Jan,13; 2015,Jan,16

40720 secondary, by recreation of defect and reclosure
EXCLUDES *Cleft lip repair with cross lip pedicle flap (Abbe-Estlander type):*
With pedicle sectioning and insertion (40761)
Without pedicle sectioning and insertion (40527)
Rhinoplasty for nasal deformity secondary to congenital cleft lip (30460, 30462)
29.8 29.8 FUD 090 J A2 80 50
AMA: 2018,Jan,8; 2017,Jan,8; 2016,Jan,13; 2015,Jan,16

40761 with cross lip pedicle flap (Abbe-Estlander type), including sectioning and inserting of pedicle
EXCLUDES *Cleft lip repair with cross lip pedicle flap (Abbe-Estlander type) without sectioning and insertion pedicle (40527)*
Cleft palate repair (42200-42225)
Other reconstructive procedures (14060-14061, 15120-15261, 15574, 15576, 15630)
31.3 31.3 FUD 090 J A2
AMA: 2014,Jan,11

40799 Unlisted procedure, lips
0.00 0.00 FUD YYY T 80
AMA: 2014,Jan,11

40800-40819 Incision and Resection of Buccal Cavity

INCLUDES Mucosal/submucosal tissue of lips/cheeks
Oral cavity outside dentoalveolar structures

40800 Drainage of abscess, cyst, hematoma, vestibule of mouth; simple
3.56 5.96 FUD 010 T P3
AMA: 2014,Jan,11

40801 complicated
5.96 8.59 FUD 010 T A2
AMA: 2014,Jan,11

40804 Removal of embedded foreign body, vestibule of mouth; simple
3.36 5.47 FUD 010 Q1 N1 80
AMA: 2014,Jan,11

40805 complicated
6.43 8.91 **FUD** 010 T P3 80
AMA: 2014,Jan,11

40806 Incision of labial frenum (frenotomy)
0.87 2.84 **FUD** 000 T P3 80
AMA: 2014,Jan,11

40808 Biopsy, vestibule of mouth
2.47 4.54 **FUD** 010 T P3
AMA: 2019,Jan,9

40810 Excision of lesion of mucosa and submucosa, vestibule of mouth; without repair
3.64 5.99 **FUD** 010 J P3
AMA: 2014,Jan,11

40812 with simple repair
5.63 8.30 **FUD** 010 J P3
AMA: 2014,Jan,11

40814 with complex repair
8.41 10.8 **FUD** 090 J A2
AMA: 2014,Jan,11

40816 complex, with excision of underlying muscle
8.81 11.4 **FUD** 090 J A2
AMA: 2014,Jan,11

40818 Excision of mucosa of vestibule of mouth as donor graft
7.78 10.4 **FUD** 090 T A2 80
AMA: 2014,Jan,11

40819 Excision of frenum, labial or buccal (frenumectomy, frenulectomy, frenectomy)
6.07 8.06 **FUD** 090 T A2 80
AMA: 2020,Aug,14

40820 Destruction of Lesion of Buccal Cavity

CMS: 100-03,140.5 Laser Procedures

INCLUDES Mucosal/submucosal tissue lips/cheeks
Oral cavity outside dentoalveolar structures

40820 Destruction of lesion or scar of vestibule of mouth by physical methods (eg, laser, thermal, cryo, chemical)
4.91 7.54 **FUD** 010 J P3
AMA: 2014,Jan,11; 1997,Nov,1

40830-40899 Repair Procedures of the Buccal Cavity

INCLUDES Mucosal/submucosal tissue lips/cheeks
Oral cavity outside dentoalveolar structures

EXCLUDES *Skin grafts (15002-15630)*

40830 Closure of laceration, vestibule of mouth; 2.5 cm or less
4.84 7.98 **FUD** 010 T G2 80
AMA: 2014,Jan,11

40831 over 2.5 cm or complex
6.64 10.1 **FUD** 010 T A2 80
AMA: 2014,Jan,11

40840 Vestibuloplasty; anterior
18.0 23.9 **FUD** 090 J A2 80
AMA: 2014,Jan,11

40842 posterior, unilateral
19.5 26.2 **FUD** 090 J A2 80
AMA: 2014,Jan,11

40843 posterior, bilateral
23.6 30.1 **FUD** 090 J A2 80
AMA: 2014,Jan,11

40844 entire arch
34.2 42.9 **FUD** 090 J A2 80
AMA: 2014,Jan,11

40845 complex (including ridge extension, muscle repositioning)
35.2 42.2 **FUD** 090 J A2 80
AMA: 2014,Jan,11

40899 Unlisted procedure, vestibule of mouth
0.00 0.00 **FUD** YYY T 80
AMA: 2014,Jan,11

41000-41018 Surgical Incision of Floor of Mouth or Tongue

EXCLUDES *Frenoplasty (41520)*

41000 Intraoral incision and drainage of abscess, cyst, or hematoma of tongue or floor of mouth; lingual
3.13 4.54 **FUD** 010 T P3
AMA: 2014,Jan,11

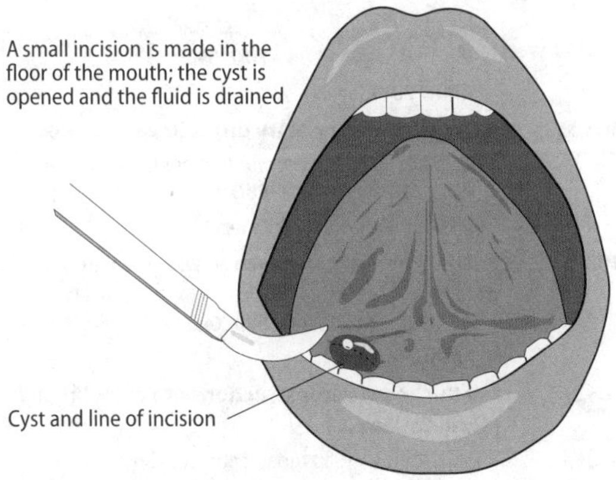

41005 sublingual, superficial
3.30 6.20 **FUD** 010 T A2 80
AMA: 2014,Jan,11

41006 sublingual, deep, supramylohyoid
6.85 9.81 **FUD** 090 T A2 80
AMA: 2014,Jan,11

41007 submental space
6.64 9.63 **FUD** 090 T A2 80
AMA: 2014,Jan,11

41008 submandibular space
7.45 10.9 **FUD** 090 J A2 80
AMA: 2014,Jan,11

41009 masticator space
8.19 11.8 **FUD** 090 T A2 80
AMA: 2014,Jan,11

41010 Incision of lingual frenum (frenotomy)
3.09 5.97 **FUD** 010 T A2 80
AMA: 2020,Aug,14; 2018,Jan,8; 2017,Nov,10; 2017,Sep,14

41015 Extraoral incision and drainage of abscess, cyst, or hematoma of floor of mouth; sublingual
8.92 11.6 **FUD** 090 T A2 80
AMA: 2014,Jan,11

41016 submental
9.92 13.0 **FUD** 090 J A2 80
AMA: 2014,Jan,11

41017 submandibular
9.86 12.9 **FUD** 090 J A2 80
AMA: 2014,Jan,11

41018 masticator space
11.4 14.5 **FUD** 090 T A2 80
AMA: 2014,Jan,11

41019 Placement of Devices for Brachytherapy

EXCLUDES *Application interstitial radioelements (77770-77772, 77778)*
Intracranial brachytherapy radiation sources with stereotactic insertion (61770)

41019 **Placement of needles, catheters, or other device(s) into the head and/or neck region (percutaneous, transoral, or transnasal) for subsequent interstitial radioelement application**
(76942, 77002, 77012, 77021)
13.9 13.9 FUD 000 J G2 80
AMA: 2018,Jan,8; 2017,Jan,8; 2016,Jan,13; 2015,Jan,16

41100-41599 Resection and Repair of the Tongue

41100 **Biopsy of tongue; anterior two-thirds**
3.07 4.94 FUD 010 T P3
AMA: 2019,Jan,9

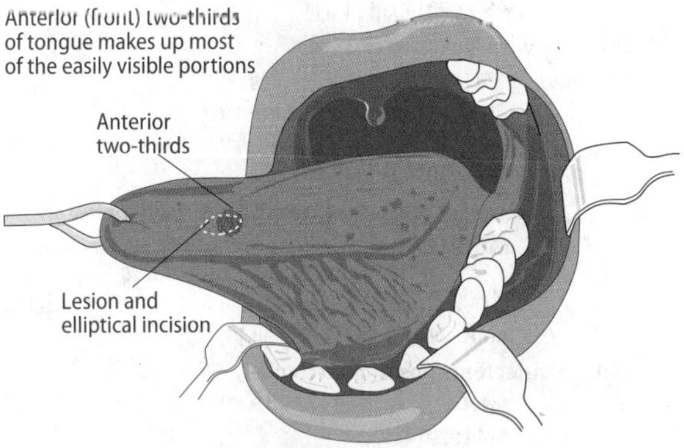

41105 **posterior one-third**
3.11 5.05 FUD 010 J P3
AMA: 2014,Jan,11

41108 **Biopsy of floor of mouth**
2.52 4.43 FUD 010 J P3
AMA: 2019,Jan,9

41110 **Excision of lesion of tongue without closure**
3.73 6.29 FUD 010 J P3
AMA: 2014,Jan,11

41112 **Excision of lesion of tongue with closure; anterior two-thirds**
7.03 9.57 FUD 090 J A2
AMA: 2014,Jan,11

41113 **posterior one-third**
7.98 10.5 FUD 090 J A2
AMA: 2014,Jan,11

41114 **with local tongue flap**
INCLUDES Excision lesion tongue with closure anterior/posterior two-thirds (41112-41113)
17.7 17.7 FUD 090 J A2 80
AMA: 2014,Jan,11

41115 **Excision of lingual frenum (frenectomy)**
4.16 7.25 FUD 010 T P3 80
AMA: 2018,Jan,8; 2017,Nov,10; 2017,Sep,14

41116 **Excision, lesion of floor of mouth**
6.18 9.50 FUD 090 J A2
AMA: 2014,Jan,11

41120 **Glossectomy; less than one-half tongue**
30.3 30.3 FUD 090 J A2 80
AMA: 2018,Jan,8; 2017,Jan,8; 2016,Jan,13; 2015,Jan,16

41130 **hemiglossectomy**
38.0 38.0 FUD 090 C 80
AMA: 2018,Jan,8; 2017,Jan,8; 2016,Jan,13; 2015,Jan,16

41135 **partial, with unilateral radical neck dissection**
62.0 62.0 FUD 090 C 80
AMA: 2018,Jan,8; 2017,Jan,8; 2016,Jan,13; 2015,Jan,16

41140 **complete or total, with or without tracheostomy, without radical neck dissection**
INCLUDES Regnoli's excision
62.3 62.3 FUD 090 C 80
AMA: 2018,Jan,8; 2017,Jan,8; 2016,Jan,13; 2015,Jan,16

41145 **complete or total, with or without tracheostomy, with unilateral radical neck dissection**
78.9 78.9 FUD 090 C 80
AMA: 2018,Jan,8; 2017,Jan,8; 2016,Jan,13; 2015,Jan,16

41150 **composite procedure with resection floor of mouth and mandibular resection, without radical neck dissection**
62.8 62.8 FUD 090 C 80
AMA: 2018,Jan,8; 2017,Jan,8; 2016,Jan,13; 2015,Jan,16

41153 **composite procedure with resection floor of mouth, with suprahyoid neck dissection**
68.8 68.8 FUD 090 C 80
AMA: 2018,Jan,8; 2017,Jan,8; 2016,Jan,13; 2015,Jan,16

41155 **composite procedure with resection floor of mouth, mandibular resection, and radical neck dissection (Commando type)**
86.1 86.1 FUD 090 C 80
AMA: 2018,Jan,8; 2017,Jan,8; 2016,Jan,13; 2015,Jan,16

41250 **Repair of laceration 2.5 cm or less; floor of mouth and/or anterior two-thirds of tongue**
4.43 7.98 FUD 010 Q1 N1 80
AMA: 2014,Jan,11

41251 **posterior one-third of tongue**
5.27 8.83 FUD 010 T A2 80
AMA: 2014,Jan,11

41252 **Repair of laceration of tongue, floor of mouth, over 2.6 cm or complex**
6.01 9.18 FUD 010 T A2 80
AMA: 2014,Jan,11

41510 **Suture of tongue to lip for micrognathia (Douglas type procedure)**
13.0 13.0 FUD 090 J A2 80
AMA: 2018,Jan,8; 2017,Jan,8; 2016,Jan,13; 2015,Jan,16

41512 **Tongue base suspension, permanent suture technique**
EXCLUDES *Suture tongue to lip for micrognathia (41510)*
18.8 18.8 FUD 090 J G2 80
AMA: 2018,Jan,8; 2017,Jan,8; 2016,Jan,13; 2015,Jan,16

41520 **Frenoplasty (surgical revision of frenum, eg, with Z-plasty)**
EXCLUDES *Frenotomy (40806, 41010)*
7.11 10.1 FUD 090 J A2 80
AMA: 2020,Aug,14; 2018,Jan,8; 2017,Nov,10; 2017,Sep,14

41530 **Submucosal ablation of the tongue base, radiofrequency, 1 or more sites, per session**
10.6 27.1 FUD 000 J P3 80
AMA: 2018,Jan,8; 2017,Jan,8; 2016,Jan,13; 2015,Jan,16

41599 **Unlisted procedure, tongue, floor of mouth**
0.00 0.00 FUD YYY T 80
AMA: 2018,Jan,8; 2017,Jan,8; 2016,Jan,13; 2015,Jan,16

41800-41899 Procedures of the Teeth and Supporting Structures

41800 **Drainage of abscess, cyst, hematoma from dentoalveolar structures**
4.35 8.29 FUD 010 Q1 N1
AMA: 2014,Jan,11

41805 **Removal of embedded foreign body from dentoalveolar structures; soft tissues**
5.42 8.45 FUD 010 T P3 80
AMA: 2014,Jan,11

41806 **bone**
7.86 11.4 FUD 010 T P3 80
AMA: 2014,Jan,11

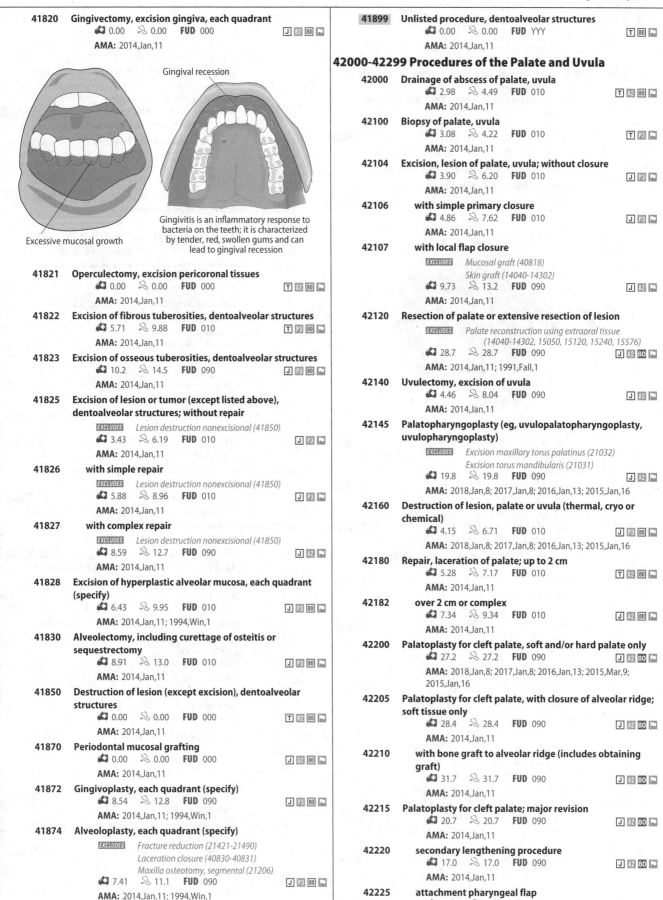

41820 **Gingivectomy, excision gingiva, each quadrant**
0.00 0.00 FUD 000 J R2 80
AMA: 2014,Jan,11

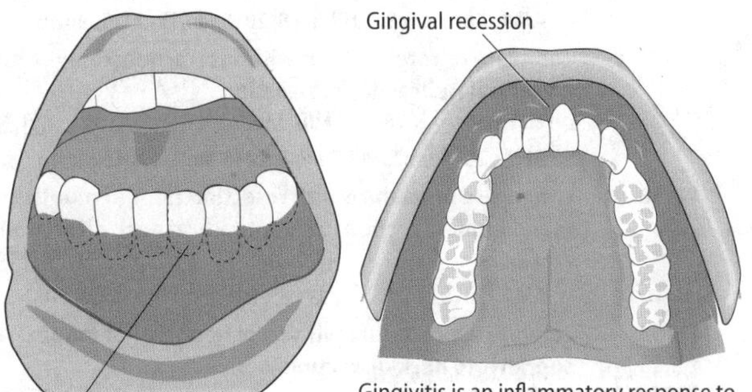

Gingivitis is an inflammatory response to bacteria on the teeth; it is characterized by tender, red, swollen gums and can lead to gingival recession

41821 **Operculectomy, excision pericoronal tissues**
0.00 0.00 FUD 000 T G2 80
AMA: 2014,Jan,11

41822 **Excision of fibrous tuberosities, dentoalveolar structures**
5.71 9.88 FUD 010 T P3 80
AMA: 2014,Jan,11

41823 **Excision of osseous tuberosities, dentoalveolar structures**
10.2 14.5 FUD 090 J P3 80
AMA: 2014,Jan,11

41825 **Excision of lesion or tumor (except listed above), dentoalveolar structures; without repair**
EXCLUDES *Lesion destruction nonexcisional (41850)*
3.43 6.19 FUD 010 J P3
AMA: 2014,Jan,11

41826 **with simple repair**
EXCLUDES *Lesion destruction nonexcisional (41850)*
5.88 8.96 FUD 010 J P3
AMA: 2014,Jan,11

41827 **with complex repair**
EXCLUDES *Lesion destruction nonexcisional (41850)*
8.59 12.7 FUD 090 J A2
AMA: 2014,Jan,11

41828 **Excision of hyperplastic alveolar mucosa, each quadrant (specify)**
6.43 9.95 FUD 010 J P3 80
AMA: 2014,Jan,11; 1994,Win,1

41830 **Alveolectomy, including curettage of osteitis or sequestrectomy**
8.91 13.0 FUD 010 J P3 80
AMA: 2014,Jan,11

41850 **Destruction of lesion (except excision), dentoalveolar structures**
0.00 0.00 FUD 000 T R2 80
AMA: 2014,Jan,11

41870 **Periodontal mucosal grafting**
0.00 0.00 FUD 000 J G2 80
AMA: 2014,Jan,11

41872 **Gingivoplasty, each quadrant (specify)**
8.54 12.8 FUD 090 J P3 80
AMA: 2014,Jan,11; 1994,Win,1

41874 **Alveoloplasty, each quadrant (specify)**
EXCLUDES *Fracture reduction (21421-21490)*
Laceration closure (40830-40831)
Maxilla osteotomy, segmental (21206)
7.41 11.1 FUD 090 J P3 80
AMA: 2014,Jan,11; 1994,Win,1

41899 **Unlisted procedure, dentoalveolar structures**
0.00 0.00 FUD YYY T 80
AMA: 2014,Jan,11

42000-42299 Procedures of the Palate and Uvula

42000 **Drainage of abscess of palate, uvula**
2.98 4.49 FUD 010 T A2 80
AMA: 2014,Jan,11

42100 **Biopsy of palate, uvula**
3.08 4.22 FUD 010 T P3
AMA: 2014,Jan,11

42104 **Excision, lesion of palate, uvula; without closure**
3.90 6.20 FUD 010 J P3
AMA: 2014,Jan,11

42106 **with simple primary closure**
4.86 7.62 FUD 010 J P3
AMA: 2014,Jan,11

42107 **with local flap closure**
EXCLUDES *Mucosal graft (40818)*
Skin graft (14040-14302)
9.73 13.2 FUD 090 J A2
AMA: 2014,Jan,11

42120 **Resection of palate or extensive resection of lesion**
EXCLUDES *Palate reconstruction using extraoral tissue (14040-14302, 15050, 15120, 15240, 15576)*
28.7 28.7 FUD 090 J A2 80
AMA: 2014,Jan,11; 1991,Fall,1

42140 **Uvulectomy, excision of uvula**
4.46 8.04 FUD 090 J A2
AMA: 2014,Jan,11

42145 **Palatopharyngoplasty (eg, uvulopalatopharyngoplasty, uvulopharyngoplasty)**
EXCLUDES *Excision maxillary torus palatinus (21032)*
Excision torus mandibularis (21031)
19.8 19.8 FUD 090 J A2
AMA: 2018,Jan,8; 2017,Jan,8; 2016,Jan,13; 2015,Jan,16

42160 **Destruction of lesion, palate or uvula (thermal, cryo or chemical)**
4.15 6.71 FUD 010 J P3 80
AMA: 2018,Jan,8; 2017,Jan,8; 2016,Jan,13; 2015,Jan,16

42180 **Repair, laceration of palate; up to 2 cm**
5.28 7.17 FUD 010 T A2 80
AMA: 2014,Jan,11

42182 **over 2 cm or complex**
7.34 9.34 FUD 010 J A2 80
AMA: 2014,Jan,11

42200 **Palatoplasty for cleft palate, soft and/or hard palate only**
27.2 27.2 FUD 090 J A2 80
AMA: 2018,Jan,8; 2017,Jan,8; 2016,Jan,13; 2015,Mar,9; 2015,Jan,16

42205 **Palatoplasty for cleft palate, with closure of alveolar ridge; soft tissue only**
28.4 28.4 FUD 090 J A2 80
AMA: 2014,Jan,11

42210 **with bone graft to alveolar ridge (includes obtaining graft)**
31.7 31.7 FUD 090 J A2 80
AMA: 2014,Jan,11

42215 **Palatoplasty for cleft palate; major revision**
20.7 20.7 FUD 090 J A2 80
AMA: 2014,Jan,11

42220 **secondary lengthening procedure**
17.0 17.0 FUD 090 J A2 80
AMA: 2014,Jan,11

42225 **attachment pharyngeal flap**
28.2 28.2 FUD 090 J G2 80
AMA: 2018,Jan,8; 2017,Jan,8; 2016,Jan,13; 2015,Jan,16

42226 **Lengthening of palate, and pharyngeal flap**
25.3 25.3 FUD 090 J A2 80
AMA: 2014,Jan,11

42227 **Lengthening of palate, with island flap**
23.6 23.6 FUD 090 J G2 80
AMA: 2014,Jan,11

42235 **Repair of anterior palate, including vomer flap**
EXCLUDES *Oronasal fistula repair (30600)*
20.7 20.7 FUD 090 J A2 80
AMA: 2018,Jan,8; 2017,Jan,8; 2016,Jan,13; 2015,Mar,9; 2015,Jan,16

42260 **Repair of nasolabial fistula**
EXCLUDES *Cleft lip repair (40700-40761)*
18.9 23.8 FUD 090 J A2 80
AMA: 2014,Jan,11

42280 **Maxillary impression for palatal prosthesis**
3.12 5.08 FUD 010 T P3 80
AMA: 2014,Jan,11

42281 **Insertion of pin-retained palatal prosthesis**
4.75 6.56 FUD 010 J G2 80
AMA: 2014,Jan,11

42299 **Unlisted procedure, palate, uvula**
0.00 0.00 FUD YYY T 80
AMA: 2018,Jan,8; 2017,Jan,8; 2016,Jan,13; 2015,Jan,16

42300-42699 Procedures of the Salivary Ducts and Glands

42300 **Drainage of abscess; parotid, simple**
4.39 6.10 FUD 010 T A2
AMA: 2014,Jan,11

42305 **parotid, complicated**
12.2 12.2 FUD 090 J A2 80
AMA: 2014,Jan,11

42310 **Drainage of abscess; submaxillary or sublingual, intraoral**
3.92 5.08 FUD 010 T A2 80
AMA: 2014,Jan,11

42320 **submaxillary, external**
5.03 7.31 FUD 010 T A2 80
AMA: 2014,Jan,11

42330 **Sialolithotomy; submandibular (submaxillary), sublingual or parotid, uncomplicated, intraoral**
4.69 6.63 FUD 010 J P3
AMA: 2014,Jan,11

42335 **submandibular (submaxillary), complicated, intraoral**
7.37 11.5 FUD 090 J P3
AMA: 2014,Jan,11

42340 **parotid, extraoral or complicated intraoral**
9.65 14.1 FUD 090 J A2 80 50
AMA: 2014,Jan,11

42400 **Biopsy of salivary gland; needle**
EXCLUDES *Fine needle aspiration (10021, [10004, 10005, 10006, 10007, 10008, 10009, 10010, 10011, 10012])*
(76942, 77002, 77012, 77021)
(88172-88173)
1.55 2.95 FUD 000 T P3
AMA: 2019,Apr,4

42405 **incisional**
(76942, 77002, 77012, 77021)
6.48 8.61 FUD 010 J A2
AMA: 2014,Jan,11

42408 **Excision of sublingual salivary cyst (ranula)**
10.0 15.0 FUD 090 J A2 80
AMA: 2014,Jan,11

42409 **Marsupialization of sublingual salivary cyst (ranula)**
6.42 10.4 FUD 090 J A2 80
AMA: 2014,Jan,11

42410 **Excision of parotid tumor or parotid gland; lateral lobe, without nerve dissection**
EXCLUDES *Facial nerve suture or graft (64864, 64865, 69740, 69745)*
17.9 17.9 FUD 090 J A2 80 50
AMA: 2014,Jan,11

42415 **lateral lobe, with dissection and preservation of facial nerve**
EXCLUDES *Facial nerve suture or graft (64864, 64865, 69740, 69745)*
30.2 30.2 FUD 090 J A2 80 50
AMA: 2014,Jan,11

42420 **total, with dissection and preservation of facial nerve**
EXCLUDES *Facial nerve suture or graft (64864, 64865, 69740, 69745)*
33.9 33.9 FUD 090 J A2 80 50
AMA: 2014,Jan,11; 2010,Aug,3-7

42425 **total, en bloc removal with sacrifice of facial nerve**
EXCLUDES *Facial nerve suture or graft (64864, 64865, 69740, 69745)*
23.9 23.9 FUD 090 J A2 80 50
AMA: 2014,Jan,11

42426 **total, with unilateral radical neck dissection**
EXCLUDES *Facial nerve suture or graft (64864, 64865, 69740, 69745)*
38.8 38.8 FUD 090 C 80 50
AMA: 2018,Jan,8; 2017,Jan,8; 2016,Jan,13; 2015,Jan,16

42440 **Excision of submandibular (submaxillary) gland**
11.8 11.8 FUD 090 J A2 80 50
AMA: 2014,Jan,11

42450 **Excision of sublingual gland**
10.3 13.1 FUD 090 J A2 80
AMA: 2014,Jan,11

42500 **Plastic repair of salivary duct, sialodochoplasty; primary or simple**
9.71 12.4 FUD 090 J A2 80
AMA: 2014,Jan,11

42505 **secondary or complicated**
12.9 15.9 FUD 090 J A2
AMA: 2014,Jan,11

42507 **Parotid duct diversion, bilateral (Wilke type procedure);**
14.4 14.4 FUD 090 J A2 80
AMA: 2014,Jan,11

42509 **with excision of both submandibular glands**
23.6 23.6 FUD 090 J A2 80
AMA: 2014,Jan,11

42510 **with ligation of both submandibular (Wharton's) ducts**
17.5 17.5 FUD 090 J A2 80
AMA: 2014,Jan,11

42550 **Injection procedure for sialography**
(70390)
1.83 4.39 FUD 000 N N1
AMA: 2014,Jan,11

42600 **Closure salivary fistula**
9.99 14.5 FUD 090 J A2 80
AMA: 2014,Jan,11

42650 **Dilation salivary duct**
1.65 2.25 FUD 000 T P3
AMA: 2014,Jan,11

42660 **Dilation and catheterization of salivary duct, with or without injection**
2.52 3.52 FUD 000 T P3 80
AMA: 2014,Jan,11

42665 **Ligation salivary duct, intraoral**
5.97 9.82 FUD 090 J A2 80
AMA: 2014,Jan,11

Digestive System *(left margin)*

42699 — 42860 *(left margin)*

42699 Unlisted procedure, salivary glands or ducts
🚑 0.00 ⚕ 0.00 **FUD** YYY
T 80 ▢
AMA: 2014,Jan,11

42700-42999 Procedures of the Adenoids/Throat/Tonsils

42700 Incision and drainage abscess; peritonsillar
🚑 3.88 ⚕ 5.43 **FUD** 010
T A2 ▢
AMA: 2014,Jan,11

42720 retropharyngeal or parapharyngeal, intraoral approach
🚑 11.1 ⚕ 12.9 **FUD** 010
J A2 80 ▢
AMA: 2014,Jan,11

42725 retropharyngeal or parapharyngeal, external approach
🚑 23.0 ⚕ 23.0 **FUD** 090
J A2 80 ▢
AMA: 2014,Jan,11

42800 Biopsy; oropharynx
EXCLUDES Laryngoscopy with biopsy (31510, 31535-31536)
🚑 3.22 ⚕ 4.49 **FUD** 010
J P3 ▢
AMA: 2014,Jan,11

42804 nasopharynx, visible lesion, simple
EXCLUDES Laryngoscopy with biopsy (31510, 31535-31536)
🚑 3.27 ⚕ 5.65 **FUD** 010
J A2 ▢
AMA: 2014,Jan,11

42806 nasopharynx, survey for unknown primary lesion
EXCLUDES Laryngoscopy with biopsy (31510, 31535-31536)
🚑 3.81 ⚕ 6.33 **FUD** 010
J A2 ▢
AMA: 2014,Jan,11

42808 Excision or destruction of lesion of pharynx, any method
🚑 4.66 ⚕ 6.53 **FUD** 010
J A2 ▢
AMA: 2014,Jan,11

42809 Removal of foreign body from pharynx
🚑 3.56 ⚕ 5.76 **FUD** 010
Q1 N1 ▢
AMA: 2014,Jan,11

Choanae
Plane of view
Nasopharynx
Parotid gland
Nasal septum
Oropharynx
Submandibular gland
Root of tongue
Laryngopharynx
Epiglottis
Esophagus
Trachea

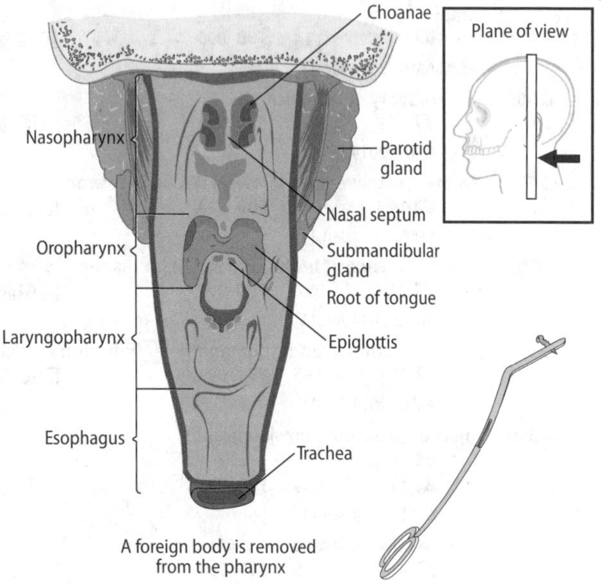

A foreign body is removed from the pharynx

42810 Excision branchial cleft cyst or vestige, confined to skin and subcutaneous tissues
🚑 8.10 ⚕ 11.0 **FUD** 090
J A2 80 50 ▢
AMA: 2014,Jan,11

42815 Excision branchial cleft cyst, vestige, or fistula, extending beneath subcutaneous tissues and/or into pharynx
🚑 15.6 ⚕ 15.6 **FUD** 090
J A2 80 50 ▢
AMA: 2014,Jan,11

42820 Tonsillectomy and adenoidectomy; younger than age 12
A
🚑 8.26 ⚕ 8.26 **FUD** 090
J A2 360 ▢
AMA: 2018,Jan,8; 2017,Jan,8; 2016,Jan,13; 2015,Jan,16

42821 age 12 or over
A
🚑 8.62 ⚕ 8.62 **FUD** 090
J A2 80 ▢
AMA: 2018,Jan,8; 2017,Jan,8; 2016,Jan,13; 2015,Jan,16

42825 Tonsillectomy, primary or secondary; younger than age 12
A
🚑 7.52 ⚕ 7.52 **FUD** 090
J A2 80 ▢
AMA: 2018,Jan,8; 2017,Jan,8; 2016,Jan,13; 2015,Jan,16

42826 age 12 or over
A
🚑 7.20 ⚕ 7.20 **FUD** 090
J A2 ▢
AMA: 2018,Jan,8; 2017,Jan,8; 2016,Jan,13; 2015,Jan,16

42830 Adenoidectomy, primary; younger than age 12
A
🚑 5.95 ⚕ 5.95 **FUD** 090
J A2 80 ▢
AMA: 2018,Jan,8; 2017,Jan,8; 2016,Jan,13; 2015,Jan,16

42831 age 12 or over
A
🚑 6.44 ⚕ 6.44 **FUD** 090
J A2 80 ▢
AMA: 2018,Jan,8; 2017,Jan,8; 2016,Jan,13; 2015,Jan,16

42835 Adenoidectomy, secondary; younger than age 12
A
🚑 5.51 ⚕ 5.51 **FUD** 090
J A2 80 ▢
AMA: 2018,Jan,8; 2017,Jan,8; 2016,Jan,13; 2015,Jan,16

42836 age 12 or over
A
🚑 6.89 ⚕ 6.89 **FUD** 090
J A2 80 ▢
AMA: 2018,Jan,8; 2017,Jan,8; 2016,Jan,13; 2015,Jan,16

42842 Radical resection of tonsil, tonsillar pillars, and/or retromolar trigone; without closure
🚑 28.7 ⚕ 28.7 **FUD** 090
J 80 ▢
AMA: 2018,Jan,8; 2017,Jan,8; 2016,Jan,13; 2015,Jan,16

42844 closure with local flap (eg, tongue, buccal)
🚑 39.9 ⚕ 39.9 **FUD** 090
J 80 ▢
AMA: 2018,Jan,8; 2017,Jan,8; 2016,Jan,13; 2015,Jan,16

42845 closure with other flap
Code also closure with other flap(s)
Code also radical neck dissection when combined (38720)
🚑 63.9 ⚕ 63.9 **FUD** 090
C 80 ▢
AMA: 2018,Jan,8; 2017,Jan,8; 2016,Jan,13; 2015,Jan,16

42860 Excision of tonsil tags
🚑 5.40 ⚕ 5.40 **FUD** 090
J A2 80 ▢
AMA: 2014,Jan,11

Tonsillar tags or polyps are removed

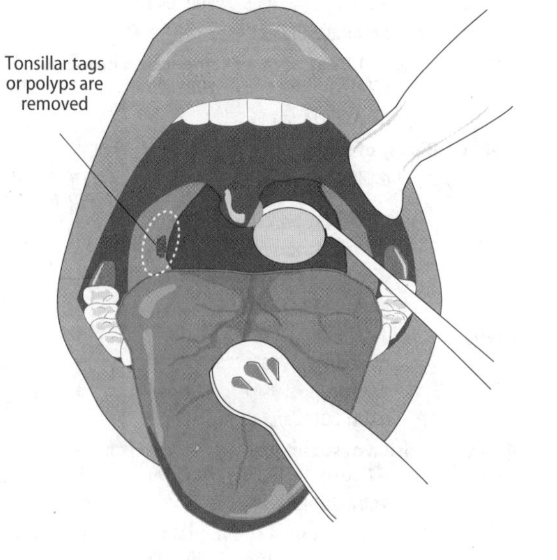

42870 **Excision or destruction lingual tonsil, any method (separate procedure)**

EXCLUDES *Nasopharynx resection (juvenile angiofibroma) by transzygomatic/bicoronal approach (61586, 61600)*

17.0 17.0 FUD 090 J A2 80

AMA: 2014,Jan,11

42890 **Limited pharyngectomy**

Code also radical neck dissection when combined (38720)

40.7 40.7 FUD 090 J A2 80

AMA: 2014,Jan,11; 2010,Aug,3-7

42892 **Resection of lateral pharyngeal wall or pyriform sinus, direct closure by advancement of lateral and posterior pharyngeal walls**

Code also radical neck dissection when combined (38720)

53.6 53.6 FUD 090 J A2 80

AMA: 2018,Jan,8; 2017,Jan,8; 2016,Jan,13; 2015,Jan,16

42894 **Resection of pharyngeal wall requiring closure with myocutaneous or fasciocutaneous flap or free muscle, skin, or fascial flap with microvascular anastomosis**

EXCLUDES *Flap used for reconstruction (15730, 15733-15734, 15756-15758)*

Code also radical neck dissection when combined (38720)

67.7 67.7 FUD 090 C 80

AMA: 2018,Jan,8; 2017,Jan,8; 2016,Jan,13; 2015,Jan,16

42900 **Suture pharynx for wound or injury**

9.56 9.56 FUD 010 T A2 80

AMA: 2014,Jan,11

42950 **Pharyngoplasty (plastic or reconstructive operation on pharynx)**

EXCLUDES *Pharyngeal flap (42225)*

22.8 22.8 FUD 090 J A2 80

AMA: 2019,Oct,10; 2018,Jan,8; 2017,Jan,8; 2016,Apr,8

42953 **Pharyngoesophageal repair**

Code also closure using myocutaneous or other flap

27.3 27.3 FUD 090 C 80

AMA: 2014,Jan,11

42955 **Pharyngostomy (fistulization of pharynx, external for feeding)**

21.7 21.7 FUD 090 T A2 80

AMA: 2014,Jan,11

42960 **Control oropharyngeal hemorrhage, primary or secondary (eg, post-tonsillectomy); simple**

4.83 4.83 FUD 010 T A2 80

AMA: 2014,Jan,11

42961 **complicated, requiring hospitalization**

11.9 11.9 FUD 090 C 80

AMA: 2014,Jan,11

42962 **with secondary surgical intervention**

14.7 14.7 FUD 090 J A2

AMA: 2014,Jan,11

42970 **Control of nasopharyngeal hemorrhage, primary or secondary (eg, postadenoidectomy); simple, with posterior nasal packs, with or without anterior packs and/or cautery**

11.7 11.7 FUD 090 T R2

AMA: 2014,Jan,11; 2002,May,7

42971 **complicated, requiring hospitalization**

12.9 12.9 FUD 090 C 80

AMA: 2014,Jan,11

42972 **with secondary surgical intervention**

14.5 14.5 FUD 090 J A2 80

AMA: 2014,Jan,11

42999 **Unlisted procedure, pharynx, adenoids, or tonsils**

0.00 0.00 FUD YYY T 80

AMA: 2018,Jan,8; 2017,Jan,8; 2016,Jan,13; 2015,Jan,16

43020-43135 Incision/Resection of Esophagus

43020 **Esophagotomy, cervical approach, with removal of foreign body**

EXCLUDES *Laparotomy with esophageal intubation (43510)*

16.2 16.2 FUD 090 T 80

AMA: 2014,Jan,11

43030 **Cricopharyngeal myotomy**

EXCLUDES *Laparotomy with esophageal intubation (43510)*

14.8 14.8 FUD 090 J G2 80

AMA: 2020,Jul,13

43045 **Esophagotomy, thoracic approach, with removal of foreign body**

EXCLUDES *Laparotomy with esophageal intubation (43510)*

37.6 37.6 FUD 090 C 80

AMA: 2014,Jan,11; 1994,Win,1

43100 **Excision of lesion, esophagus, with primary repair; cervical approach**

EXCLUDES *Gastrointestinal reconstruction for previous esophagectomy (43360-43361)*
Wide excision malignant lesion cervical esophagus, with total laryngectomy:
With radical neck dissection (31365, 43107, 43116, 43124)
Without radical neck dissection (31360, 43107, 43116, 43124)

18.0 18.0 FUD 090 C 80

AMA: 2014,Jan,11; 1994,Win,1

43101 **thoracic or abdominal approach**

EXCLUDES *Gastrointestinal reconstruction for previous esophagectomy (43360-43361)*
Wide excision malignant lesion cervical esophagus, with total laryngectomy:
With radical neck dissection (31365, 43107, 43116, 43124)
Without radical neck dissection (31360, 43107, 43116, 43124)

29.1 29.1 FUD 090 C 80

AMA: 2018,Jan,8; 2017,Jan,8; 2016,Jan,13; 2015,Jan,16

43107 **Total or near total esophagectomy, without thoracotomy; with pharyngogastrostomy or cervical esophagogastrostomy, with or without pyloroplasty (transhiatal)**

EXCLUDES *Gastrointestinal reconstruction for previous esophagectomy (43360-43361)*

86.5 86.5 FUD 090 C 80

AMA: 2014,Jan,11; 2010,Aug,3-7

43108 **with colon interposition or small intestine reconstruction, including intestine mobilization, preparation and anastomosis(es)**

EXCLUDES *Gastrointestinal reconstruction for previous esophagectomy (43360-43361)*

129. 129. FUD 090 C 80

AMA: 2014,Jan,11; 2002,May,7

43112 **Total or near total esophagectomy, with thoracotomy; with pharyngogastrostomy or cervical esophagogastrostomy, with or without pyloroplasty (ie, McKeown esophagectomy or tri-incisional esophagectomy)**

EXCLUDES *Gastrointestinal reconstruction for previous esophagectomy (43360-43361)*

101. 101. FUD 090 C 80

AMA: 2018,Jul,7; 2018,Jan,8; 2017,Jan,8; 2016,Jan,13; 2015,Jan,16

43113 **with colon interposition or small intestine reconstruction, including intestine mobilization, preparation, and anastomosis(es)**

EXCLUDES *Gastrointestinal reconstruction for previous esophagectomy (43360-43361)*

126. 126. FUD 090 C 80

AMA: 2014,Jan,11; 2002,May,7

43116 **Partial esophagectomy, cervical, with free intestinal graft, including microvascular anastomosis, obtaining the graft and intestinal reconstruction**

INCLUDES Operating microscope (69990)

EXCLUDES *Free jejunal graft with microvascular anastomosis performed by different physician (43496)*
Gastrointestinal reconstruction for previous esophagectomy (43360-43361)

Code also modifier 52 when intestinal or free jejunal graft with microvascular anastomosis performed by another physician

145. 145. **FUD** 090 C 80

AMA: 2016,Feb,12

43117 **Partial esophagectomy, distal two-thirds, with thoracotomy and separate abdominal incision, with or without proximal gastrectomy; with thoracic esophagogastrostomy, with or without pyloroplasty (Ivor Lewis)**

EXCLUDES *Esophagogastrectomy (lower third) and vagotomy (43122)*
Gastrointestinal reconstruction for previous esophagectomy (43360-43361)
Total esophagectomy with gastropharyngostomy (43107, 43124)

94.3 94.3 **FUD** 090 C 80

AMA: 2014,Jan,11; 1994,Win,1

43118 **with colon interposition or small intestine reconstruction, including intestine mobilization, preparation, and anastomosis(es)**

EXCLUDES *Esophagogastrectomy (lower third) and vagotomy (43122)*
Gastrointestinal reconstruction for previous esophagectomy (43360-43361)
Total esophagectomy with gastropharyngostomy (43107, 43124)

105. 105. **FUD** 090 C 80

AMA: 2014,Jan,11; 2002,May,7

43121 **Partial esophagectomy, distal two-thirds, with thoracotomy only, with or without proximal gastrectomy, with thoracic esophagogastrostomy, with or without pyloroplasty**

Gastrointestinal reconstruction for previous esophagectomy (43360-43361)

82.8 82.8 **FUD** 090 C 80

AMA: 2014,Jan,11; 1994,Win,1

43122 **Partial esophagectomy, thoracoabdominal or abdominal approach, with or without proximal gastrectomy; with esophagogastrostomy, with or without pyloroplasty**

Gastrointestinal reconstruction for previous esophagectomy (43360-43361)

74.3 74.3 **FUD** 090 C 80

AMA: 2014,Jan,11; 1994,Win,1

43123 **with colon interposition or small intestine reconstruction, including intestine mobilization, preparation, and anastomosis(es)**

Gastrointestinal reconstruction for previous esophagectomy (43360-43361)

131. 131. **FUD** 090 C 80

AMA: 2014,Jan,11; 2002,May,7

43124 **Total or partial esophagectomy, without reconstruction (any approach), with cervical esophagostomy**

Gastrointestinal reconstruction for previous esophagectomy (43360-43361)

110. 110. **FUD** 090 C 80

AMA: 2018,Jan,8; 2017,Jan,8; 2016,Jan,13; 2015,Jan,16

43130 **Diverticulectomy of hypopharynx or esophagus, with or without myotomy; cervical approach**

EXCLUDES *Diverticulectomy hypopharynx or cervical esophagus, endoscopic (43180)*
Gastrointestinal reconstruction for previous esophagectomy (43360-43361)

22.6 22.6 **FUD** 090 J G2 80

AMA: 2018,Jan,8; 2017,Jan,8; 2016,Jan,13; 2015,Jan,16

43135 **thoracic approach**

EXCLUDES *Diverticulectomy hypopharynx or cervical esophagus, endoscopic (43180)*
Gastrointestinal reconstruction for previous esophagectomy (43360-43361)

42.6 42.6 **FUD** 090 C 80

AMA: 2018,Jan,8; 2017,Jan,8; 2016,Jan,13; 2015,Jan,16

43180-43233 [43210, 43211, 43212, 43213, 43214, 43233] Endoscopic Procedures: Esophagus

INCLUDES Control bleeding due to endoscopic procedure during same operative session
Diagnostic endoscopy with surgical endoscopy
Examination upper esophageal sphincter (cricopharyngeus muscle) to/including gastroesophageal junction
Retroflexion examination proximal region stomach

43180 **Esophagoscopy, rigid, transoral with diverticulectomy of hypopharynx or cervical esophagus (eg, Zenker's diverticulum), with cricopharyngeal myotomy, includes use of telescope or operating microscope and repair, when performed**

INCLUDES Operating microscope (69990)

EXCLUDES *Esophagogastroduodenoscopy, flexible, transoral; with esophagogastric fundoplasty (43210)*
Open diverticulectomy hypopharynx or esophagus (43130-43135)

15.7 15.7 **FUD** 090 J G2

AMA: 2018,Jan,8; 2017,Jan,8; 2016,Feb,12; 2016,Jan,13; 2015,Nov,8

43191 **Esophagoscopy, rigid, transoral; diagnostic, including collection of specimen(s) by brushing or washing when performed (separate procedure)**

EXCLUDES *Esophagogastroduodenoscopy, flexible, transoral; with esophagogastric fundoplasty (43210)*
Esophagoscopy:
Flexible, transnasal (43197-43198)
Flexible, transoral (43200)
Rigid, transoral (43192-43196)

4.47 4.47 **FUD** 000 J G2

AMA: 2018,Jan,8; 2017,Jan,8; 2016,Jan,13; 2015,Nov,8; 2015,Jan,16

43192 **with directed submucosal injection(s), any substance**

EXCLUDES *Esophagoscopy:*
Flexible, transnasal (43197-43198)
Flexible, transoral (43201)
Rigid, transoral (43191)
Injection sclerosis of esophageal varices:
Flexible, transoral (43204)
Rigid, transoral (43499)

4.88 4.88 **FUD** 000 J G2

AMA: 2018,Jan,8; 2017,Jan,8; 2016,Jan,13; 2015,Jan,16

43193 **with biopsy, single or multiple**

EXCLUDES *Esophagoscopy:*
Flexible, transnasal (43197-43198)
Flexible, transoral (43202)
Rigid, transoral (43191)

4.85 4.85 **FUD** 000 J G2

AMA: 2018,Jan,8; 2017,Jan,8; 2016,Jan,13; 2015,Jan,16

43194 **with removal of foreign body(s)**

EXCLUDES *Esophagoscopy:*
Flexible, transnasal (43197-43198)
Flexible, transoral (43215)
Rigid, transoral (43191)

(76000)

5.55 5.55 **FUD** 000 J G2

AMA: 2018,Jan,8; 2017,Jan,8; 2016,Jan,13; 2015,Jan,16

43195 **with balloon dilation (less than 30 mm diameter)**

EXCLUDES *Dilation of esophagus:*
Flexible, with balloon diameter 30 mm or larger (43214, 43233)
Flexible, with balloon diameter less than 30 mm (43220)
Without endoscopic visualization (43450-43453)
Esophagoscopy:
Flexible, transnasal (43197-43198)
Rigid, transoral (43191)

(74360)
5.28 5.28 FUD 000 J G2
AMA: 2018,Jan,8; 2017,Jan,8; 2016,Jan,13; 2015,Jan,16

43196 **with insertion of guide wire followed by dilation over guide wire**

EXCLUDES *Esophagoscopy:*
Flexible, transnasal (43197-43198)
Flexible, transoral (43226)
Rigid, transoral (43191)

(74360)
5.63 5.63 FUD 000 J G2
AMA: 2018,Jan,8; 2017,Jan,8; 2016,Jan,13; 2015,Jan,16

43197 **Esophagoscopy, flexible, transnasal; diagnostic, including collection of specimen(s) by brushing or washing, when performed (separate procedure)**

EXCLUDES *Esophagogastroduodenoscopy, flexible, transoral (43235-43259 [43233, 43266, 43270])*
Esophagoscopy:
Flexible, transnasal; with biopsy, single or multiple (43198)
Flexible, transoral (43200-43232 [43211, 43212, 43213, 43214])
Rigid, transoral (43191-43196)
Laryngoscopy, flexible fiberoptic; diagnostic (31575)
Nasal endoscopy, diagnostic, unless different type endoscope used (31231)
Nasopharyngoscopy with endoscope (92511)

2.40 5.34 FUD 000 T P3
AMA: 2018,Jan,8; 2017,Jul,7; 2017,Jan,8; 2016,Dec,13; 2016,Sep,6; 2016,Jan,13; 2015,Nov,8; 2015,Jan,16

43198 **with biopsy, single or multiple**

EXCLUDES *Esophagogastroduodenoscopy, flexible, transoral (43235-43259 [43233, 43266, 43270])*
Esophagoscopy:
Flexible, transnasal (43197)
Flexible, transoral (43200-43232 [43211, 43212, 43213, 43214])
Rigid, transoral (43191-43196)
Laryngoscopy, flexible fiberoptic; diagnostic (31575)
Nasal endoscopy, diagnostic, unless different type endoscope used (31231)
Nasopharyngoscopy with endoscope (92511)

2.86 6.08 FUD 000 T P3
AMA: 2018,Jan,8; 2017,Jul,7; 2017,Jan,8; 2016,Dec,13; 2016,Sep,6; 2016,Jan,13; 2015,Jan,16

43200 **Esophagoscopy, flexible, transoral; diagnostic, including collection of specimen(s) by brushing or washing, when performed (separate procedure)**

EXCLUDES *Esophagogastroduodenoscopy, flexible, transoral (43235)*
Esophagoscopy:
Flexible, transnasal (43197-43198)
Flexible, transoral (43201-43232 [43211, 43212, 43213, 43214])
Rigid, transoral (43191)

2.53 6.50 FUD 000 T A2
AMA: 2018,Jan,8; 2017,Jan,8; 2016,Jan,13; 2015,Nov,8; 2015,Jan,16

43201 **with directed submucosal injection(s), any substance**

EXCLUDES *Esophagoscopy:*
Flexible, transnasal (43197-43198)
Flexible, transoral, on same lesion (43200, 43204, 43211, 43227)
Injection sclerosis esophageal varices:
Flexible, transoral (43204)
Rigid, transoral (43192, 43499)

2.98 6.89 FUD 000 J A2
AMA: 2018,Jan,8; 2017,Jan,8; 2016,Jan,13; 2015,Jan,16

43202 **with biopsy, single or multiple**

EXCLUDES *Esophagoscopy:*
Flexible, transnasal (43197-43198)
Flexible, transoral; diagnostic (43200)
Flexible, transoral, on same lesion (43211)
Rigid, transoral (43193)

2.97 9.64 FUD 000 J A2
AMA: 2018,Jan,8; 2017,Jan,8; 2016,Jan,13; 2015,Jan,16

43204 **with injection sclerosis of esophageal varices**

EXCLUDES *Band ligation non-variceal bleeding (43227)*
Esophagoscopy:
Flexible, transnasal or transoral; diagnostic (43197-43198, 43200)
Flexible, transoral; with control bleeding, any method, on same lesion (43227)
Flexible, transoral; with directed submucosal injection(s), any substance, on same lesion (43201)
Rigid, transoral, with injection esophageal varices (43499)

3.96 3.96 FUD 000 J A2
AMA: 2018,Jan,8; 2017,Jan,8; 2016,Jan,13; 2015,Jan,16

43205 **with band ligation of esophageal varices**

EXCLUDES *Band ligation non-variceal bleeding on same lesion (43227)*
Esophagoscopy, flexible, transnasal or transoral; diagnostic (43197-43198, 43200)

4.07 4.07 FUD 000 J A2
AMA: 2018,Jan,8; 2017,Jan,8; 2016,Jan,13; 2015,Jan,16

43206 **with optical endomicroscopy**

EXCLUDES *Esophagoscopy, flexible, transnasal or transoral; diagnostic (43197-43198, 43200)*
Optical endomicroscopic image(s), interpretation and report (88375)

Code also contrast agent
3.90 7.85 FUD 000 J G2
AMA: 2018,Jan,8; 2017,Nov,10; 2017,Jan,8; 2016,Jan,13; 2015,Jan,16

43210 **Resequenced code. See code following 43259.**

43211 **Resequenced code. See code following 43217.**

43212 **Resequenced code. See code following 43217.**

43213 **Resequenced code. See code following 43220.**

43214 **Resequenced code. See code following 43220.**

43215 **with removal of foreign body(s)**

Esophagoscopy:
Flexible, transnasal or transoral; diagnostic (43197-43198, 43200)
Rigid, transoral (43194)

(76000)
4.14 10.5 FUD 000 J A2
AMA: 2018,Jan,8; 2017,Jan,8; 2016,Jan,13; 2015,Jan,16

43216 **with removal of tumor(s), polyp(s), or other lesion(s) by hot biopsy forceps**

EXCLUDES *Esophagoscopy, flexible, transnasal or transoral; diagnostic (43197-43198, 43200)*

3.86 11.1 FUD 000 J A2
AMA: 2018,Jan,8; 2017,Jan,8; 2016,Jan,13; 2015,Jan,16

43217 **with removal of tumor(s), polyp(s), or other lesion(s) by snare technique**

EXCLUDES *Esophagogastroduodenoscopy, flexible, transoral (43251)*
Esophagoscopy:
Flexible, transnasal or transoral; diagnostic (43197-43198, 43200)
Flexible, transoral; with endoscopic mucosal resection, on same lesion (43211)

4.62 11.4 FUD 000 J A2

AMA: 2020,May,13; 2018,Jan,8; 2017,Jan,8; 2016,Jan,13; 2015,Jan,16

43211 **with endoscopic mucosal resection**

EXCLUDES *Esophagoscopy:*
Flexible, transnasal or transoral; diagnostic (43197-43198, 43200)
Flexible, transoral; with directed submucosal injection(s), on same lesion (43201-43202)
Flexible, transoral; with removal tumor(s), polyp(s), or other lesion(s) by snare technique, on same lesion (43217)

6.77 6.77 FUD 000 J G2

AMA: 2019,Dec,14; 2018,Jan,8; 2017,Nov,10; 2017,Jan,8; 2016,Jan,13; 2015,Jan,16

43212 **with placement of endoscopic stent (includes pre- and post-dilation and guide wire passage, when performed)**

EXCLUDES *Esophagogastroduodenoscopy, flexible, transoral; with insertion of intraluminal tube or catheter (43241)*
Esophagoscopy:
Flexible, transnasal or transoral; diagnostic (43197-43198, 43200)
Flexible, transoral; with insertion guide wire followed by passage dilator(s) over guide wire (43226)
Flexible, transoral; with transendoscopic balloon dilation (43220)

(74360)

5.48 5.48 FUD 000 J J8

AMA: 2018,Jan,8; 2017,Jan,8; 2016,Jan,13; 2015,Jan,16

43220 **with transendoscopic balloon dilation (less than 30 mm diameter)**

EXCLUDES *Dilation esophagus:*
Rigid, with balloon diameter 30 mm or larger (43214)
Rigid, with balloon diameter less than 30mm (43195)
Without endoscopic visualization (43450, 43453)
Esophagoscopy:
Flexible, transnasal; diagnostic (43197-43198)
Flexible, transoral (43200, 43212, 43226, 43229)

(74360)

3.43 29.5 FUD 000 J A2

AMA: 2018,Jan,8; 2017,Jan,8; 2016,Jan,13; 2015,Jan,16

43213 **with dilation of esophagus, by balloon or dilator, retrograde (includes fluoroscopic guidance, when performed)**

INCLUDES Fluoroscopy (76000)

EXCLUDES *Esophagoscopy, flexible, transnasal or transoral; diagnostic (43197-43198, 43200)*
Intraluminal dilation of strictures and/or obstructions (eg, esophagus), radiological supervision and interpretation (74360)

Code also each additional stricture treated in same operative session with modifier 59 and (43213)

7.48 34.9 FUD 000 J G2

AMA: 2018,Jan,8; 2017,Jan,8; 2016,Jan,13; 2015,Jan,16

43214 **with dilation of esophagus with balloon (30 mm diameter or larger) (includes fluoroscopic guidance, when performed)**

INCLUDES Fluoroscopy (76000)

EXCLUDES *Esophagoscopy, flexible, transnasal or transoral; diagnostic (43197-43198, 43200)*
Intraluminal dilation strictures and/or obstructions (eg, esophagus), radiological supervision and interpretation (74360)

5.61 5.61 FUD 000 J G2

AMA: 2018,Jan,8; 2017,Jan,8; 2016,Jan,13; 2015,Jan,16

43226 **with insertion of guide wire followed by passage of dilator(s) over guide wire**

EXCLUDES *Esophagoscopy:*
Flexible, transnasal or transoral; diagnostic (43197-43198, 43200)
Flexible, transoral; with ablation tumor(s), polyp(s), or other lesion(s), on same lesion (43229)
Flexible, transoral; with placement endoscopic stent (43212)
Flexible, transoral; with transendoscopic balloon dilation (43220)
Rigid, transoral (43196)

(74360)

3.75 10.1 FUD 000 J A2

AMA: 2018,Jan,8; 2017,Jan,8; 2016,Jan,13; 2015,Jan,16

43227 **with control of bleeding, any method**

EXCLUDES *Esophagoscopy:*
Flexible, transnasal or transoral; diagnostic (43197-43198, 43200)
Flexible, transoral; with directed submucosal injection(s), on same lesion (43201)
Flexible, transoral; with injection sclerosis esophageal varices, on same lesion (43204-43205)

4.75 17.6 FUD 000 J A2

AMA: 2018,Jan,8; 2017,Jan,8; 2016,Jan,13; 2015,Jan,16

43229 **with ablation of tumor(s), polyp(s), or other lesion(s) (includes pre- and post-dilation and guide wire passage, when performed)**

EXCLUDES *Esophagoscopy:*
Flexible, transnasal or transoral; diagnostic (43197-43198, 43200)
Flexible, transoral; with insertion guide wire followed by passage dilator(s) over guide wire, on same lesion (43226)
Flexible, transoral; with transendoscopic balloon dilation, on same lesion (43220)

Code also esophagoscopic photodynamic therapy, when performed (96570-96571)

5.70 19.8 FUD 000 J G2

AMA: 2018,Jan,8; 2017,Jan,8; 2016,Jan,13; 2015,Jan,16

43231 **with endoscopic ultrasound examination**

INCLUDES Gastrointestinal endoscopic ultrasound, supervision, and interpretation (76975)

EXCLUDES *Esophagoscopy:*
Flexible, transnasal or transoral; diagnostic (43197-43198, 43200)
Flexible, transoral; with transendoscopic ultrasound-guided intramural or transmural fine needle aspiration/biopsy(s) (43232)
Procedure performed more than one time per operative session

4.59 4.59 FUD 000 J A2

AMA: 2018,Jan,8; 2017,Jan,8; 2016,Jan,13; 2015,Jan,16

43232 **with transendoscopic ultrasound-guided intramural or transmural fine needle aspiration/biopsy(s)**

INCLUDES Gastrointestinal endoscopic ultrasound, supervision and interpretation (76975)
Ultrasonic guidance (76942)

EXCLUDES *Esophagoscopy:*
Flexible, transnasal or transoral; diagnostic (43197-43198, 43200)
Flexible, transoral; with endoscopic ultrasound examination (43231)
Procedure performed more than one time per operative session

5.75 5.75 FUD 000 J A2

AMA: 2018,Jan,8; 2017,Jan,8; 2016,Jan,13; 2015,Jan,16

43233 **Resequenced code. See code following 43249.**

43235-43210 [43210, 43233, 43266, 43270] Endoscopic Procedures: Esophagogastroduodenoscopy (EGD)

INCLUDES Control bleeding due to endoscopic procedure during same operative session
Diagnostic endoscopy with surgical endoscopy
Exam jejunum distal to anastomosis in surgically altered stomach, including post-gastroenterostomy (Billroth II) and gastric bypass (43235-43259 [43233, 43266, 43270])

EXCLUDES *Exam upper esophageal sphincter (cricopharyngeus muscle) to/including gastroesophageal junction and/or retroflexion exam proximal region stomach (43197-43232 [43211, 43212, 43213, 43214])*

Code also modifier 52 when duodenum not examined either deliberately or due to significant issues and repeat procedure will not be performed
Code also modifier 53 when duodenum not examined either deliberately or due to significant issues and repeat procedure is planned

43235 **Esophagogastroduodenoscopy, flexible, transoral; diagnostic, including collection of specimen(s) by brushing or washing, when performed (separate procedure)**

EXCLUDES *Endoscopy small intestine (44360-44379)*
Esophagogastroduodenoscopy, flexible, transoral; with esophagogastric fundoplasty (43210)
Esophagoscopy, flexible, transnasal; diagnostic (43197-43198)
Procedure performed with surgical endoscopy (43236-43259 [43233, 43266, 43270])

3.54 7.98 FUD 000 T A2

AMA: 2019,Oct,10; 2018,Jul,14; 2018,Jan,8; 2017,Jul,10; 2017,Jan,8; 2016,Jan,13; 2015,Nov,8; 2015,Jan,16

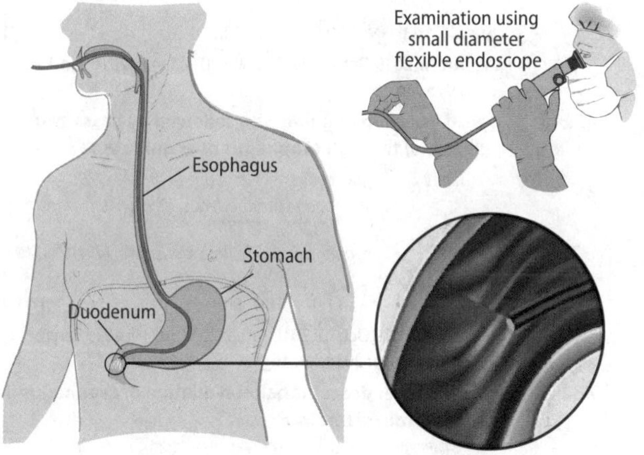

43236 **with directed submucosal injection(s), any substance**

EXCLUDES *Endoscopy small intestine (44360-44379)*
Esophagogastroduodenoscopy, on same lesion:
Flexible, transoral; with control bleeding, any method (43255)
Flexible, transoral; with endoscopic mucosal resection (43254)
Flexible, transoral; with injection sclerosis esophageal/gastric varices (43243)
Esophagoscopy, flexible, transnasal or transoral; diagnostic (43197-43198, 43235)
Injection sclerosis varices, esophageal/gastric (43243)

4.05 10.0 FUD 000 T A2

AMA: 2019,Oct,10; 2018,Jan,8; 2017,Jan,8; 2016,Jan,13; 2015,Jan,16

43237 **with endoscopic ultrasound examination limited to the esophagus, stomach or duodenum, and adjacent structures**

INCLUDES Ultrasonic guidance (76942, 76975)

EXCLUDES *Endoscopy of small intestine (44360-44379)*
Esophagogastroduodenoscopy, flexible, transoral (43238, 43242, 43253, 43259)
Esophagoscopy, flexible, transnasal; diagnostic (43197-43198)
Procedure performed more than one time per operative session

5.73 5.73 FUD 000 J A2

AMA: 2019,Oct,10; 2018,Jan,8; 2017,Jan,8; 2016,Jan,13; 2016,Jan,11; 2015,Jan,16

43238 **with transendoscopic ultrasound-guided intramural or transmural fine needle aspiration/biopsy(s), (includes endoscopic ultrasound examination limited to the esophagus, stomach or duodenum, and adjacent structures)**

INCLUDES Gastrointestinal endoscopic ultrasound, supervision and interpretation (76975)
Ultrasonic guidance (76942)

EXCLUDES *Endoscopy small intestine (44360-44379)*
Esophagogastroduodenoscopy, flexible, transoral (43237, 43242)
Esophagoscopy, flexible, transnasal (43197-43198)
Procedure performed more than one time per operative session

6.70 6.70 FUD 000 J A2

AMA: 2019,Oct,10; 2018,Jan,8; 2017,Jan,8; 2016,Jan,13; 2015,Jan,16

43239 **with biopsy, single or multiple**

EXCLUDES *Endoscopy small intestine (44360-44379)*
Esophagogastroduodenoscopy, flexible, transoral; with endoscopic mucosal resection on same lesion (43254)
Esophagoscopy, flexible, transnasal (43197-43198)

3.99 10.6 FUD 000 T A2

AMA: 2020,Jan,12; 2019,Oct,10; 2018,Jul,14; 2018,Jan,8; 2017,Jan,8; 2016,Jan,13; 2015,Jan,16

43240 **with transmural drainage of pseudocyst (includes placement of transmural drainage catheter[s]/stent[s], when performed, and endoscopic ultrasound, when performed)**

INCLUDES Gastrointestinal endoscopic ultrasound, supervision and interpretation (76975)

EXCLUDES *Endoscopic pancreatic necrosectomy (48999)*
Endoscopy small intestine (44360-44379)
Esophagogastroduodenoscopy:
Flexible, transoral (43242, [43266], 43259)
Flexible, transoral; with transendoscopic ultrasound-guided transmural injection diagnostic or therapeutic substance(s), on same lesion (43253)
Esophagoscopy, flexible, transnasal (43197-43198)
Procedure performed more than one time per operative session

11.5 | 11.5 | FUD 000 | J J8

AMA: 2019,Oct,10; 2018,Jan,8; 2017,Jan,8; 2016,Jan,13; 2015,Jan,16

43241 **with insertion of intraluminal tube or catheter**

EXCLUDES *Endoscopy small intestine (44360-44379)*
Esophagogastroduodenoscopy, flexible, transoral ([43266])
Esophagoscopy, flexible, transnasal or transoral (43197-43198, 43212)
Insertion long gastrointestinal tube (44500, 74340)
Naso or oro-gastric requiring professional skill and fluoroscopic guidance (43752)

4.17 | 4.17 | FUD 000 | J A2

AMA: 2019,Oct,10; 2018,Jan,8; 2017,Jan,8; 2016,Jan,13; 2015,Jan,16

43242 **with transendoscopic ultrasound-guided intramural or transmural fine needle aspiration/biopsy(s) (includes endoscopic ultrasound examination of the esophagus, stomach, and either the duodenum or a surgically altered stomach where the jejunum is examined distal to the anastomosis)**

INCLUDES Gastrointestinal endoscopic ultrasound, supervision and interpretation (76975)
Ultrasonic guidance (76942)

EXCLUDES *Endoscopy small intestine (44360-44379)*
Esophagogastroduodenoscopy, flexible, transoral (43237-43238, 43240, 43259)
Esophagoscopy, flexible, transnasal (43197-43198)
Procedure performed more than one time per operative session
Transmural fine needle biopsy/aspiration with ultrasound guidance, transendoscopic, esophagus/stomach/duodenum/neighboring structure (43238)

88172-88173

7.58 | 7.58 | FUD 000 | J A2

AMA: 2019,Oct,10; 2018,Jan,8; 2017,Jan,8; 2016,Jan,13; 2015,Jan,16

43243 **with injection sclerosis of esophageal/gastric varices**

EXCLUDES *Endoscopy small intestine (44360-44379)*
Esophagogastroduodenoscopy, flexible, transoral on same lesion (43236, 43255)
Esophagoscopy, flexible, transnasal (43197-43198)

6.85 | 6.85 | FUD 000 | J A2

AMA: 2019,Oct,10; 2018,Jan,8; 2017,Jan,8; 2016,Jan,13; 2015,Jan,16

43244 **with band ligation of esophageal/gastric varices**

EXCLUDES *Band ligation, non-variceal bleeding (43255)*
Endoscopy small intestine (44360-44379)
Esophagoscopy, flexible, transnasal (43197-43198)

7.08 | 7.08 | FUD 000 | J A2

AMA: 2019,Oct,10; 2018,Jan,8; 2017,Jan,8; 2016,Jan,13; 2015,Jan,16

43245 **with dilation of gastric/duodenal stricture(s) (eg, balloon, bougie)**

EXCLUDES *Endoscopy small intestine (44360-44379)*
Esophagogastroduodenoscopy, flexible, transoral ([43266])
Esophagoscopy, flexible, transnasal (43197-43198)

(74360)

5.13 | 16.2 | FUD 000 | J A2

AMA: 2019,Oct,10; 2018,Jan,8; 2017,Jan,8; 2016,Jan,13; 2015,Jan,16

43246 **with directed placement of percutaneous gastrostomy tube**

EXCLUDES *Endoscopy small intestine (44360-44372, 44376-44379)*
Esophagoscopy, flexible, transnasal (43197-43198)
Gastrostomy tube replacement without endoscopy or imaging (43762-43763)
Percutaneous insertion gastrostomy tube (49440)

5.86 | 5.86 | FUD 000 | J A2 80

AMA: 2019,Oct,10; 2019,Feb,5; 2018,Jan,8; 2017,Jan,8; 2016,Jan,13; 2015,Jan,16

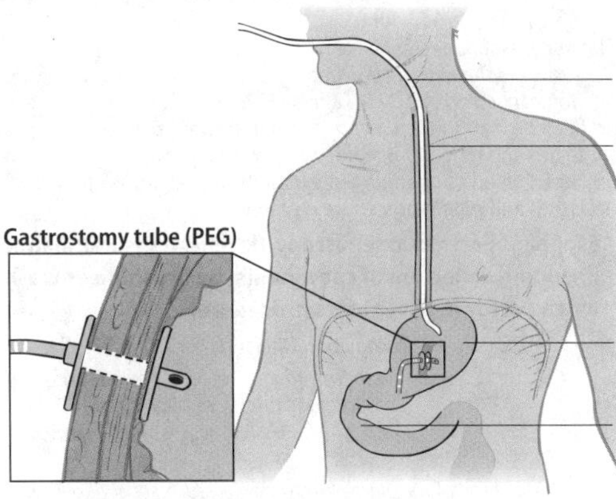

43247 **with removal of foreign body(s)**

EXCLUDES *Endoscopy small intestine (44360-44379)*
Esophagoscopy, flexible, transnasal (43197-43198)

(76000)

5.11 | 10.5 | FUD 000 | T A2

AMA: 2019,Oct,10; 2018,Jan,8; 2017,Jan,8; 2016,Jan,13; 2015,Jan,16

43248 **with insertion of guide wire followed by passage of dilator(s) through esophagus over guide wire**

EXCLUDES *Endoscopy small intestine (44360-44379)*
Esophagogastroduodenoscopy, flexible, transoral ([43266], [43270])
Esophagoscopy, flexible, transnasal (43197-43198)

(74360)

4.78 | 11.0 | FUD 000 | T A2

AMA: 2019,Oct,10; 2018,Jan,8; 2017,Jul,10; 2017,Jan,8; 2016,Jan,13; 2015,Jan,16

43249 **with transendoscopic balloon dilation of esophagus (less than 30 mm diameter)**

EXCLUDES *Endoscopy small intestine (44360-44379)*
Esophagogastroduodenoscopy:
Ablation lesion/tumor/polyp, when performed on same lesion ([43270])
With placement endoscopic stent ([43266])
Esophagoscopy, flexible, transnasal (43197-43198)

(74360)

4.42 | 31.0 | FUD 000 | J A2

AMA: 2019,Oct,10; 2018,Jul,14; 2018,Jan,8; 2017,Jan,8; 2016,Jan,13; 2015,Jan,16

43233 with dilation of esophagus with balloon (30 mm diameter or larger) (includes fluoroscopic guidance, when performed)

INCLUDES Fluoroscopy (76000)

EXCLUDES *Endoscopy small intestine (44360-44379)*
Esophagoscopy, flexible, transnasal (43197-43198)
Intraluminal dilation strictures and/or obstructions (e.g., esophagus), radiological supervision and interpretation (74360)

6.62 6.62 FUD 000 J G2

AMA: 2019,Oct,10; 2018,Jan,8; 2017,Jan,8; 2016,Jan,13; 2015,Jan,16

43250 with removal of tumor(s), polyp(s), or other lesion(s) by hot biopsy forceps

EXCLUDES *Endoscopy small intestine (44360-44379)*
Esophagoscopy, flexible, transnasal (43197-43198)

4.97 11.8 FUD 000 J A2

AMA: 2019,Oct,10; 2018,Jan,8; 2017,Jan,8; 2016,Jan,13; 2015,Jan,16

43251 with removal of tumor(s), polyp(s), or other lesion(s) by snare technique

EXCLUDES *Endoscopic mucosal resection when performed on same lesion (43254)*
Endoscopy small intestine (44360-44379)
Esophagoscopy, flexible, transnasal (43197-43198)

5.66 13.5 FUD 000 J A2

AMA: 2019,Oct,10; 2018,Jan,8; 2017,Jan,8; 2016,Jan,13; 2015,Jan,16

43252 with optical endomicroscopy

EXCLUDES *Endoscopy small intestine (44360-44379)*
Esophagoscopy, flexible, transnasal (43197-43198)
Optical endomicroscopic image(s), interpretation and report (88375)

Code also contrast agent

4.95 8.96 FUD 000 J G2

AMA: 2019,Oct,10; 2018,Jan,8; 2017,Jan,8; 2016,Jan,13; 2015,Jan,16

43253 with transendoscopic ultrasound-guided transmural injection of diagnostic or therapeutic substance(s) (eg, anesthetic, neurolytic agent) or fiducial marker(s) (includes endoscopic ultrasound examination of the esophagus, stomach, and either the duodenum or a surgically altered stomach where the jejunum is examined distal to the anastomosis)

INCLUDES Gastrointestinal endoscopic ultrasound, supervision and interpretation (76975)
Ultrasonic guidance (76942)

EXCLUDES *Endoscopy small intestine (44360-44379)*
Esophagogastroduodenoscopy:
Flexible, transoral (43237, 43259)
Flexible, transoral; with transmural drainage pseudocyst on same lesion with (43240)
Esophagoscopy, flexible, transnasal (43197-43198)
Procedure performed more than one time per operative session
Transmural fine needle biopsy/aspiration with ultrasound guidance, transendoscopic, esophagus/stomach/duodenum/neighboring structures (43238, 43242)

7.70 7.70 FUD 000 J G2

AMA: 2019,Oct,10; 2018,Apr,10; 2018,Jan,8; 2017,Jan,8; 2016,Jan,13; 2015,Jan,16

43254 with endoscopic mucosal resection

EXCLUDES *Endoscopy small intestine (44360-44379)*
Esophagogastroduodenoscopy, flexible, transoral, on same lesion (43236, 43239, 43251)
Esophagoscopy, flexible, transnasal (43197-43198)

7.80 7.80 FUD 000 J G2

AMA: 2019,Dec,14; 2019,Oct,10; 2018,Jan,8; 2017,Jan,8; 2016,Jan,13; 2015,Jan,16

43255 with control of bleeding, any method

EXCLUDES *Endoscopy small intestine (44360-44379)*
Esophagogastroduodenoscopy, flexible, transoral, on same lesion (43236, 43243-43244)
Esophagoscopy, flexible, transnasal (43197-43198)

5.79 18.6 FUD 000 J A2

AMA: 2019,Oct,10; 2018,Jan,8; 2017,Jan,8; 2016,Jan,13; 2015,Jan,16

43266 with placement of endoscopic stent (includes pre- and post-dilation and guide wire passage, when performed)

INCLUDES When performed:
Balloon dilation esophagus (43249)
Dilation gastric/duodenal stricture (43245)
Insertion guidewire/dilator (43248)

EXCLUDES *Endoscopy small intestine (44360-44379)*
Esophagogastroduodenoscopy:
Insertion intraluminal tube or catheter (43241)
Transmural drainage pseudocyst (43240)
Esophagoscopy, flexible, transnasal (43197-43198)

(74360)

6.39 6.39 FUD 000 J J8

AMA: 2019,Oct,10; 2018,Jan,8; 2017,Jan,8; 2016,Jan,13; 2015,Jan,16

43257 with delivery of thermal energy to the muscle of lower esophageal sphincter and/or gastric cardia, for treatment of gastroesophageal reflux disease

EXCLUDES *Endoscopy small intestine (44360-44379)*
Esophageal lesion ablation (43229, [43270])
Esophagoscopy, flexible, transnasal (43197-43198)

6.74 6.74 FUD 000 J A2

AMA: 2019,Oct,10; 2018,Jan,8; 2017,Jan,8; 2016,Jan,13; 2015,Jan,16

43270 with ablation of tumor(s), polyp(s), or other lesion(s) (includes pre- and post-dilation and guide wire passage, when performed)

INCLUDES Endoscopic dilation performed on same lesion (43248-43249)

EXCLUDES *Endoscopy small intestine (44360-44379)*
Esophagoscopy, flexible, transnasal (43197-43198)

Code also photodynamic therapy, when performed (96570-96571)

6.48 20.3 FUD 000 J G2

AMA: 2019,Oct,10; 2018,Jan,8; 2017,Jan,8; 2016,Jan,13; 2015,Jan,16

43259 with endoscopic ultrasound examination, including the esophagus, stomach, and either the duodenum or a surgically altered stomach where the jejunum is examined distal to the anastomosis

INCLUDES Gastrointestinal endoscopic ultrasound, supervision and interpretation (76975)

EXCLUDES *Endoscopy small intestine (44360-44379)*
Esophagogastroduodenoscopy, flexible, transoral (43237, 43240, 43242, 43253)
Esophagoscopy, flexible, transnasal (43197-43198)
Procedure performed more than one time per operative session

6.53 6.53 FUD 000 J A2

AMA: 2019,Oct,10; 2018,Jan,8; 2017,Jan,8; 2016,Jan,13; 2016,Jan,11; 2015,Jan,16

43210 with esophagogastric fundoplasty, partial or complete, includes duodenoscopy when performed

EXCLUDES *Esophagogastroduodenoscopy:*
Flexible, transnasal (43197)
Rigid, transoral (43180, 43191)
Esophagoscopy, flexible, transoral (43200)

12.5 12.5 FUD 000 J G2

AMA: 2018,Jan,8; 2017,Jan,8; 2016,Jan,13; 2015,Nov,8

43260-43278 [43266, 43270, 43274, 43275, 43276, 43277, 43278] Endoscopic Procedures: ERCP

INCLUDES Diagnostic endoscopy with surgical endoscopy
Pancreaticobiliary system:
Biliary tree (right and left hepatic ducts, cystic duct/gallbladder, and common bile ducts)
Pancreas (major and minor ducts)

EXCLUDES *ERCP via Roux-en-Y anatomy (for instance post-gastric or bariatric bypass or post total gastrectomy) or via gastrostomy (open or laparoscopic) (47999, 48999)*
Optical endomicroscopy biliary tract and pancreas, report one time per session (0397T)
Percutaneous biliary catheter procedures (47490-47544)

Code also appropriate endoscopy each anatomic site examined
Code also sphincteroplasty or ductal stricture dilation, when necessary to access debris/stones ([43277])
Code also appropriate ERCP procedure when performed on altered postoperative anatomy (i.e., Billroth II gastroenterostomy) (43260, 43262-43265, [43274], [43275], [43276], [43277], [43278], 43273)
(74328-74330)

43260 Endoscopic retrograde cholangiopancreatography (ERCP); diagnostic, including collection of specimen(s) by brushing or washing, when performed (separate procedure)

EXCLUDES *Endoscopic retrograde cholangiopancreatography (ERCP), therapeutic (43261-43265, 43274-43278 [43274, 43275, 43276, 43277, 43278])*

9.31 9.31 **FUD** 000 J A2

AMA: 2018,Jan,8; 2017,Jan,8; 2016,Jan,13; 2015,Dec,3; 2015,Jan,16

43261 with biopsy, single or multiple

INCLUDES Endoscopic retrograde cholangiopancreatography (ERCP); diagnostic (43260)

EXCLUDES *Percutaneous endoluminal biopsy biliary tree (47543)*

9.76 9.76 **FUD** 000 J A2

AMA: 2018,Jan,8; 2017,Jan,8; 2016,Jan,13; 2015,Dec,3; 2015,Jan,16

43262 with sphincterotomy/papillotomy

INCLUDES Endoscopic retrograde cholangiopancreatography (ERCP), diagnostic (43260)

EXCLUDES *Endoscopic retrograde cholangiopancreatography (ERCP):*
With exchange/insertion/removal stent in same location ([43274], [43276])
With trans-endoscopic balloon dilation ampulla/biliary or pancreatic ducts ([43277])
Percutaneous balloon dilation biliary duct or ampulla (47542)

Code also procedure performed with sphincterotomy (43261, 43263-43265, [43275], [43278])

10.3 10.3 **FUD** 000 J A2

AMA: 2018,Jan,8; 2017,Jan,8; 2016,Jan,13; 2015,Dec,3; 2015,Jan,16

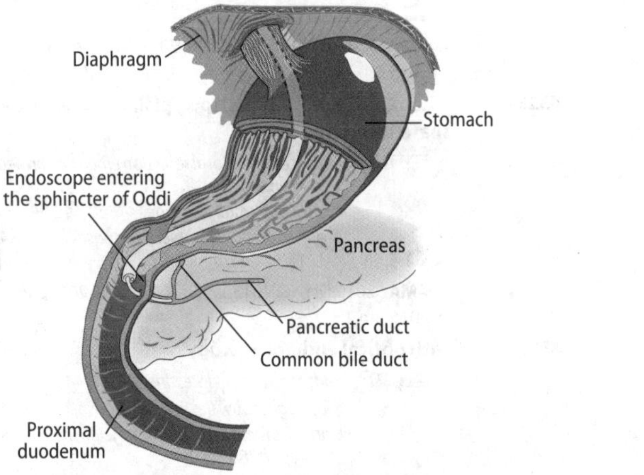

An endoscope is fed through the stomach and into the duodenum Usually a smaller sub-scope is fed up the sphincter of Oddi and into the ducts that drain the pancreas and the gallbladder (common bile)

43263 with pressure measurement of sphincter of Oddi

INCLUDES Endoscopic retrograde cholangiopancreatography (ERCP); diagnostic (43260)

EXCLUDES *Procedure performed more than one time per session*

10.4 10.4 **FUD** 000 J A2

AMA: 2018,Jan,8; 2017,Jan,8; 2016,Jan,13; 2015,Jan,16

43264 with removal of calculi/debris from biliary/pancreatic duct(s)

INCLUDES Endoscopic retrograde cholangiopancreatography (ERCP); diagnostic (43260)
Incidental dilation due to instrument passage

EXCLUDES *Endoscopic retrograde cholangiopancreatography (ERCP) with calculi destruction (43265)*
Findings without debris or calculi, even when balloon used
Percutaneous calculus/debris removal (47544)

Code also sphincteroplasty when dilation necessary to access debris/stones ([43277])

10.4 10.4 **FUD** 000 J A2

AMA: 2018,Jan,8; 2017,Jan,8; 2016,Jan,13; 2015,Dec,3; 2015,Jan,16

43265 **with destruction of calculi, any method (eg, mechanical, electrohydraulic, lithotripsy)**

INCLUDES Endoscopic retrograde cholangiopancreatography (ERCP); diagnostic (43260)
Incidental dilation due to instrument passage
Stone removal in same ductal system

EXCLUDES *Endoscopic retrograde cholangiopancreatography (ERCP) with removal of calculi/debris from biliary/pancreatic duct(s) (43264)*
Findings without debris or calculi, even when balloon used
Percutaneous calculus/debris removal (47544)

Code also sphincteroplasty when dilation necessary to access debris/stones ([43277])

12.5 12.5 FUD 000 J A2

AMA: 2018,Jan,8; 2017,Jan,8; 2016,Jan,13; 2015,Dec,3; 2015,Jan,16

43266 **Resequenced code. See code following 43255.**

43270 **Resequenced code. See code following 43257.**

\# **43274** **with placement of endoscopic stent into biliary or pancreatic duct, including pre- and post-dilation and guide wire passage, when performed, including sphincterotomy, when performed, each stent**

INCLUDES Balloon dilation in same duct
Endoscopic retrograde cholangiopancreatography (ERCP); diagnostic (43260)
Tube placement for naso-pancreatic or naso-biliary drainage

EXCLUDES *Percutaneous placement biliary stent (47538-47540)*
Procedures for stent placement or exchange in same duct (43262, [43275], [43276], [43277])

Code also for each additional stent placement in different ducts or side by side in same duct same session/day, using modifier 59 with ([43274])

13.3 13.3 FUD 000 J G2

AMA: 2018,Jan,8; 2017,Jan,8; 2016,Jan,13; 2015,Jan,16

\# **43275** **with removal of foreign body(s) or stent(s) from biliary/pancreatic duct(s)**

INCLUDES Endoscopic retrograde cholangiopancreatography (ERCP); diagnostic (43260)

EXCLUDES *Endoscopic retrograde cholangiopancreatography (ERCP) with exchange, placement, or removal of stent ([43274], [43276])*
Pancreatic or biliary duct stent removal without ERCP (43247)
Percutaneous calculus/debris removal (47544)
Procedure performed more than one time per session

11.0 11.0 FUD 000 J G2

AMA: 2018,Jan,8; 2017,Jan,8; 2016,Jan,13; 2015,Jan,16

\# **43276** **with removal and exchange of stent(s), biliary or pancreatic duct, including pre- and post-dilation and guide wire passage, when performed, including sphincterotomy, when performed, each stent exchanged**

INCLUDES Balloon dilation in same duct
Endoscopic retrograde cholangiopancreatography (ERCP); diagnostic (43260)
Stent placement or exchange one stent

EXCLUDES *Endoscopic retrograde cholangiopancreatography (ERCP) with removal foreign body(s) or stent(s) ([43275])*
Procedures for stent insertion or exchange stent in same duct (43262, [43274])

Code also each additional stent exchanged same session/day, using modifier 59 with ([43276])

13.9 13.9 FUD 000 J G2

AMA: 2018,Jan,8; 2017,Jan,8; 2016,Jan,13; 2015,Jan,16

\# **43277** **with trans-endoscopic balloon dilation of biliary/pancreatic duct(s) or of ampulla (sphincteroplasty), including sphincterotomy, when performed, each duct**

INCLUDES Endoscopic retrograde cholangiopancreatography (ERCP); diagnostic (43260)

EXCLUDES *Endoscopic retrograde cholangiopancreatography (ERCP):*
With ablation tumor(s), polyp(s), or other lesion(s) for same lesion ([43278])
With sphincterotomy/papillotomy (43262)
With stent exchange/removal same biliary/pancreatic duct ([43276])
With stent placement into same biliary/pancreatic duct ([43274])
Percutaneous dilation biliary duct/ampulla (47542)
Removal stone/debris, dilation incidental to instrument passage (43264-43265)

Code also both right and left hepatic duct (bilateral) balloon dilation, using ([43277]) and append modifier 59 to second procedure

Code also each additional balloon dilation in different ducts or side by side in same duct same session/day, using modifier 59 with ([43277])

Code also same session sphincterotomy without sphincteroplasty in different duct, using modifier 59 with (43262)

10.9 10.9 FUD 000 J G2

AMA: 2018,Jan,8; 2017,Jan,8; 2016,Jan,13; 2015,Dec,3; 2015,Jan,16

\# **43278** **with ablation of tumor(s), polyp(s), or other lesion(s), including pre- and post-dilation and guide wire passage, when performed**

INCLUDES Endoscopic retrograde cholangiopancreatography (ERCP); diagnostic (43260)

EXCLUDES *Ampullectomy (43254)*
Endoscopic retrograde cholangiopancreatography (ERCP); with trans-endoscopic balloon dilation biliary/pancreatic duct(s) or ampulla (sphincteroplasty) in same lesion with ([43277])

12.5 12.5 FUD 000 J G2

AMA: 2018,Jan,8; 2017,Jan,8; 2016,Jan,13; 2015,Jan,16

\+ **43273** **Endoscopic cannulation of papilla with direct visualization of pancreatic/common bile duct(s) (List separately in addition to code(s) for primary procedure)**

EXCLUDES *Procedure performed more than one time per session*

Code first (43260-43265, [43274], [43275], [43276], [43277], [43278])

3.47 3.47 FUD ZZZ N N1 80

AMA: 2018,Jan,8; 2017,Jan,8; 2016,Jan,13; 2015,Jan,16

43274 **Resequenced code. See code following code 43270.**

43275 **Resequenced code. See code following code 43270.**

43276 **Resequenced code. See code following code 43270.**

43277 **Resequenced code. See code following code 43270.**

43278 **Resequenced code. See code following code 43270.**

43279-43289 Laparoscopic Procedures of Esophagus

INCLUDES Diagnostic laparoscopy with surgical laparoscopy (49320)

43279 **Laparoscopy, surgical, esophagomyotomy (Heller type), with fundoplasty, when performed**

EXCLUDES *Esophagomyotomy, open method (43330-43331)*
Laparoscopy, surgical, esophagogastric fundoplasty (43280)

37.5 37.5 FUD 090 C 80

AMA: 2018,Jan,8; 2017,Aug,6; 2017,Jan,8; 2016,Jan,13; 2015,Jan,16

Digestive System

43265 — 43279

43280 **Laparoscopy, surgical, esophagogastric fundoplasty (eg, Nissen, Toupet procedures)**

EXCLUDES *Esophagogastric fundoplasty, open method (43327-43328)*
Esophagogastroduodenoscopy fundoplasty, transoral (43210)
Laparoscopy, surgical, esophageal sphincter augmentation (43284-43285)
Laparoscopy, surgical, esophagomyotomy (43279)
Laparoscopy, surgical, fundoplasty (43281-43282)

31.4 31.4 FUD 090 J 80

AMA: 2018,Jan,8; 2017,Aug,6; 2017,Jan,8; 2016,Jan,13; 2015,Nov,8; 2015,Jan,16

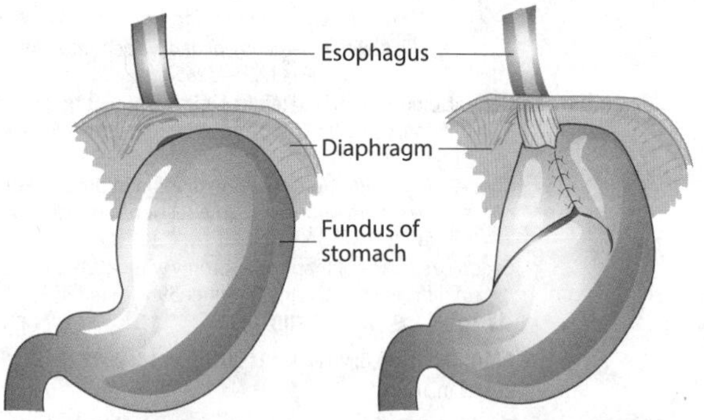

43281 **Laparoscopy, surgical, repair of paraesophageal hernia, includes fundoplasty, when performed; without implantation of mesh**

EXCLUDES *Dilation esophagus (43450, 43453)*
Implantation mesh or other prosthesis (49568)
Laparoscopy, surgical, esophagogastric fundoplasty (43280)
Transabdominal repair paraesophageal hiatal hernia (43332-43333)
Transthoracic repair diaphragmatic hernia (43334-43335)

44.7 44.7 FUD 090 J 80

AMA: 2018,Nov,11; 2018,Sep,14; 2018,Jan,8; 2017,Aug,6; 2017,Jan,8; 2016,Jan,13; 2015,Jan,16

43282 **with implantation of mesh**

EXCLUDES *Dilation esophagus (43450, 43453)*
Laparoscopy, surgical, esophagogastric fundoplasty (43280)
Transabdominal paraesophageal hernia repair (43332-43333)
Transthoracic paraesophageal hernia repair (43334-43335)

50.6 50.6 FUD 090 J 80

AMA: 2018,Jan,8; 2017,Aug,6; 2017,Jan,8; 2016,Aug,9; 2016,Jan,13; 2015,Jan,16

\+ **43283** **Laparoscopy, surgical, esophageal lengthening procedure (eg, Collis gastroplasty or wedge gastroplasty) (List separately in addition to code for primary procedure)**

Code first (43280-43282)

4.60 4.60 FUD ZZZ C 80

AMA: 2018,Jan,8; 2017,Jan,8; 2016,Jan,13; 2015,Jan,16

43284 **Laparoscopy, surgical, esophageal sphincter augmentation procedure, placement of sphincter augmentation device (ie, magnetic band), including cruroplasty when performed**

EXCLUDES *Performed during same session (43279-43282)*

18.9 18.9 FUD 090 J J8 80

AMA: 2019,Apr,10; 2018,Sep,14; 2018,Jan,8; 2017,Aug,6

43285 **Removal of esophageal sphincter augmentation device**

19.5 19.5 FUD 090 Q2 G2 80

AMA: 2018,Jan,8; 2017,Aug,6

43286 **Esophagectomy, total or near total, with laparoscopic mobilization of the abdominal and mediastinal esophagus and proximal gastrectomy, with laparoscopic pyloric drainage procedure if performed, with open cervical pharyngogastrostomy or esophagogastrostomy (ie, laparoscopic transhiatal esophagectomy)**

90.9 90.9 FUD 090 C 80

AMA: 2018,Jul,7

43287 **Esophagectomy, distal two-thirds, with laparoscopic mobilization of the abdominal and lower mediastinal esophagus and proximal gastrectomy, with laparoscopic pyloric drainage procedure if performed, with separate thoracoscopic mobilization of the middle and upper mediastinal esophagus and thoracic esophagogastrostomy (ie, laparoscopic thoracoscopic esophagectomy, Ivor Lewis esophagectomy)**

EXCLUDES *Right tube thoracostomy (32551)*

104. 104. FUD 090 C 80

AMA: 2018,Jul,7

43288 **Esophagectomy, total or near total, with thoracoscopic mobilization of the upper, middle, and lower mediastinal esophagus, with separate laparoscopic proximal gastrectomy, with laparoscopic pyloric drainage procedure if performed, with open cervical pharyngogastrostomy or esophagogastrostomy (ie, thoracoscopic, laparoscopic and cervical incision esophagectomy, McKeown esophagectomy, tri-incisional esophagectomy)**

EXCLUDES *Right tube thoracostomy (32551)*

109. 109. FUD 090 C 80

AMA: 2018,Jul,7

43289 **Unlisted laparoscopy procedure, esophagus**

0.00 0.00 FUD YYY J 80 50

AMA: 2018,Jul,7; 2018,Jan,8; 2017,Jan,8; 2016,Jan,13; 2015,Jan,16

43300-43425 Open Esophageal Repair Procedures

43300 **Esophagoplasty (plastic repair or reconstruction), cervical approach; without repair of tracheoesophageal fistula**

17.6 17.6 FUD 090 C 80

AMA: 2014,Jan,11; 2013,Jan,11-12

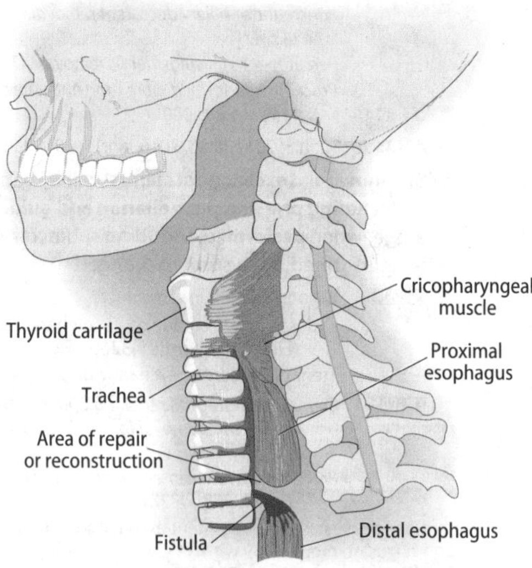

Example of esophageal atresia where the proximal esophagus fails to communicate with the lower portion; note that a fistula has developed from the trachea

43305 **with repair of tracheoesophageal fistula**

31.3 31.3 FUD 090 C 80

AMA: 2014,Jan,11; 2013,Jan,11-12

43310 Esophagoplasty (plastic repair or reconstruction), thoracic approach; without repair of tracheoesophageal fistula
42.9 42.9 FUD 090 C 80
AMA: 2014,Jan,11; 2013,Jan,11-12

43312 with repair of tracheoesophageal fistula
46.1 46.1 FUD 090 C 80
AMA: 2014,Jan,11; 2013,Jan,11-12

43313 Esophagoplasty for congenital defect (plastic repair or reconstruction), thoracic approach; without repair of congenital tracheoesophageal fistula
79.3 79.3 FUD 090 63 C 80
AMA: 2014,Jan,11; 2013,Jan,11-12

43314 with repair of congenital tracheoesophageal fistula
85.2 85.2 FUD 090 63 C 80
AMA: 2014,Jan,11; 2013,Jan,11-12

43320 Esophagogastrostomy (cardioplasty), with or without vagotomy and pyloroplasty, transabdominal or transthoracic approach
EXCLUDES *Laparoscopic approach (43280)*
40.7 40.7 FUD 090 C 80
AMA: 2014,Jan,11; 2013,Jan,11-12

43325 Esophagogastric fundoplasty, with fundic patch (Thal-Nissen procedure)
EXCLUDES *Myotomy, cricopharyngeal (43030)*
39.6 39.6 FUD 090 C 80
AMA: 2014,Jan,11; 2013,Jan,11-12

43327 Esophagogastric fundoplasty partial or complete; laparotomy
23.9 23.9 FUD 090 C 80
AMA: 2018,Jan,8; 2017,Jan,8; 2016,Jan,13; 2015,Nov,8; 2015,Jan,16

43328 thoracotomy
EXCLUDES *Esophagogastroduodenoscopy fundoplasty, transoral (43210)*
32.6 32.6 FUD 090 C 80
AMA: 2018,Jan,8; 2017,Jan,8; 2016,Jan,13; 2015,Nov,8; 2015,Jan,16

43330 Esophagomyotomy (Heller type); abdominal approach
EXCLUDES *Esophagomyotomy, laparoscopic method (43279)*
38.9 38.9 FUD 090 C 80
AMA: 2018,Jan,8; 2017,Jan,8; 2016,Jan,13; 2015,Jan,16

43331 thoracic approach
EXCLUDES *Thoracoscopy with esophagomyotomy (32665)*
38.7 38.7 FUD 090 C 80
AMA: 2018,Jan,8; 2017,Jan,8; 2016,Jan,13; 2015,Jan,16

43332 Repair, paraesophageal hiatal hernia (including fundoplication), via laparotomy, except neonatal; without implantation of mesh or other prosthesis
EXCLUDES *Neonatal diaphragmatic hernia repair (39503)*
33.7 33.7 FUD 090 C 80
AMA: 2018,Jan,8; 2017,Jan,8; 2016,Jan,13; 2015,Jan,16

43333 with implantation of mesh or other prosthesis
EXCLUDES *Neonatal diaphragmatic hernia repair (39503)*
36.8 36.8 FUD 090 C 80
AMA: 2018,Jan,8; 2017,Jan,8; 2016,Jan,13; 2015,Jan,16

43334 Repair, paraesophageal hiatal hernia (including fundoplication), via thoracotomy, except neonatal; without implantation of mesh or other prosthesis
EXCLUDES *Neonatal diaphragmatic hernia repair (39503)*
36.2 36.2 FUD 090 C 80
AMA: 2018,Jan,8; 2017,Jan,8; 2016,Jan,13; 2015,Jan,16

43335 with implantation of mesh or other prosthesis
EXCLUDES *Neonatal diaphragmatic hernia repair (39503)*
38.7 38.7 FUD 090 C 80
AMA: 2018,Jan,8; 2017,Jan,8; 2016,Jan,13; 2015,Jan,16

43336 Repair, paraesophageal hiatal hernia, (including fundoplication), via thoracoabdominal incision, except neonatal; without implantation of mesh or other prosthesis
EXCLUDES *Neonatal diaphragmatic hernia repair (39503)*
42.0 42.0 FUD 090 C 80
AMA: 2018,Jan,8; 2017,Jan,8; 2016,Jan,13; 2015,Jan,16

43337 with implantation of mesh or other prosthesis
EXCLUDES *Neonatal diaphragmatic hernia repair (39503)*
44.8 44.8 FUD 090 C 80
AMA: 2018,Jan,8; 2017,Jan,8; 2016,Jan,13; 2015,Jan,16

+ **43338 Esophageal lengthening procedure (eg, Collis gastroplasty or wedge gastroplasty) (List separately in addition to code for primary procedure)**
Code first (43280, 43327-43337)
3.37 3.37 FUD ZZZ C 80
AMA: 2018,Jan,8; 2017,Jan,8; 2016,Jan,13; 2015,Jan,16

43340 Esophagojejunostomy (without total gastrectomy); abdominal approach
40.0 40.0 FUD 090 C 80
AMA: 2014,Jan,11; 2013,Jan,11-12

43341 thoracic approach
40.5 40.5 FUD 090 C 80
AMA: 2014,Jan,11; 2013,Jan,11-12

43351 Esophagostomy, fistulization of esophagus, external; thoracic approach
38.0 38.0 FUD 090 C 80
AMA: 2014,Jan,11; 2013,Jan,11-12

43352 cervical approach
30.8 30.8 FUD 090 C 80
AMA: 2014,Jan,11; 2013,Jan,11-12

43360 Gastrointestinal reconstruction for previous esophagectomy, for obstructing esophageal lesion or fistula, or for previous esophageal exclusion; with stomach, with or without pyloroplasty
65.3 65.3 FUD 090 C 80
AMA: 2014,Jan,11; 2013,Jan,11-12

43361 with colon interposition or small intestine reconstruction, including intestine mobilization, preparation, and anastomosis(es)
78.6 78.6 FUD 090 C 80
AMA: 2014,Jan,11; 2013,Jan,11-12

43400 Ligation, direct, esophageal varices
44.4 44.4 FUD 090 C 80
AMA: 2014,Jan,11; 2013,Jan,11-12

43405 Ligation or stapling at gastroesophageal junction for pre-existing esophageal perforation
41.9 41.9 FUD 090 C 80
AMA: 2014,Jan,11; 2013,Jan,11-12

43410 Suture of esophageal wound or injury; cervical approach
29.3 29.3 FUD 090 C 80
AMA: 2018,Jan,8; 2017,Jan,8; 2016,Jan,13; 2015,Jan,16

43415 transthoracic or transabdominal approach
74.5 74.5 FUD 090 C 80
AMA: 2014,Jan,11; 2013,Jan,11-12

43420 Closure of esophagostomy or fistula; cervical approach
EXCLUDES *Paraesophageal hiatal hernia repair:*
Transabdominal (43332-43333)
Transthoracic (43334-43335)
29.1 29.1 FUD 090 J 80
AMA: 2014,Jan,11; 2013,Jan,11-12

43425 transthoracic or transabdominal approach
EXCLUDES *Paraesophageal hiatal hernia repair:*
Transabdominal (43332-43333)
Transthoracic (43334-43335)
41.8 41.8 FUD 090 C 80
AMA: 2014,Jan,11; 2013,Jan,11-12

43450-43453 Esophageal Dilation

43450 Dilation of esophagus, by unguided sound or bougie, single or multiple passes
(74220, 74360)
2.27 4.87 FUD 000 T A2
AMA: 2018,Jan,8; 2017,Jul,10; 2017,Jan,8; 2016,Jan,13; 2015,Jan,16

43453 Dilation of esophagus, over guide wire
EXCLUDES *Dilation performed with endoscopic visualization (43195, 43226)*
Endoscopic dilation by dilator or balloon:
Balloon diameter 30 mm or larger (43214, 43233)
Balloon diameter less than 30 mm (43195, 43220, 43249)
(74220, 74360)
2.50 25.4 FUD 000 J A2
AMA: 2018,Jan,8; 2017,Jan,8; 2016,Jan,13; 2015,Jan,16

43460-43499 Other/Unlisted Esophageal Procedures

43460 Esophagogastric tamponade, with balloon (Sengstaken type)
EXCLUDES *Removal foreign body esophagus with balloon catheter (43499, 74235)*
(74220)
6.13 6.13 FUD 000 C
AMA: 2014,Jan,11; 2013,Jan,11-12

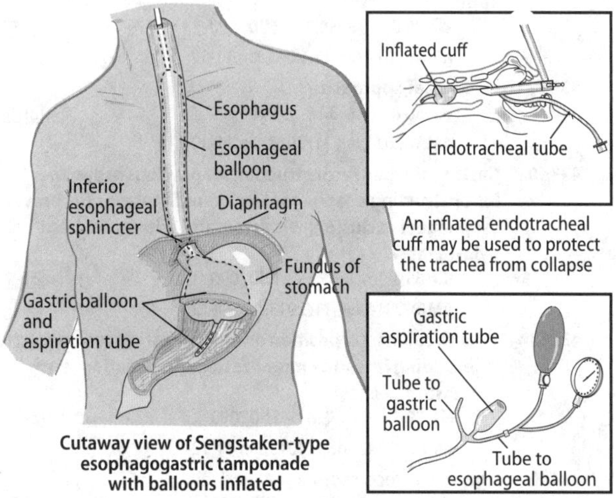

An inflated endotracheal cuff may be used to protect the trachea from collapse

Cutaway view of Sengstaken-type esophagogastric tamponade with balloons inflated

43496 Free jejunum transfer with microvascular anastomosis
INCLUDES Operating microscope (69990)
0.00 0.00 FUD 090 C 80
AMA: 2019,Dec,5; 2018,Jan,8; 2017,Jan,8; 2016,Feb,12; 2016,Jan,13; 2015,Jan,16

43499 Unlisted procedure, esophagus
0.00 0.00 FUD YYY T
AMA: 2018,Jul,7; 2018,Jan,8; 2017,Jan,8; 2016,Jan,13; 2015,Nov,10; 2015,Nov,8; 2015,Jan,16

43500-43641 Open Gastric Incisional and Resection Procedures

43500 Gastrotomy; with exploration or foreign body removal
22.7 22.7 FUD 090 C 80
AMA: 2014,Jan,11; 2013,Jan,11-12

43501 with suture repair of bleeding ulcer
39.2 39.2 FUD 090 C 80
AMA: 2014,Jan,11; 2013,Jan,11-12

43502 with suture repair of pre-existing esophagogastric laceration (eg, Mallory-Weiss)
44.5 44.5 FUD 090 C 80
AMA: 2014,Jan,11; 2013,Jan,11-12

43510 with esophageal dilation and insertion of permanent intraluminal tube (eg, Celestin or Mousseaux-Barbin)
27.6 27.6 FUD 090 T 80
AMA: 2014,Jan,11; 2013,Jan,11-12

43520 Pyloromyotomy, cutting of pyloric muscle (Fredet-Ramstedt type operation)
19.9 19.9 FUD 090 63 C 80
AMA: 2014,Jan,11; 2013,Jan,11-12

43605 Biopsy of stomach, by laparotomy
24.3 24.3 FUD 090 C 80
AMA: 2014,Jan,11; 2013,Jan,11-12

43610 Excision, local; ulcer or benign tumor of stomach
28.5 28.5 FUD 090 C 80
AMA: 2014,Jan,11; 2013,Jan,11-12

43611 malignant tumor of stomach
35.6 35.6 FUD 090 C 80
AMA: 2014,Jan,11; 2013,Jan,11-12

43620 Gastrectomy, total; with esophagoenterostomy
57.8 57.8 FUD 090 C 80
AMA: 2014,Jan,11; 2013,Jan,11-12

43621 with Roux-en-Y reconstruction
66.2 66.2 FUD 090 C 80
AMA: 2014,Jan,11; 2013,Jan,11-12

43622 with formation of intestinal pouch, any type
67.5 67.5 FUD 090 C 80
AMA: 2014,Jan,11; 2013,Jan,11-12

43631 Gastrectomy, partial, distal; with gastroduodenostomy
INCLUDES Billroth operation
42.0 42.0 FUD 090 C 80
AMA: 2014,Jan,11; 2013,Jan,11-12

43632 with gastrojejunostomy
INCLUDES Polya anastomosis
59.3 59.3 FUD 090 C 80
AMA: 2014,Jan,11; 2013,Jan,11-12

43633 with Roux-en-Y reconstruction
56.1 56.1 FUD 090 C 80
AMA: 2014,Jan,11; 2013,Jan,11-12

43634 with formation of intestinal pouch
62.0 62.0 FUD 090 C 80
AMA: 2014,Jan,11; 2013,Jan,11-12

+ **43635 Vagotomy when performed with partial distal gastrectomy (List separately in addition to code[s] for primary procedure)**
Code first as appropriate (43631-43634)
3.29 3.29 FUD ZZZ C 80
AMA: 2014,Jan,11; 2013,Jan,11-12

43640 Vagotomy including pyloroplasty, with or without gastrostomy; truncal or selective
EXCLUDES *Pyloroplasty (43800)*
Vagotomy (64755, 64760)
34.1 34.1 FUD 090 C 80
AMA: 2014,Jan,11; 2013,Jan,11-12

43641 parietal cell (highly selective)
EXCLUDES *Upper gastrointestinal endoscopy (43235-43259 [43233, 43266, 43270])*
35.1 35.1 FUD 090 C 80
AMA: 2014,Jan,11; 2013,Jan,11-12

43644-43645 Laparoscopic Gastric Bypass with Small Bowel Resection

CMS: 100-03,100.1 Bariatric Surgery for Treatment Co-morbid Conditions Due to Morbid Obesity; 100-04,32,150.1 Bariatric Surgery: Treatment of Co-Morbid Conditions Due to Morbid Obesity; 100-04,32,150.2 HCPCS Procedure Codes for Bariatric Surgery; 100-04,32,150.5 ICD Diagnosis Codes for BMI ≥35; 100-04,32,150.6 Bariatric Surgery Claims Guidance

INCLUDES Diagnostic laparoscopy (49320)

EXCLUDES *Endoscopy, upper gastrointestinal, (esophagus/stomach/duodenum/jejunum) (43235-43259 [43233, 43266, 43270])*

43644 **Laparoscopy, surgical, gastric restrictive procedure; with gastric bypass and Roux-en-Y gastroenterostomy (roux limb 150 cm or less)**

EXCLUDES *Roux limb less than 150 cm (43846)*
Roux limb greater than 150 cm (43645)

50.6 50.6 **FUD** 090 C 80

AMA: 2014,Jan,11; 2013,Jan,11-12

43645 **with gastric bypass and small intestine reconstruction to limit absorption**

EXCLUDES *Roux limb less than 150 cm (43847)*

53.9 53.9 **FUD** 090 C 80

AMA: 2018,Jan,8; 2017,Jan,8; 2016,Jan,13; 2015,Jan,16

43647-43659 Other and Unlisted Laparoscopic Gastric Procedures

INCLUDES Diagnostic laparoscopy (49320)

EXCLUDES *Endoscopy, upper gastrointestinal, (esophagus/stomach/duodenum/jejunum) (43235-43259 [43233, 43266, 43270])*

43647 **Laparoscopy, surgical; implantation or replacement of gastric neurostimulator electrodes, antrum**

EXCLUDES *Electronic analysis/programming gastric neurostimulator (95980-95982)*
Insertion gastric neurostimulator pulse generator, incisional (64590)
Laparoscopy with implantation, removal, or revision gastric neurostimulator electrodes on lesser curvature stomach (43659)
Open method (43881)
Vagus nerve blocking pulse generator and/or neurostimulator electrode array implantation, reprogramming, replacement, revision, or removal at esophagogastric junction performed laparoscopically (0312T-0317T)

0.00 0.00 **FUD** YYY J 80

AMA: 2019,Feb,6; 2018,Jan,8; 2017,Jan,8; 2016,Jan,13; 2015,Jan,16

43648 **revision or removal of gastric neurostimulator electrodes, antrum**

EXCLUDES *Electronic analysis/programming gastric neurostimulator (95980-95982)*
Laparoscopy with implantation, removal, or revision gastric neurostimulator electrodes on lesser curvature stomach (43659)
Open method (43882)
Removal or revision gastric neurostimulator pulse generator (64595)
Vagus nerve blocking pulse generator and/or neurostimulator electrode array implantation, reprogramming, replacement, revision, or removal at esophagogastric junction performed laparoscopically (0312T-0317T)

0.00 0.00 **FUD** YYY J 80

AMA: 2019,Feb,6; 2018,Jan,8; 2017,Jan,8; 2016,Jan,13; 2015,Jan,16

43651 **Laparoscopy, surgical; transection of vagus nerves, truncal**

19.0 19.0 **FUD** 090 J 80

AMA: 2018,Jan,8; 2017,Jan,8; 2016,Jan,13; 2015,Jan,16

43652 **transection of vagus nerves, selective or highly selective**

22.2 22.2 **FUD** 090 J 80

AMA: 2018,Jan,8; 2017,Jan,8; 2016,Jan,13; 2015,Jan,16

43653 **gastrostomy, without construction of gastric tube (eg, Stamm procedure) (separate procedure)**

16.6 16.6 **FUD** 090 J A2 80

AMA: 2018,Jan,8; 2017,Jan,8; 2016,Jan,13; 2015,Jan,16

43659 **Unlisted laparoscopy procedure, stomach**

0.00 0.00 **FUD** YYY J 80 50

AMA: 2018,Jul,7; 2018,Jan,8; 2017,Jan,8; 2016,Jan,13; 2015,Jan,16

43752-43763 Nonsurgical Gastric Tube Procedures

43752 **Naso- or oro-gastric tube placement, requiring physician's skill and fluoroscopic guidance (includes fluoroscopy, image documentation and report)**

EXCLUDES *Critical care services (99291-99292)*
Initial inpatient neonatal/pediatric critical care, per day (99468-99469, 99471-99472)
Insertion long gastrointestinal tube (44500, 74340)
Percutaneous insertion gastrostomy tube (43246, 49440)
Subsequent intensive care, per day, for low birth weight infant (99478-99479)

1.18 1.18 **FUD** 000 Q1 G2

AMA: 2019,Aug,8; 2018,Mar,11; 2018,Jan,8; 2017,Jan,8; 2016,Jan,13; 2015,Jan,16

43753 **Gastric intubation and aspiration(s) therapeutic, necessitating physician's skill (eg, for gastrointestinal hemorrhage), including lavage if performed**

0.63 0.63 **FUD** 000 Q1 N1 80

AMA: 2019,Aug,8; 2018,Jan,8; 2017,Jan,8; 2016,Jan,13; 2015,Jan,16

43754 **Gastric intubation and aspiration, diagnostic; single specimen (eg, acid analysis)**

EXCLUDES *Analysis gastric acid (82930)*
Naso- or oro-gastric tube placement using fluoroscopic guidance (43752)

1.03 5.18 **FUD** 000 Q1 N1 80

AMA: 2018,Jan,8; 2017,Jan,8; 2016,Jan,13; 2015,Jan,16

43755 **collection of multiple fractional specimens with gastric stimulation, single or double lumen tube (gastric secretory study) (eg, histamine, insulin, pentagastrin, calcium, secretin), includes drug administration**

EXCLUDES *Analysis gastric acid (82930)*
Naso- or oro-gastric tube placement using fluoroscopic guidance (43752)

Code also drugs or substances administered

1.74 4.43 **FUD** 000 S G2 80

AMA: 2018,Jan,8; 2017,Jan,8; 2016,Jan,13; 2015,Jan,16

43756 **Duodenal intubation and aspiration, diagnostic, includes image guidance; single specimen (eg, bile study for crystals or afferent loop culture)**

Code also drugs or substances administered

(89049-89240)

1.46 7.11 **FUD** 000 Q1 G2 80

AMA: 2018,Jan,8; 2017,Jan,8; 2016,Jan,13; 2015,Jan,16

43757 **collection of multiple fractional specimens with pancreatic or gallbladder stimulation, single or double lumen tube, includes drug administration**

Code also drugs or substances administered

(89049-89240)

2.20 9.76 **FUD** 000 T G2 80

AMA: 2018,Jan,8; 2017,Jan,8; 2016,Jan,13; 2015,Jan,16

43761 **Repositioning of a naso- or oro-gastric feeding tube, through the duodenum for enteric nutrition**

EXCLUDES *Conversion gastrostomy tube to gastro-jejunostomy tube, percutaneous (49446)*
Gastrostomy tube converted endoscopically to jejunostomy tube (44373)
Insertion long gastrointestinal tube (44500, 74340)

(76000)

2.98 3.43 **FUD** 000 T A2

AMA: 2018,Jan,8; 2017,Jan,8; 2016,Jan,13; 2015,Jan,16

43762 **Replacement of gastrostomy tube, percutaneous, includes removal, when performed, without imaging or endoscopic guidance; not requiring revision of gastrostomy tract**

1.10 6.45 **FUD** 000 G2

AMA: 2019,Feb,5

43763 **requiring revision of gastrostomy tract**

EXCLUDES *Gastrostomy tube replacement using fluoroscopy (49450)*
Percutaneous insertion gastrostomy tube (43246)

2.44 9.64 **FUD** 000 G2

AMA: 2019,Oct,10; 2019,Feb,5

43770-43775 Laparoscopic Bariatric Procedures

CMS: 100-03,100.1 Bariatric Surgery for Treatment Co-morbid Conditions Due to Morbid Obesity; 100-04,32,150.1 Bariatric Surgery: Treatment of Co-Morbid Conditions Due to Morbid Obesity; 100-04,32,150.2 HCPCS Procedure Codes for Bariatric Surgery; 100-04,32,150.5 ICD Diagnosis Codes for BMI ≥35; 100-04,32,150.6 Bariatric Surgery Claims Guidance

INCLUDES Diagnostic laparoscopy (49320)
Stomach/duodenum/jejunum/ileum
Subsequent band adjustments (change gastric band component diameter by injection/aspiration fluid through subcutaneous port component) during postoperative period

43770 **Laparoscopy, surgical, gastric restrictive procedure; placement of adjustable gastric restrictive device (eg, gastric band and subcutaneous port components)**

Code also modifier 52 for placement individual component

32.8 32.8 **FUD** 090 J 80

AMA: 2018,Jan,8; 2017,Jan,8; 2016,Jan,13; 2015,Jan,16

43771 **revision of adjustable gastric restrictive device component only**

37.2 37.2 **FUD** 090 C 80

AMA: 2018,Jan,8; 2017,Jan,8; 2016,Jan,13; 2015,Jan,16

43772 **removal of adjustable gastric restrictive device component only**

27.4 27.4 **FUD** 090 J 80

AMA: 2018,Jan,8; 2017,Jan,8; 2016,Jan,13; 2015,Jan,16

43773 **removal and replacement of adjustable gastric restrictive device component only**

EXCLUDES *Laparoscopy, surgical, gastric restrictive procedure; removal adjustable gastric restrictive device component only (43772)*

37.2 37.2 **FUD** 090 J 80

AMA: 2018,Jan,8; 2017,Jan,8; 2016,Jan,13; 2015,Jan,16

43774 **removal of adjustable gastric restrictive device and subcutaneous port components**

EXCLUDES *Removal/replacement subcutaneous port components and gastric band (43659)*

27.8 27.8 **FUD** 090 J 80

AMA: 2018,Jan,8; 2017,Jan,8; 2016,Jan,13; 2015,Jan,16

43775 **longitudinal gastrectomy (ie, sleeve gastrectomy)**

EXCLUDES *Open gastric restrictive procedure for morbid obesity, without gastric bypass, other than vertical-banded gastroplasty (43843)*
Vagus nerve blocking pulse generator and/or neurostimulator electrode array implantation, reprogramming, replacement, revision, or removal at esophagogastric junction performed laparoscopically (0312T-0317T)

32.5 32.5 **FUD** 090 C 80

AMA: 2019,Oct,10

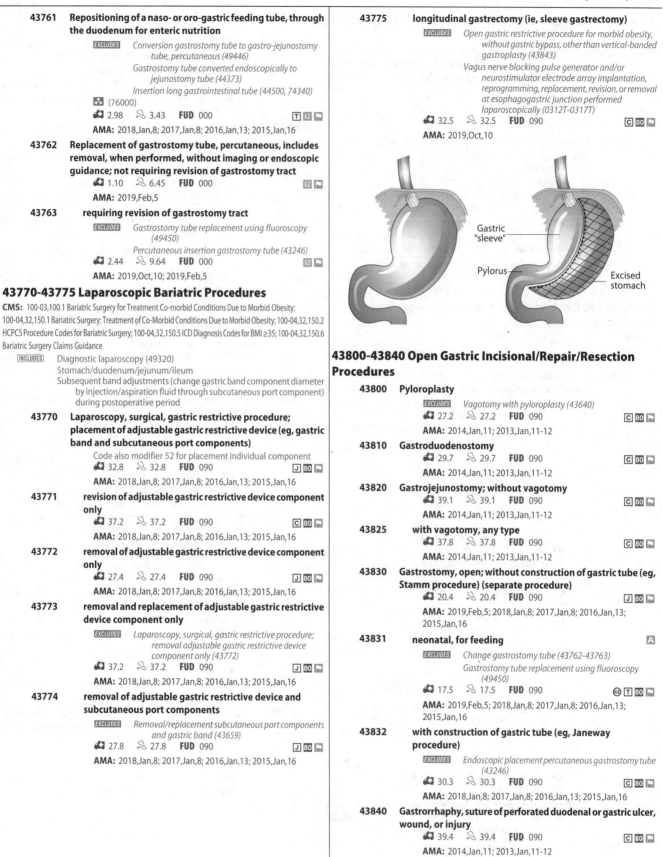

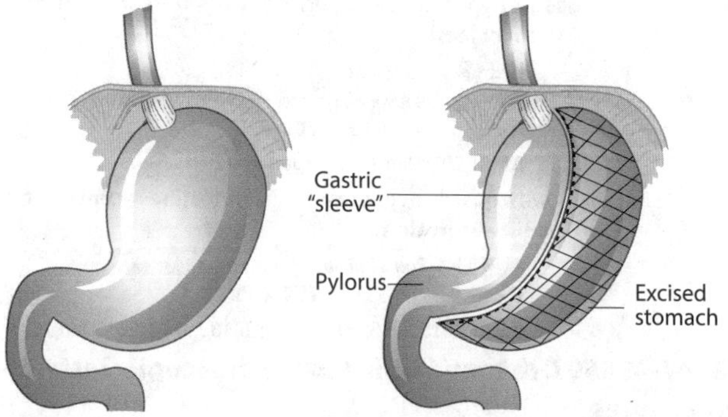

43800-43840 Open Gastric Incisional/Repair/Resection Procedures

43800 **Pyloroplasty**

EXCLUDES *Vagotomy with pyloroplasty (43640)*

27.2 27.2 **FUD** 090 C 80

AMA: 2014,Jan,11; 2013,Jan,11-12

43810 **Gastroduodenostomy**

29.7 29.7 **FUD** 090 C 80

AMA: 2014,Jan,11; 2013,Jan,11-12

43820 **Gastrojejunostomy; without vagotomy**

39.1 39.1 **FUD** 090 C 80

AMA: 2014,Jan,11; 2013,Jan,11-12

43825 **with vagotomy, any type**

37.8 37.8 **FUD** 090 C 80

AMA: 2014,Jan,11; 2013,Jan,11-12

43830 **Gastrostomy, open; without construction of gastric tube (eg, Stamm procedure) (separate procedure)**

20.4 20.4 **FUD** 090 J 80

AMA: 2019,Feb,5; 2018,Jan,8; 2017,Jan,8; 2016,Jan,13; 2015,Jan,16

43831 **neonatal, for feeding** A

EXCLUDES *Change gastrostomy tube (43762-43763)*
Gastrostomy tube replacement using fluoroscopy (49450)

17.5 17.5 **FUD** 090 63 T 80

AMA: 2019,Feb,5; 2018,Jan,8; 2017,Jan,8; 2016,Jan,13; 2015,Jan,16

43832 **with construction of gastric tube (eg, Janeway procedure)**

EXCLUDES *Endoscopic placement percutaneous gastrostomy tube (43246)*

30.3 30.3 **FUD** 090 C 80

AMA: 2018,Jan,8; 2017,Jan,8; 2016,Jan,13; 2015,Jan,16

43840 **Gastrorrhaphy, suture of perforated duodenal or gastric ulcer, wound, or injury**

39.4 39.4 **FUD** 090 C 80

AMA: 2014,Jan,11; 2013,Jan,11-12

43842-43848 Open Bariatric Procedures for Morbid Obesity

CMS: 100-03,100.1 Bariatric Surgery for Treatment Co-morbid Conditions Due to Morbid Obesity; 100-04,32,150.1 Bariatric Surgery: Treatment of Co-Morbid Conditions Due to Morbid Obesity; 100-04,32,150.2 HCPCS Procedure Codes for Bariatric Surgery; 100-04,32,150.5 ICD Diagnosis Codes for BMI ≥35; 100-04,32,150.6 Bariatric Surgery Claims Guidance

43842 Gastric restrictive procedure, without gastric bypass, for morbid obesity; vertical-banded gastroplasty
33.4 33.4 **FUD** 090 E
AMA: 2018,Jan,8; 2017,Jan,8; 2016,Jan,13; 2015,Jan,16

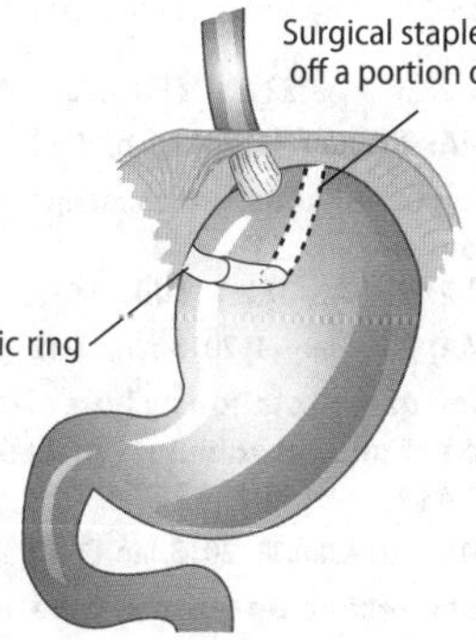

The stomach is surgically restricted to treat morbid obesity; a vertical-banded partitioning technique gives the patient a sensation of fullness, thus decreasing daily caloric intake

43843 other than vertical-banded gastroplasty
EXCLUDES *Laparoscopic longitudinal gastrectomy (e.g., sleeve gastrectomy) (43775)*
37.4 37.4 **FUD** 090 C 80
AMA: 2018,Jan,8; 2017,Jan,8; 2016,Jan,13; 2015,Jan,16

43845 Gastric restrictive procedure with partial gastrectomy, pylorus-preserving duodenoileostomy and ileoileostomy (50 to 100 cm common channel) to limit absorption (biliopancreatic diversion with duodenal switch)
EXCLUDES *Enteroenterostomy, anastomosis intestine (44130)*
Exploratory laparotomy, exploratory celiotomy (49000)
Gastrectomy, partial, distal; with Roux-en-Y reconstruction (43633)
Gastric restrictive procedure, with gastric bypass for morbid obesity; with small intestine reconstruction (43847)
56.8 56.8 **FUD** 090 C 80
AMA: 2018,Jan,8; 2017,Jan,8; 2016,Jan,13; 2015,Jan,16

43846 Gastric restrictive procedure, with gastric bypass for morbid obesity; with short limb (150 cm or less) Roux-en-Y gastroenterostomy
EXCLUDES *Performed laparoscopically (43644)*
Roux limb more than 150 cm (43847)
47.3 47.3 **FUD** 090 C 80
AMA: 2018,Jan,8; 2017,Jan,8; 2016,Jan,13; 2015,Jan,16

43847 with small intestine reconstruction to limit absorption
EXCLUDES *Performed laparoscopically (43645)*
52.4 52.4 **FUD** 090 C 80
AMA: 2018,Jan,8; 2017,Jan,8; 2016,Jan,13; 2015,Jan,16

43848 Revision, open, of gastric restrictive procedure for morbid obesity, other than adjustable gastric restrictive device (separate procedure)
EXCLUDES *Gastric restrictive port procedures (43886-43888)*
Procedures for adjustable gastric restrictive devices (43770-43774)
56.4 56.4 **FUD** 090 C 80
AMA: 2018,Jan,8; 2017,Jan,8; 2016,Jan,13; 2015,Jan,16

43850-43882 Open Gastric Procedures: Closure/Implantation/Replacement/Revision

43850 Revision of gastroduodenal anastomosis (gastroduodenostomy) with reconstruction; without vagotomy
47.5 47.5 **FUD** 090 C 80
AMA: 2014,Jan,11; 2013,Jan,11-12

43855 with vagotomy
49.1 49.1 **FUD** 090 C 80
AMA: 2014,Jan,11; 2013,Jan,11-12

43860 Revision of gastrojejunal anastomosis (gastrojejunostomy) with reconstruction, with or without partial gastrectomy or intestine resection; without vagotomy
47.7 47.7 **FUD** 090 C 80
AMA: 2014,Jan,11; 2013,Jan,11-12

43865 with vagotomy
49.9 49.9 **FUD** 090 C 80
AMA: 2014,Jan,11; 2013,Jan,11-12

43870 Closure of gastrostomy, surgical
20.6 20.6 **FUD** 090 J A2 80
AMA: 2018,Jul,14

43880 Closure of gastrocolic fistula
46.1 46.1 **FUD** 090 C 80
AMA: 2014,Jan,11; 2013,Jan,11-12

43881 Implantation or replacement of gastric neurostimulator electrodes, antrum, open
EXCLUDES *Electronic analysis and programming (95980-95982)*
Implantation/removal/revision gastric neurostimulator electrodes, lesser curvature or vagal trunk (EGJ):
Laparoscopically (43659)
Open, lesser curvature (43999)
Implantation/replacement performed laparoscopically (43647)
Insertion gastric neurostimulator pulse generator (64590)
Vagus nerve blocking pulse generator and/or neurostimulator electrode array implantation, reprogramming, replacement, revision, or removal at esophagogastric junction performed laparoscopically (0312T-0317T)
0.00 0.00 **FUD** YYY C 80
AMA: 2019,Feb,6; 2018,Jan,8; 2017,Jan,8; 2016,Jan,13; 2015,Jan,16

43882 Revision or removal of gastric neurostimulator electrodes, antrum, open
EXCLUDES *Electronic analysis and programming (95980-95982)*
Implantation/removal/revision gastric neurostimulator electrodes, lesser curvature or vagal trunk (EGJ):
Laparoscopic (43659)
Open, lesser curvature (43999)
Revision/removal gastric neurostimulator electrodes, antrum, performed laparoscopically (43648)
Revision/removal gastric neurostimulator pulse generator (64595)
Vagus nerve blocking pulse generator and/or neurostimulator electrode array implantation, reprogramming, replacement, revision, or removal at esophagogastric junction performed laparoscopically (0312T-0317T)
0.00 0.00 **FUD** YYY C 80
AMA: 2019,Feb,6; 2018,Jan,8; 2017,Jan,8; 2016,Jan,13; 2015,Jan,16

43886-43999 Bariatric Procedures: Removal/Replacement/Revision Port Components

CMS: 100-04,32,150.1 Bariatric Surgery: Treatment of Co-Morbid Conditions Due to Morbid Obesity; 100-04,32,150.2 HCPCS Procedure Codes for Bariatric Surgery; 100-04,32,150.5 ICD Diagnosis Codes for BMI ≥35; 100-04,32,150.6 Bariatric Surgery Claims Guidance

43886 **Gastric restrictive procedure, open; revision of subcutaneous port component only**
10.5 10.5 **FUD** 090 T G2 80
AMA: 2018,Jan,8; 2017,Jan,8; 2016,Jan,13; 2015,Jan,16

43887 **removal of subcutaneous port component only**
EXCLUDES *Gastric band and subcutaneous port components:*
Removal and replacement performed laparoscopically (43659)
Removal performed laparoscopically (43774)
9.52 9.52 **FUD** 090 Q2 G2 80
AMA: 2018,Jan,8; 2017,Jan,8; 2016,Jan,13; 2015,Jan,16

43888 **removal and replacement of subcutaneous port component only**
EXCLUDES *Gastric band and subcutaneous port components:*
Removal and replacement performed laparoscopically (43659)
Removal performed laparoscopically (43774)
Gastric restrictive procedure, open; removal subcutaneous port component only (43887)
13.4 13.4 **FUD** 090 T G2 80
AMA: 2018,Jan,8; 2017,Jan,8; 2016,Jan,13; 2015,Jan,16

43999 **Unlisted procedure, stomach**
0.00 0.00 **FUD** YYY T 80
AMA: 2018,Dec,10; 2018,Dec,10; 2018,Jul,14; 2018,Jan,8; 2017,Jan,8; 2016,Jan,13; 2015,Jan,16

44005-44130 Incisional and Resection Procedures of Bowel

44005 **Enterolysis (freeing of intestinal adhesion) (separate procedure)**
EXCLUDES *Enterolysis performed laparoscopically (44180)*
Excision ileoanal reservoir with ileostomy (45136)
31.7 31.7 **FUD** 090 C 80
AMA: 2018,Feb,11; 2018,Jan,8; 2017,Jan,8; 2016,Jan,13; 2015,Jan,16

44010 **Duodenotomy, for exploration, biopsy(s), or foreign body removal**
24.8 24.8 **FUD** 090 C 80
AMA: 2014,Jan,11; 2013,Jan,11-12

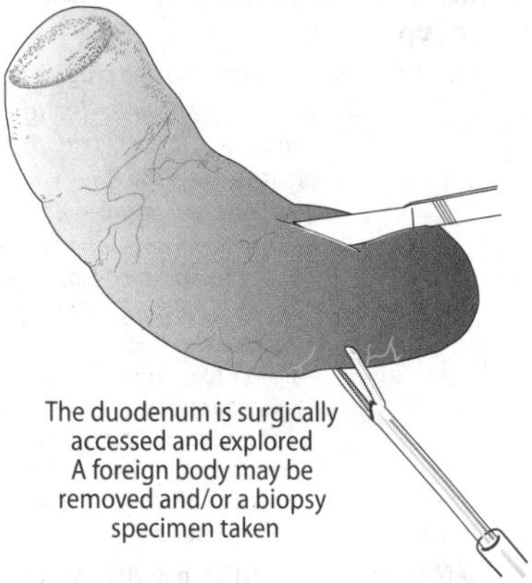

+ **44015** **Tube or needle catheter jejunostomy for enteral alimentation, intraoperative, any method (List separately in addition to primary procedure)**
Code first primary procedure
4.15 4.15 **FUD** ZZZ C 80
AMA: 2018,Jan,8; 2017,Jan,8; 2016,Jan,13; 2015,Jan,16

44020 **Enterotomy, small intestine, other than duodenum; for exploration, biopsy(s), or foreign body removal**
28.2 28.2 **FUD** 090 C 80
AMA: 2014,Jan,11; 2013,Jan,11-12

44021 **for decompression (eg, Baker tube)**
28.3 28.3 **FUD** 090 C 80
AMA: 2014,Jan,11; 2013,Jan,11-12

44025 **Colotomy, for exploration, biopsy(s), or foreign body removal**
INCLUDES Amussat's operation
EXCLUDES *Intestine exteriorization (Mikulicz resection with crushing of spur) (44602-44605)*
28.6 28.6 **FUD** 090 C 80
AMA: 2014,Jan,11; 2013,Jan,11-12

44050 **Reduction of volvulus, intussusception, internal hernia, by laparotomy**
27.2 27.2 **FUD** 090 C 80
AMA: 2014,Jan,11; 2013,Jan,11-12

44055 **Correction of malrotation by lysis of duodenal bands and/or reduction of midgut volvulus (eg, Ladd procedure)**
43.4 43.4 **FUD** 090 63 C 80
AMA: 2014,Jan,11; 2013,Jan,11-12

44100 **Biopsy of intestine by capsule, tube, peroral (1 or more specimens)**
3.11 3.11 **FUD** 000 T A2
AMA: 2014,Jan,11; 2013,Jan,11-12

44110 **Excision of 1 or more lesions of small or large intestine not requiring anastomosis, exteriorization, or fistulization; single enterotomy**
24.6 24.6 **FUD** 090 C 80
AMA: 2014,Jan,11; 2013,Jan,11-12

44111 **multiple enterotomies**
28.5 28.5 **FUD** 090 C 80
AMA: 2014,Jan,11; 2013,Jan,11-12

44120 **Enterectomy, resection of small intestine; single resection and anastomosis**
35.6 35.6 **FUD** 090 C 80
AMA: 2018,Nov,11; 2018,Jan,8; 2017,Jan,8; 2016,Jan,13; 2015,Jan,16

+ **44121** **each additional resection and anastomosis (List separately in addition to code for primary procedure)**
Code first (44120)
7.04 7.04 **FUD** ZZZ C 80
AMA: 2014,Jan,11; 2013,Jan,11-12

44125 **with enterostomy**
34.3 34.3 **FUD** 090 C 80
AMA: 2014,Jan,11; 2013,Jan,11-12

44126 **Enterectomy, resection of small intestine for congenital atresia, single resection and anastomosis of proximal segment of intestine; without tapering**
71.3 71.3 **FUD** 090 63 C 80
AMA: 2014,Jan,11; 2013,Jan,11-12

44127 **with tapering**
83.3 83.3 **FUD** 090 63 C 80
AMA: 2014,Jan,11; 2013,Jan,11-12

+ **44128** **each additional resection and anastomosis (List separately in addition to code for primary procedure)**
Code first single resection small intestine (44126, 44127)
7.10 7.10 **FUD** ZZZ 63 C 80
AMA: 2014,Jan,11; 2013,Jan,11-12

44130 **Enteroenterostomy, anastomosis of intestine, with or without cutaneous enterostomy (separate procedure)**
38.2 38.2 **FUD** 090 C 80
AMA: 2014,Jan,11; 2013,Jan,11-12

44132-44137 Intestine Transplant Procedures

CMS: 100-03,260.5 Intestinal and Multi-Visceral Transplantation; 100-04,3,90.6 Intestinal and Multi-Visceral Transplants

44132 **Donor enterectomy (including cold preservation), open; from cadaver donor**

INCLUDES Graft:
Cold preservation
Harvest

EXCLUDES *Preparation/reconstruction backbench intestinal graft (44715, 44720-44721)*

0.00 0.00 FUD XXX C 80

AMA: 2014,Jan,11; 2013,Jan,11-12

44133 **partial, from living donor**

INCLUDES Donor care
Graft:
Cold preservation
Harvest

EXCLUDES *Preparation/reconstruction backbench intestinal graft (44715, 44720-44721)*

0.00 0.00 FUD XXX C 80

AMA: 2014,Jan,11; 2013,Jan,11-12

44135 **Intestinal allotransplantation; from cadaver donor**

INCLUDES Allograft transplantation
Recipient care

0.00 0.00 FUD XXX C 80

AMA: 2014,Jan,11; 2013,Jan,11-12

44136 **from living donor**

INCLUDES Allograft transplantation
Recipient care

0.00 0.00 FUD XXX C 80

AMA: 2014,Jan,11; 2013,Jan,11-12

44137 **Removal of transplanted intestinal allograft, complete**

EXCLUDES *Partial removal transplant allograft (44120-44121, 44140)*

0.00 0.00 FUD XXX C 80

AMA: 2014,Jan,11; 2013,Jan,11-12

44139-44160 Colon Resection Procedures

+ **44139** **Mobilization (take-down) of splenic flexure performed in conjunction with partial colectomy (List separately in addition to primary procedure)**

Code first partial colectomy (44140-44147)

3.52 3.52 FUD ZZZ C 80

AMA: 2014,Jan,11; 2013,Jan,11-12

44140 **Colectomy, partial; with anastomosis**

EXCLUDES *Laparoscopic method (44204)*

39.0 39.0 FUD 090 C 80

AMA: 2020,Apr,10; 2018,Jan,8; 2017,Jan,8; 2016,Jan,13; 2015,Jan,16

44141 **with skin level cecostomy or colostomy**

53.0 53.0 FUD 090 C 80

AMA: 2018,Jan,8; 2017,Jan,8; 2016,Jan,13; 2015,Jan,16

44143 **with end colostomy and closure of distal segment (Hartmann type procedure)**

EXCLUDES *Laparoscopic method (44206)*

48.4 48.4 FUD 090 C 80

AMA: 2018,Jan,8; 2017,Jan,8; 2016,Jan,13; 2015,Jan,16

44144 **with resection, with colostomy or ileostomy and creation of mucofistula**

51.3 51.3 FUD 090 C 80

AMA: 2018,Jan,8; 2017,Jan,8; 2016,Jan,13; 2015,Jan,16

44145 **with coloproctostomy (low pelvic anastomosis)**

EXCLUDES *Laparoscopic method (44207)*

48.0 48.0 FUD 090 C 80

AMA: 2014,Jan,11; 2013,Jan,11-12

44146 **with coloproctostomy (low pelvic anastomosis), with colostomy**

EXCLUDES *Laparoscopic method (44208)*

61.2 61.2 FUD 090 C 80

AMA: 2018,Jun,11; 2018,Jan,8; 2017,Jan,8; 2016,Jan,13; 2015,Jan,16

44147 **abdominal and transanal approach**

56.3 56.3 FUD 090 C 80

AMA: 2018,Jan,8; 2017,Jan,8; 2016,Jan,13; 2015,Jan,16

44150 **Colectomy, total, abdominal, without proctectomy; with ileostomy or ileoproctostomy**

INCLUDES Lane's operation

EXCLUDES *Laparoscopic method (44210)*

54.0 54.0 FUD 090 C 80

AMA: 2014,Jan,11; 2013,Jan,11-12

44151 **with continent ileostomy**

62.9 62.9 FUD 090 C 80

AMA: 2014,Jan,11; 2013,Jan,11-12

44155 **Colectomy, total, abdominal, with proctectomy; with ileostomy**

INCLUDES Miles' colectomy

EXCLUDES *Laparoscopic method (44212)*

60.0 60.0 FUD 090 C 80

AMA: 2014,Jan,11; 2013,Jan,11-12

44156 **with continent ileostomy**

67.4 67.4 FUD 090 C 80

AMA: 2014,Jan,11; 2013,Jan,11-12

44157 **with ileoanal anastomosis, includes loop ileostomy, and rectal mucosectomy, when performed**

63.9 63.9 FUD 090 C 80

AMA: 2014,Jan,11; 2013,Jan,11-12

44158 **with ileoanal anastomosis, creation of ileal reservoir (S or J), includes loop ileostomy, and rectal mucosectomy, when performed**

EXCLUDES *Laparoscopic method (44211)*

65.5 65.5 FUD 090 C 80

AMA: 2014,Jan,11; 2013,Jan,11-12

44160 **Colectomy, partial, with removal of terminal ileum with ileocolostomy**

EXCLUDES *Laparoscopic method (44205)*

36.0 36.0 FUD 090 C 80

AMA: 2018,Jan,8; 2017,Jan,8; 2016,Jan,13; 2015,Jan,16

44180 Laparoscopic Enterolysis

INCLUDES Diagnostic laparoscopy (49320)

EXCLUDES *Laparoscopic salpingolysis/ovariolysis (58660)*

44180 **Laparoscopy, surgical, enterolysis (freeing of intestinal adhesion) (separate procedure)**

26.6 26.6 FUD 090 J 80

AMA: 2018,Feb,11; 2018,Jan,8; 2017,Jan,8; 2016,Jan,13; 2015,Jan,16

44186-44238 Laparoscopic Enterostomy Procedures

INCLUDES Diagnostic laparoscopy (49320)

44186 **Laparoscopy, surgical; jejunostomy (eg, for decompression or feeding)**

18.9 18.9 FUD 090 J 80

AMA: 2018,Jan,8; 2017,Jan,8; 2016,Jan,13; 2015,Jan,16

44187 **ileostomy or jejunostomy, non-tube**

EXCLUDES *Open method (44310)*

31.8 31.8 FUD 090 C 80

AMA: 2019,Sep,10; 2018,Jan,8; 2017,Jan,8; 2016,Jan,13; 2015,Jan,16

44188 **Laparoscopy, surgical, colostomy or skin level cecostomy**
EXCLUDES *Laparoscopy, surgical, appendectomy (44970)*
Open method (44320)
35.4 35.4 FUD 090 C 80
AMA: 2018,Jan,8; 2017,Jan,8; 2016,Jan,13; 2015,Jan,16

44202 **Laparoscopy, surgical; enterectomy, resection of small intestine, single resection and anastomosis**
EXCLUDES *Open method (44120)*
40.1 40.1 FUD 090 C 80
AMA: 2020,Jul,13; 2018,Jan,8; 2017,Jan,8; 2016,Jan,13; 2015,Jan,16

+ **44203** **each additional small intestine resection and anastomosis (List separately in addition to code for primary procedure)**
EXCLUDES *Open method (44121)*
Code first single resection small intestine (44202)
7.00 7.00 FUD ZZZ C 80
AMA: 2018,Jan,8; 2017,Jan,8; 2016,Jan,13; 2015,Jan,16

44204 **colectomy, partial, with anastomosis**
EXCLUDES *Open method (44140)*
44.7 44.7 FUD 090 C 80
AMA: 2018,Jan,8; 2017,Dec,14; 2017,Jan,8; 2016,Jan,13; 2015,Jan,16

44205 **colectomy, partial, with removal of terminal ileum with ileocolostomy**
EXCLUDES *Open method (44160)*
38.8 38.8 FUD 090 C 80
AMA: 2018,Jan,8; 2017,Jan,8; 2016,Jan,13; 2015,Jan,16

44206 **colectomy, partial, with end colostomy and closure of distal segment (Hartmann type procedure)**
EXCLUDES *Open method (44143)*
50.7 50.7 FUD 090 C 80
AMA: 2018,Jan,8; 2017,Jan,8; 2016,Jan,13; 2015,Jan,16

44207 **colectomy, partial, with anastomosis, with coloproctostomy (low pelvic anastomosis)**
EXCLUDES *Open method (44145)*
52.6 52.6 FUD 090 C 80
AMA: 2018,Jan,8; 2017,Jan,8; 2016,Jan,13; 2015,Jan,16

44208 **colectomy, partial, with anastomosis, with coloproctostomy (low pelvic anastomosis) with colostomy**
EXCLUDES *Open method (44146)*
57.4 57.4 FUD 090 C 80
AMA: 2018,Jan,8; 2017,Jan,8; 2016,Jan,13; 2015,Jan,16

44210 **colectomy, total, abdominal, without proctectomy, with ileostomy or ileoproctostomy**
EXCLUDES *Open method (44150)*
51.3 51.3 FUD 090 C 80
AMA: 2018,Jan,8; 2017,Jan,8; 2016,Jan,13; 2015,Jan,16

44211 **colectomy, total, abdominal, with proctectomy, with ileoanal anastomosis, creation of ileal reservoir (S or J), with loop ileostomy, includes rectal mucosectomy, when performed**
EXCLUDES *Open method (44157-44158)*
61.2 61.2 FUD 090 C 80
AMA: 2018,Jan,8; 2017,Jan,8; 2016,Jan,13; 2015,Jan,16

44212 **colectomy, total, abdominal, with proctectomy, with ileostomy**
EXCLUDES *Open method (44155)*
59.0 59.0 FUD 090 C 80
AMA: 2018,Jan,8; 2017,Jan,8; 2016,Jan,13, 2015,Jan,16

+ **44213** **Laparoscopy, surgical, mobilization (take-down) of splenic flexure performed in conjunction with partial colectomy (List separately in addition to primary procedure)**
EXCLUDES *Open method (44139)*
Code first partial colectomy (44204-44208)
5.43 5.43 FUD ZZZ C 80
AMA: 2018,Jan,8; 2017,Jan,8; 2016,Jan,13; 2015,Jan,16

44227 **Laparoscopy, surgical, closure of enterostomy, large or small intestine, with resection and anastomosis**
EXCLUDES *Open method (44625-44626)*
48.4 48.4 FUD 090 C 80
AMA: 2018,Jan,8; 2017,Jan,8; 2016,Jan,13; 2015,Jan,16

44238 **Unlisted laparoscopy procedure, intestine (except rectum)**
0.00 0.00 FUD YYY J 80 50
AMA: 2020,Jul,13; 2019,Oct,10; 2018,Jan,8; 2017,Jul,10; 2017,Jan,8; 2016,Jan,13; 2015,Jan,16

44300-44346 Open Enterostomy Procedures

44300 **Placement, enterostomy or cecostomy, tube open (eg, for feeding or decompression) (separate procedure)**
EXCLUDES *Intraoperative lavage, colon (44701)*
Other gastrointestinal tube(s) placed percutaneously with fluoroscopic imaging guidance (49441-49442)
24.5 24.5 FUD 090 C 80
AMA: 2018,Jan,8; 2017,Jan,8; 2016,Jan,13; 2015,Jan,16

44310 **Ileostomy or jejunostomy, non-tube**
EXCLUDES *Colectomy, partial; with resection, with colostomy or ileostomy and creation mucofistula (44144)*
Colectomy, total, abdominal (44150-44151, 44155-44156)
Excision ileoanal reservoir with ileostomy (45136)
Laparoscopic method (44187)
Proctectomy (45113, 45119)
30.2 30.2 FUD 090 C 80
AMA: 2018,Jan,8; 2017,Jan,8; 2016,Jan,13; 2015,Jan,16

44312 **Revision of ileostomy; simple (release of superficial scar) (separate procedure)**
17.1 17.1 FUD 090 T A2 80
AMA: 2014,Jan,11; 2013,Jan,11-12

44314 **complicated (reconstruction in-depth) (separate procedure)**
29.1 29.1 FUD 090 C 80
AMA: 2014,Jan,11; 2013,Jan,11-12

44316 **Continent ileostomy (Kock procedure) (separate procedure)**
EXCLUDES *Fiberoptic evaluation (44385)*
41.2 41.2 FUD 090 C 80
AMA: 2014,Jan,11; 2013,Jan,11-12

44320 **Colostomy or skin level cecostomy;**
EXCLUDES *Closure fistula (45805, 45825, 57307)*
Colectomy, partial (44141, 44144, 44146)
Exploration, repair, and presacral drainage (45563)
Laparoscopic method (44188)
Pelvic exenteration (45126, 51597, 58240)
Proctectomy (45110, 45119)
Suture large intestine (44605)
Ureterosigmoidostomy (50810)
34.9 34.9 FUD 090 C 80
AMA: 2018,Jan,8; 2017,Jan,8; 2016,Jan,13; 2015,Jan,16

44322 **with multiple biopsies (eg, for congenital megacolon) (separate procedure)**
29.2 29.2 FUD 090 C 80
AMA: 2014,Jan,11; 2013,Jan,11-12

44340 **Revision of colostomy; simple (release of superficial scar) (separate procedure)**
18.0 18.0 FUD 090 T A2
AMA: 2014,Jan,11; 2013,Jan,11-12

44345 **complicated (reconstruction in-depth) (separate procedure)**
30.4 30.4 FUD 090 C 80
AMA: 2014,Jan,11; 2013,Jan,11-12

44346 **with repair of paracolostomy hernia (separate procedure)**
34.3 34.3 FUD 090 C 80
AMA: 2018,Jan,8; 2017,Jan,8; 2016,Jan,13; 2015,Jan,16

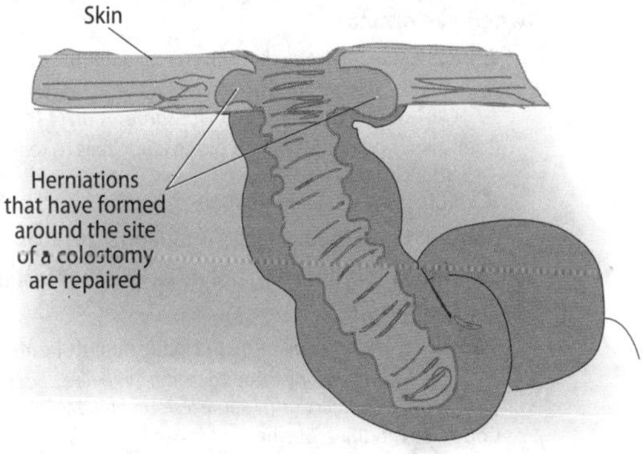
Skin
Herniations that have formed around the site of a colostomy are repaired

The colon is mobilized, trimmed if necessary, and a new stoma is often created

44360-44379 Endoscopy of Small Intestine

INCLUDES Control bleeding due to endoscopic procedure during same operative session

44360 **Small intestinal endoscopy, enteroscopy beyond second portion of duodenum, not including ileum; diagnostic, including collection of specimen(s) by brushing or washing, when performed (separate procedure)**
EXCLUDES *Esophagogastroduodenoscopy, flexible, transoral (43235-43259 [43233, 43266, 43270])*
4.14 4.14 FUD 000 J A2
AMA: 2019,Oct,10; 2018,Jan,8; 2017,Jan,8; 2016,Jan,13; 2015,Jan,16

44361 **with biopsy, single or multiple**
EXCLUDES *Esophagogastroduodenoscopy, flexible, transoral (43235-43259 [43233, 43266, 43270])*
4.65 4.65 FUD 000 J A2
AMA: 2019,Oct,10

44363 **with removal of foreign body(s)**
EXCLUDES *Esophagogastroduodenoscopy, flexible, transoral (43235-43259 [43233, 43266, 43270])*
5.54 5.54 FUD 000 J A2 80
AMA: 2019,Oct,10

44364 **with removal of tumor(s), polyp(s), or other lesion(s) by snare technique**
EXCLUDES *Esophagogastroduodenoscopy, flexible, transoral (43235-43259 [43233, 43266, 43270])*
5.90 5.90 FUD 000 J A2 80
AMA: 2019,Oct,10

44365 **with removal of tumor(s), polyp(s), or other lesion(s) by hot biopsy forceps or bipolar cautery**
EXCLUDES *Esophagogastroduodenoscopy, flexible, transoral (43235-43259 [43233, 43266, 43270])*
5.24 5.24 FUD 000 J A2 80
AMA: 2019,Oct,10

44366 **with control of bleeding (eg, injection, bipolar cautery, unipolar cautery, laser, heater probe, stapler, plasma coagulator)**
EXCLUDES *Esophagogastroduodenoscopy, flexible, transoral (43235-43259 [43233, 43266, 43270])*
6.93 6.93 FUD 000 J A2
AMA: 2019,Oct,10; 2018,Jan,8; 2017,Jan,8; 2016,Jan,13; 2015,Jan,16

44369 **with ablation of tumor(s), polyp(s), or other lesion(s) not amenable to removal by hot biopsy forceps, bipolar cautery or snare technique**
EXCLUDES *Esophagogastroduodenoscopy, flexible, transoral (43235-43259 [43233, 43266, 43270])*
7.10 7.10 FUD 000 J A2 80
AMA: 2019,Oct,10

44370 **with transendoscopic stent placement (includes predilation)**
EXCLUDES *Esophagogastroduodenoscopy, flexible, transoral (43235-43259 [43233, 43266, 43270])*
7.69 7.69 FUD 000 J J8 80
AMA: 2019,Oct,10; 2018,Jan,8; 2017,Jan,8; 2016,Jan,13; 2015,Jan,16

44372 **with placement of percutaneous jejunostomy tube**
EXCLUDES *Esophagogastroduodenoscopy, flexible, transoral (43235-43259 [43233, 43266, 43270])*
7.02 7.02 FUD 000 J A2
AMA: 2019,Oct,10; 2018,Jan,8; 2017,Jan,8; 2016,Jan,13; 2015,Jan,16

44373 **with conversion of percutaneous gastrostomy tube to percutaneous jejunostomy tube**
EXCLUDES *Esophagogastroduodenoscopy, flexible, transoral (43235-43259 [43233, 43266, 43270])*
5.62 5.62 FUD 000 J A2
AMA: 2019,Oct,10; 2018,Jan,8; 2017,Jan,8; 2016,Jan,13; 2015,Jan,16

44376 **Small intestinal endoscopy, enteroscopy beyond second portion of duodenum, including ileum; diagnostic, with or without collection of specimen(s) by brushing or washing (separate procedure)**
EXCLUDES *Small intestinal endoscopy, enteroscopy (44360-44373)*
8.33 8.33 FUD 000 J A2 80
AMA: 2018,Jan,8; 2017,Jan,8; 2016,Jan,13; 2015,Jan,16

44377 **with biopsy, single or multiple**
EXCLUDES *Small intestinal endoscopy, enteroscopy (44360-44373)*
8.63 8.63 FUD 000 J A2 80
AMA: 2018,Jan,8; 2017,Jan,8; 2016,Jan,13; 2015,Jan,16

44378 **with control of bleeding (eg, injection, bipolar cautery, unipolar cautery, laser, heater probe, stapler, plasma coagulator)**
EXCLUDES *Small intestinal endoscopy, enteroscopy (44360-44373)*
11.2 11.2 FUD 000 J A2 80
AMA: 2018,Jan,8; 2017,Jan,8; 2016,Jan,13; 2015,Jan,16

44379 **with transendoscopic stent placement (includes predilation)**
EXCLUDES *Small intestinal endoscopy, enteroscopy (44360-44373)*
11.8 11.8 FUD 000 J A2 80
AMA: 2018,Jan,8; 2017,Jan,8; 2016,Jan,13; 2015,Jan,16

44380-44384 [44381] Ileoscopy Via Stoma

INCLUDES Control bleeding due to endoscopic procedure during same operative session

EXCLUDES *Computed tomographic colonography (74261-74263)*

Code also exam nonfunctional distal colon/rectum, when performed, with:
Anoscopy (46600, 46604-46606, 46608-46615)
Proctosigmoidoscopy (45300-45327)
Sigmoidoscopy (45330-45347 [45346])

44380 **Ileoscopy, through stoma; diagnostic, including collection of specimen(s) by brushing or washing, when performed (separate procedure)**
EXCLUDES *Ileoscopy, through stoma (44382-44384 [44381])*
1.61 5.20 FUD 000 T A2
AMA: 2018,Jan,8; 2017,Jan,8; 2016,Jan,13; 2015,Jan,16

44381 **Resequenced code. See code following 44382.**

44382 **with biopsy, single or multiple**
EXCLUDES *Ileoscopy, through stoma; diagnostic (44380)*
2.10 8.14 FUD 000 T A2
AMA: 2018,Jan,8; 2017,Jan,8; 2016,Jan,13; 2015,Jan,16

44381 **with transendoscopic balloon dilation**

EXCLUDES *Ileoscopy, through stoma (44380, 44384)*

Code also each additional stricture dilated in same session, using modifier 59 with (44381)

(74360)

2.44 27.0 FUD 000 J G2

AMA: 2018,Jan,8; 2017,Jan,8; 2016,Jan,13; 2015,Jan,16

44384 **with placement of endoscopic stent (includes pre- and post-dilation and guide wire passage, when performed)**

EXCLUDES *Ileoscopy, through stoma (44380-44381)*

(74360)

4.44 4.44 FUD 000 J G2

AMA: 2018,Jan,8; 2017,Jan,8; 2016,Jan,13; 2015,Jan,16

44385-44386 Endoscopy of Small Intestinal Pouch

INCLUDES Control bleeding due to endoscopic procedure during same operative session

EXCLUDES *Computed tomographic colonography (74261-74263)*

44385 **Endoscopic evaluation of small intestinal pouch (eg, Kock pouch, ileal reservoir [S or J]); diagnostic, including collection of specimen(s) by brushing or washing, when performed (separate procedure)**

EXCLUDES *Endoscopic evaluation small intestinal pouch (44386)*

2.09 5.60 FUD 000 T A2

AMA: 2018,Jan,8; 2017,Jan,8; 2016,Jan,13; 2015,Jan,16

44386 **with biopsy, single or multiple**

EXCLUDES *Endoscopic evaluation small intestinal pouch (44385)*

2.57 8.54 FUD 000 T A2

AMA: 2018,Jan,8; 2017,Jan,8; 2016,Jan,13; 2015,Jan,16

44388-44408 [44401] Colonoscopy Via Stoma

INCLUDES Control bleeding due to endoscopic procedure during same operative session

EXCLUDES *Colonoscopy via rectum (45378, 45392-45393 [45390, 45398])*
Computed tomographic colonography (74261-74263)

Code also exam nonfunctional distal colon/rectum, when performed, with:
Anoscopy (46600, 46604-46606, 46608-46615)
Proctosigmoidoscopy (45300-45327)
Sigmoidoscopy (45330-45347 [45346])

44388 **Colonoscopy through stoma; diagnostic, including collection of specimen(s) by brushing or washing, when performed (separate procedure)**

EXCLUDES *Colonoscopy through stoma (44389-44408 [44401])*

Code also modifier 53 when planned total colonoscopy cannot be completed

4.52 8.69 FUD 000 T A2

AMA: 2018,Jan,8; 2017,Jan,8; 2016,Jan,13; 2015,Jan,16

44389 **with biopsy, single or multiple**

EXCLUDES *Colonoscopy through stoma; diagnostic (44388)*
Colonoscopy through stoma; with endoscopic mucosal resection on same lesion (44403)

Code also modifier 52 when colonoscope fails to reach junction small intestine

4.97 11.4 FUD 000 T A2

AMA: 2018,Jan,8; 2017,Jan,8; 2016,Jan,13; 2015,Jan,16

44390 **with removal of foreign body(s)**

EXCLUDES *Colonoscopy through stoma; diagnostic (44388)*

Code also modifier 52 when colonoscope fails to reach junction small intestine

(76000)

6.07 11.2 FUD 000 T A2

AMA: 2018,Jan,8; 2017,Jan,8; 2016,Jan,13; 2015,Jan,16

44391 **with control of bleeding, any method**

EXCLUDES *Colonoscopy through stoma; diagnostic (44388)*
Colonoscopy through stoma; with directed submucosal injection(s) in same lesion (44404)

Code also modifier 52 when colonoscope fails to reach junction small intestine

6.65 19.2 FUD 000 T A2

AMA: 2018,Jan,8; 2017,Jan,8; 2016,Jan,13; 2015,Jan,16

44392 **with removal of tumor(s), polyp(s), or other lesion(s) by hot biopsy forceps**

EXCLUDES *Colonoscopy through stoma; diagnostic (44388)*

Code also modifier 52 when colonoscope fails to reach junction small intestine

5.82 10.2 FUD 000 T A2

AMA: 2018,Jan,8; 2017,Jan,8; 2016,Jan,13; 2015,Jan,16

44401 **with ablation of tumor(s), polyp(s), or other lesion(s) (includes pre-and post-dilation and guide wire passage, when performed)**

EXCLUDES *Colonoscopy through stoma; diagnostic (44388)*
Colonoscopy through stoma; with transendoscopic balloon dilation for same lesion (44405)

Code also modifier 52 when colonoscope fails to reach junction small intestine

7.00 80.2 FUD 000 T G2

AMA: 2018,Jan,8; 2017,Jan,8; 2016,Jan,13; 2015,Jan,16

44394 **with removal of tumor(s), polyp(s), or other lesion(s) by snare technique**

EXCLUDES *Colonoscopy through stoma; diagnostic (44388)*
Colonoscopy through stoma; with directed submucosal injection(s) same lesion (44403)

Code also modifier 52 when colonoscope fails to reach junction small intestine

6.60 11.7 FUD 000 T A2

AMA: 2018,Jan,8; 2017,Jan,8; 2016,Jan,13; 2015,Jan,16

44401 **Resequenced code. See code following 44392.**

44402 **with endoscopic stent placement (including pre- and post-dilation and guide wire passage, when performed)**

EXCLUDES *Colonoscopy through stoma (44388, 44405)*

Code also modifier 52 when colonoscope fails to reach junction small intestine

(74360)

7.56 7.56 FUD 000 J J8

AMA: 2018,Jan,8; 2017,Jan,8; 2016,Jan,13; 2015,Jan,16

44403 **with endoscopic mucosal resection**

EXCLUDES *Colonoscopy through stoma; diagnostic (44388)*
Colonoscopy through stoma for same lesion (44389, 44394, 44404)

Code also modifier 52 when colonoscope fails to reach junction small intestine

8.77 8.77 FUD 000 T G2

AMA: 2019,Dec,14; 2018,Jan,8; 2017,Jan,8; 2016,Jan,13; 2015,Jan,16

44404 **with directed submucosal injection(s), any substance**

EXCLUDES *Colonoscopy through stoma; diagnostic (44388)*
Colonoscopy through stoma for same lesion (44391, 44403)

Code also modifier 52 when colonoscope fails to reach small intestine junction

4.97 11.3 FUD 000 T G2

AMA: 2018,Jan,8; 2017,Jan,8; 2016,Jan,13; 2015,Jan,16

44405 **with transendoscopic balloon dilation**

EXCLUDES *Colonoscopy through stoma (44388, [44401], 44402)*

Code also each additional stricture dilated same session, using modifier 59 with (44405)

Code also modifier 52 when colonoscope fails to reach small intestine junction

(74360)

5.28 15.9 FUD 000 T G2

AMA: 2018,Jan,8; 2017,Jan,8; 2016,Jan,13; 2015,Jan,16

44406 **with endoscopic ultrasound examination, limited to the sigmoid, descending, transverse, or ascending colon and cecum and adjacent structures**

INCLUDES Gastrointestinal endoscopic ultrasound, supervision and interpretation (76975)

EXCLUDES *Colonoscopy through stoma (44388, 44407)*

Procedure performed more than one time per operative session

Code also modifier 52 when colonoscope fails to reach small intestine junction

6.62 6.62 FUD 000 T G2

AMA: 2018,Jan,8; 2017,Jan,8; 2016,Jan,13; 2015,Jan,16

44407 **with transendoscopic ultrasound guided intramural or transmural fine needle aspiration/biopsy(s), includes endoscopic ultrasound examination limited to the sigmoid, descending, transverse, or ascending colon and cecum and adjacent structures**

INCLUDES Gastrointestinal endoscopic ultrasound, supervision and interpretation (76975)

Ultrasonic guidance (76942)

EXCLUDES *Colonoscopy through stoma (44388, 44406)*

Procedure performed more than one time per operative session

Code also modifier 52 when colonoscope fails to reach small intestine junction

8.08 8.08 FUD 000 T G2

AMA: 2018,Jan,8; 2017,Jan,8; 2016,Jan,13; 2015,Jan,16

44408 **with decompression (for pathologic distention) (eg, volvulus, megacolon), including placement of decompression tube, when performed**

EXCLUDES *Colonoscopy through stoma; diagnostic (44388)*

Procedure performed more than one time per operative session

6.68 6.68 FUD 000 T G2

AMA: 2018,Jan,8; 2017,Jan,8; 2016,Jan,13; 2015,Jan,16

44500 Gastrointestinal Intubation

44500 **Introduction of long gastrointestinal tube (eg, Miller-Abbott) (separate procedure)**

EXCLUDES *Placement oro- or naso-gastric tube (43752)*

(74340)

0.56 0.56 FUD 000 T G2 80

AMA: 2020,Aug,9; 2018,Jan,8; 2017,Jan,8; 2016,Sep,9; 2016,Jan,13; 2015,Jan,16

44602-44680 Open Repair Procedures of Intestines

44602 **Suture of small intestine (enterorrhaphy) for perforated ulcer, diverticulum, wound, injury or rupture; single perforation**

41.0 41.0 FUD 090 C 80

AMA: 2020,Feb,13

44603 **multiple perforations**

47.1 47.1 FUD 090 C 80

AMA: 2014,Jan,11; 2013,Dec,3

44604 **Suture of large intestine (colorrhaphy) for perforated ulcer, diverticulum, wound, injury or rupture (single or multiple perforations); without colostomy**

30.7 30.7 FUD 090 C 80

AMA: 2014,Jan,11; 2013,Dec,3

44605 **with colostomy**

37.9 37.9 FUD 090 C 80

AMA: 2014,Jan,11; 2013,Dec,3

44615 **Intestinal stricturoplasty (enterotomy and enterorrhaphy) with or without dilation, for intestinal obstruction**

31.1 31.1 FUD 090 C 80

AMA: 2014,Jan,11; 2013,Dec,3

44620 **Closure of enterostomy, large or small intestine;**

EXCLUDES *Laparoscopic method (44227)*

25.1 25.1 FUD 090 C 80

AMA: 2014,Jan,11; 2013,Dec,3

44625 **with resection and anastomosis other than colorectal**

EXCLUDES *Laparoscopic method (44227)*

29.3 29.3 FUD 090 C 80

AMA: 2014,Jan,11; 2013,Dec,3

44626 **with resection and colorectal anastomosis (eg, closure of Hartmann type procedure)**

EXCLUDES *Laparoscopic method (44227)*

46.5 46.5 FUD 090 C 80

AMA: 2014,Jan,11; 2013,Dec,3

44640 **Closure of intestinal cutaneous fistula**

40.6 40.6 FUD 090 C 80

AMA: 2014,Jan,11; 2013,Dec,3

44650 **Closure of enteroenteric or enterocolic fistula**

42.0 42.0 FUD 090 C 80

AMA: 2014,Jan,11; 2013,Dec,3

44660 **Closure of enterovesical fistula; without intestinal or bladder resection**

EXCLUDES *Closure fistula:*

Gastrocolic (43880)

Rectovesical (45800, 45805)

Renocolic (50525-50526)

38.7 38.7 FUD 090 C 80

AMA: 2014,Jan,11; 2013,Dec,3

44661 **with intestine and/or bladder resection**

EXCLUDES *Closure fistula:*

Gastrocolic (43880)

Rectovesical (45800, 45805)

Renocolic (50525-50526)

45.0 45.0 FUD 090 C 80

AMA: 2014,Jan,11; 2013,Dec,3

44680 **Intestinal plication (separate procedure)**

INCLUDES Noble intestinal plication

30.8 30.8 FUD 090 C 80

AMA: 2014,Jan,11; 2013,Dec,3

44700-44705 Other Intestinal Procedures

44700 **Exclusion of small intestine from pelvis by mesh or other prosthesis, or native tissue (eg, bladder or omentum)**

EXCLUDES *Therapeutic radiation clinical treatment (77261-77799 [77295, 77385, 77386, 77387, 77424, 77425])*

29.1 29.1 FUD 090 C 80

AMA: 2014,Jan,11; 2013,Dec,3

\+ **44701** **Intraoperative colonic lavage (List separately in addition to code for primary procedure)**

EXCLUDES *Appendectomy (44950-44960)*

Code first as appropriate (44140, 44145, 44150, 44604)

4.94 4.94 FUD ZZZ N N1 80

AMA: 2014,Jan,11; 2013,Dec,3

44705 **Preparation of fecal microbiota for instillation, including assessment of donor specimen**

EXCLUDES *Fecal instillation by enema or oro-nasogastric tube (44799)*

Therapeutic enema (74283)

2.16 3.25 FUD XXX B

AMA: 2018,Jan,8; 2017,Jan,8; 2016,Jan,13; 2015,Jan,16

44715-44799 Backbench Transplant Procedures

CMS: 100-04,3,90.6 Intestinal and Multi-Visceral Transplants

44715 **Backbench standard preparation of cadaver or living donor intestine allograft prior to transplantation, including mobilization and fashioning of the superior mesenteric artery and vein**

INCLUDES Mobilization/fashioning of superior mesenteric vein/artery

0.00 0.00 FUD XXX C 80

AMA: 2014,Jan,11; 2013,Dec,3

Digestive System

44720 — 45116

44720 **Backbench reconstruction of cadaver or living donor intestine allograft prior to transplantation; venous anastomosis, each**
8.02 8.02 FUD XXX C 80
AMA: 2014,Jan,11; 2013,Dec,3

44721 **arterial anastomosis, each**
11.2 11.2 FUD XXX C 80
AMA: 2018,Jan,8; 2017,Jan,8; 2016,Jan,13; 2015,Jan,16

44799 **Unlisted procedure, small intestine**
EXCLUDES *Unlisted colon procedure (45399)*
Unlisted intestinal procedure performed laparoscopically (44238)
Unlisted rectal procedure (45499, 45999)
0.00 0.00 FUD YYY T
AMA: 2018,Jan,8; 2017,Jan,8; 2016,Jan,13; 2015,Jan,16

44800-44899 Meckel's Diverticulum and Mesentery Procedures

44800 **Excision of Meckel's diverticulum (diverticulectomy) or omphalomesenteric duct**
22.3 22.3 FUD 090 C 80
AMA: 2014,Jan,11; 2013,Dec,3

44820 **Excision of lesion of mesentery (separate procedure)**
EXCLUDES *Resection intestine (44120-44128, 44140-44160)*
24.3 24.3 FUD 090 C 80
AMA: 2014,Jan,11; 2013,Dec,3

44850 **Suture of mesentery (separate procedure)**
EXCLUDES *Internal hernia repair/reduction (44050)*
21.7 21.7 FUD 090 C 80
AMA: 2014,Jan,11; 2013,Dec,3

44899 **Unlisted procedure, Meckel's diverticulum and the mesentery**
0.00 0.00 FUD YYY C 80
AMA: 2020,Jul,13

44900-44979 Open and Endoscopic Appendix Procedures

44900 **Incision and drainage of appendiceal abscess, open**
EXCLUDES *Image guided percutaneous catheter drainage (49406)*
22.4 22.4 FUD 090 C 80
AMA: 2014,Jan,11; 2013,Nov,9

44950 **Appendectomy;**
INCLUDES Battle's operation
EXCLUDES *Procedure performed with other intra-abdominal procedure(s) when appendectomy incidental*
18.7 18.7 FUD 090 J 80
AMA: 2018,Jan,8; 2017,Jan,8; 2016,Jan,13; 2015,Jan,16

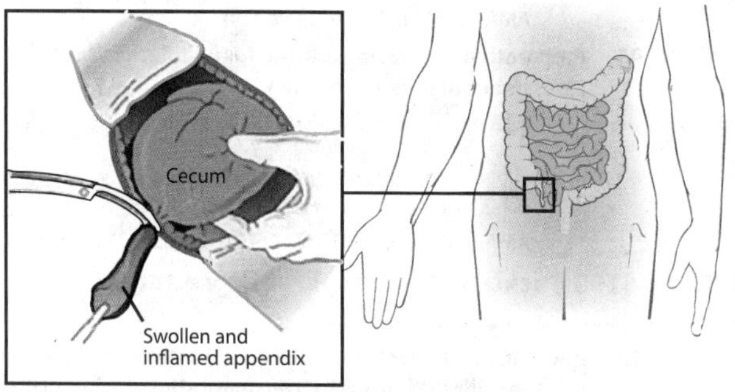

\+ **44955** **when done for indicated purpose at time of other major procedure (not as separate procedure) (List separately in addition to code for primary procedure)**
Code first primary procedure
2.45 2.45 FUD ZZZ N 80
AMA: 2018,Jan,8; 2017,Jan,8; 2016,Jan,13; 2015,Jan,16

44960 **for ruptured appendix with abscess or generalized peritonitis**
INCLUDES Battle's operation
25.5 25.5 FUD 090 C 80
AMA: 2019,Dec,12; 2018,Jan,8; 2017,Jan,8; 2016,Jan,13; 2015,Jan,16

44970 **Laparoscopy, surgical, appendectomy**
INCLUDES Diagnostic laparoscopy
17.4 17.4 FUD 090 J 80
AMA: 2019,Dec,12; 2018,Jan,8; 2017,Jan,8; 2016,Jan,13; 2015,Mar,3; 2015,Jan,16

44979 **Unlisted laparoscopy procedure, appendix**
0.00 0.00 FUD YYY J 80 50
AMA: 2018,Jan,8; 2017,Jan,8; 2016,Jan,13; 2015,Jan,16

45000-45190 Open and Transrectal Procedures of Rectum

45000 **Transrectal drainage of pelvic abscess**
EXCLUDES *Image guided transrectal catheter drainage (49407)*
12.2 12.2 FUD 090 T A2
AMA: 2014,Jan,11; 2013,Nov,9

45005 **Incision and drainage of submucosal abscess, rectum**
4.69 8.38 FUD 010 T A2
AMA: 2014,Jan,11; 2013,Dec,3

45020 **Incision and drainage of deep supralevator, pelvirectal, or retrorectal abscess**
EXCLUDES *Incision and drainage perianal, ischiorectal, intramural abscess (46050, 46060)*
16.5 16.5 FUD 090 J A2
AMA: 2014,Jan,11; 2013,Dec,3

45100 **Biopsy of anorectal wall, anal approach (eg, congenital megacolon)**
EXCLUDES *Biopsy performed endoscopically (45305)*
8.65 8.65 FUD 090 J A2
AMA: 2014,Jan,11; 2013,Dec,3

45108 **Anorectal myomectomy**
10.7 10.7 FUD 090 J A2
AMA: 2014,Jan,11; 2013,Dec,3

45110 **Proctectomy; complete, combined abdominoperineal, with colostomy**
EXCLUDES *Laparoscopic method (45395)*
53.1 53.1 FUD 090 C 80
AMA: 2014,Jan,11; 2013,Dec,3

45111 **partial resection of rectum, transabdominal approach**
INCLUDES Luschka proctectomy
31.4 31.4 FUD 090 C 80
AMA: 2014,Jan,11; 2013,Dec,3

45112 **Proctectomy, combined abdominoperineal, pull-through procedure (eg, colo-anal anastomosis)**
EXCLUDES *Proctectomy for colo-anal anastomosis with colonic pouch or reservoir creation (45119)*
53.9 53.9 FUD 090 C 80
AMA: 2014,Jan,11; 2013,Dec,3

45113 **Proctectomy, partial, with rectal mucosectomy, ileoanal anastomosis, creation of ileal reservoir (S or J), with or without loop ileostomy**
54.7 54.7 FUD 090 C 80
AMA: 2014,Jan,11; 2013,Dec,3

45114 **Proctectomy, partial, with anastomosis; abdominal and transsacral approach**
53.0 53.0 FUD 090 C 80
AMA: 2014,Jan,11; 2013,Dec,3

45116 **transsacral approach only (Kraske type)**
45.1 45.1 FUD 090 C 80
AMA: 2014,Jan,11; 2013,Dec,3

45119 **Proctectomy, combined abdominoperineal pull-through procedure (eg, colo-anal anastomosis), with creation of colonic reservoir (eg, J-pouch), with diverting enterostomy when performed**

EXCLUDES *Laparoscopic method (45397)*

55.9 55.9 **FUD** 090 C 80

AMA: 2018,Jan,8; 2017,Jan,8; 2016,Jan,13; 2015,Jan,16

45120 **Proctectomy, complete (for congenital megacolon), abdominal and perineal approach; with pull-through procedure and anastomosis (eg, Swenson, Duhamel, or Soave type operation)**

46.5 46.5 **FUD** 090 C 80

AMA: 2014,Jan,11; 2013,Dec,3

45121 **with subtotal or total colectomy, with multiple biopsies**

50.5 50.5 **FUD** 090 C 80

AMA: 2014,Jan,11; 2013,Dec,3

45123 **Proctectomy, partial, without anastomosis, perineal approach**

32.4 32.4 **FUD** 090 C 80

AMA: 2014,Jan,11; 2013,Dec,3

45126 **Pelvic exenteration for colorectal malignancy, with proctectomy (with or without colostomy), with removal of bladder and ureteral transplantations, and/or hysterectomy, or cervicectomy, with or without removal of tube(s), with or without removal of ovary(s), or any combination thereof**

80.1 80.1 **FUD** 090 C 80

AMA: 2014,Jan,11; 2013,Dec,3

45130 **Excision of rectal procidentia, with anastomosis; perineal approach**

INCLUDES Altemeier procedure

31.3 31.3 **FUD** 090 C 80

AMA: 2014,Jan,11; 2013,Dec,3

45135 **abdominal and perineal approach**

INCLUDES Altemeier procedure

37.6 37.6 **FUD** 090 C 80

AMA: 2014,Jan,11; 2013,Dec,3

45136 **Excision of ileoanal reservoir with ileostomy**

EXCLUDES *Enterolysis (44005)*
Ileostomy or jejunostomy, non-tube (44310)

51.8 51.8 **FUD** 090 C 80

AMA: 2014,Jan,11; 2013,Dec,3

45150 **Division of stricture of rectum**

12.1 12.1 **FUD** 090 T A2 80

AMA: 2014,Jan,11; 2013,Dec,3

45160 **Excision of rectal tumor by proctotomy, transsacral or transcoccygeal approach**

29.7 29.7 **FUD** 090 J A2 80

AMA: 2014,Jan,11; 2013,Dec,3

45171 **Excision of rectal tumor, transanal approach; not including muscularis propria (ie, partial thickness)**

EXCLUDES *Transanal destruction rectal tumor (45190)*
Transanal endoscopic microsurgical tumor excision (TEMS) (0184T)

17.5 17.5 **FUD** 090 J G2 80

AMA: 2018,Jan,8; 2017,Jan,8; 2016,Jan,13; 2015,Jan,16

45172 **including muscularis propria (ie, full thickness)**

EXCLUDES *Transanal destruction rectal tumor (45190)*
Transanal endoscopic microsurgical tumor excision (TEMS) (0184T)

23.5 23.5 **FUD** 090 J G2 80

AMA: 2018,Feb,11; 2018,Jan,8; 2017,Jan,8; 2016,Jan,13; 2015,Jan,16

45190 **Destruction of rectal tumor (eg, electrodesiccation, electrosurgery, laser ablation, laser resection, cryosurgery) transanal approach**

EXCLUDES *Transanal endoscopic microsurgical tumor excision (TEMS) (0184T)*
Transanal excision rectal tumor (45171-45172)

20.2 20.2 **FUD** 090 J A2

AMA: 2018,Jan,8; 2017,Jan,8; 2016,Jan,13; 2015,Jan,16

45300-45327 Rigid Proctosigmoidoscopy Procedures

INCLUDES Control bleeding due to endoscopic procedure during same operative session
Exam:
Entire rectum
Portion sigmoid colon

EXCLUDES *Computed tomographic colonography (74261-74263)*

Code also examination colon through stoma:
Colonoscopy via stoma (44388-44408 [44401])
Ileoscopy via stoma (44380-44384 [44381])

45300 **Proctosigmoidoscopy, rigid; diagnostic, with or without collection of specimen(s) by brushing or washing (separate procedure)**

(74360)

1.38 3.52 **FUD** 000 T P3

AMA: 2018,Jan,8; 2017,Jan,8; 2016,Jan,13; 2015,Jan,16

45303 **with dilation (eg, balloon, guide wire, bougie)**

(74360)

2.45 27.2 **FUD** 000 T P2

AMA: 2018,Jan,8; 2017,Jan,8; 2016,Jan,13; 2015,Jan,16

45305 **with biopsy, single or multiple**

2.10 4.63 **FUD** 000 T A2

AMA: 2018,Jan,8; 2017,Jan,8; 2016,Jan,13; 2015,Jan,16

45307 **with removal of foreign body**

2.81 5.33 **FUD** 000 J A2 80

AMA: 2018,Jan,8; 2017,Jan,8; 2016,Jan,13; 2015,Jan,16

45308 **with removal of single tumor, polyp, or other lesion by hot biopsy forceps or bipolar cautery**

2.44 5.25 **FUD** 000 J A2

AMA: 2018,Jan,8; 2017,Jan,8; 2016,Jan,13; 2015,Jan,16

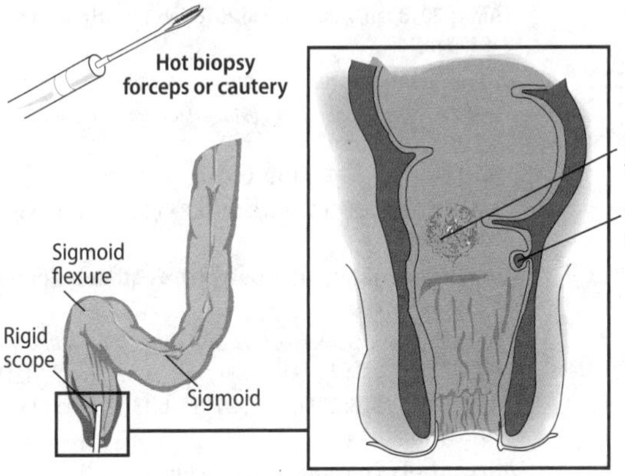

A rigid proctosigmoid procedure of the rectum and sigmoid is performed

45309 **with removal of single tumor, polyp, or other lesion by snare technique**

2.60 5.43 **FUD** 000 T A2

AMA: 2018,Jan,8; 2017,Jan,8; 2016,Jan,13; 2015,Jan,16

45315 **with removal of multiple tumors, polyps, or other lesions by hot biopsy forceps, bipolar cautery or snare technique**

3.08 5.93 **FUD** 000 T A2

AMA: 2018,Jan,8; 2017,Jan,8; 2016,Jan,13; 2015,Jan,16

45317 **with control of bleeding (eg, injection, bipolar cautery, unipolar cautery, laser, heater probe, stapler, plasma coagulator)**
3.24 | 5.52 | FUD 000 | T A2
AMA: 2018,Jan,8; 2017,Jan,8; 2016,Jan,13; 2015,Jan,16

45320 **with ablation of tumor(s), polyp(s), or other lesion(s) not amenable to removal by hot biopsy forceps, bipolar cautery or snare technique (eg, laser)**
3.05 | 5.78 | FUD 000 | J A2
AMA: 2018,Jan,8; 2017,Jan,8; 2016,Jan,13; 2015,Jan,16

45321 **with decompression of volvulus**
3.01 | 3.01 | FUD 000 | J A2
AMA: 2018,Jan,8; 2017,Jan,8; 2016,Jan,13; 2015,Jan,16

45327 **with transendoscopic stent placement (includes predilation)**
3.41 | 3.41 | FUD 000 | J J8
AMA: 2018,Jan,8; 2017,Jan,8; 2016,Jan,13; 2015,Jan,16

45330-45350 [45346] Flexible Sigmoidoscopy Procedures

INCLUDES Control bleeding due to endoscopic procedure during same operative session
Exam:
- Entire rectum
- Entire sigmoid colon
- Portion descending colon (when performed)

EXCLUDES *Computed tomographic colonography (74261-74263)*

Code also examination colon through stoma when appropriate:
- Colonoscopy (44388-44408 [44401])
- Ileoscopy (44380-44384 [44381])

45330 **Sigmoidoscopy, flexible; diagnostic, including collection of specimen(s) by brushing or washing, when performed (separate procedure)**
EXCLUDES *Sigmoidoscopy, flexible (45331-45350 [45346])*
1.61 | 4.98 | FUD 000 | T P3
AMA: 2018,Jan,8; 2017,Jan,8; 2016,Feb,13; 2016,Jan,13; 2015,Sep,12; 2015,Jan,16

45331 **with biopsy, single or multiple**
EXCLUDES *Sigmoidoscopy, flexible; with endoscopic mucosal resection same lesion (45349)*
2.08 | 7.60 | FUD 000 | T A2
AMA: 2018,Jan,8; 2017,Jan,8; 2016,Feb,13; 2016,Jan,13; 2015,Jan,16

45332 **with removal of foreign body(s)**
EXCLUDES *Sigmoidoscopy, flexible; diagnostic (45330)*
(76000)
3.06 | 7.36 | FUD 000 | T A2
AMA: 2018,Jan,8; 2017,Jan,8; 2016,Feb,13; 2016,Jan,13; 2015,Jan,16

45333 **with removal of tumor(s), polyp(s), or other lesion(s) by hot biopsy forceps**
EXCLUDES *Sigmoidoscopy, flexible; diagnostic (45330)*
2.71 | 8.92 | FUD 000 | T A2
AMA: 2018,Jan,8; 2017,Jan,8; 2016,Feb,13; 2016,Jan,13; 2015,Jan,16

45334 **with control of bleeding, any method**
EXCLUDES *Sigmoidoscopy, flexible; diagnostic (45330)*
Sigmoidoscopy, flexible; with band ligation same lesion (45350)
Sigmoidoscopy, flexible; with directed submucosal injection same lesion (45335)
3.44 | 15.3 | FUD 000 | T A2
AMA: 2018,Jan,8; 2017,Jan,8; 2016,Feb,13; 2016,Jan,13; 2015,Jan,16

45335 **with directed submucosal injection(s), any substance**
EXCLUDES *Sigmoidoscopy, flexible; diagnostic (45330)*
Sigmoidoscopy, flexible; with control bleeding same lesion (45334)
Sigmoidoscopy, flexible; with endoscopic mucosal resection same lesion (45349)
1.91 | 7.58 | FUD 000 | T A2
AMA: 2018,Jan,8; 2017,Jan,8; 2016,Feb,13; 2016,Jan,13; 2015,Jan,16

45337 **with decompression (for pathologic distention) (eg, volvulus, megacolon), including placement of decompression tube, when performed**
EXCLUDES *Procedure performed more than one time per operative session*
Sigmoidoscopy, flexible; diagnostic (45330)
3.37 | 3.37 | FUD 000 | T A2
AMA: 2018,Jan,8; 2017,Jan,8; 2016,Feb,13; 2016,Jan,13; 2015,Jan,16

45338 **with removal of tumor(s), polyp(s), or other lesion(s) by snare technique**
EXCLUDES *Sigmoidoscopy, flexible; diagnostic (45330)*
Sigmoidoscopy, flexible; with endoscopic mucosal resection same lesion (45349)
3.47 | 8.07 | FUD 000 | T A2
AMA: 2018,Jan,8; 2017,Jan,8; 2016,Feb,13; 2016,Jan,13; 2015,Jan,16

45346 **with ablation of tumor(s), polyp(s), or other lesion(s) (includes pre- and post-dilation and guide wire passage, when performed)**
EXCLUDES *Sigmoidoscopy, flexible; diagnostic (45330)*
Sigmoidoscopy, flexible; with transendoscopic balloon dilation same lesion (45340)
4.70 | 82.3 | FUD 000 | T G2
AMA: 2018,Jan,8; 2017,Jan,8; 2016,Feb,13; 2016,Jan,13; 2015,Jan,16

45340 **with transendoscopic balloon dilation**
EXCLUDES *Sigmoidoscopy, flexible (45330, [45346], 45347)*
Code also each additional stricture dilated same session, using modifier 59 with (45340)
(74360)
2.24 | 12.9 | FUD 000 | T A2
AMA: 2018,Jan,8; 2017,Jan,8; 2016,Feb,13; 2016,Jan,13; 2015,Jan,16

45341 **with endoscopic ultrasound examination**
INCLUDES Gastrointestinal endoscopic ultrasound, supervision, and interpretation (76975)
Ultrasound, transrectal (76872)
EXCLUDES *Procedure performed more than one time per operative session*
Sigmoidoscopy, flexible (45330, 45342)
3.57 | 3.57 | FUD 000 | T A2
AMA: 2018,Jan,8; 2017,Jan,8; 2016,Feb,13; 2016,Jan,13; 2015,Jan,16

45342 **with transendoscopic ultrasound guided intramural or transmural fine needle aspiration/biopsy(s)**
INCLUDES Gastrointestinal endoscopic ultrasound, supervision and interpretation (76975)
Ultrasonic guidance (76942)
Ultrasound, transrectal (76872)
EXCLUDES *Sigmoidoscopy, flexible (45330, 45341)*
Procedure performed more than one time per operative session
4.89 | 4.89 | FUD 000 | T A2
AMA: 2018,Jan,8; 2017,Jan,8; 2016,Feb,13; 2016,Jan,13; 2015,Jan,16

45346 **Resequenced code. See code following 45338.**

45347 **with placement of endoscopic stent (includes pre- and post-dilation and guide wire passage, when performed)**

EXCLUDES *Sigmoidoscopy, flexible (45330, 45340)*

(74360)

4.44 4.44 FUD 000 J J8

AMA: 2018,Jan,8; 2017,Jan,8; 2016,Feb,13; 2016,Jan,13; 2015,Jan,16

45349 **with endoscopic mucosal resection**

EXCLUDES *Procedure performed same lesion with (45331, 45335, 45338, 45350)*

Sigmoidoscopy, flexible; diagnostic (45330)

5.73 5.73 FUD 000 T G2

AMA: 2020,May,13; 2019,Dec,14; 2018,Jan,8; 2017,Jan,8; 2016,Jan,13; 2015,Jan,16

45350 **with band ligation(s) (eg, hemorrhoids)**

EXCLUDES *Hemorrhoidectomy, internal, by rubber band ligation (46221)*

Procedure performed more than one time per operative session

Sigmoidoscopy, flexible; diagnostic (45330)

Sigmoidoscopy, flexible; with control bleeding same lesion (45334)

Sigmoidoscopy, flexible; with endoscopic mucosal resection (45349)

2.92 17.8 FUD 000 T G2

AMA: 2020,Feb,11; 2018,Jan,8; 2017,Jan,8; 2016,Jan,13; 2015,Jan,16

45378-45398 [45388, 45390, 45398] Flexible and Rigid Colonoscopy Procedures

INCLUDES Control bleeding due to endoscopic procedure during same operative session

Exam:

Entire colon (rectum to cecum)

Terminal ileum (when performed)

EXCLUDES *Computed tomographic colonography (74261-74263)*

Code also modifier 53 (physician), or 73, 74 (facility) for incomplete colonoscopy

45378 **Colonoscopy, flexible; diagnostic, including collection of specimen(s) by brushing or washing, when performed (separate procedure)**

EXCLUDES *Colonoscopy, flexible (45379-45393 [45388, 45390, 45398])*

Decompression for pathological distention (45393)

5.35 9.42 FUD 000 T A2

AMA: 2018,Jan,7; 2018,Jan,8; 2017,Sep,14; 2017,Jan,8; 2016,Jan,13; 2015,Sep,12; 2015,Jan,16

45379 **with removal of foreign body(s)**

EXCLUDES *Colonoscopy, flexible; diagnostic (45378)*

Code also modifier 52 when colonoscope fails to reach small intestine junction

(76000)

6.91 12.1 FUD 000 T A2

AMA: 2018,Jan,8; 2017,Jan,8; 2016,Jan,13; 2015,Jan,16

45380 **with biopsy, single or multiple**

EXCLUDES *Colonoscopy, flexible; diagnostic (45378)*

Colonoscopy, flexible; with endoscopic mucosal resection same lesion (45390)

Code also modifier 52 when colonoscope fails to reach small intestine junction

5.87 11.7 FUD 000 T A2

AMA: 2018,Jan,8; 2017,Jan,8; 2016,Jan,13; 2015,Jan,16

45381 **with directed submucosal injection(s), any substance**

EXCLUDES *Colonoscopy, flexible; diagnostic (45378)*

Colonoscopy, flexible; with control bleeding same lesion (45382)

Colonoscopy, flexible; with endoscopic mucosal resection same lesion (45390)

Code also modifier 52 when colonoscope fails to reach small intestine junction

5.87 11.5 FUD 000 T A2

AMA: 2018,Jan,8; 2017,Jan,8; 2017,Jan,6; 2016,Jan,13; 2015,Jan,16

45382 **with control of bleeding, any method**

EXCLUDES *Colonoscopy, flexible; diagnostic (45378)*

Colonoscopy, flexible; with band ligation same lesion ([45398])

Colonoscopy, flexible; with directed submucosal injection same lesion (45381)

Code also modifier 52 when colonoscope fails to reach small intestine junction

7.48 20.0 FUD 000 T A2

AMA: 2018,Jan,8; 2017,Jan,8; 2016,Jan,13; 2015,Jan,16

\# **45388** **with ablation of tumor(s), polyp(s), or other lesion(s) (includes pre- and post-dilation and guide wire passage, when performed)**

EXCLUDES *Colonoscopy, flexible (45378, 45386)*

7.83 82.9 FUD 000 T G2

AMA: 2018,Jan,8; 2017,Jan,8; 2016,Jan,13; 2015,Jan,16

45384 **with removal of tumor(s), polyp(s), or other lesion(s) by hot biopsy forceps**

EXCLUDES *Colonoscopy, flexible; diagnostic (45378)*

Code also modifier 52 when colonoscope fails to reach small intestine junction

6.68 13.1 FUD 000 T A2

AMA: 2018,Jan,8; 2017,Jan,8; 2016,Jan,13; 2015,Jun,10; 2015,Jan,16

45385 **with removal of tumor(s), polyp(s), or other lesion(s) by snare technique**

EXCLUDES *Colonoscopy, flexible; diagnostic (45378)*

Colonoscopy, flexible; with endoscopic mucosal resection same lesion (45390)

7.35 12.6 FUD 000 T A2

AMA: 2018,Jan,8; 2017,Jan,8; 2017,Jan,6; 2016,Jan,13; 2015,Jan,16

45386 **with transendoscopic balloon dilation**

EXCLUDES *Colonoscopy, flexible (45378, [45388], 45389)*

Code also each additional stricture dilated same operative session, using modifier 59 with (45386)

(74360)

6.20 17.0 FUD 000 T A2

AMA: 2018,Jan,8; 2017,Jan,8; 2016,Jan,13; 2015,Jan,16

45388 **Resequenced code. See code following 45382.**

45389 **with endoscopic stent placement (includes pre- and post-dilation and guide wire passage, when performed)**

EXCLUDES *Colonoscopy, flexible (45378, 45386)*

(74360)

8.37 8.37 FUD 000 J J8

AMA: 2018,Jan,8; 2017,Jan,8; 2016,Jan,13; 2015,Jan,16

45390 **Resequenced code. See code following 45392.**

45391 **with endoscopic ultrasound examination limited to the rectum, sigmoid, descending, transverse, or ascending colon and cecum, and adjacent structures**

INCLUDES Gastrointestinal endoscopic ultrasound, supervision and interpretation (76975)

Ultrasound, transrectal (76872)

EXCLUDES *Colonoscopy, flexible (45378, 45392)*

Procedure performed more than one time per operative session

7.43 7.43 FUD 000 T A2

AMA: 2018,Jan,8; 2017,Jan,8; 2016,Jan,13; 2015,Jan,16

45392 **with transendoscopic ultrasound guided intramural or transmural fine needle aspiration/biopsy(s), includes endoscopic ultrasound examination limited to the rectum, sigmoid, descending, transverse, or ascending colon and cecum, and adjacent structures**

INCLUDES Gastrointestinal endoscopic ultrasound, supervision and interpretation (76975)
Ultrasonic guidance (76942)
Ultrasound, transrectal (76872)

EXCLUDES *Colonoscopy, flexible (45378, 45391)*
Procedure performed more than one time per operative session

8.78 8.78 **FUD** 000 T A2

AMA: 2018,Jan,8; 2017,Jan,8; 2016,Jan,13; 2015,Jan,16

45390 **with endoscopic mucosal resection**

EXCLUDES *Colonoscopy, flexible; diagnostic (45378)*
Colonoscopy, flexible; with band ligation same lesion ([45398])
Colonoscopy, flexible; with biopsy same lesion (45380-45381)
Colonoscopy, flexible; with removal tumor(s), polyp(s), or other lesion(s) by snare technique same lesion (45385)

9.74 9.74 **FUD** 000 T G2

AMA: 2020,May,13; 2019,Dec,14; 2018,Jan,8; 2017,Jan,6; 2017,Jan,8; 2016,Jan,13; 2015,Jan,16

45393 **with decompression (for pathologic distention) (eg, volvulus, megacolon), including placement of decompression tube, when performed**

EXCLUDES *Colonoscopy, flexible; diagnostic (45378)*
Procedure performed more than one time per operative session

7.31 7.31 **FUD** 000 T G2

AMA: 2018,Jan,8; 2017,Jan,8; 2016,Jan,13; 2015,Jan,16

45398 **with band ligation(s) (eg, hemorrhoids)**

EXCLUDES *Bleeding control by band ligation (45382)*
Colonoscopy, flexible (45378, 45390)
Hemorrhoidectomy, internal, by rubber band ligation (46221)
Procedure performed more than one time per operative session

Code also modifier 52 when colonoscope fails to reach small intestine junction

6.83 22.3 **FUD** 000 T G2

AMA: 2020,Feb,11; 2018,Jan,8; 2018,Jan,7; 2017,Sep,14; 2017,Jan,8; 2016,Jan,13; 2015,Jan,16

45395-45499 [45398, 45399] Laparoscopic Procedures of Rectum

INCLUDES Diagnostic laparoscopy

45395 **Laparoscopy, surgical; proctectomy, complete, combined abdominoperineal, with colostomy**

EXCLUDES *Open method (45110)*

56.8 56.8 **FUD** 090 C 80

AMA: 2018,Jan,8; 2017,Jan,8; 2016,Jan,13; 2015,Jan,16

45397 **proctectomy, combined abdominoperineal pull-through procedure (eg, colo-anal anastomosis), with creation of colonic reservoir (eg, J-pouch), with diverting enterostomy, when performed**

EXCLUDES *Open method (45119)*

61.8 61.8 **FUD** 090 C 80

AMA: 2018,Jan,8; 2017,Jan,8; 2016,Jan,13; 2015,Jan,16

45398 **Resequenced code. See code following 45393.**

45399 **Resequenced code. See code before 45990.**

45400 **Laparoscopy, surgical; proctopexy (for prolapse)**

EXCLUDES *Open method (45540-45541)*

32.8 32.8 **FUD** 090 C 80

AMA: 2018,Jan,8; 2017,Jan,8; 2016,Jan,13; 2015,Jan,16

45402 **proctopexy (for prolapse), with sigmoid resection**

EXCLUDES *Open method (45550)*

43.8 43.8 **FUD** 090 C 80

AMA: 2018,Jan,8; 2017,Jan,8; 2016,Jan,13; 2015,Jan,16

45499 **Unlisted laparoscopy procedure, rectum**

EXCLUDES *Unlisted rectal procedure performed via open technique (45999)*

0.00 0.00 **FUD** YYY J 80

AMA: 2014,Jan,11; 2013,Jan,11-12

45500-45825 Open Repairs of Rectum

45500 **Proctoplasty; for stenosis**

16.3 16.3 **FUD** 090 J A2 80

AMA: 2014,Jan,11; 2013,Jan,11-12

45505 **for prolapse of mucous membrane**

17.2 17.2 **FUD** 090 J A2

AMA: 2018,Jan,8; 2017,Jan,8; 2016,Jan,13; 2015,Mar,9; 2015,Jan,16

45520 **Perirectal injection of sclerosing solution for prolapse**

1.16 4.41 **FUD** 000 Q1 N1

AMA: 2018,Jan,8; 2017,Jan,8; 2016,Jan,13; 2015,Jan,16

45540 **Proctopexy (eg, for prolapse); abdominal approach**

EXCLUDES *Laparoscopic method (45400)*

30.6 30.6 **FUD** 090 C 80

AMA: 2014,Jan,11; 2013,Jan,11-12

45541 **perineal approach**

27.3 27.3 **FUD** 090 J G2 80

AMA: 2014,Jan,11; 2013,Jan,11-12

45550 **with sigmoid resection, abdominal approach**

INCLUDES Frickman proctopexy

EXCLUDES *Laparoscopic method (45402)*

42.3 42.3 **FUD** 090 C 80

AMA: 2014,Jan,11; 2013,Jan,11-12

45560 **Repair of rectocele (separate procedure)**

EXCLUDES *Posterior colporrhaphy with rectocele repair (57250)*

19.8 19.8 **FUD** 090 J A2 80

AMA: 2014,Jan,11; 2013,Jan,11-12

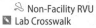

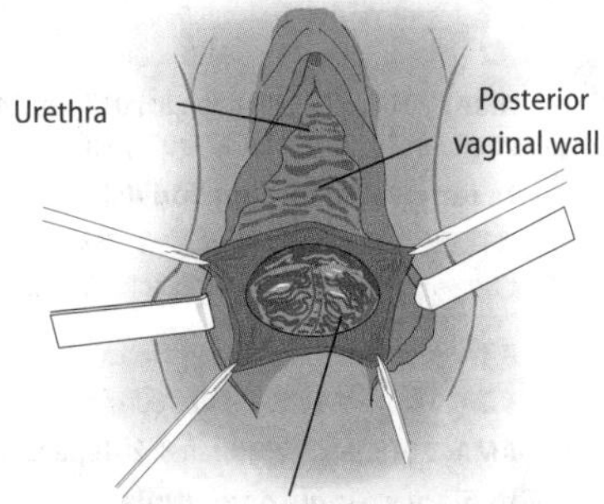

The posterior wall of the vagina is opened directly over the rectocele; the walls of both structures are repaired; a rectocele is a herniated protrusion of part of the rectum into the vagina

45562 **Exploration, repair, and presacral drainage for rectal injury;**

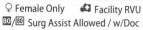

32.7 32.7 **FUD** 090 C 80

AMA: 2014,Jan,11; 2013,Jan,11-12

45563 **with colostomy**

INCLUDES Maydl colostomy

48.3 48.3 **FUD** 090 C 80

AMA: 2014,Jan,11; 2013,Jan,11-12

45800 **Closure of rectovesical fistula;**

36.4 36.4 **FUD** 090 C 80

AMA: 2014,Jan,11; 2013,Jan,11-12

45805 **with colostomy**

42.8 42.8 **FUD** 090 C 80

AMA: 2014,Jan,11; 2013,Jan,11-12

45820 **Closure of rectourethral fistula;**

EXCLUDES *Closure fistula, rectovaginal (57300-57308)*

37.0 37.0 FUD 090 C 80

AMA: 2014,Jan,11; 2013,Jan,11-12

45825 **with colostomy**

EXCLUDES *Closure fistula, rectovaginal (57300-57308)*

44.4 44.4 FUD 090 C 80

AMA: 2014,Jan,11; 2013,Jan,11-12

45900-45999 [45399] Closed Procedures of Rectum With Anesthesia

45900 **Reduction of procidentia (separate procedure) under anesthesia**

6.14 6.14 FUD 010 T A2 80

AMA: 2014,Jan,11; 2013,Jan,11-12

45905 **Dilation of anal sphincter (separate procedure) under anesthesia other than local**

4.86 4.86 FUD 010 T A2

AMA: 2014,Jan,11; 2013,Jan,11-12

45910 **Dilation of rectal stricture (separate procedure) under anesthesia other than local**

5.54 5.54 FUD 010 T A2

AMA: 2014,Jan,11; 2013,Jan,11-12

45915 **Removal of fecal impaction or foreign body (separate procedure) under anesthesia**

6.65 9.90 FUD 010 T A2

AMA: 2018,Jan,8; 2017,Jan,8; 2016,Jan,13; 2015,Jan,16

45399 **Unlisted procedure, colon**

0.00 0.00 FUD YYY T

AMA: 2018,Jan,8; 2017,Jan,8; 2016,Jan,13; 2015,Jan,16

45990 **Anorectal exam, surgical, requiring anesthesia (general, spinal, or epidural), diagnostic**

INCLUDES Diagnostic:
- Anoscopy
- Proctoscopy, rigid

Exam:
- Pelvic (when performed)
- Perineal, external
- Rectal, digital

EXCLUDES *Anogenital examination (99170)*
Anoscopy; diagnostic (46600)
Pelvic examination under anesthesia (57410)
Proctosigmoidoscopy, rigid (45300-45327)

3.09 3.09 FUD 000 J A2 80

AMA: 2018,Jan,8; 2017,Jan,8; 2016,Jan,13; 2015,Jan,16

45999 **Unlisted procedure, rectum**

EXCLUDES *Unlisted rectal procedure performed laparoscopically (45499)*

0.00 0.00 FUD YYY T 80

AMA: 2018,Jan,8; 2017,Jan,8; 2016,Jan,13; 2015,Jan,16

46020-46083 Surgical Incision of Anus

EXCLUDES *Cryosurgical destruction hemorrhoid(s) (46999)*
Fistulotomy, subcutaneous (46270)
Hemorrhoidopexy ([46947])
Injection hemorrhoid(s) (46500)
Thermal energy destruction internal hemorrhoid(s) (46930)

46020 **Placement of seton**

EXCLUDES *Anoscopy; diagnostic (46600)*
Incision and drainage ischiorectal or intramural abscess (46060)
Surgical anal fistula treatment (46280)

6.82 8.10 FUD 010 J A2

AMA: 2014,Jan,11; 2013,Jan,11-12

46030 **Removal of anal seton, other marker**

2.59 4.13 FUD 010 T A2 80

AMA: 2014,Jan,11; 2013,Jan,11-12

46040 **Incision and drainage of ischiorectal and/or perirectal abscess (separate procedure)**

12.1 15.7 FUD 090 T A2

AMA: 2014,Jan,11; 2013,Jan,11-12

46045 **Incision and drainage of intramural, intramuscular, or submucosal abscess, transanal, under anesthesia**

12.6 12.6 FUD 090 J A2

AMA: 2014,Jan,11; 2013,Jan,11-12

46050 **Incision and drainage, perianal abscess, superficial**

EXCLUDES *Incision and drainage abscess:*
Ischiorectal/intramural (46060)
Supralevator/pelvirectal/retrorectal (45020)

2.85 6.27 FUD 010 T A2

AMA: 2014,Jan,11; 2013,Jan,11-12

46060 **Incision and drainage of ischiorectal or intramural abscess, with fistulectomy or fistulotomy, submuscular, with or without placement of seton**

EXCLUDES *Incision and drainage abscess:*
Supralevator/pelvirectal/retrorectal (45020)
Placement seton (46020)

13.8 13.8 FUD 090 J A2

AMA: 2014,Jan,11; 2013,Jan,11-12

46070 **Incision, anal septum (infant)** A

EXCLUDES *Anoplasty (46700-46705)*

7.52 7.52 FUD 090 63 J G2 80

AMA: 2014,Jan,11; 2013,Jan,11-12

46080 **Sphincterotomy, anal, division of sphincter (separate procedure)**

4.60 7.74 FUD 010 J A2

AMA: 2014,Jan,11; 2013,Jan,11-12

46083 **Incision of thrombosed hemorrhoid, external**

3.08 5.24 FUD 010 T P2

AMA: 2018,Jan,8; 2017,Jan,8; 2016,Jan,13; 2015,Jan,16

46200-46262 [46220, 46320, 46945, 46946, 46948] Anal Resection and Hemorrhoidectomies

EXCLUDES *Cryosurgical destruction hemorrhoid(s) (46999)*
Hemorrhoidopexy ([46947])
Injection hemorrhoid(s) (46500)
Thermal energy destruction internal hemorrhoid(s) (46930)

46200 **Fissurectomy, including sphincterotomy, when performed**

9.45 13.0 FUD 090 J A2

AMA: 2014,Jan,11; 2013,Jan,11-12

46220 **Resequenced code. See code before 46230.**

46221 **Hemorrhoidectomy, internal, by rubber band ligation(s)**

EXCLUDES *Colonoscopy or sigmoidoscopy, flexible; with band ligation (45350, [45398])*
Transanal hemorrhoidal dearterialization, two or more columns/groups ([46948])

5.51 7.77 FUD 010 T P3

AMA: 2020,Feb,11; 2018,Jan,8; 2018,Jan,7; 2017,Sep,14; 2017,Jan,8; 2016,Jan,13; 2015,Apr,10; 2015,Jan,16

46945 **Hemorrhoidectomy, internal, by ligation other than rubber band; single hemorrhoid column/group, without imaging guidance**

EXCLUDES *Transanal hemorrhoidal dearterialization, two or more columns/groups ([46948])*
Ultrasonic guidance (76942)
Ultrasonic guidance, intraoperative (76998)
Ultrasound, transrectal (76872)

6.54 9.08 FUD 090 J R2

AMA: 2020,Feb,11; 2018,Jan,8; 2017,Jan,8; 2016,Jan,13; 2015,Apr,10

\# **46946** **2 or more hemorrhoid columns/groups, without imaging guidance**

EXCLUDES *Transanal hemorrhoidal dearterialization, two or more columns/groups ([46948])*
Ultrasonic guidance (76942)
Ultrasonic guidance, intraoperative (76998)
Ultrasound, transrectal (76872)

6.50   9.17   **FUD** 090   J A2

AMA: 2020,Feb,11; 2018,Jan,8; 2017,Jan,8; 2016,Jan,13; 2015,Apr,10

\# **46948** **Hemorrhoidectomy, internal, by transanal hemorrhoidal dearterialization, 2 or more hemorrhoid columns/groups, including ultrasound guidance, with mucopexy, when performed**

INCLUDES Ultrasonic guidance (76872, 76942, 76998)

EXCLUDES *Transanal hemorrhoidal dearterialization, single column/group (46999)*

12.7   12.7   **FUD** 090   G2

AMA: 2020,Feb,11

\# **46220** **Excision of single external papilla or tag, anus**

3.43   6.54   **FUD** 010   T A2

AMA: 2014,Jan,11; 2013,Jan,11-12

46230 **Excision of multiple external papillae or tags, anus**

5.00   8.43   **FUD** 010   J A2

AMA: 2014,Jan,11; 2013,Jan,11-12

\# **46320** **Excision of thrombosed hemorrhoid, external**

3.22   5.65   **FUD** 010   T P3

AMA: 2014,Jan,11; 2013,Jan,11-12

46250 **Hemorrhoidectomy, external, 2 or more columns/groups**

EXCLUDES *Hemorrhoidectomy, external, single column/group (46999)*
Transanal hemorrhoidal dearterialization, two or more columns/groups ([46948])

9.19   13.6   **FUD** 090   J A2

AMA: 2014,Jan,11; 2013,Jan,11-12

46255 **Hemorrhoidectomy, internal and external, single column/group;**

EXCLUDES *Transanal hemorrhoidal dearterialization, two or more columns/groups ([46948])*

10.3   14.8   **FUD** 090   J A2

AMA: 2018,Jan,8; 2017,Jan,8; 2016,Jan,13; 2015,Jan,16

46257 **with fissurectomy**

EXCLUDES *Transanal hemorrhoidal dearterialization, two or more columns/groups ([46948])*

12.3   12.3   **FUD** 090   J A2

AMA: 2014,Jan,11; 2013,Jan,11-12

46258 **with fistulectomy, including fissurectomy, when performed**

EXCLUDES *Transanal hemorrhoidal dearterialization, two or more columns/groups ([46948])*

13.7   13.7   **FUD** 090   J A2 80

AMA: 2014,Jan,11; 2013,Jan,11-12

46260 **Hemorrhoidectomy, internal and external, 2 or more columns/groups;**

INCLUDES Whitehead hemorrhoidectomy

EXCLUDES *Transanal hemorrhoidal dearterialization, two or more columns/groups ([46948])*

13.8   13.8   **FUD** 090   J A2

AMA: 2014,Jan,11; 2013,Jan,11-12

46261 **with fissurectomy**

EXCLUDES *Transanal hemorrhoidal dearterialization, two or more columns/groups ([46948])*

15.1   15.1   **FUD** 090   J A2

AMA: 2014,Jan,11; 2013,Jan,11-12

46262 **with fistulectomy, including fissurectomy, when performed**

EXCLUDES *Transanal hemorrhoidal dearterialization, two or more columns/groups ([46948])*

16.0   16.0   **FUD** 090   J A2

AMA: 2018,Jan,8; 2017,Jan,8; 2016,Jan,13; 2015,Jan,16

46270-46320 [46320] Resection of Anal Fistula

46270 **Surgical treatment of anal fistula (fistulectomy/fistulotomy); subcutaneous**

11.3   14.8   **FUD** 090   J A2

AMA: 2014,Jan,11; 2013,Jan,11-12

46275 **intersphincteric**

11.9   15.6   **FUD** 090   J A2

AMA: 2014,Jan,11; 2013,Jan,11-12

46280 **transsphincteric, suprasphincteric, extrasphincteric or multiple, including placement of seton, when performed**

EXCLUDES *Placement seton (46020)*

13.7   13.7   **FUD** 090   J A2

AMA: 2014,Jan,11; 2013,Jan,11-12

46285 **second stage**

12.0   15.7   **FUD** 090   J A2

AMA: 2014,Jan,11; 2013,Jan,11-12

46288 **Closure of anal fistula with rectal advancement flap**

15.8   15.8   **FUD** 090   J A2

AMA: 2014,Jan,11; 2013,Jan,11-12

46320 **Resequenced code. See code following 46230.**

46500 Other Hemorrhoid Procedures

EXCLUDES *Anoscopic injection bulking agent, submucosal, for fecal incontinence (46999)*

46500 **Injection of sclerosing solution, hemorrhoids**

5.20   8.54   **FUD** 010   T P3

AMA: 2018,Jan,8; 2017,Jan,8; 2016,Jan,13; 2015,Jan,16

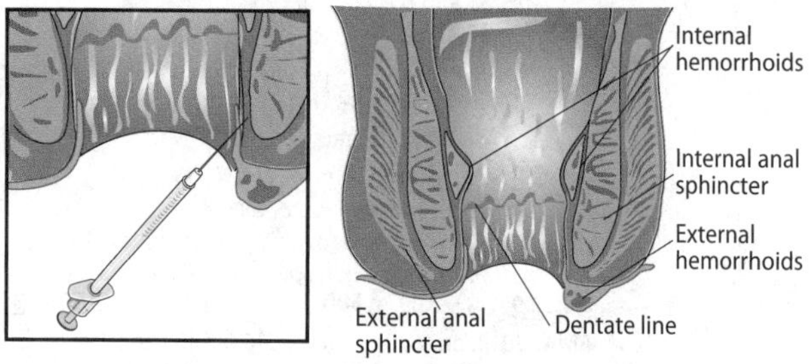

A sclerosing agent is injected into the tissues underlying hemorrhoids

46505 Chemodenervation Anal Sphincter

EXCLUDES *Chemodenervation:*
Extremity muscles (64642-64645)
Muscles/facial nerve (64612)
Neck muscles (64616)
Other peripheral nerve/branch (64640)
Pudendal nerve (64630)
Trunk muscles (64646-64647)

Code also drug(s)/substance(s) given

46505 **Chemodenervation of internal anal sphincter**

7.00   8.55   **FUD** 010   T G2 50

AMA: 2019,Apr,9; 2018,Jan,8; 2017,Jan,8; 2016,Jan,13; 2015,Jan,16

46600-46615 Anoscopic Procedures

EXCLUDES *Delivery thermal energy via anoscope to anal canal muscle (46999)*
Injection bulking agent, submucosal, for fecal incontinence (46999)

46600 Anoscopy; diagnostic, including collection of specimen(s) by brushing or washing, when performed (separate procedure)
EXCLUDES *Excision rectal tumor, transanal endoscopic microsurgical approach (i.e., TEMS) (0184T)*
High-resolution anoscopy (HRA), diagnostic (46601)
Surgical incision anus (46020-46761 [46220, 46320, 46320, 46945, 46946, 46947, 46948])
1.17 2.94 FUD 000 Q1 N1
AMA: 2018,Jan,7; 2018,Jan,8; 2017,Jan,8; 2016,Jan,13; 2015,Jan,16

46601 diagnostic, with high-resolution magnification (HRA) (eg, colposcope, operating microscope) and chemical agent enhancement, including collection of specimen(s) by brushing or washing, when performed
INCLUDES Operating microscope (69990)
2.70 3.97 FUD 000 Q1 N1
AMA: 2018,Oct,11; 2016,Feb,12

46604 with dilation (eg, balloon, guide wire, bougie)
1.90 18.3 FUD 000 T P2
AMA: 2018,Jan,8; 2017,Jan,8; 2016,Jan,13; 2015,Jan,16

46606 with biopsy, single or multiple
EXCLUDES *High resolution anoscopy (HRA) with biopsy (46607)*
2.17 7.31 FUD 000 T P3
AMA: 2019,Sep,10; 2018,Jan,8; 2017,Jan,8; 2016,Jan,13; 2015,Jan,16

46607 with high-resolution magnification (HRA) (eg, colposcope, operating microscope) and chemical agent enhancement, with biopsy, single or multiple
INCLUDES Operating microscope (69990)
3.65 5.75 FUD 000 T G2
AMA: 2019,Dec,12; 2018,Oct,11; 2016,Feb,12

46608 with removal of foreign body
2.44 7.68 FUD 000 T A2
AMA: 2018,Jan,8; 2017,Jan,8; 2016,Jan,13; 2015,Jan,16

46610 with removal of single tumor, polyp, or other lesion by hot biopsy forceps or bipolar cautery
2.34 7.30 FUD 000 J A2
AMA: 2018,Jan,8; 2017,Jan,8; 2016,Jan,13; 2015,Jan,16

46611 with removal of single tumor, polyp, or other lesion by snare technique
2.31 5.78 FUD 000 T A2
AMA: 2018,Jan,8; 2017,Jan,8; 2016,Jan,13; 2015,Jan,16

46612 with removal of multiple tumors, polyps, or other lesions by hot biopsy forceps, bipolar cautery or snare technique
2.76 8.90 FUD 000 J A2
AMA: 2018,Jan,8; 2017,Jan,8; 2016,Jan,13; 2015,Jan,16

46614 with control of bleeding (eg, injection, bipolar cautery, unipolar cautery, laser, heater probe, stapler, plasma coagulator)
1.85 4.21 FUD 000 T P3
AMA: 2018,Jan,8; 2017,Jan,8; 2016,Jan,13; 2015,Jan,16

46615 with ablation of tumor(s), polyp(s), or other lesion(s) not amenable to removal by hot biopsy forceps, bipolar cautery or snare technique
2.64 4.34 FUD 000 J A2
AMA: 2018,Jan,8; 2017,Jan,8; 2016,Jan,13; 2015,Jan,16

46700-46947 [46947] Anal Repairs and Stapled Hemorrhoidopexy

46700 Anoplasty, plastic operation for stricture; adult
18.9 18.9 FUD 090 J A2
AMA: 2014,Jan,11; 2013,Jan,11-12

46705 infant A
EXCLUDES *Anal septum incision (46070)*
16.1 16.1 FUD 090 63 C 80
AMA: 2014,Jan,11; 2013,Jan,11-12

46706 Repair of anal fistula with fibrin glue
5.14 5.14 FUD 010 J A2
AMA: 2014,Jan,11; 2013,Jan,11-12

46707 Repair of anorectal fistula with plug (eg, porcine small intestine submucosa [SIS])
14.4 14.4 FUD 090 J G2 80
AMA: 2018,Jan,8; 2017,Jan,8; 2016,Jan,13; 2015,Jan,16

46710 Repair of ileoanal pouch fistula/sinus (eg, perineal or vaginal), pouch advancement; transperineal approach
32.3 32.3 FUD 090 C 80
AMA: 2018,Jan,8; 2017,Jan,8; 2016,Jan,13; 2015,Jan,16

46712 combined transperineal and transabdominal approach
65.0 65.0 FUD 090 C 80
AMA: 2018,Jan,8; 2017,Jan,8; 2016,Jan,13; 2015,Jan,16

46715 Repair of low imperforate anus; with anoperineal fistula (cut-back procedure)
15.9 15.9 FUD 090 63 C 80
AMA: 2014,Jan,11; 2013,Jan,11-12

46716 with transposition of anoperineal or anovestibular fistula
35.4 35.4 FUD 090 63 C 80
AMA: 2014,Jan,11; 2013,Jan,11-12

46730 Repair of high imperforate anus without fistula; perineal or sacroperineal approach
57.4 57.4 FUD 090 63 C 80
AMA: 2014,Jan,11; 2013,Jan,11-12

46735 combined transabdominal and sacroperineal approaches
66.2 66.2 FUD 090 63 C 80
AMA: 2014,Jan,11; 2013,Jan,11-12

46740 Repair of high imperforate anus with rectourethral or rectovaginal fistula; perineal or sacroperineal approach
62.7 62.7 FUD 090 63 C 80
AMA: 2014,Jan,11; 2013,Jan,11-12

46742 combined transabdominal and sacroperineal approaches
72.7 72.7 FUD 090 63 C 80
AMA: 2014,Jan,11; 2013,Jan,11-12

46744 Repair of cloacal anomaly by anorectovaginoplasty and urethroplasty, sacroperineal approach ♀
103. 103. FUD 090 63 C 80
AMA: 2014,Jan,11; 2013,Jan,11-12

46746 Repair of cloacal anomaly by anorectovaginoplasty and urethroplasty, combined abdominal and sacroperineal approach; ♀
113. 113. FUD 090 C 80
AMA: 2014,Jan,11; 2013,Jan,11-12

46748 with vaginal lengthening by intestinal graft or pedicle flaps ♀
123. 123. FUD 090 C 80
AMA: 2014,Jan,11; 2013,Jan,11-12

46750 Sphincteroplasty, anal, for incontinence or prolapse; adult
21.7 21.7 FUD 090 J A2 80
AMA: 2014,Jan,11; 2013,Jan,11-12

46751 child A
19.2 19.2 FUD 090 C 80
AMA: 2014,Jan,11; 2013,Jan,11-12

46753 Graft (Thiersch operation) for rectal incontinence and/or prolapse
17.7 17.7 FUD 090 J A2
AMA: 2014,Jan,11; 2013,Jan,11-12

46754 **Removal of Thiersch wire or suture, anal canal**
Facility RVU 6.76 Non-Facility RVU 9.30 FUD 010 J A2 80 CCI
AMA: 2014,Jan,11; 2013,Jan,11-12

46760 **Sphincteroplasty, anal, for incontinence, adult; muscle transplant**
Facility RVU 31.6 Non-Facility RVU 31.6 FUD 090 J A2 80 CCI
AMA: 2014,Jan,11; 2013,Jan,11-12

46761 **levator muscle imbrication (Park posterior anal repair)**
Facility RVU 26.6 Non-Facility RVU 26.6 FUD 090 J A2 80 CCI
AMA: 2014,Jan,11; 2013,Jan,11-12

46947 **Hemorrhoidopexy (eg, for prolapsing internal hemorrhoids) by stapling**
Facility RVU 11.1 Non-Facility RVU 11.1 FUD 090 J A2 CCI
AMA: 2018,Jan,8; 2017,Jan,8; 2016,Jan,13; 2015,Jan,16

46900-46999 [46945, 46946, 46947, 46948] Destruction Procedures: Anus

46900 **Destruction of lesion(s), anus (eg, condyloma, papilloma, molluscum contagiosum, herpetic vesicle), simple; chemical**
Facility RVU 3.92 Non-Facility RVU 6.76 FUD 010 T P2 CCI
AMA: 2014,Jan,11; 2013,Jan,11-12

46910 **electrodesiccation**
Facility RVU 3.84 Non-Facility RVU 7.39 FUD 010 T P3 CCI
AMA: 2019,Dec,12

46916 **cryosurgery**
Facility RVU 4.06 Non-Facility RVU 7.00 FUD 010 T P2 CCI
AMA: 2014,Jan,11; 2013,Jan,11-12

46917 **laser surgery**
Facility RVU 3.68 Non-Facility RVU 11.9 FUD 010 J A2 CCI
AMA: 2014,Jan,11; 2013,Jan,11-12

46922 **surgical excision**
Facility RVU 3.92 Non-Facility RVU 8.00 FUD 010 J A2 CCI
AMA: 2014,Jan,11; 2013,Jan,11-12

46924 **Destruction of lesion(s), anus (eg, condyloma, papilloma, molluscum contagiosum, herpetic vesicle), extensive (eg, laser surgery, electrosurgery, cryosurgery, chemosurgery)**
Facility RVU 5.21 Non-Facility RVU 15.1 FUD 010 J A2 CCI
AMA: 2014,Jan,11; 2013,Jan,11-12

46930 **Destruction of internal hemorrhoid(s) by thermal energy (eg, infrared coagulation, cautery, radiofrequency)**
EXCLUDES *Other hemorrhoid procedures:*
Cryosurgery destruction (46999)
Excision ([46320], 46250-46262)
Hemorrhoidopexy ([46947])
Incision (46083)
Injection sclerosing solution (46500)
Ligation (46221, [46945, 46946])
Facility RVU 4.33 Non-Facility RVU 6.12 FUD 090 T P3 80 CCI
AMA: 2018,Jan,8; 2017,Jan,8; 2016,Jul,8; 2016,Jan,13; 2015,Apr,10

46940 **Curettage or cautery of anal fissure, including dilation of anal sphincter (separate procedure); initial**
Facility RVU 4.20 Non-Facility RVU 6.79 FUD 010 J P3 CCI
AMA: 2014,Jan,11; 2013,Jan,11-12

46942 **subsequent**
Facility RVU 3.74 Non-Facility RVU 6.72 FUD 010 T P3 80 CCI
AMA: 2014,Jan,11; 2013,Jan,11-12

46945 **Resequenced code. See code following 46221.**

46946 **Resequenced code. See code following resequenced code 46945.**

46947 **Resequenced code. See code following 46761.**

46948 **Resequenced code. See code before resequenced code 46220.**

46999 **Unlisted procedure, anus**
Facility RVU 0.00 Non-Facility RVU 0.00 FUD YYY T 80 CCI
AMA: 2020,Feb,11; 2018,Oct,11; 2018,Jan,8; 2017,Jan,8; 2016,Jan,13; 2015,Apr,10; 2015,Jan,16

47000-47001 Needle Biopsy of Liver

EXCLUDES *Fine needle aspiration (10021, [10004, 10005, 10006, 10007, 10008, 10009, 10010, 10011, 10012])*

47000 **Biopsy of liver, needle; percutaneous**
Radiology Crosswalk (76942, 77002, 77012, 77021)
Lab Crosswalk (88172-88173)
Facility RVU 2.56 Non-Facility RVU 8.85 FUD 000 J A2 CCI
AMA: 2019,Apr,4; 2018,Jan,8; 2017,Jan,8; 2016,Jan,13; 2015,Jan,16

+ **47001** **when done for indicated purpose at time of other major procedure (List separately in addition to code for primary procedure)**
Code first primary procedure
Radiology Crosswalk (76942, 77002)
Lab Crosswalk (88172-88173)
Facility RVU 3.04 Non-Facility RVU 3.04 FUD ZZZ N N1 CCI
AMA: 2018,Jan,8; 2017,Jan,8; 2016,Jan,13; 2015,Jan,16

47010-47130 Open Incisional and Resection Procedures of Liver

47010 **Hepatotomy, for open drainage of abscess or cyst, 1 or 2 stages**
EXCLUDES *Image guided percutaneous catheter drainage (49505)*
Facility RVU 35.2 Non-Facility RVU 35.2 FUD 090 C 80 CCI
AMA: 2014,Jan,11; 2013,Nov,9

47015 **Laparotomy, with aspiration and/or injection of hepatic parasitic (eg, amoebic or echinococcal) cyst(s) or abscess(es)**
Facility RVU 33.9 Non-Facility RVU 33.9 FUD 090 C 80 CCI
AMA: 2014,Jan,11; 2013,Jan,11-12

47100 **Biopsy of liver, wedge**
Facility RVU 24.6 Non-Facility RVU 24.6 FUD 090 C 80 CCI
AMA: 2014,Jan,11; 2013,Jan,11-12

47120 **Hepatectomy, resection of liver; partial lobectomy**
Facility RVU 68.0 Non-Facility RVU 68.0 FUD 090 C 80 CCI
AMA: 2018,Jan,8; 2017,Jan,8; 2016,Oct,11; 2016,Jan,13; 2015,Jan,16

47122 **trisegmentectomy**
Facility RVU 100. Non-Facility RVU 100. FUD 090 C 80 CCI
AMA: 2014,Jan,11; 2013,Jan,11-12

47125 **total left lobectomy**
Facility RVU 89.8 Non-Facility RVU 89.8 FUD 090 C 80 CCI
AMA: 2014,Jan,11; 2013,Jan,11-12

47130 **total right lobectomy**
Facility RVU 96.4 Non-Facility RVU 96.4 FUD 090 C 80 CCI
AMA: 2014,Jan,11; 2013,Jan,11-12

47133-47147 Liver Transplant Procedures

CMS: 100-03,260.1 Adult Liver Transplantation; 100-03,260.2 Pediatric Liver Transplantation; 100-04,3,90.4 Liver Transplants; 100-04,3,90.4.1 Standard Liver Acquisition Charge; 100-04,3,90.4.2 Billing for Liver Transplant and Acquisition Services; 100-04,3,90.6 Intestinal and Multi-Visceral Transplants

47133 **Donor hepatectomy (including cold preservation), from cadaver donor**
INCLUDES Graft:
Cold preservation
Harvest
Facility RVU 0.00 Non-Facility RVU 0.00 FUD XXX C CCI
AMA: 2014,Jan,11; 2013,Jan,11-12

47135 **Liver allotransplantation, orthotopic, partial or whole, from cadaver or living donor, any age**

INCLUDES Partial/whole recipient hepatectomy
Partial/whole transplant allograft
Recipient care

157. 157. FUD 090 C 80

AMA: 2018,Jan,8; 2017,Jan,8; 2016,Jan,13; 2015,Jan,16

47140 **Donor hepatectomy (including cold preservation), from living donor; left lateral segment only (segments II and III)**

INCLUDES Donor care
Graft:
Cold preservation
Harvest

103. 103. FUD 090 C 80

AMA: 2018,Jan,8; 2017,Jan,8; 2016,Jan,13; 2015,Jan,16

47141 **total left lobectomy (segments II, III and IV)**

INCLUDES Donor care
Graft:
Cold preservation
Harvest

124. 124. FUD 090 C 80

AMA: 2014,Jan,11; 2013,Jan,11-12

47142 **total right lobectomy (segments V, VI, VII and VIII)**

INCLUDES Donor care
Graft:
Cold preservation
Harvest

136. 136. FUD 090 C 80

AMA: 2014,Jan,11; 2013,Jan,11-12

47143 **Backbench standard preparation of cadaver donor whole liver graft prior to allotransplantation, including cholecystectomy, if necessary, and dissection and removal of surrounding soft tissues to prepare the vena cava, portal vein, hepatic artery, and common bile duct for implantation; without trisegment or lobe split**

EXCLUDES *Cholecystectomy (47600, 47610)*
Hepatectomy (47120-47125)

0.00 0.00 FUD XXX C 80

AMA: 2018,Jan,8; 2017,Jan,8; 2016,Jan,13; 2015,Jan,16

47144 **with trisegment split of whole liver graft into 2 partial liver grafts (ie, left lateral segment [segments II and III] and right trisegment [segments I and IV through VIII])**

EXCLUDES *Cholecystectomy (47600, 47610)*
Hepatectomy (47120-47125)

0.00 0.00 FUD 090 C 80

AMA: 2014,Jan,11; 2013,Jan,11-12

47145 **with lobe split of whole liver graft into 2 partial liver grafts (ie, left lobe [segments II, III, and IV] and right lobe [segments I and V through VIII])**

EXCLUDES *Cholecystectomy (47600, 47610)*
Hepatectomy (47120-47125)

0.00 0.00 FUD XXX C 80

AMA: 2014,Jan,11; 2013,Jan,11-12

47146 **Backbench reconstruction of cadaver or living donor liver graft prior to allotransplantation; venous anastomosis, each**

EXCLUDES *Cholecystectomy (47600, 47610)*
Hepatectomy (47120-47125)

9.43 9.43 FUD XXX C 80

AMA: 2014,Jan,11; 2013,Jan,11-12

47147 **arterial anastomosis, each**

EXCLUDES *Cholecystectomy (47600, 47610)*
Hepatectomy (47120-47125)

11.1 11.1 FUD XXX C 80

AMA: 2014,Jan,11; 2013,Jan,11-12

47300-47362 Open Repair of Liver

47300 **Marsupialization of cyst or abscess of liver**

32.9 32.9 FUD 090 C 80

AMA: 2014,Jan,11; 2013,Jan,11-12

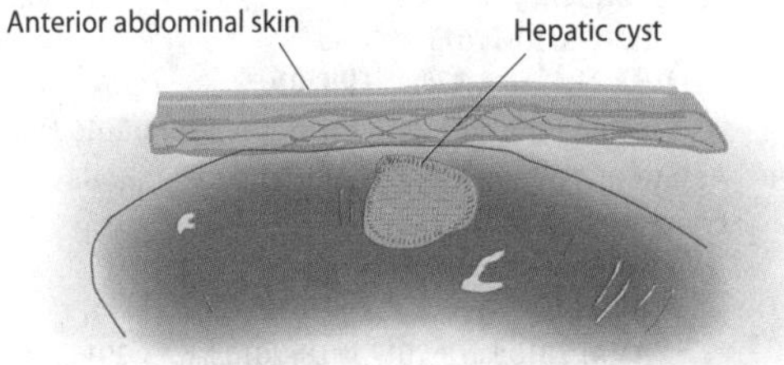

Cutaway view of liver

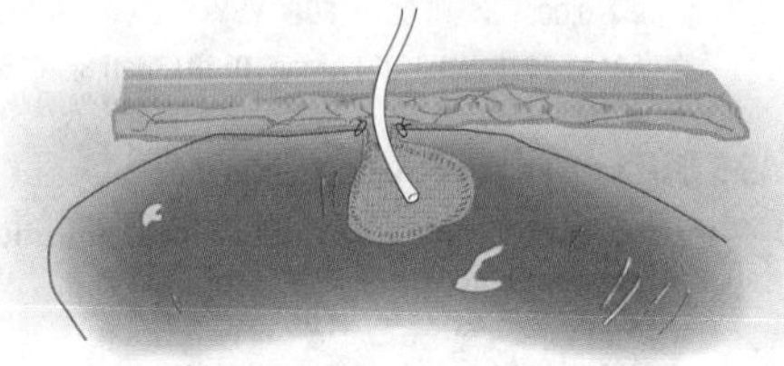

Marsupialization of cyst

A liver cyst or abscess is marsupialized; this method involves surgical access to the cyst and making an incision into it; the edges of the cyst are sutured to the abdominal wall and drainage, open or closed, is placed into the cyst

47350 **Management of liver hemorrhage; simple suture of liver wound or injury**

39.7 39.7 FUD 090 C 80

AMA: 2014,Jan,11; 2013,Jan,11-12

47360 **complex suture of liver wound or injury, with or without hepatic artery ligation**

54.8 54.8 FUD 090 C 80

AMA: 2014,Jan,11; 2013,Jan,11-12

47361 **exploration of hepatic wound, extensive debridement, coagulation and/or suture, with or without packing of liver**

88.0 88.0 FUD 090 C 80

AMA: 2014,Jan,11; 2013,Jan,11-12

47362 **re-exploration of hepatic wound for removal of packing**

42.1 42.1 FUD 090 C 80

AMA: 2020,Jan,6

47370-47379 Laparoscopic Ablation Liver Tumors

INCLUDES Diagnostic laparoscopy (49320)

47370 **Laparoscopy, surgical, ablation of 1 or more liver tumor(s); radiofrequency**

(76940)

36.4 36.4 FUD 090 J 80

AMA: 2018,Jan,8; 2017,Jan,8; 2016,Jan,13; 2015,Jan,16

47371 **cryosurgical**

(76940)

36.5 36.5 FUD 090 J 80

AMA: 2014,Jan,11; 2013,Jan,11-12

47379 **Unlisted laparoscopic procedure, liver**

0.00 0.00 FUD YYY J 80

AMA: 2018,Aug,10; 2018,Jan,8; 2017,Jan,8; 2016,Jan,13; 2015,Jan,16

47380-47399 Open/Percutaneous Ablation Liver Tumors

47380 **Ablation, open, of 1 or more liver tumor(s); radiofrequency**

(76940)

42.1 42.1 FUD 090 C 80

AMA: 2018,Jan,8; 2017,Jan,8; 2016,Jan,13; 2015,Jan,16

47381 cryosurgical
(76940)
43.2 43.2 FUD 090 C 80
AMA: 2014,Jan,11; 2013,Jan,11-12

47382 **Ablation, 1 or more liver tumor(s), percutaneous, radiofrequency**
(76940, 77013, 77022)
21.4 125. FUD 010 J G2
AMA: 2018,Jan,8; 2017,Jan,8; 2016,Jan,13; 2015,Jan,16

47383 **Ablation, 1 or more liver tumor(s), percutaneous, cryoablation**
(76940, 77013, 77022)
13.1 195. FUD 010 J J8
AMA: 2018,Jan,8; 2017,Jan,8; 2016,Jan,13; 2015,Jan,16

47399 **Unlisted procedure, liver**
0.00 0.00 FUD YYY T
AMA: 2018,Jan,8; 2017,Mar,10; 2017,Jan,8; 2016,Jan,13; 2015,Jan,16

47400-47490 Biliary Tract Procedures

47400 **Hepaticotomy or hepaticostomy with exploration, drainage, or removal of calculus**
62.9 62.9 FUD 090 C 80
AMA: 2014,Jan,11; 2013,Jan,11-12

47420 **Choledochotomy or choledochostomy with exploration, drainage, or removal of calculus, with or without cholecystotomy; without transduodenal sphincterotomy or sphincteroplasty**
39.1 39.1 FUD 090 C 80
AMA: 2014,Jan,11; 2013,Jan,11-12

47425 **with transduodenal sphincterotomy or sphincteroplasty**
39.9 39.9 FUD 090 C 80
AMA: 2014,Jan,11; 2013,Jan,11-12

47460 **Transduodenal sphincterotomy or sphincteroplasty, with or without transduodenal extraction of calculus (separate procedure)**
37.0 37.0 FUD 090 C 80
AMA: 2014,Jan,11; 2013,Jan,11-12

47480 **Cholecystotomy or cholecystostomy, open, with exploration, drainage, or removal of calculus (separate procedure)**
EXCLUDES *Percutaneous cholecystostomy (47490)*
25.4 25.4 FUD 090 C 80
AMA: 2018,Jan,8; 2017,Jan,8; 2016,Jan,13; 2015,Jan,16

47490 **Cholecystostomy, percutaneous, complete procedure, including imaging guidance, catheter placement, cholecystogram when performed, and radiological supervision and interpretation**
INCLUDES Radiological guidance (75989, 76942, 77002, 77012, 77021)
EXCLUDES *Injection procedure for cholangiography (47531-47532)*
Open cholecystostomy (47480)
9.56 9.56 FUD 010 J
AMA: 2018,Jan,8; 2017,Jan,8; 2016,Jan,13; 2015,Dec,3; 2015,Jan,16

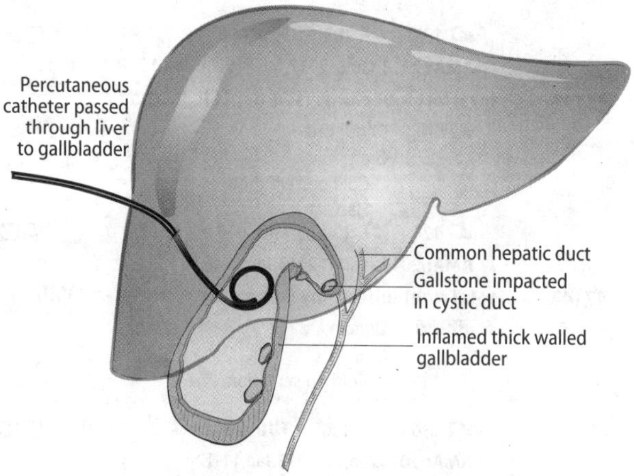

47531-47532 Injection/Insertion Procedures of Biliary Tract

INCLUDES Contrast material injection
Radiologic supervision and interpretation
EXCLUDES *Intraoperative cholangiography (74300-74301)*
Procedures performed via same access (47490, 47533-47541)

47531 **Injection procedure for cholangiography, percutaneous, complete diagnostic procedure including imaging guidance (eg, ultrasound and/or fluoroscopy) and all associated radiological supervision and interpretation; existing access**
2.07 9.00 FUD 000 Q2 N1
AMA: 2018,Jan,8; 2017,Jan,8; 2015,Dec,3

47532 **new access (eg, percutaneous transhepatic cholangiogram)**
6.18 22.6 FUD 000 Q2 N1
AMA: 2018,Jan,8; 2017,Jan,8; 2015,Dec,3

47533-47544 Percutaneous Procedures of the Biliary Tract

47533 **Placement of biliary drainage catheter, percutaneous, including diagnostic cholangiography when performed, imaging guidance (eg, ultrasound and/or fluoroscopy), and all associated radiological supervision and interpretation; external**
EXCLUDES *Conversion to internal-external drainage catheter (47535)*
Percutaneous placement stent bile duct (47538)
Placement stent bile duct, new access (47540)
Replacement existing internal drainage catheter (47536)
7.77 35.0 FUD 000 J G2
AMA: 2018,Jan,8; 2017,Jan,8; 2015,Dec,3

47534 **internal-external**
EXCLUDES *Conversion to external only drainage catheter (47536)*
Percutaneous placement stent bile duct (47538)
Placement stent bile duct, new access (47540)
10.8 41.0 FUD 000 J G2
AMA: 2018,Jan,8; 2017,Jan,8; 2015,Dec,3

47535 Conversion of external biliary drainage catheter to internal-external biliary drainage catheter, percutaneous, including diagnostic cholangiography when performed, imaging guidance (eg, fluoroscopy), and all associated radiological supervision and interpretation

5.76 28.8 FUD 000 J G2

AMA: 2018,Jan,8; 2017,Jan,8; 2015,Dec,3

47536 Exchange of biliary drainage catheter (eg, external, internal-external, or conversion of internal-external to external only), percutaneous, including diagnostic cholangiography when performed, imaging guidance (eg, fluoroscopy), and all associated radiological supervision and interpretation

INCLUDES Exchange one drainage catheter

EXCLUDES *Placement stent(s) into bile duct, percutaneous (47538)*

Code also exchange additional catheters same session with modifier 59 (47536)

3.86 19.5 FUD 000 J G2

AMA: 2018,Jan,8; 2017,Jan,8; 2015,Dec,3

47537 Removal of biliary drainage catheter, percutaneous, requiring fluoroscopic guidance (eg, with concurrent indwelling biliary stents), including diagnostic cholangiography when performed, imaging guidance (eg, fluoroscopy), and all associated radiological supervision and interpretation

EXCLUDES *Placement stent(s) into bile duct via same access (47538)*

Removal without fluoroscopic guidance; report with appropriate E/M service code

2.80 10.4 FUD 000 Q2 G2

AMA: 2018,Jan,8; 2017,Jan,8; 2015,Dec,3

47538 Placement of stent(s) into a bile duct, percutaneous, including diagnostic cholangiography, imaging guidance (eg, fluoroscopy and/or ultrasound), balloon dilation, catheter exchange(s) and catheter removal(s) when performed, and all associated radiological supervision and interpretation; existing access

EXCLUDES *Drainage catheter inserted following stent placement (47536)*

Procedures performed via same access (47536-47537)

Treatment same lesion same operative session ([43277], 47542, 47555-47556)

Code also multiple stents placed during same session when: (47538-47540)

- Serial stents placed within same bile duct
- Stent placement via two or more percutaneous access sites or space between two other stents
- Two or more stents inserted through same percutaneous access

6.88 121. FUD 000 J J8

AMA: 2018,Jan,8; 2017,Jan,8; 2016,Mar,10; 2015,Dec,3

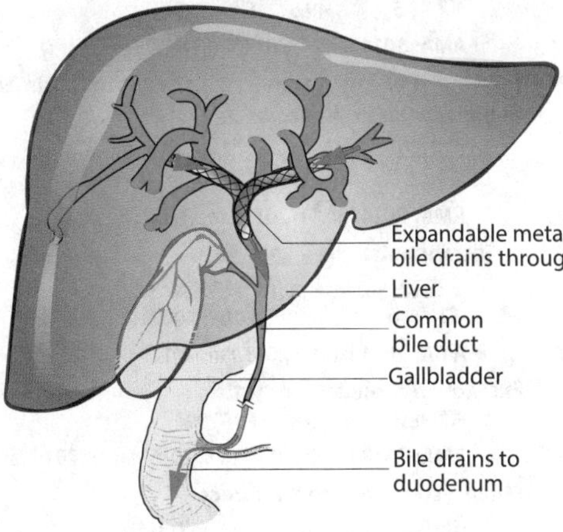

47539 new access, without placement of separate biliary drainage catheter

EXCLUDES *Treatment same lesion same operative session ([43277], 47542, 47555-47556)*

Code also multiple stents placed during same session when: (47538-47540)

- Serial stents placed within same bile duct
- Stent placement via two or more percutaneous access sites or space between two other stents
- Two or more stents inserted through same percutaneous access

12.4 135. FUD 000 J G2

AMA: 2018,Jan,8; 2017,Jan,8; 2016,Mar,10; 2015,Dec,3

47540 new access, with placement of separate biliary drainage catheter (eg, external or internal-external)

EXCLUDES *Procedures performed via same access (47533-47534)*

Treatment same lesion same operative session ([43277], 47542, 47555-47556)

Code also multiple stents placed during same session when: (47538-47540)

- Serial stents placed within same bile duct
- Stent placement via two or more percutaneous access sites or space between two other stents
- Two or more stents inserted through same percutaneous access

12.8 139. FUD 000 J J8

AMA: 2018,Jan,8; 2017,Jan,8; 2016,Mar,10; 2015,Dec,3

47541 Placement of access through the biliary tree and into small bowel to assist with an endoscopic biliary procedure (eg, rendezvous procedure), percutaneous, including diagnostic cholangiography when performed, imaging guidance (eg, ultrasound and/or fluoroscopy), and all associated radiological supervision and interpretation, new access

EXCLUDES *Access through biliary tree into small bowel for endoscopic biliary procedure (47535-47537)*

Conversion, exchange, or removal external biliary drainage catheter (47535-47537)

Injection procedure for cholangiography (47531-47532)

Placement biliary drainage catheter (47533-47534)

Placement stent(s) into bile duct (47538-47540)

Procedure performed when previous catheter access exists

9.69 33.3 FUD 000 J G2

AMA: 2018,Jan,8; 2017,Jan,8; 2015,Dec,3

+ **47542 Balloon dilation of biliary duct(s) or of ampulla (sphincteroplasty), percutaneous, including imaging guidance (eg, fluoroscopy), and all associated radiological supervision and interpretation, each duct (List separately in addition to code for primary procedure)**

EXCLUDES *Biliary endoscopy, with dilation of biliary duct stricture (47555-47556)*

Endoscopic balloon dilation ([43277], 47555-47556)

Endoscopic retrograde cholangiopancreatography (ERCP) (43262, [43277])

Placement stent(s) into a bile duct (47538-47540)

Procedure performed with balloon to remove calculi, debris, sludge without dilation (47544)

Code also one additional dilation code when more than one dilation performed same session, using modifier 59 with (47542)

Code first (47531-47537, 47541)

3.95 13.1 FUD ZZZ N N1

AMA: 2018,Jan,8; 2017,Jan,8; 2015,Dec,3

\+ **47543** **Endoluminal biopsy(ies) of biliary tree, percutaneous, any method(s) (eg, brush, forceps, and/or needle), including imaging guidance (eg, fluoroscopy), and all associated radiological supervision and interpretation, single or multiple (List separately in addition to code for primary procedure)**

EXCLUDES *Endoscopic biopsy (46261, 47553)*
Endoscopic brushings (43260, 47552)
Procedure performed more than one time per session

Code first (47531-47540)

4.20 | 13.3 | **FUD** ZZZ | N N1

AMA: 2018,Jan,8; 2017,Jan,8; 2015,Dec,3

\+ **47544** **Removal of calculi/debris from biliary duct(s) and/or gallbladder, percutaneous, including destruction of calculi by any method (eg, mechanical, electrohydraulic, lithotripsy) when performed, imaging guidance (eg, fluoroscopy), and all associated radiological supervision and interpretation (List separately in addition to code for primary procedure)**

EXCLUDES *Device deployment without finding calculi/debris*
Endoscopic calculi removal/destruction (43264-43265, 47554)
Endoscopic retrograde cholangiopancreatography (ERCP); with removal calculi/debris from biliary/pancreatic duct(s) (43264)
Procedures with removal incidental debris (47531-47543)

Code first when debris removal not incidental, as appropriate (47531-47540)

4.61 | 29.2 | **FUD** ZZZ | N N1

AMA: 2018,Jan,8; 2017,Jan,8; 2015,Dec,3

47550-47556 Endoscopic Procedures of the Biliary Tract

INCLUDES Diagnostic endoscopy (49320)

EXCLUDES *Endoscopic retrograde cholangiopancreatography (ERCP) (43260-43265, [43274], [43275], [43276], [43277], [43278], 74328-74330, 74363)*

\+ **47550** **Biliary endoscopy, intraoperative (choledochoscopy) (List separately in addition to code for primary procedure)**

Code first primary procedure

4.80 | 4.80 | **FUD** ZZZ | C 80

AMA: 2014,Jan,11; 2013,Jan,11-12

47552 **Biliary endoscopy, percutaneous via T-tube or other tract; diagnostic, with collection of specimen(s) by brushing and/or washing, when performed (separate procedure)**

9.01 | 9.01 | **FUD** 000 | J A2

AMA: 2018,Jan,8; 2017,Jan,8; 2016,Jan,13; 2015,Dec,3; 2015,Jan,16

47553 **with biopsy, single or multiple**

8.91 | 8.91 | **FUD** 000 | J A2

AMA: 2018,Jan,8; 2017,Jan,8; 2016,Jan,13; 2015,Dec,3; 2015,Jan,16

47554 **with removal of calculus/calculi**

14.9 | 14.9 | **FUD** 000 | J A2

AMA: 2018,Jan,8; 2017,Jan,8; 2016,Jan,13; 2015,Dec,3; 2015,Jan,16

47555 **with dilation of biliary duct stricture(s) without stent**

(74363)

9.46 | 9.46 | **FUD** 000 | J A2

AMA: 2018,Jan,8; 2017,Jan,8; 2016,Jan,13; 2015,Dec,3; 2015,Jan,16

47556 **with dilation of biliary duct stricture(s) with stent**

(74363)

10.7 | 10.7 | **FUD** 000 | J J8

AMA: 2018,Jan,8; 2017,Jan,8; 2016,Jan,13; 2015,Dec,3; 2015,Jan,16

47562-47579 Laparoscopic Gallbladder Procedures

INCLUDES Diagnostic laparoscopy (49320)

47562 **Laparoscopy, surgical; cholecystectomy**

19.0 | 19.0 | **FUD** 090 | J G2 80

AMA: 2020,Aug,14; 2018,Jan,8; 2017,Jan,8; 2016,Jan,13; 2015,Jan,16

47563 **cholecystectomy with cholangiography**

EXCLUDES *Percutaneous cholangiography (47531-47532)*

Code also intraoperative radiology supervision and interpretation (74300-74301)

20.7 | 20.7 | **FUD** 090 | J G2 80

AMA: 2019,Mar,10; 2018,Jan,8; 2017,Jan,8; 2016,Jan,13; 2015,Jan,16

47564 **cholecystectomy with exploration of common duct**

32.2 | 32.2 | **FUD** 090 | J G2 80

AMA: 2018,Jan,8; 2017,Jan,8; 2016,Jan,13; 2015,Jan,16

47570 **cholecystoenterostomy**

22.5 | 22.5 | **FUD** 090 | C 80

AMA: 2018,Jan,8; 2017,Jan,8; 2016,Jan,13; 2015,Jan,16

47579 **Unlisted laparoscopy procedure, biliary tract**

0.00 | 0.00 | **FUD** YYY | J 80 50

AMA: 2018,Jan,8; 2017,Jan,8; 2016,Jan,13; 2015,Jan,16

47600-47620 Open Gallbladder Procedures

47600 **Cholecystectomy;**

EXCLUDES *Laparoscopic method (47562-47564)*

30.9 | 30.9 | **FUD** 090 | C 80

AMA: 2018,Jan,8; 2017,Jan,8; 2016,Jan,13; 2015,Jan,16

47605 **with cholangiography**

EXCLUDES *Laparoscopic method (47563-47564)*

32.6 | 32.6 | **FUD** 090 | C 80

AMA: 2018,Jan,8; 2017,Jan,8; 2016,Jan,13; 2015,Jan,16

47610 **Cholecystectomy with exploration of common duct;**

EXCLUDES *Laparoscopic method (47564)*

Code also biliary endoscopy when performed in conjunction with cholecystectomy with exploration common duct (47550)

36.3 | 36.3 | **FUD** 090 | C 80

AMA: 2018,Jan,8; 2017,Jan,8; 2016,Jan,13; 2015,Jan,16

47612 **with choledochoenterostomy**

36.6 | 36.6 | **FUD** 090 | C 80

AMA: 2014,Jan,11; 2013,Jan,11-12

47620 **with transduodenal sphincterotomy or sphincteroplasty, with or without cholangiography**

40.0 | 40.0 | **FUD** 090 | C 80

AMA: 2014,Jan,11; 2013,Jan,11-12

47700-47999 Open Resection and Repair of Biliary Tract

47700 **Exploration for congenital atresia of bile ducts, without repair, with or without liver biopsy, with or without cholangiography**

30.6 | 30.6 | **FUD** 090 | 63 C 80

AMA: 2014,Jan,11; 2013,Jan,11-12

47701 **Portoenterostomy (eg, Kasai procedure)**

49.5 | 49.5 | **FUD** 090 | 63 C 80

AMA: 2014,Jan,11; 2013,Jan,11-12

47711 **Excision of bile duct tumor, with or without primary repair of bile duct; extrahepatic**

EXCLUDES *Anastomosis (47760-47800)*

45.1 | 45.1 | **FUD** 090 | C 80

AMA: 2014,Jan,11; 2013,Jan,11-12

47712 **intrahepatic**

EXCLUDES *Anastomosis (47760-47800)*

58.1 | 58.1 | **FUD** 090 | C 80

AMA: 2014,Jan,11; 2013,Jan,11-12

47715 **Excision of choledochal cyst**

38.8 | 38.8 | **FUD** 090 | C 80

AMA: 2018,Jan,8; 2017,Jan,8; 2016,Jan,13; 2015,Jan,16

47720 **Cholecystoenterostomy; direct**

EXCLUDES *Laparoscopic method (47570)*

33.4 | 33.4 | **FUD** 090 | C 80

AMA: 2018,Jan,8; 2017,Jan,8; 2016,Jan,13; 2015,Jan,16

47721 with gastroenterostomy
39.3 39.3 FUD 090 C 80
AMA: 2014,Jan,11; 2013,Jan,11-12

47740 Roux-en-Y
37.7 37.7 FUD 090 C 80
AMA: 2014,Jan,11; 2013,Jan,11-12

47741 Roux-en-Y with gastroenterostomy
42.8 42.8 FUD 090 C 80
AMA: 2014,Jan,11; 2013,Jan,11-12

47760 Anastomosis, of extrahepatic biliary ducts and gastrointestinal tract
65.4 65.4 FUD 090 C 80
AMA: 2014,Jan,11; 2013,Jan,11-12

47765 Anastomosis, of intrahepatic ducts and gastrointestinal tract
INCLUDES Longmire anastomosis
87.9 87.9 FUD 090 C 80
AMA: 2014,Jan,11; 2013,Jan,11-12

47780 Anastomosis, Roux-en-Y, of extrahepatic biliary ducts and gastrointestinal tract
71.8 71.8 FUD 090 C 80
AMA: 2014,Jan,11; 2013,Jan,11-12

47785 Anastomosis, Roux-en-Y, of intrahepatic biliary ducts and gastrointestinal tract
94.4 94.4 FUD 090 C 80
AMA: 2014,Jan,11; 2013,Jan,11-12

47800 Reconstruction, plastic, of extrahepatic biliary ducts with end-to-end anastomosis
45.5 45.5 FUD 090 C 80
AMA: 2014,Jan,11; 2013,Jan,11-12

47801 Placement of choledochal stent
32.3 32.3 FUD 090 C 80
AMA: 2018,Jan,8; 2017,Jan,8; 2016,Jan,13; 2015,Jan,16

47802 U-tube hepaticoenterostomy
44.3 44.3 FUD 090 C 80
AMA: 2014,Jan,11; 2013,Jan,11-12

47900 Suture of extrahepatic biliary duct for pre-existing injury (separate procedure)
39.7 39.7 FUD 090 C 80
AMA: 2014,Jan,11; 2013,Jan,11-12

47999 Unlisted procedure, biliary tract
0.00 0.00 FUD YYY T
AMA: 2018,Jan,8; 2017,Jan,8; 2016,Jan,13; 2015,Jan,16

48000-48548 Open Procedures of the Pancreas

EXCLUDES *Peroral pancreatic procedures performed endoscopically (43260-43265, [43274], [43275], [43276], [43277], [43278])*

48000 Placement of drains, peripancreatic, for acute pancreatitis;
54.6 54.6 FUD 090 C 80
AMA: 2014,Jan,11; 2013,Jan,11-12

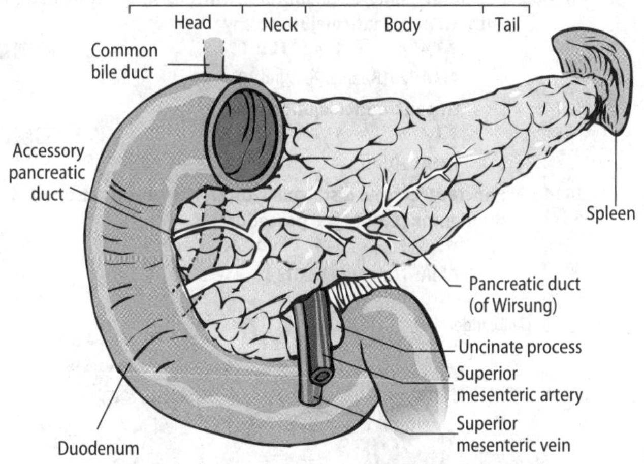

48001 with cholecystostomy, gastrostomy, and jejunostomy
67.1 67.1 FUD 090 C 80
AMA: 2014,Jan,11; 2013,Jan,11-12

48020 Removal of pancreatic calculus
34.1 34.1 FUD 090 C 80
AMA: 2014,Jan,11; 2013,Jan,11-12

48100 Biopsy of pancreas, open (eg, fine needle aspiration, needle core biopsy, wedge biopsy)
25.8 25.8 FUD 090 C 80
AMA: 2014,Jan,11; 2013,Jan,11-12

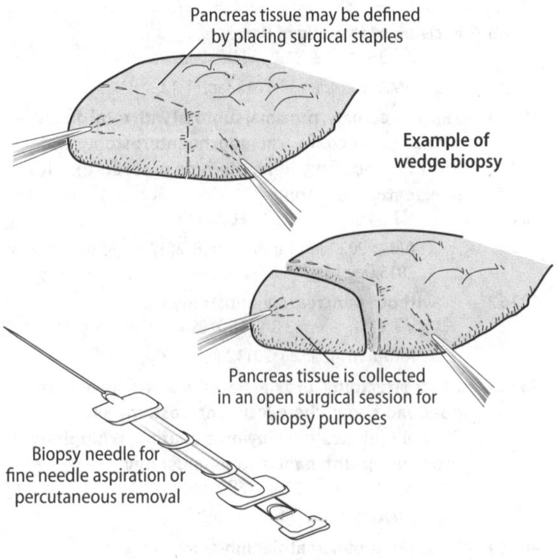

48102 Biopsy of pancreas, percutaneous needle
EXCLUDES *Fine needle aspiration ([10005, 10006, 10007, 10008, 10009, 10010, 10011, 10012])*
(76942, 77002, 77012, 77021)
(88172-88173)
6.95 15.2 FUD 010 J A2
AMA: 2019,Apr,4

48105 Resection or debridement of pancreas and peripancreatic tissue for acute necrotizing pancreatitis
82.4 82.4 FUD 090 C 80
AMA: 2014,Jan,11; 2013,Jan,11-12

48120 Excision of lesion of pancreas (eg, cyst, adenoma)
32.0 32.0 FUD 090 C 80
AMA: 2014,Jan,11; 2013,Jan,11-12

48140 Pancreatectomy, distal subtotal, with or without splenectomy; without pancreaticojejunostomy
45.4 45.4 FUD 090 C 80
AMA: 2018,Jan,8; 2017,Jul,10

48145 with pancreaticojejunostomy
47.3 47.3 FUD 090 C 80
AMA: 2014,Jan,11; 2013,Jan,11-12

48146 Pancreatectomy, distal, near-total with preservation of duodenum (Child-type procedure)
54.5 54.5 FUD 090 C 80
AMA: 2014,Jan,11; 2013,Jan,11-12

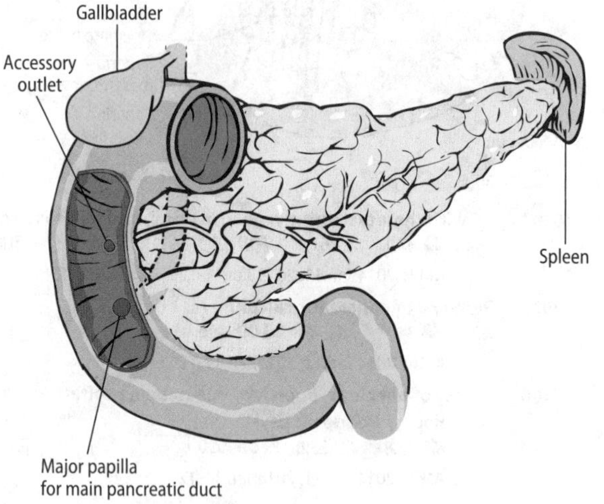

48148 Excision of ampulla of Vater
36.1 36.1 FUD 090 C 80
AMA: 2014,Jan,11; 2013,Jan,11-12

48150 Pancreatectomy, proximal subtotal with total duodenectomy, partial gastrectomy, choledochoenterostomy and gastrojejunostomy (Whipple-type procedure); with pancreatojejunostomy
90.6 90.6 FUD 090 C 80
AMA: 2020,Jun,14; 2018,Jan,8; 2017,Jan,8; 2016,Jan,13; 2015,Dec,16

48152 without pancreatojejunostomy
83.8 83.8 FUD 090 C 80
AMA: 2014,Jan,11; 2013,Jan,11-12

48153 Pancreatectomy, proximal subtotal with near-total duodenectomy, choledochoenterostomy and duodenojejunostomy (pylorus-sparing, Whipple-type procedure); with pancreatojejunostomy
90.1 90.1 FUD 090 C 80
AMA: 2014,Jan,11; 2013,Jan,11-12

48154 without pancreatojejunostomy
84.3 84.3 FUD 090 C 80
AMA: 2014,Jan,11; 2013,Jan,11-12

48155 Pancreatectomy, total
52.6 52.6 FUD 090 C 80
AMA: 2014,Jan,11; 2013,Jan,11-12

48160 Pancreatectomy, total or subtotal, with autologous transplantation of pancreas or pancreatic islet cells
EXCLUDES *Laparoscopic pancreatic islet cell transplantation (0585T)*
Open pancreatic islet cell transplantation (0586T)
Percutaneous pancreatic islet cell transplantation (0584T)
0.00 0.00 FUD XXX E
AMA: 2014,Jan,11; 2013,Jan,11-12

+ **48400** Injection procedure for intraoperative pancreatography (List separately in addition to code for primary procedure)
Code first primary procedure
(74300-74301)
3.12 3.12 FUD ZZZ C 80
AMA: 2018,Jan,8; 2017,Jan,8; 2016,Jan,13; 2015,Jan,16

48500 Marsupialization of pancreatic cyst
33.4 33.4 FUD 090 C 80
AMA: 2014,Jan,11; 2013,Jan,11-12

48510 External drainage, pseudocyst of pancreas, open
EXCLUDES *Image guided percutaneous catheter drainage (49405)*
31.8 31.8 FUD 090 C 80
AMA: 2014,Jan,11; 2013,Nov,9

48520 Internal anastomosis of pancreatic cyst to gastrointestinal tract; direct
31.5 31.5 FUD 090 C 80
AMA: 2014,Jan,11; 2013,Jan,11-12

48540 Roux-en-Y
37.8 37.8 FUD 090 C 80
AMA: 2014,Jan,11; 2013,Jan,11-12

48545 Pancreatorrhaphy for injury
39.0 39.0 FUD 090 C 80
AMA: 2014,Jan,11; 2013,Jan,11-12

48547 Duodenal exclusion with gastrojejunostomy for pancreatic injury
51.9 51.9 FUD 090 C 80
AMA: 2014,Jan,11; 2013,Jan,11-12

48548 Pancreaticojejunostomy, side-to-side anastomosis (Puestow-type operation)
48.5 48.5 FUD 090 C 80
AMA: 2014,Jan,11; 2013,Jan,11-12

48550-48999 Pancreas Transplant Procedures

CMS: 100-03,260.3 Pancreas Transplants; 100-04,3,90.5 Pancreas Transplants with Kidney Transplants; 100-04,3,90.5.1 Pancreas Transplants Alone

48550 Donor pancreatectomy (including cold preservation), with or without duodenal segment for transplantation
INCLUDES Graft:
Cold preservation
Harvest (with or without duodenal segment)
0.00 0.00 FUD XXX E
AMA: 2018,Jan,8; 2017,Jan,8; 2016,Jan,13; 2015,Jan,16

48551 Backbench standard preparation of cadaver donor pancreas allograft prior to transplantation, including dissection of allograft from surrounding soft tissues, splenectomy, duodenotomy, ligation of bile duct, ligation of mesenteric vessels, and Y-graft arterial anastomoses from iliac artery to superior mesenteric artery and to splenic artery

EXCLUDES *Biopsy pancreas (48100-48102)*
Bypass graft, with vein (35531, 35563)
Duodenotomy (44010)
Endoscopic procedures biliary tract (47550-47556)
Excision lesion mesentery (44820)
Excision lesion pancreas (48120)
Pancreatorrhaphy for injury (48545)
Placement vein patch or cuff at distal anastomosis bypass graft (35685)
Resection or debridement pancreas (48105)
Splenectomy (38100-38102)
Suture mesentery (44850)
Transduodenal sphincterotomy, sphincteroplasty (47460)

0.00 0.00 **FUD** XXX C 80

AMA: 2014,Jan,11; 2013,Jan,11-12

48552 Backbench reconstruction of cadaver donor pancreas allograft prior to transplantation, venous anastomosis, each

EXCLUDES *Biopsy pancreas (48100-48102)*
Bypass graft, with vein (35531, 35563)
Duodenotomy (44010)
Endoscopic procedures biliary tract (47550-47556)
Excision lesion mesentery (44820)
Excision lesion pancreas (48120)
Pancreatorrhaphy for injury (48545)
Placement vein patch or cuff at distal anastomosis bypass graft (35685)
Resection or debridement pancreas (48105)
Splenectomy (38100-38102)
Suture mesentery (44850)
Transduodenal sphincterotomy, sphincteroplasty (47460)

6.87 6.87 **FUD** XXX C 80

AMA: 2014,Jan,11; 2013,Jan,11-12

48554 Transplantation of pancreatic allograft

INCLUDES Allograft transplant
Recipient care

74.4 74.4 **FUD** 090 C 80

AMA: 2014,Jan,11; 2013,Jan,11-12

48556 Removal of transplanted pancreatic allograft

37.1 37.1 **FUD** 090 C 80

AMA: 2014,Jan,11; 2013,Jan,11-12

48999 Unlisted procedure, pancreas

0.00 0.00 **FUD** YYY T 80

AMA: 2018,Jan,8; 2017,Jan,8; 2016,Jan,13; 2015,Jan,16

49000-49084 Exploratory and Drainage Procedures: Abdomen/Peritoneum

49000 Exploratory laparotomy, exploratory celiotomy with or without biopsy(s) (separate procedure)

EXCLUDES *Exploration penetrating wound without laparotomy (20102)*

22.3 22.3 **FUD** 090 C 80

AMA: 2020,Jan,6; 2019,Dec,5; 2018,Jan,8; 2017,Dec,3; 2017,Jan,8; 2016,Jan,13; 2015,Jan,16

49002 Reopening of recent laparotomy

EXCLUDES *Hepatic wound re-exploration for packing removal (47362)*
Pelvic wound re-exploration for packing removal/repacking (49014)

30.4 30.4 **FUD** 090 C 80

AMA: 2020,Jan,6; 2018,Jan,8; 2017,Jan,8; 2016,Jan,13; 2015,Jan,16

49010 Exploration, retroperitoneal area with or without biopsy(s) (separate procedure)

EXCLUDES *Exploration penetrating wound without laparotomy (20102)*

26.8 26.8 **FUD** 090 C 80

AMA: 2020,Jan,6; 2019,Dec,5

49013 Preperitoneal pelvic packing for hemorrhage associated with pelvic trauma, including local exploration

12.7 12.7 **FUD** 000

AMA: 2020,Jan,6

49014 Re-exploration of pelvic wound with removal of preperitoneal pelvic packing, including repacking, when performed

10.5 10.5 **FUD** 000

AMA: 2020,Jan,6

49020 Drainage of peritoneal abscess or localized peritonitis, exclusive of appendiceal abscess, open

EXCLUDES *Appendiceal abscess (44900)*
Image guided percutaneous catheter drainage abscess/peritonitis via catheter (49406)
Image-guided transrectal/transvaginal drainage peritoneal abscess via catheter (49407)

46.3 46.3 **FUD** 090 C 80

AMA: 2014,Jan,11; 2013,Nov,9

49040 Drainage of subdiaphragmatic or subphrenic abscess, open

EXCLUDES *Image-guided percutaneous drainage subdiaphragmatic/subphrenic abscess via catheter (49406)*

29.1 29.1 **FUD** 090 C 80

AMA: 2014,Jan,11; 2013,Nov,9

49060 Drainage of retroperitoneal abscess, open

EXCLUDES *Image-guided percutaneous drainage retroperitoneal abscess via catheter (49406)*
Transrectal/transvaginal image-guided drainage retroperitoneal abscess via catheter (49407)

32.0 32.0 **FUD** 090 C

AMA: 2018,Jan,8; 2017,Jan,8; 2016,Jan,13; 2015,Jan,16

49062 Drainage of extraperitoneal lymphocele to peritoneal cavity, open

EXCLUDES *Drainage lymphocele to peritoneal cavity, laparoscopic (49323)*
Image-guided percutaneous drainage retroperitoneal lymphocele via catheter (49406)

21.3 21.3 **FUD** 090 C 80

AMA: 2018,Jan,8; 2017,Jan,8; 2016,Jan,13; 2015,Jan,16

49082 Abdominal paracentesis (diagnostic or therapeutic); without imaging guidance

2.12 5.67 **FUD** 000 T 62

AMA: 2018,Jan,8; 2017,Jan,8; 2016,Jan,13; 2015,Jan,16

49083 with imaging guidance

INCLUDES Radiological guidance (76942, 77002, 77012, 77021)

EXCLUDES *Image-guided percutaneous drainage retroperitoneal abscess via catheter (49406)*

3.11 8.44 **FUD** 000 T 62

AMA: 2018,Jan,8; 2017,Jan,8; 2016,Jan,13; 2015,Jan,16

49084 Peritoneal lavage, including imaging guidance, when performed

INCLUDES Radiological guidance (76942, 77002, 77012, 77021)

EXCLUDES *Image-guided percutaneous drainage retroperitoneal abscess via catheter (49406)*

3.13 3.13 **FUD** 000 T 62

AMA: 2018,Jan,8; 2017,Jan,8; 2016,Jan,13; 2015,Jan,16

49180 Biopsy of Mass: Abdomen/Retroperitoneum

EXCLUDES *Fine needle aspiration (10021, [10004, 10005, 10006, 10007, 10008, 10009, 10010, 10011, 10012])*
Lysis intestinal adhesions (44005)

49180 **Biopsy, abdominal or retroperitoneal mass, percutaneous needle**

(76942, 77002, 77012, 77021)
(88172-88173)
2.43 4.86 **FUD** 000 J A2
AMA: 2019,Feb,8; 2019,Apr,4; 2018,Jan,8; 2017,Jan,8; 2016,Jan,13; 2015,Jan,16

49185 Sclerotherapy of a Fluid Collection

49185 **Sclerotherapy of a fluid collection (eg, lymphocele, cyst, or seroma), percutaneous, including contrast injection(s), sclerosant injection(s), diagnostic study, imaging guidance (eg, ultrasound, fluoroscopy) and radiological supervision and interpretation when performed**

INCLUDES Multiple lesions treated via same access

EXCLUDES *Contrast injection for assessment abscess or cyst (49424)*
Pleurodesis (32560)
Radiologic examination, abscess, fistula or sinus tract stud (76080)
Sclerosis veins/endovenous ablation incompetent veins extremity (36468, 36470-36471, 36475-36476, 36478-36479)
Sclerotherapy lymphatic/vascular malformation (37241)

Code also access or drainage via needle or catheter (10030, 10160, 49405-49407, 50390)
Code also existing catheter exchange pre- or post-sclerosant injection (49423, 75984)
Code also modifier 59 for treatment multiple lesions same session via separate access
3.47 33.4 **FUD** 000 T
AMA: 2018,Jan,8; 2017,Jan,8; 2016,Mar,10

49203-49205 Open Destruction or Excision: Abdominal Tumors

EXCLUDES *Ablation, open, one or more renal mass lesion(s), cryosurgical*
Biopsy kidney or ovary (50205, 58900)
Cryoablation renal tumor (50250, 50593)
Excision perinephric cyst (50290)
Excision presacral or sacrococcygeal tumor (49215)
Exploration, renal or retroperitoneal area (49010, 50010)
Exploratory laparotomy (49000)
Laparotomy, for staging or restaging ovarian, tubal, or primary peritoneal malignancy (58960)
Nephrectomy (50225, 50236)
Oophorectomy (58940-58958)
Ovarian cystectomy (58925)
Pelvic or retroperitoneal lymphadenectomy (38770, 38780)
Primary, recurrent ovarian, uterine, or tubal resection (58957-58958)
Wedge resection or bisection ovary (58920)

Code also colectomy (44140)
Code also nephrectomy (50220, 50240)
Code also small bowel resection (44120)
Code also vena caval resection with reconstruction (37799)

49203 **Excision or destruction, open, intra-abdominal tumors, cysts or endometriomas, 1 or more peritoneal, mesenteric, or retroperitoneal primary or secondary tumors; largest tumor 5 cm diameter or less**
34.7 34.7 **FUD** 090 C 80
AMA: 2018,Jan,8; 2017,Jan,8; 2016,Jan,13; 2015,Jan,16

49204 **largest tumor 5.1-10.0 cm diameter**
44.2 44.2 **FUD** 090 C 80
AMA: 2018,Jan,8; 2017,Jan,8; 2016,Jan,13; 2015,Jan,16

49205 **largest tumor greater than 10.0 cm diameter**
50.6 50.6 **FUD** 090 C 80
AMA: 2018,Jan,8; 2017,Jan,8; 2016,Jan,13; 2015,Jan,16

49215 Resection Presacral/Sacrococcygeal Tumor

49215 **Excision of presacral or sacrococcygeal tumor**
64.2 64.2 **FUD** 090 63 C 80
AMA: 2014,Jan,11; 2013,Jan,11-12

49220-49255 Other Open Abdominal Procedures

EXCLUDES *Lysis intestinal adhesions (44005)*

49220 ~~**Staging laparotomy for Hodgkins disease or lymphoma (includes splenectomy, needle or open biopsies of both liver lobes, possibly also removal of abdominal nodes, abdominal node and/or bone marrow biopsies, ovarian repositioning)**~~

49250 **Umbilectomy, omphalectomy, excision of umbilicus (separate procedure)**
16.9 16.9 **FUD** 090 J A2
AMA: 2014,Jan,11; 2013,Jan,11-12

49255 **Omentectomy, epiploectomy, resection of omentum (separate procedure)**
22.8 22.8 **FUD** 090 C 80
AMA: 2018,Mar,11; 2018,Jan,8; 2017,Jan,8; 2016,Jan,13; 2015,Jan,16

49320-49329 Laparoscopic Procedures of the Abdomen/Peritoneum/Omentum

INCLUDES Diagnostic laparoscopy (49320)

EXCLUDES *Fulguration/excision lesions ovary/pelvic viscera/peritoneal surface, performed laparoscopically (58662)*

49320 **Laparoscopy, abdomen, peritoneum, and omentum, diagnostic, with or without collection of specimen(s) by brushing or washing (separate procedure)**
9.54 9.54 **FUD** 010 J A2 80
AMA: 2018,Jan,8; 2017,Apr,7; 2017,Jan,8; 2016,Jan,13; 2015,Dec,16; 2015,Jan,16

49321 **Laparoscopy, surgical; with biopsy (single or multiple)**
10.0 10.0 **FUD** 010 J A2 80
AMA: 2018,Aug,10; 2018,Jan,8; 2017,Jan,8; 2016,Jan,13; 2015,Jan,16

49322 **with aspiration of cavity or cyst (eg, ovarian cyst) (single or multiple)**
10.8 10.8 **FUD** 010 J A2 80
AMA: 2018,Jan,8; 2017,Jan,8; 2016,Jan,13; 2015,Jan,16

49323 **with drainage of lymphocele to peritoneal cavity**

EXCLUDES *Open drainage lymphocele to peritoneal cavity (49062)*

18.3 18.3 **FUD** 090 J 80
AMA: 2018,Jan,8; 2017,Jan,8; 2016,Jan,13; 2015,Jan,16

49324 **with insertion of tunneled intraperitoneal catheter**

EXCLUDES *Open approach (49421)*

Code also insertion subcutaneous extension to intraperitoneal cannula with remote chest exit site, when appropriate (49435)
11.3 11.3 **FUD** 010 J G2 80
AMA: 2014,Jan,11; 2013,Jan,11-12

49325 **with revision of previously placed intraperitoneal cannula or catheter, with removal of intraluminal obstructive material if performed**
12.1 12.1 **FUD** 010 J G2 80
AMA: 2014,Jan,11; 2013,Jan,11-12

\+ **49326** **with omentopexy (omental tacking procedure) (List separately in addition to code for primary procedure)**

Code first laparoscopy with permanent intraperitoneal cannula or catheter insertion or revision previously placed catheter/cannula (49324, 49325)
5.52 5.52 **FUD** ZZZ N N1 80
AMA: 2014,Jan,11; 2013,Jan,11-12

+ **49327** **with placement of interstitial device(s) for radiation therapy guidance (eg, fiducial markers, dosimeter), intra-abdominal, intrapelvic, and/or retroperitoneum, including imaging guidance, if performed, single or multiple (List separately in addition to code for primary procedure)**

EXCLUDES *Open approach (49412)*
Percutaneous approach (49411)

Code first laparoscopic abdominal, pelvic or retroperitoneal procedures

3.81 3.81 **FUD** ZZZ N N1 80

AMA: 2014,Jan,11; 2013,Jan,11-12

49329 **Unlisted laparoscopy procedure, abdomen, peritoneum and omentum**

0.00 0.00 **FUD** YYY J 80 50

AMA: 2020,Feb,13; 2019,Mar,10; 2018,Jan,8; 2017,Jan,8; 2016,Jan,13; 2015,Jan,16

49400-49436 Peritoneal and Visceral Procedures: Drainage/Insertion/Modifications/Removal

49400 **Injection of air or contrast into peritoneal cavity (separate procedure)**

(74190)

2.68 3.93 **FUD** 000 N N1

AMA: 2018,Jan,8; 2017,Jan,8; 2016,Jan,13; 2015,Jan,16

49402 **Removal of peritoneal foreign body from peritoneal cavity**

EXCLUDES *Enterolysis (44005)*
Percutaneous or open drainage or lavage (49020, 49040, 49082-49084, 49406)
Percutaneous tunneled intraperitoneal catheter insertion without subcutaneous port (49418)

24.9 24.9 **FUD** 090 J A2

AMA: 2014,Jan,11; 2013,Jan,11-12

49405 **Image-guided fluid collection drainage by catheter (eg, abscess, hematoma, seroma, lymphocele, cyst); visceral (eg, kidney, liver, spleen, lung/mediastinum), percutaneous**

INCLUDES Radiological guidance (75989, 76942, 77002-77003, 77012, 77021)

EXCLUDES *Open drainage (47010, 48510, 50020)*
Percutaneous cholecystostomy (47490)
Percutaneous pleural drainage (32556-32557)
Pneumonostomy (32200)
Thoracentesis (32554-32555)

Code also each individual collection drained per separate catheter

5.71 25.1 **FUD** 000 J

AMA: 2020,Feb,13; 2018,Jan,8; 2017,Jan,8; 2016,Jan,13; 2015,Jan,16

49406 **peritoneal or retroperitoneal, percutaneous**

INCLUDES Radiological guidance (75989, 76942, 77002-77003, 77012, 77021)

EXCLUDES *Diagnostic or therapeutic percutaneous abdominal paracentesis (49082-49083)*
Open peritoneal/retroperitoneal drainage (44900, 49020-49062, 49084, 50020, 58805, 58822)
Open transrectal drainage pelvic abscess (45000)
Percutaneous tunneled intraperitoneal catheter insertion without subcutaneous port (49418)
Transrectal/transvaginal image-guided peritoneal/retroperitoneal drainage via catheter (49407)

Code also each individual collection drained per separate catheter

5.70 25.1 **FUD** 000 J G2

AMA: 2020,Feb,13; 2018,Jan,8; 2017,Jan,8; 2016,Jan,13; 2015,Jan,16

49407 **peritoneal or retroperitoneal, transvaginal or transrectal**

INCLUDES Radiological guidance (75989, 76942, 77002-77003, 77012, 77021)

EXCLUDES *Image-guided percutaneous catheter drainage soft tissue (eg, abdominal wall, neck, extremity) (10030)*
Open transrectal/transvaginal drainage (45000, 58800, 58820)
Percutaneous pleural drainage (32556-32557)
Peritoneal drainage or lavage, open or percutaneous (49020, 49040, 49060)
Thoracentesis (32554-32555)

Code also each individual collection drained per separate catheter

6.05 20.6 **FUD** 000 J G2

AMA: 2018,Jan,8; 2017,Jan,8; 2016,Jan,13; 2015,Jan,16

49411 **Placement of interstitial device(s) for radiation therapy guidance (eg, fiducial markers, dosimeter), percutaneous, intra-abdominal, intra-pelvic (except prostate), and/or retroperitoneum, single or multiple**

EXCLUDES *Placement (percutaneous) interstitial device(s) for intrathoracic radiation therapy guidance (32553)*

Code also supply device

(76942, 77002, 77012, 77021)

5.33 13.9 **FUD** 000 S P3 80

AMA: 2018,Jan,8; 2017,Jan,8; 2016,Jun,3; 2016,Jan,13; 2015,Jan,16

+ **49412** **Placement of interstitial device(s) for radiation therapy guidance (eg, fiducial markers, dosimeter), open, intra-abdominal, intrapelvic, and/or retroperitoneum, including image guidance, if performed, single or multiple (List separately in addition to code for primary procedure)**

EXCLUDES *Laparoscopic approach (49327)*
Percutaneous approach (49411)

Code first open abdominal, pelvic or retroperitoneal procedure(s)

2.41 2.41 **FUD** ZZZ C 80

AMA: 2014,Jan,11; 2013,Jan,11-12

49418 **Insertion of tunneled intraperitoneal catheter (eg, dialysis, intraperitoneal chemotherapy instillation, management of ascites), complete procedure, including imaging guidance, catheter placement, contrast injection when performed, and radiological supervision and interpretation, percutaneous**

5.88 34.1 **FUD** 000 J G2 80

AMA: 2014,Jan,11; 2013,Nov,9

49419 **Insertion of tunneled intraperitoneal catheter, with subcutaneous port (ie, totally implantable)**

EXCLUDES *Removal catheter/cannula (49422)*

12.5 12.5 **FUD** 090 T A2

AMA: 2014,Jan,11; 2013,Jan,11-12

49421 **Insertion of tunneled intraperitoneal catheter for dialysis, open**

EXCLUDES *Laparoscopic approach (49324)*

Code also insertion subcutaneous extension to intraperitoneal cannula with remote chest exit site, when appropriate (49435)

6.65 6.65 **FUD** 000 J G2

AMA: 2018,Jan,8; 2017,Jan,8; 2016,Jan,13; 2015,Jan,16

49422 **Removal of tunneled intraperitoneal catheter**

EXCLUDES *Removal temporary catheter or cannula (Report appropriate E/M code)*

6.46 6.46 **FUD** 000 Q2 A2

AMA: 2014,Jan,11; 2013,Jan,11-12

49423 **Exchange of previously placed abscess or cyst drainage catheter under radiological guidance (separate procedure)**

(75984)

2.05 16.9 **FUD** 000 J G2 80

AMA: 2018,Jan,8; 2017,Jan,8; 2016,Jan,13; 2015,Jan,16

49424 **Contrast injection for assessment of abscess or cyst via previously placed drainage catheter or tube (separate procedure)**

(76080)

1.10 4.35 **FUD** 000 N N1 80

AMA: 2018,Jan,8; 2017,Jan,8; 2016,Jan,13; 2015,Jan,16

49425 **Insertion of peritoneal-venous shunt**

20.7 20.7 **FUD** 090 C 80

AMA: 2014,Jan,11; 2013,Jan,11-12

49426 **Revision of peritoneal-venous shunt**

EXCLUDES *Shunt patency test (78291)*

19.4 19.4 **FUD** 090 J A2

AMA: 2014,Jan,11; 2013,Jan,11-12

49427 **Injection procedure (eg, contrast media) for evaluation of previously placed peritoneal-venous shunt**

(75809, 78291)

1.13 1.13 **FUD** 000 N N1 80

AMA: 2014,Jan,11; 2013,Jan,11-12

49428 **Ligation of peritoneal-venous shunt**

12.5 12.5 **FUD** 010 C

AMA: 2014,Jan,11; 2013,Jan,11-12

49429 **Removal of peritoneal-venous shunt**

13.3 13.3 **FUD** 010 Q2 G2

AMA: 2014,Jan,11; 2013,Jan,11-12

\+ **49435** **Insertion of subcutaneous extension to intraperitoneal cannula or catheter with remote chest exit site (List separately in addition to code for primary procedure)**

Code first permanent insertion intraperitoneal catheter/cannula (49324, 49421)

3.50 3.50 **FUD** ZZZ N N1 80

AMA: 2014,Jan,11; 2013,Jan,11-12

49436 **Delayed creation of exit site from embedded subcutaneous segment of intraperitoneal cannula or catheter**

5.42 5.42 **FUD** 010 J G2 80

AMA: 2014,Jan,11; 2013,Jan,11-12

49440-49442 Insertion of Percutaneous Gastrointestinal Tube

EXCLUDES *Naso- or oro-gastric tube placement (43752)*

49440 **Insertion of gastrostomy tube, percutaneous, under fluoroscopic guidance including contrast injection(s), image documentation and report**

INCLUDES Needle placement with fluoroscopic guidance (77002)

Code also gastrostomy to gastro-jejunostomy tube conversion with initial gastrostomy tube insertion, when performed (49446)

5.93 26.6 **FUD** 010 J G2 80

AMA: 2018,Jan,8; 2017,Jan,8; 2016,Jan,13; 2015,Jan,16

49441 **Insertion of duodenostomy or jejunostomy tube, percutaneous, under fluoroscopic guidance including contrast injection(s), image documentation and report**

EXCLUDES *Gastrostomy tube to gastrojejunostomy tube conversion (49446)*

7.00 30.6 **FUD** 010 J G2 80

AMA: 2018,Jan,8; 2017,Jan,8; 2016,Jan,13; 2015,Jan,16

49442 **Insertion of cecostomy or other colonic tube, percutaneous, under fluoroscopic guidance including contrast injection(s), image documentation and report**

6.00 25.2 **FUD** 010 T G2 80

AMA: 2018,Jan,8; 2017,Jan,8; 2016,Jan,13; 2015,Jan,16

49446 Percutaneous Conversion: Gastrostomy to Gastro-jejunostomy Tube

EXCLUDES *Code also initial gastrostomy tube insertion (49440) when conversion performed same time*

49446 **Conversion of gastrostomy tube to gastro-jejunostomy tube, percutaneous, under fluoroscopic guidance including contrast injection(s), image documentation and report**

4.30 25.6 **FUD** 000 J G2 80

AMA: 2018,Jan,8; 2017,Jan,8; 2016,Jan,13; 2015,Jan,16

49450-49452 Replacement Gastrointestinal Tube

EXCLUDES *Placement new tube whether gastrostomy, jejunostomy, duodenostomy, gastro-jejunostomy, or cecostomy different percutaneous site (49440-49442)*

49450 **Replacement of gastrostomy or cecostomy (or other colonic) tube, percutaneous, under fluoroscopic guidance including contrast injection(s), image documentation and report**

EXCLUDES *Change gastrostomy tube, percutaneous, without imaging or endoscopic guidance (43762-43763)*

1.91 18.7 **FUD** 000 T G2 80

AMA: 2019,Feb,5; 2018,Jan,8; 2017,Jan,8; 2016,Jan,13; 2015,Jan,16

49451 **Replacement of duodenostomy or jejunostomy tube, percutaneous, under fluoroscopic guidance including contrast injection(s), image documentation and report**

2.61 20.3 **FUD** 000 T G2 80

AMA: 2018,Jan,8; 2017,Jan,8; 2016,Jan,13; 2015,Jan,16

49452 **Replacement of gastro-jejunostomy tube, percutaneous, under fluoroscopic guidance including contrast injection(s), image documentation and report**

4.01 25.1 **FUD** 000 T G2 80

AMA: 2018,Jan,8; 2017,Jan,8; 2016,Jan,13; 2015,Jan,16

49460-49465 Removal of Obstruction/Injection for Contrast Through Gastrointestinal Tube

49460 **Mechanical removal of obstructive material from gastrostomy, duodenostomy, jejunostomy, gastro-jejunostomy, or cecostomy (or other colonic) tube, any method, under fluoroscopic guidance including contrast injection(s), if performed, image documentation and report**

INCLUDES Contrast injection (49465)

EXCLUDES *Replacement gastrointestinal tube (49450-49452)*

1.39 20.4 **FUD** 000 T G2 80

AMA: 2018,Jan,8; 2017,Jan,8; 2016,Jan,13; 2015,Jan,16

49465 **Contrast injection(s) for radiological evaluation of existing gastrostomy, duodenostomy, jejunostomy, gastro-jejunostomy, or cecostomy (or other colonic) tube, from a percutaneous approach including image documentation and report**

EXCLUDES *Mechanical removal obstructive material from gastrointestinal tube (49460)*

Replacement gastrointestinal tube (49450-49452)

0.89 4.48 **FUD** 000 Q1 G2 80

AMA: 2018,Jan,8; 2017,Jan,8; 2016,Jan,13; 2015,Jan,16

49491-49492 Inguinal Hernia Repair on Premature Infant

INCLUDES Hernia repairs done on preterm infants younger than or equal to 50 weeks postconception age and younger than 6 months

Initial repair: no previous repair required

Mesh or other prosthesis

EXCLUDES *Abdominal wall debridement (11042, 11043)*

Intra-abdominal hernia repair/reduction (44050)

Code also repair or excision testicle(s), intestine, ovaries, when performed (44120, 54520, 58940)

49491 **Repair, initial inguinal hernia, preterm infant (younger than 37 weeks gestation at birth), performed from birth up to 50 weeks postconception age, with or without hydrocelectomy; reducible** A

23.2 23.2 **FUD** 090 63 J 80 50

AMA: 2018,Jan,8; 2017,Jan,8; 2016,Jan,13; 2015,Jan,16

26/TC PC/TC Only · A2-Z3 ASC Payment · 50 Bilateral · ♂ Male Only · ♀ Female Only · Facility RVU · Non-Facility RVU · CCI · CLIA
FUD Follow-up Days · CMS: IOM · AMA: CPT Asst · A-Y OPPSI · 80/80 Surg Assist Allowed / w/Doc · Lab Crosswalk · Radiology Crosswalk

49492 **incarcerated or strangulated** A
27.9 27.9 **FUD** 090 63 J 80 50
AMA: 2018,Jan,8; 2017,Jan,8; 2016,Jan,13; 2015,Jan,16

49495-49557 Hernia Repair: Femoral/Inguinal /Lumbar

INCLUDES Initial repair: no previous repair required
Mesh or other prosthesis
Recurrent repair: required previous repair(s)

EXCLUDES *Abdominal wall debridement (11042, 11043)*
Intra-abdominal hernia repair/reduction (44050)

Code also repair or excision testicle(s), intestine, ovaries, when performed (44120, 54520, 58940)

49495 **Repair, initial inguinal hernia, full term infant younger than age 6 months, or preterm infant older than 50 weeks postconception age and younger than age 6 months at the time of surgery, with or without hydrocelectomy; reducible** A
INCLUDES Hernia repairs done on preterm infants older than 50 weeks postconception age and younger than 6 months
11.8 11.8 **FUD** 090 63 J A2 80 50
AMA: 2018,Jan,8; 2017,Jan,8; 2016,Jan,13; 2015,Jan,16

49496 **incarcerated or strangulated** A
INCLUDES Hernia repairs done on preterm infants older than 50 weeks postconception age and younger than 6 months
17.7 17.7 **FUD** 090 63 J A2 80 50
AMA: 2018,Jan,8; 2017,Jan,8; 2016,Jan,13; 2015,Jan,16

49500 **Repair initial inguinal hernia, age 6 months to younger than 5 years, with or without hydrocelectomy; reducible** A
INCLUDES Repairs performed on patients 6 months to younger than 5 years old
11.9 11.9 **FUD** 090 J A2 80 50
AMA: 2018,Jan,8; 2017,Jan,8; 2016,Jan,13; 2015,Jan,16

49501 **incarcerated or strangulated** A
INCLUDES Repairs performed on patients 6 months to younger than 5 years old
17.6 17.6 **FUD** 090 J A2 80 50
AMA: 2018,Jan,8; 2017,Jan,8; 2016,Jan,13; 2015,Jan,16

49505 **Repair initial inguinal hernia, age 5 years or older; reducible** A
INCLUDES MacEwen hernia repair
Code also when performed:
Excision hydrocele (55040)
Excision spermatocele (54840)
Simple orchiectomy (54520)
15.0 15.0 **FUD** 090 J A2 80 50
AMA: 2018,Jan,8; 2017,Jan,8; 2016,Jan,13; 2015,Jan,16

49507 **incarcerated or strangulated** A
Code also when performed:
Excision hydrocele (55040)
Excision spermatocele (54840)
Simple orchiectomy (54520)
17.0 17.0 **FUD** 090 J A2 80 50
AMA: 2018,Jan,8; 2017,Jan,8; 2016,Jan,13; 2015,Jan,16

49520 **Repair recurrent inguinal hernia, any age; reducible**
18.3 18.3 **FUD** 090 J A2 80 50
AMA: 2018,Jan,8; 2017,Jan,8; 2016,Jan,13; 2015,Jan,16

49521 **incarcerated or strangulated**
20.8 20.8 **FUD** 090 J A2 80 50
AMA: 2018,Jan,8; 2017,Jan,8; 2016,Jan,13; 2015,Jan,16

49525 **Repair inguinal hernia, sliding, any age**
EXCLUDES *Inguinal hernia repair, incarcerated/strangulated (49496, 49501, 49507, 49521)*
16.7 16.7 **FUD** 090 J A2 80 50
AMA: 2018,Jan,8; 2017,Jan,8; 2016,Jan,13; 2015,Jan,16

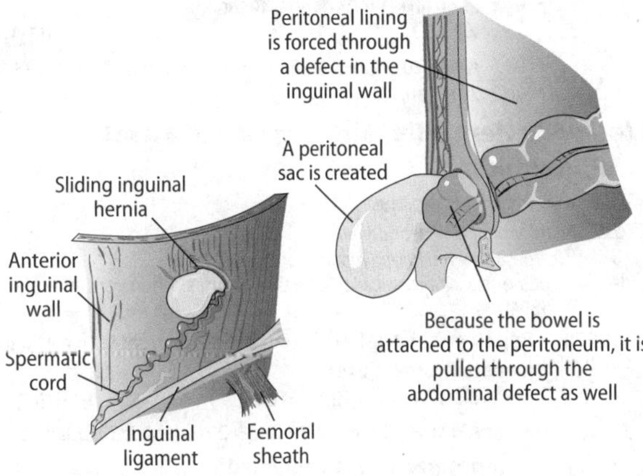

49540 **Repair lumbar hernia**
19.5 19.5 **FUD** 090 J A2 80 50
AMA: 2018,Jan,8; 2017,Jan,8; 2016,Jan,13; 2015,Jan,16

49550 **Repair initial femoral hernia, any age; reducible**
16.7 16.7 **FUD** 090 J A2 80 50
AMA: 2018,Jan,8; 2017,Jan,8; 2016,Jan,13; 2015,Jan,16

49553 **incarcerated or strangulated**
18.3 18.3 **FUD** 090 J A2 80 50
AMA: 2018,Jan,8; 2017,Jan,8; 2016,Jan,13; 2015,Jan,16

49555 **Repair recurrent femoral hernia; reducible**
17.5 17.5 **FUD** 090 J A2 80 50
AMA: 2018,Jan,8; 2017,Jan,8; 2016,Jan,13; 2015,Jan,16

49557 **incarcerated or strangulated**
21.0 21.0 **FUD** 090 J A2 80 50
AMA: 2018,Jan,8; 2017,Jan,8; 2016,Jan,13; 2015,Jan,16

49560-49568 Hernia Repair: Incisional/Ventral

INCLUDES Initial repair: no previous repair required
Recurrent repair: required previous repair(s)

EXCLUDES *Abdominal wall debridement (11042, 11043)*
Intra-abdominal hernia repair/reduction (44050)

Code also repair or excision testicle(s), intestine, ovaries, when performed (44120, 54520, 58940)

49560 **Repair initial incisional or ventral hernia; reducible**
Code also implantation mesh or other prosthesis, when performed (49568)
21.5 21.5 **FUD** 090 J A2 80 50
AMA: 2019,Nov,14; 2018,Jan,8; 2017,Jan,8; 2016,Jan,13; 2015,Jan,16

49561 **incarcerated or strangulated**
Code also implantation mesh or other prosthesis, when performed (49568)
27.0 27.0 **FUD** 090 J A2 80 50
AMA: 2019,Nov,14; 2018,Jul,14; 2018,Mar,11; 2018,Jan,8; 2017,Jan,8; 2016,Jan,13; 2015,Jan,16

49565 **Repair recurrent incisional or ventral hernia; reducible**
Code also implantation mesh or other prosthesis, when performed (49568)
22.3 22.3 **FUD** 090 J A2 80 50
AMA: 2019,Nov,14; 2018,Jan,8; 2017,Jan,8; 2016,Jan,13; 2015,Jan,16

49566 **incarcerated or strangulated**
Code also implantation mesh or other prosthesis, when performed (49568)
27.3 27.3 **FUD** 090 J A2 80 50
AMA: 2019,Nov,14; 2018,Jan,8; 2017,Jan,8; 2016,Jan,13; 2015,Jan,16

\+ **49568** **Implantation of mesh or other prosthesis for open incisional or ventral hernia repair or mesh for closure of debridement for necrotizing soft tissue infection (List separately in addition to code for the incisional or ventral hernia repair)**

EXCLUDES *Reporting with modifier 50. Report once for each side when performed bilaterally*

Code first (11004-11006, 49560-49566)

7.77 7.77 **FUD** ZZZ N N1 80

AMA: 2019,Nov,14; 2018,Jan,8; 2017,Jan,8; 2016,Jan,13; 2015,Jan,16

49570-49590 Hernia Repair: Epigastric/Lateral Ventral/Umbilical

INCLUDES Mesh or other prosthesis

EXCLUDES *Abdominal wall debridement (11042, 11043)*
Intra-abdominal hernia repair/reduction (44050)

Code also repair or excision testicle(s), intestine, ovaries, when performed (44120, 54520, 58940)

49570 **Repair epigastric hernia (eg, preperitoneal fat); reducible (separate procedure)**

12.1 12.1 **FUD** 090 J A2 80 50

AMA: 2018,Jan,8; 2017,Jan,8; 2016,Jan,13; 2015,Jan,16

49572 **incarcerated or strangulated**

14.9 14.9 **FUD** 090 J A2 80 50

AMA: 2018,Jan,8; 2017,Jan,8; 2016,Jan,13; 2015,Jan,16

49580 **Repair umbilical hernia, younger than age 5 years; reducible** A

9.69 9.69 **FUD** 090 J A2 80

AMA: 2018,Jan,8; 2017,Jan,8; 2016,Jan,13; 2015,Jan,16

49582 **incarcerated or strangulated** A

14.0 14.0 **FUD** 090 J A2 80

AMA: 2018,Jan,8; 2017,Jan,8; 2016,Jan,13; 2015,Jan,16

49585 **Repair umbilical hernia, age 5 years or older; reducible** A

INCLUDES Mayo hernia repair

12.9 12.9 **FUD** 090 J A2 80

AMA: 2018,Jan,8; 2017,Jan,8; 2016,Jan,13; 2015,Jan,16

49587 **incarcerated or strangulated** A

13.7 13.7 **FUD** 090 J A2 80

AMA: 2018,Jan,8; 2017,Jan,8; 2016,Jan,13; 2015,Jan,16

49590 **Repair spigelian hernia**

16.5 16.5 **FUD** 090 J A2 80 50

AMA: 2018,Jan,8; 2017,Jan,8; 2016,Jan,13; 2015,Jan,16

49600-49611 Repair Birth Defect Abdominal Wall: Omphalocele/Gastroschisis

INCLUDES Mesh or other prosthesis

EXCLUDES *Abdominal wall debridement (11042, 11043)*
Intra-abdominal hernia repair/reduction (44050)
Repair:
Diaphragmatic or hiatal hernia (39503, 43332-43337)
Omentum (49999)

49600 **Repair of small omphalocele, with primary closure**

21.2 21.2 **FUD** 090 63 J A2 80

AMA: 2018,Jan,8; 2017,Jan,8; 2016,Jan,13; 2015,Jan,16

49605 **Repair of large omphalocele or gastroschisis; with or without prosthesis**

144. 144. **FUD** 090 63 C 80

AMA: 2018,Jan,8; 2017,Jan,8; 2016,Jan,13; 2015,Jan,16

49606 **with removal of prosthesis, final reduction and closure, in operating room**

32.9 32.9 **FUD** 090 63 C 80

AMA: 2018,Jan,8; 2017,Jan,8; 2016,Jan,13; 2015,Jan,16

49610 **Repair of omphalocele (Gross type operation); first stage**

20.1 20.1 **FUD** 090 63 C 80

AMA: 2018,Jan,8; 2017,Jan,8; 2016,Jan,13; 2015,Jan,16

49611 **second stage**

17.7 17.7 **FUD** 090 63 C 80

AMA: 2018,Jan,8; 2017,Jan,8; 2016,Jan,13; 2015,Jan,16

49650-49659 Laparoscopic Hernia Repair

INCLUDES Diagnostic laparoscopy (49320)
Mesh or other prosthesis (49568)

49650 **Laparoscopy, surgical; repair initial inguinal hernia**

12.5 12.5 **FUD** 090 J A2 80 50

AMA: 2018,Jan,8; 2017,Jan,8; 2016,Jan,13; 2015,Jan,16

49651 **repair recurrent inguinal hernia**

16.2 16.2 **FUD** 090 J A2 80 50

AMA: 2018,Jan,8; 2017,Jan,8; 2016,Jan,13; 2015,Jan,16

49652 **Laparoscopy, surgical, repair, ventral, umbilical, spigelian or epigastric hernia (includes mesh insertion, when performed); reducible**

INCLUDES Laparoscopy, surgical, enterolysis (44180)

21.5 21.5 **FUD** 090 J G2 80 50

AMA: 2014,Jan,11; 2013,Jan,11-12

49653 **incarcerated or strangulated**

INCLUDES Laparoscopy, surgical, enterolysis (44180)

27.0 27.0 **FUD** 090 J G2 80 50

AMA: 2014,Jan,11; 2013,Jan,11-12

49654 **Laparoscopy, surgical, repair, incisional hernia (includes mesh insertion, when performed); reducible**

INCLUDES Laparoscopy, surgical, enterolysis (44180)

24.6 24.6 **FUD** 090 J G2 80 50

AMA: 2018,Jan,7

49655 **incarcerated or strangulated**

INCLUDES Laparoscopy, surgical, enterolysis (44180)

29.9 29.9 **FUD** 090 J G2 80 50

AMA: 2018,Jan,7

49656 **Laparoscopy, surgical, repair, recurrent incisional hernia (includes mesh insertion, when performed); reducible**

INCLUDES Laparoscopy, surgical, enterolysis (44180)

26.7 26.7 **FUD** 090 J G2 80 50

AMA: 2014,Jan,11; 2013,Jan,11-12

49657 **incarcerated or strangulated**

INCLUDES Laparoscopy, surgical, enterolysis (44180)

38.2 38.2 **FUD** 090 J G2 80 50

AMA: 2014,Jan,11; 2013,Jan,11-12

49659 **Unlisted laparoscopy procedure, hernioplasty, herniorrhaphy, herniotomy**

0.00 0.00 **FUD** YYY J 80 50

AMA: 2018,Jan,8; 2017,Jul,10; 2017,Jan,8; 2016,Jan,13; 2015,Jan,16

49900 Surgical Repair Abdominal Wall

EXCLUDES *Abdominal wall debridement (11042, 11043)*
Suture ruptured diaphragm (39540-39541)

49900 **Suture, secondary, of abdominal wall for evisceration or dehiscence**

23.7 23.7 **FUD** 090 C 80

AMA: 2018,Jan,8; 2017,Jan,8; 2016,Jan,13; 2015,Jan,16

49904-49999 Harvesting of Omental Flap

49904 **Omental flap, extra-abdominal (eg, for reconstruction of sternal and chest wall defects)**

INCLUDES Harvest and transfer

EXCLUDES *Omental flap harvest by second surgeon: both surgeons report code with modifier 62*

40.5 40.5 **FUD** 090 C

AMA: 2014,Jan,11; 2013,Jan,11-12

\+ **49905** **Omental flap, intra-abdominal (List separately in addition to code for primary procedure)**

EXCLUDES *Exclusion small intestine from pelvis by mesh, other prosthesis, or native tissue (44700)*

Code first primary procedure

10.3 10.3 **FUD** ZZZ C 80

AMA: 2020,Feb,13; 2018,Jan,8; 2017,Jan,8; 2016,Jan,13; 2015,Jan,16

49906 Free omental flap with microvascular anastomosis

INCLUDES Operating microscope (69990)

0.00 0.00 **FUD** 090 C

AMA: 2019,Dec,5; 2018,Jan,8; 2017,Jan,8; 2016,Feb,12; 2016,Jan,13; 2015,Jan,16

49999 Unlisted procedure, abdomen, peritoneum and omentum

0.00 0.00 **FUD** YYY T

AMA: 2020,Jun,14; 2019,Nov,14; 2018,Jan,8; 2017,Jan,8; 2016,Jan,13; 2015,Jan,16

50010-50045 Kidney Procedures for Exploration or Drainage

EXCLUDES Donor nephrectomy performed laparoscopically (50547)
Retroperitoneal
Abscess drainage (49060)
Exploration (49010)
Tumor/cyst excision (49203-49205)

50010 Renal exploration, not necessitating other specific procedures
EXCLUDES Laparoscopic ablation mass lesions of kidney (50542)
21.2 21.2 FUD 090 C 80 50
AMA: 2014,Jan,11; 2008,Aug,7-9

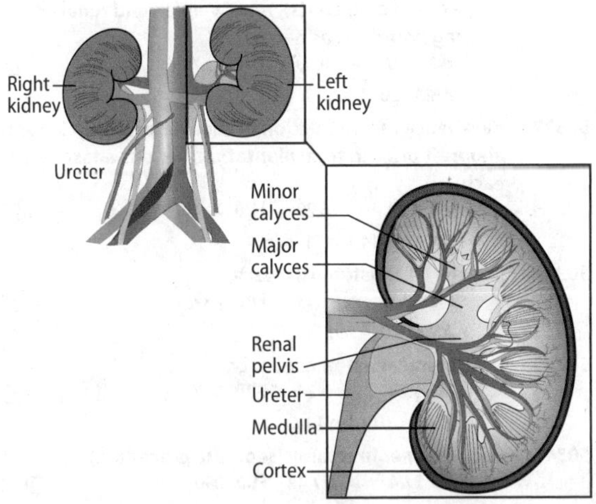

50020 Drainage of perirenal or renal abscess, open
EXCLUDES Image-guided percutaneous drainage perirenal or renal abscess (49405)
29.2 29.2 FUD 090 J
AMA: 2018,Jan,8; 2017,Jan,8; 2016,Jan,13; 2015,Jan,16

50040 Nephrostomy, nephrotomy with drainage
26.6 26.6 FUD 090 C 50
AMA: 2018,Jan,8; 2017,Jan,8; 2016,Jan,13; 2015,Jan,16

50045 Nephrotomy, with exploration
EXCLUDES Renal endoscopy through nephrotomy (50570-50580)
26.9 26.9 FUD 090 C 80 50
AMA: 2018,Jan,8; 2017,Jan,8; 2016,Jan,13; 2015,Jan,16

50060-50081 Treatment of Kidney Stones

CMS: 100-03,230.1 NCD for Treatment of Kidney Stones
EXCLUDES Retroperitoneal:
Abscess drainage (49060)
Exploration (49010)
Tumor/cyst excision (49203-49205)

50060 Nephrolithotomy; removal of calculus
32.9 32.9 FUD 090 C 80 50
AMA: 2018,Jan,8; 2017,Jan,8; 2016,Jan,13; 2015,Jan,16

50065 secondary surgical operation for calculus
34.9 34.9 FUD 090 C 80 50
AMA: 2018,Jan,8; 2017,Jan,8; 2016,Jan,13; 2015,Jan,16

50070 complicated by congenital kidney abnormality
34.2 34.2 FUD 090 C 80 50
AMA: 2018,Jan,8; 2017,Jan,8; 2016,Jan,13; 2015,Jan,16

50075 removal of large staghorn calculus filling renal pelvis and calyces (including anatrophic pyelolithotomy)
42.1 42.1 FUD 090 C 80 50
AMA: 2018,Jan,8; 2017,Jan,8; 2016,Jan,13; 2015,Jan,16

50080 Percutaneous nephrostolithotomy or pyelostolithotomy, with or without dilation, endoscopy, lithotripsy, stenting, or basket extraction; up to 2 cm
EXCLUDES Dilation existing tract by same provider ([50436, 50437])
Nephrostomy without nephrostolithotomy (50040, [50432, 50433], 52334)
(76000)
25.0 25.0 FUD 090 J G2 50
AMA: 2018,Jan,8; 2017,Jan,8; 2016,Jan,13; 2015,Jan,16

50081 over 2 cm
EXCLUDES Dilation existing tract by same provider ([50436, 50437])
Nephrostomy without nephrostolithotomy (50040, [50432, 50433], 52334)
(76000)
36.9 36.9 FUD 090 J G2 80 50
AMA: 2018,Jan,8; 2017,Jan,8; 2016,Jan,13; 2015,Jan,16

50100 Repair of Anomalous Vessels of the Kidney

EXCLUDES Retroperitoneal:
Abscess drainage (49060)
Exploration (49010)
Tumor/cyst excision (49203-49205)

50100 Transection or repositioning of aberrant renal vessels (separate procedure)
31.4 31.4 FUD 090 C 80 50
AMA: 2018,Jan,8; 2017,Jan,8; 2016,Jan,13; 2015,Jan,16

50120-50135 Procedures of Renal Pelvis

EXCLUDES Retroperitoneal:
Abscess drainage (49060)
Exploration (49010)
Tumor/cyst excision (49203-49205)

50120 Pyelotomy; with exploration
INCLUDES Gol-Vernet pyelotomy
EXCLUDES Renal endoscopy through pyelotomy (50570-50580)
27.4 27.4 FUD 090 C 80 50
AMA: 2018,Jan,8; 2017,Jan,8; 2016,Jan,13; 2015,Jan,16

50125 with drainage, pyelostomy
28.3 28.3 FUD 090 C 80 50
AMA: 2018,Jan,8; 2017,Jan,8; 2016,Jan,13; 2015,Jan,16

50130 with removal of calculus (pyelolithotomy, pelviolithotomy, including coagulum pyelolithotomy)
29.8 29.8 FUD 090 C 80 50
AMA: 2018,Jan,8; 2017,Jan,8; 2016,Jan,13; 2015,Jan,16

50135 complicated (eg, secondary operation, congenital kidney abnormality)
32.4 32.4 FUD 090 C 80 50
AMA: 2018,Jan,8; 2017,Jan,8; 2016,Jan,13; 2015,Jan,16

50200-50205 Biopsy of Kidney

EXCLUDES Laparoscopic renal mass lesion ablation (50542)
Retroperitoneal tumor/cyst excision (49203-49205)

50200 Renal biopsy; percutaneous, by trocar or needle
EXCLUDES Fine needle aspiration ([10005, 10006, 10007, 10008, 10009, 10010, 10011, 10012])
(76942, 77002, 77012, 77021)
(88172-88173)
3.70 15.4 FUD 000 J A2 50
AMA: 2019,Apr,4; 2018,Jan,8; 2017,Jan,8; 2016,Jan,13; 2015,Jan,16

50205 by surgical exposure of kidney
21.9 21.9 FUD 090 C 80 50
AMA: 2018,Jan,8; 2017,Jan,8; 2016,Jan,13; 2015,Jan,16

50220-50240 Nephrectomy Procedures

EXCLUDES Laparoscopic renal mass lesion ablation (50542)
Retroperitoneal tumor/cyst excision (49203-49205)

50220 Nephrectomy, including partial ureterectomy, any open approach including rib resection;
30.3 30.3 FUD 090 C 80 50
AMA: 2018,Jan,8; 2017,Jan,8; 2016,Jan,13; 2015,Jan,16

50225 **complicated because of previous surgery on same kidney**
34.7 34.7 **FUD** 090 C 80 50
AMA: 2018,Jan,8; 2017,Jan,8; 2016,Jan,13; 2015,Jan,16

50230 **radical, with regional lymphadenectomy and/or vena caval thrombectomy**
EXCLUDES *Vena caval resection with reconstruction (37799)*
37.0 37.0 **FUD** 090 C 80 50
AMA: 2018,Jan,8; 2017,Jan,8; 2016,Jan,13; 2015,Jan,16

50234 **Nephrectomy with total ureterectomy and bladder cuff; through same incision**
37.6 37.6 **FUD** 090 C 80 50
AMA: 2018,Jan,8; 2017,Jan,8; 2016,Jan,13; 2015,Jan,16

50236 **through separate incision**
42.3 42.3 **FUD** 090 C 80 50
AMA: 2018,Jan,8; 2017,Jan,8; 2016,Jan,13; 2015,Jan,16

50240 **Nephrectomy, partial**
EXCLUDES *Laparoscopic partial nephrectomy (50543)*
38.2 38.2 **FUD** 090 C 80 50
AMA: 2018,Jan,8; 2017,Jan,8; 2016,Jan,13; 2015,Jan,16

50250-50290 Open Removal Kidney Lesions

EXCLUDES *Open destruction or excision intra-abdominal tumors (49203-49205)*

50250 **Ablation, open, 1 or more renal mass lesion(s), cryosurgical, including intraoperative ultrasound guidance and monitoring, if performed**
EXCLUDES *Laparoscopic renal mass lesion ablation (50542)*
Percutaneous renal tumor ablation (50592-50593)
35.1 35.1 **FUD** 090 C 80
AMA: 2018,Jan,8; 2017,Jan,8; 2016,Jan,13; 2015,Jan,16

50280 **Excision or unroofing of cyst(s) of kidney**
EXCLUDES *Renal cyst laparoscopic ablation (50541)*
27.6 27.6 **FUD** 090 C 80 50
AMA: 2018,Jan,8; 2017,Jan,8; 2016,Jan,13; 2015,Jan,16

50290 **Excision of perinephric cyst**
25.9 25.9 **FUD** 090 C 80
AMA: 2018,Jan,8; 2017,Jan,8; 2016,Jan,13; 2015,Jan,16

50300-50380 Kidney Transplant Procedures

CMS: 100-04,3,90.1 Kidney Transplant - General; 100-04,3,90.1.1 Standard Kidney Acquisition Charge; 100-04,3,90.1.2 Billing for Kidney Transplant and Acquisition Services; 100-04,3,90.5 Pancreas Transplants with Kidney Transplants

EXCLUDES *Dialysis procedures (90935-90999)*
Lymphocele drainage to peritoneal cavity performed laparoscopically (49323)

50300 **Donor nephrectomy (including cold preservation); from cadaver donor, unilateral or bilateral**
INCLUDES Graft:
Cold preservation
Harvesting
EXCLUDES *Donor nephrectomy performed laparoscopically (50547)*
0.00 0.00 **FUD** XXX C
AMA: 2018,Jan,8; 2017,Jan,8; 2016,Jan,13; 2015,Jan,16

50320 **open, from living donor**
INCLUDES Donor care
Graft:
Cold preservation
Harvesting
EXCLUDES *Donor nephrectomy performed laparoscopically (50547)*
43.7 43.7 **FUD** 090 C 80 50
AMA: 2018,Jan,8; 2017,Jan,8; 2016,Jan,13; 2015,Jan,16

50323 **Backbench standard preparation of cadaver donor renal allograft prior to transplantation, including dissection and removal of perinephric fat, diaphragmatic and retroperitoneal attachments, excision of adrenal gland, and preparation of ureter(s), renal vein(s), and renal artery(s), ligating branches, as necessary**
EXCLUDES *Adrenalectomy (60540, 60545)*
0.00 0.00 **FUD** XXX C 80
AMA: 2018,Jan,8; 2017,Jan,8; 2016,Jan,13; 2015,Jan,16

50325 **Backbench standard preparation of living donor renal allograft (open or laparoscopic) prior to transplantation, including dissection and removal of perinephric fat and preparation of ureter(s), renal vein(s), and renal artery(s), ligating branches, as necessary**
0.00 0.00 **FUD** XXX C 80
AMA: 2014,Jan,11

50327 **Backbench reconstruction of cadaver or living donor renal allograft prior to transplantation; venous anastomosis, each**
6.29 6.29 **FUD** XXX C 80
AMA: 2014,Jan,11

50328 **arterial anastomosis, each**
5.53 5.53 **FUD** XXX C 80
AMA: 2014,Jan,11

50329 **ureteral anastomosis, each**
5.24 5.24 **FUD** XXX C 80
AMA: 2014,Jan,11

50340 **Recipient nephrectomy (separate procedure)**
27.4 27.4 **FUD** 090 C 80 50
AMA: 2014,Jan,11

50360 **Renal allotransplantation, implantation of graft; without recipient nephrectomy**
INCLUDES Allograft transplantation
Recipient care
Code also backbench work (50323, 50325, 50327-50329)
Code also donor nephrectomy (cadaver or living donor) (50300, 50320, 50547)
70.0 70.0 **FUD** 090 C 80
AMA: 2014,Jan,11; 1994,Win,1

50365 **with recipient nephrectomy**
INCLUDES Allograft transplantation
Recipient care
83.5 83.5 **FUD** 090 C 80 50
AMA: 2018,Jan,8; 2017,Jan,8; 2016,Jan,13; 2015,Jan,16

50370 **Removal of transplanted renal allograft**
35.0 35.0 **FUD** 090 C 80
AMA: 2014,Jan,11; 2002,Oct,5

50380 **Renal autotransplantation, reimplantation of kidney**
INCLUDES Reimplantation autograft
EXCLUDES *Secondary procedures:*
Nephrolithotomy (50060-50075)
Partial nephrectomy (50240, 50543)
58.4 58.4 **FUD** 090 C 80
AMA: 2019,Sep,10; 2018,Jan,8; 2017,Jan,8; 2016,Jan,13; 2015,Jan,16

50382-50386 Removal With/Without Replacement Internal Ureteral Stent

INCLUDES Radiological supervision and interpretation

50382 Removal (via snare/capture) and replacement of internally dwelling ureteral stent via percutaneous approach, including radiological supervision and interpretation

EXCLUDES *Dilation existing tract, percutaneous for endourologic procedure ([50436, 50437])*
Removal and replacement internally dwelling ureteral stent using transurethral approach (50385)

7.46 31.3 FUD 000 J G2 50

AMA: 2018,Jan,8; 2017,Jan,8; 2016,Jan,13; 2016,Jan,3; 2015,Jan,16

50384 Removal (via snare/capture) of internally dwelling ureteral stent via percutaneous approach, including radiological supervision and interpretation

EXCLUDES *Dilation existing tract, percutaneous for endourologic procedure ([50436, 50437])*
Removal internally dwelling ureteral stent using transurethral approach (50386)

6.71 24.8 FUD 000 Q2 G2 50

AMA: 2018,Jan,8; 2017,Jan,8; 2016,Jan,13; 2016,Jan,3; 2015,Jan,16

50385 Removal (via snare/capture) and replacement of internally dwelling ureteral stent via transurethral approach, without use of cystoscopy, including radiological supervision and interpretation

6.34 30.7 FUD 000 J G2 80 50

AMA: 2018,Jan,8; 2017,Jan,8; 2016,Jan,13; 2016,Jan,3; 2015,Jan,16

50386 Removal (via snare/capture) of internally dwelling ureteral stent via transurethral approach, without use of cystoscopy, including radiological supervision and interpretation

4.70 20.3 FUD 000 Q2 P3 80 50

AMA: 2018,Jan,8; 2017,Jan,8; 2016,Jan,3; 2016,Jan,13; 2015,Jan,16

50387 Remove/Replace Accessible Ureteral Stent

EXCLUDES *Removal and replacement ureteral stent through ureterostomy tube or ileal conduit (50688)*
Removal without replacement externally accessible ureteral stent without fluoroscopic guidance, report with appropriate E/M code

50387 Removal and replacement of externally accessible nephroureteral catheter (eg, external/internal stent) requiring fluoroscopic guidance, including radiological supervision and interpretation

2.43 14.6 FUD 000 J G2 80 50

AMA: 2018,Jan,8; 2017,Jan,8; 2016,Mar,10; 2016,Jan,13; 2016,Jan,3; 2015,Oct,5; 2015,Jan,16

50389-50435 [50430, 50431, 50432, 50433, 50434, 50435, 50436, 50437] Percutaneous and Injection Procedures With/Without Indwelling Tube/Catheter Access

50389 Removal of nephrostomy tube, requiring fluoroscopic guidance (eg, with concurrent indwelling ureteral stent)

EXCLUDES *Nephrostomy tube removal without fluoroscopic guidance, report with appropriate E/M code*

1.56 9.49 FUD 000 Q2 G2 50

AMA: 2018,Jan,8; 2017,Jan,8; 2016,Jan,13; 2016,Jan,3; 2015,Oct,5; 2015,Jan,16

50390 Aspiration and/or injection of renal cyst or pelvis by needle, percutaneous

EXCLUDES *Antegrade nephrostogram/pyelogram ([50430, 50431])*

(74425, 74470, 76942, 77002, 77012, 77021)

2.78 2.78 FUD 000 T A2 50

AMA: 2018,Jan,8; 2017,Jan,8; 2016,Jan,13; 2015,Oct,5; 2015,Jan,16

50391 Instillation(s) of therapeutic agent into renal pelvis and/or ureter through established nephrostomy, pyelostomy or ureterostomy tube (eg, anticarcinogenic or antifungal agent)

Code also therapeutic agent

2.84 3.52 FUD 000 T P3 50

AMA: 2018,Jan,8; 2017,Jan,8; 2016,Jan,13; 2015,Oct,5; 2015,Jan,16

\# **50436 Dilation of existing tract, percutaneous, for an endourologic procedure including imaging guidance (eg, ultrasound and/or fluoroscopy) and all associated radiological supervision and interpretation, with postprocedure tube placement, when performed**

EXCLUDES *Percutaneous nephrostolithotomy (50080-50081)*
Procedure performed for same renal collecting system/ureter ([50430, 50431, 50432, 50433], 52334, 74485)
Removal, replacement internally dwelling ureteral stent (50382, 50384)

4.35 4.35 FUD 000 G2 50

\# **50437 including new access into the renal collecting system**

EXCLUDES *Percutaneous nephrostolithotomy (50080-50081)*
Procedure performed for same renal collecting system/ureter ([50430, 50431, 50432, 50433], 52334, 74485)
Removal, replacement internally dwelling ureteral stent (50382, 50384)

7.29 7.29 FUD 000 G2 50

50396 Manometric studies through nephrostomy or pyelostomy tube, or indwelling ureteral catheter

(74425)

3.38 3.38 FUD 000 J A2 80 50

AMA: 2018,Jan,8; 2017,Jan,8; 2016,Jan,13; 2015,Jan,16

\# **50430 Injection procedure for antegrade nephrostogram and/or ureterogram, complete diagnostic procedure including imaging guidance (eg, ultrasound and fluoroscopy) and all associated radiological supervision and interpretation; new access**

INCLUDES Renal pelvis and associated ureter as single element

EXCLUDES *Procedure performed for same renal collecting system/ureter ([50432, 50433, 50434, 50435], 50693-50695, 74425)*

4.47 13.0 FUD 000 Q2 N1 80 50

AMA: 2018,Jan,8; 2017,Jan,8; 2016,Jan,3; 2016,Jan,13; 2015,Oct,5

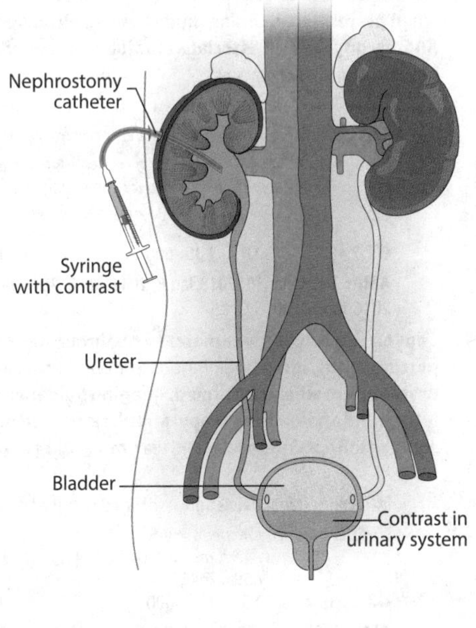

50431 **existing access**

INCLUDES Renal pelvis and associated ureter as single element

EXCLUDES *Procedure performed for same renal collecting system/ureter ([50432, 50433, 50434, 50435], 50693-50695, 74425)*

1.90 6.03 FUD 000 Q2 N1 50

AMA: 2018,Jan,8; 2017,Jan,8; 2016,Jan,3; 2016,Jan,13; 2015,Oct,5

50432 **Placement of nephrostomy catheter, percutaneous, including diagnostic nephrostogram and/or ureterogram when performed, imaging guidance (eg, ultrasound and/or fluoroscopy) and all associated radiological supervision and interpretation**

INCLUDES Renal pelvis and associated ureter as single element

EXCLUDES *Dilation nephroureteral catheter tract ([50436, 50437])*

Procedure performed for same renal collecting system/ureter ([50430, 50431], [50433], 50694-50695, 74425)

5.99 21.9 FUD 000 J G2 50

AMA: 2018,Mar,11; 2018,Jan,8; 2017,Jan,8; 2016,Jan,3; 2016,Jan,13; 2015,Oct,5

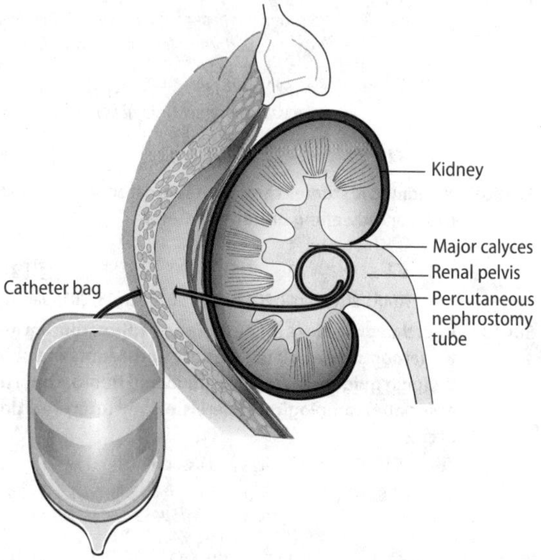

50433 **Placement of nephroureteral catheter, percutaneous, including diagnostic nephrostogram and/or ureterogram when performed, imaging guidance (eg, ultrasound and/or fluoroscopy) and all associated radiological supervision and interpretation, new access**

INCLUDES Renal pelvis and associated ureter as single element

EXCLUDES *Dilation nephroureteral catheter tract ([50436, 50437])*

Nephroureteral catheter removal/replacement (50387)

Procedures performed for same renal collecting system/ureter ([50430, 50431, 50432], 50693-50695, 74425)

7.48 30.0 FUD 000 J G2 50

AMA: 2018,Mar,11; 2018,Jan,8; 2017,Jan,8; 2016,Jan,3; 2016,Jan,13; 2015,Oct,5

50434 **Convert nephrostomy catheter to nephroureteral catheter, percutaneous, including diagnostic nephrostogram and/or ureterogram when performed, imaging guidance (eg, ultrasound and/or fluoroscopy) and all associated radiological supervision and interpretation, via pre-existing nephrostomy tract**

INCLUDES Renal pelvis and associated ureter as single element

EXCLUDES *Procedure performed for same renal collecting system/ureter ([50430, 50431], [50435], 50684, 50693, 74425)*

5.63 23.5 FUD 000 J J8 50

AMA: 2018,Jan,8; 2017,Jan,8; 2016,Jan,3; 2016,Jan,13; 2015,Oct,5

50435 **Exchange nephrostomy catheter, percutaneous, including diagnostic nephrostogram and/or ureterogram when performed, imaging guidance (eg, ultrasound and/or fluoroscopy) and all associated radiological supervision and interpretation**

INCLUDES Renal pelvis and associated ureter as single element

EXCLUDES *Procedure performed for same renal collecting system/ureter ([50430, 50431], [50434], 50693, 74425)*

Removal nephrostomy catheter requiring fluoroscopic guidance (50389)

2.91 13.4 FUD 000 J G2 50

AMA: 2018,Mar,11; 2018,Jan,8; 2017,Jan,8; 2016,Jan,3; 2016,Jan,13; 2015,Oct,5

50400-50540 [50430, 50431, 50432, 50433, 50434, 50435, 50436, 50437] Open Surgical Procedures of Kidney

50400 **Pyeloplasty (Foley Y-pyeloplasty), plastic operation on renal pelvis, with or without plastic operation on ureter, nephropexy, nephrostomy, pyelostomy, or ureteral splinting; simple**

EXCLUDES *Laparoscopic pyeloplasty (50544)*

33.5 33.5 FUD 090 C 80 50

AMA: 2018,Jan,8; 2017,Jan,8; 2016,Jan,13; 2015,Jan,16

50405 **complicated (congenital kidney abnormality, secondary pyeloplasty, solitary kidney, calycoplasty)**

EXCLUDES *Laparoscopic pyeloplasty (50544)*

40.3 40.3 FUD 090 C 80 50

AMA: 2018,Jan,8; 2017,Jan,8; 2016,Jan,13; 2015,Jan,16

50430 **Resequenced code. See code following 50396.**

50431 **Resequenced code. See code following 50396.**

50432 **Resequenced code. See code following 50396.**

50433 **Resequenced code. See code following 50396.**

50434 **Resequenced code. See code following 50396.**

50435 **Resequenced code. See code following 50396.**

50436 **Resequenced code. See code following 50391.**

50437 **Resequenced code. See code following 50391.**

50500 **Nephrorrhaphy, suture of kidney wound or injury**

37.3 37.3 FUD 090 C 80

AMA: 2014,Jan,11

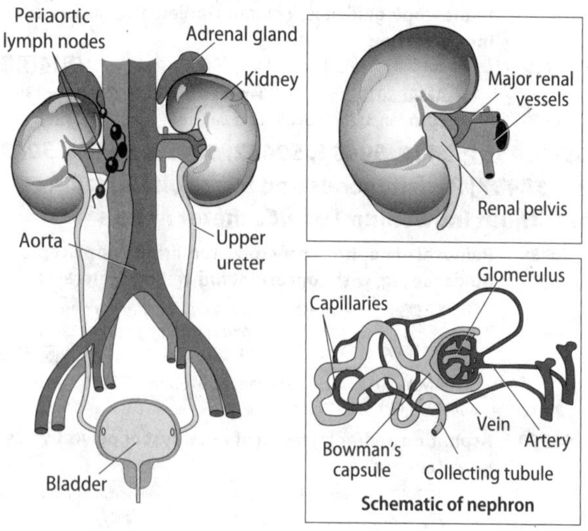

50520 **Closure of nephrocutaneous or pyelocutaneous fistula**

33.6 33.6 FUD 090 C 80

AMA: 2014,Jan,11; 2000,Oct,8

50525 **Closure of nephrovisceral fistula (eg, renocolic), including visceral repair; abdominal approach**
42.6 42.6 **FUD** 090 C 80
AMA: 2014,Jan,11

50526 **thoracic approach**
45.7 45.7 **FUD** 090 C 80
AMA: 2014,Jan,11

50540 **Symphysiotomy for horseshoe kidney with or without pyeloplasty and/or other plastic procedure, unilateral or bilateral (1 operation)**
33.2 33.2 **FUD** 090 C 80
AMA: 2014,Jan,11; 2000,Oct,8

50541-50549 Laparoscopic Surgical Procedures of the Kidney

INCLUDES Diagnostic laparoscopy (49320)
EXCLUDES *Laparoscopic drainage lymphocele to peritoneal cavity (49323)*

50541 **Laparoscopy, surgical; ablation of renal cysts**
26.5 26.5 **FUD** 090 J 80 50
AMA: 2018,Jan,8; 2017,Jan,8; 2016,Jan,13; 2015,Jan,16

50542 **ablation of renal mass lesion(s), including intraoperative ultrasound guidance and monitoring, when performed**
EXCLUDES *Open ablation renal mass lesions (50250)*
Percutaneous ablation renal tumors (50592-50593)
33.7 33.7 **FUD** 090 J 80 50
AMA: 2018,Jan,8; 2017,Jan,8; 2016,Jan,13; 2015,Jan,16

50543 **partial nephrectomy**
EXCLUDES *Partial nephrectomy, open approach (50240)*
43.0 43.0 **FUD** 090 J 80 50
AMA: 2018,Jan,8; 2017,Jan,8; 2016,Jan,13; 2015,Jan,16

50544 **pyeloplasty**
36.0 36.0 **FUD** 090 J 80 50
AMA: 2018,Jan,8; 2017,Jan,8; 2016,Jan,13; 2015,Jan,16

50545 **radical nephrectomy (includes removal of Gerota's fascia and surrounding fatty tissue, removal of regional lymph nodes, and adrenalectomy)**
EXCLUDES *Radical nephrectomy, open approach (50230)*
38.7 38.7 **FUD** 090 C 80 50
AMA: 2018,Jan,8; 2017,Jan,8; 2016,Jan,13; 2015,Jan,16

50546 **nephrectomy, including partial ureterectomy**
34.8 34.8 **FUD** 090 C 80 50
AMA: 2018,Jan,8; 2017,Jan,8; 2016,Jan,13; 2015,Jan,16

50547 **donor nephrectomy (including cold preservation), from living donor**
INCLUDES Donor care
Graft:
Cold preservation
Harvesting
EXCLUDES *Backbench reconstruction renal allograft prior to transplantation (50327-50329)*
Backbench standard preparation living donor renal allograft prior to transplantation (50325)
Donor nephrectomy, open approach (50320)
46.4 46.4 **FUD** 090 C 80 50
AMA: 2018,Jan,8; 2017,Jan,8; 2016,Jan,13; 2015,Jan,16

50548 **nephrectomy with total ureterectomy**
EXCLUDES *Nephrectomy, open approach (50234, 50236)*
38.9 38.9 **FUD** 090 C 80 50
AMA: 2018,Jan,8; 2017,Jan,8; 2016,Jan,13; 2015,Jan,16

50549 **Unlisted laparoscopy procedure, renal**
0.00 0.00 **FUD** YYY J 80 50
AMA: 2018,Jan,8; 2017,Jan,8; 2016,Jan,13; 2015,Jan,16

50551-50562 Endoscopic Procedures of Kidney via Established Nephrostomy/Pyelostomy Access

50551 **Renal endoscopy through established nephrostomy or pyelostomy, with or without irrigation, instillation, or ureteropyelography, exclusive of radiologic service;**
8.54 10.4 **FUD** 000 J A2 80 50
AMA: 2018,Jan,8; 2017,Jan,8; 2016,Jan,13; 2015,Jan,16

50553 **with ureteral catheterization, with or without dilation of ureter**
EXCLUDES *Image-guided ureter dilation without endoscopic guidance (50706)*
9.09 11.1 **FUD** 000 J A2 50
AMA: 2018,Jan,8; 2017,Jan,8; 2016,Jan,3; 2016,Jan,13; 2015,Jan,16

50555 **with biopsy**
EXCLUDES *Image-guided biopsy ureter/renal pelvis without endoscopic guidance (50606)*
9.88 11.9 **FUD** 000 J A2 80 50
AMA: 2018,Jan,8; 2017,Jan,8; 2016,Jan,3; 2016,Jan,13; 2015,Jan,16

50557 **with fulguration and/or incision, with or without biopsy**
10.0 12.1 **FUD** 000 J A2 80 50
AMA: 2018,Jan,8; 2017,Jan,8; 2016,Jan,13; 2015,Jan,16

50561 **with removal of foreign body or calculus**
11.4 13.7 **FUD** 000 J A2 80 50
AMA: 2018,Jan,8; 2017,Jan,8; 2016,Jan,13; 2015,Jan,16

50562 **with resection of tumor**
16.8 16.8 **FUD** 090 J G2 80
AMA: 2018,Jan,8; 2017,Jan,8; 2016,Jan,13; 2015,Jan,16

50570-50580 Endoscopic Procedures of Kidney via Nephrotomy/Pyelotomy Access

Code also when provided service significant and identifiable (50045, 50120)

50570 **Renal endoscopy through nephrotomy or pyelotomy, with or without irrigation, instillation, or ureteropyelography, exclusive of radiologic service;**
14.2 14.2 **FUD** 000 J G2 80 50
AMA: 2018,Jan,8; 2017,Jan,8; 2016,Jan,13; 2015,Jan,16

50572 **with ureteral catheterization, with or without dilation of ureter**
EXCLUDES *Image-guided ureter dilation without endoscopic guidance (50706)*
15.3 15.3 **FUD** 000 T G2 80 50
AMA: 2018,Jan,8; 2017,Jan,8; 2016,Jan,3; 2016,Jan,13; 2015,Jan,16

50574 **with biopsy**
EXCLUDES *Image-guide ureter/renal pelvis biopsy without endoscopic guidance (50606)*
16.3 16.3 **FUD** 000 J G2 80 50
AMA: 2018,Jan,8; 2017,Jan,8; 2016,Jan,3; 2016,Jan,13; 2015,Jan,16

50575 **with endopyelotomy (includes cystoscopy, ureteroscopy, dilation of ureter and ureteral pelvic junction, incision of ureteral pelvic junction and insertion of endopyelotomy stent)**
20.6 20.6 **FUD** 000 J G2 50
AMA: 2018,Jan,8; 2017,Jan,8; 2016,Jan,13; 2015,Jan,16

50576 **with fulguration and/or incision, with or without biopsy**
16.3 16.3 **FUD** 000 J G2 80 50
AMA: 2018,Jan,8; 2017,Jan,8; 2016,Jan,13; 2015,Jan,16

50580 **with removal of foreign body or calculus**
17.5 17.5 **FUD** 000 J G2 80 50
AMA: 2018,Jan,8; 2017,Jan,8; 2016,Jan,13; 2015,Jan,16

50590-50593 Noninvasive and Minimally Invasive Procedures of the Kidney

50590 Lithotripsy, extracorporeal shock wave
16.4 21.1 **FUD** 090 J G2 50
AMA: 2018,Jan,8; 2017,Jan,8; 2016,Jan,13; 2015,Jan,16

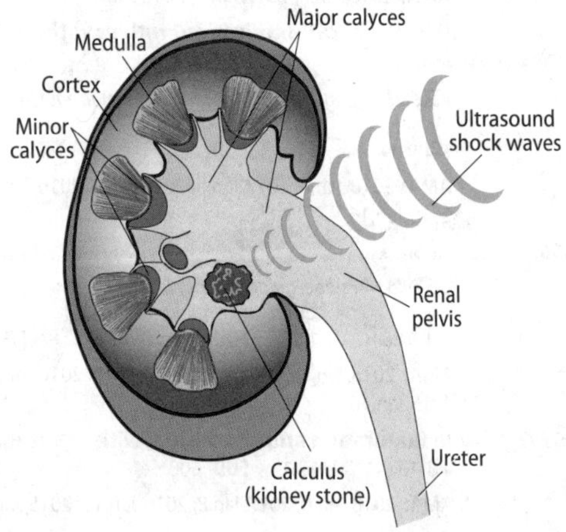

50592 Ablation, 1 or more renal tumor(s), percutaneous, unilateral, radiofrequency
(76940, 77013, 77022)
9.93 92.3 **FUD** 010 J G2 50
AMA: 2014,Jan,11

50593 Ablation, renal tumor(s), unilateral, percutaneous, cryotherapy
(76940, 77013, 77022)
13.3 125. **FUD** 010 J J8 80 50
AMA: 2018,Jan,8

50600-50940 Open and Injection Procedures of Ureter

50600 Ureterotomy with exploration or drainage (separate procedure)
Code also ureteral endoscopy through ureterotomy when procedures constitute significant identifiable service (50970-50980)
27.1 27.1 **FUD** 090 C 80 50
AMA: 2014,Jan,11; 2000,Oct,8

50605 Ureterotomy for insertion of indwelling stent, all types
28.6 28.6 **FUD** 090 C 80 50
AMA: 2018,Jan,8; 2017,Jan,8; 2016,Jan,13; 2015,Jan,16

\+ **50606 Endoluminal biopsy of ureter and/or renal pelvis, non-endoscopic, including imaging guidance (eg, ultrasound and/or fluoroscopy) and all associated radiological supervision and interpretation (List separately in addition to code for primary procedure)**
INCLUDES Renal pelvis and associated ureter as single element
EXCLUDES *Procedure performed for same renal collecting system/associated ureter with (50555, 50574, 50955, 50974, 52007, 74425)*
Code first (50382-50389, [50430, 50431, 50432, 50433, 50434, 50435], 50684, 50688, 50690, 50693-50695, 51610)
4.46 19.9 **FUD** ZZZ N N1 50
AMA: 2018,Jan,8; 2017,Jan,8; 2016,Jan,3

50610 Ureterolithotomy; upper one-third of ureter
EXCLUDES *Cystotomy with calculus basket extraction ureteral calculus (51065)*
Transvesical ureterolithotomy (51060)
Ureteral calculus manipulation/extraction performed endoscopically (50080-50081, 50561, 50961, 50980, 52320-52330, 52352-52353, [52356])
Ureterolithotomy performed laparoscopically (50945)
27.3 27.3 **FUD** 090 C 80 50
AMA: 2018,Jan,8; 2017,Jan,8; 2016,Jan,13; 2015,Jan,16

50620 middle one-third of ureter
EXCLUDES *Cystotomy with calculus basket extraction ureteral calculus (51065)*
Transvesical ureterolithotomy (51060)
Ureteral calculus manipulation/extraction performed endoscopically (50080-50081, 50561, 50961, 50980, 52320-52330, 52352-52353, [52356])
Ureterolithotomy performed laparoscopically (50945)
26.1 26.1 **FUD** 090 C 80 50
AMA: 2018,Jan,8; 2017,Jan,8; 2016,Jan,13; 2015,Jan,16

50630 lower one-third of ureter
EXCLUDES *Cystotomy with calculus basket extraction ureteral calculus (51065)*
Transvesical ureterolithotomy (51060)
Ureteral calculus manipulation/extraction performed endoscopically (50080-50081, 50561, 50961, 50980, 52320-52330, 52352-52353, [52356])
Ureterolithotomy performed laparoscopically (50945)
25.8 25.8 **FUD** 090 C 80 50
AMA: 2018,Jan,8; 2017,Jan,8; 2016,Jan,13; 2015,Jan,16

50650 Ureterectomy, with bladder cuff (separate procedure)
EXCLUDES *Ureterocele (51535, 52300)*
30.0 30.0 **FUD** 090 C 80 50
AMA: 2014,Jan,11

50660 Ureterectomy, total, ectopic ureter, combination abdominal, vaginal and/or perineal approach
EXCLUDES *Ureterocele (51535, 52300)*
33.0 33.0 **FUD** 090 C 80
AMA: 2014,Jan,11

50684 Injection procedure for ureterography or ureteropyelography through ureterostomy or indwelling ureteral catheter
EXCLUDES *Placement nephroureteral catheter ([50433, 50434])*
Placement ureteral stent (50693-50695)
(74425)
1.45 3.10 **FUD** 000 N N1 50
AMA: 2018,Jan,8; 2017,Jan,8; 2016,Jan,3; 2015,Oct,5

50686 Manometric studies through ureterostomy or indwelling ureteral catheter
2.55 3.99 **FUD** 000 S P2 80
AMA: 2014,Jan,11

50688 Change of ureterostomy tube or externally accessible ureteral stent via ileal conduit
(75984)
2.25 2.25 **FUD** 010 J A2
AMA: 2018,Jan,8; 2017,Jan,8; 2016,Jan,3

50690 Injection procedure for visualization of ileal conduit and/or ureteropyelography, exclusive of radiologic service
Code also radiological supervision and interpretation:
antegrade (74425)
retrograde (74420)
(74420, 74425)
2.02 2.87 **FUD** 000 N N1
AMA: 2018,Jan,8; 2017,Jan,8; 2016,Jan,3

50693 Placement of ureteral stent, percutaneous, including diagnostic nephrostogram and/or ureterogram when performed, imaging guidance (eg, ultrasound and/or fluoroscopy), and all associated radiological supervision and interpretation; pre-existing nephrostomy tract

INCLUDES Renal pelvis and associated ureter as single element

EXCLUDES *Procedure performed for same renal collecting system/ureter ([50430, 50431, 50432, 50433, 50434, 50435], 50684, 74425)*

5.94 28.0 **FUD** 000 J G2 50

AMA: 2018,Jan,8; 2017,Jan,8; 2016,Jan,3; 2016,Jan,13; 2015,Oct,5

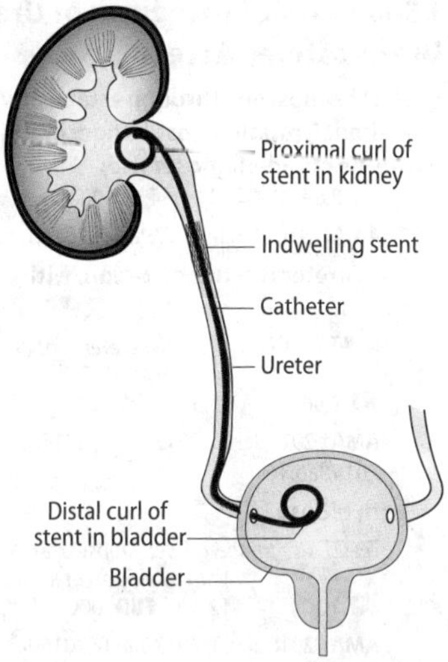

50694 new access, without separate nephrostomy catheter

INCLUDES Renal pelvis and associated ureter as single element

EXCLUDES *Procedure performed for same renal collecting system/ureter ([50430, 50431, 50432, 50433, 50434, 50435], 50684, 74425)*

7.78 30.8 **FUD** 000 J G2 50

AMA: 2018,Jan,8; 2017,Jan,8; 2016,Jan,3; 2016,Jan,13; 2015,Oct,5

50695 new access, with separate nephrostomy catheter

INCLUDES Placement separate ureteral stent and nephrostomy catheter into ureter/associated renal pelvis through new access
Renal pelvis and associated ureter as single element

EXCLUDES *Procedure performed for same renal collecting system/ureter ([50430, 50431, 50432, 50433, 50434, 50435], 50684, 74425)*

9.96 37.8 **FUD** 000 J G2 50

AMA: 2018,Jan,8; 2017,Jan,8; 2016,Jan,3; 2016,Jan,13; 2015,Oct,5

50700 Ureteroplasty, plastic operation on ureter (eg, stricture)

26.7 26.7 **FUD** 090 C 80 50

AMA: 2014,Jan,11

\+ **50705 Ureteral embolization or occlusion, including imaging guidance (eg, ultrasound and/or fluoroscopy) and all associated radiological supervision and interpretation (List separately in addition to code for primary procedure)**

INCLUDES Renal pelvis and associated ureter as single element

Code also when performed:
- Additional catheter insertions
- Diagnostic pyelography/ureterography
- Other interventions

Code first (50382-50389, [50430, 50431, 50432, 50433, 50434, 50435], 50684, 50688, 50690, 50693-50695, 51610)

5.70 54.9 **FUD** ZZZ N N1 50

AMA: 2018,Jan,8; 2017,Jan,8; 2016,Jan,3

\+ **50706 Balloon dilation, ureteral stricture, including imaging guidance (eg, ultrasound and/or fluoroscopy) and all associated radiological supervision and interpretation (List separately in addition to code for primary procedure)**

INCLUDES Dilation nephrostomy, ureters, or urethra (74485)
Renal pelvis and associated ureter as single element

EXCLUDES *Cystourethroscopy (52341, 52344-52345)*
Renal endoscopy (50553, 50572)
Ureteral endoscopy (50953, 50972)

Code also when performed:
- Additional catheter insertions
- Diagnostic pyelography/ureterography
- Other interventions

Code first (50382-50389, [50430, 50431, 50432, 50433, 50434, 50435], 50684, 50688, 50690, 50693-50695, 51610)

5.33 28.0 **FUD** ZZZ N N1 50

AMA: 2018,Jan,8; 2017,Jan,8; 2016,Jan,3

50715 Ureterolysis, with or without repositioning of ureter for retroperitoneal fibrosis

35.2 35.2 **FUD** 090 C 80 50

AMA: 2014,Jan,11

50722 Ureterolysis for ovarian vein syndrome ♀

29.0 29.0 **FUD** 090 C 80

AMA: 2014,Jan,11

50725 Ureterolysis for retrocaval ureter, with reanastomosis of upper urinary tract or vena cava

31.9 31.9 **FUD** 090 C 80

AMA: 2014,Jan,11

50727 Revision of urinary-cutaneous anastomosis (any type urostomy);

14.7 14.7 **FUD** 090 J G2 80

AMA: 2014,Jan,11; 1992,Win,1

50728 with repair of fascial defect and hernia

21.2 21.2 **FUD** 090 C 80

AMA: 2014,Jan,11; 1992,Win,1

50740 Ureteropyelostomy, anastomosis of ureter and renal pelvis

35.4 35.4 **FUD** 090 C 80 50

AMA: 2018,Jan,8; 2017,Jan,8; 2016,Jan,13; 2015,Jan,16

50750 Ureterocalycostomy, anastomosis of ureter to renal calyx

33.3 33.3 **FUD** 090 C 80 50

AMA: 2018,Jan,8; 2017,Jan,8; 2016,Jan,13; 2015,Jan,16

50760 Ureteroureterostomy

32.6 32.6 **FUD** 090 C 80 50

AMA: 2018,Jan,8; 2017,Jan,8; 2016,Jan,13; 2015,Jan,16

50770 Transureteroureterostomy, anastomosis of ureter to contralateral ureter

33.3 33.3 **FUD** 090 C 80

AMA: 2014,Jan,11

50780 Ureteroneocystostomy; anastomosis of single ureter to bladder

INCLUDES Minor procedures to prevent vesicoureteral reflux

EXCLUDES *Cystourethroplasty with ureteroneocystostomy (51820)*

31.9 31.9 **FUD** 090 C 80 50

AMA: 2018,Feb,11; 2018,Jan,8; 2017,Jan,8; 2016,Jan,13; 2015,Jan,16

50782 anastomosis of duplicated ureter to bladder

INCLUDES Minor procedures to prevent vesicoureteral reflux

31.1 31.1 **FUD** 090 C 80 50

AMA: 2018,Jan,8; 2017,Jan,8; 2016,Jan,13; 2015,Jan,16

50783 with extensive ureteral tailoring

INCLUDES Minor procedures to prevent vesicoureteral reflux

32.6 32.6 **FUD** 090 C 80 50

AMA: 2018,Jan,8; 2017,Jan,8; 2016,Jan,13; 2015,Jan,16

50785 with vesico-psoas hitch or bladder flap

INCLUDES Minor procedures to prevent vesicoureteral reflux

35.1 35.1 **FUD** 090 C 80 50

AMA: 2018,Jan,8; 2017,Jan,8; 2016,Jan,13; 2015,Jan,16

50800 **Ureteroenterostomy, direct anastomosis of ureter to intestine**

EXCLUDES *Cystectomy with ureterosigmoidostomy/ureteroileal conduit (51580-51595)*

26.7 26.7 **FUD** 090 C 80 50

AMA: 2018,Jan,8; 2017,Jan,8; 2016,Jan,13; 2015,Jan,16

50810 **Ureterosigmoidostomy, with creation of sigmoid bladder and establishment of abdominal or perineal colostomy, including intestine anastomosis**

EXCLUDES *Cystectomy with ureterosigmoidostomy/ureteroileal conduit (51580-51595)*

40.5 40.5 **FUD** 090 C 80

AMA: 2018,Jan,8; 2017,Jan,8; 2016,Jan,13; 2015,Jan,16

50815 **Ureterocolon conduit, including intestine anastomosis**

EXCLUDES *Cystectomy with ureterosigmoidostomy/ureteroileal conduit (51580-51595)*

35.3 35.3 **FUD** 090 C 80 50

AMA: 2018,Jan,8; 2017,Jan,8; 2016,Jan,13; 2015,Jan,16

50820 **Ureteroileal conduit (ileal bladder), including intestine anastomosis (Bricker operation)**

EXCLUDES *Cystectomy with ureterosigmoidostomy/ureteroileal conduit (51580-51595)*

38.0 38.0 **FUD** 090 C 80 50

AMA: 2018,Jan,8; 2017,Jan,8; 2016,Jan,13; 2015,Jan,16

50825 **Continent diversion, including intestine anastomosis using any segment of small and/or large intestine (Kock pouch or Camey enterocystoplasty)**

48.0 48.0 **FUD** 090 C 80

AMA: 2018,Jan,8; 2017,Jan,8; 2016,Jan,13; 2015,Jan,16

50830 **Urinary undiversion (eg, taking down of ureteroileal conduit, ureterosigmoidostomy or ureteroenterostomy with ureteroureterostomy or ureteroneocystostomy)**

52.0 52.0 **FUD** 090 C 80

AMA: 2018,Jan,8; 2017,Jan,8; 2016,Jan,13; 2015,Jan,16

50840 **Replacement of all or part of ureter by intestine segment, including intestine anastomosis**

35.5 35.5 **FUD** 090 C 80 50

AMA: 2018,Jan,8; 2017,Jan,8; 2016,Jan,13; 2015,Jan,16

50845 **Cutaneous appendico-vesicostomy**

INCLUDES Mitrofanoff operation

36.1 36.1 **FUD** 090 C 80

AMA: 2014,Jan,11; 1993,Win,1

50860 **Ureterostomy, transplantation of ureter to skin**

27.3 27.3 **FUD** 090 C 80 50

AMA: 2014,Jan,11; 2001,Oct,8

50900 **Ureterorrhaphy, suture of ureter (separate procedure)**

24.3 24.3 **FUD** 090 C 80 50

AMA: 2014,Jan,11; 2001,Oct,8

50920 **Closure of ureterocutaneous fistula**

25.3 25.3 **FUD** 090 C 80

AMA: 2014,Jan,11; 2001,Oct,8

50930 **Closure of ureterovisceral fistula (including visceral repair)**

31.8 31.8 **FUD** 090 C 80

AMA: 2014,Jan,11; 2001,Oct,8

50940 **Deligation of ureter**

EXCLUDES *Ureteroplasty/ureterolysis (50700-50860)*

25.6 25.6 **FUD** 090 C 80 50

AMA: 2014,Jan,11; 2001,Oct,8

50945-50949 Laparoscopic Procedures of Ureter

INCLUDES Diagnostic laparoscopy (49320)

EXCLUDES *Ureteroneocystostomy, open approach (50780-50785)*

50945 **Laparoscopy, surgical; ureterolithotomy**

28.1 28.1 **FUD** 090 J 80 50

AMA: 2018,Jan,8; 2017,Jan,8; 2016,Jan,13; 2015,Jan,16

50947 **ureteroneocystostomy with cystoscopy and ureteral stent placement**

40.1 40.1 **FUD** 090 J A2 80 50

AMA: 2018,Jan,8; 2017,Jan,8; 2016,Jan,13; 2015,Jan,16

50948 **ureteroneocystostomy without cystoscopy and ureteral stent placement**

36.9 36.9 **FUD** 090 J A2 80 50

AMA: 2018,Jan,8; 2017,Jan,8; 2016,Jan,13; 2015,Jan,16

50949 **Unlisted laparoscopy procedure, ureter**

0.00 0.00 **FUD** YYY J 80 50

AMA: 2018,Jan,8; 2017,Jan,8; 2016,Jan,13; 2015,Jan,16

50951-50961 Endoscopic Procedures of Ureter via Established Ureterostomy Access

50951 **Ureteral endoscopy through established ureterostomy, with or without irrigation, instillation, or ureteropyelography, exclusive of radiologic service;**

8.89 10.9 **FUD** 000 J A2 80 50

AMA: 2018,Jan,8; 2017,Jan,8; 2016,Jan,13; 2015,Jan,16

50953 **with ureteral catheterization, with or without dilation of ureter**

EXCLUDES *Image-guided ureter dilation without endoscopic guidance (50706)*

9.46 11.5 **FUD** 000 J A2 80 50

AMA: 2018,Jan,8; 2017,Jan,8; 2016,Jan,13; 2016,Jan,3; 2015,Jan,16

50955 **with biopsy**

EXCLUDES *Image-guided biopsy of ureter and/or renal pelvis without endoscopic guidance (50606)*

10.2 12.3 **FUD** 000 J A2 80 50

AMA: 2018,Jan,8; 2017,Jan,8; 2016,Jan,13; 2016,Jan,3; 2015,Jan,16

50957 **with fulguration and/or incision, with or without biopsy**

10.2 12.4 **FUD** 000 J A2 80 50

AMA: 2018,Jan,8; 2017,Jan,8; 2016,Jan,13; 2015,Jan,16

50961 **with removal of foreign body or calculus**

9.17 11.1 **FUD** 000 J A2 80 50

AMA: 2018,Jan,8; 2017,Jan,8; 2016,Jan,13; 2015,Jan,16

50970-50980 Endoscopic Procedures of Ureter via Ureterotomy

EXCLUDES *Ureterotomy (50600)*

50970 **Ureteral endoscopy through ureterotomy, with or without irrigation, instillation, or ureteropyelography, exclusive of radiologic service;**

10.7 10.7 **FUD** 000 J A2 80 50

AMA: 2018,Jan,8; 2017,Jan,8; 2016,Jan,13; 2015,Jan,16

50972 **with ureteral catheterization, with or without dilation of ureter**

EXCLUDES *Image-guided ureter dilation without endoscopic guidance (50706)*

10.3 10.3 **FUD** 000 J A2 80 50

AMA: 2018,Jan,8; 2017,Jan,8; 2016,Jan,3; 2016,Jan,13; 2015,Jan,16

50974 **with biopsy**

EXCLUDES *Image-guided biopsy of ureter and/or renal pelvis without endoscopic guidance (50606)*

13.6 13.6 **FUD** 000 J A2 80 50

AMA: 2018,Jan,8; 2017,Jan,8; 2016,Jan,3; 2016,Jan,13; 2015,Jan,16

50976 **with fulguration and/or incision, with or without biopsy**

13.5 13.5 **FUD** 000 J A2 80 50

AMA: 2018,Jan,8; 2017,Jan,8; 2016,Jan,13; 2015,Jan,16

50980 **with removal of foreign body or calculus**

10.3 10.3 **FUD** 000 J A2 80 50

AMA: 2018,Jan,8; 2017,Jan,8; 2016,Jan,13; 2015,Jan,16

51020-51080 Open Incisional Procedures of Bladder

51020 **Cystotomy or cystostomy; with fulguration and/or insertion of radioactive material**
13.5 13.5 FUD 090 J A2 80
AMA: 2014,Jan,11

51030 **with cryosurgical destruction of intravesical lesion**
13.6 13.6 FUD 090 J A2 80
AMA: 2014,Jan,11

51040 **Cystostomy, cystotomy with drainage**
8.36 8.36 FUD 090 J A2 80
AMA: 2014,Jan,11

51045 **Cystotomy, with insertion of ureteral catheter or stent (separate procedure)**
14.2 14.2 FUD 090 J A2 80
AMA: 2014,Jan,11

51050 **Cystolithotomy, cystotomy with removal of calculus, without vesical neck resection**
13.6 13.6 FUD 090 J A2 80
AMA: 2014,Jan,11

51060 **Transvesical ureterolithotomy**
16.8 16.8 FUD 090 J 80
AMA: 2014,Jan,11

51065 **Cystotomy, with calculus basket extraction and/or ultrasonic or electrohydraulic fragmentation of ureteral calculus**
16.7 16.7 FUD 090 J A2 80
AMA: 2014,Jan,11; 2002,May,7

51080 **Drainage of perivesical or prevesical space abscess**
EXCLUDES *Image-guided percutaneous catheter drainage (49406)*
11.8 11.8 FUD 090 J A2 80
AMA: 2014,Jan,11

51100-51102 Bladder Aspiration Procedures

51100 **Aspiration of bladder; by needle**
(76942, 77002, 77012)
1.12 1.95 FUD 000 T P3
AMA: 2018,Jan,8; 2017,Jan,8; 2016,Jan,13; 2015,Jan,16

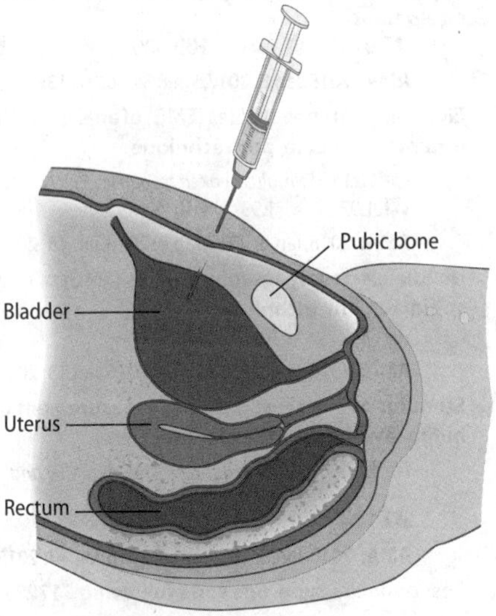

51101 **by trocar or intracatheter**
(76942, 77002, 77012)
1.50 3.79 FUD 000 S P3
AMA: 2018,Jan,8; 2017,Jan,8; 2016,Jan,13; 2015,Jan,16

51102 **with insertion of suprapubic catheter**
(76942, 77002, 77012)
4.18 6.60 FUD 000 J A2
AMA: 2018,Jan,8; 2017,Jan,8; 2016,Jan,13; 2015,Jan,16

51500-51597 Open Excisional Procedures of Bladder

51500 **Excision of urachal cyst or sinus, with or without umbilical hernia repair**
18.4 18.4 FUD 090 J A2 80
AMA: 2014,Jan,11

51520 **Cystotomy; for simple excision of vesical neck (separate procedure)**
17.2 17.2 FUD 090 J A2 80
AMA: 2014,Jan,11

51525 **for excision of bladder diverticulum, single or multiple (separate procedure)**
EXCLUDES *Transurethral resection (52305)*
24.8 24.8 FUD 090 C 80
AMA: 2014,Jan,11

51530 **for excision of bladder tumor**
EXCLUDES *Transurethral resection (52234-52240, 52305)*
22.2 22.2 FUD 090 C 80
AMA: 2014,Jan,11

51535 **Cystotomy for excision, incision, or repair of ureterocele**
EXCLUDES *Transurethral excision (52300)*
22.5 22.5 FUD 090 J 62 80 50
AMA: 2014,Jan,11; 1993,Sum,25

51550 **Cystectomy, partial; simple**
27.9 27.9 FUD 090 C 80
AMA: 2014,Jan,11

51555 **complicated (eg, postradiation, previous surgery, difficult location)**
36.6 36.6 FUD 090 C 80
AMA: 2014,Jan,11

51565 **Cystectomy, partial, with reimplantation of ureter(s) into bladder (ureteroneocystostomy)**
37.5 37.5 FUD 090 C 80
AMA: 2014,Jan,11

51570 **Cystectomy, complete; (separate procedure)**
42.6 42.6 FUD 090 C 80
AMA: 2014,Jan,11; 1993,Spr,34

51575 **with bilateral pelvic lymphadenectomy, including external iliac, hypogastric, and obturator nodes**
52.7 52.7 FUD 090 C 80
AMA: 2014,Jan,11; 1993,Spr,34

51580 **Cystectomy, complete, with ureterosigmoidostomy or ureterocutaneous transplantations;**
54.8 54.8 FUD 090 C 80
AMA: 2014,Jan,11; 1993,Spr,34

51585 **with bilateral pelvic lymphadenectomy, including external iliac, hypogastric, and obturator nodes**
61.0 61.0 FUD 090 C 80
AMA: 2014,Jan,11; 1993,Spr,34

51590 **Cystectomy, complete, with ureteroileal conduit or sigmoid bladder, including intestine anastomosis;**
55.9 55.9 FUD 090 C 80
AMA: 2014,Jan,11; 2002,May,7

51595 **with bilateral pelvic lymphadenectomy, including external iliac, hypogastric, and obturator nodes**
63.3 63.3 FUD 090 C 80
AMA: 2014,Jan,11; 2002,May,7

51596 **Cystectomy, complete, with continent diversion, any open technique, using any segment of small and/or large intestine to construct neobladder**
68.1 68.1 FUD 090 C 80
AMA: 2014,Jan,11; 2002,May,7

51597 Pelvic exenteration, complete, for vesical, prostatic or urethral malignancy, with removal of bladder and ureteral transplantations, with or without hysterectomy and/or abdominoperineal resection of rectum and colon and colostomy, or any combination thereof

EXCLUDES *Pelvic exenteration for gynecologic malignancy (58240)*

66.3 66.3 FUD 090 C 80

AMA: 2014,Jan,11

51600-51720 Injection/Insertion/Instillation Procedures of Bladder

51600 Injection procedure for cystography or voiding urethrocystography

(74430, 74455)

1.29 5.57 FUD 000 N N1

AMA: 2019,Oct,10

51605 Injection procedure and placement of chain for contrast and/or chain urethrocystography

(74430)

1.12 1.12 FUD 000 N N1

AMA: 2014,Jan,11

51610 Injection procedure for retrograde urethrocystography

(74450)

1.85 3.21 FUD 000 N N1

AMA: 2019,Oct,10; 2018,Jan,8; 2017,Jan,8; 2016,Jan,3

51700 Bladder irrigation, simple, lavage and/or instillation

0.87 2.12 FUD 000 T P3

AMA: 2014,Jan,11

51701 Insertion of non-indwelling bladder catheter (eg, straight catheterization for residual urine)

EXCLUDES *Catheterization for specimen collection (P9612)*
Insertion catheter as another procedure component

0.73 1.27 FUD 000 Q1 N1

AMA: 2018,Jan,8; 2017,Jan,8; 2016,Jan,13; 2015,Jan,16

51702 Insertion of temporary indwelling bladder catheter; simple (eg, Foley)

EXCLUDES *Focused ultrasound ablation uterine leiomyomata (0071T-0072T)*
Insertion catheter as another procedure component

0.73 1.76 FUD 000 Q1 N1

AMA: 2018,Jan,8; 2017,Jan,8; 2016,Jan,13; 2015,Jan,16

51703 complicated (eg, altered anatomy, fractured catheter/balloon)

2.23 3.78 FUD 000 S P2

AMA: 2018,Jan,8; 2017,Jan,8; 2016,Jan,13; 2015,Jan,16

51705 Change of cystostomy tube; simple

1.50 2.67 FUD 000 T P3

AMA: 2018,Jan,8; 2017,Jan,8; 2016,Jan,13; 2015,Jan,16

51710 complicated

(75984)

2.30 3.69 FUD 000 T A2

AMA: 2018,Jan,8; 2017,Jan,8; 2016,Jan,13; 2015,Jan,16

51715 Endoscopic injection of implant material into the submucosal tissues of the urethra and/or bladder neck

EXCLUDES *Injection bulking agent (submucosal) for fecal incontinence, via anoscope (46999)*

5.76 9.07 FUD 000 J J8 80

AMA: 2014,Jan,11; 1993,Win,1

51720 Bladder instillation of anticarcinogenic agent (including retention time)

Code also bacillus Calmette-Guerin vaccine (BCG) (90586)

1.27 2.40 FUD 000 T P3

AMA: 2020,Jan,11; 2018,Jan,8; 2017,Jan,8; 2016,Jan,13; 2015,Jan,16

51725-51798 [51797] Uroflowmetric Evaluations

INCLUDES Equipment
Fees for technician services
Medications
Supplies

Code also modifier 26 when physician/other qualified health care professional provides only interpretation results and/or operates equipment

51725 Simple cystometrogram (CMG) (eg, spinal manometer)

5.69 5.69 FUD 000 T P2 80

AMA: 2018,Jan,8; 2017,Jan,8; 2016,Jan,13; 2015,Jan,16

51726 Complex cystometrogram (ie, calibrated electronic equipment);

8.23 8.23 FUD 000 T A2

AMA: 2018,Jan,8; 2017,Jan,8; 2016,Jan,13; 2015,Jan,16

51727 with urethral pressure profile studies (ie, urethral closure pressure profile), any technique

9.88 9.88 FUD 000 T P3 80

AMA: 2018,Jan,8; 2017,Jan,8; 2016,Jan,13; 2015,Jan,16

51728 with voiding pressure studies (ie, bladder voiding pressure), any technique

9.55 9.55 FUD 000 T P3 80

AMA: 2018,Jan,8; 2017,Jan,8; 2016,Jan,13; 2015,Jan,16

51729 with voiding pressure studies (ie, bladder voiding pressure) and urethral pressure profile studies (ie, urethral closure pressure profile), any technique

10.6 10.6 FUD 000 T P3 80

AMA: 2018,Jan,8; 2017,Jan,8; 2016,Jan,13; 2015,Jan,16

\+ # **51797 Voiding pressure studies, intra-abdominal (ie, rectal, gastric, intraperitoneal) (List separately in addition to code for primary procedure)**

Code first (51728-51729)

4.61 4.61 FUD ZZZ N N1 80

AMA: 2018,Jan,8; 2017,Jan,8; 2016,Jan,13; 2015,Jan,16

51736 Simple uroflowmetry (UFR) (eg, stop-watch flow rate, mechanical uroflowmeter)

0.40 0.40 FUD XXX Q1 N1 80

AMA: 2018,Jan,8; 2017,Jan,8; 2016,Jan,13; 2015,Jan,16

51741 Complex uroflowmetry (eg, calibrated electronic equipment)

0.41 0.41 FUD XXX Q1 N1

AMA: 2018,Jan,8; 2017,Jan,8; 2016,Jan,13; 2015,Jan,16

51784 Electromyography studies (EMG) of anal or urethral sphincter, other than needle, any technique

EXCLUDES *Stimulus evoked response (51792)*

1.93 1.93 FUD XXX S P3

AMA: 2018,Jan,8; 2017,Jan,8; 2016,Jan,13; 2015,Jan,16

51785 Needle electromyography studies (EMG) of anal or urethral sphincter, any technique

9.17 9.17 FUD XXX T A2 80

AMA: 2018,Jan,8; 2017,Jan,8; 2016,Jan,13; 2015,Jan,16

51792 Stimulus evoked response (eg, measurement of bulbocavernosus reflex latency time)

EXCLUDES *Electromyography studies (EMG) anal or urethral sphincter (51784)*

7.04 7.04 FUD 000 Q1 N1 80

AMA: 2018,Jan,8; 2017,Jan,8; 2016,Jan,13; 2015,Jan,16

51797 **Resequenced code. See code following 51729.**

51798 Measurement of post-voiding residual urine and/or bladder capacity by ultrasound, non-imaging

0.36 0.36 FUD XXX Q1 N1 80 TC

AMA: 2018,Jun,11; 2018,Jan,8; 2017,Jan,8; 2016,Jan,13; 2015,Jan,16

51800-51980 Open Repairs Urinary System

51800 Cystoplasty or cystourethroplasty, plastic operation on bladder and/or vesical neck (anterior Y-plasty, vesical fundus resection), any procedure, with or without wedge resection of posterior vesical neck
30.3 30.3 FUD 090 C 80
AMA: 2014,Jan,11

51820 Cystourethroplasty with unilateral or bilateral ureteroneocystostomy
31.3 31.3 FUD 090 C 80
AMA: 2014,Jan,11

51840 Anterior vesicourethropexy, or urethropexy (eg, Marshall-Marchetti-Krantz, Burch); simple
EXCLUDES *Pereyra type urethropexy (57289)*
19.3 19.3 FUD 090 C 80
AMA: 2018,Jan,8; 2017,Jan,8; 2016,Jan,13; 2015,Jan,16

51841 complicated (eg, secondary repair)
EXCLUDES *Pereyra type urethropexy (57289)*
22.4 22.4 FUD 090 C 80
AMA: 2018,Jan,8; 2017,Jan,8; 2016,Jan,13; 2015,Jan,16

51845 Abdomino-vaginal vesical neck suspension, with or without endoscopic control (eg, Stamey, Raz, modified Pereyra) ♀
16.8 16.8 FUD 090 J 80
AMA: 2018,Jan,8; 2017,Jan,8; 2016,Jan,13; 2015,Jan,16

51860 Cystorrhaphy, suture of bladder wound, injury or rupture; simple
21.5 21.5 FUD 090 J 80
AMA: 2014,Jan,11

51865 complicated
25.9 25.9 FUD 090 C 80
AMA: 2014,Jan,11

51880 Closure of cystostomy (separate procedure)
13.5 13.5 FUD 090 J A2 80
AMA: 2014,Jan,11

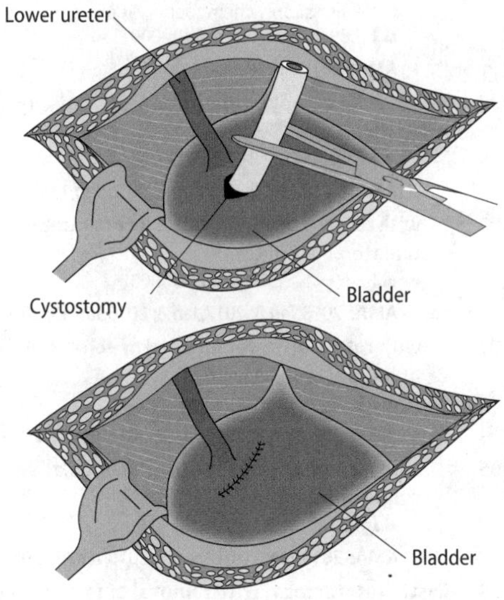

Physician removes a cystostomy tube

51900 Closure of vesicovaginal fistula, abdominal approach ♀
EXCLUDES *Vesicovaginal fistula closure, vaginal approach (57320-57330)*
23.9 23.9 FUD 090 C 80
AMA: 2014,Jan,11

51920 Closure of vesicouterine fistula; ♀
EXCLUDES *Enterovesical fistula closure (44660-44661)*
Rectovesical fistula closure (45800-45805)
22.0 22.0 FUD 090 C 80
AMA: 2014,Jan,11

51925 with hysterectomy ♀
EXCLUDES *Enterovesical fistula closure (44660-44661)*
Rectovesical fistula closure (45800-45805)
29.5 29.5 FUD 090 C 80
AMA: 2014,Jan,11

51940 Closure, exstrophy of bladder
EXCLUDES *Epispadias reconstruction with exstrophy bladder (54390)*
47.5 47.5 FUD 090 C 80
AMA: 2014,Jan,11; 2002,May,7

51960 Enterocystoplasty, including intestinal anastomosis
40.1 40.1 FUD 090 C 80
AMA: 2014,Jan,11; 2002,May,7

51980 Cutaneous vesicostomy
20.6 20.6 FUD 090 C 80
AMA: 2014,Jan,11

51990-51999 Laparoscopic Procedures of Urinary System

CMS: 100-03,230.10 Incontinence Control Devices
INCLUDES Diagnostic laparoscopy (49320)

51990 Laparoscopy, surgical; urethral suspension for stress incontinence
21.6 21.6 FUD 090 J 80
AMA: 2019,Feb,10; 2018,Jan,8; 2017,Jan,8; 2016,Jan,13; 2015,Jan,16

51992 sling operation for stress incontinence (eg, fascia or synthetic)
EXCLUDES *Removal/revision sling for stress incontinence (57287)*
Sling operation for stress incontinence, open approach (57288)
24.0 24.0 FUD 090 J J8 80
AMA: 2019,Feb,10; 2018,Jan,8; 2017,Jan,8; 2016,Jan,13; 2015,Jan,16

51999 Unlisted laparoscopy procedure, bladder
0.00 0.00 FUD YYY J 80
AMA: 2018,Jan,8; 2017,Dec,14

52000-52318 Endoscopic Procedures via Urethra: Bladder and Urethra

INCLUDES Diagnostic and therapeutic endoscopy bowel segments utilized as replacements for native bladder

52000 Cystourethroscopy (separate procedure)
EXCLUDES *Cystourethroscopy (52001, 52320, 52325, 52327, 52330, 52332, 52334, 52341-52343, [52356], 57240, 57260, 57265)*
2.34 5.39 FUD 000 T A2
AMA: 2019,Feb,10; 2018,Nov,10; 2018,Jan,8; 2017,Oct,9; 2017,Jan,8; 2016,Jan,13; 2015,Jan,16

52001 Cystourethroscopy with irrigation and evacuation of multiple obstructing clots
INCLUDES Cystourethroscopy (separate procedure) (52000)
8.31 11.3 FUD 000 J A2
AMA: 2014,Jan,11; 2001,May,5

52005 Cystourethroscopy, with ureteral catheterization, with or without irrigation, instillation, or ureteropyelography, exclusive of radiologic service;
INCLUDES Howard test
3.81 8.37 FUD 000 J A2
AMA: 2019,Mar,10; 2018,Jan,8; 2017,Jan,8; 2016,Jan,13; 2015,Jan,16

52007 **with brush biopsy of ureter and/or renal pelvis**
EXCLUDES *Image-guided ureter/renal pelvis biopsy without endoscopic guidance (50606)*
4.80 13.1 FUD 000 J A2 50
AMA: 2018,Jan,8; 2017,Jan,8; 2016,Jan,13; 2016,Jan,3; 2015,Jan,16

52010 **Cystourethroscopy, with ejaculatory duct catheterization, with or without irrigation, instillation, or duct radiography, exclusive of radiologic service** ♂
(74440)
4.79 10.9 FUD 000 T A2
AMA: 2018,Jan,8; 2017,Jan,8; 2016,Jan,13; 2015,Jan,16

52204 **Cystourethroscopy, with biopsy(s)**
4.08 10.8 FUD 000 J A2
AMA: 2018,Jan,8; 2017,Jan,8; 2016,May,12; 2016,Jan,13; 2015,Jan,16

52214 **Cystourethroscopy, with fulguration (including cryosurgery or laser surgery) of trigone, bladder neck, prostatic fossa, urethra, or periurethral glands**
Code also modifier 78 when performed by same physician:
During postoperative period (52601, 52630)
During postoperative period related surgical procedure
For postoperative bleeding
5.10 20.0 FUD 000 J A2
AMA: 2018,Jan,8; 2017,Jan,8; 2016,May,12; 2016,Jan,13; 2015,Jan,16

52224 **Cystourethroscopy, with fulguration (including cryosurgery or laser surgery) or treatment of MINOR (less than 0.5 cm) lesion(s) with or without biopsy**
5.89 20.9 FUD 000 J A2
AMA: 2018,Jan,8; 2017,Jan,8; 2016,May,12; 2016,Jan,13; 2015,Jan,16

52234 **Cystourethroscopy, with fulguration (including cryosurgery or laser surgery) and/or resection of; SMALL bladder tumor(s) (0.5 up to 2.0 cm)**
EXCLUDES *Bladder tumor excision through cystotomy (51530)*
7.12 7.12 FUD 000 J A2
AMA: 2018,Jan,8; 2017,Jan,8; 2016,May,12; 2016,Jan,13; 2015,Jan,16

52235 **MEDIUM bladder tumor(s) (2.0 to 5.0 cm)**
EXCLUDES *Bladder tumor excision through cystotomy (51530)*
8.34 8.34 FUD 000 J A2
AMA: 2018,Jan,8; 2017,Jan,8; 2016,May,12; 2016,Jan,13; 2015,Jan,16

52240 **LARGE bladder tumor(s)**
EXCLUDES *Bladder tumor excision through cystotomy (51530)*
11.3 11.3 FUD 000 J A2
AMA: 2018,Jan,8; 2017,Jan,8; 2016,May,12; 2016,Jan,13; 2015,Jan,16

52250 **Cystourethroscopy with insertion of radioactive substance, with or without biopsy or fulguration**
6.92 6.92 FUD 000 J A2
AMA: 2018,Jan,8; 2017,Jan,8; 2016,Jan,13; 2015,Jan,16

52260 **Cystourethroscopy, with dilation of bladder for interstitial cystitis; general or conduction (spinal) anesthesia**
6.07 6.07 FUD 000 J A2
AMA: 2018,Jan,8; 2017,Jan,8; 2016,Jan,13; 2015,Jan,16

52265 **local anesthesia**
4.67 10.6 FUD 000 J P3
AMA: 2018,Jan,8; 2017,Jan,8; 2016,Jan,13; 2015,Jan,16

52270 **Cystourethroscopy, with internal urethrotomy; female** ♀
5.27 10.9 FUD 000 J A2
AMA: 2018,Jan,8; 2017,Jan,8; 2016,Jan,13; 2015,Jan,16

52275 **male** ♂
7.19 14.4 FUD 000 J A2
AMA: 2018,Jan,8; 2017,Jan,8; 2016,Jan,13; 2015,Jan,16

52276 **Cystourethroscopy with direct vision internal urethrotomy**
7.65 7.65 FUD 000 J A2
AMA: 2019,Feb,10; 2018,Jan,8; 2017,Jan,8; 2016,Jan,13; 2015,Jan,16

52277 **Cystourethroscopy, with resection of external sphincter (sphincterotomy)**
9.35 9.35 FUD 000 J A2 80
AMA: 2018,Jan,8; 2017,Jan,8; 2016,Jan,13; 2015,Jan,16

52281 **Cystourethroscopy, with calibration and/or dilation of urethral stricture or stenosis, with or without meatotomy, with or without injection procedure for cystography, male or female**
EXCLUDES *Urethral delivery therapeutic drug (0499T)*
4.40 8.53 FUD 000 J A2
AMA: 2018,Jan,8; 2017,Oct,9; 2017,Jan,8; 2016,Jan,13; 2015,Jan,16

52282 **Cystourethroscopy, with insertion of permanent urethral stent**
EXCLUDES *Placement temporary prostatic urethral stent (53855)*
9.76 9.76 FUD 000 J A2
AMA: 2018,Jan,8; 2017,Jan,8; 2016,Jan,13; 2015,Jun,5; 2015,Jan,16

52283 **Cystourethroscopy, with steroid injection into stricture**
5.83 8.68 FUD 000 J A2
AMA: 2019,Feb,10; 2018,Jan,8; 2017,Jan,8; 2016,Jan,13; 2015,Mar,9; 2015,Jan,16

52285 **Cystourethroscopy for treatment of the female urethral syndrome with any or all of the following: urethral meatotomy, urethral dilation, internal urethrotomy, lysis of urethrovaginal septal fibrosis, lateral incisions of the bladder neck, and fulguration of polyp(s) of urethra, bladder neck, and/or trigone** ♀
5.66 8.66 FUD 000 J A2
AMA: 2018,Jan,8; 2017,Jan,8; 2016,Jan,13; 2015,Jan,16

52287 **Cystourethroscopy, with injection(s) for chemodenervation of the bladder**
Code also supply chemodenervation agent
4.89 9.65 FUD 000 J G2
AMA: 2019,Apr,9

52290 **Cystourethroscopy; with ureteral meatotomy, unilateral or bilateral**
7.10 7.10 FUD 000 J A2
AMA: 2018,Jan,8; 2017,Jan,8; 2016,Jan,13; 2015,Jan,16

52300 **with resection or fulguration of orthotopic ureterocele(s), unilateral or bilateral**
8.09 8.09 FUD 000 J A2 80
AMA: 2018,Jan,8; 2017,Jan,8; 2016,Jan,13; 2015,Jan,16

52301 **with resection or fulguration of ectopic ureterocele(s), unilateral or bilateral**
8.38 8.38 FUD 000 J A2 80
AMA: 2018,Jan,8; 2017,Jan,8; 2016,Jan,13; 2015,Jan,16

52305 **with incision or resection of orifice of bladder diverticulum, single or multiple**
8.06 8.06 FUD 000 J A2
AMA: 2018,Jan,8; 2017,Jan,8; 2016,Jan,13; 2015,Jan,16

52310 **Cystourethroscopy, with removal of foreign body, calculus, or ureteral stent from urethra or bladder (separate procedure); simple**
Code also modifier 58 for removal self-retaining, indwelling ureteral stent
4.39 7.03 FUD 000 J A2
AMA: 2018,Jan,8; 2017,Jan,8; 2016,Jan,13; 2015,Jun,5; 2015,Jan,16

52315 **complicated**
Code also modifier 58 for removal self-retaining, indwelling ureteral stent
7.94 12.6 FUD 000 J A2
AMA: 2018,Jan,8; 2017,Jan,8; 2016,Jan,13; 2015,Jan,16

52317 **Litholapaxy: crushing or fragmentation of calculus by any means in bladder and removal of fragments; simple or small (less than 2.5 cm)**

10.0 24.1 **FUD** 000 J A2

AMA: 2018,Jan,8; 2017,Jan,8; 2016,Jan,13; 2015,Jan,16

52318 **complicated or large (over 2.5 cm)**

13.7 13.7 **FUD** 000 J A2

AMA: 2018,Jan,8; 2017,Jan,8; 2016,Jan,13; 2015,Jan,16

52320-52356 [52356] Endoscopic Procedures via Urethra: Renal Pelvis and Ureter

INCLUDES Diagnostic cystourethroscopy when performed with therapeutic cystourethroscopy

Insertion/removal temporary ureteral catheter (52005)

EXCLUDES *Self-retaining/indwelling ureteral stent removal by cystourethroscope, with modifier 58 when appropriate (52310, 52315)*

Code also insertion indwelling stent performed in addition to other procedures within this section (52332)

52320 **Cystourethroscopy (including ureteral catheterization); with removal of ureteral calculus**

INCLUDES Cystourethroscopy (separate procedure) (52000)

7.13 7.13 **FUD** 000 J A2 50

AMA: 2018,Jan,8; 2017,Jan,8; 2016,Jan,13; 2015,Jan,16

52325 **with fragmentation of ureteral calculus (eg, ultrasonic or electro-hydraulic technique)**

INCLUDES Cystourethroscopy (separate procedure) (52000)

9.27 9.27 **FUD** 000 J A2 50

AMA: 2018,Jan,8; 2017,Jan,8; 2016,Jan,13; 2015,Jan,16

52327 **with subureteric injection of implant material**

INCLUDES Cystourethroscopy (separate procedure) (52000)

7.59 7.59 **FUD** 000 J J8 50

AMA: 2018,Jan,8; 2017,Jan,8; 2016,Jan,13; 2015,Jan,16

52330 **with manipulation, without removal of ureteral calculus**

INCLUDES Cystourethroscopy (separate procedure) (52000)

7.63 15.4 **FUD** 000 J A2 50

AMA: 2018,Jan,8; 2017,Jan,8; 2016,Jan,13; 2015,Jan,16

52332 **Cystourethroscopy, with insertion of indwelling ureteral stent (eg, Gibbons or double-J type)**

INCLUDES Cystourethroscopy (separate procedure) (52000)

EXCLUDES *Cystourethroscopy, with ureteroscopy and/or pyeloscopy; with lithotripsy when performed on same side with (52353, [52356])*

4.50 13.5 **FUD** 000 J A2 50

AMA: 2019,Dec,12; 2018,Jan,8; 2017,Jan,8; 2016,Jan,13; 2015,Jan,16

52334 **Cystourethroscopy with insertion of ureteral guide wire through kidney to establish a percutaneous nephrostomy, retrograde**

INCLUDES Cystourethroscopy (separate procedure) (52000)

EXCLUDES *Cystourethroscopy with incision/fulguration/resection congenital posterior urethral valves/obstructive hypertrophic mucosal folds (52400)*

Cystourethroscopy with pyeloscopy and/or ureteroscopy (52351-52353 [52356])

Dilation nephroureteral catheter tract ([50436], [50437])

Nephrostomy tract establishment only ([50432, 50433])

Percutaneous nephrostolithotomy (50080, 50081)

5.30 5.30 **FUD** 000 J A2

AMA: 2018,Jan,8; 2017,Jan,8; 2016,Jan,13; 2015,Jan,16

52341 **Cystourethroscopy; with treatment of ureteral stricture (eg, balloon dilation, laser, electrocautery, and incision)**

INCLUDES Diagnostic cystourethroscopy (52351)

EXCLUDES *Balloon dilation with imaging guidance (50706)*

Cystourethroscopy, separate procedure (52000)

(74485)

8.21 8.21 **FUD** 000 J A2 50

AMA: 2018,Jan,8; 2017,Jan,8; 2016,Jan,13; 2016,Jan,3; 2015,Jan,16

52342 **with treatment of ureteropelvic junction stricture (eg, balloon dilation, laser, electrocautery, and incision)**

INCLUDES Diagnostic cystourethroscopy (52351)

EXCLUDES *Balloon dilation with imaging guidance (50706)*

Cystourethroscopy (separate procedure) (52000)

(74485)

8.93 8.93 **FUD** 000 J A2 50

AMA: 2018,Jan,8; 2017,Jan,8; 2016,Jan,13; 2015,Jan,16

52343 **with treatment of intra-renal stricture (eg, balloon dilation, laser, electrocautery, and incision)**

INCLUDES Diagnostic cystourethroscopy (52351)

EXCLUDES *Balloon dilation with imaging guidance (50706)*

Cystourethroscopy (separate procedure) (52000)

(74485)

9.96 9.96 **FUD** 000 J A2 50

AMA: 2018,Jan,8; 2017,Jan,8; 2016,Jan,13; 2015,Jan,16

52344 **Cystourethroscopy with ureteroscopy; with treatment of ureteral stricture (eg, balloon dilation, laser, electrocautery, and incision)**

INCLUDES Diagnostic cystourethroscopy (52351)

EXCLUDES *Balloon dilation, ureteral stricture (50706)*

Cystourethroscopy with transurethral resection or incision ejaculatory ducts (52402)

(74485)

10.6 10.6 **FUD** 000 J A2 50

AMA: 2018,Jan,8; 2017,Jan,8; 2016,Jan,13; 2016,Jan,3; 2015,Jan,16

52345 **with treatment of ureteropelvic junction stricture (eg, balloon dilation, laser, electrocautery, and incision)**

INCLUDES Diagnostic cystourethroscopy (52351)

EXCLUDES *Balloon dilation, ureteral stricture (50706)*

Cystourethroscopy with transurethral resection or incision ejaculatory ducts (52402)

(74485)

11.4 11.4 **FUD** 000 J A2 80 50

AMA: 2018,Jan,8; 2017,Jan,8; 2016,Jan,13; 2016,Jan,3; 2015,Jan,16

52346 **with treatment of intra-renal stricture (eg, balloon dilation, laser, electrocautery, and incision)**

INCLUDES Diagnostic cystourethroscopy (52351)

EXCLUDES *Balloon dilation with imaging guidance (50706)*

Cystourethroscopy with transurethral resection or incision ejaculatory ducts (52402)

(74485)

12.9 12.9 **FUD** 000 J A2 80 50

AMA: 2018,Jan,8; 2017,Jan,8; 2016,Jan,13; 2015,Jan,16

52351 **Cystourethroscopy, with ureteroscopy and/or pyeloscopy; diagnostic**

EXCLUDES *Cystourethroscopy (52341-52346, 52352-52353 [52356])*

8.75 8.75 **FUD** 000 J A2

AMA: 2018,Jan,8; 2017,Jan,8; 2016,Jan,13; 2015,Jan,16

52352 **with removal or manipulation of calculus (ureteral catheterization is included)**

INCLUDES Diagnostic cystourethroscopy (52351)

Facility RVU 10.2 Non-Facility RVU 10.2 FUD 000 J A2 50

AMA: 2018,Jan,8; 2017,Jan,8; 2016,Jan,13; 2015,Jan,16

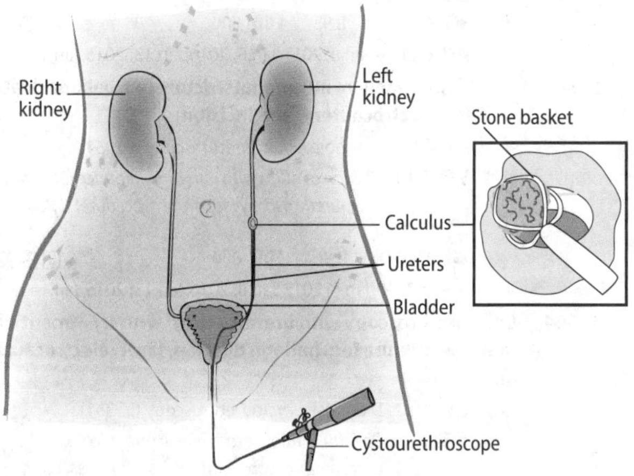

52353 **with lithotripsy (ureteral catheterization is included)**

INCLUDES Diagnostic cystourethroscopy (52351)

EXCLUDES *Cystourethroscopy when performed on same side (52332, [52356])*

Facility RVU 11.3 Non-Facility RVU 11.3 FUD 000 J A2 50

AMA: 2019,Dec,12; 2018,Jan,8; 2017,Jan,8; 2016,Jan,13; 2015,Jan,16

52356 **with lithotripsy including insertion of indwelling ureteral stent (eg, Gibbons or double-J type)**

INCLUDES Diagnostic cystourethroscopy (52351)

EXCLUDES *Cystourethroscopy (separate procedure) (52000)*

When performed on same side:

Cystourethroscopy, with insertion indwelling ureteral stent (e.g., Gibbons or double-J type) (52332)

Cystourethroscopy, with ureteroscopy and/or pyeloscopy; with lithotripsy (ureteral catheterization is included) (52353)

Facility RVU 12.0 Non-Facility RVU 12.0 FUD 000 J G2 50

AMA: 2019,Dec,12; 2018,Jan,8; 2017,Jan,8; 2016,Jan,13; 2015,Jan,16

52354 **with biopsy and/or fulguration of ureteral or renal pelvic lesion**

INCLUDES Diagnostic cystourethroscopy (52351)

EXCLUDES *Image guided biopsy without endoscopic guidance (50606)*

Facility RVU 12.0 Non-Facility RVU 12.0 FUD 000 J A2 50

AMA: 2018,Jan,8; 2017,Jan,8; 2016,Jan,13; 2015,Jan,16

52355 **with resection of ureteral or renal pelvic tumor**

INCLUDES Diagnostic cystourethroscopy (52351)

Facility RVU 13.5 Non-Facility RVU 13.5 FUD 000 J A2 50

AMA: 2018,Jan,8; 2017,Jan,8; 2016,Jan,13; 2015,Jan,16

52356 **Resequenced code. See code following 52353.**

52400-52700 Endoscopic Procedures via Urethra: Prostate and Vesical Neck

52400 **Cystourethroscopy with incision, fulguration, or resection of congenital posterior urethral valves, or congenital obstructive hypertrophic mucosal folds**

Facility RVU 13.8 Non-Facility RVU 13.8 FUD 090 J A2

AMA: 2018,Jan,8; 2017,Jan,8; 2016,Jan,13; 2015,Jan,16

52402 **Cystourethroscopy with transurethral resection or incision of ejaculatory ducts** ♂

Facility RVU 7.73 Non-Facility RVU 7.73 FUD 000 J A2

AMA: 2014,Jan,11; 2001,Apr,4

52441 **Cystourethroscopy, with insertion of permanent adjustable transprostatic implant; single implant**

Facility RVU 6.55 Non-Facility RVU 36.1 FUD 000 B

AMA: 2018,Jan,8; 2017,Jan,8; 2016,Jan,13; 2015,Jun,5

+ **52442** **each additional permanent adjustable transprostatic implant (List separately in addition to code for primary procedure)**

EXCLUDES *Permanent urethral stent insertion (52282)*

Removal stent, calculus, or foreign body (implant) (52310)

Temporary prostatic urethral stent insertion (53855)

Code first (52441)

Facility RVU 1.75 Non-Facility RVU 27.1 FUD ZZZ B

AMA: 2018,Jan,8; 2017,Jan,8; 2016,Jan,13; 2015,Jun,5

52450 **Transurethral incision of prostate** ♂

Facility RVU 13.5 Non-Facility RVU 13.5 FUD 090 J A2

AMA: 2018,Jan,8; 2017,Jan,8; 2016,Jan,13; 2015,Jun,5; 2015,Jan,16

52500 **Transurethral resection of bladder neck (separate procedure)**

Facility RVU 14.1 Non-Facility RVU 14.1 FUD 090 J A2

AMA: 2018,Jan,8; 2017,Jan,8; 2016,Jan,13; 2015,Jan,16

52601 **Transurethral electrosurgical resection of prostate, including control of postoperative bleeding, complete (vasectomy, meatotomy, cystourethroscopy, urethral calibration and/or dilation, and internal urethrotomy are included)** ♂

INCLUDES Stage 1 partial transurethral resection prostate

EXCLUDES *Ablation by waterjet (0421T)*

Excision prostate (55801-55845)

Transurethral fulguration prostate (52214)

Code also modifier 58 for stage 2 partial transurethral resection prostate

Facility RVU 21.0 Non-Facility RVU 21.0 FUD 090 J A2

AMA: 2018,Jan,8; 2017,Jan,8; 2016,Jan,13; 2015,Jun,5; 2015,Jan,16

52630 **Transurethral resection; residual or regrowth of obstructive prostate tissue including control of postoperative bleeding, complete (vasectomy, meatotomy, cystourethroscopy, urethral calibration and/or dilation, and internal urethrotomy are included)** ♂

EXCLUDES *Ablation by waterjet (0421T)*

Excision prostate (55801-55845)

Code also modifier 78 when performed by same physician within postoperative period related procedure

Facility RVU 11.5 Non-Facility RVU 11.5 FUD 090 J A2

AMA: 2018,Jan,8; 2017,Jan,8; 2016,Jan,13; 2015,Jan,16

52640 **of postoperative bladder neck contracture**

EXCLUDES *Excision prostate (55801-55845)*

Facility RVU 9.14 Non-Facility RVU 9.14 FUD 090 J A2

AMA: 2018,Jan,8; 2017,Jan,8; 2016,Jan,13; 2015,Jan,16

52647 **Laser coagulation of prostate, including control of postoperative bleeding, complete (vasectomy, meatotomy, cystourethroscopy, urethral calibration and/or dilation, and internal urethrotomy are included if performed)** ♂

Facility RVU 18.7 Non-Facility RVU 46.2 FUD 090 J A2

AMA: 2018,Jan,8; 2017,Jan,8; 2016,Jan,13; 2015,Jan,16

52648 **Laser vaporization of prostate, including control of postoperative bleeding, complete (vasectomy, meatotomy, cystourethroscopy, urethral calibration and/or dilation, internal urethrotomy and transurethral resection of prostate are included if performed)** ♂

Facility RVU 19.9 Non-Facility RVU 47.7 FUD 090 J A2

AMA: 2018,Jan,8; 2017,Jan,8; 2016,Jan,13; 2015,Jun,5; 2015,Jan,16

52649 Laser enucleation of the prostate with morcellation, including control of postoperative bleeding, complete (vasectomy, meatotomy, cystourethroscopy, urethral calibration and/or dilation, internal urethrotomy and transurethral resection of prostate are included if performed) ♂

INCLUDES Cystourethroscopy (52000, 52276, 52281)
Laser coagulation prostate (52647-52648)
Meatotomy (53020)
Transurethral resection of prostate (52601)
Vasectomy (55250)

23.8 23.8 **FUD** 090 J G2 80

AMA: 2018,Jan,8; 2017,Jan,8; 2016,Jan,13; 2015,Jun,5

52700 Transurethral drainage of prostatic abscess ♂

EXCLUDES *Litholapaxy (52317, 52318)*

12.7 12.7 **FUD** 090 J A2 80

AMA: 2018,Jan,8; 2017,Jan,8; 2016,Jan,13; 2015,Jan,16

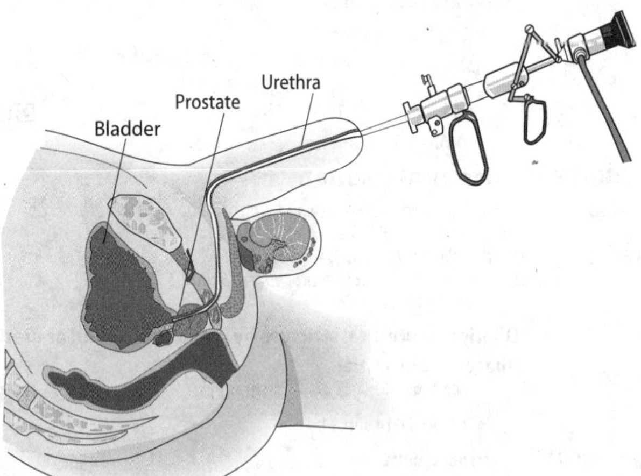

53000-53520 Open Surgical Procedures of Urethra

EXCLUDES *Endoscopic procedures; cystoscopy, urethroscopy, cystourethroscopy (52000-52700 [52356])*
Urethrocystography injection procedure (51600-51610)

53000 Urethrotomy or urethrostomy, external (separate procedure); pendulous urethra

4.28 4.28 **FUD** 010 J A2

AMA: 2014,Jan,11

53010 perineal urethra, external

8.51 8.51 **FUD** 090 J A2

AMA: 2014,Jan,11

53020 Meatotomy, cutting of meatus (separate procedure); except infant

2.80 2.80 **FUD** 000 J A2

AMA: 2014,Jan,11

53025 infant A

1.97 1.97 **FUD** 000 63 J R2 80

AMA: 2014,Jan,11

53040 Drainage of deep periurethral abscess

EXCLUDES *Incision and drainage subcutaneous abscess (10060-10061)*

11.3 11.3 **FUD** 090 J A2 80

AMA: 2014,Jan,11

53060 Drainage of Skene's gland abscess or cyst

4.70 5.25 **FUD** 010 J P3

AMA: 2014,Jan,11

53080 Drainage of perineal urinary extravasation; uncomplicated (separate procedure)

12.1 12.1 **FUD** 090 J A2

AMA: 2014,Jan,11

53085 complicated

18.7 18.7 **FUD** 090 J G2 80

AMA: 2014,Jan,11

53200 Biopsy of urethra

4.12 4.55 **FUD** 000 J A2

AMA: 2014,Jan,11

53210 Urethrectomy, total, including cystostomy; female ♀

22.2 22.2 **FUD** 090 J A2 80

AMA: 2014,Jan,11

53215 male ♂

26.8 26.8 **FUD** 090 J A2 80

AMA: 2014,Jan,11

53220 Excision or fulguration of carcinoma of urethra

13.0 13.0 **FUD** 090 J A2 80

AMA: 2014,Jan,11

53230 Excision of urethral diverticulum (separate procedure); female ♀

17.5 17.5 **FUD** 090 J A2 80

AMA: 2014,Jan,11

53235 male ♂

18.3 18.3 **FUD** 090 J A2 80

AMA: 2014,Jan,11

53240 Marsupialization of urethral diverticulum, male or female

12.2 12.2 **FUD** 090 J A2

AMA: 2014,Jan,11

53250 Excision of bulbourethral gland (Cowper's gland)

11.4 11.4 **FUD** 090 J A2

AMA: 2014,Jan,11

53260 Excision or fulguration; urethral polyp(s), distal urethra

EXCLUDES *Endoscopic method (52214, 52224)*

5.20 5.83 **FUD** 010 J A2

AMA: 2014,Jan,11

53265 urethral caruncle

EXCLUDES *Endoscopic method (52214, 52224)*

5.38 6.36 **FUD** 010 J A2

AMA: 2014,Jan,11

53270 Skene's glands

EXCLUDES *Endoscopic method (52214, 52224)*

5.32 5.98 **FUD** 010 J A2

AMA: 2014,Jan,11

53275 urethral prolapse

EXCLUDES *Endoscopic method (52214, 52224)*

7.58 7.58 **FUD** 010 J A2

AMA: 2014,Jan,11

53400 Urethroplasty; first stage, for fistula, diverticulum, or stricture (eg, Johannsen type)

EXCLUDES *Hypospadias repair (54300-54352)*

23.1 23.1 **FUD** 090 J A2 80

AMA: 2014,Jan,11

53405 second stage (formation of urethra), including urinary diversion

EXCLUDES *Hypospadias repair (54300-54352)*

25.2 25.2 **FUD** 090 J A2 80

AMA: 2014,Jan,11

53410 Urethroplasty, 1-stage reconstruction of male anterior urethra ♂

EXCLUDES *Hypospadias repair (54300-54352)*

28.3 28.3 **FUD** 090 J A2 80

AMA: 2014,Jan,11

53415 Urethroplasty, transpubic or perineal, 1-stage, for reconstruction or repair of prostatic or membranous urethra ♂

32.8 32.8 **FUD** 090 C 80

AMA: 2014,Jan,11

53420 **Urethroplasty, 2-stage reconstruction or repair of prostatic or membranous urethra; first stage** ♂
24.3 24.3 **FUD** 090 J A2
AMA: 2014,Jan,11

53425 **second stage** ♂
27.1 27.1 **FUD** 090 J A2 80
AMA: 2014,Jan,11

53430 **Urethroplasty, reconstruction of female urethra** ♀
27.9 27.9 **FUD** 090 J A2 80
AMA: 2014,Jan,11

53431 **Urethroplasty with tubularization of posterior urethra and/or lower bladder for incontinence (eg, Tenago, Leadbetter procedure)**
33.3 33.3 **FUD** 090 J A2 80
AMA: 2014,Jan,11

53440 **Sling operation for correction of male urinary incontinence (eg, fascia or synthetic)** ♂
21.7 21.7 **FUD** 090 J J8 80
AMA: 2020,Aug,6

53442 **Removal or revision of sling for male urinary incontinence (eg, fascia or synthetic)** ♂
22.6 22.6 **FUD** 090 J A2 80
AMA: 2020,Aug,6

53444 **Insertion of tandem cuff (dual cuff)**
22.9 22.9 **FUD** 090 J J8 80
AMA: 2014,Jan,11

53445 **Insertion of inflatable urethral/bladder neck sphincter, including placement of pump, reservoir, and cuff**
21.7 21.7 **FUD** 090 J J8 80
AMA: 2020,Aug,6

53446 **Removal of inflatable urethral/bladder neck sphincter, including pump, reservoir, and cuff**
18.5 18.5 **FUD** 090 Q2 A2 80
AMA: 2020,Aug,6

53447 **Removal and replacement of inflatable urethral/bladder neck sphincter including pump, reservoir, and cuff at the same operative session**
23.3 23.3 **FUD** 090 J J8 80
AMA: 2020,Aug,6

53448 **Removal and replacement of inflatable urethral/bladder neck sphincter including pump, reservoir, and cuff through an infected field at the same operative session including irrigation and debridement of infected tissue**
INCLUDES Debridement (11042, 11043)
36.9 36.9 **FUD** 090 C 80
AMA: 2020,Aug,6

53449 **Repair of inflatable urethral/bladder neck sphincter, including pump, reservoir, and cuff**
17.6 17.6 **FUD** 090 J A2 80
AMA: 2020,Aug,6

53450 **Urethromeatoplasty, with mucosal advancement**
EXCLUDES *Meatotomy (53020, 53025)*
11.8 11.8 **FUD** 090 J A2
AMA: 2018,Jan,8; 2017,Jan,8; 2016,Jan,13; 2015,Jan,16

53460 **Urethromeatoplasty, with partial excision of distal urethral segment (Richardson type procedure)**
13.2 13.2 **FUD** 090 J A2 80
AMA: 2014,Jan,11

53500 **Urethrolysis, transvaginal, secondary, open, including cystourethroscopy (eg, postsurgical obstruction, scarring)**
INCLUDES Cystourethroscopy (separate procedure) (52000)
EXCLUDES *Retropubic approach (53899)*
21.5 21.5 **FUD** 090 J 80
AMA: 2018,Jan,8; 2017,Jan,8; 2016,Jan,13; 2015,Jan,16

53502 **Urethrorrhaphy, suture of urethral wound or injury, female** ♀
14.0 14.0 **FUD** 090 J A2
AMA: 2014,Jan,11

53505 **Urethrorrhaphy, suture of urethral wound or injury; penile** ♂
14.0 14.0 **FUD** 090 J A2 80
AMA: 2014,Jan,11

53510 **perineal** ♂
18.2 18.2 **FUD** 090 J A2 80
AMA: 2014,Jan,11

53515 **prostatomembranous** ♂
23.0 23.0 **FUD** 090 J A2 80
AMA: 2014,Jan,11

53520 **Closure of urethrostomy or urethrocutaneous fistula, male (separate procedure)** ♂
EXCLUDES *Closure fistula:*
Urethrorectal (45820, 45825)
Urethrovaginal (57310)
16.1 16.1 **FUD** 090 J A2
AMA: 2014,Jan,11

53600-53665 Urethral Dilation

EXCLUDES *Endoscopic procedures; cystoscopy, urethroscopy, cystourethroscopy (52000-52700 [52356])*
Urethral catheterization (51701-51703)
Urethrocystography injection procedure (51600-51610)
(74485)

53600 **Dilation of urethral stricture by passage of sound or urethral dilator, male; initial** ♂
1.84 2.39 **FUD** 000 T P3
AMA: 2014,Jan,11

53601 **subsequent** ♂
1.55 2.29 **FUD** 000 Q1 N1
AMA: 2014,Jan,11

53605 **Dilation of urethral stricture or vesical neck by passage of sound or urethral dilator, male, general or conduction (spinal) anesthesia** ♂
EXCLUDES *Procedure performed under local anesthesia (53600-53601, 53620-53621)*
1.87 1.87 **FUD** 000 J A2
AMA: 2014,Jan,11

53620 **Dilation of urethral stricture by passage of filiform and follower, male; initial** ♂
2.52 3.79 **FUD** 000 T P3
AMA: 2014,Jan,11; 1996,Nov,1

53621 **subsequent** ♂
2.09 3.56 **FUD** 000 T P3
AMA: 2014,Jan,11

53660 **Dilation of female urethra including suppository and/or instillation; initial** ♀
1.20 2.02 **FUD** 000 S P3
AMA: 2014,Jan,11

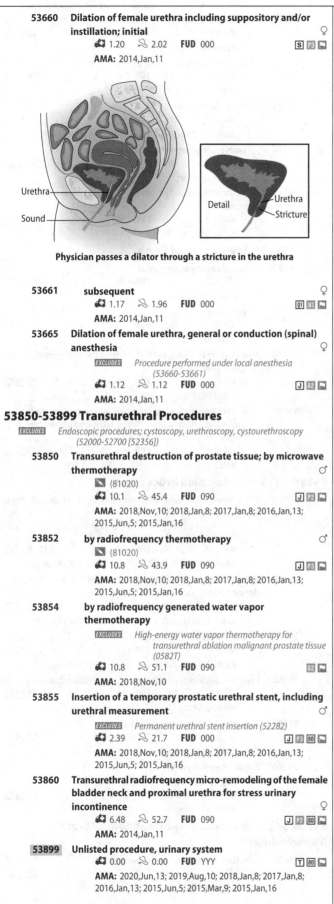

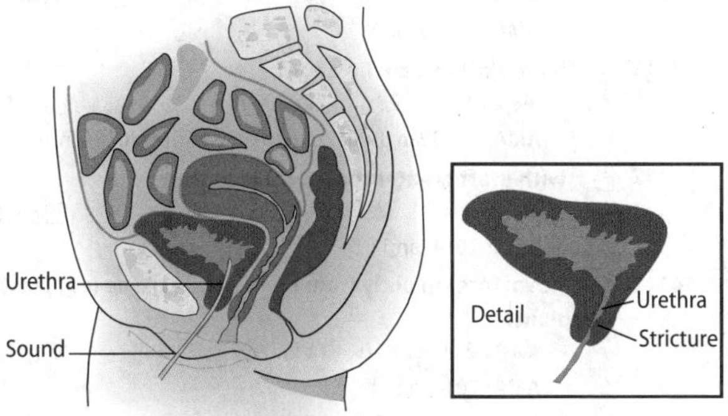

Physician passes a dilator through a stricture in the urethra

53661 **subsequent** ♀
1.17 1.96 **FUD** 000 Q1 N1
AMA: 2014,Jan,11

53665 **Dilation of female urethra, general or conduction (spinal) anesthesia** ♀
EXCLUDES *Procedure performed under local anesthesia (53660-53661)*
1.12 1.12 **FUD** 000 J A2
AMA: 2014,Jan,11

53850-53899 Transurethral Procedures

EXCLUDES *Endoscopic procedures; cystoscopy, urethroscopy, cystourethroscopy (52000-52700 [52356])*

53850 **Transurethral destruction of prostate tissue; by microwave thermotherapy** ♂
(81020)
10.1 45.4 **FUD** 090 J P2
AMA: 2018,Nov,10; 2018,Jan,8; 2017,Jan,8; 2016,Jan,13; 2015,Jun,5; 2015,Jan,16

53852 **by radiofrequency thermotherapy** ♂
(81020)
10.8 43.9 **FUD** 090 J P3
AMA: 2018,Nov,10; 2018,Jan,8; 2017,Jan,8; 2016,Jan,13; 2015,Jun,5; 2015,Jan,16

53854 **by radiofrequency generated water vapor thermotherapy**
EXCLUDES *High-energy water vapor thermotherapy for transurethral ablation malignant prostate tissue (0582T)*
10.8 51.1 **FUD** 090 G2
AMA: 2018,Nov,10

53855 **Insertion of a temporary prostatic urethral stent, including urethral measurement** ♂
EXCLUDES *Permanent urethral stent insertion (52282)*
2.39 21.7 **FUD** 000 J P3 80
AMA: 2018,Nov,10; 2018,Jan,8; 2017,Jan,8; 2016,Jan,13; 2015,Jun,5; 2015,Jan,16

53860 **Transurethral radiofrequency micro-remodeling of the female bladder neck and proximal urethra for stress urinary incontinence** ♀
6.48 52.7 **FUD** 090 J P2 80
AMA: 2014,Jan,11

53899 **Unlisted procedure, urinary system**
0.00 0.00 **FUD** YYY T 80
AMA: 2020,Jun,13; 2019,Aug,10; 2018,Jan,8; 2017,Jan,8; 2016,Jan,13; 2015,Jun,5; 2015,Mar,9; 2015,Jan,16

54000-54015 Procedures of Penis: Incisional

EXCLUDES *Debridement abdominal perineal gangrene (11004-11006)*

54000 Slitting of prepuce, dorsal or lateral (separate procedure); newborn A ♂
3.14 4.40 FUD 010 63 J A2 80
AMA: 2014,Jan,11

54001 except newborn ♂
4.02 5.44 FUD 010 J A2
AMA: 2014,Jan,11

54015 Incision and drainage of penis, deep ♂
EXCLUDES *Abscess, skin/subcutaneous (10060-10160)*
8.92 8.92 FUD 010 J A2 80
AMA: 2014,Jan,11

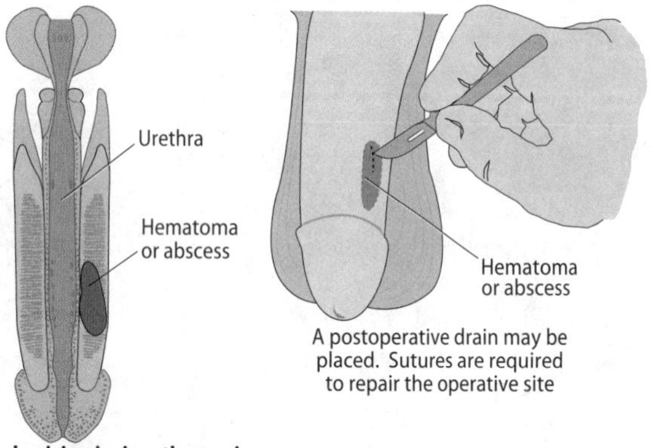

The physician incises the penis to drain an abscess or hematoma

54050-54065 Destruction of Penis Lesions: Multiple Methods

EXCLUDES *Excision/destruction other lesions (11420-11426, 11620-11626, 17000-17250, 17270-17276)*

54050 Destruction of lesion(s), penis (eg, condyloma, papilloma, molluscum contagiosum, herpetic vesicle), simple; chemical ♂
3.05 3.80 FUD 010 Q1 N1
AMA: 2014,Jan,11; 1997,Nov,1

54055 electrodesiccation ♂
2.69 3.49 FUD 010 T P3
AMA: 2014,Jan,11; 1997,Nov,1

54056 cryosurgery ♂
3.18 4.03 FUD 010 Q1 N1
AMA: 2014,Jan,11; 1997,Nov,1

54057 laser surgery ♂
2.76 3.97 FUD 010 T A2
AMA: 2014,Jan,11; 1997,Nov,1

54060 surgical excision ♂
3.76 5.29 FUD 010 T A2
AMA: 2014,Jan,11

54065 Destruction of lesion(s), penis (eg, condyloma, papilloma, molluscum contagiosum, herpetic vesicle), extensive (eg, laser surgery, electrosurgery, cryosurgery, chemosurgery) ♂
4.90 6.27 FUD 010 T A2
AMA: 2014,Jan,11; 1997,Nov,1

54100-54115 Procedures of Penis: Excisional

54100 Biopsy of penis; (separate procedure) ♂
3.50 5.67 FUD 000 J A2
AMA: 2019,Jan,9; 2018,Jan,8; 2017,Jan,8; 2016,Jan,13; 2015,Jan,16

54105 deep structures ♂
6.16 7.68 FUD 010 J A2
AMA: 2014,Jan,11

54110 Excision of penile plaque (Peyronie disease); ♂
18.0 18.0 FUD 090 J A2 80
AMA: 2014,Jan,11

54111 with graft to 5 cm in length ♂
23.1 23.1 FUD 090 J A2 80
AMA: 2018,Jan,8; 2017,Jan,8; 2016,Jan,13; 2015,Jan,16

54112 with graft greater than 5 cm in length ♂
27.0 27.0 FUD 090 J A2 80
AMA: 2014,Jan,11

54115 Removal foreign body from deep penile tissue (eg, plastic implant) ♂
12.2 13.0 FUD 090 J A2 80
AMA: 2014,Jan,11

54120-54135 Amputation of Penis

54120 Amputation of penis; partial ♂
18.2 18.2 FUD 090 J A2 80
AMA: 2014,Jan,11

54125 complete ♂
23.5 23.5 FUD 090 C 80
AMA: 2014,Jan,11

54130 Amputation of penis, radical; with bilateral inguinofemoral lymphadenectomy ♂
34.5 34.5 FUD 090 C 80
AMA: 2014,Jan,11

54135 in continuity with bilateral pelvic lymphadenectomy, including external iliac, hypogastric and obturator nodes ♂
43.6 43.6 FUD 090 C 80
AMA: 2014,Jan,11

54150-54164 Circumcision Procedures

54150 Circumcision, using clamp or other device with regional dorsal penile or ring block ♂
Code also modifier 52 when performed without dorsal penile or ring block
2.84 4.40 FUD 000 63 J A2 80
AMA: 2018,Jan,8; 2017,Jan,8; 2016,Jan,13; 2015,Jan,16

54160 Circumcision, surgical excision other than clamp, device, or dorsal slit; neonate (28 days of age or less) A ♂
4.17 6.29 FUD 010 63 J A2
AMA: 2018,Jan,8; 2017,Jan,8; 2016,Jan,13; 2015,Jan,16

54161 older than 28 days of age A ♂
5.70 5.70 FUD 010 J A2
AMA: 2018,Jan,8; 2017,Jan,8; 2016,Jan,13; 2015,Jan,16

54162 Lysis or excision of penile post-circumcision adhesions ♂
5.77 7.42 FUD 010 J A2
AMA: 2014,Jan,11

54163 Repair incomplete circumcision ♂
6.31 6.31 FUD 010 J A2
AMA: 2014,Jan,11

54164 Frenulotomy of penis ♂
EXCLUDES *Circumcision (54150-54163)*
5.54 5.54 FUD 010 J A2
AMA: 2014,Jan,11

54200-54250 Evaluation and Treatment of Erectile Abnormalities

54200 Injection procedure for Peyronie disease; ♂
2.41 3.17 FUD 010 T P3
AMA: 2014,Jan,11

54205 with surgical exposure of plaque ♂
15.4 15.4 FUD 090 J A2 80
AMA: 2014,Jan,11

54220 Irrigation of corpora cavernosa for priapism ♂
3.86 6.07 FUD 000 T A2
AMA: 2014,Jan,11

54230 Injection procedure for corpora cavernosography ♂
(74445)
2.28 2.87 FUD 000 N N1
AMA: 2014,Jan,11

54231 Dynamic cavernosometry, including intracavernosal injection of vasoactive drugs (eg, papaverine, phentolamine) ♂
3.34 4.07 FUD 000 J P3
AMA: 2014,Jan,11; 1994,Sum,29

54235 Injection of corpora cavernosa with pharmacologic agent(s) (eg, papaverine, phentolamine) ♂
2.10 2.53 FUD 000 T P3
AMA: 2018,Jan,8; 2017,Jan,8; 2016,Jan,13; 2015,Jan,16

54240 Penile plethysmography ♂
2.97 2.97 FUD 000 S P3 80
AMA: 2014,Jan,11

54250 Nocturnal penile tumescence and/or rigidity test ♂
3.50 3.50 FUD 000 T P3 80
AMA: 2014,Jan,11

54300-54390 Hypospadias Repair and Related Procedures

EXCLUDES *Other urethroplasties (53400-53430)*
Revascularization penis (37788)

54300 Plastic operation of penis for straightening of chordee (eg, hypospadias), with or without mobilization of urethra ♂
18.6 18.6 FUD 090 J A2 80
AMA: 2018,Jan,8; 2017,Jan,8; 2016,Jan,13; 2015,Jan,16

54304 Plastic operation on penis for correction of chordee or for first stage hypospadias repair with or without transplantation of prepuce and/or skin flaps ♂
21.6 21.6 FUD 090 J A2 80
AMA: 2014,Jan,11

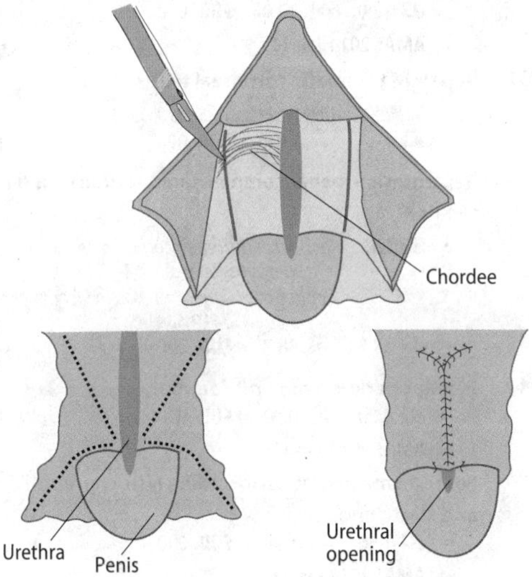

The foreskin is used in either a free graft or a flap graft to cover the ventral skin defects created to correct the chordee

54308 Urethroplasty for second stage hypospadias repair (including urinary diversion); less than 3 cm ♂
20.6 20.6 FUD 090 J A2 80
AMA: 2014,Jan,11

54312 greater than 3 cm ♂
23.6 23.6 FUD 090 J A2 80
AMA: 2014,Jan,11

54316 Urethroplasty for second stage hypospadias repair (including urinary diversion) with free skin graft obtained from site other than genitalia ♂
28.8 28.8 FUD 090 J A2 80
AMA: 2014,Jan,11

54318 Urethroplasty for third stage hypospadias repair to release penis from scrotum (eg, third stage Cecil repair) ♂
20.5 20.5 FUD 090 J A2 80
AMA: 2014,Jan,11

54322 1-stage distal hypospadias repair (with or without chordee or circumcision); with simple meatal advancement (eg, Magpi, V-flap) ♂
22.5 22.5 FUD 090 J A2 80
AMA: 2014,Jan,11

54324 with urethroplasty by local skin flaps (eg, flip-flap, prepucial flap) ♂
INCLUDES Browne's operation
27.9 27.9 FUD 090 J A2 80
AMA: 2014,Jan,11

54326 with urethroplasty by local skin flaps and mobilization of urethra ♂
27.2 27.2 FUD 090 J A2 80
AMA: 2014,Jan,11

54328 with extensive dissection to correct chordee and urethroplasty with local skin flaps, skin graft patch, and/or island flap ♂
EXCLUDES *Urethroplasty/straightening chordee (54308)*
27.1 27.1 FUD 090 J A2 80
AMA: 2018,Jan,8; 2017,Jan,8; 2016,Jan,13; 2015,Jan,16

54332 1-stage proximal penile or penoscrotal hypospadias repair requiring extensive dissection to correct chordee and urethroplasty by use of skin graft tube and/or island flap ♂
29.3 29.3 FUD 090 J 80
AMA: 2018,Jan,8; 2017,Jan,8; 2016,Jan,13; 2015,Jan,16

54336 1-stage perineal hypospadias repair requiring extensive dissection to correct chordee and urethroplasty by use of skin graft tube and/or island flap ♂
34.4 34.4 FUD 090 J 80
AMA: 2018,Jan,8; 2017,Jan,8; 2016,Jan,13; 2015,Jan,16

54340 Repair of hypospadias complications (ie, fistula, stricture, diverticula); by closure, incision, or excision, simple ♂
16.4 16.4 FUD 090 J A2 80
AMA: 2014,Jan,11

54344 requiring mobilization of skin flaps and urethroplasty with flap or patch graft ♂
27.3 27.3 FUD 090 J A2 80
AMA: 2014,Jan,11

54348 requiring extensive dissection and urethroplasty with flap, patch or tubed graft (includes urinary diversion) ♂
29.2 29.2 FUD 090 J A2 80
AMA: 2014,Jan,11

54352 Repair of hypospadias cripple requiring extensive dissection and excision of previously constructed structures including re-release of chordee and reconstruction of urethra and penis by use of local skin as grafts and island flaps and skin brought in as flaps or grafts ♂
40.9 40.9 FUD 090 J A2 80
AMA: 2014,Jan,11

54360 Plastic operation on penis to correct angulation ♂
20.8 20.8 FUD 090 J A2 80
AMA: 2014,Jan,11

54380 **Plastic operation on penis for epispadias distal to external sphincter;** ♂
INCLUDES Lowsley's operation
23.1 23.1 **FUD** 090 J A2 80
AMA: 2014,Jan,11

54385 **with incontinence** ♂
26.8 26.8 **FUD** 090 J A2 80
AMA: 2014,Jan,11

54390 **with exstrophy of bladder** ♂
35.8 35.8 **FUD** 090 C 80
AMA: 2014,Jan,11

54400-54417 Procedures to Treat Impotence

CMS: 100-03,230.4 Diagnosis and Treatment of Impotence
EXCLUDES *Other urethroplasties (53400-53430)*
Revascularization penis (37788)

54400 **Insertion of penile prosthesis; non-inflatable (semi-rigid)** ♂
EXCLUDES *Replacement/removal penile prosthesis (54415, 54416)*
15.3 15.3 **FUD** 090 J J8
AMA: 2014,Jan,11

54401 **inflatable (self-contained)** ♂
EXCLUDES *Replacement/removal penile prosthesis (54415, 54416)*
18.9 18.9 **FUD** 090 J J8
AMA: 2014,Jan,11

54405 **Insertion of multi-component, inflatable penile prosthesis, including placement of pump, cylinders, and reservoir** ♂
Code also modifier 52 for reduced services
23.4 23.4 **FUD** 090 J J8 80
AMA: 2014,Jan,11

54406 **Removal of all components of a multi-component, inflatable penile prosthesis without replacement of prosthesis** ♂
Code also modifier 52 for reduced services
21.1 21.1 **FUD** 090 Q2 A2 80
AMA: 2014,Jan,11

54408 **Repair of component(s) of a multi-component, inflatable penile prosthesis** ♂
22.8 22.8 **FUD** 090 J A2 80
AMA: 2014,Jan,11

54410 **Removal and replacement of all component(s) of a multi-component, inflatable penile prosthesis at the same operative session** ♂
24.8 24.8 **FUD** 090 J J8 80
AMA: 2014,Jan,11

54411 **Removal and replacement of all components of a multi-component inflatable penile prosthesis through an infected field at the same operative session, including irrigation and debridement of infected tissue** ♂
INCLUDES Debridement (11042, 11043)
Code also modifier 52 for reduced services
29.7 29.7 **FUD** 090 J 80
AMA: 2014,Jan,11

54415 **Removal of non-inflatable (semi-rigid) or inflatable (self-contained) penile prosthesis, without replacement of prosthesis** ♂
15.3 15.3 **FUD** 090 Q2 A2 80
AMA: 2014,Jan,11

54416 **Removal and replacement of non-inflatable (semi-rigid) or inflatable (self-contained) penile prosthesis at the same operative session** ♂
20.5 20.5 **FUD** 090 J J8 80
AMA: 2014,Jan,11

54417 **Removal and replacement of non-inflatable (semi-rigid) or inflatable (self-contained) penile prosthesis through an infected field at the same operative session, including irrigation and debridement of infected tissue** ♂
INCLUDES Debridement (11042, 11043)
25.9 25.9 **FUD** 090 J 80
AMA: 2014,Jan,11

54420-54450 Other Procedures of the Penis

EXCLUDES *Other urethroplasties (53400-53430)*
Revascularization penis (37788)

54420 **Corpora cavernosa-saphenous vein shunt (priapism operation), unilateral or bilateral** ♂
20.3 20.3 **FUD** 090 J A2 80
AMA: 2014,Jan,11

54430 **Corpora cavernosa-corpus spongiosum shunt (priapism operation), unilateral or bilateral** ♂
18.5 18.5 **FUD** 090 C 80
AMA: 2014,Jan,11

Cross section of penis

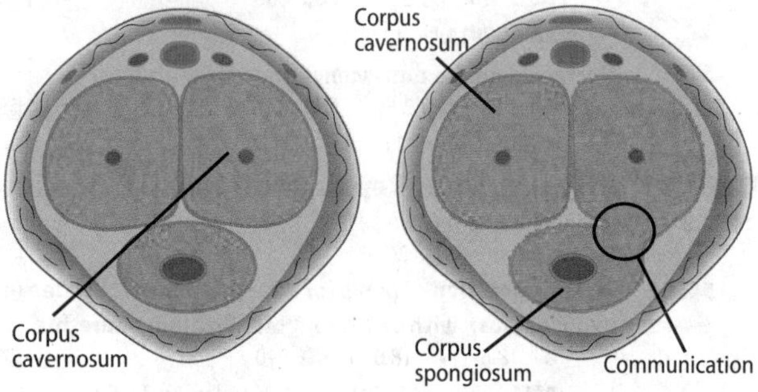

The physician creates a communication between the corpus cavernosum and the corpus spongiosum

54435 **Corpora cavernosa-glans penis fistulization (eg, biopsy needle, Winter procedure, rongeur, or punch) for priapism** ♂
12.0 12.0 **FUD** 090 J A2
AMA: 2014,Jan,11

54437 **Repair of traumatic corporeal tear(s)** ♂
EXCLUDES *Urethral repair (53410, 53415)*
19.4 19.4 **FUD** 090 J G2 80

54438 **Replantation, penis, complete amputation including urethral repair** ♂
EXCLUDES *Replantation/repair corporeal tear in incomplete amputation penis (54437)*
Replantation/urethral repair in incomplete amputation penis (53410-53415)
38.7 38.7 **FUD** 090 C 80

54440 **Plastic operation of penis for injury** ♂
0.00 0.00 **FUD** 090 J A2 80
AMA: 2014,Jan,11

54450 **Foreskin manipulation including lysis of preputial adhesions and stretching** ♂
1.66 1.98 **FUD** 000 T A2
AMA: 2014,Jan,11

54500-54560 Testicular Procedures: Incisional

EXCLUDES *Debridement abdominal perineal gangrene (11004-11006)*

54500 **Biopsy of testis, needle (separate procedure)** ♂
EXCLUDES *Fine needle aspiration (10021, [10004, 10005, 10006, 10007, 10008, 10009, 10010, 10011, 10012])*
(88172-88173)
2.15 2.15 **FUD** 000 J A2 80 50
AMA: 2019,Apr,4

54505 Biopsy of testis, incisional (separate procedure) ♂

Code also when combined with epididymogram, seminal vesiculogram or vasogram (55300)

6.07 6.07 **FUD** 010 J A2 80 50

AMA: 2018,Jan,8; 2017,Jan,8; 2016,Jan,13; 2015,Jan,16

54512 Excision of extraparenchymal lesion of testis ♂

15.6 15.6 **FUD** 090 J A2 50

AMA: 2018,Jan,8; 2017,Jan,8; 2016,Jan,13; 2015,Jan,16

54520 Orchiectomy, simple (including subcapsular), with or without testicular prosthesis, scrotal or inguinal approach ♂

INCLUDES Huggins' orchiectomy

EXCLUDES *Lymphadenectomy, radical retroperitoneal (38780)*

Code also hernia repair, when performed (49505, 49507)

9.45 9.45 **FUD** 090 J A2 50

AMA: 2018,Jan,8; 2017,Jan,8; 2016,Jan,13; 2015,Jan,16

54522 Orchiectomy, partial ♂

EXCLUDES *Lymphadenectomy, radical retroperitoneal (38780)*

17.0 17.0 **FUD** 090 J A2 80 50

AMA: 2018,Jan,8; 2017,Jan,8; 2016,Jan,13; 2015,Jan,16

54530 Orchiectomy, radical, for tumor; inguinal approach ♂

EXCLUDES *Lymphadenectomy, radical retroperitoneal (38780)*

14.6 14.6 **FUD** 090 J A2 80 50

AMA: 2018,Jan,8; 2017,Jan,8; 2016,Jan,13; 2015,Jan,16

54535 with abdominal exploration ♂

EXCLUDES *Lymphadenectomy, radical retroperitoneal (38780)*

21.4 21.4 **FUD** 090 J 80 50

AMA: 2018,Jan,8; 2017,Jan,8; 2016,Jan,13; 2015,Jan,16

54550 Exploration for undescended testis (inguinal or scrotal area) ♂

14.2 14.2 **FUD** 090 J A2 80 50

AMA: 2018,Jan,8; 2017,Mar,10; 2017,Jan,8; 2016,Jan,13; 2015,Jan,16

54560 Exploration for undescended testis with abdominal exploration ♂

19.8 19.8 **FUD** 090 J G2 80 50

AMA: 2018,Jan,8; 2017,Jan,8; 2016,Jan,13; 2015,Jan,16

54600-54699 Open and Laparoscopic Testicular Procedures

54600 Reduction of torsion of testis, surgical, with or without fixation of contralateral testis ♂

13.1 13.1 **FUD** 090 J A2 50

AMA: 2018,Jan,8; 2017,Jan,8; 2016,Jan,13; 2015,Jan,16

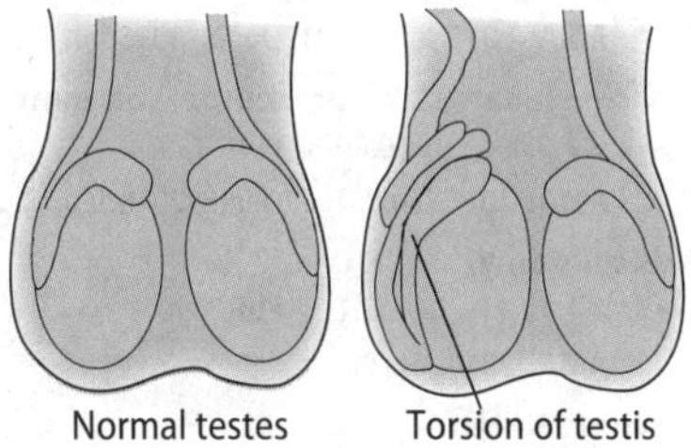

Normal testes Torsion of testis

54620 Fixation of contralateral testis (separate procedure) ♂

8.64 8.64 **FUD** 010 J A2 50

AMA: 2014,Jan,11

54640 Orchiopexy, inguinal or scrotal approach ♂

INCLUDES Bevan's operation
Koop inguinal orchiopexy
Prentice orchiopexy

EXCLUDES *Repair inguinal hernia with inguinal orchiopexy (49495-49525)*

13.8 13.8 **FUD** 090 J A2 80 50

AMA: 2018,Jan,8; 2017,Mar,10; 2017,Jan,8; 2016,Jan,13; 2015,Jan,16

54650 Orchiopexy, abdominal approach, for intra-abdominal testis (eg, Fowler-Stephens) ♂

EXCLUDES *Laparoscopic orchiopexy (54692)*

20.5 20.5 **FUD** 090 J 80 50

AMA: 2018,Jan,8; 2017,Jan,8; 2016,Jan,13; 2015,Jan,16

54660 Insertion of testicular prosthesis (separate procedure) ♂

10.3 10.3 **FUD** 090 J J8 80 50

AMA: 2018,Jan,8; 2017,Jan,8; 2016,Jan,13; 2015,Jan,16

54670 Suture or repair of testicular injury ♂

11.7 11.7 **FUD** 090 J A2 80 50

AMA: 2018,Jan,8; 2017,Jan,8; 2016,Jan,13; 2015,Jan,16

54680 Transplantation of testis(es) to thigh (because of scrotal destruction) ♂

22.7 22.7 **FUD** 090 J A2 80 50

AMA: 2018,Jan,8; 2017,Jan,8; 2016,Jan,13; 2015,Jan,16

54690 Laparoscopy, surgical; orchiectomy ♂

INCLUDES Diagnostic laparoscopy (49320)

18.9 18.9 **FUD** 090 J A2 80 50

AMA: 2019,Feb,10; 2018,Jan,8; 2017,Jan,8; 2016,Jan,13; 2015,Jan,16

54692 orchiopexy for intra-abdominal testis ♂

INCLUDES Diagnostic laparoscopy (49320)

21.9 21.9 **FUD** 090 J G2 50

AMA: 2018,Jan,8; 2017,Jan,8; 2016,Jan,13; 2015,Jan,16

54699 Unlisted laparoscopy procedure, testis ♂

0.00 0.00 **FUD** YYY J 80 50

AMA: 2018,Jan,8; 2017,Jan,8; 2016,Jan,13; 2015,Jan,16

54700-54901 Open Procedures of the Epididymis

54700 Incision and drainage of epididymis, testis and/or scrotal space (eg, abscess or hematoma) ♂

EXCLUDES *Debridement genitalia for necrotizing soft tissue infection (11004-11006)*

6.16 6.16 **FUD** 010 J A2 50

AMA: 2018,Jan,8; 2017,Jan,8; 2016,Jan,13; 2015,Jan,16

54800 Biopsy of epididymis, needle ♂

EXCLUDES *Fine needle aspiration (10021, [10004, 10005, 10006, 10007, 10008, 10009, 10010, 10011, 10012])*

88172-88173

3.64 3.64 **FUD** 000 J A2 80 50

AMA: 2019,Apr,4; 2018,Jan,8; 2017,Jan,8; 2016,Jan,13; 2015,Jan,16

54830 Excision of local lesion of epididymis ♂

10.7 10.7 **FUD** 090 J A2 80 50

AMA: 2018,Jan,8; 2017,Jan,8; 2016,Jan,13; 2015,Jan,16

54840 Excision of spermatocele, with or without epididymectomy ♂

9.29 9.29 **FUD** 090 J A2 50

AMA: 2018,Jan,8; 2017,Jan,8; 2016,Jan,13; 2015,Jan,16

54860 Epididymectomy; unilateral ♂

12.1 12.1 **FUD** 090 J A2

AMA: 2014,Jan,11

54861 bilateral ♂

16.3 16.3 **FUD** 090 J A2 80

AMA: 2014,Jan,11

54865 Exploration of epididymis, with or without biopsy ♂

10.3 10.3 **FUD** 090 J A2 80

AMA: 2014,Jan,11; 2007,Jul,5

54900 Epididymovasostomy, anastomosis of epididymis to vas deferens; unilateral ♂

EXCLUDES *Operating microscope (69990)*

23.1 23.1 **FUD** 090 J A2 80

AMA: 2018,Jan,8; 2017,Jan,8; 2016,Jan,13; 2015,Jan,16

54901 **bilateral** ♂
EXCLUDES *Operating microscope (69990)*
Facility RVU 30.5 Non-Facility RVU 30.5 FUD 090 J A2 80
AMA: 2018,Jan,8; 2017,Jan,8; 2016,Jan,13; 2015,Jan,16

55000-55180 Procedures of the Tunica Vaginalis and Scrotum

55000 **Puncture aspiration of hydrocele, tunica vaginalis, with or without injection of medication** ♂
Facility RVU 2.44 Non-Facility RVU 3.39 FUD 000 T P3 50
AMA: 2014,Jan,11

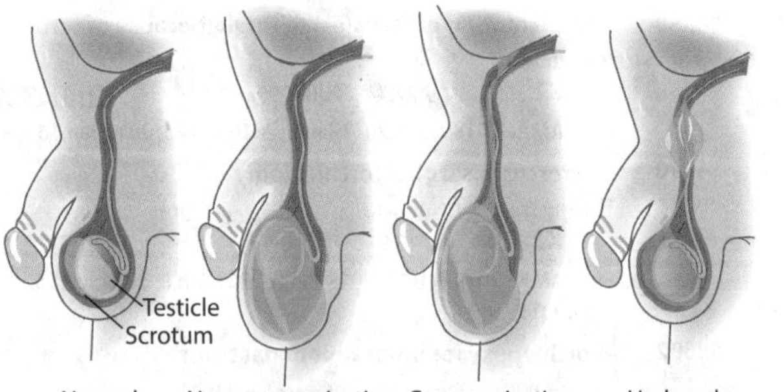

55040 **Excision of hydrocele; unilateral** ♂
EXCLUDES *Repair hernia with hydrocelectomy (49495-49501)*
Facility RVU 9.77 Non-Facility RVU 9.77 FUD 090 J A2
AMA: 2018,Jan,8; 2017,Nov,10; 2017,Jan,8; 2016,Jan,13; 2015,Jan,16

55041 **bilateral** ♂
EXCLUDES *Repair hernia with hydrocelectomy (49495-49501)*
Facility RVU 14.7 Non-Facility RVU 14.7 FUD 090 J A2
AMA: 2014,Jan,11

55060 **Repair of tunica vaginalis hydrocele (Bottle type)** ♂
Facility RVU 11.0 Non-Facility RVU 11.0 FUD 090 J A2 80 50
AMA: 2018,Jan,8; 2017,Jan,8; 2016,Jan,13; 2015,Jan,16

55100 **Drainage of scrotal wall abscess** ♂
EXCLUDES *Debridement genitalia for necrotizing soft tissue infection (11004-11006)*
Incision and drainage scrotal space (54700)
Facility RVU 4.80 Non-Facility RVU 6.28 FUD 010 J A2
AMA: 2014,Jan,11

55110 **Scrotal exploration** ♂
Facility RVU 11.1 Non-Facility RVU 11.1 FUD 090 J A2
AMA: 2014,Jan,11

55120 **Removal of foreign body in scrotum** ♂
Facility RVU 10.1 Non-Facility RVU 10.1 FUD 090 J A2 80
AMA: 2014,Jan,11

55150 **Resection of scrotum** ♂
EXCLUDES *Lesion excision skin, scrotum (11420-11426, 11620-11626)*
Facility RVU 14.2 Non-Facility RVU 14.2 FUD 090 J A2 80
AMA: 2014,Jan,11

55175 **Scrotoplasty; simple** ♂
Facility RVU 10.5 Non-Facility RVU 10.5 FUD 090 J A2 80
AMA: 2018,Jan,8; 2017,Jan,8; 2016,Jan,13; 2015,Jan,16

55180 **complicated** ♂
Facility RVU 20.0 Non-Facility RVU 20.0 FUD 090 J A2 80
AMA: 2014,Jan,11

55200-55680 Procedures of Other Male Genital Ducts and Glands

55200 **Vasotomy, cannulization with or without incision of vas, unilateral or bilateral (separate procedure)** ♂
Facility RVU 8.00 Non-Facility RVU 11.7 FUD 090 J A2 80
AMA: 2014,Jan,11

55250 **Vasectomy, unilateral or bilateral (separate procedure), including postoperative semen examination(s)** ♂
Facility RVU 6.58 Non-Facility RVU 10.6 FUD 090 J A2
AMA: 2018,Jan,8; 2017,Jan,8; 2016,Jan,13; 2015,Jan,16

55300 **Vasotomy for vasograms, seminal vesiculograms, or epididymograms, unilateral or bilateral** ♂
Code also biopsy testis and modifier 51 when combined (54505)
Radiology Crosswalk (74440)
Facility RVU 5.39 Non-Facility RVU 5.39 FUD 000 N N1 80
AMA: 2014,Jan,11

55400 **Vasovasostomy, vasovasorrhaphy** ♂
EXCLUDES *Operating microscope (69990)*
Facility RVU 14.4 Non-Facility RVU 14.4 FUD 090 J A2 80 50
AMA: 2018,Jan,8; 2017,Jan,8; 2016,Jan,13; 2015,Jan,16

55500 **Excision of hydrocele of spermatic cord, unilateral (separate procedure)** ♂
Facility RVU 11.3 Non-Facility RVU 11.3 FUD 090 J A2 80 50
AMA: 2018,Jan,8; 2017,Jan,8; 2016,Jan,13; 2015,Jan,16

55520 **Excision of lesion of spermatic cord (separate procedure)** ♂
Facility RVU 13.2 Non-Facility RVU 13.2 FUD 090 J A2 80 50
AMA: 2018,Jan,8; 2017,Jan,8; 2016,Jan,13; 2015,Jan,16

55530 **Excision of varicocele or ligation of spermatic veins for varicocele; (separate procedure)** ♂
Facility RVU 10.1 Non-Facility RVU 10.1 FUD 090 J A2 50
AMA: 2018,Jan,8; 2017,Jan,8; 2016,Jan,13; 2015,Jan,16

55535 **abdominal approach** ♂
Facility RVU 12.4 Non-Facility RVU 12.4 FUD 090 J A2 80 50
AMA: 2018,Jan,8; 2017,Jan,8; 2016,Jan,13; 2015,Jan,16

55540 **with hernia repair** ♂
Facility RVU 16.0 Non-Facility RVU 16.0 FUD 090 J A2 50
AMA: 2018,Jan,8; 2017,Jan,8; 2016,Jan,13; 2015,Jan,16

55550 **Laparoscopy, surgical, with ligation of spermatic veins for varicocele** ♂
INCLUDES Diagnostic laparoscopy (49320)
Facility RVU 12.3 Non-Facility RVU 12.3 FUD 090 J A2 80 50
AMA: 2018,Jan,8; 2017,Jan,8; 2016,Jan,13; 2015,Jan,16

55559 **Unlisted laparoscopy procedure, spermatic cord** ♂
Facility RVU 0.00 Non-Facility RVU 0.00 FUD YYY J 80 50
AMA: 2018,Jan,8; 2017,Jan,8; 2016,Jan,13; 2015,Jan,16

55600 **Vesiculotomy;** ♂
Facility RVU 12.1 Non-Facility RVU 12.1 FUD 090 J R2 80 50
AMA: 2014,Jan,11

55605 **complicated** ♂
Facility RVU 15.0 Non-Facility RVU 15.0 FUD 090 C 80 50
AMA: 2014,Jan,11

55650 **Vesiculectomy, any approach** ♂
Facility RVU 20.7 Non-Facility RVU 20.7 FUD 090 C 80 50
AMA: 2014,Jan,11

55680 **Excision of Mullerian duct cyst** ♂
EXCLUDES *Injection procedure (52010, 55300)*
Facility RVU 9.99 Non-Facility RVU 9.99 FUD 090 J A2 80 50
AMA: 2014,Jan,11

54901 — 55680

55700-55725 Procedures of Prostate: Incisional

55700 **Biopsy, prostate; needle or punch, single or multiple, any approach** ♂

EXCLUDES *Fine needle aspiration (10021, [10004, 10005, 10006, 10007, 10008, 10009, 10010, 10011, 10012])*
Needle biopsy prostate, saturation sampling for prostate mapping (55706)

(76942, 77002, 77012, 77021)

(88172-88173)

3.77 7.12 **FUD** 000 J A2

AMA: 2018,Jul,11; 2018,Jan,8; 2017,Jan,8; 2016,Jan,13; 2015,Jan,16

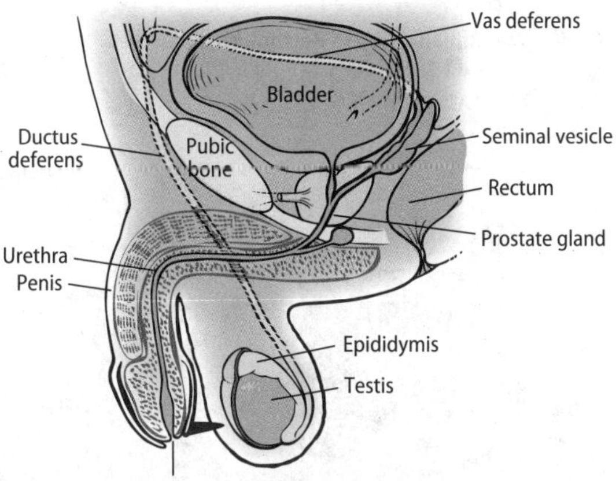

55705 **incisional, any approach** ♂

7.67 7.67 **FUD** 010 J A2

AMA: 2014,Jan,11

55706 **Biopsies, prostate, needle, transperineal, stereotactic template guided saturation sampling, including imaging guidance** ♂

EXCLUDES *Biopsy, prostate; needle or punch (55700)*

10.7 10.7 **FUD** 010 J G2 80

AMA: 2018,Jan,8; 2017,Jan,8; 2016,Jan,13; 2015,Jan,16

55720 **Prostatotomy, external drainage of prostatic abscess, any approach; simple** ♂

EXCLUDES *Drainage prostatic abscess, transurethral (52700)*

13.0 13.0 **FUD** 090 J A2 80

AMA: 2014,Jan,11

55725 **complicated** ♂

EXCLUDES *Drainage prostatic abscess, transurethral (52700)*

17.1 17.1 **FUD** 090 J A2 80

AMA: 2014,Jan,11

55801-55845 Open Prostatectomy

EXCLUDES *Limited pelvic lymphadenectomy for staging (separate procedure) (38562)*
Node dissection, independent (38770-38780)
Transurethral prostate:
Destruction (53850-53852)
Resection (52601-52640)

55801 **Prostatectomy, perineal, subtotal (including control of postoperative bleeding, vasectomy, meatotomy, urethral calibration and/or dilation, and internal urethrotomy)** ♂

31.6 31.6 **FUD** 090 C 80

AMA: 2014,Jan,11; 2003,Jun,6

55810 **Prostatectomy, perineal radical;** ♂

INCLUDES Walsh modified radical prostatectomy

37.8 37.8 **FUD** 090 C 80

AMA: 2014,Jan,11; 2003,Jun,6

55812 **with lymph node biopsy(s) (limited pelvic lymphadenectomy)** ♂

46.4 46.4 **FUD** 090 C 80

AMA: 2014,Jan,11

55815 **with bilateral pelvic lymphadenectomy, including external iliac, hypogastric and obturator nodes** ♂

EXCLUDES *When performed on separate days, report:*
Pelvic lymphadenectomy, bilateral, and append modifier 50 (38770)
Perineal radical prostatectomy (55810)

50.9 50.9 **FUD** 090 C 80

AMA: 2014,Jan,11

55821 **Prostatectomy (including control of postoperative bleeding, vasectomy, meatotomy, urethral calibration and/or dilation, and internal urethrotomy); suprapubic, subtotal, 1 or 2 stages** ♂

25.2 25.2 **FUD** 090 C 80

AMA: 2014,Jan,11; 2003,Jun,6

55831 **retropubic, subtotal** ♂

27.3 27.3 **FUD** 090 C 80

AMA: 2014,Jan,11; 2003,Jun,6

55840 **Prostatectomy, retropubic radical, with or without nerve sparing;** ♂

EXCLUDES *Prostatectomy, radical retropubic, performed laparoscopically (55866)*

33.8 33.8 **FUD** 090 C 80

AMA: 2014,Jan,11; 2003,Jun,6

55842 **with lymph node biopsy(s) (limited pelvic lymphadenectomy)** ♂

EXCLUDES *Prostatectomy, retropubic radical, performed laparoscopically (55866)*

33.8 33.8 **FUD** 090 C 80

AMA: 2014,Jan,11; 2003,Jun,6

55845 **with bilateral pelvic lymphadenectomy, including external iliac, hypogastric, and obturator nodes** ♂

EXCLUDES *Prostatectomy, retropubic radical, performed laparoscopically (55866)*
When performed on separate days, report:
Pelvic lymphadenectomy, bilateral, and append modifier 50 (38770)
Radical prostatectomy, retropubic, with or without nerve sparing (55840)

39.3 39.3 **FUD** 090 C 80

AMA: 2014,Jan,11; 2003,Jun,6

55860-55865 Prostate Exposure for Radiation Source Application

55860 **Exposure of prostate, any approach, for insertion of radioactive substance;** ♂

EXCLUDES *Interstitial radioelement application (77770-77772, 77778)*

25.3 25.3 **FUD** 090 J G2

AMA: 2014,Jan,11

55862 **with lymph node biopsy(s) (limited pelvic lymphadenectomy)** ♂

31.6 31.6 **FUD** 090 C 80

AMA: 2014,Jan,11

55865 **with bilateral pelvic lymphadenectomy, including external iliac, hypogastric and obturator nodes** ♂

38.5 38.5 **FUD** 090 C 80

AMA: 2014,Jan,11

55866 Laparoscopic Prostatectomy

55866 **Laparoscopy, surgical prostatectomy, retropubic radical, including nerve sparing, includes robotic assistance, when performed** ♂

INCLUDES Diagnostic laparoscopy (49320)

EXCLUDES *Open method (55840)*

41.6 41.6 **FUD** 090 J 80

AMA: 2018,Jan,8; 2017,Jan,8; 2016,Jan,13; 2015,Jan,16

55870-55899 Miscellaneous Prostate Procedures

55870 Electroejaculation ♂

EXCLUDES *Artificial insemination (58321-58322)*

4.10 | 5.04 | **FUD** 000 | T P3

AMA: 2014,Jan,11; 1991,Win,1

55873 Cryosurgical ablation of the prostate (includes ultrasonic guidance and monitoring) ♂

22.0 | 175. | **FUD** 090 | J J8

AMA: 2019,Sep,10; 2018,Jan,8; 2017,Jan,8; 2016,Jan,13; 2015,Sep,12; 2015,Jan,16

55874 Transperineal placement of biodegradable material, peri-prostatic, single or multiple injection(s), including image guidance, when performed ♂

INCLUDES Ultrasound guidance (76942)

4.77 | 87.0 | **FUD** 000 | T G2

55875 Transperineal placement of needles or catheters into prostate for interstitial radioelement application, with or without cystoscopy ♂

EXCLUDES *Placement needles/catheters for interstitial radioelement application, pelvic organs/genitalia, except prostate (55920)*

Code also interstitial radioelement application (77770-77772, 77778)

(76965)

22.2 | 22.2 | **FUD** 090 | J A2 80

AMA: 2018,Jan,8; 2017,Jan,8; 2016,Jan,13; 2015,Jan,16

55876 Placement of interstitial device(s) for radiation therapy guidance (eg, fiducial markers, dosimeter), prostate (via needle, any approach), single or multiple ♂

Code also supply device

(76942, 77002, 77012, 77021)

2.91 | 4.16 | **FUD** 000 | S P3

AMA: 2018,Jan,8; 2017,Jan,8; 2016,Jun,3; 2016,Jan,13; 2015,Jan,16

● **55880 Ablation of malignant prostate tissue, transrectal, with high intensity-focused ultrasound (HIFU), including ultrasound guidance**

55899 Unlisted procedure, male genital system ♂

0.00 | 0.00 | **FUD** YYY | T 80

AMA: 2020,Aug,6; 2019,Dec,12; 2019,Jun,14; 2018,Jan,8; 2017,Jan,8; 2017,Jan,6; 2016,Jan,13; 2015,Jun,5; 2015,Jan,16

55920 Insertion Brachytherapy Catheters/Needles Pelvis/Genitalia, Male/Female

55920 Placement of needles or catheters into pelvic organs and/or genitalia (except prostate) for subsequent interstitial radioelement application

EXCLUDES *Insertion Heyman capsules for brachytherapy (58346)*
Insertion vaginal ovoids and/or uterine tandems for brachytherapy (57155)
Placement catheters or needles, prostate (55875)

13.0 | 13.0 | **FUD** 000 | J G2 80

AMA: 2018,Jan,8; 2017,Jan,8; 2016,Jan,13; 2015,Jan,16

55970-55980 Transsexual Surgery

CMS: 100-02,16,10 Exclusions from Coverage; 100-02,16,180 Services Related to Noncovered Procedures

55970 Intersex surgery; male to female ♂

0.00 | 0.00 | **FUD** YYY | J

AMA: 2014,Jan,11

55980 female to male ♀

0.00 | 0.00 | **FUD** YYY | J

AMA: 2014,Jan,11

56405-56420 Incision and Drainage of Abscess

EXCLUDES *Incision and drainage Skene's gland cyst/abscess (53060)*
Incision and drainage subcutaneous abscess/cyst/furuncle (10040, 10060, 10061)

56405 Incision and drainage of vulva or perineal abscess ♀

3.43 | 3.69 | **FUD** 010 | T P3

AMA: 2019,Jul,6

56420 Incision and drainage of Bartholin's gland abscess ♀

2.97 | 4.47 | **FUD** 010 | T P2

AMA: 2019,Jul,6

56440-56442 Other Female Genital Incisional Procedures

EXCLUDES *Incision and drainage subcutaneous abscess/cyst/furuncle (10040, 10060, 10061)*

56440 Marsupialization of Bartholin's gland cyst ♀

5.25 | 5.25 | **FUD** 010 | J A2

AMA: 2019,Jul,6

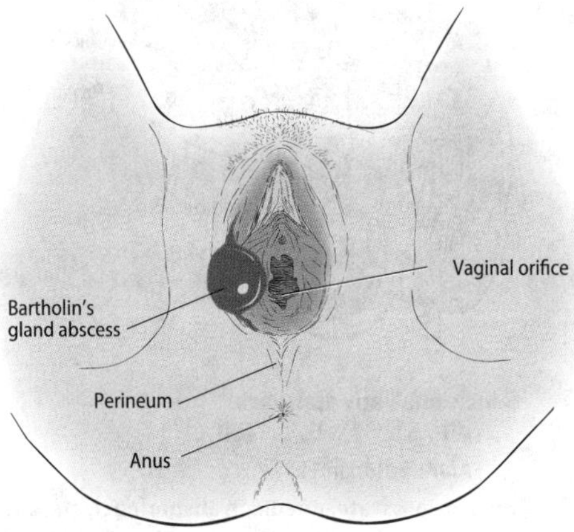

56441 Lysis of labial adhesions ♀

4.09 | 4.33 | **FUD** 010 | J A2 80

AMA: 2019,Jul,6

56442 Hymenotomy, simple incision ♀

1.36 | 1.36 | **FUD** 000 | J A2 80

AMA: 2019,Jul,6

56501-56515 Destruction of Vulvar Lesions, Any Method

EXCLUDES *Excision/fulguration/destruction:*
Skene's glands (53270)
Urethral caruncle (53265)

56501 Destruction of lesion(s), vulva; simple (eg, laser surgery, electrosurgery, cryosurgery, chemosurgery) ♀

3.60 | 4.69 | **FUD** 010 | T P3

AMA: 2019,Aug,10; 2019,Jul,6

56515 extensive (eg, laser surgery, electrosurgery, cryosurgery, chemosurgery) ♀

5.97 | 7.25 | **FUD** 010 | T A2

AMA: 2019,Aug,10; 2019,Jul,6

56605-56606 Vulvar and Perineal Biopsies

EXCLUDES *Excision local lesion (11420-11426, 11620-11626)*

56605 Biopsy of vulva or perineum (separate procedure); 1 lesion ♀

1.71 | 2.43 | **FUD** 000 | T P3

AMA: 2019,Jul,6; 2019,Jan,9; 2018,Jan,8; 2017,Jan,8; 2016,Jan,13; 2015,Jan,16

\+ **56606 each separate additional lesion (List separately in addition to code for primary procedure)** ♀

Code first (56605)

0.86 | 1.11 | **FUD** ZZZ | N N1

AMA: 2019,Jul,6; 2019,Jan,9

56620-56640 Vulvectomy Procedures

INCLUDES Removal:
Greater than 80% vulvar area - complete procedure
Less than 80% vulvar area - partial procedure
Skin and deep subcutaneous tissue - radical procedure
Skin and superficial subcutaneous tissues - simple procedure

EXCLUDES *Skin graft (15004-15005, 15120-15121, 15240-15241)*

56620 Vulvectomy simple; partial ♀
15.9 15.9 FUD 090 J A2 80
AMA: 2019,Jul,6; 2019,Jan,14; 2018,Jan,8; 2017,Jan,8; 2016,Jan,13; 2015,Jan,16

56625 complete ♀
18.6 18.6 FUD 090 J A2 80
AMA: 2019,Jul,6

56630 Vulvectomy, radical, partial; ♀
Code also lymph node biopsy/excision when partial radical vulvectomy with inguinofemoral lymph node biopsy without inguinofemoral lymphadenectomy performed (38531)
27.0 27.0 FUD 090 C 80
AMA: 2019,Jul,6; 2019,Feb,8

56631 with unilateral inguinofemoral lymphadenectomy ♀
INCLUDES Bassett's operation
34.4 34.4 FUD 090 C 80
AMA: 2019,Jul,6; 2019,Feb,8

56632 with bilateral inguinofemoral lymphadenectomy ♀
INCLUDES Bassett's operation
40.2 40.2 FUD 090 C 80
AMA: 2019,Jul,6; 2019,Feb,8

56633 Vulvectomy, radical, complete; ♀
INCLUDES Bassett's operation
34.9 34.9 FUD 090 C 80
AMA: 2019,Jul,6; 2019,Feb,8

56634 with unilateral inguinofemoral lymphadenectomy ♀
INCLUDES Bassett's operation
36.8 36.8 FUD 090 C 80
AMA: 2019,Jul,6; 2019,Feb,8

56637 with bilateral inguinofemoral lymphadenectomy ♀
INCLUDES Bassett's operation
Code also lymph node biopsy/excision when complete radical vulvectomy with inguinofemoral lymph node biopsy without inguinofemoral lymphadenectomy performed (38531)
43.9 43.9 FUD 090 C 80
AMA: 2019,Jul,6; 2019,Feb,8

56640 Vulvectomy, radical, complete, with inguinofemoral, iliac, and pelvic lymphadenectomy ♀
INCLUDES Bassett's operation
EXCLUDES *Lymphadenectomy (38760-38780)*
43.3 43.3 FUD 090 C 80 50

AMA: 2019,Jul,6; 2019,Feb,8

56700-56740 Other Excisional Procedures: External Female Genitalia

56700 Partial hymenectomy or revision of hymenal ring ♀
5.38 5.38 FUD 010 J A2 80
AMA: 2019,Jul,6

56740 Excision of Bartholin's gland or cyst ♀
EXCLUDES *Excision/fulguration/marsupialization:*
Skene's glands (53270)
Urethral carcinoma (53220)
Urethral caruncle (53265)
Urethral diverticulum (53230, 53240)
8.92 8.92 FUD 010 J A2 50
AMA: 2019,Jul,6

56800-56810 Repair/Reconstruction External Female Genitalia

EXCLUDES *Repair urethra for mucosal prolapse (53275)*

56800 Plastic repair of introitus ♀
INCLUDES Emmet's operation
7.17 7.17 FUD 010 J A2 80
AMA: 2019,Jul,6

56805 Clitoroplasty for intersex state ♀
33.6 33.6 FUD 090 J G2 80
AMA: 2019,Jul,6

56810 Perineoplasty, repair of perineum, nonobstetrical (separate procedure) ♀
INCLUDES Emmet's operation
EXCLUDES *Genitalia wound repair (12001-12007, 12041-12047, 13131-13133)*
Introitus plastic repair (56800)
Sphincteroplasty, anal (46750-46751)
Vaginal/perineum recent injury repair, nonobstetrical (57210)
7.72 7.72 FUD 010 J A2 80
AMA: 2019,Jul,6

56820-56821 Vulvar Colposcopy with/without Biopsy

EXCLUDES *Colposcopic procedures and/or examinations:*
Cervix (57452-57461)
Vagina (57420-57421)

56820 Colposcopy of the vulva; ♀
2.46 3.28 FUD 000 T P3
AMA: 2019,Jul,6; 2018,Jan,8; 2017,Jan,8; 2016,Jan,13; 2015,Jan,16

56821 with biopsy(s) ♀
3.28 4.36 FUD 000 T P3
AMA: 2019,Jul,6; 2018,Jan,8; 2017,Jan,8; 2016,Jan,13; 2015,Jan,16

57000-57023 Incisional Procedures: Vagina

57000 Colpotomy; with exploration ♀
5.44 5.44 FUD 010 J A2 80
AMA: 2019,Jul,6; 2018,Jan,8; 2017,Jan,8; 2016,Jan,13; 2015,Jan,16

57010 with drainage of pelvic abscess ♀
INCLUDES Laroyenne operation
12.9 12.9 FUD 090 J A2 80
AMA: 2019,Jul,6

57020 Colpocentesis (separate procedure) ♀
2.35 3.17 FUD 000 J A2 80
AMA: 2019,Jul,6

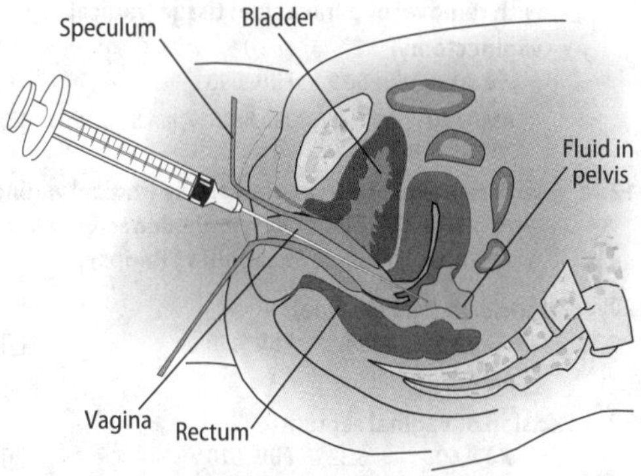

The physician aspirates matter from the pelvis through a needle inserted through the vaginal wall

57022 **Incision and drainage of vaginal hematoma; obstetrical/postpartum** ♀
4.86 4.86 **FUD** 010 J R2 80
AMA: 2019,Jul,6

57023 **non-obstetrical (eg, post-trauma, spontaneous bleeding)** ♀
9.16 9.16 **FUD** 010 J A2 80
AMA: 2019,Jul,6

57061-57065 Destruction of Vaginal Lesions, Any Method

CMS: 100-03,140.5 Laser Procedures

57061 **Destruction of vaginal lesion(s); simple (eg, laser surgery, electrosurgery, cryosurgery, chemosurgery)** ♀
3.09 4.05 **FUD** 010 J P3
AMA: 2019,Jul,6; 2018,Jan,8; 2017,Jan,8; 2016,Jan,13; 2015,Jan,16

57065 **extensive (eg, laser surgery, electrosurgery, cryosurgery, chemosurgery)** ♀
5.08 5.88 **FUD** 010 J A2
AMA: 2019,Jul,6; 2018,Jan,8; 2017,Jan,8; 2016,Jan,13; 2015,Jan,16

57100-57135 Excisional Procedures: Vagina

57100 **Biopsy of vaginal mucosa; simple (separate procedure)** ♀
1.90 2.76 **FUD** 000 T P3
AMA: 2019,Jul,6

57105 **extensive, requiring suture (including cysts)** ♀
3.75 4.19 **FUD** 010 J A2
AMA: 2019,Jul,6

57106 **Vaginectomy, partial removal of vaginal wall;** ♀
14.5 14.5 **FUD** 090 J 80
AMA: 2019,Jul,6; 2018,Jan,8; 2017,Jan,8; 2016,Jan,13; 2015,Jan,16

57107 **with removal of paravaginal tissue (radical vaginectomy)** ♀
41.5 41.5 **FUD** 090 J 80
AMA: 2019,Jul,6; 2018,Jan,8; 2017,Jan,8; 2016,Jan,13; 2015,Jan,16

57109 **with removal of paravaginal tissue (radical vaginectomy) with bilateral total pelvic lymphadenectomy and para-aortic lymph node sampling (biopsy)** ♀
50.8 50.8 **FUD** 090 J 80
AMA: 2019,Jul,6; 2018,Jan,8; 2017,Jan,8; 2016,Jan,13; 2015,Jan,16

57110 **Vaginectomy, complete removal of vaginal wall;** ♀
25.3 25.3 **FUD** 090 C 80
AMA: 2019,Jul,6; 2018,Jan,8; 2017,Jan,8; 2016,Jan,13; 2015,Jan,16

57111 **with removal of paravaginal tissue (radical vaginectomy)** ♀
50.9 50.9 **FUD** 090 C 80
AMA: 2019,Jul,6; 2018,Jan,8; 2017,Jan,8; 2016,Jan,13; 2015,Jan,16

~~**57112**~~ ~~**with removal of paravaginal tissue (radical vaginectomy) with bilateral total pelvic lymphadenectomy and para-aortic lymph node sampling (biopsy)**~~

57120 **Colpocleisis (Le Fort type)** ♀
14.6 14.6 **FUD** 090 J G2 80
AMA: 2019,Jul,6

57130 **Excision of vaginal septum** ♀
4.60 5.32 **FUD** 010 J A2 80
AMA: 2019,Jul,6

57135 **Excision of vaginal cyst or tumor** ♀
5.05 5.80 **FUD** 010 J A2
AMA: 2019,Jul,6

57150-57180 Irrigation/Insertion/Introduction Vaginal Medication or Supply

57150 **Irrigation of vagina and/or application of medicament for treatment of bacterial, parasitic, or fungoid disease** ♀
0.78 1.54 **FUD** 000 Q1 N1
AMA: 2019,Jul,6

57155 **Insertion of uterine tandem and/or vaginal ovoids for clinical brachytherapy** ♀
EXCLUDES *Insertion radioelement sources or ribbons (77761-77763, 77770-77772)*
Placement needles or catheters into pelvic organs and/or genitalia (except prostate) for interstitial radioelement application (55920)
8.09 10.6 **FUD** 000 J A2
AMA: 2019,Jul,6; 2018,Jan,8; 2017,Jan,8; 2016,Jan,13; 2015,Jan,16

57156 **Insertion of a vaginal radiation afterloading apparatus for clinical brachytherapy** ♀
4.27 5.92 **FUD** 000 T G2 80
AMA: 2019,Jul,6

57160 **Fitting and insertion of pessary or other intravaginal support device** ♀
1.33 1.79 **FUD** 000 T P3
AMA: 2019,Jul,6; 2018,Jan,8; 2017,Jan,8; 2016,Jan,13; 2015,Jan,16

57170 **Diaphragm or cervical cap fitting with instructions** ♀
1.37 1.85 **FUD** 000 T P3 80
AMA: 2019,Jul,6

57180 **Introduction of any hemostatic agent or pack for spontaneous or traumatic nonobstetrical vaginal hemorrhage (separate procedure)** ♀
3.11 4.37 **FUD** 010 T A2
AMA: 2019,Jul,6; 2018,Jan,8; 2017,Jan,8; 2016,Jan,13; 2015,Jan,16

57200-57335 Vaginal Repair and Reconstruction

EXCLUDES *Marshall-Marchetti-Kranz type urethral suspension, abdominal approach (51840-51841)*
Urethral suspension performed laparoscopically (51990)

57200 **Colporrhaphy, suture of injury of vagina (nonobstetrical)** ♀
8.87 8.87 **FUD** 090 J A2 80
AMA: 2019,Jul,6

57210 **Colpoperineorrhaphy, suture of injury of vagina and/or perineum (nonobstetrical)** ♀
10.6 10.6 **FUD** 090 J A2 80
AMA: 2019,Jul,6

57220 **Plastic operation on urethral sphincter, vaginal approach (eg, Kelly urethral plication)** ♀
9.24 9.24 **FUD** 090 J A2 80
AMA: 2019,Jul,6

57230 **Plastic repair of urethrocele** ♀
11.3 11.3 **FUD** 090 J A2 80
AMA: 2019,Jul,6

57240 **Anterior colporrhaphy, repair of cystocele with or without repair of urethrocele, including cystourethroscopy, when performed** ♀
INCLUDES Cystourethroscopy (52000)
17.0 17.0 **FUD** 090 J A2 80
AMA: 2019,Jul,6; 2018,Jan,8; 2017,Jan,8; 2016,Jan,13; 2015,Jan,16

57250 **Posterior colporrhaphy, repair of rectocele with or without perineorrhaphy** ♀

INCLUDES Rectocele repair (separate procedure) without posterior colporrhaphy (45560)

17.0 17.0 FUD 090 J A2 80

AMA: 2019,Jul,6; 2018,Jan,8; 2017,Jan,8; 2016,Jan,13; 2015,Jan,16

57260 **Combined anteroposterior colporrhaphy, including cystourethroscopy, when performed;** ♀

INCLUDES Cystourethroscopy (52000)

21.7 21.7 FUD 090 J A2 80

AMA: 2019,Jul,6; 2018,Jan,8; 2017,Jan,8; 2016,Jan,13; 2015,Jan,16

57265 **with enterocele repair** ♀

INCLUDES Cystourethroscopy (52000)

24.4 24.4 FUD 090 J A2 80

AMA: 2019,Jul,6; 2018,Jan,8; 2017,Jan,8; 2016,Jan,13; 2015,Jan,16

\+ **57267** **Insertion of mesh or other prosthesis for repair of pelvic floor defect, each site (anterior, posterior compartment), vaginal approach (List separately in addition to code for primary procedure)** ♀

Code first (45560, 57240-57265, 57285)

7.25 7.25 FUD ZZZ N N1 80

AMA: 2019,Jul,6; 2018,Jan,8; 2017,Jan,8; 2016,Jan,13; 2015,Jan,16

57268 **Repair of enterocele, vaginal approach (separate procedure)** ♀

13.9 13.9 FUD 090 J A2 80

AMA: 2019,Jul,6; 2018,Jan,8; 2017,Jan,8; 2016,Jan,13; 2015,Jan,16

57270 **Repair of enterocele, abdominal approach (separate procedure)** ♀

23.0 23.0 FUD 090 C 80

AMA: 2019,Jul,6; 2018,Jan,8; 2017,Jan,8; 2016,Jan,13; 2015,Jan,16

57280 **Colpopexy, abdominal approach** ♀

27.2 27.2 FUD 090 C 80

AMA: 2019,Jul,6; 2018,Jan,8; 2017,Jan,8; 2016,Jan,13; 2015,Jan,16

57282 **Colpopexy, vaginal; extra-peritoneal approach (sacrospinous, iliococcygeus)** ♀

15.1 15.1 FUD 090 J 80

AMA: 2019,Jul,6; 2018,Jan,8; 2017,Jan,8; 2016,Jan,13; 2015,Jan,16

57283 **intra-peritoneal approach (uterosacral, levator myorrhaphy)** ♀

EXCLUDES *Excision cervical stump (57556)*

Vaginal hysterectomy (58263, 58270, 58280, 58292, 58294)

19.6 19.6 FUD 090 J 80

AMA: 2019,Jul,6; 2018,Jan,8; 2017,Jan,8; 2016,Jan,13; 2015,Jan,16

57284 **Paravaginal defect repair (including repair of cystocele, if performed); open abdominal approach** ♀

EXCLUDES *Anterior colporrhaphy (57240)*

Anterior vesicourethropexy (51840-51841)

Combined anteroposterior colporrhaphy (57260-57265)

Hysterectomy (58152, 58267)

Laparoscopy, surgical; urethral suspension for stress incontinence (51990)

23.8 23.8 FUD 090 J 80

AMA: 2019,Jul,6; 2018,Jan,8; 2017,Jan,8; 2016,Jan,13; 2015,Jan,16

57285 **vaginal approach** ♀

EXCLUDES *Anterior colporrhaphy (57240)*

Combined anteroposterior colporrhaphy (57260-57265)

Laparoscopy, surgical; urethral suspension for stress incontinence (51990)

Vaginal hysterectomy (58267)

19.2 19.2 FUD 090 J 80

AMA: 2019,Jul,6; 2018,Jan,8; 2017,Jan,8; 2016,Jan,13; 2015,Jan,16

57287 **Removal or revision of sling for stress incontinence (eg, fascia or synthetic)** ♀

20.6 20.6 FUD 090 Q2 G2 80

AMA: 2019,Jul,6; 2018,Jan,8; 2017,Jan,8; 2016,Jan,13; 2015,Jan,16

57288 **Sling operation for stress incontinence (eg, fascia or synthetic)** ♀

INCLUDES Millin-Read operation

EXCLUDES *Sling operation for stress incontinence performed laparoscopically (51992)*

21.1 21.1 FUD 090 J J8 80

AMA: 2019,Jul,6; 2019,Feb,10; 2018,Jan,8; 2017,Jan,8; 2016,Jan,13; 2015,Jan,16

57289 **Pereyra procedure, including anterior colporrhaphy** ♀

21.7 21.7 FUD 090 J A2 80

AMA: 2019,Jul,6; 2018,Jan,8; 2017,Jan,8; 2016,Jan,13; 2015,Jan,16

57291 **Construction of artificial vagina; without graft** ♀

INCLUDES McIndoe vaginal construction

15.6 15.6 FUD 090 J A2 80

AMA: 2019,Jul,6

57292 **with graft** ♀

23.9 23.9 FUD 090 J 80

AMA: 2019,Jul,6

57295 **Revision (including removal) of prosthetic vaginal graft; vaginal approach** ♀

EXCLUDES *Laparoscopic approach (57426)*

14.2 14.2 FUD 090 J G2 80

AMA: 2019,Jul,6

57296 **open abdominal approach** ♀

EXCLUDES *Laparoscopic approach (57426)*

27.4 27.4 FUD 090 C 80

AMA: 2019,Jul,6

57300 **Closure of rectovaginal fistula; vaginal or transanal approach** ♀

17.0 17.0 FUD 090 J A2 80

AMA: 2019,Jul,6

57305 **abdominal approach** ♀

27.9 27.9 FUD 090 C 80

AMA: 2019,Jul,6

57307 **abdominal approach, with concomitant colostomy** ♀

30.3 30.3 FUD 090 C 80

AMA: 2019,Jul,6

57308 **transperineal approach, with perineal body reconstruction, with or without levator plication** ♀

19.0 19.0 FUD 090 C 80

AMA: 2019,Jul,6

57310 **Closure of urethrovaginal fistula;** ♀

13.8 13.8 FUD 090 J G2 80

AMA: 2019,Jul,6

57311 **with bulbocavernosus transplant** ♀

15.6 15.6 FUD 090 C 80

AMA: 2019,Jul,6

57320 **Closure of vesicovaginal fistula; vaginal approach** ♀

EXCLUDES *Cystostomy, concomitant (51020-51040, 51101-51102)*

15.8 15.8 **FUD** 090 J G2 80

AMA: 2019,Jul,6

57330 **transvesical and vaginal approach** ♀

EXCLUDES *Vesicovaginal fistula closure, abdominal approach (51900)*

21.8 21.8 **FUD** 090 J 80

AMA: 2019,Jul,6

57335 **Vaginoplasty for intersex state** ♀

33.9 33.9 **FUD** 090 J 80

AMA: 2019,Jul,6

57400-57415 Treatment of Vaginal Disorders Under Anesthesia

57400 **Dilation of vagina under anesthesia (other than local)** ♀

3.81 3.81 **FUD** 000 J A2 80

AMA: 2019,Jul,6

57410 **Pelvic examination under anesthesia (other than local)** ♀

3.05 3.05 **FUD** 000 J A2

AMA: 2019,Jul,6; 2018,Jan,8; 2017,Jan,8; 2016,Jan,13; 2015,Jan,16

57415 **Removal of impacted vaginal foreign body (separate procedure) under anesthesia (other than local)** ♀

EXCLUDES *Removal impacted vaginal foreign body without anesthesia, report with appropriate E/M code*

4.89 4.89 **FUD** 010 J A2 80

AMA: 2019,Jul,6

57420-57426 Endoscopic Vaginal Procedures

57420 **Colposcopy of the entire vagina, with cervix if present;** ♀

EXCLUDES *Colposcopic procedures and/or examinations:*
Cervix (57452-57461)
Vulva (56820-56821)

Code also computer-aided cervical mapping during colposcopy (57465)

Code also endometrial sampling (biopsy) performed same time as colposcopy (58110)

Code also modifier 51 for colposcopic procedures different sites, as appropriate

2.62 3.61 **FUD** 000 T P3

AMA: 2019,Jul,6; 2018,Jan,8; 2017,Jan,8; 2016,Jan,13; 2015,Jan,16

57421 **with biopsy(s) of vagina/cervix** ♀

EXCLUDES *Colposcopic procedures and/or examinations:*
Cervix (57452-57461)
Vulva (56820-56821)

Code also computer-aided cervical mapping during colposcopy (57465)

Code also endometrial sampling (biopsy) performed same time as colposcopy (58110)

Code also modifier 51 for colposcopic procedures multiple sites, as appropriate

3.55 4.86 **FUD** 000 T P3

AMA: 2019,Jul,6; 2018,Jan,8; 2017,Jan,8; 2016,Jan,13; 2015,Jan,16

57423 **Paravaginal defect repair (including repair of cystocele, if performed), laparoscopic approach** ♀

EXCLUDES *Anterior colporrhaphy (57240)*
Anterior vesicourethropexy (51840-51841)
Combined anteroposterior colporrhaphy (57260)
Diagnostic laparoscopy (49320)
Hysterectomy (58152, 58267)
Laparoscopy, surgical; urethral suspension for stress incontinence (51990)

26.8 26.8 **FUD** 090 J 80

AMA: 2019,Jul,6; 2018,Jan,8; 2017,Jan,8; 2016,Jan,13; 2015,Jan,16

57425 **Laparoscopy, surgical, colpopexy (suspension of vaginal apex)** ♀

27.6 27.6 **FUD** 090 J 80

AMA: 2019,Jul,6

57426 **Revision (including removal) of prosthetic vaginal graft, laparoscopic approach** ♀

EXCLUDES *Open abdominal approach (57296)*
Vaginal approach (57295)

24.8 24.8 **FUD** 090 J G2 80

AMA: 2019,Jul,6

57452-57465 Endoscopic Cervical Procedures

EXCLUDES *Colposcopic procedures and/or examinations:*
Vagina (57420-57421)
Vulva (56820-56821)

Code also endometrial sampling (biopsy) performed same time as colposcopy (58110)

57452 **Colposcopy of the cervix including upper/adjacent vagina;** ♀

Code also computer-aided cervical mapping during colposcopy (57465)

2.64 3.45 **FUD** 000 T P3

AMA: 2019,Jul,6; 2018,Jan,8; 2017,Jan,8; 2016,Jan,13; 2015,Jan,16

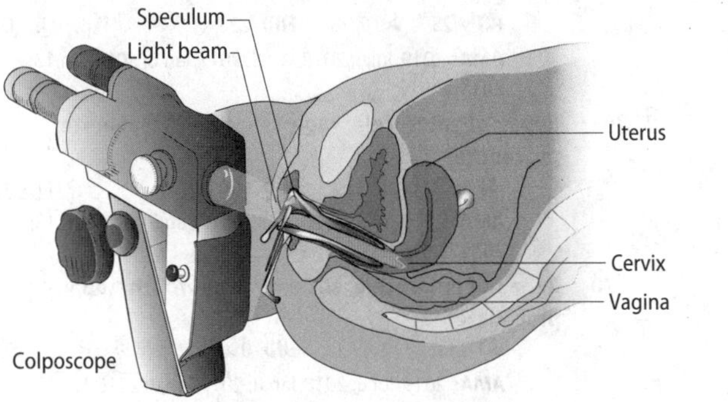

57454 **with biopsy(s) of the cervix and endocervical curettage** ♀

INCLUDES Colposcopy cervix (57452)

Code also computer-aided cervical mapping during colposcopy (57465)

3.89 4.71 **FUD** 000 T P3

AMA: 2019,Jul,6; 2018,Jan,8; 2017,Jan,8; 2016,Jan,13; 2015,Jan,16

57455 **with biopsy(s) of the cervix** ♀

INCLUDES Colposcopy cervix (57452)

Code also computer-aided cervical mapping during colposcopy (57465)

3.19 4.44 **FUD** 000 T P3

AMA: 2019,Jul,6; 2018,Jan,8; 2017,Jan,8; 2016,Jan,13; 2015,Jan,16

57456 **with endocervical curettage** ♀

INCLUDES Colposcopy cervix (57452)

EXCLUDES *Colposcopy cervix including upper/adjacent vagina; with loop electrode conization cervix (57461)*

Code also computer-aided cervical mapping during colposcopy (57465)

2.90 3.95 **FUD** 000 T P3

AMA: 2019,Jul,6; 2018,Jan,8; 2017,Jan,8; 2016,Jan,13; 2015,Jan,16

57460 **with loop electrode biopsy(s) of the cervix** ♀

INCLUDES Colposcopy cervix (57452)

Code also computer-aided cervical mapping during colposcopy (57465)

4.66 8.78 **FUD** 000 J P3

AMA: 2019,Jul,6; 2018,Jan,8; 2017,Jan,8; 2016,Jan,13; 2015,Jan,16

57461 **with loop electrode conization of the cervix** ♀

INCLUDES Colposcopy cervix (57452)

EXCLUDES *Colposcopy cervix including upper/adjacent vagina; with endocervical curettage (57456)*

Code also computer-aided cervical mapping during colposcopy (57465)

5.39 | 9.85 | FUD 000 | J P3

AMA: 2019,Jul,6; 2018,Jan,8; 2017,Jan,8; 2016,Jan,13; 2015,Jan,16

● + 57465 **Computer-aided mapping of cervix uteri during colposcopy, including optical dynamic spectral imaging and algorithmic quantification of the acetowhitening effect (List separately in addition to code for primary procedure)**

Code first (57420-57421, 57452-57461)

0.00 | 0.00 | FUD 000

57500-57556 Cervical Procedures: Multiple Techniques

EXCLUDES *Radical surgical procedures (58200-58240)*

57500 **Biopsy of cervix, single or multiple, or local excision of lesion, with or without fulguration (separate procedure)** ♀

2.17 | 4.11 | FUD 000 | T P3

AMA: 2019,Jul,6

57505 **Endocervical curettage (not done as part of a dilation and curettage)** ♀

2.90 | 3.69 | FUD 010 | T P3

AMA: 2019,Jul,6; 2018,Jan,8; 2017,Jan,8; 2016,Jan,13; 2015,Jan,16

57510 **Cautery of cervix; electro or thermal** ♀

3.29 | 4.33 | FUD 010 | J P3

AMA: 2019,Jul,6

57511 **cryocautery, initial or repeat** ♀

3.86 | 4.43 | FUD 010 | T P3

AMA: 2019,Jul,6

57513 **laser ablation** ♀

4.05 | 5.08 | FUD 010 | J A2

AMA: 2019,Jul,6

57520 **Conization of cervix, with or without fulguration, with or without dilation and curettage, with or without repair; cold knife or laser** ♀

EXCLUDES *Dilation and curettage, diagnostic/therapeutic, nonobstetrical (58120)*

8.23 | 9.59 | FUD 090 | J A2

AMA: 2019,Jul,6; 2018,Jan,8; 2017,Jan,8; 2016,Jan,13; 2015,Jan,16

57522 **loop electrode excision** ♀

7.21 | 8.25 | FUD 090 | J A2

AMA: 2019,Jul,6; 2018,Jan,8; 2017,Jan,8; 2016,Jan,13; 2015,Jan,16

57530 **Trachelectomy (cervicectomy), amputation of cervix (separate procedure)** ♀

10.0 | 10.0 | FUD 090 | J A2 80

AMA: 2019,Jul,6

57531 **Radical trachelectomy, with bilateral total pelvic lymphadenectomy and para-aortic lymph node sampling biopsy, with or without removal of tube(s), with or without removal of ovary(s)** ♀

EXCLUDES *Radical hysterectomy (58210)*

52.9 | 52.9 | FUD 090 | C 80

AMA: 2019,Jul,6

57540 **Excision of cervical stump, abdominal approach;** ♀

22.8 | 22.8 | FUD 090 | C 80

AMA: 2019,Jul,6

57545 **with pelvic floor repair** ♀

24.0 | 24.0 | FUD 090 | C 80

AMA: 2019,Jul,6

57550 **Excision of cervical stump, vaginal approach;** ♀

12.1 | 12.1 | FUD 090 | J A2 80

AMA: 2019,Jul,6

57555 **with anterior and/or posterior repair** ♀

17.7 | 17.7 | FUD 090 | J 80

AMA: 2019,Jul,6

57556 **with repair of enterocele** ♀

EXCLUDES *Insertion hemostatic agent/pack for spontaneous/traumatic nonobstetrical vaginal hemorrhage (57180)*

Intrauterine device insertion (58300)

16.8 | 16.8 | FUD 090 | J A2 80

AMA: 2019,Jul,6

57558-57800 Cervical Procedures: Dilation, Suturing, or Instrumentation

57558 **Dilation and curettage of cervical stump** ♀

EXCLUDES *Radical surgical procedures (58200-58240)*

3.33 | 3.80 | FUD 010 | J A2

AMA: 2019,Jul,6

57700 **Cerclage of uterine cervix, nonobstetrical** ♀

INCLUDES McDonald cerclage

Shirodker operation

9.13 | 9.13 | FUD 090 | J A2 80

AMA: 2019,Jul,6

57720 **Trachelorrhaphy, plastic repair of uterine cervix, vaginal approach** ♀

INCLUDES Emmet operation

9.33 | 9.33 | FUD 090 | J A2 80

AMA: 2019,Jul,6

57800 **Dilation of cervical canal, instrumental (separate procedure)** ♀

1.39 | 2.01 | FUD 000 | J P3

AMA: 2019,Jul,6

58100-58120 Procedures Involving the Endometrium

58100 **Endometrial sampling (biopsy) with or without endocervical sampling (biopsy), without cervical dilation, any method (separate procedure)** ♀

EXCLUDES *Endocervical curettage only (57505)*

Endometrial sampling (biopsy) performed in conjunction with colposcopy (58110)

1.86 | 2.80 | FUD 000 | T P3

AMA: 2019,Jul,6

+ 58110 **Endometrial sampling (biopsy) performed in conjunction with colposcopy (List separately in addition to code for primary procedure)** ♀

Code first colposcopy (57420-57421, 57452-57461)

1.19 | 1.46 | FUD ZZZ | N N1 80

AMA: 2019,Jul,6; 2018,Jan,8; 2017,Jan,8; 2016,Jan,13; 2015,Jan,16

58120 Dilation and curettage, diagnostic and/or therapeutic (nonobstetrical) ♀

EXCLUDES *Postpartum hemorrhage (59160)*

6.35 7.66 **FUD** 010 J A2

AMA: 2019,Jul,6; 2018,Jan,8; 2017,Jan,8; 2016,Jan,13; 2015,Jan,16

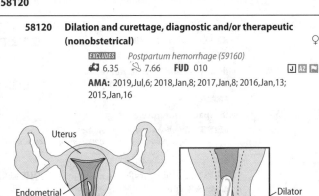

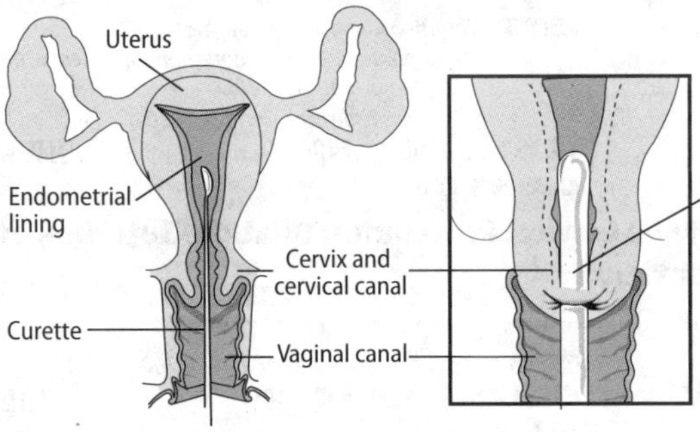

58140-58146 Myomectomy Procedures

58140 Myomectomy, excision of fibroid tumor(s) of uterus, 1 to 4 intramural myoma(s) with total weight of 250 g or less and/or removal of surface myomas; abdominal approach ♀

26.9 26.9 **FUD** 090 C 80

AMA: 2019,Jul,6; 2018,Jan,8; 2017,Jan,8; 2016,Jan,13; 2015,Jan,16

58145 vaginal approach ♀

16.2 16.2 **FUD** 090 J A2 80

AMA: 2019,Jul,6

58146 Myomectomy, excision of fibroid tumor(s) of uterus, 5 or more intramural myomas and/or intramural myomas with total weight greater than 250 g, abdominal approach ♀

EXCLUDES *Hysterectomy (58150-58240)*
Myomectomy procedures (58140-58145)

33.5 33.5 **FUD** 090 C 80

AMA: 2019,Jul,6; 2018,Jan,8; 2017,Jan,8; 2016,Jan,13; 2015,Jan,16

58150-58294 Abdominal and Vaginal Hysterectomies

CMS: 100-03,230.3 Sterilization

EXCLUDES *Destruction/excision endometriomas, open method (49203-49205, 58957-58958)*
Paracentesis (49082-49083)
Pelvic laparotomy (49000)
Secondary closure disruption evisceration abdominal wall (49900)

58150 Total abdominal hysterectomy (corpus and cervix), with or without removal of tube(s), with or without removal of ovary(s); ♀

29.2 29.2 **FUD** 090 C 80

AMA: 2019,Jul,6; 2018,Jan,8; 2017,Jan,8; 2016,Jan,13; 2015,Jan,16

58152 with colpo-urethrocystopexy (eg, Marshall-Marchetti-Krantz, Burch) ♀

EXCLUDES *Urethrocystopexy without hysterectomy (51840-51841)*

36.3 36.3 **FUD** 090 C 80

AMA: 2019,Jul,6; 2018,Jan,8; 2017,Jan,8; 2016,Jan,13; 2015,Jan,16

58180 Supracervical abdominal hysterectomy (subtotal hysterectomy), with or without removal of tube(s), with or without removal of ovary(s) ♀

27.3 27.3 **FUD** 090 C 80

AMA: 2019,Jul,6

58200 Total abdominal hysterectomy, including partial vaginectomy, with para-aortic and pelvic lymph node sampling, with or without removal of tube(s), with or without removal of ovary(s) ♀

39.0 39.0 **FUD** 090 C 80

AMA: 2019,Jul,6

58210 Radical abdominal hysterectomy, with bilateral total pelvic lymphadenectomy and para-aortic lymph node sampling (biopsy), with or without removal of tube(s), with or without removal of ovary(s) ♀

INCLUDES Wertheim hysterectomy

EXCLUDES *Chemotherapy (96401-96549)*
Hysterectomy, radical, with transposition ovary(s) (58825)

53.4 53.4 **FUD** 090 C 80

AMA: 2019,Jul,6; 2018,Jan,8; 2017,Jan,8; 2016,Jan,13; 2015,Jan,16

58240 Pelvic exenteration for gynecologic malignancy, with total abdominal hysterectomy or cervicectomy, with or without removal of tube(s), with or without removal of ovary(s), with removal of bladder and ureteral transplantations, and/or abdominoperineal resection of rectum and colon and colostomy, or any combination thereof ♀

EXCLUDES *Chemotherapy (96401-96549)*
Pelvic exenteration for male genital malignancy or lower urinary tract (51597)

83.8 83.8 **FUD** 090 C 80

AMA: 2019,Jul,6

58260 Vaginal hysterectomy, for uterus 250 g or less; ♀

24.2 24.2 **FUD** 090 J G2 80

AMA: 2019,Jul,6; 2018,Jan,8; 2017,Jan,8; 2016,Jan,13; 2015,Jan,16

58262 with removal of tube(s), and/or ovary(s) ♀

26.1 26.1 **FUD** 090 J G2 80

AMA: 2019,Jul,6

58263 with removal of tube(s), and/or ovary(s), with repair of enterocele ♀

28.8 28.8 **FUD** 090 J 80

AMA: 2019,Jul,6

58267 with colpo-urethrocystopexy (Marshall-Marchetti-Krantz type, Pereyra type) with or without endoscopic control ♀

30.9 30.9 **FUD** 090 C 80

AMA: 2019,Jul,6; 2018,Jan,8; 2017,Jan,8; 2016,Jan,13; 2015,Jan,16

58270 **with repair of enterocele** ♀

EXCLUDES *Vaginal hysterectomy with repair enterocele and removal tubes and/or ovaries (58263)*

25.8 25.8 **FUD** 090 J 80

AMA: 2019,Jul,6

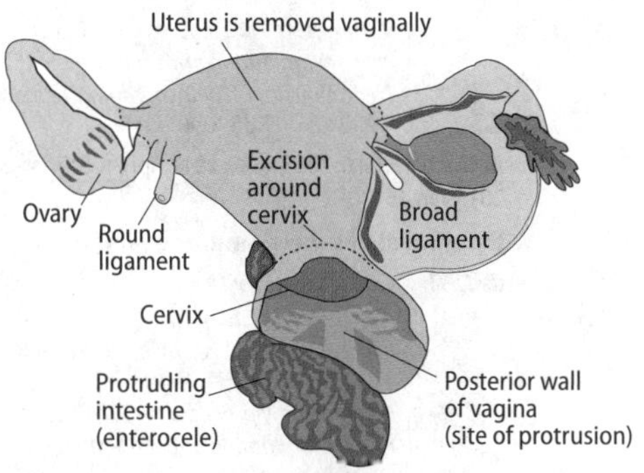

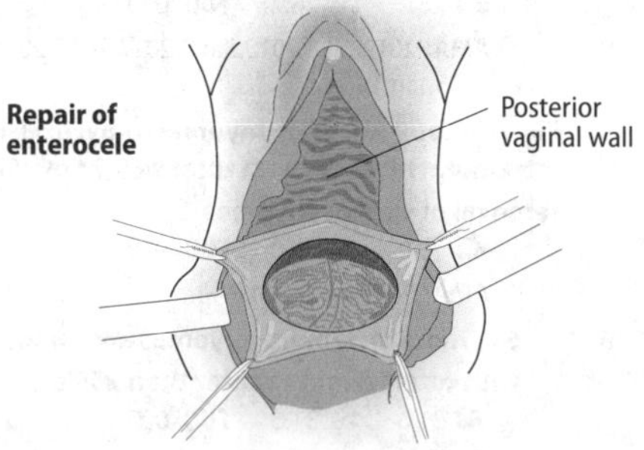

58275 **Vaginal hysterectomy, with total or partial vaginectomy;** ♀

28.6 28.6 **FUD** 090 C 80

AMA: 2019,Jul,6

58280 **with repair of enterocele** ♀

29.7 29.7 **FUD** 090 C 80

AMA: 2019,Jul,6

58285 **Vaginal hysterectomy, radical (Schauta type operation)** ♀

41.8 41.8 **FUD** 090 C 80

AMA: 2019,Jul,6; 2018,Jan,8; 2017,Jan,8; 2016,Jan,13; 2015,Jan,16

58290 **Vaginal hysterectomy, for uterus greater than 250 g;** ♀

33.4 33.4 **FUD** 090 J 80

AMA: 2019,Jul,6

58291 **with removal of tube(s) and/or ovary(s)** ♀

36.2 36.2 **FUD** 090 J 80

AMA: 2019,Jul,6

58292 **with removal of tube(s) and/or ovary(s), with repair of enterocele** ♀

38.2 38.2 **FUD** 090 J 80

AMA: 2019,Jul,6

~~58293~~ ~~**with colpo-urethrocystopexy (Marshall-Marchetti-Krantz type, Pereyra type) with or without endoscopic control**~~

58294 **with repair of enterocele** ♀

34.2 34.2 **FUD** 090 J 80

AMA: 2019,Jul,6

58300-58323 Contraception and Reproduction Procedures

58300 **Insertion of intrauterine device (IUD)** ♀

EXCLUDES *Insertion and/or removal implantable contraceptive capsules (11976, 11981-11983)*

1.49 2.60 **FUD** XXX E

AMA: 2019,Jul,6; 2018,Jan,8; 2017,Jan,8; 2016,Jan,13; 2015,Jan,16

58301 **Removal of intrauterine device (IUD)** ♀

EXCLUDES *Insertion and/or removal implantable contraceptive capsules (11976, 11981-11983)*

1.95 2.91 **FUD** 000 Q2 P3 80

AMA: 2019,Jul,6; 2018,Jan,8; 2017,Jan,8; 2016,Jan,13; 2015,Jan,16

58321 **Artificial insemination; intra-cervical** ♀

1.40 2.26 **FUD** 000 T P3 80

AMA: 2019,Jul,6

58322 **intra-uterine** ♀

1.70 2.56 **FUD** 000 T P3 80

AMA: 2019,Jul,6

58323 **Sperm washing for artificial insemination** ♀

0.37 0.45 **FUD** 000 T P3 80

AMA: 2019,Jul,6

58340-58350 Fallopian Tube Patency and Brachytherapy Procedures

58340 **Catheterization and introduction of saline or contrast material for saline infusion sonohysterography (SIS) or hysterosalpingography** ♀

(74740, 76831)

1.65 5.53 **FUD** 000 N N1

AMA: 2019,Jul,6; 2018,Jan,8; 2017,Jan,8; 2016,Jan,13; 2015,Jan,16

58345 **Transcervical introduction of fallopian tube catheter for diagnosis and/or re-establishing patency (any method), with or without hysterosalpingography** ♀

(74742)

8.27 8.27 **FUD** 010 J R2 80 50

AMA: 2019,Jul,6; 2018,Jan,8; 2017,Jan,8; 2016,Jan,13; 2015,Jan,16

58346 **Insertion of Heyman capsules for clinical brachytherapy** ♀

EXCLUDES *Insertion radioelement sources or ribbons (77761-77763, 77770-77772)*

Placement needles or catheters into pelvic organs and/or genitalia (except prostate) for interstitial radioelement application (55920)

13.2 13.2 **FUD** 090 J A2

AMA: 2019,Jul,6; 2018,Jan,8; 2017,Jan,8; 2016,Jan,13; 2015,Jan,16

58350 **Chromotubation of oviduct, including materials** ♀

2.51 3.62 **FUD** 010 J A2 50

AMA: 2019,Jul,6; 2018,Jan,8; 2017,Jan,8; 2016,Jan,13; 2015,Jan,16

58353-58356 Ablation of Endometrium

EXCLUDES *Destruction/excision endometriomas, open method (49203-49205)*

58353 **Endometrial ablation, thermal, without hysteroscopic guidance** ♀

EXCLUDES *Endometrial ablation performed hysteroscopically (58563)*

6.54 28.5 **FUD** 010 J A2

AMA: 2019,Jul,6; 2018,Jan,8; 2017,Jan,8; 2016,Jan,13; 2015,Jan,16

58356 **Endometrial cryoablation with ultrasonic guidance, including endometrial curettage, when performed** ♀

EXCLUDES *Dilation and curettage (58120)*

Endometrial biopsy (58100)

Hysterosalpingography (58340)

Ultrasound (76700, 76856)

10.2 52.0 **FUD** 010 J P3 80

AMA: 2019,Jul,6

58400-58540 Uterine Repairs: Vaginal and Abdominal

58400 Uterine suspension, with or without shortening of round ligaments, with or without shortening of sacrouterine ligaments; (separate procedure) ♀

INCLUDES Alexander's operation
Baldy-Webster operation
Manchester colporrhaphy

EXCLUDES *Anastomosis tubes to uterus (58752)*

13.1 13.1 FUD 090 C 80

AMA: 2019,Jul,6

58410 with presacral sympathectomy ♀

INCLUDES Alexander's operation

EXCLUDES *Anastomosis tubes to uterus (58752)*

23.5 23.5 FUD 090 C 80

AMA: 2019,Jul,6; 2018,Jan,8; 2017,Jan,8; 2016,Jan,13; 2015,Jan,16

58520 Hysterorrhaphy, repair of ruptured uterus (nonobstetrical) ♀

23.0 23.0 FUD 090 C 80

AMA: 2019,Jul,6

58540 Hysteroplasty, repair of uterine anomaly (Strassman type) ♀

INCLUDES Strassman type

EXCLUDES *Vesicouterine fistula closure (51920)*

26.5 26.5 FUD 090 C 80

AMA: 2019,Jul,6

58674-58554 [58674] Laparoscopic Procedures of the Uterus

INCLUDES Diagnostic laparoscopy

EXCLUDES *Hysteroscopy (58555-58565)*

58674 Laparoscopy, surgical, ablation of uterine fibroid(s) including intraoperative ultrasound guidance and monitoring, radiofrequency ♀

INCLUDES Intraoperative ultrasound (76998)

EXCLUDES *Laparoscopy (49320, 58541-58554, 58570-58573)*

23.6 23.6 FUD 090 J G2 80

AMA: 2019,Jul,6; 2018,Jan,8; 2017,Apr,7; 2017,Feb,14

58541 Laparoscopy, surgical, supracervical hysterectomy, for uterus 250 g or less; ♀

EXCLUDES *Colpotomy (57000)*
Hysteroscopy (58561)
Laparoscopy (49320, 58545-58546, 58661, 58670-58671)
Myomectomy procedures (58140-58146)
Pelvic examination under anesthesia (57410)
Treatment nonobstetrical vaginal hemorrhage (57180)

21.0 21.0 FUD 090 J G2 80

AMA: 2019,Jul,6; 2018,Jan,8; 2017,Apr,7; 2017,Jan,8; 2016,Jan,13; 2015,Jan,16

58542 with removal of tube(s) and/or ovary(s) ♀

EXCLUDES *Colpotomy (57000)*
Hysteroscopy (58561)
Laparoscopy (49320, 58545-58546, 58661, 58670-58671)
Myomectomy procedures (58140-58146)
Pelvic examination under anesthesia (57410)
Treatment nonobstetrical vaginal hemorrhage (57180)

23.9 23.9 FUD 090 J G2 80

AMA: 2019,Jul,6; 2018,Jan,8; 2017,Apr,7; 2017,Jan,8; 2016,Jan,13; 2015,Jan,16

58543 Laparoscopy, surgical, supracervical hysterectomy, for uterus greater than 250 g; ♀

EXCLUDES *Colpotomy (57000)*
Hysteroscopy (58561)
Laparoscopy (49320, 58545-58546, 58661, 58670-58671)
Myomectomy procedures (58140-58146)
Pelvic examination under anesthesia (57410)
Treatment nonobstetrical vaginal hemorrhage (57180)

24.3 24.3 FUD 090 J G2 80

AMA: 2019,Jul,6; 2018,Jan,8; 2017,Apr,7; 2017,Jan,8; 2016,Jan,13; 2015,Jan,16

58544 with removal of tube(s) and/or ovary(s) ♀

EXCLUDES *Colpotomy (57000)*
Hysteroscopy (58561)
Laparoscopy (49320, 58545-58546, 58661, 58670-58671)
Myomectomy procedures (58140-58146)
Pelvic examination under anesthesia (57410)
Treatment nonobstetrical vaginal hemorrhage (57180)

26.2 26.2 FUD 090 J G2 80

AMA: 2019,Jul,6; 2018,Jan,8; 2017,Apr,7; 2017,Jan,8; 2016,Jan,13; 2015,Jan,16

58545 Laparoscopy, surgical, myomectomy, excision; 1 to 4 intramural myomas with total weight of 250 g or less and/or removal of surface myomas ♀

26.0 26.0 FUD 090 J A2 80

AMA: 2019,Jul,6; 2017,Apr,7

58546 5 or more intramural myomas and/or intramural myomas with total weight greater than 250 g ♀

31.6 31.6 FUD 090 J A2 80

AMA: 2019,Jul,6; 2018,Jan,8; 2017,Apr,7; 2017,Jan,8; 2016,Jan,13; 2015,Jan,16

58548 Laparoscopy, surgical, with radical hysterectomy, with bilateral total pelvic lymphadenectomy and para-aortic lymph node sampling (biopsy), with removal of tube(s) and ovary(s), if performed ♀

EXCLUDES *Laparoscopy (38570-38572, 58550-58554)*
Radical hysterectomy (58210, 58285)

53.9 53.9 FUD 090 C 80

AMA: 2019,Jul,6; 2019,Mar,5; 2018,Jan,8; 2017,Apr,7; 2017,Jan,8; 2016,Jan,13; 2015,Sep,12; 2015,Jan,16

58550 Laparoscopy, surgical, with vaginal hysterectomy, for uterus 250 g or less; ♀

EXCLUDES *Colpotomy (57000)*
Hysteroscopy (58561)
Laparoscopy (49320, 58545-58546, 58661, 58670-58671)
Myomectomy procedures (58140-58146)
Pelvic examination under anesthesia (57410)
Treatment nonobstetrical vaginal hemorrhage (57180)

25.5 25.5 FUD 090 J A2 80

AMA: 2019,Jul,6; 2018,Jan,8; 2017,Apr,7; 2017,Jan,8; 2016,Jan,13; 2015,Jan,16

58552 with removal of tube(s) and/or ovary(s) ♀

EXCLUDES *Colpotomy (57000)*
Hysteroscopy (58561)
Laparoscopy (49320, 58545-58546, 58661, 58670-58671)
Myomectomy procedures (58140-58146)
Pelvic examination under anesthesia (57410)
Treatment nonobstetrical vaginal hemorrhage (57180)

28.0 28.0 FUD 090 J G2 80

AMA: 2019,Jul,6; 2018,Jan,8; 2017,Apr,7; 2017,Jan,8; 2016,Jan,13; 2015,Jan,16

58553 **Laparoscopy, surgical, with vaginal hysterectomy, for uterus greater than 250 g;** ♀

EXCLUDES *Colpotomy (57000)*
Hysteroscopy (58561)
Laparoscopy (49320, 58545-58546, 58661, 58670-58671)
Myomectomy procedures (58140-58146)
Pelvic examination under anesthesia (57410)
Treatment nonobstetrical vaginal hemorrhage (57180)

31.8 31.8 **FUD** 090 J G2 80

AMA: 2019,Jul,6; 2018,Jan,8; 2017,Apr,7

58554 **with removal of tube(s) and/or ovary(s)** ♀

EXCLUDES *Colpotomy (57000)*
Hysteroscopy (58561)
Laparoscopy (49320, 58545-58546, 58661, 58670-58671)
Myomectomy procedures (58140-58146)
Pelvic examination under anesthesia (57410)
Treatment nonobstetrical vaginal hemorrhage (57180)

38.1 38.1 **FUD** 090 J G2 80

AMA: 2019,Jul,6; 2018,Jan,8; 2017,Apr,7

58555-58565 Hysteroscopy

INCLUDES Diagnostic hysteroscopy (58555)
EXCLUDES *Laparoscopy (58541-58554, 58570-58578)*

58555 **Hysteroscopy, diagnostic (separate procedure)** ♀

4.35 8.40 **FUD** 000 J A2 80

AMA: 2019,Jul,6; 2018,Jan,8; 2017,Jan,8; 2016,Jan,13; 2015,Jan,16

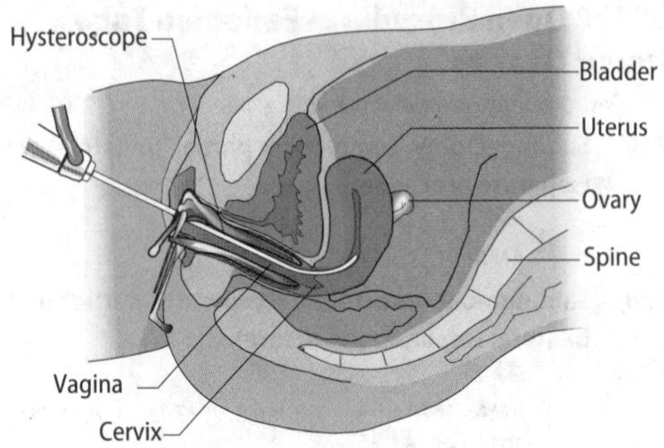

58558 **Hysteroscopy, surgical; with sampling (biopsy) of endometrium and/or polypectomy, with or without D & C** ♀

6.74 39.6 **FUD** 000 J A2

AMA: 2019,Jul,6; 2018,Jan,8; 2017,Jan,8; 2016,Jan,13; 2015,Jan,16

58559 **with lysis of intrauterine adhesions (any method)** ♀

8.33 8.33 **FUD** 000 J A2

AMA: 2019,Jul,6; 2018,Jan,8; 2017,Jan,8; 2016,Jan,13; 2015,Jan,16

58560 **with division or resection of intrauterine septum (any method)** ♀

9.16 9.16 **FUD** 000 J A2 80

AMA: 2019,Jul,6; 2018,Jan,8; 2017,Jan,8; 2016,Jan,13; 2015,Jan,16

58561 **with removal of leiomyomata** ♀

10.4 10.4 **FUD** 000 J A2 80

AMA: 2019,Jul,6; 2018,Jan,8; 2017,Jan,8; 2016,Jan,13; 2015,Jan,16

58562 **with removal of impacted foreign body** ♀

6.34 10.3 **FUD** 000 J A2

AMA: 2019,Jul,6; 2018,Jan,8; 2017,Jan,8; 2016,Jan,13; 2015,Jan,16

58563 **with endometrial ablation (eg, endometrial resection, electrosurgical ablation, thermoablation)** ♀

7.18 55.6 **FUD** 000 J A2 80

AMA: 2019,Jul,6; 2018,Jan,8; 2017,Jan,8; 2016,Jan,13; 2015,Jan,16; 2015,Jan,13

58565 **with bilateral fallopian tube cannulation to induce occlusion by placement of permanent implants** ♀

EXCLUDES *Diagnostic hysteroscopy (58555)*
Dilation cervical canal (57800)

Code also modifier 52 when unilateral procedure performed

12.9 51.6 **FUD** 090 J A2

AMA: 2019,Jul,6; 2018,Jan,8; 2017,Jan,8; 2016,Jan,13; 2015,Jan,16

58570-58579 Other Uterine Endoscopy

INCLUDES Diagnostic laparoscopy
EXCLUDES *Hysteroscopy (58555-58565)*

58570 **Laparoscopy, surgical, with total hysterectomy, for uterus 250 g or less;** ♀

EXCLUDES *Colpotomy (57000)*
Hysteroscopy (58561)
Laparoscopy (49320, 58545-58546, 58661, 58670-58671)
Myomectomy procedures (58140-58146)
Pelvic examination under anesthesia (57410)
Total abdominal hysterectomy (58150)
Treatment nonobstetrical vaginal hemorrhage (57180)

22.9 22.9 **FUD** 090 J G2 80

AMA: 2019,Jul,6; 2018,Jan,8; 2017,Apr,7

58571 **with removal of tube(s) and/or ovary(s)** ♀

EXCLUDES *Colpotomy (57000)*
Hysteroscopy (58561)
Laparoscopy (49320, 58545-58546, 58661, 58670-58671)
Myomectomy procedures (58140-58146)
Pelvic examination under anesthesia (57410)
Total abdominal hysterectomy (58150)
Treatment nonobstetrical vaginal hemorrhage (57180)

25.9 25.9 **FUD** 090 J G2 80

AMA: 2019,Jul,6; 2018,Feb,11; 2018,Jan,8; 2017,Apr,7; 2017,Jan,8; 2016,Jan,13; 2015,Jan,16

58572 **Laparoscopy, surgical, with total hysterectomy, for uterus greater than 250 g;** ♀

EXCLUDES *Colpotomy (57000)*
Hysteroscopy (58561)
Laparoscopy (49320, 58545-58546, 58661, 58670-58671)
Myomectomy procedures (58140-58146)
Pelvic examination under anesthesia (57410)
Total abdominal hysterectomy (58150)
Treatment nonobstetrical vaginal hemorrhage (57180)

29.3 29.3 **FUD** 090 J G2 80

AMA: 2019,Jul,6; 2018,Jan,8; 2017,Apr,7

58573 **with removal of tube(s) and/or ovary(s)** ♀

EXCLUDES *Colpotomy (57000)*
Hysteroscopy (58561)
Laparoscopy (49320, 58545-58546, 58661, 58670-58671)
Myomectomy procedures (58140-58146)
Pelvic examination under anesthesia (57410)
Total abdominal hysterectomy (58150)
Treatment nonobstetrical vaginal hemorrhage (57180)

35.0 35.0 **FUD** 090 J G2 80

AMA: 2019,Jul,6; 2019,Mar,5; 2018,Apr,10; 2018,Feb,11; 2018,Jan,8; 2017,Apr,7; 2017,Jan,8; 2016,Jan,13; 2015,Jan,16

58575 **Laparoscopy, surgical, total hysterectomy for resection of malignancy (tumor debulking), with omentectomy including salpingo-oophorectomy, unilateral or bilateral, when performed** ♀

EXCLUDES *Laparoscopy (49320-49321, 58570-58573, 58661)*
Omentectomy (49255)

54.9 54.9 **FUD** 090 C 80

AMA: 2019,Jul,6; 2019,Mar,5

58578 **Unlisted laparoscopy procedure, uterus** ♀

0.00 0.00 **FUD** YYY J 80 50

AMA: 2019,Jul,6; 2018,Jan,8; 2017,Jan,8; 2016,Jan,13; 2015,Jan,16

58579 **Unlisted hysteroscopy procedure, uterus** ♀

0.00 0.00 **FUD** YYY T 80 50

AMA: 2019,Jul,6; 2018,Jan,8; 2017,Jan,8; 2016,Jan,13; 2015,Jan,16

58600-58615 Sterilization by Tubal Interruption

CMS: 100-03,230.3 Sterilization

EXCLUDES *Destruction/excision endometriomas, open method (49203-49205)*

58600 **Ligation or transection of fallopian tube(s), abdominal or vaginal approach, unilateral or bilateral** ♀

INCLUDES Madlener operation

10.6 10.6 **FUD** 090 J G2 80

AMA: 2019,Jul,6; 2018,Jan,8; 2017,Jan,8; 2016,Jan,13; 2015,Jan,16

58605 **Ligation or transection of fallopian tube(s), abdominal or vaginal approach, postpartum, unilateral or bilateral, during same hospitalization (separate procedure)** ♀

EXCLUDES *Laparoscopic methods (58670-58671)*

9.65 9.65 **FUD** 090 C 80

AMA: 2019,Jul,6; 2018,Jan,8; 2017,Jan,8; 2016,Jan,13; 2015,Jan,16

\+ **58611** **Ligation or transection of fallopian tube(s) when done at the time of cesarean delivery or intra-abdominal surgery (not a separate procedure) (List separately in addition to code for primary procedure)** ♀

Code first primary procedure

2.24 2.24 **FUD** ZZZ C 80

AMA: 2019,Jul,6

58615 **Occlusion of fallopian tube(s) by device (eg, band, clip, Falope ring) vaginal or suprapubic approach** ♀

EXCLUDES *Laparoscopic method (58671)*
Lysis adnexal adhesions (58740)

7.24 7.24 **FUD** 010 J G2 80

AMA: 2019,Jul,6; 2018,Jan,8; 2017,Jan,8; 2016,Jan,13; 2015,Jan,16

58660-58679 [58674] Endoscopic Procedures Fallopian Tubes and/or Ovaries

CMS: 100-03,230.3 Sterilization

INCLUDES Diagnostic laparoscopy (49320)

EXCLUDES *Laparoscopy with biopsy fallopian tube or ovary (49321)*
Laparoscopy with ovarian cyst aspiration (49322)

58660 **Laparoscopy, surgical; with lysis of adhesions (salpingolysis, ovariolysis) (separate procedure)** ♀

19.6 19.6 **FUD** 090 J A2 80

AMA: 2019,Jul,6; 2018,Jan,8; 2017,Jan,8; 2016,Jan,13; 2015,Jan,16

58661 **with removal of adnexal structures (partial or total oophorectomy and/or salpingectomy)** ♀

18.8 18.8 **FUD** 010 J A2 80 50

AMA: 2020,Jan,12; 2019,Jul,6; 2018,Jan,8; 2017,Jan,8; 2016,Jan,13; 2015,Jan,16

58662 **with fulguration or excision of lesions of the ovary, pelvic viscera, or peritoneal surface by any method** ♀

20.6 20.6 **FUD** 090 J A2 80

AMA: 2019,Jul,6; 2018,Jan,8; 2017,Dec,14; 2017,Jan,8; 2016,Jan,13; 2015,Jan,16

58670 **with fulguration of oviducts (with or without transection)** ♀

10.3 10.3 **FUD** 090 J A2

AMA: 2019,Jul,6; 2018,Jan,8; 2017,Jan,8; 2016,Jan,13; 2015,Jan,16

58671 **with occlusion of oviducts by device (eg, band, clip, or Falope ring)** ♀

10.6 10.6 **FUD** 090 J A2

AMA: 2019,Jul,6; 2018,Jan,8; 2017,Jan,8; 2016,Jan,13; 2015,Jan,16

58672 **with fimbrioplasty** ♀

21.3 21.3 **FUD** 090 J A2 80 50

AMA: 2019,Jul,6; 2018,Jan,8; 2017,Jan,8; 2016,Jan,13; 2015,Jan,16

58673 **with salpingostomy (salpingoneostomy)** ♀

23.1 23.1 **FUD** 090 J A2 80 50

AMA: 2019,Jul,6; 2018,Jan,8; 2017,Jan,8; 2016,Jan,13; 2015,Jan,16

58674 **Resequenced code. See code before 58541.**

58679 **Unlisted laparoscopy procedure, oviduct, ovary** ♀

0.00 0.00 **FUD** YYY J 80 50

AMA: 2019,Jul,6; 2018,Jan,8; 2017,Jan,8; 2016,Jan,13; 2015,Jan,16

58700-58770 Open Procedures Fallopian Tubes, with/without Ovaries

EXCLUDES *Destruction/excision endometriomas, open method (49203-49205)*

58700 **Salpingectomy, complete or partial, unilateral or bilateral (separate procedure)** ♀

22.3 22.3 **FUD** 090 C 80

AMA: 2019,Jul,6; 2018,Sep,14

58720 **Salpingo-oophorectomy, complete or partial, unilateral or bilateral (separate procedure)** ♀

21.5 21.5 **FUD** 090 C 80

AMA: 2019,Jul,6; 2018,Jan,8; 2017,Jan,8; 2016,Jan,13; 2015,Jan,16

58740 **Lysis of adhesions (salpingolysis, ovariolysis)** ♀

EXCLUDES *Excision/fulguration lesions performed laparoscopically (58662)*
Laparoscopic method (58660)

25.9 25.9 **FUD** 090 C 80

AMA: 2019,Jul,6; 2018,Jan,8; 2017,Jan,8; 2016,Jan,13; 2015,Jan,16

58750 **Tubotubal anastomosis** ♀
26.3 26.3 **FUD** 090 C 80 50
AMA: 2019,Jul,6

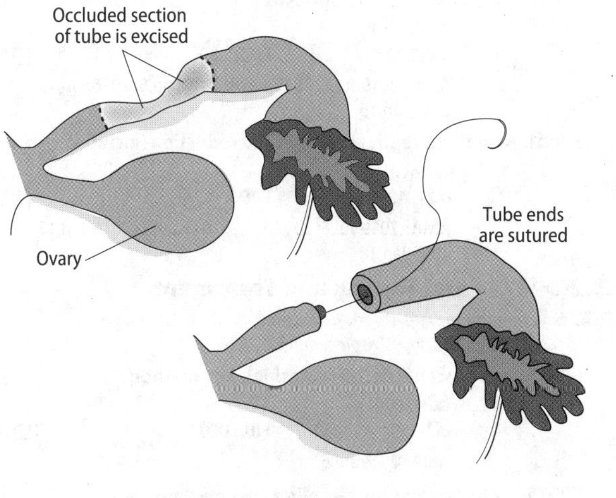

58752 **Tubouterine implantation** ♀
25.4 25.4 **FUD** 090 C 80 50
AMA: 2019,Jul,6

58760 **Fimbrioplasty** ♀
EXCLUDES *Laparoscopic method (58672)*
23.7 23.7 **FUD** 090 C 80 50
AMA: 2019,Jul,6; 2018,Jan,8; 2017,Jan,8; 2016,Jan,13; 2015,Jan,16

58770 **Salpingostomy (salpingoneostomy)** ♀
EXCLUDES *Laparoscopic method (58673)*
24.9 24.9 **FUD** 090 J 80 50
AMA: 2019,Jul,6; 2018,Jan,8; 2017,Jan,8; 2016,Jan,13; 2015,Jan,16

58800-58925 Open Procedures: Ovary

CMS: 100-03,230.3 Sterilization
EXCLUDES *Destruction/excision endometriomas, open method (49203-49205)*

58800 **Drainage of ovarian cyst(s), unilateral or bilateral (separate procedure); vaginal approach** ♀
8.92 9.96 **FUD** 090 J A2
AMA: 2019,Jul,6

58805 **abdominal approach** ♀
12.1 12.1 **FUD** 090 J G2 80
AMA: 2019,Jul,6

58820 **Drainage of ovarian abscess; vaginal approach, open** ♀
EXCLUDES *Transrectal fluid drainage using catheter, image guided (49407)*
9.02 9.02 **FUD** 090 J A2 80 50
AMA: 2019,Jul,6

58822 **abdominal approach** ♀
EXCLUDES *Transrectal fluid drainage using catheter, image guided (49407)*
20.5 20.5 **FUD** 090 C 80 50
AMA: 2019,Jul,6

58825 **Transposition, ovary(s)** ♀
20.4 20.4 **FUD** 090 C 80
AMA: 2019,Jul,6

58900 **Biopsy of ovary, unilateral or bilateral (separate procedure)** ♀
EXCLUDES *Laparoscopy with biopsy fallopian tube or ovary (49321)*
11.8 11.8 **FUD** 090 J A2 80
AMA: 2019,Jul,6; 2018,Jan,8; 2017,Jan,8; 2016,Jan,13; 2015,Jan,16

58920 **Wedge resection or bisection of ovary, unilateral or bilateral** ♀
19.8 19.8 **FUD** 090 J 80
AMA: 2019,Jul,6

58925 **Ovarian cystectomy, unilateral or bilateral** ♀
21.9 21.9 **FUD** 090 J 80
AMA: 2019,Jul,6

58940-58960 Removal Ovary(s) with/without Multiple Procedures for Malignancy

CMS: 100-03,230.3 Sterilization
EXCLUDES *Chemotherapy (96401-96549)*
Destruction/excision tumors, cysts, or endometriomas, open method (49203-49205)

58940 **Oophorectomy, partial or total, unilateral or bilateral;** ♀
EXCLUDES *Oophorectomy with tumor debulking for ovarian malignancy (58952)*
15.6 15.6 **FUD** 090 C 80
AMA: 2019,Jul,6; 2018,Jan,8; 2017,Jan,8; 2016,Jan,13; 2015,Jan,16

58943 **for ovarian, tubal or primary peritoneal malignancy, with para-aortic and pelvic lymph node biopsies, peritoneal washings, peritoneal biopsies, diaphragmatic assessments, with or without salpingectomy(s), with or without omentectomy** ♀
33.6 33.6 **FUD** 090 C 80
AMA: 2019,Jul,6

58950 **Resection (initial) of ovarian, tubal or primary peritoneal malignancy with bilateral salpingo-oophorectomy and omentectomy;** ♀
EXCLUDES *Resection/tumor debulking recurrent ovarian/tubal/primary peritoneal/uterine malignancy (58957-58958)*
32.6 32.6 **FUD** 090 C 80
AMA: 2019,Jul,6

58951 **with total abdominal hysterectomy, pelvic and limited para-aortic lymphadenectomy** ♀
EXCLUDES *Resection/tumor debulking recurrent ovarian/tubal/primary peritoneal/uterine malignancy (58957-58958)*
42.1 42.1 **FUD** 090 C 80
AMA: 2019,Jul,6; 2018,Jan,8; 2017,Jan,8; 2016,Jan,13; 2015,Jan,16

58952 **with radical dissection for debulking (ie, radical excision or destruction, intra-abdominal or retroperitoneal tumors)** ♀
EXCLUDES *Resection/tumor debulking recurrent ovarian/tubal/primary peritoneal/uterine malignancy (58957-58958)*
46.9 46.9 **FUD** 090 C 80
AMA: 2019,Jul,6; 2018,Jan,8; 2017,Jan,8; 2016,Jan,13; 2015,Jan,16

58953 **Bilateral salpingo-oophorectomy with omentectomy, total abdominal hysterectomy and radical dissection for debulking;** ♀
57.6 57.6 **FUD** 090 C 80
AMA: 2019,Jul,6; 2018,Jan,8; 2017,Jan,8; 2016,Jan,13; 2015,Jan,16

58954 **with pelvic lymphadenectomy and limited para-aortic lymphadenectomy** ♀
62.4 62.4 **FUD** 090 C 80
AMA: 2019,Jul,6; 2018,Jan,8; 2017,Jan,8; 2016,Jan,13; 2015,Jan,16

58956 **Bilateral salpingo-oophorectomy with total omentectomy, total abdominal hysterectomy for malignancy** ♀

EXCLUDES *Biopsy ovary (58900)*
Hysterectomy (58150, 58180, 58262-58263)
Laparoscopy (58550, 58661)
Omentectomy (49255)
Oophorectomy (58940)
Ovarian cystectomy (58925)
Resection malignancy (58957-58958)
Salpingectomy salpingo-oophorectomy, (58700, 58720)

39.1 39.1 FUD 090 C 80

AMA: 2019,Jul,6; 2018,Jan,8; 2017,Jan,8; 2016,Jan,13; 2015,Jan,16

58957 **Resection (tumor debulking) of recurrent ovarian, tubal, primary peritoneal, uterine malignancy (intra-abdominal, retroperitoneal tumors), with omentectomy, if performed;** ♀

EXCLUDES *Biopsy ovary (58900)*
Destruction, excision cysts, endometriomas, or tumors (49203-49215)
Enterolysis (44005)
Exploratory laparotomy (49000)
Lymphadenectomy (38770, 38780)
Omentectomy (49255)

45.4 45.4 FUD 090 C 80

AMA: 2019,Jul,6

58958 **with pelvic lymphadenectomy and limited para-aortic lymphadenectomy** ♀

EXCLUDES *Biopsy ovary (58900)*
Destruction, excision cysts, endometriomas, or tumors (49203-49215)
Enterolysis (44005)
Exploratory laparotomy (49000)
Lymphadenectomy (38770, 38780)
Omentectomy (49255)

51.2 51.2 FUD 090 C 80

AMA: 2019,Jul,6

58960 **Laparotomy, for staging or restaging of ovarian, tubal, or primary peritoneal malignancy (second look), with or without omentectomy, peritoneal washing, biopsy of abdominal and pelvic peritoneum, diaphragmatic assessment with pelvic and limited para-aortic lymphadenectomy** ♀

EXCLUDES *Resection malignancy (58957-58958)*

27.9 27.9 FUD 090 C 80

AMA: 2019,Jul,6

58970-58999 Procedural Components: In Vitro Fertilization

58970 **Follicle puncture for oocyte retrieval, any method** M ♀

(76948)

5.62 6.43 FUD 000 T A2 80

AMA: 2019,Jul,6

58974 **Embryo transfer, intrauterine** M ♀

0.00 0.00 FUD 000 T A2 80

AMA: 2019,Jul,6

58976 **Gamete, zygote, or embryo intrafallopian transfer, any method** M ♀

EXCLUDES *Adnexal procedures performed laparoscopically (58660-58673)*

6.06 7.05 FUD 000 T A2 80

AMA: 2019,Jul,6; 2018,Jan,8; 2017,Jan,8; 2016,Jan,13; 2015,Jan,16

58999 **Unlisted procedure, female genital system (nonobstetrical)** ♀

0.00 0.00 FUD YYY T

AMA: 2019,Jul,6; 2018,Jan,8; 2017,Jan,8; 2016,Jan,13; 2015,Jan,16

59000-59001 Aspiration of Amniotic Fluid

EXCLUDES *Intrauterine fetal transfusion (36460)*
Unlisted fetal invasive procedure (59897)

59000 **Amniocentesis; diagnostic** M ♀

(76946)

2.33 3.47 FUD 000 T P3

AMA: 2019,Jul,6; 2018,Jan,8; 2017,Jan,8; 2016,Jan,13; 2015,Jan,16

59001 **therapeutic amniotic fluid reduction (includes ultrasound guidance)** M ♀

5.18 5.18 FUD 000 T R2

AMA: 2019,Jul,6; 2018,Jan,8; 2017,Jan,8; 2016,Jan,13; 2015,Jan,16

59012-59076 Fetal Testing and Treatment

EXCLUDES *Intrauterine fetal transfusion (36460)*
Unlisted fetal invasive procedures (59897)

59012 **Cordocentesis (intrauterine), any method** M ♀

(76941)

5.87 5.87 FUD 000 T G2 80

AMA: 2019,Jul,6

59015 **Chorionic villus sampling, any method** M ♀

(76945)

3.82 4.51 FUD 000 T P3 80

AMA: 2019,Jul,6; 2018,Jan,8; 2017,Jan,8; 2016,Jan,13; 2015,Jan,16

59020 **Fetal contraction stress test** M ♀

1.99 1.99 FUD 000 T P3 80

AMA: 2019,Jul,6; 2018,Jan,8; 2017,Jan,8; 2016,Jan,13; 2015,Jan,16

59025 **Fetal non-stress test** M ♀

1.37 1.37 FUD 000 T P3 80

AMA: 2019,Jul,6; 2018,Jan,8; 2017,Jan,8; 2016,Jan,13; 2015,Jan,16

59030 **Fetal scalp blood sampling** M ♀

Code also modifier 76 or 77, as appropriate, for repeat fetal scalp blood sampling

3.28 3.28 FUD 000 T 80

AMA: 2019,Jul,6

59050 **Fetal monitoring during labor by consulting physician (ie, non-attending physician) with written report; supervision and interpretation** M ♀

1.49 1.49 FUD XXX M 80

AMA: 2019,Jul,6

59051 **interpretation only** M ♀

1.23 1.23 FUD XXX B 80

AMA: 2019,Jul,6

59070 **Transabdominal amnioinfusion, including ultrasound guidance** M ♀

8.99 11.6 FUD 000 T G2 80

AMA: 2019,Jul,6; 2018,Jan,8; 2017,Jan,8; 2016,Jan,13; 2015,Jan,16

59072 **Fetal umbilical cord occlusion, including ultrasound guidance** M ♀

15.0 15.0 FUD 000 T J8

AMA: 2019,Jul,6; 2018,Jan,8; 2017,Jan,8; 2016,Jan,13; 2015,Jan,16

59074 **Fetal fluid drainage (eg, vesicocentesis, thoracocentesis, paracentesis), including ultrasound guidance** M ♀

8.92 11.1 FUD 000 T G2 80

AMA: 2019,Jul,6; 2018,Jan,8; 2017,Jan,8; 2016,Jan,13; 2015,Jan,16

59076 **Fetal shunt placement, including ultrasound guidance** M ♀

15.2 15.2 FUD 000 T G2 80

AMA: 2019,Jul,6; 2018,Jan,8; 2017,Jan,8; 2016,Jan,13; 2015,Jan,16

59100-59151 Tubal Pregnancy/Hysterotomy Procedures

CMS: 100-03,230.3 Sterilization

59100 **Hysterotomy, abdominal (eg, for hydatidiform mole, abortion)** M ♀
Code also ligation fallopian tubes when performed same time as hysterotomy (58611)
24.1 24.1 FUD 090 J R2 80
AMA: 2019,Jul,6

59120 **Surgical treatment of ectopic pregnancy; tubal or ovarian, requiring salpingectomy and/or oophorectomy, abdominal or vaginal approach** M ♀
23.4 23.4 FUD 090 C 80
AMA: 2019,Jul,6

59121 **tubal or ovarian, without salpingectomy and/or oophorectomy** M ♀
23.0 23.0 FUD 090 C 80
AMA: 2019,Jul,6

59130 **abdominal pregnancy** M ♀
26.8 26.8 FUD 090 C 80
AMA: 2019,Jul,6

59135 **interstitial, uterine pregnancy requiring total hysterectomy** M ♀
27.0 27.0 FUD 090 C 80
AMA: 2019,Jul,6

59136 **interstitial, uterine pregnancy with partial resection of uterus** M ♀
25.9 25.9 FUD 090 C 80
AMA: 2019,Jul,6

59140 **cervical, with evacuation** M ♀
11.9 11.9 FUD 090 C 80
AMA: 2019,Jul,6

59150 **Laparoscopic treatment of ectopic pregnancy; without salpingectomy and/or oophorectomy** M ♀
22.7 22.7 FUD 090 J G2 80
AMA: 2019,Jul,6; 2018,Jan,8; 2017,Jan,8; 2016,Jan,13; 2015,Jan,16

59151 **with salpingectomy and/or oophorectomy** M ♀
21.7 21.7 FUD 090 J G2 80
AMA: 2019,Jul,6

59160-59200 Procedures of Uterus Prior To/After Delivery

59160 **Curettage, postpartum** M ♀
5.11 6.21 FUD 010 J A2 80
AMA: 2019,Jul,6; 2018,Jan,8; 2017,Jan,8; 2016,Jan,13; 2015,Jan,16

59200 **Insertion of cervical dilator (eg, laminaria, prostaglandin) (separate procedure)** M ♀
EXCLUDES *Fetal transfusion, intrauterine (36460)*
Hypertonic solution/prostaglandin introduction for labor initiation (59850-59857)
1.30 2.56 FUD 000 T P3
AMA: 2019,Jul,6; 2018,Jan,8; 2017,Dec,14; 2017,Jan,8; 2016,Jan,13; 2015,Jan,16

59300-59350 Postpartum Vaginal/Cervical/Uterine Repairs

EXCLUDES *Nonpregnancy-related cerclage (57700)*

59300 **Episiotomy or vaginal repair, by other than attending** M ♀
4.26 6.15 FUD 000 J P3 80
AMA: 2019,Jul,6

59320 **Cerclage of cervix, during pregnancy; vaginal** M ♀
4.37 4.37 FUD 000 J A2 80
AMA: 2019,Jul,6; 2018,Jan,8; 2017,Jan,8; 2016,Jan,13; 2015,Jan,16

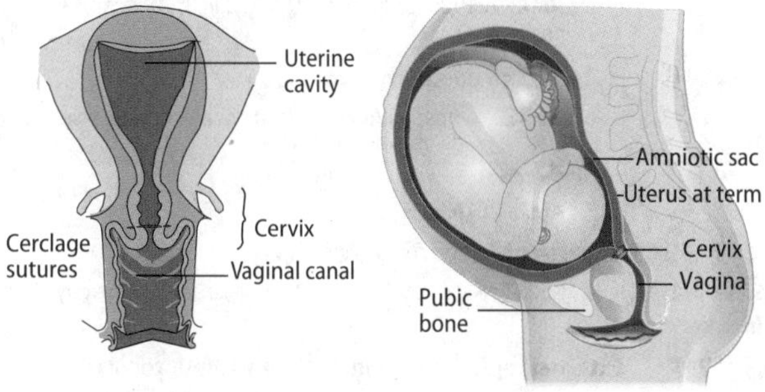

59325 **abdominal** M ♀
6.96 6.96 FUD 000 C 80
AMA: 2019,Jul,6; 2018,Jan,8; 2017,Jan,8; 2016,Jan,13; 2015,Jan,16

59350 **Hysterorrhaphy of ruptured uterus** M ♀
8.08 8.08 FUD 000 C 80
AMA: 2019,Jul,6

59400-59410 Vaginal Delivery: Comprehensive and Component Services

CMS: 100-02,15,180 Nurse-Midwife (CNM) Services; 100-02,15,20.1 Physician Expense for Surgery, Childbirth, and Treatment for Infertility

INCLUDES Care provided for uncomplicated pregnancy including delivery, antepartum, and postpartum care:
- Admission history
- Admission to hospital
- Artificial rupture membranes
- Management uncomplicated labor
- Physical exam
- Vaginal delivery with or without episiotomy or forceps

EXCLUDES *Medical complications pregnancy, labor, and delivery:*
- *Cardiac problems*
- *Diabetes*
- *Hyperemesis*
- *Hypertension*
- *Neurological problems*
- *Premature rupture membranes*
- *Pre-term labor*
- *Toxemia*
- *Trauma*

Newborn circumcision (54150, 54160)
Services incidental to or unrelated to pregnancy

59400 **Routine obstetric care including antepartum care, vaginal delivery (with or without episiotomy, and/or forceps) and postpartum care** M ♀
INCLUDES Fetal heart tones
Hospital/office visits following cesarean section or vaginal delivery
Initial/subsequent history
Physical exams
Recording weight/blood pressures
Routine chemical urinalysis
Routine prenatal visits:
- Each month up to 28 weeks gestation
- Every other week from 29 to 36 weeks gestation
- Weekly from 36 weeks until delivery

60.4 60.4 FUD MMM B
AMA: 2019,Jul,6; 2018,Jan,8; 2017,Jan,8; 2016,Jan,13; 2015,Jan,16

59409 **Vaginal delivery only (with or without episiotomy and/or forceps);** M ♀

Code also inpatient management after delivery/discharge services (99217-99239 [99224, 99225, 99226])

23.3 23.3 **FUD** MMM J 80

AMA: 2019,Jul,6; 2018,Jan,8; 2017,Jan,8; 2016,Jan,13; 2015,Jan,16

59410 **including postpartum care** M ♀

INCLUDES Hospital/office visits following cesarean section or vaginal delivery

29.9 29.9 **FUD** MMM B

AMA: 2019,Jul,6

59412-59414 Other Maternity Services

CMS: 100-02,15,180 Nurse-Midwife (CNM) Services; 100-02,15,20.1 Physician Expense for Surgery, Childbirth, and Treatment for Infertility

59412 **External cephalic version, with or without tocolysis** M ♀

Code also delivery code(s)

2.95 2.95 **FUD** MMM J G2 80

AMA: 2019,Jul,6

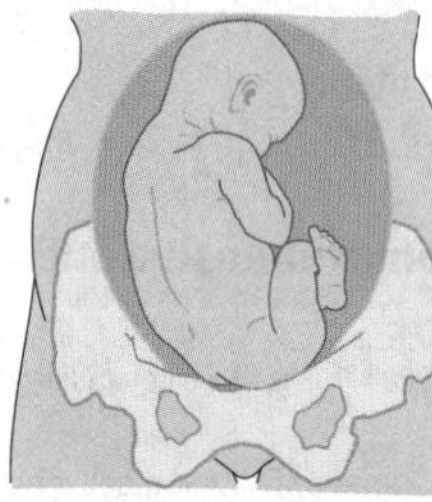
Complete breech presentation at term

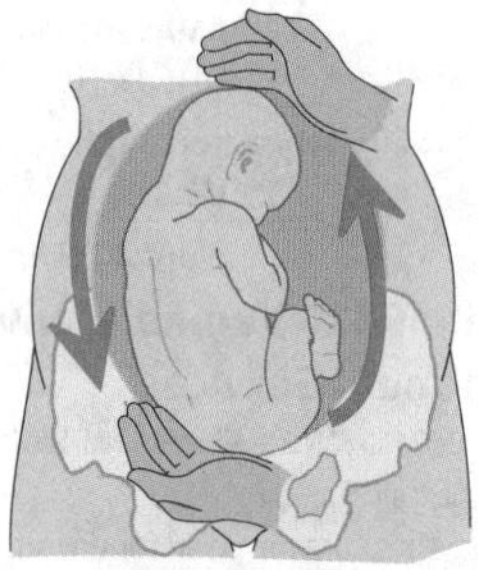
The physician feels for the baby's head and bottom externally

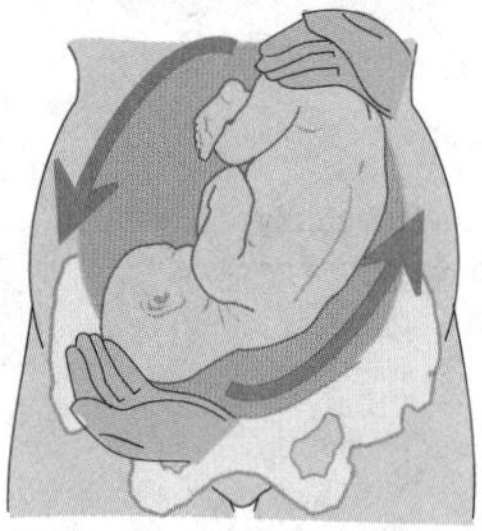
Turning the baby by applying external pressure

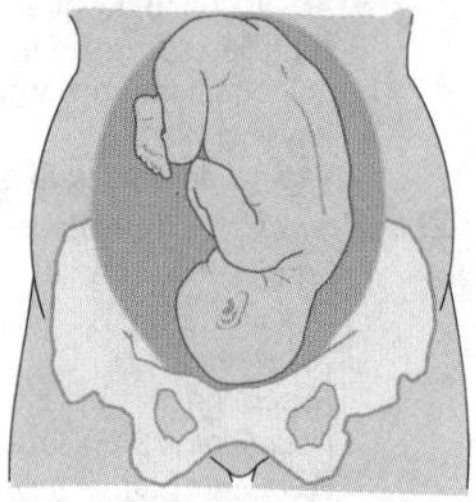
Baby is in cephalic presentation, engaged for normal delivery

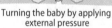

59414 **Delivery of placenta (separate procedure)** M ♀

2.66 2.66 **FUD** MMM J G2 80

AMA: 2019,Jul,6; 2018,Jan,8; 2017,Jan,8; 2016,Jan,13; 2015,Jan,16

59425-59430 Prenatal and Postpartum Visits

CMS: 100-02,15,180 Nurse-Midwife (CNM) Services; 100-02,15,20.1 Physician Expense for Surgery, Childbirth, and Treatment for Infertility

INCLUDES Physician/other qualified health care professional providing all or portion antepartum/postpartum care, but no delivery due to:
- Referral to another physician for delivery
- Termination pregnancy by abortion

EXCLUDES *Antepartum care, one to three visits, report with appropriate E/M service code*
Medical complications pregnancy, labor, and delivery:
- *Cardiac problems*
- *Diabetes*
- *Hyperemesis*
- *Hypertension*
- *Neurological problems*
- *Premature rupture membranes*
- *Pre-term labor*
- *Toxemia*
- *Trauma*

Newborn circumcision (54150, 54160)
Services incidental to or unrelated to pregnancy

59425 **Antepartum care only; 4-6 visits** M ♀

INCLUDES Fetal heart tones
Initial/subsequent history
Physical exams
Recording weight/blood pressures
Routine chemical urinalysis
Routine prenatal visits:
- Each month up to 28 weeks gestation
- Every other week from 29 to 36 weeks gestation
- Weekly from 36 weeks until delivery

10.3 13.5 **FUD** MMM B 80

AMA: 2019,Jul,6; 2018,Jan,8; 2017,Jan,8; 2016,Jan,13; 2015,Jan,16

59426 **7 or more visits** M ♀

INCLUDES Biweekly visits to 36 weeks gestation
Fetal heart tones
Initial/subsequent history
Monthly visits up to 28 weeks gestation
Physical exams
Recording weight/blood pressures
Routine chemical urinalysis
Weekly visits until delivery

17.9 23.5 **FUD** MMM B 80

AMA: 2019,Jul,6; 2018,Jan,8; 2017,Jan,8; 2016,Jan,13; 2015,Jan,16

59430 **Postpartum care only (separate procedure)** M ♀

INCLUDES Office/other outpatient visits following cesarean section or vaginal delivery

4.05 5.96 **FUD** MMM B

AMA: 2019,Jul,6; 2018,Jan,8; 2017,Jan,8; 2016,Jan,13; 2015,Jan,16

59510-59525 Cesarean Section Delivery: Comprehensive and Components of Care

CMS: 100-02,15,20.1 Physician Expense for Surgery, Childbirth, and Treatment for Infertility

INCLUDES Classic cesarean section
Low cervical cesarean section

EXCLUDES *Infant standby attendance (99360)*
Medical complications pregnancy, labor, and delivery:
Cardiac problems
Diabetes
Hyperemesis
Hypertension
Neurological problems
Premature rupture membranes
Pre-term labor
Toxemia
Trauma
Newborn circumcision (54150, 54160)
Services incidental to or unrelated to pregnancy
Vaginal delivery after prior cesarean section (59610-59614)

59510 Routine obstetric care including antepartum care, cesarean delivery, and postpartum care M ♀

INCLUDES Admission history
Admission to hospital
Cesarean delivery
Fetal heart tones
Hospital/office visits following cesarean section
Initial/subsequent history
Management uncomplicated labor
Physical exam
Recording weight/blood pressures
Routine chemical urinalysis
Routine prenatal visits:
Each month up to 28 weeks gestation
Every other week 29 to 36 weeks gestation
Weekly from 36 weeks until delivery

67.0 67.0 **FUD** MMM B

AMA: 2019,Jul,6; 2018,Jan,8; 2017,Jan,8; 2016,Jan,13; 2015,Jan,16

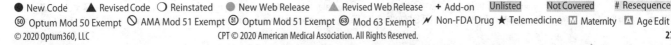

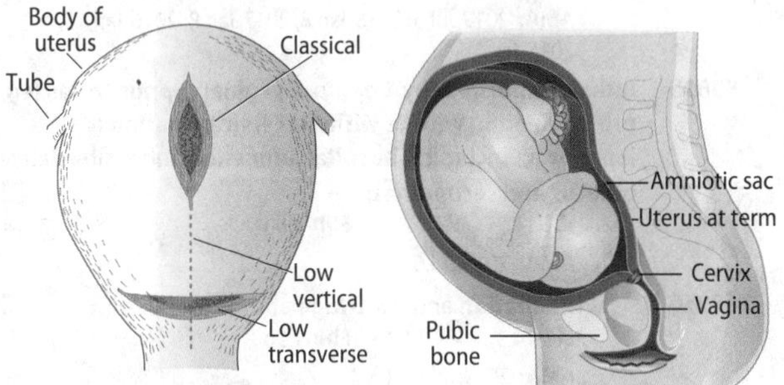

Types of Cesarean section are classified by uterine incision

59514 Cesarean delivery only; M ♀

INCLUDES Admission history
Admission to hospital
Cesarean delivery
Management uncomplicated labor
Physical exam

Code also inpatient management after delivery/discharge services (99217-99239 [99224, 99225, 99226])

26.5 26.5 **FUD** MMM C 80

AMA: 2019,Jul,6; 2018,Jan,8; 2017,Jan,8; 2016,Jan,13; 2015,Jan,16

59515 including postpartum care M ♀

INCLUDES Admission history
Admission to hospital
Cesarean delivery
Hospital/office visits following cesarean section or vaginal delivery
Management uncomplicated labor
Physical exam

36.8 36.8 **FUD** MMM B

AMA: 2019,Jul,6; 2018,Jan,8; 2017,Jan,8; 2016,Jan,13; 2015,Jan,16

+ **59525 Subtotal or total hysterectomy after cesarean delivery (List separately in addition to code for primary procedure)** M ♀

Code first cesarean delivery (59510, 59514, 59515, 59618, 59620, 59622)

14.1 14.1 **FUD** ZZZ C 80

AMA: 2019,Jul,6

59610-59614 Vaginal Delivery After Prior Cesarean Section: Comprehensive and Components of Care

CMS: 100-02,15,180 Nurse-Midwife (CNM) Services; 100-02,15,20.1 Physician Expense for Surgery, Childbirth, and Treatment for Infertility

INCLUDES Admission history
Admission to hospital
Management uncomplicated labor
Patients with previous cesarean delivery who present with vaginal delivery expectation
Physical exam
Successful vaginal delivery after previous cesarean delivery (VBAC)
Vaginal delivery with or without episiotomy or forceps

EXCLUDES *Elective cesarean delivery (59510, 59514, 59515)*
Medical complications pregnancy, labor, and delivery:
Cardiac problems
Diabetes
Hyperemesis
Hypertension
Neurological problems
Premature rupture membranes
Pre-term labor
Toxemia
Trauma
Newborn circumcision (54150, 54160)
Services incidental to or unrelated to pregnancy

59610 Routine obstetric care including antepartum care, vaginal delivery (with or without episiotomy, and/or forceps) and postpartum care, after previous cesarean delivery M ♀

INCLUDES Fetal heart tones
Hospital/office visits following cesarean section or vaginal delivery
Initial/subsequent history
Physical exams
Recording weight/blood pressures
Routine chemical urinalysis
Routine prenatal visits:
Each month up to 28 weeks gestation
Every other week 29 to 36 weeks gestation
Weekly from 36 weeks until delivery

63.4 63.4 **FUD** MMM B 80

AMA: 2019,Jul,6; 2018,Jan,8; 2017,Jan,8; 2016,Jan,13; 2015,Jan,16

59612 Vaginal delivery only, after previous cesarean delivery (with or without episiotomy and/or forceps); M ♀

Code also inpatient management after delivery/discharge services (99217-99239 [99224, 99225, 99226])

26.3 26.3 **FUD** MMM J 80

AMA: 2019,Jul,6; 2018,Jan,8; 2017,Jan,8; 2016,Jan,13; 2015,Jan,16

59614 including postpartum care M ♀

INCLUDES Hospital/office visits following cesarean section or vaginal delivery

32.6 32.6 **FUD** MMM B 80

AMA: 2019,Jul,6; 2018,Jan,8; 2017,Jan,8; 2016,Jan,13; 2015,Jan,16

59618-59622 Cesarean Section After Attempted Vaginal Birth/Prior C-Section

CMS: 100-02,15,20.1 Physician Expense for Surgery, Childbirth, and Treatment for Infertility

INCLUDES Admission history
Admission to hospital
Cesarean delivery
Cesarean delivery following unsuccessful vaginal delivery attempt after previous cesarean delivery
Management uncomplicated labor
Patients with previous cesarean delivery who present with vaginal delivery expectation
Physical exam

EXCLUDES *Elective cesarean delivery (59510, 59514, 59515)*
Medical complications of pregnancy, labor, and delivery:
Cardiac problems
Diabetes
Hyperemesis
Hypertension
Neurological problems
Premature rupture of membranes
Pre-term labor
Toxemia
Trauma
Newborn circumcision (54150, 54160)
Services incidental to or unrelated to the pregnancy

59618 **Routine obstetric care including antepartum care, cesarean delivery, and postpartum care, following attempted vaginal delivery after previous cesarean delivery** M ♀
INCLUDES Fetal heart tones
Hospital/office visits following cesarean section or vaginal delivery
Initial/subsequent history
Physical exams
Recording weight/blood pressures
Routine chemical urinalysis
Routine prenatal visits:
Each month up to 28 weeks gestation
Every two weeks 29 to 36 weeks gestation
Weekly from 36 weeks until delivery
69.1 69.1 **FUD** MMM B 80
AMA: 2019,Jul,6; 2018,Jan,8; 2017,Jan,8; 2016,Jan,13; 2015,Jan,16

59620 **Cesarean delivery only, following attempted vaginal delivery after previous cesarean delivery;** M ♀
Code also inpatient management after delivery/discharge services (99217-99239 [99224, 99225, 99226])
27.0 27.0 **FUD** MMM C 80
AMA: 2019,Jul,6; 2018,Jan,8; 2017,Jan,8; 2016,Jan,13; 2015,Jan,16

59622 **including postpartum care** M ♀
INCLUDES Hospital/office visits following cesarean section or vaginal delivery
37.4 37.4 **FUD** MMM B 80
AMA: 2019,Jul,6; 2018,Jan,8; 2017,Jan,8; 2016,Jan,13; 2015,Jan,16

59812-59830 Treatment of Miscarriage

CMS: 100-02,15,20.1 Physician Expense for Surgery, Childbirth, and Treatment for Infertility

EXCLUDES *Medical treatment spontaneous complete abortion, any trimester (99202-99233 [99224, 99225, 99226])*

59812 **Treatment of incomplete abortion, any trimester, completed surgically** M ♀
INCLUDES Surgical treatment spontaneous abortion
8.79 9.89 **FUD** 090 J A2
AMA: 2019,Jul,6; 2018,Jan,8; 2017,Jan,8; 2016,Jan,13; 2015,Jan,16

59820 **Treatment of missed abortion, completed surgically; first trimester** M ♀
10.4 11.2 **FUD** 090 J A2
AMA: 2019,Jul,6; 2018,Jan,8; 2017,Jan,8; 2016,Jan,13; 2015,Jan,16

59821 **second trimester** M ♀
10.6 11.8 **FUD** 090 J A2 80
AMA: 2019,Jul,6; 2018,Jan,8; 2017,Jan,8; 2016,Jan,13; 2015,Jan,16

59830 **Treatment of septic abortion, completed surgically** M ♀
12.7 12.7 **FUD** 090 C 80
AMA: 2019,Jul,6; 2018,Jan,8; 2017,Jan,8; 2016,Jan,13; 2015,Jan,16

59840-59866 Elective Abortions

CMS: 100-02,1,90 Termination of Pregnancy; 100-02,15,20.1 Physician Expense for Surgery, Childbirth, and Treatment for Infertility; 100-03,140.1 Abortion; 100-04,3,100.1 Billing for Abortion Services

59840 **Induced abortion, by dilation and curettage** M ♀
6.08 6.50 **FUD** 010 J A2 80
AMA: 2019,Jul,6; 2018,Jan,8; 2017,Jan,8; 2016,Jan,13; 2015,Jan,16

59841 **Induced abortion, by dilation and evacuation** M ♀
10.6 11.7 **FUD** 010 J A2 80
AMA: 2019,Jul,6; 2018,Jan,8; 2017,Jan,8; 2016,Jan,13; 2015,Jan,16

59850 **Induced abortion, by 1 or more intra-amniotic injections (amniocentesis-injections), including hospital admission and visits, delivery of fetus and secundines;** M ♀
EXCLUDES *Cervical dilator insertion (59200)*
10.1 10.1 **FUD** 090 C 80
AMA: 2019,Jul,6; 2018,Jan,8; 2017,Jan,8; 2016,Jan,13; 2015,Jan,16

59851 **with dilation and curettage and/or evacuation** M ♀
EXCLUDES *Cervical dilator insertion (59200)*
10.9 10.9 **FUD** 090 C 80
AMA: 2019,Jul,6; 2018,Jan,8; 2017,Jan,8; 2016,Jan,13; 2015,Jan,16

59852 **with hysterotomy (failed intra-amniotic injection)** M ♀
EXCLUDES *Cervical dilator insertion (59200)*
15.0 15.0 **FUD** 090 C 80
AMA: 2019,Jul,6; 2018,Jan,8; 2017,Jan,8; 2016,Jan,13; 2015,Jan,16

59855 **Induced abortion, by 1 or more vaginal suppositories (eg, prostaglandin) with or without cervical dilation (eg, laminaria), including hospital admission and visits, delivery of fetus and secundines;** M ♀
12.2 12.2 **FUD** 090 C 80
AMA: 2019,Jul,6

59856 **with dilation and curettage and/or evacuation** M ♀
14.3 14.3 **FUD** 090 C 80
AMA: 2019,Jul,6

59857 **with hysterotomy (failed medical evacuation)** M ♀
15.0 15.0 **FUD** 090 C 80
AMA: 2019,Jul,6

59866 **Multifetal pregnancy reduction(s) (MPR)** M ♀
6.22 6.22 **FUD** 000 T G2 80
AMA: 2019,Jul,6

59870-59899 Miscellaneous Obstetrical Procedures

CMS: 100-02,15,20.1 Physician Expense for Surgery, Childbirth, and Treatment for Infertility

59870 **Uterine evacuation and curettage for hydatidiform mole** M ♀
14.7 14.7 **FUD** 090 J A2 80
AMA: 2019,Jul,6; 2018,Jan,8; 2017,Jan,8; 2016,Jan,13; 2015,Jan,16

59871 **Removal of cerclage suture under anesthesia (other than local)** M ♀
3.82 3.82 **FUD** 000 02 A2 80
AMA: 2019,Jul,6; 2018,Jan,8; 2017,Jan,8; 2016,Jan,13; 2015,Jan,16

59897 **Unlisted fetal invasive procedure, including ultrasound guidance, when performed** [M] ♀
🚑 0.00 ⚕ 0.00 **FUD** YYY [T] ⚑
AMA: 2019,Jul,6

59898 **Unlisted laparoscopy procedure, maternity care and delivery** [M] ♀
🚑 0.00 ⚕ 0.00 **FUD** YYY [J] [80] [50] ⚑
AMA: 2019,Jul,6; 2018,Jan,8; 2017,Jan,8; 2016,Jan,13; 2015,Jan,16

59899 **Unlisted procedure, maternity care and delivery** [M] ♀
🚑 0.00 ⚕ 0.00 **FUD** YYY [T] [80] ⚑
AMA: 2019,Jul,6; 2018,Jan,8; 2017,Jan,8; 2016,Jan,13; 2015,Jan,16

60000 I&D of Infected Thyroglossal Cyst

60000 Incision and drainage of thyroglossal duct cyst, infected
4.37 4.99 **FUD** 010 T A2 80
AMA: 2014,Jan,11; 2002,May,7

60100 Core Needle Biopsy: Thyroid

EXCLUDES *Fine needle aspiration (10021, [10004, 10005, 10006, 10007, 10008, 10009, 10010, 10011, 10012])*

60100 Biopsy thyroid, percutaneous core needle
(76942, 77002, 77012, 77021)
(88172-88173)
2.25 3.18 **FUD** 000 T P3
AMA: 2019,Apr,4; 2018,Jan,8; 2017,Jan,8; 2016,Jan,13; 2015,Jan,16

60200 Surgical Removal Thyroid Cyst or Mass; Division of Isthmus

60200 Excision of cyst or adenoma of thyroid, or transection of isthmus
19.0 19.0 **FUD** 090 J A2 80
AMA: 2018,Jan,8; 2017,Jan,8; 2016,Jan,13; 2015,Jan,16

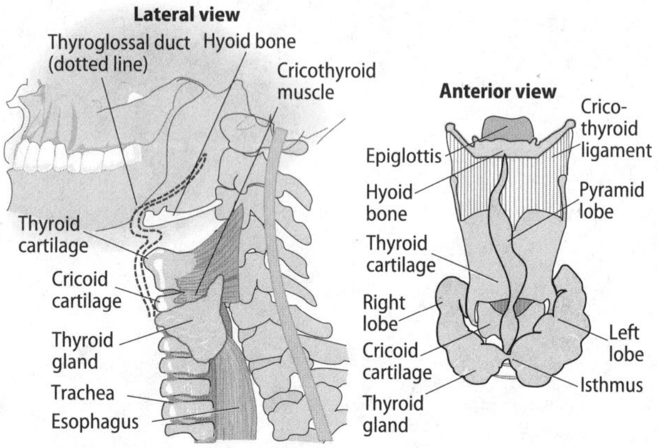

60210-60225 Subtotal Thyroidectomy

60210 Partial thyroid lobectomy, unilateral; with or without isthmusectomy
20.3 20.3 **FUD** 090 J G2 80
AMA: 2018,Jan,8; 2017,Jan,8; 2016,Jan,13; 2015,Jan,16

60212 with contralateral subtotal lobectomy, including isthmusectomy
29.0 29.0 **FUD** 090 J G2 80
AMA: 2018,Jan,8; 2017,Jan,8; 2016,Jan,13; 2015,Jan,16

60220 Total thyroid lobectomy, unilateral; with or without isthmusectomy
20.3 20.3 **FUD** 090 J G2 80
AMA: 2020,Aug,14; 2018,Jan,8; 2017,Jan,8; 2016,Jan,13; 2015,Jan,16

60225 with contralateral subtotal lobectomy, including isthmusectomy
26.8 26.8 **FUD** 090 J G2 80
AMA: 2018,Jan,8; 2017,Jan,8; 2016,Jan,13; 2015,Jan,16

60240-60271 Complete Thyroidectomy Procedures

60240 Thyroidectomy, total or complete
EXCLUDES *Subtotal or partial thyroidectomy (60271)*
26.5 26.5 **FUD** 090 J G2 80
AMA: 2018,Jan,8; 2017,Jan,8; 2016,Jan,13; 2015,Jan,16

60252 Thyroidectomy, total or subtotal for malignancy; with limited neck dissection
38.0 38.0 **FUD** 090 J 80
AMA: 2018,Jan,8; 2017,Jan,8; 2016,Jan,13; 2015,Jan,16

60254 with radical neck dissection
48.1 48.1 **FUD** 090 C 80
AMA: 2018,Jan,8; 2017,Jan,8; 2016,Jan,13; 2015,Jan,16

60260 Thyroidectomy, removal of all remaining thyroid tissue following previous removal of a portion of thyroid
31.4 31.4 **FUD** 090 J 80 50
AMA: 2018,Jan,8; 2017,Jan,8; 2016,Jan,13; 2015,Jan,16

60270 Thyroidectomy, including substernal thyroid; sternal split or transthoracic approach
39.4 39.4 **FUD** 090 C 80
AMA: 2018,Jan,8; 2017,Jan,8; 2016,Jan,13; 2015,Jan,16

60271 cervical approach
30.4 30.4 **FUD** 090 J 80
AMA: 2020,Aug,14; 2018,Jan,8; 2017,Jan,8; 2016,Jan,13; 2015,Jan,16

60280-60300 Treatment of Cyst/Sinus of Thyroid

60280 Excision of thyroglossal duct cyst or sinus;
EXCLUDES *Thyroid ultrasound (76536)*
12.6 12.6 **FUD** 090 J A2 80
AMA: 2014,Jan,11

60281 recurrent
EXCLUDES *Thyroid ultrasound (76536)*
16.8 16.8 **FUD** 090 J A2 80
AMA: 2014,Jan,11; 1994,Win,1

60300 Aspiration and/or injection, thyroid cyst
EXCLUDES *Fine needle aspiration (10021, [10004, 10005, 10006, 10007, 10008, 10009, 10010, 10011, 10012])*
(76942, 77012)
1.42 3.24 **FUD** 000 T P3
AMA: 2014,Jan,11

60500-60512 Parathyroid Procedures

60500 Parathyroidectomy or exploration of parathyroid(s);
27.9 27.9 **FUD** 090 J G2 80
AMA: 2018,Jan,8; 2017,Jan,8; 2016,Jan,13; 2015,Jan,16

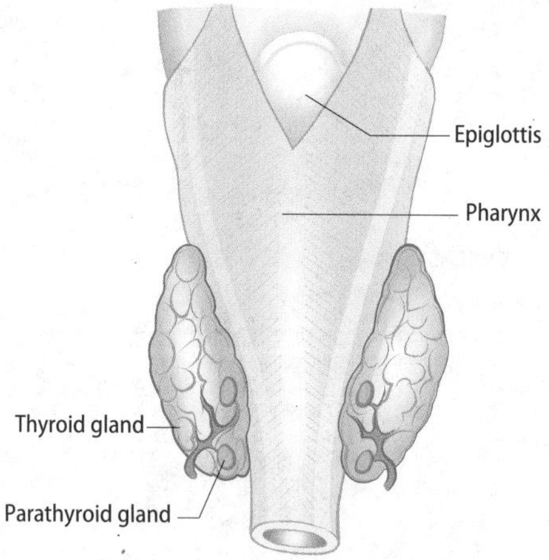

Posterior view of pharynx, thyroid glands, and parathyroid glands

60502 re-exploration
37.2 37.2 **FUD** 090 J 80
AMA: 2018,Jan,8; 2017,Jan,8; 2016,Jan,13; 2015,Jan,16

60505 with mediastinal exploration, sternal split or transthoracic approach
40.1 40.1 **FUD** 090 C 80
AMA: 2018,Jan,8; 2017,Jan,8; 2016,Jan,13; 2015,Jan,16

+ **60512** **Parathyroid autotransplantation (List separately in addition to code for primary procedure)**
Code first (60212, 60225, 60240, 60252, 60254, 60260, 60270-60271, 60500, 60502, 60505)
7.03 7.03 FUD ZZZ N 80
AMA: 2018,Jan,8; 2017,Jan,8; 2017,Jan,6; 2016,Jan,13; 2015,Jan,16

60520-60522 Thymus Procedures

EXCLUDES *Surgical thoracoscopy (video-assisted thoracic surgery (VATS) thymectomy (32673)*

60520 **Thymectomy, partial or total; transcervical approach (separate procedure)**
30.2 30.2 FUD 090 J 80
AMA: 2019,Mar,10

60521 **sternal split or transthoracic approach, without radical mediastinal dissection (separate procedure)**
32.4 32.4 FUD 090 C 80
AMA: 2018,Jan,8; 2017,Jan,8; 2016,Jan,13; 2015,Jan,16

60522 **sternal split or transthoracic approach, with radical mediastinal dissection (separate procedure)**
39.5 39.5 FUD 090 C 80
AMA: 2014,Jan,11; 2012,Oct,9-11

60540-60545 Adrenal Gland Procedures

EXCLUDES *Laparoscopic approach (60650)*
Removal remote or disseminated pheochromocytoma (49203-49205)
Standard backbench preparation cadaver donor (50323)

60540 **Adrenalectomy, partial or complete, or exploration of adrenal gland with or without biopsy, transabdominal, lumbar or dorsal (separate procedure);**
30.8 30.8 FUD 090 C 80 50
AMA: 2014,Jan,11; 1998,Nov,1

60545 **with excision of adjacent retroperitoneal tumor**
35.3 35.3 FUD 090 C 80 50
AMA: 2014,Jan,11; 1998,Nov,1

60600-60605 Carotid Body Procedures

60600 **Excision of carotid body tumor; without excision of carotid artery**
39.6 39.6 FUD 090 C 80
AMA: 2014,Jan,11

60605 **with excision of carotid artery**
48.2 48.2 FUD 090 C 80
AMA: 2018,Sep,9; 2017,Sep,13; 2016,Nov,8; 2016,Oct,10; 2016,Sep,8; 2016,Jul,10

60650-60699 Laparoscopic and Unlisted Procedures

INCLUDES Diagnostic laparoscopy (49320)

60650 **Laparoscopy, surgical, with adrenalectomy, partial or complete, or exploration of adrenal gland with or without biopsy, transabdominal, lumbar or dorsal**
EXCLUDES *Peritoneoscopy performed as separate procedure (49320)*
34.5 34.5 FUD 090 C 80 50
AMA: 2018,Jan,8; 2017,Jan,8; 2016,Jan,13; 2015,Jan,16

60659 **Unlisted laparoscopy procedure, endocrine system**
0.00 0.00 FUD YYY J 80 50
AMA: 2018,Jan,8; 2017,Jan,8; 2016,Jan,13; 2015,Jan,16

60699 **Unlisted procedure, endocrine system**
0.00 0.00 FUD YYY J 80
AMA: 2018,Jan,8; 2017,Jan,8; 2016,Jan,13; 2015,Jan,16

61000-61253 Transcranial Access via Puncture, Burr Hole, Twist Hole, or Trephine

EXCLUDES *Injection for cerebral angiography (36100-36218)*

61000 **Subdural tap through fontanelle, or suture, infant, unilateral or bilateral; initial** A

EXCLUDES *Injection for:*
Pneumoencephalography (61055)
Ventriculography (61026, 61120)

3.33 3.33 FUD 000 T R2

AMA: 2014,Jan,11

Overhead view of newborn skull

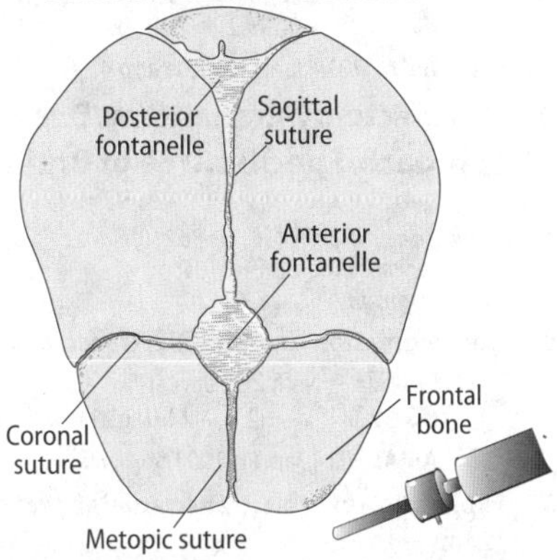

An initial tap through to the subdural level is performed on an infant via a fontanelle or suture, either unilateral or bilateral

61001 **subsequent taps** A

3.16 3.16 FUD 000 T R2

AMA: 2014,Jan,11

61020 **Ventricular puncture through previous burr hole, fontanelle, suture, or implanted ventricular catheter/reservoir; without injection**

2.87 2.87 FUD 000 T A2

AMA: 2014,Jan,11

61026 **with injection of medication or other substance for diagnosis or treatment**

INCLUDES Injection for ventriculography

3.05 3.05 FUD 000 T A2

AMA: 2014,Jan,11; 2002,May,7

61050 **Cisternal or lateral cervical (C1-C2) puncture; without injection (separate procedure)**

2.44 2.44 FUD 000 T A2 80

AMA: 2014,Jan,11; 1991,Win,1

61055 **with injection of medication or other substance for diagnosis or treatment**

INCLUDES Injection for pneumoencephalography

EXCLUDES *Myelography via lumbar injection (62302-62305)*
Radiology procedures except when furnished by different provider

3.62 3.62 FUD 000 T A2

AMA: 2014,Sep,3; 2014,Jan,11

61070 **Puncture of shunt tubing or reservoir for aspiration or injection procedure**

(75809)

1.63 1.63 FUD 000 T A2

AMA: 2018,Jan,8; 2017,Jan,8; 2016,Jan,13; 2015,Jan,16

61105 **Twist drill hole for subdural or ventricular puncture**

13.5 13.5 FUD 090 C 80

AMA: 2014,Jan,11

61107 **Twist drill hole(s) for subdural, intracerebral, or ventricular puncture; for implanting ventricular catheter, pressure recording device, or other intracerebral monitoring device**

Code also intracranial neuroendoscopic ventricular catheter insertion or reinsertion, when performed (62160)

9.20 9.20 FUD 000 ⊘ C

AMA: 2014,Jan,11; 2007,Jun,10-11

61108 **for evacuation and/or drainage of subdural hematoma**

25.8 25.8 FUD 090 C

AMA: 2014,Jan,11

61120 **Burr hole(s) for ventricular puncture (including injection of gas, contrast media, dye, or radioactive material)**

INCLUDES Injection for ventriculography

21.8 21.8 FUD 090 C 80

AMA: 2014,Jan,11

61140 **Burr hole(s) or trephine; with biopsy of brain or intracranial lesion**

36.9 36.9 FUD 090 C 80

AMA: 2014,Jan,11

61150 **with drainage of brain abscess or cyst**

39.8 39.8 FUD 090 C

AMA: 2014,Jan,11

61151 **with subsequent tapping (aspiration) of intracranial abscess or cyst**

29.1 29.1 FUD 090 C

AMA: 2014,Jan,11

61154 **Burr hole(s) with evacuation and/or drainage of hematoma, extradural or subdural**

36.6 36.6 FUD 090 C 80 50

AMA: 2014,Jan,11

61156 **Burr hole(s); with aspiration of hematoma or cyst, intracerebral**

36.5 36.5 FUD 090 C 80

AMA: 2014,Jan,11

61210 **for implanting ventricular catheter, reservoir, EEG electrode(s), pressure recording device, or other cerebral monitoring device (separate procedure)**

Code also intracranial neuroendoscopic ventricular catheter insertion or reinsertion, when performed (62160)

10.8 10.8 FUD 000 C

AMA: 2018,Jan,8; 2017,Jan,8; 2016,Jan,13; 2015,Jan,16

61215 **Insertion of subcutaneous reservoir, pump or continuous infusion system for connection to ventricular catheter**

EXCLUDES *Chemotherapy (96450)*
Refilling and maintenance implantable infusion pump (95990)

14.8 14.8 FUD 090 J A2

AMA: 2018,Jan,8; 2017,Jan,8; 2016,Jan,13; 2015,Jan,16

61250 **Burr hole(s) or trephine, supratentorial, exploratory, not followed by other surgery**

EXCLUDES *Burr hole or trephine followed by craniotomy same operative session (61304-61321)*

25.2 25.2 FUD 090 C 80 50

AMA: 2014,Jan,11

61253 **Burr hole(s) or trephine, infratentorial, unilateral or bilateral**

EXCLUDES *Burr hole or trephine followed by craniotomy same operative session (61304-61321)*

28.8 28.8 FUD 090 C 80

AMA: 2018,Jan,8; 2017,Jan,8; 2016,Jan,13; 2015,Jan,16

61304-61323 Craniectomy/Craniotomy: By Indication/Specific Area of Brain

EXCLUDES *Injection for:*
Cerebral angiography (36100-36218)
Pneumoencephalography (61055)
Ventriculography (61026, 61120)

61304 Craniectomy or craniotomy, exploratory; supratentorial
EXCLUDES *Other craniectomy/craniotomy procedures when performed same anatomical site and during same surgical encounter*
48.1 48.1 **FUD** 090 C 80
AMA: 2014,Jan,11; 2002,Sep,10

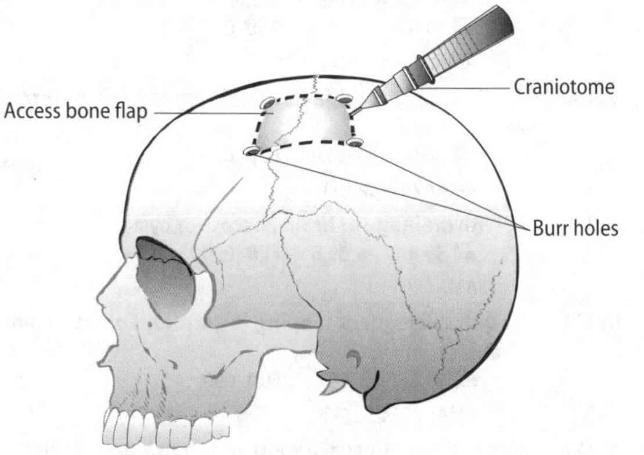

61305 infratentorial (posterior fossa)
EXCLUDES *Other craniectomy/craniotomy procedures when performed same anatomical site and during same surgical encounter*
58.6 58.6 **FUD** 090 C 80
AMA: 2014,Jan,11; 2002,Sep,10

61312 Craniectomy or craniotomy for evacuation of hematoma, supratentorial; extradural or subdural
60.8 60.8 **FUD** 090 C 80
AMA: 2018,Jan,8; 2017,Jan,8; 2016,Jan,13; 2015,Jan,16

61313 intracerebral
58.0 58.0 **FUD** 090 C 80
AMA: 2014,Jan,11; 2002,Sep,10

61314 Craniectomy or craniotomy for evacuation of hematoma, infratentorial; extradural or subdural
53.2 53.2 **FUD** 090 C 80
AMA: 2014,Jan,11; 2002,Sep,10

61315 intracerebellar
60.4 60.4 **FUD** 090 C 80
AMA: 2014,Jan,11; 2002,Sep,10

\+ **61316 Incision and subcutaneous placement of cranial bone graft (List separately in addition to code for primary procedure)**
Code first (61304, 61312-61313, 61322-61323, 61340, 61570-61571, 61680-61705)
2.60 2.60 **FUD** ZZZ C
AMA: 2014,Jan,11; 2002,Sep,10

61320 Craniectomy or craniotomy, drainage of intracranial abscess; supratentorial
55.5 55.5 **FUD** 090 C 80
AMA: 2014,Jan,11; 2002,Sep,10

61321 infratentorial
61.7 61.7 **FUD** 090 C 80
AMA: 2014,Jan,11; 2002,Sep,10

61322 Craniectomy or craniotomy, decompressive, with or without duraplasty, for treatment of intracranial hypertension, without evacuation of associated intraparenchymal hematoma; without lobectomy
EXCLUDES *Craniectomy or craniotomy for evacuation hematoma (61313)*
Subtemporal decompression (61340)
69.7 69.7 **FUD** 090 C 80
AMA: 2020,May,13; 2018,Aug,10

61323 with lobectomy
EXCLUDES *Craniectomy or craniotomy for evacuation hematoma (61313)*
Subtemporal decompression (61340)
69.2 69.2 **FUD** 090 C 80
AMA: 2014,Jan,11; 1991,Sum,4

61330-61530 Craniectomy/Craniotomy/Decompression Brain By Surgical Approach/Specific Area of Brain

EXCLUDES *Injection for:*
Cerebral angiography (36100-36218)
Pneumoencephalography (61055)
Ventriculography (61026, 61120)

61330 Decompression of orbit only, transcranial approach
INCLUDES Naffziger operation
52.8 52.8 **FUD** 090 J G2 80 50
AMA: 2014,Jan,11; 1991,Sum,4

61333 Exploration of orbit (transcranial approach); with removal of lesion
59.6 59.6 **FUD** 090 C 80 50
AMA: 2014,Jan,11; 1991,Sum,4

61340 Subtemporal cranial decompression (pseudotumor cerebri, slit ventricle syndrome)
EXCLUDES *Decompression craniotomy or craniectomy for intracranial hypertension, without hematoma removal (61322-61323)*
42.4 42.4 **FUD** 090 C 80 50
AMA: 2020,May,13

61343 Craniectomy, suboccipital with cervical laminectomy for decompression of medulla and spinal cord, with or without dural graft (eg, Arnold-Chiari malformation)
63.4 63.4 **FUD** 090 C 80
AMA: 2014,Jan,11; 1991,Sum,4

61345 Other cranial decompression, posterior fossa
EXCLUDES *Kroenlein procedure*
Orbital decompression using lateral wall approach (67445)
60.1 60.1 **FUD** 090 C 80
AMA: 2014,Jan,11; 1991,Sum,4

61450 Craniectomy, subtemporal, for section, compression, or decompression of sensory root of gasserian ganglion
INCLUDES Frazier-Spiller procedure
Hartley-Krause
Krause decompression
Taarnhoj procedure
56.0 56.0 **FUD** 090 C 80
AMA: 2014,Jan,11; 1991,Sum,4

61458 Craniectomy, suboccipital; for exploration or decompression of cranial nerves
INCLUDES Jannetta decompression
58.8 58.8 **FUD** 090 C 80
AMA: 2014,Jan,11; 1991,Sum,4

61460 **for section of 1 or more cranial nerves**
61.7 61.7 **FUD** 090 C 80
AMA: 2014,Jan,11; 1991,Sum,4

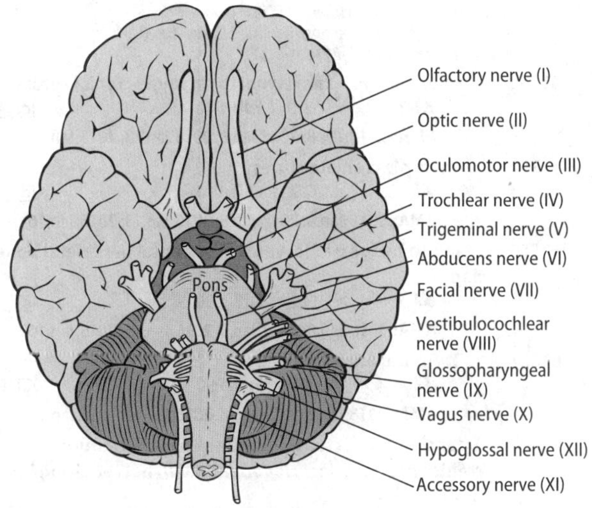

61500 **Craniectomy; with excision of tumor or other bone lesion of skull**
38.2 38.2 **FUD** 090 C 80
AMA: 2018,Jan,8; 2017,Jan,8; 2016,Jan,13; 2015,Jan,16

61501 **for osteomyelitis**
32.8 32.8 **FUD** 090 C 80
AMA: 2018,Jan,8; 2017,Jan,8; 2016,Jan,13; 2015,Jan,16

61510 **Craniectomy, trephination, bone flap craniotomy; for excision of brain tumor, supratentorial, except meningioma**
64.0 64.0 **FUD** 090 C 80
AMA: 2014,Jan,11; 1991,Sum,4

61512 **for excision of meningioma, supratentorial**
74.8 74.8 **FUD** 090 C 80
AMA: 2014,Jan,11; 1991,Sum,4

61514 **for excision of brain abscess, supratentorial**
55.9 55.9 **FUD** 090 C 80
AMA: 2014,Jan,11; 1991,Sum,4

61516 **for excision or fenestration of cyst, supratentorial**
EXCLUDES *Craniopharyngioma (61545)*
Pituitary tumor removal (61546, 61548)
54.4 54.4 **FUD** 090 C 80
AMA: 2014,Jan,11; 1991,Sum,4

\+ **61517** **Implantation of brain intracavitary chemotherapy agent (List separately in addition to code for primary procedure)**
EXCLUDES *Intracavity radioelement source or ribbon implantation (77770-77772)*
Code first (61510, 61518)
2.59 2.59 **FUD** ZZZ C
AMA: 2014,Jan,11; 1991,Sum,4

61518 **Craniectomy for excision of brain tumor, infratentorial or posterior fossa; except meningioma, cerebellopontine angle tumor, or midline tumor at base of skull**
79.9 79.9 **FUD** 090 C 80
AMA: 2014,Jan,11; 1991,Sum,4

61519 **meningioma**
86.7 86.7 **FUD** 090 C 80
AMA: 2014,Jan,11; 1991,Sum,4

61520 **cerebellopontine angle tumor**
110. 110. **FUD** 090 C 80
AMA: 2014,Jan,11; 1991,Sum,4

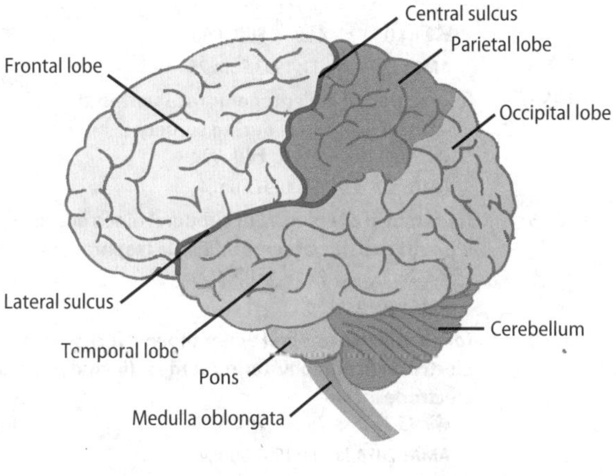

61521 **midline tumor at base of skull**
93.7 93.7 **FUD** 090 C 80
AMA: 2018,Jan,8; 2017,Jan,8; 2016,Jan,13; 2015,Jan,16

61522 **Craniectomy, infratentorial or posterior fossa; for excision of brain abscess**
62.9 62.9 **FUD** 090 C 80
AMA: 2014,Jan,11; 1991,Sum,4

61524 **for excision or fenestration of cyst**
60.1 60.1 **FUD** 090 C 80
AMA: 2014,Jan,11; 1991,Sum,4

61526 **Craniectomy, bone flap craniotomy, transtemporal (mastoid) for excision of cerebellopontine angle tumor;**
97.9 97.9 **FUD** 090 C
AMA: 2018,Mar,11; 2018,Jan,8; 2017,Jan,8; 2016,Jan,13; 2015,Jan,16

61530 **combined with middle/posterior fossa craniotomy/craniectomy**
91.0 91.0 **FUD** 090 C
AMA: 2014,Jan,11; 1991,Sum,4

61531-61545 Procedures for Seizures/Implanted Electrodes/Choroid Plexus/Craniopharyngioma

EXCLUDES *Craniotomy for:*
Multiple subpial transections during procedure (61567)
Selective amygdalohippocampectomy (61566)
Injection for:
Cerebral angiography (36100-36218)
Pneumoencephalography (61055)
Ventriculography (61026, 61120)

61531 **Subdural implantation of strip electrodes through 1 or more burr or trephine hole(s) for long-term seizure monitoring**
EXCLUDES *Continuous EEG observation ([95700, 95705, 95706, 95707, 95708, 95709, 95710, 95711, 95712, 95713, 95714, 95715, 95716, 95717, 95718, 95719, 95720, 95721, 95722, 95723, 95724, 95725, 95726])*
Craniotomy for intracranial arteriovenous malformation removal (61680-61692)
Stereotactic insertion electrodes (61760)
35.2 35.2 **FUD** 090 C 80
AMA: 2019,Jul,10

61533 **Craniotomy with elevation of bone flap; for subdural implantation of an electrode array, for long-term seizure monitoring**

EXCLUDES *Continuous EEG monitoring ([95700, 95705, 95706, 95707, 95708, 95709, 95710, 95711, 95712, 95713, 95714, 95715, 95716, 95717, 95718, 95719, 95720, 95721, 95722, 95723, 95724, 95725, 95726])*

44.0 44.0 **FUD** 090 C 80

AMA: 2014,Jan,11; 1993,Sum,25

61534 **for excision of epileptogenic focus without electrocorticography during surgery**

47.4 47.4 **FUD** 090 C 80

AMA: 2014,Jan,11; 1991,Sum,4

61535 **for removal of epidural or subdural electrode array, without excision of cerebral tissue (separate procedure)**

29.1 29.1 **FUD** 090 C 80

AMA: 2019,Jul,10

61536 **for excision of cerebral epileptogenic focus, with electrocorticography during surgery (includes removal of electrode array)**

75.2 75.2 **FUD** 090 C 80

AMA: 2014,Jan,11; 1991,Sum,4

61537 **for lobectomy, temporal lobe, without electrocorticography during surgery**

72.4 72.4 **FUD** 090 C 80

AMA: 2014,Jan,11; 1991,Sum,4

61538 **for lobectomy, temporal lobe, with electrocorticography during surgery**

77.1 77.1 **FUD** 090 C 80

AMA: 2019,Mar,6

61539 **for lobectomy, other than temporal lobe, partial or total, with electrocorticography during surgery**

68.2 68.2 **FUD** 090 C 80

AMA: 2019,Mar,6

61540 **for lobectomy, other than temporal lobe, partial or total, without electrocorticography during surgery**

62.9 62.9 **FUD** 090 C 80

AMA: 2014,Jan,11; 1991,Sum,4

61541 **for transection of corpus callosum**

63.3 63.3 **FUD** 090 C 80

AMA: 2014,Jan,11; 1991,Sum,4

61543 **for partial or subtotal (functional) hemispherectomy**

64.0 64.0 **FUD** 090 C 80

AMA: 2014,Jan,11; 1991,Sum,4

61544 **for excision or coagulation of choroid plexus**

54.8 54.8 **FUD** 090 C 80

AMA: 2014,Jan,11; 1991,Sum,4

61545 **for excision of craniopharyngioma**

92.3 92.3 **FUD** 090 C 80

AMA: 2014,Jan,11; 1991,Sum,4

61546-61548 Removal Pituitary Gland/Tumor

EXCLUDES *Injection for:*
Cerebral angiography (36100-36218)
Pneumoencephalography (61055)
Ventriculography (61026, 61120)

61546 **Craniotomy for hypophysectomy or excision of pituitary tumor, intracranial approach**

67.4 67.4 **FUD** 090 C 80

AMA: 2014,Jan,11; 1991,Sum,4

61548 **Hypophysectomy or excision of pituitary tumor, transnasal or transseptal approach, nonstereotactic**

INCLUDES Operating microscope (69990)

45.8 45.8 **FUD** 090 C 80

AMA: 2019,Dec,12; 2016,Feb,12

61550-61559 Craniosynostosis Procedures

EXCLUDES *Injection for:*
Cerebral angiography (36100-36218)
Pneumoencephalography (61055)
Ventriculography (61026, 61120)
Orbital hypertelorism reconstruction (21260-21263)
Reconstruction (21172-21180)

61550 **Craniectomy for craniosynostosis; single cranial suture**

32.1 32.1 **FUD** 090 C 80

AMA: 2018,Jan,8; 2017,Jan,8; 2016,Jan,13; 2015,Jan,16

61552 **multiple cranial sutures**

42.7 42.7 **FUD** 090 C 80

AMA: 2018,Jan,8; 2017,Jan,8; 2016,Jan,13; 2015,Jan,16

61556 **Craniotomy for craniosynostosis; frontal or parietal bone flap**

49.2 49.2 **FUD** 090 C 80

AMA: 2018,Jan,8; 2017,Jan,8; 2016,Jan,13; 2015,Jan,16

61557 **bifrontal bone flap**

49.4 49.4 **FUD** 090 C 80

AMA: 2018,Jan,8; 2017,Jan,8; 2016,Jan,13; 2015,Jan,16

61558 **Extensive craniectomy for multiple cranial suture craniosynostosis (eg, cloverleaf skull); not requiring bone grafts**

55.2 55.2 **FUD** 090 C 80

AMA: 2018,Jan,8; 2017,Jan,8; 2016,Jan,13; 2015,Jan,16

61559 **recontouring with multiple osteotomies and bone autografts (eg, barrel-stave procedure) (includes obtaining grafts)**

70.5 70.5 **FUD** 090 C 80

AMA: 2018,Jan,8; 2017,Jan,8; 2016,Jan,13; 2015,Jan,16

61563-61564 Removal Cranial Bone Tumor With/Without Optic Nerve Decompression

EXCLUDES *Injection for:*
Cerebral angiography (36100-36218)
Pneumoencephalography (61055)
Ventriculography (61026, 61120)
Reconstruction (21181-21183)

61563 **Excision, intra and extracranial, benign tumor of cranial bone (eg, fibrous dysplasia); without optic nerve decompression**

57.5 57.5 **FUD** 090 C 80

AMA: 2014,Jan,11; 1991,Sum,4

61564 **with optic nerve decompression**

69.5 69.5 **FUD** 090 C 80 50

AMA: 2014,Jan,11; 1991,Sum,4

61566-61567 Craniotomy for Seizures

EXCLUDES *Injection for:*
Cerebral angiography (36100-36218)
Pneumoencephalography (61055)
Ventriculography (61026, 61120)

61566 **Craniotomy with elevation of bone flap; for selective amygdalohippocampectomy**

64.8 64.8 **FUD** 090 C 80

AMA: 2018,Nov,7

61567 **for multiple subpial transections, with electrocorticography during surgery**

72.9 72.9 **FUD** 090 C 80

AMA: 2014,Jan,11; 1991,Sum,4

61570-61571 Removal of Foreign Body from Brain

EXCLUDES *Injection for:*
Cerebral angiography (36100-36218)
Pneumoencephalography (61055)
Ventriculography (61026, 61120)
Sequestrectomy for osteomyelitis (61501)

61570 **Craniectomy or craniotomy; with excision of foreign body from brain**

53.9 53.9 **FUD** 090 C 80

AMA: 2014,Jan,11; 1991,Sum,4

61571 **with treatment of penetrating wound of brain**
57.4 57.4 FUD 090 C 80
AMA: 2014,Jan,11; 1991,Sum,4

61575-61576 Transoral Approach Posterior Cranial Fossa/Upper Cervical Cord

EXCLUDES *Arthrodesis (22548)*
Injection for:
Cerebral angiography (36100-36218)
Pneumoencephalography (61055)
Ventriculography (61026, 61120)

61575 **Transoral approach to skull base, brain stem or upper spinal cord for biopsy, decompression or excision of lesion;**
72.4 72.4 FUD 090 C 80
AMA: 2014,Jan,11; 1991,Sum,4

61576 **requiring splitting of tongue and/or mandible (including tracheostomy)**
121. 121. FUD 090 C 80
AMA: 2014,Jan,11; 1991,Sum,4

61580-61598 Surgical Approach: Cranial Fossae

EXCLUDES *Definitive surgery (61600-61616)*
Dural repair and/or reconstruction (61618-61619)
Injection for:
Cerebral angiography (36100-36218)
Pneumoencephalography (61055)
Ventriculography (61026, 61120)
Primary closure (15730, 15733, 15756-15758)

61580 **Craniofacial approach to anterior cranial fossa; extradural, including lateral rhinotomy, ethmoidectomy, sphenoidectomy, without maxillectomy or orbital exenteration**
70.3 70.3 FUD 090 C 50
AMA: 2018,Jan,8; 2017,Jan,8; 2016,Jan,13; 2015,Jan,16

61581 **extradural, including lateral rhinotomy, orbital exenteration, ethmoidectomy, sphenoidectomy and/or maxillectomy**
76.6 76.6 FUD 090 C 50
AMA: 2018,Jan,8; 2017,Jan,8; 2016,Jan,13; 2015,Jan,16

61582 **extradural, including unilateral or bifrontal craniotomy, elevation of frontal lobe(s), osteotomy of base of anterior cranial fossa**
88.5 88.5 FUD 090 C 80
AMA: 2018,Jan,8; 2017,Jan,8; 2016,Jan,13; 2015,Jan,16

61583 **intradural, including unilateral or bifrontal craniotomy, elevation or resection of frontal lobe, osteotomy of base of anterior cranial fossa**
84.2 84.2 FUD 090 C 80
AMA: 2018,Jan,8; 2017,Dec,13; 2017,Jan,8; 2016,Jan,13; 2015,Jan,16

61584 **Orbitocranial approach to anterior cranial fossa, extradural, including supraorbital ridge osteotomy and elevation of frontal and/or temporal lobe(s); without orbital exenteration**
83.7 83.7 FUD 090 C 80 50
AMA: 2018,Jan,8; 2017,Jan,8; 2016,Jan,13; 2015,Jan,16

61585 **with orbital exenteration**
95.1 95.1 FUD 090 C 80 50
AMA: 2018,Jan,8; 2017,Jan,8; 2016,Jan,13; 2015,Jan,16

61586 **Bicoronal, transzygomatic and/or LeFort I osteotomy approach to anterior cranial fossa with or without internal fixation, without bone graft**
70.5 70.5 FUD 090 C 80
AMA: 2014,Jan,11; 1997,Nov,1

61590 **Infratemporal pre-auricular approach to middle cranial fossa (parapharyngeal space, infratemporal and midline skull base, nasopharynx), with or without disarticulation of the mandible, including parotidectomy, craniotomy, decompression and/or mobilization of the facial nerve and/or petrous carotid artery**
88.1 88.1 FUD 090 C 80 50
AMA: 2020,Apr,10; 2018,Jan,8; 2017,Jan,8; 2016,Jan,13; 2015,Jan,16

61591 **Infratemporal post-auricular approach to middle cranial fossa (internal auditory meatus, petrous apex, tentorium, cavernous sinus, parasellar area, infratemporal fossa) including mastoidectomy, resection of sigmoid sinus, with or without decompression and/or mobilization of contents of auditory canal or petrous carotid artery**
89.1 89.1 FUD 090 C 80 50
AMA: 2018,Jan,8; 2017,Jan,8; 2016,Jan,13; 2015,Jan,16

61592 **Orbitocranial zygomatic approach to middle cranial fossa (cavernous sinus and carotid artery, clivus, basilar artery or petrous apex) including osteotomy of zygoma, craniotomy, extra- or intradural elevation of temporal lobe**
92.5 92.5 FUD 090 C 80 50
AMA: 2018,Jan,8; 2017,Jan,8; 2016,Jan,13; 2015,Jan,16

61595 **Transtemporal approach to posterior cranial fossa, jugular foramen or midline skull base, including mastoidectomy, decompression of sigmoid sinus and/or facial nerve, with or without mobilization**
68.1 68.1 FUD 090 C 50
AMA: 2018,Mar,11; 2018,Jan,8; 2017,Jan,8; 2016,Jan,13; 2015,Jan,16

61596 **Transcochlear approach to posterior cranial fossa, jugular foramen or midline skull base, including labyrinthectomy, decompression, with or without mobilization of facial nerve and/or petrous carotid artery**
70.1 70.1 FUD 090 C 80 50
AMA: 2018,Jan,8; 2017,Jan,8; 2016,Jan,13; 2015,Jan,16

61597 **Transcondylar (far lateral) approach to posterior cranial fossa, jugular foramen or midline skull base, including occipital condylectomy, mastoidectomy, resection of C1-C3 vertebral body(s), decompression of vertebral artery, with or without mobilization**
85.5 85.5 FUD 090 C 80 50
AMA: 2018,Jan,8; 2017,Jan,8; 2016,Jan,13; 2015,Jan,16

61598 **Transpetrosal approach to posterior cranial fossa, clivus or foramen magnum, including ligation of superior petrosal sinus and/or sigmoid sinus**
82.9 82.9 FUD 090 C 80
AMA: 2018,Jan,8; 2017,Jan,8; 2016,Jan,13; 2015,Jan,16

61600-61616 Definitive Procedures: Cranial Fossae

EXCLUDES *Dural repair and/or reconstruction (61618-61619)*
Injection for:
Cerebral angiography (36100-36218)
Pneumoencephalography (61055)
Ventriculography (61026, 61120)
Primary closure (15730, 15733, 15756-15758)
Surgical approach (61580-61598)

61600 **Resection or excision of neoplastic, vascular or infectious lesion of base of anterior cranial fossa; extradural**
61.5 61.5 FUD 090 C 80
AMA: 2018,Jan,8; 2017,Jan,8; 2016,Jan,13; 2015,Jan,16

61601 **intradural, including dural repair, with or without graft**
70.1 70.1 FUD 090 C 80
AMA: 2018,Jan,8; 2017,Jan,8; 2016,Jan,13; 2015,Jan,16

61605 **Resection or excision of neoplastic, vascular or infectious lesion of infratemporal fossa, parapharyngeal space, petrous apex; extradural**
62.1 62.1 FUD 090 C 80
AMA: 2020,Apr,10; 2018,Jan,8; 2017,Jan,8; 2016,Jan,13; 2015,Jan,16

61606 **intradural, including dural repair, with or without graft**
85.7 85.7 **FUD** 090 C 80
AMA: 2018,Jan,8; 2017,Jan,8; 2016,Jan,13; 2015,Jan,16

61607 **Resection or excision of neoplastic, vascular or infectious lesion of parasellar area, cavernous sinus, clivus or midline skull base; extradural**
77.8 77.8 **FUD** 090 C 80
AMA: 2018,Jan,8; 2017,Jan,8; 2016,Jan,13; 2015,Jan,16

61608 **intradural, including dural repair, with or without graft**
95.7 95.7 **FUD** 090 C 80
AMA: 2018,Jan,8; 2017,Jan,8; 2016,Jan,13; 2015,Jan,16

+ 61611 **Transection or ligation, carotid artery in petrous canal; without repair (List separately in addition to code for primary procedure)**
Code first (61605-61608)
13.8 13.8 **FUD** ZZZ C 80
AMA: 2018,Jan,8; 2017,Jan,8; 2016,Jan,13; 2015,Jan,16

61613 **Obliteration of carotid aneurysm, arteriovenous malformation, or carotid-cavernous fistula by dissection within cavernous sinus**
96.9 96.9 **FUD** 090 C 80 50
AMA: 2018,Jan,8; 2017,Jan,8; 2016,Jan,13; 2015,Jan,16

61615 **Resection or excision of neoplastic, vascular or infectious lesion of base of posterior cranial fossa, jugular foramen, foramen magnum, or C1-C3 vertebral bodies; extradural**
81.9 81.9 **FUD** 090 C 80
AMA: 2018,Jan,8; 2017,Jan,8; 2016,Jan,13; 2015,Jan,16

61616 **intradural, including dural repair, with or without graft**
96.0 96.0 **FUD** 090 C 80
AMA: 2018,Mar,11; 2018,Jan,8; 2017,Jan,8; 2016,Jan,13; 2015,Jan,16

61618-61619 Reconstruction Post-Surgical Cranial Fossae Defects

EXCLUDES *Definitive surgery (61600-61616)*
Injection for:
Cerebral angiography (36100-36218)
Pneumoencephalography (61055)
Ventriculography (61026, 61120)
Primary closure (15730, 15733, 15756-15758)
Surgical approach (61580-61598)

61618 **Secondary repair of dura for cerebrospinal fluid leak, anterior, middle or posterior cranial fossa following surgery of the skull base; by free tissue graft (eg, pericranium, fascia, tensor fascia lata, adipose tissue, homologous or synthetic grafts)**
37.5 37.5 **FUD** 090 C 80
AMA: 2018,Jan,8; 2017,Jan,8; 2016,Jan,13; 2015,Jan,16

61619 **by local or regionalized vascularized pedicle flap or myocutaneous flap (including galea, temporalis, frontalis or occipitalis muscle)**
41.3 41.3 **FUD** 090 C 80
AMA: 2018,Jan,8; 2017,Jan,8; 2016,Jan,13; 2015,Jan,16

61623-61651 Neurovascular Interventional Procedures

61623 **Endovascular temporary balloon arterial occlusion, head or neck (extracranial/intracranial) including selective catheterization of vessel to be occluded, positioning and inflation of occlusion balloon, concomitant neurological monitoring, and radiologic supervision and interpretation of all angiography required for balloon occlusion and to exclude vascular injury post occlusion**
EXCLUDES *Diagnostic angiography target artery just before temporary occlusion; report only radiological supervision and interpretation*
Selective catheterization and angiography artery besides the target artery; report catheterization and radiological supervision and interpretation codes as appropriate
16.6 16.6 **FUD** 000 J
AMA: 2018,Jan,8; 2017,Jan,8; 2016,Jan,13; 2015,Jan,16

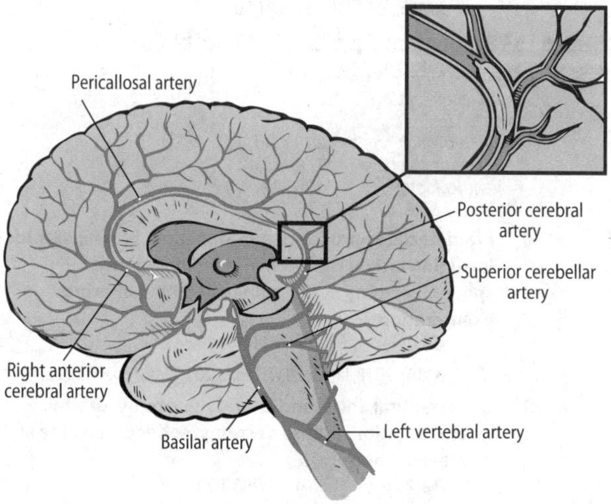

61624 **Transcatheter permanent occlusion or embolization (eg, for tumor destruction, to achieve hemostasis, to occlude a vascular malformation), percutaneous, any method; central nervous system (intracranial, spinal cord)**
EXCLUDES *Non-central nervous system transcatheter occlusion or embolization other than head or neck (37241-37244)*
(75894)
33.3 33.3 **FUD** 000 C
AMA: 2019,Sep,6; 2018,Jan,8; 2017,Jan,8; 2016,Jan,13; 2015,Jan,16

61626 **non-central nervous system, head or neck (extracranial, brachiocephalic branch)**
EXCLUDES *Non-central nervous system transcatheter occlusion or embolization other than head or neck (37241-37244)*
(75894)
25.5 25.5 **FUD** 000 J
AMA: 2019,Sep,6; 2018,Jan,8; 2017,Jan,8; 2016,Jan,13; 2015,Jan,16

61630 Balloon angioplasty, intracranial (eg, atherosclerotic stenosis), percutaneous

INCLUDES Diagnostic arteriogram when stent or angioplasty necessary
Radiology services for arteriography target vascular territory
Selective catheterization target vascular territory

EXCLUDES *Diagnostic arteriogram when stent or angioplasty not necessary (report applicable code for selective catheterization and radiology services)*
Percutaneous arterial transluminal mechanical thrombectomy and/or infusion for thrombolysis performed same vascular territory (61645)

40.6 40.6 FUD XXX C 80

AMA: 2018,Jan,8; 2017,Jul,3; 2017,Apr,9; 2017,Jan,8; 2016,Mar,3; 2016,Jan,13; 2015,Nov,3; 2015,Jan,16

61635 Transcatheter placement of intravascular stent(s), intracranial (eg, atherosclerotic stenosis), including balloon angioplasty, if performed

INCLUDES Diagnostic arteriogram when stent or angioplasty necessary
Radiology services for arteriography target vascular territory
Selective catheterization target vascular territory

EXCLUDES *Diagnostic arteriogram when stent or angioplasty not necessary (report applicable code for selective catheterization and radiology services)*
Percutaneous arterial transluminal mechanical thrombectomy and/or infusion for thrombolysis performed same vascular territory (61645)

42.6 42.6 FUD XXX C 80

AMA: 2018,Jan,8; 2017,Jul,3; 2017,Jan,8; 2016,Mar,3; 2016,Jan,13; 2015,Nov,3; 2015,Jan,16

61640 Balloon dilatation of intracranial vasospasm, percutaneous; initial vessel

INCLUDES Angiography after dilation vessel
Fluoroscopic guidance
Injection contrast material
Roadmapping
Selective catheterization target vessel
Vessel analysis

EXCLUDES *Endovascular intracranial prolonged administration pharmacologic agent performed same vascular territory (61650-61651)*

Code first (61640)

14.0 14.0 FUD 000 E

AMA: 2018,Jan,8; 2017,Jan,8; 2016,Mar,3; 2016,Jan,13; 2015,Nov,3; 2015,Jan,16

\+ **61641 each additional vessel in same vascular territory (List separately in addition to code for primary procedure)**

INCLUDES Angiography after dilation vessel
Fluoroscopic guidance
Injection contrast material
Roadmapping
Selective catheterization target vessel
Vessel analysis

EXCLUDES *Endovascular intracranial prolonged administration pharmacologic agent performed same vascular territory (61640)*

Code first (61640)

4.92 4.92 FUD ZZZ E

AMA: 2018,Jan,8; 2017,Jan,8; 2016,Mar,3; 2016,Jan,13; 2015,Nov,3; 2015,Jan,16

\+ **61642 each additional vessel in different vascular territory (List separately in addition to code for primary procedure))**

INCLUDES Angiography after dilation vessel
Fluoroscopic guidance
Injection contrast material
Roadmapping
Selective catheterization target vessel
Vessel analysis

EXCLUDES *Endovascular intracranial prolonged administration pharmacologic agent performed same vascular territory (61650-61651)*

Code first (61640)

9.84 9.84 FUD ZZZ E

AMA: 2018,Jan,8; 2017,Jan,8; 2016,Mar,3; 2016,Jan,13; 2015,Nov,3; 2015,Jan,16

61645 Percutaneous arterial transluminal mechanical thrombectomy and/or infusion for thrombolysis, intracranial, any method, including diagnostic angiography, fluoroscopic guidance, catheter placement, and intraprocedural pharmacological thrombolytic injection(s)

INCLUDES Interventions performed in intracranial artery including:
Angiography with radiologic supervision and interpretation (diagnostic and subsequent)
Closure arteriotomy by any method
Fluoroscopy
Patient monitoring
Procedures performed in vascular territories:
Left carotid
Right carotid
Vertebro-basilar

EXCLUDES *Procedure performed same vascular target area:*
Balloon angioplasty, intracranial (61630)
Diagnostic studies: aortic arch, carotid, and vertebral arteries (36221-36226)
Endovascular intracranial prolonged administration pharmacologic agent (61650-61651)
Transcatheter placement intravascular stent (61635)
Transluminal thrombectomy (37184, 37186)
Reporting code more than one time for treatment each intracranial vascular territory
Venous thrombectomy or thrombolysis (37187-37188, 37212, 37214)

24.0 24.0 FUD 000 C 80 50

AMA: 2019,Sep,6; 2019,Sep,5; 2018,Jan,8; 2017,Jan,8; 2016,Mar,3; 2016,Jan,13; 2015,Dec,18; 2015,Nov,3

61650 **Endovascular intracranial prolonged administration of pharmacologic agent(s) other than for thrombolysis, arterial, including catheter placement, diagnostic angiography, and imaging guidance; initial vascular territory**

INCLUDES Interventions performed in intracranial artery, including:
- Angiography with radiologic supervision and interpretation (diagnostic and subsequent)
- Closure arteriotomy by any method
- Fluoroscopy
- Patient monitoring
- Procedures performed in vascular territories:
  - Left carotid
  - Right carotid
  - Vertebro-basilar

Prolonged (at least 10 minutes) arterial administration nonthrombolytic agents

EXCLUDES *Procedure performed same vascular target area:*
- *Balloon dilatation intracranial vasospasm (61640-61642)*
- *Chemotherapy administration (96420-96425)*
- *Diagnostic studies: aortic arch, carotid, and vertebral arteries (36221-36228)*
- *Transluminal thrombectomy (37184, 37186, 61645)*

Reporting code more than one time for treatment each intracranial vascular territory

Treatment iatrogenic condition

Venous thrombectomy or thrombolysis

15.6 15.6 **FUD** 000 C

AMA: 2019,Sep,6; 2018,Jan,8; 2017,Jan,8; 2016,Mar,3; 2016,Jan,13; 2015,Nov,3

\+ **61651** **each additional vascular territory (List separately in addition to code for primary procedure)**

INCLUDES Interventions performed in intracranial artery, including:
- Angiography with radiologic supervision and interpretation (diagnostic and subsequent)
- Closure arteriotomy by any method
- Fluoroscopy
- Patient monitoring
- Procedures performed in vascular territories:
  - Left carotid
  - Right carotid
  - Vertebro-basilar

Prolonged (at least 10 minutes) arterial administration nonthrombolytic agents

EXCLUDES *Procedure performed same vascular target area:*
- *Balloon dilatation intracranial vasospasm (61640-61642)*
- *Chemotherapy administration (96420-96425)*
- *Diagnostic studies: aortic arch, carotid, and vertebral arteries (36221-36228)*
- *Transluminal thrombectomy (37184, 37186, 61645)*

Reporting code more than one time for treatment each intracranial vascular territory

Treatment iatrogenic condition

Venous thrombectomy or thrombolysis

Code first (61650)

6.65 6.65 **FUD** ZZZ C

AMA: 2019,Sep,6; 2018,Jan,8; 2017,Jan,8; 2016,Mar,3; 2016,Jan,13; 2015,Nov,3

61680-61692 Surgical Treatment of Arteriovenous Malformation of the Brain

INCLUDES Craniotomy

61680 **Surgery of intracranial arteriovenous malformation; supratentorial, simple**

65.1 65.1 **FUD** 090 C 80

AMA: 2014,Jan,11

61682 **supratentorial, complex**

123. 123. **FUD** 090 C 80

AMA: 2018,Jan,8; 2017,Jan,8; 2016,Jan,13; 2015,Jan,16

61684 **infratentorial, simple**

84.0 84.0 **FUD** 090 C 80

AMA: 2014,Jan,11

61686 **infratentorial, complex**

134. 134. **FUD** 090 C 80

AMA: 2018,Jan,8; 2017,Jan,8; 2016,Jan,13; 2015,Jan,16

61690 **dural, simple**

63.0 63.0 **FUD** 090 C 80

AMA: 2014,Jan,11

61692 **dural, complex**

106. 106. **FUD** 090 C 80

AMA: 2018,Jan,8; 2017,Jan,8; 2016,Jan,13; 2015,Jan,16

61697-61703 Surgical Treatment Brain Aneurysm

INCLUDES Craniotomy

61697 **Surgery of complex intracranial aneurysm, intracranial approach; carotid circulation**

INCLUDES Aneurysms bigger than 15 mm
- Calcification aneurysm neck
- Inclusion normal vessels in aneurysm neck
- Surgery needing temporary vessel occlusion, trapping, or cardiopulmonary bypass to treat aneurysm

125. 125. **FUD** 090 C 80

AMA: 2018,Jan,8; 2017,Dec,13

61698 **vertebrobasilar circulation**

INCLUDES Aneurysm bigger than 15 mm
- Calcification aneurysm neck
- Inclusion normal vessels in aneurysm neck
- Surgery needing temporary vessel occlusion, trapping, or cardiopulmonary bypass to treat aneurysm

141. 141. **FUD** 090 C 80

AMA: 2014,Jan,11

61700 **Surgery of simple intracranial aneurysm, intracranial approach; carotid circulation**

100. 100. **FUD** 090 C 80

AMA: 2018,Jan,8; 2017,Dec,13; 2017,Jan,8; 2016,Jan,13; 2015,Jan,16

61702 **vertebrobasilar circulation**

117. 117. **FUD** 090 C 80

AMA: 2014,Jan,11

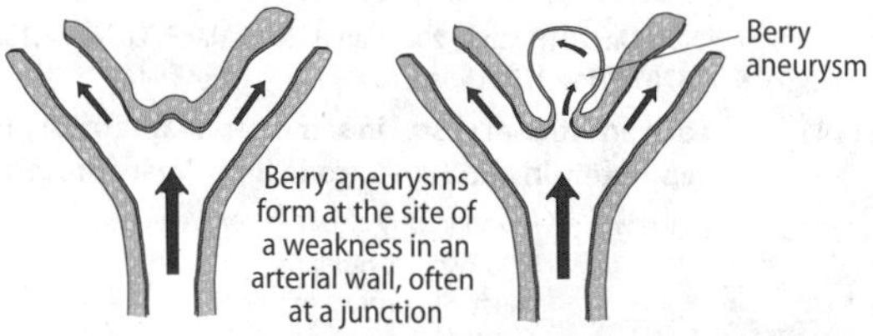

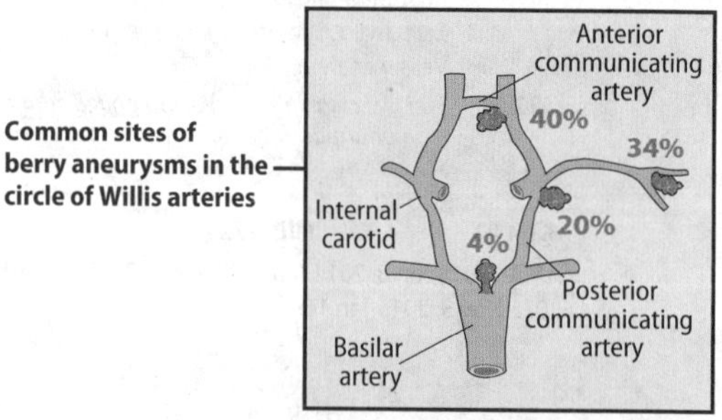

61703 **Surgery of intracranial aneurysm, cervical approach by application of occluding clamp to cervical carotid artery (Selverstone-Crutchfield type)**

EXCLUDES *Cervical approach for direct ligation carotid artery (37600-37606)*

39.0 39.0 **FUD** 090 C 80

AMA: 2014,Jan,11

61705-61710 Other Procedures for Aneurysm, Arteriovenous Malformation, and Carotid-Cavernous Fistula

INCLUDES Craniotomy

61705 **Surgery of aneurysm, vascular malformation or carotid-cavernous fistula; by intracranial and cervical occlusion of carotid artery**
73.6 73.6 **FUD** 090 C 80
AMA: 2014,Jan,11

61708 **by intracranial electrothrombosis**
EXCLUDES *Ligation or gradual occlusion internal or common carotid artery (37605-37606)*
75.1 75.1 **FUD** 090 C 80
AMA: 2014,Jan,11; 2000,Sep,11

61710 **by intra-arterial embolization, injection procedure, or balloon catheter**
63.3 63.3 **FUD** 090 C 80
AMA: 2018,Jan,8; 2017,Jan,8; 2016,Jan,13; 2015,Jan,16

61711 Extracranial-Intracranial Bypass

CMS: 100-02,16,10 Exclusions from Coverage; 100-03,20.2 Extracranial-intracranial (EC-IC) Arterial Bypass Surgery

INCLUDES Craniotomy
EXCLUDES *Carotid or vertebral thromboendarterectomy (35301)*
Code also operating microscope when appropriate (69990)

61711 **Anastomosis, arterial, extracranial-intracranial (eg, middle cerebral/cortical) arteries**
75.8 75.8 **FUD** 090 C 80
AMA: 2014,Jan,11

61720-61791 Stereotactic Procedures of the Brain

61720 **Creation of lesion by stereotactic method, including burr hole(s) and localizing and recording techniques, single or multiple stages; globus pallidus or thalamus**
37.3 37.3 **FUD** 090 J
AMA: 2018,Jan,8; 2017,Jan,8; 2016,Jan,13; 2015,Jan,16

61735 **subcortical structure(s) other than globus pallidus or thalamus**
46.8 46.8 **FUD** 090 C
AMA: 2014,Jul,8; 2014,Jan,11

61750 **Stereotactic biopsy, aspiration, or excision, including burr hole(s), for intracranial lesion;**
40.6 40.6 **FUD** 090 C
AMA: 2018,Jan,8; 2017,Jan,8; 2016,Jan,13; 2015,Jan,16

61751 **with computed tomography and/or magnetic resonance guidance**
(70450, 70460, 70470, 70551-70553)
39.7 39.7 **FUD** 090 C
AMA: 2018,Jan,8; 2017,Jan,8; 2016,Jan,13; 2015,Jan,16

61760 **Stereotactic implantation of depth electrodes into the cerebrum for long-term seizure monitoring**
46.0 46.0 **FUD** 090 C
AMA: 2014,Jul,8; 2014,Jan,11

61770 **Stereotactic localization, including burr hole(s), with insertion of catheter(s) or probe(s) for placement of radiation source**
46.8 46.8 **FUD** 090 J G2
AMA: 2018,Jan,8; 2017,Jan,8; 2016,Jan,13; 2015,Jan,16

\+ **61781** **Stereotactic computer-assisted (navigational) procedure; cranial, intradural (List separately in addition to code for primary procedure)**
EXCLUDES *Creation lesion by stereotactic method (61720-61791)*
Extradural stereotactic computer-assisted procedure for same surgical session by same individual (61782)
Radiation treatment delivery, stereotactic radiosurgery (SRS) (77371-77373)
Stereotactic implantation neurostimulator electrode array (61863-61868)
Stereotactic radiation treatment management (77432)
Stereotactic radiosurgery (61796-61799)
Ventriculocisternostomy (62201)
Code first primary procedure
6.94 6.94 **FUD** ZZZ N N1 80
AMA: 2018,Jan,8; 2017,Jan,8; 2016,Jan,13; 2015,Jan,16

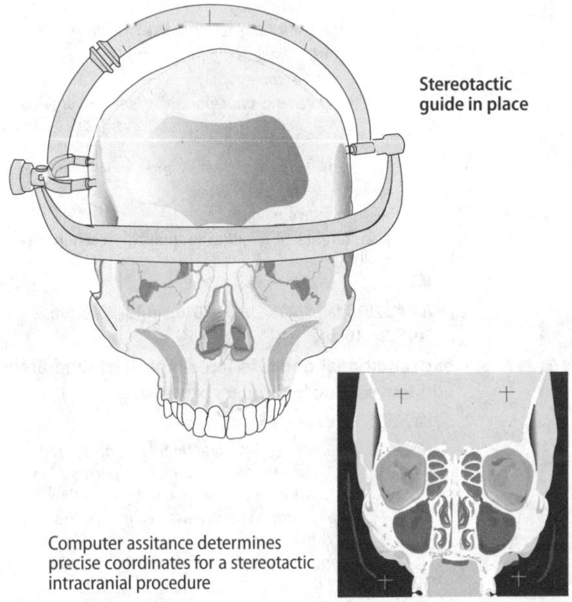

\+ **61782** **cranial, extradural (List separately in addition to code for primary procedure)**
EXCLUDES *Intradural stereotactic computer-assisted procedure for same surgical session by same individual (61781)*
Stereotactic radiosurgery (61796-61799)
Code first primary procedure
5.02 5.02 **FUD** ZZZ N N1 80
AMA: 2018,Apr,3; 2018,Jan,8; 2017,Jan,8; 2016,Jan,13; 2015,Jan,16

\+ **61783** **spinal (List separately in addition to code for primary procedure)**
EXCLUDES *Stereotactic radiosurgery (61796-61799, 63620-63621)*
Code first primary procedure
6.80 6.80 **FUD** ZZZ N N1 80
AMA: 2018,Jan,8; 2017,Jan,8; 2016,Jan,13; 2015,Jan,16

61790 **Creation of lesion by stereotactic method, percutaneous, by neurolytic agent (eg, alcohol, thermal, electrical, radiofrequency); gasserian ganglion**
25.7 25.7 **FUD** 090 J A2 50
AMA: 2014,Jul,8; 2014,Jan,11

61791 **trigeminal medullary tract**
32.4 32.4 **FUD** 090 J A2 80 50
AMA: 2018,Jan,8; 2017,Jan,8; 2016,Jan,13; 2015,Jan,16

61796-61800 Stereotactic Radiosurgery (SRS): Brain

INCLUDES Planning, dosimetry, targeting, positioning, or blocking performed by neurosurgeon

EXCLUDES *Application cranial tongs, caliper, or stereotactic frame (20660)*
Intensity modulated beam delivery plan and treatment (77301, 77385-77386)
Radiation treatment management and radiosurgery by same provider (77427-77435)
Stereotactic body radiation therapy (77373, 77435)
Stereotactic radiosurgery more than once per lesion per treatment course
Treatment planning, physics and dosimetry, and treatment delivery performed by radiation oncologist

61796 Stereotactic radiosurgery (particle beam, gamma ray, or linear accelerator); 1 simple cranial lesion

INCLUDES Lesions < 3.5 cm

EXCLUDES *Reporting code more than one time per treatment course*
Stereotactic computer-assisted procedures (61781-61783)
Stereotactic radiosurgery (61798)
Treatment complex lesions: (61798-61799)
Arteriovenous malformations (AVM)
Brainstem lesions
Cavernous sinus/parasellar/petroclival tumors, glomus tumors, pituitary tumors, and tumors pineal region
Lesions located <= 5 mm from optic nerve, chasm, or tract
Schwannomas

Code also stereotactic headframe application, when performed (61800)

Facility RVU 29.2 Non-Facility RVU 29.2 **FUD** 090 B 80 CCI

AMA: 2018,Jan,8; 2017,Jan,8; 2016,Jan,13; 2015,Jun,6; 2015,Jan,16

\+ **61797 each additional cranial lesion, simple (List separately in addition to code for primary procedure)**

INCLUDES Lesions < 3.5 cm

EXCLUDES *Reporting code for additional stereotactic radiosurgery more than four times in total per treatment course when used alone or in combination with (61799)*
Stereotactic computer-assisted procedures (61781-61783)
Treatment complex lesions: (61798-61799)
Arteriovenous malformations (AVM)
Brainstem lesion
Cavernous sinus/parasellar/petroclival tumors, glomus tumors, pituitary tumors, and tumors pineal region
Lesions located <= 5 mm from optic nerve, chasm, or tract
Schwannomas

Code first (61796, 61798)

Facility RVU 6.35 Non-Facility RVU 6.35 **FUD** ZZZ B 80 CCI

AMA: 2018,Jan,8; 2017,Jan,8; 2016,Jan,13; 2015,Jun,6; 2015,Jan,16

61798 1 complex cranial lesion

INCLUDES All therapeutic lesion creation procedures
Treatment complex lesions:
Arteriovenous malformations (AVM)
Brainstem lesions
Cavernous sinus, parasellar, petroclival, glomus, pineal region, and pituitary tumors
Lesions located <= 5 mm from optic nerve, chasm, or tract
Lesions >= 3.5 cm
Schwannomas
Treatment multiple lesions when at least one considered complex

EXCLUDES *Reporting code more than one time per treatment course*
Stereotactic computer-assisted procedures (61781-61783)
Stereotactic radiosurgery (61796)

Code also stereotactic headframe application, when performed (61800)

Facility RVU 40.5 Non-Facility RVU 40.5 **FUD** 090 B 80 CCI

AMA: 2018,Jan,8; 2017,Jan,8; 2016,Jan,13; 2015,Jun,6; 2015,Jan,16

\+ **61799 each additional cranial lesion, complex (List separately in addition to code for primary procedure)**

INCLUDES All therapeutic lesion creation procedures
Treatment complex lesions:
Arteriovenous malformations (AVM)
Brainstem lesions
Cavernous sinus, parasellar, petroclival, glomus, pineal region, and pituitary tumors
Lesions located <= 5 mm from optic nerve, chasm, or tract
Lesions >= 3.5 cm
Schwannomas

EXCLUDES *Reporting code for additional stereotactic radiosurgery more than four times in total per treatment course when used alone or in combination with (61797)*
Stereotactic computer-assisted procedures (61781-61783)

Code first (61798)

Facility RVU 8.98 Non-Facility RVU 8.98 **FUD** ZZZ B 80 CCI

AMA: 2018,Jan,8; 2017,Jan,8; 2016,Jan,13; 2015,Jun,6; 2015,Jan,16

\+ **61800 Application of stereotactic headframe for stereotactic radiosurgery (List separately in addition to code for primary procedure)**

Code first (61796, 61798)

Facility RVU 4.40 Non-Facility RVU 4.40 **FUD** ZZZ B 80 CCI

AMA: 2018,Jan,8; 2017,Jan,8; 2016,Jan,13; 2015,Jun,6; 2015,Jan,16

61850-61888 Intracranial Neurostimulation

INCLUDES Analysis system at implantation (95970)
Microelectrode recording by operating surgeon

EXCLUDES *Electronic analysis and reprogramming neurostimulator pulse generator (95970, 95976-95977, [95983, 95984])*
Neurophysiological mapping by another physician/qualified health care professional (95961-95962)

61850 Twist drill or burr hole(s) for implantation of neurostimulator electrodes, cortical

Facility RVU 28.1 Non-Facility RVU 28.1 **FUD** 090 C 80 CCI

AMA: 2019,Feb,6; 2018,Jan,8; 2017,Jan,8; 2016,Jan,13; 2015,Jan,16

61860 Craniectomy or craniotomy for implantation of neurostimulator electrodes, cerebral, cortical

Facility RVU 45.7 Non-Facility RVU 45.7 **FUD** 090 C 80 CCI

AMA: 2019,Feb,6; 2018,Jan,8; 2017,Jan,8; 2016,Jan,13; 2015,Jan,16

61863 **Twist drill, burr hole, craniotomy, or craniectomy with stereotactic implantation of neurostimulator electrode array in subcortical site (eg, thalamus, globus pallidus, subthalamic nucleus, periventricular, periaqueductal gray), without use of intraoperative microelectrode recording; first array**
43.3 43.3 FUD 090 C 80 50
AMA: 2019,Feb,6; 2018,Jan,8; 2017,Jan,8; 2016,Jan,13; 2015,Jan,16

\+ **61864** **each additional array (List separately in addition to primary procedure)**
Code first (61863)
8.36 8.36 FUD ZZZ C 80
AMA: 2019,Feb,6

61867 **Twist drill, burr hole, craniotomy, or craniectomy with stereotactic implantation of neurostimulator electrode array in subcortical site (eg, thalamus, globus pallidus, subthalamic nucleus, periventricular, periaqueductal gray), with use of intraoperative microelectrode recording; first array**
65.9 65.9 FUD 090 C 80 50
AMA: 2019,Feb,6

\+ **61868** **each additional array (List separately in addition to primary procedure)**
Code first (61867)
14.7 14.7 FUD ZZZ C 80
AMA: 2019,Feb,6; 2018,Jan,8; 2017,Jan,8; 2016,Jan,13; 2015,Jan,16

~~**61870** **Craniectomy for implantation of neurostimulator electrodes, cerebellar, cortical**~~

61880 **Revision or removal of intracranial neurostimulator electrodes**
16.6 16.6 FUD 090 Q2 G2 80 50
AMA: 2019,Feb,6

61885 **Insertion or replacement of cranial neurostimulator pulse generator or receiver, direct or inductive coupling; with connection to a single electrode array**
EXCLUDES *Percutaneous procedure to place cranial nerve neurostimulator electrode(s) (64553)*
Revision or replacement cranial nerve neurostimulator electrode array (64569)
14.9 14.9 FUD 090 J J8 80 50
AMA: 2019,Feb,6; 2018,Jan,8; 2017,Jan,8; 2016,Jan,13; 2015,Jan,16

61886 **with connection to 2 or more electrode arrays**
EXCLUDES *Percutaneous procedure to place cranial nerve neurostimulator electrode(s) (64553)*
Revision or replacement cranial nerve neurostimulator electrode array (64569)
24.7 24.7 FUD 090 J J8 80
AMA: 2019,Feb,6; 2018,Jan,8; 2017,Jan,8; 2016,Jan,13; 2015,Jan,16

61888 **Revision or removal of cranial neurostimulator pulse generator or receiver**
EXCLUDES *Insertion or replacement cranial neurostimulator pulse generator or receiver (61885-61886)*
11.5 11.5 FUD 010 J J8 50
AMA: 2019,Feb,6; 2018,Jan,8; 2017,Jan,8; 2016,Jan,13; 2015,Jan,16

62000-62148 Repair of Skull and/or Cerebrospinal Fluid Leaks

62000 **Elevation of depressed skull fracture; simple, extradural**
29.7 29.7 FUD 090 J
AMA: 2014,Jan,11

62005 **compound or comminuted, extradural**
36.6 36.6 FUD 090 C 80
AMA: 2014,Jan,11

62010 **with repair of dura and/or debridement of brain**
44.2 44.2 FUD 090 C 80
AMA: 2014,Jan,11

62100 **Craniotomy for repair of dural/cerebrospinal fluid leak, including surgery for rhinorrhea/otorrhea**
EXCLUDES *Repair spinal fluid leak (63707, 63709)*
46.4 46.4 FUD 090 C 80
AMA: 2014,Jan,11; 2002,May,7

62115 **Reduction of craniomegalic skull (eg, treated hydrocephalus); not requiring bone grafts or cranioplasty**
48.4 48.4 FUD 090 C 80
AMA: 2014,Jan,11

62117 **requiring craniotomy and reconstruction with or without bone graft (includes obtaining grafts)**
57.8 57.8 FUD 090 C 80
AMA: 2014,Jan,11

62120 **Repair of encephalocele, skull vault, including cranioplasty**
61.9 61.9 FUD 090 C 80
AMA: 2014,Jan,11

62121 **Craniotomy for repair of encephalocele, skull base**
45.7 45.7 FUD 090 C 80
AMA: 2014,Jan,11

62140 **Cranioplasty for skull defect; up to 5 cm diameter**
29.9 29.9 FUD 090 C 80
AMA: 2018,Jan,8; 2017,Jan,8; 2016,Jan,13; 2015,Jan,16

62141 **larger than 5 cm diameter**
33.1 33.1 FUD 090 C 80
AMA: 2018,Jan,8; 2017,Jan,8; 2016,Jan,13; 2015,Jan,16

62142 **Removal of bone flap or prosthetic plate of skull**
25.8 25.8 FUD 090 C 80
AMA: 2018,Jan,8; 2017,Jan,8; 2016,Jan,13; 2015,Jan,16

62143 **Replacement of bone flap or prosthetic plate of skull**
30.0 30.0 FUD 090 C 80
AMA: 2018,Jan,8; 2017,Jan,8; 2016,Jan,13; 2015,Jan,16

62145 **Cranioplasty for skull defect with reparative brain surgery**
41.0 41.0 FUD 090 C 80
AMA: 2018,Jan,8; 2017,Jan,8; 2016,Jan,13; 2015,Jan,16

62146 **Cranioplasty with autograft (includes obtaining bone grafts); up to 5 cm diameter**
34.2 34.2 FUD 090 C 80
AMA: 2018,Jan,8; 2017,Jan,8; 2016,Jan,13; 2015,Jan,16

62147 **larger than 5 cm diameter**
41.9 41.9 FUD 090 C 80
AMA: 2018,Jan,8; 2017,Jan,8; 2016,Jan,13; 2015,Jan,16

\+ **62148** **Incision and retrieval of subcutaneous cranial bone graft for cranioplasty (List separately in addition to code for primary procedure)**
Code first (62140-62147)
3.73 3.73 FUD ZZZ C
AMA: 2014,Jan,11

62160-62165 Neuroendoscopic Brain Procedures

INCLUDES Diagnostic endoscopy

\+ **62160** **Neuroendoscopy, intracranial, for placement or replacement of ventricular catheter and attachment to shunt system or external drainage (List separately in addition to code for primary procedure)**
Code first (61107, 61210, 62220-62230, 62258)
5.61 5.61 FUD ZZZ N N1
AMA: 2018,Jan,8; 2017,Jan,8; 2016,Jan,13; 2015,Jan,16

62161 **Neuroendoscopy, intracranial; with dissection of adhesions, fenestration of septum pellucidum or intraventricular cysts (including placement, replacement, or removal of ventricular catheter)**
44.1 44.1 FUD 090 C 80
AMA: 2014,Jan,11

62162 **with fenestration or excision of colloid cyst, including placement of external ventricular catheter for drainage**
55.3 55.3 FUD 090 C 80
AMA: 2014,Jan,11

~~62163 with retrieval of foreign body~~

62164 **with excision of brain tumor, including placement of external ventricular catheter for drainage**
61.0 61.0 FUD 090 C 80
AMA: 2014,Jan,11

62165 **with excision of pituitary tumor, transnasal or trans-sphenoidal approach**
44.6 44.6 FUD 090 C 80
AMA: 2019,Dec,12; 2018,Jan,8; 2017,Dec,14

62180-62258 Cerebrospinal Fluid Diversion Procedures

62180 **Ventriculocisternostomy (Torkildsen type operation)**
47.0 47.0 FUD 090 C 80
AMA: 2014,Jan,11

62190 **Creation of shunt; subarachnoid/subdural-atrial, -jugular, -auricular**
27.1 27.1 FUD 090 C
AMA: 2014,Jan,11; 2000,Dec,12

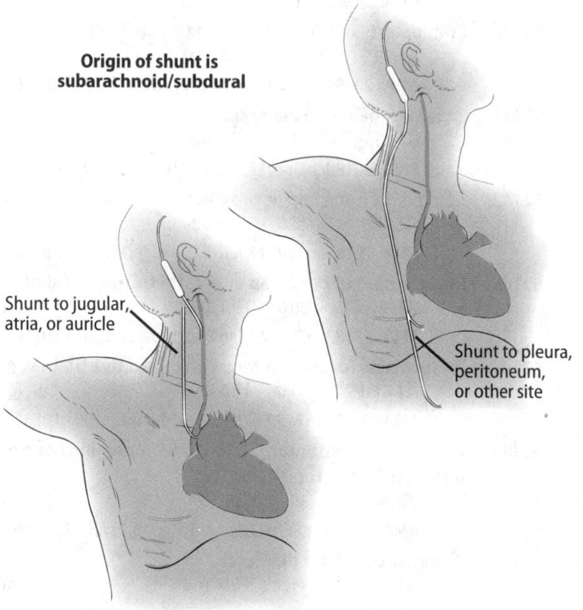

62192 **subarachnoid/subdural-peritoneal, -pleural, other terminus**
28.5 28.5 FUD 090 C 80
AMA: 2014,Jan,11

62194 **Replacement or irrigation, subarachnoid/subdural catheter**
14.1 14.1 FUD 010 J A2 80
AMA: 2018,Jan,8; 2017,Jan,8; 2016,Jan,13; 2015,Jan,16

62200 **Ventriculocisternostomy, third ventricle;**
INCLUDES Dandy ventriculocisternostomy
40.2 40.2 FUD 090 C 80
AMA: 2014,Jan,11

62201 **stereotactic, neuroendoscopic method**
EXCLUDES *Intracranial neuroendoscopic surgery (62161-62165)*
34.8 34.8 FUD 090 C
AMA: 2018,Jan,8; 2017,Jan,8; 2016,Jan,13; 2015,Jan,16

62220 **Creation of shunt; ventriculo-atrial, -jugular, -auricular**
Code also intracranial neuroendoscopic ventricular catheter insertion, when performed (62160)
29.2 29.2 FUD 090 C 80
AMA: 2014,Jan,11; 2007,Jun,10-11

62223 **ventriculo-peritoneal, -pleural, other terminus**
Code also intracranial neuroendoscopic ventricular catheter insertion, when performed (62160)
30.0 30.0 FUD 090 C 80
AMA: 2014,Jan,11; 2007,Jun,10-11

62225 **Replacement or irrigation, ventricular catheter**
Code also intracranial neuroendoscopic ventricular catheter insertion, when performed (62160)
15.3 15.3 FUD 090 J A2
AMA: 2018,Jan,8; 2017,Jan,8; 2016,Jan,13; 2015,Jan,16

62230 **Replacement or revision of cerebrospinal fluid shunt, obstructed valve, or distal catheter in shunt system**
Code also intracranial neuroendoscopic ventricular catheter insertion, when performed (62160)
Code also when proximal catheter and valve replaced (62225)
24.5 24.5 FUD 090 J A2 80
AMA: 2018,Jan,8; 2017,Jan,8; 2016,Jan,13; 2015,Jan,16

62252 **Reprogramming of programmable cerebrospinal shunt**
2.34 2.34 FUD XXX S P3 80
AMA: 2014,Jan,11; 2002,May,7

62256 **Removal of complete cerebrospinal fluid shunt system; without replacement**
EXCLUDES *Reprogramming cerebrospinal fluid (CSF) shunt (62252)*
17.3 17.3 FUD 090 C 80
AMA: 2014,Jan,11; 2002,May,7

62258 **with replacement by similar or other shunt at same operation**
EXCLUDES *Aspiration or irrigation shunt reservoir (61070)*
Reprogramming cerebrospinal fluid (CSF) shunt (62252)
Code also intracranial neuroendoscopic ventricular catheter insertion, when performed (62160)
32.5 32.5 FUD 090 C 80
AMA: 2018,Jan,8; 2017,Jan,8; 2016,Jan,13; 2015,Jan,16

62263-62264 Lysis of Epidural Lesions with Injection of Solution/Mechanical Methods

INCLUDES Epidurography (72275)
Fluoroscopic guidance (77003)
Percutaneous mechanical lysis

62263 **Percutaneous lysis of epidural adhesions using solution injection (eg, hypertonic saline, enzyme) or mechanical means (eg, catheter) including radiologic localization (includes contrast when administered), multiple adhesiolysis sessions; 2 or more days**
INCLUDES All adhesiolysis treatments, injections, and infusions during treatment course
Percutaneous epidural catheter insertion and removal for neurolytic agent injections during treatment sessions series
EXCLUDES *Procedure performed more than one time for complete series spanning two or more treatment days*
8.92 17.1 FUD 010 T A2
AMA: 2018,Jan,8; 2017,Jan,8; 2016,Jan,13; 2015,Jan,16

62264 **1 day**
INCLUDES Multiple treatment sessions performed same day
EXCLUDES *Percutaneous lysis epidural adhesions using solution injection,two or more treatment days (62263)*
6.89 12.2 FUD 010 T A2
AMA: 2018,Jan,8; 2017,Jan,8; 2016,Jan,13; 2015,Jan,16

62267-62269 Percutaneous Procedures of Spinal Cord

62267 Percutaneous aspiration within the nucleus pulposus, intervertebral disc, or paravertebral tissue for diagnostic purposes

EXCLUDES *Bone biopsy (20225)*
Decompression intervertebral disc (62287)
Fine needle aspiration ([10005, 10006, 10007, 10008, 10009, 10010, 10011, 10012])
Injection for discography (62290-62291)

Code also fluoroscopic guidance (77003)

4.54 7.60 **FUD** 000 T G2 80

AMA: 2019,Apr,4; 2018,Jan,8; 2017,Feb,12; 2017,Jan,8; 2016,Jan,13; 2015,Jan,16

62268 Percutaneous aspiration, spinal cord cyst or syrinx

(76942, 77002, 77012)

7.40 7.40 **FUD** 000 T A2

AMA: 2018,Jan,8; 2017,Dec,13

62269 Biopsy of spinal cord, percutaneous needle

EXCLUDES *Fine needle aspiration [(10005, 1006, 1007, 1008, 1009, 10010, 10011, 10012)]*

(76942, 77002, 77012)

(88172-88173)

7.66 7.66 **FUD** 000 J A2 80

AMA: 2019,Apr,4

62270-62329 [62328, 62329] Spinal Puncture, Subarachnoid Space, Diagnostic/Therapeutic

62270 Spinal puncture, lumbar, diagnostic;

EXCLUDES *Radiological guidance (77003, 77012)*

Code also ultrasound or MRI guidance (76942, 77021)

2.23 4.22 **FUD** 000 T A2

AMA: 2020,Jun,10; 2018,Jan,8; 2017,Jan,8; 2016,Jan,13; 2015,Jan,16

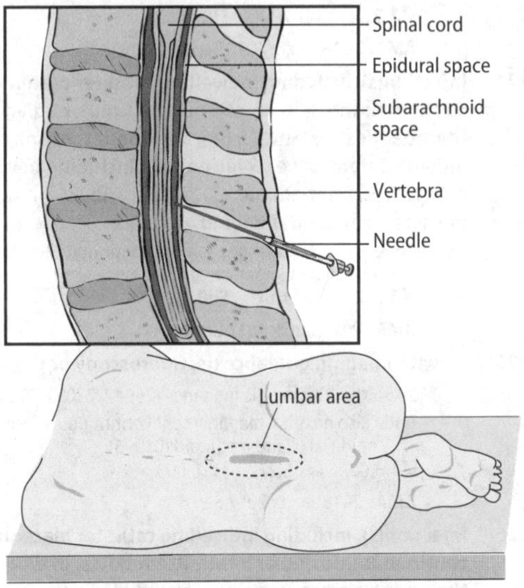

Common position to access vertebral interspace

\# **62328 with fluoroscopic or CT guidance**

INCLUDES Radiological guidance (77003, 77012)

Code also ultrasound or MRI guidance (76942, 77021)

2.59 7.40 **FUD** 000 G2

AMA: 2020,Jun,10

62272 Spinal puncture, therapeutic, for drainage of cerebrospinal fluid (by needle or catheter);

EXCLUDES *Radiological guidance (77003, 77012)*

Code also ultrasound or MRI guidance (76942, 77021)

2.41 5.57 **FUD** 000 T A2

AMA: 2020,Jun,10; 2018,Jan,8; 2017,Jan,8; 2016,Jan,13; 2015,Jan,16

\# **62329 with fluoroscopic or CT guidance**

INCLUDES Radiological guidance (77003, 77012)

Code also ultrasound or MRI guidance (76942, 77021)

3.26 9.19 **FUD** 000 G2

AMA: 2020,Jul,15; 2020,Jun,10

62273 Epidural Blood Patch

CMS: 100-03,10.5 NCD for Autogenous Epidural Blood Graft (10.5)

EXCLUDES *Injection diagnostic or therapeutic material (62320-62327)*

Code also fluoroscopic guidance (77003)

62273 Injection, epidural, of blood or clot patch

3.26 4.93 **FUD** 000 T A2

AMA: 2018,Jan,8; 2017,Jan,8; 2016,Jan,13; 2015,Jan,16

62280-62282 Neurolysis

INCLUDES Contrast injection during fluoroscopic guidance/localization

EXCLUDES *Injection diagnostic or therapeutic material only (62320-62327)*

Code also fluoroscopic guidance and localization unless formal contrast study performed (77003)

62280 Injection/infusion of neurolytic substance (eg, alcohol, phenol, iced saline solutions), with or without other therapeutic substance; subarachnoid

4.76 9.45 **FUD** 010 T A2

AMA: 2018,Jan,8; 2017,Jan,8; 2016,Jan,13; 2015,Jan,16

62281 epidural, cervical or thoracic

4.58 6.94 **FUD** 010 T A2

AMA: 2018,Jan,8; 2017,Jan,8; 2016,Jan,13; 2015,Jan,16

62282 epidural, lumbar, sacral (caudal)

4.16 8.63 **FUD** 010 T A2

AMA: 2018,Jan,8; 2017,Jan,8; 2016,Jan,13; 2015,Jan,16

62284-62294 Injection/Aspiration of Spine, Diagnostic/Therapeutic

62284 Injection procedure for myelography and/or computed tomography, lumbar

EXCLUDES *Injection C1-C2 (61055)*
Myelography (62302-62305, 72240, 72255, 72265, 72270)

Code also fluoroscopic guidance (77003)

2.54 5.61 **FUD** 000 N N1

AMA: 2018,Jan,8; 2017,Jan,8; 2016,Jan,13; 2015,Jan,16

62287 **Decompression procedure, percutaneous, of nucleus pulposus of intervertebral disc, any method utilizing needle based technique to remove disc material under fluoroscopic imaging or other form of indirect visualization, with discography and/or epidural injection(s) at the treated level(s), when performed, single or multiple levels, lumbar**

INCLUDES Endoscopic approach

EXCLUDES *Injection for discography (62290)*
Injection diagnostic or therapeutic substance(s) (62322)
Lumbar discography (72295)
Percutaneous aspiration, diagnostic (62267)
Percutaneous decompression nucleus pulposus intervertebral disc, non-needle based technique (0274T-0275T)
Radiological guidance (77003, 77012)

16.7 16.7 **FUD** 090 J A2

AMA: 2019,Dec,12; 2018,Jan,8; 2017,Feb,12; 2017,Jan,8; 2016,Jan,13; 2015,Mar,9; 2015,Jan,16

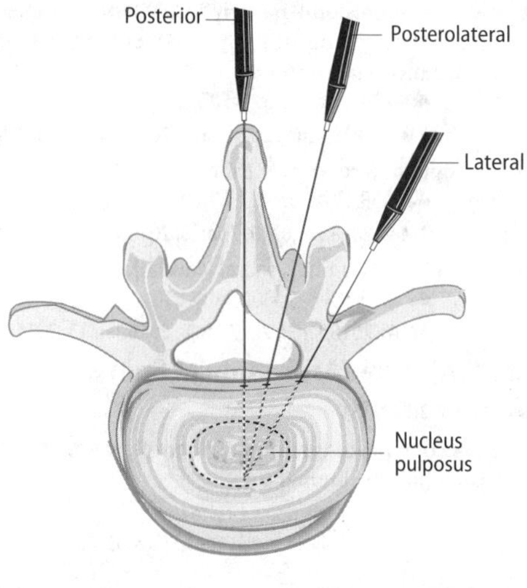

62290 **Injection procedure for discography, each level; lumbar**

(72295)

4.81 9.62 **FUD** 000 N N1

AMA: 2018,Jan,8; 2017,Feb,12; 2017,Jan,8; 2016,Jan,13; 2015,Jan,16

62291 **cervical or thoracic**

(72285)

4.65 9.28 **FUD** 000 N N1

AMA: 2018,Jan,8; 2017,Jan,8; 2016,Jan,13; 2015,Jan,16

62292 **Injection procedure for chemonucleolysis, including discography, intervertebral disc, single or multiple levels, lumbar**

16.4 16.4 **FUD** 090 J R2 80

AMA: 2018,Jan,8; 2017,Jan,8; 2016,Jan,13; 2015,Jan,16

62294 **Injection procedure, arterial, for occlusion of arteriovenous malformation, spinal**

27.8 27.8 **FUD** 090 T A2

AMA: 2014,Jan,11; 2000,Jan,1

62302-62305 Myelography

EXCLUDES *Injection C1-C2 (61055)*
Lumbar myelogram furnished by other providers (62284, 72240, 72255, 72265, 72270)

62302 **Myelography via lumbar injection, including radiological supervision and interpretation; cervical**

EXCLUDES *Myelography (62303-62305)*

3.51 7.13 **FUD** 000 Q2 N1

62303 **thoracic**

EXCLUDES *Myelography (62302, 62304-62305)*

3.51 7.29 **FUD** 000 Q2 N1

62304 **lumbosacral**

EXCLUDES *Myelography (62302-62303, 62305)*

3.45 7.04 **FUD** 000 Q2 N1

62305 **2 or more regions (eg, lumbar/thoracic, cervical/thoracic, lumbar/cervical, lumbar/thoracic/cervical)**

EXCLUDES *Myelography (62302-62305)*

3.60 7.65 **FUD** 000 Q2 N1

62320-62329 [62328, 62329] Injection/Infusion Diagnostic/Therapeutic Material

EXCLUDES *Epidurography (72275)*
Reporting code more than one time even when catheter tip or injected drug travels into different spinal area
Transforaminal epidural injection (64479-64484)

62320 **Injection(s), of diagnostic or therapeutic substance(s) (eg, anesthetic, antispasmodic, opioid, steroid, other solution), not including neurolytic substances, including needle or catheter placement, interlaminar epidural or subarachnoid, cervical or thoracic; without imaging guidance**

2.87 4.73 **FUD** 000 T G2

AMA: 2018,Jan,8; 2017,Sep,6

62321 **with imaging guidance (ie, fluoroscopy or CT)**

INCLUDES Radiologic guidance (76942, 77003, 77012)

3.08 7.05 **FUD** 000 T G2

AMA: 2018,Jan,8; 2017,Sep,6

62322 **Injection(s), of diagnostic or therapeutic substance(s) (eg, anesthetic, antispasmodic, opioid, steroid, other solution), not including neurolytic substances, including needle or catheter placement, interlaminar epidural or subarachnoid, lumbar or sacral (caudal); without imaging guidance**

2.49 4.44 **FUD** 000 T G2

AMA: 2018,Jan,8; 2017,Sep,6; 2017,Feb,12

62323 **with imaging guidance (ie, fluoroscopy or CT)**

INCLUDES Radiologic guidance (76942, 77003, 77012)

2.84 7.11 **FUD** 000 T G2

AMA: 2018,Jan,8; 2017,Sep,6

62324 **Injection(s), including indwelling catheter placement, continuous infusion or intermittent bolus, of diagnostic or therapeutic substance(s) (eg, anesthetic, antispasmodic, opioid, steroid, other solution), not including neurolytic substances, interlaminar epidural or subarachnoid, cervical or thoracic; without imaging guidance**

Code also hospital management continuous infusion drug, epidural or subarachnoid (01996)

2.60 4.14 **FUD** 000 T G2

AMA: 2018,Jan,8; 2017,Sep,6

62325 **with imaging guidance (ie, fluoroscopy or CT)**

INCLUDES Radiologic guidance (76942, 77003, 77012)

Code also hospital management continuous infusion drug, epidural or subarachnoid (01996)

3.00 6.27 **FUD** 000 T G2

AMA: 2018,Jan,8; 2017,Sep,6

62326 **Injection(s), including indwelling catheter placement, continuous infusion or intermittent bolus, of diagnostic or therapeutic substance(s) (eg, anesthetic, antispasmodic, opioid, steroid, other solution), not including neurolytic substances, interlaminar epidural or subarachnoid, lumbar or sacral (caudal); without imaging guidance**

Code also hospital management continuous infusion drug, epidural or subarachnoid (01996)

2.58 4.36 **FUD** 000 T G2

AMA: 2018,Jan,8; 2017,Sep,6

62327 **with imaging guidance (ie, fluoroscopy or CT)**

INCLUDES Radiologic guidance (76942, 77003, 77012)

Code also hospital management continuous infusion drug, epidural or subarachnoid (01996)

2.78 6.69 **FUD** 000 T G2

AMA: 2018,Jan,8; 2017,Sep,6

62328 **Resequenced code. See code following 62270.**

62329 Resequenced code. See code following 62272.

62350-62370 Procedures Related to Epidural and Intrathecal Catheters

EXCLUDES *Epidural blood patch (62273)*
Injection epidural/subarachnoid diagnostic/therapeutic drugs ([62328], [62329], 62320-62327)
Injection for lumbar computed tomography/myelography (62284)
Injection/infusion neurolytic substances (62280-62282)
Spinal puncture (62270-62272)

62350 Implantation, revision or repositioning of tunneled intrathecal or epidural catheter, for long-term medication administration via an external pump or implantable reservoir/infusion pump; without laminectomy
EXCLUDES *Maintenance and refilling infusion pumps for CNS drug therapy (95990-95991)*
11.5 11.5 FUD 010 J J8
AMA: 2018,Jan,8; 2017,Jan,8; 2016,Jan,13; 2015,Jan,16

62351 with laminectomy
EXCLUDES *Maintenance and refilling infusion pumps for CNS drug therapy (95990-95991)*
24.8 24.8 FUD 090 J 80
AMA: 2018,Jan,8; 2017,Jan,8; 2016,Jan,13; 2015,Jan,16

62355 Removal of previously implanted intrathecal or epidural catheter
7.73 7.73 FUD 010 Q2 A2 80
AMA: 2014,Jan,11; 1995,Win,1

62360 Implantation or replacement of device for intrathecal or epidural drug infusion; subcutaneous reservoir
9.13 9.13 FUD 010 J J8 80
AMA: 2014,Jan,11; 1995,Win,1

62361 nonprogrammable pump
12.4 12.4 FUD 010 J J8 80
AMA: 2014,Jan,11; 1995,Win,1

62362 programmable pump, including preparation of pump, with or without programming
11.0 11.0 FUD 010 J J8 80
AMA: 2018,Jan,8; 2017,Jan,8; 2016,Jan,13; 2015,Jan,16

62365 Removal of subcutaneous reservoir or pump, previously implanted for intrathecal or epidural infusion
8.52 8.52 FUD 010 Q2 A2 80
AMA: 2014,Jan,11; 1995,Win,1

62367 Electronic analysis of programmable, implanted pump for intrathecal or epidural drug infusion (includes evaluation of reservoir status, alarm status, drug prescription status); without reprogramming or refill
EXCLUDES *Maintenance and refilling infusion pumps for CNS drug therapy (95990-95991)*
0.72 1.14 FUD XXX S P3
AMA: 2018,Jan,8; 2017,Jan,8; 2016,Jan,13; 2015,Jan,16

62368 with reprogramming
EXCLUDES *Maintenance and refilling infusion pumps for CNS drug therapy (95990-95991)*
1.01 1.57 FUD XXX S P3
AMA: 2018,Jan,8; 2017,Jan,8; 2016,Jan,13; 2015,Jan,16

62369 with reprogramming and refill
EXCLUDES *Maintenance and refilling infusion pumps for CNS drug therapy (95990-95991)*
1.01 3.34 FUD XXX S P3
AMA: 2018,Jan,8; 2017,Jan,8; 2016,Jan,13; 2015,Jan,16

62370 with reprogramming and refill (requiring skill of a physician or other qualified health care professional)
EXCLUDES *Maintenance and refilling infusion pumps for CNS drug therapy (95990-95991)*
1.33 3.47 FUD XXX S P3
AMA: 2018,Jan,8; 2017,Jan,8; 2016,Jan,13; 2015,Jan,16

62380 Endoscopic Decompression/Laminectomy/Laminotomy

EXCLUDES *Open decompression (63030, 63056)*
Percutaneous decompression (62267, 0274T-0275T)

62380 Endoscopic decompression of spinal cord, nerve root(s), including laminotomy, partial facetectomy, foraminotomy, discectomy and/or excision of herniated intervertebral disc, 1 interspace, lumbar
0.00 0.00 FUD 090 J G2 80 50
AMA: 2018,Jan,8; 2017,Feb,12

63001-63048 Posterior Midline Approach: Laminectomy/Laminotomy/Decompression

INCLUDES Endoscopic assistance through open and direct visualization
EXCLUDES *Arthrodesis (22590-22614)*
Percutaneous decompression (62287, 0274T, 0275T)

63001 Laminectomy with exploration and/or decompression of spinal cord and/or cauda equina, without facetectomy, foraminotomy or discectomy (eg, spinal stenosis), 1 or 2 vertebral segments; cervical
36.0 36.0 FUD 090 J G2 80
AMA: 2018,Jan,8; 2017,Mar,7; 2017,Jan,8; 2016,Jan,13; 2015,Jan,16

63003 thoracic
36.0 36.0 FUD 090 J G2 80
AMA: 2018,Jan,8; 2017,Mar,7; 2017,Jan,8; 2016,Jan,13; 2015,Jan,16

63005 lumbar, except for spondylolisthesis
34.4 34.4 FUD 090 J G2 80
AMA: 2018,Jan,8; 2017,Mar,7; 2017,Feb,9; 2017,Jan,8; 2016,Jan,13; 2015,Jan,16

63011 sacral
31.6 31.6 FUD 090 J 80
AMA: 2018,Jan,8; 2017,Mar,7; 2017,Jan,8; 2016,Jan,13; 2015,Jan,16

63012 Laminectomy with removal of abnormal facets and/or pars inter-articularis with decompression of cauda equina and nerve roots for spondylolisthesis, lumbar (Gill type procedure)
34.6 34.6 FUD 090 J 80
AMA: 2019,Dec,12; 2018,Jan,8; 2017,Mar,7; 2017,Feb,9; 2017,Jan,8; 2016,Jan,13; 2015,Jan,16

63015 Laminectomy with exploration and/or decompression of spinal cord and/or cauda equina, without facetectomy, foraminotomy or discectomy (eg, spinal stenosis), more than 2 vertebral segments; cervical
43.2 43.2 FUD 090 J 80
AMA: 2018,Jan,8; 2017,Mar,7; 2017,Jan,8; 2016,Jan,13; 2015,Jan,16

63016 thoracic
44.0 44.0 FUD 090 J 80
AMA: 2018,Jan,8; 2017,Mar,7; 2017,Jan,8; 2016,Jan,13; 2015,Jan,16

63017 **lumbar**
36.7 36.7 FUD 090 J 80
AMA: 2018,Jan,8; 2017,Mar,7; 2017,Feb,9; 2017,Jan,8; 2016,Jan,13; 2015,Jan,16

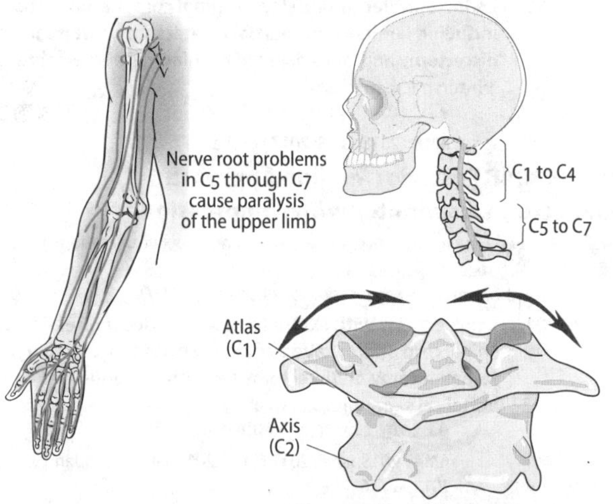

The specialized atlas allows for rotary motion, which turns the head

63020 **Laminotomy (hemilaminectomy), with decompression of nerve root(s), including partial facetectomy, foraminotomy and/or excision of herniated intervertebral disc; 1 interspace, cervical**
33.6 33.6 FUD 090 J G2 80 50
AMA: 2018,Jan,8; 2017,Mar,7; 2017,Jan,8; 2016,Jan,13; 2015,Jan,16

63030 **1 interspace, lumbar**
28.2 28.2 FUD 090 J G2 80 50
AMA: 2020,May,13; 2019,Nov,14; 2018,Jan,8; 2017,Mar,7; 2017,Feb,12; 2017,Feb,9; 2017,Jan,8; 2016,May,13; 2016,Jan,13; 2015,Jan,16

\+ **63035** **each additional interspace, cervical or lumbar (List separately in addition to code for primary procedure)**
EXCLUDES *Reporting with modifier 50. Report once for each side when performed bilaterally*
Code first (63020-63030)
5.58 5.58 FUD ZZZ N 80 50
AMA: 2018,Jan,8; 2017,Feb,9; 2017,Jan,8; 2016,Jan,13; 2015,Jan,16

63040 **Laminotomy (hemilaminectomy), with decompression of nerve root(s), including partial facetectomy, foraminotomy and/or excision of herniated intervertebral disc, reexploration, single interspace; cervical**
40.4 40.4 FUD 090 J 80 50
AMA: 2020,May,13; 2018,Jan,8; 2017,Mar,7; 2017,Jan,8; 2016,Jan,13; 2015,Jan,16

63042 **lumbar**
37.5 37.5 FUD 090 J G2 80 50
AMA: 2020,May,13; 2018,Jan,8; 2017,Mar,7; 2017,Feb,9; 2017,Jan,8; 2016,Jan,13; 2015,Jan,16

\+ **63043** **each additional cervical interspace (List separately in addition to code for primary procedure)**
EXCLUDES *Reporting with modifier 50. Report once for each side when performed bilaterally*
Code first (63040)
0.00 0.00 FUD ZZZ N 80 50
AMA: 2020,May,13; 2018,Jan,8; 2017,Jan,8; 2016,Jan,13; 2015,Jan,16

\+ **63044** **each additional lumbar interspace (List separately in addition to code for primary procedure)**
EXCLUDES *Reporting with modifier 50. Report once for each side when performed bilaterally*
Code first (63042)
0.00 0.00 FUD ZZZ N N1 80 50
AMA: 2020,May,13; 2018,Jan,8; 2017,Feb,9; 2017,Jan,8; 2016,Jan,13; 2015,Jan,16

63045 **Laminectomy, facetectomy and foraminotomy (unilateral or bilateral with decompression of spinal cord, cauda equina and/or nerve root[s], [eg, spinal or lateral recess stenosis]), single vertebral segment; cervical**
37.1 37.1 FUD 090 J G2 80
AMA: 2018,Jan,8; 2017,Mar,7; 2017,Jan,8; 2016,Jan,13; 2015,Jan,16

63046 **thoracic**
35.4 35.4 FUD 090 J G2 80
AMA: 2018,Jan,8; 2017,Mar,7; 2017,Jan,8; 2016,Jan,13; 2015,Jan,16

63047 **lumbar**
31.9 31.9 FUD 090 J G2 80
AMA: 2020,May,13; 2019,Dec,12; 2018,May,10; 2018,May,9; 2018,Jan,8; 2017,Mar,7; 2017,Feb,9; 2017,Feb,12; 2017,Jan,8; 2016,Oct,11; 2016,Jan,13; 2015,Jan,16

\+ **63048** **each additional segment, cervical, thoracic, or lumbar (List separately in addition to code for primary procedure)**
Code first (63045-63047)
6.13 6.13 FUD ZZZ N 80
AMA: 2018,Jan,8; 2017,Feb,9; 2017,Jan,8; 2016,Jan,13; 2015,Jan,16

63050-63051 Cervical Laminoplasty: Posterior Midline Approach

EXCLUDES *Procedure performed on same vertebral segment(s) (22600, 22614, 22840-22842, 63001, 63015, 63045, 63048, 63295)*

63050 **Laminoplasty, cervical, with decompression of the spinal cord, 2 or more vertebral segments;**
43.5 43.5 FUD 090 C 80
AMA: 2018,Jan,8; 2017,Mar,7; 2017,Jan,8; 2016,Jan,13; 2015,Jan,16

63051 **with reconstruction of the posterior bony elements (including the application of bridging bone graft and non-segmental fixation devices [eg, wire, suture, mini-plates], when performed)**
49.3 49.3 FUD 090 C 80
AMA: 2018,Jan,8; 2017,Mar,7; 2017,Jan,8; 2016,Jan,13; 2015,Jan,16

63055-63066 Spinal Cord/Nerve Root Decompression: Costovertebral or Transpedicular Approach

63055 **Transpedicular approach with decompression of spinal cord, equina and/or nerve root(s) (eg, herniated intervertebral disc), single segment; thoracic**
47.0 47.0 FUD 090 J G2 80
AMA: 2018,Jan,8; 2017,Mar,7; 2017,Jan,8; 2016,Jan,13; 2015,Jan,16

63056 **lumbar (including transfacet, or lateral extraforaminal approach) (eg, far lateral herniated intervertebral disc)**
43.2 43.2 FUD 090 J G2 80
AMA: 2019,Nov,14; 2018,Jan,8; 2017,Mar,7; 2017,Feb,12; 2017,Jan,8; 2016,Jan,13; 2015,Jan,16

\+ **63057** **each additional segment, thoracic or lumbar (List separately in addition to code for primary procedure)**
Code first (63055-63056)
9.28 9.28 FUD ZZZ N 80
AMA: 2018,Jan,8; 2017,Jan,8; 2016,Jan,13; 2015,Jan,16

63064 **Costovertebral approach with decompression of spinal cord or nerve root(s) (eg, herniated intervertebral disc), thoracic; single segment**

EXCLUDES *Laminectomy with intraspinal thoracic lesion removal (63266, 63271, 63276, 63281, 63286)*

51.5 51.5 FUD 090 J 80

AMA: 2018,Jan,8; 2017,Mar,7; 2017,Jan,8; 2016,Jan,13; 2015,Jan,16

\+ 63066 **each additional segment (List separately in addition to code for primary procedure)**

EXCLUDES *Laminectomy with intraspinal thoracic lesion removal (63266, 63271, 63276, 63281, 63286)*

Code first (63064)

5.97 5.97 FUD ZZZ N 80

AMA: 2014,Jan,11; 1996,Feb,6

63075-63078 Discectomy: Anterior or Anterolateral Approach

INCLUDES Operating microscope (69990)

63075 **Discectomy, anterior, with decompression of spinal cord and/or nerve root(s), including osteophytectomy; cervical, single interspace**

EXCLUDES *Anterior cervical discectomy and anterior interbody fusion at same level during same operative session (22551)*

Anterior interbody arthrodesis (even by another provider) (22554)

39.1 39.1 FUD 090 J 80

AMA: 2018,Jan,8; 2017,Mar,7; 2017,Jan,8; 2016,Feb,12; 2016,Jan,13; 2015,Apr,7; 2015,Jan,16

\+ 63076 **cervical, each additional interspace (List separately in addition to code for primary procedure)**

EXCLUDES *Anterior cervical discectomy and anterior interbody fusion at same level during same operative session (22552)*

Anterior interbody arthrodesis (even by another provider) (22554)

Code first (63075)

7.20 7.20 FUD ZZZ N 80

AMA: 2018,Jan,8; 2017,Jan,8; 2016,Feb,12; 2016,Jan,13; 2015,Jan,16

63077 **thoracic, single interspace**

43.6 43.6 FUD 090 C 80

AMA: 2018,Jan,8; 2017,Mar,7; 2017,Jan,8; 2016,Feb,12; 2016,Jan,13; 2015,Jan,16

\+ 63078 **thoracic, each additional interspace (List separately in addition to code for primary procedure)**

Code first (63077)

6.01 6.01 FUD ZZZ C 80

AMA: 2018,Jan,8; 2017,Jan,8; 2016,Feb,12; 2016,Jan,13; 2015,Jan,16

63081-63091 Vertebral Corpectomy, All Levels, Anterior Approach

INCLUDES Disc removal level below and/or above vertebral segment

Partial removal:

- Cervical: Removal ≥ 1/2 vertebral body
- Lumbar: Removal ≥ 1/3 vertebral body
- Thoracic: Removal ≥ 1/3 vertebral body

EXCLUDES *Arthrodesis (22548-22812)*

Code also reconstruction (20930-20938, 22548-22812, 22840-22855 [22859])

63081 **Vertebral corpectomy (vertebral body resection), partial or complete, anterior approach with decompression of spinal cord and/or nerve root(s); cervical, single segment**

EXCLUDES *Transoral approach (61575-61576)*

50.9 50.9 FUD 090 C 80

AMA: 2018,Jan,8; 2017,Mar,7; 2017,Jan,8; 2016,Apr,8; 2016,Jan,13; 2015,Jun,10; 2015,Jan,16

\+ 63082 **cervical, each additional segment (List separately in addition to code for primary procedure)**

EXCLUDES *Transoral approach (61575-61576)*

Code first (63081)

7.72 7.72 FUD ZZZ C 80

AMA: 2018,Jan,8; 2017,Jan,8; 2016,Apr,8; 2016,Jan,13; 2015,Jan,16

63085 **Vertebral corpectomy (vertebral body resection), partial or complete, transthoracic approach with decompression of spinal cord and/or nerve root(s); thoracic, single segment**

55.7 55.7 FUD 090 C 80

AMA: 2018,Jan,8; 2017,Mar,7; 2017,Jan,8; 2016,Apr,8; 2016,Jan,13; 2015,Jan,16

\+ 63086 **thoracic, each additional segment (List separately in addition to code for primary procedure)**

Code first (63085)

5.53 5.53 FUD ZZZ C 80

AMA: 2018,Jan,8; 2017,Jan,8; 2016,Apr,8; 2016,Jan,13; 2015,Jan,16

63087 **Vertebral corpectomy (vertebral body resection), partial or complete, combined thoracolumbar approach with decompression of spinal cord, cauda equina or nerve root(s), lower thoracic or lumbar; single segment**

69.8 69.8 FUD 090 C 80

AMA: 2018,Jan,8; 2017,Mar,7; 2017,Jan,8; 2016,Apr,8; 2016,Jan,13; 2015,Jan,16

\+ 63088 **each additional segment (List separately in addition to code for primary procedure)**

Code first (63087)

7.43 7.43 FUD ZZZ C 80

AMA: 2018,Jan,8; 2017,Jan,8; 2016,Apr,8; 2016,Jan,13; 2015,Jan,16

63090 **Vertebral corpectomy (vertebral body resection), partial or complete, transperitoneal or retroperitoneal approach with decompression of spinal cord, cauda equina or nerve root(s), lower thoracic, lumbar, or sacral; single segment**

56.8 56.8 FUD 090 C 80

AMA: 2018,Jan,8; 2017,Mar,7; 2017,Jan,8; 2016,Apr,8; 2016,Jan,13; 2015,Jan,16

\+ 63091 **each additional segment (List separately in addition to code for primary procedure)**

Code first (63090)

5.18 5.18 FUD ZZZ C 80

AMA: 2018,Jan,8; 2017,Jan,8; 2016,Apr,8; 2016,Jan,13; 2015,Jan,16

63101-63103 Corpectomy: Lateral Extracavitary Approach

INCLUDES Partial removal:

- Cervical: Removal ≥ 1/2 vertebral body
- Lumbar: Removal ≥ 1/3 vertebral body
- Thoracic: Removal ≥ 1/3 vertebral body

63101 **Vertebral corpectomy (vertebral body resection), partial or complete, lateral extracavitary approach with decompression of spinal cord and/or nerve root(s) (eg, for tumor or retropulsed bone fragments); thoracic, single segment**

67.2 67.2 FUD 090 C 80

AMA: 2018,Jan,8; 2017,Mar,7; 2017,Jan,8; 2016,Jan,13; 2015,Jan,16

63102 **lumbar, single segment**

65.5 65.5 FUD 090 C 80

AMA: 2018,Jan,8; 2017,Mar,7; 2017,Jan,8; 2016,Jan,13; 2015,Jan,16

\+ 63103 **thoracic or lumbar, each additional segment (List separately in addition to code for primary procedure)**

Code first (63101-63102)

8.53 8.53 FUD ZZZ C 80

AMA: 2014,Jan,11

63170-63295 Laminectomies

63170 **Laminectomy with myelotomy (eg, Bischof or DREZ type), cervical, thoracic, or thoracolumbar**
45.9 45.9 **FUD** 090 C 80
AMA: 2018,Jan,8; 2017,Mar,7; 2017,Jan,8; 2016,Jan,13; 2015,Jan,16

63172 **Laminectomy with drainage of intramedullary cyst/syrinx; to subarachnoid space**
40.0 40.0 **FUD** 090 C 80
AMA: 2018,Jan,8; 2017,Mar,7; 2017,Jan,8; 2016,Jan,13; 2015,Jan,16

63173 **to peritoneal or pleural space**
49.7 49.7 **FUD** 090 C 80
AMA: 2018,Jan,8; 2017,Mar,7; 2017,Jan,8; 2016,Jan,13; 2015,Jan,16

~~**63180** **Laminectomy and section of dentate ligaments, with or without dural graft, cervical; 1 or 2 segments**~~

~~**63182** **more than 2 segments**~~

63185 **Laminectomy with rhizotomy; 1 or 2 segments**
INCLUDES Dana rhizotomy
Stoffel rhizotomy
33.1 33.1 **FUD** 090 C 80
AMA: 2018,Jan,8; 2017,Mar,7; 2017,Jan,8; 2016,Jan,13; 2015,Jan,16

63190 **more than 2 segments**
36.0 36.0 **FUD** 090 C 80
AMA: 2018,Jan,8; 2017,Mar,7; 2017,Jan,8; 2016,Jan,13; 2015,Jan,16

63191 **Laminectomy with section of spinal accessory nerve**
EXCLUDES *Division sternocleidomastoid muscle for torticollis (21720)*
39.7 39.7 **FUD** 090 C 80 50
AMA: 2018,Jan,8; 2017,Mar,7; 2017,Jan,8; 2016,Jan,13; 2015,Jan,16

63194 **Laminectomy with cordotomy, with section of 1 spinothalamic tract, 1 stage; cervical**
46.0 46.0 **FUD** 090 C 80
AMA: 2018,Jan,8; 2017,Mar,7; 2017,Jan,8; 2016,Jan,13; 2015,Jan,16

63195 **thoracic**
44.2 44.2 **FUD** 090 C 80
AMA: 2018,Jan,8; 2017,Mar,7; 2017,Jan,8; 2016,Jan,13; 2015,Jan,16

63196 **Laminectomy with cordotomy, with section of both spinothalamic tracts, 1 stage; cervical**
51.3 51.3 **FUD** 090 C 80
AMA: 2018,Jan,8; 2017,Mar,7; 2017,Jan,8; 2016,Jan,13; 2015,Jan,16

63197 **thoracic**
49.3 49.3 **FUD** 090 C 80
AMA: 2018,Jan,8; 2017,Mar,7; 2017,Jan,8; 2016,Jan,13; 2015,Jan,16

63198 **Laminectomy with cordotomy with section of both spinothalamic tracts, 2 stages within 14 days; cervical**
INCLUDES Keen laminectomy
60.3 60.3 **FUD** 090 C 80
AMA: 2018,Jan,8; 2017,Mar,7; 2017,Jan,8; 2016,Jan,13; 2015,Jan,16

63199 **thoracic**
63.2 63.2 **FUD** 090 C 80
AMA: 2018,Jan,8; 2017,Mar,7; 2017,Jan,8; 2016,Jan,13; 2015,Jan,16

63200 **Laminectomy, with release of tethered spinal cord, lumbar**
44.1 44.1 **FUD** 090 C 80
AMA: 2018,Jan,8; 2017,Mar,7; 2017,Jan,8; 2016,Jan,13; 2015,Jan,16

63250 **Laminectomy for excision or occlusion of arteriovenous malformation of spinal cord; cervical**
87.8 87.8 **FUD** 090 C 80
AMA: 2018,Jan,8; 2017,Mar,7; 2017,Jan,8; 2016,Jan,13; 2015,Jan,16

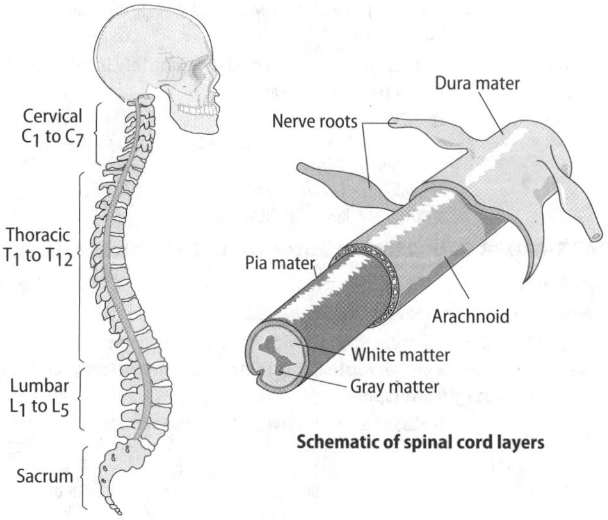

Schematic of spinal cord layers

63251 **thoracic**
87.8 87.8 **FUD** 090 C 80
AMA: 2018,Jan,8; 2017,Mar,7; 2017,Jan,8; 2016,Jan,13; 2015,Jan,16

63252 **thoracolumbar**
87.8 87.8 **FUD** 090 C 80
AMA: 2018,Jan,8; 2017,Mar,7; 2017,Jan,8; 2016,Jan,13; 2015,Jan,16

63265 **Laminectomy for excision or evacuation of intraspinal lesion other than neoplasm, extradural; cervical**
48.2 48.2 **FUD** 090 C 80
AMA: 2018,Jan,8; 2017,Mar,7; 2017,Jan,8; 2016,Jan,13; 2015,Jan,16

63266 **thoracic**
49.7 49.7 **FUD** 090 C 80
AMA: 2017,Mar,7

63267 **lumbar**
39.6 39.6 **FUD** 090 C 80
AMA: 2018,Jan,8; 2017,Mar,7; 2017,Jan,8; 2016,Jan,13; 2015,Jan,16

63268 **sacral**
40.9 40.9 **FUD** 090 C 80
AMA: 2018,Jan,8; 2017,Mar,7; 2017,Jan,8; 2016,Jan,13; 2015,Jan,16

63270 **Laminectomy for excision of intraspinal lesion other than neoplasm, intradural; cervical**
61.1 61.1 **FUD** 090 C 80
AMA: 2018,Jan,8; 2017,Mar,7; 2017,Jan,8; 2016,Jan,13; 2015,Jan,16

63271 **thoracic**
59.8 59.8 **FUD** 090 C 80
AMA: 2018,Jan,8; 2017,Mar,7; 2017,Jan,8; 2016,Jan,13; 2015,Jan,16

63272 **lumbar**
54.5 54.5 **FUD** 090 C 80
AMA: 2018,Jan,8; 2017,Mar,7; 2017,Jan,8; 2016,Jan,13; 2015,Jan,16

63273 **sacral**
53.8 53.8 **FUD** 090 C 80
AMA: 2018,Jan,8; 2017,Mar,7; 2017,Jan,8; 2016,Jan,13; 2015,Jan,16

63275 **Laminectomy for biopsy/excision of intraspinal neoplasm; extradural, cervical**
52.1 52.1 FUD 090 C 80
AMA: 2018,Jan,8; 2017,Mar,7; 2017,Jan,8; 2016,Jan,13; 2015,Jan,16

63276 **extradural, thoracic**
51.7 51.7 FUD 090 C 80
AMA: 2018,Jan,8; 2017,Mar,7; 2017,Jan,8; 2016,Jan,13; 2015,Jan,16

63277 **extradural, lumbar**
45.3 45.3 FUD 090 C 80
AMA: 2018,Jan,8; 2017,Mar,7; 2017,Jan,8; 2016,Jan,13; 2015,Jan,16

63278 **extradural, sacral**
45.9 45.9 FUD 090 C 80
AMA: 2018,Jan,8; 2017,Mar,7; 2017,Jan,8; 2016,Jan,13; 2015,Jan,16

63280 **intradural, extramedullary, cervical**
61.2 61.2 FUD 090 C 80
AMA: 2018,Jan,8; 2017,Mar,7; 2017,Jan,8; 2016,Jan,13; 2015,Jan,16

63281 **intradural, extramedullary, thoracic**
60.5 60.5 FUD 090 C 80
AMA: 2018,Jan,8; 2017,Mar,7; 2017,Jan,8; 2016,Jan,13; 2015,Jan,16

63282 **intradural, extramedullary, lumbar**
57.7 57.7 FUD 090 C 80
AMA: 2018,Jan,8; 2017,Mar,7; 2017,Jan,8; 2016,Jan,13; 2015,Jan,16

63283 **intradural, sacral**
54.8 54.8 FUD 090 C 80
AMA: 2018,Jan,8; 2017,Mar,7; 2017,Jan,8; 2016,Jan,13; 2015,Jan,16

63285 **intradural, intramedullary, cervical**
77.2 77.2 FUD 090 C 80
AMA: 2018,Jan,8; 2017,Mar,7; 2017,Jan,8; 2016,Jan,13; 2015,Jan,16

63286 **intradural, intramedullary, thoracic**
74.7 74.7 FUD 090 C 80
AMA: 2018,Jan,8; 2017,Mar,7; 2017,Jan,8; 2016,Jan,13; 2015,Jan,16

63287 **intradural, intramedullary, thoracolumbar**
81.0 81.0 FUD 090 C 80
AMA: 2018,Jan,8; 2017,Mar,7; 2017,Jan,8; 2016,Jan,13; 2015,Jan,16

63290 **combined extradural-intradural lesion, any level**
EXCLUDES *Drainage intramedullary cyst or syrinx (63172-63173)*
80.7 80.7 FUD 090 C 80
AMA: 2018,Jan,8; 2017,Mar,7; 2017,Jan,8; 2016,Jan,13; 2015,Jan,16

\+ 63295 **Osteoplastic reconstruction of dorsal spinal elements, following primary intraspinal procedure (List separately in addition to code for primary procedure)**
EXCLUDES *Procedure performed same vertebral segment(s) (22590-22614, 22840-22844, 63050-63051)*
Code first (63172-63173, 63185, 63190, 63200-63290)
9.55 9.55 FUD ZZZ C 80
AMA: 2014,Jan,11

63300-63308 Vertebral Corpectomy for Intraspinal Lesion: Anterior/Anterolateral Approach

INCLUDES Partial removal:
- Cervical: Removal ≥ 1/2 vertebral body
- Lumbar: Removal ≥ 1/3 vertebral body
- Thoracic: Removal ≥ 1/3 vertebral body

EXCLUDES *Arthrodesis (22548-22585)*
Spinal reconstruction (20930-20938)

63300 **Vertebral corpectomy (vertebral body resection), partial or complete, for excision of intraspinal lesion, single segment; extradural, cervical**
53.1 53.1 FUD 090 C 80
AMA: 2018,Jan,8; 2017,Mar,7; 2017,Jan,8; 2016,Jan,13; 2015,Jan,16

63301 **extradural, thoracic by transthoracic approach**
63.7 63.7 FUD 090 C 80
AMA: 2018,Jan,8; 2017,Mar,7; 2017,Jan,8; 2016,Jan,13; 2015,Jan,16

63302 **extradural, thoracic by thoracolumbar approach**
62.9 62.9 FUD 090 C 80
AMA: 2018,Jan,8; 2017,Mar,7; 2017,Jan,8; 2016,Jan,13; 2015,Jan,16

63303 **extradural, lumbar or sacral by transperitoneal or retroperitoneal approach**
63.1 63.1 FUD 090 C 80
AMA: 2018,Jan,8; 2017,Mar,7; 2017,Jan,8; 2016,Jan,13; 2015,Jan,16

63304 **intradural, cervical**
67.8 67.8 FUD 090 C 80
AMA: 2018,Jan,8; 2017,Mar,7; 2017,Jan,8; 2016,Jan,13; 2015,Jan,16

63305 **intradural, thoracic by transthoracic approach**
73.7 73.7 FUD 090 C 80
AMA: 2018,Jan,8; 2017,Mar,7; 2017,Jan,8; 2016,Jan,13; 2015,Jan,16

63306 **intradural, thoracic by thoracolumbar approach**
71.0 71.0 FUD 090 C 80
AMA: 2018,Jan,8; 2017,Mar,7; 2017,Jan,8; 2016,Jan,13; 2015,Jan,16

63307 **intradural, lumbar or sacral by transperitoneal or retroperitoneal approach**
69.5 69.5 FUD 090 C 80
AMA: 2018,Jan,8; 2017,Mar,7; 2017,Jan,8; 2016,Jan,13; 2015,Jan,16

\+ 63308 **each additional segment (List separately in addition to codes for single segment)**
Code first (63300-63307)
9.37 9.37 FUD ZZZ C 80
AMA: 2014,Jan,11; 2002,Feb,4

63600-63610 Stereotactic Procedures of the Spinal Cord

63600 **Creation of lesion of spinal cord by stereotactic method, percutaneous, any modality (including stimulation and/or recording)**
32.0 32.0 FUD 090 J A2 80
AMA: 2014,Jan,11; 2000,Dec,12

63610 **Stereotactic stimulation of spinal cord, percutaneous, separate procedure not followed by other surgery**
17.1 17.1 FUD 000 J J8 80
AMA: 2014,Jan,11

63620-63621 Stereotactic Radiosurgery (SRS): Spine

INCLUDES Computer assisted planning
Planning dosimetry, targeting, positioning, or blocking by neurosurgeon

EXCLUDES *Arteriovenous malformations (see Radiation Oncology Section)*
Intensity modulated beam delivery plan and treatment (77301, 77385-77386)
Radiation treatment management by same provider (77427-77432)
Stereotactic body radiation therapy (77373, 77435)
Stereotactic computer-assisted procedures (61781-61783)
Treatment planning, physics, dosimetry, treatment delivery and management provided by radiation oncologist (77261-77790 [77295, 77385, 77386, 77387, 77424, 77425])

63620 Stereotactic radiosurgery (particle beam, gamma ray, or linear accelerator); 1 spinal lesion

EXCLUDES *Reporting code more than one time per entire treatment course*

32.2 32.2 **FUD** 090 B 80

AMA: 2018,Jan,8; 2017,Jan,8; 2016,Jan,13; 2015,Jun,6; 2015,Jan,16

\+ **63621 each additional spinal lesion (List separately in addition to code for primary procedure)**

EXCLUDES *Reporting code more than one time per lesion*
Reporting code more than two times per entire treatment course

Code first (63620)

7.30 7.30 **FUD** ZZZ B 80

AMA: 2018,Jan,8; 2017,Jan,8; 2016,Jan,13; 2015,Jun,6; 2015,Jan,16

63650-63688 Spinal Neurostimulation

INCLUDES Analysis system at implantation (95970)
Complex and simple neurostimulators

EXCLUDES *Analysis and programming neurostimulator pulse generator (95970-95972)*

63650 Percutaneous implantation of neurostimulator electrode array, epidural

INCLUDES Neurostimulator system components:
Multiple contacts which four or more provide electrical stimulation in epidural space
Contacts on catheter-type lead (array)
Extension
External controller
Implanted neurostimulator

11.9 54.1 **FUD** 010 J J8

AMA: 2019,Feb,6; 2018,Oct,11; 2018,Jan,8; 2017,Dec,13; 2017,Jan,8; 2016,Jan,13; 2016,Jan,11; 2015,Dec,18; 2015,Jan,16

63655 Laminectomy for implantation of neurostimulator electrodes, plate/paddle, epidural

INCLUDES Neurostimulator system components:
Multiple contacts which four or more provide electrical stimulation in epidural space
Contacts on catheter-type lead (array)
Extension
External controller
Implanted neurostimulator

24.0 24.0 **FUD** 090 J J8 80

AMA: 2019,Feb,6; 2018,Jan,8; 2017,Jan,8; 2016,Jan,13; 2015,Jan,16

63661 Removal of spinal neurostimulator electrode percutaneous array(s), including fluoroscopy, when performed

INCLUDES Neurostimulator system components:
Multiple contacts which four or more provide electrical stimulation in epidural space
Contacts on catheter-type lead (array)
Extension
External controller
Implanted neurostimulator

EXCLUDES *Reporting code when removing or replacing temporary array placed percutaneously for external generator*

9.33 18.3 **FUD** 010 Q2 G2 80

AMA: 2019,Feb,6; 2018,Jan,8; 2017,Jan,8; 2016,Jan,13; 2015,Jan,16

63662 Removal of spinal neurostimulator electrode plate/paddle(s) placed via laminotomy or laminectomy, including fluoroscopy, when performed

INCLUDES Neurostimulator system components:
Multiple contacts which four or more provide electrical stimulation in epidural space
Contacts on catheter-type lead (array)
Extension
External controller
Implanted neurostimulator

24.3 24.3 **FUD** 090 Q2 G2 80

AMA: 2019,Feb,6; 2018,Jan,8; 2017,Jan,8; 2016,Jan,13; 2015,Jan,16

63663 Revision including replacement, when performed, of spinal neurostimulator electrode percutaneous array(s), including fluoroscopy, when performed

INCLUDES Neurostimulator system components:
Multiple contacts which four or more provide electrical stimulation in epidural space
Contacts on catheter-type lead (array)
Extension
External controller
Implanted neurostimulator

EXCLUDES *Removal of spinal neurostimulator electrode percutaneous array(s), plate/paddle(s) at same level (63661-63662)*
Reporting code when removing or replacing temporary array placed percutaneously for external generator

12.9 23.4 **FUD** 010 J J8 80

AMA: 2019,Feb,6; 2018,Jan,8; 2017,Jan,8; 2016,Jan,13; 2015,Jan,16

63664 Revision including replacement, when performed, of spinal neurostimulator electrode plate/paddle(s) placed via laminotomy or laminectomy, including fluoroscopy, when performed

INCLUDES Neurostimulator system components:
Multiple contacts which four or more provide electrical stimulation in epidural space
Contacts on catheter-type lead (array)
Extension
External controller
Implanted neurostimulator

EXCLUDES *Removal spinal neurostimulator electrode percutaneous array(s), plate/paddle(s) at same level (63661-63662)*

25.2 25.2 **FUD** 090 J J8 80

AMA: 2019,Feb,6; 2018,Jan,8; 2017,Jan,8; 2016,Jan,13; 2015,Jan,16

63685 Insertion or replacement of spinal neurostimulator pulse generator or receiver, direct or inductive coupling

EXCLUDES *Reporting code for insertion/replacement with code for revision/removal (63688)*

10.3 10.3 **FUD** 010 J J8 80

AMA: 2019,Feb,6; 2018,Jan,8; 2017,Dec,13; 2017,Jan,8; 2016,Jan,13; 2015,Jan,16

63688 Revision or removal of implanted spinal neurostimulator pulse generator or receiver

EXCLUDES *Reporting code for revision/removal with code for insertion/replacement (63685)*

10.7 10.7 **FUD** 010 Q2 A2

AMA: 2019,Feb,6; 2018,Jan,8; 2017,Jan,8; 2016,Jan,13; 2015,Jan,16

63700-63706 Repair Congenital Neural Tube Defects

EXCLUDES *Complex skin repair (see appropriate integumentary closure code)*

63700 **Repair of meningocele; less than 5 cm diameter**
37.6 37.6 **FUD** 090 ⑥③ C 80
AMA: 2014,Jan,11

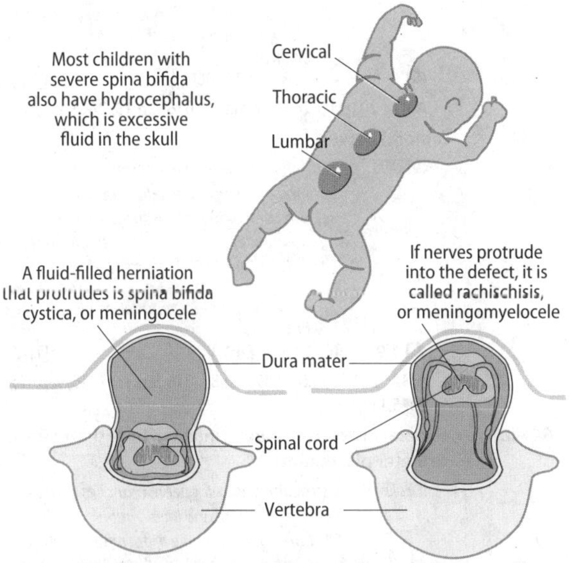

63702 **larger than 5 cm diameter**
41.8 41.8 **FUD** 090 ⑥③ C 80
AMA: 2014,Jan,11

63704 **Repair of myelomeningocele; less than 5 cm diameter**
47.7 47.7 **FUD** 090 ⑥③ C 80
AMA: 2014,Jan,11

63706 **larger than 5 cm diameter**
53.1 53.1 **FUD** 090 ⑥③ C 80
AMA: 2014,Jan,11

63707-63710 Repair Dural Cerebrospinal Fluid Leak

63707 **Repair of dural/cerebrospinal fluid leak, not requiring laminectomy**
26.8 26.8 **FUD** 090 C 80
AMA: 2014,Jan,11; 2002,May,7

63709 **Repair of dural/cerebrospinal fluid leak or pseudomeningocele, with laminectomy**
32.0 32.0 **FUD** 090 C 80
AMA: 2014,Jan,11; 2002,May,7

63710 **Dural graft, spinal**
31.6 31.6 **FUD** 090 C 80
AMA: 2014,Jan,11

63740-63746 Cerebrospinal Fluid (CSF) Shunt: Lumbar

EXCLUDES *Placement subarachnoid catheter with reservoir and/or pump:*
Not requiring laminectomy (62350, 62360-62362)
With laminectomy (62351, 62360-62362)

63740 **Creation of shunt, lumbar, subarachnoid-peritoneal, -pleural, or other; including laminectomy**
28.1 28.1 **FUD** 090 C 80
AMA: 2014,Jan,11; 2000,Dec,12

63741 **percutaneous, not requiring laminectomy**
19.7 19.7 **FUD** 090 J 80
AMA: 2014,Jan,11; 1990,Win,4

63744 **Replacement, irrigation or revision of lumbosubarachnoid shunt**
19.1 19.1 **FUD** 090 J A2 80
AMA: 2014,Jan,11

63746 **Removal of entire lumbosubarachnoid shunt system without replacement**
17.6 17.6 **FUD** 090 Q2 A2 80
AMA: 2014,Jan,11

64400-64463 [64461, 64462, 64463] Nerve Blocks

EXCLUDES *Epidural or subarachnoid injection (62320-62327)*
Nerve destruction (62280-62282, 64600-64681 [64624, 64625, 64633, 64634, 64635, 64636])

64400 **Injection(s), anesthetic agent(s) and/or steroid; trigeminal nerve, each branch (ie, ophthalmic, maxillary, mandibular)**
EXCLUDES *Destruction genicular nerve branches ([64624])*
Imaging guidance and localization
Injection genicular nerve branches (64454)
Reporting code more than one time per encounter when multiple injections required to block nerve and branches
1.44 3.05 **FUD** 000 T P3 50
AMA: 2018,Jan,8; 2017,Jan,8; 2016,Jan,13; 2015,Jan,16

64405 **greater occipital nerve**
EXCLUDES *Destruction genicular nerve branches ([64624])*
Imaging guidance and localization
Injection genicular nerve branches (64454)
Reporting code more than one time per encounter when multiple injections required to block nerve and branches
1.55 2.07 **FUD** 000 T P3 50
AMA: 2018,Jan,8; 2017,Jan,8; 2016,Oct,11; 2016,Jan,13; 2015,Jan,16

64408 **vagus nerve**
EXCLUDES *Destruction genicular nerve branches ([64624])*
Imaging guidance and localization
Injection genicular nerve branches (64454)
Reporting code more than one time per encounter when multiple injections required to block nerve and branches
2.44 3.35 **FUD** 000 T P3 80 50
AMA: 2018,Jan,8; 2017,Jan,8; 2016,Jan,13; 2015,Jan,16

64415 **brachial plexus**
EXCLUDES *Destruction genicular nerve branches ([64624])*
Imaging guidance and localization
Injection genicular nerve branches (64454)
Reporting code more than one time per encounter when multiple injections required to block nerve and branches
1.83 3.22 **FUD** 000 T A2 50
AMA: 2018,Jan,8; 2017,Jan,8; 2016,Jan,13; 2015,Jan,16

64416 **brachial plexus, continuous infusion by catheter (including catheter placement)**
EXCLUDES *Destruction genicular nerve branches ([64624])*
Imaging guidance and localization
Injection genicular nerve branches (64454)
Management epidural or subarachnoid continuous drug administration (01996)
Reporting code more than one time per encounter when multiple injections required to block nerve and branches
1.85 1.85 **FUD** 000 T G2 50
AMA: 2018,Jan,8; 2017,Jan,8; 2016,Jan,13; 2015,Jan,16

64417 **axillary nerve**
EXCLUDES *Destruction genicular nerve branches ([64624])*
Imaging guidance and localization
Injection genicular nerve branches (64454)
Reporting code more than one time per encounter when multiple injections required to block nerve and branches
2.02 3.76 **FUD** 000 T A2 50
AMA: 2018,Jan,8; 2017,Jan,8; 2016,Jan,13; 2015,Jan,16

64418 **suprascapular nerve**

EXCLUDES *Destruction genicular nerve branches ([64624])*
Imaging guidance and localization
Injection genicular nerve branches (64454)
Reporting code more than one time per encounter when multiple injections required to block nerve and branches

1.64 2.42 FUD 000 T P3 50

AMA: 2018,Jan,8; 2017,Jan,8; 2016,Jan,13; 2015,Jan,16

64420 **intercostal nerve, single level**

EXCLUDES *Destruction genicular nerve branches ([64624])*
Imaging guidance and localization
Injection genicular nerve branches (64454)
Reporting code more than one time per encounter when multiple injections required to block nerve and branches

1.72 2.85 FUD 000 T A2 50

AMA: 2018,Jan,8; 2017,Jan,8; 2016,Jan,9; 2016,Jan,13; 2015,Jun,3; 2015,Jan,16

+ **64421** **intercostal nerve, each additional level (List separately in addition to code for primary procedure)**

EXCLUDES *Destruction genicular nerve branches ([64624])*
Imaging guidance and localization
Injection genicular nerve branches (64454)
Reporting code more than one time per encounter when multiple injections required to block nerve and branches
Reporting with modifier 50. Report once for each side when performed bilaterally

Code first (64420)

0.73 0.97 FUD ZZZ T A2 50

AMA: 2018,Jan,8; 2017,Jan,8; 2016,Jan,9; 2016,Jan,13; 2015,Jun,3; 2015,Jan,16

64425 **ilioinguinal, iliohypogastric nerves**

EXCLUDES *Destruction genicular nerve branches ([64624])*
Imaging guidance and localization
Injection genicular nerve branches (64454)
Reporting code more than one time per encounter when multiple injections required to block nerve and branches

1.60 3.19 FUD 000 T P3 50

AMA: 2018,Jan,8; 2017,Jan,8; 2016,Jan,13; 2015,Jun,3; 2015,Jan,16

64430 **pudendal nerve**

EXCLUDES *Destruction genicular nerve branches ([64624])*
Imaging guidance and localization
Injection genicular nerve branches (64454)
Reporting code more than one time per encounter when multiple injections required to block nerve and branches

2.30 4.14 FUD 000 T A2 50

AMA: 2018,Jan,8; 2017,Jan,8; 2016,Jan,13; 2015,Jan,16

64435 **paracervical (uterine) nerve** ♀

EXCLUDES *Destruction genicular nerve branches ([64624])*
Imaging guidance and localization
Injection genicular nerve branches (64454)
Reporting code more than one time per encounter when multiple injections required to block nerve and branches

2.35 4.00 FUD 000 T P3 50

AMA: 2018,Jan,8; 2017,Jan,8; 2016,Jan,13; 2015,Jan,16

64445 **sciatic nerve**

EXCLUDES *Destruction genicular nerve branches ([64624])*
Imaging guidance and localization
Injection genicular nerve branches (64454)
Reporting code more than one time per encounter when multiple injections required to block nerve and branches

2.09 3.89 FUD 000 T P3 50

AMA: 2018,Jan,8; 2017,Jan,8; 2016,Jan,13; 2015,Jan,16

64446 **sciatic nerve, continuous infusion by catheter (including catheter placement)**

EXCLUDES *Destruction genicular nerve branches ([64624])*
Imaging guidance and localization
Injection genicular nerve branches (64454)
Management epidural or subarachnoid continuous drug administration (01996)
Reporting code more than one time per encounter when multiple injections required to block nerve and branches

2.28 2.28 FUD 000 T G2 50

AMA: 2018,Jan,8; 2017,Jan,8; 2016,Jan,13; 2015,Jan,16

64447 **femoral nerve**

EXCLUDES *Destruction genicular nerve branches ([64624])*
Imaging guidance and localization
Injection genicular nerve branches (64454)
Management epidural or subarachnoid continuous drug administration (01996)
Reporting code more than one time per encounter when multiple injections required to block nerve and branches

1.91 3.46 FUD 000 T P3 50

AMA: 2018,Jan,8; 2017,Jan,8; 2016,Jan,13; 2015,Sep,12; 2015,Jan,16

64448 **femoral nerve, continuous infusion by catheter (including catheter placement)**

EXCLUDES *Destruction genicular nerve branches ([64624])*
Imaging guidance and localization
Injection genicular nerve branches (64454)
Management epidural or subarachnoid continuous drug administration (01996)
Reporting code more than one time per encounter when multiple injections required to block nerve and branches

2.05 2.05 FUD 000 T G2 50

AMA: 2018,Jan,8; 2017,Jan,8; 2016,Jan,13; 2015,Sep,12; 2015,Jan,16

64449 **lumbar plexus, posterior approach, continuous infusion by catheter (including catheter placement)**

EXCLUDES *Destruction genicular nerve branches ([64624])*
Imaging guidance and localization
Injection genicular nerve branches (64454)
Management epidural or subarachnoid continuous drug administration (01996)
Reporting code more than one time per encounter when multiple injections required to block nerve and branches

2.44 2.44 FUD 000 T G2 50

AMA: 2018,Jan,8; 2017,Jan,8; 2016,Jan,13; 2015,Jan,16

64450 **other peripheral nerve or branch**

EXCLUDES *Destruction genicular nerve branches ([64624])*
Imaging guidance and localization
Injection genicular nerve branches (64454)
Injection nerves innervating the sacroiliac joint (64451)
Reporting code more than one time per encounter when multiple injections required to block nerve and branches

1.28 2.19 FUD 000 T P3 50

AMA: 2019,Nov,14; 2018,Nov,10; 2018,Jan,8; 2017,Jan,8; 2016,Oct,11; 2016,Jan,13; 2015,Nov,10; 2015,Sep,12; 2015,Jun,3; 2015,Jan,16

64451 **nerves innervating the sacroiliac joint, with image guidance (ie, fluoroscopy or computed tomography)**

INCLUDES Imaging guidance and any contrast injection

EXCLUDES *Destruction genicular nerve branches ([64624])*
Injection genicular nerve branches (64454)
Injection nerves innervating paravertebral facet joint (64493-64495)
Injection with ultrasound (76999)
Reporting code more than one time per encounter when multiple injections required to block nerve and branches

2.29 5.99 **FUD** 000 G2 50

AMA: 2020,Jul,13

64454 **genicular nerve branches, including imaging guidance, when performed**

INCLUDES Imaging guidance and any contrast injection

EXCLUDES *Destruction genicular nerve branches ([64624])*
Injection genicular nerve branches (64454)
Reporting code more than one time per encounter when multiple injections required to block nerve and branches

Code also modifier 52 for injection fewer than following all genicular nerve branches: superolateral, superomedial, and inferomedial

2.36 6.05 **FUD** 000 P3 50

AMA: 2019,Dec,8

▲ **64455** **plantar common digital nerve(s) (eg, Morton's neuroma)**

INCLUDES Single or multiple injections on the same site

EXCLUDES *Destruction by neurolytic agent; plantar common digital nerve (64632)*
Destruction genicular nerve branches ([64624])
Imaging guidance and localization
Injection genicular nerve branches (64454)
Reporting code more than one time per encounter when multiple injections required to block nerve and branches

1.00 1.36 **FUD** 000 T P3 80 50

AMA: 2018,Jan,8; 2017,Jan,8; 2016,Jan,13; 2015,Jan,16

64461 **Resequenced code. See code following 64484.**

64462 **Resequenced code. See code following 64484.**

64463 **Resequenced code. See code following 64484.**

64479-64484 Transforaminal Injection

INCLUDES Imaging guidance (fluoroscopy or CT) and contrast injection

EXCLUDES *Epidural or subarachnoid injection (62320-62327)*
Nerve destruction (62280-62282, 64600-64681 [64624, 64625, 64633, 64634, 64635, 64636])

▲ **64479** **transforaminal epidural, with imaging guidance (fluoroscopy or CT), cervical or thoracic, single level**

INCLUDES Imaging guidance and any contrast injection
Single or multiple injections same site
Transforaminal epidural injection T12-L1 level

3.76 6.95 **FUD** 000 T A2 50

AMA: 2018,Jan,8; 2017,Jan,8; 2016,Jan,13; 2016,Jan,9; 2015,Jan,16

Thoracic vertebra (superior view)

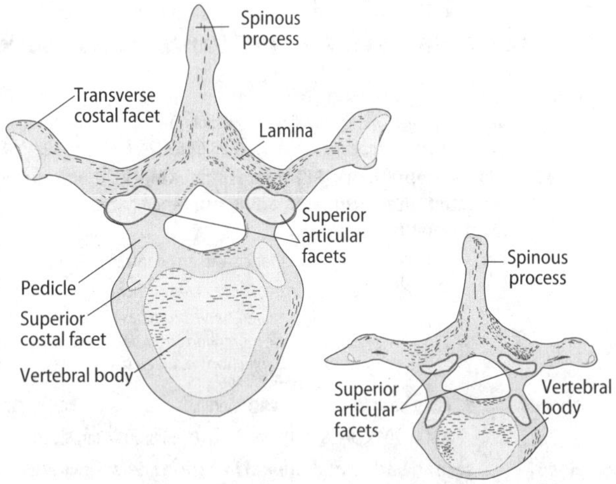

Superior view of C7

▲ + **64480** **transforaminal epidural, with imaging guidance (fluoroscopy or CT), cervical or thoracic, each additional level (List separately in addition to code for primary procedure)**

INCLUDES Imaging guidance and any contrast injection
Single or multiple injections same site

EXCLUDES *Destruction genicular nerve branches ([64624])*
Injection genicular nerve branches (64454)
Reporting with modifier 50. Report once for each side when performed bilaterally
Transforaminal epidural injection T12-L1 level
Reporting code more than one time per encounter when multiple injections required to block nerve and branches

Code first (64479)

1.80 3.42 **FUD** ZZZ N N1 50

AMA: 2018,Jan,8; 2017,Jan,8; 2016,Jan,9; 2016,Jan,13; 2015,Jan,16

▲ **64483** **transforaminal epidural, with imaging guidance (fluoroscopy or CT), lumbar or sacral, single level**

INCLUDES Imaging guidance and any contrast injection
Single or multiple injections same site

EXCLUDES *Destruction genicular nerve branches ([64624])*
Injection genicular nerve branches (64454)
Reporting code more than one time per encounter when multiple injections required to block nerve and branches

3.19 6.44 **FUD** 000 T A2 50

AMA: 2018,Jan,8; 2017,Jan,8; 2016,Oct,11; 2016,Jan,13; 2016,Jan,9; 2015,Jan,16

▲ + 64484 **transforaminal epidural, with imaging guidance (fluoroscopy or CT), lumbar or sacral, each additional level (List separately in addition to code for primary procedure)**

INCLUDES Imaging guidance and any contrast injection

Single or multiple injections same site

EXCLUDES *Destruction genicular nerve branches ([64624])*

Injection genicular nerve branches (64454)

Reporting code more than one time per encounter when multiple injections required to block nerve and branches

Reporting with modifier 50. Report once for each side when performed bilaterally

Code first (64483)

1.49 2.79 **FUD** ZZZ N N1 50

AMA: 2018,Jan,8; 2017,Jan,8; 2016,Jan,9; 2016,Jan,13; 2015,Jan,16

64461-64463 [64461, 64462, 64463] Paravertebral Blocks

INCLUDES Radiological guidance (76942, 77002-77003)

EXCLUDES *Injection:*

Anesthetic agent (64420-64421, 64479-64480)

Diagnostic or therapeutic substance (62320, 62324, 64490-64492)

\# 64461 **Paravertebral block (PVB) (paraspinous block), thoracic; single injection site (includes imaging guidance, when performed)**

INCLUDES Imaging guidance and any contrast injection

EXCLUDES *Destruction genicular nerve branches ([64624])*

Injection genicular nerve branches (64454)

Reporting code more than one time per encounter when multiple injections required to block nerve and branches

2.50 4.22 **FUD** 000 T G2 50

AMA: 2018,Dec,8; 2018,Dec,8; 2018,Jan,8; 2017,Jan,8; 2016,Jan,9

\+ # 64462 **second and any additional injection site(s) (includes imaging guidance, when performed) (List separately in addition to code for primary procedure)**

INCLUDES Imaging guidance and any contrast injection

EXCLUDES *Destruction genicular nerve branches ([64624])*

Injection genicular nerve branches (64454)

Procedure performed more than one time per day

Reporting with modifier 50. Report once for each side when performed bilaterally

Code first (64461)

1.54 2.32 **FUD** ZZZ N N1 50

AMA: 2018,Dec,8; 2018,Dec,8; 2018,Jan,8; 2017,Jan,8; 2016,Jan,9

\# 64463 **continuous infusion by catheter (includes imaging guidance, when performed)**

INCLUDES Imaging guidance and any contrast injection

EXCLUDES *Destruction genicular nerve branches ([64624])*

Injection genicular nerve branches (64454)

Reporting code more than one time per encounter when multiple injections required to block nerve and branches

2.47 4.51 **FUD** 000 T G2 50

AMA: 2018,Dec,8; 2018,Dec,8; 2018,Jan,8; 2017,Jan,8; 2016,Jan,9

64486-64489 Transversus Abdominis Plane (TAP) Block

64486 **Transversus abdominis plane (TAP) block (abdominal plane block, rectus sheath block) unilateral; by injection(s) (includes imaging guidance, when performed)**

INCLUDES Imaging guidance and any contrast injection

EXCLUDES *Destruction genicular nerve branches ([64624])*

Injection genicular nerve branches (64454)

Reporting code more than one time per encounter when multiple injections required to block nerve and branches

1.61 3.12 **FUD** 000 N N1 50

AMA: 2018,Jan,8; 2017,Jan,8; 2016,Jan,13; 2015,Jun,3

64487 **by continuous infusion(s) (includes imaging guidance, when performed)**

INCLUDES Imaging guidance and any contrast injection

EXCLUDES *Destruction genicular nerve branches ([64624])*

Injection genicular nerve branches (64454)

Reporting code more than one time per encounter when multiple injections required to block nerve and branches

1.87 4.49 **FUD** 000 N N1 50

AMA: 2018,Jan,8; 2017,Jan,8; 2016,Jan,13; 2015,Jun,3

64488 **Transversus abdominis plane (TAP) block (abdominal plane block, rectus sheath block) bilateral; by injections (includes imaging guidance, when performed)**

INCLUDES Imaging guidance and any contrast injection

EXCLUDES *Destruction genicular nerve branches ([64624])*

Injection genicular nerve branches (64454)

Reporting code more than one time per encounter when multiple injections required to block nerve and branches

2.02 3.83 **FUD** 000 N N1

AMA: 2018,Jan,8; 2017,Jan,8; 2016,Jan,13; 2015,Jun,3

64489 **by continuous infusions (includes imaging guidance, when performed)**

INCLUDES Imaging guidance and any contrast injection

EXCLUDES *Destruction genicular nerve branches ([64624])*

Injection genicular nerve branches (64454)

Reporting code more than one time per encounter when multiple injections required to block nerve and branches

2.27 6.65 **FUD** 000 N N1

AMA: 2018,Jan,8; 2017,Jan,8; 2016,Jan,13; 2015,Jun,3

64490-64495 Paraspinal Nerve Injections

INCLUDES Image guidance (CT or fluoroscopy) and any contrast injection

EXCLUDES *Injection without imaging (20552-20553)*

Ultrasonic guidance (0213T-0218T)

64490 **Injection(s), diagnostic or therapeutic agent, paravertebral facet (zygapophyseal) joint (or nerves innervating that joint) with image guidance (fluoroscopy or CT), cervical or thoracic; single level**

INCLUDES Injection T12-L1 joint and nerves that innervate joint

3.03 5.39 **FUD** 000 T G2 80 50

AMA: 2018,Jan,8; 2017,Jan,8; 2016,Jan,9; 2016,Jan,13; 2015,Jan,16

\+ 64491 **second level (List separately in addition to code for primary procedure)**

EXCLUDES *Reporting with modifier 50. Report once for each side when performed bilaterally*

Code first (64490)

1.72 2.68 **FUD** ZZZ N N1 80 50

AMA: 2018,Jan,8; 2017,Jan,8; 2016,Jan,9; 2016,Jan,13; 2015,Jan,16

\+ 64492 **third and any additional level(s) (List separately in addition to code for primary procedure)**

EXCLUDES *Procedure performed more than one time per day*

Reporting with modifier 50. Report once for each side when performed bilaterally

Code also when appropriate (64491)

Code first (64490)

1.74 2.70 **FUD** ZZZ N N1 80 50

AMA: 2018,Jan,8; 2017,Jan,8; 2016,Jan,9; 2016,Jan,13; 2015,Jan,16

64493 **Injection(s), diagnostic or therapeutic agent, paravertebral facet (zygapophyseal) joint (or nerves innervating that joint) with image guidance (fluoroscopy or CT), lumbar or sacral; single level**

EXCLUDES *Injection nerves innervating sacroiliac joint (64451)*

2.58 4.91 **FUD** 000 T G2 80 50

AMA: 2020,Jul,13; 2018,May,10; 2018,Jan,8; 2017,Jan,8; 2016,Jan,13; 2015,Jan,16

\+ 64494 **second level (List separately in addition to code for primary procedure)**

EXCLUDES *Reporting with modifier 50. Report once for each side when performed bilaterally*

Code first (64493)

1.49 2.49 FUD ZZZ N N1 80 50

AMA: 2020,Jul,13; 2018,May,10; 2018,Jan,8; 2017,Jan,8; 2016,Jan,13; 2015,Jan,16

\+ 64495 **third and any additional level(s) (List separately in addition to code for primary procedure)**

EXCLUDES *Procedure performed more than one time per day*

Reporting with modifier 50. Report once for each side when performed bilaterally

Code also when appropriate (64494)

Code first (64493)

1.51 2.49 FUD ZZZ N N1 80 50

AMA: 2018,May,10; 2018,Jan,8; 2017,Jan,8; 2016,Jan,13; 2015,Jan,16

64505-64530 Sympathetic Nerve Blocks

64505 **Injection, anesthetic agent; sphenopalatine ganglion**

2.69 3.36 FUD 000 T P3 50

AMA: 2018,Jan,8; 2017,Jan,8; 2016,Jan,13; 2015,Jan,16

64510 **stellate ganglion (cervical sympathetic)**

2.13 3.78 FUD 000 T A2 50

AMA: 2018,Jan,8; 2017,Jan,8; 2016,Jan,13; 2015,Jan,16

64517 **superior hypogastric plexus**

3.60 5.47 FUD 000 T A2

AMA: 2018,Jan,8; 2017,Jan,8; 2016,Jan,13; 2015,Jan,16

64520 **lumbar or thoracic (paravertebral sympathetic)**

2.34 5.75 FUD 000 T A2 50

AMA: 2018,Jan,8; 2017,Jan,8; 2016,Jan,13; 2015,Jan,16

64530 **celiac plexus, with or without radiologic monitoring**

EXCLUDES *Transmural anesthetic injection with transendoscopic ultrasound-guidance (43253)*

2.63 5.73 FUD 000 T A2

AMA: 2018,Jan,8; 2017,Jan,8; 2016,Jan,13; 2015,Jan,16

64553-64570 Electrical Nerve Stimulation: Insertion/Replacement/Removal/Revision

INCLUDES Analysis system at implantation (95970)

Simple and complex neurostimulators

EXCLUDES *Analysis and programming neurostimulator pulse generator (95970-95972)*

TENS therapy (97014, 97032)

64553 **Percutaneous implantation of neurostimulator electrode array; cranial nerve**

INCLUDES Temporary and permanent percutaneous array placement

EXCLUDES *Open procedure (61885-61886)*

Percutaneous electrical stimulation peripheral nerve with needle or needle electrodes (64999)

10.1 48.8 FUD 010 J J8 80

AMA: 2019,Feb,6; 2018,Oct,8; 2018,Jan,8; 2017,Jan,8; 2016,Jan,13; 2015,Jan,16

64555 **peripheral nerve (excludes sacral nerve)**

INCLUDES Temporary and permanent percutaneous array placement

EXCLUDES *Percutaneous electrical stimulation cranial nerve with needle or needle electrodes (64999)*

Posterior tibial neurostimulation (64566)

9.85 44.3 FUD 010 J J8

AMA: 2019,Feb,6; 2018,Oct,8; 2018,Aug,10; 2018,Jan,8; 2017,Dec,13; 2017,Jan,8; 2016,Feb,13; 2016,Jan,13; 2015,Jan,16; 2015,Jan,13

64561 **sacral nerve (transforaminal placement) including image guidance, if performed**

INCLUDES Temporary and permanent percutaneous array placement

EXCLUDES *Percutaneous electrical stimulation or neuromodulation with needle or needle electrodes (64999)*

8.75 20.9 FUD 010 J J8 50

AMA: 2019,Feb,6; 2018,Oct,8; 2018,Jan,8; 2017,Jan,8; 2016,Jan,13; 2015,Jan,16

64566 **Posterior tibial neurostimulation, percutaneous needle electrode, single treatment, includes programming**

EXCLUDES *Electronic analysis implanted neurostimulator pulse generator system (95970-95972)*

Percutaneous implantation neurostimulator electrode array; peripheral nerve (64555)

0.87 3.62 FUD 000 T P3 80

AMA: 2019,Feb,6; 2018,Oct,8; 2018,Jan,8; 2017,Jan,8; 2016,Jan,13; 2015,Jan,16

64568 **Incision for implantation of cranial nerve (eg, vagus nerve) neurostimulator electrode array and pulse generator**

EXCLUDES *Insertion chest wall respiratory sensor electrode or array with pulse generator connection (0466T)*

Insertion, replacement cranial neurostimulator pulse generator or receiver (61885-61886)

Removal neurostimulator electrode array and pulse generator (64570)

18.4 18.4 FUD 090 J J8 80 50

AMA: 2019,Feb,6; 2018,Mar,9; 2018,Jan,8; 2017,Jan,8; 2016,Nov,6; 2016,Jan,13; 2015,Jan,16

64569 **Revision or replacement of cranial nerve (eg, vagus nerve) neurostimulator electrode array, including connection to existing pulse generator**

EXCLUDES *Removal neurostimulator electrode array and pulse generator (64570)*

Replacement pulse generator (61885)

Revision or replacement chest wall respiratory sensor electrode with pulse generator connection (0467T)

Revision, removal pulse generator (61888)

22.1 22.1 FUD 090 J J8 80 50

AMA: 2019,Feb,6; 2018,Mar,9; 2018,Jan,8; 2017,Jan,8; 2016,Nov,6; 2016,Jan,13; 2015,Jan,16

64570 **Removal of cranial nerve (eg, vagus nerve) neurostimulator electrode array and pulse generator**

EXCLUDES *Laparoscopic revision, replacement, removal, or implantation vagus nerve blocking neurostimulator pulse generator and/or electrode array at esophagogastric junction (0312T-0317T)*

Removal chest wall respiratory sensor electrode or array (0468T)

Revision, removal pulse generator (61888)

21.2 21.2 FUD 090 Q2 G2 80 50

AMA: 2019,Feb,6; 2018,Mar,9; 2018,Jan,8; 2017,Jan,8; 2016,Nov,6; 2016,Jan,13; 2015,Jan,16

64575-64595 Implantation/Revision/Removal Neurostimulators: Incisional

INCLUDES Simple and complex neurostimulators

EXCLUDES *Analysis and programming neurostimulator pulse generator (95970-95972)*

64575 **Incision for implantation of neurostimulator electrode array; peripheral nerve (excludes sacral nerve)**

9.60 9.60 FUD 090 J J8

AMA: 2019,Feb,6

64580 **neuromuscular**

8.97 8.97 FUD 090 J J8 80

AMA: 2019,Feb,6

64581 **sacral nerve (transforaminal placement)**

19.0 19.0 FUD 090 J J8

AMA: 2019,Feb,6; 2018,Jan,8; 2017,Jan,8; 2016,Jan,13; 2015,Jan,16

64585 **Revision or removal of peripheral neurostimulator electrode array**

4.14 7.03 **FUD** 010 Q2 A2

AMA: 2019,Feb,6

64590 **Insertion or replacement of peripheral or gastric neurostimulator pulse generator or receiver, direct or inductive coupling**

EXCLUDES *Revision, removal neurostimulator pulse generator (64595)*

4.64 7.60 **FUD** 010 J J8

AMA: 2019,Feb,6; 2018,Aug,10; 2018,Jan,8; 2017,Dec,13; 2017,Jan,8; 2016,Jan,13; 2015,Jan,13; 2015,Jan,16

64595 **Revision or removal of peripheral or gastric neurostimulator pulse generator or receiver**

EXCLUDES *Insertion, replacement neurostimulator pulse generator (64590)*

3.63 6.89 **FUD** 010 Q2 A2

AMA: 2019,Feb,6; 2018,Jan,8; 2017,Jan,8; 2016,Jan,13; 2015,Jan,16

64600-64610 Chemical Denervation Trigeminal Nerve

INCLUDES Injection therapeutic medication

EXCLUDES *Electromyography or muscle electric stimulation guidance (95873-95874)*
Nerve destruction:
Anal sphincter (46505)
Bladder (52287)
Strabismus involving extraocular muscles (67345)
Treatments that do not destroy target nerve (64999)

Code also chemodenervation agent

64600 **Destruction by neurolytic agent, trigeminal nerve; supraorbital, infraorbital, mental, or inferior alveolar branch**

6.66 12.3 **FUD** 010 T A2

AMA: 2019,Apr,9; 2018,Jan,8; 2017,Jan,8; 2016,Jan,13; 2015,Jan,16

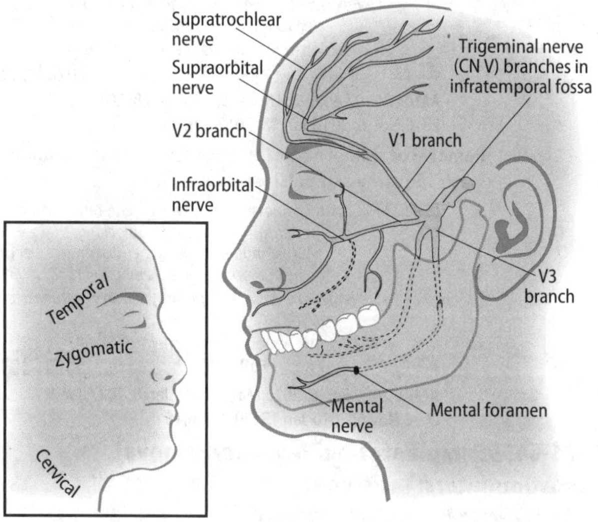

64605 **second and third division branches at foramen ovale**

10.1 17.8 **FUD** 010 J A2 80 50

AMA: 2019,Apr,9; 2018,Jan,8; 2017,Jan,8; 2016,Jan,13; 2015,Jan,16

64610 **second and third division branches at foramen ovale under radiologic monitoring**

14.2 22.0 **FUD** 010 J A2 50

AMA: 2019,Apr,9; 2018,Jan,8; 2017,Apr,9; 2017,Jan,8; 2016,Jan,13; 2015,Jan,16

64624 [64624] Chemical Denervation Genicular Nerve Branches

64624 **Destruction by neurolytic agent, genicular nerve branches including imaging guidance, when performed**

EXCLUDES *Injection genicular nerve branches (64454)*

Code also modifier 52 for destruction fewer than all genicular nerve branches: superolateral, superomedial, and inferomedial

4.23 11.5 **FUD** 010 P3 80 50

AMA: 2019,Dec,8

64625 [64625] Radiofrequency Ablation Sacroiliac Joint Nerves

64625 **Radiofrequency ablation, nerves innervating the sacroiliac joint, with image guidance (ie, fluoroscopy or computed tomography)**

INCLUDES CT needle guidance (77012)
Electrical stimulation or needle electromyelograph for guidance (95873-95874)
Fluoroscopic needle guidance or localization (77002-77003)

EXCLUDES *Destruction by neurolytic agent, paravertebral facet joint nerve ([64635])*
Radiofrequency ablation with ultrasound (76999)

5.59 14.1 **FUD** 010 G2 50

AMA: 2020,Jun,14; 2019,Dec,8

64611-64617 Chemical Denervation Procedures Head and Neck

INCLUDES Injection therapeutic medication

EXCLUDES *Electromyography or muscle electric stimulation guidance (95873-95874)*
Nerve destruction:
Anal sphincter (46505)
Bladder (52287)
Extraocular muscles to treat strabismus (67345)
Treatments that do not destroy target nerve (64999)

64611 **Chemodenervation of parotid and submandibular salivary glands, bilateral**

Code also modifier 52 for injection of fewer than four salivary glands

3.03 3.45 **FUD** 010 T P3 80

AMA: 2019,Apr,9; 2018,Jan,8; 2017,Jan,8; 2016,Jan,13; 2015,Jan,16

64612 **Chemodenervation of muscle(s); muscle(s) innervated by facial nerve, unilateral (eg, for blepharospasm, hemifacial spasm)**

3.39 3.83 **FUD** 010 T P3 50

AMA: 2019,Apr,9; 2018,Jan,8; 2017,Jan,8; 2016,Jan,13; 2015,Jan,16

64615 **muscle(s) innervated by facial, trigeminal, cervical spinal and accessory nerves, bilateral (eg, for chronic migraine)**

EXCLUDES *Chemodenervation (64612, 64616-64617, 64642-64647)*
Procedure performed more than one time per session

Code also any guidance by muscle electrical stimulation or needle electromyography but report only once (95873-95874)

3.58 4.27 **FUD** 010 T P3

AMA: 2019,Apr,9; 2018,Jan,8; 2017,Jan,8; 2016,Jan,13; 2015,Jan,16

64616 **neck muscle(s), excluding muscles of the larynx, unilateral (eg, for cervical dystonia, spasmodic torticollis)**

Code also guidance by muscle electrical stimulation or needle electromyography, but report only once (95873-95874)

3.18 3.80 **FUD** 010 T P3 50

AMA: 2019,Apr,9; 2018,Jan,8; 2017,Jan,8; 2016,Jan,13; 2015,Jan,16

64617 **larynx, unilateral, percutaneous (eg, for spasmodic dysphonia), includes guidance by needle electromyography, when performed**

EXCLUDES *Chemodenervation larynx via direct laryngoscopy (31570-31571)*
Diagnostic needle electromyography larynx (95865)
Electrical stimulation guidance for chemodenervation (95873-95874)

3.14 4.62 **FUD** 010 T P3 50

AMA: 2019,Apr,9; 2018,Jan,8; 2017,Jan,8; 2016,Jan,13; 2015,Jan,16

64620-64640 [64624, 64625, 64633, 64634, 64635, 64636] Chemical Denervation Intercostal, Facet Joint, Plantar, and Pudendal Nerve(s)

INCLUDES Injection therapeutic medication

64620 **Destruction by neurolytic agent, intercostal nerve**

5.00 5.91 **FUD** 010 T A2

AMA: 2019,Nov,14; 2019,Apr,9; 2018,Jan,8; 2017,Jan,8; 2016,Jan,13; 2015,Jan,16

64624 **Resequenced code. See code following 64610.**

64625 **Resequenced code. See code before 64611.**

\# 64633 **Destruction by neurolytic agent, paravertebral facet joint nerve(s), with imaging guidance (fluoroscopy or CT); cervical or thoracic, single facet joint**

INCLUDES Paravertebral facet destruction T12-L1 joint or nerve(s) that innervate joint
Radiological guidance (77003, 77012)

EXCLUDES *Denervation performed using chemical, low grade thermal, or pulsed radiofrequency methods (64999)*
Destruction paravertebral facet joint nerve(s) without imaging guidance (64999)

6.43 11.8 **FUD** 010 J G2 50

AMA: 2019,Apr,9; 2018,Jan,8; 2017,Jan,8; 2016,Jan,13; 2015,Feb,9; 2015,Jan,16

\+ # 64634 **cervical or thoracic, each additional facet joint (List separately in addition to code for primary procedure)**

INCLUDES Radiological guidance (77003, 77012)

EXCLUDES *Denervation performed using chemical, low grade thermal, or pulsed radiofrequency methods (64999)*
Destruction paravertebral facet joint nerve(s) without imaging guidance (64999)
Reporting with modifier 50. Report once for each side when performed bilaterally

Code first ([64633])

1.95 5.34 **FUD** ZZZ N N1 50

AMA: 2019,Apr,9; 2018,Jan,8; 2017,Jan,8; 2016,Jan,13; 2015,Feb,9; 2015,Jan,16

\# 64635 **lumbar or sacral, single facet joint**

INCLUDES Radiological guidance (77003, 77012)

EXCLUDES *Denervation performed using chemical, low grade thermal, or pulsed radiofrequency methods (64999)*
Destruction individual nerves, sacroiliac joint, by neurolytic agent (64640)
Destruction paravertebral facet joint nerve(s) without imaging guidance (64999)

6.34 11.7 **FUD** 010 J G2 50

AMA: 2020,May,13; 2019,Dec,8; 2019,Apr,9; 2018,Jan,8; 2017,Jan,8; 2016,Jan,13; 2015,Feb,9; 2015,Jan,16

\+ # 64636 **lumbar or sacral, each additional facet joint (List separately in addition to code for primary procedure)**

INCLUDES Radiological guidance (77003, 77012)

EXCLUDES *Denervation performed using chemical, low grade thermal, or pulsed radiofrequency methods (64999)*
Destruction individual nerves, sacroiliac joint, by neurolytic agent (64640)
Destruction paravertebral facet joint nerve(s) without imaging guidance (64999)
Radiofrequency ablation nerves innervating sacroiliac joint with imaging ([64625])
Reporting with modifier 50. Report once for each side when performed bilaterally

Code first ([64635])

1.71 4.85 **FUD** ZZZ N N1 50

AMA: 2020,May,13; 2019,Apr,9; 2018,Jan,8; 2017,Jan,8; 2016,Jan,13; 2015,Feb,9; 2015,Jan,16

64630 **Destruction by neurolytic agent; pudendal nerve**

5.44 6.94 **FUD** 010 T A2 80

AMA: 2019,Apr,9; 2018,Jan,8; 2017,Oct,9; 2017,Jan,8; 2016,Jan,13; 2015,Jan,16

64632 **plantar common digital nerve**

EXCLUDES *Injection(s), anesthetic agent and/or steroid (64455)*

1.96 2.45 **FUD** 010 T P3 80 50

AMA: 2019,Apr,9; 2018,Jan,8; 2017,Oct,9; 2017,Jan,8; 2016,Jan,13; 2015,Jul,10; 2015,Jan,16

64633 **Resequenced code. See code following 64620.**

64634 **Resequenced code. See code following 64620.**

64635 **Resequenced code. See code following 64620.**

64636 **Resequenced code. See code before 64630.**

64640 **other peripheral nerve or branch**

INCLUDES Neurolytic destruction of nerves of sacroiliac joint

2.69 3.86 **FUD** 010 T P3 50

AMA: 2019,Apr,9; 2018,Jan,8; 2018,Jan,7; 2017,Oct,9; 2017,Jan,8; 2016,Jan,13; 2015,Jan,16

64642-64645 Chemical Denervation Extremity Muscles

INCLUDES Trunk muscles include erector spine, obliques, paraspinal, and rectus abdominus. Remaining muscles considered neck, head or extremity muscles

EXCLUDES *Chemodenervation with needle-guided electromyography or with guidance provided by muscle electrical stimulation (95873-95874)*
Procedure performed more than once per extremity

Code also other extremities when appropriate, up to total four units per patient (when all extremities injected) (64642-64645)

64642 **Chemodenervation of one extremity; 1-4 muscle(s)**

EXCLUDES *Reporting more than one base code per session (64642)*

3.12 4.15 **FUD** 000 T P3

AMA: 2019,Aug,10; 2019,Apr,9; 2018,Jan,8; 2017,Jan,8; 2016,Jan,13; 2015,Jan,16

\+ 64643 **each additional extremity, 1-4 muscle(s) (List separately in addition to code for primary procedure)**

Code first (64642, 64644)

2.08 2.65 **FUD** ZZZ N N1

AMA: 2019,Aug,10; 2019,Apr,9; 2018,Jan,8; 2017,Jan,8; 2016,Jan,13; 2015,Jan,16

64644 **Chemodenervation of one extremity; 5 or more muscles**

EXCLUDES *Reporting more than one base code per session (64644)*

3.42 4.82 **FUD** 000 T P3

AMA: 2019,Aug,10; 2019,Apr,9; 2018,Jan,8; 2017,Jan,8; 2016,Jan,13; 2015,Jan,16

\+ 64645 **each additional extremity, 5 or more muscles (List separately in addition to code for primary procedure)**

Code first (64644)

2.40 3.33 **FUD** ZZZ N N1

AMA: 2019,Aug,10; 2019,Apr,9; 2018,Jan,8; 2017,Jan,8; 2016,Jan,13; 2015,Jan,16

64646-64647 Chemical Denervation Trunk Muscles

EXCLUDES *Procedure performed more than once per session*

64646 Chemodenervation of trunk muscle(s); 1-5 muscle(s)
3.34 4.35 **FUD** 000 T P3
AMA: 2019,Apr,9; 2018,Jan,8; 2017,Jan,8; 2016,Jan,13; 2015,Jan,16

64647 6 or more muscles
3.96 5.12 **FUD** 000 T P3
AMA: 2019,Apr,9; 2018,Jan,8; 2017,Jan,8; 2016,Jan,13; 2015,Jan,16

64650-64653 Chemical Denervation Eccrine Glands

INCLUDES Injection therapeutic medication
EXCLUDES *Bladder chemodenervation (52287)*
Chemodenervation extremities (64999)
Code also drugs or other substances used

64650 Chemodenervation of eccrine glands; both axillae
1.21 2.25 **FUD** 000 T P3 80
AMA: 2019,Apr,9; 2018,Jan,8; 2017,Jan,8; 2016,Jan,13; 2015,Jan,16

64653 other area(s) (eg, scalp, face, neck), per day
1.53 2.79 **FUD** 000 T P3 80
AMA: 2019,Apr,9; 2018,Jan,8; 2017,Jan,8; 2016,Jan,13; 2015,Jan,16

64680-64681 Neurolysis: Celiac Plexus, Superior Hypogastric Plexus

INCLUDES Injection therapeutic medication

64680 Destruction by neurolytic agent, with or without radiologic monitoring; celiac plexus
EXCLUDES *Transmural neurolytic agent injection with transendoscopic ultrasound guidance (43253)*
4.66 9.55 **FUD** 010 T A2
AMA: 2019,Apr,9; 2018,Jan,8; 2017,Jan,8; 2016,Jan,13; 2015,Jan,16

64681 superior hypogastric plexus
7.87 16.4 **FUD** 010 T A2
AMA: 2019,Apr,9; 2018,Jan,8; 2017,Jan,8; 2016,Jan,13; 2015,Jan,16

64702-64727 Decompression and/or Transposition of Nerve

INCLUDES External neurolysis and/or transposition to repair or restore nerve
Neuroplasty with nerve wrapping
Surgical decompression/freeing nerve from scar tissue
EXCLUDES *Facial nerve decompression (69720)*
Percutaneous neurolysis (62263-62264, 62280-62282)
Reporting with tissue expander insertion (11960)

64702 Neuroplasty; digital, 1 or both, same digit
14.4 14.4 **FUD** 090 J A2
AMA: 2018,Jan,8; 2017,Jan,8; 2016,Jan,13; 2015,Jan,16

64704 nerve of hand or foot
9.23 9.23 **FUD** 090 J A2 80
AMA: 2018,Jan,8; 2017,Jan,8; 2016,Jan,13; 2015,Jan,16

64708 Neuroplasty, major peripheral nerve, arm or leg, open; other than specified
14.4 14.4 **FUD** 090 J G2 80
AMA: 2018,Jan,8; 2017,Nov,10; 2017,Jan,8; 2016,Jan,13; 2015,Jan,16

64712 sciatic nerve
16.9 16.9 **FUD** 090 J G2 80 50
AMA: 2018,Jan,8; 2017,Jan,8; 2016,Jan,13; 2015,Jan,16

64713 brachial plexus
22.5 22.5 **FUD** 090 J G2 80 50
AMA: 2018,Jan,8; 2017,Jan,8; 2016,Jan,13; 2015,Jan,16

64714 lumbar plexus
21.1 21.1 **FUD** 090 J G2 80 50
AMA: 2018,Jan,8; 2017,Jan,8; 2016,Jan,13; 2015,Jan,16

64716 Neuroplasty and/or transposition; cranial nerve (specify)
15.0 15.0 **FUD** 090 J A2 80
AMA: 2018,Jan,8; 2017,Jan,8; 2016,Jan,13; 2015,Jan,16

64718 ulnar nerve at elbow
17.0 17.0 **FUD** 090 J A2 80 50
AMA: 2020,Jun,14; 2018,Jan,8; 2017,Jan,8; 2016,Jan,13; 2015,Jan,16

64719 ulnar nerve at wrist
11.5 11.5 **FUD** 090 J A2 50
AMA: 2018,Jan,8; 2017,Jan,8; 2016,Jan,13; 2015,Jan,16

64721 median nerve at carpal tunnel
EXCLUDES *Endoscopic procedure (29848)*
12.3 12.4 **FUD** 090 J A2 50
AMA: 2018,Jan,8; 2017,Jan,8; 2016,Jan,13; 2015,Jul,10; 2015,Jan,16

64722 Decompression; unspecified nerve(s) (specify)
10.3 10.3 **FUD** 090 J A2 80
AMA: 2018,Jan,8; 2017,Jan,8; 2016,Jan,13; 2015,Jan,16

64726 plantar digital nerve
7.80 7.80 **FUD** 090 J A2
AMA: 2018,Jan,8; 2017,Jan,8; 2016,Jan,13; 2015,Jan,16

\+ **64727 Internal neurolysis, requiring use of operating microscope (List separately in addition to code for neuroplasty) (Neuroplasty includes external neurolysis)**
INCLUDES Operating microscope (69990)
Code first neuroplasty (64702-64721)
5.31 5.31 **FUD** ZZZ N N1
AMA: 2018,Jan,8; 2017,Jan,8; 2016,Feb,12; 2016,Jan,13; 2015,Jan,16

64732-64772 Surgical Avulsion/Transection of Nerve

EXCLUDES *Stereotactic lesion gasserian ganglion (61790)*

64732 Transection or avulsion of; supraorbital nerve
12.7 12.7 **FUD** 090 J A2 80 50
AMA: 2018,Jan,8; 2017,Jan,8; 2016,Jan,13; 2015,Jan,16

64734 infraorbital nerve
14.5 14.5 **FUD** 090 J A2 80 50
AMA: 2014,Jan,11

64736 mental nerve
10.7 10.7 **FUD** 090 J A2 80 50
AMA: 2014,Jan,11

64738 inferior alveolar nerve by osteotomy
13.0 13.0 **FUD** 090 J A2 80 50
AMA: 2014,Jan,11

64740 lingual nerve
14.0 14.0 **FUD** 090 J A2 80 50
AMA: 2014,Jan,11

64742 facial nerve, differential or complete
14.0 14.0 **FUD** 090 J A2 80 50
AMA: 2014,Jan,11

64744 greater occipital nerve
14.2 14.2 **FUD** 090 J A2 80 50
AMA: 2014,Jan,11

64746 phrenic nerve
12.4 12.4 **FUD** 090 J A2 80 50
AMA: 2014,Jan,11

64755 vagus nerves limited to proximal stomach (selective proximal vagotomy, proximal gastric vagotomy, parietal cell vagotomy, supra- or highly selective vagotomy)
EXCLUDES *Laparoscopic procedure (43652)*
26.8 26.8 **FUD** 090 C 80
AMA: 2018,Jan,8; 2017,Jan,8; 2016,Jan,13; 2015,Jan,16

64760 vagus nerve (vagotomy), abdominal
EXCLUDES *Laparoscopic procedure (43651)*
14.7 14.7 **FUD** 090 C 80
AMA: 2018,Jan,8; 2017,Jan,8; 2016,Jan,13; 2015,Jan,16

64763 **Transection or avulsion of obturator nerve, extrapelvic, with or without adductor tenotomy**
14.8 14.8 FUD 090 J G2 80 50
AMA: 2014,Jan,11

64766 **Transection or avulsion of obturator nerve, intrapelvic, with or without adductor tenotomy**
18.2 18.2 FUD 090 J G2 80 50
AMA: 2014,Jan,11

64771 **Transection or avulsion of other cranial nerve, extradural**
17.5 17.5 FUD 090 J A2 80
AMA: 2014,Jan,11

64772 **Transection or avulsion of other spinal nerve, extradural**
EXCLUDES *Removal tender scar and soft tissue including neuroma when necessary (11400-11446, 13100-13153)*
16.2 16.2 FUD 090 J A2 80
AMA: 2018,Jan,8; 2017,Jan,8; 2016,Jan,13; 2015,Apr,10

64774-64823 Excisional Nerve Procedures

EXCLUDES *Morton neuroma excision (28080)*

64774 **Excision of neuroma; cutaneous nerve, surgically identifiable**
11.7 11.7 FUD 090 J A2
AMA: 2014,Jan,11

64776 **digital nerve, 1 or both, same digit**
11.1 11.1 FUD 090 J A2 80
AMA: 2014,Jan,11

+ **64778** **digital nerve, each additional digit (List separately in addition to code for primary procedure)**
Code first (64776)
5.30 5.30 FUD ZZZ N N1
AMA: 2014,Jan,11

64782 **hand or foot, except digital nerve**
13.2 13.2 FUD 090 J A2
AMA: 2014,Jan,11

+ **64783** **hand or foot, each additional nerve, except same digit (List separately in addition to code for primary procedure)**
Code first (64782)
6.33 6.33 FUD ZZZ N N1
AMA: 2014,Jan,11

64784 **major peripheral nerve, except sciatic**
20.9 20.9 FUD 090 J A2 80
AMA: 2014,Jan,11

64786 **sciatic nerve**
29.2 29.2 FUD 090 J A2 80 50
AMA: 2014,Jan,11

+ **64787** **Implantation of nerve end into bone or muscle (List separately in addition to neuroma excision)**
Code also, when appropriate (64774-64786)
6.96 6.96 FUD ZZZ N N1 80
AMA: 2014,Jan,11

64788 **Excision of neurofibroma or neurolemmoma; cutaneous nerve**
11.5 11.5 FUD 090 J A2
AMA: 2018,Jan,8; 2017,Jan,8; 2016,Apr,3

64790 **major peripheral nerve**
24.1 24.1 FUD 090 J A2 80
AMA: 2018,Jan,8; 2017,Jan,8; 2016,Apr,3

64792 **extensive (including malignant type)**
EXCLUDES *Destruction neurofibroma skin (0419T-0420T)*
31.4 31.4 FUD 090 J A2 80
AMA: 2018,Jan,8; 2017,Jan,8; 2016,Apr,3

64795 **Biopsy of nerve**
5.64 5.64 FUD 000 J A2
AMA: 2014,Jan,11

64802 **Sympathectomy, cervical**
24.3 24.3 FUD 090 J A2 80 50
AMA: 2014,Jan,11

64804 **Sympathectomy, cervicothoracic**
34.1 34.1 FUD 090 J 80 50
AMA: 2014,Jan,11

64809 **Sympathectomy, thoracolumbar**
INCLUDES Leriche sympathectomy
31.8 31.8 FUD 090 C 80 50
AMA: 2014,Jan,11

64818 **Sympathectomy, lumbar**
22.5 22.5 FUD 090 C 80 50
AMA: 2014,Jan,11

64820 **Sympathectomy; digital arteries, each digit**
INCLUDES Operating microscope (69990)
21.0 21.0 FUD 090 J G2
AMA: 2018,Jan,8; 2017,Jan,8; 2016,Feb,12; 2016,Jan,13; 2015,Jan,16

64821 **radial artery**
INCLUDES Operating microscope (69990)
20.0 20.0 FUD 090 J A2 50
AMA: 2016,Feb,12

64822 **ulnar artery**
INCLUDES Operating microscope (69990)
20.0 20.0 FUD 090 J G2 50
AMA: 2016,Feb,12

64823 **superficial palmar arch**
INCLUDES Operating microscope (69990)
22.7 22.7 FUD 090 J G2 50
AMA: 2016,Feb,12

64831-64907 Nerve Repair: Suture and Nerve Grafts

64831 **Suture of digital nerve, hand or foot; 1 nerve**
19.7 19.7 FUD 090 J A2 50
AMA: 2018,Jan,8; 2017,Jan,8; 2016,Jan,13; 2015,Jan,16

+ **64832** **each additional digital nerve (List separately in addition to code for primary procedure)**
Code first (64831)
9.73 9.73 FUD ZZZ N N1 80
AMA: 2018,Jan,8; 2017,Jan,8; 2016,Jan,13; 2015,Jan,16

64834 **Suture of 1 nerve; hand or foot, common sensory nerve**
21.3 21.3 FUD 090 J A2 80 50
AMA: 2014,Jan,11

64835 **median motor thenar**
23.4 23.4 FUD 090 J A2 80 50
AMA: 2014,Jan,11

64836 **ulnar motor**
23.5 23.5 FUD 090 J A2 80 50
AMA: 2014,Jan,11

+ **64837** **Suture of each additional nerve, hand or foot (List separately in addition to code for primary procedure)**
Code first (64834-64836)
10.6 10.6 FUD ZZZ N N1 80
AMA: 2014,Jan,11

64840 **Suture of posterior tibial nerve**
27.8 27.8 FUD 090 J A2 80 50
AMA: 2014,Jan,11

64856 **Suture of major peripheral nerve, arm or leg, except sciatic; including transposition**
29.2 29.2 FUD 090 J A2
AMA: 2014,Jan,11

64857 **without transposition**
30.4 30.4 FUD 090 J A2 80
AMA: 2014,Jan,11

64858 **Suture of sciatic nerve**
34.0 34.0 FUD 090 J A2 80 50
AMA: 2014,Jan,11

+ **64859** **Suture of each additional major peripheral nerve (List separately in addition to code for primary procedure)**
Code first (64856-64857)
7.19 7.19 FUD ZZZ N N1 80
AMA: 2014,Jan,11

64861 **Suture of; brachial plexus**
43.7 43.7 FUD 090 J A2 80 50
AMA: 2014,Jan,11

64862 **lumbar plexus**
39.3 39.3 FUD 090 J A2 80 50
AMA: 2014,Jan,11

64864 **Suture of facial nerve; extracranial**
24.9 24.9 FUD 090 J A2 80
AMA: 2014,Jan,11

64865 **infratemporal, with or without grafting**
31.4 31.4 FUD 090 J A2 80
AMA: 2014,Jan,11

64866 **Anastomosis; facial-spinal accessory**
36.7 36.7 FUD 090 C 80
AMA: 2014,Jan,11

64868 **facial-hypoglossal**
INCLUDES Korte-Ballance anastomosis
28.8 28.8 FUD 090 C 80
AMA: 2014,Jan,11

+ **64872** **Suture of nerve; requiring secondary or delayed suture (List separately in addition to code for primary neurorrhaphy)**
Code first (64831-64865)
3.39 3.39 FUD ZZZ N N1 80
AMA: 2014,Jan,11

+ **64874** **requiring extensive mobilization, or transposition of nerve (List separately in addition to code for nerve suture)**
Code first (64831-64865)
5.05 5.05 FUD ZZZ N N1 80
AMA: 2014,Jan,11

+ **64876** **requiring shortening of bone of extremity (List separately in addition to code for nerve suture)**
Code first (64831-64865)
5.71 5.71 FUD ZZZ N N1 80
AMA: 2014,Jan,11; 2003,Jan,1

64885 **Nerve graft (includes obtaining graft), head or neck; up to 4 cm in length**
32.1 32.1 FUD 090 J A2 80
AMA: 2018,Jan,8; 2017,Dec,12; 2017,Jan,8; 2016,Jan,13; 2015,Jan,16

64886 **more than 4 cm length**
37.2 37.2 FUD 090 J A2 80
AMA: 2018,Jan,8; 2017,Dec,12; 2017,Jan,8; 2016,Jan,13; 2015,Jan,16

64890 **Nerve graft (includes obtaining graft), single strand, hand or foot; up to 4 cm length**
31.2 31.2 FUD 090 J A2 80
AMA: 2018,Jan,8; 2017,Dec,12; 2017,Jan,8; 2016,Jan,13; 2015,Aug,8; 2015,Apr,10

64891 **more than 4 cm length**
33.2 33.2 FUD 090 J J8 80
AMA: 2018,Jan,8; 2017,Dec,12

64892 **Nerve graft (includes obtaining graft), single strand, arm or leg; up to 4 cm length**
30.1 30.1 FUD 090 J A2 80
AMA: 2018,Jan,8; 2017,Dec,12

64893 **more than 4 cm length**
32.4 32.4 FUD 090 J G2 80
AMA: 2018,Jan,8; 2017,Dec,12

64895 **Nerve graft (includes obtaining graft), multiple strands (cable), hand or foot; up to 4 cm length**
38.2 38.2 FUD 090 J A2 80
AMA: 2018,Jan,8; 2017,Dec,12; 2017,Jan,8; 2016,Jan,13; 2015,Jan,16

64896 **more than 4 cm length**
41.4 41.4 FUD 090 J A2 80
AMA: 2018,Jan,8; 2017,Dec,12; 2017,Jan,8; 2016,Jan,13; 2015,Jan,16

64897 **Nerve graft (includes obtaining graft), multiple strands (cable), arm or leg; up to 4 cm length**
36.4 36.4 FUD 090 J G2 80
AMA: 2018,Jan,8; 2017,Dec,12; 2017,Jan,8; 2016,Jan,13; 2015,Jan,16

64898 **more than 4 cm length**
39.6 39.6 FUD 090 J A2 80
AMA: 2018,Jan,8; 2017,Dec,12; 2017,Jan,8; 2016,Jan,13; 2015,Jan,16

+ **64901** **Nerve graft, each additional nerve; single strand (List separately in addition to code for primary procedure)**
Code first (64885-64893)
17.4 17.4 FUD ZZZ N N1 80
AMA: 2018,Jan,8; 2017,Dec,12; 2017,Jan,8; 2016,Jan,13; 2015,Jan,16

+ **64902** **multiple strands (cable) (List separately in addition to code for primary procedure)**
Code first (64885-64886, 64895-64898)
20.1 20.1 FUD ZZZ N N1 80
AMA: 2018,Jan,8; 2017,Dec,12; 2017,Jan,8; 2016,Jan,13; 2015,Jan,16

64905 **Nerve pedicle transfer; first stage**
29.4 29.4 FUD 090 J A2 80
AMA: 2018,Jan,8; 2017,Dec,12

64907 **second stage**
37.7 37.7 FUD 090 J A2 80
AMA: 2018,Jan,8; 2017,Dec,12

64910-64999 Nerve Repair: Synthetic and Vein Grafts

64910 Nerve repair; with synthetic conduit or vein allograft (eg, nerve tube), each nerve

INCLUDES Operating microscope (69990)

22.7 22.7 FUD 090 J J8 80

AMA: 2018,Jan,8; 2017,Dec,12; 2017,Jan,8; 2016,Jan,13; 2015,Aug,8; 2015,Apr,10; 2015,Jan,16

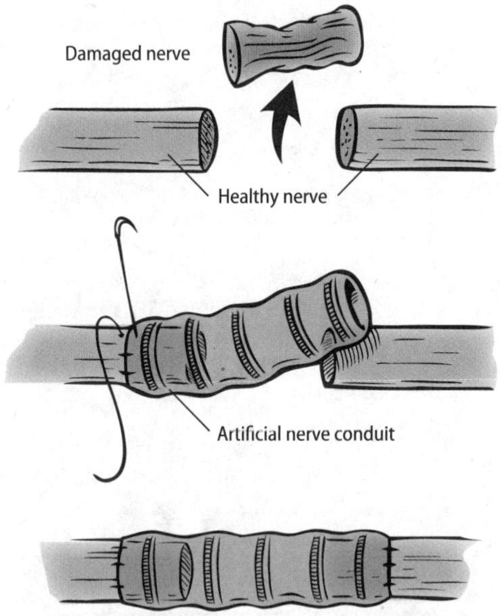

A synthetic "bridge" is affixed to each end of a severed nerve with sutures
The procedure is performed using an operating microscope

64911 with autogenous vein graft (includes harvest of vein graft), each nerve

INCLUDES Operating microscope (69990)

29.5 29.5 FUD 090 J 80

AMA: 2018,Jan,8; 2017,Dec,12; 2017,Jan,8; 2016,Jan,13; 2015,Jan,16

64912 with nerve allograft, each nerve, first strand (cable)

INCLUDES Operating microscope (69990)

26.3 26.3 FUD 090 J J8 80

AMA: 2018,Jan,8; 2017,Dec,12

\+ **64913 with nerve allograft, each additional strand (List separately in addition to code for primary procedure)**

INCLUDES Operating microscope (69990)

Code first (64912)

5.16 5.16 FUD ZZZ N N1 80

AMA: 2018,Jan,8; 2017,Dec,12

64999 Unlisted procedure, nervous system

0.00 0.00 FUD YYY T 80

AMA: 2020,Jun,14; 2020,Feb,13; 2019,Dec,12; 2019,Jul,10; 2019,May,10; 2019,Apr,9; 2018,Dec,8; 2018,Dec,8; 2018,Oct,11; 2018,Oct,8; 2018,Aug,10; 2018,Mar,9; 2018,Jan,8; 2018,Jan,7; 2017,Dec,12; 2017,Dec,13; 2017,Dec,14; 2017,Jan,8; 2016,Nov,6; 2016,Oct,11; 2016,Feb,13; 2016,Jan,13; 2015,Oct,9; 2015,Aug,8; 2015,Jul,10; 2015,Apr,10; 2015,Feb,9; 2015,Jan,16

65091-65093 Surgical Removal of Eyeball Contents

INCLUDES Operating microscope (69990)

65091 Evisceration of ocular contents; without implant
18.4 18.4 **FUD** 090 J A2 80 50
AMA: 2016,Feb,12

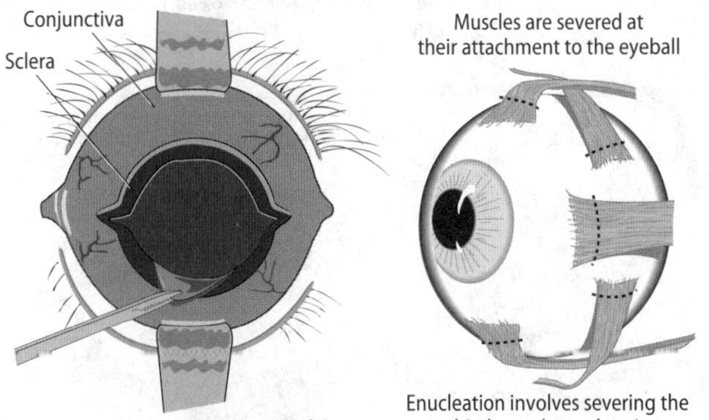

Evisceration involves removal of the contents of the eyeball: the vitreous; retina; choroid; lens; iris; and ciliary muscle. Only the scleral shell remains. A temporary or permanent implant is usually inserted

Enucleation involves severing the extraorbital muscles and optic nerve with removal of the eyeball. An implant is usually inserted and, if permanent, may involve attachment to the severed extraorbital muscles

65093 with implant
18.2 18.2 **FUD** 090 J A2 50
AMA: 2016,Feb,12

65101-65105 Surgical Removal of Eyeball

INCLUDES Operating microscope (69990)
EXCLUDES *Conjunctivoplasty following enucleation (68320-68328)*

65101 Enucleation of eye; without implant
21.3 21.3 **FUD** 090 J A2 50
AMA: 2016,Feb,12

65103 with implant, muscles not attached to implant
22.2 22.2 **FUD** 090 J A2 50
AMA: 2016,Feb,12

65105 with implant, muscles attached to implant
24.4 24.4 **FUD** 090 J A2 80 50
AMA: 2016,Feb,12

65110-65114 Surgical Removal of Orbital Contents

INCLUDES Operating microscope (69990)
EXCLUDES *Free full thickness graft (15260-15261)*
Repair more extensive than skin (67930-67975)
Skin graft (15120-15121)

65110 Exenteration of orbit (does not include skin graft), removal of orbital contents; only
36.0 36.0 **FUD** 090 J A2 80 50
AMA: 2016,Feb,12

65112 with therapeutic removal of bone
40.5 40.5 **FUD** 090 J A2 80 50
AMA: 2016,Feb,12

65114 with muscle or myocutaneous flap
43.4 43.4 **FUD** 090 J A2 80 50
AMA: 2016,Feb,12

65125-65175 Implant Procedures: Insertion, Removal, and Revision

INCLUDES Ocular implant procedures (inside muscle cone)
Operating microscope (69990)
EXCLUDES *Orbital implant insertion (outside muscle cone) (67550)*
Orbital implant removal or revision (outside muscle cone) (67560)

65125 Modification of ocular implant with placement or replacement of pegs (eg, drilling receptacle for prosthesis appendage) (separate procedure)
8.26 12.9 **FUD** 090 J G2 50
AMA: 2016,Feb,12

65130 Insertion of ocular implant secondary; after evisceration, in scleral shell
21.1 21.1 **FUD** 090 J A2 50
AMA: 2016,Feb,12

65135 after enucleation, muscles not attached to implant
22.6 22.6 **FUD** 090 J A2 50
AMA: 2016,Feb,12

65140 after enucleation, muscles attached to implant
23.3 23.3 **FUD** 090 J A2 50
AMA: 2016,Feb,12

65150 Reinsertion of ocular implant; with or without conjunctival graft
18.0 18.0 **FUD** 090 J A2 80 50
AMA: 2016,Feb,12

65155 with use of foreign material for reinforcement and/or attachment of muscles to implant
24.4 24.4 **FUD** 090 J A2 50
AMA: 2016,Feb,12

65175 Removal of ocular implant
19.0 19.0 **FUD** 090 J A2 50
AMA: 2016,Feb,12

65205-65265 Foreign Body Removal By Area of Eye

INCLUDES Operating microscope (69990)
EXCLUDES *Removal foreign body:*
Eyelid (67938)
Lacrimal system (68530)
Orbit:
Frontal approach (67413)
Lateral approach (67430)
Removal implant:
Anterior segment (65920)
Ocular (65175)
Orbital (67560)
Posterior segment (67120)

65205 Removal of foreign body, external eye; conjunctival superficial
(70030, 76529)
1.02 1.31 **FUD** 000 Q1 N1 50
AMA: 2018,Jan,8; 2017,Jan,8; 2016,Feb,12; 2016,Jan,13; 2015,Jan,16

65210 conjunctival embedded (includes concretions), subconjunctival, or scleral nonperforating
(70030, 76529)
1.04 1.30 **FUD** 000 Q1 N1 50
AMA: 2016,Feb,12

65220 corneal, without slit lamp
EXCLUDES *Repair corneal wound with foreign body (65275)*
(70030, 76529)
1.19 1.68 **FUD** 000 Q1 N1 50
AMA: 2018,Jan,8; 2017,Jan,8; 2016,Feb,12; 2016,Jan,13; 2015,Jan,16

65222 corneal, with slit lamp
EXCLUDES *Repair corneal wound with foreign body (65275)*
(70030, 76529)
1.48 1.93 **FUD** 000 Q1 N1 50
AMA: 2018,Jan,8; 2017,Jan,8; 2016,Feb,12; 2016,Jan,13; 2015,Jan,16

65235 Removal of foreign body, intraocular; from anterior chamber of eye or lens
EXCLUDES *Removal implanted material from anterior segment (65920)*
(70030, 76529)
20.2 20.2 **FUD** 090 J A2 80 50
AMA: 2018,Jan,8; 2017,Jan,8; 2016,Feb,12; 2016,Jan,13; 2015,Jan,16

65260 **from posterior segment, magnetic extraction, anterior or posterior route**

EXCLUDES *Removal implanted material from posterior segment (67120)*

(70030, 76529)

27.4 27.4 FUD 090 J A2 80 50

AMA: 2016,Feb,12

65265 **from posterior segment, nonmagnetic extraction**

EXCLUDES *Removal implanted material from posterior segment (67120)*

(70030, 76529)

30.9 30.9 FUD 090 J A2 80 50

AMA: 2016,Feb,12

65270-65290 Laceration Repair External Eye

INCLUDES Conjunctival flap
Operating microscope (69990)
Restoration anterior chamber with air or saline injection

EXCLUDES *Repair:*
Ciliary body or iris (66680)
Eyelid laceration (12011-12018, 12051-12057, 13151-13160, 67930, 67935)
Lacrimal system injury (68700)
Surgical wound (66250)
Treatment orbit fracture (21385-21408)

65270 **Repair of laceration; conjunctiva, with or without nonperforating laceration sclera, direct closure**

4.01 7.79 FUD 010 J A2 80 50

AMA: 2018,Jan,8; 2017,Jan,8; 2016,Feb,12; 2016,Jan,13; 2015,Jan,16

65272 **conjunctiva, by mobilization and rearrangement, without hospitalization**

10.0 14.5 FUD 090 J A2 50

AMA: 2016,Feb,12

65273 **conjunctiva, by mobilization and rearrangement, with hospitalization**

10.8 10.8 FUD 090 C 50

AMA: 2016,Feb,12

65275 **cornea, nonperforating, with or without removal foreign body**

13.1 16.5 FUD 090 J A2 80 50

AMA: 2016,Feb,12

65280 **cornea and/or sclera, perforating, not involving uveal tissue**

EXCLUDES *Procedure performed for surgical wound repair*

19.1 19.1 FUD 090 J A2 80 50

AMA: 2018,Jan,8; 2017,Jan,8; 2016,Feb,12; 2016,Jan,13; 2015,Jan,16

65285 **cornea and/or sclera, perforating, with reposition or resection of uveal tissue**

EXCLUDES *Procedure performed for surgical wound repair*

31.4 31.4 FUD 090 J A2 50

AMA: 2018,Jan,8; 2017,Jan,8; 2016,Feb,12; 2016,Jan,13; 2015,Jan,16

65286 **application of tissue glue, wounds of cornea and/or sclera**

14.1 20.0 FUD 090 J P3 50

AMA: 2018,Jan,8; 2017,Jan,8; 2016,Feb,12; 2016,Jan,13; 2015,Jan,16

65290 **Repair of wound, extraocular muscle, tendon and/or Tenon's capsule**

13.9 13.9 FUD 090 J A2 50

AMA: 2016,Feb,12

65400-65600 Removal Corneal Lesions

INCLUDES Operating microscope (69990)

65400 **Excision of lesion, cornea (keratectomy, lamellar, partial), except pterygium**

17.1 19.4 FUD 090 T A2 50

AMA: 2018,Jan,8; 2017,Jan,8; 2016,Feb,12; 2016,Jan,13; 2015,Jan,16

65410 **Biopsy of cornea**

2.96 4.11 FUD 000 J A2 80 50

AMA: 2018,Jan,8; 2017,Jan,8; 2016,Feb,12; 2016,Jan,13; 2015,Jan,16

65420 **Excision or transposition of pterygium; without graft**

10.7 14.9 FUD 090 J A2 50

AMA: 2018,Jan,8; 2017,Jan,8; 2016,Feb,12; 2016,Jan,13; 2015,Jan,16

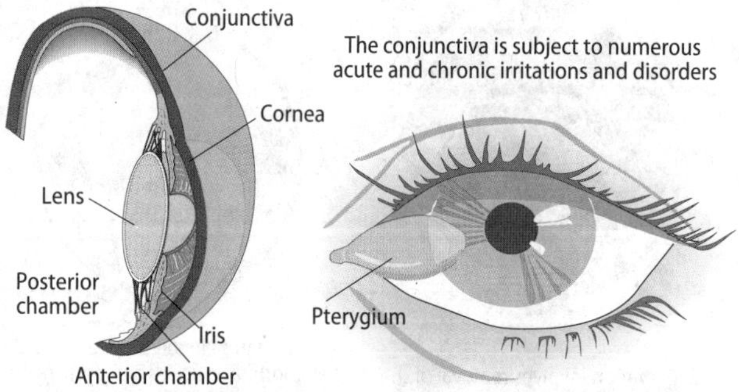

The conjunctiva is subject to numerous acute and chronic irritations and disorders

65426 **with graft**

13.6 18.7 FUD 090 J A2 50

AMA: 2018,May,10; 2018,Jan,8; 2017,Jan,8; 2016,Feb,12; 2016,Jan,13; 2015,Jan,16

65430 **Scraping of cornea, diagnostic, for smear and/or culture**

2.90 3.28 FUD 000 Q1 N1 50

AMA: 2016,Feb,12

65435 **Removal of corneal epithelium; with or without chemocauterization (abrasion, curettage)**

EXCLUDES *Collagen cross-linking, cornea (0402T)*

1.98 2.32 FUD 000 T P3 50

AMA: 2018,Jan,8; 2017,Jan,8; 2016,Feb,12; 2016,Jan,13; 2015,Jan,16

65436 **with application of chelating agent (eg, EDTA)**

10.4 10.9 FUD 090 J P3 50

AMA: 2016,Feb,12

65450 **Destruction of lesion of cornea by cryotherapy, photocoagulation or thermocauterization**

9.15 9.30 FUD 090 T G2 50

AMA: 2016,Feb,12

65600 **Multiple punctures of anterior cornea (eg, for corneal erosion, tattoo)**

9.74 11.3 FUD 090 J P3 50

AMA: 2016,Feb,12

65710-65757 Corneal Transplants

CMS: 100-03,80.7 Refractive Keratoplasty

INCLUDES Operating microscope (69990)

EXCLUDES *Computerized corneal topography (92025)*
Processing, preserving, and transporting corneal tissue (V2785)

65710 **Keratoplasty (corneal transplant); anterior lamellar**

INCLUDES Use and preparation fresh or preserved graft

EXCLUDES *Refractive keratoplasty surgery (65760-65767)*

31.7 31.7 FUD 090 J A2 80 50

AMA: 2018,Jan,8; 2017,Jan,8; 2016,Feb,12; 2016,Jan,13; 2015,Jan,16

65730 **penetrating (except in aphakia or pseudophakia)**

INCLUDES Use and preparation fresh or preserved graft

EXCLUDES *Refractive keratoplasty surgery (65760-65767)*

35.1 35.1 FUD 090 J A2 80 50

AMA: 2018,Jan,8; 2017,Jan,8; 2016,Feb,12; 2016,Jan,13; 2015,Jan,16

65750 **penetrating (in aphakia)**
INCLUDES Use and preparation fresh or preserved graft
EXCLUDES *Refractive keratoplasty surgery (65760-65767)*
35.4 35.4 FUD 090 J A2 80 50
AMA: 2018,Jan,8; 2017,Jan,8; 2016,Feb,12; 2016,Jan,13; 2015,Jan,16

65755 **penetrating (in pseudophakia)**
INCLUDES Use and preparation fresh or preserved graft
EXCLUDES *Refractive keratoplasty surgery (65760-65767)*
35.1 35.1 FUD 090 J A2 80 50
AMA: 2018,Jan,8; 2017,Jan,8; 2016,Feb,12; 2016,Jan,13; 2015,Jan,16

65756 **endothelial**
EXCLUDES *Refractive keratoplasty surgery (65760-65767)*
Code also donor material
Code also when appropriate (65757)
33.6 33.6 FUD 090 J G2 80 50
AMA: 2018,Jan,8; 2017,Jan,8; 2016,Feb,12; 2016,Jan,13; 2015,Jan,16

+ **65757** **Backbench preparation of corneal endothelial allograft prior to transplantation (List separately in addition to code for primary procedure)**
Code first (65756)
0.00 0.00 FUD ZZZ N N1 80
AMA: 2018,Jan,8; 2017,Jan,8; 2016,Feb,12; 2016,Jan,13; 2015,Jan,16

65760-65785 Corneal Refractive Procedures

CMS: 100-03,80.7 Refractive Keratoplasty
INCLUDES Operating microscope (69990)
EXCLUDES *Unlisted corneal procedures (66999)*

65760 **Keratomileusis**
EXCLUDES *Computerized corneal topography (92025)*
0.00 0.00 FUD XXX E
AMA: 2016,Feb,12

65765 **Keratophakia**
EXCLUDES *Computerized corneal topography (92025)*
0.00 0.00 FUD XXX E
AMA: 2016,Feb,12

65767 **Epikeratoplasty**
EXCLUDES *Computerized corneal topography (92025)*
0.00 0.00 FUD XXX E
AMA: 2016,Feb,12

65770 **Keratoprosthesis**
EXCLUDES *Computerized corneal topography (92025)*
39.6 39.6 FUD 090 J J8 80 50
AMA: 2016,Feb,12

65771 **Radial keratotomy**
EXCLUDES *Computerized corneal topography (92025)*
0.00 0.00 FUD XXX E
AMA: 2016,Feb,12

65772 **Corneal relaxing incision for correction of surgically induced astigmatism**
11.5 12.8 FUD 090 T A2 50
AMA: 2016,Feb,12

65775 **Corneal wedge resection for correction of surgically induced astigmatism**
EXCLUDES *Fitting contact lens to treat disease (92071-92072)*
15.8 15.8 FUD 090 J A2 50
AMA: 2018,Jan,8; 2017,Jan,8; 2016,Feb,12; 2016,Jan,13; 2015,Jan,16

65778 **Placement of amniotic membrane on the ocular surface; without sutures**
EXCLUDES *Ocular surface reconstruction (65780)*
Removal corneal epithelium (65435)
Scraping cornea, diagnostic (65430)
Using tissue glue to place amniotic membrane (66999)
1.58 40.0 FUD 000 02 N1 80 50
AMA: 2018,Feb,11; 2018,Jan,8; 2017,Jan,8; 2016,Feb,12; 2016,Jan,13; 2015,Jan,16

65779 **single layer, sutured**
EXCLUDES *Ocular surface reconstruction (65780)*
Removal corneal epithelium (65435)
Scraping cornea, diagnostic (65430)
Using tissue glue to place amniotic membrane (66999)
4.32 34.5 FUD 000 02 N1 80 50
AMA: 2018,Feb,11; 2018,Jan,8; 2017,Jan,8; 2016,Feb,12; 2016,Jan,13; 2015,Jan,16

65780 **Ocular surface reconstruction; amniotic membrane transplantation, multiple layers**
EXCLUDES *Placement amniotic membrane without reconstruction without sutures or single layer sutures (65778-65779)*
18.9 18.9 FUD 090 J A2 50
AMA: 2018,Feb,11; 2018,Jan,8; 2017,Jan,8; 2016,Feb,12; 2016,Jan,13; 2015,Jan,16

65781 **limbal stem cell allograft (eg, cadaveric or living donor)**
37.9 37.9 FUD 090 J A2 80 50
AMA: 2018,Jan,8; 2017,Jan,8; 2016,Feb,12; 2016,Jan,13; 2015,Jan,16

65782 **limbal conjunctival autograft (includes obtaining graft)**
EXCLUDES *Conjunctival allograft harvest from living donor (68371)*
32.6 32.6 FUD 090 J A2 50
AMA: 2018,Jan,8; 2017,Jan,8; 2016,Feb,12; 2016,Jan,13; 2015,Jan,16

65785 **Implantation of intrastromal corneal ring segments**
12.6 71.4 FUD 090 J P2 50
AMA: 2016,Feb,12

65800-66030 Anterior Segment Procedures

INCLUDES Operating microscope (69990)
EXCLUDES *Unlisted procedures anterior segment (66999)*

65800 **Paracentesis of anterior chamber of eye (separate procedure); with removal of aqueous**
EXCLUDES *Insertion ocular telescope prosthesis (0308T)*
2.58 3.39 FUD 000 J A2 50
AMA: 2018,Jan,8; 2017,Jan,8; 2016,Feb,12; 2016,Jan,13; 2015,Jan,16

65810 **with removal of vitreous and/or discission of anterior hyaloid membrane, with or without air injection**
EXCLUDES *Insertion ocular telescope prosthesis (0308T)*
13.2 13.2 FUD 090 J A2 50
AMA: 2018,Jan,8; 2017,Jan,8; 2016,Feb,12; 2016,Jan,13; 2015,Jan,16

65815 **with removal of blood, with or without irrigation and/or air injection**
EXCLUDES *Injection only (66020-66030)*
Insertion ocular telescope prosthesis (0308T)
Removal blood clot only (65930)
13.5 18.2 FUD 090 J A2 50
AMA: 2018,Jan,8; 2017,Jan,8; 2016,Feb,12; 2016,Jan,13; 2015,Jan,16

65820 **Goniotomy**
INCLUDES Barkan's operation
Code also ophthalmic endoscope if used (66990)
21.5 21.5 FUD 090 63 J A2 80 50
AMA: 2019,Sep,10; 2018,Dec,8; 2018,Dec,8; 2018,Jul,3; 2018,Jan,8; 2017,Jan,8; 2016,Feb,12; 2016,Jan,13; 2015,Jan,16

65850 Trabeculotomy ab externo
23.8 | 23.8 | FUD 090 | J A2 50
AMA: 2016,Feb,12

65855 Trabeculoplasty by laser surgery
EXCLUDES *Severing adhesions anterior segment (65860-65880)*
Trabeculectomy ab externo (66170)
5.87 | 6.99 | FUD 010 | T P3 50
AMA: 2018,Jan,8; 2017,Jan,8; 2016,Feb,12; 2016,Jan,13; 2015,Jan,16

65860 Severing adhesions of anterior segment, laser technique (separate procedure)
7.18 | 8.81 | FUD 090 | T P3 80 50
AMA: 2016,Feb,12

65865 Severing adhesions of anterior segment of eye, incisional technique (with or without injection of air or liquid) (separate procedure); goniosynechiae
EXCLUDES *Laser trabeculectomy (65855)*
13.4 | 13.4 | FUD 090 | J A2 50
AMA: 2016,Feb,12

65870 anterior synechiae, except goniosynechiae
16.7 | 16.7 | FUD 090 | J A2 50
AMA: 2016,Feb,12

65875 posterior synechiae
Code also ophthalmic endoscope when used (66990)
17.9 | 17.9 | FUD 090 | J A2 50
AMA: 2018,Jan,8; 2017,Jan,8; 2016,Feb,12; 2016,Jan,13; 2015,Jan,16

65880 corneovitreal adhesions
EXCLUDES *Laser procedure (66821)*
18.8 | 18.8 | FUD 090 | J A2 50
AMA: 2016,Feb,12

65900 Removal of epithelial downgrowth, anterior chamber of eye
27.6 | 27.6 | FUD 090 | J A2 80 50
AMA: 2016,Feb,12

65920 Removal of implanted material, anterior segment of eye
Code also ophthalmic endoscope when used (66990)
22.3 | 22.3 | FUD 090 | J A2 50
AMA: 2018,Jan,8; 2017,Jan,8; 2016,Feb,12; 2016,Jan,13; 2015,Jan,16

65930 Removal of blood clot, anterior segment of eye
18.1 | 18.1 | FUD 090 | J A2 50
AMA: 2016,Feb,12

66020 Injection, anterior chamber of eye (separate procedure); air or liquid
EXCLUDES *Insertion ocular telescope prosthesis (0308T)*
3.74 | 5.43 | FUD 010 | J A2 50
AMA: 2018,Jan,8; 2017,Jan,8; 2016,Feb,12; 2016,Jan,13; 2015,Jan,16

66030 medication
EXCLUDES *Insertion ocular telescope prosthesis (0308T)*
3.16 | 4.87 | FUD 010 | J A2 50
AMA: 2016,Feb,12

66130 Excision Scleral Lesion

INCLUDES Operating microscope (69990)
EXCLUDES *Removal intraocular foreign body (65235)*
Surgery on posterior sclera (67250, 67255)

66130 Excision of lesion, sclera
16.1 | 19.9 | FUD 090 | J A2 80 50
AMA: 2016,Feb,12

66150-66185 Procedures for Glaucoma

INCLUDES Operating microscope (69990)
EXCLUDES *Removal intraocular foreign body (65235)*
Surgery on posterior sclera (67250, 67255)

66150 Fistulization of sclera for glaucoma; trephination with iridectomy
24.9 | 24.9 | FUD 090 | J A2 50
AMA: 2018,Jul,3; 2016,Feb,12

66155 thermocauterization with iridectomy
24.8 | 24.8 | FUD 090 | J A2 50
AMA: 2018,Jul,3; 2016,Feb,12

66160 sclerectomy with punch or scissors, with iridectomy
INCLUDES Knapp's operation
28.1 | 28.1 | FUD 090 | J A2 50
AMA: 2018,Jul,3; 2016,Feb,12

66170 trabeculectomy ab externo in absence of previous surgery
EXCLUDES *Repair surgical wound (66250)*
Trabeculectomy ab externo (65850)
30.9 | 30.9 | FUD 090 | J A2 80 50
AMA: 2018,Dec,8; 2018,Dec,10; 2018,Dec,8; 2018,Dec,10; 2018,Jul,3; 2018,Jan,8; 2017,Jan,8; 2016,Feb,12; 2016,Jan,13; 2015,Jan,16

66172 trabeculectomy ab externo with scarring from previous ocular surgery or trauma (includes injection of antifibrotic agents)
33.9 | 33.9 | FUD 090 | J A2 80 50
AMA: 2019,Apr,7; 2018,Dec,10; 2018,Dec,10; 2018,Jul,3; 2018,Jan,8; 2017,Jan,8; 2016,Feb,12; 2016,Jan,13; 2015,Jan,16

66174 Transluminal dilation of aqueous outflow canal; without retention of device or stent
26.9 | 26.9 | FUD 090 | J A2 80 50
AMA: 2019,Sep,10; 2018,Dec,8; 2018,Dec,8; 2016,Feb,12

66175 with retention of device or stent
28.2 | 28.2 | FUD 090 | J A2 80 50
AMA: 2016,Feb,12

66179 Aqueous shunt to extraocular equatorial plate reservoir, external approach; without graft
30.6 | 30.6 | FUD 090 | J G2 80 50
AMA: 2018,Jul,3; 2018,Jan,8; 2017,Jan,8; 2016,Feb,12; 2016,Jan,13; 2015,Jan,10

66180 with graft
EXCLUDES *Scleral reinforcement (67255)*
32.3 | 32.3 | FUD 090 | J J8 80 50
AMA: 2018,Jul,3; 2018,Jan,8; 2017,Jan,8; 2016,Feb,12; 2016,Jan,13; 2015,Jan,16; 2015,Jan,10

66183 Insertion of anterior segment aqueous drainage device, without extraocular reservoir, external approach
29.2 | 29.2 | FUD 090 | J J8 80 50
AMA: 2020,Jun,14; 2018,Jul,3; 2018,Jan,8; 2017,Jan,8; 2016,Feb,12; 2016,Jan,13; 2015,Jan,16

66184 Revision of aqueous shunt to extraocular equatorial plate reservoir; without graft
22.3 | 22.3 | FUD 090 | J G2 80 50
AMA: 2018,Jan,8; 2017,Jan,8; 2016,Feb,12; 2016,Jan,13; 2015,Jan,10

66185 with graft
EXCLUDES *Removal implanted shunt (67120)*
Scleral reinforcement (67255)
23.9 | 23.9 | FUD 090 | J A2 80 50
AMA: 2018,Jan,8; 2017,Jan,8; 2016,Feb,12; 2016,Jan,13; 2015,Jan,10

66225 Staphyloma Repair

INCLUDES Operating microscope (69990)

EXCLUDES *Scleral procedures with retinal procedures (67101-67228)*
Scleral reinforcement (67250, 67255)

66225 Repair of scleral staphyloma; with graft
26.5 26.5 **FUD** 090 J A2 50
AMA: 2016,Feb,12

66250 Anterior Segment Operative Wound Revision or Repair

INCLUDES Operating microscope (69990)

EXCLUDES *Unlisted procedures anterior sclera (66999)*

66250 Revision or repair of operative wound of anterior segment, any type, early or late, major or minor procedure
15.8 21.4 **FUD** 090 J A2 50
AMA: 2018,Dec,8; 2018,Dec,8; 2018,Jan,8; 2017,Jan,8; 2016,Feb,12; 2016,Jan,13; 2015,Jan,16

66500-66505 Iridotomy With/Without Transfixion

INCLUDES Operating microscope (69990)

EXCLUDES *Photocoagulation iridotomy (66761)*

66500 Iridotomy by stab incision (separate procedure); except transfixion
10.5 10.5 **FUD** 090 J A2 50
AMA: 2016,Feb,12

66505 with transfixion as for iris bombe
11.5 11.5 **FUD** 090 J A2 50
AMA: 2016,Feb,12

66600-66635 Iridectomy Procedures

INCLUDES Operating microscope (69990)

EXCLUDES *Insertion ocular telescope prosthesis (0308T)*
Photocoagulation coreoplasty (66762)

66600 Iridectomy, with corneoscleral or corneal section; for removal of lesion
23.9 23.9 **FUD** 090 J A2 50
AMA: 2016,Feb,12

66605 with cyclectomy
30.3 30.3 **FUD** 090 J A2 50
AMA: 2016,Feb,12

66625 peripheral for glaucoma (separate procedure)
12.2 12.2 **FUD** 090 J A2 50
AMA: 2016,Feb,12

66630 sector for glaucoma (separate procedure)
16.1 16.1 **FUD** 090 J A2 50
AMA: 2016,Feb,12

66635 optical (separate procedure)
16.2 16.2 **FUD** 090 J A2 50
AMA: 2016,Feb,12

66680-66770 Other Procedures of the Uveal Tract

INCLUDES Operating microscope (69990)

EXCLUDES *Unlisted procedures ciliary body or iris (66999)*

66680 Repair of iris, ciliary body (as for iridodialysis)
EXCLUDES *Resection/repositioning uveal tissue for perforating laceration, cornea and/or sclera (65285)*
14.7 14.7 **FUD** 090 J A2 50
AMA: 2016,Feb,12

66682 Suture of iris, ciliary body (separate procedure) with retrieval of suture through small incision (eg, McCannel suture)
19.0 19.0 **FUD** 090 J A2 50
AMA: 2016,Feb,12

66700 Ciliary body destruction; diathermy
INCLUDES Heine's operation
11.1 12.8 **FUD** 090 J A2 80 50
AMA: 2016,Feb,12

66710 cyclophotocoagulation, transscleral
11.0 12.5 **FUD** 090 J A2 50
AMA: 2018,Jan,8; 2017,Jan,8; 2016,Feb,12; 2016,Jan,13; 2015,Jan,16

66711 cyclophotocoagulation, endoscopic, without concomitant removal of crystalline lens
EXCLUDES *Endoscopic cyclophotocoagulation performed in conjunction with extracapsular cataract removal with insertion lens ([66987], [66988])*
18.2 18.2 **FUD** 090 J A2 50
AMA: 2019,Dec,6; 2018,Jan,8; 2017,Jan,8; 2016,Feb,12; 2016,Jan,13; 2015,Jan,16

66720 cryotherapy
11.6 13.1 **FUD** 090 J A2 50
AMA: 2016,Feb,12

66740 cyclodialysis
11.1 12.5 **FUD** 090 J A2 50
AMA: 2016,Feb,12

66761 Iridotomy/iridectomy by laser surgery (eg, for glaucoma) (per session)
EXCLUDES *Insertion ocular telescope prosthesis (0308T)*
6.71 8.50 **FUD** 010 T P3 50
AMA: 2018,Jan,8; 2017,Jan,8; 2016,Feb,12; 2016,Jan,13; 2015,Jan,16

66762 Iridoplasty by photocoagulation (1 or more sessions) (eg, for improvement of vision, for widening of anterior chamber angle)
12.0 13.5 **FUD** 090 T P2 50
AMA: 2018,Jan,8; 2017,Jan,8; 2016,Feb,12; 2016,Jan,13; 2015,Jan,16

66770 Destruction of cyst or lesion iris or ciliary body (nonexcisional procedure)
EXCLUDES *Excision:*
Epithelial downgrowth (65900)
Iris, ciliary body lesion (66600-66605)
13.6 15.0 **FUD** 090 T P2 50
AMA: 2016,Feb,12

66820-66825 Post-Cataract Surgery Procedures

INCLUDES Operating microscope (69990)

66820 Discission of secondary membranous cataract (opacified posterior lens capsule and/or anterior hyaloid); stab incision technique (Ziegler or Wheeler knife)
12.1 12.1 **FUD** 090 J G2 50
AMA: 2016,Feb,12

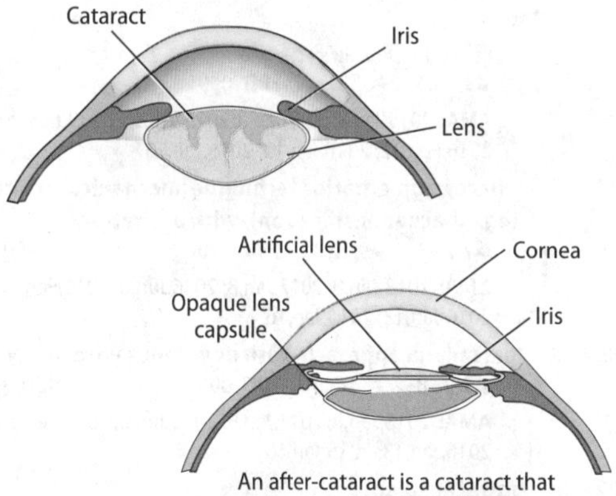

An after-cataract is a cataract that develops in a lens tissue that remains after most of the lens has already been removed

66821 laser surgery (eg, YAG laser) (1 or more stages)
8.81 9.40 **FUD** 090 T A2 50
AMA: 2016,Feb,12

66825 **Repositioning of intraocular lens prosthesis, requiring an incision (separate procedure)**

EXCLUDES *Insertion ocular telescope prosthesis (0308T)*

21.8 21.8 **FUD** 090 J A2 80 50

AMA: 2016,Feb,12

66830-66940 Cataract Extraction; Without Insertion Intraocular Lens

CMS: 100-03,80.10 Phacoemulsification Procedure--Cataract Extraction

INCLUDES Anterior and/or posterior capsulotomy
Enzymatic zonulysis
Iridectomy/iridotomy
Lateral canthotomy
Medications
Operating microscope (69990)
Subconjunctival injection
Subtenon injection
Using viscoelastic material

EXCLUDES *Removal intralenticular foreign body without lens excision (65235)*
Repair surgical laceration (66250)

66830 **Removal of secondary membranous cataract (opacified posterior lens capsule and/or anterior hyaloid) with corneo-scleral section, with or without iridectomy (iridocapsulotomy, iridocapsulectomy)**

INCLUDES Graefe's operation

20.1 20.1 **FUD** 090 J A2 50

AMA: 2016,Feb,12

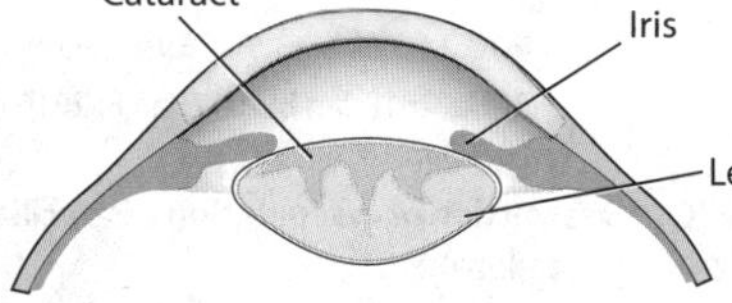

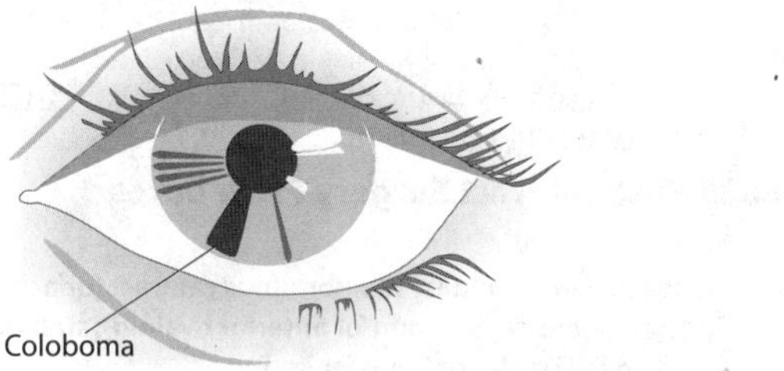

A congenital keyhole pupil is also called a coloboma of the iris

66840 **Removal of lens material; aspiration technique, 1 or more stages**

INCLUDES Fukala's operation

19.6 19.6 **FUD** 090 J A2 50

AMA: 2018,Jan,8; 2017,Jan,8; 2016,Sep,9; 2016,Jun,6; 2016,Apr,8; 2016,Feb,12; 2016,Jan,13; 2015,Jan,16

66850 **phacofragmentation technique (mechanical or ultrasonic) (eg, phacoemulsification), with aspiration**

22.3 22.3 **FUD** 090 J A2 50

AMA: 2018,Jan,8; 2017,Jan,8; 2016,Jun,6; 2016,Feb,12; 2016,Jan,13; 2015,Jan,16

66852 **pars plana approach, with or without vitrectomy**

23.8 23.8 **FUD** 090 J A2 80 50

AMA: 2018,Jan,8; 2017,Jan,8; 2016,Jun,6; 2016,Feb,12; 2016,Jan,13; 2015,Jan,16

66920 **intracapsular**

21.4 21.4 **FUD** 090 J A2 80 50

AMA: 2018,Jan,8; 2017,Jan,8; 2016,Feb,12; 2016,Jan,13; 2015,Jan,16

66930 **intracapsular, for dislocated lens**

24.3 24.3 **FUD** 090 J A2 80 50

AMA: 2018,Jan,8; 2017,Jan,8; 2016,Feb,12; 2016,Jan,13; 2015,Jan,16

66940 **extracapsular (other than 66840, 66850, 66852)**

22.1 22.1 **FUD** 090 J A2 80 50

AMA: 2018,Jan,8; 2017,Jan,8; 2016,Jun,6; 2016,Feb,12; 2016,Jan,13; 2015,Jan,16

66982-66988 [66987, 66988] Cataract Extraction: With Insertion Intraocular Lens

INCLUDES Anterior or posterior capsulotomy
Enzymatic zonulysis
Iridectomy/iridotomy
Lateral canthotomy
Medications
Operating microscope (69990)
Subconjunctival injection
Subtenon injection
Using viscoelastic material

EXCLUDES *Implanted material removal from anterior segment (65920)*
Insertion ocular telescope prosthesis (0308T)
Secondary fixation (66682)
Supply intraocular lens

66982 **Extracapsular cataract removal with insertion of intraocular lens prosthesis (1-stage procedure), manual or mechanical technique (eg, irrigation and aspiration or phacoemulsification), complex, requiring devices or techniques not generally used in routine cataract surgery (eg, iris expansion device, suture support for intraocular lens, or primary posterior capsulorrhexis) or performed on patients in the amblyogenic developmental stage; without endoscopic cyclophotocoagulation**

EXCLUDES *Complex extracapsular cataract removal in conjunction with endoscopic cyclophotocoagulation ([66987])*

(76519)

21.2 21.2 **FUD** 090 J A2 50

AMA: 2019,Dec,6; 2018,Dec,6; 2018,Dec,6; 2018,Jan,8; 2017,Dec,14; 2017,Jan,8; 2016,Mar,10; 2016,Feb,12; 2016,Jan,13; 2015,Jan,16

\# **66987** **with endoscopic cyclophotocoagulation**

EXCLUDES *Complex extracapsular cataract removal without endoscopic cyclophotocoagulation (66982)*

0.00 0.00 **FUD** 090 J8 80 50

AMA: 2019,Dec,6

66983 **Intracapsular cataract extraction with insertion of intraocular lens prosthesis (1 stage procedure)**

(76519)

21.0 21.0 **FUD** 090 J A2 50

AMA: 2019,Dec,6; 2018,Jan,8; 2017,Jan,8; 2016,Feb,12; 2016,Jan,13; 2015,Jan,16

66984 **Extracapsular cataract removal with insertion of intraocular lens prosthesis (1 stage procedure), manual or mechanical technique (eg, irrigation and aspiration or phacoemulsification); without endoscopic cyclophotocoagulation**

EXCLUDES *Complex extracapsular cataract removal (66982)*
Extracapsular cataract removal in conjunction with endoscopic cyclophotocoagulation ([66988])

(76519)

18.1 18.1 **FUD** 090 J A2 50

AMA: 2019,Dec,6; 2018,Dec,6; 2018,Dec,6; 2018,Jan,8; 2017,Jan,8; 2016,Feb,12; 2016,Jan,13; 2015,Jan,16

\# **66988** **with endoscopic cyclophotocoagulation**

EXCLUDES *Complex extracapsular cataract removal in conjunction with endoscopic cyclophotocoagulation (66987 [66987])*
Extracapsular cataract removal without endoscopic cyclophotocoagulation (66984)

0.00 0.00 **FUD** 090 J8 80 50

AMA: 2019,Dec,6

66985-66988 [66987, 66988] Secondary Insertion or Replacement of Intraocular Lens

INCLUDES Operating microscope (69990)

EXCLUDES *Implanted material removal from anterior segment (65920)*
Insertion ocular telescope prosthesis (0308T)
Secondary fixation (66682)
Supply intraocular lens

Code also ophthalmic endoscope if used (66990)

66985 Insertion of intraocular lens prosthesis (secondary implant), not associated with concurrent cataract removal

EXCLUDES *Implanted material removal from anterior segment (65920)*
Insertion lens at time of cataract procedure (66982-66984)
Insertion ocular telescope prosthesis (0308T)
Secondary fixation (66682)
Supply intraocular lens

(76519)

21.8 21.8 FUD 090 J A2 50

AMA: 2018,Jan,8; 2017,Jan,8; 2016,Feb,12; 2016,Jan,13; 2015,Jan,16

66986 Exchange of intraocular lens

(76519)

25.6 25.6 FUD 090 J A2 50

AMA: 2018,Jan,8; 2017,Jan,8; 2016,Feb,12; 2016,Jan,13; 2015,Jan,16

66987 Resequenced code. See code following 66982.

66988 Resequenced code. See code following 66984.

66990-66999 Ophthalmic Endoscopy

INCLUDES Operating microscope (69990)

\+ **66990 Use of ophthalmic endoscope (List separately in addition to code for primary procedure)**

Code first (65820, 65875, 65920, 66985-66986, 67036, 67039-67043, 67113)

2.55 2.55 FUD ZZZ N N1

AMA: 2018,Jul,3; 2018,Jan,8; 2017,Jan,8; 2016,Sep,5; 2016,Feb,12; 2016,Jan,13; 2015,Jan,16

66999 Unlisted procedure, anterior segment of eye

0.00 0.00 FUD YYY J 80 50

AMA: 2018,Jan,8; 2017,Jan,8; 2016,Apr,8; 2016,Feb,12; 2016,Jan,13; 2015,Jan,16

67005-67015 Vitrectomy: Partial and Subtotal

INCLUDES Operating microscope (69990)

67005 Removal of vitreous, anterior approach (open sky technique or limbal incision); partial removal

EXCLUDES *Anterior chamber vitrectomy by paracentesis (65810)*
Severing corneovitreal adhesions (65880)

13.4 13.4 FUD 090 J A2 50

AMA: 2018,Jan,8; 2017,Jan,8; 2016,Feb,12; 2016,Jan,13; 2015,Jan,16

67010 subtotal removal with mechanical vitrectomy

EXCLUDES *Anterior chamber vitrectomy by paracentesis (65810)*
Severing corneovitreal adhesions (65880)

15.3 15.3 FUD 090 J A2 50

AMA: 2018,Jan,8; 2017,Jan,8; 2016,Feb,12; 2016,Jan,13; 2015,Jan,16

67015 Aspiration or release of vitreous, subretinal or choroidal fluid, pars plana approach (posterior sclerotomy)

16.7 16.7 FUD 090 J A2 50

AMA: 2018,Jan,8; 2017,Jan,8; 2016,Sep,5; 2016,Jun,6; 2016,Feb,12

67025-67028 Intravitreal Injection/Implantation

INCLUDES Operating microscope (69990)

67025 Injection of vitreous substitute, pars plana or limbal approach (fluid-gas exchange), with or without aspiration (separate procedure)

17.8 20.9 FUD 090 J A2 50

AMA: 2019,Aug,10; 2018,Feb,3; 2016,Feb,12

67027 Implantation of intravitreal drug delivery system (eg, ganciclovir implant), includes concomitant removal of vitreous

EXCLUDES *Removal drug delivery system (67121)*

24.0 24.0 FUD 090 J A2 80 50

AMA: 2018,Feb,3; 2018,Jan,8; 2017,Jan,8; 2016,Feb,12; 2016,Jan,13; 2015,Jan,16

67028 Intravitreal injection of a pharmacologic agent (separate procedure)

2.79 2.86 FUD 000 S P3 50

AMA: 2018,Feb,3; 2018,Jan,8; 2017,Jan,8; 2016,Feb,12; 2016,Jan,13; 2015,Jan,16

67030-67031 Incision of Vitreous Strands/Membranes

INCLUDES Operating microscope (69990)

67030 Discission of vitreous strands (without removal), pars plana approach

15.2 15.2 FUD 090 J A2 50

AMA: 2016,Feb,12

67031 Severing of vitreous strands, vitreous face adhesions, sheets, membranes or opacities, laser surgery (1 or more stages)

10.1 11.1 FUD 090 T A2 50

AMA: 2016,Feb,12

67036-67043 Pars Plana Mechanical Vitrectomy

INCLUDES Operating microscope (69990)

EXCLUDES *Lens removal (66850)*
Removal foreign body (65260, 65265)
Unlisted vitreal procedures (67299)
Vitrectomy in retinal detachment (67108, 67113)

Code also ophthalmic endoscope if used (66990)

67036 Vitrectomy, mechanical, pars plana approach;

25.4 25.4 FUD 090 J A2 80 50

AMA: 2018,Jan,8; 2017,Jan,8; 2016,Sep,5; 2016,Feb,12; 2016,Jan,13; 2015,Jan,16

67039 with focal endolaser photocoagulation

27.2 27.2 FUD 090 J A2 80 50

AMA: 2018,Jan,8; 2017,Jan,8; 2016,Sep,5; 2016,Feb,12; 2016,Jan,13; 2015,Jan,16

67040 with endolaser panretinal photocoagulation

29.4 29.4 FUD 090 J A2 80 50

AMA: 2018,Jan,8; 2017,Jan,8; 2016,Sep,5; 2016,Feb,12; 2016,Jan,13; 2015,Jan,16

67041 with removal of preretinal cellular membrane (eg, macular pucker)

32.7 32.7 FUD 090 J G2 80 50

AMA: 2018,Jan,8; 2017,Jan,8; 2016,Sep,5; 2016,Feb,12; 2016,Jan,13; 2015,Jan,16

67042 with removal of internal limiting membrane of retina (eg, for repair of macular hole, diabetic macular edema), includes, if performed, intraocular tamponade (ie, air, gas or silicone oil)

32.7 32.7 FUD 090 J G2 80 50

AMA: 2018,Jan,8; 2017,Jan,8; 2016,Sep,5; 2016,Feb,12; 2016,Jan,13; 2015,Jan,16

67043 with removal of subretinal membrane (eg, choroidal neovascularization), includes, if performed, intraocular tamponade (ie, air, gas or silicone oil) and laser photocoagulation

34.5 34.5 FUD 090 J G2 80 50

AMA: 2018,Jan,8; 2017,Jan,8; 2016,Sep,5; 2016,Feb,12; 2016,Jan,13; 2015,Jan,16

67101-67115 Detached Retina Repair

INCLUDES Operating microscope (69990)
Primary technique when cryotherapy and/or diathermy and/or photocoagulation are used in combination

67101 Repair of retinal detachment, including drainage of subretinal fluid when performed; cryotherapy
8.10 9.40 FUD 010 J P3 50
AMA: 2018,Jan,8; 2017,Feb,14; 2017,Jan,8; 2016,Sep,5; 2016,Jun,6; 2016,Feb,12; 2016,Jan,13; 2015,Jan,16

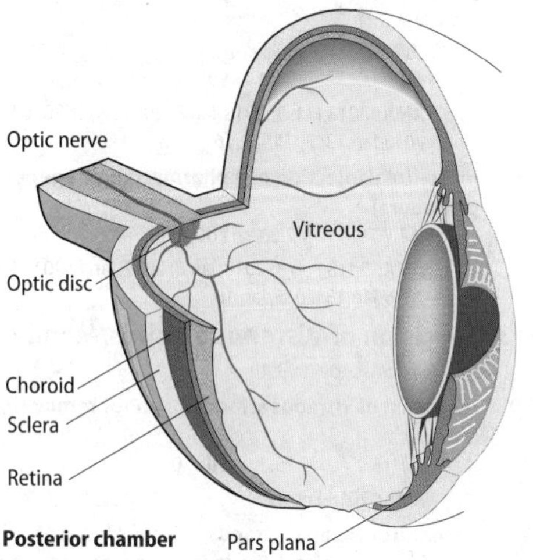

67105 photocoagulation
7.82 8.45 FUD 010 T P3 50
AMA: 2018,Jan,8; 2017,Feb,14; 2017,Jan,8; 2016,Sep,5; 2016,Jun,6; 2016,Feb,12; 2016,Jan,13; 2015,Jan,16

67107 Repair of retinal detachment; scleral buckling (such as lamellar scleral dissection, imbrication or encircling procedure), including, when performed, implant, cryotherapy, photocoagulation, and drainage of subretinal fluid
INCLUDES Gonin's operation
32.1 32.1 FUD 090 J G2 80 50
AMA: 2019,Aug,10; 2018,Jan,8; 2017,Jan,8; 2016,Sep,5; 2016,Jun,6; 2016,Feb,12

67108 with vitrectomy, any method, including, when performed, air or gas tamponade, focal endolaser photocoagulation, cryotherapy, drainage of subretinal fluid, scleral buckling, and/or removal of lens by same technique
34.1 34.1 FUD 090 J G2 80 50
AMA: 2018,Jan,8; 2017,Jan,8; 2016,Sep,5; 2016,Jun,6; 2016,Feb,12; 2016,Jan,13; 2015,Jan,16

67110 by injection of air or other gas (eg, pneumatic retinopexy)
23.1 25.0 FUD 090 J P3 50
AMA: 2018,Jan,8; 2017,Jan,8; 2016,Sep,5; 2016,Jun,6; 2016,Feb,12

67113 Repair of complex retinal detachment (eg, proliferative vitreoretinopathy, stage C-1 or greater, diabetic traction retinal detachment, retinopathy of prematurity, retinal tear of greater than 90 degrees), with vitrectomy and membrane peeling, including, when performed, air, gas, or silicone oil tamponade, cryotherapy, endolaser photocoagulation, drainage of subretinal fluid, scleral buckling, and/or removal of lens
EXCLUDES *Vitrectomy for other than retinal detachment, pars plana approach (67036-67043)*
Code also ophthalmic endoscope if used (66990)
38.0 38.0 FUD 090 J G2 80 50
AMA: 2018,Jan,8; 2017,Jan,8; 2016,Sep,5; 2016,Jun,6; 2016,Feb,12; 2016,Jan,13; 2015,Jan,16

67115 Release of encircling material (posterior segment)
14.1 14.1 FUD 090 J A2 50
AMA: 2016,Feb,12

67120-67121 Removal of Previously Implanted Prosthetic Device

INCLUDES Operating microscope (69990)
EXCLUDES *Foreign body removal (65260, 65265)*
Removal implanted material anterior segment (65920)

67120 Removal of implanted material, posterior segment; extraocular
15.8 18.8 FUD 090 J A2 50
AMA: 2016,Feb,12

67121 intraocular
25.6 25.6 FUD 090 J A2 80 50
AMA: 2016,Feb,12

67141-67145 Retinal Detachment: Preventative Procedures

INCLUDES Operating microscope (69990)
Treatment at one or more sessions that may occur at different encounters
EXCLUDES *Procedure performed more than one time during defined period of treatment*

67141 Prophylaxis of retinal detachment (eg, retinal break, lattice degeneration) without drainage, 1 or more sessions; cryotherapy, diathermy
13.8 14.9 FUD 090 T A2 50
AMA: 2018,Jan,8; 2017,Jan,8; 2016,Sep,5; 2016,Feb,12; 2016,Jan,13; 2015,Jan,16

67145 photocoagulation (laser or xenon arc)
14.0 14.9 FUD 090 T P2 50
AMA: 2018,Jan,8; 2017,Jan,8; 2016,Sep,5; 2016,Feb,12; 2016,Jan,13; 2015,Jan,16

67208-67218 Destruction of Retinal Lesions

INCLUDES Operating microscope (69990)
Treatment at one or more sessions that may occur at different encounters
EXCLUDES *Procedure performed more than one time during defined period of treatment*
Unlisted retinal procedures (67299)

67208 Destruction of localized lesion of retina (eg, macular edema, tumors), 1 or more sessions; cryotherapy, diathermy
16.4 17.0 FUD 090 T P2 50
AMA: 2018,Jan,8; 2017,Jan,8; 2016,Feb,12; 2016,Jan,13; 2015,Jan,16

67210 photocoagulation
14.1 14.6 FUD 090 T P2 50
AMA: 2018,Jan,8; 2017,Jan,8; 2016,Feb,12; 2016,Jan,13; 2015,Jan,16

67218 radiation by implantation of source (includes removal of source)
39.3 39.3 FUD 090 J A2 50
AMA: 2018,Jan,8; 2017,Jan,8; 2016,Feb,12; 2016,Jan,13; 2015,Jan,16

67220-67225 Destruction of Choroidal Lesions

INCLUDES Operating microscope (69990)

67220 Destruction of localized lesion of choroid (eg, choroidal neovascularization); photocoagulation (eg, laser), 1 or more sessions
INCLUDES Treatment at one or more sessions that may occur at different encounters
EXCLUDES *Procedure performed more than one time during defined period of treatment*
14.1 15.0 FUD 090 T P2 50
AMA: 2018,Jan,8; 2017,Jan,8; 2016,Feb,12; 2016,Jan,13; 2015,Jan,16

67221 photodynamic therapy (includes intravenous infusion)
6.05 8.07 FUD 000 T P3
AMA: 2018,Feb,10; 2018,Jan,8; 2017,Jan,8; 2016,Feb,12; 2016,Jan,13; 2015,Jan,16

\+ 67225 **photodynamic therapy, second eye, at single session (List separately in addition to code for primary eye treatment)**

Code first (67221)

0.81 0.85 **FUD** ZZZ N N1

AMA: 2018,Jan,8; 2017,Jan,8; 2016,Feb,12; 2016,Jan,13; 2015,Jan,16

67227-67229 Destruction Retinopathy

INCLUDES Operating microscope (69990)

EXCLUDES *Unlisted retinal procedures (67299)*

67227 **Destruction of extensive or progressive retinopathy (eg, diabetic retinopathy), cryotherapy, diathermy**

7.24 8.33 **FUD** 010 J P3 50

AMA: 2018,Jan,8; 2017,Jan,8; 2016,Feb,12; 2016,Jan,13; 2015,Jan,16

67228 **Treatment of extensive or progressive retinopathy (eg, diabetic retinopathy), photocoagulation**

8.72 9.73 **FUD** 010 T P3 50

AMA: 2018,Jan,8; 2017,Jan,8; 2016,Feb,12; 2016,Jan,13; 2015,Jan,16

67229 **Treatment of extensive or progressive retinopathy, 1 or more sessions, preterm infant (less than 37 weeks gestation at birth), performed from birth up to 1 year of age (eg, retinopathy of prematurity), photocoagulation or cryotherapy**

INCLUDES Treatment at one or more sessions that may occur at different encounters

EXCLUDES *Procedure performed more than one time during defined period of treatment*

33.1 33.1 **FUD** 090 T R2 50

AMA: 2018,Jan,8; 2017,Jan,8; 2016,Feb,12; 2016,Jan,13; 2015,Jan,16

67250-67255 Reinforcement of Posterior Sclera

INCLUDES Operating microscope (69990)

EXCLUDES *Removal scleral lesion (66130)*

Repair scleral staphyloma (66225)

67250 **Scleral reinforcement (separate procedure); without graft**

22.6 22.6 **FUD** 090 J A2 50

AMA: 2016,Feb,12

67255 **with graft**

EXCLUDES *Aqueous shunt to extraocular equatorial plate reservoir (66180)*

Revision aqueous shunt to extraocular equatorial plate reservoir; with graft (66185)

19.3 19.3 **FUD** 090 J A2 80 50

AMA: 2018,Jan,8; 2017,Jan,8; 2016,Feb,12; 2016,Jan,13; 2015,Jan,16; 2015,Jan,10

67299 Unlisted Posterior Segment Procedure

CMS: 100-04,4,180.3 Unlisted Service or Procedure

INCLUDES Operating microscope (69990)

67299 **Unlisted procedure, posterior segment**

0.00 0.00 **FUD** YYY J 80 50

AMA: 2018,Jan,8; 2017,Jan,8; 2016,Feb,12; 2016,Jan,13; 2015,Jan,16

67311-67334 Strabismus Procedures on Extraocular Muscles

INCLUDES Operating microscope (69990)

Code also adjustable sutures (67335)

67311 **Strabismus surgery, recession or resection procedure; 1 horizontal muscle**

16.9 16.9 **FUD** 090 J A2 50

AMA: 2018,Jan,8; 2017,Jan,8; 2017,Jan,6; 2016,Feb,12; 2016,Jan,13; 2015,Jan,16

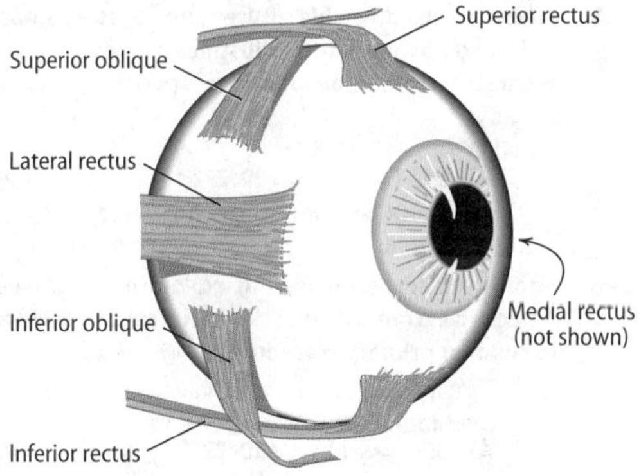

Muscles of the eyeball (right eye shown)

67312 **2 horizontal muscles**

20.3 20.3 **FUD** 090 J A2 50

AMA: 2018,Jan,8; 2017,Jan,8; 2016,Feb,12; 2016,Jan,13; 2015,Jan,16

67314 **1 vertical muscle (excluding superior oblique)**

19.1 19.1 **FUD** 090 J A2 50

AMA: 2018,Jan,8; 2017,Jan,8; 2016,Feb,12; 2016,Jan,13; 2015,Jan,16

67316 **2 or more vertical muscles (excluding superior oblique)**

22.7 22.7 **FUD** 090 J A2 80 50

AMA: 2018,Jan,8; 2017,Jan,8; 2016,Feb,12; 2016,Jan,13; 2015,Jan,16

67318 **Strabismus surgery, any procedure, superior oblique muscle**

19.9 19.9 **FUD** 090 J A2 50

AMA: 2018,Jan,8; 2017,Jan,8; 2016,Feb,12; 2016,Jan,13; 2015,Jan,16

\+ 67320 **Transposition procedure (eg, for paretic extraocular muscle), any extraocular muscle (specify) (List separately in addition to code for primary procedure)**

Code first (67311-67318)

9.10 9.10 **FUD** ZZZ N N1

AMA: 2018,Jan,8; 2017,Jan,8; 2016,Feb,12; 2016,Jan,13; 2015,Jan,16

\+ 67331 **Strabismus surgery on patient with previous eye surgery or injury that did not involve the extraocular muscles (List separately in addition to code for primary procedure)**

Code first (67311-67318)

8.70 8.70 **FUD** ZZZ N N1 50

AMA: 2018,Jan,8; 2017,Jan,8; 2016,Feb,12; 2016,Jan,13; 2015,Jan,16

\+ 67332 **Strabismus surgery on patient with scarring of extraocular muscles (eg, prior ocular injury, strabismus or retinal detachment surgery) or restrictive myopathy (eg, dysthyroid ophthalmopathy) (List separately in addition to code for primary procedure)**

Code first (67311-67318)

9.37 9.37 **FUD** ZZZ N N1 50

AMA: 2018,Jan,8; 2017,Jan,8; 2016,Feb,12; 2016,Jan,13; 2015,Jan,16

+ **67334 Strabismus surgery by posterior fixation suture technique, with or without muscle recession (List separately in addition to code for primary procedure)**

Code first (67311-67318)

8.52 8.52 **FUD** ZZZ N N1 50

AMA: 2018,Jan,8; 2017,Jan,8; 2016,Feb,12; 2016,Jan,13; 2015,Jan,16

67335-67399 Other Procedures of Extraocular Muscles

INCLUDES Operating microscope (69990)

+ **67335 Placement of adjustable suture(s) during strabismus surgery, including postoperative adjustment(s) of suture(s) (List separately in addition to code for specific strabismus surgery)**

Code first (67311-67334)

4.21 4.21 **FUD** ZZZ N N1 50

AMA: 2018,Jan,8; 2017,Jan,8; 2016,Feb,12; 2016,Jan,13; 2015,Jan,16

+ **67340 Strabismus surgery involving exploration and/or repair of detached extraocular muscle(s) (List separately in addition to code for primary procedure)**

INCLUDES Hummelsheim operation

Code first (67311-67334)

10.1 10.1 **FUD** ZZZ N N1 80

AMA: 2018,Jan,8; 2017,Jan,8; 2016,Feb,12; 2016,Jan,13; 2015,Jan,16

67343 Release of extensive scar tissue without detaching extraocular muscle (separate procedure)

Code also when performed on other than affected muscle (67311-67340)

18.5 18.5 **FUD** 090 J A2 50

AMA: 2018,Jan,8; 2017,Jan,8; 2016,Feb,12; 2016,Jan,13; 2015,Jan,16

67345 Chemodenervation of extraocular muscle

EXCLUDES *Nerve destruction for blepharospasm and other neurological disorders (64612, 64616)*

6.22 6.96 **FUD** 010 T P3 50

AMA: 2019,Apr,9; 2018,Jan,8; 2017,Jan,8; 2016,Feb,12; 2016,Jan,13; 2015,Jan,16

67346 Biopsy of extraocular muscle

EXCLUDES *Repair laceration extraocular muscle, tendon, or Tenon's capsule (65290)*

5.50 5.50 **FUD** 000 J A2 80 50

AMA: 2016,Feb,12

67399 Unlisted procedure, extraocular muscle

0.00 0.00 **FUD** YYY T 80 50

AMA: 2018,Jan,8; 2017,Jul,10; 2016,Feb,12

67400-67415 Frontal Orbitotomy

INCLUDES Operating microscope (69990)

67400 Orbitotomy without bone flap (frontal or transconjunctival approach); for exploration, with or without biopsy

27.8 27.8 **FUD** 090 J A2 50

AMA: 2016,Feb,12

67405 with drainage only

22.8 22.8 **FUD** 090 J A2 50

AMA: 2018,Jan,8; 2017,Jan,8; 2016,Feb,12; 2016,Jan,13; 2015,Jan,16

67412 with removal of lesion

24.6 24.6 **FUD** 090 J A2 50

AMA: 2016,Feb,12

67413 with removal of foreign body

25.8 25.8 **FUD** 090 J A2 80 50

AMA: 2016,Feb,12

67414 with removal of bone for decompression

38.1 38.1 **FUD** 090 J G2 80 50

AMA: 2018,Jan,8; 2017,Jan,8; 2016,Feb,12; 2016,Jan,13; 2015,Jan,16

67415 Fine needle aspiration of orbital contents

EXCLUDES *Decompression optic nerve (67570)*

Exenteration, enucleation, and repair (65101-65175)

2.96 2.96 **FUD** 000 J A2 80 50

AMA: 2016,Feb,12

67420-67450 Lateral Orbitotomy

INCLUDES Operating microscope (69990)

EXCLUDES *Orbital implant (67550, 67560)*

Surgical removal all or some orbital contents or repair after removal (65091-65175)

Transcranial approach orbitotomy (61330, 61333)

67420 Orbitotomy with bone flap or window, lateral approach (eg, Kroenlein); with removal of lesion

46.2 46.2 **FUD** 090 J A2 80 50

AMA: 2016,Feb,12

67430 with removal of foreign body

37.3 37.3 **FUD** 090 J A2 80 50

AMA: 2016,Feb,12

67440 with drainage

36.1 36.1 **FUD** 090 J A2 80 50

AMA: 2016,Feb,12

67445 with removal of bone for decompression

EXCLUDES *Decompression optic nerve sheath (67570)*

41.6 41.6 **FUD** 090 J A2 80 50

AMA: 2019,Dec,14; 2016,Feb,12

67450 for exploration, with or without biopsy

37.5 37.5 **FUD** 090 J A2 80 50

AMA: 2016,Feb,12

67500-67515 Eye Injections

INCLUDES Operating microscope (69990)

67500 Retrobulbar injection; medication (separate procedure, does not include supply of medication)

1.73 2.02 **FUD** 000 T G2 50

AMA: 2018,Jan,8; 2017,Jan,8; 2016,Feb,12; 2016,Jan,13; 2015,Jan,16

67505 alcohol

2.03 2.38 **FUD** 000 T P3 50

AMA: 2016,Feb,12

67515 Injection of medication or other substance into Tenon's capsule

EXCLUDES *Subconjunctival injection (68200)*

2.06 2.24 **FUD** 000 T P3 50

AMA: 2018,Jan,8; 2017,Jan,8; 2016,Feb,12; 2016,Jan,13; 2015,Jan,16

67550-67560 Orbital Implant

INCLUDES Operating microscope (69990)

EXCLUDES *Fracture repair malar area, orbit (21355-21408)*

Ocular implant inside muscle cone (65093-65105, 65130-65175)

67550 Orbital implant (implant outside muscle cone); insertion

27.8 27.8 **FUD** 090 J A2 50

AMA: 2016,Feb,12

67560 removal or revision

28.5 28.5 **FUD** 090 J A2 80 50

AMA: 2016,Feb,12

67570-67599 Other and Unlisted Orbital Procedures

INCLUDES Operating microscope (69990)

67570 Optic nerve decompression (eg, incision or fenestration of optic nerve sheath)

33.9 33.9 **FUD** 090 J A2 80 50

AMA: 2016,Feb,12

67599 Unlisted procedure, orbit

0.00 0.00 **FUD** YYY T 80 50

AMA: 2016,Feb,12

67700-67810 [67810] Incisional Procedures of Eyelids

INCLUDES Operating microscope (69990)

67700 Blepharotomy, drainage of abscess, eyelid
3.31 7.82 FUD 010 T P2 50
AMA: 2018,Jan,8; 2017,Jan,8; 2016,Feb,12; 2016,Jan,13; 2015,Jan,16

67710 Severing of tarsorrhaphy
2.77 6.56 FUD 010 T P3 50
AMA: 2018,Jan,8; 2017,Jan,8; 2016,Feb,12; 2016,Jan,13; 2015,Jan,16

67715 Canthotomy (separate procedure)
EXCLUDES *Canthoplasty (67950)*
Symblepharon division (68340)
3.08 7.07 FUD 010 J A2 50
AMA: 2018,Jan,8; 2017,Jan,8; 2016,Feb,12; 2016,Jan,13; 2015,Jan,16

\# **67810 Incisional biopsy of eyelid skin including lid margin**
EXCLUDES *Biopsy eyelid skin (11102-11107)*
2.03 4.99 FUD 000 T P2 50
AMA: 2019,Jan,9; 2018,Jan,8; 2017,Jan,8; 2016,Feb,12; 2016,Jan,13; 2015,Jan,16

67800-67808 Excision of Chalazion (Meibomian Cyst)

INCLUDES Lesion removal requiring more than skin:
Lid margin
Palpebral conjunctiva
Tarsus
Operating microscope (69990)

EXCLUDES *Blepharoplasty, graft, or reconstructive procedures (67930-67975)*
Excision/destruction skin lesion eyelid (11310-11313, 11440-11446, 11640-11646, 17000-17004)

67800 Excision of chalazion; single
2.93 3.64 FUD 010 T P3
AMA: 2018,Jan,8; 2017,Jan,8; 2016,Feb,12; 2016,Jan,13; 2015,Jan,16

67801 multiple, same lid
3.79 4.64 FUD 010 T P3
AMA: 2016,Feb,12

67805 multiple, different lids
4.67 5.76 FUD 010 T P3
AMA: 2018,Jan,8; 2017,Jan,8; 2016,Feb,12; 2016,Jan,13; 2015,Jan,16

67808 under general anesthesia and/or requiring hospitalization, single or multiple
10.4 10.4 FUD 090 J A2
AMA: 2016,Feb,12

67810-67850 [67810] Other Eyelid Procedures

INCLUDES Operating microscope (69990)

67810 **Resequenced code. See code following 67715.**

67820 Correction of trichiasis; epilation, by forceps only
0.99 0.93 FUD 000 Q1 N1 50
AMA: 2018,Jan,8; 2017,Jan,8; 2016,Feb,12; 2016,Jan,13; 2015,Jan,16

67825 epilation by other than forceps (eg, by electrosurgery, cryotherapy, laser surgery)
3.43 3.77 FUD 010 T P3 50
AMA: 2018,Jan,8; 2017,Jan,8; 2016,Feb,12; 2016,Jan,13; 2015,Jan,16

67830 incision of lid margin
3.92 7.64 FUD 010 T A2 50
AMA: 2016,Feb,12

67835 incision of lid margin, with free mucous membrane graft
12.4 12.4 FUD 090 J A2 80 50
AMA: 2016,Feb,12

67840 Excision of lesion of eyelid (except chalazion) without closure or with simple direct closure
EXCLUDES *Eyelid resection and reconstruction (67961, 67966)*
4.49 7.91 FUD 010 T P3 50
AMA: 2019,Jan,14; 2016,Feb,12

67850 Destruction of lesion of lid margin (up to 1 cm)
EXCLUDES *Mohs micro procedures (17311-17315)*
Topical chemotherapy (99202-99215)
3.84 6.13 FUD 010 T P3 50
AMA: 2016,Feb,12

67875-67882 Suturing of the Eyelids

INCLUDES Operating microscope (69990)
EXCLUDES *Canthoplasty (67950)*
Canthotomy (67715)
Severing of tarsorrhaphy (67710)

67875 Temporary closure of eyelids by suture (eg, Frost suture)
2.72 5.01 FUD 000 T G2 50
AMA: 2016,Feb,12

67880 Construction of intermarginal adhesions, median tarsorrhaphy, or canthorrhaphy;
10.3 13.1 FUD 090 J A2 50
AMA: 2016,Feb,12

67882 with transposition of tarsal plate
13.4 16.1 FUD 090 J A2 50
AMA: 2016,Feb,12

67900-67912 Repair of Ptosis/Retraction Eyelids, Eyebrows

INCLUDES Operating microscope (69990)

67900 Repair of brow ptosis (supraciliary, mid-forehead or coronal approach)
EXCLUDES *Forehead rhytidectomy (15824)*
14.4 18.2 FUD 090 J A2 50
AMA: 2018,Jan,8; 2017,Jan,8; 2016,Feb,12; 2016,Jan,13; 2015,Jan,16

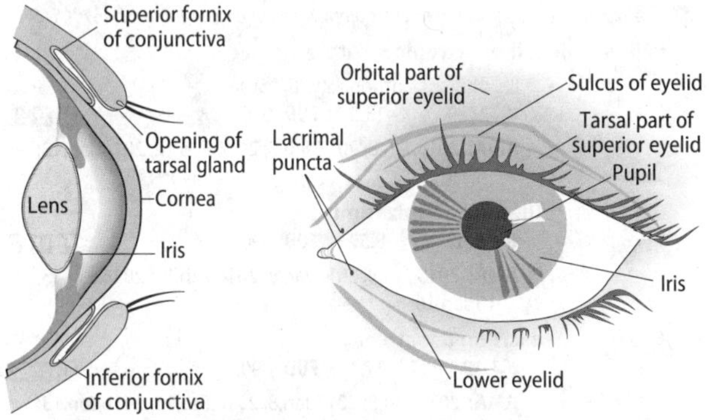

67901 Repair of blepharoptosis; frontalis muscle technique with suture or other material (eg, banked fascia)
16.5 21.9 FUD 090 J A2 50
AMA: 2018,Jan,8; 2017,Jul,10; 2017,Jan,8; 2016,Feb,12; 2016,Jan,13; 2015,Jan,16

67902 frontalis muscle technique with autologous fascial sling (includes obtaining fascia)
20.5 20.5 FUD 090 J A2 50
AMA: 2018,Jan,8; 2017,Jan,8; 2016,Feb,12; 2016,Jan,13; 2015,Jan,16

67903 (tarso) levator resection or advancement, internal approach
13.7 16.9 FUD 090 J A2 50
AMA: 2018,Jan,8; 2017,Jan,8; 2016,Feb,12; 2016,Jan,13; 2015,Jan,16

Eye, Ocular Adnexa, and Ear
67700 — 67903

67904 **(tarso) levator resection or advancement, external approach**

INCLUDES Everbusch's operation

Facility RVU 16.9 Non-Facility RVU 20.9 FUD 090 J A2 50

AMA: 2018,Jan,8; 2017,Jan,8; 2016,Feb,12; 2016,Jan,13; 2015,Jan,16

67906 **superior rectus technique with fascial sling (includes obtaining fascia)**

Facility RVU 14.4 Non-Facility RVU 14.4 FUD 090 J A2 50

AMA: 2018,Jan,8; 2017,Jan,8; 2016,Feb,12; 2016,Jan,13; 2015,Jan,16

67908 **conjunctivo-tarso-Muller's muscle-levator resection (eg, Fasanella-Servat type)**

Facility RVU 12.1 Non-Facility RVU 14.1 FUD 090 J A2 50

AMA: 2018,Jan,8; 2017,Jan,8; 2016,Feb,12; 2016,Jan,13; 2015,Jan,16

67909 **Reduction of overcorrection of ptosis**

Facility RVU 12.4 Non-Facility RVU 15.3 FUD 090 J A2 50

AMA: 2018,Jan,8; 2017,Jan,8; 2016,Feb,12; 2016,Jan,13; 2015,Jan,16

67911 **Correction of lid retraction**

EXCLUDES *Autologous graft harvest ([15769], 20920, 20922)*
Lid defect correction using fat obtained via liposuction (15773-15774)
Mucous membrane graft repair trichiasis (67835)

Facility RVU 15.8 Non-Facility RVU 15.8 FUD 090 J A2 50

AMA: 2018,Jan,8; 2017,Jan,8; 2016,Feb,12; 2016,Jan,13; 2015,Jan,16

67912 **Correction of lagophthalmos, with implantation of upper eyelid lid load (eg, gold weight)**

Facility RVU 13.8 Non-Facility RVU 25.4 FUD 090 J A2 50

AMA: 2018,Jan,8; 2017,Jan,8; 2016,Feb,12; 2016,Jan,13; 2015,Jan,16

67914-67924 Repair Ectropion/Entropion

INCLUDES Operating microscope (69990)

EXCLUDES *Cicatricial ectropion or entropion with scar excision or graft (67961-67966)*

67914 **Repair of ectropion; suture**

INCLUDES Canthoplasty (67950)

Facility RVU 9.29 Non-Facility RVU 13.5 FUD 090 J A2 50

AMA: 2018,Jan,8; 2017,Jan,8; 2016,Feb,12; 2016,Jan,13; 2015,Jan,16

67915 **thermocauterization**

Facility RVU 5.62 Non-Facility RVU 8.52 FUD 090 J P3 50

AMA: 2018,Jan,8; 2017,Jan,8; 2016,Feb,12; 2016,Jan,13; 2015,Jan,16

67916 **excision tarsal wedge**

Facility RVU 12.1 Non-Facility RVU 17.1 FUD 090 J A2 50

AMA: 2018,Jan,8; 2017,Jan,8; 2016,Feb,12; 2016,Jan,13; 2015,Jan,16

67917 **extensive (eg, tarsal strip operations)**

EXCLUDES *Repair everted punctum (68705)*

Facility RVU 13.0 Non-Facility RVU 17.3 FUD 090 J A2 50

AMA: 2020,Feb,13; 2018,Jan,8; 2017,Jan,8; 2016,Feb,12; 2016,Jan,13; 2015,Jan,16

67921 **Repair of entropion; suture**

Facility RVU 8.82 Non-Facility RVU 13.2 FUD 090 J A2 50

AMA: 2018,Jan,8; 2017,Jan,8; 2016,Feb,12; 2016,Jan,13; 2015,Jan,16

67922 **thermocauterization**

Facility RVU 5.52 Non-Facility RVU 8.42 FUD 090 J P3 50

AMA: 2018,Jan,8; 2017,Jan,8; 2016,Feb,12; 2016,Jan,13; 2015,Jan,16

67923 **excision tarsal wedge**

Facility RVU 12.1 Non-Facility RVU 17.1 FUD 090 J A2 50

AMA: 2018,Jan,8; 2017,Jan,8; 2016,Feb,12; 2016,Jan,13; 2015,Jan,16

67924 **extensive (eg, tarsal strip or capsulopalpebral fascia repairs operation)**

INCLUDES Canthoplasty (67950)

Facility RVU 12.9 Non-Facility RVU 18.2 FUD 090 J A2 50

AMA: 2018,Jan,8; 2017,Jan,8; 2016,Feb,12; 2016,Jan,13; 2015,Jan,16

67930-67935 Repair Eyelid Wound

INCLUDES Operating microscope (69990)
Repairs involving more than skin:
- Lid margin
- Palpebral conjunctiva
- Tarsus

EXCLUDES *Blepharoplasty for entropion or ectropion (67916-67917, 67923-67924)*
Correction lid retraction and blepharoptosis (67901-67911)
Free graft (15120-15121, 15260-15261)
Graft preparation (15004)
Plastic repair lacrimal canaliculi (68700)
Removal eyelid lesion (67800 [67810], 67840-67850)
Repair blepharochalasis (15820-15823)
Repair involving eyelid skin (12011-12018, 12051-12057, 13151-13153)
Skin adjacent tissue transfer (14060-14061)
Tarsorrhaphy, canthorrhaphy (67880, 67882)

67930 **Suture of recent wound, eyelid, involving lid margin, tarsus, and/or palpebral conjunctiva direct closure; partial thickness**

Facility RVU 6.78 Non-Facility RVU 10.4 FUD 010 J P3 50

AMA: 2016,Feb,12

67935 **full thickness**

Facility RVU 12.5 Non-Facility RVU 16.9 FUD 090 J A2 50

AMA: 2016,Feb,12

67938-67999 Eyelid Reconstruction/Repair/Removal Deep Foreign Body

INCLUDES Operating microscope (69990)

EXCLUDES *Blepharoplasty for entropion or ectropion (67916-67917, 67923-67924)*
Correction lid retraction and blepharoptosis (67901-67911)
Free graft (15120-15121, 15260-15261)
Graft preparation (15004)
Plastic repair lacrimal canaliculi (68700)
Removal eyelid lesion (67800-67808, 67840-67850)
Repair blepharochalasis (15820-15823)
Repair involving eyelid skin (12011-12018, 12051-12057, 13151-13153)
Skin adjacent tissue transfer (14060-14061)
Tarsorrhaphy, canthorrhaphy (67880, 67882)

67938 **Removal of embedded foreign body, eyelid**

Facility RVU 3.28 Non-Facility RVU 7.36 FUD 010 T P2 50

AMA: 2018,Jan,8; 2017,Jan,8; 2016,Feb,12; 2016,Jan,13; 2015,Jan,16

67950 **Canthoplasty (reconstruction of canthus)**

Facility RVU 13.1 Non-Facility RVU 16.4 FUD 090 J A2 50

AMA: 2016,Feb,12

67961 **Excision and repair of eyelid, involving lid margin, tarsus, conjunctiva, canthus, or full thickness, may include preparation for skin graft or pedicle flap with adjacent tissue transfer or rearrangement; up to one-fourth of lid margin**

INCLUDES Canthoplasty (67950)

EXCLUDES *Delay flap (15630)*
Flap attachment (15650)
Free skin grafts (15120-15121, 15260-15261)
Tubed pedicle flap preparation (15576)

Facility RVU 12.8 Non-Facility RVU 16.4 FUD 090 J A2 80 50

AMA: 2018,Jan,8; 2017,Jan,8; 2016,Feb,12; 2016,Jan,13; 2015,Jan,16

67966 **over one-fourth of lid margin**

INCLUDES Canthoplasty (67950)

EXCLUDES *Delay flap (15630)*
Flap attachment (15650)
Free skin grafts (15120-15121, 15260-15261)
Tubed pedicle flap preparation (15576)

Facility RVU 18.7 Non-Facility RVU 21.9 FUD 090 J A2 50

AMA: 2018,Jan,8; 2017,Jan,8; 2016,Feb,12; 2016,Jan,13; 2015,Jan,16

67971 Reconstruction of eyelid, full thickness by transfer of tarsoconjunctival flap from opposing eyelid; up to two-thirds of eyelid, 1 stage or first stage
INCLUDES Dupuy-Dutemp reconstruction
Landboldt's operation
20.4 20.4 FUD 090 J A2 50
AMA: 2016,Feb,12

67973 total eyelid, lower, 1 stage or first stage
INCLUDES Landboldt's operation
26.3 26.3 FUD 090 J A2 80 50
AMA: 2016,Feb,12

67974 total eyelid, upper, 1 stage or first stage
INCLUDES Landboldt's operation
26.2 26.2 FUD 090 J A2 80 50
AMA: 2016,Feb,12

67975 second stage
INCLUDES Landboldt's operation
19.4 19.4 FUD 090 J A2 50
AMA: 2016,Feb,12

67999 Unlisted procedure, eyelids
0.00 0.00 FUD YYY T 80 50
AMA: 2018,Jan,8; 2017,Jul,10; 2017,Jan,8; 2016,Feb,12; 2016,Jan,13; 2015,Jan,16

68020-68200 Conjunctival Biopsy/Injection/Treatment of Lesions

INCLUDES Operating microscope (69990)
EXCLUDES *Foreign body removal (65205-65265)*

68020 Incision of conjunctiva, drainage of cyst
3.11 3.41 FUD 010 T P3 50
AMA: 2016,Feb,12

68040 Expression of conjunctival follicles (eg, for trachoma)
EXCLUDES *Automated evacuation meibomian glands with heat/pressure (0207T)*
Manual evacuation meibomian glands ([0563T])
1.40 1.78 FUD 000 T P3 50
AMA: 2018,Jan,8; 2017,Jan,8; 2016,Feb,12; 2016,Jan,13; 2015,Jan,16

68100 Biopsy of conjunctiva
2.75 4.97 FUD 000 J P3 50
AMA: 2019,Jan,9; 2016,Feb,12

68110 Excision of lesion, conjunctiva; up to 1 cm
4.18 6.63 FUD 010 J P3 50
AMA: 2018,Feb,11; 2018,Jan,8; 2017,Jan,6; 2016,Feb,12

68115 over 1 cm
5.18 9.19 FUD 010 J A2 50
AMA: 2018,Feb,11; 2016,Feb,12

68130 with adjacent sclera
11.6 15.5 FUD 090 J A2 50
AMA: 2016,Feb,12

68135 Destruction of lesion, conjunctiva
4.24 4.46 FUD 010 J P3 50
AMA: 2016,Feb,12

68200 Subconjunctival injection
EXCLUDES *Retrobulbar or Tenon's capsule injection (67500-67515)*
0.99 1.19 FUD 000 Q1 N1 50
AMA: 2018,Jan,8; 2017,Jan,8; 2016,Feb,12; 2016,Jan,13; 2015,Jan,16

68320-68340 Conjunctivoplasty Procedures

INCLUDES Operating microscope (69990)
EXCLUDES *Conjunctival foreign body removal (65205, 65210)*
Laceration repair (65270-65273)

68320 Conjunctivoplasty; with conjunctival graft or extensive rearrangement
15.3 20.8 FUD 090 J A2 50
AMA: 2018,Jan,8; 2017,Jan,8; 2016,Feb,12; 2016,Jan,13; 2015,Jan,16

68325 with buccal mucous membrane graft (includes obtaining graft)
18.5 18.5 FUD 090 J A2 50
AMA: 2016,Feb,12

68326 Conjunctivoplasty, reconstruction cul-de-sac; with conjunctival graft or extensive rearrangement
18.3 18.3 FUD 090 J A2 50
AMA: 2016,Feb,12

68328 with buccal mucous membrane graft (includes obtaining graft)
20.1 20.1 FUD 090 J A2 80 50
AMA: 2016,Feb,12

68330 Repair of symblepharon; conjunctivoplasty, without graft
13.0 17.4 FUD 090 J A2 80 50
AMA: 2016,Feb,12

68335 with free graft conjunctiva or buccal mucous membrane (includes obtaining graft)
18.4 18.4 FUD 090 J A2 50
AMA: 2016,Feb,12

68340 division of symblepharon, with or without insertion of conformer or contact lens
11.2 16.4 FUD 090 J A2 80 50
AMA: 2016,Feb,12

68360-68399 Conjunctival Flaps and Unlisted Procedures

INCLUDES Operating microscope (69990)

68360 Conjunctival flap; bridge or partial (separate procedure)
EXCLUDES *Conjunctival flap for injury (65280, 65285)*
Conjunctival foreign body removal (65205, 65210)
Surgical wound repair (66250)
11.7 15.3 FUD 090 J A2 50
AMA: 2016,Feb,12

68362 total (such as Gunderson thin flap or purse string flap)
EXCLUDES *Conjunctival flap for injury (65280, 65285)*
Conjunctival foreign body removal (65205, 65210)
Surgical wound repair (66250)
18.5 18.5 FUD 090 J A2 50
AMA: 2018,Jan,8; 2017,Jan,8; 2016,Feb,12; 2016,Jan,13; 2015,Jan,16

68371 Harvesting conjunctival allograft, living donor
11.7 11.7 FUD 010 J A2 50
AMA: 2018,Jan,8; 2017,Jan,8; 2016,Feb,12; 2016,Jan,13; 2015,Jan,16

68399 Unlisted procedure, conjunctiva
0.00 0.00 FUD YYY T 80 50
AMA: 2018,Jan,8; 2017,Jan,8; 2016,Feb,12; 2016,Jan,13; 2015,Jan,16

68400-68899 Nasolacrimal System Procedures

INCLUDES Operating microscope (69990)

68400 Incision, drainage of lacrimal gland
3.76 8.24 **FUD** 010 T P3 50
AMA: 2016,Feb,12

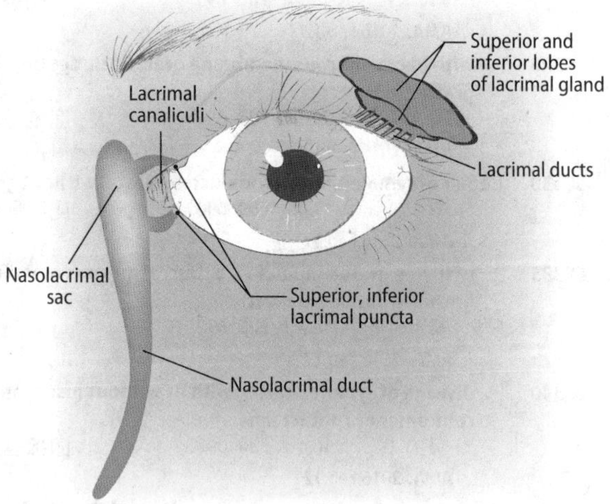

68420 Incision, drainage of lacrimal sac (dacryocystotomy or dacryocystostomy)
4.75 9.35 **FUD** 010 J P3 50
AMA: 2016,Feb,12

68440 Snip incision of lacrimal punctum
2.80 2.92 **FUD** 010 T P3 50
AMA: 2016,Feb,12

68500 Excision of lacrimal gland (dacryoadenectomy), except for tumor; total
28.6 28.6 **FUD** 090 J A2 50
AMA: 2016,Feb,12

68505 partial
28.5 28.5 **FUD** 090 J A2 50
AMA: 2016,Feb,12

68510 Biopsy of lacrimal gland
8.26 12.9 **FUD** 000 J A2 80 50
AMA: 2016,Feb,12

68520 Excision of lacrimal sac (dacryocystectomy)
20.0 20.0 **FUD** 090 J A2 80 50
AMA: 2016,Feb,12

68525 Biopsy of lacrimal sac
7.52 7.52 **FUD** 000 J A2 50
AMA: 2016,Feb,12

68530 Removal of foreign body or dacryolith, lacrimal passages
INCLUDES Meller's excision
7.23 12.2 **FUD** 010 T P2 50
AMA: 2016,Feb,12

68540 Excision of lacrimal gland tumor; frontal approach
27.0 27.0 **FUD** 090 J A2 50
AMA: 2016,Feb,12

68550 involving osteotomy
33.3 33.3 **FUD** 090 J A2 50
AMA: 2016,Feb,12

68700 Plastic repair of canaliculi
17.0 17.0 **FUD** 090 J A2 50
AMA: 2016,Feb,12

68705 Correction of everted punctum, cautery
4.68 7.19 **FUD** 010 T P2 50
AMA: 2020,Feb,13; 2018,Jan,8; 2017,Jan,8; 2016,Feb,12; 2016,Jan,13; 2015,Jan,16

68720 Dacryocystorhinostomy (fistulization of lacrimal sac to nasal cavity)
22.1 22.1 **FUD** 090 J A2 80 50
AMA: 2018,Jan,8; 2017,Jan,8; 2016,Feb,12; 2016,Jan,13; 2015,Jan,16

68745 Conjunctivorhinostomy (fistulization of conjunctiva to nasal cavity); without tube
22.2 22.2 **FUD** 090 J A2 80 50
AMA: 2016,Feb,12

68750 with insertion of tube or stent
22.4 22.4 **FUD** 090 J A2 80 50
AMA: 2018,Jan,8; 2017,Jan,8; 2016,Feb,12; 2016,Jan,13; 2015,Jan,16

68760 Closure of the lacrimal punctum; by thermocauterization, ligation, or laser surgery
4.11 6.07 **FUD** 010 T P2 50
AMA: 2016,Feb,12

68761 by plug, each
EXCLUDES *Drug-eluting lacrimal implant (0356T)*
Drug-eluting ocular insert (0444T-0445T)
3.32 4.20 **FUD** 010 T P3 80 50
AMA: 2018,Jan,8; 2017,Jan,8; 2016,Feb,12; 2016,Jan,13; 2015,Jan,16

68770 Closure of lacrimal fistula (separate procedure)
17.7 17.7 **FUD** 090 J A2 80 50
AMA: 2016,Feb,12

68801 Dilation of lacrimal punctum, with or without irrigation
2.18 2.60 **FUD** 010 Q1 N1 50
AMA: 2016,Feb,12

68810 Probing of nasolacrimal duct, with or without irrigation;
EXCLUDES *Ophthalmological exam under anesthesia (92018)*
3.64 4.47 **FUD** 010 T A2 50
AMA: 2018,Jan,8; 2017,Jan,8; 2016,Feb,12; 2016,Jan,13; 2015,Jan,16

68811 requiring general anesthesia
EXCLUDES *Ophthalmological exam under anesthesia (92018)*
3.82 3.82 **FUD** 010 J A2 50
AMA: 2018,Jan,8; 2017,Jan,8; 2016,Feb,12; 2016,Jan,13; 2015,Jan,16

68815 with insertion of tube or stent
EXCLUDES *Drug-eluting lacrimal implant (0356T)*
Drug-eluting ocular insert (0444T-0445T)
Ophthalmological exam under anesthesia (92018)
6.27 11.0 **FUD** 010 J A2 50
AMA: 2018,Jan,8; 2017,Jan,8; 2016,Feb,12; 2016,Jan,13; 2015,Jan,16

68816 with transluminal balloon catheter dilation
EXCLUDES *Probing nasolacrimal duct (68810-68811, 68815)*
4.45 22.2 **FUD** 010 J G2 50
AMA: 2018,Jan,8; 2017,Jan,8; 2016,Feb,12; 2016,Jan,13; 2015,Jan,16

68840 Probing of lacrimal canaliculi, with or without irrigation
3.27 3.70 **FUD** 010 T P3 50
AMA: 2016,Feb,12

68850 Injection of contrast medium for dacryocystography
(70170, 78660)
1.59 1.80 **FUD** 000 N N1 50
AMA: 2018,Jan,8; 2017,Jan,8; 2016,Feb,12; 2016,Jan,13; 2015,Jan,16

68899 Unlisted procedure, lacrimal system
0.00 0.00 **FUD** YYY T 80 50
AMA: 2014,Jan,11; 1991,Sum,17

69000-69020 Treatment External Abscess/Hematoma

69000 Drainage external ear, abscess or hematoma; simple
3.47 | 5.34 | FUD 010 | T P3 50
AMA: 2018,Jan,8; 2017,Jan,8; 2016,Jan,13; 2015,Jan,16

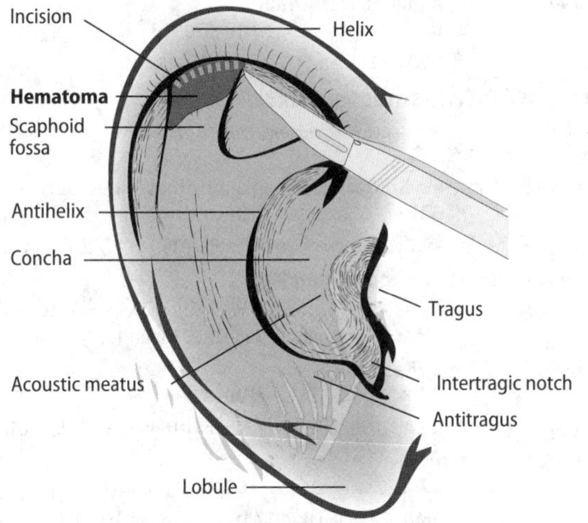

An incision is made to drain the contents of an abscess or hematoma

69005 complicated
4.50 | 6.13 | FUD 010 | J P3 50
AMA: 2014,Jan,11; 1999,Oct,10

69020 Drainage external auditory canal, abscess
4.03 | 6.57 | FUD 010 | T P3 50
AMA: 2018,Jan,8; 2017,Jan,8; 2016,Jan,13; 2015,Jan,16

69090 Cosmetic Ear Piercing

CMS: 100-02,16,10 Exclusions from Coverage; 100-02,16,120 Cosmetic Procedures

69090 Ear piercing
0.00 | 0.00 | FUD XXX | E
AMA: 2014,Jan,11; 1999,Oct,10

69100-69222 External Ear/Auditory Canal Procedures

EXCLUDES *Reconstruction ear (see integumentary section codes)*

69100 Biopsy external ear
1.37 | 2.79 | FUD 000 | T P3
AMA: 2019,Jan,9

69105 Biopsy external auditory canal
1.78 | 4.00 | FUD 000 | T P3 50
AMA: 2014,Jan,11; 1999,Oct,10

69110 Excision external ear; partial, simple repair
9.21 | 13.0 | FUD 090 | J A2 50
AMA: 2014,Jan,11; 1999,Oct,10

69120 complete amputation
11.1 | 11.1 | FUD 090 | J A2
AMA: 2014,Jan,11; 1999,Oct,10

69140 Excision exostosis(es), external auditory canal
24.8 | 24.8 | FUD 090 | J A2 80 50
AMA: 2014,Jan,11; 1999,Oct,10

69145 Excision soft tissue lesion, external auditory canal
7.04 | 11.1 | FUD 090 | J A2 50
AMA: 2019,Dec,14

69150 Radical excision external auditory canal lesion; without neck dissection
EXCLUDES *Skin graft (15004-15261)*
Temporal bone resection (69535)
29.5 | 29.5 | FUD 090 | J A2
AMA: 2014,Jan,11; 2003,Jan,1

69155 with neck dissection
EXCLUDES *Skin graft (15004-15261)*
Temporal bone resection (69535)
47.0 | 47.0 | FUD 090 | C 80
AMA: 2014,Jan,11; 1999,Oct,10

69200 Removal foreign body from external auditory canal; without general anesthesia
1.35 | 2.31 | FUD 000 | Q1 N1 50
AMA: 2014,Jan,11; 1999,Oct,10

69205 with general anesthesia
2.77 | 2.77 | FUD 010 | J A2 50
AMA: 2018,Jan,8; 2017,Jan,8; 2016,Jan,13; 2015,Jan,16

69209 Removal impacted cerumen using irrigation/lavage, unilateral
EXCLUDES *Removal impacted cerumen using instrumentation (69210)*
Removal nonimpacted cerumen (see appropriate E/M code(s)) (99202-99233 [99224, 99225, 99226], 99241-99255, 99281-99285, 99304-99318, 99324-99337, 99341-99350)
0.40 | 0.40 | FUD 000 | Q1 N1 50
AMA: 2018,Jan,8; 2017,Jan,8; 2016,Mar,10; 2016,Feb,13; 2016,Jan,7

69210 Removal impacted cerumen requiring instrumentation, unilateral
EXCLUDES *Removal impacted cerumen using irrigation or lavage (69209)*
Removal nonimpacted cerumen (see appropriate E/M code(s)) (99202-99233 [99224, 99225, 99226], 99241-99255, 99281-99285, 99304-99318, 99324-99337, 99341-99350)
0.96 | 1.36 | FUD 000 | Q1 N1
AMA: 2018,Jan,8; 2017,Jan,8; 2016,Mar,10; 2016,Feb,13; 2016,Jan,13; 2016,Jan,7; 2015,Jan,16

69220 Debridement, mastoidectomy cavity, simple (eg, routine cleaning)
1.46 | 2.25 | FUD 000 | Q1 N1 50
AMA: 2014,Jan,11; 1999,Oct,10

69222 Debridement, mastoidectomy cavity, complex (eg, with anesthesia or more than routine cleaning)
3.81 | 6.02 | FUD 010 | T P3 50
AMA: 2014,Jan,11; 1999,Oct,10

69300 Plastic Surgery for Prominent Ears

CMS: 100-02,16,120 Cosmetic Procedures; 100-02,16,180 Services Related to Noncovered Procedures

EXCLUDES *Suture laceration external ear (12011-14302)*

69300 Otoplasty, protruding ear, with or without size reduction
13.8 | 18.1 | FUD YYY | J A2 80 50
AMA: 2014,Jan,11; 1999,Oct,10

69310-69399 Reconstruction Auditory Canal: Postaural Approach

EXCLUDES *Suture laceration external ear (12011-14302)*

69310 Reconstruction of external auditory canal (meatoplasty) (eg, for stenosis due to injury, infection) (separate procedure)
30.9 | 30.9 | FUD 090 | J A2 50
AMA: 2018,Jan,8; 2017,Jan,8; 2016,Jan,13; 2015,Jan,16

69320 Reconstruction external auditory canal for congenital atresia, single stage
EXCLUDES *Other reconstruction surgery with graft (13151-15760, 21230-21235)*
Tympanoplasty (69631, 69641)
43.4 | 43.4 | FUD 090 | J A2 80 50
AMA: 2014,Jan,11; 1999,Oct,10

69399 Unlisted procedure, external ear
EXCLUDES *Otoscopy under general anesthesia (92502)*
0.00 | 0.00 | FUD YYY | T 80
AMA: 2014,Jan,11; 1999,Oct,10

69420-69450 Ear Drum Procedures

69420 Myringotomy including aspiration and/or eustachian tube inflation
3.39 | 5.31 | **FUD** 010 | T P2 50
AMA: 2018,Jan,8; 2017,Jan,8; 2016,Jan,13; 2015,Jan,16

69421 Myringotomy including aspiration and/or eustachian tube inflation requiring general anesthesia
4.21 | 4.21 | **FUD** 010 | J A2 50
AMA: 2018,Jan,8; 2017,Jan,8; 2016,Jan,13; 2015,Jan,16

69424 Ventilating tube removal requiring general anesthesia
EXCLUDES *Cochlear device implantation (69930)*
Eardrum repair (69610-69646)
Foreign body removal (69205)
Implantation, replacement electromagnetic bone conduction hearing device in temporal bone (69710-69745)
Labyrinth procedures (69801-69915)
Mastoid obliteration (69670)
Myringotomy (69420-69421)
Polyp, glomus tumor removal (69535-69554)
Removal impacted cerumen requiring instrumentation (69210)
Repair window (69666-69667)
Revised mastoidectomy (69601-69604)
Stapes procedures (69650-69662)
Transmastoid excision (69501-69530)
Tympanic neurectomy (69676)
Tympanostomy, tympanolysis (69433-69450)
1.73 | 3.62 | **FUD** 000 | Q2 P3 50
AMA: 2018,Jan,8; 2017,Jan,8; 2016,Jan,13; 2015,Jan,16

69433 Tympanostomy (requiring insertion of ventilating tube), local or topical anesthesia
EXCLUDES *Tympanostomy with tube insertion using iontophoresis and automated tube delivery system (0583T)*
3.72 | 5.62 | **FUD** 010 | T P3 50
AMA: 2018,Feb,11; 2018,Jan,8; 2017,Jan,8; 2016,Jan,13; 2015,Jan,16

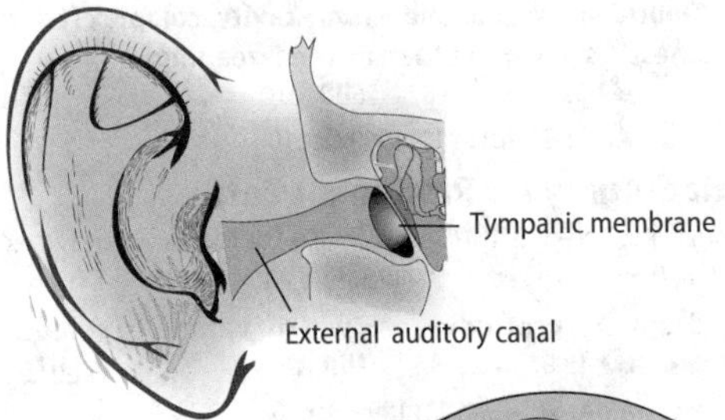

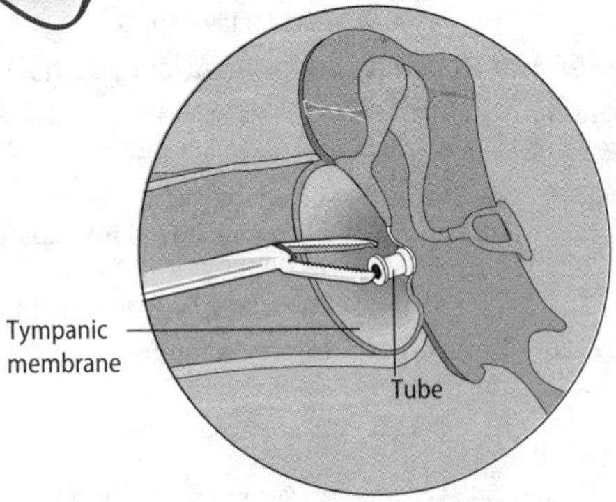

69436 Tympanostomy (requiring insertion of ventilating tube), general anesthesia
4.51 | 4.51 | **FUD** 010 | T A2 50
AMA: 2018,Feb,11; 2018,Jan,8; 2017,Jan,8; 2016,Jan,13; 2015,Jan,16

69440 Middle ear exploration through postauricular or ear canal incision
EXCLUDES *Atticotomy (69601-69604)*
19.5 | 19.5 | **FUD** 090 | J A2 50
AMA: 2014,Jan,11; 2008,Sep,10 -11

69450 Tympanolysis, transcanal
15.4 | 15.4 | **FUD** 090 | J A2 80 50
AMA: 2014,Jan,11; 2008,Sep,10 -11

69501-69530 Transmastoid Excision

EXCLUDES *Mastoidectomy cavity debridement (69220, 69222)*
Skin graft (15004-15770)

69501 Transmastoid antrotomy (simple mastoidectomy)
20.3 | 20.3 | **FUD** 090 | J A2 50
AMA: 2018,Jan,8; 2017,Jan,8; 2016,Jan,13; 2015,Jan,16

69502 Mastoidectomy; complete
27.3 | 27.3 | **FUD** 090 | J A2 80 50
AMA: 2018,Jan,8; 2017,Jan,8; 2016,Jan,13; 2015,Jan,16

69505 modified radical
34.2 | 34.2 | **FUD** 090 | J A2 80 50
AMA: 2018,Jan,8; 2017,Jan,8; 2016,Jan,13; 2015,Jan,16

69511 radical
35.0 | 35.0 | **FUD** 090 | J A2 80 50
AMA: 2018,Jan,8; 2017,Jan,8; 2016,Jan,13; 2015,Jan,16

69530 Petrous apicectomy including radical mastoidectomy
47.1 | 47.1 | **FUD** 090 | J A2 80 50
AMA: 2014,Jan,11; 1999,Oct,10

69535-69554 Polyp and Glomus Tumor Removal

69535 Resection temporal bone, external approach
EXCLUDES *Middle fossa approach (69950-69970)*
75.4 | 75.4 | **FUD** 090 | C 50
AMA: 2014,Jan,11; 1999,Oct,10

69540 Excision aural polyp
3.58 | 5.83 | **FUD** 010 | T P3 50
AMA: 2014,Jan,11; 1999,Oct,10

69550 Excision aural glomus tumor; transcanal
29.5 | 29.5 | **FUD** 090 | J A2 80 50
AMA: 2014,Jan,11; 1999,Oct,10

69552 transmastoid
44.6 | 44.6 | **FUD** 090 | J A2 80 50
AMA: 2014,Jan,11; 1999,Oct,10

69554 extended (extratemporal)
71.5 | 71.5 | **FUD** 090 | C 80 50
AMA: 2014,Jan,11; 1999,Oct,10

69601-69605 Revised Mastoidectomy

EXCLUDES *Skin graft (15120-15121, 15260-15261)*

69601 Revision mastoidectomy; resulting in complete mastoidectomy
29.5 | 29.5 | **FUD** 090 | J A2 80 50
AMA: 2018,Jan,8; 2017,Jan,8; 2016,Jan,13; 2015,Jan,16

69602 resulting in modified radical mastoidectomy
30.8 | 30.8 | **FUD** 090 | J A2 80 50
AMA: 2018,Jan,8; 2017,Jan,8; 2016,Jan,13; 2015,Jan,16

69603 resulting in radical mastoidectomy
35.9 | 35.9 | **FUD** 090 | J A2 80 50
AMA: 2018,Jan,8; 2017,Jan,8; 2016,Jan,13; 2015,Jan,16

69604 resulting in tympanoplasty
EXCLUDES *Secondary tympanoplasty following mastoidectomy (69631-69632)*
31.5 | 31.5 | **FUD** 090 | J A2 50
AMA: 2018,Jan,8; 2017,Jan,8; 2016,Jan,13; 2015,Jan,16

69605 ~~**with apicectomy**~~

69610-69646 Eardrum Repair with/without Other Procedures

69610 **Tympanic membrane repair, with or without site preparation of perforation for closure, with or without patch**
8.27 10.8 FUD 010 J P3 50
AMA: 2018,Jan,8; 2017,Jan,8; 2016,Jan,13; 2015,May,10; 2015,Apr,10; 2015,Jan,16

69620 **Myringoplasty (surgery confined to drumhead and donor area)**
13.9 20.0 FUD 090 J A2 50
AMA: 2018,Jan,8; 2017,Jan,8; 2016,Jan,13; 2015,May,10; 2015,Apr,10; 2015,Jan,16

69631 **Tympanoplasty without mastoidectomy (including canalplasty, atticotomy and/or middle ear surgery), initial or revision; without ossicular chain reconstruction**
25.0 25.0 FUD 090 J A2 50
AMA: 2018,Jan,8; 2017,Jan,8; 2016,Jan,13; 2015,Jan,16

69632 **with ossicular chain reconstruction (eg, postfenestration)**
30.5 30.5 FUD 090 J A2 50
AMA: 2018,Jan,8; 2017,Jan,8; 2016,Jan,13; 2015,Jan,16

69633 **with ossicular chain reconstruction and synthetic prosthesis (eg, partial ossicular replacement prosthesis [PORP], total ossicular replacement prosthesis [TORP])**
29.6 29.6 FUD 090 J A2 50
AMA: 2018,Jan,8; 2017,Jan,8; 2016,Jan,13; 2015,Jan,16

69635 **Tympanoplasty with antrotomy or mastoidotomy (including canalplasty, atticotomy, middle ear surgery, and/or tympanic membrane repair); without ossicular chain reconstruction**
35.3 35.3 FUD 090 J A2 50
AMA: 2018,Jan,8; 2017,Jan,8; 2016,Jan,13; 2015,Jan,16

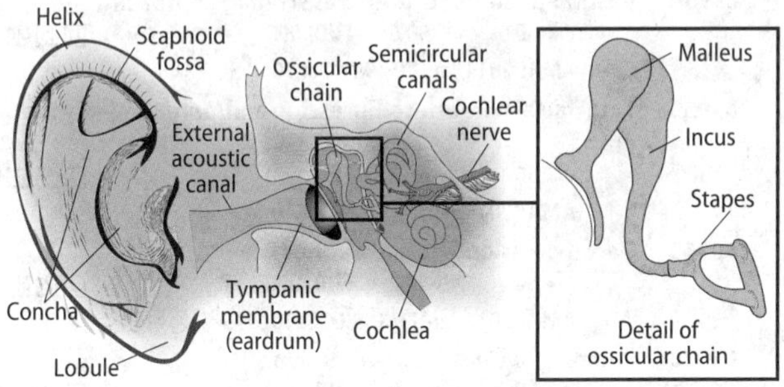

69636 **with ossicular chain reconstruction**
39.3 39.3 FUD 090 J A2 80 50
AMA: 2018,Jan,8; 2017,Jan,8; 2016,Jan,13; 2015,Jan,16

69637 **with ossicular chain reconstruction and synthetic prosthesis (eg, partial ossicular replacement prosthesis [PORP], total ossicular replacement prosthesis [TORP])**
39.9 39.9 FUD 090 J A2 80 50
AMA: 2018,Jan,8; 2017,Jan,8; 2016,Jan,13; 2015,Jan,16

69641 **Tympanoplasty with mastoidectomy (including canalplasty, middle ear surgery, tympanic membrane repair); without ossicular chain reconstruction**
29.6 29.6 FUD 090 J A2 50
AMA: 2018,Jan,8; 2017,Jan,8; 2016,Jan,13; 2015,Jan,16

69642 **with ossicular chain reconstruction**
38.0 38.0 FUD 090 J A2 50
AMA: 2018,Jan,8; 2017,Jan,8; 2016,Jan,13; 2015,Jan,16

69643 **with intact or reconstructed wall, without ossicular chain reconstruction**
34.7 34.7 FUD 090 J A2 50
AMA: 2018,Jan,8; 2017,Jan,8; 2016,Jan,13; 2015,Jan,16

69644 **with intact or reconstructed canal wall, with ossicular chain reconstruction**
42.1 42.1 FUD 090 J A2 50
AMA: 2018,Jan,8; 2017,Jan,8; 2016,Jan,13; 2015,Jan,16

69645 **radical or complete, without ossicular chain reconstruction**
41.4 41.4 FUD 090 J A2 50
AMA: 2018,Jan,8; 2017,Jan,8; 2016,Jan,13; 2015,Jan,16

69646 **radical or complete, with ossicular chain reconstruction**
44.1 44.1 FUD 090 J A2 80 50
AMA: 2018,Jan,8; 2017,Jan,8; 2016,Jan,13; 2015,Jan,16

69650-69662 Stapes Procedures

69650 **Stapes mobilization**
22.8 22.8 FUD 090 J A2 50
AMA: 2014,Jan,11; 1999,Oct,10

69660 **Stapedectomy or stapedotomy with reestablishment of ossicular continuity, with or without use of foreign material;**
26.3 26.3 FUD 090 J A2 50
AMA: 2014,Jan,11; 1999,Oct,10

69661 **with footplate drill out**
34.3 34.3 FUD 090 J A2 80 50
AMA: 2014,Jan,11; 1999,Oct,10

69662 **Revision of stapedectomy or stapedotomy**
32.9 32.9 FUD 090 J A2 50
AMA: 2014,Jan,11; 1999,Oct,10

69666-69706 Other Inner Ear Procedures

69666 **Repair oval window fistula**
22.9 22.9 FUD 090 J A2 80 50
AMA: 2014,Jan,11; 1999,Oct,10

69667 **Repair round window fistula**
23.0 23.0 FUD 090 J A2 80 50
AMA: 2014,Jan,11; 1999,Oct,10

69670 **Mastoid obliteration (separate procedure)**
26.8 26.8 FUD 090 J A2 80 50
AMA: 2014,Jan,11; 1999,Oct,10

69676 **Tympanic neurectomy**
23.6 23.6 FUD 090 J A2 50
AMA: 2014,Jan,11; 1999,Oct,10

69700 **Closure postauricular fistula, mastoid (separate procedure)**
19.3 19.3 FUD 090 T A2 50
AMA: 2014,Jan,11; 1999,Oct,10

● **69705** **Nasopharyngoscopy, surgical, with dilation of eustachian tube (ie, balloon dilation); unilateral**
EXCLUDES *Nasal endoscopy, diagnostic (31231)*
Nasopharyngoscopy with endoscope (92511)

● **69706** **bilateral**
EXCLUDES *Nasal endoscopy, diagnostic (31231)*
Nasopharyngoscopy with endoscope (92511)

69710-69718 Procedures Related to Hearing Aids/Auditory Implants

CMS: 100-02,16,100 Hearing Devices

69710 **Implantation or replacement of electromagnetic bone conduction hearing device in temporal bone**
INCLUDES Removal existing device when performing replacement procedure
0.00 0.00 FUD XXX E
AMA: 2014,Jan,11; 1999,Oct,10

69711 **Removal or repair of electromagnetic bone conduction hearing device in temporal bone**
24.2 24.2 FUD 090 J A2 80 50
AMA: 2014,Jan,11; 1999,Oct,10

69714 **Implantation, osseointegrated implant, temporal bone, with percutaneous attachment to external speech processor/cochlear stimulator; without mastoidectomy**
30.4 30.4 FUD 090 J J8 50
AMA: 2018,Jan,8; 2017,Jan,8; 2016,Jan,13; 2015,Jan,16

69715 with mastoidectomy
37.6 37.6 **FUD** 090 J J8 50
AMA: 2014,Jan,11; 1999,Oct,10

69717 Replacement (including removal of existing device), osseointegrated implant, temporal bone, with percutaneous attachment to external speech processor/cochlear stimulator; without mastoidectomy
31.9 31.9 **FUD** 090 J J8 50
AMA: 2014,Jan,11; 1999,Oct,10

69718 with mastoidectomy
38.0 38.0 **FUD** 090 J G2 50
AMA: 2014,Jan,11; 1999,Oct,10

69720-69799 Procedures of the Facial Nerve

EXCLUDES *Extracranial suture facial nerve (64864)*

69720 Decompression facial nerve, intratemporal; lateral to geniculate ganglion
34.1 34.1 **FUD** 090 J A2 80 50
AMA: 2014,Jan,11; 1999,Oct,10

69725 including medial to geniculate ganglion
53.5 53.5 **FUD** 090 J 80 50
AMA: 2014,Jan,11; 1999,Oct,10

69740 Suture facial nerve, intratemporal, with or without graft or decompression; lateral to geniculate ganglion
33.2 33.2 **FUD** 090 J A2 80 50
AMA: 2014,Jan,11; 1999,Oct,10

69745 including medial to geniculate ganglion
35.2 35.2 **FUD** 090 J A2 80 50
AMA: 2014,Jan,11; 1999,Oct,10

69799 Unlisted procedure, middle ear
0.00 0.00 **FUD** YYY T 80 50
AMA: 2019,Jan,14; 2018,Jan,8; 2017,Jan,8; 2016,Jan,13; 2015,Jan,16

69801-69915 Procedures of the Labyrinth

69801 Labyrinthotomy, with perfusion of vestibuloactive drug(s), transcanal
EXCLUDES *Myringotomy, tympanostomy on same ear (69420-69421, 69433, 69436)*
Procedure performed more than one time per day
3.55 6.05 **FUD** 000 T P3 80 50
AMA: 2018,Jan,8; 2017,Jan,8; 2016,Jan,13; 2015,Jan,16

69805 Endolymphatic sac operation; without shunt
29.8 29.8 **FUD** 090 J A2 80 50
AMA: 2014,Jan,11; 1999,Oct,10

69806 with shunt
26.6 26.6 **FUD** 090 J A2 50
AMA: 2014,Jan,11; 1999,Oct,10

69905 Labyrinthectomy; transcanal
26.0 26.0 **FUD** 090 J A2 50
AMA: 2014,Jan,11; 1999,Oct,10

69910 with mastoidectomy
28.7 28.7 **FUD** 090 J A2 80 50
AMA: 2014,Jan,11; 1999,Oct,10

69915 Vestibular nerve section, translabyrinthine approach
EXCLUDES *Transcranial approach (69950)*
43.6 43.6 **FUD** 090 J A2 80 50
AMA: 2014,Jan,11; 1999,Oct,10

69930-69949 Cochlear Implantation

CMS: 100-02,16,100 Hearing Devices

69930 Cochlear device implantation, with or without mastoidectomy
34.8 34.8 **FUD** 090 J J8 80 50
AMA: 2014,Jan,11; 1999,Oct,10

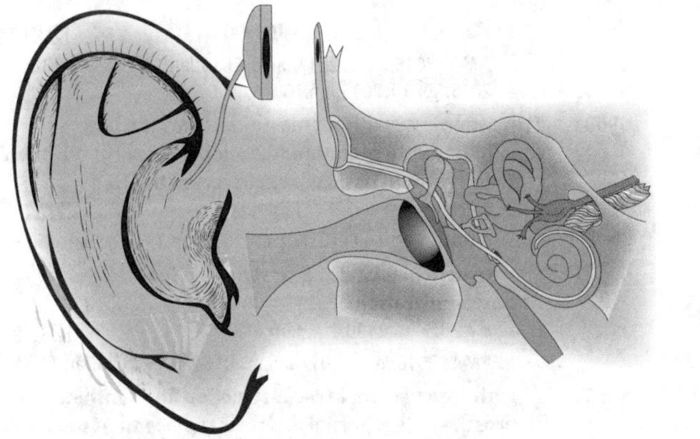

The internal coil is secured to the temporal bone and an electrode is fed through the round window into the cochlea

69949 Unlisted procedure, inner ear
0.00 0.00 **FUD** YYY T 80 50
AMA: 2014,Jan,11; 1999,Oct,10

69950-69979 Inner Ear Procedures via Craniotomy

EXCLUDES *External approach (69535)*

69950 Vestibular nerve section, transcranial approach
50.6 50.6 **FUD** 090 C 80 50
AMA: 2014,Jan,11; 1999,Oct,10

69955 Total facial nerve decompression and/or repair (may include graft)
56.1 56.1 **FUD** 090 J 80 50
AMA: 2014,Jan,11; 1999,Oct,10

69960 Decompression internal auditory canal
54.2 54.2 **FUD** 090 J 80 50
AMA: 2014,Jan,11; 1999,Oct,10

69970 Removal of tumor, temporal bone
60.8 60.8 **FUD** 090 J 80 50
AMA: 2014,Jan,11; 1999,Oct,10

69979 Unlisted procedure, temporal bone, middle fossa approach
0.00 0.00 **FUD** YYY T 80 50
AMA: 2018,Jan,8; 2017,Jan,8; 2016,Jan,13; 2015,Jan,16

69990 Operating Microscope

EXCLUDES *Magnifying loupes*
Reporting code with (15756-15758, 15842, 19364, 19368, 20955-20962, 20969-20973, 22551-22552, 22856-22857 [22858], 22861, 26551-26554, 26556, 31526, 31531, 31536, 31541-31546, 31561, 31571, 43116, 43180, 43496, 46601, 46607, 49906, 61548, 63075-63078, 64727, 64820-64823, 64912-64913, 65091-68850 [66987, 66988, 67810], 0184T, 0308T, 0402T, 0583T)

\+ **69990** Microsurgical techniques, requiring use of operating microscope (List separately in addition to code for primary procedure)
Code first primary procedure
6.30 6.30 **FUD** ZZZ N N1 80
AMA: 2018,Feb,11; 2018,Jan,8; 2017,Dec,12; 2017,Dec,13; 2017,Dec,14; 2017,Jan,8; 2016,Feb,12; 2016,Jan,13; 2015,Jan,16

70010-70015 Radiography: Neurodiagnostic

70010 Myelography, posterior fossa, radiological supervision and interpretation
1.73 1.73 FUD XXX Q2 N1 80
AMA: 2018,Jan,8; 2017,Jan,8; 2016,Jan,13; 2015,Jan,16

70015 Cisternography, positive contrast, radiological supervision and interpretation
4.35 4.35 FUD XXX Q2 N1 80
AMA: 2014,Jan,11; 2012,Feb,9-10

70030-70390 Radiography: Head, Neck, Orofacial Structures

INCLUDES Minimum number views or more views when needed to adequately complete study
Radiographs repeated during encounter due to substandard quality; only one unit reported

EXCLUDES *Obtaining more films after initial film review, based on radiologist discretion, order for test, and change in patient's condition*

70030 Radiologic examination, eye, for detection of foreign body
0.87 0.87 FUD XXX Q1 N1 80
AMA: 2014,Jan,11; 2012,Feb,9-10

70100 Radiologic examination, mandible; partial, less than 4 views
1.03 1.03 FUD XXX Q1 N1 80
AMA: 2014,Jan,11; 2012,Feb,9-10

70110 complete, minimum of 4 views
1.13 1.13 FUD XXX Q1 N1 80
AMA: 2014,Jan,11; 2012,Feb,9-10

70120 Radiologic examination, mastoids; less than 3 views per side
1.03 1.03 FUD XXX Q1 N1 80
AMA: 2014,Jan,11; 2012,Feb,9-10

70130 complete, minimum of 3 views per side
1.68 1.68 FUD XXX Q1 N1 80
AMA: 2014,Jan,11; 2012,Feb,9-10

70134 Radiologic examination, internal auditory meati, complete
1.59 1.59 FUD XXX Q1 N1 80
AMA: 2014,Jan,11; 2012,Feb,9-10

70140 Radiologic examination, facial bones; less than 3 views
0.88 0.88 FUD XXX Q1 N1 80
AMA: 2014,Jan,11; 2012,Feb,9-10

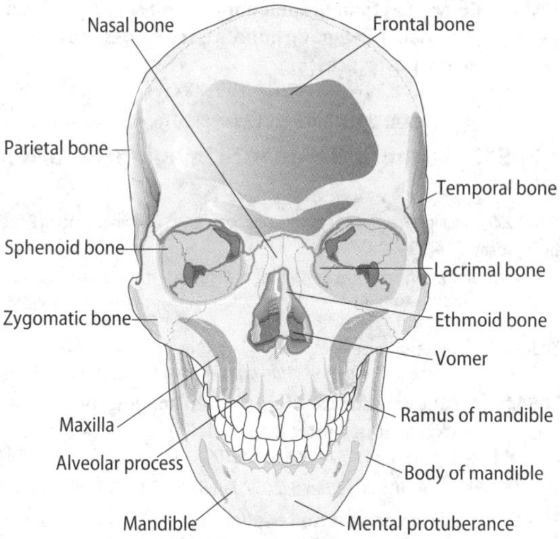

70150 complete, minimum of 3 views
1.23 1.23 FUD XXX Q1 N1 80
AMA: 2014,Jan,11; 2012,Feb,9-10

70160 Radiologic examination, nasal bones, complete, minimum of 3 views
1.02 1.02 FUD XXX Q1 N1 80
AMA: 2014,Jan,11; 2012,Feb,9-10

70170 Dacryocystography, nasolacrimal duct, radiological supervision and interpretation
EXCLUDES *Injection contrast (68850)*
0.00 0.00 FUD XXX Q2 N1 80
AMA: 2014,Jan,11; 2012,Feb,9-10

70190 Radiologic examination; optic foramina
1.08 1.08 FUD XXX Q1 N1 80
AMA: 2014,Jan,11; 2012,Feb,9-10

70200 orbits, complete, minimum of 4 views
1.31 1.31 FUD XXX Q1 N1 80
AMA: 2014,Jan,11; 2012,Feb,9-10

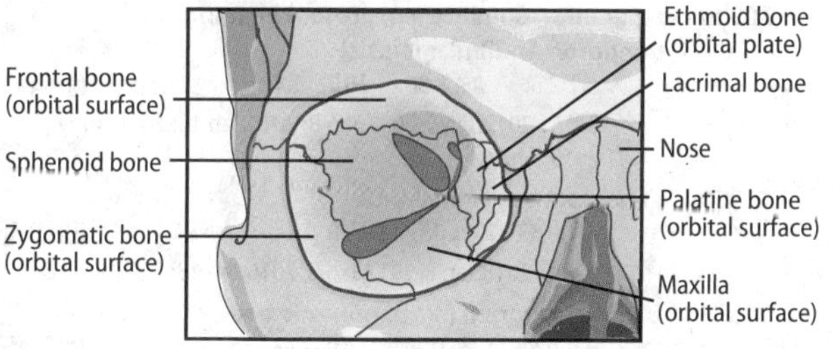

70210 Radiologic examination, sinuses, paranasal, less than 3 views
0.89 0.89 FUD XXX Q1 N1 80
AMA: 2014,Jan,11; 2012,Feb,9-10

70220 Radiologic examination, sinuses, paranasal, complete, minimum of 3 views
1.10 1.10 FUD XXX Q1 N1 80
AMA: 2014,Jan,11; 2012,Feb,9-10

70240 Radiologic examination, sella turcica
0.94 0.94 FUD XXX Q1 N1 80
AMA: 2014,Jan,11; 2012,Feb,9-10

70250 X-ray of skull, fewer than 4 views
1.07 1.07 FUD XXX Q1 N1 80
AMA: 2014,Jan,11; 2012,Feb,9-10

70260 complete, minimum of 4 views
1.24 1.24 FUD XXX Q1 N1 80
AMA: 2014,Jan,11; 2012,Feb,9-10

70300 Radiologic examination, teeth; single view
0.39 0.39 FUD XXX Q1 N1 80
AMA: 2014,Jan,11; 2012,Feb,9-10

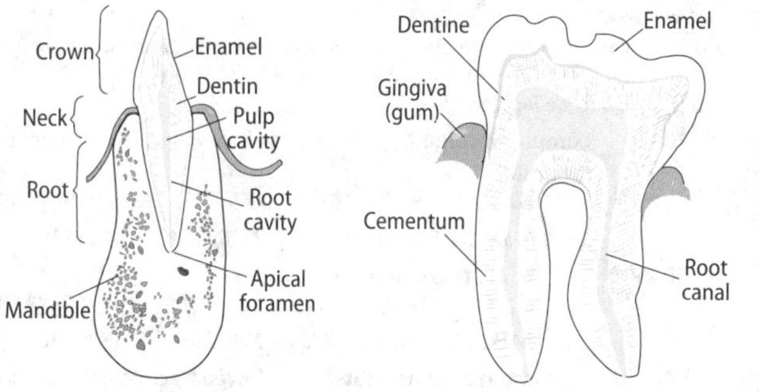

Section of incisor Section of molar

70310 partial examination, less than full mouth
1.10 1.10 FUD XXX Q1 N1 80
AMA: 2014,Jan,11; 2012,Feb,9-10

70320 complete, full mouth
1.56 1.56 FUD XXX Q1 N1 80
AMA: 2014,Jan,11; 2012,Feb,9-10

70328 **Radiologic examination, temporomandibular joint, open and closed mouth; unilateral**
Facility RVU 0.94 Non-Facility RVU 0.94 FUD XXX Q1 N1 80
AMA: 2014,Jan,11; 2012,Feb,9-10

70330 **bilateral**
1.45 1.45 FUD XXX Q1 N1 80
AMA: 2018,Jan,8; 2017,Jan,8; 2016,Jan,13; 2015,Jan,16

70332 **Temporomandibular joint arthrography, radiological supervision and interpretation**
INCLUDES Fluoroscopic guidance (77002)
2.15 2.15 FUD XXX Q2 N1 80
AMA: 2018,Jan,8; 2017,Jan,8; 2016,Jan,13; 2015,Jan,16

70336 **Magnetic resonance (eg, proton) imaging, temporomandibular joint(s)**
8.86 8.86 FUD XXX Q3 Z2 80
AMA: 2018,Jan,8; 2017,Jan,8; 2016,Jan,13; 2015,Aug,6; 2015,Jan,16

70350 **Cephalogram, orthodontic**
0.53 0.53 FUD XXX Q1 N1 80
AMA: 2018,Jan,8; 2017,Jan,8; 2016,Jan,13; 2015,Jan,16

70355 **Orthopantogram (eg, panoramic x-ray)**
0.54 0.54 FUD XXX Q1 N1 80
AMA: 2014,Jan,11; 2012,Feb,9-10

70360 **Radiologic examination; neck, soft tissue**
0.86 0.86 FUD XXX Q1 N1 80
AMA: 2014,Jan,11; 2012,Feb,9-10

70370 **pharynx or larynx, including fluoroscopy and/or magnification technique**
2.49 2.49 FUD XXX Q1 N1 80
AMA: 2014,Jan,11; 2012,Feb,9-10

70371 **Complex dynamic pharyngeal and speech evaluation by cine or video recording**
EXCLUDES *Laryngeal computed tomography (70490-70492)*
3.03 3.03 FUD XXX Q1 N1 80
AMA: 2018,Jan,8; 2017,Jan,8; 2016,Jan,13; 2015,Jan,16

70380 **Radiologic examination, salivary gland for calculus**
0.95 0.95 FUD XXX Q1 N1 80
AMA: 2014,Jan,11; 2012,Feb,9-10

70390 **Sialography, radiological supervision and interpretation**
3.16 3.16 FUD XXX Q2 N1 80
AMA: 2014,Jan,11; 2012,Feb,9-10

70450-70492 Computerized Tomography: Head, Neck, Face

CMS: 100-04,4,250.16 Multiple Procedure Payment Reduction: Certain Diagnostic Imaging Procedures Rendered by Physicians

INCLUDES Imaging using tomographic technique enhanced by computer imaging to create cross-sectional body plane view
EXCLUDES *3D rendering (76376-76377)*

70450 **Computed tomography, head or brain; without contrast material**
3.26 3.26 FUD XXX Q3 Z2 80
AMA: 2018,Jan,8; 2017,Jan,8; 2016,Jan,13; 2015,Jan,16

70460 **with contrast material(s)**
4.61 4.61 FUD XXX Q3 Z2 80
AMA: 2018,Jan,8; 2017,Jan,8; 2016,Jan,13; 2015,Jan,16

70470 **without contrast material, followed by contrast material(s) and further sections**
5.38 5.38 FUD XXX Q3 Z2 80
AMA: 2018,Jan,8; 2017,Jan,8; 2016,Jan,13; 2015,Jan,16

70480 **Computed tomography, orbit, sella, or posterior fossa or outer, middle, or inner ear; without contrast material**
5.64 5.64 FUD XXX Q3 Z2 80
AMA: 2018,Jan,8; 2017,Jan,8; 2016,Jan,13; 2015,Jan,16

70481 **with contrast material(s)**
7.76 7.76 FUD XXX Q3 Z2 80
AMA: 2018,Jan,8; 2017,Jan,8; 2016,Jan,13; 2015,Jan,16

70482 **without contrast material, followed by contrast material(s) and further sections**
6.97 6.97 FUD XXX Q3 Z2 80
AMA: 2014,Jan,11; 2012,Feb,9-10

70486 **Computed tomography, maxillofacial area; without contrast material**
3.92 3.92 FUD XXX Q3 Z2 80
AMA: 2018,Jan,8; 2017,Jan,8; 2016,Jan,13; 2015,Jan,16

70487 **with contrast material(s)**
4.70 4.70 FUD XXX Q3 Z2 80
AMA: 2014,Jan,11; 2012,Feb,9-10

70488 **without contrast material, followed by contrast material(s) and further sections**
5.73 5.73 FUD XXX Q3 Z2 80
AMA: 2014,Jan,11; 2012,Feb,9-10

70490 **Computed tomography, soft tissue neck; without contrast material**
EXCLUDES *CT cervical spine (72125)*
4.63 4.63 FUD XXX Q3 Z2 80
AMA: 2014,Jan,11; 2012,Feb,9-10

70491 **with contrast material(s)**
EXCLUDES *CT cervical spine (72125)*
5.71 5.71 FUD XXX Q3 Z2 80
AMA: 2014,Jan,11; 2012,Feb,9-10

70492 **without contrast material followed by contrast material(s) and further sections**
EXCLUDES *CT cervical spine (72125)*
6.89 6.89 FUD XXX Q3 Z2 80
AMA: 2014,Jan,11; 2012,Feb,9-10

70496-70498 Computerized Tomographic Angiography: Head and Neck

CMS: 100-04,4,250.16 Multiple Procedure Payment Reduction: Certain Diagnostic Imaging Procedures Rendered by Physicians

INCLUDES Computed tomography to visualize arterial and venous vessels

70496 **Computed tomographic angiography, head, with contrast material(s), including noncontrast images, if performed, and image postprocessing**
8.31 8.31 FUD XXX Q3 Z2 80
AMA: 2018,Jan,8; 2017,Jan,8; 2016,Jan,13; 2015,Jan,16

70498 **Computed tomographic angiography, neck, with contrast material(s), including noncontrast images, if performed, and image postprocessing**
8.29 8.29 FUD XXX Q3 Z2 80
AMA: 2018,Jan,8; 2017,Jan,8; 2016,Jan,13; 2015,Jan,16

70540-70543 Magnetic Resonance Imaging: Face, Neck, Orbits

CMS: 100-04,4,250.16 Multiple Procedure Payment Reduction: Certain Diagnostic Imaging Procedures Rendered by Physicians

INCLUDES Three-dimensional imaging that measures response oatomic nuclei in soft tissues to high-frequency radio waves when strong magnetic field applied
EXCLUDES *Magnetic resonance angiography head/neck (70544-70549)*
Procedure performed more than one time per session

70540 **Magnetic resonance (eg, proton) imaging, orbit, face, and/or neck; without contrast material(s)**
7.34 7.34 FUD XXX Q3 Z2 80
AMA: 2018,Jan,8; 2017,Jan,8; 2016,Jan,13; 2015,Jan,16

70542 **with contrast material(s)**
8.72 8.72 FUD XXX Q3 Z2 80
AMA: 2018,Jan,8; 2017,Jan,8; 2016,Jan,13; 2015,Jan,16

70543 **without contrast material(s), followed by contrast material(s) and further sequences**
11.1 11.1 FUD XXX Q3 Z2 80
AMA: 2018,Jan,8; 2017,Jan,8; 2016,Jan,13; 2015,Jan,16

70544-70549 Magnetic Resonance Angiography: Head and Neck

CMS: 100-04,13,40.1.1 Magnetic Resonance Angiography; 100-04,13,40.1.2 HCPCS Coding Requirements; 100-04,4,250.16 Multiple Procedure Payment Reduction: Certain Diagnostic Imaging Procedures Rendered by Physicians

INCLUDES Magnetic fields and radio waves to produce detailed cross-sectional internal body structure images

EXCLUDES *Reporting code with following unless separate diagnostic MRI performed (70551-70553)*

70544 Magnetic resonance angiography, head; without contrast material(s)
7.84 7.84 FUD XXX 03 Z2 80
AMA: 2018,Jan,8; 2017,Jan,8; 2016,Jan,13; 2015,Jan,16

70545 with contrast material(s)
7.21 7.21 FUD XXX 03 Z2 80
AMA: 2018,Jan,8; 2017,Jan,8; 2016,Jan,13; 2015,Jan,16

70546 without contrast material(s), followed by contrast material(s) and further sequences
10.4 10.4 FUD XXX 03 Z2 80
AMA: 2018,Jan,8; 2017,Jan,8; 2016,Jan,13; 2015,Jan,16

70547 Magnetic resonance angiography, neck; without contrast material(s)
6.93 6.93 FUD XXX 03 Z2 80
AMA: 2018,Jan,8; 2017,Jan,8; 2016,Jan,13; 2015,Jan,16

70548 with contrast material(s)
7.74 7.74 FUD XXX 03 Z2 80
AMA: 2018,Jan,8; 2017,Jan,8; 2016,Jan,13; 2015,Jan,16

70549 without contrast material(s), followed by contrast material(s) and further sequences
10.9 10.9 FUD XXX 03 Z2 80
AMA: 2018,Jan,8; 2017,Jan,8; 2016,Jan,13; 2015,Jan,16

70551-70553 Magnetic Resonance Imaging: Brain and Brain Stem

CMS: 100-04,4,200.3.2 Multi-Source Photon Stereotactic RadiosurgeryPlanning and Delivery; 100-04,4,250.16 Multiple Procedure Payment Reduction: Certain Diagnostic Imaging Procedures Rendered by Physicians

INCLUDES Three-dimensional imaging that measures response oatomic nuclei in soft tissues to high-frequency radio waves when strong magnetic field applied

EXCLUDES *Magnetic spectroscopy (76390)*

70551 Magnetic resonance (eg, proton) imaging, brain (including brain stem); without contrast material
6.28 6.28 FUD XXX 03 Z2 80
AMA: 2018,Jan,8; 2017,Jan,8; 2016,Jan,13; 2015,Jan,16

70552 with contrast material(s)
8.69 8.69 FUD XXX 03 Z2 80
AMA: 2018,Jan,8; 2017,Jan,8; 2016,Jan,13; 2015,Jan,16

70553 without contrast material, followed by contrast material(s) and further sequences
10.4 10.4 FUD XXX 03 Z2 80
AMA: 2018,Jan,8; 2017,Jan,8; 2016,Jan,13; 2015,Jan,16

70554-70555 Magnetic Resonance Imaging: Brain Mapping

INCLUDES Neuroimaging technique using MRI to identify and map signals related to brain activity

EXCLUDES *Reporting code with following unless separate diagnostic MRI performed (70551-70553)*

70554 Magnetic resonance imaging, brain, functional MRI; including test selection and administration of repetitive body part movement and/or visual stimulation, not requiring physician or psychologist administration
EXCLUDES *Functional brain mapping (96020)*
Testing performed by physician or psychologist (70555)
12.4 12.4 FUD XXX 03 Z2 80
AMA: 2018,Jan,8; 2017,Jan,8; 2016,Jan,13; 2015,Jan,16

70555 requiring physician or psychologist administration of entire neurofunctional testing
EXCLUDES *Testing performed by technologist, nonphysician, or nonpsychologist (70554)*
Code also (96020)
0.00 0.00 FUD XXX S Z2 80
AMA: 2018,Jan,8; 2017,Jan,8; 2016,Jan,13; 2015,Jan,16

70557-70559 Magnetic Resonance Imaging: Intraoperative

EXCLUDES *Intracranial lesion stereotaxic biopsy with magnetic resonance guidance (61751, 77021-77022)*
Procedures performed more than one time per surgical encounter
Reporting codes unless separate report generated

Code also stereotactic biopsy, aspiration, or excision, when performed with MRI (61751)

70557 Magnetic resonance (eg, proton) imaging, brain (including brain stem and skull base), during open intracranial procedure (eg, to assess for residual tumor or residual vascular malformation); without contrast material
0.00 0.00 FUD XXX S Z2 80
AMA: 2014,Jan,11; 2012,Feb,9-10

70558 with contrast material(s)
0.00 0.00 FUD XXX S Z2 80
AMA: 2014,Jan,11; 2012,Feb,9-10

70559 without contrast material(s), followed by contrast material(s) and further sequences
0.00 0.00 FUD XXX S Z2 80
AMA: 2014,Jan,11; 2012,Feb,9-10

71045-71130 Radiography: Thorax

71045 Radiologic examination, chest; single view
EXCLUDES *Acute abdomen series, complete (2 or more views) including chest view (74022)*
Remotely performed CAD (0175T)
Code also concurrent computer-aided detection (CAD) (0174T)
0.70 0.70 FUD XXX 03 Z3 80
AMA: 2019,Aug,8; 2019,May,10; 2019,Mar,10; 2018,Apr,7

71046 2 views
EXCLUDES *Acute abdomen series, complete (2 or more views) including chest view (74022)*
Remotely performed CAD (0175T)
Code also concurrent computer-aided detection (CAD) (0174T)
0.89 0.89 FUD XXX 03 Z3 80
AMA: 2019,Aug,8; 2019,Mar,10; 2018,Apr,7

71047 3 views
EXCLUDES *Acute abdomen series, complete (2 or more views) including chest view (74022)*
Remotely performed CAD (0175T)
Code also concurrent computer-aided detection (CAD) (0174T)
1.12 1.12 FUD XXX Q1 N1 80
AMA: 2019,Mar,10; 2018,Apr,7

71048 4 or more views
EXCLUDES *Acute abdomen series, complete (2 or more views) including chest view (74022)*
Remotely performed CAD (0175T)
Code also concurrent computer-aided detection (CAD) (0174T)
1.21 1.21 FUD XXX Q1 N1 80
AMA: 2019,Mar,10; 2018,Apr,7

Radiology

70544 — 71048

71100 **Radiologic examination, ribs, unilateral; 2 views**
1.00 1.00 **FUD** XXX Q1 N1 80
AMA: 2014,Jan,11; 2012,Feb,9-10

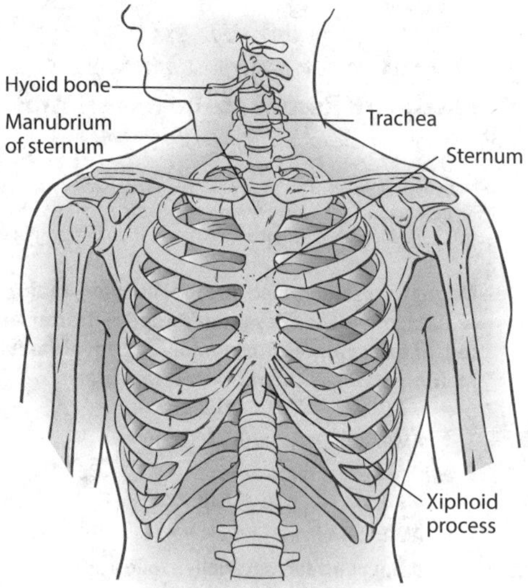

71101 **including posteroanterior chest, minimum of 3 views**
1.11 1.11 **FUD** XXX Q1 N1 80
AMA: 2014,Jan,11; 2012,Feb,9-10

71110 **Radiologic examination, ribs, bilateral; 3 views**
1.21 1.21 **FUD** XXX Q1 N1 80
AMA: 2014,Jan,11; 2012,Feb,9-10

71111 **including posteroanterior chest, minimum of 4 views**
1.38 1.38 **FUD** XXX Q1 N1 80
AMA: 2014,Jan,11; 2012,Feb,9-10

71120 **Radiologic examination; sternum, minimum of 2 views**
0.88 0.88 **FUD** XXX Q1 N1 80
AMA: 2014,Jan,11; 2012,Feb,9-10

71130 **sternoclavicular joint or joints, minimum of 3 views**
1.12 1.12 **FUD** XXX Q1 N1 80
AMA: 2014,Jan,11; 2012,Feb,9-10

71250-71271 Computerized Tomography: Thorax

INCLUDES Imaging using tomographic technique enhanced by computer imaging to create cross-sectional body plane view

EXCLUDES *3D rendering (76376-76377)*
CT breast (0633T-0638T)
CT heart (75571-75574)

▲ **71250** **Computed tomography, thorax, diagnostic; without contrast material**
CT thorax with contrast (71260-71270)
EXCLUDES *CT thorax for lung cancer screening (71271)*
4.47 4.47 **FUD** XXX Q3 Z2 80
AMA: 2020,Sep,11; 2018,Jan,8; 2017,Jan,8; 2016,Jan,13; 2015,Jan,16

▲ **71260** **with contrast material(s)**
EXCLUDES *CT thorax for lung cancer screening (71271)*
CT thorax without contrast (71250, 71270)
5.52 5.52 **FUD** XXX Q3 Z2 80
AMA: 2020,Sep,11; 2018,Jan,8; 2017,Jan,8; 2016,Jan,13; 2015,Jan,16

▲ **71270** **without contrast material, followed by contrast material(s) and further sections**
EXCLUDES *CT thorax for lung cancer screening (71271)*
CT thorax with or without contrast only (71250, 71260)
6.53 6.53 **FUD** XXX Q3 Z2 80
AMA: 2020,Sep,11; 2018,Jan,8; 2017,Jan,8; 2016,Jan,13; 2015,Jan,16

● **71271** **Computed tomography, thorax, low dose for lung cancer screening, without contrast material(s)**
EXCLUDES *CT thorax not for lung cancer screening (71250, 71260, 71270)*

71275 Computerized Tomographic Angiography: Thorax

CMS: 100-04,4,250.16 Multiple Procedure Payment Reduction: Certain Diagnostic Imaging Procedures Rendered by Physicians

INCLUDES Multiple rapid thin section CT scans to create cross-sectional bone, organ, and tissue images

EXCLUDES *CT angiography coronary arteries including calcification score and/or cardiac morphology (75574)*

71275 **Computed tomographic angiography, chest (noncoronary), with contrast material(s), including noncontrast images, if performed, and image postprocessing**
8.53 8.53 **FUD** XXX Q3 Z2 80
AMA: 2020,Sep,11; 2018,Jan,8; 2017,Jan,8; 2016,Jan,13; 2015,Jan,16

71550-71552 Magnetic Resonance Imaging: Thorax

CMS: 100-04,4,250.16 Multiple Procedure Payment Reduction: Certain Diagnostic Imaging Procedures Rendered by Physicians

INCLUDES Three-dimensional imaging that measures response atomic nuclei in soft tissues to high-frequency radio waves when strong magnetic field applied

EXCLUDES *MRI of the breast (77046-77049)*

71550 **Magnetic resonance (eg, proton) imaging, chest (eg, for evaluation of hilar and mediastinal lymphadenopathy); without contrast material(s)**
11.1 11.1 **FUD** XXX Q3 Z2 80
AMA: 2018,Jan,8; 2017,Jan,8; 2016,Jan,13; 2015,Jan,16

71551 **with contrast material(s)**
12.3 12.3 **FUD** XXX Q3 Z2 80
AMA: 2018,Jan,8; 2017,Jan,8; 2016,Jan,13; 2015,Jan,16

71552 **without contrast material(s), followed by contrast material(s) and further sequences**
15.5 15.5 **FUD** XXX Q3 Z2 80
AMA: 2018,Jan,8; 2017,Jan,8; 2016,Jan,13; 2015,Jan,16

71555 Magnetic Resonance Angiography: Thorax

CMS: 100-04,13,40.1.1 Magnetic Resonance Angiography; 100-04,13,40.1.2 HCPCS Coding Requirements; 100-04,4,250.16 Multiple Procedure Payment Reduction: Certain Diagnostic Imaging Procedures Rendered by Physicians

71555 **Magnetic resonance angiography, chest (excluding myocardium), with or without contrast material(s)**
10.8 10.8 **FUD** XXX B 80
AMA: 2018,Jan,8; 2017,Jan,8; 2016,Jan,13; 2015,Jan,16

72020-72120 Radiography: Spine

INCLUDES Minimum number views or more views when needed to adequately complete study
Radiographs repeated during encounter due to substandard quality; only one unit reported

EXCLUDES *Obtaining more films after initial film review, based on the radiologist discretion, an order for the test, and change in patient's condition*

72020 **Radiologic examination, spine, single view, specify level**
EXCLUDES *Single view entire thoracic and lumbar spine (72081)*
0.65 0.65 **FUD** XXX Q1 N1 80
AMA: 2018,Jan,8; 2017,Jan,8; 2016,Sep,4; 2016,Jan,13; 2015,Oct,9; 2015,Jan,16

72040 **Radiologic examination, spine, cervical; 2 or 3 views**
1.03 1.03 FUD XXX Q1 N1 80
AMA: 2018,Aug,10; 2018,Jan,8; 2017,Jan,8; 2016,Jan,13; 2015,Jan,16

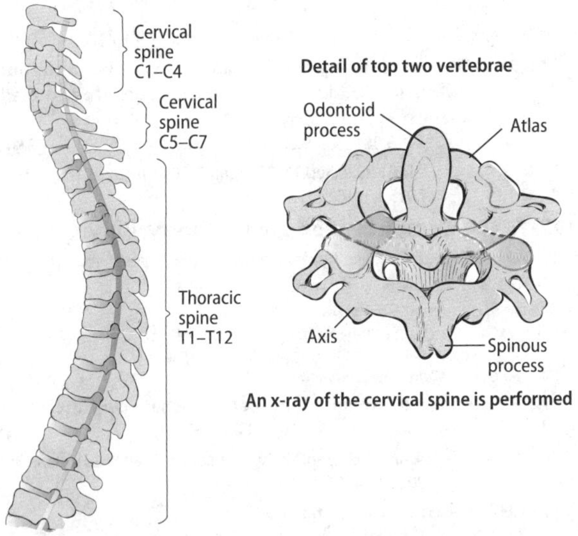

An x-ray of the cervical spine is performed

72050 **4 or 5 views**
1.42 1.42 FUD XXX Q1 N1 80
AMA: 2014,Jan,11; 2012,Feb,9-10

72052 **6 or more views**
1.69 1.69 FUD XXX Q1 N1 80
AMA: 2014,Jan,11; 2012,Feb,9-10

72070 **Radiologic examination, spine; thoracic, 2 views**
0.89 0.89 FUD XXX Q1 N1 80
AMA: 2018,Jan,8; 2017,Jan,8; 2016,Jan,13; 2015,Jan,16

72072 **thoracic, 3 views**
1.08 1.08 FUD XXX Q1 N1 80
AMA: 2018,Jan,8; 2017,Jan,8; 2016,Jan,13; 2015,Jan,16

72074 **thoracic, minimum of 4 views**
1.21 1.21 FUD XXX Q1 N1 80
AMA: 2018,Jan,8; 2017,Jan,8; 2016,Jan,13; 2015,Jan,16

72080 **thoracolumbar junction, minimum of 2 views**
EXCLUDES *Single view thoracolumbar junction (72020)*
0.95 0.95 FUD XXX Q1 N1 80
AMA: 2018,Jan,8; 2017,Jan,8; 2016,Sep,4; 2016,Jan,13; 2015,Oct,9; 2015,Jan,16

72081 **Radiologic examination, spine, entire thoracic and lumbar, including skull, cervical and sacral spine if performed (eg, scoliosis evaluation); one view**
1.17 1.17 FUD XXX Q1 N1 80
AMA: 2018,Jan,8; 2017,Jan,8; 2016,Sep,4

72082 **2 or 3 views**
1.90 1.90 FUD XXX Q1 N1 80
AMA: 2018,Jan,8; 2017,Jan,8; 2016,Sep,4

72083 **4 or 5 views**
2.21 2.21 FUD XXX S Z2 80
AMA: 2018,Jan,8; 2017,Jan,8; 2016,Sep,4

72084 **minimum of 6 views**
2.62 2.62 FUD XXX S Z2 80
AMA: 2018,Jan,8; 2017,Jan,8; 2016,Sep,4

72100 **Radiologic examination, spine, lumbosacral; 2 or 3 views**
1.07 1.07 FUD XXX Q1 N1 80
AMA: 2018,Jan,8; 2017,Jan,8; 2016,Jan,13; 2015,Jan,16

72110 **minimum of 4 views**
1.36 1.36 FUD XXX Q1 N1 80
AMA: 2018,Jan,8; 2017,Jan,8; 2016,Jan,13; 2015,Jan,16

72114 **complete, including bending views, minimum of 6 views**
1.64 1.64 FUD XXX Q1 N1 80
AMA: 2014,Jan,11; 2012,Feb,9-10

72120 **bending views only, 2 or 3 views**
1.11 1.11 FUD XXX Q1 N1 80
AMA: 2018,Jan,8; 2017,Jan,8; 2016,Aug,7

72125-72133 Computerized Tomography: Spine

CMS: 100-04,12,20.4.7 Services Not Meeting National Electrical Manufacturers Association (NEMA) Standard; 100-04,4,20.6.12 Use of HCPCS Modifier – CT; 100-04,4,250.16 Multiple Procedure Payment Reduction: Certain Diagnostic Imaging Procedures Rendered by Physicians

INCLUDES Imaging using tomographic technique enhanced by computer imaging to create cross-sectional body plane view

EXCLUDES *3D rendering (76376-76377)*

Code also intrathecal injection procedure when performed (61055, 62284)

72125 **Computed tomography, cervical spine; without contrast material**
5.18 5.18 FUD XXX Q3 Z2 80
AMA: 2020,Sep,11

72126 **with contrast material**
6.40 6.40 FUD XXX Q3 Z3 80
AMA: 2020,Sep,11; 2018,Jan,8; 2017,Jan,8; 2016,Jan,13; 2015,Jan,16

72127 **without contrast material, followed by contrast material(s) and further sections**
6.48 6.48 FUD XXX Q3 Z2 80
AMA: 2020,Sep,11

72128 **Computed tomography, thoracic spine; without contrast material**
5.08 5.08 FUD XXX Q3 Z2 80
AMA: 2020,Sep,11

72129 **with contrast material**
5.54 5.54 FUD XXX Q3 Z2 80
AMA: 2020,Sep,11; 2019,Jan,14; 2018,Jan,8; 2017,Jan,8; 2016,Jan,13; 2015,Jan,16

72130 **without contrast material, followed by contrast material(s) and further sections**
7.59 7.59 FUD XXX Q3 Z2 80
AMA: 2020,Sep,11

72131 **Computed tomography, lumbar spine; without contrast material**
4.36 4.36 FUD XXX Q3 Z2 80
AMA: 2020,Sep,11

72132 **with contrast material**
5.51 5.51 FUD XXX Q3 Z3 80
AMA: 2020,Sep,11; 2019,Jan,14; 2018,Jan,8; 2017,Jan,8; 2016,Jan,13; 2015,Jan,16

72133 **without contrast material, followed by contrast material(s) and further sections**
6.45 6.45 FUD XXX Q3 Z2 80
AMA: 2020,Sep,11

72141-72158 Magnetic Resonance Imaging: Spine

CMS: 100-04,4,250.16 Multiple Procedure Payment Reduction: Certain Diagnostic Imaging Procedures Rendered by Physicians

INCLUDES Three-dimensional imaging that measures response atomic nuclei in soft tissues to high-frequency radio waves when strong magnetic field applied

EXCLUDES *MR spectroscopy (0609T-0610T)*

Code also intrathecal injection procedure when performed (61055, 62284)

72141 **Magnetic resonance (eg, proton) imaging, spinal canal and contents, cervical; without contrast material**
6.11 6.11 FUD XXX Q3 Z2 80
AMA: 2018,Jan,8; 2017,Jan,8; 2016,Jan,13; 2015,Jan,16

72142 **with contrast material(s)**
EXCLUDES *MRI cervical spinal canal performed without contrast followed by repeating study with contrast (72156)*
8.88 8.88 FUD XXX Q3 Z2 80
AMA: 2018,Jan,8; 2017,Jan,8; 2016,Jan,13; 2015,Jan,16

72146 **Magnetic resonance (eg, proton) imaging, spinal canal and contents, thoracic; without contrast material**
6.23 6.23 **FUD** XXX Q3 Z2 80
AMA: 2018,Jan,8; 2017,Jan,8; 2016,Jan,13; 2015,Jan,16

72147 **with contrast material(s)**
EXCLUDES *MRI thoracic spinal canal performed without contrast followed by repeating study with contrast (72157)*
8.82 8.82 **FUD** XXX Q3 Z2 80
AMA: 2018,Jan,8; 2017,Jan,8; 2016,Jan,13; 2015,Jan,16

72148 **Magnetic resonance (eg, proton) imaging, spinal canal and contents, lumbar; without contrast material**
6.23 6.23 **FUD** XXX Q3 Z2 80
AMA: 2018,Jan,8; 2017,Jan,8; 2016,Jan,13; 2015,Jan,16

72149 **with contrast material(s)**
EXCLUDES *MRI lumbar spinal canal performed without contrast followed by repeating study with contrast (72158)*
8.92 8.92 **FUD** XXX Q3 Z2 80
AMA: 2014,Jan,11; 2012,Feb,9-10

72156 **Magnetic resonance (eg, proton) imaging, spinal canal and contents, without contrast material, followed by contrast material(s) and further sequences; cervical**
10.3 10.3 **FUD** XXX Q3 Z2 80
AMA: 2014,Jan,11; 2012,Feb,9-10

72157 **thoracic**
10.5 10.5 **FUD** XXX Q3 Z2 80
AMA: 2014,Jan,11; 2012,Feb,9-10

72158 **lumbar**
10.3 10.3 **FUD** XXX Q3 Z2 80
AMA: 2014,Jan,11; 2012,Feb,9-10

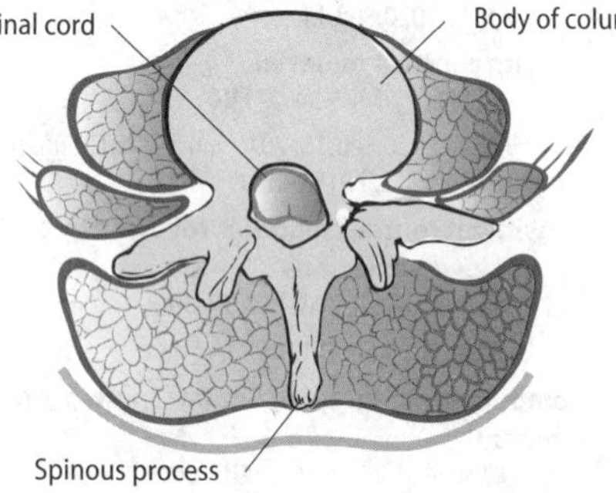

Superior view of thoracic spine and surrounding paraspinal muscles

72159 Magnetic Resonance Angiography: Spine

CMS: 100-04,13,40.1.1 Magnetic Resonance Angiography; 100-04,13,40.1.2 HCPCS Coding Requirements; 100-04,4,250.16 Multiple Procedure Payment Reduction: Certain Diagnostic Imaging Procedures Rendered by Physicians

72159 **Magnetic resonance angiography, spinal canal and contents, with or without contrast material(s)**
11.2 11.2 **FUD** XXX B 80
AMA: 2018,Jan,8; 2017,Jan,8; 2016,Jan,13; 2015,Jan,16

72170-72190 Radiography: Pelvis

INCLUDES Minimum number views or more views when needed to adequately complete study
Radiographs repeated during encounter due to substandard quality; only one unit reported

EXCLUDES *Combined CT or CT angiography abdomen and pelvis (74174, 74176-74178)*
Obtaining more films after initial film review, based on radiologist discretion, order for test, and change in patient's condition
Pelvimetry (74710)
Second interpretation by requesting physician (included in E/M service)

72170 **Radiologic examination, pelvis; 1 or 2 views**
0.80 0.80 **FUD** XXX Q1 N1 80
AMA: 2018,Jan,8; 2017,Jan,8; 2016,Aug,7; 2016,Jun,5; 2016,Jan,13; 2015,Jan,16

72190 **complete, minimum of 3 views**
1.12 1.12 **FUD** XXX Q1 N1 80
AMA: 2016,Jun,5

72191 Computerized Tomographic Angiography: Pelvis

CMS: 100-04,4,250.16 Multiple Procedure Payment Reduction: Certain Diagnostic Imaging Procedures Rendered by Physicians

EXCLUDES *Computed tomographic angiography (73706, 74174-74175, 75635)*

72191 **Computed tomographic angiography, pelvis, with contrast material(s), including noncontrast images, if performed, and image postprocessing**
9.08 9.08 **FUD** XXX Q3 Z2 80
AMA: 2020,Sep,11; 2018,Jan,8; 2017,Jan,8; 2016,Jan,13; 2015,Jan,16

72192-72194 Computerized Tomography: Pelvis

CMS: 100-04,4,250.16 Multiple Procedure Payment Reduction: Certain Diagnostic Imaging Procedures Rendered by Physicians

EXCLUDES *3D rendering (76376-76377)*
Combined CT abdomen and pelvis (74176-74178)
CT colonography, diagnostic (74261-74262)
CT colonography, screening (74263)

72192 **Computed tomography, pelvis; without contrast material**
4.10 4.10 **FUD** XXX Q3 Z2 80
AMA: 2020,Sep,11; 2018,Jan,8; 2017,Jan,8; 2016,Jan,13; 2015,Jan,16

72193 **with contrast material(s)**
6.59 6.59 **FUD** XXX Q3 Z2 80
AMA: 2020,Sep,11; 2018,Jan,8; 2017,Jan,8; 2016,Jan,13; 2015,Jan,16

72194 **without contrast material, followed by contrast material(s) and further sections**
7.48 7.48 **FUD** XXX Q3 Z2 80
AMA: 2020,Sep,11; 2018,Jan,8; 2017,Jan,8; 2016,Jan,13; 2015,Jan,16

72195-72197 Magnetic Resonance Imaging: Pelvis

CMS: 100-04,4,250.16 Multiple Procedure Payment Reduction: Certain Diagnostic Imaging Procedures Rendered by Physicians

INCLUDES Three-dimensional imaging that measures response atomic nuclei in soft tissues to high-frequency radio waves when strong magnetic field applied

EXCLUDES *MRI fetus(es) (74712-74713)*

72195 **Magnetic resonance (eg, proton) imaging, pelvis; without contrast material(s)**
7.62 7.62 **FUD** XXX Q3 Z2 80
AMA: 2018,Jul,11; 2018,Jan,8; 2017,Jan,8; 2016,Jun,5; 2016,Jan,13; 2015,Jan,16

72196 **with contrast material(s)**
8.74 8.74 **FUD** XXX Q3 Z2 80
AMA: 2018,Jul,11; 2018,Jan,8; 2017,Jan,8; 2016,Jun,5; 2016,Jan,13; 2015,Jan,16

72197 **without contrast material(s), followed by contrast material(s) and further sequences**
10.9 10.9 **FUD** XXX Q3 Z2 80
AMA: 2018,Jul,11; 2018,Jan,8; 2017,Jan,8; 2016,Jun,5; 2016,Jan,13; 2015,Jan,16

72198 Magnetic Resonance Angiography: Pelvis

CMS: 100-04,13,40.1.1 Magnetic Resonance Angiography; 100-04,13,40.1.2 HCPCS Coding Requirements; 100-04,4,250.16 Multiple Procedure Payment Reduction: Certain Diagnostic Imaging Procedures Rendered by Physicians

INCLUDES Magnetic fields and radio waves to produce detailed cross-sectional images arteries and veins

72198 **Magnetic resonance angiography, pelvis, with or without contrast material(s)**
11.0 11.0 **FUD** XXX B 80
AMA: 2018,Jan,8; 2017,Jan,8; 2016,Jan,13; 2015,Jan,16

72200-72220 Radiography: Pelvisacral

INCLUDES Minimum number views or more views when needed to adequately complete study
Radiographs repeated during encounter due to substandard quality; only one unit reported

EXCLUDES *Obtaining more films after initial film review, based on radiologist discretion, order for, and change in patient's condition*
Second interpretation by requesting physician (included in E/M service)

72200 Radiologic examination, sacroiliac joints; less than 3 views
0.90 0.90 FUD XXX Q1 N1 80
AMA: 2014,Jan,11; 2012,Feb,9-10

72202 3 or more views
0.98 0.98 FUD XXX Q1 N1 80
AMA: 2014,Jan,11; 2012,Feb,9-10

72220 Radiologic examination, sacrum and coccyx, minimum of 2 views
0.88 0.88 FUD XXX Q1 N1 80
AMA: 2014,Jan,11; 2012,Feb,9-10

72240-72270 Myelography with Contrast: Spinal Cord

CMS: 100-04,13,30.1.3.1 Payment for Low Osmolar Contrast Material

EXCLUDES *Injection procedure for myelography (62284)*
Myelography (62302-62305)

Code also injection at C1-C2 for complete myelography (61055)

72240 Myelography, cervical, radiological supervision and interpretation
3.14 3.14 FUD XXX Q2 N1 80
AMA: 2018,Jan,8; 2017,Jan,8; 2016,Jan,13; 2015,Jan,16

72255 Myelography, thoracic, radiological supervision and interpretation
3.19 3.19 FUD XXX Q2 N1 80
AMA: 2018,Jan,8; 2017,Jan,8; 2016,Jan,13; 2015,Jan,16

72265 Myelography, lumbosacral, radiological supervision and interpretation
2.90 2.90 FUD XXX Q2 N1 80
AMA: 2018,Jan,8; 2017,Jan,8; 2016,Jan,13; 2015,Jan,16

72270 Myelography, 2 or more regions (eg, lumbar/thoracic, cervical/thoracic, lumbar/cervical, lumbar/thoracic/cervical), radiological supervision and interpretation
4.00 4.00 FUD XXX Q2 N1 80
AMA: 2018,Jan,8; 2017,Jan,8; 2016,Jan,13; 2015,Jan,16

72275 Radiography: Epidural Space

INCLUDES Epidurogram, image documentation, and formal written report
Fluoroscopic guidance (77003)

EXCLUDES *Arthrodesis (22586)*
Second interpretation by requesting physician (included in E/M service)

Code also injection procedure as appropriate (62280-62282, 62320-62327, 64479-64480, 64483-64484)

72275 Epidurography, radiological supervision and interpretation
3.48 3.48 FUD XXX N N1 80
AMA: 2018,Jan,8; 2017,Jan,8; 2016,Jan,13; 2015,Jan,16

72285 Radiography: Intervertebral Disc (Cervical/Thoracic)

CMS: 100-04,13,30.1.3.1 Payment for Low Osmolar Contrast Material

Code also discography injection procedure (62291)

72285 Discography, cervical or thoracic, radiological supervision and interpretation
3.32 3.32 FUD XXX Q2 N1 80
AMA: 2018,Jan,8; 2017,Jan,8; 2016,Jan,13; 2015,Jan,16

72295 Radiography: Intervertebral Disc (Lumbar)

CMS: 100-04,13,30.1.3.1 Payment for Low Osmolar Contrast Material

Code also discography injection procedure (62290)

72295 Discography, lumbar, radiological supervision and interpretation
2.90 2.90 FUD XXX Q2 N1 80
AMA: 2018,Jan,8; 2017,Feb,12; 2017,Jan,8; 2016,Jan,13; 2015,Jan,16

73000-73085 Radiography: Shoulder and Upper Arm

INCLUDES Minimum number views or more views when needed to adequately complete study
Radiographs repeated during encounter due to substandard quality; only one unit reported

EXCLUDES *Obtaining more films after initial film review, based on radiologist discretion, order for test, and change in patient's condition*
Second interpretation by requesting physician (included in E/M service)
Stress views upper body joint(s), when performed (77071)

73000 Radiologic examination; clavicle, complete
0.88 0.88 FUD XXX Q1 N1 80
AMA: 2014,Jan,11; 2012,Feb,9-10

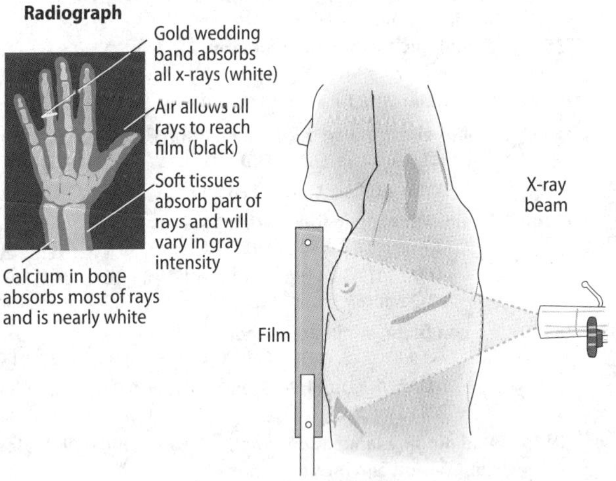

Posterioranterior (PA) chest study; lateral views also common

73010 scapula, complete
0.90 0.90 FUD XXX Q1 N1 80
AMA: 2014,Jan,11; 2012,Feb,9-10

73020 Radiologic examination, shoulder; 1 view
0.67 0.67 FUD XXX Q1 N1 80
AMA: 2014,Jan,11; 2012,Feb,9-10

73030 complete, minimum of 2 views
0.85 0.85 FUD XXX Q1 N1 80
AMA: 2014,Jan,11; 2012,Feb,9-10

73040 Radiologic examination, shoulder, arthrography, radiological supervision and interpretation
INCLUDES Fluoroscopic guidance (77002)
Code also arthrography injection procedure (23350)
3.12 3.12 FUD XXX Q2 N1 80
AMA: 2018,Jan,8; 2017,Jan,8; 2016,Jan,13; 2015,Jan,16

73050 Radiologic examination; acromioclavicular joints, bilateral, with or without weighted distraction
1.05 1.05 FUD XXX Q1 N1 80
AMA: 2014,Jan,11; 2012,Feb,9-10

73060 humerus, minimum of 2 views
0.88 0.88 FUD XXX Q1 N1 80
AMA: 2014,Jan,11; 2012,Feb,9-10

73070 Radiologic examination, elbow; 2 views
0.76 0.76 FUD XXX Q1 N1 80
AMA: 2018,Jan,8; 2017,Jan,8; 2016,Jan,13; 2015,Jan,16

73080 complete, minimum of 3 views
0.84 0.84 FUD XXX Q1 N1 80
AMA: 2014,Jan,11; 2012,Feb,9-10

73085 **Radiologic examination, elbow, arthrography, radiological supervision and interpretation**

INCLUDES Fluoroscopic guidance (77002)

Code also arthrography injection procedure (24220)

3.18 3.18 **FUD** XXX Q2 N1 80

AMA: 2018,Jan,8; 2017,Jan,8; 2016,Jan,13; 2015,Jan,16

73090-73140 Radiography: Forearm and Hand

INCLUDES Minimum number views or more views when needed to adequately complete study

Radiographs repeated during encounter due to substandard quality; only one unit reported

EXCLUDES *Obtaining more films after initial film review, based on radiologist discretion, order for test, and change in patient's condition*

Second interpretation by requesting physician (included in E/M service)

Stress views upper body joint(s), when performed (77071)

73090 **Radiologic examination; forearm, 2 views**

0.79 0.79 **FUD** XXX Q1 N1 80

AMA: 2018,Jan,8; 2017,Jan,8; 2016,Jan,13; 2015,Jan,16

73092 **upper extremity, infant, minimum of 2 views** A

0.81 0.81 **FUD** XXX Q1 N1 80

AMA: 2014,Jan,11; 2012,Feb,9-10

73100 **Radiologic examination, wrist; 2 views**

0.92 0.92 **FUD** XXX Q1 N1 80

AMA: 2018,Oct,11; 2018,Jan,8; 2017,Jan,8; 2016,Jan,13; 2015,Jan,16

73110 **complete, minimum of 3 views**

1.03 1.03 **FUD** XXX Q1 N1 80

AMA: 2018,Oct,11; 2018,Jan,8; 2017,Jan,8; 2016,Jan,13; 2015,Jan,16

73115 **Radiologic examination, wrist, arthrography, radiological supervision and interpretation**

INCLUDES Fluoroscopic guidance (77002)

Code also arthrography injection procedure (25246)

3.33 3.33 **FUD** XXX Q2 N1 80

AMA: 2018,Jan,8; 2017,Jan,8; 2016,Jan,13; 2015,Jan,16

73120 **Radiologic examination, hand; 2 views**

0.85 0.85 **FUD** XXX Q1 N1 80

AMA: 2018,Oct,11

73130 **minimum of 3 views**

0.98 0.98 **FUD** XXX Q1 N1 80

AMA: 2014,Jan,11; 2012,Feb,9-10

73140 **Radiologic examination, finger(s), minimum of 2 views**

1.00 1.00 **FUD** XXX Q1 N1 80

AMA: 2018,Jan,8; 2017,Jan,8; 2016,Jan,13; 2015,Jan,16

73200-73202 Computerized Tomography: Shoulder, Arm, Hand

CMS: 100-04,4,250.16 Multiple Procedure Payment Reduction: Certain Diagnostic Imaging Procedures Rendered by Physicians

INCLUDES Imaging using tomographic technique enhanced by computer imaging to create cross-sectional body plane view

Intravascular, intrathecal, or intra-articular contrast materials when noted in code descriptor

EXCLUDES *3D rendering (76376-76377)*

73200 **Computed tomography, upper extremity; without contrast material**

5.03 5.03 **FUD** XXX Q3 Z2 80

AMA: 2018,Jan,8; 2017,Jan,8; 2016,Jan,13; 2015,Jan,16

73201 **with contrast material(s)**

6.26 6.26 **FUD** XXX Q3 Z3 80

AMA: 2018,Jan,8; 2017,Jan,8; 2016,Jan,13; 2015,Aug,6; 2015,Jan,16

73202 **without contrast material, followed by contrast material(s) and further sections**

7.82 7.82 **FUD** XXX Q3 Z2 80

AMA: 2014,Jan,11; 2012,Feb,9-10

73206 Computerized Tomographic Angiography: Shoulder, Arm, and Hand

CMS: 100-04,4,250.16 Multiple Procedure Payment Reduction: Certain Diagnostic Imaging Procedures Rendered by Physicians

INCLUDES Intravascular, intrathecal, or intra-articular contrast materials when noted in code descriptor

Multiple rapid thin section CT scans to create cross-sectional images arteries and veins

73206 **Computed tomographic angiography, upper extremity, with contrast material(s), including noncontrast images, if performed, and image postprocessing**

9.24 9.24 **FUD** XXX Q3 Z2 80

AMA: 2018,Jan,8; 2017,Jan,8; 2016,Jan,13; 2015,Jan,16

73218-73223 Magnetic Resonance Imaging: Shoulder, Arm, Hand

CMS: 100-04,4,250.16 Multiple Procedure Payment Reduction: Certain Diagnostic Imaging Procedures Rendered by Physicians

INCLUDES Three-dimensional imaging that measures response atomic nuclei in soft tissues to high-frequency radio waves when strong magnetic field applied

Intravascular, intrathecal, or intra-articular contrast materials when noted in code descriptor

73218 **Magnetic resonance (eg, proton) imaging, upper extremity, other than joint; without contrast material(s)**

9.93 9.93 **FUD** XXX Q3 Z2 80

AMA: 2018,Jan,8; 2017,Jan,8; 2016,Jan,13; 2015,Jan,16

73219 **with contrast material(s)**

10.9 10.9 **FUD** XXX Q3 Z2 80

AMA: 2018,Jan,8; 2017,Jan,8; 2016,Jan,13; 2015,Jan,16

73220 **without contrast material(s), followed by contrast material(s) and further sequences**

13.7 13.7 **FUD** XXX Q3 Z2 80

AMA: 2018,Jan,8; 2017,Jan,8; 2016,Jan,13; 2015,Jan,16

73221 **Magnetic resonance (eg, proton) imaging, any joint of upper extremity; without contrast material(s)**

6.57 6.57 **FUD** XXX Q3 Z2 80

AMA: 2018,Jan,8; 2017,Jan,8; 2016,Jan,13; 2015,Jan,16

73222 **with contrast material(s)**

10.2 10.2 **FUD** XXX Q3 Z3 80

AMA: 2018,Jan,8; 2017,Jan,8; 2016,Jan,13; 2015,Aug,6; 2015,Jan,16

73223 **without contrast material(s), followed by contrast material(s) and further sequences**

12.7 12.7 **FUD** XXX Q3 Z2 80

AMA: 2018,Jan,8; 2017,Jan,8; 2016,Jan,13; 2015,Jan,16

73225 Magnetic Resonance Angiography: Shoulder, Arm, Hand

CMS: 100-04,13,40.1.1 Magnetic Resonance Angiography; 100-04,4,250.16 Multiple Procedure Payment Reduction: Certain Diagnostic Imaging Procedures Rendered by Physicians

INCLUDES Intravascular, intrathecal, or intra-articular contrast materials when noted in code descriptor

Magnetic fields and radio waves to produce detailed cross-sectional images arteries and veins

73225 **Magnetic resonance angiography, upper extremity, with or without contrast material(s)**

11.1 11.1 **FUD** XXX B 80

AMA: 2018,Jan,8; 2017,Jan,8; 2016,Jan,13; 2015,Jan,16

73501-73552 Radiography: Pelvic Region and Thigh

EXCLUDES *Stress views lower body joint(s), when performed (77071)*

73501 **Radiologic examination, hip, unilateral, with pelvis when performed; 1 view**

0.89 0.89 **FUD** XXX Q1 N1 80

AMA: 2018,Jan,8; 2017,Jan,8; 2016,Aug,7; 2016,Jun,8; 2016,Jan,13; 2015,Oct,9

73502 2-3 views
1.27 1.27 FUD XXX Q1 N1 80
AMA: 2018,Jan,8; 2017,Jan,8; 2016,Aug,7; 2016,Jun,8; 2016,Jan,13; 2015,Oct,9

73503 minimum of 4 views
1.57 1.57 FUD XXX Q1 N1 80
AMA: 2018,Jan,8; 2017,Jan,8; 2016,Aug,7; 2016,Jun,8; 2016,Jan,13; 2015,Oct,9

73521 **Radiologic examination, hips, bilateral, with pelvis when performed; 2 views**
1.12 1.12 FUD XXX Q1 N1 80
AMA: 2018,Jan,8; 2017,Jan,8; 2016,Aug,7; 2016,Jun,8; 2016,Jan,13; 2015,Oct,9

73522 3-4 views
1.46 1.46 FUD XXX Q1 N1 80
AMA: 2018,Jan,8; 2017,Jan,8; 2016,Aug,7; 2016,Jun,8; 2016,Jan,13; 2015,Oct,9

73523 minimum of 5 views
1.66 1.66 FUD XXX S N1 80
AMA: 2018,Jan,8; 2017,Jan,8; 2016,Aug,7; 2016,Jun,8; 2016,Jan,13; 2015,Oct,9

73525 **Radiologic examination, hip, arthrography, radiological supervision and interpretation**
INCLUDES Fluoroscopic guidance (77002)
3.47 3.47 FUD XXX Q2 N1 80
AMA: 2018,Jan,8; 2017,Jan,8; 2016,Nov,10; 2016,Aug,7; 2016,Jan,13; 2015,Jan,16

73551 **Radiologic examination, femur; 1 view**
0.82 0.82 FUD XXX Q1 N1 80
AMA: 2018,Jan,8; 2017,Jan,8; 2016,Aug,7

73552 minimum 2 views
0.97 0.97 FUD XXX Q1 N1 80
AMA: 2018,Jan,8; 2017,Nov,10; 2017,Jan,8; 2016,Aug,7

73560-73660 Radiography: Lower Leg, Ankle, and Foot

EXCLUDES *Stress views lower body joint(s), when performed (77071)*

73560 **Radiologic examination, knee; 1 or 2 views**
0.94 0.94 FUD XXX Q1 N1 80
AMA: 2018,Jan,8; 2017,Jan,8; 2016,Jan,13; 2015,May,10; 2015,Feb,10

73562 3 views
1.05 1.05 FUD XXX Q1 N1 80
AMA: 2014,Jan,11; 2012,Feb,9-10

73564 complete, 4 or more views
1.17 1.17 FUD XXX Q1 N1 80
AMA: 2018,Jan,8; 2017,Jan,8; 2016,Jan,13; 2015,May,10; 2015,Feb,10; 2015,Jan,16

73565 both knees, standing, anteroposterior
1.05 1.05 FUD XXX Q1 N1 80
AMA: 2018,Jan,8; 2017,Jan,8; 2016,Jan,13; 2015,May,10; 2015,Feb,10

73580 **Radiologic examination, knee, arthrography, radiological supervision and interpretation**
INCLUDES Fluoroscopic guidance (77002)
3.59 3.59 FUD XXX Q2 N1 80
AMA: 2019,Aug,7; 2018,Jan,8; 2017,Jan,8; 2016,Jan,13; 2015,Aug,6; 2015,Jan,16

73590 **Radiologic examination; tibia and fibula, 2 views**
0.86 0.86 FUD XXX Q1 N1 80
AMA: 2018,Jan,8; 2017,Nov,10; 2017,Jan,8; 2016,Jan,13; 2015,Jan,16

73592 lower extremity, infant, minimum of 2 views A
0.81 0.81 FUD XXX Q1 N1 80
AMA: 2018,Jan,8; 2017,Nov,10

73600 **Radiologic examination, ankle; 2 views**
0.87 0.87 FUD XXX Q1 N1 80
AMA: 2018,Jan,8; 2017,Jan,8; 2016,Jan,13; 2015,Jan,16

73610 complete, minimum of 3 views
0.98 0.98 FUD XXX Q1 N1 80
AMA: 2018,Jan,8; 2017,Jan,8; 2016,Jan,13; 2015,Jan,16

73615 **Radiologic examination, ankle, arthrography, radiological supervision and interpretation**
INCLUDES Fluoroscopic guidance (77002)
3.34 3.34 FUD XXX Q2 N1 80
AMA: 2018,Jan,8; 2017,Jan,8; 2016,Jan,13; 2015,Jan,16

73620 **Radiologic examination, foot; 2 views**
0.78 0.78 FUD XXX Q1 N1 80
AMA: 2018,Jan,8; 2017,Jan,8; 2016,Jan,13; 2015,Jan,16

73630 complete, minimum of 3 views
0.88 0.88 FUD XXX Q1 N1 80
AMA: 2014,Jan,11; 2012,Feb,9-10

73650 **Radiologic examination; calcaneus, minimum of 2 views**
0.76 0.76 FUD XXX Q1 N1 80
AMA: 2014,Jan,11; 2012,Feb,9-10

73660 toe(s), minimum of 2 views
0.79 0.79 FUD XXX Q1 N1 80
AMA: 2014,Jan,11; 2012,Feb,9-10

73700-73702 Computerized Tomography: Leg, Ankle, and Foot

CMS: 100-04,4,250.16 Multiple Procedure Payment Reduction: Certain Diagnostic Imaging Procedures Rendered by Physicians

EXCLUDES *3D rendering (76376-76377)*

73700 **Computed tomography, lower extremity; without contrast material**
4.36 4.36 FUD XXX Q3 Z2 80
AMA: 2018,Jan,8; 2017,Jan,8; 2016,Jan,13; 2015,Jan,16

73701 with contrast material(s)
6.36 6.36 FUD XXX Q3 Z2 80
AMA: 2019,Aug,7; 2018,Jan,8; 2017,Jan,8; 2016,Jan,13; 2015,Jan,16

73702 without contrast material, followed by contrast material(s) and further sections
6.56 6.56 FUD XXX Q3 Z2 80
AMA: 2019,Aug,7; 2018,Jan,8; 2017,Jan,8; 2016,Jan,13; 2015,Jan,16

73706 Computerized Tomographic Angiography: Leg, Ankle, and Foot

CMS: 100-04,4,250.16 Multiple Procedure Payment Reduction: Certain Diagnostic Imaging Procedures Rendered by Physicians

EXCLUDES *CT angiography for aorto-iliofemoral runoff (75635)*

73706 **Computed tomographic angiography, lower extremity, with contrast material(s), including noncontrast images, if performed, and image postprocessing**
10.0 10.0 FUD XXX Q3 Z2 80
AMA: 2018,Jan,8; 2017,Jan,8; 2016,Jan,13; 2015,Jan,16

73718-73723 Magnetic Resonance Imaging: Leg, Ankle, and Foot

CMS: 100-04,4,250.16 Multiple Procedure Payment Reduction: Certain Diagnostic Imaging Procedures Rendered by Physicians

73718 **Magnetic resonance (eg, proton) imaging, lower extremity other than joint; without contrast material(s)**
7.39 7.39 FUD XXX Q3 Z2 80
AMA: 2018,Jan,8; 2017,Jan,8; 2016,Jan,13; 2015,Jan,16

73719 with contrast material(s)
8.58 8.58 FUD XXX Q3 Z2 80
AMA: 2019,Aug,7; 2018,Jan,8; 2017,Jan,8; 2016,Jan,13; 2015,Jan,16

73720 without contrast material(s), followed by contrast material(s) and further sequences
11.2 11.2 FUD XXX Q3 Z2 80
AMA: 2019,Aug,7; 2018,Jan,8; 2017,Jan,8; 2016,Jan,13; 2015,Jan,16

73721 **Magnetic resonance (eg, proton) imaging, any joint of lower extremity; without contrast material**
6.44 6.44 **FUD** XXX Q3 Z2 80
AMA: 2018,Jan,8; 2017,Jan,8; 2016,Jan,13; 2015,Jan,16

73722 **with contrast material(s)**
10.5 10.5 **FUD** XXX Q3 Z3 80
AMA: 2019,Aug,7; 2018,Jan,8; 2017,Jan,8; 2016,Jan,13; 2015,Aug,6; 2015,Jan,16

73723 **without contrast material(s), followed by contrast material(s) and further sequences**
12.7 12.7 **FUD** XXX Q3 Z2 80
AMA: 2019,Aug,7; 2018,Jan,8; 2017,Jan,8; 2016,Jan,13; 2015,Jan,16

73725 Magnetic Resonance Angiography: Leg, Ankle, and Foot

CMS: 100-04,13,40.1.2 HCPCS Coding Requirements; 100-04,4,250.16 Multiple Procedure Payment Reduction: Certain Diagnostic Imaging Procedures Rendered by Physicians

73725 **Magnetic resonance angiography, lower extremity, with or without contrast material(s)**
11.1 11.1 **FUD** XXX B 80
AMA: 2018,Jan,8; 2017,Jan,8; 2016,Jan,13; 2015,Jan,16

74018-74022 Radiography: Abdomen--General

74018 **Radiologic examination, abdomen; 1 view**
0.80 0.80 **FUD** XXX Q1 N1 80
AMA: 2020,Apr,10; 2019,May,10; 2018,Apr,7

74019 **2 views**
0.98 0.98 **FUD** XXX Q1 N1 80
AMA: 2018,Apr,7

74021 **3 or more views**
1.17 1.17 **FUD** XXX Q1 N1 80
AMA: 2018,Apr,7

74022 **Radiologic examination, complete acute abdomen series, including 2 or more views of the abdomen (eg, supine, erect, decubitus), and a single view chest**
1.36 1.36 **FUD** XXX Q1 N1 80
AMA: 2019,May,10; 2018,Apr,7; 2016,Jun,5

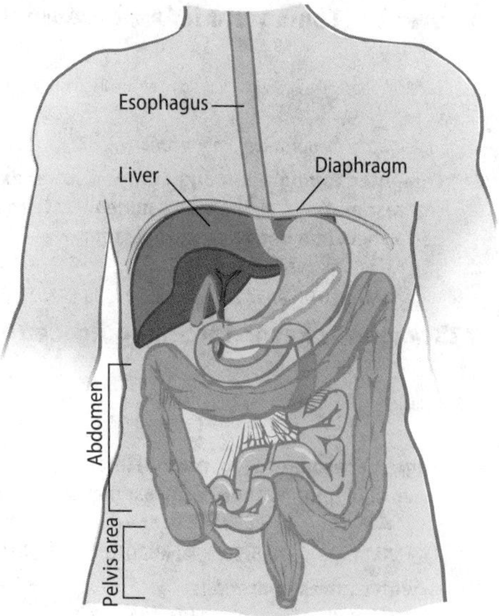

74150-74170 Computerized Tomography: Abdomen–General

CMS: 100-04,4,250.16 Multiple Procedure Payment Reduction: Certain Diagnostic Imaging Procedures Rendered by Physicians

EXCLUDES *3D rendering (76376-76377)*
Combined CT abdomen and pelvis (74176-74178)
CT colonography, diagnostic (74261-74262)
CT colonography, screening (74263)

74150 **Computed tomography, abdomen; without contrast material**
4.20 4.20 **FUD** XXX Q3 Z2 80
AMA: 2020,Sep,11; 2018,Jan,8; 2017,Jan,8; 2016,Jun,5; 2016,Jan,13; 2015,Jan,16

74160 **with contrast material(s)**
6.72 6.72 **FUD** XXX Q3 Z2 80
AMA: 2020,Sep,11; 2018,Jan,8; 2017,Jan,8; 2016,Jun,5; 2016,Jan,13; 2015,Jan,16

74170 **without contrast material, followed by contrast material(s) and further sections**
7.62 7.62 **FUD** XXX Q3 Z2 80
AMA: 2020,Sep,11; 2018,Jan,8; 2017,Jan,8; 2016,Jun,5; 2016,Jan,13; 2015,Jan,16

74174-74175 Computerized Tomographic Angiography: Abdomen and Pelvis

CMS: 100-04,4,250.16 Multiple Procedure Payment Reduction: Certain Diagnostic Imaging Procedures Rendered by Physicians

EXCLUDES *CT angiography for aorto-iliofemoral runoff (75635)*
CT angiography, lower extremity (73706)
CT angiography, pelvis (72191)

74174 **Computed tomographic angiography, abdomen and pelvis, with contrast material(s), including noncontrast images, if performed, and image postprocessing**
EXCLUDES *3D rendering (76376-76377)*
CT angiography abdomen (74175)
11.1 11.1 **FUD** XXX S Z2 80
AMA: 2020,Sep,11

74175 **Computed tomographic angiography, abdomen, with contrast material(s), including noncontrast images, if performed, and image postprocessing**
9.10 9.10 **FUD** XXX Q3 Z2 80
AMA: 2020,Sep,11; 2018,Jan,8; 2017,Jan,8; 2016,Jan,13; 2015,Jan,16

74176-74178 Computerized Tomography: Abdomen and Pelvis

CMS: 100-04,4,250.16 Multiple Procedure Payment Reduction: Certain Diagnostic Imaging Procedures Rendered by Physicians

EXCLUDES *CT abdomen or pelvis alone (72192-72194, 74150-74170)*
Procedure performed more than one time for each combined abdomen and pelvis examination

74176 **Computed tomography, abdomen and pelvis; without contrast material**
5.63 5.63 **FUD** XXX Q3 Z3
AMA: 2020,Sep,11; 2018,Jan,8; 2017,Jan,8; 2016,Jan,13; 2015,Jan,16

74177 **with contrast material(s)**
8.99 8.99 **FUD** XXX Q3 Z2
AMA: 2020,Sep,11; 2018,Jan,8; 2017,Jan,8; 2016,Jan,13; 2015,Jan,16

74178 **without contrast material in one or both body regions, followed by contrast material(s) and further sections in one or both body regions**
10.3 10.3 **FUD** XXX Q3 Z2
AMA: 2020,Sep,11; 2018,Jan,8; 2017,Jan,8; 2016,Jan,13; 2015,Jan,16

74181-74183 Magnetic Resonance Imaging: Abdomen–General

CMS: 100-04,4,250.16 Multiple Procedure Payment Reduction: Certain Diagnostic Imaging Procedures Rendered by Physicians

74181 **Magnetic resonance (eg, proton) imaging, abdomen; without contrast material(s)**

6.34 6.34 FUD XXX 03 Z2 80

AMA: 2018,Mar,11; 2018,Jan,8; 2017,Jan,8; 2016,Jan,13; 2015,Jan,16

74182 **with contrast material(s)**

9.90 9.90 FUD XXX 03 Z2 80

AMA: 2018,Mar,11; 2018,Jan,8; 2017,Jan,8; 2016,Jan,13; 2015,Jan,16

74183 **without contrast material(s), followed by with contrast material(s) and further sequences**

11.0 11.0 FUD XXX 03 Z2 80

AMA: 2018,Mar,11; 2018,Jan,8; 2017,Jan,8; 2016,Jan,13; 2015,Jan,16

74185 Magnetic Resonance Angiography: Abdomen–General

CMS: 100-04,13,40.1.1 Magnetic Resonance Angiography; 100-04,13,40.1.2 HCPCS Coding Requirements; 100-04,4,250.16 Multiple Procedure Payment Reduction: Certain Diagnostic Imaging Procedures Rendered by Physicians

74185 **Magnetic resonance angiography, abdomen, with or without contrast material(s)**

11.1 11.1 FUD XXX B 80

AMA: 2018,Jan,8; 2017,Jan,8; 2016,Jan,13; 2015,Jan,16

74190 Peritoneography

74190 **Peritoneogram (eg, after injection of air or contrast), radiological supervision and interpretation**

EXCLUDES *CT pelvis or abdomen (72192, 74150)*

Code also injection procedure (49400)

0.00 0.00 FUD XXX Q2 N1 80

AMA: 2018,Jan,8; 2017,Jan,8; 2016,Jan,13; 2015,Jan,16

74210-74235 Radiography: Throat and Esophagus

EXCLUDES *Percutaneous placement gastrostomy tube, endoscopic (43246)*
Percutaneous placement gastrostomy tube, fluoroscopic guidance (49440)

74210 **Radiologic examination, pharynx and/or cervical esophagus, including scout neck radiograph(s) and delayed image(s), when performed, contrast (eg, barium) study**

2.49 2.49 FUD XXX Q1 N1 80

AMA: 2020,Aug,9

74220 **Radiologic examination, esophagus, including scout chest radiograph(s) and delayed image(s), when performed; single-contrast (eg, barium) study**

EXCLUDES *Double-contrast study (74221)*
Small bowel follow-through (74248)
Upper GI tract studies (74240-74246)

2.71 2.71 FUD XXX Q1 N1 80

AMA: 2020,Aug,9

74221 **double-contrast (eg, high-density barium and effervescent agent) study**

EXCLUDES *Single-contrast study (74220)*
Small bowel follow-through (74248)
Upper GI tract studies (74240-74246)

3.06 3.06 FUD XXX 80

AMA: 2020,Aug,9

74230 **Radiologic examination, swallowing function, with cineradiography/videoradiography, including scout neck radiograph(s) and delayed image(s), when performed, contrast (eg, barium) study**

EXCLUDES *Swallowing function motion fluoroscopic examination (92611)*

3.64 3.64 FUD XXX Q1 Z2 80

AMA: 2020,Aug,9; 2018,Jan,8; 2017,Jan,8; 2016,Jan,13; 2015,Jan,16

74235 **Removal of foreign body(s), esophageal, with use of balloon catheter, radiological supervision and interpretation**

Code also procedure (43499)

0.00 0.00 FUD XXX N N1 80

AMA: 2014,Jan,11; 2012,Feb,9-10

74240-74283 Radiography: Intestines

EXCLUDES *Percutaneous placement gastrostomy tube, endoscopic (43246)*
Percutaneous placement gastrostomy tube, fluoroscopic guidance (49440)

74240 **Radiologic examination, upper gastrointestinal tract, including scout abdominal radiograph(s) and delayed image(s), when performed; single-contrast (eg, barium) study**

INCLUDES Upper GI with KUB

EXCLUDES *Double-contrast study (74246)*
Esophagus studies (74220-74221)

Code also small bowel follow-through when performed (74248)

3.45 3.45 FUD XXX Q1 Z3 80

AMA: 2020,Aug,9; 2018,Jan,8; 2017,Jan,8; 2016,Sep,7

74246 **double-contrast (eg, high-density barium and effervescent agent) study, including glucagon, when administered**

INCLUDES Upper GI with KUB

EXCLUDES *Esophagus studies (74220-74221)*
Single-contrast study (74240)

3.84 3.84 FUD XXX Q1 Z2 80

AMA: 2020,Aug,9; 2018,Jan,8; 2017,Jan,8; 2016,Sep,7

+ **74248** **Radiologic small intestine follow-through study, including multiple serial images (List separately in addition to code for primary procedure for upper GI radiologic examination)**

EXCLUDES *Single- or double-contrast small intestine studies (74250-74251)*

Code first (74240, 74246)

2.32 2.32 FUD ZZZ 80

AMA: 2020,Aug,9

74250 **Radiologic examination, small intestine, including multiple serial images and scout abdominal radiograph(s), when performed; single-contrast (eg, barium) study**

EXCLUDES *Double-contrast study (74251)*
Small bowel follow-through (74248)

3.41 3.41 FUD XXX Q1 Z3 80

AMA: 2020,Aug,9; 2018,Jan,8; 2017,Jan,8; 2016,Sep,7

74251 **double-contrast (eg, high-density barium and air via enteroclysis tube) study, including glucagon, when administered**

EXCLUDES *Single-contrast study (74250)*
Small bowel follow-through (74248)

Code also insertion long gastrointestinal tube (44500, 74340)

11.3 11.3 FUD XXX S Z2 80

AMA: 2020,Aug,9; 2018,Jan,8; 2017,Jan,8; 2016,Sep,7

74261 **Computed tomographic (CT) colonography, diagnostic, including image postprocessing; without contrast material**

EXCLUDES *3D rendering (76376-76377)*
CT abdomen or pelvis alone (72192-72194, 74150-74170)
Screening CT colonography (74263)

13.4 13.4 FUD XXX 03 Z2 80

AMA: 2020,Sep,11; 2020,Feb,13; 2018,Jan,8; 2017,Jan,8; 2016,Jan,13; 2015,Jan,16

74262 **with contrast material(s) including non-contrast images, if performed**

EXCLUDES *3D rendering (76376-76377)*
CT abdomen or pelvis alone (72192-72194, 74150-74170)
Screening CT colonography (74263)

15.1 15.1 FUD XXX 03 Z2 80

AMA: 2020,Sep,11; 2020,Feb,13; 2018,Jan,8; 2017,Jan,8; 2016,Jan,13; 2015,Jan,16

74263 **Computed tomographic (CT) colonography, screening, including image postprocessing**

EXCLUDES *3D rendering (76376-76377)*
CT abdomen or pelvis alone (72192-72194, 74150-74170)
CT colonography (74261-74262)

21.1 21.1 FUD XXX E

AMA: 2020,Sep,11; 2020,Feb,13; 2018,Jan,8; 2017,Jan,8; 2016,Jan,13; 2015,Jan,16

74270 **Radiologic examination, colon, including scout abdominal radiograph(s) and delayed image(s), when performed; single-contrast (eg, barium) study**

EXCLUDES *Double-contrast study (74280)*

4.34 4.34 FUD XXX Q1 N1 80

AMA: 2020,Aug,9; 2018,Jan,8; 2017,Jan,8; 2016,Jan,13; 2015,Jan,16

74280 **double-contrast (eg, high density barium and air) study, including glucagon, when administered**

EXCLUDES *Single-contrast study (74270)*

6.41 6.41 FUD XXX S N1 80

AMA: 2020,Aug,9

74283 **Therapeutic enema, contrast or air, for reduction of intussusception or other intraluminal obstruction (eg, meconium ileus)**

7.00 7.00 FUD XXX S Z2 80

AMA: 2014,Jan,11; 2012,Feb,9-10

74290-74330 Radiography: Biliary Tract

74290 **Cholecystography, oral contrast**

2.15 2.15 FUD XXX Q1 N1 80

AMA: 2014,Jan,11; 2012,Feb,9-10

74300 **Cholangiography and/or pancreatography; intraoperative, radiological supervision and interpretation**

0.00 0.00 FUD XXX N N1 80

AMA: 2018,Jan,8; 2017,Jan,8; 2016,Jan,13; 2015,Dec,3; 2015,Jan,16

+ **74301** **additional set intraoperative, radiological supervision and interpretation (List separately in addition to code for primary procedure)**

Code first (74300)

0.00 0.00 FUD ZZZ N N1 80

AMA: 2015,Dec,3

74328 **Endoscopic catheterization of the biliary ductal system, radiological supervision and interpretation**

Code also ERCP (43261-43265, 43274-43278 [43274, 43275, 43276, 43277, 43278])

0.00 0.00 FUD XXX N N1 80

AMA: 2018,Jan,8; 2017,Jan,8; 2016,Jan,13; 2015,Jan,16

74329 **Endoscopic catheterization of the pancreatic ductal system, radiological supervision and interpretation**

Code also ERCP (43261-43265, 43274-43278 [43274, 43275, 43276, 43277, 43278])

0.00 0.00 FUD XXX N N1 80

AMA: 2014,Jan,11; 2012,Feb,9-10

74330 **Combined endoscopic catheterization of the biliary and pancreatic ductal systems, radiological supervision and interpretation**

Code also ERCP (43261-43265, 43274-43278 [43274, 43275, 43276, 43277, 43278])

0.00 0.00 FUD XXX N N1 80

AMA: 2014,Jan,11; 2012,Feb,9-10

74340-74363 Radiography: Bilidigestive Intubation

EXCLUDES *Percutaneous placement gastrostomy tube, endoscopic (43246)*
Percutaneous placement gastrotomy tube, fluoroscopic guidance (49440)

74340 **Introduction of long gastrointestinal tube (eg, Miller-Abbott), including multiple fluoroscopies and images, radiological supervision and interpretation**

Code also placement tube (44500)

0.00 0.00 FUD XXX N N1 80

AMA: 2020,Aug,9; 2018,Jan,8; 2017,Jan,8; 2016,Sep,9

74355 **Percutaneous placement of enteroclysis tube, radiological supervision and interpretation**

INCLUDES Fluoroscopic guidance (77002)

0.00 0.00 FUD XXX N N1 80

AMA: 2018,Jan,8; 2017,Jan,8; 2016,Jan,13; 2015,Jan,16

74360 **Intraluminal dilation of strictures and/or obstructions (eg, esophagus), radiological supervision and interpretation**

EXCLUDES *Esophagogastroduodenoscopy, flexible, transoral; with dilation esophagus (43233)*
Esophagoscopy, flexible, transoral; with dilation esophagus (43213-43214)

0.00 0.00 FUD XXX N N1 80

AMA: 2018,Jan,8; 2017,Jan,8; 2016,Jan,13; 2015,Jan,16

74363 **Percutaneous transhepatic dilation of biliary duct stricture with or without placement of stent, radiological supervision and interpretation**

EXCLUDES *Surgical procedure (47555-47556)*

0.00 0.00 FUD XXX N N1 80

AMA: 2014,Jan,11; 2012,Feb,9-10

74400-74775 Radiography: Urogenital

74400 **Urography (pyelography), intravenous, with or without KUB, with or without tomography**

3.36 3.36 FUD XXX S Z2 80

AMA: 2014,Jan,11; 2012,Feb,9-10

74410 **Urography, infusion, drip technique and/or bolus technique;**

3.66 3.66 FUD XXX S Z2 80

AMA: 2014,Jan,11; 2012,Feb,9-10

74415 **with nephrotomography**

4.28 4.28 FUD XXX S Z2 80

AMA: 2014,Jan,11; 2012,Feb,9-10

74420 **Urography, retrograde, with or without KUB**

2.08 2.08 FUD XXX S Z2 80

AMA: 2018,Jan,8; 2017,Jan,8; 2016,Jan,13; 2015,Jan,16

▲ **74425 Urography, antegrade, radiological supervision and interpretation**

EXCLUDES *Injection for antegrade nephrostogram and/or ureterogram ([50430, 50431, 50432, 50433, 50434, 50435])*
Ureteral stent placement (50693-50695)

Code also aspiration/injection renal cyst or pelvis, percutaneous (50390)
Code also injection procedure:
ureterography or ureteropyelography (50684)
visualization ileal conduit/ureteropyelography (50690)
Code also manometric study through nephrostomy or pyelostomy tube (50396)

3.66 3.66 FUD XXX Q2 N1 80

AMA: 2018,Jan,8; 2017,Jan,8; 2016,Jan,13; 2016,Jan,3; 2015,Oct,5; 2015,Jan,16

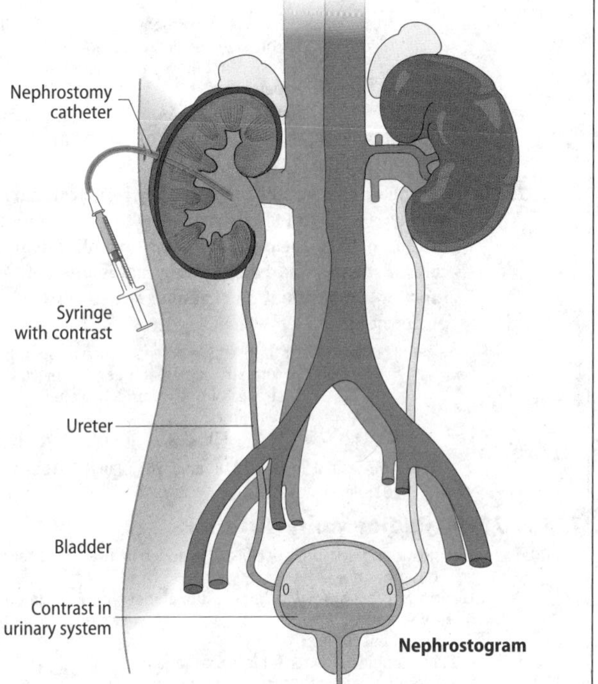

74430 Cystography, minimum of 3 views, radiological supervision and interpretation

1.13 1.13 FUD XXX Q2 N1 80

AMA: 2014,Jan,11; 2012,Feb,9-10

74440 Vasography, vesiculography, or epididymography, radiological supervision and interpretation ♂

2.44 2.44 FUD XXX Q2 N1 80

AMA: 2014,Jan,11; 2012,Feb,9-10

74445 Corpora cavernosography, radiological supervision and interpretation ♂

INCLUDES Needle placement with fluoroscopic guidance (77002)

0.00 0.00 FUD XXX Q2 N1 80

AMA: 2018,Jan,8; 2017,Jan,8; 2016,Jan,13; 2015,Jan,16

74450 Urethrocystography, retrograde, radiological supervision and interpretation

0.00 0.00 FUD XXX Q2 N1 80

AMA: 2019,Oct,10

74455 Urethrocystography, voiding, radiological supervision and interpretation

2.55 2.55 FUD XXX Q2 N1 80

AMA: 2019,Oct,10

74470 Radiologic examination, renal cyst study, translumbar, contrast visualization, radiological supervision and interpretation

INCLUDES Needle placement with fluoroscopic guidance (77002)

0.00 0.00 FUD XXX Q2 N1 80

AMA: 2018,Jan,8; 2017,Jan,8; 2016,Jan,13; 2015,Jan,16

74485 Dilation of ureter(s) or urethra, radiological supervision and interpretation

EXCLUDES *Change pyelostomy/nephrostomy tube ([50435])*
Nephrostomy tract dilation for procedure ([50436, 50437])
Ureter dilation without radiologic guidance (52341, 52344)

3.19 3.19 FUD XXX Q2 N1 80

AMA: 2018,Jan,8; 2017,Jan,8; 2016,Jan,13; 2016,Jan,3; 2015,Oct,5; 2015,Jan,16

74710 Pelvimetry, with or without placental localization ♀

EXCLUDES *Imaging procedures on abdomen and pelvis (72170-72190, 74018-74019, 74021-74022, 74150-74170)*

1.08 1.08 FUD XXX Q1 N1 80

AMA: 2014,Jan,11; 2012,Feb,9-10

74712 Magnetic resonance (eg, proton) imaging, fetal, including placental and maternal pelvic imaging when performed; single or first gestation ♀

EXCLUDES *Imaging maternal pelvis or placenta without fetal imaging (72195-72197)*

13.3 13.3 FUD XXX S Z2 80

AMA: 2018,Jan,8; 2017,Jan,8; 2016,Jun,5

\+ **74713 each additional gestation (List separately in addition to code for primary procedure)** ♀

EXCLUDES *Imaging maternal pelvis or placenta without fetal imaging (72195-72197)*

Code first (74712)

6.46 6.46 FUD ZZZ N N1 80

AMA: 2018,Jan,8; 2017,Jan,8; 2016,Jun,5

74740 Hysterosalpingography, radiological supervision and interpretation ♀

EXCLUDES *Imaging procedures abdomen and pelvis (72170-72190, 74018-74019, 74021-74022, 74150-74170)*

Code also injection saline/contrast (58340)

2.32 2.32 FUD XXX Q2 N1 80

AMA: 2018,Jan,8; 2017,Jan,8; 2016,Jan,13; 2015,Jan,16

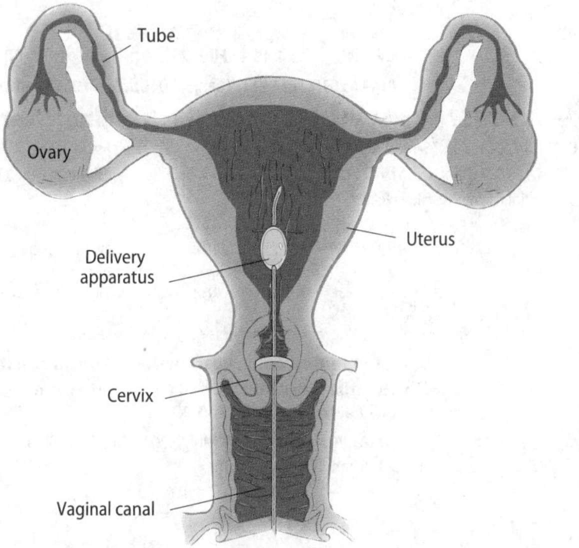

Hysterosalpingography (imaging of the uterus and tubes) is performed. Report for radiological supervision and interpretation

74742 **Transcervical catheterization of fallopian tube, radiological supervision and interpretation** ♀

EXCLUDES *Imaging procedures abdomen and pelvis (72170-72190, 74018-74019, 74021-74022, 74150-74170)*

Code also transcervical fallopian tube catheter (58345)

0.00 0.00 **FUD** XXX N N1 80

AMA: 2018,Jan,8; 2017,Jan,8; 2016,Jan,13; 2015,Jan,16

74775 **Perineogram (eg, vaginogram, for sex determination or extent of anomalies)** M ♀

EXCLUDES *Imaging procedures abdomen and pelvis (72170-72190, 74018-74019, 74021-74022, 74150-74170)*

0.00 0.00 **FUD** XXX S Z2 80

AMA: 2014,Jan,11; 2012,Feb,9-10

75557-75565 Magnetic Resonance Imaging: Heart Structure and Physiology

INCLUDES Physiologic evaluation cardiac function

EXCLUDES *3D rendering (76376-76377)*
Cardiac catheterization procedures (93451-93572)
Reporting more than one code in this group per session

Code also separate vascular injection (36000-36299)

75557 **Cardiac magnetic resonance imaging for morphology and function without contrast material;**

9.01 9.01 **FUD** XXX 03 Z2 80

AMA: 2018,Jan,8; 2017,Jan,8; 2016,Jan,13; 2015,Jan,16

75559 **with stress imaging**

INCLUDES Pharmacologic wall motion stress evaluation without contrast

Code also stress testing when performed (93015-93018)

12.7 12.7 **FUD** XXX 03 Z2 80

AMA: 2018,Jan,8; 2017,Jan,8; 2016,Jan,13; 2015,Jan,16

75561 **Cardiac magnetic resonance imaging for morphology and function without contrast material(s), followed by contrast material(s) and further sequences;**

12.0 12.0 **FUD** XXX 03 Z2 80

AMA: 2018,Jan,8; 2017,Jan,8; 2016,Jan,13; 2015,Jan,16

75563 **with stress imaging**

INCLUDES Pharmacologic perfusion stress evaluation with contrast

Code also stress testing when performed (93015-93018)

14.2 14.2 **FUD** XXX 03 Z2 80

AMA: 2018,Jan,8; 2017,Jan,8; 2016,Jan,13; 2015,Jan,16

\+ **75565** **Cardiac magnetic resonance imaging for velocity flow mapping (List separately in addition to code for primary procedure)**

Code first (75557, 75559, 75561, 75563)

1.48 1.48 **FUD** ZZZ N N1 80

AMA: 2018,Jan,8; 2017,Jan,8; 2016,Jan,13; 2015,Jan,16

75571-75574 Computed Tomographic Imaging: Heart

CMS: 100-04,12,20.4.7 Services Not Meeting National Electrical Manufacturers Association (NEMA) Standard; 100-04,4,20.6.12 Use of HCPCS Modifier – CT; 100-04,4,250.16 Multiple Procedure Payment Reduction: Certain Diagnostic Imaging Procedures Rendered by Physicians

EXCLUDES *3D rendering (76376-76377)*
Automated quantification/characterization coronary atherosclerotic plaque ([0623T, 0624T, 0625T, 0626T])
Fractional flow reserve (FFR) from coronary CT angiography data (0501T-0504T)
Reporting more than one code in this group per session

75571 **Computed tomography, heart, without contrast material, with quantitative evaluation of coronary calcium**

2.92 2.92 **FUD** XXX 01 N1 80

AMA: 2020,Sep,11; 2020,Jul,5; 2018,Jan,8; 2017,Jan,8; 2016,Jan,13; 2015,Jan,16

75572 **Computed tomography, heart, with contrast material, for evaluation of cardiac structure and morphology (including 3D image postprocessing, assessment of cardiac function, and evaluation of venous structures, if performed)**

INCLUDES Quantitative assessment(s) such as quantification coronary percentage stenosis, ejection fraction, stroke volume, ventricular volume, when performed

7.01 7.01 **FUD** XXX S Z2 80

AMA: 2020,Sep,11; 2018,Jan,8; 2017,Jan,8; 2016,Jan,13; 2015,Jan,16

75573 **Computed tomography, heart, with contrast material, for evaluation of cardiac structure and morphology in the setting of congenital heart disease (including 3D image postprocessing, assessment of LV cardiac function, RV structure and function and evaluation of venous structures, if performed)**

INCLUDES Quantitative assessment(s) such as quantification coronary percentage stenosis, ejection fraction, stroke volume, ventricular volume, when performed

9.43 9.43 **FUD** XXX S Z2 80

AMA: 2020,Sep,11; 2018,Jan,8; 2017,Jan,8; 2016,Jan,13; 2015,Jan,16

75574 **Computed tomographic angiography, heart, coronary arteries and bypass grafts (when present), with contrast material, including 3D image postprocessing (including evaluation of cardiac structure and morphology, assessment of cardiac function, and evaluation of venous structures, if performed)**

INCLUDES Quantitative assessment(s) such as quantification coronary percentage stenosis, ejection fraction, stroke volume, ventricular volume, when performed

11.0 11.0 **FUD** XXX S Z2 80

AMA: 2020,Sep,11; 2018,Jan,8; 2017,Jan,8; 2016,Jan,13; 2015,Jan,16

75600-75774 Radiography: Arterial

INCLUDES Diagnostic angiography specifically included in interventional code description
Diagnostic procedures with interventional supervision and interpretation:
- Angiography
- Contrast injection
- Fluoroscopic guidance for intervention
- Post-angioplasty/atherectomy/stent angiography
- Roadmapping
- Vessel measurement

EXCLUDES *Catheterization codes for diagnostic angiography lower extremity when access site other than site used for therapy required*
Diagnostic angiogram during separate encounter from interventional procedure
Diagnostic angiography with interventional procedure if:
1. No previous catheter-based angiogram accessible and complete diagnostic procedure performed, and decision to proceed with interventional procedure based on diagnostic service, OR
2. Previous diagnostic angiogram accessible but documentation in medical record specifies that:
A. patient's condition has changed
B. insufficient imaging patient's anatomy and/or disease, OR
C. clinical change during procedure that necessitates new examination away from intervention site
3. Modifier 59 appended to code(s) for diagnostic radiological supervision and interpretation service to indicate guidelines were met
Intra-arterial procedures (36100-36248)
Intravenous procedures (36000, 36005-36015)

75600 **Aortography, thoracic, without serialography, radiological supervision and interpretation**

EXCLUDES *Supravalvular aortography (93567)*

5.63 5.63 **FUD** XXX 02 N1 80

AMA: 2014,Jan,11; 2012,Feb,9-10

75605 **Aortography, thoracic, by serialography, radiological supervision and interpretation**

EXCLUDES *Supravalvular aortography (93567)*

3.67 3.67 **FUD** XXX 02 N1 80

AMA: 2018,Jan,8; 2017,Jan,8; 2016,Jan,13; 2015,Jan,16

75625 Aortography, abdominal, by serialography, radiological supervision and interpretation

EXCLUDES *Supravalvular aortography (93567)*

3.73 3.73 FUD XXX Q2 N1 80

AMA: 2020,Sep,14; 2018,Jan,8; 2017,Jan,8; 2016,Jan,13; 2015,Jan,16

75630 Aortography, abdominal plus bilateral iliofemoral lower extremity, catheter, by serialography, radiological supervision and interpretation

EXCLUDES *Supravalvular aortography (93567)*

4.81 4.81 FUD XXX Q2 N1 80

AMA: 2020,Sep,14; 2018,Jan,8; 2017,Jan,8; 2016,Jan,13; 2015,Jan,16

75635 Computed tomographic angiography, abdominal aorta and bilateral iliofemoral lower extremity runoff, with contrast material(s), including noncontrast images, if performed, and image postprocessing

EXCLUDES *3D rendering (76376-76377)*
CT angiography, abdomen, lower extremity, pelvis (72191, 73706, 74174-74175)

12.4 12.4 FUD XXX Q2 N1 80

AMA: 2020,Sep,11; 2018,Jan,8; 2017,Jan,8; 2016,Jan,13; 2015,Jan,16

75705 Angiography, spinal, selective, radiological supervision and interpretation

7.09 7.09 FUD XXX Q2 N1 80

AMA: 2014,Jan,11; 2012,Feb,9-10

75710 Angiography, extremity, unilateral, radiological supervision and interpretation

4.63 4.63 FUD XXX Q2 N1 80

AMA: 2018,Jan,8; 2017,Mar,3; 2017,Jan,8; 2016,Jan,13; 2015,Jan,16

75716 Angiography, extremity, bilateral, radiological supervision and interpretation

5.04 5.04 FUD XXX Q2 N1 80

AMA: 2020,Sep,14; 2018,Jan,8; 2017,Jan,8; 2016,Jan,13; 2015,Jan,16

75726 Angiography, visceral, selective or supraselective (with or without flush aortogram), radiological supervision and interpretation

EXCLUDES *Selective angiography, each additional visceral vessel examined after basic examination (75774)*

5.20 5.20 FUD XXX Q2 N1 80

AMA: 2014,Jan,11; 2012,Feb,9-10

75731 Angiography, adrenal, unilateral, selective, radiological supervision and interpretation

4.73 4.73 FUD XXX Q2 Z3 80

AMA: 2014,Jan,11; 2012,Feb,9-10

75733 Angiography, adrenal, bilateral, selective, radiological supervision and interpretation

5.09 5.09 FUD XXX Q2 N1 80

AMA: 2014,Jan,11; 2012,Feb,9-10

75736 Angiography, pelvic, selective or supraselective, radiological supervision and interpretation

4.38 4.38 FUD XXX Q2 N1 80

AMA: 2014,Jan,11; 2012,Feb,9-10

75741 Angiography, pulmonary, unilateral, selective, radiological supervision and interpretation

4.03 4.03 FUD XXX Q2 N1 80

AMA: 2019,Jun,3; 2018,Jan,8; 2017,Jan,8; 2016,Jan,13; 2015,Jan,16

75743 Angiography, pulmonary, bilateral, selective, radiological supervision and interpretation

4.55 4.55 FUD XXX Q2 N1 80

AMA: 2019,Jun,3; 2018,Jan,8; 2017,Jan,8; 2016,Jan,13; 2015,Jan,16

75746 Angiography, pulmonary, by nonselective catheter or venous injection, radiological supervision and interpretation

EXCLUDES *Nonselective injection procedure or catheter introduction with cardiac cath (93568)*

4.07 4.07 FUD XXX Q2 Z3 80

AMA: 2019,Jun,3

75756 Angiography, internal mammary, radiological supervision and interpretation

EXCLUDES *Internal mammary angiography with cardiac cath (93455, 93457, 93459, 93461, 93564)*

4.62 4.62 FUD XXX Q2 N1 80

AMA: 2018,Jan,8; 2017,Jan,8; 2016,Jan,13; 2015,Jan,16

+ **75774 Angiography, selective, each additional vessel studied after basic examination, radiological supervision and interpretation (List separately in addition to code for primary procedure)**

EXCLUDES *Angiography (75600-75756)*
Cardiac cath procedures (93452-93462, 93531-93533, 93563-93568)
Catheterizations (36215-36248)
Dialysis circuit angiography (current access), report modifier 52 with (36901)
Nonselective catheter placement, thoracic aorta (36221-36228)

Code also diagnostic angiography upper extremities and other vascular beds (except cervicocerebral vessels), when appropriate

Code first initial vessel

3.04 3.04 FUD ZZZ N N1 80

AMA: 2020,Sep,14; 2018,Jan,8; 2017,Jan,8; 2016,Jan,13; 2015,Jan,16

75801-75893 Radiography: Lymphatic and Venous

INCLUDES Diagnostic venography specifically included in interventional code description
Diagnostic procedures with interventional supervision and interpretation:
- Contrast injection
- Fluoroscopic guidance for intervention
- Post-angioplasty/venography
- Roadmapping
- Venography
- Vessel measurement

EXCLUDES *Diagnostic venogram during separate encounter from interventional procedure*
Diagnostic venography with interventional procedure if:
1. No previous catheter-based venogram accessible and complete diagnostic procedure performed and decision to proceed with interventional procedure based on diagnostic service, OR
2. Previous diagnostic venogram accessible but documentation in medical record specifies that:
A. patient's condition has changed
B. insufficient imaging patient's anatomy and/or disease, OR
C. clinical change during procedure that necessitates new examination away from intervention site
Intravenous procedures (36000-36015, 36400-36510 [36465, 36466, 36482, 36483])
Lymphatic injection procedures (38790)

75801 Lymphangiography, extremity only, unilateral, radiological supervision and interpretation

0.00 0.00 FUD XXX Q2 N1 80

AMA: 2014,Jan,11; 2012,Feb,9-10

75803 Lymphangiography, extremity only, bilateral, radiological supervision and interpretation

0.00 0.00 FUD XXX Q2 Z2 80

AMA: 2014,Jan,11; 2012,Feb,9-10

75805 Lymphangiography, pelvic/abdominal, unilateral, radiological supervision and interpretation

0.00 0.00 FUD XXX Q2 Z2 80

AMA: 2014,Jan,11; 2012,Feb,9-10

75807 Lymphangiography, pelvic/abdominal, bilateral, radiological supervision and interpretation

0.00 0.00 FUD XXX Q2 N1 80

AMA: 2014,Jan,11; 2012,Feb,9-10

75809 Shuntogram for investigation of previously placed indwelling nonvascular shunt (eg, LeVeen shunt, ventriculoperitoneal shunt, indwelling infusion pump), radiological supervision and interpretation

Code also surgical procedure (49427, 61070)

2.69 2.69 FUD XXX Q2 N1 80

AMA: 2018,Jan,8; 2017,Jan,8; 2016,Jan,13; 2015,Jan,16

75810 Splenoportography, radiological supervision and interpretation

0.00 0.00 FUD XXX Q2 Z2 80

AMA: 2018,Jan,8; 2017,Jan,8; 2016,Jan,13; 2015,Jan,16

75820 Venography, extremity, unilateral, radiological supervision and interpretation

3.15 3.15 FUD XXX Q2 N1 80

AMA: 2019,Mar,6; 2018,Jan,8; 2017,Jan,8; 2016,May,5; 2016,Jan,13; 2015,May,3; 2015,Jan,16

75822 Venography, extremity, bilateral, radiological supervision and interpretation

3.56 3.56 FUD XXX Q2 Z3 80

AMA: 2014,Jan,11; 2012,Feb,9-10

75825 Venography, caval, inferior, with serialography, radiological supervision and interpretation

3.55 3.55 FUD XXX Q2 N1 80

AMA: 2018,Jan,8; 2017,Feb,14; 2017,Jan,8; 2016,Jan,13; 2015,Jan,16

75827 Venography, caval, superior, with serialography, radiological supervision and interpretation

3.82 3.82 FUD XXX Q2 N1 80

AMA: 2018,Jan,8; 2017,Jan,8; 2016,Jan,13; 2015,Jan,16

75831 Venography, renal, unilateral, selective, radiological supervision and interpretation

3.70 3.70 FUD XXX Q2 N1 80

AMA: 2014,Jan,11; 2012,Feb,9-10

75833 Venography, renal, bilateral, selective, radiological supervision and interpretation

4.55 4.55 FUD XXX Q2 N1 80

AMA: 2014,Jan,11; 2012,Feb,9-10

75840 Venography, adrenal, unilateral, selective, radiological supervision and interpretation

4.08 4.08 FUD XXX Q2 N1 80

AMA: 2014,Jan,11; 2012,Feb,9-10

75842 Venography, adrenal, bilateral, selective, radiological supervision and interpretation

4.95 4.95 FUD XXX Q2 N1 80

AMA: 2014,Jan,11; 2012,Feb,9-10

75860 Venography, venous sinus (eg, petrosal and inferior sagittal) or jugular, catheter, radiological supervision and interpretation

3.99 3.99 FUD XXX Q2 N1 80

AMA: 2014,Jan,11; 2012,Feb,9-10

75870 Venography, superior sagittal sinus, radiological supervision and interpretation

5.30 5.30 FUD XXX Q2 Z3 80

AMA: 2014,Jan,11; 2012,Feb,9-10

75872 Venography, epidural, radiological supervision and interpretation

4.08 4.08 FUD XXX Q2 N1 80

AMA: 2014,Jan,11; 2012,Feb,9-10

75880 Venography, orbital, radiological supervision and interpretation

3.44 3.44 FUD XXX Q2 N1 80

AMA: 2014,Jan,11; 2012,Feb,9-10

75885 Percutaneous transhepatic portography with hemodynamic evaluation, radiological supervision and interpretation

4.21 4.21 FUD XXX Q2 N1 80

AMA: 2018,Jan,8; 2017,Jan,8; 2016,Jan,13; 2015,Jan,16

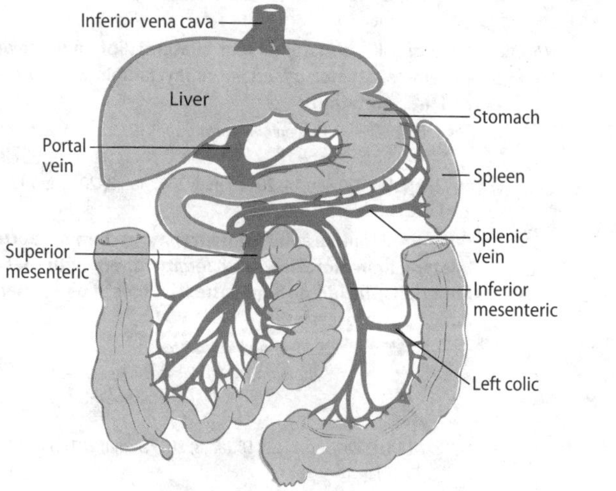

Schematic showing the portal vein

75887 Percutaneous transhepatic portography without hemodynamic evaluation, radiological supervision and interpretation

4.24 4.24 FUD XXX Q2 Z3 80

AMA: 2018,Jan,8; 2017,Jan,8; 2016,Jan,13; 2015,Jan,16

75889 Hepatic venography, wedged or free, with hemodynamic evaluation, radiological supervision and interpretation

3.81 3.81 FUD XXX Q2 N1 80

AMA: 2014,Jan,11; 2012,Feb,9-10

75891 Hepatic venography, wedged or free, without hemodynamic evaluation, radiological supervision and interpretation

3.87 3.87 FUD XXX Q2 N1 80

AMA: 2014,Jan,11; 2012,Feb,9-10

75893 Venous sampling through catheter, with or without angiography (eg, for parathyroid hormone, renin), radiological supervision and interpretation

Code also surgical procedure (36500)

3.32 3.32 FUD XXX Q2 N1 80

AMA: 2014,Jan,11; 2012,Feb,9-10

75894-75902 Transcatheter Procedures

INCLUDES Diagnostic procedures with interventional supervision and interpretation:
- Angiography/venography
- Completion angiography/venography except for those services allowed by (75898)
- Contrast injection
- Fluoroscopic guidance for intervention
- Roadmapping
- Vessel measurement

EXCLUDES *Diagnostic angiography/venography performed same session as transcatheter therapy unless specifically included in code descriptor or excluded in venography/angiography notes (75600-75893)*

75894 Transcatheter therapy, embolization, any method, radiological supervision and interpretation

EXCLUDES *Endovenous ablation therapy incompetent vein (36478-36479)*
Transluminal balloon angioplasty (36475-36476)
Vascular embolization or occlusion (37241-37244)

0.00 0.00 FUD XXX N N1 80

AMA: 2018,Mar,3; 2018,Jan,8; 2017,Jan,8; 2016,Nov,3; 2016,Jan,13; 2015,Jan,16

75898 **Angiography through existing catheter for follow-up study for transcatheter therapy, embolization or infusion, other than for thrombolysis**

EXCLUDES *Percutaneous arterial transluminal mechanical thrombectomy (61645)*
Prolonged endovascular intracranial administration pharmacologic agent(s) (61650-61651)
Transcatheter therapy, arterial infusion for thrombolysis (37211-37214)
Vascular embolization or occlusion (37241-37244)

0.00 0.00 **FUD** XXX Q2 Z2 80

AMA: 2019,Sep,6; 2018,Jan,8; 2017,Jan,8; 2016,Jan,13; 2015,Nov,3; 2015,Jan,16

75901 **Mechanical removal of pericatheter obstructive material (eg, fibrin sheath) from central venous device via separate venous access, radiologic supervision and interpretation**

EXCLUDES *Venous catheterization (36010-36012)*

Code also surgical procedure (36595)

6.15 6.15 **FUD** XXX N N1 80

AMA: 2018,Jan,8; 2017,Jan,8; 2016,Jan,13; 2015,Jan,16

75902 **Mechanical removal of intraluminal (intracatheter) obstructive material from central venous device through device lumen, radiologic supervision and interpretation**

EXCLUDES *Venous catheterization (36010-36012)*

Code also surgical procedure (36596)

2.40 2.40 **FUD** XXX N N1 80

AMA: 2018,Jan,8; 2017,Jan,8; 2016,Jan,13; 2015,Jan,16

75956-75959 Endovascular Aneurysm Repair

INCLUDES Diagnostic procedures with interventional supervision and interpretation:
Angiography/venography
Completion angiography/venography except for those services allowed by (75898)
Contrast injection
Fluoroscopic guidance for intervention
Injection procedure only for transcatheter therapy or biopsy (36100-36299)
Percutaneous needle biopsy;
Pancreas (48102)
Retroperitoneal lymph node/mass (49180)
Roadmapping
Vessel measurement

EXCLUDES *Diagnostic angiography/venography performed same session as transcatheter therapy unless specifically included in code descriptor (75600-75893)*
Radiological supervision and interpretation for transluminal angioplasty in:
Femoral/popliteal arteries (37224-37227)
Iliac artery (37220-37223)
Tibial/peroneal artery (37228-37235)

75956 **Endovascular repair of descending thoracic aorta (eg, aneurysm, pseudoaneurysm, dissection, penetrating ulcer, intramural hematoma, or traumatic disruption); involving coverage of left subclavian artery origin, initial endoprosthesis plus descending thoracic aortic extension(s), if required, to level of celiac artery origin, radiological supervision and interpretation**

Code also endovascular graft implantation (33880)

0.00 0.00 **FUD** XXX C 80

AMA: 2018,Jan,8; 2017,Jan,8; 2016,Jan,13; 2015,Jan,16

75957 **not involving coverage of left subclavian artery origin, initial endoprosthesis plus descending thoracic aortic extension(s), if required, to level of celiac artery origin, radiological supervision and interpretation**

Code also endovascular graft implantation (33881)

0.00 0.00 **FUD** XXX C 80

AMA: 2018,Jan,8; 2017,Jan,8; 2016,Jan,13; 2015,Jan,16

75958 **Placement of proximal extension prosthesis for endovascular repair of descending thoracic aorta (eg, aneurysm, pseudoaneurysm, dissection, penetrating ulcer, intramural hematoma, or traumatic disruption), radiological supervision and interpretation**

Code also placement each additional proximal extension(s) (75958)

Code also proximal endovascular extension implantation (33883-33884)

0.00 0.00 **FUD** XXX C 80

AMA: 2018,Jan,8; 2017,Jan,8; 2016,Jan,13; 2015,Jan,16

75959 **Placement of distal extension prosthesis(s) (delayed) after endovascular repair of descending thoracic aorta, as needed, to level of celiac origin, radiological supervision and interpretation**

INCLUDES Corresponding services for placement distal thoracic endovascular extension(s) placed during procedure following principal procedure

EXCLUDES *Endovascular repair descending thoracic aorta (75956-75957)*
Reporting code more than one time no matter how many modules are deployed

Code also placement distal endovascular extension (33886)

0.00 0.00 **FUD** XXX C 80

AMA: 2018,Jan,8; 2017,Jan,8; 2016,Jan,13; 2015,Jan,16

75970 Percutaneous Transluminal Angioplasty

INCLUDES Diagnostic procedures with interventional supervision and interpretation:
Angiography/venography
Completion angiography/venography except for those services allowed by (75898)
Contrast injection
Fluoroscopic guidance for intervention
Roadmapping
Vessel measurement

EXCLUDES *Diagnostic angiography/venography performed same session as transcatheter therapy unless specifically included in code descriptor (75600-75893)*
Injection procedure only for transcatheter therapy or biopsy (36100-36299)
Percutaneous needle biopsy (48102)
Pancreas (48102)
Retroperitoneal lymph node/mass (49180)
Radiological supervision and interpretation for transluminal balloon angioplasty in:
Femoral/popliteal arteries (37224-37227)
Iliac artery (37220-37223)
Tibial/peroneal artery (37228-37235)
Transcatheter renal/ureteral biopsy (52007)

75970 **Transcatheter biopsy, radiological supervision and interpretation**

0.00 0.00 **FUD** XXX N N1 80

AMA: 2018,Jan,8

75984-75989 Percutaneous Drainage

75984 **Change of percutaneous tube or drainage catheter with contrast monitoring (eg, genitourinary system, abscess), radiological supervision and interpretation**

EXCLUDES *Change only nephrostomy/pyelostomy tube ([50435])*
Cholecystostomy, percutaneous (47490)
Introduction procedure only for percutaneous biliary drainage (47531-47544)
Nephrostolithotomy/pyelostolithotomy, percutaneous (50080-50081)
Percutaneous replacement gastrointestinal tube using fluoroscopic guidance (49450-49452)
Removal and/or replacement internal ureteral stent using transurethral approach (50385-50386)

2.89 2.89 **FUD** XXX N N1 80

AMA: 2014,Jan,11; 2012,Feb,9-10

75989 **Radiological guidance (ie, fluoroscopy, ultrasound, or computed tomography), for percutaneous drainage (eg, abscess, specimen collection), with placement of catheter, radiological supervision and interpretation**

INCLUDES Imaging guidance

EXCLUDES *Cholecystostomy (47490)*
Image-guided fluid collection drainage by catheter (10030, 49405-49407)
Pericardial drainage (33017-33019)
Thoracentesis (32554-32557)

3.42 3.42 FUD XXX N N1 80

AMA: 2020,Jan,7; 2018,Jan,8; 2017,Jan,8; 2016,Jan,13; 2015,Dec,3; 2015,Jan,16

76000-76145 Miscellaneous Techniques

EXCLUDES *Arthrography:*
Ankle (73615)
Elbow (73085)
Hip (73525)
Knee (73580)
Shoulder (73040)
Wrist (73115)
CT cerebral perfusion test (0042T)

76000 **Fluoroscopy (separate procedure), up to 1 hour physician or other qualified health care professional time**

EXCLUDES *Extracorporeal membrane oxygenation (ECMO)/extracorporeal life support (ECLS) (33957-33959, [33962, 33963, 33964])*
Insertion/removal/replacement wireless cardiac stimulator (0515T-0520T)
Insertion/replacement/removal leadless pacemaker ([33274, 33275])

1.18 1.18 FUD XXX S Z3 80

AMA: 2019,Sep,10; 2019,Sep,5; 2019,Jun,3; 2019,Mar,6; 2018,Apr,7; 2018,Mar,3; 2018,Jan,8; 2017,Jan,8; 2016,Nov,3; 2016,Aug,5; 2016,May,5; 2016,May,13; 2016,Mar,5; 2016,Jan,11; 2016,Jan,13; 2015,Nov,3; 2015,Sep,3; 2015,May,3; 2015,Jan,16

76010 **Radiologic examination from nose to rectum for foreign body, single view, child** A

0.77 0.77 FUD XXX Q1 N1 80

AMA: 2018,Jan,8; 2017,Jan,8; 2016,Jan,13; 2015,Jan,16

76080 **Radiologic examination, abscess, fistula or sinus tract study, radiological supervision and interpretation**

EXCLUDES *Contrast injections, radiology evaluation, and guidance via fluoroscopy for gastrostomy, duodenostomy, jejunostomy, gastro-jejunostomy, or cecostomy tube (49465)*

1.67 1.67 FUD XXX Q2 N1 80

AMA: 2018,Jan,8; 2017,Jan,8; 2016,Jan,13; 2015,Jan,16

76098 **Radiological examination, surgical specimen**

EXCLUDES *Breast biopsy with placement breast localization device(s) (19081-19086)*

0.47 0.47 FUD XXX Q2 N1 80

AMA: 2012,Feb,9-10; 1997,Nov,1

76100 **Radiologic examination, single plane body section (eg, tomography), other than with urography**

2.75 2.75 FUD XXX Q1 N1 80

AMA: 2012,Feb,9-10; 1997,Nov,1

76101 **Radiologic examination, complex motion (ie, hypercycloidal) body section (eg, mastoid polytomography), other than with urography; unilateral**

EXCLUDES *Nephrotomography (74415)*
Panoramic x-ray (70355)
Procedure performed more than one time per day

2.77 2.77 FUD XXX Q1 Z2 80

AMA: 2012,Feb,9-10; 1997,Nov,1

76102 **bilateral**

EXCLUDES *Nephrotomography (74415)*
Panoramic x-ray (70355)
Procedure performed more than one time per day

4.88 4.88 FUD XXX S Z2 80

AMA: 2012,Feb,9-10; 1997,Nov,1

76120 **Cineradiography/videoradiography, except where specifically included**

2.87 2.87 FUD XXX Q1 N1 80

AMA: 2018,Jan,8; 2017,Jan,8; 2016,Jan,13; 2015,Jan,16

\+ **76125** **Cineradiography/videoradiography to complement routine examination (List separately in addition to code for primary procedure)**

Code first primary procedure

0.00 0.00 FUD ZZZ N N1 80

AMA: 2018,Jan,8; 2017,Jan,8; 2016,Jan,13; 2015,Jan,16

76140 **Consultation on X-ray examination made elsewhere, written report**

0.00 0.00 FUD XXX E

AMA: 2018,Jan,8; 2017,Jan,8; 2016,Jan,13; 2015,Jan,16

● **76145** **Medical physics dose evaluation for radiation exposure that exceeds institutional review threshold, including report**

76376-76377 Three-dimensional Manipulation

INCLUDES 3D manipulation volumetric data set
Concurrent physician supervision image postprocessing
Rendering image

EXCLUDES *Anatomic guide 3D-printed and designed from image data set (0561T-0562T)*
Anatomic model 3D-printed from image data set (0559T-0560T)
Arthrography:
Ankle (73615)
Elbow (73085)
Hip (73525)
Knee (73580)
Shoulder (73040)
Wrist (73115)
Automated quantification/characterization coronary atherosclerotic plaque ([0623T, 0624T, 0625T, 0626T])
Cardiac MRI (75557, 75559, 75561, 75563, 75565)
Computer-aided detection MRI data for lesion, breast MRI (77046-77049)
CT angiography (70496, 70498, 71275, 72191, 73206, 73706, 74174-74175, 74261-74263, 75571-75574, 75635)
CT breast (0633T-0638T)
CT cerebral perfusion test (0042T)
Digital breast tomosynthesis (77061-77063)
Echocardiography, transesophageal (TEE) for guidance (93355)
Magnetic resonance angiography (70544-70549, 71555, 72198, 73225, 73725, 74185)
Nuclear radiology procedures (78012-78999 [78429, 78430, 78431, 78432, 78433, 78434, 78804, 78830, 78831, 78832, 78835])
Physician planning patient-specific fenestrated visceral aortic endograft (34839)

Code also base imaging procedure(s)

76376 **3D rendering with interpretation and reporting of computed tomography, magnetic resonance imaging, ultrasound, or other tomographic modality with image postprocessing under concurrent supervision; not requiring image postprocessing on an independent workstation**

EXCLUDES *3D rendering (76377)*
Bronchoscopy, with computer-assisted, image-guided navigation (31627)

0.65 0.65 FUD XXX N N1 80

AMA: 2019,Oct,10; 2019,Sep,10; 2019,Aug,5; 2018,Jul,11; 2018,Jan,8; 2017,Jan,8; 2016,Apr,8; 2016,Jan,13; 2015,Jan,16

76377 **requiring image postprocessing on an independent workstation**

EXCLUDES *3D rendering (76376)*

2.01 2.01 FUD XXX N N1 80

AMA: 2019,Oct,10; 2019,Sep,10; 2019,Aug,5; 2018,Jul,11; 2018,Jan,8; 2017,Jan,8; 2016,Apr,8; 2016,Jan,13; 2015,Jan,16

76380 Computerized Tomography: Delimited

EXCLUDES *Arthrography:*
Ankle (73615)
Elbow (73085)
Hip (73525)
Knee (73580)
Shoulder (73040)
Wrist (73115)
CT cerebral perfusion test (0042T)

76380 Computed tomography, limited or localized follow-up study
4.07 4.07 FUD XXX Q1 N1 80
AMA: 2019,Mar,10; 2018,Jan,8; 2017,Jan,8; 2016,Jan,13; 2015,Jan,16

76390-76391 Magnetic Resonance Spectroscopy

EXCLUDES *Arthrography:*
Ankle (73615)
Elbow (73085)
Hip (73525)
Knee (73580)
Shoulder (73040)
Wrist (73115)
CT cerebral perfusion test (0042T)

76390 Magnetic resonance spectroscopy
EXCLUDES *MRI*
MR spectroscopy for discogenic pain (0609T-0610T)
11.9 11.9 FUD XXX E
AMA: 2012,Feb,9-10; 1997,Nov,1

76391 Magnetic resonance (eg, vibration) elastography
6.54 6.54 FUD XXX Z2 80
AMA: 2019,Aug,3

76496-76499 Unlisted Radiology Procedures

76496 Unlisted fluoroscopic procedure (eg, diagnostic, interventional)
0.00 0.00 FUD XXX Q1 N1 80
AMA: 2012,Feb,9-10; 1997,Nov,1

76497 Unlisted computed tomography procedure (eg, diagnostic, interventional)
0.00 0.00 FUD XXX Q1 N1 80
AMA: 2018,Sep,10; 2018,Jan,8; 2017,Jan,8; 2016,Jan,13; 2015,Jan,16

76498 Unlisted magnetic resonance procedure (eg, diagnostic, interventional)
0.00 0.00 FUD XXX S Z2 80
AMA: 2019,Aug,5; 2018,Jul,11; 2018,Jan,8; 2017,Jan,8; 2016,Jan,13; 2015,Jan,16

76499 Unlisted diagnostic radiographic procedure
0.00 0.00 FUD XXX Q1 N1 80
AMA: 2018,Jan,8; 2017,Jan,8; 2016,Dec,15; 2016,Jul,8; 2016,Jan,13; 2015,Jan,16

76506 Ultrasound: Brain

INCLUDES Required permanent documentation ultrasound images except when diagnostic purpose is biometric measurement
Written documentation

EXCLUDES *Noninvasive vascular studies, diagnostic (93880-93990)*
Ultrasound not including thorough assessment organ or site, recorded image, and written report

76506 Echoencephalography, real time with image documentation (gray scale) (for determination of ventricular size, delineation of cerebral contents, and detection of fluid masses or other intracranial abnormalities), including A-mode encephalography as secondary component where indicated
3.25 3.25 FUD XXX Q1 N1 80
AMA: 2018,Jan,8; 2017,Jan,8; 2016,Jan,13; 2015,Jan,16

76510-76529 Ultrasound: Eyes

INCLUDES Required permanent documentation ultrasound images except when diagnostic purpose is biometric measurement
Written documentation

76510 Ophthalmic ultrasound, diagnostic; B-scan and quantitative A-scan performed during the same patient encounter
2.56 2.56 FUD XXX Q1 N1 80
AMA: 2018,Jan,8; 2017,Jan,8; 2016,Jan,13; 2015,Jan,16

76511 quantitative A-scan only
1.75 1.75 FUD XXX Q1 N1 80
AMA: 2019,Jan,12; 2018,Jan,8; 2017,Jan,8; 2016,Jan,13; 2015,Jan,16

76512 B-scan (with or without superimposed non-quantitative A-scan)
1.73 1.73 FUD XXX Q1 N1 80
AMA: 2019,Jan,12; 2018,Jan,8; 2017,Jan,8; 2016,Jan,13; 2015,Jan,16

▲ **76513 anterior segment ultrasound, immersion (water bath) B-scan or high resolution biomicroscopy, unilateral or bilateral**
EXCLUDES *Computerized ophthalmic testing other than by ultrasound (92132-92134)*
2.78 2.78 FUD XXX Q1 N1 80
AMA: 2019,Jan,12; 2018,Jan,8; 2017,Jan,8; 2016,Jan,13; 2015,Jan,16

76514 corneal pachymetry, unilateral or bilateral (determination of corneal thickness)
INCLUDES Biometric measurement for which permanent image documentation not required
EXCLUDES *Collagen cross-linking cornea (0402T)*
0.34 0.34 FUD XXX Q1 80
AMA: 2019,Jan,12; 2018,Jan,8; 2017,Jan,8; 2016,Feb,12; 2016,Jan,13; 2015,Jan,16

76516 Ophthalmic biometry by ultrasound echography, A-scan;
INCLUDES Biometric measurement for which permanent image documentation not required
1.36 1.36 FUD XXX Q1 N1 80
AMA: 2019,Jan,12; 2018,Jan,8; 2017,Jan,8; 2016,Jan,13; 2015,Jan,16

76519 with intraocular lens power calculation
INCLUDES Biometric measurement for which permanent image documentation not required
Written prescription that satisfies requirement for written report
EXCLUDES *Partial coherence interferometry (92136)*
1.88 1.88 FUD XXX Q1 N1 80
AMA: 2019,Jan,12; 2018,Jan,8; 2017,Jan,8; 2016,Jan,13; 2015,Jan,16

76529 Ophthalmic ultrasonic foreign body localization
2.33 2.33 FUD XXX Q1 N1 80
AMA: 2019,Jan,12; 2018,Jan,8; 2017,Jan,8; 2016,Jan,13; 2015,Jan,16

76536-76800 Ultrasound: Neck, Thorax, Abdomen, and Spine

INCLUDES Required permanent documentation ultrasound images except when diagnostic purpose is biometric measurement
Written documentation

EXCLUDES *Focused ultrasound ablation uterine leiomyomata (0071T-0072T)*
Ultrasound exam not including thorough assessment organ or site, recorded image, and written report

76536 Ultrasound, soft tissues of head and neck (eg, thyroid, parathyroid, parotid), real time with image documentation
3.27 3.27 FUD XXX Q1 N1 80
AMA: 2018,Jan,8; 2017,Oct,9; 2017,Jan,8; 2016,Jan,13; 2015,Jan,16

76604 Ultrasound, chest (includes mediastinum), real time with image documentation
2.23 2.23 FUD XXX Q1 N1 80
AMA: 2018,Jan,8; 2017,Oct,9; 2017,Jan,8; 2016,Jan,13; 2015,Jan,16

76641 **Ultrasound, breast, unilateral, real time with image documentation, including axilla when performed; complete**

INCLUDES Complete examination all four quadrants, retroareolar region, and axilla when performed

EXCLUDES *Procedure performed more than one time per breast per session*

3.02 3.02 **FUD** XXX Q1 N1 80 50

AMA: 2018,Jan,8; 2017,Oct,9; 2017,Jan,8; 2016,Jan,13; 2015,Aug,8

76642 **limited**

INCLUDES Examination not including all complete examination elements

EXCLUDES *Procedure performed more than one time per breast per session*

2.47 2.47 **FUD** XXX Q1 N1 80 50

AMA: 2018,Jan,8; 2017,Oct,9

76700 **Ultrasound, abdominal, real time with image documentation; complete**

INCLUDES Real time scans:
- Common bile duct
- Gallbladder
- Inferior vena cava
- Kidneys
- Liver
- Pancreas
- Spleen
- Upper abdominal aorta

3.47 3.47 **FUD** XXX Q3 Z2 80

AMA: 2018,Jan,8; 2017,Oct,9; 2017,Jan,8; 2016,Jan,13; 2015,Jan,16

76705 **limited (eg, single organ, quadrant, follow-up)**

2.56 2.56 **FUD** XXX Q3 Z2 80

AMA: 2018,Jan,8; 2017,Oct,9; 2017,Jan,8; 2016,Jan,13; 2015,Jan,16

76706 **Ultrasound, abdominal aorta, real time with image documentation, screening study for abdominal aortic aneurysm (AAA)**

EXCLUDES *Diagnostic ultrasound aorta (76770-76775)*
Duplex scan aorta (93978-93979)

3.21 3.21 **FUD** XXX S 80

AMA: 2018,Jan,8; 2017,Sep,11

76770 **Ultrasound, retroperitoneal (eg, renal, aorta, nodes), real time with image documentation; complete**

INCLUDES Complete assessment kidneys and bladder when history indicates urinary pathology
Real time scans:
- Abdominal aorta
- Common iliac artery origins
- Inferior vena cava
- Kidneys

3.18 3.18 **FUD** XXX Q3 Z2 80

AMA: 2018,Jan,8; 2017,Oct,9; 2017,Jan,8; 2016,Jan,13; 2015,Jan,16

76775 **limited**

1.66 1.66 **FUD** XXX Q1 N1 80

AMA: 2018,Jan,8; 2017,Oct,9; 2017,Jan,8; 2016,Jan,13; 2015,Jan,16

76776 **Ultrasound, transplanted kidney, real time and duplex Doppler with image documentation**

EXCLUDES *Abdominal/pelvic/scrotal contents/retroperitoneal duplex scan (93975-93976)*
Transplanted kidney ultrasound without duplex doppler (76775)

4.41 4.41 **FUD** XXX Q3 Z2 80

AMA: 2018,Jan,8; 2017,Jan,8; 2016,Jan,13; 2015,Jan,16

76800 **Ultrasound, spinal canal and contents**

4.04 4.04 **FUD** XXX Q1 N1 80

AMA: 2018,Jan,8; 2017,Jan,8; 2016,Jan,13; 2015,Jan,16

76801-76802 Ultrasound: Pregnancy Less Than 14 Weeks

INCLUDES Determination number gestational sacs and fetuses
Gestational sac/fetal measurement appropriate for gestational age (younger than 14 weeks 0 days)
Inspection maternal uterus and adnexa
Quality analysis amniotic fluid volume/gestational sac shape
Visualization fetal and placental anatomic formation
Written documentation each exam component

EXCLUDES *Focused ultrasound ablation uterine leiomyomata (0071T-0072T)*
Ultrasound exam not including thorough assessment organ or site, recorded image, and written report

76801 **Ultrasound, pregnant uterus, real time with image documentation, fetal and maternal evaluation, first trimester (< 14 weeks 0 days), transabdominal approach; single or first gestation** M ♀

EXCLUDES *Fetal nuchal translucency measurement, first trimester (76813)*

3.45 3.45 **FUD** XXX S Z2 80

AMA: 2018,Jan,8; 2017,Jan,8; 2016,Jan,13; 2015,Jan,16

+ **76802** **each additional gestation (List separately in addition to code for primary procedure)** M ♀

EXCLUDES *Fetal nuchal translucency measurement, first trimester (76814)*

Code first (76801)

1.78 1.78 **FUD** ZZZ N N1 80

AMA: 2018,Jan,8; 2017,Jan,8; 2016,Jan,13; 2015,Jan,16

76805-76810 Ultrasound: Pregnancy of 14 Weeks or More

INCLUDES Determination number gestational/chorionic sacs and fetuses
Evaluation:
- Amniotic fluid
- Four chambered heart
- Intracranial, spinal, abdominal anatomy
- Placenta location
- Umbilical cord insertion site

Examination maternal adnexa if visible
Gestational sac/fetal measurement appropriate for gestational age (older than or equal to 14 weeks 0 days)
Written documentation each exam component

EXCLUDES *Focused ultrasound ablation uterine leiomyomata (0071T-0072T)*
Ultrasound exam not including thorough assessment organ or site, recorded image, and written report

76805 **Ultrasound, pregnant uterus, real time with image documentation, fetal and maternal evaluation, after first trimester (> or = 14 weeks 0 days), transabdominal approach; single or first gestation** M ♀

3.97 3.97 **FUD** XXX S Z2 80

AMA: 2018,Jan,8; 2017,Jan,8; 2016,Jan,13; 2015,Jan,16

+ **76810** **each additional gestation (List separately in addition to code for primary procedure)** M ♀

Code first (76805)

2.59 2.59 **FUD** ZZZ N N1 80

AMA: 2018,Jan,8; 2017,Jan,8; 2016,Jan,13; 2015,Jan,16

76811-76812 Ultrasound: Pregnancy, with Additional Studies of Fetus

INCLUDES Determination number gestational/chorionic sacs and fetuses
Evaluation:
- Amniotic fluid
- Examination maternal adnexa if visible
- Focused ultrasound ablation uterine leiomyomata (0071T-0072T)
- Four-chambered heart
- Gestational sac/fetal measurement appropriate for gestational age (older than or equal to 14 weeks 0 days)
- Intracranial, spinal, abdominal anatomy
- Placenta location
- Ultrasound exam not including thorough assessment organ or site, recorded image, and written report
- Umbilical cord insertion site
- Written documentation each exam component

Examination of maternal adnexa if visible
Gestational sac/fetal measurement appropriate for gestational age (older than or equal to 14 weeks 0 days)
Written documentation of each component of exam, including reason for nonvisualization, when applicable

EXCLUDES *Focused ultrasound ablation of uterine leiomyomata (0071T-0072T)*
Ultrasound exam that does not include thorough assessment organ or site, recorded image, and written report

76811 Ultrasound, pregnant uterus, real time with image documentation, fetal and maternal evaluation plus detailed fetal anatomic examination, transabdominal approach; single or first gestation M ♀
5.12 5.12 FUD XXX S Z3 80
AMA: 2018,Jan,8; 2017,Jan,8; 2016,Jan,13; 2015,Jan,16

+ **76812 each additional gestation (List separately in addition to code for primary procedure)** M ♀
Code first (76811)
5.72 5.72 FUD ZZZ N N1 80
AMA: 2018,Jan,8; 2017,Jan,8; 2016,Jan,13; 2015,Jan,16

76813-76828 Ultrasound: Other Fetal Evaluations

INCLUDES Required permanent documentation ultrasound images except when diagnostic purpose is biometric measurement
Written documentation

EXCLUDES *Focused ultrasound ablation uterine leiomyomata (0071T-0072T)*
Ultrasound exam not including thorough assessment organ or site, recorded image, and written report

76813 Ultrasound, pregnant uterus, real time with image documentation, first trimester fetal nuchal translucency measurement, transabdominal or transvaginal approach; single or first gestation M ♀
3.45 3.45 FUD XXX Q1 N1 80
AMA: 2018,Jan,8; 2017,Jan,8; 2016,Jan,13; 2015,Jan,16

+ **76814 each additional gestation (List separately in addition to code for primary procedure)** M ♀
Code first (76813)
2.27 2.27 FUD XXX N N1 80
AMA: 2018,Jan,8; 2017,Jan,8; 2016,Jan,13; 2015,Jan,16

76815 Ultrasound, pregnant uterus, real time with image documentation, limited (eg, fetal heart beat, placental location, fetal position and/or qualitative amniotic fluid volume), 1 or more fetuses M ♀
INCLUDES Exam concentrating on one or more elements
Reporting only one time per exam, not per element
EXCLUDES *Fetal nuchal translucency measurement, first trimester (76813-76814)*
2.37 2.37 FUD XXX Q1 N1 80
AMA: 2018,Jan,8; 2017,Jan,8; 2016,Jan,13; 2015,Jan,16

76816 Ultrasound, pregnant uterus, real time with image documentation, follow-up (eg, re-evaluation of fetal size by measuring standard growth parameters and amniotic fluid volume, re-evaluation of organ system(s) suspected or confirmed to be abnormal on a previous scan), transabdominal approach, per fetus M ♀
INCLUDES Re-evaluation fetal size, interval growth, or aberrancies noted on prior ultrasound
Code also modifier 59 for examination each additional fetus
3.19 3.19 FUD XXX Q1 N1 80
AMA: 2018,Jan,8; 2017,Jan,8; 2016,Jan,13; 2015,Jan,16

76817 Ultrasound, pregnant uterus, real time with image documentation, transvaginal M ♀
EXCLUDES *Transvaginal ultrasound, non-obstetrical (76830)*
Code also transabdominal obstetrical ultrasound, when performed
2.73 2.73 FUD XXX Q1 N1 80
AMA: 2018,Jan,8; 2017,Jan,8; 2016,Jan,13; 2015,Jan,16

76818 Fetal biophysical profile; with non-stress testing M ♀
Code also modifier 59 for each additional fetus
3.44 3.44 FUD XXX S Z2 80
AMA: 2018,Jan,8; 2017,Jan,8; 2016,Jan,13; 2015,Jan,16

76819 without non-stress testing M ♀
EXCLUDES *Amniotic fluid index without non-stress test (76815)*
Code also modifier 59 for each additional fetus
2.45 2.45 FUD XXX S Z3 80
AMA: 2018,Jan,8; 2017,Jan,8; 2016,Jan,13; 2015,Jan,16

76820 Doppler velocimetry, fetal; umbilical artery M
1.35 1.35 FUD XXX Q1 N1 80
AMA: 2018,Jan,8; 2017,Jan,8; 2016,Jul,8; 2016,Jan,13; 2015,Jan,16

76821 middle cerebral artery M
2.55 2.55 FUD XXX Q1 N1 80
AMA: 2018,Jan,8; 2017,Jan,8; 2016,Jan,13; 2015,Jan,16

76825 Echocardiography, fetal, cardiovascular system, real time with image documentation (2D), with or without M-mode recording; M ♀
7.79 7.79 FUD XXX S Z3 80
AMA: 2018,Jan,8; 2017,Sep,14; 2017,Jan,8; 2016,Jan,13; 2015,Jan,16

76826 follow-up or repeat study M ♀
4.58 4.58 FUD XXX S Z2 80
AMA: 2018,Jan,8; 2017,Sep,14

76827 Doppler echocardiography, fetal, pulsed wave and/or continuous wave with spectral display; complete M ♀
2.07 2.07 FUD XXX Q1 N1 80
AMA: 2018,Jan,8; 2017,Jan,8; 2016,Jan,13; 2015,Jan,16

76828 follow-up or repeat study M ♀
EXCLUDES *Color mapping (93325)*
1.47 1.47 FUD XXX Q1 N1 80
AMA: 2018,Jan,8; 2017,Jan,8; 2016,Jan,13; 2015,Jan,16

76830-76873 Ultrasound: Male and Female Genitalia

INCLUDES Required permanent documentation ultrasound images except when diagnostic purpose is biometric measurement
Written documentation

EXCLUDES *Focused ultrasound ablation uterine leiomyomata (0071T-0072T)*
Ultrasound exam not including thorough assessment organ or site, recorded image, and written report

76830 Ultrasound, transvaginal ♀

EXCLUDES *Transvaginal ultrasound, obstetric (76817)*

Code also transabdominal nonobstetrical ultrasound, when performed

3.47 3.47 **FUD** XXX S Z2 80

AMA: 2018,Jan,8; 2017,Oct,9; 2017,Jan,8; 2016,Jan,13; 2015,Jan,16

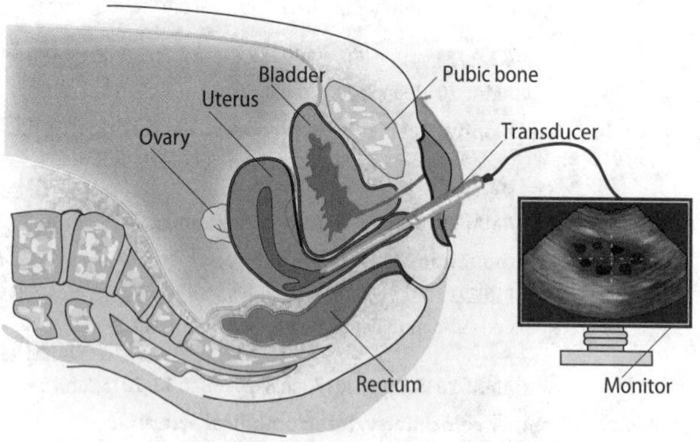

Ultrasound is performed in real time with image documentation by a transvaginal approach

76831 Saline infusion sonohysterography (SIS), including color flow Doppler, when performed ♀

Code also saline introduction for saline infusion sonohysterography (58340)

3.36 3.36 **FUD** XXX 03 Z3 80

AMA: 2018,Jan,8; 2017,Jan,8; 2016,Jan,13; 2015,Jan,16

76856 Ultrasound, pelvic (nonobstetric), real time with image documentation; complete

INCLUDES Total examination female pelvic anatomy including:
- Bladder measurement
- Description and measurement uterus and adnexa
- Description any pelvic pathology
- Measurement, endometrium

Total examination male pelvis including:
- Bladder measurement
- Description any pelvic pathology
- Evaluation prostate and seminal vesicles

3.09 3.09 **FUD** XXX 03 Z2 80

AMA: 2018,Jan,8; 2017,Oct,9; 2017,Jan,8; 2016,Aug,9; 2016,Jan,13; 2015,Jan,16

76857 limited or follow-up (eg, for follicles)

INCLUDES Focused evaluation limited to:
- Evaluation one or more elements listed in 76856 and/or
- Re-evaluation one or more pelvic aberrancies noted on prior ultrasound

Urinary bladder alone

EXCLUDES *Bladder volume or post-voided residual measurement without bladder imaging (51798)*
Urinary bladder and kidneys (76770)

1.38 1.38 **FUD** XXX 03 Z3 80

AMA: 2018,Jan,8; 2017,Oct,9; 2017,Jan,8; 2016,Jan,13; 2015,Jan,16

76870 Ultrasound, scrotum and contents ♂

2.97 2.97 **FUD** XXX 01 N1 80

AMA: 2018,Jan,8; 2017,Oct,9

76872 Ultrasound, transrectal;

EXCLUDES *Colonoscopy (45391-45392)*
Cystourethroscopy with transurethral anterior prostate commissurotomy/drug dellivery (0619T)
Hemorrhoidectomy by transanal hemorrhoidal dearterialization ([46948])
Sigmoidoscopy (45341-45342)
Transurethral prostate ablation (0421T)

4.43 4.43 **FUD** XXX S Z2 80

AMA: 2020,Feb,11; 2018,Nov,10; 2018,Jul,11; 2018,Jan,8; 2017,Oct,9; 2017,Jan,8; 2016,Jan,13; 2015,Jan,16

76873 prostate volume study for brachytherapy treatment planning (separate procedure) ♂

4.91 4.91 **FUD** XXX S Z2 80

AMA: 2018,Jan,8; 2017,Jan,8; 2016,Jan,13; 2015,Jan,16

76881-76886 Ultrasound: Extremities

EXCLUDES *Doppler studies extremities (93925-93926, 93930-93931, 93970-93971)*

76881 Ultrasound, complete joint (ie, joint space and peri-articular soft tissue structures) real-time with image documentation

INCLUDES Real-time scans specific joint including assessment:
- Joint space
- Muscles
- Other soft tissue
- Tendons

Required permanent image documentation
Stress manipulations and dynamic imaging when performed
Written documentation including explanation any joint components not visualized

2.51 2.51 **FUD** XXX S Z3 80

AMA: 2018,Jan,8; 2017,Oct,9; 2017,Jan,8; 2016,Sep,9

76882 Ultrasound, limited, joint or other nonvascular extremity structure(s) (eg, joint space, peri-articular tendon[s], muscle[s], nerve[s], other soft tissue structure[s], or soft tissue mass[es]), real-time with image documentation

INCLUDES Limited joint examination or evaluation due to mass or other abnormality not requiring all complete joint evaluation components (76881)

Real-time scans specific joint including assessment:
- Joint space
- Muscles
- Other soft tissue
- Tendons

Required permanent image documentation
Written documentation including explanation any joint components not visualized

1.61 1.61 **FUD** XXX 01 N1 80

AMA: 2018,Jan,8; 2017,Oct,9; 2017,Jan,8; 2016,Sep,9

76885 Ultrasound, infant hips, real time with imaging documentation; dynamic (requiring physician or other qualified health care professional manipulation) A

4.05 4.05 **FUD** XXX 01 N1 80

AMA: 2012,Feb,9-10; 2002,May,7

76886 limited, static (not requiring physician or other qualified health care professional manipulation) A

2.97 2.97 **FUD** XXX 01 N1 80

AMA: 2012,Feb,9-10; 2002,May,7

76932-76970 Imaging Guidance: Ultrasound

INCLUDES Required permanent documentation ultrasound images except when diagnostic purpose is biometric measurement
Written documentation

EXCLUDES *Focused ultrasound ablation uterine leiomyomata (0071T-0072T)*
Ultrasound exam not including thorough assessment organ or site, recorded image, and written report

76932 Ultrasonic guidance for endomyocardial biopsy, imaging supervision and interpretation

0.00 0.00 **FUD** YYY N N1 80

AMA: 2012,Feb,9-10; 2001,Sep,4

76936 **Ultrasound guided compression repair of arterial pseudoaneurysm or arteriovenous fistulae (includes diagnostic ultrasound evaluation, compression of lesion and imaging)**

7.60 7.60 FUD XXX S Z2 80

AMA: 2012,Feb,9-10; 2002,May,7

\+ **76937** **Ultrasound guidance for vascular access requiring ultrasound evaluation of potential access sites, documentation of selected vessel patency, concurrent realtime ultrasound visualization of vascular needle entry, with permanent recording and reporting (List separately in addition to code for primary procedure)**

INCLUDES Ultrasound guidance, needle placement (76942)

EXCLUDES *Endovascular venous arterialization, tibial or peroneal vein ([0620T])*
Endovenous femoral-popliteal arterial revascularization (0505T)
Extremity venous noninvasive vascular diagnostic study performed separately from venous access guidance (93970-93971)
Insertion or replacement peripherally inserted central venous catheter (36568-36569, [36572, 36573], 36584)
Insertion, removal, or replacement permanent leadless pacemaker ([33274, 33275])
Insertion, removal, or repositioning vena cava filter (37191-37193)
Ligation perforator veins (37760-37761)

Code first primary procedure

0.96 0.96 FUD ZZZ N N1 80

AMA: 2019,May,3; 2019,Mar,6; 2018,Mar,3; 2018,Jan,8; 2017,Dec,3; 2017,Aug,10; 2017,Jul,3; 2017,Mar,3; 2017,Jan,8; 2016,Nov,3; 2016,Jul,6; 2016,Jan,13; 2015,Jul,10; 2015,Jan,16

76940 **Ultrasound guidance for, and monitoring of, parenchymal tissue ablation**

EXCLUDES *Ablation (20982-20983, [32994], 32998, 47370-47383, 50250, 50542, 50592-50593, 0582T, 0600T-0601T)*
Ultrasound guidance:
Intraoperative (76998)
Needle placement (76942)

0.00 0.00 FUD YYY N N1 80

AMA: 2018,Jan,8; 2017,Nov,8; 2017,Jan,8; 2016,Jan,13; 2015,Jul,8; 2015,Jan,16

76941 **Ultrasonic guidance for intrauterine fetal transfusion or cordocentesis, imaging supervision and interpretation** M ♀

Code also surgical procedure (36460, 59012)

0.00 0.00 FUD XXX N N1 80

AMA: 2012,Feb,9-10; 2001,Sep,4

76942 **Ultrasonic guidance for needle placement (eg, biopsy, aspiration, injection, localization device), imaging supervision and interpretation**

EXCLUDES *Arthrocentesis (20604, 20606, 20611)*
Autologous WBC injection (0481T)
Breast biopsy with placement localization device(s) (19083)
Core needle biopsy, lung or mediastinum (32408)
Esophagogastroduodenoscopy (43237, 43242)
Esophagoscopy (43232)
Fine needle aspiration biopsy ([10004, 10005, 10006], 10021)
Gastrointestinal endoscopic ultrasound (76975)
Hemorrhoidectomy by transanal hemorrhoidal dearterialization ([46948])
Image-guided fluid collection drainage by catheter (10030)
Injection procedures (27096, 64479-64484, 0232T)
Ligation (37760-37761)
Paravertebral facet joint injections (64490-64491, 64493-64495, 0213T-0218T)
Placement breast localization device(s) (19285)
Sigmoidoscopy (45341-45342)
Thoracentesis (32554-32557)
Transperineal placement, periprostatic biodegradable material (55874)
Transurethral ablation, malignant prostate tissue (0582T)

1.61 1.61 FUD XXX N N1 80

AMA: 2020,Jun,10; 2020,Feb,11; 2020,Feb,9; 2020,Jan,7; 2019,Aug,10; 2019,Apr,4; 2019,Feb,8; 2018,Jul,11; 2018,Mar,3; 2018,Jan,8; 2017,Dec,13; 2017,Sep,6; 2017,Jun,10; 2017,Jan,8; 2016,Nov,3; 2016,Jun,3; 2016,Jan,13; 2016,Jan,9; 2015,Dec,3; 2015,Nov,10; 2015,Aug,8; 2015,Feb,6; 2015,Jan,16

76945 **Ultrasonic guidance for chorionic villus sampling, imaging supervision and interpretation** M ♀

Code also surgical procedure (59015)

0.00 0.00 FUD XXX N N1 80

AMA: 2012,Feb,9-10; 2001,Sep,4

76946 **Ultrasonic guidance for amniocentesis, imaging supervision and interpretation** M ♀

0.91 0.91 FUD XXX N N1 80

AMA: 2012,Feb,9-10; 2001,Sep,4

76948 **Ultrasonic guidance for aspiration of ova, imaging supervision and interpretation** M ♀

2.15 2.15 FUD XXX N N1 80

AMA: 2012,Feb,9-10; 2001,Sep,4

76965 **Ultrasonic guidance for interstitial radioelement application**

2.62 2.62 FUD XXX N N1 80

AMA: 2012,Feb,9-10; 1997,Nov,1

~~**76970** **Ultrasound study follow-up (specify)**~~

76975 Endoscopic Ultrasound

INCLUDES Required permanent documentation ultrasound images except when diagnostic purpose is biometric measurement
Written documentation

EXCLUDES *Focused ultrasound ablation uterine leiomyomata (0071T-0072T)*
Ultrasound exam not including thorough assessment organ or site, recorded image, and written report

76975 **Gastrointestinal endoscopic ultrasound, supervision and interpretation**

INCLUDES Ultrasonic guidance (76942)

EXCLUDES *Colonoscopy (44406-44407, 45391-45392)*
Esophagogastroduodenoscopy (43237-43238, 43240, 43242, 43259)
Esophagoscopy (43231-43232)
Sigmoidoscopy (45341-45342)

0.00 0.00 FUD XXX Q2 N1 80

AMA: 2018,Jan,8; 2017,Jan,8; 2016,Jan,13; 2015,Jan,16

Radiology

76936 — 76975

76977 Bone Density Measurements: Ultrasound

CMS: 100-02,15,80.5.5 Frequency Standards

INCLUDES Required permanent documentation ultrasound images except when diagnostic purpose is biometric measurement
Written documentation

EXCLUDES *Ultrasound exam not including thorough assessment organ or site, recorded image, and written report*

76977 **Ultrasound bone density measurement and interpretation, peripheral site(s), any method**
0.21 0.21 **FUD** XXX S Z3 80
AMA: 2012,Feb,9-10; 1998,Nov,1

76978-76979 Targeted Dynamic Microbubble Sonographic Contrast Characterization: Ultrasound

INCLUDES Intravenous injection (96374)

76978 **Ultrasound, targeted dynamic microbubble sonographic contrast characterization (non-cardiac); initial lesion**
9.21 9.21 **FUD** XXX Z2 80
AMA: 2019,Jun,9

\+ **76979** **each additional lesion with separate injection (List separately in addition to code for primary procedure)**
Code first (76978)
6.23 6.23 **FUD** ZZZ N1 80
AMA: 2019,Jun,9

76981-76983 Elastography: Ultrasound

EXCLUDES *Shear wave liver elastography (91200)*

76981 **Ultrasound, elastography; parenchyma (eg, organ)**
EXCLUDES *Reporting code more than one time each session for same parenchymal organ and/or parenchymal organ and lesion*
3.04 3.04 **FUD** XXX Z2 80
AMA: 2019,Aug,3

76982 **first target lesion**
2.71 2.71 **FUD** XXX Z2 80
AMA: 2019,Aug,3

\+ **76983** **each additional target lesion (List separately in addition to code for primary procedure)**
EXCLUDES *Reporting code more than one time each session for same parenchymal organ and/or parenchymal organ and lesion*
Code first (76982)
1.67 1.67 **FUD** ZZZ N1 80
AMA: 2019,Aug,3

76998-76999 Imaging Guidance During Surgery: Ultrasound

INCLUDES Required permanent documentation ultrasound images except when diagnostic purpose is biometric measurement
Written documentation

EXCLUDES *Focused ultrasound ablation uterine leiomyomata (0071T-0072T)*
Ultrasound exam not including thorough assessment organ or site, recorded image, and written report

76998 **Ultrasonic guidance, intraoperative**
EXCLUDES *Ablation (47370-47371, 47380-47382)*
Endovenous ablation therapy incompetent vein (36475, 36479)
Hemorrhoidectomy by transanal hemorrhoidal dearterialization ([46948])
Ligation (37760-37761)
Wireless cardiac stimulator (0515T-0520T)
0.00 0.00 **FUD** XXX N N1 80
AMA: 2020,Feb,11; 2018,Mar,3; 2018,Jan,8; 2017,Apr,7; 2017,Jan,8; 2016,Nov,3; 2016,Jan,13; 2015,Aug,8; 2015,Jan,16

76999 **Unlisted ultrasound procedure (eg, diagnostic, interventional)**
0.00 0.00 **FUD** XXX Q1 N1 80
AMA: 2019,Dec,8; 2018,Jul,11; 2018,Jan,8; 2017,Jan,8; 2016,Jan,13; 2015,Jan,16

77001-77022 Imaging Guidance Techniques

EXCLUDES *Imaging guidance, breast localization device(s) (19081, 19281, 19283)*

\+ **77001** **Fluoroscopic guidance for central venous access device placement, replacement (catheter only or complete), or removal (includes fluoroscopic guidance for vascular access and catheter manipulation, any necessary contrast injections through access site or catheter with related venography radiologic supervision and interpretation, and radiographic documentation of final catheter position) (List separately in addition to code for primary procedure)**
INCLUDES Fluoroscopic guidance for needle placement (77002)
EXCLUDES *Any procedure codes that include fluoroscopic guidance in code descriptor*
Extracorporeal membrane oxygenation (ECMO)/extracorporeal life support (ECLS) (33957-33959, [33962, 33963, 33964])
Formal extremity venography performed separately from venous access and interpreted separately (36005, 75820, 75822, 75825, 75827)
Insertion peripherally inserted central venous catheter (PICC) (36568-36569, [36572, 36573])
Replacement peripherally inserted central venous catheter (PICC) (36584)
Code first primary procedure
2.71 2.71 **FUD** ZZZ N N1 80
AMA: 2019,May,3; 2018,Jan,8; 2017,Jan,8; 2016,Jan,13; 2015,Jan,16

\+ **77002** **Fluoroscopic guidance for needle placement (eg, biopsy, aspiration, injection, localization device) (List separately in addition to code for primary procedure)**
EXCLUDES *Ablation therapy (20982-20983)*
Any procedure codes that include fluoroscopic guidance in code descriptor:
Radiological guidance for percutaneous drainage by catheter (75989)
Transhepatic portography (75885, 75887)
Arthrography procedure(s) (70332, 73040, 73085, 73115, 73525, 73580, 73615)
Biopsy, breast, with placement breast localization device(s) (19081-19086)
Image-guided fluid collection drainage by catheter (10030)
Placement breast localization device(s) (19281-19288)
Platelet rich plasma injection(s) (0232T)
Thoracentesis (32554-32557)
Code first surgical procedure (10160, 20206, 20220, 20225, 20520, 20525-20526, 20550, 20551, 20552, 20553, 20555, 20600, 20605, 20610, 20612, 20615, 21116, 21550, 23350, 24220, 25246, 27093-27095, 27369, 27648, 32400, 32553, 36002, 38220-38222, 38505, 38794, 41019, 42400-42405, 47000-47001, 48102, 49180, 49411, 50200, 50390, 51100-51102, 55700, 55876, 60100, 62268-62269, 64400-64448, 64450, 64455, 64505, 64600-64605)
2.86 2.86 **FUD** ZZZ N N1 80
AMA: 2020,Feb,9; 2020,Jan,7; 2019,Dec,8; 2019,Dec,12; 2019,Aug,7; 2019,Mar,6; 2019,Apr,4; 2019,Feb,8; 2018,Dec,10; 2018,Dec,10; 2018,Jan,8; 2017,Jun,10; 2017,Jan,8; 2016,Sep,9; 2016,Aug,7; 2016,Jun,3; 2016,Jan,9; 2016,Jan,13; 2015,Dec,3; 2015,Aug,6; 2015,Jul,8; 2015,Feb,6; 2015,Feb,10; 2015,Jan,16

+ **77003** **Fluoroscopic guidance and localization of needle or catheter tip for spine or paraspinous diagnostic or therapeutic injection procedures (epidural or subarachnoid) (List separately in addition to code for primary procedure)**

EXCLUDES *Any procedure codes that include fluoroscopic guidance in code descriptor*
Arthrodesis (22586)
Image-guided fluid collection drainage by catheter (10030)
Injection allogenic cellular and/or tissue-based product, intervertebral disc (0627T-0628T)
Injection medication (subarachnoid/interlaminar epidural) (62320-62327)
Spinal puncture (62270, [62328], 62272, [62329])

Code first (61050-61055, 62267, 62273, 62280-62284, 64449, 64510, 64517, 64520, 64610, 96450)

2.85 2.85 FUD ZZZ N N1 80

AMA: 2020,Jun,10; 2019,Dec,8; 2018,Jan,8; 2017,Dec,13; 2017,Sep,6; 2017,Feb,9; 2017,Feb,12; 2017,Jan,8; 2016,Jan,11; 2016,Jan,9; 2016,Jan,13; 2015,Jan,16

77011 **Computed tomography guidance for stereotactic localization**

EXCLUDES *Arthrodesis (22586)*

6.47 6.47 FUD XXX N N1

AMA: 2018,Jan,8; 2017,Jan,8; 2016,Jan,13; 2015,Jan,16

77012 **Computed tomography guidance for needle placement (eg, biopsy, aspiration, injection, localization device), radiological supervision and interpretation**

EXCLUDES *Arthrodesis (22586)*
Autologous white blood cell concentrate (0481T)
Core needle biopsy, lung or mediastinum (32408)
Destruction paravertebral facet joint nerve by neurolysis ([64633, 64634, 64635, 64636])
Fine needle aspiration biopsy using CT guidance ([10009, 10010])
Image-guided fluid collection drainage by catheter (10030)
Injection allogenic cellular and/or tissue-based product, intervertebral disc (0629T-0630T)
Injection, paravertebral facet joint (64490-64495)
Platelet rich plasma injection(s) (0232T)
Sacroiliac joint arthrography (27096)
Spinal puncture (62270, [62328], 62272, [62329])
Thoracentesis (32554-32557)
Transforaminal epidural needle placement/injection (64479-64480, 64483-64484)

4.27 4.27 FUD XXX N N1

AMA: 2020,Jun,10; 2020,Jan,7; 2019,Dec,8; 2019,Apr,4; 2019,Feb,8; 2018,Jan,8; 2017,Sep,6; 2017,Feb,12; 2017,Jan,8; 2016,Jun,3; 2016,Jan,13; 2015,Dec,3; 2015,Feb,6; 2015,Jan,16

77013 **Computed tomography guidance for, and monitoring of, parenchymal tissue ablation**

EXCLUDES *Ablation therapy (20982-20983, [32994], 32998, 47382-47383, 50592-50593)*
Ablation, irreversible electroporation (0600T)

0.00 0.00 FUD XXX N N1 80

AMA: 2018,Jan,8; 2017,Nov,8; 2017,Jan,8; 2016,Jan,13; 2015,Jul,8; 2015,Jan,16

77014 **Computed tomography guidance for placement of radiation therapy fields**

Code also placement interstitial device(s) for radiation therapy guidance (31627, 32553, 49411, 55876)

3.45 3.45 FUD XXX N N1

AMA: 2018,Jan,8; 2017,Jan,8; 2016,Feb,3; 2016,Jan,13; 2015,Apr,10; 2015,Jan,16

77021 **Magnetic resonance imaging guidance for needle placement (eg, for biopsy, needle aspiration, injection, or placement of localization device) radiological supervision and interpretation**

EXCLUDES *Autologous white blood cell concentrate (0481T)*
Biopsy, breast, with placement breast localization device(s) (19085)
Core needle biopsy, lung or mediastinum (32408)
Fine needle aspiration biopsy using MR guidance ([10011, 10012])
Image-guided fluid collection drainage by catheter (10030)
Placement breast localization device(s) (19287)
Platelet rich plasma injection(s) (0232T)
Surgical procedure
Thoracentesis (32554-32557)

13.1 13.1 FUD XXX N N1

AMA: 2020,Jun,10; 2020,Feb,9; 2020,Jan,7; 2019,Apr,4; 2019,Feb,8; 2018,Jul,11; 2018,Jan,8; 2017,Jun,10; 2017,Jan,8; 2016,Jun,3; 2016,Jan,13; 2015,Dec,3; 2015,Feb,6; 2015,Jan,16

77022 **Magnetic resonance imaging guidance for, and monitoring of, parenchymal tissue ablation**

EXCLUDES *Ablation:*
Irreversible electroporation (0600T)
Percutaneous radiofrequency ([32994], 32998, 47382-47383, 50592-50593)
Reduction or eradication one or more bone tumors (20982-20983)
Uterine leiomyomata by focused ablation (0071T-0072T)

0.00 0.00 FUD XXX N N1 80

AMA: 2019,Sep,10; 2018,Mar,3; 2018,Jan,8; 2017,Nov,8; 2017,Jan,8; 2016,Nov,3; 2016,Jan,13; 2015,Jul,8; 2015,Jan,16

77046-77067 Radiography: Breast

77046 **Magnetic resonance imaging, breast, without contrast material; unilateral**

7.02 7.02 FUD XXX Z2 80

AMA: 2019,Aug,5

77047 **bilateral**

7.08 7.08 FUD XXX Z2 80

AMA: 2019,Aug,5

77048 **Magnetic resonance imaging, breast, without and with contrast material(s), including computer-aided detection (CAD real-time lesion detection, characterization and pharmacokinetic analysis), when performed; unilateral**

11.1 11.1 FUD XXX 80

AMA: 2019,Dec,14; 2019,Aug,5

77049 **bilateral**

11.1 11.1 FUD XXX 80

AMA: 2019,Dec,14; 2019,Aug,5

77053 **Mammary ductogram or galactogram, single duct, radiological supervision and interpretation**

Code also injection procedure (19030)

1.60 1.60 FUD XXX Q2 N1

AMA: 2018,Jan,8; 2017,Jan,8; 2016,Jan,13; 2015,Jan,16

77054 **Mammary ductogram or galactogram, multiple ducts, radiological supervision and interpretation**

2.07 2.07 FUD XXX Q2 N1

AMA: 2018,Jan,8; 2017,Jan,8; 2016,Jan,13; 2015,Jan,16

77061 **Diagnostic digital breast tomosynthesis; unilateral**

EXCLUDES *3D rendering (76376-76377)*
Screening mammography (77067)

0.00 0.00 FUD XXX E

AMA: 2020,Sep,14; 2018,Jan,8

77062 **bilateral**

EXCLUDES *3D rendering (76376-76377)*
Screening mammography (77067)

0.00 0.00 FUD XXX E

AMA: 2020,Sep,14; 2018,Jan,8; 2017,Jan,8; 2016,Dec,15

+ **77063 Screening digital breast tomosynthesis, bilateral (List separately in addition to code for primary procedure)**
EXCLUDES *3D rendering (76376-76377)*
Diagnostic mammography (77065-77066)
Code first (77067)
1.55 1.55 FUD ZZZ A
AMA: 2020,Sep,14; 2018,Jan,8; 2017,Jan,8; 2016,Dec,15

77065 Diagnostic mammography, including computer-aided detection (CAD) when performed; unilateral
3.78 3.78 FUD XXX A 80
AMA: 2020,Sep,14; 2019,Aug,5; 2018,Jan,8; 2017,Jan,8; 2016,Dec,15

77066 bilateral
4.76 4.76 FUD XXX A 80
AMA: 2020,Sep,14; 2019,Aug,5; 2018,Jan,8; 2017,Jan,8; 2016,Dec,15

77067 Screening mammography, bilateral (2-view study of each breast), including computer-aided detection (CAD) when performed
EXCLUDES *Breast scan, electrical impedance (76499)*
3.86 3.86 FUD XXX A 80
AMA: 2020,Sep,14; 2019,Aug,5; 2018,Jan,8; 2017,Jan,8; 2016,Dec,15

77071-77086 [77085, 77086] Additional Evaluations of Bones and Joints

77071 Manual application of stress performed by physician or other qualified health care professional for joint radiography, including contralateral joint if indicated
Code also interpretation stressed images according to anatomical site and number of views
1.43 1.43 FUD XXX Q1 N1 80 26
AMA: 2018,Jan,8; 2017,Jan,8; 2016,Jan,13; 2015,Jan,16

77072 Bone age studies
0.71 0.71 FUD XXX Q1 N1 80
AMA: 2018,Jan,8; 2017,Jan,8; 2016,Jan,13; 2015,Jan,16

77073 Bone length studies (orthoroentgenogram, scanogram)
1.06 1.06 FUD XXX Q1 N1 80
AMA: 2018,Jan,8; 2017,Jan,8; 2016,Jan,13; 2015,Jan,16

77074 Radiologic examination, osseous survey; limited (eg, for metastases)
1.78 1.78 FUD XXX Q1 N1 80
AMA: 2018,Jan,8; 2017,Jan,8; 2016,Jan,13; 2015,Jan,16

77075 complete (axial and appendicular skeleton)
2.60 2.60 FUD XXX Q1 N1 80
AMA: 2018,Jan,8; 2017,Jan,8; 2016,Jan,13; 2015,Jan,16

77076 Radiologic examination, osseous survey, infant
2.85 2.85 FUD XXX Q1 N1 80
AMA: 2018,Jan,8; 2017,Jan,8; 2016,Jan,13; 2015,Jan,16

77077 Joint survey, single view, 2 or more joints (specify)
1.29 1.29 FUD XXX Q1 N1 80
AMA: 2018,Jan,8; 2017,Jan,8; 2016,Jan,13; 2015,Jan,16

77078 Computed tomography, bone mineral density study, 1 or more sites, axial skeleton (eg, hips, pelvis, spine)
3.24 3.24 FUD XXX S Z2 80
AMA: 2018,Jan,8; 2017,Jan,8; 2016,Jan,13; 2015,Jan,16

77080 Dual-energy X-ray absorptiometry (DXA), bone density study, 1 or more sites; axial skeleton (eg, hips, pelvis, spine)
EXCLUDES *Dual-energy x-ray absorptiometry (DXA), bone density study ([77085])*
Vertebral fracture assessment via dual-energy x-ray absorptiometry (DXA) ([77086])
1.13 1.13 FUD XXX S Z3 80
AMA: 2018,Jan,8; 2017,Jan,8; 2016,Jan,13; 2015,Jan,16

77081 appendicular skeleton (peripheral) (eg, radius, wrist, heel)
0.91 0.91 FUD XXX S Z3 80
AMA: 2018,Jan,8; 2017,Jan,8; 2016,Jan,13; 2015,Jan,16

\# **77085 axial skeleton (eg, hips, pelvis, spine), including vertebral fracture assessment**
EXCLUDES *Dual-energy x-ray absorptiometry (DXA), bone density study (77080)*
Vertebral fracture assessment via dual-energy x-ray absorptiometry (DXA) ([77086])
1.54 1.54 FUD XXX Q1 N1 80

\# **77086 Vertebral fracture assessment via dual-energy X-ray absorptiometry (DXA)**
EXCLUDES *Dual-energy x-ray absorptiometry (DXA), bone density study (77080)*
Therapy performed more than one time for treatment to specific area
Vertebral fracture assessment via dual-energy X-ray absorptiometry (DXA) ([77085])
0.99 0.99 FUD XXX Q1 N1 80

77084 Magnetic resonance (eg, proton) imaging, bone marrow blood supply
10.7 10.7 FUD XXX S Z2 80
AMA: 2018,Jan,8; 2017,Jan,8; 2016,Jan,13; 2015,Jan,16

77085 **Resequenced code. See code following 77081.**

77086 **Resequenced code. See code before 77084.**

77261-77263 Therapeutic Radiology: Treatment Planning

INCLUDES Determination:
- Appropriate treatment devices
- Number and size treatment ports
- Treatment method
- Treatment time/dosage
- Treatment volume

Interpretation special testing
Tumor localization

EXCLUDES *Brachytherapy (0394T-0395T)*
Radiation treatment delivery, superficial (77401)

77261 Therapeutic radiology treatment planning; simple
INCLUDES Planning for single treatment area included in single port or simple parallel opposed ports with simple or no blocking
2.03 2.03 FUD XXX B 80 26
AMA: 2018,Jan,8; 2017,Jan,8; 2016,Feb,3; 2016,Jan,13; 2015,Jan,16

77262 intermediate
INCLUDES Planning for three or more converging ports, two separate treatment sites, multiple blocks, or special time dose constraints
3.06 3.06 FUD XXX B 80 26
AMA: 2018,Jan,8; 2017,Jan,8; 2016,Feb,3; 2016,Jan,13; 2015,Jan,16

77263 complex
INCLUDES Planning for very complex blocking, custom shielding blocks, tangential ports, special wedges or compensators, three or more separate treatment areas, rotational or special beam considerations, treatment modality combinations
4.78 4.78 FUD XXX B 80 26
AMA: 2018,Jan,8; 2017,Jan,8; 2016,Feb,3; 2016,Jan,13; 2015,Jan,16

77280-77299 [77295] Radiation Therapy Simulation

77280 Therapeutic radiology simulation-aided field setting; simple
INCLUDES Simulation single treatment site
7.85 7.85 FUD XXX S Z2 80
AMA: 2018,Jan,8; 2017,Jan,8; 2016,Jan,13; 2015,Apr,10; 2015,Jan,16

77285 intermediate
INCLUDES Two different treatment sites
12.9 12.9 FUD XXX S Z2 80
AMA: 2018,Jan,8; 2017,Jan,8; 2016,Jan,13; 2015,Apr,10; 2015,Jan,16

77290 **complex**

INCLUDES Brachytherapy
Complex blocking
Contrast material
Custom shielding blocks
Hyperthermia probe verification
Rotation, arc or particle therapy
Simulation to ≥ 3 treatment sites

14.4 14.4 FUD XXX S Z2 80

AMA: 2018,Jan,8; 2017,Jan,8; 2016,Sep,9; 2016,Jan,13; 2015,Apr,10; 2015,Jan,16

+ **77293** **Respiratory motion management simulation (List separately in addition to code for primary procedure)**

Code first (77295, 77301)

12.7 12.7 FUD ZZZ N N1 80

AMA: 2018,Jan,8; 2017,Jan,8; 2016,Jan,13; 2015,Dec,16

77295 **Resequenced code. See code before 77300.**

77299 **Unlisted procedure, therapeutic radiology clinical treatment planning**

0.00 0.00 FUD XXX S Z2 80

AMA: 2018,Jan,8; 2017,Jan,8; 2016,Jan,13; 2015,Jan,16

77295-77370 [77295] Radiation Physics Services

\# **77295** **3-dimensional radiotherapy plan, including dose-volume histograms**

13.9 13.9 FUD XXX S Z3 80

AMA: 2018,Jan,8; 2017,Jan,8; 2016,Jan,13; 2015,Dec,16; 2015,Jun,6; 2015,Jan,16

77300 **Basic radiation dosimetry calculation, central axis depth dose calculation, TDF, NSD, gap calculation, off axis factor, tissue inhomogeneity factors, calculation of non-ionizing radiation surface and depth dose, as required during course of treatment, only when prescribed by the treating physician**

EXCLUDES *Brachytherapy (77316-77318, 77767-77772, 0394T-0395T)*
Teletherapy plan (77306-77307, 77321)

1.88 1.88 FUD XXX S Z3 80

AMA: 2018,Jan,8; 2017,Jan,8; 2016,Jan,13; 2015,Jan,16

77301 **Intensity modulated radiotherapy plan, including dose-volume histograms for target and critical structure partial tolerance specifications**

55.0 55.0 FUD XXX S Z2 80

AMA: 2018,Jan,8; 2017,Jan,8; 2016,Jan,13; 2015,Jan,16

77306 **Teletherapy isodose plan; simple (1 or 2 unmodified ports directed to a single area of interest), includes basic dosimetry calculation(s)**

EXCLUDES *Brachytherapy (0394T-0395T)*
Radiation dosimetry calculation (77300)
Radiation treatment delivery (77401)
Therapy performed more than one time for treatment to specific area

4.25 4.25 FUD XXX S Z3 80

AMA: 2018,Jan,8; 2017,Jan,8; 2016,Feb,3

77307 **complex (multiple treatment areas, tangential ports, the use of wedges, blocking, rotational beam, or special beam considerations), includes basic dosimetry calculation(s)**

EXCLUDES *Brachytherapy (0394T-0395T)*
Radiation dosimetry calculation (77300)
Radiation treatment delivery (77401)
Therapy performed more than one time for treatment to specific area

8.20 8.20 FUD XXX S Z3 80

AMA: 2018,Jan,8; 2017,Jan,8; 2016,Feb,3

77316 **Brachytherapy isodose plan; simple (calculation[s] made from 1 to 4 sources, or remote afterloading brachytherapy, 1 channel), includes basic dosimetry calculation(s)**

EXCLUDES *Brachytherapy (0394T-0395T)*
Radiation dosimetry calculation (77300)
Radiation treatment delivery (77401)

6.17 6.17 FUD XXX S Z3 80

AMA: 2018,Jan,8; 2017,Jan,8; 2016,Feb,3

77317 **intermediate (calculation[s] made from 5 to 10 sources, or remote afterloading brachytherapy, 2-12 channels), includes basic dosimetry calculation(s)**

EXCLUDES *Brachytherapy (0394T-0395T)*
Radiation dosimetry calculation (77300)
Radiation treatment delivery (77401)

8.09 8.09 FUD XXX S Z2 80

AMA: 2018,Jan,8; 2017,Jan,8

77318 **complex (calculation[s] made from over 10 sources, or remote afterloading brachytherapy, over 12 channels), includes basic dosimetry calculation(s)**

EXCLUDES *Brachytherapy (0394T-0395T)*
Radiation dosimetry calculation (77300)
Radiation treatment delivery (77401)

11.5 11.5 FUD XXX S Z2 80

AMA: 2018,Jan,8; 2017,Jan,8; 2016,Feb,3

77321 **Special teletherapy port plan, particles, hemibody, total body**

2.68 2.68 FUD XXX S Z3 80

AMA: 2018,Jan,8; 2017,Jan,8; 2016,Jan,13; 2015,Jan,16

77331 **Special dosimetry (eg, TLD, microdosimetry) (specify), only when prescribed by the treating physician**

1.84 1.84 FUD XXX S Z3 80

AMA: 2018,Jan,8; 2017,Jan,8; 2016,Jan,13; 2015,Jun,6; 2015,Jan,16

77332 **Treatment devices, design and construction; simple (simple block, simple bolus)**

EXCLUDES *Brachytherapy (0394T-0395T)*
Radiation treatment delivery (77401)

1.49 1.49 FUD XXX S Z3 80

AMA: 2018,Jan,8; 2017,Jan,8; 2016,Feb,3; 2016,Jan,13; 2015,Jan,16

77333 **intermediate (multiple blocks, stents, bite blocks, special bolus)**

EXCLUDES *Brachytherapy (0394T-0395T)*
Radiation treatment delivery (77401)

3.10 3.10 FUD XXX S Z2 80

AMA: 2018,Jan,8; 2017,Jan,8; 2016,Feb,3; 2016,Jan,13; 2015,Jan,16

77334 **complex (irregular blocks, special shields, compensators, wedges, molds or casts)**

EXCLUDES *Brachytherapy (0394T-0395T)*
Radiation treatment delivery (77401)

3.61 3.61 FUD XXX S Z3 80

AMA: 2018,Jan,8; 2017,Jan,8; 2016,Sep,9; 2016,Feb,3; 2016,Jan,13; 2015,Dec,16; 2015,Jan,16

77336 **Continuing medical physics consultation, including assessment of treatment parameters, quality assurance of dose delivery, and review of patient treatment documentation in support of the radiation oncologist, reported per week of therapy**

EXCLUDES *Brachytherapy (0394T-0395T)*
Radiation treatment delivery (77401)

2.26 2.26 FUD XXX S Z2 80 TC

AMA: 2018,Jan,8; 2017,Jan,8; 2016,Feb,3; 2016,Jan,13; 2015,Jan,16

77338 **Multi-leaf collimator (MLC) device(s) for intensity modulated radiation therapy (IMRT), design and construction per IMRT plan**

EXCLUDES *Immobilization in IMRT treatment (77332-77334)*
Intensity modulated radiation treatment delivery (IMRT) (77385)
Reporting code more than one time per IMRT plan

13.7 13.7 **FUD** XXX S Z2 80

AMA: 2018,Jan,8; 2017,Jan,8; 2016,Jan,13; 2015,Jan,16

77370 **Special medical radiation physics consultation**

3.52 3.52 **FUD** XXX S Z2 80 TC

AMA: 2018,Jan,8; 2017,Jan,8; 2016,Feb,3; 2016,Jan,13; 2015,Jun,6; 2015,Jan,16

77371-77399 [77385, 77386, 77387] Stereotactic Radiosurgery (SRS) Planning and Delivery

77371 **Radiation treatment delivery, stereotactic radiosurgery (SRS), complete course of treatment of cranial lesion(s) consisting of 1 session; multi-source Cobalt 60 based**

EXCLUDES *Guidance with computed tomography for radiation therapy field placement (77014)*

0.00 0.00 **FUD** XXX J 80 TC

AMA: 2018,Jan,8; 2017,Jan,8; 2016,Jan,13; 2015,Jan,16

77372 **linear accelerator based**

EXCLUDES *Guidance with computed tomography for radiation therapy field placement (77014)*
Radiation treatment supervision (77432)

30.2 30.2 **FUD** XXX J 80 TC

AMA: 2018,Jan,8; 2017,Jan,8; 2016,Jan,13; 2015,Jan,16

77373 **Stereotactic body radiation therapy, treatment delivery, per fraction to 1 or more lesions, including image guidance, entire course not to exceed 5 fractions**

EXCLUDES *Guidance with computed tomography for radiation therapy field placement (77014)*
Intensity modulated radiation treatment delivery (IMRT) (77385-77386)
Radiation treatment delivery (77401-77402, 77407, 77412)
Single fraction cranial lesion(s) (77371-77372)

36.6 36.6 **FUD** XXX S 80 TC

AMA: 2018,Jan,8; 2017,Jan,8; 2016,Jan,13; 2015,Jun,6; 2015,Jan,16

77385 **Resequenced code. See code following 77417.**

77386 **Resequenced code. See code following 77417.**

77387 **Resequenced code. See code following 77417.**

77399 **Unlisted procedure, medical radiation physics, dosimetry and treatment devices, and special services**

0.00 0.00 **FUD** XXX S Z2 80

AMA: 2018,Jan,8; 2017,Jan,8; 2016,Jan,13; 2015,Jan,16

77401-77425 [77385, 77386, 77387, 77424, 77425] Radiation Treatment

INCLUDES Technical component and assorted energy levels

77401 **Radiation treatment delivery, superficial and/or ortho voltage, per day**

EXCLUDES *Continuing medical physics consultation (77336)*
Isodose plan:
Brachytherapy (77316-77318)
Teletherapy (77306-77307)
Management:
Intraoperative radiation treatment (77469-77470)
Radiation therapy (77431-77432)
Radiation treatment (77427)
Stereotactic body radiation therapy (77435)
Stereotactic body radiation therapy, treatment delivery (77373)
Unlisted procedure, therapeutic radiology treatment management (77499)
Therapeutic radiology treatment planning (77261-77263)
Treatment devices, design and construction (77332-77334)

Code also E/M services when performed alone, as appropriate

0.70 0.70 **FUD** XXX S Z3 80 TC

AMA: 2018,Jan,8; 2017,Jan,8; 2016,Feb,3; 2016,Jan,13; 2015,Dec,14; 2015,Jan,16

77402 **Radiation treatment delivery, ≥1 MeV; simple**

EXCLUDES *Stereotactic body radiation therapy, treatment delivery (77373)*

0.00 0.00 **FUD** XXX S Z2 80 TC

AMA: 2018,Jan,8; 2017,Jan,8; 2016,Jun,9; 2016,Mar,7; 2016,Feb,3; 2016,Jan,13; 2015,Dec,14; 2015,Jan,16

77407 **intermediate**

EXCLUDES *Stereotactic body radiation therapy, treatment delivery (77373)*

0.00 0.00 **FUD** XXX S Z2 80 TC

AMA: 2018,Jan,8; 2017,Jan,8; 2016,Jun,9; 2016,Mar,7; 2016,Feb,3; 2016,Jan,13; 2015,Dec,14; 2015,Jan,16

77412 **complex**

0.00 0.00 **FUD** XXX S Z2 80 TC

AMA: 2018,Jan,8; 2017,Jan,8; 2016,Jun,9; 2016,Mar,7; 2016,Feb,3; 2016,Jan,13; 2015,Dec,14; 2015,Jan,16

77417 **Therapeutic radiology port image(s)**

0.32 0.32 **FUD** XXX N N1 80 TC

AMA: 2018,Jan,8; 2017,Dec,14; 2017,Jan,8; 2016,Jan,13; 2015,Dec,14; 2015,Jan,16

\# **77385** **Intensity modulated radiation treatment delivery (IMRT), includes guidance and tracking, when performed; simple**

0.00 0.00 **FUD** XXX S Z2 80 TC

AMA: 2018,Jan,8; 2017,Jan,8; 2016,Feb,3

\# **77386** **complex**

0.00 0.00 **FUD** XXX S Z2 80 TC

AMA: 2018,Jan,8; 2017,Jan,8; 2016,Feb,3

\# **77387** **Guidance for localization of target volume for delivery of radiation treatment, includes intrafraction tracking, when performed**

0.00 0.00 **FUD** XXX N N1 80

AMA: 2018,Jan,8; 2017,Jan,8; 2016,Feb,3; 2016,Jan,13; 2015,Dec,16; 2015,Dec,14

\# **77424** **Intraoperative radiation treatment delivery, x-ray, single treatment session**

0.00 0.00 **FUD** XXX J Z2

AMA: 2018,Jan,8; 2017,Jan,8; 2016,Jan,13; 2015,Dec,14

\# **77425** **Intraoperative radiation treatment delivery, electrons, single treatment session**

0.00 0.00 **FUD** XXX J Z2

AMA: 2018,Jan,8; 2017,Jan,8; 2016,Jan,13; 2015,Dec,14; 2015,Jan,16

77423-77425 [77424, 77425] Neutron Therapy

77423 **High energy neutron radiation treatment delivery, 1 or more isocenter(s) with coplanar or non-coplanar geometry with blocking and/or wedge, and/or compensator(s)**
0.00 0.00 FUD XXX S Z3 80 TC
AMA: 2018,Jan,8; 2017,Jan,8; 2016,Jan,13; 2015,Dec,14; 2015,Jan,16

77424 **Resequenced code. See code following 77417.**

77425 **Resequenced code. See code following 77417.**

77427-77499 Radiation Therapy Management

INCLUDES Assessment patient for medical evaluation and management (at least one per treatment management service) including:
Coordination care/treatment
Evaluation patient's response to treatment
Review:
Dose delivery
Dosimetry
Lab tests
Patient treatment set-up
Port film
Treatment parameters
X-rays
Five fractions or treatment sessions regardless of time. Two or more fractions performed same day can be reported separately provided a distinct break in service exists between sessions and fractions are usually furnished on different days

EXCLUDES *High dose rate electronic brachytherapy (0394T-0395T)*
Radiation treatment delivery (77401)

77427 **Radiation treatment management, 5 treatments**
5.37 5.37 FUD XXX B 26
AMA: 2018,Jan,8; 2017,Jan,8; 2016,Feb,3; 2016,Jan,13; 2015,Jun,6; 2015,Jan,16

77431 **Radiation therapy management with complete course of therapy consisting of 1 or 2 fractions only**
2.96 2.96 FUD XXX B 80 26
AMA: 2018,Jan,8; 2017,Jan,8; 2016,Feb,3; 2016,Jan,13; 2015,Jun,6; 2015,Jan,16

77432 **Stereotactic radiation treatment management of cranial lesion(s) (complete course of treatment consisting of 1 session)**
12.0 12.0 FUD XXX B 80 26
AMA: 2018,Jan,8; 2017,Jan,8; 2016,Feb,3; 2016,Jan,13; 2015,Dec,14; 2015,Dec,16; 2015,Jun,6; 2015,Jan,16

77435 **Stereotactic body radiation therapy, treatment management, per treatment course, to 1 or more lesions, including image guidance, entire course not to exceed 5 fractions**
18.1 18.1 FUD XXX N N1 80 26
AMA: 2018,Jan,8; 2017,Jan,8; 2016,Feb,3; 2016,Jan,13; 2015,Dec,14; 2015,Jun,6; 2015,Jan,16

77469 **Intraoperative radiation treatment management**
9.00 9.00 FUD XXX B 80
AMA: 2018,Jan,8; 2017,Jan,8; 2016,Feb,3; 2015,Jun,6

77470 **Special treatment procedure (eg, total body irradiation, hemibody radiation, per oral or endocavitary irradiation)**
3.75 3.75 FUD XXX S Z3 80
AMA: 2018,Jan,8; 2017,Jan,8; 2016,Feb,3; 2016,Jan,13; 2015,Jun,6; 2015,Jan,16

77499 **Unlisted procedure, therapeutic radiology treatment management**
0.00 0.00 FUD XXX B 80
AMA: 2018,Jan,8; 2017,Jan,8; 2016,Feb,3; 2016,Jan,13; 2015,Jun,6; 2015,Jan,16

77520-77525 Proton Therapy

EXCLUDES *High dose rate electronic brachytherapy, per fraction (0394T-0395T)*

77520 **Proton treatment delivery; simple, without compensation**
0.00 0.00 FUD XXX S Z2 80 TC
AMA: 2018,Jan,8; 2017,Jan,8; 2016,Jan,13; 2015,Jan,16

77522 **simple, with compensation**
0.00 0.00 FUD XXX S Z2 80 TC
AMA: 2012,Feb,9-10; 2010,Oct,3-4

77523 **intermediate**
0.00 0.00 FUD XXX S Z2 80 TC
AMA: 2018,Jan,8; 2017,Jan,8; 2016,Jan,13; 2015,Jan,16

77525 **complex**
0.00 0.00 FUD XXX S Z2 80 TC
AMA: 2012,Feb,9-10; 2010,Oct,3-4

77600-77620 Hyperthermia Treatment

CMS: 100-03,110.1 Hyperthermia for Treatment of Cancer

INCLUDES Heat generating devices
Interstitial insertion temperature sensors
Management during course therapy
Normal follow-up care for three months after completion
Physics planning

EXCLUDES *Initial E/M service*
Radiation therapy treatment (77371-77373, 77401-77412, 77423)

77600 **Hyperthermia, externally generated; superficial (ie, heating to a depth of 4 cm or less)**
13.1 13.1 FUD XXX S Z2 80
AMA: 2018,Jan,8; 2017,Jan,8; 2016,Jan,13; 2015,Jan,16

77605 **deep (ie, heating to depths greater than 4 cm)**
24.0 24.0 FUD XXX S Z2 80
AMA: 2018,Jan,8; 2017,Jan,8; 2016,Jan,13; 2015,Jan,16

77610 **Hyperthermia generated by interstitial probe(s); 5 or fewer interstitial applicators**
19.2 19.2 FUD XXX S Z2 80
AMA: 2018,Jan,8; 2017,Jan,8; 2016,Jan,13; 2015,Jan,16

77615 **more than 5 interstitial applicators**
30.0 30.0 FUD XXX S Z2 80
AMA: 2018,Jan,8; 2017,Jan,8; 2016,Jan,13; 2015,Jan,16

77620 **Hyperthermia generated by intracavitary probe(s)**
14.6 14.6 FUD XXX S Z2 80
AMA: 2018,Jan,8; 2017,Jan,8; 2016,Jan,13; 2015,Jan,16

77750-77799 Brachytherapy

CMS: 100-04,13,70.4 Clinical Brachytherapy; 100-04,13,70.5 Radiation Physics Services; 100-04,4,61.4.4 Billing for Brachytherapy Source Supervision, Handling and Loading Costs

INCLUDES Hospital admission and daily visits

EXCLUDES *Placement:*
Heyman capsules (58346)
Ovoids and tandems (57155)

77750 **Infusion or instillation of radioelement solution (includes 3-month follow-up care)**
10.7 10.7 FUD 090 S Z2 80
AMA: 2018,Jan,8; 2017,Jan,8; 2016,Jan,13; 2015,Jan,16

77761 **Intracavitary radiation source application; simple**
11.4 11.4 FUD 090 S Z3 80
AMA: 2018,Jan,8; 2017,Jan,8; 2016,Jan,13; 2015,Jan,16

77762 **intermediate**
15.0 15.0 FUD 090 S Z3 80
AMA: 2018,Jan,8; 2017,Jan,8; 2016,Jan,13; 2015,Jan,16

77763 **complex**
21.4 21.4 FUD 090 S Z3 80
AMA: 2018,Jan,8; 2017,Jan,8; 2016,Jan,13; 2015,Jan,16

77767 **Remote afterloading high dose rate radionuclide skin surface brachytherapy, includes basic dosimetry, when performed; lesion diameter up to 2.0 cm or 1 channel**
6.78 6.78 FUD XXX S Z2 80

77768 **lesion diameter over 2.0 cm and 2 or more channels, or multiple lesions**
10.1 10.1 FUD XXX S Z2 80

77770 **Remote afterloading high dose rate radionuclide interstitial or intracavitary brachytherapy, includes basic dosimetry, when performed; 1 channel**
9.51 9.51 FUD XXX S Z3 80

77771 **2-12 channels**
16.9 | 16.9 | FUD XXX | S Z2 80

77772 **over 12 channels**
25.5 | 25.5 | FUD XXX | S Z2 80

77778 **Interstitial radiation source application, complex, includes supervision, handling, loading of radiation source, when performed**
24.0 | 24.0 | FUD 000 | S Z2 80
AMA: 2018,Jan,8; 2017,Jan,8; 2016,Jan,13; 2015,Jan,16

77789 **Surface application of low dose rate radionuclide source**
3.49 | 3.49 | FUD 000 | S Z2 80
AMA: 2018,Jan,8; 2017,Jan,8; 2016,Jan,13; 2015,Jan,16

77790 **Supervision, handling, loading of radiation source**
0.43 | 0.43 | FUD XXX | N N1 80 TC
AMA: 2018,Jan,8; 2017,Jan,8; 2016,Jan,13; 2015,Jan,16

77799 **Unlisted procedure, clinical brachytherapy**
0.00 | 0.00 | FUD XXX | S Z2 80
AMA: 2018,Jan,8; 2017,Jan,8; 2016,Jan,13; 2015,Jan,16

78012-78099 Nuclear Radiology: Thyroid, Parathyroid, Adrenal

EXCLUDES *Diagnostic services (see appropriate sections)*
Follow-up care (see appropriate section)
Code also radiopharmaceutical(s) and/or drug(s) supplied

78012 **Thyroid uptake, single or multiple quantitative measurement(s) (including stimulation, suppression, or discharge, when performed)**
2.34 | 2.34 | FUD XXX | S Z2 80
AMA: 2018,Jan,8; 2017,Jan,8; 2016,Jan,13; 2015,Jan,16

78013 **Thyroid imaging (including vascular flow, when performed);**
5.54 | 5.54 | FUD XXX | S Z2 80
AMA: 2018,Jan,8; 2017,Jan,8; 2016,Jan,13; 2015,Jan,16

78014 **with single or multiple uptake(s) quantitative measurement(s) (including stimulation, suppression, or discharge, when performed)**
6.95 | 6.95 | FUD XXX | S Z2 80
AMA: 2018,Jan,8; 2017,Jan,8; 2016,Jan,13; 2015,Jan,16

78015 **Thyroid carcinoma metastases imaging; limited area (eg, neck and chest only)**
6.47 | 6.47 | FUD XXX | S Z2 80
AMA: 2018,Jan,8; 2017,Jan,8; 2016,Jan,13; 2015,Jan,16

78016 **with additional studies (eg, urinary recovery)**
8.08 | 8.08 | FUD XXX | S Z2 80
AMA: 2018,Jan,8; 2017,Jan,8; 2016,Jan,13; 2015,Jan,16

78018 **whole body**
8.96 | 8.96 | FUD XXX | S Z2 80
AMA: 2018,Jan,8; 2017,Jan,8; 2016,Jan,13; 2015,Jan,16

\+ **78020** **Thyroid carcinoma metastases uptake (List separately in addition to code for primary procedure)**
2.41 | 2.41 | FUD ZZZ | N N1 80
AMA: 2018,Jan,8; 2017,Jan,8; 2016,Jan,13; 2015,Jan,16

78070 **Parathyroid planar imaging (including subtraction, when performed);**
EXCLUDES *Distribution radiopharmaceutical agents or tumor localization (78800-78802, [78804], 78803)*
Radiopharmaceutical quantification measurements ([78835])
SPECT with concurrently acquired CT transmission scan ([78830, 78831, 78832])
8.48 | 8.48 | FUD XXX | S Z2 80
AMA: 2018,Jan,8; 2017,Jan,8; 2016,Dec,9; 2016,Dec,16; 2016,Jan,13; 2015,Jan,16

78071 **with tomographic (SPECT)**
EXCLUDES *Distribution radiopharmaceutical agents or tumor localization (78800-78802, [78804], 78803)*
Radiopharmaceutical quantification measurements ([78835])
SPECT with concurrently acquired CT transmission scan ([78830, 78831, 78832])
10.1 | 10.1 | FUD XXX | S Z2 80
AMA: 2018,Jan,8; 2017,Jan,8; 2016,Dec,16; 2016,Dec,9

78072 **with tomographic (SPECT), and concurrently acquired computed tomography (CT) for anatomical localization**
EXCLUDES *Distribution radiopharmaceutical agents or tumor localization (78800-78802, [78804], 78803)*
Radiopharmaceutical quantification measurements ([78835])
SPECT with concurrently acquired CT transmission scan ([78830, 78831, 78832])
11.2 | 11.2 | FUD XXX | S Z2 80
AMA: 2018,Jan,8; 2017,Jan,8; 2016,Dec,16; 2016,Dec,9

78075 **Adrenal imaging, cortex and/or medulla**
13.0 | 13.0 | FUD XXX | S Z2 80
AMA: 2018,Jan,8; 2017,Jan,8; 2016,Jan,13; 2015,Jan,16

78099 **Unlisted endocrine procedure, diagnostic nuclear medicine**
0.00 | 0.00 | FUD XXX | S Z2 80
AMA: 2018,Jan,8; 2017,Jan,8; 2016,Dec,9; 2016,Jan,13; 2015,Jan,16

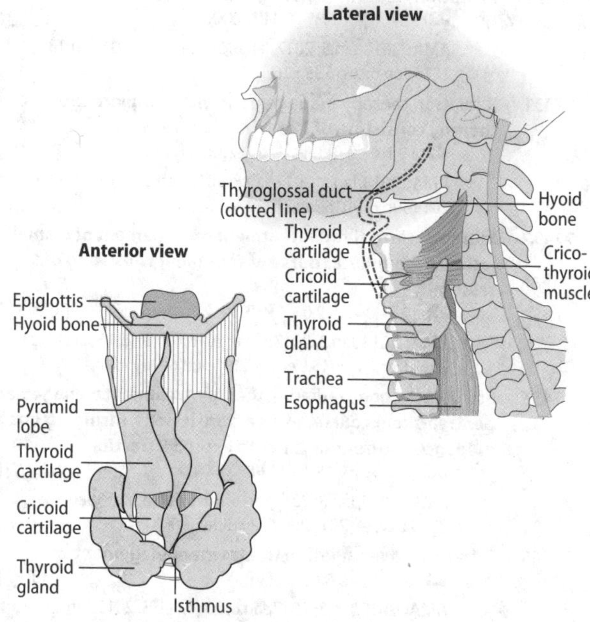

78102-78199 Nuclear Radiology: Blood Forming Organs

EXCLUDES *Diagnostic services (see appropriate sections)*
Follow-up care (see appropriate section)
Radioimmunoassays (82009-84999 [82042, 82652])
Code also radiopharmaceutical(s) and/or drug(s) supplied

78102 **Bone marrow imaging; limited area**
4.89 | 4.89 | FUD XXX | S Z2 80
AMA: 2018,Jan,8; 2017,Jan,8; 2016,Jan,13; 2015,Jan,16

78103 **multiple areas**
6.20 | 6.20 | FUD XXX | S Z2 80
AMA: 2012,Feb,9-10; 2007,Jan,28-31

78104 **whole body**
7.14 | 7.14 | FUD XXX | S Z2 80
AMA: 2012,Feb,9-10; 2007,Jan,28-31

78110 **Plasma volume, radiopharmaceutical volume-dilution technique (separate procedure); single sampling**
1.99 1.99 FUD XXX S Z2 80
AMA: 2012,Feb,9-10; 2007,Jan,28-31

78111 **multiple samplings**
2.11 2.11 FUD XXX S Z2 80
AMA: 2012,Feb,9-10; 2007,Jan,28-31

78120 **Red cell volume determination (separate procedure); single sampling**
2.04 2.04 FUD XXX S Z2 80
AMA: 2012,Feb,9-10; 2007,Jan,28-31

78121 **multiple samplings**
2.23 2.23 FUD XXX S Z2 80
AMA: 2012,Feb,9-10; 2007,Jan,28-31

78122 **Whole blood volume determination, including separate measurement of plasma volume and red cell volume (radiopharmaceutical volume-dilution technique)**
2.75 2.75 FUD XXX S Z2 80
AMA: 2012,Feb,9-10; 2007,Jan,28-31

▲ **78130** **Red cell survival study**
3.59 3.59 FUD XXX S Z2 80
AMA: 2012,Feb,9-10; 2007,Jan,28-31

~~**78135** **differential organ/tissue kinetics (eg, splenic and/or hepatic sequestration)**~~

78140 **Labeled red cell sequestration, differential organ/tissue (eg, splenic and/or hepatic)**
3.19 3.19 FUD XXX S Z2 80
AMA: 2012,Feb,9-10; 2007,Jan,28-31

78185 **Spleen imaging only, with or without vascular flow**
EXCLUDES *Liver imaging (78215-78216)*
4.87 4.87 FUD XXX S Z2 80
AMA: 2012,Feb,9-10; 2007,Jan,28-31

78191 **Platelet survival study**
3.56 3.56 FUD XXX S Z2 80
AMA: 2012,Feb,9-10; 2007,Jan,28-31

78195 **Lymphatics and lymph nodes imaging**
EXCLUDES *Sentinel node identification without scintigraphy (38792)*
Sentinel node removal (38500-38542)
10.2 10.2 FUD XXX S Z2 80
AMA: 2018,Jan,8; 2017,Jan,8; 2016,Jan,13; 2015,Jan,16

78199 **Unlisted hematopoietic, reticuloendothelial and lymphatic procedure, diagnostic nuclear medicine**
0.00 0.00 FUD XXX S Z2 80
AMA: 2018,Jan,8; 2017,Jan,8; 2016,Jan,13; 2015,Jan,16

78201-78299 Nuclear Radiology: Digestive System

EXCLUDES *Diagnostic services (see appropriate sections)*
Follow-up care (see appropriate section)
Code also radiopharmaceutical(s) and/or drug(s) supplied

78201 **Liver imaging; static only**
EXCLUDES *Spleen imaging only (78185)*
5.49 5.49 FUD XXX S Z2 80
AMA: 2018,Jan,8; 2017,Jan,8; 2016,Jan,13; 2015,Jan,16

78202 **with vascular flow**
EXCLUDES *Spleen imaging only (78185)*
5.82 5.82 FUD XXX S Z2 80
AMA: 2012,Feb,9-10; 2007,Jan,28-31

78215 **Liver and spleen imaging; static only**
5.59 5.59 FUD XXX S Z2 80
AMA: 2012,Feb,9-10; 2007,Jan,28-31

78216 **with vascular flow**
3.68 3.68 FUD XXX S Z2 80
AMA: 2012,Feb,9-10; 2007,Jan,28-31

78226 **Hepatobiliary system imaging, including gallbladder when present;**
9.38 9.38 FUD XXX S Z2 80
AMA: 2012,Feb,9-10

78227 **with pharmacologic intervention, including quantitative measurement(s) when performed**
12.8 12.8 FUD XXX S Z2 80
AMA: 2012,Feb,9-10

78230 **Salivary gland imaging;**
4.99 4.99 FUD XXX S Z2 80
AMA: 2012,Feb,9-10; 2007,Jan,28-31

78231 **with serial images**
2.98 2.98 FUD XXX S Z2 80
AMA: 2012,Feb,9-10; 2007,Jan,28-31

78232 **Salivary gland function study**
2.96 2.96 FUD XXX S Z2 80
AMA: 2012,Feb,9-10; 2007,Jan,28-31

78258 **Esophageal motility**
6.19 6.19 FUD XXX S Z2 80
AMA: 2012,Feb,9-10; 2007,Jan,28-31

78261 **Gastric mucosa imaging**
5.83 5.83 FUD XXX S Z2 80
AMA: 2012,Feb,9-10; 2007,Jan,28-31

78262 **Gastroesophageal reflux study**
6.86 6.86 FUD XXX S Z2 80
AMA: 2018,Jan,8; 2017,Jan,8; 2016,Jan,13; 2015,Dec,11

78264 **Gastric emptying imaging study (eg, solid, liquid, or both);**
EXCLUDES *Procedure performed more than one time per study*
9.65 9.65 FUD XXX S Z2 80
AMA: 2018,Jan,8; 2017,Jan,8; 2016,Jan,13; 2015,Dec,11

78265 **with small bowel transit**
EXCLUDES *Procedure performed more than one time per study*
11.2 11.2 FUD XXX S Z2 80
AMA: 2018,Jan,8; 2017,Jan,8; 2015,Dec,11

78266 **with small bowel and colon transit, multiple days**
EXCLUDES *Procedure performed more than one time per study*
12.3 12.3 FUD XXX S Z2 80
AMA: 2018,Jan,8; 2017,Jan,8; 2015,Dec,11

78267 **Urea breath test, C-14 (isotopic); acquisition for analysis**
EXCLUDES *Breath hydrogen/methane test (91065)*
0.00 0.00 FUD XXX A
AMA: 2020,OctSE,1; 2018,Jan,8; 2017,Jan,8; 2016,Jan,13; 2015,Jan,16

78268 **analysis**
EXCLUDES *Breath hydrogen/methane test (91065)*
0.00 0.00 FUD XXX A
AMA: 2020,OctSE,1; 2018,Jan,8; 2017,Jan,8; 2016,Jan,13; 2015,Jan,16

78278 **Acute gastrointestinal blood loss imaging**
9.97 9.97 FUD XXX S Z2 80
AMA: 2012,Feb,9-10; 2007,Jan,28-31

78282 **Gastrointestinal protein loss**
0.00 0.00 FUD XXX S Z2 80
AMA: 2018,Jul,14

78290 **Intestine imaging (eg, ectopic gastric mucosa, Meckel's localization, volvulus)**
9.44 9.44 FUD XXX S Z2 80
AMA: 2012,Feb,9-10; 2007,Jan,28-31

78291 **Peritoneal-venous shunt patency test (eg, for LeVeen, Denver shunt)**
Code also (49427)
7.39 7.39 FUD XXX S Z2 80
AMA: 2012,Feb,9-10; 2007,Jan,28-31

78299 **Unlisted gastrointestinal procedure, diagnostic nuclear medicine**
0.00 0.00 FUD XXX S Z2 80
AMA: 2018,Jan,8; 2017,Jan,8; 2016,Jan,13; 2015,Jan,16

78300-78399 Nuclear Radiology: Bones and Joints

EXCLUDES *Diagnostic services (see appropriate sections)*
Follow-up care (see appropriate section)
Code also radiopharmaceutical(s) and/or drug(s) supplied

78300 **Bone and/or joint imaging; limited area**
6.56 6.56 FUD XXX S Z2 80
AMA: 2018,Jan,8; 2017,Jan,8; 2016,Jan,13; 2015,Jan,16

78305 **multiple areas**
7.95 7.95 FUD XXX S Z2 80
AMA: 2018,Jan,8; 2017,Jan,8; 2016,Jan,13; 2015,Jan,16

78306 **whole body**
8.62 8.62 FUD XXX S Z2 80
AMA: 2018,Jan,8; 2017,Jan,8; 2016,Jan,13; 2015,Jan,16

78315 **3 phase study**
9.98 9.98 FUD XXX S Z2 80
AMA: 2018,Jan,8; 2017,Jan,8; 2016,Jan,13; 2015,Jan,16

78350 **Bone density (bone mineral content) study, 1 or more sites; single photon absorptiometry**
0.91 0.91 FUD XXX E
AMA: 2012,Feb,9-10; 2007,Jan,28-31

78351 **dual photon absorptiometry, 1 or more sites**
0.44 0.44 FUD XXX E
AMA: 2012,Feb,9-10; 2007,Jan,28-31

78399 **Unlisted musculoskeletal procedure, diagnostic nuclear medicine**
0.00 0.00 FUD XXX S Z2 80
AMA: 2018,Jan,8; 2017,Jan,8; 2016,Jan,13; 2015,Jan,16

78414-78499 [78429, 78430, 78431, 78432, 78433, 78434] Nuclear Radiology: Heart and Vascular

EXCLUDES *Diagnostic services (see appropriate sections)*
Follow-up care (see appropriate section)
Code also radiopharmaceutical(s) and/or drug(s) supplied

78414 **Determination of central c-v hemodynamics (non-imaging) (eg, ejection fraction with probe technique) with or without pharmacologic intervention or exercise, single or multiple determinations**
0.00 0.00 FUD XXX S Z2 80
AMA: 2018,Jan,8; 2017,Jan,8; 2016,Jan,13; 2015,Jan,16

78428 **Cardiac shunt detection**
5.29 5.29 FUD XXX S Z2 80
AMA: 2018,Jan,8; 2017,Jan,8; 2016,Jan,13; 2015,Jan,16

78429 **Resequenced code. See code following 78459.**

78430 **Resequenced code. See code following 78491.**

78431 **Resequenced code. See code following 78492.**

78432 **Resequenced code. See code following 78492.**

78433 **Resequenced code. See code following 78492.**

78434 **Resequenced code. See code following 78492.**

78445 **Non-cardiac vascular flow imaging (ie, angiography, venography)**
5.38 5.38 FUD XXX S Z2 80
AMA: 2018,Jan,8; 2017,Jan,8; 2016,Jan,13; 2015,Jan,16

78451 **Myocardial perfusion imaging, tomographic (SPECT) (including attenuation correction, qualitative or quantitative wall motion, ejection fraction by first pass or gated technique, additional quantification, when performed); single study, at rest or stress (exercise or pharmacologic)**

EXCLUDES *Distribution radiopharmaceutical agents or tumor localization (78800-78802, [78804], 78803)*
Radiopharmaceutical quantification measurements ([78835])
SPECT with concurrently acquired CT transmission scan ([78830, 78831, 78832])
Code also stress testing when performed (93015-93018)
9.63 9.63 FUD XXX S Z2 80
AMA: 2020,Jul,5; 2018,Jan,8; 2017,Jan,8; 2016,Jan,13; 2015,Jan,16

78452 **multiple studies, at rest and/or stress (exercise or pharmacologic) and/or redistribution and/or rest reinjection**

EXCLUDES *Distribution radiopharmaceutical agents or tumor localization (78800-78802, [78804], 78803)*
Radiopharmaceutical quantification measurements ([78835])
SPECT with concurrently acquired CT transmission scan ([78830, 78831, 78832])
Code also stress testing when performed (93015-93018)
13.4 13.4 FUD XXX S Z2 80
AMA: 2020,Jul,5; 2018,Jan,8; 2017,Jan,8; 2016,Jan,13; 2015,Jan,16

78453 **Myocardial perfusion imaging, planar (including qualitative or quantitative wall motion, ejection fraction by first pass or gated technique, additional quantification, when performed); single study, at rest or stress (exercise or pharmacologic)**
Code also stress testing when performed (93015-93018)
8.66 8.66 FUD XXX S Z2 80
AMA: 2020,Jul,5; 2018,Jan,8; 2017,Jan,8; 2016,Jan,13; 2015,Jan,16

78454 **multiple studies, at rest and/or stress (exercise or pharmacologic) and/or redistribution and/or rest reinjection**
Code also stress testing when performed (93015-93018)
12.5 12.5 FUD XXX S Z2 80
AMA: 2020,Jul,5; 2018,Jan,8; 2017,Jan,8; 2016,Jan,13; 2015,Jan,16

78456 **Acute venous thrombosis imaging, peptide**
8.93 8.93 FUD XXX S Z2
AMA: 2018,Jan,8; 2017,Jan,8; 2016,Jan,13; 2015,Jan,16

78457 **Venous thrombosis imaging, venogram; unilateral**
5.52 5.52 FUD XXX S Z2 80
AMA: 2018,Jan,8; 2017,Jan,8; 2016,Jan,13; 2015,Jan,16

78458 **bilateral**
5.88 5.88 FUD XXX S Z2 80
AMA: 2018,Jan,8; 2017,Jan,8; 2016,Jan,13; 2015,Jan,16

78459 **Myocardial imaging, positron emission tomography (PET), metabolic evaluation study (including ventricular wall motion[s] and/or ejection fraction[s], when performed), single study;**

INCLUDES Examination CT transmission images for field of view anatomy review

EXCLUDES *CT coronary calcium scoring (75571)*
CT for other than attenuation correction/anatomical localization; report site-specific CT code with modifier 59
Myocardial perfusion studies (78491-78492)
0.00 0.00 FUD XXX S Z2 80
AMA: 2020,Jul,5; 2018,Jan,8; 2017,Jan,8; 2016,Jan,13; 2015,Jan,16

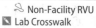

\# **78429** **with concurrently acquired computed tomography transmission scan**

INCLUDES Examination CT transmission images for field of view anatomy review

EXCLUDES *CT coronary calcium scoring (75571)*

CT for other than attenuation correction/anatomical localization; report site-specific CT code with modifier 59

0.00 0.00 FUD XXX Z2 80

AMA: 2020,Jul,5

78466 **Myocardial imaging, infarct avid, planar; qualitative or quantitative**

5.72 5.72 FUD XXX S Z2 80

AMA: 2012,Feb,9-10; 2010,May,5-6

78468 **with ejection fraction by first pass technique**

5.88 5.88 FUD XXX S Z2 80

AMA: 2018,Jan,8; 2017,Jan,8; 2016,Jan,13; 2015,Jan,16

78469 **tomographic SPECT with or without quantification**

EXCLUDES *Distribution radiopharmaceutical agents or tumor localization (78800-78802, [78804], 78803)*

Myocardial sympathetic innervation imaging (0331T-0332T)

Radiopharmaceutical quantification measurements ([78835])

SPECT with concurrently acquired CT transmission scan ([78830, 78831, 78832])

6.39 6.39 FUD XXX S Z2 80

AMA: 2018,Nov,11; 2018,Jan,8; 2017,Jan,8; 2016,Jan,13; 2015,Jan,16

78472 **Cardiac blood pool imaging, gated equilibrium; planar, single study at rest or stress (exercise and/or pharmacologic), wall motion study plus ejection fraction, with or without additional quantitative processing**

EXCLUDES *Cardiac blood pool imaging (78481, 78483, 78494)*

Myocardial perfusion imaging (78451-78454)

Right ventricular ejection fraction by first pass technique (78496)

Code also stress testing when performed (93015-93018)

6.59 6.59 FUD XXX S Z2 80

AMA: 2018,Jan,8; 2017,Jan,8; 2016,Jan,13; 2015,Jan,16

78473 **multiple studies, wall motion study plus ejection fraction, at rest and stress (exercise and/or pharmacologic), with or without additional quantification**

EXCLUDES *Cardiac blood pool imaging (78481, 78483, 78494)*

Myocardial perfusion imaging (78451-78454)

Code also stress testing when performed (93015-93018)

8.32 8.32 FUD XXX S Z2 80

AMA: 2018,Jan,8; 2017,Jan,8; 2016,Jan,13; 2015,Jan,16

78481 **Cardiac blood pool imaging (planar), first pass technique; single study, at rest or with stress (exercise and/or pharmacologic), wall motion study plus ejection fraction, with or without quantification**

EXCLUDES *Myocardial perfusion imaging (78451-78454)*

Code also stress testing when performed (93015-93018)

5.03 5.03 FUD XXX S Z2 80

AMA: 2018,Jan,8; 2017,Jan,8; 2016,Jan,13; 2015,Jan,16

78483 **multiple studies, at rest and with stress (exercise and/or pharmacologic), wall motion study plus ejection fraction, with or without quantification**

EXCLUDES *Blood flow studies brain (78610)*

Myocardial perfusion imaging (78451-78454)

Code also stress testing when performed (93015-93018)

6.89 6.89 FUD XXX S Z2 80

AMA: 2018,Jan,8; 2017,Jan,8; 2016,Jan,13; 2015,Jan,16

78491 **Myocardial imaging, positron emission tomography (PET), perfusion study (including ventricular wall motion[s] and/or ejection fraction[s], when performed); single study, at rest or stress (exercise or pharmacologic)**

Code also stress testing when performed (93015-93018)

0.00 0.00 FUD XXX S Z2 80

AMA: 2020,Jul,5; 2018,Jan,8; 2017,Jan,8; 2016,Jan,13; 2015,Jan,16

\# **78430** **single study, at rest or stress (exercise or pharmacologic), with concurrently acquired computed tomography transmission scan**

INCLUDES Examination CT transmission images for field of view anatomy review

Code also stress testing when performed (93015-93018)

0.00 0.00 FUD XXX Z2 80

AMA: 2020,Jul,5

78492 **multiple studies at rest and stress (exercise or pharmacologic)**

Code also stress testing when performed (93015-93018)

0.00 0.00 FUD XXX S Z2 80

AMA: 2020,Jul,5; 2018,Jan,8; 2017,Jan,8; 2016,Jan,13; 2015,Jan,16

\# **78431** **multiple studies at rest and stress (exercise or pharmacologic), with concurrently acquired computed tomography transmission scan**

INCLUDES Examination CT transmission images for field of view anatomy review

Code also stress testing when performed (93015-93018)

2.62 2.62 FUD XXX Z2 80

AMA: 2020,Jul,5

\# **78432** **Myocardial imaging, positron emission tomography (PET), combined perfusion with metabolic evaluation study (including ventricular wall motion[s] and/or ejection fraction[s], when performed), dual radiotracer (eg, myocardial viability);**

Code also stress testing when performed (93015-93018)

0.00 0.00 FUD XXX Z2 80

AMA: 2020,Jul,5

\# **78433** **with concurrently acquired computed tomography transmission scan**

INCLUDES Examination CT transmission images for field of view anatomy review

EXCLUDES *CT for other than attenuation correction/anatomical localization; use site-specific CT code with modifier 59*

Code also stress testing when performed (93015-93018)

0.00 0.00 FUD XXX Z2 80

AMA: 2020,Jul,5

\+ # **78434** **Absolute quantitation of myocardial blood flow (AQMBF), positron emission tomography (PET), rest and pharmacologic stress (List separately in addition to code for primary procedure)**

EXCLUDES *CT coronary calcium scoring (75571)*

Myocardial imaging by planar or SPECT (78451-78454)

Code first ([78431], 78492)

0.00 0.00 FUD ZZZ N1 80

AMA: 2020,Jul,5

78494 **Cardiac blood pool imaging, gated equilibrium, SPECT, at rest, wall motion study plus ejection fraction, with or without quantitative processing**

EXCLUDES *Distribution radiopharmaceutical agents or tumor localization (78800-78802, [78804], 78803)*

Radiopharmaceutical quantification measurements ([78835])

SPECT with concurrently acquired CT transmission scan ([78830, 78831, 78832])

6.51 6.51 FUD XXX S Z2 80

AMA: 2018,Jan,8; 2017,Jan,8; 2016,Jan,13; 2015,Jan,16

+ **78496 Cardiac blood pool imaging, gated equilibrium, single study, at rest, with right ventricular ejection fraction by first pass technique (List separately in addition to code for primary procedure)**

Code first (78472)

1.25 1.25 FUD ZZZ N N1 80

AMA: 2018,Jan,8; 2017,Jan,8; 2016,Jan,13; 2015,Jan,16

78499 Unlisted cardiovascular procedure, diagnostic nuclear medicine

0.00 0.00 FUD XXX S Z2 80

AMA: 2018,Jan,8; 2017,Jan,8; 2016,Jan,13; 2015,Jan,16

78579-78599 Nuclear Radiology: Lungs

EXCLUDES *Diagnostic services (see appropriate sections)*
Follow-up care (see appropriate sections)

Code also radiopharmaceutical(s) and/or drug(s) supplied

78579 Pulmonary ventilation imaging (eg, aerosol or gas)

EXCLUDES *Procedure performed more than one time per imaging session*

5.36 5.36 FUD XXX S Z2 80

AMA: 2012,Feb,9-10

78580 Pulmonary perfusion imaging (eg, particulate)

EXCLUDES *Myocardial perfusion imaging (78451-78454)*
Procedure performed more than one time per imaging session

6.87 6.87 FUD XXX S Z2 80

AMA: 2018,Jan,8; 2017,Jan,8; 2016,Jan,13; 2015,Jan,16

78582 Pulmonary ventilation (eg, aerosol or gas) and perfusion imaging

EXCLUDES *Myocardial perfusion imaging (78451-78454)*
Procedure performed more than one time per imaging session

9.54 9.54 FUD XXX S Z2 80

AMA: 2012,Feb,9-10

78597 Quantitative differential pulmonary perfusion, including imaging when performed

EXCLUDES *Myocardial perfusion imaging (78451-78454)*
Procedure performed more than one time per imaging session

5.74 5.74 FUD XXX S Z2 80

AMA: 2012,Feb,9-10

78598 Quantitative differential pulmonary perfusion and ventilation (eg, aerosol or gas), including imaging when performed

EXCLUDES *Myocardial perfusion imaging (78451-78454)*
Procedure performed more than one time per imaging session

8.80 8.80 FUD XXX S Z2 80

AMA: 2012,Feb,9-10

78599 Unlisted respiratory procedure, diagnostic nuclear medicine

0.00 0.00 FUD XXX S Z2 80

AMA: 2018,Jan,8; 2017,Jan,8; 2016,Jan,13; 2015,Jan,16

78600-78650 Nuclear Radiology: Brain/Cerebrospinal Fluid

EXCLUDES *Diagnostic services (see appropriate sections)*
Follow-up care (see appropriate section)

Code also radiopharmaceutical(s) and/or drug(s) supplied

78600 Brain imaging, less than 4 static views;

5.32 5.32 FUD XXX S Z2 80

AMA: 2018,Jan,8; 2017,Jan,8; 2016,Jan,13; 2015,Jan,16

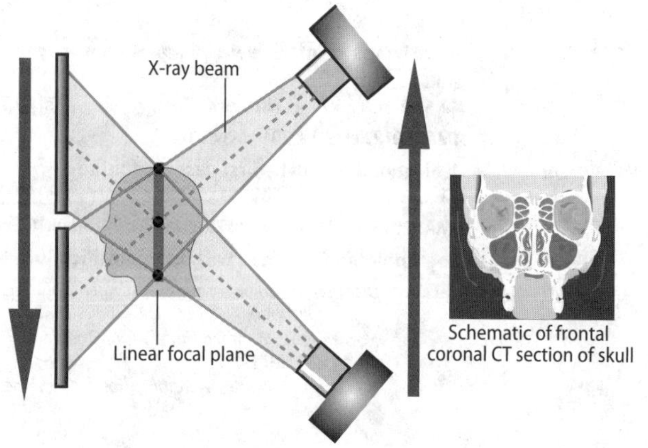

78601 with vascular flow

6.25 6.25 FUD XXX S Z2 80

AMA: 2012,Feb,9-10; 2007,Jan,28-31

78605 Brain imaging, minimum 4 static views;

5.71 5.71 FUD XXX S Z2 80

AMA: 2012,Feb,9-10; 2007,Jan,28-31

78606 with vascular flow

9.45 9.45 FUD XXX S Z2 80

AMA: 2012,Feb,9-10; 2007,Jan,28-31

78608 Brain imaging, positron emission tomography (PET); metabolic evaluation

0.00 0.00 FUD XXX S Z2 80

AMA: 2012,Feb,9-10; 2007,Jan,28-31

78609 perfusion evaluation

2.16 2.16 FUD XXX E

AMA: 2012,Feb,9-10; 2007,Jan,28-31

78610 Brain imaging, vascular flow only

5.04 5.04 FUD XXX S Z2 80

AMA: 2012,Feb,9-10; 2007,Jan,28-31

78630 Cerebrospinal fluid flow, imaging (not including introduction of material); cisternography

Code also injection procedure (61000-61070, 62270-62327)

9.74 9.74 FUD XXX S Z2 80

AMA: 2018,Jan,8

78635 ventriculography

Code also injection procedure (61000-61070, 62270-62294)

9.77 9.77 FUD XXX S Z2 80

AMA: 2012,Feb,9-10; 2007,Jan,28-31

78645 shunt evaluation

Code also injection procedure (61000-61070, 62270-62294)

9.28 9.28 FUD XXX S Z2 80

AMA: 2012,Feb,9-10; 2007,Jan,28-31

78650 Cerebrospinal fluid leakage detection and localization

Code also injection procedure (61000-61070, 62270-62294)

7.89 7.89 FUD XXX S Z2 80

AMA: 2012,Feb,9-10; 2007,Jan,28-31

78660-78699 Nuclear Radiology: Lacrimal Duct System

Code also radiopharmaceutical(s) and/or drug(s) supplied

78660 Radiopharmaceutical dacryocystography

5.26 5.26 FUD XXX S Z2 80

AMA: 2012,Feb,9-10; 2007,Jan,28-31

78699 **Unlisted nervous system procedure, diagnostic nuclear medicine**
0.00 0.00 FUD XXX S Z2 80
AMA: 2018,Jan,8; 2017,Jan,8; 2016,Jan,13; 2015,Jan,16

78700-78725 Nuclear Radiology: Renal Anatomy and Function

EXCLUDES *Diagnostic services (see appropriate sections)*
Follow-up care (see appropriate section)
Renal endoscopy with insertion radioactive substances (77778)
Code also radiopharmaceutical(s) and/or drug(s) supplied

78700 **Kidney imaging morphology;**
4.92 4.92 FUD XXX S Z2 80
AMA: 2018,Jan,8; 2017,Jan,8; 2016,Jan,13; 2015,Jan,16

78701 **with vascular flow**
6.25 6.25 FUD XXX S Z2 80
AMA: 2012,Feb,9-10; 2007,Mar,7-8

78707 **with vascular flow and function, single study without pharmacological intervention**
6.66 6.66 FUD XXX S Z2 80
AMA: 2018,Jan,8; 2017,Jan,8; 2016,Jan,13; 2015,Jan,16

78708 **with vascular flow and function, single study, with pharmacological intervention (eg, angiotensin converting enzyme inhibitor and/or diuretic)**
5.09 5.09 FUD XXX S Z2 80
AMA: 2018,Jan,8; 2017,Jan,8; 2016,Jan,13; 2015,Jan,16

78709 **with vascular flow and function, multiple studies, with and without pharmacological intervention (eg, angiotensin converting enzyme inhibitor and/or diuretic)**
10.5 10.5 FUD XXX S Z2 80
AMA: 2018,Jan,8; 2017,Jan,8; 2016,Jan,13; 2015,Jan,16

78725 **Kidney function study, non-imaging radioisotopic study**
3.10 3.10 FUD XXX S Z2 80
AMA: 2012,Feb,9-10; 2007,Jan,28-31

78730-78799 Nuclear Radiology: Urogenital

EXCLUDES *Diagnostic services (see appropriate sections)*
Follow-up care (see appropriate section)
Code also radiopharmaceutical(s) and/or drug(s) supplied

\+ **78730** **Urinary bladder residual study (List separately in addition to code for primary procedure)**
EXCLUDES *Measurement postvoid residual urine and /or bladder capacity using ultrasound (51798)*
Ultrasound imaging bladder only with measurement postvoid residual urine (76857)
Code first (78740)
2.22 2.22 FUD ZZZ N N1 80
AMA: 2018,Jan,8; 2017,Jan,8; 2016,Jan,13; 2015,Jan,16

78740 **Ureteral reflux study (radiopharmaceutical voiding cystogram)**
EXCLUDES *Catheterization (51701-51703)*
Code also urinary bladder residual study (78730)
6.29 6.29 FUD XXX S Z2 80
AMA: 2012,Feb,9-10; 2007,Jan,28-31

78761 **Testicular imaging with vascular flow** ♂
6.08 6.08 FUD XXX S Z2 80
AMA: 2018,Jan,8; 2017,Jan,8; 2016,Jan,13; 2015,Jan,16

78799 **Unlisted genitourinary procedure, diagnostic nuclear medicine**
0.00 0.00 FUD XXX S Z2 80
AMA: 2018,Jan,8; 2017,Jan,8; 2016,Jan,13; 2015,Jan,16

78800-78835 [78804, 78830, 78831, 78832, 78835] Nuclear Radiology: Tumor Localization

EXCLUDES *CSF studies requiring injection procedure (61055, 61070, 62320-62323)*
Code also radiopharmaceutical(s) and/or drug(s) supplied

78800 **Radiopharmaceutical localization of tumor, inflammatory process or distribution of radiopharmaceutical agent(s) (includes vascular flow and blood pool imaging, when performed); planar, single area (eg, head, neck, chest, pelvis), single day imaging**
INCLUDES Ocular radiophosphorus tumor identification
EXCLUDES *Specific organ (see appropriate site)*
5.61 5.61 FUD XXX S Z2 80
AMA: 2018,Nov,11; 2018,Jan,8; 2017,Jan,8; 2016,Jan,13; 2015,Jan,16

78801 **planar, 2 or more areas (eg, abdomen and pelvis, head and chest), 1 or more days imaging or single area imaging over 2 or more days**
7.42 7.42 FUD XXX S Z2 80
AMA: 2018,Jan,8; 2017,Jan,8; 2016,Jan,13; 2015,Jan,16

78802 **planar, whole body, single day imaging**
9.29 9.29 FUD XXX S Z2 80
AMA: 2012,Feb,9-10; 2007,Jan,28-31

\# **78804** **planar, whole body, requiring 2 or more days imaging**
16.3 16.3 FUD XXX S Z2 80
AMA: 2012,Feb,9-10; 2007,Jan,28-31

78803 **tomographic (SPECT), single area (eg, head, neck, chest, pelvis), single day imaging**
11.1 11.1 FUD XXX S Z2 80
AMA: 2018,Nov,11; 2018,Jan,8; 2017,Jan,8; 2016,Dec,9; 2016,Dec,16; 2016,Jan,13; 2015,Oct,9

78804 **Resequenced code. See code following 78802.**

\# **78830** **tomographic (SPECT) with concurrently acquired computed tomography (CT) transmission scan for anatomical review, localization and determination/detection of pathology, single area (eg, head, neck, chest, pelvis), single day imaging**
14.0 14.0 FUD XXX Z2 80

\# **78831** **tomographic (SPECT), minimum 2 areas (eg, pelvis and knees, abdomen and pelvis), single day imaging, or single area imaging over 2 or more days**
20.3 20.3 FUD XXX Z2 80

\# **78832** **tomographic (SPECT) with concurrently acquired computed tomography (CT) transmission scan for anatomical review, localization and determination/detection of pathology, minimum 2 areas (eg, pelvis and knees, abdomen and pelvis), single day imaging, or single area imaging over 2 or more days**
26.4 26.4 FUD XXX Z2 80

\+ # **78835** **Radiopharmaceutical quantification measurement(s) single area (List separately in addition to code for primary procedure)**
2.95 2.95 FUD ZZZ 80

78808 Intravenous Injection for Radiopharmaceutical Localization

Code also radiopharmaceutical(s) and/or drug(s) supplied

78808 **Injection procedure for radiopharmaceutical localization by non-imaging probe study, intravenous (eg, parathyroid adenoma)**
1.12 1.12 FUD XXX Q1 N1 80
AMA: 2018,Jan,8; 2017,Jan,8; 2016,Dec,9

Radiology

78699 — 78808

78811-78999 [78830, 78831, 78832, 78835] Nuclear Radiology: Diagnosis, Staging, Restaging or Monitoring Cancer

CMS: 100-03,220.6.17 Positron Emission Tomography (FDG) for Oncologic Conditions; 100-03,220.6.19 NaF-18 PET to Identify Bone Metastasis of Cancer; 100-03,220.6.9 FDG PET for Refractory Seizures; 100-04,13,60 Positron Emission Tomography (PET) Scans - General Information; 100-04,13,60.13 Billing for PET Scans for Specific Indications of Cervical Cancer; 100-04,13,60.15 Billing for CMS-Approved Clinical Trials for PET Scans; 100-04,13,60.16 Billing and Coverage for PET Scans; 100-04,13,60.17 Billing and Coverage Changes for PET Scans for Cervical Cancer; 100-04,13,60.18 Billing and Coverage for PET (NaF-18) Scans to Identify Bone Metastasis; 100-04,13,60.2 Use of Gamma Cameras, Full and Partial Ring PET Scanners; 100-04,13,60.3 PET Scan Qualifying Conditions; 100-04,13,60.3.1 Appropriate Codes for PET Scans; 100-04,13,60.3.2 Tracer Codes Required for Positron Emission Tomography (PET) Scans

EXCLUDES *CT scan performed for other than attenuation correction and anatomical localization (report with appropriate site-specific CT code and modifier 59)*
Ocular radiophosphorus tumor identification (78800)
PET brain scan (78608-78609)
PET myocardial imaging (78459, 78491-78492)
Procedure performed more than one time per imaging session

Code also radiopharmaceutical(s) and/or drug(s) supplied

78811 **Positron emission tomography (PET) imaging; limited area (eg, chest, head/neck)**
Facility RVU 0.00 Non-Facility RVU 0.00 **FUD** XXX S Z2 80
AMA: 2018,Jan,8; 2017,Jan,8; 2016,Jan,13; 2015,Jan,16

78812 **skull base to mid-thigh**
Facility RVU 0.00 Non-Facility RVU 0.00 **FUD** XXX S Z2 80
AMA: 2018,Jan,8; 2017,Jan,8; 2016,Jan,13; 2015,Jan,16

78813 **whole body**
Facility RVU 0.00 Non-Facility RVU 0.00 **FUD** XXX S Z2 80
AMA: 2018,Jan,8; 2017,Jan,8; 2016,Jan,13; 2015,Jan,16

78814 **Positron emission tomography (PET) with concurrently acquired computed tomography (CT) for attenuation correction and anatomical localization imaging; limited area (eg, chest, head/neck)**
Facility RVU 0.00 Non-Facility RVU 0.00 **FUD** XXX S Z2 80
AMA: 2018,Jan,8; 2017,Jan,8; 2016,Jan,13; 2015,Jan,16

78815 **skull base to mid-thigh**
Facility RVU 0.00 Non-Facility RVU 0.00 **FUD** XXX S Z2 80
AMA: 2018,Jan,8; 2017,Jan,8; 2016,Jan,13; 2015,Jan,16

78816 **whole body**
Facility RVU 0.00 Non-Facility RVU 0.00 **FUD** XXX S Z2 80
AMA: 2020,Sep,11; 2018,Jan,8; 2017,Jan,8; 2016,Jan,13; 2015,Jan,16

78830 **Resequenced code. See code following code 78803.**

78831 **Resequenced code. See code following code 78803.**

78832 **Resequenced code. See code following code 78803.**

78835 **Resequenced code. See code following code 78803.**

78999 **Unlisted miscellaneous procedure, diagnostic nuclear medicine**
Facility RVU 0.00 Non-Facility RVU 0.00 **FUD** XXX S Z2 80
AMA: 2018,Jan,8; 2017,Jan,8; 2016,Dec,9; 2016,Dec,16; 2016,Jan,13; 2015,Oct,9; 2015,Jan,16

79005-79999 Systemic Radiopharmaceutical Therapy

EXCLUDES *Imaging guidance*
Injection into artery, body cavity, or joint (see appropriate injection codes)
Radiological supervision and interpretation

79005 **Radiopharmaceutical therapy, by oral administration**
EXCLUDES *Monoclonal antibody treatment (79403)*
Facility RVU 3.92 Non-Facility RVU 3.92 **FUD** XXX S Z3 80
AMA: 2018,Jan,8; 2017,Jan,8; 2016,Jan,13; 2015,Jan,16

79101 **Radiopharmaceutical therapy, by intravenous administration**
EXCLUDES *Administration nonantibody radioelement solution including follow-up care (77750)*
Hydration infusion (96360)
Intravenous injection, IV push (96374-96375, 96409)
Radiolabeled monoclonal antibody IV infusion (79403)
Venipuncture (36400, 36410)
Facility RVU 4.18 Non-Facility RVU 4.18 **FUD** XXX S Z3 80
AMA: 2018,Jan,8; 2017,Jan,8; 2016,Jan,13; 2015,Jan,16

79200 **Radiopharmaceutical therapy, by intracavitary administration**
Facility RVU 3.86 Non-Facility RVU 3.86 **FUD** XXX S Z3 80
AMA: 2018,Jan,8; 2017,Jan,8; 2016,Jan,13; 2015,Jan,16

79300 **Radiopharmaceutical therapy, by interstitial radioactive colloid administration**
Facility RVU 0.00 Non-Facility RVU 0.00 **FUD** XXX S Z2 80
AMA: 2018,Jan,8; 2017,Jan,8; 2016,Jan,13; 2015,Jan,16

79403 **Radiopharmaceutical therapy, radiolabeled monoclonal antibody by intravenous infusion**
EXCLUDES *Intravenous radiopharmaceutical therapy (79101)*
Facility RVU 5.39 Non-Facility RVU 5.39 **FUD** XXX S Z3 80
AMA: 2018,Jan,8; 2017,Jan,8; 2016,Jan,13; 2015,Jan,16

79440 **Radiopharmaceutical therapy, by intra-articular administration**
Facility RVU 3.48 Non-Facility RVU 3.48 **FUD** XXX S Z3 80
AMA: 2018,Jan,8; 2017,Jan,8; 2016,Jan,13; 2015,Jan,16

79445 **Radiopharmaceutical therapy, by intra-arterial particulate administration**
EXCLUDES *Intra-arterial injections (96373, 96420)*
Procedural and radiological supervision and interpretation for angiographic and interventional procedures before intra-arterial radiopharmaceutical therapy
Facility RVU 0.00 Non-Facility RVU 0.00 **FUD** XXX S Z2 80
AMA: 2018,Jan,8; 2017,Jan,8; 2016,Jan,13; 2015,Jan,16

79999 **Radiopharmaceutical therapy, unlisted procedure**
Facility RVU 0.00 Non-Facility RVU 0.00 **FUD** XXX S Z2 80
AMA: 2018,Jan,8; 2017,Jan,8; 2016,Jan,13; 2015,Jan,16

80047-80081 [80081] Multi-test Laboratory Panels

INCLUDES Specified test grous that may be reported in a panel

EXCLUDES *Reporting two or more panel codes including same tests; report panel with most tests in common to meet panel code definition*

Code also individual tests not part included in panel, when appropriate

80047 Basic metabolic panel (Calcium, ionized)

INCLUDES Calcium, ionized (82330)
Carbon dioxide (bicarbonate) (82374)
Chloride (82435)
Creatinine (82565)
Glucose (82947)
Potassium (84132)
Sodium (84295)
Urea nitrogen (BUN) (84520)

0.00 0.00 FUD XXX

AMA: 2020,Jun,3; 2018,Jan,8; 2017,Jan,8; 2016,Jan,13; 2015,Jan,16

80048 Basic metabolic panel (Calcium, total)

INCLUDES Calcium, total (82310)
Carbon dioxide (bicarbonate) (82374)
Chloride (82435)
Creatinine (82565)
Glucose (82947)
Potassium (84132)
Sodium (84295)
Urea nitrogen (BUN) (84520)

0.00 0.00 FUD XXX

AMA: 2018,Jan,8; 2017,Jan,8; 2016,Jan,13; 2015,Jan,16

80050 General health panel

INCLUDES Complete blood count (CBC), automated, with:
Manual differential WBC count
Blood smear with manual differential AND complete (CBC), automated (85007, 85027)
Manual differential WBC count, buffy coat AND complete (CBC), automated (85009, 85027)
OR
Automated differential WBC count
Automated differential WBC count AND complete (CBC), automated/automated differential WBC count (85004, 85025)
Automated differential WBC count AND complete (CBC), automated (85004, 85027)
Comprehensive metabolic profile (80053)
Thyroid stimulating hormone (84443)

0.00 0.00 FUD XXX

AMA: 2018,Jan,8; 2017,Jan,8; 2016,Jan,13; 2015,Jan,16

80051 Electrolyte panel

INCLUDES Carbon dioxide (bicarbonate) (82374)
Chloride (82435)
Potassium (84132)
Sodium (84295)

0.00 0.00 FUD XXX

AMA: 2018,Jan,8; 2017,Jan,8; 2016,Jan,13; 2015,Jan,16

80053 Comprehensive metabolic panel

INCLUDES Albumin (82040)
Bilirubin, total (82247)
Calcium, total (82310)
Carbon dioxide (bicarbonate) (82374)
Chloride (82435)
Creatinine (82565)
Glucose (82947)
Phosphatase, alkaline (84075)
Potassium (84132)
Protein, total (84155)
Sodium (84295)
Transferase, alanine amino (ALT) (SGPT) (84460)
Transferase, aspartate amino (AST) (SGOT) (84450)
Urea nitrogen (BUN) (84520)

0.00 0.00 FUD XXX

AMA: 2018,Jan,8; 2017,Jan,8; 2016,Jan,13; 2015,Jan,16

80055 Obstetric panel M ♀

INCLUDES Complete blood count (CBC), automated, with:
Manual differential WBC count
Blood smear with manual differential AND complete (CBC), automated (85007, 85027)
Manual differential WBC count, buffy coat AND complete (CBC), automated (85009, 85027)
OR
Automated differential WBC count
Automated differential WBC count AND complete (CBC), automated/automated differential WBC count (85004, 85025)
Automated differential WBC count AND complete (CBC), automated (85004, 85027)
Blood typing, ABO and Rh (86900-86901)
Hepatitis B surface antigen (HBsAg) (87340)
RBC antibody screen, each serum technique (86850)
Rubella antibody (86762)
Syphilis test, non-treponemal antibody qualitative (86592)

EXCLUDES *Reporting code when syphilis screening provided using treponemal antibody approach. Instead, assign individual codes for tests performed in OB panel (86780)*

0.00 0.00 FUD XXX

AMA: 2018,Jan,8; 2017,Jan,8; 2016,Jan,13; 2015,Jan,16

80081 Obstetric panel (includes HIV testing) M ♀

INCLUDES Complete blood count (CBC), automated, with:
Manual differential WBC count
Blood smear with manual differential AND complete (CBC), automated (85007, 85027)
Manual differential WBC count, buffy count AND complete (CBC), automated (85009, 85027)
OR
Automated differential WBC count
Automated differential WBC count AND complete (CBC), automated/automated differential WBC count (85004, 85025)
Automated differential WBC count AND complete (CBC), automated (85004, 85027)
Blood typing, ABO and Rh (86900-86901)
Hepatitis B surface antigen (HBsAg) (87340)
HIV-1 antigens, with HIV-1 and HIV-2 antibodies, single result (87389)
RBC antibody screen, each serum technique (86850)
Rubella antibody (86762)
Syphilis test, non-treponemal antibody qualitative (86592)

EXCLUDES *Reporting code when syphilis screening provided using treponemal antibody approach. Instead, assign individual codes for tests performed in OB panel (86780)*

0.00 0.00 FUD XXX

AMA: 2018,Jan,8; 2017,Jan,8; 2016,Jan,13

80061 Lipid panel

INCLUDES Cholesterol, serum, total (82465)
Lipoprotein, direct measurement, high density cholesterol (HDL cholesterol) (83718)
Triglycerides (84478)

0.00 0.00 FUD XXX

AMA: 2018,Jan,8; 2017,Sep,11; 2017,Jan,8; 2016,Jan,13; 2015,Jan,16

80069 Renal function panel

INCLUDES Albumin (82040)
Calcium, total (82310)
Carbon dioxide (bicarbonate) (82374)
Chloride (82435)
Creatinine (82565)
Glucose (82947)
Phosphorus inorganic (phosphate) (84100)
Potassium (84132)
Sodium (84295)
Urea nitrogen (BUN) (84520)

0.00 0.00 FUD XXX

AMA: 2018,Jan,8; 2017,Jan,8; 2016,Jan,13; 2015,Jan,16

80074 **Acute hepatitis panel**

INCLUDES Hepatitis A antibody (HAAb) IgM (86709)
Hepatitis B core antibody (HBcAb), IgM (86705)
Hepatitis B surface antigen (HBsAg) (87340)
Hepatitis C antibody (86803)

0.00 0.00 **FUD** XXX Q

AMA: 2018,Jan,8; 2017,Jan,8; 2016,Jan,13; 2015,Jan,16

80076 **Hepatic function panel**

INCLUDES Albumin (82040)
Bilirubin, direct (82248)
Bilirubin, total (82247)
Phosphatase, alkaline (84075)
Protein, total (84155)
Transferase, alanine amino (ALT) (SGPT) (84460)
Transferase, aspartate amino (AST) (SGOT) (84450)

0.00 0.00 **FUD** XXX Q

AMA: 2018,Jan,8; 2017,Jan,8; 2016,Jan,13; 2015,Jan,16

80081 **Resequenced code. See code following 80055.**

80305-80307 [80305, 80306, 80307] Nonspecific Drug Screening

INCLUDES All class testing procedures performed per modality
Validation testing

EXCLUDES *Confirmatory drug testing ([80320, 80321, 80322, 80323, 80324, 80325, 80326, 80327, 80328, 80329, 80330, 80331, 80332, 80333, 80334, 80335, 80336, 80337, 80338, 80339, 80340, 80341, 80342, 80343, 80344, 80345, 80346, 80347, 80348, 80349, 80350, 80351, 80352, 80353, 80354, 80355, 80356, 80357, 80358, 80359, 80360, 80361, 80362, 80363, 80364, 80365, 80366, 80367, 80368, 80369, 80370, 80371, 80372, 80373, 80374, 80375, 80376, 80377, 83992], [83992])*

\# **80305** **Drug test(s), presumptive, any number of drug classes, any number of devices or procedures; capable of being read by direct optical observation only (eg, utilizing immunoassay [eg, dipsticks, cups, cards, or cartridges]), includes sample validation when performed, per date of service**

0.00 0.00 **FUD** XXX Q

AMA: 2018,Jul,14; 2018,Jan,8; 2017,Mar,6

\# **80306** **read by instrument assisted direct optical observation (eg, utilizing immunoassay [eg, dipsticks, cups, cards, or cartridges]), includes sample validation when performed, per date of service**

0.00 0.00 **FUD** XXX Q

AMA: 2018,Jan,8; 2017,Mar,6

\# **80307** **by instrument chemistry analyzers (eg, utilizing immunoassay [eg, EIA, ELISA, EMIT, FPIA, IA, KIMS, RIA]), chromatography (eg, GC, HPLC), and mass spectrometry either with or without chromatography, (eg, DART, DESI, GC-MS, GC-MS/MS, LC-MS, LC-MS/MS, LDTD, MALDI, TOF) includes sample validation when performed, per date of service**

0.00 0.00 **FUD** XXX Q

AMA: 2018,Jan,8; 2017,Mar,6

80320-80377 [80320, 80321, 80322, 80323, 80324, 80325, 80326, 80327, 80328, 80329, 80330, 80331, 80332, 80333, 80334, 80335, 80336, 80337, 80338, 80339, 80340, 80341, 80342, 80343, 80344, 80345, 80346, 80347, 80348, 80349, 80350, 80351, 80352, 80353, 80354, 80355, 80356, 80357, 80358, 80359, 80360, 80361, 80362, 80363, 80364, 80365, 80366, 80367, 80368, 80369, 80370, 80371, 80372, 80373, 80374, 80375, 80376, 80377, 83992] Confirmatory Drug Testing

INCLUDES Antihistamine drug tests ([80375, 80376, 80377])
Detection specific drugs using methods other than immunoassay or enzymatic technique

EXCLUDES *Definitive drug testing for any drug class not specified; report with NOS codes ([80375, 80376, 80377])*
Metabolites separate from code for drug except when distinct code available

\# **80320** **Alcohols**

EXCLUDES *Alcohol (ethanol) therapeutic drug assay (82077)*

0.00 0.00 **FUD** XXX B

AMA: 2018,Jan,8; 2017,Jan,8; 2016,Jan,13; 2015,Apr,3

\# **80321** **Alcohol biomarkers; 1 or 2**

0.00 0.00 **FUD** XXX B

AMA: 2015,Apr,3

\# **80322** **3 or more**

0.00 0.00 **FUD** XXX B

AMA: 2015,Apr,3

\# **80323** **Alkaloids, not otherwise specified**

0.00 0.00 **FUD** XXX B

AMA: 2015,Apr,3

\# **80324** **Amphetamines; 1 or 2**

0.00 0.00 **FUD** XXX B

AMA: 2015,Apr,3

\# **80325** **3 or 4**

0.00 0.00 **FUD** XXX B

AMA: 2015,Apr,3

\# **80326** **5 or more**

0.00 0.00 **FUD** XXX B

AMA: 2015,Apr,3

\# **80327** **Anabolic steroids; 1 or 2**

0.00 0.00 **FUD** XXX B

AMA: 2015,Apr,3

\# **80328** **3 or more**

EXCLUDES *Analysis dihydrotestosterone for monitoring, endogenous levels of hormone (82642)*

0.00 0.00 **FUD** XXX B

AMA: 2015,Apr,3

\# **80329** **Analgesics, non-opioid; 1 or 2**

EXCLUDES *Acetaminophen therapeutic drug assay (80143)*
Salicylate therapeutic drug assay ([80179])

0.00 0.00 **FUD** XXX B

AMA: 2015,Apr,3

\# **80330** **3-5**

EXCLUDES *Acetaminophen therapeutic drug assay (80143)*
Salicylate therapeutic drug assay ([80179])

0.00 0.00 **FUD** XXX B

AMA: 2015,Apr,3

\# **80331** **6 or more**

EXCLUDES *Acetaminophen therapeutic drug assay (80143)*
Salicylate therapeutic drug assay ([80179])

0.00 0.00 **FUD** XXX B

AMA: 2015,Apr,3

\# **80332** **Antidepressants, serotonergic class; 1 or 2**

0.00 0.00 **FUD** XXX B

AMA: 2015,Apr,3

80333 3-5
0.00 0.00 FUD XXX B
AMA: 2015,Apr,3

80334 6 or more
0.00 0.00 FUD XXX B
AMA: 2015,Apr,3

80335 Antidepressants, tricyclic and other cyclicals; 1 or 2
0.00 0.00 FUD XXX B
AMA: 2015,Apr,3

80336 3-5
0.00 0.00 FUD XXX B
AMA: 2015,Apr,3

80337 6 or more
0.00 0.00 FUD XXX B
AMA: 2015,Apr,3

80338 Antidepressants, not otherwise specified
0.00 0.00 FUD XXX B
AMA: 2015,Apr,3

80339 Antiepileptics, not otherwise specified; 1-3
0.00 0.00 FUD XXX B
AMA: 2015,Apr,3

80340 4-6
0.00 0.00 FUD XXX B
AMA: 2015,Apr,3

80341 7 or more
EXCLUDES *Carbamazepine therapeutic drug assay (80156, 80157, [80161])*
Definitive drug testing for antihistamines ([80375, 80376, 80377])
0.00 0.00 FUD XXX B
AMA: 2015,Apr,3

80342 Antipsychotics, not otherwise specified; 1-3
0.00 0.00 FUD XXX B
AMA: 2015,Apr,3

80343 4-6
0.00 0.00 FUD XXX B
AMA: 2015,Apr,3

80344 7 or more
0.00 0.00 FUD XXX B
AMA: 2015,Apr,3

80345 Barbiturates
0.00 0.00 FUD XXX B
AMA: 2015,Apr,3

80346 Benzodiazepines; 1-12
0.00 0.00 FUD XXX B
AMA: 2015,Apr,3

80347 13 or more
0.00 0.00 FUD XXX B
AMA: 2015,Apr,3

80348 Buprenorphine
0.00 0.00 FUD XXX B
AMA: 2015,Apr,3

80349 Cannabinoids, natural
0.00 0.00 FUD XXX B
AMA: 2015,Apr,3

80350 Cannabinoids, synthetic; 1-3
0.00 0.00 FUD XXX B
AMA: 2015,Apr,3

80351 4-6
0.00 0.00 FUD XXX B
AMA: 2015,Apr,3

80352 7 or more
0.00 0.00 FUD XXX B
AMA: 2015,Apr,3

80353 Cocaine
0.00 0.00 FUD XXX B
AMA: 2015,Apr,3

80354 Fentanyl
0.00 0.00 FUD XXX B
AMA: 2015,Apr,3

80355 Gabapentin, non-blood
EXCLUDES *Therapeutic drug assay ([80171])*
0.00 0.00 FUD XXX B
AMA: 2018,Jan,8; 2017,Jan,8; 2016,Jan,13; 2015,Apr,3

80356 Heroin metabolite
0.00 0.00 FUD XXX B
AMA: 2015,Apr,3

80357 Ketamine and norketamine
0.00 0.00 FUD XXX B
AMA: 2015,Apr,3

80358 Methadone
0.00 0.00 FUD XXX B
AMA: 2015,Apr,3

80359 Methylenedioxyamphetamines (MDA, MDEA, MDMA)
0.00 0.00 FUD XXX B
AMA: 2015,Apr,3

80360 Methylphenidate
0.00 0.00 FUD XXX B
AMA: 2015,Apr,3

80361 Opiates, 1 or more
0.00 0.00 FUD XXX B
AMA: 2015,Apr,3

80362 Opioids and opiate analogs; 1 or 2
0.00 0.00 FUD XXX B
AMA: 2015,Apr,3

80363 3 or 4
0.00 0.00 FUD XXX B
AMA: 2015,Apr,3

80364 5 or more
0.00 0.00 FUD XXX B
AMA: 2015,Apr,3

80365 Oxycodone
0.00 0.00 FUD XXX B
AMA: 2015,Apr,3

83992 Phencyclidine (PCP)
0.00 0.00 FUD XXX E
AMA: 2018,Jan,8; 2017,Jan,8; 2016,Jan,13; 2015,Jun,10; 2015,Apr,3

80366 Pregabalin
0.00 0.00 FUD XXX B
AMA: 2015,Apr,3

80367 Propoxyphene
0.00 0.00 FUD XXX B
AMA: 2015,Apr,3

80368 Sedative hypnotics (non-benzodiazepines)
0.00 0.00 FUD XXX B
AMA: 2015,Apr,3

80369 Skeletal muscle relaxants; 1 or 2
0.00 0.00 FUD XXX B
AMA: 2015,Apr,3

80370 3 or more
0.00 0.00 FUD XXX B
AMA: 2015,Apr,3

\# **80371** **Stimulants, synthetic**
0.00 0.00 FUD XXX B
AMA: 2015,Apr,3

\# **80372** **Tapentadol**
0.00 0.00 FUD XXX B
AMA: 2015,Apr,3

\# **80373** **Tramadol**
0.00 0.00 FUD XXX B
AMA: 2015,Apr,3

\# **80374** **Stereoisomer (enantiomer) analysis, single drug class**
Code also index drug analysis when appropriate
0.00 0.00 FUD XXX B
AMA: 2015,Apr,3

\# **80375** **Drug(s) or substance(s), definitive, qualitative or quantitative, not otherwise specified; 1-3**
0.00 0.00 FUD XXX B
AMA: 2018,Jan,8; 2017,Jan,8; 2016,Jan,13; 2015,Apr,3

\# **80376** **4-6**
0.00 0.00 FUD XXX B
AMA: 2018,Jan,8; 2017,Jan,8; 2016,Jan,13; 2015,Apr,3

\# **80377** **7 or more**
EXCLUDES *Definitive drug testing for antihistamines ([80375, 80376, 80377])*
0.00 0.00 FUD XXX B
AMA: 2018,Jan,8; 2017,Jan,8; 2016,Jan,13; 2015,Apr,3

80143-80377 [80161, 80164, 80165, 80167, 80171, 80176, 80179, 80181, 80189, 80193, 80204, 80210, 80230, 80235, 80280, 80285, 80305, 80306, 80307, 80320, 80321, 80322, 80323, 80324, 80325, 80326, 80327, 80328, 80329, 80330, 80331, 80332, 80333, 80334, 80335, 80336, 80337, 80338, 80339, 80340, 80341, 80342, 80343, 80344, 80345, 80346, 80347, 80348, 80349, 80350, 80351, 80352, 80353, 80354, 80355, 80356, 80357, 80358, 80359, 80360, 80361, 80362, 80363, 80364, 80365, 80366, 80367, 80368, 80369, 80370, 80371, 80372, 80373, 80374, 80375, 80376, 80377]

Therapeutic Drug Levels

INCLUDES Monitoring known, prescribed or over-the-counter medication levels
Testing drug and metabolite(s) in primary code
Tests on specimens from blood, blood components, and spinal fluid

● **80143** **Acetaminophen**
EXCLUDES *Acetaminophen confirmatory drug testing ([80329, 80330, 80331])*

80145 **Adalimumab**
0.00 0.00 FUD XXX

80150 **Amikacin**
0.00 0.00 FUD XXX Q
AMA: 2018,Jan,8; 2017,Jan,8; 2016,Jan,13; 2015,Apr,3; 2015,Jan,16

● **80151** **Amiodarone**

80155 **Caffeine**
0.00 0.00 FUD XXX Q
AMA: 2015,Apr,3

80156 **Carbamazepine; total**
0.00 0.00 FUD XXX Q
AMA: 2018,Jan,8; 2017,Jan,8; 2016,Jan,13; 2015,Apr,3; 2015,Jan,16

80157 **free**
0.00 0.00 FUD XXX Q
AMA: 2018,Jan,8; 2017,Jan,8; 2016,Jan,13; 2015,Apr,3; 2015,Jan,16

● # **80161** **Carbamazepine; -10,11-epoxide**
0.00 0.00 FUD 000

80158 **Cyclosporine**
0.00 0.00 FUD XXX Q
AMA: 2018,Jan,8; 2017,Jan,8; 2016,Jan,13; 2015,Apr,3; 2015,Jan,16

80159 **Clozapine**
0.00 0.00 FUD XXX Q
AMA: 2015,Apr,3

80161 **Resequenced code. See code following 80157.**

80162 **Digoxin; total**
0.00 0.00 FUD XXX Q
AMA: 2018,Jan,8; 2017,Jan,8; 2016,Jan,13; 2015,Apr,3; 2015,Jan,16

80163 **free**
0.00 0.00 FUD XXX Q
AMA: 2018,Jan,8; 2017,Jan,8; 2016,Jan,13; 2015,Apr,3

80164 **Resequenced code. See code following 80201.**

80165 **Resequenced code. See code following 80201.**

80167 **Resequenced code. See code following 80169.**

80168 **Ethosuximide**
0.00 0.00 FUD XXX Q
AMA: 2018,Jan,8; 2017,Jan,8; 2016,Jan,13; 2015,Apr,3; 2015,Jan,16

80169 **Everolimus**
0.00 0.00 FUD XXX Q
AMA: 2015,Apr,3

● # **80167** **Felbamate**
0.00 0.00 FUD 000

● # **80181** **Flecainide**
0.00 0.00 FUD 000

\# **80171** **Gabapentin, whole blood, serum, or plasma**
0.00 0.00 FUD XXX Q
AMA: 2018,Jan,8; 2017,Jan,8; 2016,Jan,13; 2015,Apr,3

80170 **Gentamicin**
0.00 0.00 FUD XXX Q
AMA: 2018,Jan,8; 2017,Jan,8; 2016,Jan,13; 2015,Apr,3; 2015,Jan,16

80171 **Resequenced code. See code before 80170.**

80173 **Haloperidol**
0.00 0.00 FUD XXX Q
AMA: 2018,Jan,8; 2017,Jan,8; 2016,Jan,13; 2015,Apr,3; 2015,Jan,16

\# **80230** **Infliximab**
0.00 0.00 FUD XXX

● # **80189** **Itraconazole**
0.00 0.00 FUD 000

\# **80235** **Lacosamide**
0.00 0.00 FUD XXX

80175 **Lamotrigine**
0.00 0.00 FUD XXX Q
AMA: 2015,Apr,3

80176 **Resequenced code. See code following 80177.**

● # **80193** **Leflunomide**
0.00 0.00 FUD 000

80177 **Levetiracetam**
0.00 0.00 FUD XXX Q
AMA: 2015,Apr,3

\# **80176** **Lidocaine**
0.00 0.00 FUD XXX Q
AMA: 2018,Jan,8; 2017,Jan,8; 2016,Jan,13; 2015,Apr,3; 2015,Jan,16

80178 Lithium
0.00 0.00 FUD XXX
AMA: 2018,Jan,8; 2017,Jan,8; 2016,Jan,13; 2015,Apr,3; 2015,Jan,16

● # **80204 Methotrexate**
0.00 0.00 FUD 000

80179 **Resequenced code. See code before 80195.**

80180 Mycophenolate (mycophenolic acid)
0.00 0.00 FUD XXX
AMA: 2015,Apr,3

80181 **Resequenced code. See code following resequenced code 80167.**

80183 Oxcarbazepine
0.00 0.00 FUD XXX
AMA: 2015,Apr,3

80184 Phenobarbital
0.00 0.00 FUD XXX
AMA: 2018,Jan,8; 2017,Jan,8; 2016,Jan,13; 2015,Apr,3; 2015,Jan,16

80185 Phenytoin; total
0.00 0.00 FUD XXX
AMA: 2018,Jan,8; 2017,Jan,8; 2016,Jan,13; 2015,Apr,3; 2015,Jan,16

80186 free
0.00 0.00 FUD XXX
AMA: 2018,Jan,8; 2017,Jan,8; 2016,Jan,13; 2015,Apr,3; 2015,Jan,16

80187 Posaconazole
0.00 0.00 FUD XXX

80188 Primidone
0.00 0.00 FUD XXX
AMA: 2018,Jan,8; 2017,Jan,8; 2016,Jan,13; 2015,Apr,3; 2015,Jan,16

80189 **Resequenced code. See code following resequenced code 80230.**

80190 Procainamide;
0.00 0.00 FUD XXX
AMA: 2018,Jan,8; 2017,Jan,8; 2016,Jan,13; 2015,Apr,3; 2015,Jan,16

80192 with metabolites (eg, n-acetyl procainamide)
0.00 0.00 FUD XXX
AMA: 2018,Jan,8; 2017,Jan,8; 2016,Jan,13; 2015,Apr,3; 2015,Jan,16

80193 **Resequenced code. See code before 80177.**

80194 Quinidine
0.00 0.00 FUD XXX
AMA: 2018,Jan,8; 2017,Jan,8; 2016,Jan,13; 2015,Apr,3; 2015,Jan,16

● # **80210 Rufinamide**
0.00 0.00 FUD 000

● # **80179 Salicylate**
EXCLUDES *Salicylate confirmatory drug testing ([80329, 80330, 80331])*
0.00 0.00 FUD 000

80195 Sirolimus
0.00 0.00 FUD XXX
AMA: 2018,Jan,8; 2017,Jan,8; 2016,Jan,13; 2015,Apr,3; 2015,Jan,16

80197 Tacrolimus
0.00 0.00 FUD XXX
AMA: 2018,Jan,8; 2017,Jan,8; 2016,Jan,13; 2015,Apr,3; 2015,Jan,16

80198 Theophylline
0.00 0.00 FUD XXX
AMA: 2018,Jan,8; 2017,Jan,8; 2016,Jan,13; 2015,Apr,3; 2015,Jan,16

80199 Tiagabine
0.00 0.00 FUD XXX
AMA: 2015,Apr,3

80200 Tobramycin
0.00 0.00 FUD XXX
AMA: 2018,Jan,8; 2017,Jan,8; 2016,Jan,13; 2015,Apr,3; 2015,Jan,16

80201 Topiramate
0.00 0.00 FUD XXX
AMA: 2018,Jan,8; 2017,Jan,8; 2016,Jan,13; 2015,Apr,3; 2015,Jan,16

80164 Valproic acid (dipropylacetic acid); total
0.00 0.00 FUD XXX
AMA: 2018,Jan,8; 2017,Jan,8; 2016,Jan,13; 2015,Apr,3; 2015,Jan,16

80165 free
0.00 0.00 FUD XXX
AMA: 2018,Jan,8; 2017,Jan,8; 2016,Jan,13; 2015,Apr,3

80202 Vancomycin
0.00 0.00 FUD XXX
AMA: 2018,Jan,8; 2017,Jan,8; 2016,Jan,13; 2015,Apr,3; 2015,Jan,16

80280 Vedolizumab
0.00 0.00 FUD XXX

80285 Voriconazole
0.00 0.00 FUD XXX

80203 Zonisamide
0.00 0.00 FUD XXX
AMA: 2015,Apr,3

80204 **Resequenced code. See code following 80178.**

80210 **Resequenced code. See code following 80194.**

80230 **Resequenced code. See code following 80173.**

80235 **Resequenced code. See code before 80175.**

80280 **Resequenced code. See code following 80202.**

80285 **Resequenced code. See code before 80203.**

80299 Quantitation of therapeutic drug, not elsewhere specified
0.00 0.00 FUD XXX
AMA: 2018,Jan,8; 2017,Jan,8; 2016,Jan,13; 2015,Apr,3; 2015,Jan,16

80305 **Resequenced code. See code before 80143.**

80306 **Resequenced code. See code before 80143.**

80307 **Resequenced code. See code before 80143.**

80320 **Resequenced code. See code before 80143.**

80321 **Resequenced code. See code before 80143.**

80322 **Resequenced code. See code before 80143.**

80323 **Resequenced code. See code before 80143.**

80324 **Resequenced code. See code before 80143.**

80325 **Resequenced code. See code before 80143.**

80326 **Resequenced code. See code before 80143.**

80327 **Resequenced code. See code before 80143.**

80328 **Resequenced code. See code before 80143.**

80329 **Resequenced code. See code before 80143.**

80330 **Resequenced code. See code before 80143.**

80331 **Resequenced code. See code before 80143.**

80332 **Resequenced code. See code before 80143.**

80333 **Resequenced code. See code before 80143.**

80334 **Resequenced code. See code before 80143.**

80335 **Resequenced code. See code before 80143.**

80336 **Resequenced code. See code before 80143.**

80337 **Resequenced code. See code before 80143.**

80338 **Resequenced code. See code before 80143.**

80339 **Resequenced code. See code before 80143.**

80340 **Resequenced code. See code before 80143.**

80341 **Resequenced code. See code before 80143.**

80342 **Resequenced code. See code before 80143.**

80343 **Resequenced code. See code before 80143.**

80344 **Resequenced code. See code before 80143.**

80345 **Resequenced code. See code before 80143.**

80346 **Resequenced code. See code before 80143.**

80347 **Resequenced code. See code before 80143.**

80348 **Resequenced code. See code before 80143.**

80349 **Resequenced code. See code before 80143.**

80350 **Resequenced code. See code before 80143.**

80351 **Resequenced code. See code before 80143.**

80352 **Resequenced code. See code before 80143.**

80353 **Resequenced code. See code before 80143.**

80354 **Resequenced code. See code before 80143.**

80355 **Resequenced code. See code before 80143.**

80356 **Resequenced code. See code before 80143.**

80357 **Resequenced code. See code before 80143.**

80358 **Resequenced code. See code before 80143.**

80359 **Resequenced code. See code before 80143.**

80360 **Resequenced code. See code before 80143.**

80361 **Resequenced code. See code before 80143.**

80362 **Resequenced code. See code before 80143.**

80363 **Resequenced code. See code before 80143.**

80364 **Resequenced code. See code before 80143.**

80365 **Resequenced code. See code before 80143.**

80366 **Resequenced code. See code before 80143.**

80367 **Resequenced code. See code before 80143.**

80368 **Resequenced code. See code before 80143.**

80369 **Resequenced code. See code before 80143.**

80370 **Resequenced code. See code before 80143.**

80371 **Resequenced code. See code before 80143.**

80372 **Resequenced code. See code before 80143.**

80373 **Resequenced code. See code before 80143.**

80374 **Resequenced code. See code before 80143.**

80375 **Resequenced code. See code before 80143.**

80376 **Resequenced code. See code before 80143.**

80377 **Resequenced code. See code before 80143.**

80400-80439 Stimulation and Suppression Test Panels

EXCLUDES *Administration evocative or suppressive material (96365-96368, 96372, 96374-96376, C8957)*
Evocative or suppression test substances, when applicable
Physician monitoring and attendance during test (see E/M services)

80400 **ACTH stimulation panel; for adrenal insufficiency**

INCLUDES Cortisol x 2 (82533)
0.00 0.00 **FUD** XXX
AMA: 2018,Jan,8; 2017,Jan,8; 2016,Jan,13; 2015,Jan,16

80402 **for 21 hydroxylase deficiency**

INCLUDES 17 hydroxyprogesterone X 2 (83498)
Cortisol x 2 (82533)
0.00 0.00 **FUD** XXX
AMA: 2014,Jan,11; 2005,Jul,11-12

80406 **for 3 beta-hydroxydehydrogenase deficiency**

INCLUDES 17 hydroxypregnenolone x 2 (84143)
Cortisol x 2 (82533)
0.00 0.00 **FUD** XXX
AMA: 2014,Jan,11; 2005,Jul,11-12

80408 **Aldosterone suppression evaluation panel (eg, saline infusion)**

INCLUDES Aldosterone x 2 (82088)
Renin x 2 (84244)
0.00 0.00 **FUD** XXX
AMA: 2014,Jan,11; 2005,Jul,11-12

80410 **Calcitonin stimulation panel (eg, calcium, pentagastrin)**

INCLUDES Calcitonin x 3 (82308)
0.00 0.00 **FUD** XXX
AMA: 2014,Jan,11; 2005,Jul,11-12

80412 **Corticotropic releasing hormone (CRH) stimulation panel**

INCLUDES Adrenocorticotropic hormone (ACTH) x 6 (82024)
Cortisol x 6 (82533)
0.00 0.00 **FUD** XXX
AMA: 2014,Jan,11; 2005,Jul,11-12

80414 **Chorionic gonadotropin stimulation panel; testosterone response**

INCLUDES Testosterone x 2 on three pooled blood samples (84403)
0.00 0.00 **FUD** XXX
AMA: 2014,Jan,11; 2005,Jul,11-12

▲ **80415** **estradiol response**

INCLUDES Estradiol x 2 on three pooled blood samples (82670)
0.00 0.00 **FUD** XXX
AMA: 2014,Jan,11; 2005,Jul,11-12

80416 **Renal vein renin stimulation panel (eg, captopril)**

INCLUDES Renin x 6 (84244)
0.00 0.00 **FUD** XXX
AMA: 2014,Jan,11; 2005,Jul,11-12

80417 **Peripheral vein renin stimulation panel (eg, captopril)**

INCLUDES Renin x 2 (84244)
0.00 0.00 **FUD** XXX
AMA: 2014,Jan,11; 2005,Jul,11-12

80418 **Combined rapid anterior pituitary evaluation panel**

INCLUDES Adrenocorticotropic hormone (ACTH) x 4 (82024)
Cortisol x 4 (82533)
Follicle stimulating hormone (FSH) x 4 (83001)
Human growth hormone x 4 (83003)
Luteinizing hormone (LH) x 4 (83002)
Prolactin x 4 (84146)
Thyroid stimulating hormone (TSH) x 4 (84443)
0.00 0.00 **FUD** XXX
AMA: 2014,Jan,11; 2005,Jul,11-12

80420 **Dexamethasone suppression panel, 48 hour**

INCLUDES Cortisol x 2 (82533)
Free cortisol, urine x 2 (82530)
Volume measurement for timed collection x 2 (81050)
EXCLUDES *Single dose dexamethasone (82533)*
0.00 0.00 **FUD** XXX
AMA: 2014,Jan,11; 2005,Jul,11-12

80422 **Glucagon tolerance panel; for insulinoma**

INCLUDES Glucose x 3 (82947)
Insulin x 3 (83525)
0.00 0.00 **FUD** XXX
AMA: 2014,Jan,11; 2005,Jul,11-12

80424 **for pheochromocytoma**

INCLUDES Catecholamines, fractionated x 2 (82384)

0.00 0.00 **FUD** XXX

AMA: 2014,Jan,11; 2005,Jul,11-12

80426 **Gonadotropin releasing hormone stimulation panel**

INCLUDES Follicle stimulating hormone (FSH) x 4 (83001)
Luteinizing hormone (LH) x 4 (83002)

0.00 0.00 **FUD** XXX

AMA: 2014,Jan,11; 2005,Jul,11-12

80428 **Growth hormone stimulation panel (eg, arginine infusion, l-dopa administration)**

INCLUDES Human growth hormone (HGH) x 4 (83003)

0.00 0.00 **FUD** XXX

AMA: 2014,Jan,11; 2005,Jul,11-12

80430 **Growth hormone suppression panel (glucose administration)**

INCLUDES Glucose x 3 (82947)
Human growth hormone (HGH) x 4 (83003)

0.00 0.00 **FUD** XXX

AMA: 2014,Jan,11; 2005,Jul,11-12

80432 **Insulin-induced C-peptide suppression panel**

INCLUDES C-peptide x 5 (84681)
Glucose x 5 (82947)
Insulin (83525)

0.00 0.00 **FUD** XXX

AMA: 2014,Jan,11; 2005,Jul,11-12

80434 **Insulin tolerance panel; for ACTH insufficiency**

INCLUDES Cortisol x 5 (82533)
Glucose x 5 (82947)

0.00 0.00 **FUD** XXX

AMA: 2014,Jan,11; 2005,Jul,11-12

80435 **for growth hormone deficiency**

INCLUDES Glucose x 5 (82947)
Human growth hormone (HGH) x 5 (83003)

0.00 0.00 **FUD** XXX

AMA: 2014,Jan,11; 2005,Aug,9-10

80436 **Metyrapone panel**

INCLUDES 11 deoxycortisol x 2 (82634)
Cortisol x 2 (82533)

0.00 0.00 **FUD** XXX

AMA: 2014,Jan,11; 2005,Jul,11-12

80438 **Thyrotropin releasing hormone (TRH) stimulation panel; 1 hour**

INCLUDES Thyroid stimulating hormone (TSH) x 3 (84443)

0.00 0.00 **FUD** XXX

AMA: 2014,Jan,11; 2005,Jul,11-12

80439 **2 hour**

INCLUDES Thyroid stimulating hormone (TSH) x 4 (84443)

0.00 0.00 **FUD** XXX

AMA: 2014,Jan,11; 2005,Jul,11-12

80500-80502 Consultation By Clinical Pathologist

INCLUDES Pharmacokinetic consultations
Written report by pathologist for tests requiring additional medical judgment and requested by physician or other qualified health care professional

EXCLUDES *Consultations including patient examination*
Reporting code when medical interpretive assessment not provided

80500 **Clinical pathology consultation; limited, without review of patient's history and medical records**

0.56 0.65 **FUD** XXX

AMA: 2018,Jan,8; 2017,Jan,8; 2016,Jan,13; 2015,Jan,16

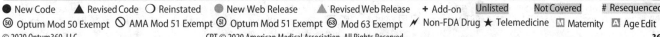

80502 **comprehensive, for a complex diagnostic problem, with review of patient's history and medical records**

2.02 2.11 **FUD** XXX

AMA: 2018,Jan,8; 2017,Jan,8; 2016,Jan,13; 2015,Jan,16

81000-81099 Urine Tests

81000 **Urinalysis, by dip stick or tablet reagent for bilirubin, glucose, hemoglobin, ketones, leukocytes, nitrite, pH, protein, specific gravity, urobilinogen, any number of these constituents; non-automated, with microscopy**

0.00 0.00 **FUD** XXX

AMA: 2018,Jul,14; 2018,Jan,8; 2017,Jan,8; 2016,Jan,13; 2015,Jan,16

81001 **automated, with microscopy**

0.00 0.00 **FUD** XXX

AMA: 2014,Jan,11; 2005,Jul,11-12

81002 **non-automated, without microscopy**

INCLUDES Mosenthal test

0.00 0.00 **FUD** XXX

AMA: 2018,Jan,8; 2017,Jan,8; 2016,Jan,13; 2015,Jan,16

81003 **automated, without microscopy**

0.00 0.00 **FUD** XXX

AMA: 2018,Jan,8; 2017,Jan,8; 2016,Jan,13; 2015,Jan,16

81005 **Urinalysis; qualitative or semiquantitative, except immunoassays**

INCLUDES Benedict test for dextrose

EXCLUDES *Immunoassay, qualitative or semiquantitative (83518)*
Microalbumin (82043-82044)
Nonimmunoassay reagent strip analysis (81000, 81002)

0.00 0.00 **FUD** XXX

AMA: 2018,Jan,8; 2017,Jan,8; 2016,Jan,13; 2015,Jan,16

81007 **bacteriuria screen, except by culture or dipstick**

EXCLUDES *Culture (87086-87088)*
Dipstick (81000, 81002)

0.00 0.00 **FUD** XXX

AMA: 2014,Jan,11; 2005,Jul,11-12

81015 **microscopic only**

EXCLUDES *Sperm evaluation for retrograde ejaculation (89331)*

0.00 0.00 **FUD** XXX

AMA: 2018,Jan,8; 2017,Nov,10

81020 **2 or 3 glass test**

INCLUDES Valentine's test

0.00 0.00 **FUD** XXX

AMA: 2014,Jan,11; 2005,Jul,11-12

81025 **Urine pregnancy test, by visual color comparison methods** M ♀

0.00 0.00 **FUD** XXX

AMA: 2018,Jan,8; 2017,Jan,8; 2016,Jan,13; 2015,Jan,16

81050 **Volume measurement for timed collection, each**

0.00 0.00 **FUD** XXX

AMA: 2014,Jan,11; 2005,Jul,11-12

81099 **Unlisted urinalysis procedure**

0.00 0.00 **FUD** XXX

AMA: 2018,Jan,8; 2017,Jan,8; 2016,Jan,13; 2015,Jan,16

Pathology and Laboratory

80424 — 81099

81105-81364 [81105, 81106, 81107, 81108, 81109, 81110, 81111, 81112, 81120, 81121, 81161, 81162, 81163, 81164, 81165, 81166, 81167, 81168, 81173, 81174, 81184, 81185, 81186, 81187, 81188, 81189, 81190, 81191, 81192, 81193, 81194, 81200, 81201, 81202, 81203, 81204, 81205, 81206, 81207, 81208, 81209, 81210, 81219, 81227, 81230, 81231, 81233, 81234, 81238, 81239, 81245, 81246, 81250, 81257, 81258, 81259, 81261, 81262, 81263, 81264, 81265, 81266, 81267, 81268, 81269, 81271, 81274, 81277, 81278, 81279, 81283, 81284, 81285, 81286, 81287, 81288, 81289, 81291, 81292, 81293, 81294, 81295, 81301, 81302, 81303, 81304, 81306, 81307, 81308, 81309, 81312, 81320, 81324, 81325, 81326, 81332, 81334, 81336, 81337, 81338, 81339, 81343, 81344, 81345, 81347, 81348, 81351, 81352, 81353, 81357, 81361, 81362, 81363, 81364] Gene Analysis: Tier 1 Procedures

INCLUDES All analytical procedures in evaluation:
- Amplification
- Cell lysis
- Detection
- Digestion
- Extraction
- Nucleic acid stabilization

Code selection based on specific gene being reviewed
Evaluation constitutional or somatic gene variations
Evaluation gene variant presence using common gene variant name
Gene specific and genomic testing
Generally, all listed gene variants in code description (lists not all inclusive)
Genes described using Human Genome Organization (HUGO) approved names
Protein or disease examples in code description not all inclusive
Qualitative results unless otherwise stated
Tier 1 molecular pathology codes (81105-81254 [81161, 81162, 81163, 81164, 81165, 81166, 81167, 81173, 81174, 81184, 81185, 81186, 81187, 81188, 81189, 81190, 81200, 81201, 81202, 81203, 81204, 81205, 81206, 81207, 81208, 81209, 81210, 81219, 81227, 81230, 81231, 81233, 81234, 81238, 81239, 81245, 81246, 81250, 81257, 81258, 81259, 81265, 81266, 81267, 81268, 81269, 81284, 81285, 81286, 81289, 81361, 81362, 81363, 81364])

EXCLUDES *Full gene sequencing using separate gene variant assessment codes unless specifically stated in code description*
In situ hybridization analyses (88271-88275, 88365-88368 [88364, 88373, 88374])
Microbial identification (87149-87153, 87471-87801 [87623, 87624, 87625], 87900-87904 [87906, 87910, 87912])
Other related gene variants not listed in code description
Tier 1 molecular pathology codes (81370-81383)
Tier 2 codes (81400-81408)
Unlisted molecular pathology procedures ([81479])

Code also modifier 26 when only interpretation and report performed
Code also services required before cell lysis

81105 **Resequenced code. See code before 81260.**

81106 **Resequenced code. See code before 81260.**

81107 **Resequenced code. See code before 81260.**

81108 **Resequenced code. See code before 81260.**

81109 **Resequenced code. See code before 81260.**

81110 **Resequenced code. See code before 81260.**

81111 **Resequenced code. See code before 81260.**

81112 **Resequenced code. See code before 81260.**

81120 **Resequenced code. See code before 81260.**

81121 **Resequenced code. See code before 81260.**

81161 **Resequenced code. See code following 81231.**

81162 **Resequenced code. See code following resequenced code 81210.**

81163 **Resequenced code. See code following resequenced code 81210.**

81164 **Resequenced code. See code before 81212.**

81165 **Resequenced code. See code following 81212.**

81166 **Resequenced code. See code following 81212.**

81167 **Resequenced code. See code following 81216.**

81168 **Resequenced code. See code before 81218.**

81170 ***ABL1 (ABL proto-oncogene 1, non-receptor tyrosine kinase)* (eg, acquired imatinib tyrosine kinase inhibitor resistance), gene analysis, variants in the kinase domain**
0.00 0.00 FUD XXX A
AMA: 2018,Jan,8; 2017,Jan,8; 2016,Aug,9

81171 ***AFF2 (AF4/FMR2 family, member 2 [FMR2])* (eg, fragile X mental retardation 2 [FRAXE]) gene analysis; evaluation to detect abnormal (eg, expanded) alleles**
0.00 0.00 FUD XXX

81172 **characterization of alleles (eg, expanded size and methylation status)**
0.00 0.00 FUD XXX

81173 **Resequenced code. See code following resequenced code 81204.**

81174 **Resequenced code. See code following resequenced code 81204.**

\# 81201 ***APC (adenomatous polyposis coli)* (eg, familial adenomatosis polyposis [FAP], attenuated FAP) gene analysis; full gene sequence**
0.00 0.00 FUD XXX A
AMA: 2020,OctSE,1; 2018,Nov,9; 2018,Jan,8; 2017,Jan,8; 2016,Aug,9; 2016,Jan,13; 2015,Jan,16

\# 81202 **known familial variants**
0.00 0.00 FUD XXX A
AMA: 2020,OctSE,1; 2018,Nov,9; 2018,Jan,8; 2017,Jan,8; 2016,Aug,9; 2016,Jan,13; 2015,Jan,16

\# 81203 **duplication/deletion variants**
0.00 0.00 FUD XXX A
AMA: 2020,OctSE,1; 2018,Nov,9; 2018,Jan,8; 2017,Jan,8; 2016,Aug,9; 2016,Jan,13; 2015,Jan,16

\# 81204 ***AR (androgen receptor)* (eg, spinal and bulbar muscular atrophy, Kennedy disease, X chromosome inactivation) gene analysis; characterization of alleles (eg, expanded size or methylation status)**
0.00 0.00 FUD XXX
AMA: 2020,OctSE,1; 2018,Nov,9

\# 81173 **full gene sequence**
0.00 0.00 FUD XXX

\# 81174 **known familial variant**
0.00 0.00 FUD XXX

\# 81200 ***ASPA (aspartoacylase)* (eg, Canavan disease) gene analysis, common variants (eg, E285A, Y231X)**
0.00 0.00 FUD XXX A
AMA: 2020,OctSE,1; 2018,Nov,9; 2018,Jan,8; 2017,Jan,8; 2016,Aug,9; 2016,Jan,13; 2015,Jan,16

81175 ***ASXL1 (additional sex combs like 1, transcriptional regulator)* (eg, myelodysplastic syndrome, myeloproliferative neoplasms, chronic myelomonocytic leukemia), gene analysis; full gene sequence**
0.00 0.00 FUD XXX A

81176 **targeted sequence analysis (eg, exon 12)**
0.00 0.00 FUD XXX A

81177 ***ATN1 (atrophin 1)* (eg, dentatorubral-pallidoluysian atrophy) gene analysis, evaluation to detect abnormal (eg, expanded) alleles**
0.00 0.00 FUD XXX

81178 ***ATXN1 (ataxin 1)* (eg, spinocerebellar ataxia) gene analysis, evaluation to detect abnormal (eg, expanded) alleles**
0.00 0.00 FUD XXX
AMA: 2019,Sep,7

81179 ***ATXN2 (ataxin 2)*** **(eg, spinocerebellar ataxia) gene analysis, evaluation to detect abnormal (eg, expanded) alleles**
0.00 0.00 FUD XXX
AMA: 2019,Sep,7

81180 ***ATXN3 (ataxin 3)*** **(eg, spinocerebellar ataxia, Machado-Joseph disease) gene analysis, evaluation to detect abnormal (eg, expanded) alleles**
0.00 0.00 FUD XXX
AMA: 2019,Sep,7

81181 ***ATXN7 (ataxin 7)*** **(eg, spinocerebellar ataxia) gene analysis, evaluation to detect abnormal (eg, expanded) alleles**
0.00 0.00 FUD XXX
AMA: 2019,Sep,7

81182 ***ATXN8OS (ATXN8 opposite strand [non-protein coding])*** **(eg, spinocerebellar ataxia) gene analysis, evaluation to detect abnormal (eg, expanded) alleles**
0.00 0.00 FUD XXX
AMA: 2019,Sep,7

81183 ***ATXN10 (ataxin 10)*** **(eg, spinocerebellar ataxia) gene analysis, evaluation to detect abnormal (eg, expanded) alleles**
0.00 0.00 FUD XXX
AMA: 2019,Sep,7

81184 **Resequenced code. See code following resequenced code 81233.**

81185 **Resequenced code. See code following resequenced code 81233.**

81186 **Resequenced code. See code following resequenced code 81233.**

81187 **Resequenced code. See code following resequenced code 81268.**

81188 **Resequenced code. See code following resequenced code 81266.**

81189 **Resequenced code. See code following resequenced code 81266.**

81190 **Resequenced code. See code following resequenced code 81266.**

81191 **Resequenced code. See code following numeric code 81312.**

81192 **Resequenced code. See code following numeric code 81312.**

81193 **Resequenced code. See code following numeric code 81312.**

81194 **Resequenced code. See code following numeric code 81312.**

81200 **Resequenced code. See code before 81175.**

81201 **Resequenced code. See code following code 81174.**

81202 **Resequenced code. See code following code 81174.**

81203 **Resequenced code. See code following code 81174.**

81204 **Resequenced code. See code following code 81174.**

81205 **Resequenced code. See code following code 81210.**

81206 **Resequenced code. See code following code 81210.**

81207 **Resequenced code. See code following code 81210.**

81208 **Resequenced code. See code following code 81210.**

81209 **Resequenced code. See code following code 81210.**

81210 **Resequenced code. See code following resequenced code 81209.**

81205 ***BCKDHB (branched-chain keto acid dehydrogenase E1, beta polypeptide)*** **(eg, maple syrup urine disease) gene analysis, common variants (eg, R183P, G278S, E422X)**
0.00 0.00 FUD XXX A
AMA: 2020,OctSE,1; 2018,Nov,9; 2018,Jan,8; 2017,Jan,8; 2016,Aug,9; 2016,Jan,13; 2015,Jan,16

81206 ***BCR/ABL1 (t(9;22))*** **(eg, chronic myelogenous leukemia) translocation analysis; major breakpoint, qualitative or quantitative**
0.00 0.00 FUD XXX A
AMA: 2020,OctSE,1; 2018,Nov,9; 2018,Jan,8; 2017,Jan,8; 2016,Aug,9; 2016,Jan,13; 2015,Jan,16

81207 **minor breakpoint, qualitative or quantitative**
0.00 0.00 FUD XXX A
AMA: 2020,OctSE,1; 2018,Nov,9; 2018,Jan,8; 2017,Jan,8; 2016,Aug,9; 2016,Jan,13; 2015,Jan,16

81208 **other breakpoint, qualitative or quantitative**
0.00 0.00 FUD XXX A
AMA: 2020,OctSE,1; 2018,Nov,9; 2018,Jan,8; 2017,Jan,8; 2016,Aug,9; 2016,Jan,13; 2015,Jan,16

81209 ***BLM (Bloom syndrome, RecQ helicase-like)*** **(eg, Bloom syndrome) gene analysis, 2281del6ins7 variant**
0.00 0.00 FUD XXX A
AMA: 2020,OctSE,1; 2018,Nov,9; 2018,Jan,8; 2017,Jan,8; 2016,Aug,9; 2016,Jan,13; 2015,Jan,16

81210 ***BRAF (B-Raf proto-oncogene, serine/threonine kinase)*** **(eg, colon cancer, melanoma), gene analysis, V600 variant(s)**
0.00 0.00 FUD XXX A
AMA: 2020,OctSE,1; 2018,Nov,9; 2018,Jan,8; 2017,Jan,8; 2016,Aug,9; 2016,Jan,13; 2015,Jan,16

81162 ***BRCA1 (BRCA1, DNA repair associated), BRCA2 (BRCA2, DNA repair associated)*** **(eg, hereditary breast and ovarian cancer) gene analysis; full sequence analysis and full duplication/deletion analysis (ie, detection of large gene rearrangements)**

EXCLUDES *BRCA1 common duplication/deletion variant ([81479])*
BRCA1, BRCA2 full duplication/deletion analysis only (81164, 81166-81167, 81216)
BRCA1, BRCA2 full sequence analysis only (81163, 81165)
BRCA1, BRCA2 known familial variant only (81215, 81217)
Hereditary breast cancer genomic sequence analysis panel (81432)

0.00 0.00 FUD XXX A
AMA: 2019,May,5; 2018,Jan,8; 2017,Jan,8; 2016,Aug,9

81163 **full sequence analysis**

EXCLUDES *BRCA1 common duplication/deletion variant ([81479])*
BRCA1, BRCA2 full duplication/deletion analysis only (81164, 81216)
BRCA1, BRCA2 full sequence analysis and full duplication/deletion analysis (81162)
BRCA1, BRCA2 full sequence analysis only (81165)
Hereditary breast cancer genomic sequence analysis panel (81432)

0.00 0.00 FUD XXX
AMA: 2019,May,5

81164 **full duplication/deletion analysis (ie, detection of large gene rearrangements)**

EXCLUDES *BRCA1 common duplication/deletion variant ([81479])*
BRCA1, BRCA2 full sequence analysis and full duplication/deletion analysis (81162)
BRCA1, BRCA2 full sequence analysis only (81163)
BRCA1, BRCA2 full duplication/deletion analysis only (81166-81167)
BRCA1, BRCA2 known familial variant only (81217)

0.00 0.00 FUD XXX
AMA: 2019,May,5

81212 **185delAG, 5385insC, 6174delT variants**
0.00 0.00 FUD XXX A
AMA: 2020,OctSE,1; 2019,May,5; 2018,Nov,9; 2018,Jan,8; 2017,Jan,8; 2016,Aug,9; 2016,Jan,13; 2015,Jan,16

\# **81165** ***BRCA1 (BRCA1, DNA repair associated)*** **(eg, hereditary breast and ovarian cancer) gene analysis; full sequence analysis**

EXCLUDES *BRCA1 common duplication/deletion variant ([81479])*
BRCA1, BRCA2 full sequence analysis and full duplication/deletion analysis (81162)
BRCA1, BRCA2 full sequence analysis only (81163)
Hereditary breast cancer genomic sequence analysis panel (81432)

0.00 0.00 FUD XXX

AMA: 2019,May,5

\# **81166** **full duplication/deletion analysis (ie, detection of large gene rearrangements)**

EXCLUDES *BRCA1 common duplication/deletion variant ([81479])*
BRCA1, BRCA2 full duplication/deletion analysis only (81164)
BRCA1, BRCA2 full sequence analysis and full duplication/deletion analysis (81162)

0.00 0.00 FUD XXX

AMA: 2019,May,5

81215 **known familial variant**

EXCLUDES *BRCA1 common duplication/deletion variant ([81479])*

0.00 0.00 FUD XXX A

AMA: 2020,OctSE,1; 2019,May,5; 2018,Nov,9; 2018,Jan,8; 2017,Jan,8; 2016,Aug,9; 2016,Jan,13; 2015,Jan,16

81216 ***BRCA2 (BRCA2, DNA repair associated)*** **(eg, hereditary breast and ovarian cancer) gene analysis; full sequence analysis**

EXCLUDES *BRCA1, BRCA2 full sequence analysis only (81163)*
BRCA1, BRCA2 full sequence analysis and full duplication/deletion analysis (81162)
Hereditary breast cancer genomic sequence analysis panel (81432)

0.00 0.00 FUD XXX A

AMA: 2020,OctSE,1; 2019,May,5; 2018,Nov,9; 2018,Jan,8; 2017,Jan,8; 2016,Aug,9; 2016,Jan,13; 2015,Jan,16

\# **81167** **full duplication/deletion analysis (ie, detection of large gene rearrangements)**

EXCLUDES *BRCA1, BRCA2 full duplication/deletion analysis only (81164, 81167)*
BRCA1, BRCA2 full sequence analysis and full duplication/deletion analysis (81162)

0.00 0.00 FUD XXX

AMA: 2019,May,5

81217 **known familial variant**

EXCLUDES *BRCA1, BRCA2 full duplication/deletion analysis only (81164, 81167)*
BRCA1, BRCA2 full sequence analysis and full duplication/deletion analysis (81162)

0.00 0.00 FUD XXX A

AMA: 2020,OctSE,1; 2019,May,5; 2018,Nov,9; 2018,Jan,8; 2017,Jan,8; 2016,Aug,9; 2016,Jan,13; 2015,Jan,16

\# **81233** ***BTK (Bruton's tyrosine kinase)*** **(eg, chronic lymphocytic leukemia) gene analysis, common variants (eg, C481S, C481R, C481F)**

0.00 0.00 FUD XXX

AMA: 2020,OctSE,1; 2018,Nov,9

\# **81184** ***CACNA1A (calcium voltage-gated channel subunit alpha1 A)*** **(eg, spinocerebellar ataxia) gene analysis; evaluation to detect abnormal (eg, expanded) alleles**

0.00 0.00 FUD XXX

\# **81185** **full gene sequence**

0.00 0.00 FUD XXX

\# **81186** **known familial variant**

0.00 0.00 FUD XXX

\# **81219** ***CALR (calreticulin)*** **(eg, myeloproliferative disorders), gene analysis, common variants in exon 9**

0.00 0.00 FUD XXX A

AMA: 2020,OctSE,1; 2018,Nov,9; 2018,Jan,8; 2017,Jan,8; 2016,Aug,9

● # **81168** ***CCND1/IGH (t(11;14))*** **(eg, mantle cell lymphoma) translocation analysis, major breakpoint, qualitative and quantitative, if performed**

0.00 0.00 FUD 000

81218 ***CEBPA (CCAAT/enhancer binding protein [C/EBP], alpha)*** **(eg, acute myeloid leukemia), gene analysis, full gene sequence**

0.00 0.00 FUD XXX A

AMA: 2020,OctSE,1; 2018,Nov,9; 2018,Jan,8; 2017,Jan,8; 2016,Aug,9

81219 **Resequenced code. See code before 81218.**

81220 ***CFTR (cystic fibrosis transmembrane conductance regulator)*** **(eg, cystic fibrosis) gene analysis; common variants (eg, ACMG/ACOG guidelines)**

EXCLUDES *Excludes Intron 8 poly-T analysis performed in conjunction with 81220 in R117H positive patient*

0.00 0.00 FUD XXX A

AMA: 2020,OctSE,1; 2018,Nov,9; 2018,Jan,8; 2017,Jan,8; 2016,Aug,9; 2016,Jan,13; 2015,Jan,16

81221 **known familial variants**

0.00 0.00 FUD XXX A

AMA: 2020,OctSE,1; 2018,Nov,9; 2018,Jan,8; 2017,Jan,8; 2016,Aug,9; 2016,Jan,13; 2015,Jan,16

81222 **duplication/deletion variants**

0.00 0.00 FUD XXX A

AMA: 2020,OctSE,1; 2018,Nov,9; 2018,Jan,8; 2017,Jan,8; 2016,Aug,9; 2016,Jan,13; 2015,Jan,16

81223 **full gene sequence**

0.00 0.00 FUD XXX A

AMA: 2020,OctSE,1; 2018,Nov,9; 2018,Jan,8; 2017,Jan,8; 2016,Aug,9; 2016,Jan,13; 2015,Jan,16

81224 **intron 8 poly-T analysis (eg, male infertility)**

0.00 0.00 FUD XXX A

AMA: 2020,OctSE,1; 2018,Nov,9; 2018,Jan,8; 2017,Jan,8; 2016,Aug,9; 2016,Jan,13; 2015,Jan,16

\# **81267** **Chimerism (engraftment) analysis, post transplantation specimen (eg, hematopoietic stem cell), includes comparison to previously performed baseline analyses; without cell selection**

0.00 0.00 FUD XXX A

AMA: 2020,OctSE,1; 2018,Nov,9; 2018,Jan,8; 2017,Jan,8; 2016,Aug,9; 2016,Jan,13; 2015,Jan,16

\# **81268** **with cell selection (eg, CD3, CD33), each cell type**

0.00 0.00 FUD XXX A

AMA: 2020,OctSE,1; 2018,Nov,9; 2018,Jan,8; 2017,Jan,8; 2016,Aug,9; 2016,Jan,13; 2015,Jan,16

\# **81187** ***CNBP (CCHC-type zinc finger nucleic acid binding protein)*** **(eg, myotonic dystrophy type 2) gene analysis, evaluation to detect abnormal (eg, expanded) alleles**

0.00 0.00 FUD XXX

\# **81265** **Comparative analysis using Short Tandem Repeat (STR) markers; patient and comparative specimen (eg, pre-transplant recipient and donor germline testing, post-transplant non-hematopoietic recipient germline [eg, buccal swab or other germline tissue sample] and donor testing, twin zygosity testing, or maternal cell contamination of fetal cells)**

0.00 0.00 FUD XXX A

AMA: 2020,OctSE,1; 2018,Nov,9; 2018,Jan,8; 2017,Jan,8; 2016,Aug,9; 2016,Jan,13; 2015,Jan,16

\+ # **81266** **each additional specimen (eg, additional cord blood donor, additional fetal samples from different cultures, or additional zygosity in multiple birth pregnancies) (List separately in addition to code for primary procedure)**

0.00 0.00 FUD XXX A

AMA: 2020,OctSE,1; 2018,Nov,9; 2018,Jan,8; 2017,Jan,8; 2016,Aug,9; 2016,Jan,13; 2015,Jan,16

\# **81188** ***CSTB (cystatin B)*** **(eg, Unverricht-Lundborg disease) gene analysis; evaluation to detect abnormal (eg, expanded) alleles**
0.00 0.00 FUD XXX

\# **81189** **full gene sequence**
0.00 0.00 FUD XXX

\# **81190** **known familial variant(s)**
0.00 0.00 FUD XXX

\# **81227** ***CYP2C9 (cytochrome P450, family 2, subfamily C, polypeptide 9)*** **(eg, drug metabolism), gene analysis, common variants (eg, *2, *3, *5, *6)**
0.00 0.00 FUD XXX A
AMA: 2020,OctSE,1; 2018,Nov,9; 2018,Jan,8; 2017,Jan,8; 2016,Aug,9; 2016,Jan,13; 2015,Jan,16

81225 ***CYP2C19 (cytochrome P450, family 2, subfamily C, polypeptide 19)*** **(eg, drug metabolism), gene analysis, common variants (eg, *2, *3, *4, *8, *17)**
0.00 0.00 FUD XXX A
AMA: 2020,OctSE,1; 2018,Nov,9; 2018,Jan,8; 2017,Jan,8; 2016,Aug,9; 2016,Jan,13; 2015,Jan,16

81226 ***CYP2D6 (cytochrome P450, family 2, subfamily D, polypeptide 6)*** **(eg, drug metabolism), gene analysis, common variants (eg, *2, *3, *4, *5, *6, *9, *10, *17, *19, *29, *35, *41, *1XN, *2XN, *4XN)**
0.00 0.00 FUD XXX A
AMA: 2020,OctSE,1; 2018,Nov,9; 2018,Jan,8; 2017,Jan,8; 2016,Aug,9; 2016,Jan,13; 2015,Jan,16

81227 **Resequenced code. See code following resequenced code 81190.**

\# **81230** ***CYP3A4 (cytochrome P450 family 3 subfamily A member 4)*** **(eg, drug metabolism), gene analysis, common variant(s) (eg, *2, *22)**
0.00 0.00 FUD XXX A
AMA: 2020,OctSE,1; 2018,Nov,9

\# **81231** ***CYP3A5 (cytochrome P450 family 3 subfamily A member 5)*** **(eg, drug metabolism), gene analysis, common variants (eg, *2, *3, *4, *5, *6, *7)**
0.00 0.00 FUD XXX A
AMA: 2020,OctSE,1; 2018,Nov,9

81228 **Cytogenomic constitutional (genome-wide) microarray analysis; interrogation of genomic regions for copy number variants (eg, bacterial artificial chromosome [BAC] or oligo-based comparative genomic hybridization [CGH] microarray analysis)**
EXCLUDES *Analyte-specific molecular pathology procedures included in microarray analysis*
When performed in conjunction with single nucleotide polymorphism interrogation (81229)
0.00 0.00 FUD XXX A
AMA: 2020,OctSE,1; 2018,Nov,9; 2018,Jan,8; 2017,Apr,3; 2017,Jan,8; 2016,Aug,9; 2016,Jan,13; 2015,Jan,16

81229 **interrogation of genomic regions for copy number and single nucleotide polymorphism (SNP) variants for chromosomal abnormalities**
EXCLUDES *Analyte-specific molecular pathology procedures included in microarray analysis*
Copy number variant detection using oligonucleotide interrogation only (81228)
Fetal genomic sequencing or other molecular multianalyte assays using circulating cell-free DNA in maternal blood ([81479], 81420, 81422)
Molecular cytogenetics; DNA probe (88271)
Specific code for targeted cytogenomic constitutional microarray analysis
Unlisted molecular pathology procedures ([81479])
0.00 0.00 FUD XXX A
AMA: 2020,OctSE,1; 2018,Nov,9; 2018,Jan,8; 2017,Apr,3; 2017,Jan,8; 2016,Aug,9; 2016,Jan,13; 2015,Jan,16

\# **81277** **Cytogenomic neoplasia (genome-wide) microarray analysis, interrogation of genomic regions for copy number and loss-of-heterozygosity variants for chromosomal abnormalities**
EXCLUDES *Analyte-specific molecular pathology procedures included in microarray analysis for neoplasia*
Molecular cytogenetics; DNA probe (88271)
0.00 0.00 FUD XXX
AMA: 2020,OctSE,1; 2020,Feb,10

81230 **Resequenced code. See code following code 81227.**

81231 **Resequenced code. See code following code 81227.**

\# **81161** ***DMD (dystrophin)*** **(eg, Duchenne/Becker muscular dystrophy) deletion analysis, and duplication analysis, if performed**
0.00 0.00 FUD XXX A
AMA: 2020,OctSE,1; 2018,Nov,9; 2018,Jan,8; 2017,Jan,8; 2016,Aug,9

\# **81234** ***DMPK (DM1 protein kinase)*** **(eg, myotonic dystrophy type 1) gene analysis; evaluation to detect abnormal (expanded) alleles**
0.00 0.00 FUD XXX
AMA: 2020,OctSE,1; 2018,Nov,9

\# **81239** **characterization of alleles (eg, expanded size)**
0.00 0.00 FUD XXX
AMA: 2020,OctSE,1; 2018,Nov,9

81232 ***DPYD (dihydropyrimidine dehydrogenase)*** **(eg, 5-fluorouracil/5-FU and capecitabine drug metabolism), gene analysis, common variant(s) (eg, *2A, *4, *5, *6)**
0.00 0.00 FUD XXX A
AMA: 2020,OctSE,1; 2018,Nov,9

81233 **Resequenced code. See code following 81217.**

81234 **Resequenced code. See code following code 81231.**

81235 ***EGFR (epidermal growth factor receptor)*** **(eg, non-small cell lung cancer) gene analysis, common variants (eg, exon 19 LREA deletion, L858R, T790M, G719A, G719S, L861Q)**
0.00 0.00 FUD XXX A
AMA: 2020,OctSE,1; 2018,Nov,9; 2018,Jan,8; 2017,Jan,8; 2016,Aug,9; 2016,Jan,13; 2015,Jan,16

81236 ***EZH2 (enhancer of zeste 2 polycomb repressive complex 2 subunit)*** **(eg, myelodysplastic syndrome, myeloproliferative neoplasms) gene analysis, full gene sequence**
0.00 0.00 FUD XXX
AMA: 2020,OctSE,1; 2019,Jul,3; 2018,Nov,9

81237 ***EZH2 (enhancer of zeste 2 polycomb repressive complex 2 subunit)*** **(eg, diffuse large B-cell lymphoma) gene analysis, common variant(s) (eg, codon 646)**
0.00 0.00 FUD XXX
AMA: 2020,OctSE,1; 2019,Jul,3; 2018,Nov,9

81238 **Resequenced code. See code following 81241.**

81239 **Resequenced code. See code before 81232.**

81240 ***F2 (prothrombin, coagulation factor II)*** **(eg, hereditary hypercoagulability) gene analysis, 20210G>A variant**
0.00 0.00 FUD XXX A
AMA: 2020,OctSE,1; 2018,Nov,9; 2018,Jan,8; 2017,Jan,8; 2016,Aug,9; 2016,Jan,13; 2015,Jan,16

81241 ***F5 (coagulation factor V)*** **(eg, hereditary hypercoagulability) gene analysis, Leiden variant**
0.00 0.00 FUD XXX A
AMA: 2020,OctSE,1; 2018,Nov,9; 2018,Jan,8; 2017,Jan,8; 2016,Aug,9; 2016,Jan,13; 2015,Jan,16

\# **81238** ***F9 (coagulation factor IX)*** **(eg, hemophilia B), full gene sequence**
0.00 0.00 FUD XXX A
AMA: 2020,OctSE,1; 2018,Nov,9

81242 ***FANCC (Fanconi anemia, complementation group C)*** **(eg, Fanconi anemia, type C) gene analysis, common variant (eg, IVS4+4A>T)**
0.00 0.00 FUD XXX
AMA: 2020,OctSE,1; 2018,Nov,9; 2018,Jan,8; 2017,Jan,8; 2016,Aug,9; 2016,Jan,13; 2015,Jan,16

\# **81245** ***FLT3 (fms-related tyrosine kinase 3)*** **(eg, acute myeloid leukemia), gene analysis; internal tandem duplication (ITD) variants (ie, exons 14, 15)**
0.00 0.00 FUD XXX
AMA: 2020,OctSE,1; 2018,Nov,9; 2018,Jan,8; 2017,Jan,8; 2016,Aug,9; 2016,Jan,13; 2015,Jan,16; 2015,Jan,3

\# **81246** **tyrosine kinase domain (TKD) variants (eg, D835, I836)**
0.00 0.00 FUD XXX
AMA: 2020,OctSE,1; 2018,Nov,9; 2018,Jan,8; 2017,Jan,8; 2016,Aug,9; 2016,Jan,13; 2015,Jan,3

81243 ***FMR1 (fragile X mental retardation 1)*** **(eg, fragile X mental retardation) gene analysis; evaluation to detect abnormal (eg, expanded) alleles**
INCLUDES Evaluation to detect and characterize abnormal alleles using single assay [i.e., PCR]
EXCLUDES *Evaluation to detect and characterize abnormal alleles (81244)*
0.00 0.00 FUD XXX
AMA: 2020,OctSE,1; 2019,Jul,3; 2018,Nov,9; 2018,Jan,8; 2017,Jan,8; 2016,Aug,9; 2016,Jan,13; 2015,Jan,16

81244 **characterization of alleles (eg, expanded size and promoter methylation status)**
EXCLUDES *Evaluation to detect and characterize abnormal alleles using single assay [i.e., PCR] (81243)*
0.00 0.00 FUD XXX
AMA: 2020,OctSE,1; 2019,Jul,3; 2018,Nov,9; 2018,Jan,8; 2017,Jan,8; 2016,Aug,9; 2016,Jan,13; 2015,Jan,16

81245 **Resequenced code. See code following 81242.**

81246 **Resequenced code. See code following 81242.**

\# **81284** ***FXN (frataxin)*** **(eg, Friedreich ataxia) gene analysis; evaluation to detect abnormal (expanded) alleles**
0.00 0.00 FUD XXX
AMA: 2020,OctSE,1; 2018,Nov,9

\# **81285** **characterization of alleles (eg, expanded size)**
0.00 0.00 FUD XXX
AMA: 2020,OctSE,1; 2018,Nov,9

\# **81286** **full gene sequence**
0.00 0.00 FUD XXX
AMA: 2020,OctSE,1; 2018,Nov,9

\# **81289** **known familial variant(s)**
0.00 0.00 FUD XXX
AMA: 2020,OctSE,1; 2018,Nov,9

\# **81250** ***G6PC (glucose-6-phosphatase, catalytic subunit)*** **(eg, Glycogen storage disease, type 1a, von Gierke disease) gene analysis, common variants (eg, R83C, Q347X)**
0.00 0.00 FUD XXX
AMA: 2020,OctSE,1; 2018,Nov,9; 2018,Jan,8; 2017,Jan,8; 2016,Aug,9; 2016,Jan,13; 2015,Jan,16

81247 ***G6PD (glucose-6-phosphate dehydrogenase)*** **(eg, hemolytic anemia, jaundice), gene analysis; common variant(s) (eg, A, A-)**
0.00 0.00 FUD XXX
AMA: 2020,OctSE,1; 2018,Nov,9

81248 **known familial variant(s)**
0.00 0.00 FUD XXX
AMA: 2020,OctSE,1; 2018,Nov,9

81249 **full gene sequence**
0.00 0.00 FUD XXX
AMA: 2020,OctSE,1; 2018,Nov,9

81250 **Resequenced code. See code before 81247.**

81251 ***GBA (glucosidase, beta, acid)*** **(eg, Gaucher disease) gene analysis, common variants (eg, N370S, 84GG, L444P, IVS2+1G>A)**
0.00 0.00 FUD XXX
AMA: 2020,OctSE,1; 2018,Nov,9; 2018,Jan,8; 2017,Jan,8; 2016,Aug,9; 2016,Jan,13; 2015,Jan,16

81252 ***GJB2 (gap junction protein, beta 2, 26kDa, connexin 26)*** **(eg, nonsyndromic hearing loss) gene analysis; full gene sequence**
0.00 0.00 FUD XXX
AMA: 2020,OctSE,1; 2018,Nov,9; 2018,Jan,8; 2017,Jan,8; 2016,Aug,9; 2016,Jan,13; 2015,Jan,16

81253 **known familial variants**
0.00 0.00 FUD XXX
AMA: 2020,OctSE,1; 2018,Nov,9; 2018,Jan,8; 2017,Jan,8; 2016,Aug,9; 2016,Jan,13; 2015,Jan,16

81254 ***GJB6 (gap junction protein, beta 6, 30kDa, connexin 30)*** **(eg, nonsyndromic hearing loss) gene analysis, common variants (eg, 309kb [del(GJB6-D13S1830)] and 232kb [del(GJB6-D13S1854)])**
0.00 0.00 FUD XXX
AMA: 2020,OctSE,1; 2018,Nov,9; 2018,Jan,8; 2017,Jan,8; 2016,Aug,9; 2016,Jan,13; 2015,Jan,16

\# **81257** ***HBA1/HBA2 (alpha globin 1 and alpha globin 2)*** **(eg, alpha thalassemia, Hb Bart hydrops fetalis syndrome, HbH disease), gene analysis; common deletions or variant (eg, Southeast Asian, Thai, Filipino, Mediterranean, alpha3.7, alpha4.2, alpha20.5, Constant Spring)**
0.00 0.00 FUD XXX
AMA: 2020,OctSE,1; 2018,Nov,9; 2018,Jan,8; 2017,Jan,8; 2016,Aug,9; 2016,Jan,13; 2015,Jan,16

\# **81258** **known familial variant**
0.00 0.00 FUD XXX
AMA: 2020,OctSE,1; 2018,Nov,9

\# **81259** **full gene sequence**
0.00 0.00 FUD XXX
AMA: 2020,OctSE,1; 2018,Nov,9

\# **81269** **duplication/deletion variants**
0.00 0.00 FUD XXX
AMA: 2020,OctSE,1; 2018,Nov,9

\# **81361** ***HBB (hemoglobin, subunit beta)*** **(eg, sickle cell anemia, beta thalassemia, hemoglobinopathy); common variant(s) (eg, HbS, HbC, HbE)**
0.00 0.00 FUD XXX
AMA: 2020,OctSE,1; 2018,Nov,9

\# **81362** **known familial variant(s)**
0.00 0.00 FUD XXX
AMA: 2020,OctSE,1; 2018,Nov,9

\# **81363** **duplication/deletion variant(s)**
0.00 0.00 FUD XXX
AMA: 2020,OctSE,1; 2018,Nov,9; 2018,Sep,14

\# **81364** **full gene sequence**
0.00 0.00 FUD XXX
AMA: 2020,OctSE,1; 2018,Nov,9; 2018,Sep,14

81255 ***HEXA (hexosaminidase A [alpha polypeptide])*** **(eg, Tay-Sachs disease) gene analysis, common variants (eg, 1278insTATC, 1421+1G>C, G269S)**
0.00 0.00 FUD XXX
AMA: 2020,OctSE,1; 2018,Nov,9; 2018,Jan,8; 2017,Jan,8; 2016,Aug,9; 2016,Jan,13; 2015,Jan,16

81256 ***HFE (hemochromatosis)*** **(eg, hereditary hemochromatosis) gene analysis, common variants (eg, C282Y, H63D)**
0.00 0.00 FUD XXX
AMA: 2020,OctSE,1; 2018,Nov,9; 2018,Jan,8; 2017,Jan,8; 2016,Aug,9; 2016,Jan,13; 2015,Jan,16

81257 **Resequenced code. See code following 81254.**

81258 Resequenced code. See code following 81254.

81259 Resequenced code. See code following 81254.

\# 81271 *HTT (huntingtin)* (eg, Huntington disease) gene analysis; evaluation to detect abnormal (eg, expanded) alleles
0.00 0.00 FUD XXX
AMA: 2020,OctSE,1; 2018,Nov,9

\# 81274 characterization of alleles (eg, expanded size)
0.00 0.00 FUD XXX
AMA: 2020,OctSE,1; 2018,Nov,9

\# 81105 *Human Platelet Antigen 1 genotyping (HPA-1), ITGB3 (integrin, beta 3 [platelet glycoprotein IIIa], antigen CD61 [GPIIIa])* (eg, neonatal alloimmune thrombocytopenia [NAIT], post-transfusion purpura), gene analysis, common variant, HPA-1a/b (L33P)
0.00 0.00 FUD XXX A

\# 81106 *Human Platelet Antigen 2 genotyping (HPA-2), GP1BA (glycoprotein Ib [platelet], alpha polypeptide [GPIba])* (eg, neonatal alloimmune thrombocytopenia [NAIT], post-transfusion purpura), gene analysis, common variant, HPA-2a/b (T145M)
0.00 0.00 FUD XXX A

\# 81107 *Human Platelet Antigen 3 genotyping (HPA-3), ITGA2B (integrin, alpha 2b [platelet glycoprotein IIb of IIb/IIIa complex], antigen CD41 [GPIIb])* (eg, neonatal alloimmune thrombocytopenia [NAIT], post-transfusion purpura), gene analysis, common variant, HPA-3a/b (I843S)
0.00 0.00 FUD XXX A

\# 81108 *Human Platelet Antigen 4 genotyping (HPA-4), ITGB3 (integrin, beta 3 [platelet glycoprotein IIIa], antigen CD61 [GPIIIa])* (eg, neonatal alloimmune thrombocytopenia [NAIT], post-transfusion purpura), gene analysis, common variant, HPA-4a/b (R143Q)
0.00 0.00 FUD XXX A

\# 81109 *Human Platelet Antigen 5 genotyping (HPA-5), ITGA2 (integrin, alpha 2 [CD49B, alpha 2 subunit of VLA-2 receptor] [GPIa])* (eg, neonatal alloimmune thrombocytopenia [NAIT], post-transfusion purpura), gene analysis, common variant (eg, HPA-5a/b (K505E))
0.00 0.00 FUD XXX A

\# 81110 *Human Platelet Antigen 6 genotyping (HPA-6w), ITGB3 (integrin, beta 3 [platelet glycoprotein IIIa, antigen CD61] [GPIIIa])* (eg, neonatal alloimmune thrombocytopenia [NAIT], post-transfusion purpura), gene analysis, common variant, HPA-6a/b (R489Q)
0.00 0.00 FUD XXX A

\# 81111 *Human Platelet Antigen 9 genotyping (HPA-9w), ITGA2B (integrin, alpha 2b [platelet glycoprotein IIb of IIb/IIIa complex, antigen CD41] [GPIIb])* (eg, neonatal alloimmune thrombocytopenia [NAIT], post-transfusion purpura), gene analysis, common variant, HPA-9a/b (V837M)
0.00 0.00 FUD XXX A

\# 81112 *Human Platelet Antigen 15 genotyping (HPA-15), CD109 (CD109 molecule)* (eg, neonatal alloimmune thrombocytopenia [NAIT], post-transfusion purpura), gene analysis, common variant, HPA-15a/b (S682Y)
0.00 0.00 FUD XXX A

\# 81120 *IDH1 (isocitrate dehydrogenase 1 [NADP+], soluble)* (eg, glioma), common variants (eg, R132H, R132C)
0.00 0.00 FUD XXX A

\# 81121 *IDH2 (isocitrate dehydrogenase 2 [NADP+], mitochondrial)* (eg, glioma), common variants (eg, R140W, R172M)
0.00 0.00 FUD XXX A

\# 81283 *IFNL3 (interferon, lambda 3)* (eg, drug response), gene analysis, rs12979860 variant
0.00 0.00 FUD XXX A
AMA: 2020,OctSE,1; 2018,Nov,9

\# 81261 *IGH@ (Immunoglobulin heavy chain locus)* (eg, leukemias and lymphomas, B-cell), gene rearrangement analysis to detect abnormal clonal population(s); amplified methodology (eg, polymerase chain reaction)
0.00 0.00 FUD XXX A
AMA: 2020,OctSE,1; 2018,Nov,9; 2018,Jan,8; 2017,Jan,8; 2016,Aug,9; 2016,Jan,13; 2015,Jan,16

\# 81262 direct probe methodology (eg, Southern blot)
0.00 0.00 FUD XXX A
AMA: 2020,OctSE,1; 2018,Nov,9; 2018,Jan,8; 2017,Jan,8; 2016,Aug,9; 2016,Jan,13; 2015,Jan,16

\# 81263 *IGH@ (Immunoglobulin heavy chain locus)* (eg, leukemia and lymphoma, B-cell), variable region somatic mutation analysis
0.00 0.00 FUD XXX A
AMA: 2020,OctSE,1; 2018,Nov,9; 2018,Jan,8; 2017,Jan,8; 2016,Aug,9; 2016,Jan,13; 2015,Jan,16

● # 81278 *IGH@/BCL2 (t(14;18))* (eg, follicular lymphoma) translocation analysis, major breakpoint region (MBR) and minor cluster region (mcr) breakpoints, qualitative or quantitative
0.00 0.00 FUD 000

\# 81264 *IGK@ (Immunoglobulin kappa light chain locus)* (eg, leukemia and lymphoma, B-cell), gene rearrangement analysis, evaluation to detect abnormal clonal population(s)
0.00 0.00 FUD XXX A
AMA: 2020,OctSE,1; 2018,Nov,9; 2018,Jan,8; 2017,Jan,8; 2016,Aug,9; 2016,Jan,13; 2015,Jan,16

81260 *IKBKAP (inhibitor of kappa light polypeptide gene enhancer in B-cells, kinase complex-associated protein)* (eg, familial dysautonomia) gene analysis, common variants (eg, 2507+6T>C, R696P)
0.00 0.00 FUD XXX A
AMA: 2020,OctSE,1; 2018,Nov,9; 2018,Jan,8; 2017,Jan,8; 2016,Aug,9; 2016,Jan,13; 2015,Jan,16

81261 Resequenced code. See code before 81260.

81262 Resequenced code. See code before 81260.

81263 Resequenced code. See code following resequenced code 81262.

81264 Resequenced code. See code before 81260.

81265 Resequenced code. See code following resequenced code 81187.

81266 Resequenced code. See code following resequenced code 81265.

81267 Resequenced code. See code following 81224.

81268 Resequenced code. See code following 81224.

81269 Resequenced code. See code following resequenced code 81259.

81270 *JAK2 (Janus kinase 2)* (eg, myeloproliferative disorder) gene analysis, p.Val617Phe (V617F) variant
0.00 0.00 FUD XXX A
AMA: 2020,OctSE,1; 2018,Nov,9; 2018,Jan,8; 2017,Jan,8; 2016,Aug,9; 2016,Jan,13; 2015,Jan,16

● # 81279 *JAK2 (Janus kinase 2)* (eg, myeloproliferative disorder) targeted sequence analysis (eg, exons 12 and 13)
0.00 0.00 FUD 000

81271 Resequenced code. See code following code 81259.

81272 *KIT (v-kit Hardy-Zuckerman 4 feline sarcoma viral oncogene homolog)* (eg, gastrointestinal stromal tumor [GIST], acute myeloid leukemia, melanoma), gene analysis, targeted sequence analysis (eg, exons 8, 11, 13, 17, 18)
0.00 0.00 FUD XXX A
AMA: 2020,OctSE,1; 2018,Nov,9; 2018,Jan,8; 2017,Jan,8; 2016,Aug,9

81273 ***KIT (v-kit Hardy-Zuckerman 4 feline sarcoma viral oncogene homolog)*** **(eg, mastocytosis), gene analysis, D816 variant**
0.00 0.00 FUD XXX A
AMA: 2020,OctSE,1; 2018,Nov,9; 2018,Jan,8; 2017,Jan,8; 2016,Aug,9

81274 **Resequenced code. See code following resequenced code 81271.**

81275 ***KRAS (Kirsten rat sarcoma viral oncogene homolog)*** **(eg, carcinoma) gene analysis; variants in exon 2 (eg, codons 12 and 13)**
0.00 0.00 FUD XXX A
AMA: 2020,OctSE,1; 2018,Nov,9; 2018,Jan,8; 2017,Jan,8; 2016,Aug,9; 2016,Jan,13; 2015,Jan,16

81276 **additional variant(s) (eg, codon 61, codon 146)**
0.00 0.00 FUD XXX A
AMA: 2020,OctSE,1; 2018,Nov,9; 2018,Jan,8; 2017,Jan,8; 2016,Aug,9

81277 **Resequenced code. See code following 81229.**

81278 **Resequenced code. See code following resequenced code 81263.**

81279 **Resequenced code. See code following 81270.**

81283 **Resequenced code. See code following resequenced code 81121.**

81284 **Resequenced code. See code following code 81246.**

81285 **Resequenced code. See code following code 81246.**

81286 **Resequenced code. See code following code 81246.**

81287 **Resequenced code. See code following resequenced code 81304.**

81288 **Resequenced code. See code following resequenced code 81292.**

81289 **Resequenced code. See code following code 81246.**

81290 ***MCOLN1 (mucolipin 1)*** **(eg, Mucolipidosis, type IV) gene analysis, common variants (eg, IVS3-2A>G, del6.4kb)**
0.00 0.00 FUD XXX A
AMA: 2020,OctSE,1; 2018,Nov,9; 2018,Jan,8; 2017,Jan,8; 2016,Aug,9; 2016,Jan,13; 2015,Jan,16

\# **81302** ***MECP2 (methyl CpG binding protein 2)*** **(eg, Rett syndrome) gene analysis; full sequence analysis**
0.00 0.00 FUD XXX A
AMA: 2020,OctSE,1; 2018,Nov,9; 2018,Jan,8; 2017,Jan,8; 2016,Aug,9; 2016,Jan,13; 2015,Jan,16

\# **81303** **known familial variant**
0.00 0.00 FUD XXX A
AMA: 2020,OctSE,1; 2018,Nov,9; 2018,Jan,8; 2017,Jan,8; 2016,Aug,9; 2016,Jan,13; 2015,Jan,16

\# **81304** **duplication/deletion variants**
0.00 0.00 FUD XXX A
AMA: 2020,OctSE,1; 2018,Nov,9; 2018,Jan,8; 2017,Jan,8; 2016,Aug,9; 2016,Jan,13; 2015,Jan,16

\# **81287** ***MGMT (O-6-methylguanine-DNA methyltransferase)*** **(eg, glioblastoma multiforme), promoter methylation analysis**
0.00 0.00 FUD XXX A
AMA: 2020,OctSE,1; 2019,Jul,3; 2018,Dec,10; 2018,Dec,10; 2018,Nov,9; 2018,Jan,8; 2017,Jan,8; 2016,Aug,9

\# **81301** **Microsatellite instability analysis (eg, hereditary non-polyposis colorectal cancer, Lynch syndrome) of markers for mismatch repair deficiency (eg, BAT25, BAT26), includes comparison of neoplastic and normal tissue, if performed**
0.00 0.00 FUD XXX A
AMA: 2020,OctSE,1; 2018,Nov,9; 2018,Jan,8; 2017,Jan,8; 2016,Aug,9; 2016,Jan,13; 2015,Jan,16

\# **81292** ***MLH1 (mutL homolog 1, colon cancer, nonpolyposis type 2)*** **(eg, hereditary non-polyposis colorectal cancer, Lynch syndrome) gene analysis; full sequence analysis**
0.00 0.00 FUD XXX A
AMA: 2020,OctSE,1; 2018,Nov,9; 2018,Jan,8; 2017,Jan,8; 2016,Aug,9; 2016,Jan,13; 2015,Jan,16; 2015,Jan,3

\# **81288** **promoter methylation analysis**
0.00 0.00 FUD XXX A
AMA: 2020,OctSE,1; 2018,Nov,9; 2018,Jan,8; 2017,Jan,8; 2016,Aug,9; 2016,Jan,13; 2015,Jan,3

\# **81293** **known familial variants**
0.00 0.00 FUD XXX A
AMA: 2020,OctSE,1; 2018,Nov,9; 2018,Jan,8; 2017,Jan,8; 2016,Aug,9; 2016,Jan,13; 2015,Jan,16

\# **81294** **duplication/deletion variants**
0.00 0.00 FUD XXX A
AMA: 2020,OctSE,1; 2018,Nov,9; 2018,Jan,8; 2017,Jan,8; 2016,Aug,9; 2016,Jan,13; 2015,Jan,16

● # **81338** ***MPL (MPL proto-oncogene, thrombopoietin receptor)*** **(eg, myeloproliferative disorder) gene analysis; common variants (eg, W515A, W515K, W515L, W515R)**
0.00 0.00 FUD 000

● # **81339** **sequence analysis, exon 10**
0.00 0.00 FUD 000

\# **81295** ***MSH2 (mutS homolog 2, colon cancer, nonpolyposis type 1)*** **(eg, hereditary non-polyposis colorectal cancer, Lynch syndrome) gene analysis; full sequence analysis**
0.00 0.00 FUD XXX A
AMA: 2020,OctSE,1; 2018,Nov,9; 2018,Jan,8; 2017,Jan,8; 2016,Aug,9; 2016,Jan,13; 2015,Jan,16

81291 **Resequenced code. See code before 81305.**

81292 **Resequenced code. See code before code 81291.**

81293 **Resequenced code. See code before code 81291.**

81294 **Resequenced code. See code before code 81291.**

81295 **Resequenced code. See code before code 81291.**

81296 **known familial variants**
0.00 0.00 FUD XXX A
AMA: 2020,OctSE,1; 2018,Nov,9; 2018,Jan,8; 2017,Jan,8; 2016,Aug,9; 2016,Jan,13; 2015,Jan,16

81297 **duplication/deletion variants**
0.00 0.00 FUD XXX A
AMA: 2020,OctSE,1; 2018,Nov,9; 2018,Jan,8; 2017,Jan,8; 2016,Aug,9; 2016,Jan,13; 2015,Jan,16

81298 ***MSH6 (mutS homolog 6 [E. coli])*** **(eg, hereditary non-polyposis colorectal cancer, Lynch syndrome) gene analysis; full sequence analysis**
0.00 0.00 FUD XXX A
AMA: 2020,OctSE,1; 2018,Nov,9; 2018,Jan,8; 2017,Jan,8; 2016,Aug,9; 2016,Jan,13; 2015,Jan,16

81299 **known familial variants**
0.00 0.00 FUD XXX A
AMA: 2020,OctSE,1; 2018,Nov,9; 2018,Jan,8; 2017,Jan,8; 2016,Aug,9; 2016,Jan,13; 2015,Jan,16

81300 **duplication/deletion variants**
0.00 0.00 FUD XXX A
AMA: 2020,OctSE,1; 2018,Nov,9; 2018,Jan,8; 2017,Jan,8; 2016,Aug,9; 2016,Jan,13; 2015,Jan,16

81301 **Resequenced code. See code following resequenced code 81287.**

81302 **Resequenced code. See code following 81290.**

81303 **Resequenced code. See code following 81290.**

81304 **Resequenced code. See code following 81290.**

\# 81291 *MTHFR (5,10-methylenetetrahydrofolate reductase)* (eg, hereditary hypercoagulability) gene analysis, common variants (eg, 677T, 1298C)
0.00 0.00 FUD XXX
AMA: 2020,OctSE,1; 2018,Nov,9; 2018,Jan,8; 2017,Jan,8; 2016,Aug,9; 2016,Jan,13; 2015,Jan,16

81305 *MYD88 (myeloid differentiation primary response 88)* (eg, Waldenstrom's macroglobulinemia, lymphoplasmacytic leukemia) gene analysis, p.Leu265Pro (L265P) variant
0.00 0.00 FUD XXX
AMA: 2020,OctSE,1; 2019,Jul,3; 2018,Nov,9

81306 Resequenced code. See code following code 81312.

81307 Resequenced code. See code before 81313.

81308 Resequenced code. See code before 81313.

81309 Resequenced code. See code following 81314.

81310 *NPM1 (nucleophosmin)* (eg, acute myeloid leukemia) gene analysis, exon 12 variants
0.00 0.00 FUD XXX
AMA: 2020,OctSE,1; 2018,Nov,9; 2018,Jan,8; 2017,Jan,8; 2016,Aug,9; 2016,Jan,13; 2015,Jan,16

81311 *NRAS (neuroblastoma RAS viral [v-ras] oncogene homolog)* (eg, colorectal carcinoma), gene analysis, variants in exon 2 (eg, codons 12 and 13) and exon 3 (eg, codon 61)
0.00 0.00 FUD XXX
AMA: 2020,OctSE,1; 2018,Nov,9; 2018,Jan,8; 2017,Jan,8; 2016,Aug,9

81312 Resequenced code. See code before resequenced code 81307.

● # 81191 *NTRK1 (neurotrophic receptor tyrosine kinase 1)* (eg, solid tumors) translocation analysis
0.00 0.00 FUD 000

● # 81192 *NTRK2 (neurotrophic receptor tyrosine kinase 2)* (eg, solid tumors) translocation analysis
0.00 0.00 FUD 000

● # 81193 *NTRK3 (neurotrophic receptor tyrosine kinase 3)* (eg, solid tumors) translocation analysis
0.00 0.00 FUD 000

● # 81194 *NTRK (neurotrophic-tropomyosin receptor tyrosine kinase 1, 2, and 3)* (eg, solid tumors) translocation analysis
INCLUDES Analysis NTRK1, NTRK2, and NTRK3 by single assay
0.00 0.00 FUD 000

\# 81306 *NUDT15 (nudix hydrolase 15)* (eg, drug metabolism) gene analysis, common variant(s) (eg, *2, *3, *4, *5, *6)
0.00 0.00 FUD XXX
AMA: 2020,OctSE,1; 2019,Jul,3; 2018,Nov,9

\# 81312 *PABPN1 (poly[A] binding protein nuclear 1)* (eg, oculopharyngeal muscular dystrophy) gene analysis, evaluation to detect abnormal (eg, expanded) alleles
0.00 0.00 FUD XXX
AMA: 2020,OctSE,1; 2018,Nov,9

\# 81307 *PALB2 (partner and localizer of BRCA2)* (eg, breast and pancreatic cancer) gene analysis; full gene sequence
0.00 0.00 FUD XXX
AMA: 2020,OctSE,1

\# 81308 known familial variant
0.00 0.00 FUD XXX
AMA: 2020,OctSE,1

81313 *PCA3/KLK3 (prostate cancer antigen 3 [non-protein coding]/kallikrein-related peptidase 3 [prostate specific antigen])* ratio (eg, prostate cancer)
0.00 0.00 FUD XXX
AMA: 2020,OctSE,1; 2018,Nov,9; 2018,Jan,8; 2017,Jan,8; 2016,Aug,9; 2016,Jan,13; 2015,Jan,3

81314 *PDGFRA (platelet-derived growth factor receptor, alpha polypeptide)* (eg, gastrointestinal stromal tumor [GIST]), gene analysis, targeted sequence analysis (eg, exons 12, 18)
0.00 0.00 FUD XXX
AMA: 2020,OctSE,1; 2018,Nov,9; 2018,Jan,8; 2017,Jan,8; 2016,Aug,9

\# 81309 *PIK3CA (phosphatidylinositol-4, 5-biphosphate 3-kinase, catalytic subunit alpha)* (eg, colorectal and breast cancer) gene analysis, targeted sequence analysis (eg, exons 7, 9, 20)
0.00 0.00 FUD XXX
AMA: 2020,OctSE,1; 2020,Apr,10

\# 81320 *PLCG2 (phospholipase C gamma 2)* (eg, chronic lymphocytic leukemia) gene analysis, common variants (eg, R665W, S707F, L845F)
0.00 0.00 FUD XXX
AMA: 2020,OctSE,1; 2019,Jul,3; 2018,Nov,9

81315 *PML/RARalpha, (t(15;17)), (promyelocytic leukemia/retinoic acid receptor alpha)* (eg, promyelocytic leukemia) translocation analysis; common breakpoints (eg, intron 3 and intron 6), qualitative or quantitative
0.00 0.00 FUD XXX
AMA: 2020,OctSE,1; 2018,Nov,9; 2018,Jan,8; 2017,Jan,8; 2016,Aug,9; 2016,Jan,13; 2015,Jan,16

81316 single breakpoint (eg, intron 3, intron 6 or exon 6), qualitative or quantitative
0.00 0.00 FUD XXX
AMA: 2020,OctSE,1; 2018,Nov,9; 2018,Jan,8; 2017,Jan,8; 2016,Aug,9; 2016,Jan,13; 2015,Jan,16

\# 81324 *PMP22 (peripheral myelin protein 22)* (eg, Charcot-Marie-Tooth, hereditary neuropathy with liability to pressure palsies) gene analysis; duplication/deletion analysis
0.00 0.00 FUD XXX
AMA: 2020,OctSE,1; 2018,Nov,9; 2018,Jan,8; 2017,Jan,8; 2016,Aug,9; 2016,Jan,13; 2015,Jan,16

\# 81325 full sequence analysis
0.00 0.00 FUD XXX
AMA: 2020,OctSE,1; 2018,Nov,9; 2018,May,6; 2018,Jan,8; 2017,Jan,8; 2016,Aug,9; 2016,Jan,13; 2015,Jan,16

\# 81326 known familial variant
0.00 0.00 FUD XXX
AMA: 2020,OctSE,1; 2018,Nov,9; 2018,Jan,8; 2017,Jan,8; 2016,Aug,9; 2016,Jan,13; 2015,Jan,16

81317 *PMS2 (postmeiotic segregation increased 2 [S. cerevisiae])* (eg, hereditary non-polyposis colorectal cancer, Lynch syndrome) gene analysis; full sequence analysis
0.00 0.00 FUD XXX
AMA: 2020,OctSE,1; 2018,Nov,9; 2018,Jan,8; 2017,Jan,8; 2016,Aug,9; 2016,Jan,13; 2015,Jan,16

81318 known familial variants
0.00 0.00 FUD XXX
AMA: 2020,OctSE,1; 2018,Nov,9; 2018,Jan,8; 2017,Jan,8; 2016,Aug,9; 2016,Jan,13; 2015,Jan,16

81319 duplication/deletion variants
0.00 0.00 FUD XXX
AMA: 2020,OctSE,1; 2018,Nov,9; 2018,Jan,8; 2017,Jan,8; 2016,Aug,9; 2016,Jan,13; 2015,Jan,16

81320 Resequenced code. See code before 81315.

\# 81343 *PPP2R2B (protein phosphatase 2 regulatory subunit Bbeta)* (eg, spinocerebellar ataxia) gene analysis, evaluation to detect abnormal (eg, expanded) alleles
0.00 0.00 FUD XXX
AMA: 2020,OctSE,1; 2018,Nov,9

81321 *PTEN (phosphatase and tensin homolog)* (eg, Cowden syndrome, PTEN hamartoma tumor syndrome) gene analysis; full sequence analysis
0.00 0.00 FUD XXX A
AMA: 2020,OctSE,1; 2018,Nov,9; 2018,Jan,8; 2017,Jan,8; 2016,Aug,9; 2016,Jan,13; 2015,Jan,16

81322 known familial variant
0.00 0.00 FUD XXX A
AMA: 2020,OctSE,1; 2018,Nov,9; 2018,Jan,8; 2017,Jan,8; 2016,Aug,9; 2016,Jan,13; 2015,Jan,16

81323 duplication/deletion variant
0.00 0.00 FUD XXX A
AMA: 2020,OctSE,1; 2018,Nov,9; 2018,Jan,8; 2017,Jan,8; 2016,Aug,9; 2016,Jan,13; 2015,Jan,16

81324 **Resequenced code. See code following 81316.**

81325 **Resequenced code. See code following 81316.**

81326 **Resequenced code. See code following 81316.**

81334 *RUNX1 (runt related transcription factor 1)* (eg, acute myeloid leukemia, familial platelet disorder with associated myeloid malignancy), gene analysis, targeted sequence analysis (eg, exons 3-8)
0.00 0.00 FUD XXX A
AMA: 2020,OctSE,1; 2018,Nov,9

81327 *SEPT9 (Septin9)* (eg, colorectal cancer) promoter methylation analysis
0.00 0.00 FUD XXX A
AMA: 2020,OctSE,1; 2019,Jul,3; 2018,Nov,9

81332 *SERPINA1 (serpin peptidase inhibitor, clade A, alpha-1 antiproteinase, antitrypsin, member 1)* (eg, alpha-1-antitrypsin deficiency), gene analysis, common variants (eg, *S and *Z)
0.00 0.00 FUD XXX A
AMA: 2020,OctSE,1; 2018,Nov,9; 2018,Jan,8; 2017,Jan,8; 2016,Aug,9; 2016,Jan,13; 2015,Jan,16

● # **81347** *SF3B1 (splicing factor [3b] subunit B1)* (eg, myelodysplastic syndrome/acute myeloid leukemia) gene analysis, common variants (eg, A672T, E622D, L833F, R625C, R625L)
0.00 0.00 FUD 000

81328 *SLCO1B1 (solute carrier organic anion transporter family, member 1B1)* (eg, adverse drug reaction), gene analysis, common variant(s) (eg, *5)
0.00 0.00 FUD XXX A
AMA: 2020,OctSE,1; 2018,Nov,9

81329 *SMN1 (survival of motor neuron 1, telomeric)* (eg, spinal muscular atrophy) gene analysis; dosage/deletion analysis (eg, carrier testing), includes SMN2 (survival of motor neuron 2, centromeric) analysis, if performed
0.00 0.00 FUD XXX
AMA: 2020,OctSE,1; 2019,Jul,3; 2018,Nov,9

81336 full gene sequence
0.00 0.00 FUD XXX
AMA: 2020,OctSE,1; 2019,Jul,3; 2018,Nov,9

81337 known familial sequence variant(s)
0.00 0.00 FUD XXX
AMA: 2020,OctSE,1; 2019,Jul,3; 2018,Nov,9

81330 *SMPD1(sphingomyelin phosphodiesterase 1, acid lysosomal)* (eg, Niemann-Pick disease, Type A) gene analysis, common variants (eg, R496L, L302P, fsP330)
0.00 0.00 FUD XXX A
AMA: 2020,OctSE,1; 2018,Nov,9; 2018,Jan,8; 2017,Jan,8; 2016,Aug,9; 2016,Jan,13; 2015,Jan,16

81331 *SNRPN/UBE3A (small nuclear ribonucleoprotein polypeptide N and ubiquitin protein ligase E3A)* (eg, Prader-Willi syndrome and/or Angelman syndrome), methylation analysis
0.00 0.00 FUD XXX A
AMA: 2020,OctSE,1; 2018,Nov,9; 2018,Jan,8; 2017,Jan,8; 2016,Aug,9; 2016,Jan,13; 2015,Jan,16

81332 **Resequenced code. See code following 81327.**

● # **81348** *SRSF2 (serine and arginine-rich splicing factor 2)* (eg, myelodysplastic syndrome, acute myeloid leukemia) gene analysis, common variants (eg, P95H, P95L)
0.00 0.00 FUD 000

81344 *TBP (TATA box binding protein)* (eg, spinocerebellar ataxia) gene analysis, evaluation to detect abnormal (eg, expanded) alleles
0.00 0.00 FUD XXX
AMA: 2020,OctSE,1; 2018,Nov,9

81345 *TERT (telomerase reverse transcriptase)* (eg, thyroid carcinoma, glioblastoma multiforme) gene analysis, targeted sequence analysis (eg, promoter region)
0.00 0.00 FUD XXX
AMA: 2020,OctSE,1; 2019,Jul,3; 2018,Nov,9

81333 *TGFBI (transforming growth factor beta-induced)* (eg, corneal dystrophy) gene analysis, common variants (eg, R124H, R124C, R124L, R555W, R555Q)
0.00 0.00 FUD XXX
AMA: 2020,OctSE,1; 2019,Jul,3; 2018,Nov,9

81334 **Resequenced code. See code following code 81326.**

● # **81351** *TP53 (tumor protein 53)* (eg, Li-Fraumeni syndrome) gene analysis; full gene sequence
0.00 0.00 FUD 000

● # **81352** targeted sequence analysis (eg, 4 oncology)
0.00 0.00 FUD 000

● # **81353** known familial variant
0.00 0.00 FUD 000

81335 *TPMT (thiopurine S-methyltransferase)* (eg, drug metabolism), gene analysis, common variants (eg, *2, *3)
0.00 0.00 FUD XXX A
AMA: 2020,OctSE,1; 2018,Nov,9

81336 **Resequenced code. See code following 81329.**

81337 **Resequenced code. See code following 81329.**

81338 **Resequenced code. See code following resequenced code 81294.**

81339 **Resequenced code. See code fbefore resequenced code 81295.**

81340 *TRB@ (T cell antigen receptor, beta)* (eg, leukemia and lymphoma), gene rearrangement analysis to detect abnormal clonal population(s); using amplification methodology (eg, polymerase chain reaction)
0.00 0.00 FUD XXX A
AMA: 2020,OctSE,1; 2018,Nov,9; 2018,Jan,8; 2017,Jan,8; 2016,Aug,9; 2016,Jan,13; 2015,Jan,16

81341 using direct probe methodology (eg, Southern blot)
0.00 0.00 FUD XXX A
AMA: 2020,OctSE,1; 2018,Nov,9; 2018,Jan,8; 2017,Jan,8; 2016,Aug,9; 2016,Jan,13; 2015,Jan,16

81342 *TRG@ (T cell antigen receptor, gamma)* (eg, leukemia and lymphoma), gene rearrangement analysis, evaluation to detect abnormal clonal population(s)
0.00 0.00 FUD XXX A
AMA: 2020,OctSE,1; 2018,Nov,9; 2018,Jan,8; 2017,Jan,8; 2016,Aug,9; 2016,Jan,13; 2015,Jan,16

81343 **Resequenced code. See code following code 81320.**

81344 **Resequenced code. See code following code 81320.**

81345 **Resequenced code. See code following code 81320.**

81346 *TYMS (thymidylate synthetase)* (eg, 5-fluorouracil/5-FU drug metabolism), gene analysis, common variant(s) (eg, tandem repeat variant)
0.00 0.00 FUD XXX A
AMA: 2020,OctSE,1; 2018,Nov,9

81347 **Resequenced code. See code before 81328.**

81348 **Resequenced code. See code following 81331.**

● # **81357** ***U2AF1 (U2 small nuclear RNA auxiliary factor 1)* (eg, myelodysplastic syndrome, acute myeloid leukemia) gene analysis, common variants (eg, S34F, S34Y, Q157R, Q157P)**
0.00 0.00 FUD 000

81350 ***UGT1A1 (UDP glucuronosyltransferase 1 family, polypeptide A1)* (eg, drug metabolism, hereditary unconjugated hyperbilirubinemia [Gilbert syndrome]) gene analysis, common variants (eg, *28, *36, *37)**
0.00 0.00 FUD XXX A
AMA: 2020,OctSE,1; 2020,Apr,9; 2018,Nov,9; 2018,Jan,8; 2017,Jan,8; 2016,Aug,9; 2016,Jan,13; 2015,Jan,16

81351 **Resequenced code. See code following 81333.**

81352 **Resequenced code. See code following 81333.**

81353 **Resequenced code. See code following 81333.**

81355 ***VKORC1 (vitamin K epoxide reductase complex, subunit 1)* (eg, warfarin metabolism), gene analysis, common variant(s) (eg, -1639G>A, c.173+1000C>T)**
0.00 0.00 FUD XXX A
AMA: 2020,OctSE,1; 2018,Nov,9; 2018,Jan,8; 2017,Jan,8; 2016,Aug,9; 2016,Jan,13; 2015,Jan,16

81357 **Resequenced code. See code following 81346.**

● **81360** ***ZRSR2 (zinc finger CCCH-type, RNA binding motif and serine/arginine-rich 2)* (eg, myelodysplastic syndrome, acute myeloid leukemia) gene analysis, common variant(s) (eg, E65fs, E122fs, R448fs)**

81361 **Resequenced code. See code following resequenced code 81269.**

81362 **Resequenced code. See code following resequenced code 81269.**

81363 **Resequenced code. See code following resequenced code 81269.**

81364 **Resequenced code. See code following resequenced code 81269.**

81370-81383 Human Leukocyte Antigen (HLA) Testing

INCLUDES Additional testing performed to resolve ambiguous allele combinations for high-resolution typing
All analytical procedures in evaluation:
- Amplification
- Cell lysis
- Detection
- Digestion
- Extraction
- Nucleic acid stabilization

Analysis to identify human leukocyte antigen (HLA) alleles and allele groups connected to specific diseases and individual response to drug therapy in addition to other clinical uses
Code selection based on specific gene being reviewed
Evaluation gene variant presence using common gene variant name
Generally, all listed gene variants in code description tested (lists not all inclusive)
Genes described using Human Genome Organization (HUGO) approved names
High-resolution typing resolves common well-defined (CWD) alleles usually identified by at least four-digits. Some instances when high-resolution typing may include ambiguities for rare alleles may be reported as string of alleles or National Marrow Donor Program (NMDP) code
Histocompatibility antigen testing
Intermediate resolution HLA testing identified by string of alleles or NMDP code
Low and intermediate resolution considered low resolution for code assignment
Low-resolution HLA type reporting identified by two-digit HLA name
Multiple variant alleles or allele groups identified by typing
One or more HLA genes in specific clinical circumstances
Protein or disease examples in code description not all inclusive
Qualitative results unless otherwise stated
Typing performed to determine recipient compatibility and potential donors undergoing solid organ or hematopoietic stem cell pretransplantation testing

EXCLUDES *Full gene sequencing using separate gene variant assessment codes unless specifically stated in code description*
HLA antigen typing by nonmolecular pathology methods (86812-86821)
In situ hybridization analyses (88271-88275, 88368-88375 [88377])
Microbial identification (87149-87153, 87471-87801 [87623, 87624, 87625], 87900-87904 [87906, 87910, 87912])
Other related gene variants not listed in code description
Tier 1 molecular pathology codes (81105-81254 [81161, 81162, 81163, 81164, 81165, 81166, 81167, 81173, 81174, 81184, 81185, 81186, 81187, 81188, 81189, 81190, 81200, 81201, 81202, 81203, 81204, 81205, 81206, 81207, 81208, 81209, 81210, 81219, 81227, 81230, 81231, 81233, 81234, 81238, 81239, 81245, 81246, 81250, 81257, 81258, 81259, 81265, 81266, 81267, 81268, 81269, 81284, 81285, 81286, 81289, 81361, 81362, 81363, 81364])
Tier 2 and unlisted molecular pathology procedures (81400-81408, [81479])

Code also modifier 26 when only interpretation and report performed
Code also services required before cell lysis

81370 **HLA Class I and II typing, low resolution (eg, antigen equivalents); *HLA-A, -B, -C, -DRB1/3/4/5, and -DQB1***
0.00 0.00 FUD XXX A
AMA: 2020,OctSE,1; 2018,Nov,9; 2018,Jan,8; 2017,Jan,8; 2016,Aug,9; 2016,Jan,13; 2015,Jan,16

81371 ***HLA-A, -B, and -DRB1* (eg, verification typing)**
0.00 0.00 FUD XXX A
AMA: 2020,OctSE,1; 2018,Nov,9; 2018,Jan,8; 2017,Jan,8; 2016,Aug,9; 2016,Jan,13; 2015,Jan,16

81372 **HLA Class I typing, low resolution (eg, antigen equivalents); complete *(ie, HLA-A, -B, and -C)***
EXCLUDES *Class I and II low-resolution HLA typing for HLA-A, -B, -C, -DRB1/3/4/5, and -DQB1 (81370)*
0.00 0.00 FUD XXX A
AMA: 2020,OctSE,1; 2018,Nov,9; 2018,Jan,8; 2017,Jan,8; 2016,Aug,9; 2016,Jan,13; 2015,Jan,16

81373 **one locus *(eg, HLA-A, -B, or -C)*, each**
EXCLUDES *Complete Class 1 (HLA-A, -B, and -C) low-resolution typing (81372)*
Reporting presence or absence single antigen equivalent using low-resolution methodology (81374)
0.00 0.00 FUD XXX A
AMA: 2020,OctSE,1; 2018,Nov,9; 2018,Jan,8; 2017,Jan,8; 2016,Aug,9; 2016,Jan,13; 2015,Jan,16

Pathology and Laboratory
81348 — 81373

81374 **one antigen equivalent *(eg, B*27)*, each**

EXCLUDES *Testing for presence or absence more than two antigen equivalents at locus, report for each locus test (81373)*

0.00 0.00 FUD XXX A

AMA: 2020,OctSE,1; 2018,Nov,9; 2018,Jan,8; 2017,Jan,8; 2016,Aug,9; 2016,Jan,13; 2015,Jan,16

81375 **HLA Class II typing, low resolution (eg, antigen equivalents); *HLA-DRB1/3/4/5 and -DQB1***

EXCLUDES *Class I and II low-resolution HLA typing for HLA-A, -B, -C, -DRB 1/3/4/5, and DQB1 (81370)*

0.00 0.00 FUD XXX A

AMA: 2020,OctSE,1; 2018,Nov,9; 2018,Jan,8; 2017,Jan,8; 2016,Aug,9; 2016,Jan,13; 2015,Jan,16

81376 **one locus *(eg, HLA-DRB1, -DRB3/4/5, -DQB1, -DQA1, -DPB1, or -DPA1)*, each**

INCLUDES Low-resolution typing, HLA-DRB1/3/4/5 reported as single locus

EXCLUDES *Low-resolution typing for HLA-DRB1/3/4/5 and -DQB1 (81375)*

0.00 0.00 FUD XXX A

AMA: 2020,OctSE,1; 2018,Nov,9; 2018,Jan,8; 2017,Jan,8; 2016,Aug,9; 2016,Jan,13; 2015,Jan,16

81377 **one antigen equivalent, each**

EXCLUDES *Testing for presence or absence more than two antigen equivalents at locus (81376)*

0.00 0.00 FUD XXX A

AMA: 2020,OctSE,1; 2018,Nov,9; 2018,Jan,8; 2017,Jan,8; 2016,Aug,9; 2016,Jan,13; 2015,Jan,16

81378 **HLA Class I and II typing, high resolution (ie, alleles or allele groups), *HLA-A, -B, -C, and -DRB1***

0.00 0.00 FUD XXX A

AMA: 2020,OctSE,1; 2018,Nov,9; 2018,Jan,8; 2017,Jan,8; 2016,Aug,9; 2016,Jan,13; 2015,Jan,16

81379 **HLA Class I typing, high resolution (ie, alleles or allele groups); complete (ie, *HLA-A, -B, and -C*)**

0.00 0.00 FUD XXX A

AMA: 2020,OctSE,1; 2018,Nov,9; 2018,Jan,8; 2017,Jan,8; 2016,Aug,9; 2016,Jan,13; 2015,Jan,16

81380 **one locus (eg, *HLA-A, -B, or -C*), each**

EXCLUDES *Complete Class I high-resolution typing for HLA-A, -B, and -C (81379)*

Testing for presence or absence single allele or allele group using high-resolution methodology (81381)

0.00 0.00 FUD XXX A

AMA: 2020,OctSE,1; 2018,Nov,9; 2018,Jan,8; 2017,Jan,8; 2016,Aug,9; 2016,Jan,13; 2015,Jan,16

81381 **one allele or allele group (eg, *B*57:01P*), each**

EXCLUDES *Testing for presence or absence more than two alleles or allele groups at locus, report for each locus (81380)*

0.00 0.00 FUD XXX A

AMA: 2020,OctSE,1; 2018,Nov,9; 2018,Jan,8; 2017,Jan,8; 2016,Aug,9; 2016,Jan,13; 2015,Jan,16

81382 **HLA Class II typing, high resolution (ie, alleles or allele groups); one locus (eg, *HLA-DRB1, -DRB3/4/5, -DQB1, -DQA1, -DPB1, or -DPA1*), each**

INCLUDES Typing one or all DRB3/4/5 genes regarded as one locus

EXCLUDES *Testing for just presence or absence single allele or allele group using high-resolution methodology (81383)*

0.00 0.00 FUD XXX A

AMA: 2020,OctSE,1; 2018,Nov,9; 2018,Jan,8; 2017,Jan,8; 2016,Jan,13; 2015,Jan,16

81383 **one allele or allele group (eg, *HLA-DQB1*06:02P*), each**

EXCLUDES *Testing for presence or absence more than two alleles or allele groups at locus, report for each locus (81382)*

0.00 0.00 FUD XXX A

AMA: 2020,OctSE,1; 2018,Nov,9; 2018,Jan,8; 2017,Jan,8; 2016,Jan,13; 2015,Jan,16

81400-81479 [81479] Molecular Pathology Tier 2 Procedures

INCLUDES All analytical procedures in evaluation:
- Amplification
- Cell lysis
- Detection
- Digestion
- Extraction
- Nucleic acid stabilization

Code selection based on specific gene being reviewed
Codes arranged by technical resource level and work involved
Evaluation gene variant presence using common gene variant name
Generally, all listed gene variants in code description tested (lists not all inclusive)
Genes described using Human Genome Organization (HUGO) approved names
Histocompatibility testing
Protein or disease examples in code description (lists not all inclusive)
Qualitative results unless otherwise stated
Specific analytes listed after code description for selecting appropriate molecular pathology procedure
Targeted genomic testing (81410-81471 [81448])
Testing for more rare diseases

EXCLUDES *Full gene sequencing using separate gene variant assessment codes unless specifically stated in code description*
In situ hybridization analyses (88271-88275, 88365-88368 [88364, 88373, 88374])
Microbial identification (87149-87153, 87471-87801 [87623, 87624, 87625], 87900-87904 [87906, 87910, 87912])
Other related gene variants not listed in code description
Tier 1 molecular pathology (81105-81254 [81161, 81162, 81163, 81164, 81165, 81166, 81167, 81173, 81174, 81184, 81185, 81186, 81187, 81188, 81189, 81190, 81200, 81201, 81202, 81203, 81204, 81205, 81206, 81207, 81208, 81209, 81210, 81219, 81227, 81230, 81231, 81233, 81234, 81238, 81239, 81245, 81246, 81250, 81257, 81258, 81259, 81265, 81266, 81267, 81268, 81269, 81284, 81285, 81286, 81289, 81361, 81362, 81363, 81364])
Unlisted molecular pathology procedures ([81479])

Code also modifier 26 when only interpretation and report performed
Code also services required before cell lysis

81400 **Molecular pathology procedure, Level 1 (eg, identification of single germline variant [eg, SNP] by techniques such as restriction enzyme digestion or melt curve analysis)**

ACADM (acyl-CoA dehydrogenase, C-4 to C-12 straight chain, MCAD) (eg, medium chain acyl dehydrogenase deficiency), K304E variant

ACE (angiotensin converting enzyme) (eg, hereditary blood pressure regulation), insertion/deletion variant

AGTR1 (angiotensin II receptor, type 1) (eg, essential hypertension), 1166A>C variant

BCKDHA (branched chain keto acid dehydrogenase E1, alpha polypeptide) (eg, maple syrup urine disease, type 1A), Y438N variant

CCR5 (chemokine C-C motif receptor 5) (eg, HIV resistance), 32-bp deletion mutation/794 825del32 deletion

CLRN1 (clarin 1) (eg, Usher syndrome, type 3), N48K variant

F2 (coagulation factor 2) (eg, hereditary hypercoagulability), 1199G>A variant

F5 (coagulation factor V) (eg, hereditary hypercoagulability), HR2 variant

F7 (coagulation factor VII [serum prothrombin conversion accelerator]) (eg, hereditary hypercoagulability), R353Q variant

F13B (coagulation factor XIII, B polypeptide) (eg, hereditary hypercoagulability), V34L variant

FGB (fibrinogen beta chain) (eg, hereditary ischemic heart disease), -455G>A variant

FGFR1 (fibroblast growth factor receptor 1) (eg, Pfeiffer syndrome type 1, craniosynostosis), P252R variant

FGFR3 (fibroblast growth factor receptor 3) (eg, Muenke syndrome), P250R variant

FKTN (fukutin) (eg, Fukuyama congenital muscular dystrophy), retrotransposon insertion variant

GNE (glucosamine [UDP-N-acetyl]-2 -epimerase/N-acetylmannosamine kinase) (eg, inclusion body myopathy 2 [IBM2], Nonaka myopathy), M712T variant

IVD (isovaleryl-CoA dehydrogenase) (eg, isovaleric acidemia), A282V variant

LCT (lactase-phlorizin hydrolase) (eg, lactose intolerance), 13910 C>T variant

NEB (nebulin) (eg, nemaline myopathy 2), exon 55 deletion variant

PCDH15 (protocadherin-related 15) (eg, Usher syndrome type 1F), R245X variant

SERPINE1 (serpine peptidase inhibitor clade E, member 1, plasminogen activator inhibitor -1, PAI-1) (eg, thrombophilia), 4G variant

SHOC2 (soc-2 suppressor of clear homolog) (eg, Noonan-like syndrome with loose anagen hair), S2G variant

SRY (sex determining region Y) (eg, 46,XX testicular disorder of sex development, gonadal dysgenesis), gene analysis

TOR1A (torsin family 1, member A [torsin A]) (eg, early-onset primary dystonia [DYT1]), 907_909delGAG (904_906delGAG) variant

0.00 0.00 **FUD** XXX A

AMA: 2020,OctSE,1; 2019,Jul,3; 2018,Nov,9; 2018,Jan,8; 2017,Jan,8; 2016,Aug,9; 2016,Jan,13; 2015,Jan,16; 2015,Jan,3

▲ **81401** **Molecular pathology procedure, Level 2 (eg, 2-10 SNPs, 1 methylated variant, or 1 somatic variant [typically using nonsequencing target variant analysis], or detection of a dynamic mutation disorder/triplet repeat)**

ABCC8 (ATP-binding cassette, sub-family C [CFTR/MRP], member 8) (eg, familial hyperinsulinism), common variants (eg, c.3898-9G>A [c.3992-9G>A], F1388del)

ABL1 (ABL proto oncogene 1, non-receptor tyrosine kinase) (eg, acquired imatinib resistance), T315I variant

ACADM (acyl-CoA dehydrogenase, C-4 to C-12 straight chain, MCAD) (eg, medium chain acyl dehydrogenase deficiency), common variants (eg, K304E, Y42H)

ADRB2 (adrenergic beta-2 receptor surface) (eg, drug metabolism), common variants (eg, G16R, Q27E)

APOB (apolipoprotein B) (eg, familial hypercholesterolemia type B), common variants (eg, R3500Q, R3500W)

*APOE (apolipoprotein E) (eg, hyperlipoproteinemia type III, cardiovascular disease, Alzheimer disease), common variants (eg, *2, *3, *4)*

CBFB/MYH11 (inv(16)) (eg, acute myeloid leukemia), qualitative, and quantitative, if performed

CBS (cystathionine-beta-synthase) (eg, homocystinuria, cystathionine beta-synthase deficiency), common variants (eg, I278T, G307S)

CFH/ARMS2 (complement factor H/age-related maculopathy susceptibility 2) (eg, macular degeneration), common variants (eg, Y402H [CFH], A69S [ARMS2])

DEK/NUP214 (t(6;9))(eg, acute myeloid leukemia), translocation analysis, qualitative, and quantitative, if performed

E2A/PBX1 (t(1;19)) (eg, acute lymphocytic leukemia), translocation analysis, qualitative, and quantitative, if performed

EML4/ALK (inv(2)) (eg, non-small cell lung cancer), translocation or inversion analysis

ETV6/RUNX1 (t(12;21)) (eg, acute lymphocytic leukemia), translocation analysis, qualitative and quantitative, if performed

EWSR1/ATF1 (t(12;22)) (eg, clear cell sarcoma), translocation analysis, qualitative, and quantitative, if performed

EWSR1/ERG (t(21;22)) (eg, Ewing sarcoma/peripheral neuroectodermal tumor), translocation analysis, qualitative and quantitative, if performed

EWSR1/FLI1 (t(11;22)) (eg, Ewing sarcoma/peripheral neuroectodermal tumor), translocation analysis, qualitative and quantitative, if performed

EWSR1/WT1 (t(11;22)) (eg, desmoplastic small round cell tumor), translocation analysis, qualitative and quantitative, if performed

F11 (coagulation factor XI) (eg, coagulation disorder), common variants (eg, E117X [Type II], F283L [Type III], IVS14del14, and IVS14+1G>A [Type I])

FGFR3 (fibroblast growth factor receptor 3) (eg, achondroplasia, hypochondroplasia), common variants (eg, 1138G>A, 1138G>C, 1620C>A, 1620C>G)

FIP1L1/PDGFRA (del[4q12]) (eg, imatinib-sensitive chronic eosinophilic leukemia), qualitative and quantitative, if performed

FLG (filaggrin) (eg, ichthyosis vulgaris), common variants (eg, R501X, 2282del4, R2447X, S3247X, 3702delG)

FOXO1/PAX3 (t(2;13)) (eg, alveolar rhabdomyosarcoma), translocation analysis, qualitative and quantitative, if performed

FOXO1/PAX7 (t(1;13)) (eg, alveolar rhabdomyosarcoma), translocation analysis, qualitative and quantitative, if performed

FUS/DDIT3 (t(12;16)) (eg, myxoid liposarcoma), translocation analysis, qualitative, and quantitative, if performed

GALC (galactosylceramidase) (eg, Krabbe disease), common variants (eg, c.857G>A, 30-kb deletion)

GALT (galactose-1-phosphate uridylyltransferase) (eg, galactosemia), common variants (eg, Q188R, S135L, K285N, T138M, L195P, Y209C, IVS2-2A>G, P171S, del5kb, N314D, L218L/N314D)

H19 (imprinted maternally expressed transcript [non-protein coding]) (eg, Beckwith-Wiedemann syndrome), methylation analysis

IGH@/BCL2 (t(14;18)) (eg, follicular lymphoma), translocation and analysis; single breakpoint (eg) major breakpoint region [MBR] or minor cluster region [mcr]), qualitative or quantitative

(When both MBR and mcr breakpoints are performed, report [81278])

KCNQ1OT1 (KCNQ1 overlapping transcript 1 [non-protein coding]) (e.g, Beckwith-Wiedemann syndrome), methylation analysis

LINC00518 (long intergenic non-protein coding RNA 518) (eg, melanoma), expression analysis

LRRK2 (leucine-rich repeat kinase 2) (eg, Parkinson disease), common variants (eg, R1441G, G2019S, I2020T)

MED12 (mediator complex subunit 12) (eg, FG syndrome type 1, Lujan syndrome), common variants (eg, R961W, N1007S)

MEG3/DLK1 (maternally expressed 3 [non-protein coding]/delta-like 1 homolog [Drosophila]) (eg, intrauterine growth retardation), methylation analysis

MLL/AFF1 (t(4;11)) (eg acute lymphoblastic leukemia), translocation analysis, qualitative and quantitative, if performed

MLL/MLLT3 (t(9;11)) (eg, acute myeloid leukemia) translocation analysis, qualitative and quantitative, if performed

MT-RNR1 (mitochondrially encoded 12S RNA) (eg, nonsyndromic hearing loss), common variants (eg, m.1555>G, m1494C>T)

MUTYH (mutY homolog [E.coli]) (eg, MYH-associated polyposis), common variants (eg, Y165C, G382D)

MT-ATP6 (mitochondrially encoded ATP synthase 6) (eg, neuropathy with ataxia and retinitis pigmentosa [NARP], Leigh syndrome), common variants (eg, m.8993T>G, m.8993T>C)

MT-ND4, MT-ND6 (mitochondrially encoded NADH dehydrogenase 4, mitochondrially encoded NADH dehydrogenase 6) (eg, Leber hereditary optic neuropathy [LHON]), common variants (eg m.11778G>A, m3460G>A, m14484T>C)

MT-ND5 (mitochondrially encoded tRNA leucine 1 [UUA/G], mitochondrially encoded NADH dehydrogenase 5) (eg, mitochondrial encephalopathy with lactic acidosis and stroke-like episodes [MELAS]), common variants (eg, m.3243A>G, m.3271T>C, m.3252A>G, m.13513G>A)

MT-TK (mitochondrially encoded tRNA lysine) (eg, myoclonic epilepsy with ragged-red fibers [MERRF]), common variants (eg, m8344A>G, m.8356T>C)

MT-TL1 (mitochondrially encoded tRNA leucine 1[UUA/G]) (eg, diabetes and hearing loss), common variants (eg, m.3243A>G, m.14709 T>C) MT-TL1

MT-TS1, MT-RNR1 (mitochondrially encoded tRNA serine 1 [UCN], mitochondrially encoded 12S RNA) (eg, nonsyndromic sensorineural deafness [including aminoglycoside-induced nonsyndromic deafness]) common variants (eg, m.7445A>G, m.1555A>G)

NOD2 (nucleotide-binding oligomerization domain containing 2) (eg, Crohn's disease, Blau syndrome), common variants (eg, SNP 8, SNP 12, SNP 13)

NPM/ALK (t(2;5)) (eg, anaplastic large cell lymphoma), translocation analysis

PAX8/PPARG (t(2;3) (q13;p25)) (eg, follicular thyroid carcinoma), translocation analysis

PRAME (preferentially expressed antigen in melanoma)(eg, melanoma), expression analysis

PRSS1 (protease, serine, 1 [trypsin 1]) (eg, hereditary pancreatitis), common variants (eg, N29I, A16V, R122H)

PYGM (phosphorylase, glycogen, muscle) (eg, glycogen storage disease type V, McArdle disease), common variants (eg, R50X, G205S)

RUNX1/RUNX1T1 (t(8;21)) (eg, acute myeloid leukemia) translocation analysis, qualitative and quantitative, if performed

SS18/SSX1 (t(X;18)) (eg, synovial sarcoma), translocation analysis, qualitative and quantitative, if performed

SS18/SSX2 (t(X;18)) (eg, synovial sarcoma), translocation analysis, qualitative and quantitative, if performed

VWF (von Willebrand factor) (eg, von Willebrand disease type 2N), common variants (eg, T791M, R816W, R854Q)

0.00 0.00 **FUD** XXX A

AMA: 2020,OctSE,1; 2019,Sep,7; 2019,Jul,3; 2018,Nov,9; 2018,Jan,8; 2017,Jan,8; 2016,Aug,9; 2016,Jan,13; 2015,Jan,16; 2015,Jan,3

▲ **81402** **Molecular pathology procedure, Level 3 (eg, >10 SNPs, 2-10 methylated variants, or 2-10 somatic variants [typically using non-sequencing target variant analysis], immunoglobulin and T-cell receptor gene rearrangements, duplication/deletion variants of 1 exon, loss of heterozygosity [LOH], uniparental disomy [UPD])**

Chromosome 1p-/19q- (eg, glial tumors), deletion analysis

Chromosome 18q- (eg, D18S55, D18S58, D18S61, D18S64, and D18S69) (eg, colon cancer), allelic imbalance assessment (ie, loss of heterozygosity)

COL1A1/PDGFB (t(17;22)) (eg, dermatofibrosarcoma protuberans), translocation analysis, multiple breakpoints, qualitative, and quantitative, if performed

CYP21A2 (cytochrome P450, family 21, subfamily A, polypeptide 2) (eg, congenital adrenal hyperplasia, 21-hydroxylase deficiency), common variants (eg, IVS2-13G, P30L, I172N, exon 6 mutation cluster [I235N, V236E, M238K], V281L, L307FfsX6, Q318X, R356W, P453S, G110VfsX21, 30-kb deletion variant)

ESR1/PGR (receptor 1/progesterone receptor) ratio (eg, breast cancer)

MEFV (Mediterranean fever) (eg, familial Mediterranean fever), common variants (eg, E148Q, P369S, F479L, M680I, I692del, M694V, M694I, K695R, V726A, A744S, R761H)

TRD@ (T cell antigen receptor, delta) (eg, leukemia and lymphoma), gene rearrangement analysis, evaluation to detect abnormal clonal population

Uniparental disomy (UPD) (eg, Russell-Silver syndrome, Prader-Willi/Angelman syndrome), short tandem repeat (STR) analysis

0.00 0.00 **FUD** XXX A

AMA: 2020,OctSE,1; 2018,Nov,9; 2018,Jan,8; 2017,Jan,8; 2016,Aug,9; 2016,Jan,13; 2015,Jan,16; 2015,Jan,3

▲ **81403** **Molecular pathology procedure, Level 4 (eg, analysis of single exon by DNA sequence analysis, analysis of >10 amplicons using multiplex PCR in 2 or more independent reactions, mutation scanning or duplication/deletion variants of 2-5 exons)**

ANG (angiogenin, ribonuclease, RNase A family, 5) (eg, amyotrophic lateral sclerosis), full gene sequence

ARX (aristaless-related homeobox) (eg, X-linked lissencephaly with ambiguous genitalia, X-linked mental retardation), duplication/deletion analysis

CEL (carboxyl ester lipase [bile salt-stimulated lipase]) (eg, maturity-onset diabetes of the young [MODY]), targeted sequence analysis of exon 11 (eg, c.1785delC, c.1686delT)

CTNNB1 (catenin [cadherin-associated protein], beta 1, 88kDa) (eg, desmoid tumors), targeted sequence analysis (eg, exon 3)

DAZ/SRY (deleted in azoospermia and sex determining region Y) (eg, male infertility), common deletions (eg, AZFa, AZFb, AZFc, AZFd)

DNMT3A (DNA [cytosine-5-]-methyltransferase 3 alpha) (eg, acute myeloid leukemia), targeted sequence analysis (eg, exon 23)

EPCAM (epithelial cell adhesion molecule) (eg, Lynch syndrome), duplication/deletion analysis

F8 (coagulation factor VIII) (eg, hemophilia A), inversion analysis, intron 1 and intron 22A

F12 (coagulation factor XII [Hageman factor]) (eg, angioedema, hereditary, type III; factor XII deficiency), targeted sequence analysis of exon 9

FGFR3 (fibroblast growth factor receptor 3) (eg, isolated craniosynostosis), targeted sequence analysis (eg, exon 7)

(For targeted sequence analysis of multiple FGFR3 exons, use 81404) *(81404)*

GJB1 (gap junction protein, beta 1) (eg, Charcot-Marie-Tooth X-linked), full gene sequence

GNAQ (guanine nucleotide-binding protein G[q] subunit alpha) (eg, uveal melanoma), common variants (eg, R183, Q209)

HRAS (v-Ha-ras Harvey rat sarcoma viral oncogene homolog) (eg, Costello syndrome), exon 2 sequence

Human erythrocyte antigen gene analyses (eg, SLC14A1 [Kidd blood group], BCAM [Lutheran blood group], ICAM4 [Landsteiner-Wiener blood group], SLC4A1 [Diego blood group], AQP1 [Colton blood group], ERMAP [Scianna blood group], RHCE [Rh blood group, CcEe antigens], KEL [Kell blood group], DARC [Duffy blood group], GYPA, GYPB, GYPE [MNS blood group], ART4 [Dombrock blood group]) (eg, sickle-cell disease, thalassemia, hemolytic transfusion reactions, hemolytic disease of the fetus or newborn), common variants

KCNC3 (potassium voltage-gated channel, Shaw-related subfamily, member 3) (eg, spinocerebellar ataxia), targeted sequence analysis (eg, exon 2)

KCNJ2 (potassium inwardly-rectifying channel, subfamily J, member 2) (eg, Andersen-Tawil syndrome), full gene sequence

KCNJ11 (potassium inwardly-rectifying channel, subfamily J, member 11) (eg, familial hyperinsulinism), full gene sequence

Killer cell immunoglobulin-like receptor (KIR) gene family (eg, hematopoietic stem cell transplantation), genotyping of KIR family genes

Known familial variant, not otherwise specified, for gene listed in Tier 1 or Tier 2, or identified during a genomic sequencing procedure, DNA sequence analysis, each variant exon

(For a known familial variant that is considered a common variant, use specific common variant Tier 1 or Tier 2 code)

MC4R (melanocortin 4 receptor) (eg, obesity), full gene sequence

*MICA (MHC class I polypeptide-related sequence A) (eg, solid organ transplantation), common variants (eg, *001, *002)*

MT-RNR1 (mitochondrially encoded 12S RNA) (eg, nonsyndromic hearing loss), full gene sequence

MT-TS1 (mitochondrially encoded tRNA serine 1) (eg, nonsyndromic hearing loss), full gene sequence

NDP (Norrie disease [pseudoglioma]) (eg, Norrie disease), duplication/deletion analysis

NHLRC1 (NHL repeat containing 1) (eg, progressive myoclonus epilepsy), full gene sequence

PHOX2B (paired-like homeobox 2b) (eg, congenital central hypoventilation syndrome), duplication/deletion analysis

PLN (phospholamban) (eg, dilated cardiomyopathy, hypertrophic cardiomyopathy), full gene sequence

RHD (Rh blood group, D antigen) (eg, hemolytic disease of the fetus and newborn, Rh maternal/fetal compatibility), deletion analysis (eg, exons 4, 5, and 7, pseudogene)

RHD (Rh blood group, D antigen) (eg, hemolytic disease of the fetus and newborn, Rh maternal/fetal compatibility), deletion analysis (eg, exons 4, 5, and 7, pseudogene), performed on cell-free fetal DNA in maternal blood

(For human erythrocyte gene analysis of RHD, use a separate unit of 81403)

SH2D1A (SH2 domain containing 1A) (eg, X-linked lymphoproliferative syndrome), duplication/deletion analysis

TWIST1 (twist homolog 1 [Drosophila]) (eg, Saethre-Chotzen syndrome), duplication/deletion analysis

UBA1 (ubiquitin-like modifier activating enzyme 1) (eg, spinal muscular atrophy, X-linked), targeted sequence analysis (eg, exon 15)

VHL (von Hippel-Lindau tumor suppressor) (eg, von Hippel-Lindau familial cancer syndrome), deletion/duplication analysis

VWF (von Willebrand factor) (eg, von Willebrand disease types 2A, 2B, 2M), targeted sequence analysis (eg, exon 28)

0.00 0.00 **FUD** XXX A M

AMA: 2020,OctSE,1; 2019,Jul,3; 2018,Nov,9; 2018,May,6; 2018,Jan,8; 2017,Jan,8; 2016,Aug,9; 2016,Jan,13; 2015,Jan,16; 2015,Jan,3

▲ **81404** **Molecular pathology procedure, Level 5 (eg, analysis of 2-5 exons by DNA sequence analysis, mutation scanning or duplication/deletion variants of 6-10 exons, or characterization of a dynamic mutation disorder/triplet repeat by Southern blot analysis)**

ACADS (acyl-CoA dehydrogenase, C-2 to C-3 short chain) (eg, short chain acyl-CoA dehydrogenase deficiency), targeted sequence analysis (eg, exons 5 and 6)

AQP2 (aquaporin 2 [collecting duct]) (eg, nephrogenic diabetes insipidus), full gene sequence

ARX (aristaless related homeobox) (eg, X-linked lissencephaly with ambiguous genitalia, X-linked mental retardation), full gene sequence

AVPR2 (arginine vasopressin receptor 2) (eg, nephrogenic diabetes insipidus), full gene sequence

BBS10 (Bardet-Biedl syndrome 10) (eg, Bardet-Biedl syndrome), full gene sequence

BTD (biotinidase) (eg, biotinidase deficiency), full gene sequence

C10orf2 (chromosome 10 open reading frame 2) (eg, mitochondrial DNA depletion syndrome), full gene sequence

CAV3 (caveolin 3) (eg, CAV3-related distal myopathy, limb-girdle muscular dystrophy type 1C), full gene sequence

CD40LG (CD40 ligand) (eg, X-linked hyper IgM syndrome), full gene sequence

CDKN2A (cyclin-dependent kinase inhibitor 2A) (eg, CDKN2A-related cutaneous malignant melanoma, familial atypical mole-malignant melanoma syndrome), full gene sequence

CLRN1 (clarin 1) (eg, Usher syndrome, type 3), full gene sequence

COX6B1 (cytochrome c oxidase subunit VIb polypeptide 1) (eg, mitochondrial respiratory chain complex IV deficiency), full gene sequence

CPT2 (carnitine palmitoyltransferase 2) (eg, carnitine palmitoyltransferase II deficiency), full gene sequence

CRX (cone-rod homeobox) (eg, cone-rod dystrophy 2, Leber congenital amaurosis), full gene sequence

CYP1B1 (cytochrome P450, family 1, subfamily B, polypeptide 1) (eg, primary congenital glaucoma), full gene sequence

EGR2 (early growth response 2) (eg, Charcot-Marie-Tooth), full gene sequence

EMD (emerin) (eg, Emery-Dreifuss muscular dystrophy), duplication/deletion analysis

EPM2A (epilepsy, progressive myoclonus type 2A, Lafora disease [laforin]) (eg, progressive myoclonus epilepsy), full gene sequence

FGF23 (fibroblast growth factor 23) (eg, hypophosphatemic rickets), full gene sequence

FGFR2 (fibroblast growth factor receptor 2) (eg, craniosynostosis, Apert syndrome, Crouzon syndrome), targeted sequence analysis (eg, exons 8, 10)

FGFR3 (fibroblast growth factor receptor 3) (eg, achondroplasia, hypochondroplasia), targeted sequence analysis (eg, exons 8, 11, 12, 13)

FHL1 (four and a half LIM domains 1) (eg, Emery-Dreifuss muscular dystrophy), full gene sequence

FKRP (Fukutin related protein) (eg, congenital muscular dystrophy type 1C [MDC1C], limb-girdle muscular dystrophy [LGMD] type 2I), full gene sequence

FOXG1 (forkhead box G1) (eg, Rett syndrome), full gene sequence

FSHMD1A (facioscapulohumeral muscular dystrophy 1A) (eg, facioscapulohumeral muscular dystrophy), evaluation to detect abnormal (eg, deleted) alleles

FSHMD1A (facioscapulohumeral muscular dystrophy 1A) (eg, facioscapulohumeral muscular dystrophy), characterization of haplotype(s) (ie, chromosome 4A and 4B haplotypes)

GH1 (growth hormone 1) (eg, growth hormone deficiency), full gene sequence

GP1BB (glycoprotein Ib [platelet], beta polypeptide) (eg, Bernard-Soulier syndrome type B), full gene sequence

(For common deletion variants of alpha globin 1 and alpha globin 2 genes, use 81257)

HNF1B (HNF1 homeobox B) (eg, maturity-onset diabetes of the young [MODY]), duplication/deletion analysis

HRAS (v-Ha-ras Harvey rat sarcoma viral oncogene homolog) (eg, Costello syndrome), full gene sequence

HSD3B2 (hydroxy-delta-5-steroid dehydrogenase, 3 beta- and steroid delta-isomerase 2) (eg, 3-beta-hydroxysteroid dehydrogenase type II deficiency), full gene sequence

HSD11B2 (hydroxysteroid [11-beta] dehydrogenase 2) (eg, mineralocorticoid excess syndrome), full gene sequence

HSPB1 (heat shock 27kDa protein 1) (eg, Charcot-Marie-Tooth disease), full gene sequence

INS (insulin) (eg, diabetes mellitus), full gene sequence

KCNJ1 (potassium inwardly-rectifying channel, subfamily J, member 1) (eg, Bartter syndrome), full gene sequence

KCNJ10 (potassium inwardly-rectifying channel, subfamily J, member 10) (eg, SeSAME syndrome, EAST syndrome, sensorineural hearing loss), full gene sequence

LITAF (lipopolysaccharide-induced TNF factor) (eg, Charcot-Marie-Tooth), full gene sequence

MEFV (Mediterranean fever) (eg, familial Mediterranean fever), full gene sequence

MEN1 (multiple endocrine neoplasia I) (eg, multiple endocrine neoplasia type 1, Wermer syndrome), duplication/deletion analysis

MMACHC (methylmalonic aciduria [cobalamin deficiency] cblC type, with homocystinuria) (eg, methylmalonic acidemia and homocystinuria), full gene sequence

MPV17 (MpV17 mitochondrial inner membrane protein) (eg, mitochondrial DNA depletion syndrome), duplication/deletion analysis

NDP (Norrie disease [pseudoglioma]) (eg, Norrie disease), full gene sequence

NDUFA1 (NADH dehydrogenase [ubiquinone] 1 alpha subcomplex, 1, 7.5kDa) (eg, Leigh syndrome, mitochondrial complex I deficiency), full gene sequence

NDUFAF2 (NADH dehydrogenase [ubiquinone] 1 alpha subcomplex, assembly factor 2) (eg, Leigh syndrome, mitochondrial complex I deficiency), full gene sequence

NDUFS4 (NADH dehydrogenase [ubiquinone] Fe-S protein 4, 18kDa [NADH-coenzyme Q reductase]) (eg, Leigh syndrome, mitochondrial complex I deficiency), full gene sequence

NIPA1 (non-imprinted in Prader-Willi/Angelman syndrome 1) (eg, spastic paraplegia), full gene sequence

NLGN4X (neuroligin 4, X-linked) (eg, autism spectrum disorders), duplication/deletion analysis

NPC2 (Niemann-Pick disease, type C2 [epididymal secretory protein E1]) (eg, Niemann-Pick disease type C2), full gene sequence

NR0B1 (nuclear receptor subfamily 0, group B, member 1) (eg, congenital adrenal hypoplasia), full gene sequence

PDX1 (pancreatic and duodenal homeobox 1) (eg, maturity-onset diabetes of the young [MODY]), full gene sequence

PHOX2B (paired-like homeobox 2b) (eg, congenital central hypoventilation syndrome), full gene sequence

PIK3CA (phosphatidylinositol-4,5-bisphosphate 3-kinase, catalytic subunit alpha) (eg, colorectal cancer), targeted sequence analysis (eg, exons 9 and 20)

PLP1 (proteolipid protein 1) (eg, Pelizaeus-Merzbacher disease, spastic paraplegia), duplication/deletion analysis

PQBP1 (polyglutamine binding protein 1) (eg, Renpenning syndrome), duplication/deletion analysis

PRNP (prion protein) (eg, genetic prion disease), full gene sequence

PROP1 (PROP paired-like homeobox 1) (eg, combined pituitary hormone deficiency), full gene sequence

PRPH2 (peripherin 2 [retinal degeneration, slow]) (eg, retinitis pigmentosa), full gene sequence

PRSS1 (protease, serine, 1 [trypsin 1]) (eg, hereditary pancreatitis), full gene sequence

RAF1 (v-raf-1 murine leukemia viral oncogene homolog 1) (eg, LEOPARD syndrome), targeted sequence analysis (eg, exons 7, 12, 14, 17)

RET (ret proto-oncogene) (eg, multiple endocrine neoplasia, type 2B and familial medullary thyroid carcinoma), common variants (eg, M918T, 2647_2648delinsTT, A883F)

RHO (rhodopsin) (eg, retinitis pigmentosa), full gene sequence

RP1 (retinitis pigmentosa 1) (eg, retinitis pigmentosa), full gene sequence

SCN1B (sodium channel, voltage-gated, type I, beta) (eg, Brugada syndrome), full gene sequence

SCO2 (SCO cytochrome oxidase deficient homolog 2 [SCO1L]) (eg, mitochondrial respiratory chain complex IV deficiency), full gene sequence

SDHC (succinate dehydrogenase complex, subunit C, integral membrane protein, 15kDa) (eg, hereditary paraganglioma-pheochromocytoma syndrome), duplication/deletion analysis

SDHD (succinate dehydrogenase complex, subunit D, integral membrane protein) (eg, hereditary paraganglioma), full gene sequence

SGCG (sarcoglycan, gamma [35kDa dystrophin-associated glycoprotein]) (eg, limb-girdle muscular dystrophy), duplication/deletion analysis

SH2D1A (SH2 domain containing 1A) (eg, X-linked lymphoproliferative syndrome), full gene sequence

SLC16A2 (solute carrier family 16, member 2 [thyroid hormone transporter]) (eg, specific thyroid hormone cell transporter deficiency, Allan-Herndon-Dudley syndrome), duplication/deletion analysis

SLC25A20 (solute carrier family 25 [carnitine/acylcarnitine translocase], member 20) (eg, carnitine-acylcarnitine translocase deficiency), duplication/deletion analysis

SLC25A4 (solute carrier family 25 [mitochondrial carrier; adenine nucleotide translocation], member 4) (eg, progressive external ophthalmoplegia), full gene sequence

SOD1 (superoxide dismutase 1, soluble) (eg, amyotrophic lateral sclerosis), full gene sequence

SPINK1 (serine peptidase inhibitor, Kazal type 1) (eg, hereditary pancreatitis), full gene sequence

STK11 (serine/threonine kinase 11) (eg, Peutz-Jeghers syndrome), duplication/deletion analysis

TACO1 (translational activator of mitochondrial encoded cytochrome c oxidase I) (eg, mitochondrial respiratory chain complex IV deficiency), full gene sequence

THAP1 (THAP domain containing, apoptosis associated protein 1) (eg, torsion dystonia), full gene sequence

TOR1A (torsin family 1, member A [torsin A]) (eg, torsion dystonia), full gene sequence

TTPA (tocopherol [alpha] transfer protein) (eg, ataxia), full gene sequence

TTR (transthyretin) (eg, familial transthyretin amyloidosis), full gene sequence

TWIST1 (twist homolog 1 [Drosophila]) (eg, Saethre-Chotzen syndrome), full gene sequence

TYR (tyrosinase [oculocutaneous albinism IA]) (eg, oculocutaneous albinism IA), full gene sequence

UGT1A1 (UDP glucuronosyltransferase 1 family, polypeptide A1) (eg, hereditary unconjugated hyperbilirubinemia [Crigler-Najjar syndrome]) full gene sequence

USH1G (Usher syndrome 1G [autosomal recessive]) (eg, Usher syndrome, type 1), full gene sequence

VWF (von Willebrand factor) (eg, von Willebrand disease type 1C), targeted sequence analysis (eg, exons 26, 27, 37)

VHL (von Hippel-Lindau tumor suppressor) (eg, von Hippel-Lindau familial cancer syndrome), full gene sequence

ZEB2 (zinc finger E-box binding homeobox 2) (eg, Mowat-Wilson syndrome), duplication/deletion analysis

ZNF41 (zinc finger protein 41) (eg, X-linked mental retardation 89), full gene sequence

0.00 0.00 **FUD** XXX A

AMA: 2020,OctSE,1; 2020,Apr,9; 2019,Jul,3; 2018,Nov,9; 2018,May,6; 2018,Jan,8; 2017,Jan,8; 2016,Aug,9; 2016,Jan,13; 2015,Jan,3; 2015,Jan,16

▲ **81405** **Molecular pathology procedure, Level 6 (eg, analysis of 6-10 exons by DNA sequence analysis, mutation scanning or duplication/deletion variants of 11-25 exons, regionally targeted cytogenomic array analysis)**

ABCD1 (ATP-binding cassette, sub-family D [ALD], member 1) (eg, adrenoleukodystrophy), full gene sequence

ACADS (acyl-CoA dehydrogenase, C-2 to C-3 short chain) (eg, short chain acyl-CoA dehydrogenase deficiency), full gene sequence

ACTA2 (actin, alpha 2, smooth muscle, aorta) (eg, thoracic aortic aneurysms and aortic dissections), full gene sequence

ACTC1 (actin, alpha, cardiac muscle 1) (eg, familial hypertrophic cardiomyopathy), full gene sequence

ANKRD1 (ankyrin repeat domain 1) (eg, dilated cardiomyopathy), full gene sequence

APTX (aprataxin) (eg, ataxia with oculomotor apraxia 1), full gene sequence

ARSA (arylsulfatase A) (eg, arylsulfatase A deficiency), full gene sequence

BCKDHA (branched chain keto acid dehydrogenase E1, alpha polypeptide) (eg, maple syrup urine disease, type 1A), full gene sequence

BCS1L (BCS1-like [S. cerevisiae]) (eg, Leigh syndrome, mitochondrial complex III deficiency, GRACILE syndrome), full gene sequence

BMPR2 (bone morphogenetic protein receptor, type II [serine/threonine kinase]) (eg, heritable pulmonary arterial hypertension), duplication/deletion analysis

CASQ2 (calsequestrin 2 [cardiac muscle]) (eg, catecholaminergic polymorphic ventricular tachycardia), full gene sequence

CASR (calcium-sensing receptor) (eg, hypocalcemia), full gene sequence

CDKL5 (cyclin-dependent kinase-like 5) (eg, early infantile epileptic encephalopathy), duplication/deletion analysis

CHRNA4 (cholinergic receptor, nicotinic, alpha 4) (eg, nocturnal frontal lobe epilepsy), full gene sequence

CHRNB2 (cholinergic receptor, nicotinic, beta 2 [neuronal]) (eg, nocturnal frontal lobe epilepsy), full gene sequence

COX10 (COX10 homolog, cytochrome c oxidase assembly protein) (eg, mitochondrial respiratory chain complex IV deficiency), full gene sequence

COX15 (COX15 homolog, cytochrome c oxidase assembly protein) (eg, mitochondrial respiratory chain complex IV deficiency), full gene sequence

CPOX (coproporphyrinogen oxidase) (eg, hereditary coproporphyria), full gene sequence

CTRC (chymotrypsin C) (eg, hereditary pancreatitis), full gene sequence

CYP11B1 (cytochrome P450, family 11, subfamily B, polypeptide 1) (eg, congenital adrenal hyperplasia), full gene sequence

CYP17A1 (cytochrome P450, family 17, subfamily A, polypeptide 1) (eg, congenital adrenal hyperplasia), full gene sequence

CYP21A2 (cytochrome P450, family 21, subfamily A, polypeptide2) (eg, steroid 21-hydroxylase isoform, congenital adrenal hyperplasia), full gene sequence

Cytogenomic constitutional targeted microarray analysis of chromosome 22q13 by interrogation of genomic regions for copy number and single nucleotide polymorphism (SNP) variants for chromosomal abnormalities

(When performing genome-wide cytogenomic constitutional microarray analysis, see 81228, 81229) (81228-81229)

(Do not report analyte-specific molecular pathology procedures separately when the specific analytes are included as part of the microarray analysis of chromosome 22q13)

(Do not report 88271 when performing cytogenomic microarray analysis)

DBT (dihydrolipoamide branched chain transacylase E2) (eg, maple syrup urine disease, type 2), duplication/deletion analysis

DCX (doublecortin) (eg, X-linked lissencephaly), full gene sequence

DES (desmin) (eg, myofibrillar myopathy), full gene sequence

DFNB59 (deafness, autosomal recessive 59) (eg, autosomal recessive nonsyndromic hearing impairment), full gene sequence

DGUOK (deoxyguanosine kinase) (eg, hepatocerebral mitochondrial DNA depletion syndrome), full gene sequence

DHCR7 (7-dehydrocholesterol reductase) (eg, Smith-Lemli-Opitz syndrome), full gene sequence

EIF2B2 (eukaryotic translation initiation factor 2B, subunit 2 beta, 39kDa) (eg, leukoencephalopathy with vanishing white matter), full gene sequence

EMD (emerin) (eg, Emery-Dreifuss muscular dystrophy), full gene sequence

ENG (endoglin) (eg, hereditary hemorrhagic telangiectasia, type 1), duplication/deletion analysis

EYA1 (eyes absent homolog 1 [Drosophila]) (eg, branchio-oto-renal [BOR] spectrum disorders), duplication/deletion analysis

FGFR1 (fibroblast growth factor receptor 1) (eg, Kallmann syndrome 2), full gene sequence

FH (fumarate hydratase) (eg, fumarate hydratase deficiency, hereditary leiomyomatosis with renal cell cancer), full gene sequence

FKTN (fukutin) (eg, limb-girdle muscular dystrophy [LGMD] type 2M or 2L), full gene sequence

FTSJ1 (FtsJ RNA methyltransferase homolog 1 [E. coli]) (eg, X-linked mental retardation 9), duplication/deletion analysis

GABRG2 (gamma-aminobutyric acid [GABA] A receptor, gamma 2) (eg, generalized epilepsy with febrile seizures), full gene sequence

GCH1 (GTP cyclohydrolase 1) (eg, autosomal dominant dopa-responsive dystonia), full gene sequence

GDAP1 (ganglioside-induced differentiation-associated protein 1) (eg, Charcot-Marie-Tooth disease), full gene sequence

GFAP (glial fibrillary acidic protein) (eg, Alexander disease), full gene sequence

GHR (growth hormone receptor) (eg, Laron syndrome), full gene sequence

GHRHR (growth hormone releasing hormone receptor) (eg, growth hormone deficiency), full gene sequence

GLA (galactosidase, alpha) (eg, Fabry disease), full gene sequence

HNF1A (HNF1 homeobox A) (eg, maturity-onset diabetes of the young [MODY]), full gene sequence

HNF1B (HNF1 homeobox B) (eg, maturity-onset diabetes of the young [MODY]), full gene sequence

HTRA1 (HtrA serine peptidase 1) (eg, macular degeneration), full gene sequence

IDS (iduronate 2-sulfatase) (eg, mucopolysaccharidosis, type II), full gene sequence

IL2RG (interleukin 2 receptor, gamma) (eg, X-linked severe combined immunodeficiency), full gene sequence

ISPD (isoprenoid synthase domain containing) (eg, muscle-eye-brain disease, Walker-Warburg syndrome), full gene sequence

KRAS (Kirsten rat sarcoma viral oncogene homolog) (eg, Noonan syndrome), full gene sequence

LAMP2 (lysosomal-associated membrane protein 2) (eg, Danon disease), full gene sequence

LDLR (low density lipoprotein receptor) (eg, familial hypercholesterolemia), duplication/deletion analysis

MEN1 (multiple endocrine neoplasia I) (eg, multiple endocrine neoplasia type 1, Wermer syndrome), full gene sequence

MMAA (methylmalonic aciduria [cobalamine deficiency] type A) (eg, MMAA-related methylmalonic acidemia), full gene sequence

MMAB (methylmalonic aciduria [cobalamine deficiency] type B) (eg, MMAA-related methylmalonic acidemia), full gene sequence

MPI (mannose phosphate isomerase) (eg, congenital disorder of glycosylation 1b), full gene sequence

Pathology and Laboratory

81405 — 81405

MPV17 (MpV17 mitochondrial inner membrane protein) (eg, mitochondrial DNA depletion syndrome), full gene sequence

MPZ (myelin protein zero) (eg, Charcot-Marie-Tooth), full gene sequence

MTM1 (myotubularin 1) (eg, X-linked centronuclear myopathy), duplication/deletion analysis

MYL2 (myosin, light chain 2, regulatory, cardiac, slow) (eg, familial hypertrophic cardiomyopathy), full gene sequence

MYL3 (myosin, light chain 3, alkali, ventricular, skeletal, slow) (eg, familial hypertrophic cardiomyopathy), full gene sequence

MYOT (myotilin) (eg, limb-girdle muscular dystrophy), full gene sequence

NDUFS7 (NADH dehydrogenase [ubiquinone] Fe-S protein 7, 20kDa [NADH-coenzyme Q reductase]) (eg, Leigh syndrome, mitochondrial complex I deficiency), full gene sequence

NDUFS8 (NADH dehydrogenase [ubiquinone] Fe-S protein 8, 23kDa [NADH-coenzyme Q reductase]) (eg, Leigh syndrome, mitochondrial complex I deficiency), full gene sequence

NDUFV1 (NADH dehydrogenase [ubiquinone] flavoprotein 1, 51kDa) (eg, Leigh syndrome, mitochondrial complex I deficiency), full gene sequence

NEFL (neurofilament, light polypeptide) (eg, Charcot-Marie-Tooth), full gene sequence

NF2 (neurofibromin 2 [merlin]) (eg, neurofibromatosis, type 2), duplication/deletion analysis

NLGN3 (neuroligin 3) (eg, autism spectrum disorders), full gene sequence

NLGN4X (neuroligin 4, X-linked) (eg, autism spectrum disorders), full gene sequence

NPHP1 (nephronophthisis 1 [juvenile]) (eg, Joubert syndrome), deletion analysis, and duplication analysis, if performed

NPHS2 (nephrosis 2, idiopathic, steroid-resistant [podocin]) (eg, steroid-resistant nephrotic syndrome), full gene sequence

NSD1 (nuclear receptor binding SET domain protein 1) (eg, Sotos syndrome), duplication/deletion analysis

OTC (ornithine carbamoyltransferase) (eg, ornithine transcarbamylase deficiency), full gene sequence

PAFAH1B1 (platelet-activating factor acetylhydrolase 1b, regulatory subunit 1 [45kDa]) (eg, lissencephaly, Miller-Dieker syndrome), duplication/deletion analysis

PARK2 (Parkinson protein 2, E3 ubiquitin protein ligase [parkin]) (eg, Parkinson disease), duplication/deletion analysis

PCCA (propionyl CoA carboxylase, alpha polypeptide) (eg, propionic acidemia, type 1), duplication/deletion analysis

PCDH19 (protocadherin 19) (eg, epileptic encephalopathy), full gene sequence

PDHA1 (pyruvate dehydrogenase [lipoamide] alpha 1) (eg, lactic acidosis), duplication/deletion analysis

PDHB (pyruvate dehydrogenase [lipoamide] beta) (eg, lactic acidosis), full gene sequence

PINK1 (PTEN induced putative kinase 1) (eg, Parkinson disease), full gene sequence

PKLR (pyruvate kinase, liver and RBC) (eg, pyruvate kinase deficiency), full gene sequence

PLP1 (proteolipid protein 1) (eg, Pelizaeus-Merzbacher disease, spastic paraplegia), full gene sequence

POU1F1 (POU class 1 homeobox 1) (eg, combined pituitary hormone deficiency), full gene sequence

PQBP1 (polyglutamine binding protein 1) (eg, Renpenning syndrome), full gene sequence

PRX (periaxin) (eg, Charcot-Marie-Tooth disease), full gene sequence

PSEN1 (presenilin 1) (eg, Alzheimer's disease), full gene sequence

RAB7A (RAB7A, member RAS oncogene family) (eg, Charcot-Marie-Tooth disease), full gene sequence

RAI1 (retinoic acid induced 1) (eg, Smith-Magenis syndrome), full gene sequence

REEP1 (receptor accessory protein 1) (eg, spastic paraplegia), full gene sequence

RET (ret proto-oncogene) (eg, multiple endocrine neoplasia, type 2A and familial medullary thyroid carcinoma), targeted sequence analysis (eg, exons 10, 11, 13-16)

RPS19 (ribosomal protein S19) (eg, Diamond-Blackfan anemia), full gene sequence

RRM2B (ribonucleotide reductase M2 B [TP53 inducible]) (eg, mitochondrial DNA depletion), full gene sequence

SCO1 (SCO cytochrome oxidase deficient homolog 1) (eg, mitochondrial respiratory chain complex IV deficiency), full gene sequence

SDHB (succinate dehydrogenase complex, subunit B, iron sulfur) (eg, hereditary paraganglioma), full gene sequence

SDHC (succinate dehydrogenase complex, subunit C, integral membrane protein, 15kDa) (eg, hereditary paraganglioma-pheochromocytoma syndrome), full gene sequence

SGCA (sarcoglycan, alpha [50kDa dystrophin-associated glycoprotein]) (eg, limb-girdle muscular dystrophy), full gene sequence

SGCB (sarcoglycan, beta [43kDa dystrophin-associated glycoprotein]) (eg, limb-girdle muscular dystrophy), full gene sequence

SGCD (sarcoglycan, delta [35kDa dystrophin-associated glycoprotein]) (eg, limb-girdle muscular dystrophy), full gene sequence

SGCE (sarcoglycan, epsilon) (eg, myoclonic dystonia), duplication/deletion analysis

SGCG (sarcoglycan, gamma [35kDa dystrophin-associated glycoprotein]) (eg, limb-girdle muscular dystrophy), full gene sequence

SHOC2 (soc-2 suppressor of clear homolog) (eg, Noonan-like syndrome with loose anagen hair), full gene sequence

SHOX (short stature homeobox) (eg, Langer mesomelic dysplasia), full gene sequence

SIL1 (SIL1 homolog, endoplasmic reticulum chaperone [S. cerevisiae]) (eg, ataxia), full gene sequence

SLC2A1 (solute carrier family 2 [facilitated glucose transporter], member 1) (eg, glucose transporter type 1 [GLUT 1] deficiency syndrome), full gene sequence

SLC16A2 (solute carrier family 16, member 2 [thyroid hormone transporter]) (eg, specific thyroid hormone cell transporter deficiency, Allan-Herndon-Dudley syndrome), full gene sequence

SLC22A5 (solute carrier family 22 [organic cation/carnitine transporter], member 5) (eg, systemic primary carnitine deficiency), full gene sequence

SLC25A20 (solute carrier family 25 [carnitine/acylcarnitine translocase], member 20) (eg, carnitine-acylcarnitine translocase deficiency), full gene sequence

SMAD4 (SMAD family member 4) (eg, hemorrhagic telangiectasia syndrome, juvenile polyposis), duplication/deletion analysis

SPAST (spastin) (eg, spastic paraplegia), duplication/deletion analysis

SPG7 (spastic paraplegia 7 [pure and complicated autosomal recessive]) (eg, spastic paraplegia), duplication/deletion analysis

SPRED1 (sprouty-related, EVH1 domain containing 1) (eg, Legius syndrome), full gene sequence

STAT3 (signal transducer and activator of transcription 3 [acute-phase response factor]) (eg, autosomal dominant hyper-IgE syndrome), targeted sequence analysis (eg, exons 12, 13, 14, 16, 17, 20, 21)

STK11 (serine/threonine kinase 11) (eg, Peutz-Jeghers syndrome), full gene sequence

SURF1 (surfeit 1) (eg, mitochondrial respiratory chain complex IV deficiency), full gene sequence

TARDBP (TAR DNA binding protein) (eg, amyotrophic lateral sclerosis), full gene sequence

TBX5 (T-box 5) (eg, Holt-Oram syndrome), full gene sequence

TCF4 (transcription factor 4) (eg, Pitt-Hopkins syndrome), duplication/deletion analysis

TGFBR1 (transforming growth factor, beta receptor 1) (eg, Marfan syndrome), full gene sequence

TGFBR2 (transforming growth factor, beta receptor 2) (eg, Marfan syndrome), full gene sequence

THRB (thyroid hormone receptor, beta) (eg, thyroid hormone resistance, thyroid hormone beta receptor deficiency), full gene sequence or targeted sequence analysis of >5 exons

TK2 (thymidine kinase 2, mitochondrial) (eg, mitochondrial DNA depletion syndrome), full gene sequence

TNNC1 (troponin C type 1 [slow]) (eg, hypertrophic cardiomyopathy or dilated cardiomyopathy), full gene sequence

TNNI3 (troponin 1, type 3 [cardiac]) (eg, familial hypertrophic cardiomyopathy), full gene sequence

TPM1 (tropomyosin 1 [alpha]) (eg, familial hypertrophic cardiomyopathy), full gene sequence

TSC1 (tuberous sclerosis 1) (eg, tuberous sclerosis), duplication/deletion analysis

TYMP (thymidine phosphorylase) (eg, mitochondrial DNA depletion syndrome), full gene sequence

VWF (von Willebrand factor) (eg, von Willebrand disease type 2N), targeted sequence analysis (eg, exons 18-20, 23-25)

WT1 (Wilms tumor 1) (eg, Denys-Drash syndrome, familial Wilms tumor), full gene sequence

ZEB2 (zinc finger E-box binding homeobox 2) (eg, Mowat-Wilson syndrome), full gene sequence

0.00 0.00 **FUD** XXX A

AMA: 2020,OctSE,1; 2019,Jul,3; 2018,Nov,9; 2018,Sep,14; 2018,May,6; 2018,Jan,8; 2017,Jan,8; 2016,Aug,9; 2016,Jan,13; 2015,Jan,3; 2015,Jan,16

81406 Molecular pathology procedure, Level 7 (eg, analysis of 11-25 exons by DNA sequence analysis, mutation scanning or duplication/deletion variants of 26-50 exons)

ACADVL (acyl-CoA dehydrogenase, very long chain) (eg, very long chain acyl-coenzyme A dehydrogenase deficiency), full gene sequence

ACTN4 (actinin, alpha 4) (eg, focal segmental glomerulosclerosis), full gene sequence

AFG3L2 (AFG3 ATPase family gene 3-like 2 [S. cerevisiae]) (eg, spinocerebellar ataxia), full gene sequence

AIRE (autoimmune regulator) (eg, autoimmune polyendocrinopathy syndrome type 1), full gene sequence

ALDH7A1 (aldehyde dehydrogenase 7 family, member A1) (eg, pyridoxine-dependent epilepsy), full gene sequence

ANO5 (anoctamin 5) (eg, limb-girdle muscular dystrophy), full gene sequence

ANOS1 (anosim-1) (eg, Kallmann syndrome 1), full gene sequence

APP (amyloid beta [A4] precursor protein) (eg, Alzheimer's disease), full gene sequence

ASS1 (argininosuccinate synthase 1) (eg, citrullinemia type I), full gene sequence

ATL1 (atlastin GTPase 1) (eg, spastic paraplegia), full gene sequence

ATP1A2 (ATPase, Na+/K+ transporting, alpha 2 polypeptide) (eg, familial hemiplegic migraine), full gene sequence

ATP7B (ATPase, Cu++ transporting, beta polypeptide) (eg, Wilson disease), full gene sequence

BBS1 (Bardet-Biedl syndrome 1) (eg, Bardet-Biedl syndrome), full gene sequence

BBS2 (Bardet-Biedl syndrome 2) (eg, Bardet-Biedl syndrome), full gene sequence

BCKDHB (branched-chain keto acid dehydrogenase E1, beta polypeptide) (eg, maple syrup urine disease, type 1B), full gene sequence

BEST1 (bestrophin 1) (eg, vitelliform macular dystrophy), full gene sequence

BMPR2 (bone morphogenetic protein receptor, type II [serine/threonine kinase]) (eg, heritable pulmonary arterial hypertension), full gene sequence

BRAF (B-Raf proto-oncogene, serine/threonine kinase) (eg, Noonan syndrome), full gene sequence

BSCL2 (Berardinelli-Seip congenital lipodystrophy 2 [seipin]) (eg, Berardinelli-Seip congenital lipodystrophy), full gene sequence

BTK (Bruton agammaglobulinemia tyrosine kinase) (eg, X-linked agammaglobulinemia), full gene sequence

CACNB2 (calcium channel, voltage-dependent, beta 2 subunit) (eg, Brugada syndrome), full gene sequence

CAPN3 (calpain 3) (eg, limb-girdle muscular dystrophy [LGMD] type 2A, calpainopathy), full gene sequence

CBS (cystathionine-beta-synthase) (eg, homocystinuria, cystathionine beta-synthase deficiency), full gene sequence

CDH1 (cadherin 1, type 1, E-cadherin [epithelial]) (eg, hereditary diffuse gastric cancer), full gene sequence

CDKL5 (cyclin-dependent kinase-like 5) (eg, early infantile epileptic encephalopathy), full gene sequence

CLCN1 (chloride channel 1, skeletal muscle) (eg, myotonia congenita), full gene sequence

CLCNKB (chloride channel, voltage-sensitive Kb) (eg, Bartter syndrome 3 and 4b), full gene sequence

CNTNAP2 (contactin-associated protein-like 2) (eg, Pitt-Hopkins-like syndrome 1), full gene sequence

COL6A2 (collagen, type VI, alpha 2) (eg, collagen type VI-related disorders), duplication/deletion analysis

CPT1A (carnitine palmitoyltransferase 1A [liver]) (eg, carnitine palmitoyltransferase 1A [CPT1A] deficiency), full gene sequence

CRB1 (crumbs homolog 1 [Drosophila]) (eg, Leber congenital amaurosis), full gene sequence

CREBBP (CREB binding protein) (eg, Rubinstein-Taybi syndrome), duplication/deletion analysis

DBT (dihydrolipoamide branched chain transacylase E2) (eg, maple syrup urine disease, type 2), full gene sequence

DLAT (dihydrolipoamide S-acetyltransferase) (eg, pyruvate dehydrogenase E2 deficiency), full gene sequence

DLD (dihydrolipoamide dehydrogenase) (eg, maple syrup urine disease, type III), full gene sequence

DSC2 (desmocollin) (eg, arrhythmogenic right ventricular dysplasia/cardiomyopathy 11), full gene sequence

DSG2 (desmoglein 2) (eg, arrhythmogenic right ventricular dysplasia/cardiomyopathy 10), full gene sequence

DSP (desmoplakin) (eg, arrhythmogenic right ventricular dysplasia/cardiomyopathy 8), full gene sequence

EFHC1 (EF-hand domain [C-terminal] containing 1) (eg, juvenile myoclonic epilepsy), full gene sequence

EIF2B3 (eukaryotic translation initiation factor 2B, subunit 3 gamma, 58kDa) (eg, leukoencephalopathy with vanishing white matter), full gene sequence

EIF2B4 (eukaryotic translation initiation factor 2B, subunit 4 delta, 67kDa) (eg, leukoencephalopathy with vanishing white matter), full gene sequence

EIF2B5 (eukaryotic translation initiation factor 2B, subunit 5 epsilon, 82kDa) (eg, childhood ataxia with central nervous system hypomyelination/vanishing white matter), full gene sequence

ENG (endoglin) (eg, hereditary hemorrhagic telangiectasia, type 1), full gene sequence

EYA1 (eyes absent homolog 1 [Drosophila]) (eg, branchio-oto-renal [BOR] spectrum disorders), full gene sequence

F8 (coagulation factor VIII) (eg, hemophilia A), duplication/deletion analysis

FAH (fumarylacetoacetate hydrolase [fumarylacetoacetase]) (eg, tyrosinemia, type 1), full gene sequence

FASTKD2 (FAST kinase domains 2) (eg, mitochondrial respiratory chain complex IV deficiency), full gene sequence

FIG4 (FIG4 homolog, SAC1 lipid phosphatase domain containing [S. cerevisiae]) (eg, Charcot-Marie-Tooth disease), full gene sequence

FTSJ1 (FtsJ RNA methyltransferase homolog 1 [E. coli]) (eg, X-linked mental retardation 9), full gene sequence

FUS (fused in sarcoma) (eg, amyotrophic lateral sclerosis), full gene sequence

GAA (glucosidase, alpha; acid) (eg, glycogen storage disease type II [Pompe disease]), full gene sequence

GALC (galactosylceramidase) (eg, Krabbe disease), full gene sequence

GALT (galactose-1-phosphate uridylyltransferase) (eg, galactosemia), full gene sequence

GARS (glycyl-tRNA synthetase) (eg, Charcot-Marie-Tooth disease), full gene sequence

GCDH (glutaryl-CoA dehydrogenase) (eg, glutaricacidemia type 1), full gene sequence

GCK (glucokinase [hexokinase 4]) (eg, maturity-onset diabetes of the young [MODY]), full gene sequence

GLUD1 (glutamate dehydrogenase 1) (eg, familial hyperinsulinism), full gene sequence

GNE (glucosamine [UDP-N-acetyl]-2-epimerase/N-acetylmannosamine kinase) (eg, inclusion body myopathy 2 [IBM2], Nonaka myopathy), full gene sequence

GRN (granulin) (eg, frontotemporal dementia), full gene sequence

HADHA (hydroxyacyl-CoA dehydrogenase/3-ketoacyl-CoA thiolase/enoyl-CoA hydratase [trifunctional protein] alpha subunit) (eg, long chain acyl-coenzyme A dehydrogenase deficiency), full gene sequence

HADHB (hydroxyacyl-CoA dehydrogenase/3-ketoacyl-CoA thiolase/enoyl-CoA hydratase [trifunctional protein], beta subunit) (eg, trifunctional protein deficiency), full gene sequence

HEXA (hexosaminidase A, alpha polypeptide) (eg, Tay-Sachs disease), full gene sequence

HLCS (HLCS holocarboxylase synthetase) (eg, holocarboxylase synthetase deficiency), full gene sequence

HMBS (hydroxymethylbilane synthase) (eg, acute intermittent porphyria), full gene sequence

HNF4A (hepatocyte nuclear factor 4, alpha) (eg, maturity-onset diabetes of the young [MODY]), full gene sequence

IDUA (iduronidase, alpha-L-) (eg, mucopolysaccharidosis type I), full gene sequence

INF2 (inverted formin, FH2 and WH2 domain containing) (eg, focal segmental glomerulosclerosis), full gene sequence

IVD (isovaleryl-CoA dehydrogenase) (eg, isovaleric acidemia), full gene sequence

JAG1 (jagged 1) (eg, Alagille syndrome), duplication/deletion analysis

JUP (junction plakoglobin) (eg, arrhythmogenic right ventricular dysplasia/cardiomyopathy 11), full gene sequence

KCNH2 (potassium voltage-gated channel, subfamily H [eag-related], member 2) (eg, short QT syndrome, long QT syndrome), full gene sequence

KCNQ1 (potassium voltage-gated channel, KQT-like subfamily, member 1) (eg, short QT syndrome, long QT syndrome), full gene sequence

KCNQ2 (potassium voltage-gated channel, KQT-like subfamily, member 2) (eg, epileptic encephalopathy), full gene sequence

LDB3 (LIM domain binding 3) (eg, familial dilated cardiomyopathy, myofibrillar myopathy), full gene sequence

LDLR (low density lipoprotein receptor) (eg, familial hypercholesterolemia), full gene sequence

LEPR (leptin receptor(eg, obesity with hypogonadism), full gene sequence

LHCGR (luteinizing hormone/choriogonadotropin receptor) (eg, precocious male puberty), full gene sequence

LMNA (lamin A/C) (eg, Emery-Dreifuss muscular dystrophy [EDMD1, 2 and 3] limb-girdle muscular dystrophy [LGMD] type 1B, dilated cardiomyopathy [CMD1A], familial partial lipodystrophy [FPLD2]), full gene sequence

LRP5 (low density lipoprotein receptor-related protein 5) (eg, osteopetrosis), full gene sequence

MAP2K1 (mitogen-activated protein kinase 1) (eg, cardiofaciocutaneous syndrome), full gene sequence

MAP2K2 (mitogen-activated protein kinase 2) (eg, cardiofaciocutaneous syndrome), full gene sequence

MAPT (microtubule-associated protein tau) (eg, frontotemporal dementia), full gene sequence

MCCC1 (methylcrotonoyl-CoA carboxylase 1 [alpha]) (eg, 3-methylcrotonyl-CoA carboxylase deficiency), full gene sequence

MCCC2 (methylcrotonoyl-CoA carboxylase 2 [beta]) (eg, 3-methylcrotonyl carboxylase deficiency), full gene sequence

MFN2 (mitofusin 2) (eg, Charcot-Marie-Tooth disease), full gene sequence

MTM1 (myotubularin 1) (eg, X-linked centronuclear myopathy), full gene sequence

MUT (methylmalonyl CoA mutase) (eg, methylmalonic acidemia), full gene sequence

MUTYH (mutY homolog [E. coli]) (eg, MYH-associated polyposis), full gene sequence

NDUFS1 (NADH dehydrogenase [ubiquinone] Fe-S protein 1, 75kDa [NADH-coenzyme Q reductase]) (eg, Leigh syndrome, mitochondrial complex I deficiency), full gene sequence

NF2 (neurofibromin 2 [merlin]) (eg, neurofibromatosis, type 2), full gene sequence

NOTCH3 (notch 3) (eg, cerebral autosomal dominant arteriopathy with subcortical infarcts and leukoencephalopathy [CADASIL]), targeted sequence analysis (eg, exons 1-23)

NPC1 (Niemann-Pick disease, type C1) (eg, Niemann-Pick disease), full gene sequence

NPHP1 (nephronophthisis 1 [juvenile]) (eg, Joubert syndrome), full gene sequence

NSD1 (nuclear receptor binding SET domain protein 1) (eg, Sotos syndrome), full gene sequence

OPA1 (optic atrophy 1) (eg, optic atrophy), duplication/deletion analysis

OPTN (optineurin) (eg, amyotrophic lateral sclerosis), full gene sequence

PAFAH1B1 (platelet-activating factor acetylhydrolase 1b, regulatory subunit 1 [45kDa]) (eg, lissencephaly, Miller-Dieker syndrome), full gene sequence

PAH (phenylalanine hydroxylase) (eg, phenylketonuria), full gene sequence

PALB2 (partner and localizer of BRCA2) (eg, breast and pancreatic cancer), full gene sequence

PARK2 (Parkinson protein 2, E3 ubiquitin protein ligase [parkin]) (eg, Parkinson disease), full gene sequence

PAX2 (paired box 2) (eg, renal coloboma syndrome), full gene sequence

PC (pyruvate carboxylase) (eg, pyruvate carboxylase deficiency), full gene sequence

PCCA (propionyl CoA carboxylase, alpha polypeptide) (eg, propionic acidemia, type 1), full gene sequence

PCCB (propionyl CoA carboxylase, beta polypeptide) (eg, propionic acidemia), full gene sequence

PCDH15 (protocadherin-related 15) (eg, Usher syndrome type 1F), duplication/deletion analysis

PCSK9 (proprotein convertase subtilisin/kexin type 9) (eg familial hypercholesterolemia), full gene sequence

PDHA1 (pyruvate dehydrogenase [lipoamide] alpha 1) (eg, lactic acidosis), full gene sequence

PDHX (pyruvate dehydrogenase complex, component X) (eg, lactic acidosis), full gene sequence

PHEX (phosphate-regulating endopeptidase homolog, X-linked) (eg, hypophosphatemic rickets), full gene sequence

PKD2 (polycystic kidney disease 2 [autosomal dominant]) (eg, polycystic kidney disease), full gene sequence

PKP2 (plakophilin 2) (eg, arrhythmogenic right ventricular dysplasia/cardiomyopathy 9), full gene sequence

PNKD (eg, paroxysmal nonkinesigenic dyskinesia), full gene sequence

POLG (polymerase [DNA directed], gamma) (eg, Alpers-Huttenlocher syndrome, autosomal dominant progressive external ophthalmoplegia), full gene sequence

POMGNT1 (protein O-linked mannose beta1, 2-N acetylglucosaminyltransferase) (eg, muscle-eye-brain disease, Walker-Warburg syndrome), full gene sequence

POMT1 (protein-O-mannosyltransferase 1) (eg, limb-girdle muscular dystrophy [LGMD] type 2K, Walker-Warburg syndrome), full gene sequence

POMT2 (protein-O-mannosyltransferase 2) (eg, limb-girdle muscular dystrophy [LGMD] type 2N, Walker-Warburg syndrome), full gene sequence

PPOX (protoporphyrinogen oxidase) (eg, variegate porphyria), full gene sequence

PRKAG2 (protein kinase, AMP-activated, gamma 2 non-catalytic subunit) (eg, familial hypertrophic cardiomyopathy with Wolff-Parkinson-White syndrome, lethal congenital glycogen storage disease of heart), full gene sequence

PRKCG (protein kinase C, gamma) (eg, spinocerebellar ataxia), full gene sequence

PSEN2 (presenilin 2[Alzheimer's disease 4]) (eg, Alzheimer's disease), full gene sequence

PTPN11 (protein tyrosine phosphatase, non-receptor type 11) (eg, Noonan syndrome, LEOPARD syndrome), full gene sequence

PYGM (phosphorylase, glycogen, muscle) (eg, glycogen storage disease type V, McArdle disease), full gene sequence

RAF1 (v-raf-1 murine leukemia viral oncogene homolog 1) (eg, LEOPARD syndrome), full gene sequence

RET (ret proto-oncogene) (eg, Hirschsprung disease), full gene sequence

RPE65 (retinal pigment epithelium-specific protein 65kDa) (eg, retinitis pigmentosa, Leber congenital amaurosis), full gene sequence

RYR1 (ryanodine receptor 1, skeletal) (eg, malignant hyperthermia), targeted sequence analysis of exons with functionally-confirmed mutations

SCN4A (sodium channel, voltage-gated, type IV, alpha subunit) (eg, hyperkalemic periodic paralysis), full gene sequence

SCNN1A (sodium channel, nonvoltage-gated 1 alpha) (eg, pseudohypoaldosteronism), full gene sequence

SCNN1B (sodium channel, nonvoltage-gated 1, beta) (eg, Liddle syndrome, pseudohypoaldosteronism), full gene sequence

SCNN1G (sodium channel, nonvoltage-gated 1, gamma) (eg, Liddle syndrome, pseudohypoaldosteronism), full gene sequence

SDHA (succinate dehydrogenase complex, subunit A, flavoprotein [Fp]) (eg, Leigh syndrome, mitochondrial complex II deficiency), full gene sequence

SETX (senataxin) (eg, ataxia), full gene sequence

SGCE (sarcoglycan, epsilon) (eg, myoclonic dystonia), full gene sequence

SH3TC2 (SH3 domain and tetratricopeptide repeats 2) (eg, Charcot-Marie-Tooth disease), full gene sequence

SLC9A6 (solute carrier family 9 [sodium/hydrogen exchanger], member 6) (eg, Christianson syndrome), full gene sequence

SLC26A4 (solute carrier family 26, member 4) (eg, Pendred syndrome), full gene sequence

SLC37A4 (solute carrier family 37 [glucose-6-phosphate transporter], member 4) (eg, glycogen storage disease type Ib), full gene sequence

SMAD4 (SMAD family member 4) (eg, hemorrhagic telangiectasia syndrome, juvenile polyposis), full gene sequence

SOS1 (son of sevenless homolog 1) (eg, Noonan syndrome, gingival fibromatosis), full gene sequence

SPAST (spastin) (eg, spastic paraplegia), full gene sequence

SPG7 (spastic paraplegia 7 [pure and complicated autosomal recessive]) (eg, spastic paraplegia), full gene sequence

STXBP1 (syntaxin-binding protein 1) (eg, epileptic encephalopathy), full gene sequence

TAZ (tafazzin) (eg, methylglutaconic aciduria type 2, Barth syndrome), full gene sequence

TCF4 (transcription factor 4) (eg, Pitt-Hopkins syndrome), full gene sequence

TH (tyrosine hydroxylase) (eg, Segawa syndrome), full gene sequence

TMEM43 (transmembrane protein 43) (eg, arrhythmogenic right ventricular cardiomyopathy), full gene sequence

TNNT2 (troponin T, type 2 [cardiac]) (eg, familial hypertrophic cardiomyopathy), full gene sequence

TRPC6 (transient receptor potential cation channel, subfamily C, member 6) (eg, focal segmental glomerulosclerosis), full gene sequence

TSC1 (tuberous sclerosis 1) (eg, tuberous sclerosis), full gene sequence

TSC2 (tuberous sclerosis 2) (eg, tuberous sclerosis), duplication/deletion analysis

UBE3A (ubiquitin protein ligase E3A) (eg, Angelman syndrome) full gene sequence

UMOD (uromodulin) (eg, glomerulocystic kidney disease with hyperuricemia and isosthenuria), full gene sequence

VWF (von Willebrand factor) (von Willebrand disease type 2A), extended targeted sequence analysis (eg, exons 11-16, 24-26, 51, 52)

WAS (Wiskott-Aldrich syndrome [eczema-thrombocytopenia]) (eg, Wiskott-Aldrich syndrome), full gene sequence

0.00 0.00 **FUD** XXX A

AMA: 2020,OctSE,1; 2020,Feb,10; 2018,Nov,9; 2018,May,6; 2018,Jan,8; 2017,Apr,9; 2017,Jan,8; 2016,Aug,9; 2016,Jan,13; 2015,Jan,3; 2015,Jan,16

81407 Molecular pathology procedure, Level 8 (eg, analysis of 26-50 exons by DNA sequence analysis, mutation scanning or duplication/deletion variants of >50 exons, sequence analysis of multiple genes on one platform)

ABCC8 (ATP-binding cassette, sub-family C [CFTR/MRP], member 8) (eg, familial hyperinsulinism), full gene sequence

AGL (amylo-alpha-1, 6-glucosidase, 4-alpha-glucanotransferase) (eg, glycogen storage disease type III), full gene sequence

AHI1 (Abelson helper integration site 1) (eg, Joubert syndrome), full gene sequence

APOB (apolipoprotein B) (eg, familial hypercholesterolemia type B) full gene sequence

ASPM (asp [abnormal spindle] homolog, microcephaly associated [Drosophila]) (eg, primary microcephaly), full gene sequence

CHD7 (chromodomain helicase DNA binding protein 7) (eg, CHARGE syndrome), full gene sequence

COL4A4 (collagen, type IV, alpha 4) (eg, Alport syndrome), full gene sequence

COL4A5 (collagen, type IV, alpha 5) (eg, Alport syndrome), duplication/deletion analysis

COL6A1 (collagen, type VI, alpha 1) (eg, collagen type VI-related disorders), full gene sequence

COL6A2 (collagen, type VI, alpha 2) (eg, collagen type VI-related disorders), full gene sequence

COL6A3 (collagen, type VI, alpha 3) (eg, collagen type VI-related disorders), full gene sequence

CREBBP (CREB binding protein) (eg, Rubinstein-Taybi syndrome), full gene sequence

F8 (coagulation factor VIII) (eg, hemophilia A), full gene sequence

JAG1 (jagged 1) (eg, Alagille syndrome), full gene sequence

KDM5C (lysine [K]-specific demethylase 5C) (eg, X-linked mental retardation), full gene sequence

KIAA0196 (KIAA0196) (eg, spastic paraplegia), full gene sequence

L1CAM (L1 cell adhesion molecule) (eg, MASA syndrome, X-linked hydrocephaly), full gene sequence

LAMB2 (laminin, beta 2 [laminin S]) (eg, Pierson syndrome), full gene sequence

MYBPC3 (myosin binding protein C, cardiac) (eg, familial hypertrophic cardiomyopathy), full gene sequence

MYH6 (myosin, heavy chain 6, cardiac muscle, alpha) (eg, familial dilated cardiomyopathy), full gene sequence

MYH7 (myosin, heavy chain 7, cardiac muscle, beta) (eg, familial hypertrophic cardiomyopathy, Liang distal myopathy), full gene sequence

MYO7A (myosin VIIA) (eg, Usher syndrome, type 1), full gene sequence

NOTCH1 (notch 1) (eg, aortic valve disease), full gene sequence

NPHS1 (nephrosis 1, congenital, Finnish type [nephrin]) (eg, congenital Finnish nephrosis), full gene sequence

OPA1 (optic atrophy 1) (eg, optic atrophy), full gene sequence

PCDH15 (protocadherin-related 15) (eg, Usher syndrome, type 1), full gene sequence

PKD1 (polycystic kidney disease 1 [autosomal dominant]) (eg, polycystic kidney disease), full gene sequence

PLCE1 (phospholipase C, epsilon 1) (eg, nephrotic syndrome type 3), full gene sequence

SCN1A (sodium channel, voltage-gated, type 1, alpha subunit) (eg, generalized epilepsy with febrile seizures), full gene sequence

SCN5A (sodium channel, voltage-gated, type V, alpha subunit) (eg, familial dilated cardiomyopathy), full gene sequence

SLC12A1 (solute carrier family 12 [sodium/potassium/chloride transporters], member 1) (eg, Bartter syndrome), full gene sequence

SLC12A3 (solute carrier family 12 [sodium/chloride transporters], member 3) (eg, Gitelman syndrome), full gene sequence

SPG11 (spastic paraplegia 11 [autosomal recessive]) (eg, spastic paraplegia), full gene sequence

SPTBN2 (spectrin, beta, non-erythrocytic 2) (eg, spinocerebellar ataxia), full gene sequence

TMEM67 (transmembrane protein 67) (eg, Joubert syndrome), full gene sequence

TSC2 (tuberous sclerosis 2) (eg, tuberous sclerosis), full gene sequence

USH1C (Usher syndrome 1C [autosomal recessive, severe]) (eg, Usher syndrome, type 1), full gene sequence

VPS13B (vacuolar protein sorting 13 homolog B [yeast]) (eg, Cohen syndrome), duplication/deletion analysis

WDR62 (WD repeat domain 62) (eg, primary autosomal recessive microcephaly), full gene sequence

0.00 0.00 **FUD** XXX A

AMA: 2020,OctSE,1; 2019,Jul,3; 2018,Nov,9; 2018,May,6; 2018,Jan,8; 2017,Jan,8; 2016,Aug,9; 2016,Jan,13; 2015,Jan,16; 2015,Jan,3

81408 Molecular pathology procedure, Level 9 (eg, analysis of >50 exons in a single gene by DNA sequence analysis)

ABCA4 (ATP-binding cassette, sub-family A [ABC1], member 4) (eg, Stargardt disease, age-related macular degeneration), full gene sequence

ATM (ataxia telangiectasia mutated) (eg, ataxia telangiectasia), full gene sequence

CDH23 (cadherin-related 23) (eg, Usher syndrome, type 1), full gene sequence

CEP290 (centrosomal protein 290kDa) (eg, Joubert syndrome), full gene sequence

COL1A1 (collagen, type I, alpha 1) (eg, osteogenesis imperfecta, type I), full gene sequence

COL1A2 (collagen, type I, alpha 2) (eg, osteogenesis imperfecta, type I), full gene sequence

COL4A1 (collagen, type IV, alpha 1) (eg, brain small-vessel disease with hemorrhage), full gene sequence

COL4A3 (collagen, type IV, alpha 3 [Goodpasture antigen]) (eg, Alport syndrome), full gene sequence

COL4A5 (collagen, type IV, alpha 5) (eg, Alport syndrome), full gene sequence

DMD (dystrophin) (eg, Duchenne/Becker muscular dystrophy), full gene sequence

DYSF (dysferlin, limb girdle muscular dystrophy 2B [autosomal recessive]) (eg, limb-girdle muscular dystrophy), full gene sequence

FBN1 (fibrillin 1) (eg, Marfan syndrome), full gene sequence

ITPR1 (inositol 1,4,5-trisphosphate receptor, type 1) (eg, spinocerebellar ataxia), full gene sequence

LAMA2 (laminin, alpha 2) (eg, congenital muscular dystrophy), full gene sequence

LRRK2 (leucine-rich repeat kinase 2) (eg, Parkinson disease), full gene sequence

MYH11 (myosin, heavy chain 11, smooth muscle) (eg, thoracic aortic aneurysms and aortic dissections), full gene sequence

NEB (nebulin) (eg, nemaline myopathy 2), full gene sequence

NF1 (neurofibromin 1) (eg, neurofibromatosis, type 1), full gene sequence

PKHD1 (polycystic kidney and hepatic disease 1) (eg, autosomal recessive polycystic kidney disease), full gene sequence

RYR1 (ryanodine receptor 1, skeletal) (eg, malignant hyperthermia), full gene sequence

RYR2 (ryanodine receptor 2 [cardiac]) (eg, catecholaminergic polymorphic ventricular tachycardia, arrhythmogenic right ventricular dysplasia), full gene sequence or targeted sequence analysis of > 50 exons

USH2A (Usher syndrome 2A [autosomal recessive, mild]) (eg, Usher syndrome, type 2), full gene sequence

VPS13B (vacuolar protein sorting 13 homolog B [yeast]) (eg, Cohen syndrome), full gene sequence

VWF (von Willebrand factor) (eg, von Willebrand disease types 1 and 3), full gene sequence

0.00 0.00 FUD XXX A

AMA: 2020,OctSE,1; 2018,Nov,9; 2018,May,6; 2018,Jan,8; 2017,Jan,8; 2016,Aug,9; 2016,Jan,13; 2015,Jan,16; 2015,Jan,3

81479 **Unlisted molecular pathology procedure**

0.00 0.00 FUD XXX A

AMA: 2019,Jun,11; 2019,May,5; 2018,Dec,10; 2018,Dec,10; 2018,Nov,9; 2018,Sep,14; 2018,Jun,8; 2018,May,6; 2018,Jan,8; 2017,Apr,9; 2017,Jan,8; 2016,Sep,9; 2016,Aug,9; 2016,Apr,4; 2016,Jan,13; 2015,Jan,3; 2015,Jan,16

81410-81479 [81419, 81443, 81448, 81479] Genomic Sequencing

EXCLUDES *In situ hybridization analyses (88271-88275, 88365-88368 [88364, 88373, 88374])*
Microbial identification (87149-87153, 87471-87801 [87623, 87624, 87625], 87900-87904 [87906, 87910, 87912])

81410 **Aortic dysfunction or dilation (eg, Marfan syndrome, Loeys Dietz syndrome, Ehler Danlos syndrome type IV, arterial tortuosity syndrome); genomic sequence analysis panel, must include sequencing of at least 9 genes, including *FBN1, TGFBR1, TGFBR2, COL3A1, MYH11, ACTA2, SLC2A10, SMAD3,* and *MYLK***

0.00 0.00 FUD XXX A

AMA: 2018,Jan,8; 2017,Jan,8; 2016,Jan,13; 2015,Jan,3

81411 **duplication/deletion analysis panel, must include analyses for *TGFBR1, TGFBR2, MYH11, and COL3A1***

0.00 0.00 FUD XXX A

AMA: 2018,Jan,8; 2017,Jan,8; 2016,Jan,13; 2015,Jan,3

81412 **Ashkenazi Jewish associated disorders (eg, Bloom syndrome, Canavan disease, cystic fibrosis, familial dysautonomia, Fanconi anemia group C, Gaucher disease, Tay-Sachs disease), genomic sequence analysis panel, must include sequencing of at least 9 genes, including *ASPA, BLM, CFTR, FANCC, GBA, HEXA, IKBKAP, MCOLN1,* and *SMPD1***

0.00 0.00 FUD XXX A

AMA: 2018,Nov,9; 2018,Jan,8; 2017,Jan,8; 2016,Apr,4

81413 **Cardiac ion channelopathies (eg, Brugada syndrome, long QT syndrome, short QT syndrome, catecholaminergic polymorphic ventricular tachycardia); genomic sequence analysis panel, must include sequencing of at least 10 genes, including ANK2, CASQ2, CAV3, KCNE1, KCNE2, KCNH2, KCNJ2, KCNQ1, RYR2, and SCN5A**

EXCLUDES *Evaluation cardiomyopathy (81439)*

0.00 0.00 FUD XXX A

AMA: 2018,Jan,8; 2017,Apr,3

81414 **duplication/deletion gene analysis panel, must include analysis of at least 2 genes, including KCNH2 and KCNQ1**

EXCLUDES *Evaluation cardiomyopathy (81439)*

0.00 0.00 FUD XXX A

AMA: 2018,Jan,8; 2017,Apr,3

● # **81419** **Epilepsy genomic sequence analysis panel, must include analyses for *ALDH7A1, CACNA1A, CDKL5, CHD2, GABRG2, GRIN2A, KCNQ2, MECP2, PCDH19, POLG, PRRT2, SCN1A, SCN1B, SCN2A, SCN8A, SLC2A1, SLC9A6, STXBP1, SYNGAP1, TCF4, TPP1, TSC1, TSC2,* and *ZEB2***

0.00 0.00 FUD 000

81415 **Exome (eg, unexplained constitutional or heritable disorder or syndrome); sequence analysis**

0.00 0.00 FUD XXX A

AMA: 2018,Jan,8; 2017,Jan,8; 2016,Jan,13; 2015,Jan,3

+ **81416** **sequence analysis, each comparator exome (eg, parents, siblings) (List separately in addition to code for primary procedure)**

Code first (81415)

0.00 0.00 FUD XXX A

AMA: 2018,Jan,8; 2017,Jan,8; 2016,Jan,13; 2015,Jan,3

81417 **re-evaluation of previously obtained exome sequence (eg, updated knowledge or unrelated condition/syndrome)**

EXCLUDES *Incidental results*
Microarray assessment (81228-81229)

0.00 0.00 FUD XXX A

AMA: 2018,Jan,8; 2017,Jan,8; 2016,Jan,13; 2015,Jan,3

81419 **Resequenced code. See code following 81414.**

81420 **Fetal chromosomal aneuploidy (eg, trisomy 21, monosomy X) genomic sequence analysis panel, circulating cell-free fetal DNA in maternal blood, must include analysis of chromosomes 13, 18, and 21** M

EXCLUDES *Genome-wide microarray analysis (81228-81229)*
Molecular cytogenetics (88271)

0.00 0.00 FUD XXX A

AMA: 2018,Apr,10; 2018,Jan,8; 2017,Jan,8; 2016,Jan,13; 2015,Dec,18; 2015,Jan,3

81422 **Fetal chromosomal microdeletion(s) genomic sequence analysis (eg, DiGeorge syndrome, Cri-du-chat syndrome), circulating cell-free fetal DNA in maternal blood**

EXCLUDES *Genome-wide microarray analysis (81228-81229)*
Molecular cytogenetics (88271)

0.00 0.00 FUD XXX A

AMA: 2018,Jan,8; 2017,Apr,3

81443 **Genetic testing for severe inherited conditions (eg, cystic fibrosis, Ashkenazi Jewish-associated disorders [eg, Bloom syndrome, Canavan disease, Fanconi anemia type C, mucolipidosis type VI, Gaucher disease, Tay-Sachs disease], beta hemoglobinopathies, phenylketonuria, galactosemia), genomic sequence analysis panel, must include sequencing of at least 15 genes (eg, *ACADM, ARSA, ASPA, ATP7B, BCKDHA, BCKDHB, BLM, CFTR, DHCR7, FANCC, G6PC, GAA, GALT, GBA, GBE1, HBB, HEXA, IKBKAP, MCOLN1, PAH*)**

EXCLUDES *When performed separately:*
Ashkenazi Jewish-associated disorder analysis only (81412)
Fragile X mental retardation (FMR1) analysis (81243)
Hemoglobin A testing ([81257])
Spinal muscular atrophy (SMN1) analysis (81329)

0.00 0.00 FUD XXX

AMA: 2019,Jul,3; 2018,Nov,9

81425 **Genome (eg, unexplained constitutional or heritable disorder or syndrome); sequence analysis**

0.00 0.00 FUD XXX A

AMA: 2018,Jan,8; 2017,Jan,8; 2016,Jan,13; 2015,Jan,3

+ **81426** **sequence analysis, each comparator genome (eg, parents, siblings) (List separately in addition to code for primary procedure)**

Code first (81425)

0.00 0.00 FUD XXX A

AMA: 2018,Jan,8; 2017,Jan,8; 2016,Jan,13; 2015,Jan,3

81427 **re-evaluation of previously obtained genome sequence (eg, updated knowledge or unrelated condition/syndrome)**

EXCLUDES *Genome-wide microarray analysis (81228-81229)*
Incidental results

0.00 0.00 FUD XXX A

AMA: 2018,Jan,8; 2017,Jan,8; 2016,Jan,13; 2015,Jan,3

81430 **Hearing loss (eg, nonsyndromic hearing loss, Usher syndrome, Pendred syndrome); genomic sequence analysis panel, must include sequencing of at least 60 genes, including *CDH23, CLRN1, GJB2, GPR98, MTRNR1, MYO7A, MYO15A, PCDH15, OTOF, SLC26A4, TMC1, TMPRSS3, USH1C, USH1G, USH2A,* and *WFS1***
0.00 0.00 FUD XXX
AMA: 2018,Jan,8; 2017,Jan,8; 2016,Jan,13; 2015,Jan,3

81431 **duplication/deletion analysis panel, must include copy number analyses for *STRC* and *DFNB1* deletions in *GJB2* and *GJB6* genes**
0.00 0.00 FUD XXX
AMA: 2018,Jan,8; 2017,Jan,8; 2016,Jan,13; 2015,Jan,3

81432 **Hereditary breast cancer-related disorders (eg, hereditary breast cancer, hereditary ovarian cancer, hereditary endometrial cancer); genomic sequence analysis panel, must include sequencing of at least 10 genes, always including *BRCA1, BRCA2, CDH1, MLH1, MSH2, MSH6, PALB2, PTEN, STK11, and TP53***
0.00 0.00 FUD XXX
AMA: 2019,May,5; 2018,Jan,8; 2017,Jan,8; 2016,Apr,4

81433 **duplication/deletion analysis panel, must include analyses for *BRCA1, BRCA2, MLH1, MSH2,* and *STK11***
0.00 0.00 FUD XXX
AMA: 2018,Jan,8; 2017,Jan,8; 2016,Apr,4

81434 **Hereditary retinal disorders (eg, retinitis pigmentosa, Leber congenital amaurosis, cone-rod dystrophy), genomic sequence analysis panel, must include sequencing of at least 15 genes, including *ABCA4, CNGA1, CRB1, EYS, PDE6A, PDE6B, PRPF31, PRPH2, RDH12, RHO, RP1, RP2, RPE65, RPGR,* and *USH2A***
0.00 0.00 FUD XXX
AMA: 2018,Jan,8; 2017,Jan,8; 2016,Apr,4

81435 **Hereditary colon cancer disorders (eg, Lynch syndrome, PTEN hamartoma syndrome, Cowden syndrome, familial adenomatosis polyposis); genomic sequence analysis panel, must include sequencing of at least 10 genes, including *APC, BMPR1A, CDH1, MLH1, MSH2, MSH6, MUTYH, PTEN, SMAD4,* and *STK11***
0.00 0.00 FUD XXX
AMA: 2018,Jan,8; 2017,Jan,8; 2016,Apr,4; 2016,Jan,13; 2015,Jan,3

81436 **duplication/deletion analysis panel, must include analysis of at least 5 genes, including *MLH1, MSH2, EPCAM, SMAD4,* and *STK11***
0.00 0.00 FUD XXX
AMA: 2018,Jan,8; 2017,Jan,8; 2016,Apr,4; 2016,Jan,13; 2015,Jan,3

81437 **Hereditary neuroendocrine tumor disorders (eg, medullary thyroid carcinoma, parathyroid carcinoma, malignant pheochromocytoma or paraganglioma); genomic sequence analysis panel, must include sequencing of at least 6 genes, including *MAX, SDHB, SDHC, SDHD, TMEM127,* and *VHL***
0.00 0.00 FUD XXX
AMA: 2018,Jan,8; 2017,Jan,8; 2016,Apr,4

81438 **duplication/deletion analysis panel, must include analyses for *SDHB, SDHC, SDHD,* and *VHL***
0.00 0.00 FUD XXX
AMA: 2018,Jan,8; 2017,Jan,8; 2016,Apr,4

\# **81448** **Hereditary peripheral neuropathies (eg, Charcot-Marie-Tooth, spastic paraplegia), genomic sequence analysis panel, must include sequencing of at least 5 peripheral neuropathy-related genes (eg, *BSCL2, GJB1, MFN2, MPZ, REEP1, SPAST, SPG11, SPTLC1*)**
0.00 0.00 FUD XXX
AMA: 2018,May,6

81439 **Hereditary cardiomyopathy (eg, hypertrophic cardiomyopathy, dilated cardiomyopathy, arrhythmogenic right ventricular cardiomyopathy), genomic sequence analysis panel, must include sequencing of at least 5 cardiomyopathy-related genes (eg, *DSG2, MYBPC3, MYH7, PKP2, TTN*)**
EXCLUDES *Genetic sequencing for cardiac ion channelopathies (81413-81414)*
0.00 0.00 FUD XXX
AMA: 2018,Sep,14; 2018,Jan,8; 2017,Apr,3

81440 **Nuclear encoded mitochondrial genes (eg, neurologic or myopathic phenotypes), genomic sequence panel, must include analysis of at least 100 genes, including *BCS1L, C10orf2, COQ2, COX10, DGUOK, MPV17, OPA1, PDSS2, POLG, POLG2, RRM2B, SCO1, SCO2, SLC25A4, SUCLA2, SUCLG1, TAZ, TK2,* and *TYMP***
0.00 0.00 FUD XXX
AMA: 2018,Jan,8; 2017,Jan,8; 2016,Jan,13; 2015,Jan,3

81442 **Noonan spectrum disorders (eg, Noonan syndrome, cardio-facio-cutaneous syndrome, Costello syndrome, LEOPARD syndrome, Noonan-like syndrome), genomic sequence analysis panel, must include sequencing of at least 12 genes, including *BRAF, CBL, HRAS, KRAS, MAP2K1, MAP2K2, NRAS, PTPN11, RAF1, RIT1, SHOC2,* and *SOS1***
0.00 0.00 FUD XXX
AMA: 2018,Jan,8; 2017,Jan,8; 2016,Apr,4

81443 **Resequenced code. See code following 81422.**

81445 **Targeted genomic sequence analysis panel, solid organ neoplasm, DNA analysis, and RNA analysis when performed, 5-50 genes (eg, *ALK, BRAF, CDKN2A, EGFR, ERBB2, KIT, KRAS, NRAS, MET, PDGFRA, PDGFRB, PGR, PIK3CA, PTEN, RET*), interrogation for sequence variants and copy number variants or rearrangements, if performed**
EXCLUDES *Microarray copy number assessment (81406)*
0.00 0.00 FUD XXX
AMA: 2018,Jan,8; 2017,Jan,8; 2016,Apr,4; 2016,Jan,13; 2015,Jan,3

81448 **Resequenced code. See code following 81438.**

81450 **Targeted genomic sequence analysis panel, hematolymphoid neoplasm or disorder, DNA analysis, and RNA analysis when performed, 5-50 genes (eg, *BRAF, CEBPA, DNMT3A, EZH2, FLT3, IDH1, IDH2, JAK2, KRAS, KIT, MLL, NRAS, NPM1, NOTCH1*), interrogation for sequence variants, and copy number variants or rearrangements, or isoform expression or mRNA expression levels, if performed**
EXCLUDES *Microarray copy number assessment (81406)*
0.00 0.00 FUD XXX
AMA: 2018,Jan,8; 2017,Jan,8; 2016,Apr,4; 2016,Jan,13; 2015,Jan,3

81455 **Targeted genomic sequence analysis panel, solid organ or hematolymphoid neoplasm, DNA analysis, and RNA analysis when performed, 51 or greater genes (eg, *ALK, BRAF, CDKN2A, CEBPA, DNMT3A, EGFR, ERBB2, EZH2, FLT3, IDH1, IDH2, JAK2, KIT, KRAS, MLL, NPM1, NRAS, MET, NOTCH1, PDGFRA, PDGFRB, PGR, PIK3CA, PTEN, RET*), interrogation for sequence variants and copy number variants or rearrangements, if performed**
EXCLUDES *Microarray copy number assessment (81406)*
0.00 0.00 FUD XXX
AMA: 2018,Jan,8; 2017,Jan,8; 2016,Apr,4; 2016,Jan,13; 2015,Jan,3

81460 **Whole mitochondrial genome (eg, Leigh syndrome, mitochondrial encephalomyopathy, lactic acidosis, and stroke-like episodes [MELAS], myoclonic epilepsy with ragged-red fibers [MERFF], neuropathy, ataxia, and retinitis pigmentosa [NARP], Leber hereditary optic neuropathy [LHON]), genomic sequence, must include sequence analysis of entire mitochondrial genome with heteroplasmy detection**
0.00 0.00 FUD XXX
AMA: 2018,Jan,8; 2017,Jan,8; 2016,Jan,13; 2015,Jan,3

81465 Whole mitochondrial genome large deletion analysis panel (eg, Kearns-Sayre syndrome, chronic progressive external ophthalmoplegia), including heteroplasmy detection, if performed
0.00 0.00 FUD XXX A
AMA: 2018,Jan,8; 2017,Jan,8; 2016,Jan,13; 2015,Jan,3

81470 X-linked intellectual disability (XLID) (eg, syndromic and non-syndromic XLID); genomic sequence analysis panel, must include sequencing of at least 60 genes, including *ARX, ATRX, CDKL5, FGD1, FMR1, HUWE1, IL1RAPL, KDM5C, L1CAM, MECP2, MED12, MID1, OCRL, RPS6KA3,* and *SLC16A2*
0.00 0.00 FUD XXX A
AMA: 2018,Jan,8; 2017,Jan,8; 2016,Jan,13; 2015,Jan,3

81471 duplication/deletion gene analysis, must include analysis of at least 60 genes, including *ARX, ATRX, CDKL5, FGD1, FMR1, HUWE1, IL1RAPL, KDM5C, L1CAM, MECP2, MED12, MID1, OCRL, RPS6KA3,* and *SLC16A2*
0.00 0.00 FUD XXX A
AMA: 2018,Jan,8; 2017,Jan,8; 2016,Jan,13; 2015,Jan,3

***81479* Resequenced code. See code following 81408.**

81490-81599 [81500, 81503, 81504, 81522, 81540, 81546, 81595, 81596] Multianalyte Assays

INCLUDES Procedures using multiple assay panel results (eg, molecular pathology, fluorescent in situ hybridization, non-nucleic acid-based) and other patient information to perform algorithmic analysis
Required analytical services (eg, amplification, cell lysis, detection, digestion, extraction, hybridization, nucleic acid stabilization) and algorithmic analysis

EXCLUDES *Genomic resequencing tests (81410-81471 [81448])*
In situ hybridization analyses (88271-88275, 88365-88368 [88364, 88373, 88374])
Microbial identification (87149-87153, 87471-87801 [87623, 87624, 87625], 87900-87904 [87906, 87910, 87912])
Multianalyte assays with algorithmic analyses without a Category I code (0002M-0007M, 0011M-0013M)

Code also procedures performed prior to cell lysis (eg, microdissection) (88380-88381)

81490 Autoimmune (rheumatoid arthritis), analysis of 12 biomarkers using immunoassays, utilizing serum, prognostic algorithm reported as a disease activity score
EXCLUDES *C-reactive protein (86140)*
0.00 0.00 FUD XXX Q

\# **81595 Cardiology (heart transplant), mRNA, gene expression profiling by real-time quantitative PCR of 20 genes (11 content and 9 housekeeping), utilizing subfraction of peripheral blood, algorithm reported as a rejection risk score**
0.00 0.00 FUD XXX A
AMA: 2019,Jun,11

81493 Coronary artery disease, mRNA, gene expression profiling by real-time RT-PCR of 23 genes, utilizing whole peripheral blood, algorithm reported as a risk score
0.00 0.00 FUD XXX A

***81500* Resequenced code. See code following 81538.**

***81503* Resequenced code. See code before 81539.**

***81504* Resequenced code. See code following resequenced code 81546.**

81506 Endocrinology (type 2 diabetes), biochemical assays of seven analytes (glucose, HbA1c, insulin, hs-CRP, adiponectin, ferritin, interleukin 2-receptor alpha), utilizing serum or plasma, algorithm reporting a risk score
EXCLUDES *C-reactive protein; high sensitivity (hsCRP) (86141)*
Ferritin (82728)
Glucose (82947)
Hemoglobin; glycosylated (A1C) (83036)
Immunoassay for analyte other than infectious agent antibody or infectious agent antigen (83520)
Insulin; total (83525)
Unlisted chemistry procedure (84999)
0.00 0.00 FUD XXX E
AMA: 2019,Jun,11; 2015,Jan,3

81507 Fetal aneuploidy (trisomy 21, 18, and 13) DNA sequence analysis of selected regions using maternal plasma, algorithm reported as a risk score for each trisomy ♀
EXCLUDES *Genome-wide microarray analysis (81228-81229)*
Molecular cytogenetics (88271)
0.00 0.00 FUD XXX A
AMA: 2019,Jun,11; 2018,Apr,10; 2015,Jan,3

81508 Fetal congenital abnormalities, biochemical assays of two proteins (PAPP-A, hCG [any form]), utilizing maternal serum, algorithm reported as a risk score ♀
EXCLUDES *Gonadotropin, chorionic (hCG) (84702)*
Pregnancy-associated plasma protein-A (PAPP-A) (84163)
0.00 0.00 FUD XXX E
AMA: 2019,Jun,11; 2015,Jan,3

81509 Fetal congenital abnormalities, biochemical assays of three proteins (PAPP-A, hCG [any form], DIA), utilizing maternal serum, algorithm reported as a risk score ♀
EXCLUDES *Gonadotropin, chorionic (hCG) (84702)*
Inhibin A (86336)
Pregnancy-associated plasma protein-A (PAPP-A) (84163)
0.00 0.00 FUD XXX E
AMA: 2019,Jun,11; 2015,Jan,3

81510 Fetal congenital abnormalities, biochemical assays of three analytes (AFP, uE3, hCG [any form]), utilizing maternal serum, algorithm reported as a risk score ♀
EXCLUDES *Alpha-fetoprotein (AFP) (82105)*
Estriol (82677)
Gonadotropin, chorionic (hCG) (84702)
0.00 0.00 FUD XXX E
AMA: 2019,Jun,11; 2015,Jan,3

81511 Fetal congenital abnormalities, biochemical assays of four analytes (AFP, uE3, hCG [any form], DIA) utilizing maternal serum, algorithm reported as a risk score (may include additional results from previous biochemical testing) ♀
EXCLUDES *Alpha-fetoprotein (AFP) (82105)*
Estriol (82677)
Gonadotropin, chorionic (hCG) (84702)
Inhibin A (86336)
0.00 0.00 FUD XXX E
AMA: 2019,Jun,11; 2015,Jan,3

81512 Fetal congenital abnormalities, biochemical assays of five analytes (AFP, uE3, total hCG, hyperglycosylated hCG, DIA) utilizing maternal serum, algorithm reported as a risk score ♀
EXCLUDES *Alpha-fetoprotein (AFP) (82105)*
Estriol (82677)
Gonadotropin, chorionic (hCG) (84702)
Inhibin A (86336)
0.00 0.00 FUD XXX E
AMA: 2019,Jun,11; 2015,Jan,3

● **81513** **Infectious disease, bacterial vaginosis, quantitative real-time amplification of RNA markers for Atopobium vaginae, Gardnerella vaginalis, and Lactobacillus species, utilizing vaginal-fluid specimens, algorithm reported as a positive or negative result for bacterial vaginosis**

● **81514** **Infectious disease, bacterial vaginosis and vaginitis, quantitative real-time amplification of DNA markers for Gardnerella vaginalis, Atopobium vaginae, Megasphaera type 1, Bacterial Vaginosis Associated Bacteria-2 (BVAB-2), and Lactobacillus species (L. crispatus and L. jensenii), utilizing vaginal-fluid specimens, algorithm reported as a positive or negative for high likelihood of bacterial vaginosis, includes separate detection of Trichomonas vaginalis and/or Candida species (C. albicans, C. tropicalis, C. parapsilosis, C. dubliniensis), Candida glabrata, Candida krusei, when reported**

EXCLUDES *Candida (87480-87482)*
Gardnerella vaginalis (87510-87512)
Trichomonas vaginalis (87660-87661)

81596 **Infectious disease, chronic hepatitis C virus (HCV) infection, six biochemical assays (ALT, A2-macroglobulin, apolipoprotein A-1, total bilirubin, GGT, and haptoglobin) utilizing serum, prognostic algorithm reported as scores for fibrosis and necroinflammatory activity in liver**

0.00 0.00 **FUD** XXX

AMA: 2019,Jun,11; 2019,Jul,3

81518 **Oncology (breast), mRNA, gene expression profiling by real-time RT-PCR of 11 genes (7 content and 4 housekeeping), utilizing formalin-fixed paraffin-embedded tissue, algorithms reported as percentage risk for metastatic recurrence and likelihood of benefit from extended endocrine therapy**

0.00 0.00 **FUD** XXX

AMA: 2019,Jun,11; 2019,Jul,3

81522 **Oncology (breast), mRNA, gene expression profiling by RT-PCR of 12 genes (8 content and 4 housekeeping), utilizing formalin-fixed paraffin-embedded tissue, algorithm reported as recurrence risk score**

0.00 0.00 **FUD** XXX

81519 **Oncology (breast), mRNA, gene expression profiling by real-time RT-PCR of 21 genes, utilizing formalin-fixed paraffin embedded tissue, algorithm reported as recurrence score**

0.00 0.00 **FUD** XXX A

AMA: 2019,Jun,11; 2018,Jan,8; 2017,Jan,8; 2016,Jan,13; 2015,Jan,3

81520 **Oncology (breast), mRNA gene expression profiling by hybrid capture of 58 genes (50 content and 8 housekeeping), utilizing formalin-fixed paraffin-embedded tissue, algorithm reported as a recurrence risk score**

0.00 0.00 **FUD** XXX A

AMA: 2019,Jun,11; 2018,Jun,8

81521 **Oncology (breast), mRNA, microarray gene expression profiling of 70 content genes and 465 housekeeping genes, utilizing fresh frozen or formalin-fixed paraffin-embedded tissue, algorithm reported as index related to risk of distant metastasis**

0.00 0.00 **FUD** XXX A

AMA: 2019,Jun,11; 2018,Jun,8

81522 **Resequenced code. See code following 81518.**

81525 **Oncology (colon), mRNA, gene expression profiling by real-time RT-PCR of 12 genes (7 content and 5 housekeeping), utilizing formalin-fixed paraffin-embedded tissue, algorithm reported as a recurrence score**

0.00 0.00 **FUD** XXX A

AMA: 2019,Jun,11

81528 **Oncology (colorectal) screening, quantitative real-time target and signal amplification of 10 DNA markers (*KRAS* mutations, promoter methylation of *NDRG4* and *BMP3*) and fecal hemoglobin, utilizing stool, algorithm reported as a positive or negative result**

EXCLUDES *Blood, occult, by fecal hemoglobin (82274)*
KRAS (Kirsten rat sarcoma viral oncogene homolog) (81275)

0.00 0.00 **FUD** XXX A

AMA: 2019,Jun,11

● **81529** **Oncology (cutaneous melanoma), mRNA, gene expression profiling by real-time RT-PCR of 31 genes (28 content and 3 housekeeping), utilizing formalin-fixed paraffin-embedded tissue, algorithm reported as recurrence risk, including likelihood of sentinel lymph node metastasis**

81535 **Oncology (gynecologic), live tumor cell culture and chemotherapeutic response by DAPI stain and morphology, predictive algorithm reported as a drug response score; first single drug or drug combination**

0.00 0.00 **FUD** XXX Q

AMA: 2019,Jun,11

+ **81536** **each additional single drug or drug combination (List separately in addition to code for primary procedure)**

Code first (81535)

0.00 0.00 **FUD** XXX Q

AMA: 2019,Jun,11

81538 **Oncology (lung), mass spectrometric 8-protein signature, including amyloid A, utilizing serum, prognostic and predictive algorithm reported as good versus poor overall survival**

0.00 0.00 **FUD** XXX Q

AMA: 2019,Jun,11

81500 **Oncology (ovarian), biochemical assays of two proteins (CA-125 and HE4), utilizing serum, with menopausal status, algorithm reported as a risk score** ♀

EXCLUDES *Human epididymis protein 4 (HE4) (86305)*
Immunoassay for tumor antigen, quantitative; CA 125 (86304)

0.00 0.00 **FUD** XXX E

AMA: 2019,Jun,11; 2015,Jan,3

81503 **Oncology (ovarian), biochemical assays of five proteins (CA-125, apolipoprotein A1, beta-2 microglobulin, transferrin, and pre-albumin), utilizing serum, algorithm reported as a risk score** ♀

EXCLUDES *Apolipoprotein (82172)*
Beta-2 microglobulin (82232)
Immunoassay for tumor antigen, quantitative; CA 125 (86304)
Prealbumin (84134)
Transferrin (84466)

0.00 0.00 **FUD** XXX Q

AMA: 2019,Jun,11; 2015,Jan,3

81539 **Oncology (high-grade prostate cancer), biochemical assay of four proteins (Total PSA, Free PSA, Intact PSA, and human kallikrein-2 [hK2]), utilizing plasma or serum, prognostic algorithm reported as a probability score** ♂

0.00 0.00 **FUD** XXX Q

AMA: 2019,Jun,11; 2018,Jan,8; 2017,Apr,3

81540 **Resequenced code. See code before 81552.**

81541 **Oncology (prostate), mRNA gene expression profiling by real-time RT-PCR of 46 genes (31 content and 15 housekeeping), utilizing formalin-fixed paraffin-embedded tissue, algorithm reported as a disease-specific mortality risk score**

0.00 0.00 **FUD** XXX A

AMA: 2019,Jun,11; 2018,Aug,8

26/TC PC/TC Only A2-Z3 ASC Payment 50 Bilateral ♂ Male Only ♀ Female Only Facility RVU Non-Facility RVU CCI CLIA
FUD Follow-up Days **CMS:** IOM **AMA:** CPT Asst A-Y OPPSI 80/80 Surg Assist Allowed / w/Doc Lab Crosswalk Radiology Crosswalk

81542 **Oncology (prostate), mRNA, microarray gene expression profiling of 22 content genes, utilizing formalin-fixed paraffin-embedded tissue, algorithm reported as metastasis risk score** ♂
0.00 0.00 FUD XXX

~~**81545** **Oncology (thyroid), gene expression analysis of 142 genes, utilizing fine needle aspirate, algorithm reported as a categorical result (eg, benign or suspicious)**~~

81546 **Resequenced code. See code following 81551.**

81551 **Oncology (prostate), promoter methylation profiling by real-time PCR of 3 genes (*GSTP1, APC, RASSF1*), utilizing formalin-fixed paraffin-embedded tissue, algorithm reported as a likelihood of prostate cancer detection on repeat biopsy**
0.00 0.00 FUD XXX A
AMA: 2019,Jun,11; 2018,Aug,8

● # **81546** **Oncology (thyroid), mRNA, gene expression analysis of 10,196 genes, utilizing fine needle aspirate, algorithm reported as a categorical result (eg, benign or suspicious)**
0.00 0.00 FUD 000

81504 **Oncology (tissue of origin), microarray gene expression profiling of > 2000 genes, utilizing formalin-fixed paraffin-embedded tissue, algorithm reported as tissue similarity scores**
0.00 0.00 FUD XXX A
AMA: 2019,Jun,11; 2015,Jan,3

81540 **Oncology (tumor of unknown origin), mRNA, gene expression profiling by real-time RT-PCR of 92 genes (87 content and 5 housekeeping) to classify tumor into main cancer type and subtype, utilizing formalin-fixed paraffin-embedded tissue, algorithm reported as a probability of a predicted main cancer type and subtype**
0.00 0.00 FUD XXX A
AMA: 2019,Jun,11

81552 **Oncology (uveal melanoma), mRNA, gene expression profiling by real-time RT-PCR of 15 genes (12 content and 3 housekeeping), utilizing fine needle aspirate or formalin-fixed paraffin-embedded tissue, algorithm reported as risk of metastasis**
0.00 0.00 FUD XXX
AMA: 2020,Jan,10

● **81554** **Pulmonary disease (idiopathic pulmonary fibrosis [IPF]), mRNA, gene expression analysis of 190 genes, utilizing transbronchial biopsies, diagnostic algorithm reported as categorical result (eg, positive or negative for high probability of usual interstitial pneumonia [UIP])**

81595 **Resequenced code. See code following 81490.**

81596 **Resequenced code. See code following 81514.**

81599 **Unlisted multianalyte assay with algorithmic analysis**
0.00 0.00 FUD XXX E
AMA: 2019,Jun,11; 2018,Jun,8; 2018,Apr,10; 2015,Jan,3

82009-82030 Chemistry: Acetaldehyde—Adenosine

INCLUDES Clinical information not requested by ordering physician
Mathematically calculated results
Quantitative analysis unless otherwise specified
Specimens from any source unless otherwise specified

EXCLUDES *Analytes from nonrequested laboratory analysis*
Calculated results representing score or probability derived by algorithm
Drug testing ([80305, 80306, 80307], [80324, 80325, 80326, 80327, 80328, 80329, 80330, 80331, 80332, 80333, 80334, 80335, 80336, 80337, 80338, 80339, 80340, 80341, 80342, 80343, 80344, 80345, 80346, 80347, 80348, 80349, 80350, 80351, 80352, 80353, 80354, 80355, 80356, 80357, 80358, 80359, 80360, 80361, 80362, 80363, 80364, 80365, 80366, 80367, 80368, 80369, 80370, 80371, 80372, 80373, 80374, 80375, 80376, 80377, 83992])
Organ or disease panels (80048-80076 [80081])
Therapeutic drug assays (80150-80299 [80164, 80165, 80171])

82009 **Ketone body(s) (eg, acetone, acetoacetic acid, beta-hydroxybutyrate); qualitative**
0.00 0.00 FUD XXX Q
AMA: 2018,Jan,8; 2017,Jan,8; 2016,Jan,13; 2015,Jun,10; 2015,Apr,3; 2015,Jan,16

82010 **quantitative**
0.00 0.00 FUD XXX Q
AMA: 2018,Jan,8; 2017,Jan,8; 2016,Jan,13; 2015,Jun,10; 2015,Apr,3; 2015,Jan,16

82013 **Acetylcholinesterase**
EXCLUDES *Acid phosphatase (84060-84066)*
Gastric acid analysis (82930)
0.00 0.00 FUD XXX Q
AMA: 2015,Jun,10; 2015,Apr,3

82016 **Acylcarnitines; qualitative, each specimen**
0.00 0.00 FUD XXX Q
AMA: 2015,Jun,10; 2015,Apr,3

82017 **quantitative, each specimen**
EXCLUDES *Carnitine (82379)*
0.00 0.00 FUD XXX Q
AMA: 2015,Jun,10; 2015,Apr,3

82024 **Adrenocorticotropic hormone (ACTH)**
0.00 0.00 FUD XXX Q
AMA: 2015,Jun,10; 2015,Apr,3

82030 **Adenosine, 5-monophosphate, cyclic (cyclic AMP)**
0.00 0.00 FUD XXX Q
AMA: 2015,Jun,10; 2015,Apr,3

82040-82042 [82042] Chemistry: Albumin

INCLUDES Clinical information not requested by ordering physician
Mathematically calculated results
Quantitative analysis unless otherwise specified
Specimens from any other sources unless otherwise specified

EXCLUDES *Analytes from nonrequested laboratory analysis*
Calculated results representing score or probability derived by algorithm
Drug testing ([80305, 80306, 80307], [80324, 80325, 80326, 80327, 80328, 80329, 80330, 80331, 80332, 80333, 80334, 80335, 80336, 80337, 80338, 80339, 80340, 80341, 80342, 80343, 80344, 80345, 80346, 80347, 80348, 80349, 80350, 80351, 80352, 80353, 80354, 80355, 80356, 80357, 80358, 80359, 80360, 80361, 80362, 80363, 80364, 80365, 80366, 80367, 80368, 80369, 80370, 80371, 80372, 80373, 80374, 80375, 80376, 80377, 83992])
Organ or disease panels (80048-80076 [80081])
Therapeutic drug assays (80150-80299 [80164, 80165, 80171])

82040 **Albumin; serum, plasma or whole blood**
0.00 0.00 FUD XXX Q
AMA: 2018,Jan,8; 2017,Jan,8; 2016,Jan,13; 2015,Jun,10; 2015,Apr,3; 2015,Jan,16

82042 **Resequenced code. See code following 82045.**

82043 **urine (eg, microalbumin), quantitative**
0.00 0.00 FUD XXX Q
AMA: 2018,Jan,8; 2017,Jan,8; 2016,Jan,13; 2015,Jun,10; 2015,Apr,3; 2015,Jan,16

	82044	**urine (eg, microalbumin), semiquantitative (eg, reagent strip assay)**
		EXCLUDES *Prealbumin (84134)*
		🚚 0.00 ✂ 0.00 **FUD** XXX ☒ ◙ ▣
		AMA: 2018,Jan,8; 2017,Jan,8; 2016,Jan,13; 2015,Jun,10; 2015,Apr,3; 2015,Jan,16
	82045	**ischemia modified**
		🚚 0.00 ✂ 0.00 **FUD** XXX ◙ ▣
		AMA: 2015,Jun,10; 2015,Apr,3
#	82042	**other source, quantitative, each specimen**
		EXCLUDES *Total protein (84155-84157, 84160)*
		🚚 0.00 ✂ 0.00 **FUD** XXX ◙ ▣
		AMA: 2015,Jun,10; 2015,Apr,3

82075-82107 Chemistry: Alcohol—Alpha-fetoprotein (AFP)

INCLUDES   Clinical information not requested by ordering physician
Mathematically calculated results
Quantitative analysis unless otherwise specified
Specimens from any source unless otherwise specified

EXCLUDES   *Analytes from nonrequested laboratory analysis*
Calculated results representing score or probability derived by algorithm
Drug testing ([80305, 80306, 80307], [80324, 80325, 80326, 80327, 80328, 80329, 80330, 80331, 80332, 80333, 80334, 80335, 80336, 80337, 80338, 80339, 80340, 80341, 80342, 80343, 80344, 80345, 80346, 80347, 80348, 80349, 80350, 80351, 80352, 80353, 80354, 80355, 80356, 80357, 80358, 80359, 80360, 80361, 80362, 80363, 80364, 80365, 80366, 80367, 80368, 80369, 80370, 80371, 80372, 80373, 80374, 80375, 80376, 80377, 83992])
Organ or disease panels (80048-80076 [80081])
Therapeutic drug assays (80150-80299 [80164, 80165, 80171])

▲	82075	**Alcohol (ethanol); breath**
		🚚 0.00 ✂ 0.00 **FUD** XXX ◙ ▣
		AMA: 2015,Jun,10; 2015,Apr,3
●	82077	**any specimen except urine and breath, immunoassay (eg, IA, EIA, ELISA, RIA, EMIT, FPIA) and enzymatic methods (eg, alcohol dehydrogenase)**
		EXCLUDES *Alcohol (ethanol) confirmatory drug testing ([80320])*
	82085	**Aldolase**
		🚚 0.00 ✂ 0.00 **FUD** XXX ◙ ▣
		AMA: 2015,Jun,10; 2015,Apr,3
	82088	**Aldosterone**
		EXCLUDES *Alkaline phosphatase (84075, 84080)*
		Alphaketoglutarate (82009-82010)
		Alphatocopherol (VitaminE) (84446)
		🚚 0.00 ✂ 0.00 **FUD** XXX ◙ ▣
		AMA: 2015,Jun,10; 2015,Apr,3
	82103	**Alpha-1-antitrypsin; total**
		🚚 0.00 ✂ 0.00 **FUD** XXX ◙ ▣
		AMA: 2015,Jun,10; 2015,Apr,3
	82104	**phenotype**
		🚚 0.00 ✂ 0.00 **FUD** XXX ◙ ▣
		AMA: 2015,Jun,10; 2015,Apr,3
	82105	**Alpha-fetoprotein (AFP); serum**
		🚚 0.00 ✂ 0.00 **FUD** XXX ◙ ▣
		AMA: 2015,Jun,10; 2015,Apr,3
	82106	**amniotic fluid** Ⓜ
		🚚 0.00 ✂ 0.00 **FUD** XXX ◙ ▣
		AMA: 2015,Jun,10; 2015,Apr,3
	82107	**AFP-L3 fraction isoform and total AFP (including ratio)**
		🚚 0.00 ✂ 0.00 **FUD** XXX ◙ ▣
		AMA: 2015,Jun,10; 2015,Apr,3

82108 Chemistry: Aluminum

CMS: 100-02,11,20.2 ESRD Laboratory Services

INCLUDES   Clinical information not requested by ordering physician
Mathematically calculated results
Quantitative analysis unless otherwise specified
Specimens from any source unless otherwise specified

EXCLUDES   *Analytes from nonrequested laboratory analysis*
Calculated results representing score or probability derived by algorithm
Drug testing ([80305, 80306, 80307], [80324, 80325, 80326, 80327, 80328, 80329, 80330, 80331, 80332, 80333, 80334, 80335, 80336, 80337, 80338, 80339, 80340, 80341, 80342, 80343, 80344, 80345, 80346, 80347, 80348, 80349, 80350, 80351, 80352, 80353, 80354, 80355, 80356, 80357, 80358, 80359, 80360, 80361, 80362, 80363, 80364, 80365, 80366, 80367, 80368, 80369, 80370, 80371, 80372, 80373, 80374, 80375, 80376, 80377, 83992])
Organ or disease panels (80048-80076 [80081])
Therapeutic drug assays (80150-80299 [80164, 80165, 80171])

	82108	**Aluminum**
		🚚 0.00 ✂ 0.00 **FUD** XXX ◙ ▣
		AMA: 2015,Jun,10; 2015,Apr,3

82120-82261 Chemistry: Amines—Biotinidase

INCLUDES   Clinical information not requested by ordering physician
Mathematically calculated results
Quantitative analysis unless otherwise specified
Specimens from any source unless otherwise specified

EXCLUDES   *Analytes from nonrequested laboratory analysis*
Calculated results representing score or probability derived by algorithm
Drug testing ([80305, 80306, 80307], [80324, 80325, 80326, 80327, 80328, 80329, 80330, 80331, 80332, 80333, 80334, 80335, 80336, 80337, 80338, 80339, 80340, 80341, 80342, 80343, 80344, 80345, 80346, 80347, 80348, 80349, 80350, 80351, 80352, 80353, 80354, 80355, 80356, 80357, 80358, 80359, 80360, 80361, 80362, 80363, 80364, 80365, 80366, 80367, 80368, 80369, 80370, 80371, 80372, 80373, 80374, 80375, 80376, 80377, 83992])
Organ or disease panels (80048-80076 [80081])
Therapeutic drug assays (80150-80299 [80164, 80165, 80171])

	82120	**Amines, vaginal fluid, qualitative** ♀
		EXCLUDES *Combined pH and amines test for vaginitis (82120, 83986)*
		🚚 0.00 ✂ 0.00 **FUD** XXX ☒ ◙ ▣
		AMA: 2018,Jan,8; 2017,Jan,8; 2016,Jan,13; 2015,Jun,10; 2015,Apr,3; 2015,Jan,16
	82127	**Amino acids; single, qualitative, each specimen**
		🚚 0.00 ✂ 0.00 **FUD** XXX ◙ ▣
		AMA: 2015,Jun,10; 2015,Apr,3
	82128	**multiple, qualitative, each specimen**
		🚚 0.00 ✂ 0.00 **FUD** XXX ◙ ▣
		AMA: 2015,Jun,10; 2015,Apr,3
	82131	**single, quantitative, each specimen**
		INCLUDES Van Slyke method
		🚚 0.00 ✂ 0.00 **FUD** XXX ◙ ▣
		AMA: 2018,Jan,8; 2017,Jan,8; 2016,Jan,13; 2015,Jun,10; 2015,Apr,3; 2015,Jan,16
	82135	**Aminolevulinic acid, delta (ALA)**
		🚚 0.00 ✂ 0.00 **FUD** XXX ◙ ▣
		AMA: 2015,Jun,10; 2015,Apr,3
	82136	**Amino acids, 2 to 5 amino acids, quantitative, each specimen**
		🚚 0.00 ✂ 0.00 **FUD** XXX ◙ ▣
		AMA: 2015,Jun,10; 2015,Apr,3
	82139	**Amino acids, 6 or more amino acids, quantitative, each specimen**
		🚚 0.00 ✂ 0.00 **FUD** XXX ◙ ▣
		AMA: 2015,Jun,10; 2015,Apr,3
	82140	**Ammonia**
		🚚 0.00 ✂ 0.00 **FUD** XXX ◙ ▣
		AMA: 2015,Jun,10; 2015,Apr,3
	82143	**Amniotic fluid scan (spectrophotometric)** Ⓜ ♀
		EXCLUDES *Amobarbital ([80345])*
		L/S ratio (83661)
		🚚 0.00 ✂ 0.00 **FUD** XXX ◙ ▣
		AMA: 2015,Jun,10; 2015,Apr,3

26/TC PC/TC Only   A2-Z3 ASC Payment   50 Bilateral   ♂ Male Only   ♀ Female Only   🚚 Facility RVU   ✂ Non-Facility RVU   ▣ CCI   ☒ CLIA
FUD Follow-up Days   **CMS:** IOM   **AMA:** CPT Asst   A-Y OPPSI   80/80 Surg Assist Allowed / w/Doc   ◩ Lab Crosswalk   ⊠ Radiology Crosswalk

82150 **Amylase**
0.00 0.00 **FUD** XXX
AMA: 2015,Jun,10; 2015,Apr,3

82154 **Androstanediol glucuronide**
0.00 0.00 **FUD** XXX
AMA: 2018,Jan,8; 2017,Jan,8; 2016,Jan,13; 2015,Jun,10; 2015,Apr,3; 2015,Jan,16

82157 **Androstenedione**
0.00 0.00 **FUD** XXX
AMA: 2015,Jun,10; 2015,Apr,3

82160 **Androsterone**
0.00 0.00 **FUD** XXX
AMA: 2015,Jun,10; 2015,Apr,3

82163 **Angiotensin II**
0.00 0.00 **FUD** XXX
AMA: 2015,Jun,10; 2015,Apr,3

82164 **Angiotensin I - converting enzyme (ACE)**
EXCLUDES *Antidiuretic hormone (ADH) (84588)*
Antimony (83015)
Antitrypsin, alpha-1- (82103-82104)
0.00 0.00 **FUD** XXX
AMA: 2015,Jun,10; 2015,Apr,3

82172 **Apolipoprotein, each**
0.00 0.00 **FUD** XXX
AMA: 2015,Jun,10; 2015,Apr,3

82175 **Arsenic**
EXCLUDES *Heavy metal screening (83015)*
0.00 0.00 **FUD** XXX
AMA: 2015,Jun,10; 2015,Apr,3

82180 **Ascorbic acid (Vitamin C), blood**
EXCLUDES *Aspirin (acetylsalicylic acid) ([80329, 80330, 80331])*
Atherogenic index, blood, ultracentrifugation, quantitative (83701)
Salicylate therapeutic drug assay ([80179])
0.00 0.00 **FUD** XXX
AMA: 2015,Jun,10; 2015,Apr,3

82190 **Atomic absorption spectroscopy, each analyte**
0.00 0.00 **FUD** XXX
AMA: 2015,Jun,10; 2015,Apr,3

82232 **Beta-2 microglobulin**
0.00 0.00 **FUD** XXX
AMA: 2015,Jun,10; 2015,Apr,3

82239 **Bile acids; total**
0.00 0.00 **FUD** XXX
AMA: 2015,Jun,10; 2015,Apr,3

82240 **cholylglycine**
EXCLUDES *Bile pigments, urine (81000-81005)*
0.00 0.00 **FUD** XXX
AMA: 2015,Jun,10; 2015,Apr,3

82247 **Bilirubin; total**
INCLUDES Van Den Bergh test
0.00 0.00 **FUD** XXX
AMA: 2018,Jan,8; 2017,Jan,8; 2016,Jan,13; 2015,Jun,10; 2015,Apr,3; 2015,Jan,16

82248 **direct**
0.00 0.00 **FUD** XXX
AMA: 2018,Jan,8; 2017,Jan,8; 2016,Jan,13; 2015,Jun,10; 2015,Apr,3; 2015,Jan,16

82252 **feces, qualitative**
0.00 0.00 **FUD** XXX
AMA: 2015,Jun,10; 2015,Apr,3

82261 **Biotinidase, each specimen**
0.00 0.00 **FUD** XXX
AMA: 2015,Jun,10; 2015,Apr,3

82270-82274 Chemistry: Occult Blood

CMS: 100-04,16,70.8 CLIA Waived Tests; 100-04,18,60 Colorectal Cancer Screening

INCLUDES Clinical information not requested by ordering physician
Mathematically calculated results
Quantitative analysis unless otherwise specified
Specimens from any source unless otherwise specified

EXCLUDES *Analytes from nonrequested laboratory analysis*
Calculated results representing score or probability derived by algorithm
Drug testing ([80305, 80306, 80307], [80324, 80325, 80326, 80327, 80328, 80329, 80330, 80331, 80332, 80333, 80334, 80335, 80336, 80337, 80338, 80339, 80340, 80341, 80342, 80343, 80344, 80345, 80346, 80347, 80348, 80349, 80350, 80351, 80352, 80353, 80354, 80355, 80356, 80357, 80358, 80359, 80360, 80361, 80362, 80363, 80364, 80365, 80366, 80367, 80368, 80369, 80370, 80371, 80372, 80373, 80374, 80375, 80376, 80377, 83992])
Organ or disease panels (80048-80076 [80081])
Therapeutic drug assays (80150-80299 [80164, 80165, 80171])

82270 **Blood, occult, by peroxidase activity (eg, guaiac), qualitative; feces, consecutive collected specimens with single determination, for colorectal neoplasm screening (ie, patient was provided 3 cards or single triple card for consecutive collection)**
INCLUDES Day test
0.00 0.00 **FUD** XXX
AMA: 2018,Jan,8; 2017,Jan,8; 2016,Jan,13; 2015,Jun,10; 2015,Apr,3; 2015,Jan,16

82271 **other sources**
0.00 0.00 **FUD** XXX
AMA: 2015,Jun,10; 2015,Apr,3

82272 **Blood, occult, by peroxidase activity (eg, guaiac), qualitative, feces, 1-3 simultaneous determinations, performed for other than colorectal neoplasm screening**
0.00 0.00 **FUD** XXX
AMA: 2018,Jan,8; 2017,Jan,8; 2016,Jan,13; 2015,Jun,10; 2015,Apr,3; 2015,Jan,16

82274 **Blood, occult, by fecal hemoglobin determination by immunoassay, qualitative, feces, 1-3 simultaneous determinations**
0.00 0.00 **FUD** XXX
AMA: 2015,Jun,10; 2015,Apr,3

82286-82308 [82652] Chemistry: Bradykinin—Calcitonin

INCLUDES Clinical information not requested by ordering physician
Mathematically calculated results
Quantitative analysis unless otherwise specified
Specimens from any source unless otherwise specified

EXCLUDES *Analytes from nonrequested laboratory analysis*
Calculated results representing score or probability derived by algorithm
Drug testing ([80305, 80306, 80307], [80324, 80325, 80326, 80327, 80328, 80329, 80330, 80331, 80332, 80333, 80334, 80335, 80336, 80337, 80338, 80339, 80340, 80341, 80342, 80343, 80344, 80345, 80346, 80347, 80348, 80349, 80350, 80351, 80352, 80353, 80354, 80355, 80356, 80357, 80358, 80359, 80360, 80361, 80362, 80363, 80364, 80365, 80366, 80367, 80368, 80369, 80370, 80371, 80372, 80373, 80374, 80375, 80376, 80377, 83992])
Organ or disease panels (80048-80076 [80081])
Therapeutic drug assays (80150-80299 [80164, 80165, 80171])

82286 **Bradykinin**
0.00 0.00 **FUD** XXX
AMA: 2015,Jun,10; 2015,Apr,3

82300 **Cadmium**
0.00 0.00 **FUD** XXX
AMA: 2015,Jun,10; 2015,Apr,3

82306 **Vitamin D; 25 hydroxy, includes fraction(s), if performed**
0.00 0.00 **FUD** XXX
AMA: 2015,Jun,10; 2015,Apr,3

\# **82652** **1, 25 dihydroxy, includes fraction(s), if performed**
0.00 0.00 **FUD** XXX
AMA: 2015,Jun,10; 2015,Apr,3

82308 **Calcitonin**
0.00 0.00 **FUD** XXX
AMA: 2015,Jun,10; 2015,Apr,3

82310-82373 Chemistry: Calcium, total; Carbohydrate Deficient Transferrin

INCLUDES Clinical information not requested by ordering physician
Mathematically calculated results
Quantitative analysis unless otherwise specified
Specimens from any source unless otherwise specified

EXCLUDES *Analytes from nonrequested laboratory analysis*
Calculated results representing score or probability derived by algorithm
Drug testing ([80305, 80306, 80307], [80324, 80325, 80326, 80327, 80328, 80329, 80330, 80331, 80332, 80333, 80334, 80335, 80336, 80337, 80338, 80339, 80340, 80341, 80342, 80343, 80344, 80345, 80346, 80347, 80348, 80349, 80350, 80351, 80352, 80353, 80354, 80355, 80356, 80357, 80358, 80359, 80360, 80361, 80362, 80363, 80364, 80365, 80366, 80367, 80368, 80369, 80370, 80371, 80372, 80373, 80374, 80375, 80376, 80377, 83992])
Organ or disease panels (80048-80076 [80081])
Therapeutic drug assays (80150-80299 [80164, 80165, 80171])

82310 Calcium; total
0.00 0.00 **FUD** XXX
AMA: 2018,Jan,8; 2017,Jan,8; 2016,Jan,13; 2015,Jun,10; 2015,Apr,3; 2015,Jan,16

82330 ionized
0.00 0.00 **FUD** XXX
AMA: 2018,Jan,8; 2017,Jan,8; 2016,Jan,13; 2015,Jun,10; 2015,Apr,3; 2015,Jan,16

82331 after calcium infusion test
0.00 0.00 **FUD** XXX
AMA: 2015,Jun,10; 2015,Apr,3

82340 urine quantitative, timed specimen
0.00 0.00 **FUD** XXX
AMA: 2015,Jun,10; 2015,Apr,3

82355 Calculus; qualitative analysis
0.00 0.00 **FUD** XXX
AMA: 2015,Jun,10; 2015,Apr,3

82360 quantitative analysis, chemical
0.00 0.00 **FUD** XXX
AMA: 2015,Jun,10; 2015,Apr,3

82365 infrared spectroscopy
0.00 0.00 **FUD** XXX
AMA: 2015,Jun,10; 2015,Apr,3

82370 X-ray diffraction
0.00 0.00 **FUD** XXX
AMA: 2015,Jun,10; 2015,Apr,3

82373 Carbohydrate deficient transferrin
0.00 0.00 **FUD** XXX
AMA: 2015,Jun,10; 2015,Apr,3

82374 Chemistry: Carbon Dioxide

CMS: 100-02,11,20.2 ESRD Laboratory Services; 100-02,11,30.2.2 Automated Multi-Channel Chemistry (AMCC) Tests; 100-04,16,40.6.1 Automated Multi-Channel Chemistry (AMCC) Tests for ESRD Beneficiaries; 100-04,16,70.8 CLIA Waived Tests; 100-04,16,90.2 Organ or Disease Oriented Panels

INCLUDES Clinical information not requested by ordering physician
Mathematically calculated results
Quantitative analysis unless otherwise specified
Specimens from any source unless otherwise specified

EXCLUDES *Analytes from nonrequested laboratory analysis*
Calculated results representing score or probability derived by algorithm
Drug testing ([80305, 80306, 80307], [80324, 80325, 80326, 80327, 80328, 80329, 80330, 80331, 80332, 80333, 80334, 80335, 80336, 80337, 80338, 80339, 80340, 80341, 80342, 80343, 80344, 80345, 80346, 80347, 80348, 80349, 80350, 80351, 80352, 80353, 80354, 80355, 80356, 80357, 80358, 80359, 80360, 80361, 80362, 80363, 80364, 80365, 80366, 80367, 80368, 80369, 80370, 80371, 80372, 80373, 80374, 80375, 80376, 80377, 83992])
Organ or disease panels (80048-80076 [80081])
Therapeutic drug assays (80150-80299 [80164, 80165, 80171])

82374 Carbon dioxide (bicarbonate)
EXCLUDES *Blood gases (82803)*
0.00 0.00 **FUD** XXX
AMA: 2018,Jan,8; 2017,Jan,8; 2016,Jan,13; 2015,Jun,10; 2015,Apr,3; 2015,Jan,16

82375-82376 Chemistry: Carboxyhemoglobin (Carbon Monoxide)

INCLUDES Clinical information not requested by ordering physician
Mathematically calculated results
Specimens from any source unless otherwise specified

EXCLUDES *Analytes from nonrequested laboratory analysis*
Calculated results representing score or probability derived by algorithm
Drug testing ([80305, 80306, 80307], [80324, 80325, 80326, 80327, 80328, 80329, 80330, 80331, 80332, 80333, 80334, 80335, 80336, 80337, 80338, 80339, 80340, 80341, 80342, 80343, 80344, 80345, 80346, 80347, 80348, 80349, 80350, 80351, 80352, 80353, 80354, 80355, 80356, 80357, 80358, 80359, 80360, 80361, 80362, 80363, 80364, 80365, 80366, 80367, 80368, 80369, 80370, 80371, 80372, 80373, 80374, 80375, 80376, 80377, 83992])
Organ or disease panels (80048-80076 [80081])
Transcutaneous measurement of carboxyhemoglobin (88740)

82375 Carboxyhemoglobin; quantitative
0.00 0.00 **FUD** XXX
AMA: 2018,Jan,8; 2017,Jan,8; 2016,Jan,13; 2015,Jun,10; 2015,Apr,3; 2015,Jan,16

82376 qualitative
0.00 0.00 **FUD** XXX
AMA: 2015,Jun,10; 2015,Apr,3

82378 Chemistry: Carcinoembryonic Antigen (CEA)

CMS: 100-03,190.26 Carcinoembryonic Antigen (CEA)

INCLUDES Clinical information not requested by ordering physician

EXCLUDES *Analytes from nonrequested laboratory analysis*
Calculated results representing score or probability derived by algorithm

82378 Carcinoembryonic antigen (CEA)
0.00 0.00 **FUD** XXX
AMA: 2018,Jan,8; 2017,Jan,8; 2016,Jan,13; 2015,Jun,10; 2015,Apr,3; 2015,Jan,16

82379-82415 Chemistry: Carnitine—Chloramphenicol

INCLUDES Clinical information not requested by ordering physician
Mathematically calculated results
Quantitative analysis unless otherwise specified
Specimens from any source unless otherwise specified

EXCLUDES *Analytes from nonrequested laboratory analysis*
Calculated results representing score or probability derived by algorithm
Drug testing ([80305, 80306, 80307], [80324, 80325, 80326, 80327, 80328, 80329, 80330, 80331, 80332, 80333, 80334, 80335, 80336, 80337, 80338, 80339, 80340, 80341, 80342, 80343, 80344, 80345, 80346, 80347, 80348, 80349, 80350, 80351, 80352, 80353, 80354, 80355, 80356, 80357, 80358, 80359, 80360, 80361, 80362, 80363, 80364, 80365, 80366, 80367, 80368, 80369, 80370, 80371, 80372, 80373, 80374, 80375, 80376, 80377, 83992])
Organ or disease panels (80048-80076 [80081])
Therapeutic drug assays (80150-80299 [80164, 80165, 80171])

82379 Carnitine (total and free), quantitative, each specimen
EXCLUDES *Acylcarnitine (82016-82017)*
0.00 0.00 **FUD** XXX
AMA: 2015,Jun,10; 2015,Apr,3

82380 Carotene
0.00 0.00 **FUD** XXX
AMA: 2015,Jun,10; 2015,Apr,3

82382 Catecholamines; total urine
0.00 0.00 **FUD** XXX
AMA: 2015,Jun,10; 2015,Apr,3

82383 blood
0.00 0.00 **FUD** XXX
AMA: 2015,Jun,10; 2015,Apr,3

82384 fractionated
EXCLUDES *Urine metabolites (83835, 84585)*
0.00 0.00 **FUD** XXX
AMA: 2015,Jun,10; 2015,Apr,3

82387 Cathepsin-D
0.00 0.00 **FUD** XXX
AMA: 2015,Jun,10; 2015,Apr,3

82390 Ceruloplasmin
0.00 0.00 **FUD** XXX
AMA: 2015,Jun,10; 2015,Apr,3

82397 **Chemiluminescent assay**
0.00 0.00 **FUD** XXX
AMA: 2018,Jan,8; 2017,Jan,8; 2016,Jan,13; 2015,Jun,10; 2015,Apr,3; 2015,Jan,16

82415 **Chloramphenicol**
0.00 0.00 **FUD** XXX
AMA: 2015,Jun,10; 2015,Apr,3

82435-82438 Chemistry: Chloride

INCLUDES Clinical information not requested by ordering physician
Mathematically calculated results
Quantitative analysis unless otherwise specified
Specimens from any source unless otherwise specified

EXCLUDES *Analytes from nonrequested laboratory analysis*
Calculated results representing score or probability derived by algorithm
Organ or disease panels (80048-80076 [80081])
Therapeutic drug assays (80150-80299 [80164, 80165, 80171])

82435 **Chloride; blood**
0.00 0.00 **FUD** XXX
AMA: 2018,Jan,8; 2017,Jan,8; 2016,Jan,13; 2015,Jun,10; 2015,Apr,3; 2015,Jan,16

82436 **urine**
0.00 0.00 **FUD** XXX
AMA: 2015,Jun,10; 2015,Apr,3

82438 **other source**
EXCLUDES *Sweat collections by iontophoresis (89230)*
0.00 0.00 **FUD** XXX
AMA: 2018,Jan,8; 2017,Jan,8; 2016,Jan,13; 2015,Jun,10; 2015,Apr,3; 2015,Jan,16

82441 Chemistry: Chlorinated Hydrocarbons

INCLUDES Clinical information not requested by ordering physician
Mathematically calculated results
Quantitative analysis unless otherwise specified
Specimens from any source unless otherwise specified

EXCLUDES *Analytes from nonrequested laboratory analysis*
Calculated results representing a score or probability derived by algorithm

82441 **Chlorinated hydrocarbons, screen**
EXCLUDES *Cholecalciferol (Vitamin D) (82306)*
0.00 0.00 **FUD** XXX
AMA: 2015,Jun,10; 2015,Apr,3

82465 Chemistry: Cholesterol, Total

CMS: 100-03,190.23 Lipid Testing; 100-04,16,40.6.1 Automated Multi-Channel Chemistry (AMCC) Tests for ESRD Beneficiaries; 100-04,16,70.8 CLIA Waived Tests; 100-04,16,90.2 Organ or Disease Oriented Panels

INCLUDES Clinical information not requested by ordering physician
Mathematically calculated results
Quantitative analysis unless otherwise specified

EXCLUDES *Analytes from nonrequested laboratory analysis*
Calculated results representing score or probability derived by algorithm
Organ or disease panels (80048-80076 [80081])

82465 **Cholesterol, serum or whole blood, total**
EXCLUDES *High density lipoprotein (HDL) (83718)*
0.00 0.00 **FUD** XXX
AMA: 2018,Jan,8; 2017,Jan,8; 2016,Jan,13; 2015,Jun,10; 2015,Apr,3; 2015,Jan,16

82480-82507 Chemistry: Cholinesterase—Citrate

INCLUDES Clinical information not requested by ordering physician
Mathematically calculated results
Quantitative analysis unless otherwise specified
Specimens from any source unless otherwise specified

EXCLUDES *Analytes from nonrequested laboratory analysis*
Calculated results representing score or probability derived by algorithm
Drug testing ([80305, 80306, 80307], [80324, 80325, 80326, 80327, 80328, 80329, 80330, 80331, 80332, 80333, 80334, 80335, 80336, 80337, 80338, 80339, 80340, 80341, 80342, 80343, 80344, 80345, 80346, 80347, 80348, 80349, 80350, 80351, 80352, 80353, 80354, 80355, 80356, 80357, 80358, 80359, 80360, 80361, 80362, 80363, 80364, 80365, 80366, 80367, 80368, 80369, 80370, 80371, 80372, 80373, 80374, 80375, 80376, 80377, 83992])
Organ or disease panels (80048-80076 [80081])
Therapeutic drug assays (80150-80299 [80164, 80165, 80171])

82480 **Cholinesterase; serum**
0.00 0.00 **FUD** XXX
AMA: 2015,Jun,10; 2015,Apr,3

82482 **RBC**
0.00 0.00 **FUD** XXX
AMA: 2015,Jun,10; 2015,Apr,3

82485 **Chondroitin B sulfate, quantitative**
EXCLUDES *Chorionic gonadotropin (84702-84703)*
0.00 0.00 **FUD** XXX
AMA: 2015,Jun,10; 2015,Apr,3

82495 **Chromium**
0.00 0.00 **FUD** XXX
AMA: 2015,Jun,10; 2015,Apr,3

82507 **Citrate**
EXCLUDES *Cocaine, qualitative analysis ([80353])*
Codeine, qualitative analysis ([80361])
Complement (86160-86162)
0.00 0.00 **FUD** XXX
AMA: 2015,Jun,10; 2015,Apr,3

82523 Chemistry: Collagen Crosslinks, Any Method

CMS: 100-03,190.19 NCD for Collagen Crosslinks, Any Method; 100-04,16,70.8 CLIA Waived Tests

INCLUDES Clinical information not requested by ordering physician
Mathematically calculated results
Quantitative analysis unless otherwise specified
Specimens from any source unless otherwise specified

EXCLUDES *Analytes from nonrequested laboratory analysis*
Calculated results representing score or probability derived by algorithm
Organ or disease panels (80048-80076 [80081])
Therapeutic drug assays (80150-80299 [80164, 80165, 80171])

82523 **Collagen cross links, any method**
0.00 0.00 **FUD** XXX
AMA: 2015,Jun,10; 2015,Apr,3

82525-82735 [82652, 82681] Chemistry: Copper—Fluoride

INCLUDES Clinical information not requested by ordering physician
Mathematically calculated results
Quantitative analysis unless otherwise specified
Specimens from any source unless otherwise specified

EXCLUDES *Analytes from nonrequested laboratory analysis*
Calculated results representing score or probability derived by algorithm
Drug testing ([80305, 80306, 80307], [80324, 80325, 80326, 80327, 80328, 80329, 80330, 80331, 80332, 80333, 80334, 80335, 80336, 80337, 80338, 80339, 80340, 80341, 80342, 80343, 80344, 80345, 80346, 80347, 80348, 80349, 80350, 80351, 80352, 80353, 80354, 80355, 80356, 80357, 80358, 80359, 80360, 80361, 80362, 80363, 80364, 80365, 80366, 80367, 80368, 80369, 80370, 80371, 80372, 80373, 80374, 80375, 80376, 80377, 83992])
Organ or disease panels (80048-80076 [80081])
Therapeutic drug assays (80150-80299 [80164, 80165, 80171])

82525 **Copper**
EXCLUDES *Coproporphyrin (84119-84120)*
Corticosteroids (83491)
0.00 0.00 **FUD** XXX
AMA: 2015,Jun,10; 2015,Apr,3

82528 **Corticosterone**
INCLUDES Porter-Silber test
0.00 0.00 **FUD** XXX
AMA: 2015,Jun,10; 2015,Apr,3

82530 **Cortisol; free**
0.00 0.00 **FUD** XXX
AMA: 2018,Jan,8; 2017,Jan,8; 2016,Jan,13; 2015,Jun,10; 2015,Apr,3; 2015,Jan,16

82533 **total**
0.00 0.00 **FUD** XXX
AMA: 2018,Jan,8; 2017,Jan,8; 2016,Jan,13; 2015,Jun,10; 2015,Apr,3; 2015,Jan,16

82540 **Creatine**
0.00 0.00 **FUD** XXX
AMA: 2015,Jun,10; 2015,Apr,3

82542 Column chromatography, includes mass spectrometry, if performed (eg, HPLC, LC, LC/MS, LC/MS-MS, GC, GC/MS-MS, GC/MS, HPLC/MS), non-drug analyte(s) not elsewhere specified, qualitative or quantitative, each specimen

EXCLUDES *Column chromatography/mass spectrometry drugs/substances ([80305, 80306, 80307], [80320, 80321, 80322, 80323, 80324, 80325, 80326, 80327, 80328, 80329, 80330, 80331, 80332, 80333, 80334, 80335, 80336, 80337, 80338, 80339, 80340, 80341, 80342, 80343, 80344, 80345, 80346, 80347, 80348, 80349, 80350, 80351, 80352, 80353, 80354, 80355, 80356, 80357, 80358, 80359, 80360, 80361, 80362, 80363, 80364, 80365, 80366, 80367, 80368, 80369, 80370, 80371, 80372, 80373, 80374, 80375, 80376, 80377, 83992])*

Procedure performed more than one time per specimen

0.00 0.00 FUD XXX

AMA: 2018,Jan,8; 2017,Jan,8; 2016,Jan,13; 2015,Jun,10; 2015,Apr,3

82550 Creatine kinase (CK), (CPK); total

0.00 0.00 FUD XXX

AMA: 2018,Jan,8; 2017,Jan,8; 2016,Jan,13; 2015,Jun,10; 2015,Apr,3; 2015,Jan,16

82552 isoenzymes

0.00 0.00 FUD XXX

AMA: 2018,Jan,8; 2017,Jan,8; 2016,Jan,13; 2015,Jun,10; 2015,Apr,3; 2015,Jan,16

82553 MB fraction only

0.00 0.00 FUD XXX

AMA: 2018,Jan,8; 2017,Jan,8; 2016,Jan,13; 2015,Jun,10; 2015,Apr,3; 2015,Jan,16

82554 isoforms

0.00 0.00 FUD XXX

AMA: 2018,Jan,8; 2017,Jan,8; 2016,Jan,13; 2015,Jun,10; 2015,Apr,3; 2015,Jan,16

82565 Creatinine; blood

0.00 0.00 FUD XXX

AMA: 2018,Jan,8; 2017,Jan,8; 2016,Jan,13; 2015,Jun,10; 2015,Apr,3; 2015,Jan,16

82570 other source

0.00 0.00 FUD XXX

AMA: 2015,Jun,10; 2015,Apr,3

82575 clearance

INCLUDES Holten test

0.00 0.00 FUD XXX

AMA: 2015,Jun,10; 2015,Apr,3

82585 Cryofibrinogen

0.00 0.00 FUD XXX

AMA: 2015,Jun,10; 2015,Apr,3

82595 Cryoglobulin, qualitative or semi-quantitative (eg, cryocrit)

EXCLUDES *Crystals, pyrophosphate vs urate (89060)*

Quantitative, cryoglobulin (82784-82785)

0.00 0.00 FUD XXX

AMA: 2015,Jun,10; 2015,Apr,3

82600 Cyanide

0.00 0.00 FUD XXX

AMA: 2015,Jun,10; 2015,Apr,3

82607 Cyanocobalamin (Vitamin B-12);

EXCLUDES *Cyclic AMP (82030)*

Cyclosporine (80158)

0.00 0.00 FUD XXX

AMA: 2015,Jun,10; 2015,Apr,3

82608 unsaturated binding capacity

EXCLUDES *Cyclic AMP (82030)*

Cyclosporine (80158)

0.00 0.00 FUD XXX

AMA: 2015,Jun,10; 2015,Apr,3

82610 Cystatin C

0.00 0.00 FUD XXX

AMA: 2018,Jan,8; 2017,Jan,8; 2016,Jan,13; 2015,Jun,10; 2015,Apr,3; 2015,Jan,16

82615 Cystine and homocystine, urine, qualitative

0.00 0.00 FUD XXX

AMA: 2015,Jun,10; 2015,Apr,3

82626 Dehydroepiandrosterone (DHEA)

EXCLUDES *Anabolic steroids ([80327, 80328])*

0.00 0.00 FUD XXX

AMA: 2018,Jan,8; 2017,Jan,8; 2016,Jan,13; 2015,Jun,10; 2015,Apr,3; 2015,Jan,16

82627 Dehydroepiandrosterone-sulfate (DHEA-S)

EXCLUDES *Delta-aminolevulinicacid (ALA) (82135)*

0.00 0.00 FUD XXX

AMA: 2018,Jan,8; 2017,Jan,8; 2016,Jan,13; 2015,Jun,10; 2015,Apr,3; 2015,Jan,16

82633 Desoxycorticosterone, 11-

0.00 0.00 FUD XXX

AMA: 2015,Jun,10; 2015,Apr,3

82634 Deoxycortisol, 11-

EXCLUDES *Dexamethasone suppression test (80420)*

Diastase, urine (82150)

0.00 0.00 FUD XXX

AMA: 2015,Jun,10; 2015,Apr,3

82638 Dibucaine number

EXCLUDES *Dichloroethane (82441)*

Dichloromethane (82441)

Diethylether (84600)

0.00 0.00 FUD XXX

AMA: 2015,Jun,10; 2015,Apr,3

82642 Dihydrotestosterone (DHT)

EXCLUDES *Anabolic drug testing analysis dihydrotestosterone ([80327, 80328])*

Dipropylaceticacid ([80164])

Dopamine (82382)

Duodenal contents, individual enzymes for intubation and collection (43756-43757)

0.00 0.00 FUD XXX

82652 **Resequenced code. See code following 82306.**

82656 Elastase, pancreatic (EL-1), fecal, qualitative or semi-quantitative

0.00 0.00 FUD XXX

AMA: 2018,Jan,8; 2017,Jan,8; 2016,Jan,13; 2015,Jun,10; 2015,Apr,3; 2015,Jan,16

82657 Enzyme activity in blood cells, cultured cells, or tissue, not elsewhere specified; nonradioactive substrate, each specimen

0.00 0.00 FUD XXX

AMA: 2015,Jun,10; 2015,Apr,3

82658 radioactive substrate, each specimen

0.00 0.00 FUD XXX

AMA: 2015,Jun,10; 2015,Apr,3

82664 Electrophoretic technique, not elsewhere specified

EXCLUDES *Endocrine receptor assays (84233-84235)*

0.00 0.00 FUD XXX

AMA: 2015,Jun,10; 2015,Apr,3

82668 Erythropoietin

0.00 0.00 FUD XXX

AMA: 2015,Jun,10; 2015,Apr,3

▲ **82670 Estradiol; total**

0.00 0.00 FUD XXX

AMA: 2015,Jun,10; 2015,Apr,3

● # **82681 free, direct measurement (eg, equilibrium dialysis)**

0.00 0.00 FUD 000

82671 Estrogens; fractionated
EXCLUDES *Estrogen receptor assay (84233)*
0.00 0.00 FUD XXX
AMA: 2015,Jun,10; 2015,Apr,3

82672 total
EXCLUDES *Estrogen receptor assay (84233)*
0.00 0.00 FUD XXX
AMA: 2015,Jun,10; 2015,Apr,3

82677 Estriol
0.00 0.00 FUD XXX
AMA: 2015,Jun,10; 2015,Apr,3

82679 Estrone
EXCLUDES *Alcohol (ethanol) definitive drug testing ([80320])*
Alcohol (ethanol) therapeutic drug assay (82077)
0.00 0.00 FUD XXX
AMA: 2015,Jun,10; 2015,Apr,3

82681 **Resequenced code. See code following 82670.**

82693 Ethylene glycol
0.00 0.00 FUD XXX
AMA: 2015,Jun,10; 2015,Apr,3

82696 Etiocholanolone
EXCLUDES *Fractionation ketosteroids (83593)*
0.00 0.00 FUD XXX
AMA: 2015,Jun,10; 2015,Apr,3

82705 Fat or lipids, feces; qualitative
0.00 0.00 FUD XXX
AMA: 2015,Jun,10; 2015,Apr,3

82710 quantitative
0.00 0.00 FUD XXX
AMA: 2015,Jun,10; 2015,Apr,3

82715 Fat differential, feces, quantitative
0.00 0.00 FUD XXX
AMA: 2015,Jun,10; 2015,Apr,3

82725 Fatty acids, nonesterified
0.00 0.00 FUD XXX
AMA: 2015,Jun,10; 2015,Apr,3

82726 Very long chain fatty acids
0.00 0.00 FUD XXX
AMA: 2015,Jun,10; 2015,Apr,3

82728 Ferritin
EXCLUDES *Fetal hemoglobin (83030, 83033, 85460)*
Fetoprotein, alpha-1 (82105-82106)
0.00 0.00 FUD XXX
AMA: 2015,Jun,10; 2015,Apr,3

82731 Fetal fibronectin, cervicovaginal secretions, semi-quantitative
M ♀
0.00 0.00 FUD XXX
AMA: 2015,Jun,10; 2015,Apr,3

82735 Fluoride
EXCLUDES *Foam stability test (83662)*
0.00 0.00 FUD XXX
AMA: 2015,Jun,10; 2015,Apr,3

82746-82941 Chemistry: Folic Acid—Gastrin

INCLUDES Clinical information not requested by ordering physician
Mathematically calculated results
Quantitative analysis unless otherwise specified
Specimens from any source unless otherwise specified

EXCLUDES *Analytes from nonrequested laboratory analysis*
Calculated results representing score or probability derived by algorithm
Drug testing ([80305, 80306, 80307], [80324, 80325, 80326, 80327, 80328, 80329, 80330, 80331, 80332, 80333, 80334, 80335, 80336, 80337, 80338, 80339, 80340, 80341, 80342, 80343, 80344, 80345, 80346, 80347, 80348, 80349, 80350, 80351, 80352, 80353, 80354, 80355, 80356, 80357, 80358, 80359, 80360, 80361, 80362, 80363, 80364, 80365, 80366, 80367, 80368, 80369, 80370, 80371, 80372, 80373, 80374, 80375, 80376, 80377, 83992])
Organ or disease panels (80048-80076 [80081])
Therapeutic drug assays (80150-80299 [80164, 80165, 80171])

82746 Folic acid; serum
0.00 0.00 FUD XXX
AMA: 2015,Jun,10; 2015,Apr,3

82747 RBC
EXCLUDES *Follicle stimulating hormone (FSH) (83001)*
0.00 0.00 FUD XXX
AMA: 2015,Jun,10; 2015,Apr,3

82757 Fructose, semen
EXCLUDES *Fructosamine (82985)*
Fructose, TLC screen (84375)
0.00 0.00 FUD XXX
AMA: 2015,Jun,10; 2015,Apr,3

82759 Galactokinase, RBC
0.00 0.00 FUD XXX
AMA: 2015,Jun,10; 2015,Apr,3

82760 Galactose
0.00 0.00 FUD XXX
AMA: 2015,Jun,10; 2015,Apr,3

82775 Galactose-1-phosphate uridyl transferase; quantitative
0.00 0.00 FUD XXX
AMA: 2015,Jun,10; 2015,Apr,3

82776 screen
0.00 0.00 FUD XXX
AMA: 2015,Jun,10; 2015,Apr,3

82777 Galectin-3
0.00 0.00 FUD XXX
AMA: 2015,Jun,10; 2015,Apr,3

82784 Gammaglobulin (immunoglobulin); IgA, IgD, IgG, IgM, each
INCLUDES Farr test
0.00 0.00 FUD XXX
AMA: 2018,Jan,8; 2017,Jan,8; 2016,Jan,13; 2015,Jun,10; 2015,Apr,3; 2015,Jan,16

82785 IgE
INCLUDES Farr test
EXCLUDES *Allergen specific, IgE (86003, 86005)*
0.00 0.00 FUD XXX
AMA: 2018,Jan,8; 2017,Jan,8; 2016,Jan,13; 2015,Jun,10; 2015,Apr,3; 2015,Jan,16

82787 immunoglobulin subclasses (eg, IgG1, 2, 3, or 4), each
EXCLUDES *Gamma-glutamyltransferase (GGT) (82977)*
0.00 0.00 FUD XXX
AMA: 2015,Jun,10; 2015,Apr,3

82800 Gases, blood, pH only
0.00 0.00 FUD XXX
AMA: 2015,Jun,10; 2015,Apr,3

82803 Gases, blood, any combination of pH, pCO2, pO2, CO2, HCO3 (including calculated O2 saturation);
INCLUDES Two or more listed analytes
0.00 0.00 FUD XXX
AMA: 2015,Jun,10; 2015,Apr,3

82805 **with O2 saturation, by direct measurement, except pulse oximetry**
0.00 0.00 **FUD** XXX
AMA: 2015,Jun,10; 2015,Apr,3

82810 **Gases, blood, O2 saturation only, by direct measurement, except pulse oximetry**
EXCLUDES *Pulse oximetry (94760)*
0.00 0.00 **FUD** XXX
AMA: 2015,Jun,10; 2015,Apr,3

82820 **Hemoglobin-oxygen affinity (pO2 for 50% hemoglobin saturation with oxygen)**
EXCLUDES *Gastric acid analysis (82930)*
0.00 0.00 **FUD** XXX
AMA: 2015,Jun,10; 2015,Apr,3

82930 **Gastric acid analysis, includes pH if performed, each specimen**
0.00 0.00 **FUD** XXX
AMA: 2018,Jan,8; 2017,Jan,8; 2016,Jan,13; 2015,Jun,10; 2015,Apr,3; 2015,Jan,16

82938 **Gastrin after secretin stimulation**
0.00 0.00 **FUD** XXX
AMA: 2015,Jun,10; 2015,Apr,3

82941 **Gastrin**
EXCLUDES *Gentamicin (80170)*
GGT (82977)
Qualitative column chromatography report specific analyte or (82542)
0.00 0.00 **FUD** XXX
AMA: 2015,Jun,10; 2015,Apr,3

82943-82962 Chemistry: Glucagon—Glucose Testing

CMS: 100-03,190.20 Blood Glucose Testing
INCLUDES Clinical information not requested by ordering physician
Mathematically calculated results
Quantitative analysis unless otherwise specified
Specimens from any source unless otherwise specified
EXCLUDES *Analytes from nonrequested laboratory analysis*
Calculated results representing score or probability derived by algorithm
Organ or disease panels (80048-80076 [80081])
Therapeutic drug assays (80150-80299 [80164, 80165, 80171])
Code also glucose administration injection (96374)

82943 **Glucagon**
0.00 0.00 **FUD** XXX
AMA: 2015,Jun,10; 2015,Apr,3

82945 **Glucose, body fluid, other than blood**
0.00 0.00 **FUD** XXX
AMA: 2015,Jun,10; 2015,Apr,3

82946 **Glucagon tolerance test**
0.00 0.00 **FUD** XXX
AMA: 2015,Jun,10; 2015,Apr,3

82947 **Glucose; quantitative, blood (except reagent strip)**
0.00 0.00 **FUD** XXX
AMA: 2018,Jan,8; 2017,Jan,8; 2016,Jan,13; 2015,Jun,10; 2015,Apr,3; 2015,Jan,16

82948 **blood, reagent strip**
0.00 0.00 **FUD** XXX
AMA: 2018,Jan,8; 2017,Jan,8; 2016,Jan,13; 2015,Jun,10; 2015,Apr,3; 2015,Jan,16

82950 **post glucose dose (includes glucose)**
0.00 0.00 **FUD** XXX
AMA: 2018,Jan,8; 2017,Jan,8; 2016,Jan,13; 2015,Jun,10; 2015,Apr,3; 2015,Jan,16

82951 **tolerance test (GTT), 3 specimens (includes glucose)**
0.00 0.00 **FUD** XXX
AMA: 2018,Jan,8; 2017,Jan,8; 2016,Jan,13; 2015,Jun,10; 2015,Apr,3; 2015,Jan,16

+ **82952** **tolerance test, each additional beyond 3 specimens (List separately in addition to code for primary procedure)**
EXCLUDES *Insulin tolerance test (80434-80435)*
Leucine tolerance test (80428)
Semiquantitative urine glucose (81000, 81002, 81005, 81099)
Code first (82951)
0.00 0.00 **FUD** XXX
AMA: 2018,Jan,8; 2017,Jan,8; 2016,Jan,13; 2015,Jun,10; 2015,Apr,3; 2015,Jan,16

82955 **Glucose-6-phosphate dehydrogenase (G6PD); quantitative**
Code also glucose tolerance test with medication, when performed (96374)
0.00 0.00 **FUD** XXX
AMA: 2015,Jun,10; 2015,Apr,3

82960 **screen**
Code also glucose tolerance test with medication, when performed (96374)
0.00 0.00 **FUD** XXX
AMA: 2015,Jun,10; 2015,Apr,3

82962 **Glucose, blood by glucose monitoring device(s) cleared by the FDA specifically for home use**
0.00 0.00 **FUD** XXX
AMA: 2018,Jan,8; 2017,Jan,8; 2016,Jan,13; 2015,Jun,10; 2015,Apr,3; 2015,Jan,16

82963-83690 Chemistry: Glucosidase—Lipase

INCLUDES Clinical information not requested by ordering physician
Mathematically calculated results
Quantitative analysis unless otherwise specified
Specimens from any source unless otherwise specified
EXCLUDES *Analytes from nonrequested laboratory analysis*
Calculated results representing score or probability derived by algorithm
Drug testing ([80305, 80306, 80307], [80324, 80325, 80326, 80327, 80328, 80329, 80330, 80331, 80332, 80333, 80334, 80335, 80336, 80337, 80338, 80339, 80340, 80341, 80342, 80343, 80344, 80345, 80346, 80347, 80348, 80349, 80350, 80351, 80352, 80353, 80354, 80355, 80356, 80357, 80358, 80359, 80360, 80361, 80362, 80363, 80364, 80365, 80366, 80367, 80368, 80369, 80370, 80371, 80372, 80373, 80374, 80375, 80376, 80377, 83992])
Organ or disease panels (80048-80076 [80081])
Therapeutic drug assays (80150-80299 [80164, 80165, 80171])

82963 **Glucosidase, beta**
0.00 0.00 **FUD** XXX
AMA: 2015,Jun,10; 2015,Apr,3

82965 **Glutamate dehydrogenase**
0.00 0.00 **FUD** XXX
AMA: 2015,Jun,10; 2015,Apr,3

82977 **Glutamyltransferase, gamma (GGT)**
0.00 0.00 **FUD** XXX
AMA: 2018,Jan,8; 2017,Jan,8; 2016,Jan,13; 2015,Jun,10; 2015,Apr,3; 2015,Jan,16

82978 **Glutathione**
0.00 0.00 **FUD** XXX
AMA: 2015,Jun,10; 2015,Apr,3

82979 **Glutathione reductase, RBC**
EXCLUDES *Glycohemoglobin (83036)*
0.00 0.00 **FUD** XXX
AMA: 2015,Jun,10; 2015,Apr,3

82985 **Glycated protein**
EXCLUDES *Gonadotropin chorionic (hCG) (84702-84703)*
0.00 0.00 **FUD** XXX
AMA: 2018,Jan,8; 2017,Jan,8; 2016,Jan,13; 2015,Jun,10; 2015,Apr,3; 2015,Jan,16

83001 **Gonadotropin; follicle stimulating hormone (FSH)**
0.00 0.00 **FUD** XXX
AMA: 2015,Jun,10; 2015,Apr,3

83002 **luteinizing hormone (LH)**
EXCLUDES *Luteinizing releasing factor (LRH) (83727)*
0.00 0.00 **FUD** XXX
AMA: 2015,Jun,10; 2015,Apr,3

83003 **Growth hormone, human (HGH) (somatotropin)**
EXCLUDES *Antibody to human growth hormone (86277)*
0.00 0.00 FUD XXX
AMA: 2015,Jun,10; 2015,Apr,3

83006 **Growth stimulation expressed gene 2 (ST2, Interleukin 1 receptor like-1)**
0.00 0.00 FUD XXX
AMA: 2015,Jun,10; 2015,Apr,3

83009 **Helicobacter pylori, blood test analysis for urease activity, non-radioactive isotope (eg, C-13)**
EXCLUDES *H. pylori, breath test analysis for urease activity (83013-83014)*
0.00 0.00 FUD XXX
AMA: 2015,Jun,10; 2015,Apr,3

83010 **Haptoglobin; quantitative**
0.00 0.00 FUD XXX
AMA: 2015,Jun,10; 2015,Apr,3

83012 **phenotypes**
0.00 0.00 FUD XXX
AMA: 2015,Jun,10; 2015,Apr,3

83013 **Helicobacter pylori; breath test analysis for urease activity, non-radioactive isotope (eg, C-13)**
0.00 0.00 FUD XXX
AMA: 2020,OctSE,1; 2018,Jan,8; 2017,Jan,8; 2016,Jan,13; 2015,Jun,10; 2015,Apr,3; 2015,Jan,16

83014 **drug administration**
EXCLUDES *H. pylori:*
Blood test analysis for urease activity (83009)
Enzyme immunoassay (87339)
Liquid scintillation counter (78267-78268)
Stool (87338)
0.00 0.00 FUD XXX
AMA: 2020,OctSE,1; 2018,Jan,8; 2017,Jan,8; 2016,Jan,13; 2015,Jun,10; 2015,Apr,3; 2015,Jan,16

83015 **Heavy metal (eg, arsenic, barium, beryllium, bismuth, antimony, mercury); qualitative, any number of analytes**
INCLUDES Reinsch test
0.00 0.00 FUD XXX
AMA: 2015,Jun,10; 2015,Apr,3

83018 **quantitative, each, not elsewhere specified**
EXCLUDES *Evaluation known heavy metal with specific code*
0.00 0.00 FUD XXX
AMA: 2015,Jun,10; 2015,Apr,3

83020 **Hemoglobin fractionation and quantitation; electrophoresis (eg, A2, S, C, and/or F)**
0.00 0.00 FUD XXX
AMA: 2015,Jun,10; 2015,Apr,3

83021 **chromatography (eg, A2, S, C, and/or F)**
EXCLUDES *Analysis glycosylated (A1c) hemoglobin by chromatography or electrophoresis without identified hemoglobin variant (83036)*
0.00 0.00 FUD XXX
AMA: 2018,Jan,8; 2017,Jan,8; 2016,Jan,13; 2015,Jun,10; 2015,Apr,3; 2015,Jan,16

83026 **Hemoglobin; by copper sulfate method, non-automated**
0.00 0.00 FUD XXX
AMA: 2015,Jun,10; 2015,Apr,3

83030 **F (fetal), chemical**
0.00 0.00 FUD XXX
AMA: 2015,Jun,10; 2015,Apr,3

83033 **F (fetal), qualitative**
0.00 0.00 FUD XXX
AMA: 2015,Jun,10; 2015,Apr,3

83036 **glycosylated (A1C)**
EXCLUDES *Analysis glycosylated (A1c) hemoglobin by chromatography or electrophoresis without identified hemoglobin variant (83020-83021)*
Detection hemoglobin, fecal, by immunoassay (82274)
0.00 0.00 FUD XXX
AMA: 2018,Jan,8; 2017,Jan,8; 2016,Jan,13; 2015,Jun,10; 2015,Apr,3; 2015,Jan,16

83037 **glycosylated (A1C) by device cleared by FDA for home use**
0.00 0.00 FUD XXX
AMA: 2018,Jan,8; 2017,Jan,8; 2016,Jan,13; 2015,Jun,10; 2015,Apr,3; 2015,Jan,16

83045 **methemoglobin, qualitative**
0.00 0.00 FUD XXX
AMA: 2015,Jun,10; 2015,Apr,3

83050 **methemoglobin, quantitative**
EXCLUDES *Transcutaneous methemoglobin test (88741)*
0.00 0.00 FUD XXX
AMA: 2018,Jan,8; 2017,Jan,8; 2016,Jan,13; 2015,Jun,10; 2015,Apr,3; 2015,Jan,16

83051 **plasma**
0.00 0.00 FUD XXX
AMA: 2015,Jun,10; 2015,Apr,3

83060 **sulfhemoglobin, quantitative**
0.00 0.00 FUD XXX
AMA: 2015,Jun,10; 2015,Apr,3

83065 **thermolabile**
0.00 0.00 FUD XXX
AMA: 2015,Jun,10; 2015,Apr,3

83068 **unstable, screen**
0.00 0.00 FUD XXX
AMA: 2015,Jun,10; 2015,Apr,3

83069 **urine**
0.00 0.00 FUD XXX
AMA: 2015,Jun,10; 2015,Apr,3

83070 **Hemosiderin, qualitative**
EXCLUDES *HIAA (83497)*
Qualitative column chromatography report specific analyte or (82542)
0.00 0.00 FUD XXX
AMA: 2015,Jun,10; 2015,Apr,3

83080 **b-Hexosaminidase, each assay**
0.00 0.00 FUD XXX
AMA: 2015,Jun,10; 2015,Apr,3

83088 **Histamine**
EXCLUDES *Hollander test (43754-43755)*
0.00 0.00 FUD XXX
AMA: 2015,Jun,10; 2015,Apr,3

83090 **Homocysteine**
0.00 0.00 FUD XXX
AMA: 2018,Jan,8; 2017,Jan,8; 2016,Jan,13; 2015,Jun,10; 2015,Apr,3; 2015,Jan,16

83150 **Homovanillic acid (HVA)**
EXCLUDES *Hormone testing report from alphabetic list in Chemistry section*
Hydrogen/methane breath test (91065)
0.00 0.00 FUD XXX
AMA: 2015,Jun,10; 2015,Apr,3

83491 **Hydroxycorticosteroids, 17- (17-OHCS)**
EXCLUDES *Cortisol (82530, 82533)*
Deoxycortisol (82634)
0.00 0.00 FUD XXX
AMA: 2015,Jun,10; 2015,Apr,3

83497   Hydroxyindolacetic acid, 5-(HIAA)
> EXCLUDES   *5-Hydroxytryptamine (84260)*
>   *Urine qualitative test (81005)*
>
> 🚑 0.00   ⚗ 0.00   **FUD** XXX   🔲 🔲
>
> AMA: 2015,Jun,10; 2015,Apr,3

83498   Hydroxyprogesterone, 17-d
> 🚑 0.00   ⚗ 0.00   **FUD** XXX   🔲 🔲
>
> AMA: 2015,Jun,10; 2015,Apr,3

83500   Hydroxyproline; free
> 🚑 0.00   ⚗ 0.00   **FUD** XXX   🔲 🔲
>
> AMA: 2015,Jun,10; 2015,Apr,3

83505   total
> 🚑 0.00   ⚗ 0.00   **FUD** XXX   🔲 🔲
>
> AMA: 2015,Jun,10; 2015,Apr,3

83516   Immunoassay for analyte other than infectious agent antibody or infectious agent antigen; qualitative or semiquantitative, multiple step method
> 🚑 0.00   ⚗ 0.00   **FUD** XXX   ❌ 🔲 🔲
>
> AMA: 2020,OctSE,1; 2020,AugSE,1; 2020,AugSE,1; 2020,AugSE,1; 2015,Jun,10; 2015,Apr,3

83518   qualitative or semiquantitative, single step method (eg, reagent strip)
> 🚑 0.00   ⚗ 0.00   **FUD** XXX   🔲 🔲
>
> AMA: 2020,OctSE,1; 2015,Jun,10; 2015,Apr,3

83519   quantitative, by radioimmunoassay (eg, RIA)
> 🚑 0.00   ⚗ 0.00   **FUD** XXX   🔲 🔲
>
> AMA: 2020,OctSE,1; 2018,Jan,8; 2017,Jan,8; 2016,Jan,13; 2015,Jun,10; 2015,Apr,3; 2015,Jan,16

83520   quantitative, not otherwise specified
> EXCLUDES   *Immunoassays for antibodies to infectious agent antigen report specific analyte/method from Immunology*
>   *Immunoassay of tumor antigens not elsewhere specified (86316)*
>   *Immunoglobulins (82784, 82785)*
>
> 🚑 0.00   ⚗ 0.00   **FUD** XXX   🔲 🔲
>
> AMA: 2020,OctSE,1; 2015,Jun,10; 2015,Apr,3

83525   Insulin; total
> EXCLUDES   *Proinsulin (84206)*
>
> 🚑 0.00   ⚗ 0.00   **FUD** XXX   🔲 🔲
>
> AMA: 2015,Jun,10; 2015,Apr,3

83527   free
> 🚑 0.00   ⚗ 0.00   **FUD** XXX   🔲 🔲
>
> AMA: 2018,Jan,8; 2017,Jan,8; 2016,Jan,13; 2015,Jun,10; 2015,Apr,3; 2015,Jan,16

83528   Intrinsic factor
> EXCLUDES   *Intrinsic factor antibodies (86340)*
>
> 🚑 0.00   ⚗ 0.00   **FUD** XXX   🔲 🔲
>
> AMA: 2015,Jun,10; 2015,Apr,3

83540   Iron
> 🚑 0.00   ⚗ 0.00   **FUD** XXX   🔲 🔲
>
> AMA: 2018,Jan,8; 2017,Jan,8; 2016,Jan,13; 2015,Jun,10; 2015,Apr,3; 2015,Jan,16

83550   Iron binding capacity
> 🚑 0.00   ⚗ 0.00   **FUD** XXX   🔲 🔲
>
> AMA: 2015,Jun,10; 2015,Apr,3

83570   Isocitric dehydrogenase (IDH)
> EXCLUDES   *Isonicotinic acid hydrazide, INH, report specific method*
>   *Isopropyl alcohol ([80320])*
>
> 🚑 0.00   ⚗ 0.00   **FUD** XXX   🔲 🔲
>
> AMA: 2015,Jun,10; 2015,Apr,3

83582   Ketogenic steroids, fractionation
> EXCLUDES   *Ketone bodies:*
>   *Serum (82009, 82010)*
>   *Urine (81000-81003)*
>
> 🚑 0.00   ⚗ 0.00   **FUD** XXX   🔲 🔲
>
> AMA: 2015,Jun,10; 2015,Apr,3

83586   Ketosteroids, 17- (17-KS); total
> 🚑 0.00   ⚗ 0.00   **FUD** XXX   🔲 🔲
>
> AMA: 2015,Jun,10; 2015,Apr,3

83593   fractionation
> 🚑 0.00   ⚗ 0.00   **FUD** XXX   🔲 🔲
>
> AMA: 2015,Jun,10; 2015,Apr,3

83605   Lactate (lactic acid)
> 🚑 0.00   ⚗ 0.00   **FUD** XXX   ❌ 🔲 🔲
>
> AMA: 2015,Jun,10; 2015,Apr,3

83615   Lactate dehydrogenase (LD), (LDH);
> 🚑 0.00   ⚗ 0.00   **FUD** XXX   🔲 🔲
>
> AMA: 2018,Jan,8; 2017,Jan,8; 2016,Jan,13; 2015,Jun,10; 2015,Apr,3; 2015,Jan,16

83625   isoenzymes, separation and quantitation
> 🚑 0.00   ⚗ 0.00   **FUD** XXX   🔲 🔲
>
> AMA: 2018,Jan,8; 2017,Jan,8; 2016,Jan,13; 2015,Jun,10; 2015,Apr,3; 2015,Jan,16

83630   Lactoferrin, fecal; qualitative
> 🚑 0.00   ⚗ 0.00   **FUD** XXX   🔲 🔲
>
> AMA: 2018,Jan,8; 2017,Jan,8; 2016,Jan,13; 2015,Jun,10; 2015,Apr,3; 2015,Jan,16

83631   quantitative
> 🚑 0.00   ⚗ 0.00   **FUD** XXX   🔲 🔲
>
> AMA: 2018,Jan,8; 2017,Jan,8; 2016,Jan,13; 2015,Jun,10; 2015,Apr,3; 2015,Jan,16

83632   Lactogen, human placental (HPL) human chorionic somatomammotropin   Ⓜ
> 🚑 0.00   ⚗ 0.00   **FUD** XXX   🔲 🔲
>
> AMA: 2015,Jun,10; 2015,Apr,3

83633   Lactose, urine, qualitative
> EXCLUDES   *Lactase deficiency breath hydrogen/methane test (91065)*
>   *Lactose tolerance test (82951, 82952)*
>
> 🚑 0.00   ⚗ 0.00   **FUD** XXX   🔲 🔲
>
> AMA: 2015,Jun,10; 2015,Apr,3

83655   Lead
> 🚑 0.00   ⚗ 0.00   **FUD** XXX   ❌ 🔲 🔲
>
> AMA: 2015,Jun,10; 2015,Apr,3

83661   Fetal lung maturity assessment; lecithin sphingomyelin (L/S) ratio   Ⓜ
> 🚑 0.00   ⚗ 0.00   **FUD** XXX   🔲 🔲
>
> AMA: 2018,Jan,8; 2017,Jan,8; 2016,Jan,13; 2015,Jun,10; 2015,Apr,3; 2015,Jan,16

83662   foam stability test   Ⓜ
> 🚑 0.00   ⚗ 0.00   **FUD** XXX   🔲 🔲
>
> AMA: 2015,Jun,10; 2015,Apr,3

83663   fluorescence polarization   Ⓜ
> 🚑 0.00   ⚗ 0.00   **FUD** XXX   🔲 🔲
>
> AMA: 2015,Jun,10; 2015,Apr,3

83664   lamellar body density   Ⓜ
> EXCLUDES   *Phosphatidylglycerol (84081)*
>
> 🚑 0.00   ⚗ 0.00   **FUD** XXX   🔲 🔲
>
> AMA: 2015,Jun,10; 2015,Apr,3

83670   Leucine aminopeptidase (LAP)
> 🚑 0.00   ⚗ 0.00   **FUD** XXX   🔲 🔲
>
> AMA: 2015,Jun,10; 2015,Apr,3

83690   Lipase
> 🚑 0.00   ⚗ 0.00   **FUD** XXX   🔲 🔲
>
> AMA: 2015,Jun,10; 2015,Apr,3

26/TC PC/TC Only	A2-Z3 ASC Payment	50 Bilateral	♂ Male Only	♀ Female Only	🚑 Facility RVU	⚗ Non-Facility RVU	🔲 CCI	❌ CLIA
FUD Follow-up Days	**CMS:** IOM	**AMA:** CPT Asst	A-Y OPPSI	80/80 Surg Assist Allowed / w/Doc		🔲 Lab Crosswalk	🔲 Radiology Crosswalk	

83695-83727 Chemistry: Lipoprotein—Luteinizing Releasing Factor

[INCLUDES] Clinical information not requested by ordering physician
Mathematically calculated results
Quantitative analysis unless otherwise specified
Specimens from any source unless otherwise specified

[EXCLUDES] *Analytes from nonrequested laboratory analysis*
Calculated results representing score or probability derived by algorithm
Organ or disease panels (80048-80076 [80081])
Therapeutic drug assays (80150-80299 [80164, 80165, 80171])

83695 Lipoprotein (a)
0.00 0.00 FUD XXX [Q]
AMA: 2018,Jan,8; 2017,Jan,8; 2016,Jan,13; 2015,Jun,10; 2015,Apr,3; 2015,Jan,16

83698 Lipoprotein-associated phospholipase A2 (Lp-PLA2)
[EXCLUDES] *Secretory type II phospholipase A2 (sPLA2-IIA) (0423T)*
0.00 0.00 FUD XXX [Q]
AMA: 2015,Jun,10; 2015,Apr,3

83700 Lipoprotein, blood; electrophoretic separation and quantitation
0.00 0.00 FUD XXX [Q]
AMA: 2018,Jan,8; 2017,Jan,8; 2016,Jan,13; 2015,Jun,10; 2015,Apr,3; 2015,Jan,16

83701 high resolution fractionation and quantitation of lipoproteins including lipoprotein subclasses when performed (eg, electrophoresis, ultracentrifugation)
0.00 0.00 FUD XXX [Q]
AMA: 2018,Jan,8; 2017,Jan,8; 2016,Jan,13; 2015,Jun,10; 2015,Apr,3; 2015,Jan,16

83704 quantitation of lipoprotein particle number(s) (eg, by nuclear magnetic resonance spectroscopy), includes lipoprotein particle subclass(es), when performed
0.00 0.00 FUD XXX [Q]
AMA: 2018,Jan,8; 2017,Jan,8; 2016,Jan,13; 2015,Jun,10; 2015,Apr,3; 2015,Jan,16

83718 Lipoprotein, direct measurement; high density cholesterol (HDL cholesterol)
0.00 0.00 FUD XXX [X] [A]
AMA: 2018,Jan,8; 2017,Jan,8; 2016,Jan,13; 2015,Jun,10; 2015,Apr,3; 2015,Jan,16

83719 VLDL cholesterol
0.00 0.00 FUD XXX [Q]
AMA: 2018,Jan,8; 2017,Jan,8; 2016,Jan,13; 2015,Jun,10; 2015,Apr,3; 2015,Jan,16

83721 LDL cholesterol
[EXCLUDES] *Fractionation by high resolution electrophoresis or ultracentrifugation (83701)*
Lipoprotein particle numbers and subclasses analysis by nuclear magnetic resonance spectroscopy (83704)
0.00 0.00 FUD XXX [X] [Q]
AMA: 2018,Jan,8; 2017,Jan,8; 2016,Jan,13; 2015,Jun,10; 2015,Apr,3; 2015,Jan,16

83722 small dense LDL cholesterol
[EXCLUDES] *Fractionation by high resolution electrophoresis or ultracentrifugation (83701)*
Lipoprotein particle numbers/subclass analysis by nuclear magnetic resonance spectroscopy (83704)
0.00 0.00 FUD XXX

83727 Luteinizing releasing factor (LRH)
[EXCLUDES] *alpha-2-Macroglobulin (86329)*
Luteinizing hormone (LH) (83002)
0.00 0.00 FUD XXX [Q]
AMA: 2015,Jun,10; 2015,Apr,3

83735-83885 Chemistry: Magnesium—Nickel

[INCLUDES] Clinical information not requested by the ordering physician
Mathematically calculated results
Quantitative analysis unless otherwise specified
Specimens from any source unless otherwise specified

[EXCLUDES] *Analytes from nonrequested laboratory analysis*
Calculated results representing a score or probability derived by algorithm
Organ or disease panels (80048-80076 [80081])
Therapeutic drug assays (80150-80299 [80164, 80165, 80171])

83735 Magnesium
0.00 0.00 FUD XXX [Q]
AMA: 2015,Jun,10; 2015,Apr,3

83775 Malate dehydrogenase
[EXCLUDES] *Maltose tolerance (82951, 82952)*
Mammotropin (84146)
0.00 0.00 FUD XXX [Q]
AMA: 2015,Jun,10; 2015,Apr,3

83785 Manganese
0.00 0.00 FUD XXX [Q]
AMA: 2015,Jun,10; 2015,Apr,3

83789 Mass spectrometry and tandem mass spectrometry (eg, MS, MS/MS, MALDI, MS-TOF, QTOF), non-drug analyte(s) not elsewhere specified, qualitative or quantitative, each specimen
[EXCLUDES] *Column chromatography/mass spectrometry drugs or substances ([80305], [80306], [80307], [80320, 80321, 80322, 80323, 80324, 80325, 80326, 80327, 80328, 80329, 80330, 80331, 80332, 80333, 80334, 80335, 80336, 80337, 80338, 80339, 80340, 80341, 80342, 80343, 80344, 80345, 80346, 80347, 80348, 80349, 80350, 80351, 80352, 80353, 80354, 80355, 80356, 80357, 80358, 80359, 80360, 80361, 80362, 80363, 80364, 80365, 80366, 80367, 80368, 80369, 80370, 80371, 80372, 80373, 80374, 80375, 80376, 80377, 83992])*
Procedure performed more than one time per specimen
Report specific analyte testing with code(s) from Chemistry section
0.00 0.00 FUD XXX [Q]
AMA: 2015,Jun,10; 2015,Apr,3

83825 Mercury, quantitative
[EXCLUDES] *Mercury screen (83015)*
0.00 0.00 FUD XXX [Q]
AMA: 2015,Jun,10; 2015,Apr,3

83835 Metanephrines
[EXCLUDES] *Catecholamines (82382-82384)*
Methamphetamine ([80324], [80325], [80326])
Methane breath test (91065)
0.00 0.00 FUD XXX [Q]
AMA: 2015,Jun,10; 2015,Apr,3

83857 Methemalbumin
[EXCLUDES] *Methemoglobin (83045, 83050)*
Methyl alcohol ([80320])
Microalbumin
Quantitative (82043)
Semiquantitative (82044)
0.00 0.00 FUD XXX [Q]
AMA: 2015,Jun,10; 2015,Apr,3

83861 Microfluidic analysis utilizing an integrated collection and analysis device, tear osmolarity
[EXCLUDES] *beta-2 Microglobulin (82232)*
Code also when performed on both eyes 83861 X 2
0.00 0.00 FUD XXX [X] [Q]
AMA: 2015,Jun,10; 2015,Apr,3

83864 Mucopolysaccharides, acid, quantitative
0.00 0.00 FUD XXX [Q]
AMA: 2015,Jun,10; 2015,Apr,3

83872 Mucin, synovial fluid (Ropes test)
0.00 0.00 FUD XXX [Q]
AMA: 2015,Jun,10; 2015,Apr,3

83873 Myelin basic protein, cerebrospinal fluid
EXCLUDES Oligoclonal bands (83916)
0.00 0.00 FUD XXX
AMA: 2015,Jun,10; 2015,Apr,3

83874 Myoglobin
0.00 0.00 FUD XXX
AMA: 2018,Jan,8; 2017,Jan,8; 2016,Jan,13; 2015,Jun,10; 2015,Apr,3; 2015,Jan,16

83876 Myeloperoxidase (MPO)
0.00 0.00 FUD XXX
AMA: 2015,Jun,10; 2015,Apr,3

83880 Natriuretic peptide
0.00 0.00 FUD XXX
AMA: 2018,Jan,8; 2017,Jan,8; 2016,Jan,13; 2015,Jun,10; 2015,Apr,3; 2015,Jan,16

83883 Nephelometry, each analyte not elsewhere specified
0.00 0.00 FUD XXX
AMA: 2015,Jun,10; 2015,Apr,3

83885 Nickel
0.00 0.00 FUD XXX
AMA: 2015,Jun,10; 2015,Apr,3

83915-84066 [83992] Chemistry: Nucleotidase 5'- —Phosphatase (Acid)

INCLUDES Clinical information not requested by ordering physician
Mathematically calculated results
Quantitative analysis unless otherwise specified
Specimens from any source unless otherwise specified
EXCLUDES Analytes from nonrequested laboratory analysis
Calculated results representing score or probability derived by algorithm
Drug testing ([80305, 80306, 80307], [80324, 80325, 80326, 80327, 80328, 80329, 80330, 80331, 80332, 80333, 80334, 80335, 80336, 80337, 80338, 80339, 80340, 80341, 80342, 80343, 80344, 80345, 80346, 80347, 80348, 80349, 80350, 80351, 80352, 80353, 80354, 80355, 80356, 80357, 80358, 80359, 80360, 80361, 80362, 80363, 80364, 80365, 80366, 80367, 80368, 80369, 80370, 80371, 80372, 80373, 80374, 80375, 80376, 80377, 83992])
Organ or disease panels (80048-80076 [80081])
Therapeutic drug assays (80150-80299 [80164, 80165, 80171])

83915 Nucleotidase 5'-
0.00 0.00 FUD XXX
AMA: 2015,Jun,10; 2015,Apr,3

83916 Oligoclonal immune (oligoclonal bands)
0.00 0.00 FUD XXX
AMA: 2015,Jun,10; 2015,Apr,3

83918 Organic acids; total, quantitative, each specimen
0.00 0.00 FUD XXX
AMA: 2018,Jan,8; 2017,Jan,8; 2016,Jan,13; 2015,Jun,10; 2015,Apr,3; 2015,Jan,16

83919 qualitative, each specimen
0.00 0.00 FUD XXX
AMA: 2015,Jun,10; 2015,Apr,3

83921 Organic acid, single, quantitative
0.00 0.00 FUD XXX
AMA: 2015,Jun,10; 2015,Apr,3

83930 Osmolality; blood
EXCLUDES Tear osmolarity (83861)
0.00 0.00 FUD XXX
AMA: 2015,Jun,10; 2015,Apr,3

83935 urine
EXCLUDES Tear osmolarity (83861)
0.00 0.00 FUD XXX
AMA: 2015,Jun,10; 2015,Apr,3

83937 Osteocalcin (bone g1a protein)
0.00 0.00 FUD XXX
AMA: 2018,Jan,8; 2017,Jan,8; 2016,Jan,13; 2015,Jun,10; 2015,Apr,3; 2015,Jan,16

83945 Oxalate
0.00 0.00 FUD XXX
AMA: 2015,Jun,10; 2015,Apr,3

83950 Oncoprotein; HER-2/neu
EXCLUDES Tissue (88342, 88365)
0.00 0.00 FUD XXX
AMA: 2015,Jun,10; 2015,Apr,3

83951 des-gamma-carboxy-prothrombin (DCP)
0.00 0.00 FUD XXX
AMA: 2015,Jun,10; 2015,Apr,3

83970 Parathormone (parathyroid hormone)
EXCLUDES Chlorinated hydrocarbon screen (82441)
Quantitative pesticide report code for specific method
0.00 0.00 FUD XXX
AMA: 2015,Jun,10; 2015,Apr,3

83986 pH; body fluid, not otherwise specified
EXCLUDES Blood pH (82800, 82803)
0.00 0.00 FUD XXX
AMA: 2018,Jan,8; 2017,Jan,8; 2016,May,13; 2016,Jan,13; 2015,Jun,10; 2015,Apr,3; 2015,Jan,16

83987 exhaled breath condensate
EXCLUDES Blood pH (82800, 82803)
Phenobarbital ([80345])
0.00 0.00 FUD XXX
AMA: 2015,Jun,10; 2015,Apr,3

83992 Resequenced code. See code following resequenced code 80365.

83993 Calprotectin, fecal
0.00 0.00 FUD XXX
AMA: 2018,Jan,8; 2017,Jan,8; 2016,Jan,13; 2015,Jun,10; 2015,Apr,3; 2015,Jan,16

84030 Phenylalanine (PKU), blood
INCLUDES Guthrie test
EXCLUDES Phenylalanine-tyrosine ratio (84030, 84510)
0.00 0.00 FUD XXX
AMA: 2015,Jun,10; 2015,Apr,3

84035 Phenylketones, qualitative
0.00 0.00 FUD XXX
AMA: 2015,Jun,10; 2015,Apr,3

84060 Phosphatase, acid; total
0.00 0.00 FUD XXX
AMA: 2015,Jun,10; 2015,Apr,3

84066 prostatic
0.00 0.00 FUD XXX
AMA: 2015,Jun,10; 2015,Apr,3

84075-84080 Chemistry: Phosphatase (Alkaline)

CMS: 100-03,160.17 Payment for L-Dopa /Associated Inpatient Hospital Services
INCLUDES Clinical information not requested by ordering physician
Mathematically calculated results
Quantitative analysis unless otherwise specified
Specimens from any source unless otherwise specified
EXCLUDES Analytes from nonrequested laboratory analysis
Calculated results representing score or probability derived by algorithm
Organ or disease panels (80048-80076 [80081])

84075 Phosphatase, alkaline;
0.00 0.00 FUD XXX
AMA: 2018,Jan,8; 2017,Jan,8; 2016,Jan,13; 2015,Jun,10; 2015,Apr,3; 2015,Jan,16

84078 heat stable (total not included)
0.00 0.00 FUD XXX
AMA: 2015,Jun,10; 2015,Apr,3

84080 isoenzymes
0.00 0.00 FUD XXX
AMA: 2015,Jun,10; 2015,Apr,3

84081-84150 Chemistry: Phosphatidylglycerol—Prostaglandin

INCLUDES Clinical information not requested by ordering physician
Mathematically calculated results
Quantitative analysis unless otherwise specified
Specimens from any source unless otherwise specified

EXCLUDES *Analytes from nonrequested laboratory analysis*
Calculated results representing score or probability derived by algorithm
Organ or disease panels (80048-80076 [80081])
Therapeutic drug assays (80150-80299 [80164, 80165, 80171])

84081 Phosphatidylglycerol

EXCLUDES *Cholinesterase (82480, 82482)*
Inorganic phosphates (84100)
Organic phosphates, report code for specific method

0.00 0.00 FUD XXX

AMA: 2015,Jun,10; 2015,Apr,3

84085 Phosphogluconate, 6-, dehydrogenase, RBC

0.00 0.00 FUD XXX

AMA: 2015,Jun,10; 2015,Apr,3

84087 Phosphohexose isomerase

0.00 0.00 FUD XXX

AMA: 2015,Jun,10; 2015,Apr,3

84100 Phosphorus inorganic (phosphate);

0.00 0.00 FUD XXX

AMA: 2018,Jan,8; 2017,Jan,8; 2016,Jan,13; 2015,Jun,10; 2015,Apr,3; 2015,Jan,16

84105 urine

EXCLUDES *Pituitary gonadotropins (83001-83002)*
PKU (84030, 84035)

0.00 0.00 FUD XXX

AMA: 2015,Jun,10; 2015,Apr,3

84106 Porphobilinogen, urine; qualitative

0.00 0.00 FUD XXX

AMA: 2015,Jun,10; 2015,Apr,3

84110 quantitative

0.00 0.00 FUD XXX

AMA: 2015,Jun,10; 2015,Apr,3

84112 Evaluation of cervicovaginal fluid for specific amniotic fluid protein(s) (eg, placental alpha microglobulin-1 [PAMG-1], placental protein 12 [PP12], alpha-fetoprotein), qualitative, each specimen ♀

0.00 0.00 FUD XXX

AMA: 2015,Jun,10; 2015,Apr,3

84119 Porphyrins, urine; qualitative

0.00 0.00 FUD XXX

AMA: 2015,Jun,10; 2015,Apr,3

84120 quantitation and fractionation

0.00 0.00 FUD XXX

AMA: 2015,Jun,10; 2015,Apr,3

84126 Porphyrins, feces, quantitative

EXCLUDES *Porphyrin precursors (82135, 84106, 84110)*
Protoporphyrin, RBC (84202, 84203)

0.00 0.00 FUD XXX

AMA: 2015,Jun,10; 2015,Apr,3

84132 Potassium; serum, plasma or whole blood

0.00 0.00 FUD XXX

AMA: 2018,Jan,8; 2017,Jan,8; 2016,Jan,13; 2015,Jun,10; 2015,Apr,3; 2015,Jan,16

84133 urine

0.00 0.00 FUD XXX

AMA: 2015,Jun,10; 2015,Apr,3

84134 Prealbumin

EXCLUDES *Microalbumin (82043-82044)*

0.00 0.00 FUD XXX

AMA: 2015,Jun,10; 2015,Apr,3

84135 Pregnanediol ♀

0.00 0.00 FUD XXX

AMA: 2015,Jun,10; 2015,Apr,3

84138 Pregnanetriol ♀

0.00 0.00 FUD XXX

AMA: 2015,Jun,10; 2015,Apr,3

84140 Pregnenolone

0.00 0.00 FUD XXX

AMA: 2018,Jan,8; 2017,Jan,8; 2016,Jan,13; 2015,Jun,10; 2015,Apr,3; 2015,Jan,16

84143 17-hydroxypregnenolone

0.00 0.00 FUD XXX

AMA: 2018,Jan,8; 2017,Jan,8; 2016,Jan,13; 2015,Jun,10; 2015,Apr,3; 2015,Jan,16

84144 Progesterone

EXCLUDES *Progesterone receptor assay (84234)*
Proinsulin (84206)

0.00 0.00 FUD XXX

AMA: 2015,Jun,10; 2015,Apr,3

84145 Procalcitonin (PCT)

0.00 0.00 FUD XXX

AMA: 2015,Jun,10; 2015,Apr,3

84146 Prolactin

0.00 0.00 FUD XXX

AMA: 2015,Jun,10; 2015,Apr,3

84150 Prostaglandin, each

0.00 0.00 FUD XXX

AMA: 2015,Jun,10; 2015,Apr,3

84152-84154 Chemistry: Prostate Specific Antigen

CMS: 100-03,190.31 Prostate Specific Antigen (PSA); 100-03,210.1 Prostate Cancer Screening Tests

INCLUDES Clinical information not requested by ordering physician
Mathematically calculated results
Quantitative analysis unless otherwise specified

EXCLUDES *Analytes from nonrequested laboratory analysis*
Calculated results representing score or probability derived by algorithm

84152 Prostate specific antigen (PSA); complexed (direct measurement) ♂

0.00 0.00 FUD XXX

AMA: 2015,Jun,10; 2015,Apr,3

84153 total ♂

0.00 0.00 FUD XXX

AMA: 2018,Jan,8; 2017,Jan,8; 2016,Jan,13; 2015,Jun,10; 2015,Apr,3; 2015,Jan,16

84154 free ♂

0.00 0.00 FUD XXX

AMA: 2018,Jan,8; 2017,Jan,8; 2016,Jan,13; 2015,Jun,10; 2015,Apr,3; 2015,Jan,16

84155-84157 Chemistry: Protein, Total (Not by Refractometry)

INCLUDES Clinical information not requested by ordering physician
Mathematically calculated results

EXCLUDES *Analytes from nonrequested laboratory analysis*
Calculated results representing score or probability derived by algorithm
Organ or disease panels (80048-80076 [80081])

84155 Protein, total, except by refractometry; serum, plasma or whole blood

0.00 0.00 FUD XXX

AMA: 2018,Jan,8; 2017,Jan,8; 2016,Jan,13; 2015,Jun,10; 2015,Apr,3; 2015,Jan,16

84156 urine

0.00 0.00 FUD XXX

AMA: 2015,Jun,10; 2015,Apr,3

84157 other source (eg, synovial fluid, cerebrospinal fluid)

0.00 0.00 FUD XXX

AMA: 2015,Jun,10; 2015,Apr,3

84160-84432 Chemistry: Protein, Total (Refractometry)—Thyroglobulin

INCLUDES Clinical information not requested by ordering physician
Mathematically calculated results
Quantitative analysis unless otherwise specified
Specimens from any source unless otherwise specified

EXCLUDES *Analytes from nonrequested laboratory analysis*
Calculated results representing score or probability derived by algorithm
Drug testing ([80305, 80306, 80307], [80324, 80325, 80326, 80327, 80328, 80329, 80330, 80331, 80332, 80333, 80334, 80335, 80336, 80337, 80338, 80339, 80340, 80341, 80342, 80343, 80344, 80345, 80346, 80347, 80348, 80349, 80350, 80351, 80352, 80353, 80354, 80355, 80356, 80357, 80358, 80359, 80360, 80361, 80362, 80363, 80364, 80365, 80366, 80367, 80368, 80369, 80370, 80371, 80372, 80373, 80374, 80375, 80376, 80377, 83992])
Organ or disease panels (80048-80076 [80081])
Therapeutic drug assays (80150-80299 [80164, 80165, 80171])

84160 Protein, total, by refractometry, any source
EXCLUDES *Urine total protein, dipstick method (81000-81003)*
0.00 0.00 FUD XXX
AMA: 2015,Jun,10; 2015,Apr,3

84163 Pregnancy-associated plasma protein-A (PAPP-A) ♀
0.00 0.00 FUD XXX
AMA: 2015,Jun,10; 2015,Apr,3

84165 Protein; electrophoretic fractionation and quantitation, serum
0.00 0.00 FUD XXX
AMA: 2015,Jun,10; 2015,Apr,3

84166 electrophoretic fractionation and quantitation, other fluids with concentration (eg, urine, CSF)
0.00 0.00 FUD XXX
AMA: 2015,Jun,10; 2015,Apr,3

84181 Western Blot, with interpretation and report, blood or other body fluid
0.00 0.00 FUD XXX
AMA: 2015,Jun,10; 2015,Apr,3

84182 Western Blot, with interpretation and report, blood or other body fluid, immunological probe for band identification, each
EXCLUDES *Western Blot tissue analysis (88371)*
0.00 0.00 FUD XXX
AMA: 2015,Jun,10; 2015,Apr,3

84202 Protoporphyrin, RBC; quantitative
0.00 0.00 FUD XXX
AMA: 2015,Jun,10; 2015,Apr,3

84203 screen
0.00 0.00 FUD XXX
AMA: 2015,Jun,10; 2015,Apr,3

84206 Proinsulin
EXCLUDES *Pseudocholinesterase (82480)*
0.00 0.00 FUD XXX
AMA: 2015,Jun,10; 2015,Apr,3

84207 Pyridoxal phosphate (Vitamin B-6)
0.00 0.00 FUD XXX
AMA: 2015,Jun,10; 2015,Apr,3

84210 Pyruvate
0.00 0.00 FUD XXX
AMA: 2015,Jun,10; 2015,Apr,3

84220 Pyruvate kinase
0.00 0.00 FUD XXX
AMA: 2015,Jun,10; 2015,Apr,3

84228 Quinine
0.00 0.00 FUD XXX
AMA: 2018,Jan,8; 2017,Jan,8; 2016,Jan,13; 2015,Jun,10; 2015,Apr,3

84233 Receptor assay; estrogen
0.00 0.00 FUD XXX
AMA: 2015,Jun,10; 2015,Apr,3

84234 progesterone
0.00 0.00 FUD XXX
AMA: 2015,Jun,10; 2015,Apr,3

84235 endocrine, other than estrogen or progesterone (specify hormone)
0.00 0.00 FUD XXX
AMA: 2015,Jun,10; 2015,Apr,3

84238 non-endocrine (specify receptor)
0.00 0.00 FUD XXX
AMA: 2018,Jan,8; 2017,Jan,8; 2016,Jan,13; 2015,Jun,10; 2015,Apr,3; 2015,Jan,16

84244 Renin
0.00 0.00 FUD XXX
AMA: 2015,Jun,10; 2015,Apr,3

84252 Riboflavin (Vitamin B-2)
EXCLUDES *Salicylates ([80329], [80330], [80331])*
Salicylate therapeutic drug assay ([80179])
Secretin test reported with appropriate analyses (43756, 43757, 99070)
0.00 0.00 FUD XXX
AMA: 2015,Jun,10; 2015,Apr,3

84255 Selenium
0.00 0.00 FUD XXX
AMA: 2015,Jun,10; 2015,Apr,3

84260 Serotonin
EXCLUDES *Urine metabolites (HIAA) (83497)*
0.00 0.00 FUD XXX
AMA: 2015,Jun,10; 2015,Apr,3

84270 Sex hormone binding globulin (SHBG)
0.00 0.00 FUD XXX
AMA: 2018,Jan,8; 2017,Jan,8; 2016,Jan,13; 2015,Jun,10; 2015,Apr,3; 2015,Jan,16

84275 Sialic acid
EXCLUDES *Sickle hemoglobin (85660)*
0.00 0.00 FUD XXX
AMA: 2015,Jun,10; 2015,Apr,3

84285 Silica
0.00 0.00 FUD XXX
AMA: 2015,Jun,10; 2015,Apr,3

84295 Sodium; serum, plasma or whole blood
0.00 0.00 FUD XXX
AMA: 2018,Jan,8; 2017,Jan,8; 2016,Jan,13; 2015,Jun,10; 2015,Apr,3; 2015,Jan,16

84300 urine
0.00 0.00 FUD XXX
AMA: 2015,Jun,10; 2015,Apr,3

84302 other source
EXCLUDES *Somatomammotropin (83632)*
Somatotropin (83003)
0.00 0.00 FUD XXX
AMA: 2018,Jan,8; 2017,Jan,8; 2016,Jan,13; 2015,Jun,10; 2015,Apr,3; 2015,Jan,16

84305 Somatomedin
0.00 0.00 FUD XXX
AMA: 2018,Jan,8; 2017,Jan,8; 2016,Jan,13; 2015,Jun,10; 2015,Apr,3; 2015,Jan,16

84307 Somatostatin
0.00 0.00 FUD XXX
AMA: 2018,Jan,8; 2017,Jan,8; 2016,Jan,13; 2015,Jun,10; 2015,Apr,3; 2015,Jan,16

84311 Spectrophotometry, analyte not elsewhere specified
0.00 0.00 FUD XXX
AMA: 2015,Jun,10; 2015,Apr,3

84315 Specific gravity (except urine)

EXCLUDES *Stone analysis (82355-82370)*
Suppression of growth stimulation expressed gene 2 [ST2] testing (83006)
Urine specific gravity (81000-81003)

0.00 0.00 FUD XXX

AMA: 2015,Jun,10; 2015,Apr,3

84375 Sugars, chromatographic, TLC or paper chromatography

0.00 0.00 FUD XXX

AMA: 2015,Jun,10; 2015,Apr,3

84376 Sugars (mono-, di-, and oligosaccharides); single qualitative, each specimen

0.00 0.00 FUD XXX

AMA: 2018,Jan,8; 2017,Jan,8; 2016,Jan,13; 2015,Jun,10; 2015,Apr,3; 2015,Jan,16

84377 multiple qualitative, each specimen

0.00 0.00 FUD XXX

AMA: 2018,Jan,8; 2017,Jan,8; 2016,Jan,13; 2015,Jun,10; 2015,Apr,3; 2015,Jan,16

84378 single quantitative, each specimen

0.00 0.00 FUD XXX

AMA: 2015,Jun,10; 2015,Apr,3

84379 multiple quantitative, each specimen

0.00 0.00 FUD XXX

AMA: 2018,Jan,8; 2017,Jan,8; 2016,Jan,13; 2015,Jun,10; 2015,Apr,3; 2015,Jan,16

84392 Sulfate, urine

EXCLUDES *Sulfhemoglobin (83060)*
T-3 (84479-84481)
T-4 (84436-84439)

0.00 0.00 FUD XXX

AMA: 2015,Jun,10; 2015,Apr,3

84402 Testosterone; free

EXCLUDES *Anabolic steroids ([80327, 80328])*

0.00 0.00 FUD XXX

AMA: 2015,Jun,10; 2015,Apr,3

84403 total

EXCLUDES *Anabolic steroids ([80327, 80328])*

0.00 0.00 FUD XXX

AMA: 2015,Jun,10; 2015,Apr,3

84410 bioavailable, direct measurement (eg, differential precipitation)

0.00 0.00 FUD XXX

84425 Thiamine (Vitamin B-1)

0.00 0.00 FUD XXX

AMA: 2015,Jun,10; 2015,Apr,3

84430 Thiocyanate

0.00 0.00 FUD XXX

AMA: 2015,Jun,10; 2015,Apr,3

84431 Thromboxane metabolite(s), including thromboxane if performed, urine

Code also determination concurrent urine creatinine (82570)

0.00 0.00 FUD XXX

AMA: 2015,Jun,10; 2015,Apr,3

84432 Thyroglobulin

EXCLUDES *Thyroglobulin antibody (86800)*
Thyrotropin releasing hormone (TRH) (80438, 80439)

0.00 0.00 FUD XXX

AMA: 2018,Jan,8; 2017,Jan,8; 2016,Jan,13; 2015,Jun,10; 2015,Apr,3; 2015,Jan,16

84436-84445 Chemistry: Thyroid Tests

CMS: 100-03,190.22 Thyroid Testing

INCLUDES Clinical information not requested by the ordering physician
Mathematically calculated results
Quantitative analysis unless otherwise specified
Specimens from any source unless otherwise specified

EXCLUDES *Analytes from nonrequested laboratory analysis*
Calculated results representing a score or probability derived by algorithm
Organ or disease panels (80048-80076 [80081])
Therapeutic drug assays (80150-80299 [80164, 80165, 80171])

84436 Thyroxine; total

0.00 0.00 FUD XXX

AMA: 2018,Jan,8; 2017,Jan,8; 2016,Jan,13; 2015,Jun,10; 2015,Apr,3; 2015,Jan,16

84437 requiring elution (eg, neonatal)

0.00 0.00 FUD XXX

AMA: 2015,Jun,10; 2015,Apr,3

84439 free

0.00 0.00 FUD XXX

AMA: 2015,Jun,10; 2015,Apr,3

84442 Thyroxine binding globulin (TBG)

0.00 0.00 FUD XXX

AMA: 2015,Jun,10; 2015,Apr,3

84443 Thyroid stimulating hormone (TSH)

0.00 0.00 FUD XXX

AMA: 2015,Jun,10; 2015,Apr,3

84445 Thyroid stimulating immune globulins (TSI)

EXCLUDES *Tobramycin (80200)*

0.00 0.00 FUD XXX

AMA: 2018,Jan,8; 2017,Jan,8; 2016,Jan,13; 2015,Jun,10; 2015,Apr,3; 2015,Jan,16

84446-84449 Chemistry: Tocopherol Alpha—Transcortin

INCLUDES Clinical information not requested by ordering physician
Mathematically calculated results
Quantitative analysis unless otherwise specified
Specimens from any source unless otherwise specified

EXCLUDES *Analytes from nonrequested laboratory analysis*
Calculated results representing score or probability derived by algorithm
Organ or disease panels (80048-80076 [80081])
Therapeutic drug assays (80150-80299 [80164, 80165, 80171])

84446 Tocopherol alpha (Vitamin E)

0.00 0.00 FUD XXX

AMA: 2015,Jun,10; 2015,Apr,3

84449 Transcortin (cortisol binding globulin)

0.00 0.00 FUD XXX

AMA: 2018,Jan,8; 2017,Jan,8; 2016,Jan,13; 2015,Jun,10; 2015,Apr,3; 2015,Jan,16

84450-84460 Chemistry: Transferase

CMS: 100-02,11,30.2.2 Automated Multi-Channel Chemistry (AMCC) Tests; 100-03,160.17 Payment for L-Dopa /Associated Inpatient Hospital Services; 100-04,16,40.6.1 Automated Multi-Channel Chemistry (AMCC) Tests for ESRD Beneficiaries; 100-04,16,70.8 CLIA Waived Tests

INCLUDES Clinical information not requested by ordering physician
Mathematically calculated results
Quantitative analysis unless otherwise specified

EXCLUDES *Analytes from nonrequested laboratory analysis*
Calculated results representing score or probability derived by algorithm

84450 Transferase; aspartate amino (AST) (SGOT)

0.00 0.00 FUD XXX

AMA: 2018,Jan,8; 2017,Jan,8; 2016,Jan,13; 2015,Jun,10; 2015,Apr,3; 2015,Jan,16

84460 alanine amino (ALT) (SGPT)

0.00 0.00 FUD XXX

AMA: 2018,Jan,8; 2017,Jan,8; 2016,Jan,13; 2015,Jun,10; 2015,Apr,3; 2015,Jan,16

84466 Chemistry: Transferrin

CMS: 100-02,11,20.2 ESRD Laboratory Services; 100-03,190.18 Serum Iron Studies

INCLUDES Clinical information not requested by ordering physician
Mathematically calculated results
Quantitative analysis unless otherwise specified

EXCLUDES *Analytes from nonrequested laboratory analysis*
Calculated results representing score or probability derived by algorithm

84466 Transferrin
EXCLUDES *Iron binding capacity (83550)*
0.00 0.00 **FUD** XXX
AMA: 2018,Jan,8; 2017,Jan,8; 2016,Jan,13; 2015,Jun,10; 2015,Apr,3; 2015,Jan,16

84478 Chemistry: Triglycerides

CMS: 100-02,11,30.2.2 Automated Multi-Channel Chemistry (AMCC) Tests; 100-03,190.23 Lipid Testing; 100-04,16,70.8 CLIA Waived Tests; 100-04,16,90.2 Organ or Disease Oriented Panels

INCLUDES Clinical information not requested by ordering physician
Mathematically calculated results

EXCLUDES *Analytes from nonrequested laboratory analysis*
Calculated results representing score or probability derived by algorithm
Organ or disease panels (80048-80076 [80081])

84478 Triglycerides
0.00 0.00 **FUD** XXX
AMA: 2018,Jan,8; 2017,Jan,8; 2016,Jan,13; 2015,Jun,10; 2015,Apr,3; 2015,Jan,16

84479-84482 Chemistry: Thyroid Hormone—Triiodothyronine

CMS: 100-03,190.22 Thyroid Testing

INCLUDES Clinical information not requested by ordering physician
Mathematically calculated results
Quantitative analysis unless otherwise specified
Specimens from any source unless otherwise specified

EXCLUDES *Analytes from nonrequested laboratory analysis*
Calculated results representing score or probability derived by algorithm
Organ or disease panels (80048-80076 [80081])

84479 Thyroid hormone (T3 or T4) uptake or thyroid hormone binding ratio (THBR)
0.00 0.00 **FUD** XXX
AMA: 2018,Jan,8; 2017,Jan,8; 2016,Jan,13; 2015,Jun,10; 2015,Apr,3; 2015,Jan,16

84480 Triiodothyronine T3; total (TT-3)
0.00 0.00 **FUD** XXX
AMA: 2015,Jun,10; 2015,Apr,3

84481 free
0.00 0.00 **FUD** XXX
AMA: 2015,Jun,10; 2015,Apr,3

84482 reverse
0.00 0.00 **FUD** XXX
AMA: 2018,Jan,8; 2017,Jan,8; 2016,Jan,13; 2015,Jun,10; 2015,Apr,3; 2015,Jan,16

84484-84512 Chemistry: Troponin (Quantitative)—Troponin (Qualitative)

INCLUDES Clinical information not requested by ordering physician
Mathematically calculated results
Specimens from any source unless otherwise specified

EXCLUDES *Analytes from nonrequested laboratory analysis*
Calculated results representing score or probability derived by algorithm
Organ or disease panels

84484 Troponin, quantitative
EXCLUDES *Qualitative troponin assay (84512)*
0.00 0.00 **FUD** XXX
AMA: 2018,Jan,8; 2017,Jan,8; 2016,Jan,13; 2015,Jun,10; 2015,Apr,3; 2015,Jan,16

84485 Trypsin; duodenal fluid
0.00 0.00 **FUD** XXX
AMA: 2015,Jun,10; 2015,Apr,3

84488 feces, qualitative
0.00 0.00 **FUD** XXX
AMA: 2015,Jun,10; 2015,Apr,3

84490 feces, quantitative, 24-hour collection
0.00 0.00 **FUD** XXX
AMA: 2015,Jun,10; 2015,Apr,3

84510 Tyrosine
EXCLUDES *Urate crystal identification (89060)*
0.00 0.00 **FUD** XXX
AMA: 2015,Jun,10; 2015,Apr,3

84512 Troponin, qualitative
EXCLUDES *Quantitative troponin assay (84484)*
0.00 0.00 **FUD** XXX
AMA: 2018,Jan,8; 2017,Jan,8; 2016,Jan,13; 2015,Jun,10; 2015,Apr,3; 2015,Jan,16

84520-84525 Chemistry: Urea Nitrogen (Blood)

CMS: 100-03,160.17 Payment for L-Dopa /Associated Inpatient Hospital Services

INCLUDES Clinical information not requested by ordering physician
Mathematically calculated results

EXCLUDES *Analytes from nonrequested laboratory analysis*
Calculated results representing score or probability derived by algorithm
Organ or disease panels (80048-80076 [80081])

84520 Urea nitrogen; quantitative
0.00 0.00 **FUD** XXX
AMA: 2018,Jan,8; 2017,Jan,8; 2016,Jan,13; 2015,Jun,10; 2015,Apr,3; 2015,Jan,16

84525 semiquantitative (eg, reagent strip test)
INCLUDES Patterson's test
0.00 0.00 **FUD** XXX
AMA: 2018,Jan,8; 2017,Jan,8; 2016,Jan,13; 2015,Jun,10; 2015,Apr,3; 2015,Jan,16

84540-84630 Chemistry: Urea Nitrogen (Urine)—Zinc

INCLUDES Clinical information not requested by ordering physician
Mathematically calculated results
Quantitative analysis unless otherwise specified
Specimens from any source unless otherwise specified

EXCLUDES *Analytes from nonrequested laboratory analysis*
Calculated results representing score or probability derived by algorithm
Organ or disease panels (80048-80076 [80081])
Therapeutic drug assays (80150-80299 [80164, 80165, 80171])

84540 Urea nitrogen, urine
0.00 0.00 **FUD** XXX
AMA: 2015,Jun,10; 2015,Apr,3

84545 Urea nitrogen, clearance
0.00 0.00 **FUD** XXX
AMA: 2015,Jun,10; 2015,Apr,3

84550 Uric acid; blood
0.00 0.00 **FUD** XXX
AMA: 2018,Jan,8; 2017,Jan,8; 2016,Jan,13; 2015,Jun,10; 2015,Apr,3; 2015,Jan,16

84560 other source
0.00 0.00 **FUD** XXX
AMA: 2015,Jun,10; 2015,Apr,3

84577 Urobilinogen, feces, quantitative
0.00 0.00 **FUD** XXX
AMA: 2015,Jun,10; 2015,Apr,3

84578 Urobilinogen, urine; qualitative
0.00 0.00 **FUD** XXX
AMA: 2015,Jun,10; 2015,Apr,3

84580 quantitative, timed specimen
0.00 0.00 **FUD** XXX
AMA: 2015,Jun,10; 2015,Apr,3

84583 semiquantitative
EXCLUDES *Uroporphyrins (84120)*
Valproic acid (dipropylacetic acid) ([80164])
0.00 0.00 **FUD** XXX
AMA: 2015,Jun,10; 2015,Apr,3

84585 Vanillylmandelic acid (VMA), urine
0.00 0.00 **FUD** XXX
AMA: 2015,Jun,10; 2015,Apr,3

84586 **Vasoactive intestinal peptide (VIP)**
0.00 0.00 FUD XXX
AMA: 2018,Jan,8; 2017,Jan,8; 2016,Jan,13; 2015,Jun,10; 2015,Apr,3; 2015,Jan,16

84588 **Vasopressin (antidiuretic hormone, ADH)**
0.00 0.00 FUD XXX
AMA: 2018,Jan,7; 2015,Jun,10; 2015,Apr,3

84590 **Vitamin A**
EXCLUDES *Vitamin B-1 (84425)*
Vitamin B-2 (84252)
Vitamin B-6 (84207)
Vitamin B-12 (82607)
Vitamin C (82180)
Vitamin D (82306, [82652])
Vitamin E (84446)
0.00 0.00 FUD XXX
AMA: 2015,Jun,10; 2015,Apr,3

84591 **Vitamin, not otherwise specified**
0.00 0.00 FUD XXX
AMA: 2015,Jun,10; 2015,Apr,3

84597 **Vitamin K**
EXCLUDES *Vanillylmandelic acid (VMA) (84585)*
0.00 0.00 FUD XXX
AMA: 2015,Jun,10; 2015,Apr,3

84600 **Volatiles (eg, acetic anhydride, diethylether)**
EXCLUDES *Carbon tetrachloride, dichloroethane, dichloromethane (82441)*
Isopropyl alcohol and methanol ([80320])
Volume, blood, RISA, or Cr-51 (78110, 78111)
0.00 0.00 FUD XXX
AMA: 2015,Jun,10; 2015,Apr,3

84620 **Xylose absorption test, blood and/or urine**
EXCLUDES *Administration (99070)*
0.00 0.00 FUD XXX
AMA: 2015,Jun,10; 2015,Apr,3

84630 **Zinc**
0.00 0.00 FUD XXX
AMA: 2015,Jun,10; 2015,Apr,3

84681-84999 Other and Unlisted Chemistry Tests

INCLUDES Clinical information not requested by ordering physician
Mathematically calculated results
Quantitative analysis unless otherwise specified
Specimens from any source unless otherwise specified

EXCLUDES *Analytes from nonrequested laboratory analysis*
Calculated results representing score or probability derived by algorithm
Confirmational testing, not otherwise specified drug ([80375, 80376, 80377], 80299)
Organ or disease panels (80048-80076 [80081])

84681 **C-peptide**
0.00 0.00 FUD XXX
AMA: 2015,Jun,10; 2015,Apr,3

84702 **Gonadotropin, chorionic (hCG); quantitative**
0.00 0.00 FUD XXX
AMA: 2015,Jun,10; 2015,Apr,3

84703 **qualitative**
EXCLUDES *Urine pregnancy test by visual color comparison (81025)*
0.00 0.00 FUD XXX
AMA: 2015,Jun,10; 2015,Apr,3

84704 **free beta chain**
0.00 0.00 FUD XXX
AMA: 2018,Jan,8; 2017,Jan,8; 2016,Jan,13; 2015,Jun,10; 2015,Apr,3; 2015,Jan,16

84830 **Ovulation tests, by visual color comparison methods for human luteinizing hormone** ♀
0.00 0.00 FUD XXX
AMA: 2018,Jan,8; 2017,Jan,8; 2016,Jan,13; 2015,Jun,10; 2015,Apr,3

84999 **Unlisted chemistry procedure**
EXCLUDES *Definitive drug testing, not otherwise specified ([80375], [80376], [80377], 80299)*
0.00 0.00 FUD XXX
AMA: 2018,Jan,8; 2017,Jan,8; 2016,Jan,13; 2015,Apr,3; 2015,Jan,16

85002 Bleeding Time Test

EXCLUDES *Agglutinins (86000, 86156, 86157)*
Antiplasmin (85410)
Antithrombin III (85300, 85301)
Blood banking procedures (86077-86079)

85002 **Bleeding time**
0.00 0.00 FUD XXX
AMA: 2018,Jan,8; 2017,Jan,8; 2016,Jan,13; 2015,Jan,16

85004-85049 Blood Counts

CMS: 100-03,190.15 Blood Counts

EXCLUDES *Agglutinins (86000, 86156-86157)*
Antiplasmin (85410)
Antithrombin III (85300-85301)
Blood banking procedures (86850-86999)

85004 **Blood count; automated differential WBC count**
0.00 0.00 FUD XXX
AMA: 2018,Jan,8; 2017,Jan,8; 2016,Jan,13; 2015,Jan,16

85007 **blood smear, microscopic examination with manual differential WBC count**
0.00 0.00 FUD XXX
AMA: 2018,Jan,8; 2017,Jan,8; 2016,Jan,13; 2015,Jan,16

85008 **blood smear, microscopic examination without manual differential WBC count**
EXCLUDES *Cell count other fluids (eg, CSF) (89050-89051)*
0.00 0.00 FUD XXX
AMA: 2018,Jan,8; 2017,Jan,8; 2016,Jan,13; 2015,Jan,16

85009 **manual differential WBC count, buffy coat**
EXCLUDES *Eosinophils, nasal smear (89190)*
0.00 0.00 FUD XXX
AMA: 2018,Jan,8; 2017,Jan,8; 2016,Jan,13; 2015,Jan,16

85013 **spun microhematocrit**
0.00 0.00 FUD XXX
AMA: 2005,Aug,7-8; 2005,Jul,11-12

85014 **hematocrit (Hct)**
0.00 0.00 FUD XXX
AMA: 2018,Jan,8; 2017,Jan,8; 2016,Jan,13; 2015,Jan,16

85018 **hemoglobin (Hgb)**
EXCLUDES *Immunoassay, hemoglobin, fecal (82274)*
Other hemoglobin determination (83020-83069)
Transcutaneous hemoglobin measurement (88738)
0.00 0.00 FUD XXX
AMA: 2018,Jan,8; 2017,Jan,8; 2016,Jan,13; 2015,Jan,16

85025 **complete (CBC), automated (Hgb, Hct, RBC, WBC and platelet count) and automated differential WBC count**
0.00 0.00 FUD XXX
AMA: 2018,Jan,8; 2017,Jan,8; 2016,Jan,13; 2015,Jan,16

85027 **complete (CBC), automated (Hgb, Hct, RBC, WBC and platelet count)**
0.00 0.00 FUD XXX
AMA: 2018,Jan,8; 2017,Jan,8; 2016,Jan,13; 2015,Jan,16

85032 **manual cell count (erythrocyte, leukocyte, or platelet) each**
0.00 0.00 FUD XXX
AMA: 2018,Jan,8; 2017,Jan,8; 2016,Jan,13; 2015,Jan,16

85041 **red blood cell (RBC), automated**
EXCLUDES *Complete blood count (85025, 85027)*
0.00 0.00 FUD XXX
AMA: 2018,Jan,8; 2017,Jan,8; 2016,Jan,13; 2015,Jan,16

85044 **reticulocyte, manual**
0.00 0.00 FUD XXX
AMA: 2018,Jan,8; 2017,Jan,8; 2016,Jan,13; 2015,Jan,16

85045 **reticulocyte, automated**
0.00 0.00 FUD XXX
AMA: 2018,Jan,8; 2017,Jan,8; 2016,Jan,13; 2015,Jan,16

85046 **reticulocytes, automated, including 1 or more cellular parameters (eg, reticulocyte hemoglobin content [CHr], immature reticulocyte fraction [IRF], reticulocyte volume [MRV], RNA content), direct measurement**
0.00 0.00 FUD XXX
AMA: 2005,Aug,7-8; 2005,Jul,11-12

85048 **leukocyte (WBC), automated**
0.00 0.00 FUD XXX
AMA: 2018,Jan,8; 2017,Jan,8; 2016,Jan,13; 2015,Jan,16

85049 **platelet, automated**
0.00 0.00 FUD XXX
AMA: 2005,Aug,7-8; 2005,Jul,11-12

85055-85705 Coagulopathy Testing

EXCLUDES *Agglutinins (86000, 86156-86157)*
Antiplasmin (85410)
Antithrombin III (85300-85301)
Blood banking procedures (86850-86999)

85055 **Reticulated platelet assay**
0.00 0.00 FUD XXX
AMA: 2005,Aug,7-8; 2005,Jul,11-12

85060 **Blood smear, peripheral, interpretation by physician with written report**
0.70 0.70 FUD XXX
AMA: 2005,Aug,7-8; 2005,Jul,11-12

85097 **Bone marrow, smear interpretation**
EXCLUDES *Bone biopsy (20220, 20225, 20240, 20245, 20250-20251)*
Special stains (88312-88313)
1.42 2.11 FUD XXX
AMA: 2018,Jan,8; 2017,Jan,8; 2016,Jan,13; 2015,Jan,16

85130 **Chromogenic substrate assay**
EXCLUDES *Circulating anticoagulant screen (mixing studies) (85611, 85732)*
0.00 0.00 FUD XXX
AMA: 2005,Aug,7-8; 2005,Jul,11-12

85170 **Clot retraction**
0.00 0.00 FUD XXX
AMA: 2005,Aug,7-8; 2005,Jul,11-12

85175 **Clot lysis time, whole blood dilution**
EXCLUDES *Clotting factor I (fibrinogen) (85384, 85385)*
0.00 0.00 FUD XXX
AMA: 2005,Aug,7-8; 2005,Jul,11-12

85210 **Clotting; factor II, prothrombin, specific**
EXCLUDES *Prothrombin time (85610-85611)*
Russell viper venom time (85612-85613)
0.00 0.00 FUD XXX
AMA: 2005,Aug,7-8; 2005,Jul,11-12

85220 **factor V (AcG or proaccelerin), labile factor**
0.00 0.00 FUD XXX
AMA: 2005,Aug,7-8; 2005,Jul,11-12

85230 **factor VII (proconvertin, stable factor)**
0.00 0.00 FUD XXX
AMA: 2005,Aug,7-8; 2005,Jul,11-12

85240 **factor VIII (AHG), 1-stage**
0.00 0.00 FUD XXX
AMA: 2005,Aug,7-8; 2005,Jul,11-12

85244 **factor VIII related antigen**
0.00 0.00 FUD XXX
AMA: 2005,Aug,7-8; 2005,Jul,11-12

85245 **factor VIII, VW factor, ristocetin cofactor**
0.00 0.00 FUD XXX
AMA: 2005,Aug,7-8; 2005,Jul,11-12

85246 **factor VIII, VW factor antigen**
0.00 0.00 FUD XXX
AMA: 2005,Aug,7-8; 2005,Jul,11-12

85247 **factor VIII, von Willebrand factor, multimetric analysis**
0.00 0.00 FUD XXX
AMA: 2005,Aug,7-8; 2005,Jul,11-12

85250 **factor IX (PTC or Christmas)**
0.00 0.00 FUD XXX
AMA: 2005,Aug,7-8; 2005,Jul,11-12

85260 **factor X (Stuart-Prower)**
0.00 0.00 FUD XXX
AMA: 2005,Aug,7-8; 2005,Jul,11-12

85270 **factor XI (PTA)**
0.00 0.00 FUD XXX
AMA: 2005,Aug,7-8; 2005,Jul,11-12

85280 **factor XII (Hageman)**
0.00 0.00 FUD XXX
AMA: 2005,Aug,7-8; 2005,Jul,11-12

85290 **factor XIII (fibrin stabilizing)**
0.00 0.00 FUD XXX
AMA: 2005,Aug,7-8; 2005,Jul,11-12

85291 **factor XIII (fibrin stabilizing), screen solubility**
0.00 0.00 FUD XXX
AMA: 2005,Aug,7-8; 2005,Jul,11-12

85292 **prekallikrein assay (Fletcher factor assay)**
0.00 0.00 FUD XXX
AMA: 2005,Aug,7-8; 2005,Jul,11-12

85293 **high molecular weight kininogen assay (Fitzgerald factor assay)**
0.00 0.00 FUD XXX
AMA: 2005,Aug,7-8; 2005,Jul,11-12

85300 **Clotting inhibitors or anticoagulants; antithrombin III, activity**
0.00 0.00 FUD XXX
AMA: 2005,Aug,7-8; 2005,Jul,11-12

85301 **antithrombin III, antigen assay**
0.00 0.00 FUD XXX
AMA: 2005,Aug,7-8; 2005,Jul,11-12

85302 **protein C, antigen**
0.00 0.00 FUD XXX
AMA: 2005,Aug,7-8; 2005,Jul,11-12

85303 **protein C, activity**
0.00 0.00 FUD XXX
AMA: 2005,Aug,7-8; 2005,Jul,11-12

85305 **protein S, total**
0.00 0.00 FUD XXX
AMA: 2005,Jul,11-12; 2005,Aug,7-8

85306 **protein S, free**
0.00 0.00 FUD XXX
AMA: 2005,Aug,7-8; 2005,Jul,11-12

85307 **Activated Protein C (APC) resistance assay**
0.00 0.00 FUD XXX
AMA: 2005,Aug,7-8; 2005,Jul,11-12

85335 **Factor inhibitor test**
0.00 0.00 FUD XXX
AMA: 2005,Aug,7-8; 2005,Jul,11-12

85337 **Thrombomodulin**
EXCLUDES *Mixing studies for inhibitors (85732)*
0.00 0.00 FUD XXX
AMA: 2005,Aug,7-8; 2005,Jul,11-12

85345 **Coagulation time; Lee and White**
0.00 0.00 FUD XXX
AMA: 2005,Aug,7-8; 2005,Jul,11-12

Pathology and Laboratory
85045 — 85345

85347 **activated**
0.00 0.00 FUD XXX
AMA: 2019,Apr,10

85348 **other methods**
EXCLUDES *Differential count (85007-85009, 85025)*
Duke bleeding time (85002)
Eosinophils, nasal smear (89190)
0.00 0.00 FUD XXX
AMA: 2005,Aug,7-8; 2005,Jul,11-12

85360 **Euglobulin lysis**
EXCLUDES *Fetal hemoglobin (83030, 83033, 85460)*
0.00 0.00 FUD XXX
AMA: 2005,Aug,7-8; 2005,Jul,11-12

85362 **Fibrin(ogen) degradation (split) products (FDP) (FSP); agglutination slide, semiquantitative**
EXCLUDES *Immunoelectrophoresis (86320)*
0.00 0.00 FUD XXX
AMA: 2005,Aug,7-8; 2005,Jul,11-12

85366 **paracoagulation**
0.00 0.00 FUD XXX
AMA: 2005,Aug,7-8; 2005,Jul,11-12

85370 **quantitative**
0.00 0.00 FUD XXX
AMA: 2005,Aug,7-8; 2005,Jul,11-12

85378 **Fibrin degradation products, D-dimer; qualitative or semiquantitative**
0.00 0.00 FUD XXX
AMA: 2018,Jan,8; 2017,Jan,8; 2016,Jan,13; 2015,Jan,16

85379 **quantitative**
INCLUDES Ultrasensitive and standard sensitivity quantitative D-dimer (85379)
0.00 0.00 FUD XXX
AMA: 2005,Aug,7-8; 2005,Jul,11-12

85380 **ultrasensitive (eg, for evaluation for venous thromboembolism), qualitative or semiquantitative**
0.00 0.00 FUD XXX
AMA: 2018,Jan,8; 2017,Jan,8; 2016,Jan,13; 2015,Jan,16

85384 **Fibrinogen; activity**
0.00 0.00 FUD XXX
AMA: 2019,Apr,10

85385 **antigen**
0.00 0.00 FUD XXX
AMA: 2005,Jul,11-12; 2005,Aug,7-8

85390 **Fibrinolysins or coagulopathy screen, interpretation and report**
0.00 0.00 FUD XXX 80
AMA: 2019,Apr,10

85396 **Coagulation/fibrinolysis assay, whole blood (eg, viscoelastic clot assessment), including use of any pharmacologic additive(s), as indicated, including interpretation and written report, per day**
0.58 0.58 FUD XXX N 80
AMA: 2019,Apr,10

85397 **Coagulation and fibrinolysis, functional activity, not otherwise specified (eg, ADAMTS-13), each analyte**
0.00 0.00 FUD XXX

85400 **Fibrinolytic factors and inhibitors; plasmin**
0.00 0.00 FUD XXX
AMA: 2005,Aug,7-8; 2005,Jul,11-12

85410 **alpha-2 antiplasmin**
0.00 0.00 FUD XXX
AMA: 2005,Aug,7-8; 2005,Jul,11-12

85415 **plasminogen activator**
0.00 0.00 FUD XXX
AMA: 2005,Aug,7-8; 2005,Jul,11-12

85420 **plasminogen, except antigenic assay**
0.00 0.00 FUD XXX
AMA: 2005,Aug,7-8; 2005,Jul,11-12

85421 **plasminogen, antigenic assay**
EXCLUDES *Fragility, red blood cell (85547, 85555-85557)*
0.00 0.00 FUD XXX
AMA: 2005,Aug,7-8; 2005,Jul,11-12

85441 **Heinz bodies; direct**
0.00 0.00 FUD XXX
AMA: 2005,Aug,7-8; 2005,Jul,11-12

85445 **induced, acetyl phenylhydrazine**
EXCLUDES *Hematocrit (PCV) (85014, 85025, 85027)*
Hemoglobin (83020-83068, 85018, 85025, 85027)
0.00 0.00 FUD XXX
AMA: 2005,Aug,7-8; 2005,Jul,11-12

85460 **Hemoglobin or RBCs, fetal, for fetomaternal hemorrhage; differential lysis (Kleihauer-Betke)** M ♀
EXCLUDES *Hemoglobin F (83030, 83033)*
Hemolysins (86940-86941)
0.00 0.00 FUD XXX
AMA: 2018,Jan,8; 2017,Jan,8; 2016,Jan,13; 2015,Jan,16

85461 **rosette** M ♀
0.00 0.00 FUD XXX
AMA: 2005,Jul,11-12; 2005,Aug,7-8

85475 **Hemolysin, acid**
INCLUDES Ham test
EXCLUDES *Hemolysins and agglutinins (86940-86941)*
0.00 0.00 FUD XXX
AMA: 2005,Aug,7-8; 2005,Jul,11-12

85520 **Heparin assay**
0.00 0.00 FUD XXX
AMA: 2005,Aug,7-8; 2005,Jul,11-12

85525 **Heparin neutralization**
0.00 0.00 FUD XXX
AMA: 2018,Jan,8; 2017,Aug,9

85530 **Heparin-protamine tolerance test**
0.00 0.00 FUD XXX
AMA: 2005,Aug,7-8; 2005,Jul,11-12

85536 **Iron stain, peripheral blood**
EXCLUDES *Iron stains on bone marrow or other tissues with physician evaluation (88313)*
0.00 0.00 FUD XXX
AMA: 2005,Aug,7-8; 2005,Jul,11-12

85540 **Leukocyte alkaline phosphatase with count**
0.00 0.00 FUD XXX
AMA: 2005,Aug,7-8; 2005,Jul,11-12

85547 **Mechanical fragility, RBC**
0.00 0.00 FUD XXX
AMA: 2005,Aug,7-8; 2005,Jul,11-12

85549 **Muramidase**
EXCLUDES *Nitroblue tetrazolium dye test (86384)*
0.00 0.00 FUD XXX
AMA: 2005,Aug,7-8; 2005,Jul,11-12

85555 **Osmotic fragility, RBC; unincubated**
0.00 0.00 FUD XXX
AMA: 2005,Aug,7-8; 2005,Jul,11-12

85557 **incubated**
EXCLUDES *Packed cell volume (85013)*
Parasites, blood (eg, malaria smears) (87207)
Partial thromboplastin time (85730, 85732)
Plasmin (85400)
Plasminogen (85420)
Plasminogen activator (85415)
0.00 0.00 FUD XXX
AMA: 2005,Aug,7-8; 2005,Jul,11-12

85576 **Platelet, aggregation (in vitro), each agent**
EXCLUDES *Thromboxane metabolite(s), including thromboxane,*
when performed, in urine (84431)
🖢 0.00   ⚖ 0.00   **FUD** XXX   ☒ ◨ 80 ▣
AMA: 2019,Apr,10; 2018,Jan,8; 2017,Jan,8; 2016,Jan,13;
2015,Jan,16

85597 **Phospholipid neutralization; platelet**
🖢 0.00   ⚖ 0.00   **FUD** XXX   ◨ ▣
AMA: 2018,Jan,8; 2017,Jan,8; 2016,Jan,13; 2015,Jan,16

85598 **hexagonal phospholipid**
🖢 0.00   ⚖ 0.00   **FUD** XXX   ◨ ▣
AMA: 2018,Jan,8; 2017,Jan,8; 2016,Jan,13; 2015,Jan,16

85610 **Prothrombin time;**
🖢 0.00   ⚖ 0.00   **FUD** XXX   ☒ ◨ ▣
AMA: 2005,Aug,7-8; 2005,Jul,11-12

85611 **substitution, plasma fractions, each**
🖢 0.00   ⚖ 0.00   **FUD** XXX   ◨ ▣
AMA: 2005,Aug,7-8; 2005,Jul,11-12

85612 **Russell viper venom time (includes venom); undiluted**
🖢 0.00   ⚖ 0.00   **FUD** XXX   ◨ ▣
AMA: 2005,Aug,7-8; 2005,Jul,11-12

85613 **diluted**
EXCLUDES *Red blood cell count (85025, 85027, 85041)*
🖢 0.00   ⚖ 0.00   **FUD** XXX   ◨ ▣
AMA: 2005,Aug,7-8; 2005,Jul,11-12

85635 **Reptilase test**
EXCLUDES *Reticulocyte count (85044-85045)*
🖢 0.00   ⚖ 0.00   **FUD** XXX   ◨ ▣
AMA: 2005,Aug,7-8; 2005,Jul,11-12

85651 **Sedimentation rate, erythrocyte; non-automated**
🖢 0.00   ⚖ 0.00   **FUD** XXX   ☒ ◨ ▣
AMA: 2005,Aug,7-8; 2005,Jul,11-12

85652 **automated**
INCLUDES Westergren test
🖢 0.00   ⚖ 0.00   **FUD** XXX   ◨ ▣
AMA: 2005,Aug,7-8; 2005,Jul,11-12

85660 **Sickling of RBC, reduction**
EXCLUDES *Hemoglobin electrophoresis (83020)*
Smears (87207)
🖢 0.00   ⚖ 0.00   **FUD** XXX   ◨ ▣
AMA: 2005,Aug,7-8; 2005,Jul,11-12

85670 **Thrombin time; plasma**
🖢 0.00   ⚖ 0.00   **FUD** XXX   ◨ ▣
AMA: 2005,Jul,11-12; 2005,Aug,7-8

85675 **titer**
🖢 0.00   ⚖ 0.00   **FUD** XXX   ◨ ▣
AMA: 2005,Jul,11-12; 2005,Aug,7-8

85705 **Thromboplastin inhibition, tissue**
EXCLUDES *Individual clotting factors (85245-85247)*
🖢 0.00   ⚖ 0.00   **FUD** XXX   ◨ ▣
AMA: 2005,Aug,7-8; 2005,Jul,11-12

85730-85732 Partial Thromboplastin Time (PTT)

EXCLUDES *Agglutinins (86000, 86156-86157)*
Antiplasmin (85410)
Antithrombin III (85300-85301)
Blood banking procedures (86850-86999)

85730 **Thromboplastin time, partial (PTT); plasma or whole blood**
INCLUDES Hicks-Pitney test
🖢 0.00   ⚖ 0.00   **FUD** XXX   ◨ ▣
AMA: 2005,Aug,7-8; 2005,Jul,11-12

85732 **substitution, plasma fractions, each**
🖢 0.00   ⚖ 0.00   **FUD** XXX   ◨ ▣
AMA: 2018,Jan,8; 2017,Jan,8; 2016,Jan,13; 2015,Jan,16

85810-85999 Blood Viscosity and Unlisted Hematology Procedures

85810 **Viscosity**
EXCLUDES *von Willebrand factor assay (85245-85247)*
WBC count (85025, 85027, 85048, 89050)
🖢 0.00   ⚖ 0.00   **FUD** XXX   ◨ ▣
AMA: 2018,Jan,8; 2017,Jan,8; 2016,Jan,13; 2015,Jan,16

85999 **Unlisted hematology and coagulation procedure**
🖢 0.00   ⚖ 0.00   **FUD** XXX   ◨ ▣
AMA: 2018,Jan,8; 2017,Aug,9; 2017,Jan,8; 2016,Jan,13;
2015,Jan,16

86000-86063 Antibody Testing

86000 **Agglutinins, febrile (eg, Brucella, Francisella, Murine typhus, Q fever, Rocky Mountain spotted fever, scrub typhus), each antigen**
EXCLUDES *Infectious agent antibodies (86602-86804)*
🖢 0.00   ⚖ 0.00   **FUD** XXX   ◨ ▣
AMA: 2018,Jan,8; 2017,Jan,8; 2016,Jan,13; 2015,Jan,16

86001 **Allergen specific IgG quantitative or semiquantitative, each allergen**
EXCLUDES *Agglutinins and autohemolysins (86940-86941)*
🖢 0.00   ⚖ 0.00   **FUD** XXX   ◨ ▣
AMA: 2005,Aug,7-8; 2005,Jul,11-12

86003 **Allergen specific IgE; quantitative or semiquantitative, crude allergen extract, each**
EXCLUDES *Total quantitative IgE (82785)*
🖢 0.00   ⚖ 0.00   **FUD** XXX   ◨ ▣
AMA: 2018,Jan,8; 2017,Jan,8; 2016,Jan,13; 2015,Jan,16

86005 **qualitative, multiallergen screen (eg, disk, sponge, card)**
EXCLUDES *Total qualitative IgE (83518)*
🖢 0.00   ⚖ 0.00   **FUD** XXX   ◨ ▣
AMA: 2018,Jan,8; 2017,Jan,8; 2016,Jan,13; 2015,Jan,16

86008 **quantitative or semiquantitative, recombinant or purified component, each**
EXCLUDES *Alpha-1 antitrypsin (82103, 82104)*
Alpha-1 feto-protein (82105, 82106)
Anti-AChR (acetylcholine receptor) antibody titer
(86255, 86256)
Anticardiolipin antibody (86147)
Anti-deoxyribonuclease titer (86215)
Anti-DNA (86225)
🖢 0.00   ⚖ 0.00   **FUD** XXX   ◨ ▣

86021 **Antibody identification; leukocyte antibodies**
🖢 0.00   ⚖ 0.00   **FUD** XXX   ◨ ▣
AMA: 2020,AugSE,1; 2020,AugSE,1; 2020,AugSE,1

86022 **platelet antibodies**
🖢 0.00   ⚖ 0.00   **FUD** XXX   ◨ ▣
AMA: 2020,AugSE,1; 2020,AugSE,1; 2020,AugSE,1

86023 **platelet associated immunoglobulin assay**
🖢 0.00   ⚖ 0.00   **FUD** XXX   ◨ ▣
AMA: 2020,AugSE,1; 2020,AugSE,1; 2020,AugSE,1

86038 **Antinuclear antibodies (ANA);**
🖢 0.00   ⚖ 0.00   **FUD** XXX   ◨ ▣
AMA: 2005,Aug,7-8; 2005,Jul,11-12

86039 **titer**
EXCLUDES *Antistreptococcal antibody, ie, anti-DNAse (86215)*
Antistreptokinase titer (86590)
🖢 0.00   ⚖ 0.00   **FUD** XXX   ◨ ▣
AMA: 2005,Aug,7-8; 2005,Jul,11-12

86060 **Antistreptolysin O; titer**
EXCLUDES *Antibodies, infectious agents (86602-86804)*
🖢 0.00   ⚖ 0.00   **FUD** XXX   ◨ ▣
AMA: 2005,Jul,11-12; 2005,Aug,7-8

| 26/TC PC/TC Only | A2-Z4 ASC Payment | 50 Bilateral | ♂ Male Only | ♀ Female Only | 🖢 Facility RVU | ⚖ Non-Facility RVU | ▣ CCI | ☒ CLIA |
| **FUD** Follow-up Days | **CMS:** IOM | **AMA:** CPT Asst | A-Y OPPSI | 80/80 Surg Assist Allowed / w/Doc | | ◧ Lab Crosswalk | ☒ Radiology Crosswalk |

414

CPT © 2020 American Medical Association. All Rights Reserved.

© 2020 Optum360, LLC

86063 **screen**

EXCLUDES *Antibodies to blastomyces (86612)*
Antibodies, infectious agents (86602-86804)

0.00 0.00 FUD XXX Q

AMA: 2005,Jul,11-12; 2005,Aug,7-8

86077-86079 Blood Bank Services

86077 **Blood bank physician services; difficult cross match and/or evaluation of irregular antibody(s), interpretation and written report**

1.46 1.57 FUD XXX Q1 80

AMA: 2005,Aug,7-8; 2005,Jul,11-12

86078 **investigation of transfusion reaction including suspicion of transmissible disease, interpretation and written report**

1.46 1.57 FUD XXX Q1 80

AMA: 2005,Aug,7-8; 2005,Jul,11-12

86079 **authorization for deviation from standard blood banking procedures (eg, use of outdated blood, transfusion of Rh incompatible units), with written report**

EXCLUDES *Brucella antibodies (86622)*
Candida antibodies (86628)
Candida skin test (86485)

1.46 1.56 FUD XXX Q1 80

AMA: 2005,Aug,7-8; 2005,Jul,11-12

86140-86344 [86152, 86153, 86328] Diagnostic Immunology Testing

86140 **C-reactive protein;**

EXCLUDES *Candidiasis (86628)*

0.00 0.00 FUD XXX Q

AMA: 2005,Aug,7-8; 2005,Jul,11-12

86141 **high sensitivity (hsCRP)**

0.00 0.00 FUD XXX Q

AMA: 2005,Aug,7-8; 2005,Jul,11-12

86146 **Beta 2 Glycoprotein I antibody, each**

0.00 0.00 FUD XXX Q

AMA: 2005,Aug,7-8; 2005,Jul,11-12

86147 **Cardiolipin (phospholipid) antibody, each Ig class**

0.00 0.00 FUD XXX Q

AMA: 2005,Aug,7-8; 2005,Jul,11-12

86152 **Cell enumeration using immunologic selection and identification in fluid specimen (eg, circulating tumor cells in blood);**

EXCLUDES *Flow cytometric immunophenotyping (88184-88189)*
Flow cytometric quantitation (86355-86357, 86359-86361, 86367)

Code also physician interpretation/report when performed ([86153])

0.00 0.00 FUD XXX Q

86153 **physician interpretation and report, when required**

EXCLUDES *Flow cytometric immunophenotyping (88184-88189)*
Flow cytometric quantitation (86355-86357, 86359-86361, 86367)

Code first cell enumeration, when performed ([86152])

0.00 0.00 FUD 000 B 80

86148 **Anti-phosphatidylserine (phospholipid) antibody**

EXCLUDES *Antiprothrombin (phospholipid cofactor) antibody (86849)*

0.00 0.00 FUD XXX Q

AMA: 2018,Jan,8; 2017,Jan,8; 2016,Jan,13; 2015,Jan,16

86152 **Resequenced code. See code following 86147.**

86153 **Resequenced code. See code before 86148.**

86155 **Chemotaxis assay, specify method**

EXCLUDES *Antibodies, coccidioides (86635)*
Clostridium difficile toxin (87230)
Skin test, coccidioides (86490)

0.00 0.00 FUD XXX Q

AMA: 2005,Aug,7-8; 2005,Jul,11-12

86156 **Cold agglutinin; screen**

0.00 0.00 FUD XXX Q

AMA: 2005,Aug,7-8; 2005,Jul,11-12

86157 **titer**

0.00 0.00 FUD XXX Q

AMA: 2005,Aug,7-8; 2005,Jul,11-12

86160 **Complement; antigen, each component**

0.00 0.00 FUD XXX Q

AMA: 2005,Aug,7-8; 2005,Jul,11-12

86161 **functional activity, each component**

0.00 0.00 FUD XXX Q

AMA: 2005,Aug,7-8; 2005,Jul,11-12

86162 **total hemolytic (CH50)**

0.00 0.00 FUD XXX Q

AMA: 2005,Aug,7-8; 2005,Jul,11-12

86171 **Complement fixation tests, each antigen**

EXCLUDES *Coombs test*

0.00 0.00 FUD XXX Q

AMA: 2005,Aug,7-8; 2005,Jul,11-12

86200 **Cyclic citrullinated peptide (CCP), antibody**

0.00 0.00 FUD XXX Q

AMA: 2018,Jan,8; 2017,Jan,8; 2016,Jan,13; 2015,Jan,16

86215 **Deoxyribonuclease, antibody**

0.00 0.00 FUD XXX Q

AMA: 2005,Aug,7-8; 2005,Jul,11-12

86225 **Deoxyribonucleic acid (DNA) antibody; native or double stranded**

EXCLUDES *Echinococcus antibodies, report code for specific method*
HIV antibody tests (86701-86703)

0.00 0.00 FUD XXX Q

AMA: 2005,Aug,7-8; 2005,Jul,11-12

86226 **single stranded**

EXCLUDES *Anti D.S, DNA, IFA, eg, using C. Lucilae (86255-86256)*

0.00 0.00 FUD XXX Q

AMA: 2005,Aug,7-8; 2005,Jul,11-12

86235 **Extractable nuclear antigen, antibody to, any method (eg, nRNP, SS-A, SS-B, Sm, RNP, Sc170, J01), each antibody**

0.00 0.00 FUD XXX Q

AMA: 2005,Aug,7-8; 2005,Jul,11-12

86255 **Fluorescent noninfectious agent antibody; screen, each antibody**

0.00 0.00 FUD XXX Q 80

AMA: 2020,AugSE,1; 2020,AugSE,1; 2020,AugSE,1

86256 **titer, each antibody**

EXCLUDES *Fluorescent technique for antigen identification in tissue (88346, [88350])*
FTA (86780)
Gel (agar) diffusion tests (86331)
Indirect fluorescence (88346, [88350])

0.00 0.00 FUD XXX Q 80

AMA: 2020,AugSE,1; 2020,AugSE,1; 2020,AugSE,1

86277 **Growth hormone, human (HGH), antibody**

0.00 0.00 FUD XXX Q

AMA: 2005,Aug,7-8; 2005,Jul,11-12

86280 **Hemagglutination inhibition test (HAI)**

EXCLUDES *Antibodies to infectious agents (86602-86804)*
Rubella (86762)

0.00 0.00 FUD XXX Q

AMA: 2005,Aug,7-8; 2005,Jul,11-12

86294 Immunoassay for tumor antigen, qualitative or semiquantitative (eg, bladder tumor antigen)

EXCLUDES *Qualitative NMP22 protein (86386)*

🚗 0.00   0.00 **FUD** XXX ❌ Ⓠ ▣

AMA: 2005,Aug,7-8; 2005,Jul,11-12

86300 Immunoassay for tumor antigen, quantitative; CA 15-3 (27.29)

🚗 0.00   0.00 **FUD** XXX Ⓠ ▣

AMA: 2005,Aug,7-8; 2005,Jul,11-12

86301 CA 19-9

🚗 0.00   0.00 **FUD** XXX Ⓠ ▣

AMA: 2005,Aug,7-8; 2005,Jul,11-12

86304 CA 125

EXCLUDES *Antibody, hepatitis delta agent (86692)*
Measurement serum HER-2/neu oncoprotein (83950)

🚗 0.00   0.00 **FUD** XXX Ⓠ ▣

AMA: 2005,Aug,7-8; 2005,Jul,11-12

86305 Human epididymis protein 4 (HE4)

🚗 0.00   0.00 **FUD** XXX Ⓠ ▣

86308 Heterophile antibodies; screening

EXCLUDES *Antibodies, infectious agents (86602-86804)*

🚗 0.00   0.00 **FUD** XXX ❌ Ⓠ ▣

AMA: 2005,Jul,11-12; 2005,Aug,7-8

86309 titer

EXCLUDES *Antibodies, infectious agents (86602-86804)*

🚗 0.00   0.00 **FUD** XXX Ⓠ ▣

AMA: 2005,Jul,11-12; 2005,Aug,7-8

86310 titers after absorption with beef cells and guinea pig kidney

EXCLUDES *Antibodies, infectious agents (86602-86804)*
Histoplasma antibodies (86698)
Histoplasmosis skin test (86510)
Human growth hormone antibody (86277)

🚗 0.00   0.00 **FUD** XXX Ⓠ ▣

AMA: 2005,Jul,11-12; 2005,Aug,7-8

86316 Immunoassay for tumor antigen, other antigen, quantitative (eg, CA 50, 72-4, 549), each

🚗 0.00   0.00 **FUD** XXX Ⓠ ▣

AMA: 2018,Jan,8; 2017,Jan,8; 2016,Jan,13; 2015,Jan,16

86317 Immunoassay for infectious agent antibody, quantitative, not otherwise specified

EXCLUDES *Immunoassay techniques for infectious antigens (87301-87451)*
Immunoassay techniques for noninfectious antigens (83516, 83518-83520)
Immunoassay techniques with direct/visual observation for infectious antigens (87802-87899 [87806, 87811])
Particle agglutination test (86403)

🚗 0.00   0.00 **FUD** XXX Ⓠ ▣

AMA: 2020,OctSE,1

▲ **86318** Immunoassay for infectious agent antibody(ies), qualitative or semiquantitative, single-step method (eg, reagent strip);

🚗 0.00   0.00 **FUD** XXX ❌ Ⓠ ▣

AMA: 2020,AugSE,1; 2020,AugSE,1; 2020,AugSE,1; 2018,Jan,8; 2017,Jan,8; 2016,Jan,13; 2015,Jan,16

● # **86328** severe acute respiratory syndrome coronavirus 2 (SARS-CoV-2) (Coronavirus disease [COVID-19])

INCLUDES Testing for antibodies only

EXCLUDES *Severe acute respiratory syndrome coronavirus 2 [SARS-CoV-2] [coronavirus disease {COVID-19}] testing via multiple-step method (86769)*
Testing for presence neutralizing antibodies that block cell infection ([86408, 86409])

🚗 0.00   0.00 **FUD** XXX

AMA: 2020,SepSE,1; 2020,AugSE,1; 2020,SepSE,1; 2020,AugSE,1; 2020,AugSE,1

86320 Immunoelectrophoresis; serum

🚗 0.00   0.00 **FUD** XXX Ⓠ 80 ▣

AMA: 2005,Jul,11-12; 2005,Aug,7-8

86325 other fluids (eg, urine, cerebrospinal fluid) with concentration

🚗 0.00   0.00 **FUD** XXX Ⓠ 80 ▣

AMA: 2005,Jul,11-12; 2005,Aug,7-8

86327 crossed (2-dimensional assay)

🚗 0.00   0.00 **FUD** XXX Ⓠ 80 ▣

AMA: 2005,Jul,11-12; 2005,Aug,7-8

86328 Resequenced code. See code following 86318.

86329 Immunodiffusion; not elsewhere specified

🚗 0.00   0.00 **FUD** XXX Ⓠ ▣

AMA: 2018,Jan,8; 2017,Jan,8; 2016,Jan,13; 2015,Jan,16

86331 gel diffusion, qualitative (Ouchterlony), each antigen or antibody

🚗 0.00   0.00 **FUD** XXX Ⓠ ▣

AMA: 2005,Aug,7-8; 2005,Jul,11-12

86332 Immune complex assay

🚗 0.00   0.00 **FUD** XXX Ⓠ ▣

AMA: 2005,Aug,7-8; 2005,Jul,11-12

86334 Immunofixation electrophoresis; serum

🚗 0.00   0.00 **FUD** XXX Ⓠ 80 ▣

AMA: 2005,Jul,11-12; 2005,Aug,7-8

86335 other fluids with concentration (eg, urine, CSF)

🚗 0.00   0.00 **FUD** XXX Ⓠ 80 ▣

AMA: 2005,Aug,7-8; 2005,Jul,11-12

86336 Inhibin A

🚗 0.00   0.00 **FUD** XXX Ⓠ ▣

AMA: 2005,Aug,7-8; 2005,Jul,11-12

86337 Insulin antibodies

🚗 0.00   0.00 **FUD** XXX Ⓠ ▣

AMA: 2005,Aug,7-8; 2005,Jul,11-12

86340 Intrinsic factor antibodies

EXCLUDES *Antibodies, leptospira (86720)*
Leukoagglutinins (86021)

🚗 0.00   0.00 **FUD** XXX Ⓠ ▣

AMA: 2005,Jul,11-12; 2005,Aug,7-8

86341 Islet cell antibody

🚗 0.00   0.00 **FUD** XXX Ⓠ ▣

AMA: 2018,Jan,8; 2017,Jan,8; 2016,Jan,13; 2015,Jan,16

86343 Leukocyte histamine release test (LHR)

🚗 0.00   0.00 **FUD** XXX Ⓠ ▣

AMA: 2005,Aug,7-8; 2005,Jul,11-12

86344 Leukocyte phagocytosis

🚗 0.00   0.00 **FUD** XXX Ⓠ ▣

AMA: 2005,Aug,7-8; 2005,Jul,11-12

86352 Assay Cellular Function

86352 Cellular function assay involving stimulation (eg, mitogen or antigen) and detection of biomarker (eg, ATP)

🚗 0.00   0.00 **FUD** XXX Ⓠ ▣

86353 Lymphocyte Mitogen Response Assay

CMS: 100-03,190.8 Lymphocyte Mitogen Response Assays

86353 Lymphocyte transformation, mitogen (phytomitogen) or antigen induced blastogenesis

EXCLUDES *Cellular function assay with stimulation and biomarker detection (86352)*
Malaria antibodies (86750)

🚗 0.00   0.00 **FUD** XXX Ⓠ ▣

AMA: 2005,Aug,7-8; 2005,Jul,11-12

26/TC PC/TC Only	A2-Z3 ASC Payment	50 Bilateral	♂ Male Only	♀ Female Only	🚗 Facility RVU	Non-Facility RVU	▣ CCI	❌ CLIA
FUD Follow-up Days	CMS: IOM	AMA: CPT Asst	A-Y OPPSI	80/80 Surg Assist Allowed / w/Doc		Ⓛ Lab Crosswalk		Radiology Crosswalk

86355-86593 [86408, 86409, 86413] Additional Diagnostic Immunology Testing

86355 **B cells, total count**
EXCLUDES *Flow cytometry interpretation (88187-88189)*
0.00 0.00 FUD XXX
AMA: 2018,Jan,8; 2017,Jan,8; 2016,Jan,13; 2015,Jan,16

86356 **Mononuclear cell antigen, quantitative (eg, flow cytometry), not otherwise specified, each antigen**
EXCLUDES *Flow cytometry interpretation (88187-88189)*
0.00 0.00 FUD XXX
AMA: 2018,Jan,8; 2017,Jan,8; 2016,Jan,13; 2015,Jan,16

86357 **Natural killer (NK) cells, total count**
EXCLUDES *Flow cytometry interpretation (88187-88189)*
0.00 0.00 FUD XXX
AMA: 2018,Jan,8; 2017,Jan,8; 2016,Jan,13; 2015,Jan,16

86359 **T cells; total count**
EXCLUDES *Flow cytometry interpretation (88187-88189)*
0.00 0.00 FUD XXX
AMA: 2018,Jan,8; 2017,Jan,8; 2016,Jan,13; 2015,Jan,16

86360 **absolute CD4 and CD8 count, including ratio**
EXCLUDES *Flow cytometry interpretation (88187-88189)*
0.00 0.00 FUD XXX
AMA: 2018,Jan,8; 2017,Jan,8; 2016,Jan,13; 2015,Jan,16

86361 **absolute CD4 count**
EXCLUDES *Flow cytometry interpretation (88187-88189)*
0.00 0.00 FUD XXX
AMA: 2018,Jan,8; 2017,Jan,8; 2016,Jan,13; 2015,Jan,16

86367 **Stem cells (ie, CD34), total count**
EXCLUDES *Flow cytometric immunophenotyping, potential hematolymphoid neoplasia assessment (88184-88189)*
Flow cytometry interpretation (88187-88189)
0.00 0.00 FUD XXX
AMA: 2018,Jan,8; 2017,Jan,8; 2016,Jan,13; 2015,Jan,16

86376 **Microsomal antibodies (eg, thyroid or liver-kidney), each**
0.00 0.00 FUD XXX
AMA: 2020,AugSE,1; 2020,AugSE,1; 2020,AugSE,1

86382 **Neutralization test, viral**
0.00 0.00 FUD XXX
AMA: 2005,Aug,7-8; 2005,Jul,11-12

● # **86408** **Neutralizing antibody, severe acute respiratory syndrome coronavirus 2 (SARS-CoV-2) (Coronavirus disease [COVID-19]); screen**
INCLUDES Testing for presence neutralizing antibodies that block cell infection
EXCLUDES *Testing for presence antibodies only ([86328])*
0.00 0.00 FUD 000
AMA: 2020,AugSE,1

● # **86409** **titer**
INCLUDES Testing for presence neutralizing antibodies that block cell infection
EXCLUDES *Testing for presence antibodies only ([86328])*
0.00 0.00 FUD 000
AMA: 2020,AugSE,1

● # **86413** **Severe acute respiratory syndrome coronavirus 2 (SARS-CoV-2) (Coronavirus disease [COVID-19]) antibody, quantitative**
INCLUDES Testing for presence and adaptive immune response to SARS-CoV-2
0.00 0.00 FUD 000
AMA: 2020,SepSE,1

86384 **Nitroblue tetrazolium dye test (NTD)**
0.00 0.00 FUD XXX
AMA: 2005,Aug,7-8; 2005,Jul,11-12

86386 **Nuclear Matrix Protein 22 (NMP22), qualitative**
EXCLUDES *Ouchterlony diffusion (86331)*
Platelet antibodies (86022, 86023)
0.00 0.00 FUD XXX

86403 **Particle agglutination; screen, each antibody**
0.00 0.00 FUD XXX
AMA: 2020,OctSE,1

86406 **titer, each antibody**
EXCLUDES *Pregnancy test (84702, 84703)*
Rapid plasma reagin test (RPR) (86592, 86593)
0.00 0.00 FUD XXX
AMA: 2005,Jul,11-12; 2005,Aug,7-8

86408 **Resequenced code. See code following 86382.**

86409 **Resequenced code. See code following 86382.**

86413 **Resequenced code. See code following resequenced code 86409.**

86430 **Rheumatoid factor; qualitative**
0.00 0.00 FUD XXX
AMA: 2005,Aug,7-8; 2005,Jul,11-12

86431 **quantitative**
EXCLUDES *Serologic syphilis testing (86592, 86593)*
0.00 0.00 FUD XXX
AMA: 2005,Aug,7-8; 2005,Jul,11-12

86480 **Tuberculosis test, cell mediated immunity antigen response measurement; gamma interferon**
0.00 0.00 FUD XXX
AMA: 2019,Dec,12; 2018,Jan,8; 2017,Jan,8; 2016,Jan,13; 2015,Jan,16

86481 **enumeration of gamma interferon-producing T-cells in cell suspension**
0.00 0.00 FUD XXX
AMA: 2019,Dec,12

86485 **Skin test; candida**
EXCLUDES *Candida antibody (86628)*
0.00 0.00 FUD XXX
AMA: 2005,Jul,11-12; 2005,Aug,7-8

86486 **unlisted antigen, each**
0.15 0.15 FUD XXX
AMA: 2008,Apr,5-7

86490 **coccidioidomycosis**
2.49 2.49 FUD XXX
AMA: 2005,Aug,7-8; 2005,Jul,11-12

86510 **histoplasmosis**
EXCLUDES *Histoplasma antibody (86698)*
0.19 0.19 FUD XXX
AMA: 2005,Aug,7-8; 2005,Jul,11-12

86580 **tuberculosis, intradermal**
INCLUDES Heaf test
Intradermal Mantoux test
EXCLUDES *Antibodies to sporothrix, report code for specific method*
Skin test for allergy (95012-95199)
Smooth muscle antibody (86255-86256)
Tuberculosis test, cell mediated immunity measurement gamma interferon antigen response (86480)
0.24 0.24 FUD XXX
AMA: 2005,Aug,7-8; 2005,Jul,11-12

86590 **Streptokinase, antibody**
EXCLUDES *Antibodies, infectious agents (86602-86804)*
Streptolysin O antibody, antistreptolysin O (86060, 86063)
0.00 0.00 FUD XXX
AMA: 2005,Jul,11-12; 2005,Aug,7-8

Pathology and Laboratory

86355 — 86590

86592 **Syphilis test, non-treponemal antibody; qualitative (eg, VDRL, RPR, ART)**

INCLUDES Wasserman test

EXCLUDES *Antibodies to infectious agents (86602-86804)*

0.00 0.00 FUD XXX A

AMA: 2005,Jul,11-12; 2005,Aug,7-8

86593 **quantitative**

EXCLUDES *Antibodies, infectious agents (86602-86804)*
Tetanus antibody (86774)
Thyroglobulin (84432)
Thyroglobulin antibody (86800)
Thyroid microsomal antibody (86376)
Toxoplasma antibody (86777-86778)

0.00 0.00 FUD XXX A

AMA: 2005,Jul,11-12; 2005,Aug,7-8

86602-86698 Testing for Antibodies to Infectious Agents: Actinomyces—Histoplasma

INCLUDES Qualitative or semiquantitative immunoassays performed by multiple-step methods for detection, antibodies to infectious agents

EXCLUDES *Detection:*
Antibodies other than those to infectious agents, see specific antibody or method
Infectious agent/antigen (87260-87899 [87623, 87624, 87625, 87806])
Immunoassays by single-step method (86318, [86328])

86602 **Antibody; actinomyces**

0.00 0.00 FUD XXX Q

AMA: 2020,OctSE,1; 2020,AugSE,1; 2020,AugSE,1; 2020,AugSE,1; 2018,Jan,8; 2017,Jan,8; 2016,Jan,13; 2015,Jan,16

86603 **adenovirus**

0.00 0.00 FUD XXX Q

AMA: 2020,OctSE,1; 2020,AugSE,1; 2020,AugSE,1; 2020,AugSE,1

86606 **Aspergillus**

0.00 0.00 FUD XXX Q

AMA: 2020,OctSE,1; 2020,AugSE,1; 2020,AugSE,1; 2020,AugSE,1

86609 **bacterium, not elsewhere specified**

0.00 0.00 FUD XXX Q

AMA: 2020,OctSE,1; 2020,AugSE,1; 2020,AugSE,1; 2020,AugSE,1

86611 **Bartonella**

0.00 0.00 FUD XXX Q

AMA: 2020,OctSE,1; 2020,AugSE,1; 2020,AugSE,1; 2020,AugSE,1

86612 **Blastomyces**

0.00 0.00 FUD XXX Q

AMA: 2020,OctSE,1; 2020,AugSE,1; 2020,AugSE,1; 2020,AugSE,1

86615 **Bordetella**

0.00 0.00 FUD XXX Q

AMA: 2020,OctSE,1; 2020,AugSE,1; 2020,AugSE,1; 2020,AugSE,1

86617 **Borrelia burgdorferi (Lyme disease) confirmatory test (eg, Western Blot or immunoblot)**

0.00 0.00 FUD XXX Q

AMA: 2020,OctSE,1; 2020,AugSE,1; 2020,AugSE,1; 2020,AugSE,1

86618 **Borrelia burgdorferi (Lyme disease)**

0.00 0.00 FUD XXX Q

AMA: 2020,OctSE,1; 2020,AugSE,1; 2020,AugSE,1; 2020,AugSE,1

86619 **Borrelia (relapsing fever)**

0.00 0.00 FUD XXX Q

AMA: 2020,OctSE,1; 2020,AugSE,1; 2020,AugSE,1; 2020,AugSE,1

86622 **Brucella**

0.00 0.00 FUD XXX Q

AMA: 2020,OctSE,1; 2020,AugSE,1; 2020,AugSE,1; 2020,AugSE,1

86625 **Campylobacter**

0.00 0.00 FUD XXX Q

AMA: 2020,OctSE,1; 2020,AugSE,1; 2020,AugSE,1; 2020,AugSE,1

86628 **Candida**

EXCLUDES *Candida skin test (86485)*

0.00 0.00 FUD XXX Q

AMA: 2020,OctSE,1; 2020,AugSE,1; 2020,AugSE,1; 2020,AugSE,1

86631 **Chlamydia**

0.00 0.00 FUD XXX A

AMA: 2020,OctSE,1; 2020,AugSE,1; 2020,AugSE,1; 2020,AugSE,1

86632 **Chlamydia, IgM**

EXCLUDES *Chlamydia antigen (87270, 87320)*
Fluorescent antibody technique (86255-86256)

0.00 0.00 FUD XXX A

AMA: 2020,OctSE,1; 2020,AugSE,1; 2020,AugSE,1; 2020,AugSE,1

86635 **Coccidioides**

EXCLUDES *Severe Acute Respiratory Syndrome Coronavirus 2 [SARS-CoV-2] [Coronavirus disease [COVID-19]] antibody testing ([86328], 86769)*

0.00 0.00 FUD XXX Q

AMA: 2020,OctSE,1; 2020,AugSE,1; 2020,AugSE,1; 2020,AugSE,1

86638 **Coxiella burnetii (Q fever)**

0.00 0.00 FUD XXX Q

AMA: 2020,OctSE,1; 2020,AugSE,1; 2020,AugSE,1; 2020,AugSE,1

86641 **Cryptococcus**

0.00 0.00 FUD XXX Q

AMA: 2020,OctSE,1; 2020,AugSE,1; 2020,AugSE,1; 2020,AugSE,1

86644 **cytomegalovirus (CMV)**

0.00 0.00 FUD XXX Q

AMA: 2020,OctSE,1; 2020,AugSE,1; 2020,AugSE,1; 2020,AugSE,1

86645 **cytomegalovirus (CMV), IgM**

0.00 0.00 FUD XXX Q

AMA: 2020,OctSE,1; 2020,AugSE,1; 2020,AugSE,1; 2020,AugSE,1; 2018,Jan,8; 2017,Jan,8; 2016,Jan,13; 2015,Jan,16

86648 **Diphtheria**

0.00 0.00 FUD XXX Q

AMA: 2020,OctSE,1; 2020,AugSE,1; 2020,AugSE,1; 2020,AugSE,1

86651 **encephalitis, California (La Crosse)**

0.00 0.00 FUD XXX Q

AMA: 2020,OctSE,1; 2020,AugSE,1; 2020,AugSE,1; 2020,AugSE,1

86652 **encephalitis, Eastern equine**

0.00 0.00 FUD XXX Q

AMA: 2020,OctSE,1; 2020,AugSE,1; 2020,AugSE,1; 2020,AugSE,1

86653 **encephalitis, St. Louis**

0.00 0.00 FUD XXX Q

AMA: 2020,OctSE,1; 2020,AugSE,1; 2020,AugSE,1; 2020,AugSE,1

86654 **encephalitis, Western equine**

0.00 0.00 FUD XXX Q

AMA: 2020,OctSE,1; 2020,AugSE,1; 2020,AugSE,1; 2020,AugSE,1

86658 **enterovirus (eg, coxsackie, echo, polio)**

EXCLUDES *Antibodies to:*
Trichinella (86784)
Trypanosoma—see code for specific methodology
Tuberculosis (86580)
Viral—see code for specific methodology

0.00 0.00 FUD XXX Q

AMA: 2020,OctSE,1; 2020,AugSE,1; 2020,AugSE,1; 2020,AugSE,1

86663 **Epstein-Barr (EB) virus, early antigen (EA)**

0.00 0.00 FUD XXX Q

AMA: 2020,OctSE,1; 2020,AugSE,1; 2020,AugSE,1; 2020,AugSE,1

86664 **Epstein-Barr (EB) virus, nuclear antigen (EBNA)**

0.00 0.00 FUD XXX Q

AMA: 2020,OctSE,1; 2020,AugSE,1; 2020,AugSE,1; 2020,AugSE,1

86665 **Epstein-Barr (EB) virus, viral capsid (VCA)**

0.00 0.00 FUD XXX Q

AMA: 2020,OctSE,1; 2020,AugSE,1; 2020,AugSE,1; 2020,AugSE,1

86666 **Ehrlichia**

0.00 0.00 FUD XXX Q

AMA: 2020,OctSE,1; 2020,AugSE,1; 2020,AugSE,1; 2020,AugSE,1

86668 **Francisella tularensis**

0.00 0.00 FUD XXX Q

AMA: 2020,OctSE,1; 2020,AugSE,1; 2020,AugSE,1; 2020,AugSE,1

86671 **fungus, not elsewhere specified**
0.00 0.00 **FUD** XXX
AMA: 2020,OctSE,1; 2020,AugSE,1; 2020,AugSE,1; 2020,AugSE,1

86674 **Giardia lamblia**
0.00 0.00 **FUD** XXX
AMA: 2020,OctSE,1; 2020,AugSE,1; 2020,AugSE,1; 2020,AugSE,1

86677 **Helicobacter pylori**
0.00 0.00 **FUD** XXX
AMA: 2020,OctSE,1; 2020,AugSE,1; 2020,AugSE,1; 2020,AugSE,1; 2018,Jan,8; 2017,Jan,8; 2016,Jan,13; 2015,Jan,16

86682 **helminth, not elsewhere specified**
0.00 0.00 **FUD** XXX
AMA: 2020,OctSE,1; 2020,AugSE,1; 2020,AugSE,1; 2020,AugSE,1

86684 **Haemophilus influenza**
0.00 0.00 **FUD** XXX
AMA: 2020,OctSE,1; 2020,AugSE,1; 2020,AugSE,1; 2020,AugSE,1

86687 **HTLV-I**
0.00 0.00 **FUD** XXX
AMA: 2020,OctSE,1; 2020,AugSE,1; 2020,AugSE,1; 2020,AugSE,1

86688 **HTLV-II**
0.00 0.00 **FUD** XXX
AMA: 2020,OctSE,1; 2020,AugSE,1; 2020,AugSE,1; 2020,AugSE,1

86689 **HTLV or HIV antibody, confirmatory test (eg, Western Blot)**
0.00 0.00 **FUD** XXX
AMA: 2020,OctSE,1; 2020,AugSE,1; 2020,AugSE,1; 2020,AugSE,1; 2018,Jan,8; 2017,Jan,8; 2016,Jan,13; 2015,Jan,16

86692 **hepatitis, delta agent**
EXCLUDES *Hepatitis delta agent, antigen (87380)*
0.00 0.00 **FUD** XXX
AMA: 2020,OctSE,1; 2020,AugSE,1; 2020,AugSE,1; 2020,AugSE,1

86694 **herpes simplex, non-specific type test**
0.00 0.00 **FUD** XXX
AMA: 2020,OctSE,1; 2020,AugSE,1; 2020,AugSE,1; 2020,AugSE,1

86695 **herpes simplex, type 1**
0.00 0.00 **FUD** XXX
AMA: 2020,OctSE,1; 2020,AugSE,1; 2020,AugSE,1; 2020,AugSE,1; 2018,Jan,8; 2017,Jan,8; 2016,Jan,13; 2015,Jan,16

86696 **herpes simplex, type 2**
0.00 0.00 **FUD** XXX
AMA: 2020,OctSE,1; 2020,AugSE,1; 2020,AugSE,1; 2020,AugSE,1

86698 **histoplasma**
0.00 0.00 **FUD** XXX
AMA: 2020,OctSE,1; 2020,AugSE,1; 2020,AugSE,1; 2020,AugSE,1

86701-86703 Testing for HIV Antibodies

CMS: 100-03,190.14 Human Immunodeficiency Virus Testing (Diagnosis); 100-03,190.9 Serologic Testing for Acquired Immunodeficiency Syndrome (AIDS)

INCLUDES Qualitative or semiquantitative immunoassays performed by multiple-step methods for detection, antibodies to infectious agents

EXCLUDES *Confirmatory test for HIV antibody (86689)*
HIV-1 antigen (87390)
HIV-1 antigen(s) with HIV 1 and 2 antibodies, single result (87389)
HIV-2 antigen (87391)
Immunoassays by single-step method (86318)

Code also modifier 92 for test performed using kit or transportable instrument comprising (all or part) single-use, disposable analytical chamber

86701 **Antibody; HIV-1**
0.00 0.00 **FUD** XXX
AMA: 2020,OctSE,1; 2020,AugSE,1; 2020,AugSE,1; 2020,AugSE,1; 2018,Jan,8; 2017,Jan,8; 2016,Jan,13; 2015,Jan,16

86702 **HIV-2**
0.00 0.00 **FUD** XXX
AMA: 2020,OctSE,1; 2020,AugSE,1; 2020,AugSE,1; 2020,AugSE,1; 2018,Jan,8; 2017,Jan,8; 2016,Jan,13; 2015,Jan,16

86703 **HIV-1 and HIV-2, single result**
0.00 0.00 **FUD** XXX
AMA: 2020,OctSE,1; 2020,AugSE,1; 2020,AugSE,1; 2020,AugSE,1; 2018,Jan,8; 2017,Jan,8; 2016,Jan,13; 2015,Jan,16

86704-86804 Testing for Infectious Disease Antibodies: Hepatitis—Yersinia

INCLUDES Qualitative or semiquantitative immunoassays performed by multiple-step methods for detection, antibodies to infectious agents

EXCLUDES *Detection of:*
Antibodies other than those to infectious agents, see specific antibody or method
Infectious agent/antigen (87260-87899 [87623, 87624, 87625, 87806])
Immunoassays by single-step method (86318)

86704 **Hepatitis B core antibody (HBcAb); total**
0.00 0.00 **FUD** XXX
AMA: 2020,OctSE,1; 2020,AugSE,1; 2020,AugSE,1; 2020,AugSE,1; 2018,Jan,8; 2017,Jan,8; 2016,Jan,13; 2015,Jan,16

86705 **IgM antibody**
0.00 0.00 **FUD** XXX
AMA: 2020,OctSE,1; 2020,AugSE,1; 2020,AugSE,1; 2020,AugSE,1; 2018,Jan,8; 2017,Jan,8; 2016,Jan,13; 2015,Jan,16

86706 **Hepatitis B surface antibody (HBsAb)**
0.00 0.00 **FUD** XXX
AMA: 2020,OctSE,1; 2020,AugSE,1; 2020,AugSE,1; 2020,AugSE,1

86707 **Hepatitis Be antibody (HBeAb)**
0.00 0.00 **FUD** XXX
AMA: 2020,OctSE,1; 2020,AugSE,1; 2020,AugSE,1; 2020,AugSE,1

86708 **Hepatitis A antibody (HAAb)**
0.00 0.00 **FUD** XXX
AMA: 2020,OctSE,1; 2020,AugSE,1; 2020,AugSE,1; 2020,AugSE,1; 2018,Jan,8; 2017,Jan,8; 2016,Jan,13; 2015,Jan,16

86709 **Hepatitis A antibody (HAAb), IgM antibody**
0.00 0.00 **FUD** XXX
AMA: 2020,OctSE,1; 2020,AugSE,1; 2020,AugSE,1; 2020,AugSE,1; 2018,Jan,8; 2017,Jan,8; 2016,Jan,13; 2015,Jan,16

86710 **Antibody; influenza virus**
0.00 0.00 **FUD** XXX
AMA: 2020,OctSE,1; 2020,AugSE,1; 2020,AugSE,1; 2020,AugSE,1; 2018,Jan,8; 2017,Jan,8; 2016,Jan,13; 2015,Jan,16

86711 **JC (John Cunningham) virus**
0.00 0.00 **FUD** XXX
AMA: 2020,OctSE,1; 2020,AugSE,1; 2020,AugSE,1; 2020,AugSE,1

86713 **Legionella**
0.00 0.00 **FUD** XXX
AMA: 2020,OctSE,1; 2020,AugSE,1; 2020,AugSE,1; 2020,AugSE,1

86717 **Leishmania**
0.00 0.00 **FUD** XXX
AMA: 2020,OctSE,1; 2020,AugSE,1; 2020,AugSE,1; 2020,AugSE,1

86720 **Leptospira**
0.00 0.00 **FUD** XXX
AMA: 2020,OctSE,1; 2020,AugSE,1; 2020,AugSE,1; 2020,AugSE,1

86723 **Listeria monocytogenes**
0.00 0.00 **FUD** XXX
AMA: 2020,OctSE,1; 2020,AugSE,1; 2020,AugSE,1; 2020,AugSE,1

86727 **lymphocytic choriomeningitis**
0.00 0.00 **FUD** XXX
AMA: 2020,OctSE,1; 2020,AugSE,1; 2020,AugSE,1; 2020,AugSE,1

86732 **mucormycosis**
0.00 0.00 **FUD** XXX
AMA: 2020,OctSE,1; 2020,AugSE,1; 2020,AugSE,1; 2020,AugSE,1

86735 **mumps**
0.00 0.00 **FUD** XXX
AMA: 2020,OctSE,1; 2020,AugSE,1; 2020,AugSE,1; 2020,AugSE,1; 2018,Jan,8; 2017,Jan,8; 2016,Jan,13; 2015,Jan,16

86738 **mycoplasma**
0.00 0.00 **FUD** XXX
AMA: 2020,OctSE,1; 2020,AugSE,1; 2020,AugSE,1; 2020,AugSE,1

86741 Neisseria meningitidis
0.00 0.00 FUD XXX
AMA: 2020,OctSE,1; 2020,AugSE,1; 2020,AugSE,1; 2020,AugSE,1

86744 Nocardia
0.00 0.00 FUD XXX
AMA: 2020,OctSE,1; 2020,AugSE,1; 2020,AugSE,1; 2020,AugSE,1

86747 parvovirus
0.00 0.00 FUD XXX
AMA: 2020,OctSE,1; 2020,AugSE,1; 2020,AugSE,1; 2020,AugSE,1

86750 Plasmodium (malaria)
0.00 0.00 FUD XXX
AMA: 2020,OctSE,1; 2020,AugSE,1; 2020,AugSE,1; 2020,AugSE,1

86753 protozoa, not elsewhere specified
0.00 0.00 FUD XXX
AMA: 2020,OctSE,1; 2020,AugSE,1; 2020,AugSE,1; 2020,AugSE,1

86756 respiratory syncytial virus
0.00 0.00 FUD XXX
AMA: 2020,OctSE,1; 2020,AugSE,1; 2020,AugSE,1; 2020,AugSE,1

86757 Rickettsia
0.00 0.00 FUD XXX
AMA: 2020,OctSE,1; 2020,AugSE,1; 2020,AugSE,1; 2020,AugSE,1

86759 rotavirus
0.00 0.00 FUD XXX
AMA: 2020,OctSE,1; 2020,AugSE,1; 2020,AugSE,1; 2020,AugSE,1

86762 rubella
0.00 0.00 FUD XXX
AMA: 2020,OctSE,1; 2020,AugSE,1; 2020,AugSE,1; 2020,AugSE,1

86765 rubeola
0.00 0.00 FUD XXX
AMA: 2020,OctSE,1; 2020,AugSE,1; 2020,AugSE,1; 2020,AugSE,1

86768 Salmonella
0.00 0.00 FUD XXX
AMA: 2020,OctSE,1; 2020,AugSE,1; 2020,AugSE,1; 2020,AugSE,1

● 86769 severe acute respiratory syndrome coronavirus 2 (SARS-CoV-2) (Coronavirus disease [COVID-19])
EXCLUDES *Antibody, severe acute respiratory syndrome coronavirus 2 (SARS-CoV-2) (coronavirus disease [COVID-19]), includes titer(s) (0224U)*
Severe acute respiratory syndrome coronavirus 2 (SARS-CoV-2) (coronavirus disease [COVID-19]) antibody testing via single-step method ([86328])
AMA: 2020,SepSE,1; 2020,OctSE,1; 2020,AugSE,1; 2020,SepSE,1; 2020,AugSE,1; 2020,AugSE,1; 2020,May,3; 2020,JuneSE,1

86771 Shigella
0.00 0.00 FUD XXX
AMA: 2020,OctSE,1; 2020,AugSE,1; 2020,AugSE,1; 2020,AugSE,1

86774 tetanus
0.00 0.00 FUD XXX
AMA: 2020,OctSE,1; 2020,AugSE,1; 2020,AugSE,1; 2020,AugSE,1

86777 Toxoplasma
0.00 0.00 FUD XXX
AMA: 2020,OctSE,1; 2020,AugSE,1; 2020,AugSE,1; 2020,AugSE,1

86778 Toxoplasma, IgM
0.00 0.00 FUD XXX
AMA: 2020,OctSE,1; 2020,AugSE,1; 2020,AugSE,1; 2020,AugSE,1

86780 Treponema pallidum
EXCLUDES *Nontreponemal antibody analysis syphilis testing (86592-86593)*
0.00 0.00 FUD XXX
AMA: 2020,OctSE,1; 2020,AugSE,1; 2020,AugSE,1; 2020,AugSE,1

86784 Trichinella
0.00 0.00 FUD XXX
AMA: 2020,OctSE,1; 2020,AugSE,1; 2020,AugSE,1; 2020,AugSE,1

86787 varicella-zoster
0.00 0.00 FUD XXX
AMA: 2020,OctSE,1; 2020,AugSE,1; 2020,AugSE,1; 2020,AugSE,1

86788 West Nile virus, IgM
0.00 0.00 FUD XXX
AMA: 2020,OctSE,1; 2020,AugSE,1; 2020,AugSE,1; 2020,AugSE,1

86789 West Nile virus
0.00 0.00 FUD XXX
AMA: 2020,OctSE,1; 2020,AugSE,1; 2020,AugSE,1; 2020,AugSE,1

86790 virus, not elsewhere specified
0.00 0.00 FUD XXX
AMA: 2020,OctSE,1; 2020,AugSE,1; 2020,AugSE,1; 2020,AugSE,1

86793 Yersinia
0.00 0.00 FUD XXX
AMA: 2020,OctSE,1; 2020,AugSE,1; 2020,AugSE,1; 2020,AugSE,1

86794 Zika virus, IgM
0.00 0.00 FUD XXX
AMA: 2020,OctSE,1; 2020,AugSE,1; 2020,AugSE,1; 2020,AugSE,1

86800 Thyroglobulin antibody
EXCLUDES *Thyroglobulin (84432)*
0.00 0.00 FUD XXX
AMA: 2020,OctSE,1; 2020,AugSE,1; 2020,AugSE,1; 2020,AugSE,1

86803 Hepatitis C antibody;
0.00 0.00 FUD XXX
AMA: 2020,OctSE,1; 2020,AugSE,1; 2020,AugSE,1; 2020,AugSE,1

86804 confirmatory test (eg, immunoblot)
0.00 0.00 FUD XXX
AMA: 2020,OctSE,1; 2020,AugSE,1; 2020,AugSE,1; 2020,AugSE,1; 2018,Jan,8; 2017,Jan,8; 2016,Jan,13; 2015,Jan,16

86805-86808 Pre-Transplant Antibody Cross Matching

86805 Lymphocytotoxicity assay, visual crossmatch; with titration
0.00 0.00 FUD XXX
AMA: 2018,Jan,8; 2017,Jan,8; 2016,Jan,13; 2015,Jan,16

86806 without titration
0.00 0.00 FUD XXX
AMA: 2005,Aug,7-8; 2005,Jul,11-12

86807 Serum screening for cytotoxic percent reactive antibody (PRA); standard method
0.00 0.00 FUD XXX
AMA: 2018,Jan,8; 2017,Jan,8; 2016,Jan,13; 2015,Jan,16

86808 quick method
0.00 0.00 FUD XXX
AMA: 2018,Jan,8; 2017,Jan,8; 2016,Jan,13; 2015,Jan,16

86812-86826 Histocompatibility Testing

CMS: 100-03,110.23 Stem Cell Transplantation; 100-03,190.1 Histocompatibility Testing; 100-04,3,90.3 Stem Cell Transplantation; 100-04,3,90.3.1 Allogeneic Stem Cell Transplantation; 100-04,3,90.3.3 Billing for Allogeneic Stem Cell Transplants; 100-04,32,90 Billing for Stem Cell Transplantation; 100-04,4,231.11 Billing for Allogeneic Stem Cell Transplants

EXCLUDES *HLA typing by molecular pathology techniques (81370-81383)*

86812 HLA typing; A, B, or C (eg, A10, B7, B27), single antigen
0.00 0.00 FUD XXX
AMA: 2018,Jan,8; 2017,Jan,8; 2016,Jan,13; 2015,Jan,16

86813 A, B, or C, multiple antigens
0.00 0.00 FUD XXX
AMA: 2018,Jan,8; 2017,Jan,8; 2016,Jan,13; 2015,Jan,16

86816 DR/DQ, single antigen
0.00 0.00 FUD XXX
AMA: 2018,Jan,8; 2017,Jan,8; 2016,Jan,13; 2015,Jan,16

86817 DR/DQ, multiple antigens
0.00 0.00 FUD XXX
AMA: 2018,Jan,8; 2017,Jan,8; 2016,Jan,13; 2015,Jan,16

86821 lymphocyte culture, mixed (MLC)
0.00 0.00 FUD XXX
AMA: 2018,Jan,8; 2017,Jan,8; 2016,Jan,13; 2015,Jan,16

86825 **Human leukocyte antigen (HLA) crossmatch, non-cytotoxic (eg, using flow cytometry); first serum sample or dilution**

INCLUDES Autologous HLA crossmatch

EXCLUDES *B cells (86355)*
Flow cytometry (88184-88189)
Lymphocytotoxicity visual crossmatch (86805-86806)
T cells (86359)

0.00 0.00 **FUD** XXX Q

AMA: 2020,Aug,14

\+ **86826** **each additional serum sample or sample dilution (List separately in addition to primary procedure)**

INCLUDES Autologous HLA crossmatch

EXCLUDES *B cells (86355)*
Flow cytometry (88184-88189)
Lymphocytotoxicity visual crossmatch (86805-86806)
T cells (86359)

Code first (86825)

0.00 0.00 **FUD** XXX U

AMA: 2020,Aug,14

86828-86849 HLA Antibodies

86828 **Antibody to human leukocyte antigens (HLA), solid phase assays (eg, microspheres or beads, ELISA, flow cytometry); qualitative assessment of the presence or absence of antibody(ies) to HLA Class I and Class II HLA antigens**

Code also solid phase testing, untreated and treated specimens, either class of HLA after treatment (86828-86833)

0.00 0.00 **FUD** XXX Q

86829 **qualitative assessment of the presence or absence of antibody(ies) to HLA Class I or Class II HLA antigens**

Code also solid phase testing, untreated and treated specimens, either class of HLA after treatment (86828-86833)

0.00 0.00 **FUD** XXX Q

86830 **antibody identification by qualitative panel using complete HLA phenotypes, HLA Class I**

Code also solid phase testing, untreated and treated specimens, either class of HLA after treatment (86828-86833)

0.00 0.00 **FUD** XXX Q

86831 **antibody identification by qualitative panel using complete HLA phenotypes, HLA Class II**

Code also solid phase testing, untreated and treated specimens, either class of HLA after treatment (86828-86833)

0.00 0.00 **FUD** XXX Q

86832 **high definition qualitative panel for identification of antibody specificities (eg, individual antigen per bead methodology), HLA Class I**

Code also solid phase testing, untreated and treated specimens, either class of HLA after treatment (86828-86833)

0.00 0.00 **FUD** XXX Q

86833 **high definition qualitative panel for identification of antibody specificities (eg, individual antigen per bead methodology), HLA Class II**

Code also solid phase testing, untreated and treated specimens, either class of HLA after treatment (86828-86833)

0.00 0.00 **FUD** XXX Q

86834 **semi-quantitative panel (eg, titer), HLA Class I**

0.00 0.00 **FUD** XXX Q

86835 **semi-quantitative panel (eg, titer), HLA Class II**

0.00 0.00 **FUD** XXX Q

86849 **Unlisted immunology procedure**

0.00 0.00 **FUD** XXX N

AMA: 2019,Dec,12; 2018,Jan,8; 2017,Jan,8; 2016,Jan,13; 2015,Jan,16

86850-86999 Transfusion Services

EXCLUDES *Apheresis (36511-36512)*
Therapeutic phlebotomy (99195)

86850 **Antibody screen, RBC, each serum technique**

0.00 0.00 **FUD** XXX Q1

AMA: 2020,AugSE,1; 2020,AugSE,1; 2020,AugSE,1; 2018,Jan,8; 2017,Jan,8; 2016,Jan,13; 2015,Jan,16

86860 **Antibody elution (RBC), each elution**

0.00 0.00 **FUD** XXX Q1

AMA: 2020,AugSE,1; 2020,AugSE,1; 2020,AugSE,1

86870 **Antibody identification, RBC antibodies, each panel for each serum technique**

0.00 0.00 **FUD** XXX Q2

AMA: 2020,AugSE,1; 2020,AugSE,1; 2020,AugSE,1; 2018,Jan,8; 2017,Jan,8; 2016,Jan,13; 2015,Jan,16

86880 **Antihuman globulin test (Coombs test); direct, each antiserum**

0.00 0.00 **FUD** XXX Q1

AMA: 2005,Aug,7-8; 2005,Jul,11-12

86885 **indirect, qualitative, each reagent red cell**

0.00 0.00 **FUD** XXX Q1

AMA: 2018,Jan,8; 2017,Jan,8; 2016,Jan,13; 2015,Jan,16

86886 **indirect, each antibody titer**

EXCLUDES *Indirect antihuman globulin (Coombs) test for RBC antibody identification using reagent red cell panels (86870)*
Indirect antihuman globulin (Coombs) test for RBC antibody screening (86850)

0.00 0.00 **FUD** XXX Q1

AMA: 2018,Jan,8; 2017,Jan,8; 2016,Jan,13; 2015,Jan,16

86890 **Autologous blood or component, collection processing and storage; predeposited**

0.00 0.00 **FUD** XXX Q1

AMA: 2018,Jan,8; 2017,Jan,8; 2016,Jan,13; 2015,Jan,16

86891 **intra- or postoperative salvage**

0.00 0.00 **FUD** XXX Q1

AMA: 2005,Aug,7-8; 2005,Jul,11-12

86900 **Blood typing, serologic; ABO**

0.00 0.00 **FUD** XXX Q1

AMA: 2005,Jul,11-12; 2005,Aug,7-8

86901 **Rh (D)**

0.00 0.00 **FUD** XXX Q1

AMA: 2018,Jan,8; 2017,Jan,8; 2016,Jan,13; 2015,Jan,16

86902 **antigen testing of donor blood using reagent serum, each antigen test**

Code also one time for each antigen, each unit blood, when multiple units tested for same antigen

0.00 0.00 **FUD** XXX Q1

AMA: 2010,Dec,7-10

86904 **antigen screening for compatible unit using patient serum, per unit screened**

0.00 0.00 **FUD** XXX Q1

AMA: 2005,Aug,7-8; 2005,Jul,11-12

86905 **RBC antigens, other than ABO or Rh (D), each**

0.00 0.00 **FUD** XXX Q1

AMA: 2005,Jul,11-12; 2005,Aug,7-8

86906 **Rh phenotyping, complete**

EXCLUDES *Reporting molecular pathology procedures for human erythrocyte antigen typing (81403)*

0.00 0.00 **FUD** XXX Q1

AMA: 2005,Jul,11-12; 2005,Aug,7-8

86910 **Blood typing, for paternity testing, per individual; ABO, Rh and MN**

0.00 0.00 **FUD** XXX E

AMA: 2005,Jul,11-12; 2005,Aug,7-8

86911 **each additional antigen system**
0.00 0.00 FUD XXX E
AMA: 2005,Jul,11-12; 2005,Aug,7-8

86920 **Compatibility test each unit; immediate spin technique**
0.00 0.00 FUD XXX Q1
AMA: 2018,Jan,8; 2017,Jan,8; 2016,Jan,13; 2015,Jan,16

86921 **incubation technique**
0.00 0.00 FUD XXX Q1
AMA: 2018,Jan,8; 2017,Jan,8; 2016,Jan,13; 2015,Jan,16

86922 **antiglobulin technique**
0.00 0.00 FUD XXX Q1
AMA: 2018,Jan,8; 2017,Jan,8; 2016,Jan,13; 2015,Jan,16

86923 **electronic**
EXCLUDES *Other compatibility test techniques (86920-86922)*
0.00 0.00 FUD XXX Q1
AMA: 2018,Jan,8; 2017,Jan,8; 2016,Jan,13; 2015,Jan,16

86927 **Fresh frozen plasma, thawing, each unit**
0.00 0.00 FUD XXX S
AMA: 2005,Aug,7-8; 2005,Jul,11-12

86930 **Frozen blood, each unit; freezing (includes preparation)**
0.00 0.00 FUD XXX Q1
AMA: 2018,Jan,8; 2017,Jan,8; 2016,Jan,13; 2015,Jan,16

86931 **thawing**
0.00 0.00 FUD XXX Q1
AMA: 2018,Jan,8; 2017,Jan,8; 2016,Jan,13; 2015,Jan,16

86932 **freezing (includes preparation) and thawing**
0.00 0.00 FUD XXX Q1
AMA: 2018,Jan,8; 2017,Jan,8; 2016,Jan,13; 2015,Jan,16

86940 **Hemolysins and agglutinins; auto, screen, each**
0.00 0.00 FUD XXX Q
AMA: 2005,Aug,7-8; 2005,Jul,11-12

86941 **incubated**
0.00 0.00 FUD XXX Q
AMA: 2005,Jul,11-12; 2005,Aug,7-8

86945 **Irradiation of blood product, each unit**
0.00 0.00 FUD XXX Q1
AMA: 2018,Jan,8; 2017,Jan,8; 2016,Jan,13; 2015,Jan,16

86950 **Leukocyte transfusion**
EXCLUDES *Infusion allogeneic lymphocytes (38242)*
Leukapheresis (36511)
0.00 0.00 FUD XXX Q1
AMA: 2018,Jan,8; 2017,Jan,8; 2016,Jan,13; 2015,Jan,16

86960 **Volume reduction of blood or blood product (eg, red blood cells or platelets), each unit**
0.00 0.00 FUD XXX Q1
AMA: 2018,Jan,8; 2017,Jan,8; 2016,Jan,13; 2015,Jan,16

86965 **Pooling of platelets or other blood products**
EXCLUDES *Autologous WBC injection (0481T)*
Injection platelet rich plasma (0232T)
0.00 0.00 FUD XXX Q1
AMA: 2018,Jan,8; 2017,Jan,8; 2016,Jan,13; 2015,Jan,16

86970 **Pretreatment of RBCs for use in RBC antibody detection, identification, and/or compatibility testing; incubation with chemical agents or drugs, each**
0.00 0.00 FUD XXX Q1
AMA: 2005,Jul,11-12; 2005,Aug,7-8

86971 **incubation with enzymes, each**
0.00 0.00 FUD XXX Q1
AMA: 2005,Jul,11-12; 2005,Aug,7-8

86972 **by density gradient separation**
0.00 0.00 FUD XXX Q1
AMA: 2005,Jul,11-12; 2005,Aug,7-8

86975 **Pretreatment of serum for use in RBC antibody identification; incubation with drugs, each**
0.00 0.00 FUD XXX Q1
AMA: 2005,Jul,11-12; 2005,Aug,7-8

86976 **by dilution**
0.00 0.00 FUD XXX Q1
AMA: 2005,Jul,11-12; 2005,Aug,7-8

86977 **incubation with inhibitors, each**
0.00 0.00 FUD XXX Q1
AMA: 2005,Jul,11-12; 2005,Aug,7-8

86978 **by differential red cell absorption using patient RBCs or RBCs of known phenotype, each absorption**
0.00 0.00 FUD XXX Q1
AMA: 2005,Jul,11-12; 2005,Aug,7-8

86985 **Splitting of blood or blood products, each unit**
0.00 0.00 FUD XXX Q1
AMA: 2018,Jan,8; 2017,Jan,8; 2016,Jan,13; 2015,Jan,16

86999 **Unlisted transfusion medicine procedure**
0.00 0.00 FUD XXX Q1
AMA: 2018,Jan,8; 2017,Jan,8; 2016,Jan,13; 2015,Jan,16

87003-87118 Identification of Microorganisms

INCLUDES Bacteriology, mycology, parasitology, and virology
EXCLUDES *Additional tests using molecular probes, chromatography, nucleic acid resequencing, or immunologic techniques (87140-87158)*
Code also modifier 59 for multiple specimens or sites
Code also modifier 91 for repeat procedures performed on same day

87003 **Animal inoculation, small animal, with observation and dissection**
0.00 0.00 FUD XXX Q
AMA: 2005,Aug,7-8; 2005,Jul,11-12

87015 **Concentration (any type), for infectious agents**
EXCLUDES *Direct smear for ova and parasites (87177)*
0.00 0.00 FUD XXX Q
AMA: 2005,Aug,7-8; 2005,Jul,11-12

87040 **Culture, bacterial; blood, aerobic, with isolation and presumptive identification of isolates (includes anaerobic culture, if appropriate)**
0.00 0.00 FUD XXX Q
AMA: 2018,Jan,8; 2017,Jan,8; 2016,Jan,13; 2015,Jan,16

87045 **stool, aerobic, with isolation and preliminary examination (eg, KIA, LIA), Salmonella and Shigella species**
0.00 0.00 FUD XXX Q
AMA: 2005,Aug,7-8; 2005,Jul,11-12

87046 **stool, aerobic, additional pathogens, isolation and presumptive identification of isolates, each plate**
0.00 0.00 FUD XXX Q
AMA: 2018,Jan,8; 2017,Jan,8; 2016,Jan,13; 2015,Jan,16

87070 **any other source except urine, blood or stool, aerobic, with isolation and presumptive identification of isolates**
EXCLUDES *Urine (87088)*
0.00 0.00 FUD XXX Q
AMA: 2018,Jan,8; 2017,Jan,8; 2016,Jan,13; 2015,Jan,16

87071 **quantitative, aerobic with isolation and presumptive identification of isolates, any source except urine, blood or stool**
EXCLUDES *Urine (87088)*
0.00 0.00 FUD XXX Q
AMA: 2018,Jan,8; 2017,Jan,8; 2016,Jan,13; 2015,Jan,16

87073 **quantitative, anaerobic with isolation and presumptive identification of isolates, any source except urine, blood or stool**
EXCLUDES *Definitive identification isolates (87076, 87077)*
Typing isolates (87140-87158)
0.00 0.00 FUD XXX Q
AMA: 2018,Jan,8; 2017,Jan,8; 2016,Jan,13; 2015,Jan,16

87075 **any source, except blood, anaerobic with isolation and presumptive identification of isolates**
0.00 0.00 FUD XXX
AMA: 2005,Aug,7-8; 2005,Jul,11-12

87076 **anaerobic isolate, additional methods required for definitive identification, each isolate**
0.00 0.00 FUD XXX
AMA: 2018,Jan,8; 2017,Jan,8; 2016,Jan,13; 2015,Jan,16

87077 **aerobic isolate, additional methods required for definitive identification, each isolate**
0.00 0.00 FUD XXX
AMA: 2018,Jan,8; 2017,Jan,8; 2016,Jan,13; 2015,Jan,16

87081 **Culture, presumptive, pathogenic organisms, screening only;**
0.00 0.00 FUD XXX
AMA: 2018,Jan,8; 2017,Jan,8; 2016,Jan,13; 2015,Jan,16

87084 **with colony estimation from density chart**
0.00 0.00 FUD XXX
AMA: 2005,Aug,7-8; 2005,Jul,11-12

87086 **Culture, bacterial; quantitative colony count, urine**
0.00 0.00 FUD XXX
AMA: 2018,Jan,8; 2017,Jan,8; 2016,Jan,13; 2015,Jan,16

87088 **with isolation and presumptive identification of each isolate, urine**
0.00 0.00 FUD XXX
AMA: 2018,Jan,8; 2017,Jan,8; 2016,Jan,13; 2015,Jan,16

87101 **Culture, fungi (mold or yeast) isolation, with presumptive identification of isolates; skin, hair, or nail**
0.00 0.00 FUD XXX
AMA: 2018,Jan,8; 2017,Jan,8; 2016,Jan,13; 2015,Jan,16

87102 **other source (except blood)**
0.00 0.00 FUD XXX
AMA: 2005,Aug,7-8; 2005,Jul,11-12

87103 **blood**
0.00 0.00 FUD XXX
AMA: 2005,Aug,7-8; 2005,Jul,11-12

87106 **Culture, fungi, definitive identification, each organism; yeast**
0.00 0.00 FUD XXX
AMA: 2005,Aug,7-8; 2005,Jul,11-12

87107 **mold**
0.00 0.00 FUD XXX
AMA: 2005,Aug,7-8; 2005,Jul,11-12

87109 **Culture, mycoplasma, any source**
0.00 0.00 FUD XXX
AMA: 2005,Aug,7-8; 2005,Jul,11-12

87110 **Culture, chlamydia, any source**
EXCLUDES *Immunofluorescence staining shell vials (87140)*
0.00 0.00 FUD XXX
AMA: 2005,Aug,7-8; 2005,Jul,11-12

87116 **Culture, tubercle or other acid-fast bacilli (eg, TB, AFB, mycobacteria) any source, with isolation and presumptive identification of isolates**
EXCLUDES *Concentration (87015)*
0.00 0.00 FUD XXX
AMA: 2005,Aug,7-8; 2005,Jul,11-12

87118 **Culture, mycobacterial, definitive identification, each isolate**
0.00 0.00 FUD XXX
AMA: 2005,Aug,7-8; 2005,Jul,11-12

87140-87158 Additional Culture Typing Techniques

INCLUDES Bacteriology, mycology, parasitology, and virology
EXCLUDES *Reporting molecular procedure codes as substitute for codes in this range (81105-81183 [81173, 81174, 81200, 81201, 81202, 81203, 81204], 81400-81408, [81479])*
Code also definitive identification
Code also modifier 59 for multiple specimens or sites
Code also modifier 91 for repeat procedures performed on same day

87140 **Culture, typing; immunofluorescent method, each antiserum**
0.00 0.00 FUD XXX
AMA: 2020,OctSE,1; 2018,Jan,8; 2017,Jan,8; 2016,Jan,13; 2015,Jan,16

87143 **gas liquid chromatography (GLC) or high pressure liquid chromatography (HPLC) method**
0.00 0.00 FUD XXX
AMA: 2020,OctSE,1

87147 **immunologic method, other than immunofluorescence (eg, agglutination grouping), per antiserum**
0.00 0.00 FUD XXX
AMA: 2020,OctSE,1; 2018,Jan,8; 2017,Jan,8; 2016,Jan,13; 2015,Jan,16

87149 **identification by nucleic acid (DNA or RNA) probe, direct probe technique, per culture or isolate, each organism probed**
0.00 0.00 FUD XXX
AMA: 2020,OctSE,1; 2018,Jan,8; 2017,Jan,8; 2016,Jan,13; 2015,Jan,16

87150 **identification by nucleic acid (DNA or RNA) probe, amplified probe technique, per culture or isolate, each organism probed**
0.00 0.00 FUD XXX
AMA: 2020,OctSE,1; 2018,Jan,8; 2017,Jan,8; 2016,Jan,13; 2015,Jan,16

87152 **identification by pulse field gel typing**
0.00 0.00 FUD XXX
AMA: 2020,OctSE,1; 2018,Jan,8; 2017,Jan,8; 2016,Jan,13; 2015,Jan,16

87153 **identification by nucleic acid sequencing method, each isolate (eg, sequencing of the 16S rRNA gene)**
0.00 0.00 FUD XXX
AMA: 2020,OctSE,1; 2018,Jan,8; 2017,Jan,8; 2016,Jan,13; 2015,Jan,16

87158 **other methods**
0.00 0.00 FUD XXX
AMA: 2020,OctSE,1; 2018,Jan,8; 2017,Jan,8; 2016,Jan,13; 2015,Jan,16

87164-87255 Identification of Organism from Primary Source and Sensitivity Studies

INCLUDES Bacteriology, mycology, parasitology, and virology
EXCLUDES *Additional tests using molecular probes, chromatography, or immunologic techniques (87140-87158)*
Code also modifier 59 for multiple specimens or sites
Code also modifier 91 for repeat procedures performed on same day

87164 **Dark field examination, any source (eg, penile, vaginal, oral, skin); includes specimen collection**
0.00 0.00 FUD XXX
AMA: 2005,Jul,11-12; 2005,Aug,7-8

87166 **without collection**
0.00 0.00 FUD XXX
AMA: 2005,Aug,7-8; 2005,Jul,11-12

87168 **Macroscopic examination; arthropod**
0.00 0.00 FUD XXX
AMA: 2005,Aug,7-8; 2005,Jul,11-12

87169 **parasite**
0.00 0.00 FUD XXX
AMA: 2005,Aug,7-8; 2005,Jul,11-12

87172 **Pinworm exam (eg, cellophane tape prep)**
0.00 0.00 **FUD** XXX
AMA: 2005,Aug,7-8; 2005,Jul,11-12

87176 **Homogenization, tissue, for culture**
0.00 0.00 **FUD** XXX
AMA: 2005,Aug,7-8; 2005,Jul,11-12

87177 **Ova and parasites, direct smears, concentration and identification**
EXCLUDES *Coccidia or microsporidia exam (87207)*
Complex special stain (trichrome, iron hematoxylin) (87209)
Concentration for infectious agents (87015)
Direct smears from primary source (87207)
Nucleic acid probes in cytologic material (88365)
0.00 0.00 **FUD** XXX
AMA: 2018,Jan,8; 2017,Jan,8; 2016,Jan,13; 2015,Jan,16

87181 **Susceptibility studies, antimicrobial agent; agar dilution method, per agent (eg, antibiotic gradient strip)**
0.00 0.00 **FUD** XXX
AMA: 2018,Jan,8; 2017,Jan,8; 2016,Jan,13; 2015,Jan,16

87184 **disk method, per plate (12 or fewer agents)**
0.00 0.00 **FUD** XXX
AMA: 2018,Jan,8; 2017,Jan,8; 2016,Jan,13; 2015,Jan,16

87185 **enzyme detection (eg, beta lactamase), per enzyme**
0.00 0.00 **FUD** XXX
AMA: 2018,Jan,8; 2017,Jan,8; 2016,Jan,13; 2015,Jan,16

87186 **microdilution or agar dilution (minimum inhibitory concentration [MIC] or breakpoint), each multi-antimicrobial, per plate**
0.00 0.00 **FUD** XXX
AMA: 2018,Jan,8; 2017,Jan,8; 2016,Jan,13; 2015,Jan,16

\+ **87187** **microdilution or agar dilution, minimum lethal concentration (MLC), each plate (List separately in addition to code for primary procedure)**
Code first (87186, 87188)
0.00 0.00 **FUD** XXX
AMA: 2018,Jan,8; 2017,Jan,8; 2016,Jan,13; 2015,Jan,16

87188 **macrobroth dilution method, each agent**
0.00 0.00 **FUD** XXX
AMA: 2018,Jan,8; 2017,Jan,8; 2016,Jan,13; 2015,Jan,16

87190 **mycobacteria, proportion method, each agent**
EXCLUDES *Other mycobacterial susceptibility studies (87181, 87184, 87186, 87188)*
0.00 0.00 **FUD** XXX
AMA: 2005,Aug,7-8; 2005,Jul,11-12

87197 **Serum bactericidal titer (Schlichter test)**
0.00 0.00 **FUD** XXX
AMA: 2005,Aug,7-8; 2005,Jul,11-12

87205 **Smear, primary source with interpretation; Gram or Giemsa stain for bacteria, fungi, or cell types**
0.00 0.00 **FUD** XXX
AMA: 2018,Jan,8; 2017,Jan,8; 2016,Jan,13; 2015,Jan,16

87206 **fluorescent and/or acid fast stain for bacteria, fungi, parasites, viruses or cell types**
0.00 0.00 **FUD** XXX
AMA: 2005,Aug,7-8; 2005,Jul,11-12

87207 **special stain for inclusion bodies or parasites (eg, malaria, coccidia, microsporidia, trypanosomes, herpes viruses)**
EXCLUDES *Direct smears with concentration and identification (87177)*
Fat, fibers, meat, nasal eosinophils, starch (89049-89240)
Thick smear preparation (87015)
0.00 0.00 **FUD** XXX 80
AMA: 2018,Jan,8; 2017,Jan,8; 2016,Jan,13; 2015,Jan,16

87209 **complex special stain (eg, trichrome, iron hemotoxylin) for ova and parasites**
0.00 0.00 **FUD** XXX
AMA: 2018,Jan,8; 2017,Jan,8; 2016,Jan,13; 2015,Jan,16

87210 **wet mount for infectious agents (eg, saline, India ink, KOH preps)**
EXCLUDES *KOH evaluation skin, hair, or nails (87220)*
0.00 0.00 **FUD** XXX
AMA: 2018,Jan,8; 2017,Jan,8; 2016,May,13

87220 **Tissue examination by KOH slide of samples from skin, hair, or nails for fungi or ectoparasite ova or mites (eg, scabies)**
0.00 0.00 **FUD** XXX
AMA: 2005,Aug,7-8; 2005,Jul,11-12

87230 **Toxin or antitoxin assay, tissue culture (eg, Clostridium difficile toxin)**
0.00 0.00 **FUD** XXX
AMA: 2005,Aug,7-8; 2005,Jul,11-12

87250 **Virus isolation; inoculation of embryonated eggs, or small animal, includes observation and dissection**
0.00 0.00 **FUD** XXX
AMA: 2020,OctSE,1

87252 **tissue culture inoculation, observation, and presumptive identification by cytopathic effect**
0.00 0.00 **FUD** XXX
AMA: 2005,Aug,7-8; 2005,Jul,11-12

87253 **tissue culture, additional studies or definitive identification (eg, hemabsorption, neutralization, immunofluorescence stain), each isolate**
EXCLUDES *Electron microscopy (88348)*
Inclusion bodies in:
Fluids (88106)
Smears (87207-87210)
Tissue sections (88304-88309)
0.00 0.00 **FUD** XXX
AMA: 2005,Aug,7-8; 2005,Jul,11-12

87254 **centrifuge enhanced (shell vial) technique, includes identification with immunofluorescence stain, each virus**
Code also (87252)
0.00 0.00 **FUD** XXX
AMA: 2018,Jan,8; 2017,Jan,8; 2016,Jan,13; 2015,Jan,16

87255 **including identification by non-immunologic method, other than by cytopathic effect (eg, virus specific enzymatic activity)**
0.00 0.00 **FUD** XXX
AMA: 2020,OctSE,1; 2018,Jan,8; 2017,Jan,8; 2016,Jan,13; 2015,Jan,16

87260-87300 Fluorescence Microscopy by Organism

INCLUDES Primary source only
EXCLUDES *Comparable tests on culture material (87140-87158)*
Identification antibodies (86602-86804)
Immunoassay techniques with direct/visual observation for infectious antigens (87260-87300)
Microscopic identification infectious agents via direct/indirect immunofluorescent assay (IFA) techniques (87301-87451, 87802-87899 [87806, 87811])
Nonspecific agent detection (87299, 87449, 87797-87799, 87899)
Code also modifier 59 for different species or strains reported by same code

87260 **Infectious agent antigen detection by immunofluorescent technique; adenovirus**
0.00 0.00 **FUD** XXX
AMA: 2020,OctSE,1; 2020,AugSE,1; 2020,AugSE,1; 2020,AugSE,1

87265 **Bordetella pertussis/parapertussis**
0.00 0.00 **FUD** XXX
AMA: 2020,OctSE,1; 2020,AugSE,1; 2020,AugSE,1; 2020,AugSE,1

87267 **Enterovirus, direct fluorescent antibody (DFA)**
0.00 0.00 **FUD** XXX
AMA: 2020,OctSE,1; 2020,AugSE,1; 2020,AugSE,1; 2020,AugSE,1; 2018,Jan,8; 2017,Jan,8; 2016,Jan,13; 2015,Jan,16

87269 giardia
0.00 0.00 FUD XXX
AMA: 2020,OctSE,1; 2020,AugSE,1; 2020,AugSE,1; 2020,AugSE,1

87270 Chlamydia trachomatis
0.00 0.00 FUD XXX
AMA: 2020,OctSE,1; 2020,AugSE,1; 2020,AugSE,1; 2020,AugSE,1

87271 Cytomegalovirus, direct fluorescent antibody (DFA)
0.00 0.00 FUD XXX
AMA: 2020,OctSE,1; 2020,AugSE,1; 2020,AugSE,1; 2020,AugSE,1; 2018,Jan,8; 2017,Jan,8; 2016,Jan,13; 2015,Jan,16

87272 cryptosporidium
0.00 0.00 FUD XXX
AMA: 2020,OctSE,1; 2020,AugSE,1; 2020,AugSE,1; 2020,AugSE,1

87273 Herpes simplex virus type 2
0.00 0.00 FUD XXX
AMA: 2020,OctSE,1; 2020,AugSE,1; 2020,AugSE,1; 2020,AugSE,1

87274 Herpes simplex virus type 1
0.00 0.00 FUD XXX
AMA: 2020,OctSE,1; 2020,AugSE,1; 2020,AugSE,1; 2020,AugSE,1

87275 influenza B virus
0.00 0.00 FUD XXX
AMA: 2020,OctSE,1; 2020,AugSE,1; 2020,AugSE,1; 2020,AugSE,1; 2018,Jan,8; 2017,Jan,8; 2016,Jan,13; 2015,Jan,16

87276 influenza A virus
0.00 0.00 FUD XXX
AMA: 2020,OctSE,1; 2020,AugSE,1; 2020,AugSE,1; 2020,AugSE,1; 2018,Jan,8; 2017,Jan,8; 2016,Jan,13; 2015,Jan,16

87278 Legionella pneumophila
0.00 0.00 FUD XXX
AMA: 2020,OctSE,1; 2020,AugSE,1; 2020,AugSE,1; 2020,AugSE,1

87279 Parainfluenza virus, each type
0.00 0.00 FUD XXX
AMA: 2020,OctSE,1; 2020,AugSE,1; 2020,AugSE,1; 2020,AugSE,1

87280 respiratory syncytial virus
0.00 0.00 FUD XXX
AMA: 2020,OctSE,1; 2020,AugSE,1; 2020,AugSE,1; 2020,AugSE,1

87281 Pneumocystis carinii
0.00 0.00 FUD XXX
AMA: 2020,OctSE,1; 2020,AugSE,1; 2020,AugSE,1; 2020,AugSE,1

87283 Rubeola
0.00 0.00 FUD XXX
AMA: 2020,OctSE,1; 2020,AugSE,1; 2020,AugSE,1; 2020,AugSE,1

87285 Treponema pallidum
0.00 0.00 FUD XXX
AMA: 2020,OctSE,1; 2020,AugSE,1; 2020,AugSE,1; 2020,AugSE,1

87290 Varicella zoster virus
0.00 0.00 FUD XXX
AMA: 2020,OctSE,1; 2020,AugSE,1; 2020,AugSE,1; 2020,AugSE,1

87299 not otherwise specified, each organism
0.00 0.00 FUD XXX
AMA: 2020,OctSE,1; 2020,AugSE,1; 2020,AugSE,1; 2020,AugSE,1; 2018,Jan,8; 2017,Jan,8; 2016,Jan,13; 2015,Jan,16

87300 **Infectious agent antigen detection by immunofluorescent technique, polyvalent for multiple organisms, each polyvalent antiserum**
EXCLUDES *Physician evaluation infectious disease agents by immunofluorescence (88346)*
0.00 0.00 FUD XXX
AMA: 2020,OctSE,1; 2020,AugSE,1; 2020,AugSE,1; 2020,AugSE,1

87301-87451 Enzyme Immunoassay Technique by Organism

INCLUDES Primary source only
EXCLUDES *Comparable tests on culture material (87140-87158)*
Identification antibodies (86602-86804)
Nonspecific agent detection (87449, 87797-87799, 87899)
Code also modifier 59 for different species or strains reported by same code

▲ 87301 **Infectious agent antigen detection by immunoassay technique, (eg, enzyme immunoassay [EIA], enzyme-linked immunosorbent assay [ELISA], fluorescence immunoassay [FIA], immunochemiluminometric assay [IMCA]) qualitative or semiquantitative; adenovirus enteric types 40/41**
0.00 0.00 FUD XXX
AMA: 2020,OctSE,1; 2020,AugSE,1; 2020,AugSE,1; 2020,AugSE,1; 2020,May,3; 2020,JuneSE,1; 2018,Jan,8; 2017,Jan,8; 2016,Jan,13; 2015,Jan,16

▲ 87305 Aspergillus
0.00 0.00 FUD XXX
AMA: 2020,OctSE,1; 2020,AugSE,1; 2020,AugSE,1; 2020,AugSE,1

▲ 87320 Chlamydia trachomatis
0.00 0.00 FUD XXX
AMA: 2020,OctSE,1; 2020,AugSE,1; 2020,AugSE,1; 2020,AugSE,1

▲ 87324 Clostridium difficile toxin(s)
0.00 0.00 FUD XXX
AMA: 2020,OctSE,1; 2020,AugSE,1; 2020,AugSE,1; 2020,AugSE,1

▲ 87327 Cryptococcus neoformans
EXCLUDES *Cryptococcus latex agglutination (86403)*
0.00 0.00 FUD XXX
AMA: 2020,OctSE,1; 2020,AugSE,1; 2020,AugSE,1; 2020,AugSE,1

▲ 87328 cryptosporidium
0.00 0.00 FUD XXX
AMA: 2020,OctSE,1; 2020,AugSE,1; 2020,AugSE,1; 2020,AugSE,1

▲ 87329 giardia
0.00 0.00 FUD XXX
AMA: 2020,OctSE,1; 2020,AugSE,1; 2020,AugSE,1; 2020,AugSE,1

▲ 87332 cytomegalovirus
0.00 0.00 FUD XXX
AMA: 2020,OctSE,1; 2020,AugSE,1; 2020,AugSE,1; 2020,AugSE,1

▲ 87335 Escherichia coli 0157
EXCLUDES *Giardia antigen (87329)*
0.00 0.00 FUD XXX
AMA: 2020,OctSE,1; 2020,AugSE,1; 2020,AugSE,1; 2020,AugSE,1

▲ 87336 Entamoeba histolytica dispar group
0.00 0.00 FUD XXX
AMA: 2020,OctSE,1; 2020,AugSE,1; 2020,AugSE,1; 2020,AugSE,1

▲ 87337 Entamoeba histolytica group
0.00 0.00 FUD XXX
AMA: 2020,OctSE,1; 2020,AugSE,1; 2020,AugSE,1; 2020,AugSE,1

▲ 87338 Helicobacter pylori, stool
0.00 0.00 FUD XXX
AMA: 2020,OctSE,1; 2020,AugSE,1; 2020,AugSE,1; 2020,AugSE,1; 2018,Jan,8; 2017,Jan,8; 2016,Jan,13; 2015,Jan,16

▲ 87339 Helicobacter pylori
EXCLUDES *H. pylori:*
Breath and blood by mass spectrometry (83013-83014)
Liquid scintillation counter (78267-78268)
Stool (87338)
0.00 0.00 FUD XXX
AMA: 2020,OctSE,1; 2020,AugSE,1; 2020,AugSE,1; 2020,AugSE,1

▲ 87340 hepatitis B surface antigen (HBsAg)
0.00 0.00 FUD XXX
AMA: 2020,OctSE,1; 2020,AugSE,1; 2020,AugSE,1; 2020,AugSE,1; 2018,Jan,8; 2017,Jan,8; 2016,Jan,13; 2015,Jan,16

▲ **87341** **hepatitis B surface antigen (HBsAg) neutralization**
0.00 0.00 **FUD** XXX
AMA: 2020,OctSE,1; 2020,AugSE,1; 2020,AugSE,1; 2020,AugSE,1

87350 **hepatitis Be antigen (HBeAg)**
0.00 0.00 **FUD** XXX
AMA: 2020,OctSE,1; 2020,AugSE,1; 2020,AugSE,1; 2020,AugSE,1

▲ **87380** **hepatitis, delta agent**
0.00 0.00 **FUD** XXX
AMA: 2020,OctSE,1; 2020,AugSE,1; 2020,AugSE,1; 2020,AugSE,1

▲ **87385** **Histoplasma capsulatum**
0.00 0.00 **FUD** XXX
AMA: 2020,OctSE,1; 2020,AugSE,1; 2020,AugSE,1; 2020,AugSE,1

▲ **87389** **HIV-1 antigen(s), with HIV-1 and HIV-2 antibodies, single result**
Code also modifier 92 for test performed using kit or transportable instrument comprising (all or part) single-use, disposable analytical chamber
0.00 0.00 **FUD** XXX
AMA: 2020,OctSE,1; 2020,AugSE,1; 2020,AugSE,1; 2020,AugSE,1

▲ **87390** **HIV-1**
0.00 0.00 **FUD** XXX
AMA: 2020,OctSE,1; 2020,AugSE,1; 2020,AugSE,1; 2020,AugSE,1

▲ **87391** **HIV-2**
0.00 0.00 **FUD** XXX
AMA: 2020,OctSE,1; 2020,AugSE,1; 2020,AugSE,1; 2020,AugSE,1

▲ **87400** **Influenza, A or B, each**
0.00 0.00 **FUD** XXX
AMA: 2020,OctSE,1; 2020,AugSE,1; 2020,AugSE,1; 2020,AugSE,1; 2018,Jan,8; 2017,Jan,8; 2016,Jan,13; 2015,Jan,16

▲ **87420** **respiratory syncytial virus**
0.00 0.00 **FUD** XXX
AMA: 2020,OctSE,1; 2020,AugSE,1; 2020,AugSE,1; 2020,AugSE,1

▲ **87425** **rotavirus**
0.00 0.00 **FUD** XXX
AMA: 2020,OctSE,1; 2020,AugSE,1; 2020,AugSE,1; 2020,AugSE,1

▲ **87426** **severe acute respiratory syndrome coronavirus (eg, SARS-CoV, SARS-CoV-2 [COVID-19])**
AMA: 2020,OctSE,1; 2020,AugSE,1; 2020,AugSE,1; 2020,AugSE,1

▲ **87427** **Shiga-like toxin**
0.00 0.00 **FUD** XXX
AMA: 2020,OctSE,1; 2020,AugSE,1; 2020,AugSE,1; 2020,AugSE,1

▲ **87430** **Streptococcus, group A**
0.00 0.00 **FUD** XXX
AMA: 2020,OctSE,1; 2020,AugSE,1; 2020,AugSE,1; 2020,AugSE,1; 2018,Jan,8; 2017,Jan,8; 2016,Jan,13; 2015,Jan,16

▲ **87449** **not otherwise specified, each organism**
0.00 0.00 **FUD** XXX
AMA: 2020,OctSE,1; 2020,AugSE,1; 2020,AugSE,1; 2020,AugSE,1; 2018,Jan,8; 2017,Jan,8; 2016,Jan,13; 2015,Jan,16

~~**87450**~~ ~~**single step method, not otherwise specified, each organism**~~
To report, see (87301-87451, 87802-87899 [87806, 87811])

▲ **87451** **polyvalent for multiple organisms, each polyvalent antiserum**
0.00 0.00 **FUD** XXX
AMA: 2020,OctSE,1; 2020,AugSE,1; 2020,AugSE,1; 2020,AugSE,1

87471-87801 [87623, 87624, 87625] Detection Infectious Agent by Probe Techniques

INCLUDES Primary source only

EXCLUDES *Comparable tests on culture material (87140-87158)*
Identification antibodies (86602-86804)
Nonspecific agent detection (87299, 87449, 87797-87799, 87899)
Reporting molecular procedure codes as substitute for codes in this range (81161-81408 [81105, 81106, 81107, 81108, 81109, 81110, 81111, 81112, 81120, 81121, 81161, 81162, 81230, 81231, 81238, 81269, 81283, 81287, 81288, 81334])

Code also modifier 59 for different species or strains reported by same code

87471 **Infectious agent detection by nucleic acid (DNA or RNA); Bartonella henselae and Bartonella quintana, amplified probe technique**
0.00 0.00 **FUD** XXX
AMA: 2020,OctSE,1; 2020,AugSE,1; 2020,AugSE,1; 2020,AugSE,1; 2018,Jan,8; 2017,Jan,8; 2016,Jan,13; 2015,Jan,16

87472 **Bartonella henselae and Bartonella quintana, quantification**
0.00 0.00 **FUD** XXX
AMA: 2020,OctSE,1; 2020,AugSE,1; 2020,AugSE,1; 2020,AugSE,1; 2018,Jan,8; 2017,Jan,8; 2016,Jan,13; 2015,Jan,16

87475 **Borrelia burgdorferi, direct probe technique**
0.00 0.00 **FUD** XXX
AMA: 2020,OctSE,1; 2020,AugSE,1; 2020,AugSE,1; 2020,AugSE,1; 2018,Jan,8; 2017,Jan,8; 2016,Jan,13; 2015,Jan,16

87476 **Borrelia burgdorferi, amplified probe technique**
0.00 0.00 **FUD** XXX
AMA: 2020,OctSE,1; 2020,AugSE,1; 2020,AugSE,1; 2020,AugSE,1; 2018,Jan,8; 2017,Jan,8; 2016,Jan,13; 2015,Jan,16

87480 **Candida species, direct probe technique**
0.00 0.00 **FUD** XXX
AMA: 2020,OctSE,1; 2020,AugSE,1; 2020,AugSE,1; 2020,AugSE,1; 2018,Jan,8; 2017,Jan,8; 2016,Jan,13; 2015,Jan,16

87481 **Candida species, amplified probe technique**
0.00 0.00 **FUD** XXX
AMA: 2020,OctSE,1; 2020,AugSE,1; 2020,AugSE,1; 2020,AugSE,1; 2018,Jan,8; 2017,Jan,8; 2016,Jan,13; 2015,Jan,16

87482 **Candida species, quantification**
0.00 0.00 **FUD** XXX
AMA: 2020,OctSE,1; 2020,AugSE,1; 2020,AugSE,1; 2020,AugSE,1; 2018,Jan,8; 2017,Jan,8; 2016,Jan,13; 2015,Jan,16

87483 **central nervous system pathogen (eg, Neisseria meningitidis, Streptococcus pneumoniae, Listeria, Haemophilus influenzae, E. coli, Streptococcus agalactiae, enterovirus, human parechovirus, herpes simplex virus type 1 and 2, human herpesvirus 6, cytomegalovirus, varicella zoster virus, Cryptococcus), includes multiplex reverse transcription, when performed, and multiplex amplified probe technique, multiple types or subtypes, 12-25 targets**
0.00 0.00 **FUD** XXX
AMA: 2020,OctSE,1; 2020,AugSE,1; 2020,AugSE,1; 2020,AugSE,1

87485 **Chlamydia pneumoniae, direct probe technique**
0.00 0.00 **FUD** XXX
AMA: 2020,OctSE,1; 2020,AugSE,1; 2020,AugSE,1; 2020,AugSE,1; 2018,Jan,8; 2017,Jan,8; 2016,Jan,13; 2015,Jan,16

87486 **Chlamydia pneumoniae, amplified probe technique**
0.00 0.00 **FUD** XXX
AMA: 2020,OctSE,1; 2020,AugSE,1; 2020,AugSE,1; 2020,AugSE,1; 2018,Jan,8; 2017,Jan,8; 2016,Jan,13; 2015,Jan,16

87487 **Chlamydia pneumoniae, quantification**
0.00 0.00 **FUD** XXX
AMA: 2020,OctSE,1; 2020,AugSE,1; 2020,AugSE,1; 2020,AugSE,1; 2018,Jan,8; 2017,Jan,8; 2016,Jan,13; 2015,Jan,16

87490 Chlamydia trachomatis, direct probe technique
0.00 0.00 FUD XXX
AMA: 2020,OctSE,1; 2020,AugSE,1; 2020,AugSE,1; 2020,AugSE,1; 2018,Jan,8; 2017,Jan,8; 2016,Jan,13; 2015,Jan,16

87491 Chlamydia trachomatis, amplified probe technique
0.00 0.00 FUD XXX
AMA: 2020,OctSE,1; 2020,AugSE,1; 2020,AugSE,1; 2020,AugSE,1; 2018,Jan,8; 2017,Jan,8; 2016,Jan,13; 2015,Jan,16

87492 Chlamydia trachomatis, quantification
0.00 0.00 FUD XXX
AMA: 2020,OctSE,1; 2020,AugSE,1; 2020,AugSE,1; 2020,AugSE,1; 2018,Jan,8; 2017,Jan,8; 2016,Jan,13; 2015,Jan,16

87493 Clostridium difficile, toxin gene(s), amplified probe technique
0.00 0.00 FUD XXX
AMA: 2020,OctSE,1; 2020,AugSE,1; 2020,AugSE,1; 2020,AugSE,1; 2018,Jan,8; 2017,Jan,8; 2016,Jan,13; 2015,Jan,16

87495 cytomegalovirus, direct probe technique
0.00 0.00 FUD XXX
AMA: 2020,OctSE,1; 2020,AugSE,1; 2020,AugSE,1; 2020,AugSE,1; 2018,Jan,8; 2017,Jan,8; 2016,Jan,13; 2015,Jan,16

87496 cytomegalovirus, amplified probe technique
0.00 0.00 FUD XXX
AMA: 2020,OctSE,1; 2020,AugSE,1; 2020,AugSE,1; 2020,AugSE,1; 2018,Jan,8; 2017,Jan,8; 2016,Jan,13; 2015,Jan,16

87497 cytomegalovirus, quantification
0.00 0.00 FUD XXX
AMA: 2020,OctSE,1; 2020,AugSE,1; 2020,AugSE,1; 2020,AugSE,1; 2018,Jan,8; 2017,Jan,8; 2016,Jan,13; 2015,Jan,16

87498 enterovirus, amplified probe technique, includes reverse transcription when performed
0.00 0.00 FUD XXX
AMA: 2020,OctSE,1; 2020,AugSE,1; 2020,AugSE,1; 2020,AugSE,1; 2018,Jan,8; 2017,Jan,8; 2016,Jan,13; 2015,Jan,16

87500 vancomycin resistance (eg, enterococcus species van A, van B), amplified probe technique
0.00 0.00 FUD XXX
AMA: 2020,OctSE,1; 2020,AugSE,1; 2020,AugSE,1; 2020,AugSE,1; 2018,Jan,8; 2017,Jan,8; 2016,Jan,13; 2015,Jan,16

87501 influenza virus, includes reverse transcription, when performed, and amplified probe technique, each type or subtype
0.00 0.00 FUD XXX
AMA: 2020,OctSE,1; 2020,AugSE,1; 2020,AugSE,1; 2020,AugSE,1; 2018,Jan,8; 2017,Jan,8; 2016,Jan,13; 2015,Jan,16

87502 influenza virus, for multiple types or sub-types, includes multiplex reverse transcription, when performed, and multiplex amplified probe technique, first 2 types or sub-types
0.00 0.00 FUD XXX
AMA: 2020,OctSE,1; 2020,AugSE,1; 2020,AugSE,1; 2020,AugSE,1; 2018,Jan,8; 2017,Jan,8; 2016,Jan,13; 2015,Jan,16

\+ **87503 influenza virus, for multiple types or sub-types, includes multiplex reverse transcription, when performed, and multiplex amplified probe technique, each additional influenza virus type or sub-type beyond 2 (List separately in addition to code for primary procedure)**
Code first (87502)
0.00 0.00 FUD XXX
AMA: 2020,OctSE,1; 2020,AugSE,1; 2020,AugSE,1; 2020,AugSE,1; 2018,Jan,8; 2017,Jan,8; 2016,Jan,13; 2015,Jan,16

87505 gastrointestinal pathogen (eg, Clostridium difficile, E. coli, Salmonella, Shigella, norovirus, Giardia), includes multiplex reverse transcription, when performed, and multiplex amplified probe technique, multiple types or subtypes, 3-5 targets
0.00 0.00 FUD XXX
AMA: 2020,OctSE,1; 2020,AugSE,1; 2020,AugSE,1; 2020,AugSE,1

87506 gastrointestinal pathogen (eg, Clostridium difficile, E. coli, Salmonella, Shigella, norovirus, Giardia), includes multiplex reverse transcription, when performed, and multiplex amplified probe technique, multiple types or subtypes, 6-11 targets
0.00 0.00 FUD XXX
AMA: 2020,OctSE,1; 2020,AugSE,1; 2020,AugSE,1; 2020,AugSE,1

87507 gastrointestinal pathogen (eg, Clostridium difficile, E. coli, Salmonella, Shigella, norovirus, Giardia), includes multiplex reverse transcription, when performed, and multiplex amplified probe technique, multiple types or subtypes, 12-25 targets
0.00 0.00 FUD XXX
AMA: 2020,OctSE,1; 2020,AugSE,1; 2020,AugSE,1; 2020,AugSE,1

87510 Gardnerella vaginalis, direct probe technique
0.00 0.00 FUD XXX
AMA: 2020,OctSE,1; 2020,AugSE,1; 2020,AugSE,1; 2020,AugSE,1; 2018,Jan,8; 2017,Jan,8; 2016,Jan,13; 2015,Jan,16

87511 Gardnerella vaginalis, amplified probe technique
0.00 0.00 FUD XXX
AMA: 2020,OctSE,1; 2020,AugSE,1; 2020,AugSE,1; 2020,AugSE,1; 2018,Jan,8; 2017,Jan,8; 2016,Jan,13; 2015,Jan,16

87512 Gardnerella vaginalis, quantification
0.00 0.00 FUD XXX
AMA: 2020,OctSE,1; 2020,AugSE,1; 2020,AugSE,1; 2020,AugSE,1; 2018,Jan,8; 2017,Jan,8; 2016,Jan,13; 2015,Jan,16

87516 hepatitis B virus, amplified probe technique
0.00 0.00 FUD XXX
AMA: 2020,OctSE,1; 2020,AugSE,1; 2020,AugSE,1; 2020,AugSE,1; 2018,Jan,8; 2017,Jan,8; 2016,Jan,13; 2015,Jan,16

87517 hepatitis B virus, quantification
0.00 0.00 FUD XXX
AMA: 2020,OctSE,1; 2020,AugSE,1; 2020,AugSE,1; 2020,AugSE,1; 2018,Jan,8; 2017,Jan,8; 2016,Jan,13; 2015,Jan,16

87520 hepatitis C, direct probe technique
0.00 0.00 FUD XXX
AMA: 2020,OctSE,1; 2020,AugSE,1; 2020,AugSE,1; 2020,AugSE,1; 2018,Jan,8; 2017,Jan,8; 2016,Jan,13; 2015,Jan,16

87521 hepatitis C, amplified probe technique, includes reverse transcription when performed
0.00 0.00 FUD XXX
AMA: 2020,OctSE,1; 2020,AugSE,1; 2020,AugSE,1; 2020,AugSE,1; 2018,Jan,8; 2017,Jan,8; 2016,Jan,13; 2015,Jan,16

87522 hepatitis C, quantification, includes reverse transcription when performed
0.00 0.00 FUD XXX
AMA: 2020,OctSE,1; 2020,AugSE,1; 2020,AugSE,1; 2020,AugSE,1; 2018,Jan,8; 2017,Jan,8; 2016,Jan,13; 2015,Jan,16

87525 hepatitis G, direct probe technique
0.00 0.00 FUD XXX
AMA: 2020,OctSE,1; 2020,AugSE,1; 2020,AugSE,1; 2020,AugSE,1; 2018,Jan,8; 2017,Jan,8; 2016,Jan,13; 2015,Jan,16

87526 hepatitis G, amplified probe technique
0.00 0.00 FUD XXX
AMA: 2020,OctSE,1; 2020,AugSE,1; 2020,AugSE,1; 2020,AugSE,1; 2018,Jan,8; 2017,Jan,8; 2016,Jan,13; 2015,Jan,16

87527 hepatitis G, quantification
0.00 0.00 FUD XXX
AMA: 2020,OctSE,1; 2020,AugSE,1; 2020,AugSE,1; 2020,AugSE,1; 2018,Jan,8; 2017,Jan,8; 2016,Jan,13; 2015,Jan,16

87528 Herpes simplex virus, direct probe technique
0.00 0.00 FUD XXX
AMA: 2020,OctSE,1; 2020,AugSE,1; 2020,AugSE,1; 2020,AugSE,1; 2018,Jan,8; 2017,Jan,8; 2016,Jan,13; 2015,Jan,16

87529 Herpes simplex virus, amplified probe technique
0.00 0.00 FUD XXX
AMA: 2020,OctSE,1; 2020,AugSE,1; 2020,AugSE,1; 2020,AugSE,1; 2018,Jan,8; 2017,Jan,8; 2016,Jan,13; 2015,Jan,16

87530 **Herpes simplex virus, quantification**
0.00 0.00 FUD XXX
AMA: 2020,OctSE,1; 2020,AugSE,1; 2020,AugSE,1; 2020,AugSE,1; 2018,Jan,8; 2017,Jan,8; 2016,Jan,13; 2015,Jan,16

87531 **Herpes virus-6, direct probe technique**
0.00 0.00 FUD XXX
AMA: 2020,OctSE,1; 2020,AugSE,1; 2020,AugSE,1; 2020,AugSE,1; 2018,Jan,8; 2017,Jan,8; 2016,Jan,13; 2015,Jan,16

87532 **Herpes virus-6, amplified probe technique**
0.00 0.00 FUD XXX
AMA: 2020,OctSE,1; 2020,AugSE,1; 2020,AugSE,1; 2020,AugSE,1; 2018,Jan,8; 2017,Jan,8; 2016,Jan,13; 2015,Jan,16

87533 **Herpes virus-6, quantification**
0.00 0.00 FUD XXX
AMA: 2020,OctSE,1; 2020,AugSE,1; 2020,AugSE,1; 2020,AugSE,1; 2018,Jan,8; 2017,Jan,8; 2016,Jan,13; 2015,Jan,16

87534 **HIV-1, direct probe technique**
0.00 0.00 FUD XXX
AMA: 2020,OctSE,1; 2020,AugSE,1; 2020,AugSE,1; 2020,AugSE,1; 2018,Jan,8; 2017,Jan,8; 2016,Jan,13; 2015,Jan,16

87535 **HIV-1, amplified probe technique, includes reverse transcription when performed**
0.00 0.00 FUD XXX
AMA: 2020,OctSE,1; 2020,AugSE,1; 2020,AugSE,1; 2020,AugSE,1; 2018,Jan,8; 2017,Jan,8; 2016,Jan,13; 2015,Jan,16

87536 **HIV-1, quantification, includes reverse transcription when performed**
0.00 0.00 FUD XXX
AMA: 2020,OctSE,1; 2020,AugSE,1; 2020,AugSE,1; 2020,AugSE,1; 2018,Jan,8; 2017,Jan,8; 2016,Jan,13; 2015,Jan,16

87537 **HIV-2, direct probe technique**
0.00 0.00 FUD XXX
AMA: 2020,OctSE,1; 2020,AugSE,1; 2020,AugSE,1; 2020,AugSE,1; 2018,Jan,8; 2017,Jan,8; 2016,Jan,13; 2015,Jan,16

87538 **HIV-2, amplified probe technique, includes reverse transcription when performed**
0.00 0.00 FUD XXX
AMA: 2020,OctSE,1; 2020,AugSE,1; 2020,AugSE,1; 2020,AugSE,1; 2018,Jan,8; 2017,Jan,8; 2016,Jan,13; 2015,Jan,16

87539 **HIV-2, quantification, includes reverse transcription when performed**
0.00 0.00 FUD XXX
AMA: 2020,OctSE,1; 2020,AugSE,1; 2020,AugSE,1; 2020,AugSE,1; 2018,Jan,8; 2017,Jan,8; 2016,Jan,13; 2015,Jan,16

87623 **Human Papillomavirus (HPV), low-risk types (eg, 6, 11, 42, 43, 44)**
0.00 0.00 FUD XXX
AMA: 2020,OctSE,1; 2020,AugSE,1; 2020,AugSE,1; 2020,AugSE,1

87624 **Human Papillomavirus (HPV), high-risk types (eg, 16, 18, 31, 33, 35, 39, 45, 51, 52, 56, 58, 59, 68)**
INCLUDES Low- and high-risk types in one assay
0.00 0.00 FUD XXX
AMA: 2020,OctSE,1; 2020,AugSE,1; 2020,AugSE,1; 2020,AugSE,1; 2018,Jan,8; 2017,Jan,8; 2016,Jan,13; 2015,Oct,9

87625 **Human Papillomavirus (HPV), types 16 and 18 only, includes type 45, if performed**
EXCLUDES *HPV detection (genotyping) (0500T)*
0.00 0.00 FUD XXX
AMA: 2020,OctSE,1; 2020,AugSE,1; 2020,AugSE,1; 2020,AugSE,1; 2018,Jan,8; 2017,Jan,8; 2016,Jan,13; 2015,Oct,9; 2015,Jun,10

87540 **Legionella pneumophila, direct probe technique**
0.00 0.00 FUD XXX
AMA: 2020,OctSE,1; 2020,AugSE,1; 2020,AugSE,1; 2020,AugSE,1; 2018,Jan,8; 2017,Jan,8; 2016,Jan,13; 2015,Jan,16

87541 **Legionella pneumophila, amplified probe technique**
0.00 0.00 FUD XXX
AMA: 2020,OctSE,1; 2020,AugSE,1; 2020,AugSE,1; 2020,AugSE,1; 2018,Jan,8; 2017,Jan,8; 2016,Jan,13; 2015,Jan,16

87542 **Legionella pneumophila, quantification**
0.00 0.00 FUD XXX
AMA: 2020,OctSE,1; 2020,AugSE,1; 2020,AugSE,1; 2020,AugSE,1; 2018,Jan,8; 2017,Jan,8; 2016,Jan,13; 2015,Jan,16

87550 **Mycobacteria species, direct probe technique**
0.00 0.00 FUD XXX
AMA: 2020,OctSE,1; 2020,AugSE,1; 2020,AugSE,1; 2020,AugSE,1; 2018,Jan,8; 2017,Jan,8; 2016,Jan,13; 2015,Jan,16

87551 **Mycobacteria species, amplified probe technique**
0.00 0.00 FUD XXX
AMA: 2020,OctSE,1; 2020,AugSE,1; 2020,AugSE,1; 2020,AugSE,1; 2018,Jan,8; 2017,Jan,8; 2016,Jan,13; 2015,Jan,16

87552 **Mycobacteria species, quantification**
0.00 0.00 FUD XXX
AMA: 2020,OctSE,1; 2020,AugSE,1; 2020,AugSE,1; 2020,AugSE,1; 2018,Jan,8; 2017,Jan,8; 2016,Jan,13; 2015,Jan,16

87555 **Mycobacteria tuberculosis, direct probe technique**
0.00 0.00 FUD XXX
AMA: 2020,OctSE,1; 2020,AugSE,1; 2020,AugSE,1; 2020,AugSE,1; 2018,Jan,8; 2017,Jan,8; 2016,Jan,13; 2015,Jan,16

87556 **Mycobacteria tuberculosis, amplified probe technique**
0.00 0.00 FUD XXX
AMA: 2020,OctSE,1; 2020,AugSE,1; 2020,AugSE,1; 2020,AugSE,1; 2018,Jan,8; 2017,Jan,8; 2016,Jan,13; 2015,Jan,16

87557 **Mycobacteria tuberculosis, quantification**
0.00 0.00 FUD XXX
AMA: 2020,OctSE,1; 2020,AugSE,1; 2020,AugSE,1; 2020,AugSE,1; 2018,Jan,8; 2017,Jan,8; 2016,Jan,13; 2015,Jan,16

87560 **Mycobacteria avium-intracellulare, direct probe technique**
0.00 0.00 FUD XXX
AMA: 2020,OctSE,1; 2020,AugSE,1; 2020,AugSE,1; 2020,AugSE,1; 2018,Jan,8; 2017,Jan,8; 2016,Jan,13; 2015,Jan,16

87561 **Mycobacteria avium-intracellulare, amplified probe technique**
0.00 0.00 FUD XXX
AMA: 2020,OctSE,1; 2020,AugSE,1; 2020,AugSE,1; 2020,AugSE,1; 2018,Jan,8; 2017,Jan,8; 2016,Jan,13; 2015,Jan,16

87562 **Mycobacteria avium-intracellulare, quantification**
0.00 0.00 FUD XXX
AMA: 2020,OctSE,1; 2020,AugSE,1; 2020,AugSE,1; 2020,AugSE,1; 2018,Jan,8; 2017,Jan,8; 2016,Jan,13; 2015,Jan,16

87563 **Mycoplasma genitalium, amplified probe technique**
0.00 0.00 FUD XXX
AMA: 2020,OctSE,1; 2020,AugSE,1; 2020,AugSE,1; 2020,AugSE,1

87580 **Mycoplasma pneumoniae, direct probe technique**
0.00 0.00 FUD XXX
AMA: 2020,OctSE,1; 2020,AugSE,1; 2020,AugSE,1; 2020,AugSE,1; 2018,Jan,8; 2017,Jan,8; 2016,Jan,13; 2015,Jan,16

87581 **Mycoplasma pneumoniae, amplified probe technique**
0.00 0.00 FUD XXX
AMA: 2020,OctSE,1; 2020,AugSE,1; 2020,AugSE,1; 2020,AugSE,1; 2018,Jan,8; 2017,Jan,8; 2016,Jan,13; 2015,Jan,16

87582 **Mycoplasma pneumoniae, quantification**
0.00 0.00 FUD XXX
AMA: 2020,OctSE,1; 2020,AugSE,1; 2020,AugSE,1; 2020,AugSE,1; 2018,Jan,8; 2017,Jan,8; 2016,Jan,13; 2015,Jan,16

87590 **Neisseria gonorrhoeae, direct probe technique**
0.00 0.00 FUD XXX
AMA: 2020,OctSE,1; 2020,AugSE,1; 2020,AugSE,1; 2020,AugSE,1; 2018,Jan,8; 2017,Jan,8; 2016,Jan,13; 2015,Jan,16

87591	**Neisseria gonorrhoeae, amplified probe technique**

🚑 0.00   ⚕ 0.00   **FUD** XXX   [A][▫]

AMA: 2020,OctSE,1; 2020,AugSE,1; 2020,AugSE,1; 2020,AugSE,1; 2018,Jan,8; 2017,Jan,8; 2016,Jan,13; 2015,Jan,16

87592	**Neisseria gonorrhoeae, quantification**

🚑 0.00   ⚕ 0.00   **FUD** XXX   [Q][▫]

AMA: 2020,OctSE,1; 2020,AugSE,1; 2020,AugSE,1; 2020,AugSE,1; 2018,Jan,8; 2017,Jan,8; 2016,Jan,13; 2015,Jan,16

87623	**Resequenced code. See code following 87539.**
87624	**Resequenced code. See code following 87539.**
87625	**Resequenced code. See code before 87540.**

87631	**respiratory virus (eg, adenovirus, influenza virus, coronavirus, metapneumovirus, parainfluenza virus, respiratory syncytial virus, rhinovirus), includes multiplex reverse transcription, when performed, and multiplex amplified probe technique, multiple types or subtypes, 3-5 targets**

> INCLUDES Detection multiple respiratory viruses with one test
>
> EXCLUDES *Assay for severe acute respiratory syndrome coronavirus 2 (SARS-CoV-2) (Coronavirus disease) (COVID-19) (87635)*
>
> *Assays for typing or subtyping influenza viruses only (87501-87503)*
>
> *Single test for detection multiple infectious organisms (87800-87801)*

🚑 0.00   ⚕ 0.00   **FUD** XXX   [X][Q][▫]

AMA: 2020,OctSE,1; 2020,AugSE,1; 2020,AugSE,1; 2020,AugSE,1; 2020,Apr,3; 2020,Mar,3; 2018,Jan,8; 2017,Jan,8; 2016,Jan,13; 2015,Jan,16

87632	**respiratory virus (eg, adenovirus, influenza virus, coronavirus, metapneumovirus, parainfluenza virus, respiratory syncytial virus, rhinovirus), includes multiplex reverse transcription, when performed, and multiplex amplified probe technique, multiple types or subtypes, 6-11 targets**

> INCLUDES Detection multiple respiratory viruses with one test
>
> EXCLUDES *Assay for severe acute respiratory syndrome coronavirus 2 (SARS-CoV-2) (Coronavirus disease) (COVID-19) (87635)*
>
> *Assays for typing or subtyping influenza viruses only (87501-87503)*
>
> *Single test to detect multiple infectious organisms (87800-87801)*

🚑 0.00   ⚕ 0.00   **FUD** XXX   [Q][▫]

AMA: 2020,OctSE,1; 2020,AugSE,1; 2020,AugSE,1; 2020,AugSE,1; 2020,Apr,3; 2020,Mar,3; 2018,Jan,8; 2017,Jan,8; 2016,Jan,13; 2015,Jan,16

87633	**respiratory virus (eg, adenovirus, influenza virus, coronavirus, metapneumovirus, parainfluenza virus, respiratory syncytial virus, rhinovirus), includes multiplex reverse transcription, when performed, and multiplex amplified probe technique, multiple types or subtypes, 12-25 targets**

> INCLUDES Detection multiple respiratory viruses with one test
>
> EXCLUDES *Assay for severe acute respiratory syndrome coronavirus 2 (SARS-CoV-2) (Coronavirus disease) (COVID-19) (87635)*
>
> *Assays for typing or subtyping influenza viruses only (87501-87503)*
>
> *Single test to detect multiple infectious organisms (87800-87801)*

🚑 0.00   ⚕ 0.00   **FUD** XXX   [X][Q][▫]

AMA: 2020,OctSE,1; 2020,AugSE,1; 2020,AugSE,1; 2020,AugSE,1; 2020,Apr,3; 2020,Mar,3; 2018,Jan,8; 2017,Jan,8; 2016,Jan,13; 2015,Jan,16

87634	**respiratory syncytial virus, amplified probe technique**

> EXCLUDES *Assays for RSV with other respiratory viruses (87631-87633)*

🚑 0.00   ⚕ 0.00   **FUD** XXX   [X][Q][▫]

AMA: 2020,OctSE,1; 2020,AugSE,1; 2020,AugSE,1; 2020,AugSE,1

● 87635	**severe acute respiratory syndrome coronavirus 2 (SARS-CoV-2) (Coronavirus disease [COVID-19]), amplified probe technique**

> EXCLUDES *HCPCS codes for reporting coronavirus testing (U0001-U0002)*
>
> *Proprietary Laboratory Analyses (PLA) used to detect multiple types or subtypes of respiratory pathogens (0098U-0100U)*
>
> *Single procedure nucleic acid assays to detect multiple respiratory viruses by multiplex reaction (87631-87633)*

Code also code 87635, with modifier 59, for assays performed on specimens from different anatomic locations, when performed

AMA: 2020,OctSE,1; 2020,AugSE,1; 2020,AugSE,1; 2020,AugSE,1; 2020,Apr,3; 2020,Mar,3

● 87636	**severe acute respiratory syndrome coronavirus 2 (SARS-CoV-2) (Coronavirus disease [COVID-19]) and influenza virus types A and B, multiplex amplified probe technique**

> EXCLUDES *Nucleic acid detection multiple respiratory infectious agents (87631-87633):*
>
> *including Severe Acute Respiratory Syndrome coronavirus 2 (SARS-CoV-2) (Coronavirus disease) (COVID-19) with additional agents beyond influenza A and B and respiratory syncytial virus*
>
> *not including Severe Acute Respiratory Syndrome coronavirus 2 (SARS-CoV-2) (Coronavirus disease) (COVID-19)*

● 87637	**severe acute respiratory syndrome coronavirus 2 (SARS-CoV-2) (Coronavirus disease [COVID-19]), influenza virus types A and B, and respiratory syncytial virus, multiplex amplified probe technique**

> EXCLUDES *Nucleic acid detection multiple respiratory infectious agents (87631-87633):*
>
> *Including severe acute respiratory syndrome coronavirus 2 (SARS-CoV-2) (coronavirus disease) (COVID-19) with additional agents beyond influenza A and B and respiratory syncytial virus*
>
> *Not including severe acute respiratory syndrome coronavirus 2 (SARS-CoV-2) (coronavirus disease) (COVID-19)*

87640	**Staphylococcus aureus, amplified probe technique**

🚑 0.00   ⚕ 0.00   **FUD** XXX   [Q][▫]

AMA: 2020,OctSE,1; 2020,AugSE,1; 2020,AugSE,1; 2020,AugSE,1; 2018,Jan,8; 2017,Jan,8; 2016,Jan,13; 2015,Jan,16

87641	**Staphylococcus aureus, methicillin resistant, amplified probe technique**

> EXCLUDES *Assays that detect methicillin resistance and identify Staphylococcus aureus using single nucleic acid sequence (87641)*

🚑 0.00   ⚕ 0.00   **FUD** XXX   [Q][▫]

AMA: 2020,OctSE,1; 2020,AugSE,1; 2020,AugSE,1; 2020,AugSE,1; 2018,Jan,8; 2017,Jan,8; 2016,Jan,13; 2015,Jan,16

87650	**Streptococcus, group A, direct probe technique**

🚑 0.00   ⚕ 0.00   **FUD** XXX   [Q][▫]

AMA: 2020,OctSE,1; 2020,AugSE,1; 2020,AugSE,1; 2020,AugSE,1; 2018,Jan,8; 2017,Jan,8; 2016,Jan,13; 2015,Jan,16

87651	**Streptococcus, group A, amplified probe technique**

🚑 0.00   ⚕ 0.00   **FUD** XXX   [X][Q][▫]

AMA: 2020,OctSE,1; 2020,AugSE,1; 2020,AugSE,1; 2020,AugSE,1; 2018,Jan,8; 2017,Jan,8; 2016,Jan,13; 2015,Jan,16

87652	**Streptococcus, group A, quantification**

🚑 0.00   ⚕ 0.00   **FUD** XXX   [Q][▫]

AMA: 2020,OctSE,1; 2020,AugSE,1; 2020,AugSE,1; 2020,AugSE,1; 2018,Jan,8; 2017,Jan,8; 2016,Jan,13; 2015,Jan,16

87653	**Streptococcus, group B, amplified probe technique**

🚑 0.00   ⚕ 0.00   **FUD** XXX   [Q][▫]

AMA: 2020,OctSE,1; 2020,AugSE,1; 2020,AugSE,1; 2020,AugSE,1; 2018,Jan,8; 2017,Jan,8; 2016,Jan,13; 2015,Jan,16

87660 **Trichomonas vaginalis, direct probe technique**
0.00 0.00 **FUD** XXX
AMA: 2020,OctSE,1; 2020,AugSE,1; 2020,AugSE,1; 2020,AugSE,1; 2018,Jan,8; 2017,Jan,8; 2016,Jan,13; 2015,Jan,16

87661 **Trichomonas vaginalis, amplified probe technique**
0.00 0.00 **FUD** XXX
AMA: 2020,OctSE,1; 2020,AugSE,1; 2020,AugSE,1; 2020,AugSE,1

87662 **Zika virus, amplified probe technique**
0.00 0.00 **FUD** XXX
AMA: 2020,OctSE,1; 2020,AugSE,1; 2020,AugSE,1; 2020,AugSE,1

87797 **Infectious agent detection by nucleic acid (DNA or RNA), not otherwise specified; direct probe technique, each organism**
0.00 0.00 **FUD** XXX
AMA: 2020,OctSE,1; 2020,AugSE,1; 2020,AugSE,1; 2020,AugSE,1; 2018,Jan,8; 2017,Jan,8; 2016,Aug,9; 2016,Jan,13; 2015,Jan,16

87798 **amplified probe technique, each organism**
0.00 0.00 **FUD** XXX
AMA: 2020,OctSE,1; 2020,AugSE,1; 2020,AugSE,1; 2020,AugSE,1; 2018,Jan,8; 2017,Jan,8; 2016,Jan,13; 2015,Jan,16

87799 **quantification, each organism**
0.00 0.00 **FUD** XXX
AMA: 2020,OctSE,1; 2020,AugSE,1; 2020,AugSE,1; 2020,AugSE,1; 2018,Jan,8; 2017,Jan,8; 2016,Jan,13; 2015,Jan,16

87800 **Infectious agent detection by nucleic acid (DNA or RNA), multiple organisms; direct probe(s) technique**
INCLUDES Single test to detect multiple infectious organisms
EXCLUDES *Detection specific infectious agents not otherwise specified (87797-87799)*
Each specific organism nucleic acid detection from primary source (87471-87660 [87623, 87624, 87625])
0.00 0.00 **FUD** XXX
AMA: 2020,OctSE,1; 2020,AugSE,1; 2020,AugSE,1; 2020,AugSE,1; 2018,Jan,8; 2017,Jan,8; 2016,Aug,9; 2016,Jan,13; 2015,Jan,16

87801 **amplified probe(s) technique**
INCLUDES Single test to detect multiple infectious organisms
EXCLUDES *Detection multiple respiratory viruses with one test (87631-87633)*
Detection specific infectious agents not otherwise specified (87797-87799)
Each specific organism nucleic acid detection from primary source (87471-87660 [87623, 87624, 87625])
0.00 0.00 **FUD** XXX
AMA: 2020,OctSE,1; 2020,AugSE,1; 2020,AugSE,1; 2020,AugSE,1; 2018,Jan,8; 2017,Jan,8; 2016,Jan,13; 2015,Jan,16

87802-87899 [87806, 87811] Detection Infectious Agent by Immunoassay with Direct Optical Observation

▲ **87802** **Infectious agent antigen detection by immunoassay with direct optical (ie, visual) observation; Streptococcus, group B**
0.00 0.00 **FUD** XXX
AMA: 2020,OctSE,1; 2020,AugSE,1; 2020,AugSE,1; 2020,AugSE,1

▲ **87803** **Clostridium difficile toxin A**
0.00 0.00 **FUD** XXX
AMA: 2020,OctSE,1; 2020,AugSE,1; 2020,AugSE,1; 2020,AugSE,1

▲ # **87806** **HIV-1 antigen(s), with HIV-1 and HIV-2 antibodies**
0.00 0.00 **FUD** XXX
AMA: 2020,OctSE,1; 2020,AugSE,1; 2020,AugSE,1; 2020,AugSE,1

▲ **87804** **Influenza**
0.00 0.00 **FUD** XXX
AMA: 2020,OctSE,1; 2020,AugSE,1; 2020,AugSE,1; 2020,AugSE,1; 2018,Jan,8; 2017,Jan,8; 2016,Jan,13; 2015,Jan,16

87806 **Resequenced code. See code following 87803.**

▲ **87807** **respiratory syncytial virus**
0.00 0.00 **FUD** XXX
AMA: 2020,OctSE,1; 2020,AugSE,1; 2020,AugSE,1; 2020,AugSE,1

● # **87811** **severe acute respiratory syndrome coronavirus 2 (SARS-CoV-2) (Coronavirus disease [COVID-19])**

▲ **87808** **Trichomonas vaginalis**
0.00 0.00 **FUD** XXX
AMA: 2020,OctSE,1; 2020,AugSE,1; 2020,AugSE,1; 2020,AugSE,1

▲ **87809** **adenovirus**
0.00 0.00 **FUD** XXX
AMA: 2020,OctSE,1; 2020,AugSE,1; 2020,AugSE,1; 2020,AugSE,1; 2018,Jan,8; 2017,Jan,8; 2016,Jan,13; 2015,Jan,16

▲ **87810** **Chlamydia trachomatis**
0.00 0.00 **FUD** XXX
AMA: 2020,OctSE,1; 2020,AugSE,1; 2020,AugSE,1; 2020,AugSE,1; 2018,Jan,8; 2017,Jan,8; 2016,Jan,13; 2015,Jan,16

87811 **Resequenced code. See code following 87807.**

▲ **87850** **Neisseria gonorrhoeae**
0.00 0.00 **FUD** XXX
AMA: 2020,OctSE,1; 2020,AugSE,1; 2020,AugSE,1; 2020,AugSE,1; 2018,Jan,8; 2017,Jan,8; 2016,Jan,13; 2015,Jan,16

▲ **87880** **Streptococcus, group A**
0.00 0.00 **FUD** XXX
AMA: 2020,OctSE,1; 2020,AugSE,1; 2020,AugSE,1; 2020,AugSE,1; 2018,Jan,8; 2017,Jan,8; 2016,Jan,13; 2015,Jan,16

▲ **87899** **not otherwise specified**
0.00 0.00 **FUD** XXX
AMA: 2020,OctSE,1; 2020,AugSE,1; 2020,AugSE,1; 2020,AugSE,1; 2018,Jan,8; 2017,Jan,8; 2016,Jan,13; 2015,Jan,16

87900-87999 [87906, 87910, 87912] Drug Sensitivity Genotype/Phenotype

87900 **Infectious agent drug susceptibility phenotype prediction using regularly updated genotypic bioinformatics**
0.00 0.00 **FUD** XXX
AMA: 2020,OctSE,1; 2018,Jan,8; 2017,Jan,8; 2016,Jan,13; 2015,Dec,18; 2015,Jan,16

87910 **Infectious agent genotype analysis by nucleic acid (DNA or RNA); cytomegalovirus**
EXCLUDES *HPV detection (genotyping) (0500T)*
HIV-1 infectious agent phenotype prediction (87900)
0.00 0.00 **FUD** XXX
AMA: 2018,Jan,8; 2017,Jan,8; 2016,Jan,13; 2015,Jan,16

87901 **HIV-1, reverse transcriptase and protease regions**
EXCLUDES *Infectious agent drug susceptibility phenotype prediction for HIV-1 (87900)*
0.00 0.00 **FUD** XXX
AMA: 2020,OctSE,1; 2018,Jan,8; 2017,Jan,8; 2016,Jan,13; 2015,Jan,16

87906 **HIV-1, other region (eg, integrase, fusion)**
EXCLUDES *HIV-1 infectious agent phenotype prediction (87900)*
0.00 0.00 **FUD** XXX
AMA: 2018,Jan,8; 2017,Jan,8; 2016,Jan,13; 2015,Jan,16

87912 **Hepatitis B virus**
0.00 0.00 **FUD** XXX
AMA: 2018,Jan,8; 2017,Jan,8; 2016,Jan,13; 2015,Jan,16

87902 **Hepatitis C virus**
0.00 0.00 **FUD** XXX
AMA: 2020,OctSE,1; 2018,Jan,8; 2017,Jan,8; 2016,Jan,13; 2015,Dec,18; 2015,Nov,10; 2015,Jan,16

87903 **Infectious agent phenotype analysis by nucleic acid (DNA or RNA) with drug resistance tissue culture analysis, HIV 1; first through 10 drugs tested**
0.00 0.00 **FUD** XXX
AMA: 2020,OctSE,1; 2018,Jan,8; 2017,Jan,8; 2016,Jan,13; 2015,Jan,16

+ **87904** **each additional drug tested (List separately in addition to code for primary procedure)**
Code first (87903)
0.00 0.00 FUD XXX Q
AMA: 2018,Jan,8; 2017,Jan,8; 2016,Jan,13; 2015,Jan,16

87905 **Infectious agent enzymatic activity other than virus (eg, sialidase activity in vaginal fluid)**
EXCLUDES *Virus isolation identified by nonimmunologic method, and by noncytopathic effect (87255)*
0.00 0.00 FUD XXX Q

87906 **Resequenced code. See code following 87901.**

87910 **Resequenced code. See code following 87900.**

87912 **Resequenced code. See code before 87902.**

87999 **Unlisted microbiology procedure**
0.00 0.00 FUD XXX N
AMA: 2018,Jan,8; 2017,Jan,8; 2016,Jan,13; 2015,Jan,16

88000-88099 Autopsy Services

CMS: 100-02,15,80.1 Payment for Clinical Laboratory Services
INCLUDES Services for physicians only

88000 **Necropsy (autopsy), gross examination only; without CNS**
0.00 0.00 FUD XXX E
AMA: 2018,Jan,8; 2017,Jan,8; 2016,Jan,13; 2015,Jan,16

88005 **with brain**
0.00 0.00 FUD XXX E
AMA: 2005,Jul,11-12; 2005,Aug,7-8

88007 **with brain and spinal cord**
0.00 0.00 FUD XXX E
AMA: 2005,Jul,11-12; 2005,Aug,7-8

88012 **infant with brain** A
0.00 0.00 FUD XXX E
AMA: 2005,Jul,11-12; 2005,Aug,7-8

88014 **stillborn or newborn with brain** A
0.00 0.00 FUD XXX E
AMA: 2005,Jul,11-12; 2005,Aug,7-8

88016 **macerated stillborn** A
0.00 0.00 FUD XXX E
AMA: 2005,Jul,11-12; 2005,Aug,7-8

88020 **Necropsy (autopsy), gross and microscopic; without CNS**
0.00 0.00 FUD XXX E
AMA: 2005,Jul,11-12; 2005,Aug,7-8

88025 **with brain**
0.00 0.00 FUD XXX E
AMA: 2005,Jul,11-12; 2005,Aug,7-8

88027 **with brain and spinal cord**
0.00 0.00 FUD XXX E
AMA: 2005,Jul,11-12; 2005,Aug,7-8

88028 **infant with brain** A
0.00 0.00 FUD XXX E
AMA: 2005,Jul,11-12; 2005,Aug,7-8

88029 **stillborn or newborn with brain** A
0.00 0.00 FUD XXX E
AMA: 2005,Jul,11-12; 2005,Aug,7-8

88036 **Necropsy (autopsy), limited, gross and/or microscopic; regional**
0.00 0.00 FUD XXX E
AMA: 2005,Jul,11-12; 2005,Aug,7-8

88037 **single organ**
0.00 0.00 FUD XXX E
AMA: 2005,Jul,11-12; 2005,Aug,7-8

88040 **Necropsy (autopsy); forensic examination**
0.00 0.00 FUD XXX E
AMA: 2005,Jul,11-12; 2005,Aug,7-8

88045 **coroner's call**
0.00 0.00 FUD XXX E
AMA: 2005,Jul,11-12; 2005,Aug,7-8

88099 **Unlisted necropsy (autopsy) procedure**
0.00 0.00 FUD XXX E
AMA: 2018,Jan,8; 2017,Jan,8; 2016,Jan,13; 2015,Jan,16

88104-88140 Cytopathology: Other Than Cervical/Vaginal

88104 **Cytopathology, fluids, washings or brushings, except cervical or vaginal; smears with interpretation**
1.93 1.93 FUD XXX Q1 80
AMA: 2018,Jan,8; 2017,Jan,8; 2016,Jan,13; 2015,Jan,16

88106 **simple filter method with interpretation**
EXCLUDES *Cytopathology smears with interpretation (88104)*
Selective cellular enhancement (nongynecological) including filter transfer techniques (88112)
1.81 1.81 FUD XXX Q1 80
AMA: 2018,Jan,8; 2017,Jan,8; 2016,Jan,13; 2015,Jan,16

88108 **Cytopathology, concentration technique, smears and interpretation (eg, Saccomanno technique)**
EXCLUDES *Cervical or vaginal smears (88150-88155)*
Gastric intubation with lavage (43754-43755)
(74340)
1.71 1.71 FUD XXX Q1 80
AMA: 2018,Jan,8; 2017,Jan,8; 2016,Jan,13; 2015,Jan,16

88112 **Cytopathology, selective cellular enhancement technique with interpretation (eg, liquid based slide preparation method), except cervical or vaginal**
EXCLUDES *Cytopathology cellular enhancement technique (88108)*
1.90 1.90 FUD XXX Q1 80
AMA: 2005,Aug,7-8; 2005,Jul,11-12

88120 **Cytopathology, in situ hybridization (eg, FISH), urinary tract specimen with morphometric analysis, 3-5 molecular probes, each specimen; manual**
EXCLUDES *More than five probes (88399)*
Morphometric in situ hybridization on specimens other than urinary tract (88367-88368 [88373, 88374])
16.3 16.3 FUD XXX Q2 80
AMA: 2010,Dec,7-10

88121 **using computer-assisted technology**
EXCLUDES *More than five probes (88399)*
Morphometric in situ hybridization on specimens other than urinary tract (88367-88368 [88373, 88374])
12.4 12.4 FUD XXX Q1 80
AMA: 2010,Dec,7-10

88125 **Cytopathology, forensic (eg, sperm)**
0.75 0.75 FUD XXX Q1 80
AMA: 2005,Aug,7-8; 2005,Jul,11-12

88130 **Sex chromatin identification; Barr bodies**
0.00 0.00 FUD XXX Q
AMA: 2005,Aug,7-8; 2005,Jul,11-12

88140 **peripheral blood smear, polymorphonuclear drumsticks**
EXCLUDES *Guard stain (88313)*
0.00 0.00 FUD XXX Q
AMA: 2018,Jan,8; 2017,Jan,8; 2016,Jan,13; 2015,Jan,16

88141-88155 Pap Smears

CMS: 100-03,210.2 Screening Pap Smears/Pelvic Examinations for Early Cancer Detection
EXCLUDES *Non-Bethesda method (88150-88153)*

88141 **Cytopathology, cervical or vaginal (any reporting system), requiring interpretation by physician** ♀
Code also (88142-88153, 88164-88167, 88174-88175)
0.90 0.90 FUD XXX N 80 26
AMA: 2018,Jan,8; 2017,Jan,8; 2016,Jan,13; 2015,Jan,16

88142 **Cytopathology, cervical or vaginal (any reporting system), collected in preservative fluid, automated thin layer preparation; manual screening under physician supervision** ♀
INCLUDES Bethesda or non-Bethesda method
0.00 0.00 FUD XXX
AMA: 2018,Jan,8; 2017,Jan,8; 2016,Jan,13; 2015,Jan,16

88143 **with manual screening and rescreening under physician supervision** ♀
INCLUDES Bethesda or non-Bethesda method
EXCLUDES *Automated screening automated thin layer preparation (88174-88175)*
0.00 0.00 FUD XXX
AMA: 2018,Jan,8; 2017,Jan,8; 2016,Jan,13; 2015,Jan,16

88147 **Cytopathology smears, cervical or vaginal; screening by automated system under physician supervision** ♀
0.00 0.00 FUD XXX
AMA: 2018,Jan,8; 2017,Jan,8; 2016,Jan,13; 2015,Jan,16

88148 **screening by automated system with manual rescreening under physician supervision** ♀
0.00 0.00 FUD XXX
AMA: 2018,Jan,8; 2017,Jan,8; 2016,Jan,13; 2015,Jan,16

88150 **Cytopathology, slides, cervical or vaginal; manual screening under physician supervision** ♀
EXCLUDES *Bethesda method Pap smears (88164-88167)*
0.00 0.00 FUD XXX
AMA: 2018,Jan,8; 2017,Jan,8; 2016,Jan,13; 2015,Jan,16

88152 **with manual screening and computer-assisted rescreening under physician supervision**
EXCLUDES *Bethesda method Pap smears (88164-88167)*
0.00 0.00 FUD XXX
AMA: 2018,Jan,8; 2017,Jan,8; 2016,Jan,13; 2015,Jan,16

88153 **with manual screening and rescreening under physician supervision** ♀
EXCLUDES *Bethesda method Pap smears (88164-88167)*
0.00 0.00 FUD XXX
AMA: 2018,Jan,8; 2017,Jan,8; 2016,Jan,13; 2015,Jan,16

\+ **88155** **Cytopathology, slides, cervical or vaginal, definitive hormonal evaluation (eg, maturation index, karyopyknotic index, estrogenic index) (List separately in addition to code[s] for other technical and interpretation services)** ♀
Code first (88142-88153, 88164-88167, 88174-88175)
0.00 0.00 FUD XXX
AMA: 2018,Jan,8; 2017,Jan,8; 2016,Jan,13; 2015,Jan,16

88160-88162 Cytopathology Smears (Other Than Pap)

88160 **Cytopathology, smears, any other source; screening and interpretation**
2.01 2.01 FUD XXX
AMA: 2006,Dec,10-12; 2005,Jul,11-12

88161 **preparation, screening and interpretation**
1.87 1.87 FUD XXX
AMA: 2018,Jan,8; 2017,Jan,8; 2016,Jan,13; 2015,Jan,16

88162 **extended study involving over 5 slides and/or multiple stains**
EXCLUDES *Aerosol collection sputum (89220)*
Special stains (88312-88314)
2.80 2.80 FUD XXX
AMA: 2005,Aug,7 8; 2005,Jul,11-12

88164-88167 Pap Smears: Bethesda System

CMS: 100-03,210.2 Screening Pap Smears/Pelvic Examinations for Early Cancer Detection
EXCLUDES *Non-Bethesda method (88150-88153)*

88164 **Cytopathology, slides, cervical or vaginal (the Bethesda System); manual screening under physician supervision** ♀
0.00 0.00 FUD XXX
AMA: 2018,Jan,8; 2017,Jan,8; 2016,Jan,13; 2015,Jan,16

88165 **with manual screening and rescreening under physician supervision** ♀
0.00 0.00 FUD XXX
AMA: 2018,Jan,8; 2017,Jan,8; 2016,Jan,13; 2015,Jan,16

88166 **with manual screening and computer-assisted rescreening under physician supervision** ♀
0.00 0.00 FUD XXX
AMA: 2018,Jan,8; 2017,Jan,8; 2016,Jan,13; 2015,Jan,16

88167 **with manual screening and computer-assisted rescreening using cell selection and review under physician supervision** ♀
EXCLUDES *Fine needle aspiration ([10004, 10005, 10006, 10007, 10008, 10009, 10010, 10011, 10012])*
0.00 0.00 FUD XXX
AMA: 2018,Jan,8; 2017,Jan,8; 2016,Jan,13; 2015,Jan,16

88172-88177 [88177] Cytopathology of Needle Biopsy

EXCLUDES *Fine needle aspiration (10021, [10004, 10005, 10006, 10007, 10008, 10009, 10010, 10011, 10012])*

88172 **Cytopathology, evaluation of fine needle aspirate; immediate cytohistologic study to determine adequacy for diagnosis, first evaluation episode, each site**
INCLUDES Submission complete set cytologic material for evaluation no matter how many needle passes performed or slides prepared from each site
EXCLUDES *Cytologic examination during intraoperative pathology consultation (88333-88334)*
1.58 1.58 FUD XXX
AMA: 2019,Feb,8; 2019,Apr,4; 2018,Jan,8; 2017,Jan,8; 2016,Jan,13; 2016,Jan,11; 2015,Jan,16

88173 **interpretation and report**
INCLUDES Interpretation and report from each anatomical site no matter how many passes or evaluation episodes performed during aspiration
EXCLUDES *Cytologic examination during intraoperative pathology consultation (88333-88334)*
4.32 4.32 FUD XXX
AMA: 2019,Feb,8; 2019,Apr,4; 2018,Jan,8; 2017,Jan,8; 2016,Jan,13; 2015,Jan,16

\+ # **88177** **immediate cytohistologic study to determine adequacy for diagnosis, each separate additional evaluation episode, same site (List separately in addition to code for primary procedure)**
Code also each additional immediate repeat evaluation episode(s) required from same site (i.e., previous sample inadequate)
Code first (88172)
0.84 0.84 FUD ZZZ
AMA: 2019,Apr,4; 2018,Jan,8; 2017,Jan,8; 2016,Jan,11

88174-88177 [88177] Pap Smears: Automated Screening

EXCLUDES *Non-Bethesda method (88150-88153)*

88174 **Cytopathology, cervical or vaginal (any reporting system), collected in preservative fluid, automated thin layer preparation; screening by automated system, under physician supervision** ♀
INCLUDES Bethesda or non-Bethesda method
0.00 0.00 FUD XXX
AMA: 2018,Jan,8; 2017,Jan,8; 2016,Jan,13; 2015,Jan,16

88175 **with screening by automated system and manual rescreening or review, under physician supervision** ♀
INCLUDES Bethesda or non-Bethesda method
EXCLUDES *Manual screening (88142-88143)*
0.00 0.00 FUD XXX
AMA: 2018,Jan,8; 2017,Jan,8; 2016,Jan,13; 2015,Jan,16

88177 **Resequenced code. See code following 88173.**

88182-88199 Cytopathology Using the Fluorescence-Activated Cell Sorter

88182 Flow cytometry, cell cycle or DNA analysis
EXCLUDES *DNA ploidy analysis by morphometric technique (88358)*
3.79 3.79 FUD XXX Q2 80
AMA: 2018,Jan,8; 2017,Jan,8; 2016,Jan,13; 2015,Jan,16

88184 Flow cytometry, cell surface, cytoplasmic, or nuclear marker, technical component only; first marker
1.88 1.88 FUD XXX Q2 80 TC
AMA: 2018,Jan,8; 2017,Jan,8; 2016,Jan,13; 2015,Jan,16

+ **88185 each additional marker (List separately in addition to code for first marker)**
Code first (88184)
0.62 0.62 FUD ZZZ N 80 TC
AMA: 2018,Jan,8; 2017,Jan,8; 2016,Jan,13; 2015,Jan,16

88187 Flow cytometry, interpretation; 2 to 8 markers
EXCLUDES *Antibody assessment by flow cytometry (83516-83520, 86000-86849 [86152, 86153])*
Cell enumeration by immunologic selection and identification ([86152, 86153])
Interpretation (86355-86357, 86359-86361, 86367)
1.08 1.08 FUD XXX B 80 26
AMA: 2018,Jan,8; 2017,Jan,8; 2016,Jan,13; 2015,Jan,16

88188 9 to 15 markers
EXCLUDES *Antibody assessment by flow cytometry (83516-83520, 86000-86849 [86152, 86153])*
Cell enumeration by immunologic selection and identification ([86152, 86153])
Interpretation (86355-86357, 86359-86361, 86367)
1.83 1.83 FUD XXX B 80 26
AMA: 2018,Jan,8; 2017,Jan,8; 2016,Jan,13; 2015,Jan,16

88189 16 or more markers
EXCLUDES *Antibody assessment by flow cytometry (83516-83520, 86000-86849 [86152, 86153])*
Cell enumeration using immunologic selection and identification in fluid sample ([86152, 86153])
Interpretation (86355-86357, 86359-86361, 86367)
2.45 2.45 FUD XXX B 80 26
AMA: 2018,Jan,8; 2017,Jan,8; 2016,Jan,13; 2015,Jan,16

88199 Unlisted cytopathology procedure
EXCLUDES *Electron microscopy (88348)*
0.00 0.00 FUD XXX Q1 80
AMA: 2018,Jan,8; 2017,Jan,8; 2016,Jan,13; 2015,Jan,16

88230-88299 Cytogenic Studies

CMS: 100-03,190.3 Cytogenic Studies
EXCLUDES *Acetylcholinesterase (82013)*
Alpha-fetoprotein (amniotic fluid or serum) (82105-82106)
Microdissection (88380)
Molecular pathology codes (81105-81383 [81105, 81106, 81107, 81108, 81109, 81110, 81111, 81112, 81120, 81121, 81161, 81162, 81163, 81164, 81165, 81166, 81167, 81173, 81174, 81184, 81185, 81186, 81187, 81188, 81189, 81190, 81200, 81201, 81202, 81203, 81204, 81205, 81206, 81207, 81208, 81209, 81210, 81219, 81227, 81230, 81231, 81233, 81234, 81238, 81239, 81245, 81246, 81250, 81257, 81258, 81259, 81261, 81262, 81263, 81264, 81265, 81266, 81267, 81268, 81269, 81271, 81274, 81283, 81284, 81285, 81286, 81287, 81288, 81289, 81291, 81292, 81293, 81294, 81295, 81301, 81302, 81303, 81304, 81306, 81312, 81320, 81324, 81325, 81326, 81332, 81334, 81336, 81337, 81343, 81344, 81345, 81361, 81362, 81363, 81364], 81400-81408, [81479], 81410-81471 [81448], 81500-81512, 81599)

88230 Tissue culture for non-neoplastic disorders; lymphocyte
0.00 0.00 FUD XXX Q
AMA: 2018,Jan,8; 2017,Jan,8; 2016,Jan,13; 2015,Jan,16

88233 skin or other solid tissue biopsy
0.00 0.00 FUD XXX Q
AMA: 2018,Jan,8; 2017,Jan,8; 2016,Jan,13; 2015,Jan,16

88235 amniotic fluid or chorionic villus cells M
0.00 0.00 FUD XXX Q
AMA: 2018,Jan,8; 2017,Jan,8; 2016,Jan,13; 2015,Jan,16

88237 Tissue culture for neoplastic disorders; bone marrow, blood cells
0.00 0.00 FUD XXX Q
AMA: 2018,Jan,8; 2017,Jan,8; 2016,Jan,13; 2015,Jan,16

88239 solid tumor
0.00 0.00 FUD XXX Q
AMA: 2018,Jan,8; 2017,Jan,8; 2016,Jan,13; 2015,Jan,16

88240 Cryopreservation, freezing and storage of cells, each cell line
EXCLUDES *Therapeutic cryopreservation and storage (38207)*
0.00 0.00 FUD XXX Q
AMA: 2018,Jan,8; 2017,Jan,8; 2016,Jan,13; 2015,Jan,16

88241 Thawing and expansion of frozen cells, each aliquot
EXCLUDES *Therapeutic thawing of prior harvest (38208)*
0.00 0.00 FUD XXX Q
AMA: 2018,Jan,8; 2017,Jan,8; 2016,Jan,13; 2015,Jan,16

88245 Chromosome analysis for breakage syndromes; baseline Sister Chromatid Exchange (SCE), 20-25 cells
0.00 0.00 FUD XXX Q
AMA: 2018,Jan,8; 2017,Jan,8; 2016,Jan,13; 2015,Jan,16

88248 baseline breakage, score 50-100 cells, count 20 cells, 2 karyotypes (eg, for ataxia telangiectasia, Fanconi anemia, fragile X)
0.00 0.00 FUD XXX Q
AMA: 2018,Jan,8; 2017,Jan,8; 2016,Jan,13; 2015,Jan,16

88249 score 100 cells, clastogen stress (eg, diepoxybutane, mitomycin C, ionizing radiation, UV radiation)
0.00 0.00 FUD XXX Q
AMA: 2018,Jan,8; 2017,Jan,8; 2016,Jan,13; 2015,Jan,16

88261 Chromosome analysis; count 5 cells, 1 karyotype, with banding
0.00 0.00 FUD XXX Q
AMA: 2018,Jan,8; 2017,Jan,8; 2016,Jan,13; 2015,Jan,16

88262 count 15-20 cells, 2 karyotypes, with banding
0.00 0.00 FUD XXX Q
AMA: 2019,Aug,10; 2018,Jan,8; 2017,Jan,8; 2016,Jan,13; 2015,Jan,16

88263 count 45 cells for mosaicism, 2 karyotypes, with banding
0.00 0.00 FUD XXX Q
AMA: 2018,Jan,8; 2017,Jan,8; 2016,Jan,13; 2015,Jan,16

88264 analyze 20-25 cells
0.00 0.00 FUD XXX Q
AMA: 2019,Aug,10; 2018,Jan,8; 2017,Jan,8; 2016,Jan,13; 2015,Jan,16

88267 Chromosome analysis, amniotic fluid or chorionic villus, count 15 cells, 1 karyotype, with banding M ♀
0.00 0.00 FUD XXX Q
AMA: 2018,Jan,8; 2017,Jan,8; 2016,Jan,13; 2015,Jan,16

88269 Chromosome analysis, in situ for amniotic fluid cells, count cells from 6-12 colonies, 1 karyotype, with banding M ♀
0.00 0.00 FUD XXX Q
AMA: 2018,Jan,8; 2017,Jan,8; 2016,Jan,13; 2015,Jan,16

88271 Molecular cytogenetics; DNA probe, each (eg, FISH)
EXCLUDES *Cytogenomic microarray analysis (81228-81229, 81405-81406, [81479])*
Fetal chromosome analysis using maternal blood (81420-81422)
0.00 0.00 FUD XXX Q
AMA: 2020,Feb,10; 2018,Jan,8; 2017,Apr,3; 2017,Jan,8; 2016,Jan,13; 2015,Jan,16

88272 chromosomal in situ hybridization, analyze 3-5 cells (eg, for derivatives and markers)
0.00 0.00 FUD XXX Q
AMA: 2018,Jan,8; 2017,Jan,8; 2016,Jan,13; 2015,Jan,16

88273 **chromosomal in situ hybridization, analyze 10-30 cells (eg, for microdeletions)**
0.00 0.00 FUD XXX Q
AMA: 2018,Jan,8; 2017,Jan,8; 2016,Jan,13; 2015,Jan,16

88274 **interphase in situ hybridization, analyze 25-99 cells**
0.00 0.00 FUD XXX Q
AMA: 2018,Jan,8; 2017,Jan,8; 2016,Jan,13; 2015,Jan,16

88275 **interphase in situ hybridization, analyze 100-300 cells**
0.00 0.00 FUD XXX Q
AMA: 2018,Jan,8; 2017,Jan,8; 2016,Jan,13; 2015,Jan,16

88280 **Chromosome analysis; additional karyotypes, each study**
0.00 0.00 FUD XXX Q
AMA: 2018,Jan,8; 2017,Jan,8; 2016,Jan,13; 2015,Jan,16

88283 **additional specialized banding technique (eg, NOR, C-banding)**
0.00 0.00 FUD XXX Q
AMA: 2018,Jan,8; 2017,Jan,8; 2016,Jan,13; 2015,Jan,16

88285 **additional cells counted, each study**
0.00 0.00 FUD XXX Q
AMA: 2018,Jan,8; 2017,Jan,8; 2016,Jan,13; 2015,Jan,16

88289 **additional high resolution study**
0.00 0.00 FUD XXX Q
AMA: 2018,Jan,8; 2017,Jan,8; 2016,Jan,13; 2015,Jan,16

88291 **Cytogenetics and molecular cytogenetics, interpretation and report**
0.94 0.94 FUD XXX M 80 26
AMA: 2018,Jan,8; 2017,Jan,8; 2016,Jan,13; 2015,Jan,16

88299 **Unlisted cytogenetic study**
0.00 0.00 FUD XXX Q1 80
AMA: 2018,Jan,8; 2017,Jan,8; 2016,Jan,13; 2015,Jan,16

88300 Evaluation of Surgical Specimen: Gross Anatomy

CMS: 100-02,15,80.1 Payment for Clinical Laboratory Services

INCLUDES Attainment, examination, and reporting
Unit of service is the specimen

EXCLUDES *Additional procedures (88311-88365 [88341, 88350], 88399)*
Microscopic exam (88302-88309)

88300 **Level I - Surgical pathology, gross examination only**
0.44 0.44 FUD XXX Q1 80
AMA: 2018,Jan,8; 2017,Jan,8; 2016,Jan,13; 2015,Jan,16

88302-88309 Evaluation of Surgical Specimens: Gross and Microscopic Anatomy

CMS: 100-02,15,80.1 Payment for Clinical Laboratory Services

INCLUDES Attainment, examination, and reporting
Unit of service is the specimen

EXCLUDES *Additional procedures (88311-88365 [88341, 88350], 88399)*
Mohs surgery (17311-17315)

88302 **Level II - Surgical pathology, gross and microscopic examination**

INCLUDES Confirming identification and disease absence:
- Appendix, incidental
- Fallopian tube, sterilization
- Fingers or toes traumatic amputation
- Foreskin, newborn
- Hernia sac, any site
- Hydrocele sac
- Nerve
- Skin, plastic repair
- Sympathetic ganglion
- Testis, castration
- Vaginal mucosa, incidental
- Vas deferens, sterilization

0.87 0.87 FUD XXX Q1 80
AMA: 2018,Jan,8; 2017,Jan,8; 2016,Jan,13; 2015,Jan,16

88304 **Level III - Surgical pathology, gross and microscopic examination**

INCLUDES
- Abortion, induced
- Abscess
- Anal tag
- Aneurysm-atrial/ventricular
- Appendix, other than incidental
- Artery, atheromatous plaque
- Bartholin's gland cyst
- Bone fragment(s), other than pathologic fracture
- Bursa/ synovial cyst
- Carpal tunnel tissue
- Cartilage, shavings
- Cholesteatoma
- Colon, colostomy stoma
- Conjunctiva-biopsy/pterygium
- Cornea
- Diverticulum-esophagus/small intestine
- Dupuytren's contracture tissue
- Femoral head, other than fracture
- Fissure/fistula
- Foreskin, other than newborn
- Gallbladder
- Ganglion cyst
- Hematoma
- Hemorrhoids
- Hydatid of Morgagni
- Intervertebral disc
- Joint, loose body
- Meniscus
- Mucocele, salivary
- Neuroma-Morton's/traumatic
- Pilonidal cyst/sinus
- Polyps, inflammatory-nasal/sinusoidal
- Skin-cyst/tag/debridement
- Soft tissue, debridement
- Soft tissue, lipoma
- Spermatocele
- Tendon/tendon sheath
- Testicular appendage
- Thrombus or embolus
- Tonsil and/or adenoids
- Varicocele
- Vas deferens, other than sterilization
- Vein, varicosity

1.16 1.16 FUD XXX Q1 80
AMA: 2018,Jan,8; 2017,Jan,8; 2016,Jan,13; 2015,Jan,16

88305 **Level IV - Surgical pathology, gross and microscopic examination**

INCLUDES
- Abortion, spontaneous/missed
- Artery, biopsy
- Bone exostosis
- Bone marrow, biopsy
- Brain/meninges, other than for tumor resection
- Breast biopsy without microscopic assessment of surgical margin
- Breast reduction mammoplasty
- Bronchus, biopsy
- Cell block, any source
- Cervix, biopsy
- Colon, biopsy
- Duodenum, biopsy
- Endocervix, curettings/biopsy
- Endometrium, curettings/biopsy
- Esophagus, biopsy
- Extremity, amputation, traumatic
- Fallopian tube, biopsy
- Fallopian tube, ectopic pregnancy
- Femoral head, fracture
- Finger/toes, amputation, nontraumatic
- Gingiva/oral mucosa, biopsy
- Heart valve
- Joint resection
- Kidney biopsy
- Larynx biopsy

Leiomyoma(s), uterine myomectomy-without uterus
Lip, biopsy/wedge resection
Lung, transbronchial biopsy
Lymph node, biopsy
Muscle, biopsy
Nasal mucosa, biopsy
Nasopharynx/oropharynx, biopsy
Nerve biopsy
Odontogenic/dental cyst
Omentum, biopsy
Ovary, biopsy/wedge resection
Ovary with or without tube, nonneoplastic
Parathyroid gland
Peritoneum, biopsy
Pituitary tumor
Placenta, other than third trimester
Pleura/pericardium-biopsy/tissue
Polyp:
  Cervical/endometrial
  Colorectal
  Stomach/small intestine
Prostate:
  Needle biopsy
  TUR
Salivary gland, biopsy
Sinus, paranasal biopsy
Skin, other than cyst/tag/debridement/plastic repair
Small intestine, biopsy
Soft tissue, other than tumor/mas/lipoma/debridement
Spleen
Stomach biopsy
Synovium
Testis, other than tumor/biopsy, castration
Thyroglossal duct/brachial cleft cyst
Tongue, biopsy
Tonsil, biopsy
Trachea biopsy
Ureter, biopsy
Urethra, biopsy
Urinary bladder, biopsy
Uterus, with or without tubes and ovaries, for prolapse
Vagina biopsy
Vulva/labial biopsy

1.98 1.98 **FUD** XXX 01 80

AMA: 2018,May,3; 2018,Jan,8; 2017,Jan,8; 2016,Jan,13; 2015,Jan,16

88307 Level V - Surgical pathology, gross and microscopic examination

INCLUDES
Adrenal resection
Bone, biopsy/curettings
Bone fragment(s), pathologic fractures
Brain, biopsy
Brain meninges, tumor resection
Breast, excision of lesion, requiring microscopic evaluation of surgical margins
Breast, mastectomy-partial/simple
Cervix, conization
Colon, segmental resection, other than for tumor
Extremity, amputation, nontraumatic
Eye, enucleation
Kidney, partial/total nephrectomy
Larynx, partial/total resection
Liver
  Biopsy, needle/wedge
  Partial resection
Lung, wedge biopsy
Lymph nodes, regional resection
Mediastinum, mass
Myocardium, biopsy
Odontogenic tumor
Ovary with or without tube, neoplastic
Pancreas, biopsy
Placenta, third trimester
Prostate, except radical resection
Salivary gland
Sentinel lymph node
Small intestine, resection, other than for tumor
Soft tissue mass (except lipoma)-biopsy/simple excision
Stomach-subtotal/total resection, other than for tumor
Testis, biopsy
Thymus, tumor
Thyroid, total/lobe
Ureter, resection
Urinary bladder, TUR
Uterus, with or without tubes and ovaries, other than neoplastic/prolapse

7.59 7.59 **FUD** XXX 02 80

AMA: 2018,Jan,8; 2017,Jan,8; 2016,Jan,13; 2015,Jan,16

88309 Level VI - Surgical pathology, gross and microscopic examination

INCLUDES
Bone resection
Breast, mastectomy-with regional lymph nodes
Colon:
  Segmental resection for tumor
  Total resection
Esophagus, partial/total resection
Extremity, disarticulation
Fetus, with dissection
Larynx, partial/total resection-with regional lymph nodes
Lung-total/lobe/segment resection
Pancreas, total/subtotal resection
Prostate, radical resection
Small intestine, resection for tumor
Soft tissue tumor, extensive resection
Stomach, subtotal/total resection for tumor
Testis, tumor
Tongue/tonsil, resection for tumor
Urinary bladder, partial/total resection
Uterus, with or without tubes and ovaries, neoplastic
Vulva, total/subtotal resection

EXCLUDES
Evaluation fine needle aspirate (88172-88173)
Fine needle aspiration (10021, [10004, 10005, 10006, 10007, 10008, 10009, 10010, 10011, 10012])

11.8 11.8 **FUD** XXX 02 80

AMA: 2018,Jan,8; 2017,Jan,8; 2016,Jan,13; 2015,Jan,16

88311-88399 [88341, 88350, 88364, 88373, 88374, 88377] Additional Surgical Pathology Services

CMS: 100-02,15,80.1 Payment for Clinical Laboratory Services

\+ **88311** **Decalcification procedure (List separately in addition to code for surgical pathology examination)**
Code first surgical pathology exam (88302-88309)
0.61 0.61 **FUD** XXX N 80
AMA: 2018,Jan,8; 2017,Jan,8; 2016,Jan,13; 2015,Jan,16

88312 **Special stain including interpretation and report; Group I for microorganisms (eg, acid fast, methenamine silver)**
INCLUDES Reporting one unit for each special stain performed on surgical pathology block, cytologic sample, or hematologic smear
2.97 2.97 **FUD** XXX Q1 80
AMA: 2018,Jan,8; 2017,Jan,8; 2016,Jan,13; 2015,Jan,16

88313 **Group II, all other (eg, iron, trichrome), except stain for microorganisms, stains for enzyme constituents, or immunocytochemistry and immunohistochemistry**
INCLUDES Reporting one unit for each special stain performed on surgical pathology block, cytologic sample, or hematologic smear
EXCLUDES *Immunocytochemistry and immunohistochemistry (88342)*
2.05 2.05 **FUD** XXX Q1 80
AMA: 2018,Jan,8; 2017,Jan,8; 2016,Jan,13; 2015,Jan,16

\+ **88314** **histochemical stain on frozen tissue block (List separately in addition to code for primary procedure)**
INCLUDES Reporting one unit for each special stain on each frozen surgical pathology block
EXCLUDES *Routine frozen section stain during Mohs surgery (17311-17315)*
Special stain performed on frozen tissue section specimen to identify enzyme constituents (88319)
Code also modifier 59 for nonroutine histochemical stain on frozen section during Mohs surgery
Code first (17311-17315, 88302-88309, 88331-88332)
2.73 2.73 **FUD** XXX N 80
AMA: 2018,Jan,8; 2017,Jan,8; 2016,Jan,13; 2015,Jan,16

88319 **Group III, for enzyme constituents**
INCLUDES Reporting one unit for each special stain on each frozen surgical pathology block
EXCLUDES *Detection of enzyme constituents by immunohistochemical or immunocytochemical methodology (88342)*
2.74 2.74 **FUD** XXX Q2 80
AMA: 2018,Jan,8; 2017,Jan,8; 2016,Jan,13; 2015,Jan,16

88321 **Consultation and report on referred slides prepared elsewhere**
2.44 2.84 **FUD** XXX Q1 80
AMA: 2018,Jan,8; 2017,Jan,8; 2016,Jan,13; 2015,Jan,16

88323 **Consultation and report on referred material requiring preparation of slides**
3.28 3.28 **FUD** XXX Q1 80
AMA: 2018,Jan,8; 2017,Jan,8; 2016,Jan,13; 2015,Jan,16

88325 **Consultation, comprehensive, with review of records and specimens, with report on referred material**
4.29 5.12 **FUD** XXX Q1 80
AMA: 2018,Jan,8; 2017,Jan,8; 2016,Jan,13; 2015,Jan,16

88329 **Pathology consultation during surgery;**
1.04 1.47 **FUD** XXX Q1 80
AMA: 2018,Jan,8; 2017,Jan,8; 2016,Jan,13; 2015,Jan,16

88331 **first tissue block, with frozen section(s), single specimen**
Code also cytologic evaluation performed at same time (88334)
2.75 2.75 **FUD** XXX Q1 80
AMA: 2018,Jan,8; 2017,Jan,8; 2016,Jan,13; 2015,Jan,16

\+ **88332** **each additional tissue block with frozen section(s) (List separately in addition to code for primary procedure)**
Code first (88331)
1.54 1.54 **FUD** XXX N 80
AMA: 2018,Jan,8; 2017,Jan,8; 2016,Jan,13; 2015,Jan,16

88333 **cytologic examination (eg, touch prep, squash prep), initial site**
EXCLUDES *Intraprocedural cytologic evaluation fine needle aspirate (88172)*
Nonintraoperative cytologic examination (88160-88162)
2.53 2.53 **FUD** XXX Q2 80
AMA: 2018,Jan,8; 2017,Jan,8; 2016,Jan,13; 2015,Jan,16

\+ **88334** **cytologic examination (eg, touch prep, squash prep), each additional site (List separately in addition to code for primary procedure)**
EXCLUDES *Intraprocedural cytologic evaluation fine needle aspirate (88172)*
Nonintraoperative cytologic examination (88160-88162)
Percutaneous needle biopsy requiring intraprocedural cytologic examination (88333)
Code first (88331, 88333)
1.58 1.58 **FUD** ZZZ N 80
AMA: 2018,Jan,8; 2017,Jan,8; 2016,Jan,13; 2015,Jan,16

88341 **Resequenced code. See code following 88342.**

88342 **Immunohistochemistry or immunocytochemistry, per specimen; initial single antibody stain procedure**
EXCLUDES *Morphometric analysis, tumor immunohistochemistry, on same antibody (88360-88361)*
Multiplex antibody stain (88344)
Reporting code more than one time for each specific antibody
3.01 3.01 **FUD** XXX Q2 80
AMA: 2018,Jan,8; 2017,Jan,8; 2016,Jan,13; 2015,Jun,10; 2015,Jan,16

\+ # **88341** **each additional single antibody stain procedure (List separately in addition to code for primary procedure)**
EXCLUDES *Morphometric analysis (88360-88361)*
Multiplex antibody stain (88344)
Reporting code more than one time for each specific antibody
Code first (88342)
2.62 2.62 **FUD** ZZZ N 80
AMA: 2018,Jan,8; 2017,Jan,8; 2016,Jan,13; 2015,Jun,10

88344 **each multiplex antibody stain procedure**
INCLUDES Staining with multiple antibodies on same slide
EXCLUDES *Morphometric analysis, tumor immunohistochemistry, on same antibody (88360-88361)*
Reporting code more than one time for each specific antibody
4.86 4.86 **FUD** XXX Q1 80
AMA: 2018,Jan,8; 2017,Jan,8; 2016,Jan,13; 2015,Jun,10

88346 **Immunofluorescence, per specimen; initial single antibody stain procedure**
EXCLUDES *Fluorescent in situ hybridization studies (88364-88369 [88364, 88373, 88374, 88377])*
Multiple immunofluorescence analysis (88399)
3.11 3.11 **FUD** XXX Q2 80
AMA: 2018,Jan,8; 2017,Jan,8; 2016,Jan,13; 2015,Jan,16

\+ # **88350** **each additional single antibody stain procedure (List separately in addition to code for primary procedure)**
EXCLUDES *Fluorescent in situ hybridization studies (88364-88369 [88364, 88373, 88374, 88377])*
Multiple immunofluorescence analysis (88399)
Code first (88346)
2.18 2.18 **FUD** ZZZ N 80

88348 **Electron microscopy, diagnostic**
10.9 10.9 **FUD** XXX Q2 80
AMA: 2011,Dec,14-18; 2005,Jul,11-12

88350 **Resequenced code. See code following 88346.**

88355 **Morphometric analysis; skeletal muscle**
3.88 3.88 FUD XXX 01 80
AMA: 2018,Jan,8; 2017,Jan,8; 2016,Jan,13; 2015,Jan,16

88356 **nerve**
6.34 6.34 FUD XXX 01 80
AMA: 2018,Jan,8; 2017,Jan,8; 2016,Jan,13; 2015,Jan,16

88358 **tumor (eg, DNA ploidy)**
EXCLUDES *Special stain, Group II (88313)*
3.61 3.61 FUD XXX 02 80
AMA: 2018,Jan,8; 2017,Jan,8; 2016,Jan,13; 2015,Jan,16

88360 **Morphometric analysis, tumor immunohistochemistry (eg, Her-2/neu, estrogen receptor/progesterone receptor), quantitative or semiquantitative, per specimen, each single antibody stain procedure; manual**
EXCLUDES *Additional stain procedures unless each test for different antibody (88341, 88342, 88344)*
Morphometric analysis using in situ hybridization techniques (88367-88368 [88373, 88374])
3.60 3.60 FUD XXX 02 80
AMA: 2018,Jan,8; 2017,Jan,8; 2016,Jan,13; 2015,Jun,10; 2015,Jan,16

88361 **using computer-assisted technology**
EXCLUDES *Additional stain procedures unless each test for different antibody (88341, 88342, 88344)*
Morphometric analysis using in situ hybridization techniques (88367-88368 [88373, 88374])
3.58 3.58 FUD XXX 02 80
AMA: 2018,Jan,8; 2017,Jan,8; 2016,Jan,13; 2015,Jun,10; 2015,Jan,16

88362 **Nerve teasing preparations**
5.92 5.92 FUD XXX 02 80
AMA: 2018,Jan,8; 2017,Jan,8; 2016,Jan,13; 2015,Jan,16

88363 **Examination and selection of retrieved archival (ie, previously diagnosed) tissue(s) for molecular analysis (eg, KRAS mutational analysis)**
INCLUDES Archival retrieval only
0.57 0.67 FUD XXX 01 80
AMA: 2018,Jan,8; 2017,Jan,8; 2016,Jan,13; 2015,Jan,16

88364 **Resequenced code. See code following 88365.**

88365 **In situ hybridization (eg, FISH), per specimen; initial single probe stain procedure**
EXCLUDES *Morphometric analysis probe stain procedures with same probe (88367, [88374], 88368, [88377])*
5.10 5.10 FUD XXX 01 80
AMA: 2018,Nov,11; 2018,Jan,8; 2017,Jan,8; 2016,Jan,13; 2015,Jan,16

+ # **88364** **each additional single probe stain procedure (List separately in addition to code for primary procedure)**
Code first (88365)
3.74 3.74 FUD ZZZ N 80

88366 **each multiplex probe stain procedure**
EXCLUDES *Morphometric analysis probe stain procedures (88367, [88374], 88368, [88377])*
7.80 7.80 FUD XXX 01 80

88367 **Morphometric analysis, in situ hybridization (quantitative or semi-quantitative), using computer-assisted technology, per specimen; initial single probe stain procedure**
EXCLUDES *In situ hybridization probe stain procedures for same probe (88365, 88366, 88368, [88377])*
Morphometric in situ hybridization evaluation urinary tract cytologic specimens (88120-88121)
3.08 3.08 FUD XXX 02 80
AMA: 2018,Jan,8; 2017,Jan,8; 2016,Jan,13; 2015,Jan,16

+ # **88373** **each additional single probe stain procedure (List separately in addition to code for primary procedure)**
Code first (88367)
2.11 2.11 FUD ZZZ N 80

88374 **each multiplex probe stain procedure**
EXCLUDES *In situ hybridization probe stain procedures for same probe (88365, 88366, 88368, [88377])*
9.65 9.65 FUD XXX 01 80

88368 **Morphometric analysis, in situ hybridization (quantitative or semi-quantitative), manual, per specimen; initial single probe stain procedure**
EXCLUDES *In situ hybridization probe stain procedures for same probe (88365, 88366-88367, [88374])*
Morphometric in situ hybridization evaluation urinary tract cytologic specimens (88120-88121)
3.59 3.59 FUD XXX 02 80
AMA: 2018,Jan,8; 2017,Jan,8; 2016,Jan,13; 2015,Jan,16

+ **88369** **each additional single probe stain procedure (List separately in addition to code for primary procedure)**
Code first (88368)
3.23 3.23 FUD ZZZ N 80

88377 **each multiplex probe stain procedure**
EXCLUDES *In situ hybridization probe stain procedures for same probe (88365, 88366-88367, [88374])*
Morphometric in situ hybridization evaluation, urinary tract cytologic specimens (88120-88121)
11.4 11.4 FUD XXX 01 80

88371 **Protein analysis of tissue by Western Blot, with interpretation and report;**
0.00 0.00 FUD XXX N 80
AMA: 2018,Jan,8; 2017,Jan,8; 2016,Jan,13; 2015,Dec,18; 2015,Jan,16

88372 **immunological probe for band identification, each**
0.00 0.00 FUD XXX N 80
AMA: 2018,Jan,8; 2017,Jan,8; 2016,Jan,13; 2015,Jan,16

88373 **Resequenced code. See code following 88367.**

88374 **Resequenced code. See code following 88367.**

88375 **Optical endomicroscopic image(s), interpretation and report, real-time or referred, each endoscopic session**
EXCLUDES *Endoscopic procedures that include optical endomicroscopy (43206, 43252, 0397T)*
1.42 1.42 FUD XXX B 80 26
AMA: 2018,Jan,8; 2017,Jan,8; 2016,Jan,13; 2015,Jan,16

88377 **Resequenced code. See code following 88369.**

88380 **Microdissection (ie, sample preparation of microscopically identified target); laser capture**
EXCLUDES *Microdissection, manual procedure (88381)*
3.78 3.78 FUD XXX N 80
AMA: 2018,Aug,3; 2018,Jan,8; 2017,Jan,8; 2016,Jan,13; 2015,Jan,16

88381 **manual**
EXCLUDES *Microdissection, laser capture procedure (88380)*
4.34 4.34 FUD XXX N 80
AMA: 2018,Aug,3; 2018,Jan,8; 2017,Jan,8; 2016,Jan,13; 2015,Jan,16

88387 **Macroscopic examination, dissection, and preparation of tissue for non-microscopic analytical studies (eg, nucleic acid-based molecular studies); each tissue preparation (eg, a single lymph node)**
EXCLUDES *Pathology consultation during surgery (88329-88334, 88388)*
Tissue preparation for microbiologic cultures or flow cytometric studies
1.00 1.00 FUD XXX N 80
AMA: 2018,Jan,8; 2017,Jan,8; 2016,Jan,13; 2015,Jan,16

\+ **88388** **in conjunction with a touch imprint, intraoperative consultation, or frozen section, each tissue preparation (eg, a single lymph node) (List separately in addition to code for primary procedure)**

EXCLUDES *Tissue preparation for microbiologic cultures or flow cytometric studies*

Code first (88329-88334)

1.00 1.00 FUD XXX N 80

AMA: 2018,Jan,8; 2017,Jan,8; 2016,Jan,13; 2015,Jan,16

88399 **Unlisted surgical pathology procedure**

0.00 0.00 FUD XXX Q1 80

AMA: 2018,Jan,8; 2017,Jan,8; 2016,Jan,13; 2015,Jan,16

88720-88749 Transcutaneous Procedures

EXCLUDES *Transcutaneous oxyhemoglobin measurement (0493T)*
Wavelength fluorescent spectroscopy advanced glycation end products (skin) (88749)

88720 **Bilirubin, total, transcutaneous**

EXCLUDES *Transdermal oxygen saturation testing (94760-94762)*

0.00 0.00 FUD XXX Q

AMA: 2020,May,13; 2018,Jan,8; 2017,Jan,8; 2016,Jan,13; 2015,Jan,16

88738 **Hemoglobin (Hgb), quantitative, transcutaneous**

EXCLUDES *In vitro hemoglobin measurement (85018)*

0.00 0.00 FUD XXX Q

AMA: 2018,Jan,8; 2017,Jan,8; 2016,Jan,13; 2015,Jan,16

88740 **Hemoglobin, quantitative, transcutaneous, per day; carboxyhemoglobin**

EXCLUDES *In vitro carboxyhemoglobin measurement (82375)*

0.00 0.00 FUD XXX Q

AMA: 2018,Jan,8; 2017,Jan,8; 2016,Jan,13; 2015,Jan,16

88741 **methemoglobin**

EXCLUDES *In vitro quantitative methemoglobin measurement (83050)*

0.00 0.00 FUD XXX Q

AMA: 2018,Jan,8; 2017,Jan,8; 2016,Jan,13; 2015,Jan,16

88749 **Unlisted in vivo (eg, transcutaneous) laboratory service**

INCLUDES All in vivo measurements not specifically listed

0.00 0.00 FUD XXX Q

AMA: 2010,Dec,7-10

89049-89240 Other Pathology Services

89049 **Caffeine halothane contracture test (CHCT) for malignant hyperthermia susceptibility, including interpretation and report**

1.77 7.06 FUD XXX Q1 80

AMA: 2018,Jan,8; 2017,Jan,8; 2016,Jan,13; 2015,Jan,16

89050 **Cell count, miscellaneous body fluids (eg, cerebrospinal fluid, joint fluid), except blood;**

0.00 0.00 FUD XXX Q

AMA: 2018,Jan,8; 2017,Jan,8; 2016,Jan,13; 2015,Jan,16

89051 **with differential count**

0.00 0.00 FUD XXX Q

AMA: 2018,Jan,8; 2017,Jan,8; 2016,Jan,13; 2015,Jan,16

89055 **Leukocyte assessment, fecal, qualitative or semiquantitative**

0.00 0.00 FUD XXX Q

AMA: 2018,Jan,8; 2017,Jan,8; 2016,Jan,13; 2015,Jan,16

89060 **Crystal identification by light microscopy with or without polarizing lens analysis, tissue or any body fluid (except urine)**

EXCLUDES *Crystal identification on paraffin embedded tissue*

0.00 0.00 FUD XXX Q 80

AMA: 2018,Jan,8; 2017,Jan,8; 2016,Jan,13; 2015,Jan,16

89125 **Fat stain, feces, urine, or respiratory secretions**

0.00 0.00 FUD XXX Q

AMA: 2018,Jan,8; 2017,Jan,8; 2016,Jan,13; 2015,Jan,16

89160 **Meat fibers, feces**

0.00 0.00 FUD XXX Q

AMA: 2018,Jan,8; 2017,Jan,8; 2016,Jan,13; 2015,Jan,16

89190 **Nasal smear for eosinophils**

EXCLUDES *Occult blood feces (82270)*
Paternity tests (86910)

0.00 0.00 FUD XXX Q

AMA: 2018,Jan,8; 2017,Jan,8; 2016,Jan,13; 2015,Jan,16

89220 **Sputum, obtaining specimen, aerosol induced technique (separate procedure)**

0.46 0.46 FUD XXX Q1 80 TC

AMA: 2018,Jan,8; 2017,Jan,8; 2016,Jan,13; 2015,Jan,16

89230 **Sweat collection by iontophoresis**

0.07 0.07 FUD XXX Q1 80 TC

AMA: 2018,Jan,8; 2017,Jan,8; 2016,Jan,13; 2015,Jan,16

89240 **Unlisted miscellaneous pathology test**

0.00 0.00 FUD XXX Q1 80

AMA: 2018,Jan,8; 2017,Jan,8; 2016,Jan,13; 2015,Jan,16

89250-89398 Infertility Treatment Services

CMS: 100-02,1,100 Treatment for Infertility

89250 **Culture of oocyte(s)/embryo(s), less than 4 days;**

0.00 0.00 FUD XXX Q1

AMA: 2018,Jan,8; 2017,Jan,8; 2016,Jan,13; 2015,Jan,16

89251 **with co-culture of oocyte(s)/embryos**

EXCLUDES *Extended culture oocyte(s)/embryo(s) (89272)*

0.00 0.00 FUD XXX Q2

AMA: 2018,Jan,8; 2017,Jan,8; 2016,Jan,13; 2015,Jan,16

89253 **Assisted embryo hatching, microtechniques (any method)**

0.00 0.00 FUD XXX Q1

AMA: 2018,Jan,8; 2017,Jan,8; 2016,Jan,13; 2015,Jan,16

89254 **Oocyte identification from follicular fluid**

0.00 0.00 FUD XXX Q1

AMA: 2018,Jan,8; 2017,Jan,8; 2016,Jan,13; 2015,Jan,16

89255 **Preparation of embryo for transfer (any method)**

0.00 0.00 FUD XXX Q1

AMA: 2018,Jan,8; 2017,Jan,8; 2016,Jan,13; 2015,Jan,16

89257 **Sperm identification from aspiration (other than seminal fluid)**

EXCLUDES *Semen analysis (89300-89320)*
Sperm identification from testis tissue (89264)

0.00 0.00 FUD XXX Q1

AMA: 2018,Jan,8; 2017,Jan,8; 2016,Jan,13; 2015,Jan,16

89258 **Cryopreservation; embryo(s)**

0.00 0.00 FUD XXX Q2

AMA: 2018,Jan,8; 2017,Jan,8; 2016,Jan,13; 2015,Jan,16

89259 **sperm**

EXCLUDES *Cryopreservation testicular reproductive tissue (89335)*

0.00 0.00 FUD XXX Q1

AMA: 2018,Jan,8; 2017,Jan,8; 2016,Jan,13; 2015,Jan,16

89260 **Sperm isolation; simple prep (eg, sperm wash and swim-up) for insemination or diagnosis with semen analysis**

0.00 0.00 FUD XXX Q1

AMA: 2018,Jan,8; 2017,Jan,8; 2016,Jan,13; 2015,Jan,16

89261 **complex prep (eg, Percoll gradient, albumin gradient) for insemination or diagnosis with semen analysis**

EXCLUDES *Semen analysis without sperm wash or swim-up (89320)*

0.00 0.00 FUD XXX Q1

AMA: 2018,Jan,8; 2017,Jan,8; 2016,Jan,13; 2015,Jan,16

89264 **Sperm identification from testis tissue, fresh or cryopreserved** ♂

EXCLUDES *Biopsy testis (54500, 54505)*
Semen analysis (89300-89320)
Sperm identification from aspiration (89257)

0.00 0.00 FUD XXX Q1

AMA: 2018,Jan,8; 2017,Jan,8; 2016,Jan,13; 2015,Jan,16

89268 Insemination of oocytes
0.00 0.00 FUD XXX Q1
AMA: 2018,Jan,8; 2017,Jan,8; 2016,Jan,13; 2015,Jan,16

89272 Extended culture of oocyte(s)/embryo(s), 4-7 days
0.00 0.00 FUD XXX Q2
AMA: 2018,Jan,8; 2017,Jan,8; 2016,Jan,13; 2015,Jan,16

89280 Assisted oocyte fertilization, microtechnique; less than or equal to 10 oocytes
0.00 0.00 FUD XXX Q2
AMA: 2018,Jan,8; 2017,Jan,8; 2016,Jan,13; 2015,Jan,16

89281 greater than 10 oocytes
0.00 0.00 FUD XXX Q1
AMA: 2018,Jan,8; 2017,Jan,8; 2016,Jan,13; 2015,Jan,16

89290 Biopsy, oocyte polar body or embryo blastomere, microtechnique (for pre-implantation genetic diagnosis); less than or equal to 5 embryos
0.00 0.00 FUD XXX Q1
AMA: 2018,Jan,8; 2017,Jan,8; 2016,Jan,13; 2015,Jan,16

89291 greater than 5 embryos
0.00 0.00 FUD XXX Q1
AMA: 2018,Jan,8; 2017,Jan,8; 2016,Jan,13; 2015,Jan,16

89300 Semen analysis; presence and/or motility of sperm including Huhner test (post coital)
0.00 0.00 FUD XXX Q
AMA: 2018,Jan,8; 2017,Jan,8; 2016,Jan,13; 2015,Jan,16

89310 motility and count (not including Huhner test) ♂
0.00 0.00 FUD XXX Q
AMA: 2018,Jan,8; 2017,Jan,8; 2016,Jan,13; 2015,Jan,16

89320 volume, count, motility, and differential ♂
EXCLUDES *Skin testing (86485-86580, 95012-95199)*
0.00 0.00 FUD XXX Q
AMA: 2018,Jan,8; 2017,Jan,8; 2016,Jan,13; 2015,Jan,16

89321 sperm presence and motility of sperm, if performed ♂
EXCLUDES *Hyaluronan binding assay (HBA) (89398)*
0.00 0.00 FUD XXX Q
AMA: 2018,Jan,8; 2017,Jan,8; 2016,Jan,13; 2015,Jan,16

89322 volume, count, motility, and differential using strict morphologic criteria (eg, Kruger) ♂
0.00 0.00 FUD XXX Q
AMA: 2018,Jan,8; 2017,Jan,8; 2016,Jan,13; 2015,Jan,16

89325 Sperm antibodies ♂
EXCLUDES *Medicolegal identification sperm (88125)*
0.00 0.00 FUD XXX Q
AMA: 2018,Jan,8; 2017,Jan,8; 2016,Jan,13; 2015,Jan,16

89329 Sperm evaluation; hamster penetration test ♂
0.00 0.00 FUD XXX Q
AMA: 2018,Jan,8; 2017,Jan,8; 2016,Jan,13; 2015,Jan,16

89330 cervical mucus penetration test, with or without spinnbarkeit test ♂
0.00 0.00 FUD XXX Q
AMA: 2018,Jan,8; 2017,Jan,8; 2016,Jan,13; 2015,Jan,16

89331 Sperm evaluation, for retrograde ejaculation, urine (sperm concentration, motility, and morphology, as indicated) ♂
EXCLUDES *Detection sperm in urine (81015)*
Code also semen analysis on concurrent sperm specimen (89300-89322)
0.00 0.00 FUD XXX Q
AMA: 2018,Jan,8; 2017,Jan,8; 2016,Jan,13; 2015,Jan,16

89335 Cryopreservation, reproductive tissue, testicular
EXCLUDES *Cryopreservation:*
Embryo(s) (89258)
Immature oocyte(s) (89398)
Mature oocytes (89337)
Ovarian reproductive tissue (89398)
Sperm (89259)
0.00 0.00 FUD XXX Q1
AMA: 2018,Jan,8; 2017,Jan,8; 2016,Jan,13; 2015,Jan,16

89337 Cryopreservation, mature oocyte(s) ♀
EXCLUDES *Cryopreservation immature oocyte[s] (89398)*
0.00 0.00 FUD XXX Q1
AMA: 2018,Jan,8; 2017,Jan,8; 2016,Jan,13; 2015,Jan,16

89342 Storage (per year); embryo(s)
0.00 0.00 FUD XXX Q1
AMA: 2018,Jan,8; 2017,Jan,8; 2016,Jan,13; 2015,Jan,16

89343 sperm/semen
0.00 0.00 FUD XXX Q1
AMA: 2018,Jan,8; 2017,Jan,8; 2016,Jan,13; 2015,Jan,16

89344 reproductive tissue, testicular/ovarian
0.00 0.00 FUD XXX Q1
AMA: 2018,Jan,8; 2017,Jan,8; 2016,Jan,13; 2015,Jan,16

89346 oocyte(s)
0.00 0.00 FUD XXX Q2
AMA: 2018,Jan,8; 2017,Jan,8; 2016,Jan,13; 2015,Jan,16

89352 Thawing of cryopreserved; embryo(s)
0.00 0.00 FUD XXX Q1
AMA: 2018,Jan,8; 2017,Jan,8; 2016,Jan,13; 2015,Jan,16

89353 sperm/semen, each aliquot
0.00 0.00 FUD XXX Q1
AMA: 2018,Jan,8; 2017,Jan,8; 2016,Jan,13; 2015,Jan,16

89354 reproductive tissue, testicular/ovarian
0.00 0.00 FUD XXX Q1
AMA: 2018,Jan,8; 2017,Jan,8; 2016,Jan,13; 2015,Jan,16

89356 oocytes, each aliquot
0.00 0.00 FUD XXX Q1
AMA: 2018,Jan,8; 2017,Jan,8; 2016,Jan,13; 2015,Jan,16

89398 Unlisted reproductive medicine laboratory procedure
INCLUDES Cryopreservation:
immature oocytes
ovarian reproductive tissue
Hyaluronan binding assay (HBA)
0.00 0.00 FUD XXX Q1

0001U-0241U Proprietary Laboratory Analysis (PLA)

In response to the Protecting Access to Medicare Act of 2014 (PAMA), which focuses on payment and coding of clinical laboratory studies paid for under the Medicare Clinical Laboratory Fee Schedule (CLFS), the AMA has developed a new category of CPT codes known as Proprietary Laboratory Analyses (PLA), which will be released on a quarterly basis. These alphanumeric codes will appear at the end of the Pathology and Laboratory chapter of the CPT book and will include a wide range of tests. Codes in this section can also be found in Appendix L along with the procedure's proprietary name and clinical laboratory or manufacturer. When multiple codes have identical code descriptors and can only be distinguished by a proprietary test name, instructional notes are provided to help ensure accurate code assignment.

INCLUDES All necessary investigative services
PLA codes take priority over other CPT codes
EXCLUDES *Additional procedures necessary before cell lysis (88380-88381)*

0001U Red blood cell antigen typing, DNA, human erythrocyte antigen gene analysis of 35 antigens from 11 blood groups, utilizing whole blood, common RBC alleles reported
INCLUDES PreciseType® HEA Test, Immucor, Inc
0.00 0.00 FUD 000 A
AMA: 2019,Jun,11

0002U Oncology (colorectal), quantitative assessment of three urine metabolites (ascorbic acid, succinic acid and carnitine) by liquid chromatography with tandem mass spectrometry (LC-MS/MS) using multiple reaction monitoring acquisition, algorithm reported as likelihood of adenomatous polyps
INCLUDES PolypDX™, Atlantic Diagnostic Laboratories, LLC, Metabolomic Technologies Inc
0.00 0.00 FUD 000 Q
AMA: 2018,Aug,3

0003U Oncology (ovarian) biochemical assays of five proteins (apolipoprotein A-1, CA 125 II, follicle stimulating hormone, human epididymis protein 4, transferrin), utilizing serum, algorithm reported as a likelihood score

INCLUDES Overa (OVA1 Next Generation), Aspira Labs, Inc, Vermillion, Inc

0.00 0.00 FUD 000 Q

0005U Oncology (prostate) gene expression profile by real-time RT-PCR of 3 genes (*ERG, PCA3,* and *SPDEF*), urine, algorithm reported as risk score

INCLUDES ExosomeDx® Prostate (IntelliScore), Exosome Diagnostics, Inc, Exosome Diagnostics, Inc

0.00 0.00 FUD 000 Q

~~**0006U Detection of interacting medications, substances, supplements and foods, 120 or more analytes, definitive chromatography with mass spectrometry, urine, description and severity of each interaction identified, per date of service**~~

0007U Drug test(s), presumptive, with definitive confirmation of positive results, any number of drug classes, urine, includes specimen verification including DNA authentication in comparison to buccal DNA, per date of service

INCLUDES ToxProtect, Genotox Laboratories Ltd

0.00 0.00 FUD 000 Q

AMA: 2018,Jan,6

0008U Helicobacter pylori detection and antibiotic resistance, DNA, 16S and 23S rRNA, gyrA, pbp1, rdxA and rpoB, next-generation sequencing, formalin-fixed paraffin-embedded or fresh tissue or fecal sample, predictive, reported as positive or negative for resistance to clarithromycin, fluoroquinolones, metronidazole, amoxicillin, tetracycline, and rifabutin

INCLUDES AmHPR® H. pylori Antibiotic Resistance Panel, American Molecular Laboratories, Inc

0.00 0.00 FUD 000 A

0009U Oncology (breast cancer), ERBB2 (HER2) copy number by FISH, tumor cells from formalin fixed paraffin embedded tissue isolated using image-based dielectrophoresis (DEP) sorting, reported as ERBB2 gene amplified or non-amplified

INCLUDES DEPArray™ HER2, PacificDx

0.00 0.00 FUD 000 Q

0010U Infectious disease (bacterial), strain typing by whole genome sequencing, phylogenetic-based report of strain relatedness, per submitted isolate

INCLUDES Bacterial Typing by Whole Genome Sequencing, Mayo Clinic

0.00 0.00 FUD 000 A

0011U Prescription drug monitoring, evaluation of drugs present by LC-MS/MS, using oral fluid, reported as a comparison to an estimated steady-state range, per date of service including all drug compounds and metabolites

INCLUDES Cordant CORE™, Cordant Health Solutions

0.00 0.00 FUD 000 Q

0012U Germline disorders, gene rearrangement detection by whole genome next-generation sequencing, DNA, whole blood, report of specific gene rearrangement(s)

INCLUDES MatePair Targeted Rearrangements, Congenital, Mayo Clinic

0.00 0.00 FUD 000 A

0013U Oncology (solid organ neoplasia), gene rearrangement detection by whole genome next-generation sequencing, DNA, fresh or frozen tissue or cells, report of specific gene rearrangement(s)

INCLUDES MatePair Targeted Rearrangements, Oncology, Mayo Clinic

0.00 0.00 FUD 000 A

0014U Hematology (hematolymphoid neoplasia), gene rearrangement detection by whole genome next-generation sequencing, DNA, whole blood or bone marrow, report of specific gene rearrangement(s)

INCLUDES MatePair Targeted Rearrangements, Hematologic, Mayo Clinic

0.00 0.00 FUD 000 A

0016U Oncology (hematolymphoid neoplasia), RNA, *BCR/ABL1* major and minor breakpoint fusion transcripts, quantitative PCR amplification, blood or bone marrow, report of fusion not detected or detected with quantitation

INCLUDES BCR-ABL1 major and minor breakpoint fusion transcripts, University of Iowa, Department of Pathology, Asuragen

0.00 0.00 FUD 000 A

0017U Oncology (hematolymphoid neoplasia), *JAK2* mutation, DNA, PCR amplification of exons 12-14 and sequence analysis, blood or bone marrow, report of *JAK2* mutation not detected or detected

INCLUDES *JAK2* Mutation, University of Iowa, Department of Pathology

0.00 0.00 FUD 000 A

0018U Oncology (thyroid), microRNA profiling by RT-PCR of 10 microRNA sequences, utilizing fine needle aspirate, algorithm reported as a positive or negative result for moderate to high risk of malignancy

INCLUDES ThyraMIR™, Interpace Diagnostics

0.00 0.00 FUD 000 A

0019U Oncology, RNA, gene expression by whole transcriptome sequencing, formalin-fixed paraffin embedded tissue or fresh frozen tissue, predictive algorithm reported as potential targets for therapeutic agents

INCLUDES OncoTarget/OncoTreat, Columbia University Department of Pathology and Cell Biology, Darwin Health

0.00 0.00 FUD 000 A

0021U Oncology (prostate), detection of 8 autoantibodies (ARF 6, NKX3-1, 5'-UTR-BMI1, CEP 164, 3'-UTR-Ropporin, Desmocollin, AURKAIP-1, CSNK2A2), multiplexed immunoassay and flow cytometry serum, algorithm reported as risk score

INCLUDES Apifiny®, Armune BioScience, Inc

0.00 0.00 FUD 000 Q

0022U Targeted genomic sequence analysis panel, non-small cell lung neoplasia, DNA and RNA analysis, 23 genes, interrogation for sequence variants and rearrangements, reported as presence/absence of variants and associated therapy(ies) to consider

INCLUDES Oncomine™ Dx Target Test, Thermo Fisher Scientific

0.00 0.00 FUD 000 A

0023U Oncology (acute myelogenous leukemia), DNA, genotyping of internal tandem duplication, p.D835, p.I836, using mononuclear cells, reported as detection or non-detection of *FLT3* mutation and indication for or against the use of midostaurin

INCLUDES LeukoStrat® CDx *FLT3* Mutation Assay, LabPMM LLC, an Invivoscribe Technologies, Inc Company, Invivoscribe Technologies, Inc

0.00 0.00 FUD 000 A

0024U Glycosylated acute phase proteins (GlycA), nuclear magnetic resonance spectroscopy, quantitative

INCLUDES GlycA, Laboratory Corporation of America, Laboratory Corporation of America

0.00 0.00 FUD 000 Q

0025U Tenofovir, by liquid chromatography with tandem mass spectrometry (LC-MS/MS), urine, quantitative

INCLUDES UrSure Tenofovir Quantification Test, Synergy Medical Laboratories, UrSure Inc

0.00 0.00 FUD 000 Q

0026U Oncology (thyroid), DNA and mRNA of 112 genes, next-generation sequencing, fine needle aspirate of thyroid nodule, algorithmic analysis reported as a categorical result ("Positive, high probability of malignancy" or "Negative, low probability of malignancy")

INCLUDES Thyroseq Genomic Classifier, CBLPath, Inc, University of Pittsburgh Medical Center

0.00 0.00 FUD 000 A

0027U *JAK2 (Janus kinase 2)* (eg, myeloproliferative disorder) gene analysis, targeted sequence analysis exons 12-15

INCLUDES *JAK2* Exons 12 to 15 Sequencing, Mayo Clinic, Mayo Clinic

0.00 0.00 FUD 000 A

0029U Drug metabolism (adverse drug reactions and drug response), targeted sequence analysis (ie, *CYP1A2, CYP2C19, CYP2C9, CYP2D6, CYP3A4, CYP3A5, CYP4F2, SLCO1B1, VKORC1* and rs12777823)

INCLUDES Focused Pharmacogenomics Panel, Mayo Clinic, Mayo Clinic

0.00 0.00 FUD 000 A

0030U Drug metabolism (warfarin drug response), targeted sequence analysis (ie, *CYP2C9, CYP4F2, VKORC1*, rs12777823)

INCLUDES Warfarin Response Genotype, Mayo Clinic, Mayo Clinic

0.00 0.00 FUD 000 A

0031U *CYP1A2 (cytochrome P450 family 1, subfamily A, member 2)*(eg, drug metabolism) gene analysis, common variants (ie, *1F, *1K, *6, *7)

INCLUDES Cytochrome P450 1A2 Genotype, Mayo Clinic, Mayo Clinic

0.00 0.00 FUD 000 A

0032U *COMT (catechol-O-methyltransferase)(drug metabolism)* gene analysis, c.472G>A (rs4680) variant

INCLUDES Catechol-O-Methyltransferase (*COMT*) Genotype, Mayo Clinic, Mayo Clinic

0.00 0.00 FUD 000 A

0033U *HTR2A (5-hydroxytryptamine receptor 2A), HTR2C (5-hydroxytryptamine receptor 2C)* (eg, citalopram metabolism) gene analysis, common variants (ie, *HTR2A* rs7997012 [c.614-2211T>C], *HTR2C* rs3813929 [c.-759C>T] and rs1414334 [c.551-3008C>G])

INCLUDES Serotonin Receptor Genotype (*HTR2A* and *HTR2C*), Mayo Clinic, Mayo Clinic

0.00 0.00 FUD 000 A

0034U *TPMT (thiopurine S-methyltransferase), NUDT15 (nudix hydroxylase 15)(eg, thiopurine metabolism)*, gene analysis, common variants (ie, *TPMT* *2, *3A, *3B, *3C, *4, *5, *6, *8, *12; *NUDT15* *3, *4, *5)

INCLUDES Thiopurine Methyltransferase (*TPMT*) and Nudix Hydrolase (*NUDT15*) Genotyping, Mayo Clinic, Mayo Clinic

0.00 0.00 FUD 000 A

0035U Neurology (prion disease), cerebrospinal fluid, detection of prion protein by quaking-induced conformational conversion, qualitative

INCLUDES Real-time quaking-induced conversion for prion detection (RT-QuIC), National Prion Disease Pathology Surveillance Center

0.00 0.00 FUD 000

0036U Exome (ie, somatic mutations), paired formalin-fixed paraffin-embedded tumor tissue and normal specimen, sequence analyses

INCLUDES EXaCT-1 Whole Exome Testing, Lab of Oncology-Molecular Detection, Weill Cornell Medicine-Clinical Genomics Laboratory

0.00 0.00 FUD 000

0037U Targeted genomic sequence analysis, solid organ neoplasm, DNA analysis of 324 genes, interrogation for sequence variants, gene copy number amplifications, gene rearrangements, microsatellite instability and tumor mutational burden

INCLUDES FoundationOne CDx™ (F1CDx), Foundation Medicine, Inc, Foundation Medicine, Inc

0.00 0.00 FUD 000

0038U Vitamin D, 25 hydroxy D2 and D3, by LC-MS/MS, serum microsample, quantitative

INCLUDES Sensieva™ Droplet 25OH Vitamin D2/D3 Microvolume LC/MS Assay, InSource Diagnostics, InSource Diagnostics

0.00 0.00 FUD 000

0039U Deoxyribonucleic acid (DNA) antibody, double stranded, high avidity

INCLUDES Anti-dsDNA, High Salt/Avidity, University of Washington, Department of Laboratory Medicine, Bio-Rad

0.00 0.00 FUD 000

0040U *BCR/ABL1 (t(9;22))* (eg, chronic myelogenous leukemia) translocation analysis, major breakpoint, quantitative

INCLUDES MRDx BCR-ABL Test, MolecularMD, MolecularMD

0.00 0.00 FUD 000

0041U Borrelia burgdorferi, antibody detection of 5 recombinant protein groups, by immunoblot, IgM

INCLUDES Lyme ImmunoBlot IgM, IGeneX Inc, ID-FISH Technology Inc. (ASR) (Lyme ImmunoBlot IgM Strips Only)

0.00 0.00 FUD 000

0042U Borrelia burgdorferi, antibody detection of 12 recombinant protein groups, by immunoblot, IgG

INCLUDES Lyme ImmunoBlot IgG, IGeneX Inc, ID-FISH Technology Inc (ASR) (Lyme ImmunoBlot IgG Strips Only)

0.00 0.00 FUD 000

0043U Tick-borne relapsing fever Borrelia group, antibody detection to 4 recombinant protein groups, by immunoblot, IgM

INCLUDES Tick-Borne Relapsing Fever (TBRF) Borrelia ImmunoBlots IgM Test, IGeneX Inc, ID-FISH Technology Inc (Provides TBRF ImmunoBlot IgM Strips)

0.00 0.00 FUD 000

0044U Tick-borne relapsing fever Borrelia group, antibody detection to 4 recombinant protein groups, by immunoblot, IgG

INCLUDES Tick-Borne Relapsing Fever (TBRF) Borrelia ImmunoBlots IgG Test, IGeneX Inc, ID-FISH Technology Inc (Provides TBRF ImmunoBlot IgG Strips)

0.00 0.00 FUD 000

0045U Oncology (breast ductal carcinoma in situ), mRNA, gene expression profiling by real-time RT-PCR of 12 genes (7 content and 5 housekeeping), utilizing formalin-fixed paraffin-embedded tissue, algorithm reported as recurrence score

INCLUDES The Oncotype DX® Breast DCIS Score™ Test, Genomic Health, Inc, Genomic Health, Inc

0.00 0.00 FUD 000

0046U *FLT3* (fms-related tyrosine kinase 3) (eg, acute myeloid leukemia) internal tandem duplication (ITD) variants, quantitative

INCLUDES FLT3 ITD MRD by NGS, LabPMM LLC, an Invivoscribe Technologies, Inc Company

0.00 0.00 FUD 000

Pathology and Laboratory

0026U — 0046U

● New Code ▲ Revised Code ○ Reinstated ● New Web Release ▲ Revised Web Release + Add-on Unlisted Not Covered # Resequenced
Optum Mod 50 Exempt AMA Mod 51 Exempt Optum Mod 51 Exempt Mod 63 Exempt Non-FDA Drug ★ Telemedicine Maternity Age Edit

0047U **Oncology (prostate), mRNA, gene expression profiling by real-time RT-PCR of 17 genes (12 content and 5 housekeeping), utilizing formalin-fixed paraffin-embedded tissue, algorithm reported as a risk score**

INCLUDES Oncotype DX Genomic Prostate Score, Genomic Health, Inc, Genomic Health, Inc

0.00 0.00 FUD 000

0048U **Oncology (solid organ neoplasia), DNA, targeted sequencing of protein-coding exons of 468 cancer-associated genes, including interrogation for somatic mutations and microsatellite instability, matched with normal specimens, utilizing formalin-fixed paraffin-embedded tumor tissue, report of clinically significant mutation(s)**

INCLUDES MSK-IMPACT (Integrated Mutation Profiling of Actionable Cancer Targets), Memorial Sloan Kettering Cancer Center

0.00 0.00 FUD 000

0049U **NPM1 (nucleophosmin) (eg, acute myeloid leukemia) gene analysis, quantitative**

INCLUDES *NPM1* MRD by NGS, LabPMM LLC, an Invivoscribe Technologies, Inc Company

0.00 0.00 FUD 000

0050U **Targeted genomic sequence analysis panel, acute myelogenous leukemia, DNA analysis, 194 genes, interrogation for sequence variants, copy number variants or rearrangements**

INCLUDES MyAML NGS Panel, LabPMM LLC, an Invivoscribe Technologies, Inc Company

0.00 0.00 FUD 000

0051U **Prescription drug monitoring, evaluation of drugs present by LC-MS/MS, urine, 31 drug panel, reported as quantitative results, detected or not detected, per date of service**

INCLUDES UCompliDx, Elite Medical Laboratory Solutions, LLC, Elite Medical Laboratory Solutions, LLC (LDT)

0.00 0.00 FUD 000

0052U **Lipoprotein, blood, high resolution fractionation and quantitation of lipoproteins, including all five major lipoprotein classes and subclasses of HDL, LDL, and VLDL by vertical auto profile ultracentrifugation**

INCLUDES VAP Cholesterol Test, VAP Diagnostics Laboratory, Inc, VAP Diagnostics Laboratory, Inc

0.00 0.00 FUD 000

0053U **Oncology (prostate cancer), FISH analysis of 4 genes (*ASAP1, HDAC9, CHD1* and *PTEN*), needle biopsy specimen, algorithm reported as probability of higher tumor grade**

INCLUDES Prostate Cancer Risk Panel, Mayo Clinic, Laboratory Developed Test

0.00 0.00 FUD 000

0054U **Prescription drug monitoring, 14 or more classes of drugs and substances, definitive tandem mass spectrometry with chromatography, capillary blood, quantitative report with therapeutic and toxic ranges, including steady-state range for the prescribed dose when detected, per date of service**

INCLUDES AssuranceRx Micro Serum, Firstox Laboratories, LLC, Firstox Laboratories, LLC

0.00 0.00 FUD 000

0055U **Cardiology (heart transplant), cell-free DNA, PCR assay of 96 DNA target sequences (94 single nucleotide polymorphism targets and two control targets), plasma**

INCLUDES myTAIHEART, TAI Diagnostics, Inc, TAI Diagnostics, Inc

0.00 0.00 FUD 000

0056U **Hematology (acute myelogenous leukemia), DNA, whole genome next-generation sequencing to detect gene rearrangement(s), blood or bone marrow, report of specific gene rearrangement(s)**

INCLUDES MatePair Acute Myeloid Leukemia Panel, Mayo Clinic, Laboratory Developed Test

0.00 0.00 FUD 000

~~**0057U** **Oncology (solid organ neoplasia), mRNA, gene expression profiling by massively parallel sequencing for analysis of 51 genes, utilizing formalin-fixed paraffin-embedded tissue, algorithm reported as a normalized percentile rank**~~

0058U **Oncology (Merkel cell carcinoma), detection of antibodies to the Merkel cell polyoma virus oncoprotein (small T antigen), serum, quantitative**

INCLUDES Merkel SmT Oncoprotein Antibody Titer, University of Washington, Department of Laboratory Medicine

0.00 0.00 FUD 000

0059U **Oncology (Merkel cell carcinoma), detection of antibodies to the Merkel cell polyoma virus capsid protein (VP1), serum, reported as positive or negative**

INCLUDES Merkel Virus VP1 Capsid Antibody, University of Washington, Department of Laboratory Medicine

0.00 0.00 FUD 000

0060U **Twin zygosity, genomic targeted sequence analysis of chromosome 2, using circulating cell-free fetal DNA in maternal blood**

INCLUDES Twins Zygosity PLA, Natera, Inc, Natera, Inc

0.00 0.00 FUD 000

0061U **Transcutaneous measurement of five biomarkers (tissue oxygenation [StO2], oxyhemoglobin [ctHbO2], deoxyhemoglobin [ctHbR], papillary and reticular dermal hemoglobin concentrations [ctHb1 and ctHb2]), using spatial frequency domain imaging (SFDI) and multi-spectral analysis**

INCLUDES Transcutaneous multispectral measurement of tissue oxygenation and hemoglobin using spatial frequency domain imaging (SFDI), Modulated Imaging, Inc, Modulated Imaging, Inc

0.00 0.00 FUD 000

0062U **Autoimmune (systemic lupus erythematosus), IgG and IgM analysis of 80 biomarkers, utilizing serum, algorithm reported with a risk score**

INCLUDES SLE-key® Rule Out, Veracis Inc, Veracis Inc

0.00 0.00 FUD 000

0063U **Neurology (autism), 32 amines by LC-MS/MS, using plasma, algorithm reported as metabolic signature associated with autism spectrum disorder**

INCLUDES NPDX ASD ADM Panel I, Stemina Biomarker Discovery, Inc, Stemina Biomarker Discovery, Inc d/b/a NeuroPointDX

0.00 0.00 FUD 000

0064U **Antibody, Treponema pallidum, total and rapid plasma reagin (RPR), immunoassay, qualitative**

INCLUDES BioPlex 2200 Syphilis Total & RPR Assay, Bio-Rad Laboratories, Bio-Rad Laboratories

0.00 0.00 FUD 000

0065U **Syphilis test, non-treponemal antibody, immunoassay, qualitative (RPR)**

INCLUDES BioPlex 2200 RPR Assay, Bio-Rad Laboratories, Bio-Rad Laboratories

0.00 0.00 FUD 000

0066U **Placental alpha-micro globulin-1 (PAMG-1), immunoassay with direct optical observation, cervico-vaginal fluid, each specimen**

INCLUDES PartoSure™ Test, Parsagen Diagnostics, Inc, Parsagen Diagnostics, Inc, a QIAGEN Company

0.00 0.00 FUD 000

0067U **Oncology (breast), immunohistochemistry, protein expression profiling of 4 biomarkers (matrix metalloproteinase-1 [MMP-1], carcinoembryonic antigen-related cell adhesion molecule 6 [CEACAM6], hyaluronoglucosaminidase [HYAL1], highly expressed in cancer protein [HEC1]), formalin-fixed paraffin-embedded precancerous breast tissue, algorithm reported as carcinoma risk score**

INCLUDES BBDRisk Dx™, Silbiotech, Inc, Silbiotech, Inc

0.00 0.00 FUD 000

0068U **Candida species panel (*C. albicans, C. glabrata, C. parapsilosis, C. kruseii, C tropicalis, and C. auris*), amplified probe technique with qualitative report of the presence or absence of each species**

INCLUDES MYCODART-PCR™ Dual Amplification Real Time PCR Panel for 6 Candida species, RealTime Laboratories, Inc/MycoDART, Inc, RealTime Laboratories, Inc

0.00 0.00 FUD 000

0069U **Oncology (colorectal), microRNA, RT-PCR expression profiling of miR-31-3p, formalin-fixed paraffin-embedded tissue, algorithm reported as an expression score**

INCLUDES miR-31*now*™, GoPath Laboratories, GoPath Laboratories

0.00 0.00 FUD 000

0070U ***CYP2D6 (cytochrome P450, family 2, subfamily D, polypeptide 6)* (eg, drug metabolism) gene analysis, common and select rare variants (ie, *2, *3, *4, *4N, *5, *6, *7, *8, *9, *10, *11, *12, *13, *14A, *14B, *15, *17, *29, *35, *36, *41, *57, *61, *63, *68, *83, *xN)**

INCLUDES *CYP2D6* Common Variants and Copy Number, Mayo Clinic, Laboratory Developed Test

0.00 0.00 FUD 000

\+ **0071U** ***CYP2D6 (cytochrome P450, family 2, subfamily D, polypeptide 6)* (eg, drug metabolism) gene analysis, full gene sequence (List separately in addition to code for primary procedure)**

INCLUDES *CYP2D6* Full Gene Sequencing, Mayo Clinic, Laboratory Developed Test

Code first (0070U)

0.00 0.00 FUD 000

\+ **0072U** ***CYP2D6 (cytochrome P450, family 2, subfamily D, polypeptide 6)* (eg, drug metabolism) gene analysis, targeted sequence analysis (ie, CYP2D6-2D7 hybrid gene) (List separately in addition to code for primary procedure)**

INCLUDES *CYP2D6-2D7* Hybrid Gene Targeted Sequence Analysis, Mayo Clinic, Laboratory Developed Test

Code first (0070U)

0.00 0.00 FUD 000

\+ **0073U** ***CYP2D6 (cytochrome P450, family 2, subfamily D, polypeptide 6)* (eg, drug metabolism) gene analysis, targeted sequence analysis (ie, CYP2D7-2D6 hybrid gene) (List separately in addition to code for primary procedure)**

INCLUDES *CYP2D7-2D6* Hybrid Gene Targeted Sequence Analysis, Mayo Clinic, Laboratory Developed Test

Code first (0070U)

0.00 0.00 FUD 000

\+ **0074U** ***CYP2D6 (cytochrome P450, family 2, subfamily D, polypeptide 6)* (eg, drug metabolism) gene analysis, targeted sequence analysis (ie, non-duplicated gene when duplication/multiplication is trans) (List separately in addition to code for primary procedure)**

INCLUDES *CYP2D6* trans-duplication/multiplication non-duplicated gene targeted sequence analysis, Mayo Clinic, Laboratory Developed Test

Code first (0070U)

0.00 0.00 FUD 000

\+ **0075U** ***CYP2D6 (cytochrome P450, family 2, subfamily D, polypeptide 6)* (eg, drug metabolism) gene analysis, targeted sequence analysis (ie, 5' gene duplication/multiplication) (List separately in addition to code for primary procedure)**

INCLUDES *CYP2D6* 5' gene duplication/multiplication targeted sequence analysis, Mayo Clinic, Laboratory Developed Test

Code first (0070U)

0.00 0.00 FUD 000

\+ **0076U** ***CYP2D6 (cytochrome P450, family 2, subfamily D, polypeptide 6)* (eg, drug metabolism) gene analysis, targeted sequence analysis (ie, 3' gene duplication/ multiplication) (List separately in addition to code for primary procedure)**

INCLUDES *CYP2D6* 3' gene duplication/multiplication targeted sequence analysis, Mayo Clinic, Laboratory Developed Test

Code first (0070U)

0.00 0.00 FUD 000

0077U **Immunoglobulin paraprotein (M-protein), qualitative, immunoprecipitation and mass spectrometry, blood or urine, including isotype**

INCLUDES M-Protein Detection and Isotyping by MALDI-TOF Mass Spectrometry, Mayo Clinic, Laboratory Developed Test

0.00 0.00 FUD 000

0078U **Pain management (opioid-use disorder) genotyping panel, 16 common variants (ie, *ABCB1, COMT, DAT1, DBH, DOR, DRD1, DRD2, DRD4, GABA, GAL, HTR2A, HTTLPR, MTHFR, MUOR, OPRK1, OPRM1*), buccal swab or other germline tissue sample, algorithm reported as positive or negative risk of opioid-use disorder**

INCLUDES INFINITI® Neural Response Panel, PersonalizeDx Labs, AutoGenomics Inc

0.00 0.00 FUD 000

0079U **Comparative DNA analysis using multiple selected single-nucleotide polymorphisms (SNPs), urine and buccal DNA, for specimen identity verification**

INCLUDES ToxLok™, InSource Diagnostics, InSource Diagnostics

0.00 0.00 FUD 000

0080U **Oncology (lung), mass spectrometric analysis of galectin-3-binding protein and scavenger receptor cysteine-rich type 1 protein M130, with five clinical risk factors (age, smoking status, nodule diameter, nodule-spiculation status and nodule location), utilizing plasma, algorithm reported as a categorical probability of malignancy**

INCLUDES BDX-XL2, Biodesix®, Inc, Biodesix®, Inc

0.00 0.00 FUD 000

0082U **Drug test(s), definitive, 90 or more drugs or substances, definitive chromatography with mass spectrometry, and presumptive, any number of drug classes, by instrument chemistry analyzer (utilizing immunoassay), urine, report of presence or absence of each drug, drug metabolite or substance with description and severity of significant interactions per date of service**

INCLUDES NextGen Precision™ Testing, Precision Diagnostics, Precision Diagnostics LBN Precision Toxicology, LLC

0.00 0.00 FUD 000

0083U **Oncology, response to chemotherapy drugs using motility contrast tomography, fresh or frozen tissue, reported as likelihood of sensitivity or resistance to drugs or drug combinations**

INCLUDES Onco4D™, Animated Dynamics, Inc, Animated Dynamics, Inc

0.00 0.00 FUD 000

0084U **Red blood cell antigen typing, DNA, genotyping of 10 blood groups with phenotype prediction of 37 red blood cell antigens**

INCLUDES BLOODchip® ID CORE XT™, Grifols Diagnostic Solutions Inc

0.00 0.00 **FUD** 000

0086U **Infectious disease (bacterial and fungal), organism identification, blood culture, using rRNA FISH, 6 or more organism targets, reported as positive or negative with phenotypic minimum inhibitory concentration (MIC)-based antimicrobial susceptibility**

INCLUDES Accelerate PhenoTest™ BC kit, Accelerate Diagnostics, Inc

0.00 0.00 **FUD** 000

0087U **Cardiology (heart transplant), mRNA gene expression profiling by microarray of 1283 genes, transplant biopsy tissue, allograft rejection and injury algorithm reported as a probability score**

INCLUDES Molecular Microscope® MMDx—Heart, Kashi Clinical Laboratories

0.00 0.00 **FUD** 000

0088U **Transplantation medicine (kidney allograft rejection), microarray gene expression profiling of 1494 genes, utilizing transplant biopsy tissue, algorithm reported as a probability score for rejection**

INCLUDES Molecular Microscope® MMDx—Kidney, Kashi Clinical Laboratories

0.00 0.00 **FUD** 000

0089U **Oncology (melanoma), gene expression profiling by RTqPCR, *PRAME* and *LINC00518*, superficial collection using adhesive patch(es)**

INCLUDES Pigmented Lesion Assay (PLA), DermTech

0.00 0.00 **FUD** 000

0090U **Oncology (cutaneous melanoma), mRNA gene expression profiling by RT-PCR of 23 genes (14 content and 9 housekeeping), utilizing formalin-fixed paraffin-embedded tissue, algorithm reported as a categorical result (ie, benign, indeterminate, malignant)**

INCLUDES myPath® Melanoma, Myriad Genetic Laboratories

0.00 0.00 **FUD** 000

0091U **Oncology (colorectal) screening, cell enumeration of circulating tumor cells, utilizing whole blood, algorithm, for the presence of adenoma or cancer, reported as a positive or negative result**

INCLUDES FirstSightCRC™, CellMax Life

0.00 0.00 **FUD** 000

0092U **Oncology (lung), three protein biomarkers, immunoassay using magnetic nanosensor technology, plasma, algorithm reported as risk score for likelihood of malignancy**

INCLUDES REVEAL Lung Nodule Characterization, MagArray, Inc

0.00 0.00 **FUD** 000

0093U **Prescription drug monitoring, evaluation of 65 common drugs by LC-MS/MS, urine, each drug reported detected or not detected**

INCLUDES ComplyRX, Claro Labs

0.00 0.00 **FUD** 000

0094U **Genome (eg, unexplained constitutional or heritable disorder or syndrome), rapid sequence analysis**

INCLUDES RCIGM Rapid Whole Genome Sequencing, Rady Children's Institute for Genomic Medicine (RCIGM)

0.00 0.00 **FUD** 000

0095U **Inflammation (eosinophilic esophagitis), ELISA analysis of eotaxin-3 *(CCL26 [C-C motif chemokine ligand 26])* and major basic protein *(PRG2 [proteoglycan 2, pro eosinophil major basic protein])*, specimen obtained by swallowed nylon string, algorithm reported as predictive probability index for active eosinophilic esophagitis**

INCLUDES Esophageal String Test™ (EST), Cambridge Biomedical, Inc

0.00 0.00 **FUD** 000

0096U **Human papillomavirus (HPV), high-risk types (ie, 16, 18, 31, 33, 35, 39, 45, 51, 52, 56, 58, 59, 66, 68), male urine**

INCLUDES HPV, High-Risk, Male Urine, Molecular Testing Labs

0.00 0.00 **FUD** 000

0097U **Gastrointestinal pathogen, multiplex reverse transcription and multiplex amplified probe technique, multiple types or subtypes, 22 targets (Campylobacter [C. jejuni/C. coli/C. upsaliensis], Clostridium difficile [C. difficile] toxin A/B, Plesiomonas shigelloides, Salmonella, Vibrio [V. parahaemolyticus/V. vulnificus/V. cholerae], including specific identification of Vibrio cholerae, Yersinia enterocolitica, Enteroaggregative Escherichia coli [EAEC], Enteropathogenic Escherichia coli [EPEC], Enterotoxigenic Escherichia coli [ETEC] lt/st, Shiga-like toxin-producing Escherichia coli [STEC] stx1/stx2 [including specific identification of the E. coli O157 serogroup within STEC], Shigella/Enteroinvasive Escherichia coli [EIEC], Cryptosporidium, Cyclospora cayetanensis, Entamoeba histolytica, Giardia lamblia [also known as G. intestinalis and G. duodenalis], adenovirus F 40/41, astrovirus, norovirus GI/GII, rotavirus A, sapovirus [Genogroups I, II, IV, and V])**

INCLUDES BioFire® FilmArray® Gastrointestinal (GI) Panel, BioFire® Diagnostics

0.00 0.00 **FUD** 000

0098U **Respiratory pathogen, multiplex reverse transcription and multiplex amplified probe technique, multiple types or subtypes, 14 targets (adenovirus, coronavirus, human metapneumovirus, influenza A, influenza A subtype H1, influenza A subtype H3, influenza A subtype H1-2009, influenza B, parainfluenza virus, human rhinovirus/enterovirus, respiratory syncytial virus, Bordetella pertussis, Chlamydophila pneumoniae, Mycoplasma pneumoniae)**

INCLUDES BioFire® FilmArray® Respiratory Panel (RP) EZ, BioFire® Diagnostics

0.00 0.00 **FUD** 000

AMA: 2020,Apr,3; 2020,Mar,3

0099U **Respiratory pathogen, multiplex reverse transcription and multiplex amplified probe technique, multiple types or subtypes, 20 targets (adenovirus, coronavirus 229E, coronavirus HKU1, coronavirus, coronavirus OC43, human metapneumovirus, influenza A, influenza A subtype, influenza A subtype H3, influenza A subtype H1-2009, influenza, parainfluenza virus, parainfluenza virus 2, parainfluenza virus 3, parainfluenza virus 4, human rhinovirus/enterovirus, respiratory syncytial virus, Bordetella pertussis, Chlamydophila pneumonia, Mycoplasma pneumoniae)**

INCLUDES BioFire® FilmArray® Respiratory Panel (RP), BioFire® Diagnostics

EXCLUDES *Assay for severe acute respiratory syndrome coronavirus 2 (SARS-CoV-2) (Coronavirus disease) (COVID-19) (87635)*

0.00 0.00 **FUD** 000

AMA: 2020,Apr,3; 2020,Mar,3

0100U Respiratory pathogen, multiplex reverse transcription and multiplex amplified probe technique, multiple types or subtypes, 21 targets (adenovirus, coronavirus 229E, coronavirus HKU1, coronavirus NL63, coronavirus OC43, human metapneumovirus, human rhinovirus/enterovirus, influenza A, including subtypes H1, H1-2009, and H3, influenza B, parainfluenza virus 1, parainfluenza virus 2, parainfluenza virus 3, parainfluenza virus 4, respiratory syncytial virus, Bordetella parapertussis [IS1001], Bordetella pertussis [ptxP], Chlamydia pneumoniae, Mycoplasma pneumoniae)

INCLUDES BioFire® FilmArray® Respiratory Panel 2 (RP2), BioFire® Diagnostics

0.00 0.00 FUD 000

AMA: 2020,Apr,3; 2020,Mar,3

0101U Hereditary colon cancer disorders (eg, Lynch syndrome, *PTEN* hamartoma syndrome, Cowden syndrome, familial adenomatosis polyposis), genomic sequence analysis panel utilizing a combination of NGS, Sanger, MLPA, and array CGH, with MRNA analytics to resolve variants of unknown significance when indicated (15 genes [sequencing and deletion/duplication], *EPCAM* and *GREM1* [deletion/duplication only])

INCLUDES ColoNext®, Ambry Genetics®, Ambry Genetics®

0.00 0.00 FUD 000

0102U Hereditary breast cancer-related disorders (eg, hereditary breast cancer, hereditary ovarian cancer, hereditary endometrial cancer), genomic sequence analysis panel utilizing a combination of NGS, Sanger, MLPA, and array CGH, with mRNA analytics to resolve variants of unknown significance when indicated (17 genes [sequencing and deletion/duplication])

INCLUDES BreastNext®, Ambry Genetics®, Ambry Genetics®

0.00 0.00 FUD 000

0103U Hereditary ovarian cancer (eg, hereditary ovarian cancer, hereditary endometrial cancer), genomic sequence analysis panel utilizing a combination of NGS, Sanger, MLPA, and array CGH, with MRNA analytics to resolve variants of unknown significance when indicated (24 genes [sequencing and deletion/duplication], *EPCAM* [deletion/duplication only])

INCLUDES OvaNext®, Ambry Genetics®, Ambry Genetics®

0.00 0.00 FUD 000

0105U Nephrology (chronic kidney disease), multiplex electrochemiluminescent immunoassay (ECLIA) of tumor necrosis factor receptor 1A, receptor superfamily 2 (*TNFR1, TNFR2*), and kidney injury molecule-1 (KIM-1) combined with longitudinal clinical data, including *APOL1* genotype if available, and plasma (isolated fresh or frozen), algorithm reported as probability score for rapid kidney function decline (RKFD)

INCLUDES KidneyIntelXT™, RenalytixAI, RenalytixAI

0.00 0.00 FUD 000

0106U Gastric emptying, serial collection of 7 timed breath specimens, non-radioisotope carbon-13 (^{13}C) spirulina substrate, analysis of each specimen by gas isotope ratio mass spectrometry, reported as rate of $^{13}CO_2$ excretion

INCLUDES 13C-Spirulina Gastric Emptying Breath Test (GEBT), Cairn Diagnostics d/b/a Advanced Breath Diagnostics, LLC, Cairn Diagnostics d/b/a Advanced Breath Diagnostics, LLC

0.00 0.00 FUD 000

0107U Clostridium difficile toxin(s) antigen detection by immunoassay technique, stool, qualitative, multiple-step method

INCLUDES Singulex Clarity C. diff toxins A/B assay, Singulex

0.00 0.00 FUD 000

0108U Gastroenterology (Barrett's esophagus), whole slide-digital imaging, including morphometric analysis, computer-assisted quantitative immunolabeling of 9 protein biomarkers (p16, AMACR, p53, CD68, COX-2, CD45RO, HIF1a, HER-2, K20) and morphology, formalin-fixed paraffin-embedded tissue, algorithm reported as risk of progression to high-grade dysplasia or cancer

INCLUDES TissueCypher® Barrett's Esophagus Assay, Cernostics, Cernostics

0.00 0.00 FUD 000

0109U Infectious disease (Aspergillus species), real-time PCR for detection of DNA from 4 species *(A. fumigatus, A. terreus, A. niger,* and *A. flavus)*, blood, lavage fluid, or tissue, qualitative reporting of presence or absence of each species

INCLUDES MYCODART-PCR™ Dual Amplification Real Time PCR Panel for 4 Aspergillus species, RealTime Laboratories, Inc/MycoDART, Inc

0.00 0.00 FUD 000

0110U Prescription drug monitoring, one or more oral oncology drug(s) and substances, definitive tandem mass spectrometry with chromatography, serum or plasma from capillary blood or venous blood, quantitative report with steady-state range for the prescribed drug(s) when detected

INCLUDES Oral OncolyticAssuranceRX, Firstox Laboratories, LLC, Firstox Laboratories, LLC

0.00 0.00 FUD 000

0111U Oncology (colon cancer), targeted *KRAS* (codons 12, 13, and 61) and *NRAS* (codons 12, 13, and 61) gene analysis utilizing formalin-fixed paraffin-embedded tissue

INCLUDES Praxis(™) Extended RAS Panel, Illumina, Illumina

0.00 0.00 FUD 000

0112U Infectious agent detection and identification, targeted sequence analysis (16S and 18S rRNA genes) with drug-resistance gene

INCLUDES MicroGenDX qPCR & NGS For Infection, MicroGenDX, MicroGenDX

0.00 0.00 FUD 000

0113U Oncology (prostate), measurement of *PCA3* and *TMPRSS2-ERG* in urine and PSA in serum following prostatic massage, by RNA amplification and fluorescence-based detection, algorithm reported as risk score

INCLUDES MiPS (Mi-Prostate Score), MLabs, Mlabs

0.00 0.00 FUD 000

0114U Gastroenterology (Barrett's esophagus), *VIM* and *CCNA1* methylation analysis, esophageal cells, algorithm reported as likelihood for Barrett's esophagus

INCLUDES EsoGuard™, Lucid Diagnostics, Lucid Diagnostics

0.00 0.00 FUD 000

0115U Respiratory infectious agent detection by nucleic acid (DNA and RNA), 18 viral types and subtypes and 2 bacterial targets, amplified probe technique, including multiplex reverse transcription for RNA targets, each analyte reported as detected or not detected

INCLUDES ePlex Respiratory Pathogen (RP) Panel, GenMark Diagnostics, Inc, GenMark Diagnostics, Inc

0.00 0.00 FUD 000

AMA: 2020,Apr,3

0116U Prescription drug monitoring, enzyme immunoassay of 35 or more drugs confirmed with LC-MS/MS, oral fluid, algorithm results reported as a patient-compliance measurement with risk of drug to drug interactions for prescribed medications

INCLUDES Snapshot Oral Fluid Compliance, Ethos Laboratories

0.00 0.00 FUD 000

0117U **Pain management, analysis of 11 endogenous analytes (methylmalonic acid, xanthurenic acid, homocysteine, pyroglutamic acid, vanilmandelate, 5-hydroxyindoleacetic acid, hydroxymethylglutarate, ethylmalonate, 3-hydroxypropyl mercapturic acid (3-HPMA), quinolinic acid, kynurenic acid), LC-MS/MS, urine, algorithm reported as a pain-index score with likelihood of atypical biochemical function associated with pain**

INCLUDES Foundation PI[SM], Ethos Laboratories

0.00 0.00 **FUD** 000

0118U **Transplantation medicine, quantification of donor-derived cell-free DNA using whole genome next-generation sequencing, plasma, reported as percentage of donor-derived cell-free DNA in the total cell-free DNA**

INCLUDES Viracor TRAC™ dd-cfDNA, Viracor Eurofins, Viracor Eurofins

0.00 0.00 **FUD** 000

0119U **Cardiology, ceramides by liquid chromatography-tandem mass spectrometry, plasma, quantitative report with risk score for major cardiovascular events**

INCLUDES MI-HEART Ceramides, Plasma, Mayo Clinic, Laboratory Developed Test

0.00 0.00 **FUD** 000

0120U **Oncology (B-cell lymphoma classification), mRNA, gene expression profiling by fluorescent probe hybridization of 58 genes (45 content and 13 housekeeping genes), formalin-fixed paraffin-embedded tissue, algorithm reported as likelihood for primary mediastinal B-cell lymphoma (PMBCL) and diffuse large B-cell lymphoma (DLBCL) with cell of origin subtyping in the latter**

INCLUDES Lymph3Cx Lymphoma Molecular Subtyping Assay, Mayo Clinic, Laboratory Developed Test

0.00 0.00 **FUD** 000

0121U **Sickle cell disease, microfluidic flow adhesion (VCAM-1), whole blood**

INCLUDES Flow Adhesion of Whole Blood on VCAM-1 (FAB-V), Functional Fluidics, Functional Fluidics

0.00 0.00 **FUD** 000

0122U **Sickle cell disease, microfluidic flow adhesion (P-Selectin), whole blood**

INCLUDES Flow Adhesion of Whole Blood to P-SELECTIN (WB-PSEL), Functional Fluidics, Functional Fluidics

0.00 0.00 **FUD** 000

0123U **Mechanical fragility, RBC, shear stress and spectral analysis profiling**

INCLUDES Mechanical Fragility, RBC by shear stress profiling and spectral analysis, Functional Fluidics, Functional Fluidics

0.00 0.00 **FUD** 000

~~**0124U** **Fetal congenital abnormalities, biochemical assays of 3 analytes (free beta-hCG, PAPP-A, AFP), time-resolved fluorescence immunoassay, maternal dried-blood spot, algorithm reported as risk scores for fetal trisomies 13/18 and 21**~~

~~**0125U** **Fetal congenital abnormalities and perinatal complications, biochemical assays of 5 analytes (free beta-hCG, PAPP-A, AFP, placental growth factor, and inhibin-A), time-resolved fluorescence immunoassay, maternal serum, algorithm reported as risk scores for fetal trisomies 13/18, 21, and preeclampsia**~~

~~**0126U** **Fetal congenital abnormalities and perinatal complications, biochemical assays of 5 analytes (free beta-hCG, PAPP-A, AFP, placental growth factor, and inhibin-A), time-resolved fluorescence immunoassay, includes qualitative assessment of Y chromosome in cell-free fetal DNA, maternal serum and plasma, predictive algorithm reported as a risk scores for fetal trisomies 13/18, 21, and preeclampsia**~~

~~**0127U** **Obstetrics (preeclampsia), biochemical assays of 3 analytes (PAPP-A, AFP, and placental growth factor), time-resolved fluorescence immunoassay, maternal serum, predictive algorithm reported as a risk score for preeclampsia**~~

~~**0128U** **Obstetrics (preeclampsia), biochemical assays of 3 analytes (PAPP-A, AFP, and placental growth factor), time-resolved fluorescence immunoassay, includes qualitative assessment of Y chromosome in cell-free fetal DNA, maternal serum and plasma, predictive algorithm reported as a risk score for preeclampsia**~~

0129U **Hereditary breast cancer-related disorders (eg, hereditary breast cancer, hereditary ovarian cancer, hereditary endometrial cancer), genomic sequence analysis and deletion/duplication analysis panel *(ATM, BRCA1, BRCA2, CDH1, CHEK2, PALB2, PTEN, and TP53)***

INCLUDES BRCAplus, Ambry Genetics

0.00 0.00 **FUD** 000

\+ **0130U** **Hereditary colon cancer disorders (eg, Lynch syndrome, PTEN hamartoma syndrome, Cowden syndrome, familial adenomatosis polyposis), targeted mRNA sequence analysis panel *(APC, CDH1, CHEK2, MLH1, MSH2, MSH6, MUTYH, PMS2, PTEN, and TP53)* (List separately in addition to code for primary procedure)**

INCLUDES +RNAinsight™ for ColoNext®, Ambry Genetics

Code first (81435, 0101U)

0.00 0.00 **FUD** 000

\+ **0131U** **Hereditary breast cancer-related disorders (eg, hereditary breast cancer, hereditary ovarian cancer, hereditary endometrial cancer), targeted mRNA sequence analysis panel (13 genes) (List separately in addition to code for primary procedure)**

INCLUDES +RNAinsight™ for BreastNext®, Ambry Genetics

Code first ([81162], 81432, 0102U)

0.00 0.00 **FUD** 000

\+ **0132U** **Hereditary ovarian cancer-related disorders (eg, hereditary breast cancer, hereditary ovarian cancer, hereditary endometrial cancer), targeted mRNA sequence analysis panel (17 genes) (List separately in addition to code for primary procedure)**

INCLUDES +RNAinsight™ for OvaNext®, Ambry Genetics

Code first ([81162], 81432, 0103U)

0.00 0.00 **FUD** 000

\+ **0133U** **Hereditary prostate cancer-related disorders, targeted mRNA sequence analysis panel (11 genes) (List separately in addition to code for primary procedure)**

INCLUDES +RNAinsight™ for ProstateNext®, Ambry Genetics

Code first ([81162])

0.00 0.00 **FUD** 000

\+ **0134U** **Hereditary pan cancer (eg, hereditary breast and ovarian cancer, hereditary endometrial cancer, hereditary colorectal cancer), targeted mRNA sequence analysis panel (18 genes) (List separately in addition to code for primary procedure)**

INCLUDES +RNAinsight™ for CancerNext®, Ambry Genetics

Code first ([81162], 81432, 81435)

0.00 0.00 **FUD** 000

\+ **0135U** **Hereditary gynecological cancer (eg, hereditary breast and ovarian cancer, hereditary endometrial cancer, hereditary colorectal cancer), targeted mRNA sequence analysis panel (12 genes) (List separately in addition to code for primary procedure)**

INCLUDES +RNAinsight™ for GYNPlus®, Ambry Genetics

Code first ([81162])

0.00 0.00 **FUD** 000

+ **0136U** ***ATM (ataxia telangiectasia mutated)*** **(eg, ataxia telangiectasia) mRNA sequence analysis (List separately in addition to code for primary procedure)**

INCLUDES +RNAinsight™ for *ATM*, Ambry Genetics

Code first (81408)

0.00 0.00 FUD 000

+ **0137U** ***PALB2 (partner and localizer of BRCA2)*** **(eg, breast and pancreatic cancer) mRNA sequence analysis (List separately in addition to code for ...**

INCLUDES +RNAinsight™ for *PALB2*, Ambry Genetics

Code first (81406)

0.00 0.00 FUD 000

+ **0138U** ***BRCA1 (BRCA1, DNA repair associated), BRCA2 (BRCA2, DNA repair associated)*** **(eg, hereditary breast and ovarian cancer) mRNA sequence analysis (List separately in addition to code for primary procedure)**

INCLUDES +RNAinsight™ for *BRCA1/2*, Ambry Genetics

Code first ([81162])

0.00 0.00 FUD 000

● **0139U** **Neurology (autism spectrum disorder [ASD]), quantitative measurements of 6 central carbon metabolites (ie, α-ketoglutarate, alanine, lactate, phenylalanine, pyruvate, and succinate), LC-MS/MS, plasma, algorithmic analysis with result reported as negative or positive (with metabolic subtypes of ASD)**

NPDX ASD Energy Metabolism, Stemina Biomarker Discovery, Inc, Stemina Biomarker Discovery, Inc.

● **0140U** **Infectious disease (fungi), fungal pathogen identification, DNA (15 fungal targets), blood culture, amplified probe technique, each target reported as detected or not detected**

INCLUDES ePlex® BCID Fungal Pathogens Panel, GenMark Diagnostics, Inc, GenMark Diagnostics, Inc

● **0141U** **Infectious disease (bacteria and fungi), gram-positive organism identification and drug resistance element detection, DNA (20 gram-positive bacterial targets, 4 resistance genes, 1 pan gram-negative bacterial target, 1 pan Candida target), blood culture, amplified probe technique, each target reported as detected or not detected**

INCLUDES ePlex® BCID Gram-Positive Panel, GenMark Diagnostics, Inc, GenMark Diagnostics, Inc

● **0142U** **Infectious disease (bacteria and fungi), gram-negative bacterial identification and drug resistance element detection, DNA (21 gram-negative bacterial targets, 6 resistance genes, 1 pan gram-positive bacterial target, 1 pan Candida target), amplified probe technique, each target reported as detected or not detected**

INCLUDES ePlex® BCID Gram-Negative Panel, GenMark Diagnostics, Inc, GenMark Diagnostics, Inc

● **0143U** **Drug assay, definitive, 120 or more drugs or metabolites, urine, quantitative liquid chromatography with tandem mass spectrometry (LC-MS/MS) using multiple reaction monitoring (MRM), with drug or metabolite description, comments including sample validation, per date of service**

INCLUDES CareViewRx, Newstar Medical Laboratories, LLC, Newstar Medical Laboratories, LLC

EXCLUDES *PsychViewRx Plus analysis by Newstar Medical Laboratories, LLC. To report, see (0150U)*

● **0144U** **Drug assay, definitive, 160 or more drugs or metabolites, urine, quantitative liquid chromatography with tandem mass spectrometry (LC-MS/MS) using multiple reaction monitoring (MRM), with drug or metabolite description, comments including sample validation, per date of service**

INCLUDES CareViewRx Plus, Newstar Medical Laboratories, LLC, Newstar Medical Laboratories, LLC

● **0145U** **Drug assay, definitive, 65 or more drugs or metabolites, urine, quantitative liquid chromatography with tandem mass spectrometry (LC-MS/MS) using multiple reaction monitoring (MRM), with drug or metabolite description, comments including sample validation, per date of service**

INCLUDES PainViewRx, Newstar Medical Laboratories, LLC, Newstar Medical Laboratories, LLC

● **0146U** **Drug assay, definitive, 80 or more drugs or metabolites, urine, by quantitative liquid chromatography with tandem mass spectrometry (LC-MS/MS) using multiple reaction monitoring (MRM), with drug or metabolite description, comments including sample validation, per date of service**

INCLUDES PainViewRx Plus, Newstar Medical Laboratories, LLC, Newstar Medical Laboratories, LLC

● **0147U** **Drug assay, definitive, 85 or more drugs or metabolites, urine, quantitative liquid chromatography with tandem mass spectrometry (LC-MS/MS) using multiple reaction monitoring (MRM), with drug or metabolite description, comments including sample validation, per date of service**

INCLUDES RiskViewRx, Newstar Medical Laboratories, LLC, Newstar Medical Laboratories, LLC

● **0148U** **Drug assay, definitive, 100 or more drugs or metabolites, urine, quantitative liquid chromatography with tandem mass spectrometry (LC-MS/MS) using multiple reaction monitoring (MRM), with drug or metabolite description, comments including sample validation, per date of service**

INCLUDES RiskViewRx Plus, Newstar Medical Laboratories, LLC, Newstar Medical Laboratories, LLC

● **0149U** **Drug assay, definitive, 60 or more drugs or metabolites, urine, quantitative liquid chromatography with tandem mass spectrometry (LC-MS/MS) using multiple reaction monitoring (MRM), with drug or metabolite description, comments including sample validation, per date of service**

INCLUDES PsychViewRx, Newstar Medical Laboratories, LLC, Newstar Medical Laboratories, LLC

● **0150U** **Drug assay, definitive, 120 or more drugs or metabolites, urine, quantitative liquid chromatography with tandem mass spectrometry (LC-MS/MS) using multiple reaction monitoring (MRM), with drug or metabolite description, comments including sample validation, per date of service**

INCLUDES PsychViewRx Plus, Newstar Medical Laboratories, LLC, Newstar Medical Laboratories, LLC

EXCLUDES *CareViewRx analysis by Newstar Medical Laboratories, LLC. To report, see (0143U)*

● **0151U** **Infectious disease (bacterial or viral respiratory tract infection), pathogen specific nucleic acid (DNA or RNA), 33 targets, real-time semi-quantitative PCR, bronchoalveolar lavage, sputum, or endotracheal aspirate, detection of 33 organismal and antibiotic resistance genes with limited semi-quantitative results**

INCLUDES BioFire® FilmArray® Pneumonia Panel, BioFire® Diagnostics, BioFire® Diagnostics

AMA: 2020,Apr,3

▲ **0152U** **Infectious disease (bacteria, fungi, parasites, and DNA viruses), microbial cell-free DNA, plasma, untargeted next-generation sequencing, report for significant positive pathogens**

INCLUDES Karius® Test, Karius Inc, Karius Inc

● **0153U** **Oncology (breast), mRNA, gene expression profiling by next-generation sequencing of 101 genes, utilizing formalin-fixed paraffin-embedded tissue, algorithm reported as a triple negative breast cancer clinical subtype(s) with information on immune cell involvement**

INCLUDES Insight TNBCtype™, Insight Molecular Labs

▲ **0154U** **Oncology (urothelial cancer), RNA, analysis by real-time RT-PCR of the *FGFR3 (fibroblast growth factor receptor3)* gene analysis (ie, p.R248C [c.742C>T], p.S249C [c.746C>G], p.G370C [c.1108G>T], p.Y373C [c.1118A>G], FGFR3-TACC3v1, and FGFR3-TACC3v3) utilizing formalin-fixed paraffin-embedded urothelial cancer tumor tissue, reported as *FGFR* gene alteration status**

INCLUDES therascreen® *FGFR* RGQ RT-PCR Kit, QIAGEN, QIAGEN GmbH

AMA: 2020,Jun,11

▲ **0155U** **Oncology (breast cancer), DNA, *PIK3CA (phosphatidylinositol-4,5-bisphosphate 3-kinase, catalytic subunit alpha)* (eg, breast cancer) gene analysis (ie, p.C420R, p.E542K, p.E545A, p.E545D [g.1635G>T only], p.E545G, p.E545K, p.Q546E, p.Q546R, p.H1047L, p.H1047R, p.H1047Y), utilizing formalin-fixed paraffin-embedded breast tumor tissue, reported as *PIK3CA* gene mutation status**

INCLUDES therascreen® *PIK3CA* RGQ PCR Kit, QIAGEN, QIAGEN GmbH

AMA: 2020,Jun,11

● **0156U** **Copy number (eg, intellectual disability, dysmorphology), sequence analysis**

INCLUDES SMASH™, New York Genome Center, Marvel Genomics™

● + **0157U** ***APC (APC regulator of WNT signaling pathway)* (eg, familial adenomatosis polyposis [FAP]) mRNA sequence analysis (List separately in addition to code for primary procedure)**

INCLUDES CustomNext + RNA: *APC*, Ambry Genetics®, Ambry Genetics®

Code first ([81201])

0.00 0.00 **FUD** 000

● + **0158U** ***MLH1 (mutL homolog 1)* (eg, hereditary non-polyposis colorectal cancer, Lynch syndrome) mRNA sequence analysis (List separately in addition to code for primary procedure)**

INCLUDES CustomNext + RNA: *MLH1*, Ambry Genetics®, Ambry Genetics®

Code first ([81292])

0.00 0.00 **FUD** 000

● + **0159U** ***MSH2 (mutS homolog 2)* (eg, hereditary colon cancer, Lynch syndrome) mRNA sequence analysis (List separately in addition to code for primary procedure)**

INCLUDES CustomNext + RNA: *MSH2*, Ambry Genetics®, Ambry Genetics®

Code first ([81295])

0.00 0.00 **FUD** 000

● + **0160U** ***MSH6 (mutS homolog 6)* (eg, hereditary colon cancer, Lynch syndrome) mRNA sequence analysis (List separately in addition to code for primary procedure)**

INCLUDES CustomNext + RNA: *MSH6*, Ambry Genetics®, Ambry Genetics®

Code first (81298)

0.00 0.00 **FUD** 000

● + **0161U** ***PMS2 (PMS1 homolog 2, mismatch repair system component)* (eg, hereditary non-polyposis colorectal cancer, Lynch syndrome) mRNA sequence analysis (List separately in addition to code for primary procedure)**

INCLUDES CustomNext + RNA: *PMS2*, Ambry Genetics®, Ambry Genetics®

Code first (81317)

0.00 0.00 **FUD** 000

● + **0162U** **Hereditary colon cancer (Lynch syndrome), targeted mRNA sequence analysis panel *(MLH1, MSH2, MSH6, PMS2)* (List separately in addition to code for primary procedure)**

INCLUDES CustomNext + RNA: Lynch *(MLH1, MSH2, MSH6, PMS2)*, Ambry Genetics®, Ambry Genetics®

Code first ([81292], [81295], 81298, 81317, 81435)

0.00 0.00 **FUD** 000

● **0163U** **Oncology (colorectal) screening, biochemical enzyme-linked immunosorbent assay (ELISA) of 3 plasma or serum proteins (teratocarcinoma derived growth factor-1 [TDGF-1, Cripto-1], carcinoembryonic antigen [CEA], extracellular matrix protein [ECM]), with demographic data (age, gender, CRC-screening compliance) using a proprietary algorithm and reported as likelihood of CRC or advanced adenomas**

INCLUDES BeScreened™-CRC, Beacon Biomedical Inc, Beacon Biomedical Inc

AMA: 2020,Jun,11

● **0164U** **Gastroenterology (irritable bowel syndrome [IBS]), immunoassay for anti-CdtB and anti-vinculin antibodies, utilizing plasma, algorithm for elevated or not elevated qualitative results**

INCLUDES ibs-smart™, Gemelli Biotech, Gemelli Biotech

AMA: 2020,Jun,11

▲ **0165U** **Peanut allergen-specific quantitative assessment of multiple epitopes using enzyme-linked immunosorbent assay (ELISA), blood, individual epitope results and probability of peanut allergy**

INCLUDES VeriMAP™ Peanut Dx – Bead-based Epitope Assay, AllerGenis™ Clinical Laboratory, AllerGenis™ LLC

AMA: 2020,Jun,11

● **0166U** **Liver disease, 10 biochemical assays (α2-macroglobulin, haptoglobin, apolipoprotein A1, bilirubin, GGT, ALT, AST, triglycerides, cholesterol, fasting glucose) and biometric and demographic data, utilizing serum, algorithm reported as scores for fibrosis, necroinflammatory activity, and steatosis with a summary interpretation**

INCLUDES LiverFASt™, Fibronostics, Fibronostics

AMA: 2020,Jun,11

● **0167U** **Gonadotropin, chorionic (hCG), immunoassay with direct optical observation, blood**

INCLUDES ADEXUSDx hCG Test, NOWDiagnostics, NOWDiagnostics

AMA: 2020,Jun,11

● **0168U** **Fetal aneuploidy (trisomy 21, 18, and 13) DNA sequence analysis of selected regions using maternal plasma without fetal fraction cutoff, algorithm reported as a risk score for each trisomy**

INCLUDES Vanadis® NIPT, PerkinElmer, Inc, PerkinElmer Genomics

AMA: 2020,Jun,11

● **0169U** ***NUDT15 (nudix hydrolase 15)* and *TPMT (thiopurine S-methyltransferase)* (eg, drug metabolism) gene analysis, common variants**

INCLUDES NT *(NUDT15* and *TPMT)* genotyping panel, RPRD Diagnostics

AMA: 2020,Jun,11

● **0170U** **Neurology (autism spectrum disorder [ASD]), RNA, next-generation sequencing, saliva, algorithmic analysis, and results reported as predictive probability of ASD diagnosis**

INCLUDES Clarifi™, Quadrant Biosciences, Inc, Quadrant Biosciences, Inc

AMA: 2020,Jun,11

● **0171U** **Targeted genomic sequence analysis panel, acute myeloid leukemia, myelodysplastic syndrome, and myeloproliferative neoplasms, DNA analysis, 23 genes, interrogation for sequence variants, rearrangements and minimal residual disease, reported as presence/absence**

INCLUDES MyMRD® NGS Panel, Laboratory for Personalized Molecular Medicine, Laboratory for Personalized Molecular Medicine

AMA: 2020,Jun,11

● **0172U** **Oncology (solid tumor as indicated by the label), somatic mutation analysis of *BRCA1 (BRCA1, DNA repair associated), BRCA2 (BRCA2, DNA repair associated)* and analysis of homologous recombination deficiency pathways, DNA, formalin-fixed paraffin-embedded tissue, algorithm quantifying tumor genomic instability score**

INCLUDES myChoice® CDx, Myriad Genetics Laboratories, Inc, Myriad Genetics Laboratories, Inc

● **0173U** **Psychiatry (ie, depression, anxiety), genomic analysis panel, includes variant analysis of 14 genes**

INCLUDES Psych HealthPGx Panel, RPRD Diagnostics, RPRD Diagnostics

● **0174U** **Oncology (solid tumor), mass spectrometric 30 protein targets, formalin-fixed paraffin-embedded tissue, prognostic and predictive algorithm reported as likely, unlikely, or uncertain benefit of 39 chemotherapy and targeted therapeutic oncology agents**

INCLUDES LC-MS/MS Targeted Proteomic Assay, OncoOmicDx Laboratory, LDT

● **0175U** **Psychiatry (eg, depression, anxiety), genomic analysis panel, variant analysis of 15 genes**

INCLUDES Genomind® Professional PGx Express™ CORE, Genomind, Inc, Genomind, Inc

● **0176U** **Cytolethal distending toxin B (CdtB) and vinculin IgG antibodies by immunoassay (ie, ELISA)**

INCLUDES IBS*Schek*®, Commonwealth Diagnostics International, Inc, Commonwealth Diagnostics International, Inc

● **0177U** **Oncology (breast cancer), DNA, *PIK3CA (phosphatidylinositol-4,5-bisphosphate 3-kinase catalytic subunit alpha)* gene analysis of 11 gene variants utilizing plasma, reported as *PIK3CA* gene mutation status**

INCLUDES therascreen® *PIK3CA* RGQ PCR Kit, QIAGEN, QIAGEN GmbH

● **0178U** **Peanut allergen-specific quantitative assessment of multiple epitopes using enzyme-linked immunosorbent assay (ELISA), blood, report of minimum eliciting exposure for a clinical reaction**

INCLUDES VeriMAP™ Peanut Sensitivity - Bead Based Epitope Assay, AllerGenis™ Clinical Laboratory, AllerGenis™ LLC

● **0179U** **Oncology (non-small cell lung cancer), cell-free DNA, targeted sequence analysis of 23 genes (single nucleotide variations, insertions and deletions, fusions without prior knowledge of partner/breakpoint, copy number variations), with report of significant mutation(s)**

INCLUDES Resolution ctDx Lung™, Resolution Bioscience, Resolution Bioscience, Inc

● **0180U** **Red cell antigen (ABO blood group) genotyping (ABO), gene analysis Sanger/chain termination/conventional sequencing, *ABO (ABO, alpha 1-3-N-acetylgalactosaminyltransferase and alpha 1-3-galactosyltransferase)* gene, including subtyping, 7 exons**

INCLUDES Navigator ABO Sequencing, Grifols Immunohematology Center, Grifols Immunohematology Center

● **0181U** **Red cell antigen (Colton blood group) genotyping (CO), gene analysis, *AQP1 (aquaporin 1 [Colton blood group])* exon 1**

INCLUDES Navigator CO Sequencing, Grifols Immunohematology Center, Grifols Immunohematology Center

● **0182U** **Red cell antigen (Cromer blood group) genotyping (CROM), gene analysis, *CD55 (CD55 molecule [Cromer blood group])* exons 1-10**

INCLUDES Navigator CROM Sequencing, Grifols Immunohematology Center, Grifols Immunohematology Center

● **0183U** **Red cell antigen (Diego blood group) genotyping (DI), gene analysis, *SLC4A1 (solute carrier family 4 member 1 [Diego blood group])* exon 19**

INCLUDES Navigator DI Sequencing, Grifols Immunohematology Center, Grifols Immunohematology Center

● **0184U** **Red cell antigen (Dombrock blood group) genotyping (DO), gene analysis, *ART4 (ADP-ribosyltransferase 4 [Dombrock blood group])* exon 2**

INCLUDES Navigator DO Sequencing, Grifols Immunohematology Center, Grifols Immunohematology Center

● **0185U** **Red cell antigen (H blood group) genotyping (FUT1), gene analysis, *FUT1 (fucosyltransferase 1 [H blood group])* exon 4**

INCLUDES Navigator FUT1 Sequencing, Grifols Immunohematology Center, Grifols Immunohematology Center

● **0186U** **Red cell antigen (H blood group) genotyping (FUT2), gene analysis, *FUT2 (fucosyltransferase 2)* exon 2**

INCLUDES Navigator FUT2 Sequencing, Grifols Immunohematology Center, Grifols Immunohematology Center

● **0187U** **Red cell antigen (Duffy blood group) genotyping (FY), gene analysis, *ACKR1 (atypical chemokine receptor 1 [Duffy blood group])* exons 1-2**

INCLUDES Navigator FY Sequencing, Grifols Immunohematology Center, Grifols Immunohematology Center

● **0188U** **Red cell antigen (Gerbich blood group) genotyping (GE), gene analysis, *GYPC (glycophorin C [Gerbich blood group])* exons 1-4**

INCLUDES Navigator GE Sequencing, Grifols Immunohematology Center, Grifols Immunohematology Center

● **0189U** **Red cell antigen (MNS blood group) genotyping (GYPA), gene analysis, *GYPA (glycophorin A [MNS blood group])* introns 1, 5, exon 2**

INCLUDES Navigator GYPA Sequencing, Grifols Immunohematology Center, Grifols Immunohematology Center

● **0190U** **Red cell antigen (MNS blood group) genotyping (GYPB), gene analysis, *GYPB (glycophorin B [MNS blood group])* introns 1, 5, pseudoexon 3**

INCLUDES Navigator GYPB Sequencing, Grifols Immunohematology Center, Grifols Immunohematology Center

● **0191U** **Red cell antigen (Indian blood group) genotyping (IN), gene analysis, *CD44 (CD44 molecule [Indian blood group])* exons 2, 3, 6**

INCLUDES Navigator IN Sequencing, Grifols Immunohematology Center, Grifols Immunohematology Center

● **0192U** **Red cell antigen (Kidd blood group) genotyping (JK), gene analysis, *SLC14A1 (solute carrier family 14 member 1 [Kidd blood group])* gene promoter, exon 9**

INCLUDES Navigator JK Sequencing, Grifols Immunohematology Center, Grifols Immunohematology Center

● **0193U** **Red cell antigen (JR blood group) genotyping (JR), gene analysis, *ABCG2 (ATP binding cassette subfamily G member 2 [Junior blood group])* exons 2-26**

INCLUDES Navigator JR Sequencing, Grifols Immunohematology Center, Grifols Immunohematology Center

● **0194U** **Red cell antigen (Kell blood group) genotyping (KEL), gene analysis, *KEL (Kell metallo-endopeptidase [Kell blood group])* exon 8**

INCLUDES Navigator KEL Sequencing, Grifols Immunohematology Center, Grifols Immunohematology Center

● **0195U** ***KLF1 (Kruppel-like factor 1)*, targeted sequencing (ie, exon 13)**

INCLUDES Navigator *KLF1* Sequencing, Grifols Immunohematology Center, Grifols Immunohematology Center

● **0196U** **Red cell antigen (Lutheran blood group) genotyping (LU), gene analysis, *BCAM (basal cell adhesion molecule [Lutheran blood group])* exon 3**

INCLUDES Navigator LU Sequencing, Grifols Immunohematology Center, Grifols Immunohematology Center

● **0197U** **Red cell antigen (Landsteiner-Wiener blood group) genotyping (LW), gene analysis, *ICAM4 (intercellular adhesion molecule 4 [Landsteiner-Wiener blood group])* exon 1**

INCLUDES Navigator LW Sequencing, Grifols Immunohematology Center, Grifols Immunohematology Center

● **0198U** **Red cell antigen (RH blood group) genotyping (RHD and RHCE), gene analysis Sanger/chain termination/conventional sequencing, *RHD (Rh blood group D antigen)* exons 1-10 and *RHCE (Rh blood group CcEe antigens)* exon 5**

INCLUDES Navigator RHD/CE Sequencing, Grifols Immunohematology Center, Grifols Immunohematology Center

● **0199U** **Red cell antigen (Scianna blood group) genotyping (SC), gene analysis, *ERMAP (erythroblast membrane associated protein [Scianna blood group])* exons 4, 12**

INCLUDES Navigator SC Sequencing, Grifols Immunohematology Center, Grifols Immunohematology Center

● **0200U** **Red cell antigen (Kx blood group) genotyping (XK), gene analysis, *XK (X-linked Kx blood group)* exons 1-3**

INCLUDES Navigator XK Sequencing, Grifols Immunohematology Center, Grifols Immunohematology Center

● **0201U** **Red cell antigen (Yt blood group) genotyping (YT), gene analysis, *ACHE (acetylcholinesterase [Cartwright blood group])* exon 2**

INCLUDES Navigator YT Sequencing, Grifols Immunohematology Center, Grifols Immunohematology Center

● **0202U** **Infectious disease (bacterial or viral respiratory tract infection), pathogen-specific nucleic acid (DNA or RNA), 22 targets including severe acute respiratory syndrome coronavirus 2 (SARS-CoV-2), qualitative RT-PCR, nasopharyngeal swab, each pathogen reported as detected or not detected**

INCLUDES BioFire® Respiratory Panel 2.1 (RP2.1), BioFire® Diagnostics, BioFire® Diagnostics, LLC

EXCLUDES *QIAstat-Dx Respiratory SARS CoV-2 Panel, QIAGEN Sciences, QIAGEN GmbH. To report, see (0223U)*

AMA: 2020,AugSE,1; 2020,AugSE,1; 2020,AugSE,1; 2020,MaySE,1; 2020,May,3; 2020,JuneSE,1

● **0203U** **Autoimmune (inflammatory bowel disease), mRNA, gene expression profiling by quantitative RT-PCR, 17 genes (15 target and 2 reference genes), whole blood, reported as a continuous risk score and classification of inflammatory bowel disease aggressiveness**

INCLUDES PredictSURE IBD™ Test, KSL Diagnostics, PredictImmune Ltd

● **0204U** **Oncology (thyroid), mRNA, gene expression analysis of 593 genes (including *BRAF, RAS, RET, PAX8,* and *NTRK*) for sequence variants and rearrangements, utilizing fine needle aspirate, reported as detected or not detected**

INCLUDES Afirma Xpression Atlas, Veracyte, Inc, Veracyte, Inc

● **0205U** **Ophthalmology (age-related macular degeneration), analysis of 3 gene variants (2 *CFH* gene, 1 *ARMS2* gene), using PCR and MALDI-TOF, buccal swab, reported as positive or negative for neovascular age-related macular-degeneration risk associated with zinc supplements**

INCLUDES Vita Risk®, Arctic Medical Laboratories, Arctic Medical Laboratories

● **0206U** **Neurology (Alzheimer disease); cell aggregation using morphometric imaging and protein kinase C-epsilon (PKCe) concentration in response to amylospheroid treatment by ELISA, cultured skin fibroblasts, each reported as positive or negative for Alzheimer disease**

INCLUDES DISCERN™, NeuroDiagnostics, NeuroDiagnostics

● + **0207U** **quantitative imaging of phosphorylated *ERK1* and *ERK2* in response to bradykinin treatment by in situ immunofluorescence, using cultured skin fibroblasts, reported as a probability index for Alzheimer disease (List separately in addition to code for primary procedure)**

INCLUDES DISCERN™, NeuroDiagnostics, NeuroDiagnostics

Code first (0206U)

0.00 0.00 **FUD** 000

● **0208U** **Oncology (medullary thyroid carcinoma), mRNA, gene expression analysis of 108 genes, utilizing fine needle aspirate, algorithm reported as positive or negative for medullary thyroid carcinoma**

INCLUDES Afirma Medullary Thyroid Carcinoma (MTC) Classifier, Veracyte, Inc, Veracyte, Inc

● **0209U** **Cytogenomic constitutional (genome-wide) analysis, interrogation of genomic regions for copy number, structural changes and areas of homozygosity for chromosomal abnormalities**

INCLUDES CNGnome™, PerkinElmer Genomics, PerkinElmer Genomics

● **0210U** **Syphilis test, non-treponemal antibody, immunoassay, quantitative (RPR)**

INCLUDES BioPlex 2200 RPR Assay - Quantitative, Bio-Rad Laboratories, Bio-Rad Laboratories

● **0211U** **Oncology (pan-tumor), DNA and RNA by next-generation sequencing, utilizing formalin-fixed paraffin-embedded tissue, interpretative report for single nucleotide variants, copy number alterations, tumor mutational burden, and microsatellite instability, with therapy association**

INCLUDES MI Cancer Seek™ - NGS Analysis, Caris MPI d/b/a Caris Life Sciences, Caris MPI d/b/a Caris Life Sciences

● **0212U** **Rare diseases (constitutional/heritable disorders), whole genome and mitochondrial DNA sequence analysis, including small sequence changes, deletions, duplications, short tandem repeat gene expansions, and variants in non-uniquely mappable regions, blood or saliva, identification and categorization of genetic variants, proband**

INCLUDES Genomic Unity® Whole Genome Analysis – Proband, Variantyx Inc, Variantyx Inc

EXCLUDES *Genome (e.g., unexplained constitutional or heritable disorder or syndrome); sequence analysis (81425)*

● **0213U** **Rare diseases (constitutional/heritable disorders), whole genome and mitochondrial DNA sequence analysis, including small sequence changes, deletions, duplications, short tandem repeat gene expansions, and variants in non-uniquely mappable regions, blood or saliva, identification and categorization of genetic variants, each comparator genome (eg, parent, sibling)**

INCLUDES Genomic Unity® Whole Genome Analysis - Comparator, Variantyx Inc, Variantyx Inc

EXCLUDES *Genome (e.g., unexplained constitutional or heritable disorder or syndrome); sequence analysis, each comparator genome (e.g., parents, siblings) (81426)*

● **0214U** **Rare diseases (constitutional/heritable disorders), whole exome and mitochondrial DNA sequence analysis, including small sequence changes, deletions, duplications, short tandem repeat gene expansions, and variants in non-uniquely mappable regions, blood or saliva, identification and categorization of genetic variants, proband**

INCLUDES Genomic Unity® Exome Plus Analysis - Proband, Variantyx Inc, Variantyx Inc

EXCLUDES *Exome (e.g., unexplained constitutional or heritable disorder or syndrome); sequence analysis (81415)*

● **0215U Rare diseases (constitutional/heritable disorders), whole exome and mitochondrial DNA sequence analysis, including small sequence changes, deletions, duplications, short tandem repeat gene expansions, and variants in non-uniquely mappable regions, blood or saliva, identification and categorization of genetic variants, each comparator exome (eg, parent, sibling)**

INCLUDES Genomic Unity® Exome Plus Analysis - Comparator, Variantyx Inc, Variantyx Inc

EXCLUDES *Exome (e.g., unexplained constitutional or heritable disorder or syndrome); sequence analysis, each comparator exome (e.g., parents, siblings) (81416)*

● **0216U Neurology (inherited ataxias), genomic DNA sequence analysis of 12 common genes including small sequence changes, deletions, duplications, short tandem repeat gene expansions, and variants in non-uniquely mappable regions, blood or saliva, identification and categorization of genetic variants**

INCLUDES Genomic Unity® Ataxia Repeat Expansion and Sequence Analysis, Variantyx Inc, Variantyx Inc

● **0217U Neurology (inherited ataxias), genomic DNA sequence analysis of 51 genes including small sequence changes, deletions, duplications, short tandem repeat gene expansions, and variants in non-uniquely mappable regions, blood or saliva, identification and categorization of genetic variants**

INCLUDES Genomic Unity® Comprehensive Ataxia Repeat Expansion and Sequence Analysis, Variantyx Inc, Variantyx Inc

● **0218U Neurology (muscular dystrophy), *DMD* gene sequence analysis, including small sequence changes, deletions, duplications, and variants in non-uniquely mappable regions, blood or saliva, identification and characterization of genetic variants**

INCLUDES Genomic Unity® DMD Analysis, Variantyx Inc, Variantyx Inc

● **0219U Infectious agent (human immunodeficiency virus), targeted viral next-generation sequence analysis (ie, protease [PR], reverse transcriptase [RT], integrase [INT]), algorithm reported as prediction of antiviral drug susceptibility**

INCLUDES *Sentosa®* SQ HIV-1 Genotyping Assay, Vela Diagnostics USA, Inc, Vela Operations Singapore Pte Ltd

● **0220U Oncology (breast cancer), image analysis with artificial intelligence assessment of 12 histologic and immunohistochemical features, reported as a recurrence score**

INCLUDES PreciseDx™ Breast Cancer Test, PreciseDx, PreciseDx

● **0221U Red cell antigen (ABO blood group) genotyping (ABO), gene analysis, next-generation sequencing, *ABO (ABO, alpha 1-3-N-acetylgalactosaminyltransferase and alpha 1-3-galactosyltransferase)* gene**

INCLUDES Navigator ABO Blood Group NGS, Grifols Immunohematology Center, Grifols Immunohematology Center

● **0222U Red cell antigen (RH blood group) genotyping (RHD and RHCE), gene analysis, next-generation sequencing, RH proximal promoter, exons 1-10, portions of introns 2-3**

INCLUDES Navigator Rh Blood Group NGS, Grifols Immunohematology Center, Grifols Immunohematology Center

● **0223U Infectious disease (bacterial or viral respiratory tract infection), pathogen-specific nucleic acid (DNA or RNA), 22 targets including severe acute respiratory syndrome coronavirus 2 (SARS-CoV-2), qualitative RT-PCR, nasopharyngeal swab, each pathogen reported as detected or not detected**

INCLUDES QIAstat-Dx Respiratory SARS CoV-2 Panel, QIAGEN Sciences, QIAGEN GmbH

EXCLUDES *BioFire® Respiratory Panel 2.1 (RP2.1), BioFire® Diagnostics, BioFire® Diagnostics, LLC. To report, see (0202U)*

AMA: 2020,AugSE,1; 2020,AugSE,1; 2020,AugSE,1

● **0224U Antibody, severe acute respiratory syndrome coronavirus 2 (SARS-CoV-2) (Coronavirus disease [COVID-19]), includes titer(s), when performed**

INCLUDES COVID-19 Antibody Test, Mt Sinai, Mount Sinai Laboratory

EXCLUDES *Antibody; severe acute respiratory syndrome coronavirus 2 (SARS-CoV-2) (coronavirus disease [COVID-19]) (86769)*

AMA: 2020,AugSE,1; 2020,AugSE,1; 2020,AugSE,1

● **0225U Infectious disease (bacterial or viral respiratory tract infection) pathogen-specific DNA and RNA, 21 targets, including severe acute respiratory syndrome coronavirus 2 (SARS-CoV-2), amplified probe technique, including multiplex reverse transcription for RNA targets, each analyte reported as detected or not detected**

INCLUDES ePlex® Respiratory Pathogen Panel 2, GenMark Dx, GenMark Diagnostics, Inc

AMA: 2020,AugSE,1

● **0226U Surrogate viral neutralization test (sVNT), severe acute respiratory syndrome coronavirus 2 (SARS-CoV-2) (Coronavirus disease [COVID-19]), ELISA, plasma, serum**

INCLUDES Tru-Immune™, Ethos Laboratories, GenScript® USA Inc

AMA: 2020,AugSE,1

● **0227U Drug assay, presumptive, 30 or more drugs or metabolites, urine, liquid chromatography with tandem mass spectrometry (LC-MS/MS) using multiple reaction monitoring (MRM), with drug or metabolite description, includes sample validation**

INCLUDES Comprehensive Screen, Aspenti Health

● **0228U Oncology (prostate), multianalyte molecular profile by photometric detection of macromolecules adsorbed on nanosponge array slides with machine learning, utilizing first morning voided urine, algorithm reported as likelihood of prostate cancer**

INCLUDES PanGIA Prostate, Genetics Institute of America, Entopsis, LLC

● **0229U *BCAT1 (Branched chain amino acid transaminase 1)* or *IKZF1 (IKAROS family zinc finger 1)* (eg, colorectal cancer) promoter methylation analysis**

INCLUDES Colvera®, Clinical Genomics Pathology Inc

● **0230U *AR (androgen receptor)* (eg, spinal and bulbar muscular atrophy, Kennedy disease, X chromosome inactivation), full sequence analysis, including small sequence changes in exonic and intronic regions, deletions, duplications, short tandem repeat (STR) expansions, mobile element insertions, and variants in non-uniquely mappable regions**

INCLUDES Genomic Unity® AR Analysis, Variantyx Inc, Variantyx Inc

● **0231U *CACNA1A (calcium voltage-gated channel subunit alpha 1A)* (eg, spinocerebellar ataxia), full gene analysis, including small sequence changes in exonic and intronic regions, deletions, duplications, short tandem repeat (STR) gene expansions, mobile element insertions, and variants in non-uniquely mappable regions**

INCLUDES Genomic Unity® CACNA1A Analysis, Variantyx Inc, Variantyx Inc

● **0232U** ***CSTB (cystatin B)*** **(eg, progressive myoclonic epilepsy type 1A, Unverricht-Lundborg disease), full gene analysis, including small sequence changes in exonic and intronic regions, deletions, duplications, short tandem repeat (STR) expansions, mobile element insertions, and variants in non-uniquely mappable regions**

INCLUDES Genomic Unity® CSTB Analysis, Variantyx Inc, Variantyx Inc

● **0233U** ***FXN (frataxin)*** **(eg, Friedreich ataxia), gene analysis, including small sequence changes in exonic and intronic regions, deletions, duplications, short tandem repeat (STR) expansions, mobile element insertions, and variants in non-uniquely mappable regions**

INCLUDES Genomic Unity® FXN Analysis, Variantyx Inc, Variantyx Inc

● **0234U** ***MECP2 (methyl CpG binding protein 2)*** **(eg, Rett syndrome), full gene analysis, including small sequence changes in exonic and intronic regions, deletions, duplications, mobile element insertions, and variants in non-uniquely mappable regions**

INCLUDES Genomic Unity® MECP2 Analysis, Variantyx Inc, Variantyx Inc

● **0235U** ***PTEN (phosphatase and tensin homolog)*** **(eg, Cowden syndrome, PTEN hamartoma tumor syndrome), full gene analysis, including small sequence changes in exonic and intronic regions, deletions, duplications, mobile element insertions, and variants in non-uniquely mappable regions**

INCLUDES Genomic Unity® PTEN Analysis, Variantyx Inc, Variantyx Inc

● **0236U** ***SMN1 (survival of motor neuron 1, telomeric)*** **and** ***SMN2 (survival of motor neuron 2, centromeric)*** **(eg, spinal muscular atrophy) full gene analysis, including small sequence changes in exonic and intronic regions, duplications and deletions, and mobile element insertions**

INCLUDES Genomic Unity® SMN1/2 Analysis, Variantyx Inc, Variantyx Inc

● **0237U** **Cardiac ion channelopathies (eg, Brugada syndrome, long QT syndrome, short QT syndrome, catecholaminergic polymorphic ventricular tachycardia), genomic sequence analysis panel including** ***ANK2, CASQ2, CAV3, KCNE1, KCNE2, KCNH2, KCNJ2, KCNQ1, RYR2,*** **and** ***SCN5A,*** **including small sequence changes in exonic and intronic regions, deletions, duplications, mobile element insertions, and variants in non-uniquely mappable regions**

INCLUDES Genomic Unity® Cardiac Ion Channelopathies Analysis, Variantyx Inc, Variantyx Inc

● **0238U** **Oncology (Lynch syndrome), genomic DNA sequence analysis of** ***MLH1, MSH2, MSH6, PMS2,*** **and** ***EPCAM,*** **including small sequence changes in exonic and intronic regions, deletions, duplications, mobile element insertions, and variants in non-uniquely mappable regions**

INCLUDES Genomic Unity® Lynch Syndrome Analysis, Variantyx Inc, Variantyx Inc

● **0239U** **Targeted genomic sequence analysis panel, solid organ neoplasm, cell-free DNA, analysis of 311 or more genes, interrogation for sequence variants, including substitutions, insertions, deletions, select rearrangements, and copy number variations**

INCLUDES FoundationOne® Liquid CDx, FOUNDATION MEDICINE, INC, FOUNDATION MEDICINE, INC

● **0240U** **Infectious disease (viral respiratory tract infection), pathogen-specific RNA, 3 targets (severe acute respiratory syndrome coronavirus 2 [SARS-CoV-2], influenza A, influenza B), upper respiratory specimen, each pathogen reported as detected or not detected**

INCLUDES Xpert® Xpress SARS-CoV-2/Flu/RSV (SARS-CoV-2 & Flu targets only), Cepheid

● **0241U** **Infectious disease (viral respiratory tract infection), pathogen-specific RNA, 4 targets (severe acute respiratory syndrome coronavirus 2 [SARS-CoV-2], influenza A, influenza B, respiratory syncytial virus [RSV]), upper respiratory specimen, each pathogen reported as detected or not detected**

INCLUDES Xpert® Xpress SARS-CoV-2/Flu/RSV (all targets), Cepheid

90281-90399 Immunoglobulin Products

[INCLUDES] Immune globulin product only
- Anti-infectives
- Antitoxins
- Isoantibodies
- Monoclonal antibodies

Code also (96365-96372, 96374-96375)

90281 Immune globulin (Ig), human, for intramuscular use
[INCLUDES] Gamastan
✚ 0.00 ⚕ 0.00 **FUD** XXX [51] [E] ⚑
AMA: 2020,Jan,11; 2018,Jan,8; 2017,Jan,8; 2016,Jan,13; 2015,Jan,16

90283 Immune globulin (IgIV), human, for intravenous use
✚ 0.00 ⚕ 0.00 **FUD** XXX [51] [E] ⚑
AMA: 2020,Jan,11; 2018,Jan,8; 2017,Jan,8; 2016,Jan,13; 2015,Jan,16

90284 Immune globulin (SCIg), human, for use in subcutaneous infusions, 100 mg, each
✚ 0.00 ⚕ 0.00 **FUD** XXX [51] [E] ⚑
AMA: 2020,Jan,11; 2018,Jan,8; 2017,Jan,8; 2016,Jan,13; 2015,Jan,16

90287 Botulinum antitoxin, equine, any route
✚ 0.00 ⚕ 0.00 **FUD** XXX [51] [E] ⚑
AMA: 2020,Jan,11; 2018,Jan,8; 2017,Jan,8; 2016,Jan,13; 2015,Jan,16

90288 Botulism immune globulin, human, for intravenous use
✚ 0.00 ⚕ 0.00 **FUD** XXX [51] [E] ⚑
AMA: 2020,Jan,11; 2018,Jan,8; 2017,Jan,8; 2016,Jan,13; 2015,Jan,16

90291 Cytomegalovirus immune globulin (CMV-IgIV), human, for intravenous use
[INCLUDES] Cytogram
✚ 0.00 ⚕ 0.00 **FUD** XXX [51] [E] ⚑
AMA: 2020,Jan,11; 2018,Jan,8; 2017,Jan,8; 2016,Jan,13; 2015,Jan,16

90296 Diphtheria antitoxin, equine, any route
✚ 0.00 ⚕ 0.00 **FUD** XXX [51] [E] ⚑
AMA: 2020,Jan,11; 2018,Jan,8; 2017,Jan,8; 2016,Jan,13; 2015,Jan,16

90371 Hepatitis B immune globulin (HBIg), human, for intramuscular use
[INCLUDES] HBIG
✚ 0.00 ⚕ 0.00 **FUD** XXX [51] [K] [K2] ⚑
AMA: 2020,Jan,11; 2018,Jan,8; 2017,Jan,8; 2016,Jan,13; 2015,Jan,16

90375 Rabies immune globulin (RIg), human, for intramuscular and/or subcutaneous use
[INCLUDES] HyperRAB
✚ 0.00 ⚕ 0.00 **FUD** XXX [51] [K] [K2] ⚑
AMA: 2020,Jan,11; 2018,Jan,8; 2017,Jan,8; 2016,Jan,13; 2015,Jan,16

90376 Rabies immune globulin, heat-treated (RIg-HT), human, for intramuscular and/or subcutaneous use
✚ 0.00 ⚕ 0.00 **FUD** XXX [51] [K] [K2] ⚑
AMA: 2020,Jan,11; 2018,Jan,8; 2017,Jan,8; 2016,Jan,13; 2015,Jan,16

● **90377 Rabies immune globulin, heat- and solvent/detergent-treated (RIg-HT S/D), human, for intramuscular and/or subcutaneous use**
✚ 0.00 ⚕ 0.00 **FUD** 000 [51]

90378 Respiratory syncytial virus, monoclonal antibody, recombinant, for intramuscular use, 50 mg, each
[INCLUDES] Synagis
✚ 0.00 ⚕ 0.00 **FUD** XXX [51] [K] [K2] ⚑
AMA: 2020,Jan,11; 2018,Jan,8; 2017,Jan,8; 2016,Jan,13; 2015,Jan,16

90384 Rho(D) immune globulin (RhIg), human, full-dose, for intramuscular use
✚ 0.00 ⚕ 0.00 **FUD** XXX [51] [E] ⚑
AMA: 2020,Jan,11; 2018,Jan,8; 2017,Jan,8; 2016,Jan,13; 2015,Jan,16

90385 Rho(D) immune globulin (RhIg), human, mini-dose, for intramuscular use
✚ 0.00 ⚕ 0.00 **FUD** XXX [51] [E] ⚑
AMA: 2020,Jan,11; 2018,Jan,8; 2017,Jan,8; 2016,Jan,13; 2015,Jan,16

90386 Rho(D) immune globulin (RhIgIV), human, for intravenous use
✚ 0.00 ⚕ 0.00 **FUD** XXX [51] [E] ⚑
AMA: 2020,Jan,11; 2018,Jan,8; 2017,Jan,8; 2016,Jan,13; 2015,Jan,16

90389 Tetanus immune globulin (TIg), human, for intramuscular use
[INCLUDES] HyperTET S/D (Tetanus Immune Globulin)
✚ 0.00 ⚕ 0.00 **FUD** XXX [51] [E] ⚑
AMA: 2020,Jan,11; 2018,Jan,8; 2017,Jan,8; 2016,Jan,13; 2015,Jan,16

90393 Vaccinia immune globulin, human, for intramuscular use
✚ 0.00 ⚕ 0.00 **FUD** XXX [51] [E] ⚑
AMA: 2020,Jan,11; 2018,Jan,8; 2017,Jan,8; 2016,Jan,13; 2015,Jan,16

90396 Varicella-zoster immune globulin, human, for intramuscular use
[INCLUDES] VariZIG
✚ 0.00 ⚕ 0.00 **FUD** XXX [51] [K] [K2] ⚑
AMA: 2020,Jan,11; 2018,Jan,8; 2017,Jan,8; 2016,Jan,13; 2015,Jan,16

90399 Unlisted immune globulin
✚ 0.00 ⚕ 0.00 **FUD** XXX [51] [E] ⚑
AMA: 2020,Jan,11; 2018,Jan,8; 2017,Jan,8; 2016,Jan,13; 2015,Jan,16

90460-90461 Injections Provided with Counseling

[INCLUDES]
- All components influenza vaccine, report one time only
- Combination vaccines which comprise multiple vaccine components
- Components (all antigens) in vaccines to prevent disease due to specific organisms
- Counseling by physician or other qualified health care professional
- Multivalent antigens or multiple antigen serotypes against single organisms considered one component
- Patient/family face-to-face counseling by doctor or qualified health care professional for patients age 18 years and younger

[EXCLUDES]
- *Administration influenza and pneumococcal vaccine for Medicare patients (G0008-G0009)*
- *Allergy testing (95004-95028)*
- *Bacterial/viral/fungal skin tests (86485-86580)*
- *Diagnostic or therapeutic injections (96365-96371, 96372-96379)*
- *Vaccines provided without face-to-face counseling from physician or qualified health care professional or to patients age 18 years and older (90471-90474)*

Code also significant, separately identifiable E/M service when appropriate
Code also toxoid/vaccine (90476-90749 [90620, 90621, 90625, 90630, 90644, 90672, 90673, 90674, 90750, 90756])

90460 Immunization administration through 18 years of age via any route of administration, with counseling by physician or other qualified health care professional; first or only component of each vaccine or toxoid administered [A]
Code also each additional component in vaccine (e.g., 5-year-old receives DtaP-IPV IM administration, and MMR/Varicella vaccines SQ administration. Report initial component two times, and additional components six times)
✚ 0.47 ⚕ 0.47 **FUD** XXX [B] [80] ⚑
AMA: 2020,Jul,11; 2020,Jan,11; 2018,Nov,7; 2018,Jan,8; 2017,Jan,8; 2016,Oct,6; 2016,Jan,13; 2015,May,6; 2015,Apr,10; 2015,Apr,9; 2015,Jan,16

+ **90461** **each additional vaccine or toxoid component administered (List separately in addition to code for primary procedure)** A

Code also each additional component in vaccine (e.g., 5-year-old receives DtaP-IPV IM administration, and MMR/Varicella vaccines SQ administration. Report initial component two times, and additional components six times)

Code first initial component in each vaccine provided (90460)

0.36 0.36 FUD ZZZ B 80

AMA: 2020,Jul,11; 2020,Jan,11; 2018,Nov,7; 2018,Jan,8; 2017,Jan,8; 2016,Oct,6; 2016,Jan,13; 2015,May,6; 2015,Apr,10; 2015,Jan,16

90471-90474 Injections and Other Routes of Administration Without Physician Counseling

CMS: 100-04,18,10.4 CWF Edits for Influenza Virus and Pneumococcal Vaccinations

EXCLUDES *Administration influenza and pneumococcal vaccine for Medicare patients (G0008-G0009)*
Administration vaccine with counseling (90460-90461)
Allergy testing (95004-95028)
Bacterial/viral/fungal skin tests (86485-86580)
Diagnostic or therapeutic injections (96365-96371, 96374)
Patient/family face-to-face counseling

Code also significant separately identifiable E/M service when appropriate

Code also toxoid/vaccine (90476-90749 [90620, 90621, 90625, 90630, 90644, 90672, 90673, 90674, 90750, 90756])

90471 **Immunization administration (includes percutaneous, intradermal, subcutaneous, or intramuscular injections); 1 vaccine (single or combination vaccine/toxoid)**

EXCLUDES *Intranasal/oral administration (90473)*

0.40 0.40 FUD XXX Q1 80

AMA: 2020,Jul,11; 2020,Jan,11; 2019,Jun,11; 2018,Nov,7; 2018,Jan,8; 2017,Jan,8; 2016,Oct,6; 2016,Jan,13; 2015,May,6; 2015,Apr,9; 2015,Apr,10; 2015,Jan,16

+ **90472** **each additional vaccine (single or combination vaccine/toxoid) (List separately in addition to code for primary procedure)**

EXCLUDES *BCG vaccine, intravesical administration (51720, 90586)*
Immune globulin administration (96365-96371, 96374)
Immune globulin product (90281-90399)

Code first initial vaccine (90460, 90471, 90473)

0.36 0.36 FUD ZZZ N 80

AMA: 2020,Jul,11; 2020,Jan,11; 2018,Nov,7; 2018,Jan,8; 2017,Jan,8; 2016,Oct,6; 2016,Jan,13; 2015,May,6; 2015,Apr,9; 2015,Apr,10; 2015,Jan,16

90473 **Immunization administration by intranasal or oral route; 1 vaccine (single or combination vaccine/toxoid)**

EXCLUDES *Administration by injection (90471)*

0.47 0.47 FUD XXX Q1 80

AMA: 2020,Jan,11; 2018,Nov,7; 2018,Jan,8; 2017,Jan,8; 2016,Jan,13; 2015,May,6; 2015,Jan,16

+ **90474** **each additional vaccine (single or combination vaccine/toxoid) (List separately in addition to code for primary procedure)**

Code first initial vaccine (90460, 90471, 90473)

0.36 0.36 FUD ZZZ N 80

AMA: 2018,Nov,7; 2018,Jan,8; 2017,Jan,8; 2016,Jan,13; 2015,May,6; 2015,Apr,9; 2015,Jan,16

90476-90756 [90619, 90620, 90621, 90625, 90630, 90644, 90672, 90673, 90674, 90694, 90750, 90756] Vaccination Products

INCLUDES Patient's age for reporting purposes, not for product license
Vaccine product only

EXCLUDES *Immune globulins and administration (90281-90399, 96365-96375)*
Reporting each combination vaccine component individually

Code also administration vaccine (90460-90474)

Code also significant separately identifiable E/M service when appropriate

90476 **Adenovirus vaccine, type 4, live, for oral use**

INCLUDES Adeno-4

0.00 0.00 FUD XXX (51) N N1

AMA: 2018,Jan,8; 2017,Jan,8; 2016,Jan,13; 2015,May,6; 2015,Jan,16

90477 **Adenovirus vaccine, type 7, live, for oral use**

INCLUDES Adeno-7

0.00 0.00 FUD XXX (51) M

AMA: 2018,Jan,8; 2017,Jan,8; 2016,Jan,13; 2015,May,6; 2015,Jan,16

90581 **Anthrax vaccine, for subcutaneous or intramuscular use**

INCLUDES BioThrax

0.00 0.00 FUD XXX (51) E

AMA: 2018,Jan,8; 2017,Jan,8; 2016,Jan,13; 2015,May,6; 2015,Jan,16

90585 **Bacillus Calmette-Guerin vaccine (BCG) for tuberculosis, live, for percutaneous use**

INCLUDES Mycobax

0.00 0.00 FUD XXX (51) M

AMA: 2018,Jan,8; 2017,Jan,8; 2016,Jan,13; 2015,May,6; 2015,Jan,16

90586 **Bacillus Calmette-Guerin vaccine (BCG) for bladder cancer, live, for intravesical use**

INCLUDES TheraCys
TICE BCG

0.00 0.00 FUD XXX (51) B

AMA: 2020,Jan,11; 2018,Jan,8; 2017,Jan,8; 2016,Jan,13; 2015,May,6; 2015,Jan,16

90587 **Dengue vaccine, quadrivalent, live, 3 dose schedule, for subcutaneous use**

0.00 0.00 FUD XXX (51) E

AMA: 2018,Nov,7; 2018,Jan,8

90619 **Resequenced code. See code following 90734.**

90620 **Resequenced code. See code following 90734.**

90621 **Resequenced code. See code following 90734.**

90625 **Resequenced code. See code following 90723.**

90630 **Resequenced code. See code following 90654.**

90632 **Hepatitis A vaccine (HepA), adult dosage, for intramuscular use** A

INCLUDES Havrix
Vaqta

0.00 0.00 FUD XXX (51) N N1

AMA: 2018,Jan,8; 2017,Jan,8; 2016,Jan,13; 2015,May,6; 2015,Jan,16

90633 **Hepatitis A vaccine (HepA), pediatric/adolescent dosage-2 dose schedule, for intramuscular use** A

INCLUDES Havrix
Vaqta

0.00 0.00 FUD XXX (51) N N1

AMA: 2018,Jan,8; 2017,Jan,8; 2016,Jan,13; 2015,May,6; 2015,Jan,16

90634 **Hepatitis A vaccine (HepA), pediatric/adolescent dosage-3 dose schedule, for intramuscular use** A

INCLUDES Havrix

0.00 0.00 FUD XXX (51) N N1

AMA: 2018,Jan,8; 2017,Jan,8; 2016,Jan,13; 2015,May,6; 2015,Jan,16

90636 **Hepatitis A and hepatitis B vaccine (HepA-HepB), adult dosage, for intramuscular use** A

INCLUDES Twinrix

0.00 0.00 FUD XXX (51) N N1

AMA: 2018,Jan,8; 2017,Jan,8; 2016,Jan,13; 2015,May,6; 2015,Jan,16

90644 **Resequenced code. See code following 90732.**

90647 **Haemophilus influenzae type b vaccine (Hib), PRP-OMP conjugate, 3 dose schedule, for intramuscular use**

INCLUDES PedvaxHIB

0.00 0.00 FUD XXX (51) N N1

AMA: 2018,Jan,8; 2017,Jan,8; 2016,Jan,13; 2015,May,6; 2015,Jan,16

90648 Haemophilus influenzae type b vaccine (Hib), PRP-T conjugate, 4 dose schedule, for intramuscular use

INCLUDES ActHIB
Hiberix
OmniHIB

0.00 0.00 FUD XXX

AMA: 2018,Jan,8; 2017,Jan,8; 2016,Jan,13; 2015,May,6; 2015,Jan,16

90649 Human Papillomavirus vaccine, types 6, 11, 16, 18, quadrivalent (4vHPV), 3 dose schedule, for intramuscular use

INCLUDES Gardasil

0.00 0.00 FUD XXX

AMA: 2018,Jan,8; 2017,Jan,8; 2016,Jan,13; 2015,May,6; 2015,Jan,16

90650 Human Papillomavirus vaccine, types 16, 18, bivalent (2vHPV), 3 dose schedule, for intramuscular use

INCLUDES Cervarix

0.00 0.00 FUD XXX

AMA: 2018,Jan,8; 2017,Jan,8; 2016,Jan,13; 2015,May,6; 2015,Jan,16

90651 Human Papillomavirus vaccine types 6, 11, 16, 18, 31, 33, 45, 52, 58, nonavalent (9vHPV), 2 or 3 dose schedule, for intramuscular use

INCLUDES GARDASIL 9

0.00 0.00 FUD XXX

AMA: 2018,Nov,7; 2018,Jan,8; 2017,Jan,8; 2016,Jan,13; 2015,May,6; 2015,Jan,16

90653 Influenza vaccine, inactivated (IIV), subunit, adjuvanted, for intramuscular use

INCLUDES Fluad

0.00 0.00 FUD XXX

AMA: 2019,Jun,11; 2018,Jan,8; 2017,Jan,8; 2016,Oct,6; 2016,Jan,13; 2015,May,6; 2015,Jan,16

90654 Influenza virus vaccine, trivalent (IIV3), split virus, preservative-free, for intradermal use

INCLUDES Fluzone intradermal

0.00 0.00 FUD XXX

AMA: 2018,Jan,8; 2017,Jan,8; 2016,Jan,13; 2015,May,6; 2015,Apr,9; 2015,Jan,16

90630 Influenza virus vaccine, quadrivalent (IIV4), split virus, preservative free, for intradermal use

INCLUDES Fluzone Intradermal Quadrivalent

0.00 0.00 FUD XXX

AMA: 2018,Jan,8; 2017,Jan,8; 2016,Jan,13; 2015,May,6; 2015,Jan,16

90655 Influenza virus vaccine, trivalent (IIV3), split virus, preservative free, 0.25 mL dosage, for intramuscular use

INCLUDES Afluria
Fluzone, no preservative, pediatric dose

0.00 0.00 FUD XXX

AMA: 2018,Jan,8; 2017,Jan,8; 2016,Oct,6; 2016,May,9; 2016,Jan,13; 2015,May,6; 2015,Jan,16

90656 Influenza virus vaccine, trivalent (IIV3), split virus, preservative free, 0.5 mL dosage, for intramuscular use

INCLUDES Afluria

0.00 0.00 FUD XXX

AMA: 2018,Jan,8; 2017,Jan,8; 2016,Oct,6; 2016,May,9; 2016,Jan,13; 2015,May,6; 2015,Jan,16

90657 Influenza virus vaccine, trivalent (IIV3), split virus, 0.25 mL dosage, for intramuscular use

INCLUDES Afluria
Flulaval
Fluvirin
Fluzone (5 ml vial [0.25ml dose])

0.00 0.00 FUD XXX

AMA: 2018,Jan,8; 2017,Jan,8; 2016,Oct,6; 2016,May,9; 2016,Jan,13; 2015,May,6; 2015,Jan,16

90658 Influenza virus vaccine, trivalent (IIV3), split virus, 0.5 mL dosage, for intramuscular use

INCLUDES Afluria
Flulaval
Fluvirin
Fluzone

0.00 0.00 FUD XXX

AMA: 2018,Jan,8; 2017,Jan,8; 2016,Oct,6; 2016,May,9; 2016,Jan,13; 2015,May,6; 2015,Jan,16

90660 Influenza virus vaccine, trivalent, live (LAIV3), for intranasal use

INCLUDES FluMist

0.00 0.00 FUD XXX

AMA: 2018,Jan,8; 2017,Jan,8; 2016,Jan,13; 2015,May,6; 2015,Jan,16

90672 Influenza virus vaccine, quadrivalent, live (LAIV4), for intranasal use

INCLUDES FluMist Quadrivalent

0.00 0.00 FUD XXX

AMA: 2018,Jan,8; 2017,Jan,8; 2016,Jan,13; 2015,May,6; 2015,Jan,16

90661 Influenza virus vaccine (ccIIV3), derived from cell cultures, subunit, preservative and antibiotic free, for intramuscular use

INCLUDES Flucelvax

0.00 0.00 FUD XXX

AMA: 2018,Jan,8; 2017,Jan,8; 2016,Oct,6; 2016,Jan,13; 2015,May,6; 2015,Jan,16

90674 Influenza virus vaccine, quadrivalent (ccIIV4), derived from cell cultures, subunit, preservative and antibiotic free, 0.5 mL dosage, for intramuscular use

INCLUDES Flucelvax Quadrivalent

0.00 0.00 FUD XXX

AMA: 2018,Jan,8; 2017,Jan,8; 2016,Oct,6

90756 Influenza virus vaccine, quadrivalent (ccIIV4), derived from cell cultures, subunit, antibiotic free, 0.5mL dosage, for intramuscular use

INCLUDES Flucelvax Quadrivalent

0.00 0.00 FUD XXX

AMA: 2018,Nov,7

90673 Influenza virus vaccine, trivalent (RIV3), derived from recombinant DNA, hemagglutinin (HA) protein only, preservative and antibiotic free, for intramuscular use

0.00 0.00 FUD XXX

AMA: 2018,Jan,8; 2017,Jan,8; 2016,Jan,13; 2015,May,6; 2015,Jan,16

90662 Influenza virus vaccine (IIV), split virus, preservative free, enhanced immunogenicity via increased antigen content, for intramuscular use

INCLUDES Fluzone high-dose Quadribalent

0.00 0.00 FUD XXX

AMA: 2018,Jan,8; 2017,Jan,8; 2016,Jan,13; 2015,May,6; 2015,Jan,16

90664 Influenza virus vaccine, live (LAIV), pandemic formulation, for intranasal use

0.00 0.00 FUD XXX

AMA: 2018,Jan,8; 2017,Jan,8; 2016,Jan,13; 2015,May,6; 2015,Jan,16

Medicine

90648 — 90664

90666 **Influenza virus vaccine (IIV), pandemic formulation, split virus, preservative free, for intramuscular use**
0.00 0.00 FUD XXX
AMA: 2018,Jan,8; 2017,Jan,8; 2016,Jan,13; 2015,May,6; 2015,Jan,16

90667 **Influenza virus vaccine (IIV), pandemic formulation, split virus, adjuvanted, for intramuscular use**
0.00 0.00 FUD XXX
AMA: 2018,Jan,8; 2017,Jan,8; 2016,Jan,13; 2015,May,6; 2015,Jan,16

90668 **Influenza virus vaccine (IIV), pandemic formulation, split virus, for intramuscular use**
0.00 0.00 FUD XXX
AMA: 2018,Jan,8; 2017,Jan,8; 2016,Jan,13; 2015,May,6; 2015,Jan,16

90670 **Pneumococcal conjugate vaccine, 13 valent (PCV13), for intramuscular use**
INCLUDES Prevnar 13
0.00 0.00 FUD XXX
AMA: 2018,Jan,8; 2017,Jan,8; 2016,Jan,13; 2015,May,6; 2015,Jan,16

90672 **Resequenced code. See code following 90660.**

90673 **Resequenced code. See code before 90662.**

90674 **Resequenced code. See code following 90661.**

90675 **Rabies vaccine, for intramuscular use**
INCLUDES Imovax
RabAvert
0.00 0.00 FUD XXX
AMA: 2018,Jan,8; 2017,Jan,8; 2016,Jan,13; 2015,May,6; 2015,Jan,16

90676 **Rabies vaccine, for intradermal use**
0.00 0.00 FUD XXX
AMA: 2018,Jan,8; 2017,Jan,8; 2016,Jan,13; 2015,May,6; 2015,Jan,16

90680 **Rotavirus vaccine, pentavalent (RV5), 3 dose schedule, live, for oral use**
INCLUDES RotaTeq
0.00 0.00 FUD XXX
AMA: 2018,Jan,8; 2017,Jan,8; 2016,Jan,13; 2015,May,6; 2015,Jan,16

90681 **Rotavirus vaccine, human, attenuated (RV1), 2 dose schedule, live, for oral use**
INCLUDES Rotarix
0.00 0.00 FUD XXX
AMA: 2018,Jan,8; 2017,Jan,8; 2016,Jan,13; 2015,May,6; 2015,Jan,16

90682 **Influenza virus vaccine, quadrivalent (RIV4), derived from recombinant DNA, hemagglutinin (HA) protein only, preservative and antibiotic free, for intramuscular use**
INCLUDES Flublok Quadrivalent
0.00 0.00 FUD XXX
AMA: 2018,Nov,7; 2018,Jan,8; 2017,Jan,8

90685 **Influenza virus vaccine, quadrivalent (IIV4), split virus, preservative free, 0.25 mL, for intramuscular use** A
INCLUDES Afluria Quadrivalent
Fluzone Quadrivalent
0.00 0.00 FUD XXX
AMA: 2018,Jan,8; 2017,Jan,8; 2016,Oct,6; 2016,May,9; 2016,Jan,13; 2015,May,6; 2015,Jan,16

90686 **Influenza virus vaccine, quadrivalent (IIV4), split virus, preservative free, 0.5 mL dosage, for intramuscular use** A
INCLUDES Afluria Quadrivalent
Fluarix Quadrivalent
FluLaval Quadrivalent
Fluzone Quadrivalent
0.00 0.00 FUD XXX
AMA: 2018,Jan,8; 2017,Jan,8; 2016,Oct,6; 2016,May,9; 2016,Jan,13; 2015,May,6; 2015,Jan,16

90687 **Influenza virus vaccine, quadrivalent (IIV4), split virus, 0.25 mL dosage, for intramuscular use** A
INCLUDES Afluria Quadrivalent
Fluzone Quadrivalent
0.00 0.00 FUD XXX
AMA: 2018,Jan,8; 2017,Jan,8; 2016,Oct,6; 2016,May,9; 2016,Jan,13; 2015,May,6; 2015,Jan,16

90688 **Influenza virus vaccine, quadrivalent (IIV4), split virus, 0.5 mL dosage, for intramuscular use** A
INCLUDES Afluria Quadrivalent
Flulaval Quadrivalent
Fluzone Quadrivalent
0.00 0.00 FUD XXX
AMA: 2020,Jul,11; 2018,Jan,8; 2017,Jan,8; 2016,Oct,6; 2016,May,9; 2016,Jan,13; 2015,May,6; 2015,Jan,16

90689 **Influenza virus vaccine quadrivalent (IIV4), inactivated, adjuvanted, preservative free, 0.25 mL dosage, for intramuscular use**
0.00 0.00 FUD XXX
AMA: 2020,Jul,11; 2019,Jul,10; 2018,Nov,7

90694 **Influenza virus vaccine, quadrivalent (aIIV4), inactivated, adjuvanted, preservative free, 0.5 mL dosage, for intramuscular use**
INCLUDES Fluad Quadrivalent
0.00 0.00 FUD XXX
AMA: 2020,Jul,11

90690 **Typhoid vaccine, live, oral**
INCLUDES Vivotif
0.00 0.00 FUD XXX
AMA: 2020,Jul,11; 2018,Jan,8; 2017,Jan,8; 2016,Jan,13; 2015,May,6; 2015,Jan,16

90691 **Typhoid vaccine, Vi capsular polysaccharide (ViCPs), for intramuscular use**
INCLUDES Typhim Vi
0.00 0.00 FUD XXX
AMA: 2020,Jul,11; 2018,Jan,8; 2017,Jan,8; 2016,Jan,13; 2015,May,6; 2015,Jan,16

90694 **Resequenced code. See code following 90689.**

90696 **Diphtheria, tetanus toxoids, acellular pertussis vaccine and inactivated poliovirus vaccine (DTaP-IPV), when administered to children 4 through 6 years of age, for intramuscular use** A
INCLUDES KINRIX
Quadracel
0.00 0.00 FUD XXX
AMA: 2018,Jan,8; 2017,Jan,8; 2016,Jan,13; 2015,May,6; 2015,Jan,16

90697 **Diphtheria, tetanus toxoids, acellular pertussis vaccine, inactivated poliovirus vaccine, Haemophilus influenzae type b PRP-OMP conjugate vaccine, and hepatitis B vaccine (DTaP-IPV-Hib-HepB), for intramuscular use**
0.00 0.00 FUD XXX
AMA: 2018,Jan,8; 2017,Jan,8; 2016,Jan,13; 2015,May,6; 2015,Jan,16

90698 **Diphtheria, tetanus toxoids, acellular pertussis vaccine, Haemophilus influenzae type b, and inactivated poliovirus vaccine, (DTaP-IPV/Hib), for intramuscular use**

[INCLUDES] Pentacel

🏥 0.00 🩺 0.00 **FUD** XXX [51] [N] [N1] ⚑

AMA: 2018,Jan,8; 2017,Jan,8; 2016,Jan,13; 2015,May,6; 2015,Jan,16

90700 **Diphtheria, tetanus toxoids, and acellular pertussis vaccine (DTaP), when administered to individuals younger than 7 years, for intramuscular use** [A]

[INCLUDES] Daptacel
Infanrix

🏥 0.00 🩺 0.00 **FUD** XXX [51] [N] ⚑

AMA: 2018,Jan,8; 2017,Jan,8; 2016,Jan,13; 2015,May,6; 2015,Jan,16

90702 **Diphtheria and tetanus toxoids adsorbed (DT) when administered to individuals younger than 7 years, for intramuscular use** [A]

[INCLUDES] Diphtheria and Tetanus Toxoids Adsorbed USP (For Pediatric Use)

🏥 0.00 🩺 0.00 **FUD** XXX [51] [N] ⚑

AMA: 2018,Jan,8; 2017,Jan,8; 2016,Jan,13; 2015,May,6; 2015,Jan,16

90707 **Measles, mumps and rubella virus vaccine (MMR), live, for subcutaneous use**

[INCLUDES] M-M-R II

🏥 0.00 🩺 0.00 **FUD** XXX [51] [N] ⚑

AMA: 2018,Jan,8; 2017,Jan,8; 2016,Jan,13; 2015,May,6; 2015,Jan,16

90710 **Measles, mumps, rubella, and varicella vaccine (MMRV), live, for subcutaneous use**

[INCLUDES] ProQuad

🏥 0.00 🩺 0.00 **FUD** XXX [51] [N] ⚑

AMA: 2018,Jan,8; 2017,Jan,8; 2016,Jan,13; 2015,May,6; 2015,Jan,16

90713 **Poliovirus vaccine, inactivated (IPV), for subcutaneous or intramuscular use**

[INCLUDES] IPOL

🏥 0.00 🩺 0.00 **FUD** XXX [51] [N] ⚑

AMA: 2018,Jan,8; 2017,Jan,8; 2016,Jan,13; 2015,May,6; 2015,Jan,16

90714 **Tetanus and diphtheria toxoids adsorbed (Td), preservative free, when administered to individuals 7 years or older, for intramuscular use** [A]

[INCLUDES] Tenivac
Tetanus-diphtheria toxoids absorbed

🏥 0.00 🩺 0.00 **FUD** XXX [51] [N] ⚑

AMA: 2018,Jan,8; 2017,Jan,8; 2016,Jan,13; 2015,May,6; 2015,Jan,16

90715 **Tetanus, diphtheria toxoids and acellular pertussis vaccine (Tdap), when administered to individuals 7 years or older, for intramuscular use** [A]

[INCLUDES] Adacel
Boostrix

🏥 0.00 🩺 0.00 **FUD** XXX [51] [N] ⚑

AMA: 2018,Jan,8; 2017,Jan,8; 2016,Jan,13; 2015,May,6; 2015,Jan,16

90716 **Varicella virus vaccine (VAR), live, for subcutaneous use**

[INCLUDES] Varivax

🏥 0.00 🩺 0.00 **FUD** XXX [51] [M] ⚑

AMA: 2018,Jan,8; 2017,Jan,8; 2016,Jan,13; 2015,May,6; 2015,Mar,3; 2015,Jan,16

90717 **Yellow fever vaccine, live, for subcutaneous use**

[INCLUDES] YF-VAX

🏥 0.00 🩺 0.00 **FUD** XXX [51] [N] [N1] ⚑

AMA: 2018,Jan,8; 2017,Jan,8; 2016,Jan,13; 2015,May,6; 2015,Jan,16

90723 **Diphtheria, tetanus toxoids, acellular pertussis vaccine, hepatitis B, and inactivated poliovirus vaccine (DTaP-HepB-IPV), for intramuscular use**

[INCLUDES] PEDIARIX

🏥 0.00 🩺 0.00 **FUD** XXX [51] [M] ⚑

AMA: 2018,Jan,8; 2017,Jan,8; 2016,Jan,13; 2015,May,6; 2015,Jan,16

\# **90625** **Cholera vaccine, live, adult dosage, 1 dose schedule, for oral use** [A]

🏥 0.00 🩺 0.00 **FUD** XXX [51] [E] ⚑

AMA: 2018,Jan,8; 2017,Jan,8; 2016,Oct,6; 2016,Jan,13

90732 **Pneumococcal polysaccharide vaccine, 23-valent (PPSV23), adult or immunosuppressed patient dosage, when administered to individuals 2 years or older, for subcutaneous or intramuscular use** [A]

[INCLUDES] Pneumovax 23

🏥 0.00 🩺 0.00 **FUD** XXX [51] [L] [L1] ⚑

AMA: 2018,Jan,8; 2017,Jan,8; 2016,Jan,13; 2015,May,6; 2015,Jan,16

\# **90644** **Meningococcal conjugate vaccine, serogroups C & Y and Haemophilus influenzae type b vaccine (Hib-MenCY), 4 dose schedule, when administered to children 6 weeks-18 months of age, for intramuscular use** [A]

[INCLUDES] MenHibrix

🏥 0.00 🩺 0.00 **FUD** XXX [51] [M] ⚑

AMA: 2018,Jan,8; 2017,Jan,8; 2016,Jan,13; 2015,May,6; 2015,Jan,16

90733 **Meningococcal polysaccharide vaccine, serogroups A, C, Y, W-135, quadrivalent (MPSV4), for subcutaneous use**

[INCLUDES] Menomune-A/C/Y/W-135

🏥 0.00 🩺 0.00 **FUD** XXX [51] [M] ⚑

AMA: 2018,Jan,8; 2017,Jan,8; 2016,Jan,13; 2015,May,6; 2015,Jan,16

90734 **Meningococcal conjugate vaccine, serogroups A, C, W, Y, quadrivalent, diphtheria toxoid carrier (MenACWY-D) or CRM197 carrier (MenACWY-CRM), for intramuscular use**

[INCLUDES] Menactra
Menveo

🏥 0.00 🩺 0.00 **FUD** XXX [51] [M] ⚑

AMA: 2020,Jan,11; 2018,Jan,8; 2017,Jan,8; 2016,Oct,6; 2016,Jan,13; 2015,May,6; 2015,Jan,16

\# **90619** **Meningococcal conjugate vaccine, serogroups A, C, W, Y, quadrivalent, tetanus toxoid carrier (MenACWY-TT), for intramuscular use**

🏥 0.00 🩺 0.00 **FUD** XXX [51] ⚑

AMA: 2020,Jan,11

\# **90620** **Meningococcal recombinant protein and outer membrane vesicle vaccine, serogroup B (MenB-4C), 2 dose schedule, for intramuscular use**

[INCLUDES] Bexsero

🏥 0.00 🩺 0.00 **FUD** XXX [51] [M] ⚑

AMA: 2018,Nov,7; 2018,Jan,8; 2017,Jan,8; 2016,Jan,13; 2015,May,6; 2015,Jan,16

\# **90621** **Meningococcal recombinant lipoprotein vaccine, serogroup B (MenB-FHbp), 2 or 3 dose schedule, for intramuscular use**

[INCLUDES] Trumenba

🏥 0.00 🩺 0.00 **FUD** XXX [51] [M] ⚑

AMA: 2018,Nov,7; 2018,Jan,8; 2017,Jan,8; 2016,Jan,13; 2015,May,6; 2015,Jan,16

90736 **Zoster (shingles) vaccine (HZV), live, for subcutaneous injection**

[INCLUDES] Zostavax

🏥 0.00 🩺 0.00 **FUD** XXX [51] [M] ⚑

AMA: 2018,Nov,7; 2018,Jan,8; 2017,Jan,8; 2016,Jan,13; 2015,May,6; 2015,Jan,16

● New Code ▲ Revised Code ○ Reinstated ● New Web Release ▲ Revised Web Release + Add-on Unlisted Not Covered # Resequenced
[50] Optum Mod 50 Exempt ⊘ AMA Mod 51 Exempt [51] Optum Mod 51 Exempt [63] Mod 63 Exempt ⍁ Non-FDA Drug ★ Telemedicine [M] Maternity [A] Age Edit

\# **90750** **Zoster (shingles) vaccine (HZV), recombinant, subunit, adjuvanted, for intramuscular use**
0.00 0.00 **FUD** XXX (51) M
AMA: 2018,Nov,7

90738 **Japanese encephalitis virus vaccine, inactivated, for intramuscular use**
INCLUDES Ixiaro
0.00 0.00 **FUD** XXX (51) M
AMA: 2018,Jan,8; 2017,Jan,8; 2016,Jan,13; 2015,May,6; 2015,Jan,16

90739 **Hepatitis B vaccine (HepB), adult dosage, 2 dose schedule, for intramuscular use**
0.00 0.00 **FUD** XXX (51) E
AMA: 2018,Nov,7; 2018,Jan,8; 2017,Jan,8; 2016,Jan,13; 2015,May,6; 2015,Jan,16

90740 **Hepatitis B vaccine (HepB), dialysis or immunosuppressed patient dosage, 3 dose schedule, for intramuscular use**
INCLUDES Recombivax HB
0.00 0.00 **FUD** XXX (51) F F4
AMA: 2018,Jan,8; 2017,Jan,8; 2016,Jan,13; 2015,May,6; 2015,Jan,16

90743 **Hepatitis B vaccine (HepB), adolescent, 2 dose schedule, for intramuscular use** A
INCLUDES Energix-B
Recombivax HB
0.00 0.00 **FUD** XXX (51) F F4
AMA: 2018,Jan,8; 2017,Jan,8; 2016,Jan,13; 2015,May,6; 2015,Jan,16

90744 **Hepatitis B vaccine (HepB), pediatric/adolescent dosage, 3 dose schedule, for intramuscular use** A
INCLUDES Energix-B
Flucelvax Quadrivalent
Recombivax HB
0.00 0.00 **FUD** XXX (51) F F4
AMA: 2018,Jan,8; 2017,Jan,8; 2016,Jan,13; 2015,May,6; 2015,Jan,16

90746 **Hepatitis B vaccine (HepB), adult dosage, 3 dose schedule, for intramuscular use**
INCLUDES Energix-B
Recombivax HB
0.00 0.00 **FUD** XXX (51) F F4
AMA: 2018,Jan,8; 2017,Jan,8; 2016,Jan,13; 2015,May,6; 2015,Jan,16

90747 **Hepatitis B vaccine (HepB), dialysis or immunosuppressed patient dosage, 4 dose schedule, for intramuscular use**
INCLUDES Energix-B
RECOMBIVAX dialysis
0.00 0.00 **FUD** XXX (51) F F4
AMA: 2018,Jan,8; 2017,Jan,8; 2016,Jan,13; 2015,May,6; 2015,Jan,16

90748 **Hepatitis B and Haemophilus influenzae type b vaccine (Hib-HepB), for intramuscular use**
INCLUDES COMVAX
0.00 0.00 **FUD** XXX (51) E
AMA: 2018,Jan,8; 2017,Jan,8; 2016,Jan,13; 2015,May,6; 2015,Jan,16

90749 **Unlisted vaccine/toxoid**
0.00 0.00 **FUD** XXX (51) N N1
AMA: 2018,Jan,8; 2017,Jan,8; 2016,Jan,13; 2015,May,6; 2015,Jan,16

90750 **Resequenced code. See code following 90736.**

90756 **Resequenced code. See code following 90661.**

90785 Complex Interactive Encounter

CMS: 100-02,15,160 Clinical Psychologist Services; 100-02,15,170 Clinical Social Worker (CSW) Services; 100-03,10.3 Inpatient Pain Rehabilitation Programs; 100-03,10.4 Outpatient Hospital Pain Rehabilitation Programs; 100-03,130.1 Inpatient Stays for Alcoholism Treatment; 100-04,12,100 Teaching Physician Services; 100-04,4,260.1 Special Partial Hospitalization Billing Requirements forHospitals, Community Mental Health Centers, and Critical Access Hospitals; 100-04,4,260.1.1 Bill Review for Partial Hospitalization Services Provided in Community Mental Health Centers (CMHC)

INCLUDES Complicated communication issues affecting psychiatric service
Involved communication with:
- Emotionally charged or dissonant family members
- Patients wanting others present during visit (e.g., family member, translator)
- Patients with impaired or undeveloped verbal skills
- Patients with third parties responsible for their care (e.g., parents, guardians)
- Third-party involvement (e.g., schools, probation and parole officers, child protective agencies)

One or more following activity:
- Discussion sentinel event demanding third-party involvement (i.e., abuse or neglect reported to state agency)
- Interference by caregiver's behavior or emotional state to understand and assist in treatment plan
- Managing discordant communication complicating care among participating members (e.g., arguing, reactivity)
- Nonverbal communication methods (e.g., toys, other devices, or translator) to eliminate communication barriers

EXCLUDES *Adaptive behavior assessment/treatment ([97151, 97152, 97153, 97154, 97155, 97156, 97157, 97158], 0362T, 0373T)*
Crisis psychotherapy (90839-90840)

\+ **90785** **Interactive complexity (List separately in addition to the code for primary procedure)**
Code first, when performed (99202-99255 [99224, 99225, 99226], 99304-99337, 99341-99350, 90791-90792, 90832-90834, 90836-90838, 90853)
0.39 0.42 **FUD** ZZZ N
AMA: 2020,Aug,3; 2018,Nov,3; 2018,Jul,12; 2018,Apr,9; 2018,Jan,8; 2017,Jan,8; 2016,Dec,11; 2016,Jan,13; 2015,Jan,16

90791-90792 Psychiatric Evaluations

CMS: 100-02,15,170 Clinical Social Worker (CSW) Services; 100-03,10.3 Inpatient Pain Rehabilitation Programs; 100-03,130.1 Inpatient Stays for Alcoholism Treatment; 100-03,130.2 Outpatient Hospital Services for Alcoholism; 100-04,12,100 Teaching Physician Services; 100-04,12,190.3 List of Telehealth Services; 100-04,12,190.6 Payment Methodology for Physician/Practitioner at the Distant Site ; 100-04,12,190.6.1 Submission of Telehealth Claims for Distant Site Practitioners; 100-04,12,190.7 Contractor Editing of Telehealth Claims; 100-04,4,260.1 Special Partial Hospitalization Billing Requirements forHospitals, Community Mental Health Centers, and Critical Access Hospitals; 100-04,4,260.1.1 Bill Review for Partial Hospitalization Services Provided in Community Mental Health Centers (CMHC)

INCLUDES Diagnostic assessment or reassessment without psychotherapy services
EXCLUDES *Adaptive behavior assessment/treatment ([97151, 97152, 97153, 97154, 97155, 97156, 97157, 97158], 0362T, 0373T)*
Crisis psychotherapy (90839-90840)
E/M services (99202-99337 [99224, 99225, 99226], 99341-99350, 99366-99368, 99401-99443 [99415, 99416, 99417, 99421, 99422, 99423, 99439])

Code also interactive complexity services when applicable (90785)

90791 **Psychiatric diagnostic evaluation**
3.54 3.89 **FUD** XXX ★ 03
AMA: 2020,Aug,3; 2018,Nov,3; 2018,Jul,12; 2018,Apr,9; 2018,Jan,8; 2017,Nov,3; 2017,Jan,8; 2016,Jan,13; 2015,Jan,16

90792 **Psychiatric diagnostic evaluation with medical services**
4.01 4.37 **FUD** XXX ★ 03
AMA: 2020,Aug,3; 2019,Dec,14; 2018,Nov,3; 2018,Jul,12; 2018,Apr,9; 2018,Jan,8; 2017,Nov,3; 2017,Jan,8; 2016,Jan,13; 2015,Jan,16

90832-90838 Psychotherapy Services

CMS: 100-02,15,160 Clinical Psychologist Services; 100-02,15,170 Clinical Social Worker (CSW) Services; 100-03,130.1 Inpatient Stays for Alcoholism Treatment; 100-03,130.2 Outpatient Hospital Services for Alcoholism; 100-03,130.3 Chemical Aversion Therapy for Treatment of Alcoholism; 100-04,12,100 Teaching Physician Services; 100-04,12,160 Independent Psychologist Services; 100-04,12,170 Clinical Psychologist Services; 100-04,12,190.3 List of Telehealth Services; 100-04,12,190.6 Payment Methodology for Physician/Practitioner at the Distant Site ; 100-04,12,190.6.1 Submission of Telehealth Claims for Distant Site Practitioners; 100-04,12,190.7 Contractor Editing of Telehealth Claims

INCLUDES Face-to-face time with patient (family, other informers may also be present)
Pharmacologic management in time allocated to psychotherapy service codes
Psychotherapy only (90832, 90834, 90837)
Psychotherapy with separately identifiable medical E/M services includes add-on codes (90833, 90836, 90838)
Service times no less than 16 minutes
Services provided in all settings
Therapeutic communication to:
Ameliorate patient's mental and behavioral symptoms
Modify behavior
Support and encourage personality growth and development
Treatment for:
Behavior disturbances
Mental illness

EXCLUDES *Adaptive behavior assessment/treatment ([97151, 97152, 97153, 97154, 97155, 97156, 97157, 97158], 0362T, 0373T)*
Crisis psychotherapy (90839-90840)
Family psychotherapy (90846-90847)

Code also interactive complexity services with time provider spends performing service reflected in time for appropriate psychotherapy code (90785)

90832 Psychotherapy, 30 minutes with patient
1.76 | 1.90 FUD XXX ★ 03
AMA: 2020,Aug,3; 2018,Nov,3; 2018,Jul,12; 2018,Jan,8; 2017,Nov,3; 2017,Sep,11; 2017,Jan,8; 2016,Dec,11; 2016,Jan,13; 2015,Oct,9; 2015,Jan,16

\+ **90833 Psychotherapy, 30 minutes with patient when performed with an evaluation and management service (List separately in addition to the code for primary procedure)**
Code first (99202-99255 [99224, 99225, 99226], 99304-99337, 99341-99350)
1.84 | 1.97 FUD ZZZ ★ N
AMA: 2020,Aug,3; 2018,Nov,3; 2018,Jul,12; 2018,Jan,8; 2017,Nov,3; 2017,Jan,8; 2016,Dec,11; 2016,Jan,13; 2015,Oct,9; 2015,Jan,16

90834 Psychotherapy, 45 minutes with patient
2.35 | 2.53 FUD XXX ★ 03
AMA: 2020,Aug,3; 2018,Nov,3; 2018,Jul,12; 2018,Jan,8; 2017,Nov,3; 2017,Jan,8; 2016,Dec,11; 2016,Jan,13; 2015,Oct,9; 2015,Jan,16

\+ **90836 Psychotherapy, 45 minutes with patient when performed with an evaluation and management service (List separately in addition to the code for primary procedure)**
Code first (99202-99255 [99224, 99225, 99226], 99304-99337, 99341-99350)
2.33 | 2.49 FUD ZZZ ★ N
AMA: 2020,Aug,3; 2018,Nov,3; 2018,Jul,12; 2018,Jan,8; 2017,Nov,3; 2017,Jan,8; 2016,Dec,11; 2016,Jan,13; 2015,Oct,9; 2015,Jan,16

90837 Psychotherapy, 60 minutes with patient
Code also prolonged service for psychotherapy performed without E/M service face-to-face with patient lasting 90 minutes or longer (99354-99357)
3.53 | 3.80 FUD XXX ★ 03
AMA: 2020,Sep,3; 2020,Aug,3; 2018,Nov,3; 2018,Jul,12; 2018,Jan,8; 2017,Nov,3; 2017,Jan,8; 2016,Dec,11; 2016,Jan,13; 2015,Oct,3; 2015,Oct,9; 2015,Jan,16

\+ **90838 Psychotherapy, 60 minutes with patient when performed with an evaluation and management service (List separately in addition to the code for primary procedure)**
Code first (99202-99255 [99224, 99225, 99226], 99304-99337, 99341-99350)
3.08 | 3.29 FUD ZZZ ★ N
AMA: 2020,Aug,3; 2018,Nov,3; 2018,Jul,12; 2018,Jan,8; 2017,Nov,3; 2017,Jan,8; 2016,Dec,11; 2016,Jan,13; 2015,Oct,9; 2015,Jan,16

90839-90840 Services for Patients in Crisis

CMS: 100-02,15,170 Clinical Social Worker (CSW) Services; 100-03,130.1 Inpatient Stays for Alcoholism Treatment; 100-03,130.3 Chemical Aversion Therapy for Treatment of Alcoholism; 100-04,12,100 Teaching Physician Services; 100-04,12,160 Independent Psychologist Services; 100-04,12,160.1 Payment of Independent Psychologist Services; 100-04,12,170 Clinical Psychologist Services

INCLUDES 30 minutes or more face-to-face time with patient (for all or part service) and/or family providing crisis psychotherapy
All time spent exclusively with patient (for all or part service) and/or family, even if time not continuous
Emergent care to patient in severe distress (e.g., life threatening or complex)
Institute interventions to minimize psychological trauma
Measures to ease crisis and reestablish safety
Psychotherapy

EXCLUDES *Adaptive behavior assessment/treatment ([97151, 97152, 97153, 97154, 97155, 97156, 97157, 97158], 0362T, 0373T)*
Other psychiatric services (90785-90899)

90839 Psychotherapy for crisis; first 60 minutes
INCLUDES First 30-74 minutes crisis psychotherapy per day
EXCLUDES *Reporting code more than one time per day, even when service not continuous on that date*
3.69 | 3.96 FUD XXX 03 80
AMA: 2020,Aug,3; 2018,Nov,3; 2018,Jul,12; 2018,Jan,8; 2017,Nov,3; 2017,Jan,8; 2016,Jan,13; 2015,Oct,9; 2015,Jan,16

\+ **90840 each additional 30 minutes (List separately in addition to code for primary service)**
INCLUDES Up to 30 minutes time beyond initial 74 minutes
Code first (90839)
1.76 | 1.90 FUD ZZZ N 80
AMA: 2020,Aug,3; 2018,Nov,3; 2018,Jul,12; 2018,Jan,8; 2017,Nov,3; 2017,Jan,8; 2016,Jan,13; 2015,Oct,9; 2015,Jan,16

90845-90863 Additional Psychotherapy Services

CMS: 100-02,15,170 Clinical Social Worker (CSW) Services; 100-03,10.3 Inpatient Pain Rehabilitation Programs; 100-03,10.4 Outpatient Hospital Pain Rehabilitation Programs

EXCLUDES *Adaptive behavior assessment/treatment ([97151, 97152, 97153, 97154, 97155, 97156, 97157, 97158], 0362T, 0373T)*
Analysis/programming neurostimulators for vagus nerve stimulation therapy (95970, 95976-95977)
Crisis psychotherapy (90839-90840)

90845 Psychoanalysis
2.53 | 2.78 FUD XXX ★ 03 80
AMA: 2020,Aug,3; 2018,Nov,3; 2018,Jul,12; 2018,Jan,8; 2017,Jan,8; 2016,Jan,13; 2015,Oct,9; 2015,Jan,16

90846 Family psychotherapy (without the patient present), 50 minutes
EXCLUDES *Service times less than 26 minutes*
2.85 | 2.87 FUD XXX ★ 03 80
AMA: 2020,Aug,3; 2018,Nov,3; 2018,Jul,12; 2018,Jan,8; 2017,Nov,3; 2017,Mar,10; 2017,Jan,8; 2016,Dec,11; 2016,Jan,13; 2015,Oct,9; 2015,Jan,16

90847 Family psychotherapy (conjoint psychotherapy) (with patient present), 50 minutes
EXCLUDES *Service times less than 26 minutes*
Service times more than 80 minutes, see prolonged services (99354-99357)
2.96 | 3.18 FUD XXX ★ 03 80
AMA: 2020,Sep,3; 2020,Aug,3; 2018,Nov,3; 2018,Jul,12; 2018,Jan,8; 2017,Nov,3; 2017,Jan,8; 2016,Dec,11; 2016,Jan,13; 2015,Oct,9; 2015,Jan,16

90849 Multiple-family group psychotherapy

Facility RVU 0.87 Non-Facility RVU 1.17 **FUD** XXX 03 80 CCI

AMA: 2020,Aug,3; 2018,Nov,3; 2018,Jul,12; 2018,Jan,8; 2017,Nov,3; 2017,Jan,8; 2016,Jan,13; 2015,Oct,9; 2015,Jan,16

90853 Group psychotherapy (other than of a multiple-family group)

Code also group psychotherapy with interactive complexity (90785)

Facility RVU 0.70 Non-Facility RVU 0.76 **FUD** XXX 03 80 CCI

AMA: 2020,Aug,3; 2018,Nov,3; 2018,Jul,12; 2018,Jan,8; 2017,Nov,3; 2017,Mar,10; 2017,Jan,8; 2016,Jan,13; 2015,Oct,9; 2015,Jan,16

\+ **90863 Pharmacologic management, including prescription and review of medication, when performed with psychotherapy services (List separately in addition to the code for primary procedure)**

INCLUDES Pharmacologic management in time allocated to psychotherapy service codes

Code first (90832, 90834, 90837)

Facility RVU 0.70 Non-Facility RVU 0.74 **FUD** XXX ★ E CCI

AMA: 2020,Aug,3; 2018,Nov,3; 2018,Jul,12; 2018,Jan,8; 2017,Jan,8; 2016,Jan,13; 2015,Jan,16

90865-90870 Other Psychiatric Treatment

EXCLUDES *Adaptive behavior assessment/treatment ([97151, 97152, 97153, 97154, 97155, 97156, 97157, 97158], 0362T, 0373T)*
Analysis/programming neurostimulators for vagus nerve stimulation therapy (95970, 95976-95977)
Crisis psychotherapy (90839-90840)

90865 Narcosynthesis for psychiatric diagnostic and therapeutic purposes (eg, sodium amobarbital (Amytal) interview)

Facility RVU 3.59 Non-Facility RVU 4.79 **FUD** XXX 03 80 CCI

AMA: 2020,Aug,3; 2018,Nov,3; 2018,Jul,12; 2018,Jan,8; 2017,Jan,8; 2016,Jan,13; 2015,Jan,16

90867 Therapeutic repetitive transcranial magnetic stimulation (TMS) treatment; initial, including cortical mapping, motor threshold determination, delivery and management

INCLUDES E/M services related directly to:
Cortical mapping
Delivery and management TMS services
Motor threshold determination

EXCLUDES *Electromyography (95860, 95870)*
Evoked potential studies (95928, 95929, [95939])
Medication management
Reporting code more than one time for each treatment course
Significant, separately identifiable E/M service
Significant, separately identifiable psychotherapy service
Subsequent transcranial magnetic stimulation (TMS) treatment:
Delivery and management (90868)
Motor threshold redetermination (90869)

Facility RVU 0.00 Non-Facility RVU 0.00 **FUD** 000 S CCI

AMA: 2020,Aug,3; 2018,Nov,3; 2018,Jul,12

90868 subsequent delivery and management, per session

INCLUDES E/M services related directly to:
Cortical mapping
Delivery and management TMS services
Motor threshold determination

EXCLUDES *Medication management*
Significant, separately identifiable E/M service
Significant, separately identifiable psychotherapy service

Facility RVU 0.00 Non-Facility RVU 0.00 **FUD** 000 S CCI

AMA: 2020,Aug,3; 2018,Nov,3; 2018,Jul,12

90869 subsequent motor threshold re-determination with delivery and management

INCLUDES E/M services related directly to:
Cortical mapping
Delivery and management TMS services
Motor threshold determination

EXCLUDES *Electromyography (95860, 95870)*
Evoked potential studies (95928-95929, [95939])
Medication management
Significant, separately identifiable E/M service
Significant, separately identifiable psychotherapy service
Transcranial magnetic stimulation (TMS) treatment:
Initial (90867)
Subsequent delivery and managment (90868)

Facility RVU 0.00 Non-Facility RVU 0.00 **FUD** 000 S CCI

AMA: 2020,Aug,3; 2018,Nov,3; 2018,Jul,12

90870 Electroconvulsive therapy (includes necessary monitoring)

Facility RVU 3.12 Non-Facility RVU 4.96 **FUD** 000 S 80 CCI

AMA: 2020,Aug,3; 2018,Nov,3; 2018,Jul,12; 2018,Jan,8; 2017,Jan,8; 2016,Jan,13; 2015,Jan,16

90875-90880 Psychiatric Therapy with Biofeedback or Hypnosis

CMS: 100-02,15,170 Clinical Social Worker (CSW) Services; 100-04,12,160 Independent Psychologist Services; 100-04,12,160.1 Payment of Independent Psychologist Services; 100-04,12,170 Clinical Psychologist Services

EXCLUDES *Adaptive behavior assessment/treatment ([97151, 97152, 97153, 97154, 97155, 97156, 97157, 97158], 0362T, 0373T)*
Analysis/programming neurostimulators for vagus nerve stimulation therapy (95970, 95976-95977)
Crisis psychotherapy (90839-90840)

90875 Individual psychophysiological therapy incorporating biofeedback training by any modality (face-to-face with the patient), with psychotherapy (eg, insight oriented, behavior modifying or supportive psychotherapy); 30 minutes

Facility RVU 1.73 Non-Facility RVU 1.80 **FUD** XXX E CCI

AMA: 2020,Aug,3; 2018,Nov,3; 2018,Jul,12; 2018,Jan,8; 2017,Jan,8; 2016,Jan,13; 2015,Jan,16

90876 45 minutes

Facility RVU 2.74 Non-Facility RVU 3.05 **FUD** XXX E CCI

AMA: 2020,Aug,3; 2018,Nov,3; 2018,Jul,12; 2018,Jan,8; 2017,Jan,8; 2016,Jan,13; 2015,Jan,16

90880 Hypnotherapy

Facility RVU 2.58 Non-Facility RVU 2.98 **FUD** XXX 03 80 CCI

AMA: 2020,Aug,3; 2018,Nov,3; 2018,Jul,12; 2018,Jan,8; 2017,Jan,8; 2016,Jan,13; 2015,Jan,16

90882-90899 Psychiatric Services without Patient Face-to-Face Contact

CMS: 100-04,12,160 Independent Psychologist Services; 100-04,12,160.1 Payment of Independent Psychologist Services

EXCLUDES *Analysis/programming neurostimulators for vagus nerve stimulation therapy (95970, 95976-95977)*
Crisis psychotherapy (90839-90840)

90882 Environmental intervention for medical management purposes on a psychiatric patient's behalf with agencies, employers, or institutions

Facility RVU 0.00 Non-Facility RVU 0.00 **FUD** XXX E CCI

AMA: 2020,Aug,3; 2018,Nov,3; 2018,Jul,12; 2018,Jan,8; 2017,Jan,8; 2016,Jan,13; 2015,Jan,16

90885 Psychiatric evaluation of hospital records, other psychiatric reports, psychometric and/or projective tests, and other accumulated data for medical diagnostic purposes

Facility RVU 1.43 Non-Facility RVU 1.43 **FUD** XXX N CCI

AMA: 2020,Aug,3; 2018,Nov,3; 2018,Jul,12; 2018,Jan,8; 2017,Jan,8; 2016,Jan,13; 2015,Jan,16

90887 **Interpretation or explanation of results of psychiatric, other medical examinations and procedures, or other accumulated data to family or other responsible persons, or advising them how to assist patient**

EXCLUDES *Adaptive behavior assessment/treatment ([97151, 97152, 97153, 97154, 97155, 97156, 97157, 97158], 0362T, 0373T)*

2.14 | 2.48 | **FUD** XXX | N

AMA: 2020,Aug,3; 2018,Nov,3; 2018,Jul,12; 2018,Jan,8; 2017,Jan,8; 2016,Jan,13; 2015,Jan,16

90889 **Preparation of report of patient's psychiatric status, history, treatment, or progress (other than for legal or consultative purposes) for other individuals, agencies, or insurance carriers**

0.00 | 0.00 | **FUD** XXX | N

AMA: 2020,Aug,3; 2018,Nov,3; 2018,Jul,12; 2018,Jan,8; 2017,Jan,8; 2016,Jan,13; 2015,Jan,16

90899 **Unlisted psychiatric service or procedure**

0.00 | 0.00 | **FUD** XXX | 03 80

AMA: 2020,Aug,3; 2018,Nov,3; 2018,Jul,12; 2018,Jan,8; 2017,Jan,8; 2016,Jan,13; 2015,Jan,16

90901-90913 Biofeedback Therapy

EXCLUDES *Psychophysiological therapy utilizing biofeedback training (90875-90876)*

90901 **Biofeedback training by any modality**

0.57 | 1.13 | **FUD** 000 | A 80

AMA: 2020,Jun,13; 2018,Jan,8; 2017,Jan,8; 2016,Jan,13; 2015,Jan,16

90912 **Biofeedback training, perineal muscles, anorectal or urethral sphincter, including EMG and/or manometry, when performed; initial 15 minutes of one-on-one physician or other qualified health care professional contact with the patient**

EXCLUDES *Incontinence treatment using pulsed magnetic neuromodulation (53899)*
Testing rectal sensation, tone, and compliance (91120)

1.26 | 2.27 | **FUD** 000 | 80

AMA: 2020,Jun,13

+ **90913** **each additional 15 minutes of one-on-one physician or other qualified health care professional contact with the patient (List separately in addition to code for primary procedure)**

EXCLUDES *Incontinence treatment using pulsed magnetic neuromodulation (53899)*
Testing rectal sensation, tone, and compliance (91120)

Code first (90912)

0.70 | 0.92 | **FUD** ZZZ | 80

AMA: 2020,Jun,13

90935-90940 Hemodialysis Services: Inpatient ESRD and Outpatient Non-ESRD

CMS: 100-02,11,20 Renal Dialysis Items and Services ; 100-04,3,100.6 Inpatient Renal Services

EXCLUDES *Attendance by physician or other qualified health care provider for prolonged period of time (99354-99360 [99415, 99416])*
Blood specimen collection from partial/complete implantable venous access device (36591)
Declotting cannula (36831, 36833, 36860-36861)
Hemodialysis home visit by non-physician health care professional (99512)
Therapeutic apheresis procedures (36511-36516)
Thrombolytic agent declotting implanted vascular access device/catheter (36593)

Code also significant separately identifiable E/M service not related to dialysis procedure or renal failure with modifier 25 (99202-99215, 99217-99223 [99224, 99225, 99226], 99231-99239, 99241-99245, 99281-99285, 99291-99292, 99304-99318, 99324-99337, 99341-99350, 99466-99467, 99468-99472, 99475-99480)

90935 **Hemodialysis procedure with single evaluation by a physician or other qualified health care professional**

INCLUDES All E/M services related to patient's renal disease rendered on day dialysis performed
Inpatient ESRD and non-ESRD procedures
Only one patient evaluation related to hemodialysis procedure
Outpatient non-ESRD dialysis

2.07 | 2.07 | **FUD** 000 | S 80

AMA: 2018,Jan,8; 2017,Jan,8; 2016,Jan,13; 2015,Jan,16

90937 **Hemodialysis procedure requiring repeated evaluation(s) with or without substantial revision of dialysis prescription**

INCLUDES All E/M services related to patient's renal disease rendered on day dialysis performed
Inpatient ESRD and non-ESRD procedures
Outpatient non-ESRD dialysis
Re-evaluation patient during hemodialysis procedure

2.95 | 2.95 | **FUD** 000 | B 80

AMA: 2018,Jan,8; 2017,Jan,8; 2016,Jan,13; 2015,Jan,16

90940 **Hemodialysis access flow study to determine blood flow in grafts and arteriovenous fistulae by an indicator method**

EXCLUDES *Hemodialysis access duplex scan (93990)*

0.00 | 0.00 | **FUD** XXX | N

AMA: 2018,Jan,8; 2017,Jan,8; 2016,Jan,13; 2015,Jan,16

90945-90947 Dialysis Techniques Other Than Hemodialysis

CMS: 100-04,12,40.3 Global Surgery Review; 100-04,3,100.6 Inpatient Renal Services

INCLUDES All E/M services related to patient's renal disease rendered on day dialysis performed
Procedures other than hemodialysis:
Continuous renal replacement therapies
Hemofiltration
Peritoneal dialysis

EXCLUDES *Attendance by physician or other qualified health care provider for prolonged time period (99354-99360 [99415, 99416])*
Hemodialysis
Tunneled intraperitoneal catheter insertion
Open (49421)
Percutaneous (49418)

Code also significant, separately identifiable E/M service not related to dialysis procedure or renal failure with modifier 25 (99202-99215, 99217-99223 [99224, 99225, 99226], 99231-99239, 99241-99245, 99281-99285, 99291-99292, 99304-99318, 99324-99337, 99341-99350, 99466-99467, 99468-99472, 99475-99480)

90945 **Dialysis procedure other than hemodialysis (eg, peritoneal dialysis, hemofiltration, or other continuous renal replacement therapies), with single evaluation by a physician or other qualified health care professional**

INCLUDES Only one patient evaluation related to procedure

EXCLUDES *Peritoneal dialysis home infusion (99601, 99602)*

2.42 | 2.42 | **FUD** 000 | V 80

AMA: 2018,Jan,8; 2017,Jan,8; 2016,Jan,13; 2015,Jan,16

90947 **Dialysis procedure other than hemodialysis (eg, peritoneal dialysis, hemofiltration, or other continuous renal replacement therapies) requiring repeated evaluations by a physician or other qualified health care professional, with or without substantial revision of dialysis prescription**

EXCLUDES *Re-evaluation during procedure*

3.51 3.51 **FUD** 000 B 80

AMA: 2018,Jan,8; 2017,Jan,8; 2016,Jan,13; 2015,Jan,16

90951-90962 End-stage Renal Disease Monthly Outpatient Services

CMS: 100-02,11,20 Renal Dialysis Items and Services ; 100-04,12,190.3 List of Telehealth Services; 100-04,12,190.3.4 ESRD-Related Services as a Telehealth Service; 100-04,8,140.1 ESRD-Related Services Under the Monthly Capitation Payment

INCLUDES Establishing dialyzing cycle
Management dialysis visits
Outpatient E/M dialysis visits
Patient management during dialysis for month
Telephone calls

EXCLUDES *ESRD/non-ESRD dialysis services performed in inpatient setting (90935-90937, 90945-90947)*
Non-ESRD dialysis services performed in outpatient setting (90935-90937, 90945-90947)
Non-ESRD related E/M services that cannot be performed during dialysis session
Services provided in same month with:
Chronic care management ([99439, 99490, 99491])
Complex chronic care management (99487-99489)

90951 **End-stage renal disease (ESRD) related services monthly, for patients younger than 2 years of age to include monitoring for the adequacy of nutrition, assessment of growth and development, and counseling of parents; with 4 or more face-to-face visits by a physician or other qualified health care professional per month** A

26.6 26.6 **FUD** XXX ★ M 80

AMA: 2018,Feb,11; 2018,Jan,8; 2017,Jan,8; 2016,Jan,13; 2015,Jan,16

90952 **with 2-3 face-to-face visits by a physician or other qualified health care professional per month** A

0.00 0.00 **FUD** XXX ★ M 80

AMA: 2018,Feb,11; 2018,Jan,8; 2017,Jan,8; 2016,Jan,13; 2015,Jan,16

90953 **with 1 face-to-face visit by a physician or other qualified health care professional per month** A

0.00 0.00 **FUD** XXX M 80

AMA: 2018,Feb,11; 2018,Jan,8; 2017,Jan,8; 2016,Jan,13; 2015,Jan,16

90954 **End-stage renal disease (ESRD) related services monthly, for patients 2-11 years of age to include monitoring for the adequacy of nutrition, assessment of growth and development, and counseling of parents; with 4 or more face-to-face visits by a physician or other qualified health care professional per month** A

22.9 22.9 **FUD** XXX ★ M 80

AMA: 2018,Feb,11; 2018,Jan,8; 2017,Jan,8; 2016,Jan,13; 2015,Jan,16

90955 **with 2-3 face-to-face visits by a physician or other qualified health care professional per month** A

12.9 12.9 **FUD** XXX ★ M 80

AMA: 2018,Feb,11; 2018,Jan,8; 2017,Jan,8; 2016,Jan,13; 2015,Jan,16

90956 **with 1 face-to-face visit by a physician or other qualified health care professional per month** A

9.00 9.00 **FUD** XXX M 80

AMA: 2018,Feb,11; 2018,Jan,8; 2017,Jan,8; 2016,Jan,13; 2015,Jan,16

90957 **End-stage renal disease (ESRD) related services monthly, for patients 12-19 years of age to include monitoring for the adequacy of nutrition, assessment of growth and development, and counseling of parents; with 4 or more face-to-face visits by a physician or other qualified health care professional per month** A

18.3 18.3 **FUD** XXX ★ M 80

AMA: 2018,Feb,11; 2018,Jan,8; 2017,Jan,8; 2016,Jan,13; 2015,Jan,16

90958 **with 2-3 face-to-face visits by a physician or other qualified health care professional per month** A

12.3 12.3 **FUD** XXX ★ M 80

AMA: 2018,Feb,11; 2018,Jan,8; 2017,Jan,8; 2016,Jan,13; 2015,Jan,16

90959 **with 1 face-to-face visit by a physician or other qualified health care professional per month** A

8.41 8.41 **FUD** XXX M 80

AMA: 2018,Feb,11; 2018,Jan,8; 2017,Jan,8; 2016,Jan,13; 2015,Jan,16

90960 **End-stage renal disease (ESRD) related services monthly, for patients 20 years of age and older; with 4 or more face-to-face visits by a physician or other qualified health care professional per month** A

8.07 8.07 **FUD** XXX ★ M 80

AMA: 2018,Feb,11; 2018,Jan,8; 2017,Jan,8; 2016,Jan,13; 2015,Jan,16

90961 **with 2-3 face-to-face visits by a physician or other qualified health care professional per month** A

6.74 6.74 **FUD** XXX ★ M 80

AMA: 2018,Feb,11; 2018,Jan,8; 2017,Jan,8; 2016,Jan,13; 2015,Jan,16

90962 **with 1 face-to-face visit by a physician or other qualified health care professional per month** A

5.21 5.21 **FUD** XXX M 80

AMA: 2018,Feb,11; 2018,Jan,8; 2017,Jan,8; 2016,Jan,13; 2015,Jan,16

90963-90966 End-stage Renal Disease Monthly Home Dialysis Services

CMS: 100-02,11,20 Renal Dialysis Items and Services ; 100-04,12,190.3.4 ESRD-Related Services as a Telehealth Service; 100-04,8,140.1 ESRD-Related Services Under the Monthly Capitation Payment; 100-04,8,140.1.1 Payment for Managing Patients on Home Dialysis

INCLUDES ESRD services for home dialysis patients
Services provided for full month

EXCLUDES *Services provided in same month with:*
Chronic care management ([99439, 99490, 99491])
Complex chronic care management (99487-99489)

90963 **End-stage renal disease (ESRD) related services for home dialysis per full month, for patients younger than 2 years of age to include monitoring for the adequacy of nutrition, assessment of growth and development, and counseling of parents** A

15.4 15.4 **FUD** XXX M 80

AMA: 2018,Feb,11; 2018,Jan,8; 2017,Jan,8; 2016,Jan,13; 2015,Jan,16

90964 **End-stage renal disease (ESRD) related services for home dialysis per full month, for patients 2-11 years of age to include monitoring for the adequacy of nutrition, assessment of growth and development, and counseling of parents** A

13.5 13.5 **FUD** XXX M 80

AMA: 2018,Feb,11; 2018,Jan,8; 2017,Jan,8; 2016,Jan,13; 2015,Jan,16

90965 **End-stage renal disease (ESRD) related services for home dialysis per full month, for patients 12-19 years of age to include monitoring for the adequacy of nutrition, assessment of growth and development, and counseling of parents** A

12.9 12.9 **FUD** XXX M 80

AMA: 2018,Feb,11; 2018,Jan,8; 2017,Jan,8; 2016,Jan,13; 2015,Jan,16

90966 **End-stage renal disease (ESRD) related services for home dialysis per full month, for patients 20 years of age and older** A

6.72 6.72 **FUD** XXX M 80

AMA: 2018,Feb,11; 2018,Jan,8; 2017,Jan,8; 2016,Jan,13; 2015,Jan,16

90967-90970 End-stage Renal Disease Services: Partial Month

CMS: 100-02,11,20 Renal Dialysis Items and Services

INCLUDES ESRD services for less than full month, such as:
- Outpatient ESRD-related services initiated prior to assessment completion
- Patient spending partial month as hospital inpatient
- Patient who is transient, dies, recovers, or undergoes kidney transplant

Services reported on daily basis, less hospitalization days

EXCLUDES *Services provided in same month with:*
- *Chronic care management ([99439, 99490, 99491])*
- *Complex chronic care management (99487-99489)*

90967 **End-stage renal disease (ESRD) related services for dialysis less than a full month of service, per day; for patients younger than 2 years of age** A

0.51 0.51 **FUD** XXX M 80

AMA: 2018,Feb,11; 2018,Jan,8; 2017,Jan,8; 2016,Jan,13; 2015,Jan,16

90968 **for patients 2-11 years of age** A

0.45 0.45 **FUD** XXX M 80

AMA: 2018,Feb,11; 2018,Jan,8; 2017,Jan,8; 2016,Jan,13; 2015,Jan,16

90969 **for patients 12-19 years of age** A

0.43 0.43 **FUD** XXX M 80

AMA: 2018,Feb,11; 2018,Jan,8; 2017,Jan,8; 2016,Jan,13; 2015,Jan,16

90970 **for patients 20 years of age and older** A

0.22 0.22 **FUD** XXX M 80

AMA: 2018,Feb,11; 2018,Jan,8; 2017,Jan,8; 2016,Jan,13; 2015,Jan,16

90989-90993 Dialysis Training Services

CMS: 100-04,3,100.6 Inpatient Renal Services

90989 **Dialysis training, patient, including helper where applicable, any mode, completed course**

0.00 0.00 **FUD** XXX B

AMA: 2018,Feb,11; 2018,Jan,8; 2017,Jan,8; 2016,Jan,13; 2015,Jan,16

90993 **Dialysis training, patient, including helper where applicable, any mode, course not completed, per training session**

0.00 0.00 **FUD** XXX B

AMA: 2018,Feb,11; 2018,Jan,8; 2017,Jan,8; 2016,Jan,13; 2015,Jan,16

90997-90999 Hemoperfusion and Unlisted Dialysis Procedures

CMS: 100-04,3,100.6 Inpatient Renal Services

90997 **Hemoperfusion (eg, with activated charcoal or resin)**

2.53 2.53 **FUD** 000 B 80

AMA: 2018,Feb,11

90999 **Unlisted dialysis procedure, inpatient or outpatient**

0.00 0.00 **FUD** XXX B 80

AMA: 2018,Feb,11

91010-91022 Esophageal Manometry

91010 **Esophageal motility (manometric study of the esophagus and/or gastroesophageal junction) study with interpretation and report;**

EXCLUDES *Esophageal motility studies with high-resolution esophageal pressure topography (91299)*

Code also for esophageal motility studies with stimulant or perfusion (91013)

5.38 5.38 **FUD** 000 S 80

AMA: 2018,Feb,11

\+ **91013** **with stimulation or perfusion (eg, stimulant, acid or alkali perfusion) (List separately in addition to code for primary procedure)**

EXCLUDES *Esophageal motility studies with high-resolution esophageal pressure topography (91299)*
Reporting code more than one time for each session

Code first (91010)

0.73 0.73 **FUD** ZZZ N 80

AMA: 2018,Feb,11

91020 **Gastric motility (manometric) studies**

EXCLUDES *Gastrointestinal imaging by wireless capsule (91112)*

7.01 7.01 **FUD** 000 S 80

AMA: 2018,Feb,11; 2018,Jan,8; 2017,Jan,8; 2016,Jan,13; 2015,Jan,16

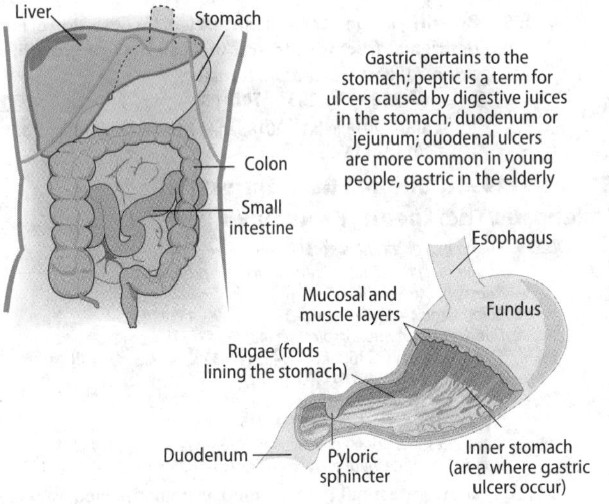

91022 **Duodenal motility (manometric) study**

EXCLUDES *Fluoroscopy (76000)*
Gastric motility study (91020)
Gastrointestinal imaging by wireless capsule (91112)

4.77 4.77 **FUD** 000 S 80

AMA: 2018,Feb,11; 2018,Jan,8; 2017,Jan,8; 2016,Jan,13; 2015,Jan,16

91030-91040 Esophageal Reflux Tests

EXCLUDES *Duodenal intubation/aspiration (43756-43757)*
Esophagoscopy (43180-43233 [43211, 43212, 43213, 43214])
Insertion:
- *Esophageal tamponade tube (43460)*
- *Insertion long gastrointestinal tube (44500)*

Radiologic services, gastrointestinal (74210-74363)
Upper gastrointestinal endoscopy (43235-43259 [43233, 43266, 43270])

91030 **Esophagus, acid perfusion (Bernstein) test for esophagitis**

3.91 3.91 **FUD** 000 S 80

AMA: 2018,Feb,11

91034 **Esophagus, gastroesophageal reflux test; with nasal catheter pH electrode(s) placement, recording, analysis and interpretation**

5.41 5.41 **FUD** 000 S 80

AMA: 2018,Feb,11; 2018,Jan,8; 2017,Jan,8; 2016,Jan,13; 2015,Jan,16

91035 with mucosal attached telemetry pH electrode placement, recording, analysis and interpretation

INCLUDES Endoscopy only to place device

🚑 13.6 ⚕ 13.6 **FUD** 000 [S] [Z2] [80] [□]

AMA: 2018,Feb,11; 2018,Jan,8; 2017,Jan,8; 2016,Jan,13; 2015,Jan,16

91037 Esophageal function test, gastroesophageal reflux test with nasal catheter intraluminal impedance electrode(s) placement, recording, analysis and interpretation;

🚑 4.66 ⚕ 4.66 **FUD** 000 [S] [80] [□]

AMA: 2018,Feb,11

91038 prolonged (greater than 1 hour, up to 24 hours)

🚑 12.4 ⚕ 12.4 **FUD** 000 [S] [80] [□]

AMA: 2018,Feb,11; 2018,Jan,8; 2017,Jan,8; 2016,Jan,13; 2015,Jan,16

91040 Esophageal balloon distension study, diagnostic, with provocation when performed

EXCLUDES Reporting code more than one time for each session

🚑 13.5 ⚕ 13.5 **FUD** 000 [S] [80] [□]

AMA: 2018,Feb,11; 2018,Jan,8; 2017,Jan,6

91065 Breath Analysis

CMS: 100-03,100.5 Diagnostic Breath Analysis

EXCLUDES H. pylori breath test analysis, radioactive (C-14) or nonradioactive (C-13) (78268, 83013)

Code also each challenge administered

91065 Breath hydrogen or methane test (eg, for detection of lactase deficiency, fructose intolerance, bacterial overgrowth, or oro-cecal gastrointestinal transit)

🚑 2.13 ⚕ 2.13 **FUD** 000 [S] [80] [□]

AMA: 2018,Feb,11; 2018,Jan,8; 2017,Jan,8; 2016,Jan,13; 2015,Jan,16

91110-91299 Additional Gastrointestinal Diagnostic/Therapeutic Procedures

EXCLUDES Abdominal paracentesis (49082-49084)
Abdominal paracentesis with medication administration (96440, 96446)
Anoscopy (46600-46615)
Colonoscopy (45378-45393 [45388, 45390, 45398])
Duodenal intubation/aspiration (43756-43757)
Esophagoscopy (43180-43233 [43211, 43212, 43213, 43214])
Proctosigmoidoscopy (45300-45327)
Radiologic services, gastrointestinal (74210-74363)
Sigmoidoscopy (45330-45350 [45346])
Small intestine/stomal endoscopy (44360-44408 [44381, 44401])
Upper gastrointestinal endoscopy (43235-43259 [43233, 43266, 43270])

91110 Gastrointestinal tract imaging, intraluminal (eg, capsule endoscopy), esophagus through ileum, with interpretation and report

EXCLUDES Imaging colon (0355T)
Imaging esophagus through ileum (91111)

Code also modifier 52 when ileum not visualized

🚑 24.9 ⚕ 24.9 **FUD** XXX [T] [80] [□]

AMA: 2018,Feb,11; 2018,Jan,8; 2017,Jan,8; 2016,Jan,13; 2015,Jan,16

91111 Gastrointestinal tract imaging, intraluminal (eg, capsule endoscopy), esophagus with interpretation and report

EXCLUDES Imaging colon (0355T)
Imaging esophagus through ileum (91111)
Wireless capsule to measure transit times or pressure in gastrointestinal tract (91112)

🚑 24.4 ⚕ 24.4 **FUD** XXX [T] [80] [□]

AMA: 2018,Feb,11; 2018,Jan,8; 2017,Jan,8; 2016,Jan,13; 2015,Jan,16

91112 Gastrointestinal transit and pressure measurement, stomach through colon, wireless capsule, with interpretation and report

EXCLUDES Colon motility study (91117)
Duodenal motility study (91022)
Gastric motility studies (91020)
pH body fluid (83986)

🚑 40.9 ⚕ 40.9 **FUD** XXX [T] [80] [□]

AMA: 2018,Feb,11; 2018,Jan,8; 2017,Jan,8; 2016,Jan,13; 2015,Jan,16

91117 Colon motility (manometric) study, minimum 6 hours continuous recording (including provocation tests, eg, meal, intracolonic balloon distension, pharmacologic agents, if performed), with interpretation and report

EXCLUDES Anal manometry (91122)
Rectal sensation, tone and compliance testing (91120)
Reporting code more than one time no matter how many provocations
Wireless capsule to measure transit times or pressure in gastrointestinal tract (91112)

🚑 3.96 ⚕ 3.96 **FUD** 000 [T] [80] [□]

AMA: 2018,Feb,11; 2018,Jan,8; 2017,Jan,8; 2016,Jan,13; 2015,Jan,16

91120 Rectal sensation, tone, and compliance test (ie, response to graded balloon distention)

EXCLUDES Anorectal manometry (91122)
Biofeedback training (90912, 90913)
Colon motility study (91117)

🚑 13.7 ⚕ 13.7 **FUD** XXX [S] [80] [□]

AMA: 2020,Jun,13; 2018,Feb,11; 2018,Jan,8; 2017,Jan,8; 2016,Jan,13; 2015,Jan,16

91122 Anorectal manometry

EXCLUDES Colon motility study (91117)

🚑 7.13 ⚕ 7.13 **FUD** 000 [T] [80] [□]

AMA: 2018,Feb,11

91132 Electrogastrography, diagnostic, transcutaneous;

🚑 6.80 ⚕ 6.80 **FUD** XXX [S] [80] [□]

AMA: 2018,Feb,11

91133 with provocative testing

🚑 9.82 ⚕ 9.82 **FUD** XXX [Q1] [80] [□]

AMA: 2018,Feb,11

91200 Liver elastography, mechanically induced shear wave (eg, vibration), without imaging, with interpretation and report

EXCLUDES Ultrasound elastography parenchyma (76981-76983)

🚑 1.05 ⚕ 1.05 **FUD** XXX [Q1] [80] [□]

AMA: 2019,Aug,3; 2018,Feb,11; 2018,Jan,8; 2017,Oct,9

91299 Unlisted diagnostic gastroenterology procedure

🚑 0.00 ⚕ 0.00 **FUD** XXX [S] [80] [□]

AMA: 2018,Feb,11; 2018,Jan,8; 2017,Jan,8; 2016,Jan,13; 2015,Jan,16

| [26]/[TC] PC/TC Only | [A2]-[Z3] ASC Payment | [50] Bilateral | ♂ Male Only | ♀ Female Only | 🚑 Facility RVU | ⚕ Non-Facility RVU | [□] CCI | [✕] CLIA |
| **FUD** Follow-up Days | **CMS:** IOM | **AMA:** CPT Asst | [A]-[Y] OPPSI | [80]/[80] Surg Assist Allowed / w/Doc | | [▨] Lab Crosswalk | | [▨] Radiology Crosswalk |

464

CPT © 2020 American Medical Association. All Rights Reserved.

© 2020 Optum360, LLC

92002-92014 Ophthalmic Medical Services

CMS: 100-02,15,30.4 Optometrist's Services

INCLUDES Routine ophthalmoscopy
Services provided to established patients who have received professional services from physician or other qualified health care provider or another physician or other qualified health care professional within same group practice/exact same specialty and subspecialty within past three years
Services provided to new patients who have received no professional services from physician or other qualified health care provider or another physician or other qualified health care professional within same group practice/exact same specialty and subspecialty within past three years

EXCLUDES *Retinal polarization scan (0469T)*
Surgical procedures on eye/ocular adnexa (65091-68899 [66987, 66988, 67810])
Visual screening tests (99173-99174 [99177])

92002 Ophthalmological services: medical examination and evaluation with initiation of diagnostic and treatment program; intermediate, new patient

INCLUDES Evaluation new/existing condition complicated by new diagnostic or management problem
Integrated services where medical decision making cannot be separated from examination methods
Intermediate services:
- External ocular/adnexal examination
- General medical observation
- History

Other diagnostic procedures:
- Biomicroscopy
- Mydriasis
- Ophthalmoscopy
- Tonometry

Problems not related to primary diagnosis

1.36 2.37 **FUD** XXX V 80

AMA: 2018,Feb,11; 2018,Feb,3; 2018,Jan,8; 2017,Sep,14; 2017,Jan,8; 2016,Jan,13; 2015,Jan,16

92004 comprehensive, new patient, 1 or more visits

INCLUDES Comprehensive services:
- Basic sensorimotor examination
- Biomicroscopy
- Dilation (cycloplegia)
- External examinations
- General medical observation
- Gross visual fields
- History
- Initiation diagnostic/treatment programs
- Mydriasis
- Ophthalmoscopic examinations
- Other diagnostic procedures
- Prescription medication
- Special diagnostic/treatment services
- Tonometry

General evaluation complete visual system
Integrated services where medical decision making cannot be separated from examination methods
Single service that need not be performed at one session

2.77 4.23 **FUD** XXX V 80

AMA: 2018,Feb,11; 2018,Feb,3; 2018,Jan,8; 2017,Sep,14; 2017,Jan,8; 2016,Nov,9; 2016,Jan,13; 2015,Jan,16

92012 Ophthalmological services: medical examination and evaluation, with initiation or continuation of diagnostic and treatment program; intermediate, established patient

INCLUDES Evaluation new/existing condition complicated by new diagnostic or management problem
Integrated services where medical decision making cannot be separated from examination methods
Problems not related to primary diagnosis
Intermediate services:
- External ocular/adnexal examination
- General medical observation
- History
- Other diagnostic procedures:
  - Biomicroscopy
  - Mydriasis
  - Ophthalmoscopy
  - Tonometry

1.49 2.49 **FUD** XXX V 80

AMA: 2018,Feb,11; 2018,Feb,3; 2018,Jan,8; 2017,Sep,14; 2017,Jan,8; 2016,Jan,13; 2015,Jan,16

92014 comprehensive, established patient, 1 or more visits

INCLUDES General evaluation complete visual system
Integrated services where medical decision making cannot be separated from examination methods
Single service that need not be performed at one session
Comprehensive services:
- Basic sensorimotor examination
- Biomicroscopy
- Dilation (cycloplegia)
- External examinations
- General medical observation
- Gross visual fields
- History
- Initiation diagnostic/treatment programs
- Mydriasis
- Ophthalmoscopic examinations
- Other diagnostic procedures
- Prescription medication
- Special diagnostic/treatment services
- Tonometry

2.23 3.55 **FUD** XXX V 80

AMA: 2018,Feb,11; 2018,Feb,3; 2018,Jan,8; 2017,Sep,14; 2017,Jan,8; 2016,Nov,9; 2016,Jan,13; 2015,Jan,16

92015-92145 Ophthalmic Special Services

INCLUDES Routine ophthalmoscopy

EXCLUDES *Surgical procedures on eye/ocular adnexa (65091-68899 [66987, 66988, 67810])*

Code also E/M services, when performed
Code also general ophthalmological services, when performed (92002-92014)

92015 Determination of refractive state

INCLUDES Lens prescription:
- Absorptive factor
- Axis
- Impact resistance
- Lens power
- Prism

Specification lens type:
- Bifocal
- Monofocal

EXCLUDES *Ocular screening, instrument based (99173-99174 [99177])*

0.55 0.56 **FUD** XXX E

AMA: 2018,Feb,11; 2018,Jan,8; 2017,Jan,8; 2016,Mar,10; 2016,Jan,13; 2015,Jan,16

92018 Ophthalmological examination and evaluation, under general anesthesia, with or without manipulation of globe for passive range of motion or other manipulation to facilitate diagnostic examination; complete

4.13 4.13 **FUD** XXX J 80

AMA: 2018,Feb,11; 2018,Jan,8; 2017,Jan,8; 2016,Jan,13; 2015,Jan,16

92019 **limited**

Facility RVU 2.05 Non-Facility RVU 2.05 **FUD** XXX J 80 CCI

AMA: 2018,Feb,11; 2018,Jan,8; 2017,Jan,8; 2016,Jan,13; 2015,Jan,16

92020 **Gonioscopy (separate procedure)**

EXCLUDES *Gonioscopy under general anesthesia (92018)*
Laser trabeculostomy ab interno (0621T-0622T)

Facility RVU 0.60 Non-Facility RVU 0.78 **FUD** XXX Q1 80 CCI

AMA: 2018,Feb,11; 2018,Jan,8; 2017,Jan,8; 2016,Jan,13; 2015,Jan,16

92025 **Computerized corneal topography, unilateral or bilateral, with interpretation and report**

EXCLUDES *Corneal transplant procedures (65710-65771)*
Manual keratoscopy

Facility RVU 1.07 Non-Facility RVU 1.07 **FUD** XXX Q1 80 CCI

AMA: 2018,Feb,11; 2018,Jan,8; 2017,Jan,8; 2016,Jan,13; 2015,Jan,16

92060 **Sensorimotor examination with multiple measurements of ocular deviation (eg, restrictive or paretic muscle with diplopia) with interpretation and report (separate procedure)**

Facility RVU 1.79 Non-Facility RVU 1.79 **FUD** XXX Q1 80 CCI

AMA: 2018,Feb,11; 2018,Jan,8; 2017,Jan,8; 2016,Jan,13; 2015,Jan,16

92065 **Orthoptic and/or pleoptic training, with continuing medical direction and evaluation**

Facility RVU 1.49 Non-Facility RVU 1.49 **FUD** XXX Q1 80 CCI

AMA: 2018,Feb,11; 2018,Jan,8; 2017,Jan,8; 2016,Jan,13; 2015,Jan,16

92071 **Fitting of contact lens for treatment of ocular surface disease**

EXCLUDES *Contact lens service for keratoconus (92072)*

Code also lens supply with appropriate supply code or (99070)

Facility RVU 0.95 Non-Facility RVU 1.07 **FUD** XXX N 80 50 CCI

AMA: 2018,Feb,11

92072 **Fitting of contact lens for management of keratoconus, initial fitting**

EXCLUDES *Contact lens service for disease ocular surface (92071)*
Subsequent fittings (99211-99215, 92012-92014)

Code also lens supply with appropriate supply code or (99070)

Facility RVU 2.84 Non-Facility RVU 3.72 **FUD** XXX N 80 CCI

AMA: 2018,Feb,11; 2018,Jan,8; 2017,Sep,14; 2017,Jan,8; 2016,Jan,13; 2015,Jan,16

92081 **Visual field examination, unilateral or bilateral, with interpretation and report; limited examination (eg, tangent screen, Autoplot, arc perimeter, or single stimulus level automated test, such as Octopus 3 or 7 equivalent)**

INCLUDES Gross visual testing/confrontation testing

Facility RVU 0.96 Non-Facility RVU 0.96 **FUD** XXX Q1 80 CCI

AMA: 2018,Feb,11; 2018,Jan,8; 2017,Jan,8; 2016,Jan,13; 2015,Jan,16

92082 **intermediate examination (eg, at least 2 isopters on Goldmann perimeter, or semiquantitative, automated suprathreshold screening program, Humphrey suprathreshold automatic diagnostic test, Octopus program 33)**

INCLUDES Gross visual testing/confrontation testing

Facility RVU 1.34 Non-Facility RVU 1.34 **FUD** XXX Q1 80 CCI

AMA: 2018,Feb,11; 2018,Jan,8; 2017,Jan,8; 2016,Jan,13; 2015,Jan,16

92083 **extended examination (eg, Goldmann visual fields with at least 3 isopters plotted and static determination within the central 30°, or quantitative, automated threshold perimetry, Octopus program G-1, 32 or 42, Humphrey visual field analyzer full threshold programs 30-2, 24-2, or 30/60-2)**

INCLUDES Gross visual field testing/confrontation testing

EXCLUDES *Assessment visual field, by data transmission, by patient to surveillance center (0378T-0379T)*

Facility RVU 1.78 Non-Facility RVU 1.78 **FUD** XXX Q1 80 CCI

AMA: 2018,Feb,11; 2018,Jan,8; 2017,Jan,8; 2016,Jan,13; 2015,Jan,16

92100 **Serial tonometry (separate procedure) with multiple measurements of intraocular pressure over an extended time period with interpretation and report, same day (eg, diurnal curve or medical treatment of acute elevation of intraocular pressure)**

EXCLUDES *Intraocular pressure monitoring for 24 hours or more (0329T)*
Ocular blood flow measurements (0198T)
Single-episode tonometry (99202-99215, 92002-92004)

Facility RVU 0.96 Non-Facility RVU 2.32 **FUD** XXX N 80 CCI

AMA: 2018,Feb,11; 2018,Jan,8; 2017,Jan,8; 2016,Jan,13; 2015,Jan,16

92132 **Scanning computerized ophthalmic diagnostic imaging, anterior segment, with interpretation and report, unilateral or bilateral**

EXCLUDES *Imaging anterior segment with specular microscopy and endothelial cell analysis (92286)*
Scanning computerized ophthalmic diagnostic imaging optic nerve and retina (92133-92134)
Tear film imaging (0330T)

Facility RVU 0.89 Non-Facility RVU 0.89 **FUD** XXX Q1 80 CCI

AMA: 2018,Feb,11; 2018,Jan,8; 2017,Jan,8; 2016,Jan,13; 2015,Jan,16

92133 **Scanning computerized ophthalmic diagnostic imaging, posterior segment, with interpretation and report, unilateral or bilateral; optic nerve**

EXCLUDES *Remote imaging for retinal disease (92227-92228)*
Scanning computerized ophthalmic imaging retina same visit (92134)

Facility RVU 1.05 Non-Facility RVU 1.05 **FUD** XXX Q1 80 CCI

AMA: 2018,Feb,11; 2018,Jan,8; 2017,Jan,8; 2016,Jan,13; 2015,Jan,16

92134 **retina**

EXCLUDES *Remote imaging for retinal disease (92227-92228)*
Scanning computerized ophthalmic imaging retina same visit (92134)

Facility RVU 1.15 Non-Facility RVU 1.15 **FUD** XXX Q1 80 CCI

AMA: 2018,Feb,11; 2018,Jan,8; 2017,Jan,8; 2016,Jan,13; 2015,Jan,16

92136 **Ophthalmic biometry by partial coherence interferometry with intraocular lens power calculation**

EXCLUDES *Tear film imaging (0330T)*

Facility RVU 1.76 Non-Facility RVU 1.76 **FUD** XXX Q1 80 CCI

AMA: 2018,Feb,11; 2018,Jan,8; 2017,Jan,8; 2016,Jan,13; 2015,Jan,16

92145 **Corneal hysteresis determination, by air impulse stimulation, unilateral or bilateral, with interpretation and report**

Facility RVU 0.42 Non-Facility RVU 0.42 **FUD** XXX Q1 80 CCI

AMA: 2018,Feb,11

92201-92287 Other Ophthalmology Services

EXCLUDES *Ophthalmological exam under anesthesia (92018)*
Prescription, fitting, and/or medical supervision ocular prosthesis adaptation by physician (99202-99215, 99241-99245, 92002-92014)
Surgical procedures on eye/ocular adnexa (65091-68899 [66987, 66988, 67810])

92201 Ophthalmoscopy, extended; with retinal drawing and scleral depression of peripheral retinal disease (eg, for retinal tear, retinal detachment, retinal tumor) with interpretation and report, unilateral or bilateral

EXCLUDES *Fundus photography with interpretation and report (92250)*

0.65 0.71 FUD XXX 80

AMA: 2019,Dec,3

92202 with drawing of optic nerve or macula (eg, for glaucoma, macular pathology, tumor) with interpretation and report, unilateral or bilateral

EXCLUDES *Fundus photography with interpretation and report (92250)*

0.42 0.45 FUD XXX 80

AMA: 2019,Dec,3

▲ **92227 Imaging of retina for detection or monitoring of disease; with remote clinical staff review and report, unilateral or bilateral**

EXCLUDES *Fundus photography with interpretation and report (92250)*
Imaging for retinal disease:
Point of care automated analysis and report (92229)
Remote interpretation and report (92228)
Scanning computerized ophthalmic imaging:
Optic nerve (92133)
Retina (92134)

0.40 0.40 FUD XXX ★ Q1 80 TC

AMA: 2019,Aug,10; 2018,Feb,11; 2018,Jan,8; 2017,Jan,8; 2016,Jul,8; 2016,Jan,13; 2015,Jan,16

▲ **92228 with remote physician or other qualified health care professional interpretation and report, unilateral or bilateral**

EXCLUDES *Fundus photography with interpretation and report (92250)*
Imaging for retinal disease:
Point of care automated analysis and report (92229)
Remote clinical staff review and report (92227)
Scanning computerized ophthalmic imaging:
Optic nerve (92133)
Retina (92134)

0.96 0.96 FUD XXX ★ Q1 80

AMA: 2018,Feb,11; 2018,Jan,8; 2017,Jan,8; 2016,Jan,13; 2015,Jan,16

● **92229 point-of-care automated analysis and report, unilateral or bilateral**

EXCLUDES *Fundus photography with interpretation and report (92250)*
Remote imaging for retinal disease (92227-92228)
Scanning computerized ophthalmic imaging:
Optic nerve (92133)
Retina (92134)

92230 Fluorescein angioscopy with interpretation and report

0.95 1.83 FUD XXX Q1 80

AMA: 2018,Feb,11; 2018,Jan,8; 2017,Jan,8; 2016,Jan,13; 2015,Jan,16

92235 Fluorescein angiography (includes multiframe imaging) with interpretation and report, unilateral or bilateral

EXCLUDES *Fluorescein and indocyanine-green angiography (92242)*

2.59 2.59 FUD XXX S 80

AMA: 2018,Feb,11; 2018,Jan,8; 2017,Jun,8; 2017,Jan,8; 2016,Jan,13; 2015,Jan,16

92240 Indocyanine-green angiography (includes multiframe imaging) with interpretation and report, unilateral or bilateral

EXCLUDES *Fluorescein and indocyanine-green angiography (92242)*

5.69 5.69 FUD XXX S 80

AMA: 2018,Feb,11; 2018,Jan,8; 2017,Jun,8; 2017,Jan,8; 2016,Jan,13; 2015,Jan,16

92242 Fluorescein angiography and indocyanine-green angiography (includes multiframe imaging) performed at the same patient encounter with interpretation and report, unilateral or bilateral

6.71 6.71 FUD XXX S 80

AMA: 2018,Feb,11; 2018,Jan,8; 2017,Jun,8

92250 Fundus photography with interpretation and report

1.27 1.27 FUD XXX Q1 80

AMA: 2019,Dec,3; 2018,Feb,11; 2018,Jan,8; 2017,Jan,8; 2016,Jul,8; 2016,Jan,13; 2015,May,9; 2015,Jan,16

92260 Ophthalmodynamometry

0.31 0.55 FUD XXX Q1 80

AMA: 2018,Feb,11; 2018,Jan,8; 2017,Jan,8; 2016,Jan,13; 2015,Jan,16

92265 Needle oculoelectromyography, 1 or more extraocular muscles, 1 or both eyes, with interpretation and report

2.48 2.48 FUD XXX Q1 80

AMA: 2018,Feb,11; 2018,Jan,8; 2017,Jan,8; 2016,Jan,13; 2015,Jan,16

92270 Electro-oculography with interpretation and report

EXCLUDES *Recording saccadic eye movement (92700)*
Vestibular function testing (92537-92538, 92540-92542, 92544-92549)

2.73 2.73 FUD XXX Q1 80

AMA: 2020,Apr,7; 2018,Feb,11; 2018,Jan,8; 2017,Jan,8; 2016,Jan,13; 2015,Sep,7; 2015,Jan,16

92273 Electroretinography (ERG), with interpretation and report; full field (ie, ffERG, flash ERG, Ganzfeld ERG)

EXCLUDES *Pattern electroretinography (PERG) (0509T)*

3.78 3.78 FUD XXX 80

AMA: 2019,Jan,12

92274 multifocal (mfERG)

EXCLUDES *Pattern electroretinography (PERG) (0509T)*

2.56 2.56 FUD XXX 80

AMA: 2019,Jan,12

92283 Color vision examination, extended, eg, anomaloscope or equivalent

1.52 1.52 FUD XXX Q1 80

AMA: 2018,Feb,11; 2018,Jan,8; 2017,Jan,8; 2016,Jan,13; 2015,Jan,16

92284 Dark adaptation examination with interpretation and report

1.74 1.74 FUD XXX Q1 80

AMA: 2018,Feb,11; 2018,Jan,8; 2017,Jan,8; 2016,Jan,13; 2015,Jan,16

92285 External ocular photography with interpretation and report for documentation of medical progress (eg, close-up photography, slit lamp photography, goniophotography, stereo-photography)

0.61 0.61 FUD XXX Q1 80

AMA: 2018,Feb,11; 2018,Jan,8; 2017,Jan,8; 2016,Jan,13; 2015,Jan,16

92286 Anterior segment imaging with interpretation and report; with specular microscopy and endothelial cell analysis

1.10 1.10 FUD XXX Q1 80

AMA: 2018,Feb,11; 2018,Jan,8; 2017,Jan,8; 2016,Jan,13; 2015,Jan,16

92287 **with fluorescein angiography**
4.46 | 4.46 | FUD XXX | Q1 80
AMA: 2018,Feb,11; 2018,Jan,8; 2017,Jan,8; 2016,Jan,13; 2015,Jan,16

92310-92326 Services Related to Contact Lenses

CMS: 100-02,15,30.4 Optometrist's Services

INCLUDES Incidental revision lens during training period
Patient training/instruction
Specification optical/physical characteristics:
- Curvature
- Flexibility
- Gas-permeability
- Power
- Size

EXCLUDES *Extended wear lenses follow up (92012-92014)*
General ophthalmological services
Therapeutic/surgical use contact lens (68340, 92071-92072)

92310 **Prescription of optical and physical characteristics of and fitting of contact lens, with medical supervision of adaptation; corneal lens, both eyes, except for aphakia**
Code also modifier 52 for prescription and fitting only one eye
1.71 | 2.86 | FUD XXX | E
AMA: 2018,Feb,11; 2018,Jan,8; 2017,Jan,8; 2016,Jan,13; 2015,Jan,16

92311 **corneal lens for aphakia, 1 eye**
1.54 | 2.95 | FUD XXX | Q1 80
AMA: 2018,Feb,11; 2018,Jan,8; 2017,Jan,8; 2016,Jan,13; 2015,Jan,16

92312 **corneal lens for aphakia, both eyes**
1.77 | 3.42 | FUD XXX | Q1 80
AMA: 2018,Feb,11; 2018,Jan,8; 2017,Jan,8; 2016,Jan,13; 2015,Jan,16

92313 **corneoscleral lens**
1.31 | 2.78 | FUD XXX | Q1 80
AMA: 2018,Feb,11; 2018,Jan,8; 2017,Jan,8; 2016,Jan,13; 2015,Jan,16

92314 **Prescription of optical and physical characteristics of contact lens, with medical supervision of adaptation and direction of fitting by independent technician; corneal lens, both eyes except for aphakia**
Code also modifier 52 for prescription and fitting only one eye
1.02 | 2.43 | FUD XXX | E
AMA: 2018,Feb,11; 2018,Jan,8; 2017,Jan,8; 2016,Jan,13; 2015,Jan,16

92315 **corneal lens for aphakia, 1 eye**
0.62 | 2.19 | FUD XXX | Q1 80
AMA: 2018,Feb,11; 2018,Jan,8; 2017,Jan,8; 2016,Jan,13; 2015,Jan,16

92316 **corneal lens for aphakia, both eyes**
0.93 | 2.72 | FUD XXX | Q1 80
AMA: 2018,Feb,11; 2018,Jan,8; 2017,Jan,8; 2016,Jan,13; 2015,Jan,16

92317 **corneoscleral lens**
0.62 | 2.29 | FUD XXX | Q1 80
AMA: 2018,Feb,11; 2018,Jan,8; 2017,Jan,8; 2016,Jan,13; 2015,Jan,16

92325 **Modification of contact lens (separate procedure), with medical supervision of adaptation**
1.24 | 1.24 | FUD XXX | Q1 80
AMA: 2018,Feb,11; 2018,Jan,8; 2017,Jan,8; 2016,Jan,13; 2015,Jan,16

92326 **Replacement of contact lens**
1.05 | 1.05 | FUD XXX | Q1 80
AMA: 2018,Feb,11; 2018,Jan,8; 2017,Jan,8; 2016,Jan,13; 2015,Jan,16

92340-92499 Services Related to Eyeglasses

CMS: 100-02,15,30.4 Optometrist's Services

INCLUDES Anatomical facial characteristics measurement
Final adjustment of spectacles to visual axes/anatomical topography
Written laboratory specifications

EXCLUDES *Materials supply*

92340 **Fitting of spectacles, except for aphakia; monofocal**
0.53 | 0.99 | FUD XXX | E
AMA: 2018,Feb,11; 2018,Jan,8; 2017,Jan,8; 2016,Jan,13; 2015,Jan,16

92341 **bifocal**
0.70 | 1.15 | FUD XXX | E
AMA: 2018,Feb,11; 2018,Jan,8; 2017,Jan,8; 2016,Jan,13; 2015,Jan,16

92342 **multifocal, other than bifocal**
0.77 | 1.23 | FUD XXX | E
AMA: 2018,Feb,11; 2018,Jan,8; 2017,Jan,8; 2016,Jan,13; 2015,Jan,16

92352 **Fitting of spectacle prosthesis for aphakia; monofocal**
0.53 | 1.17 | FUD XXX | Q1
AMA: 2018,Feb,11; 2018,Jan,8; 2017,Jan,8; 2016,Jan,13; 2015,Jan,16

92353 **multifocal**
0.72 | 1.36 | FUD XXX | Q1
AMA: 2018,Feb,11; 2018,Jan,8; 2017,Jan,8; 2016,Jan,13; 2015,Jan,16

92354 **Fitting of spectacle mounted low vision aid; single element system**
0.38 | 0.38 | FUD XXX | Q1
AMA: 2018,Feb,11; 2018,Jan,8; 2017,Jan,8; 2016,Jan,13; 2015,Jan,16

92355 **telescopic or other compound lens system**
0.58 | 0.58 | FUD XXX | Q1
AMA: 2018,Feb,11; 2018,Jan,8; 2017,Jan,8; 2016,Jan,13; 2015,Jan,16

92358 **Prosthesis service for aphakia, temporary (disposable or loan, including materials)**
0.32 | 0.32 | FUD XXX | Q1
AMA: 2018,Feb,11; 2018,Jan,8; 2017,Jan,8; 2016,Jan,13; 2015,Jan,16

92370 **Repair and refitting spectacles; except for aphakia**
0.46 | 0.88 | FUD XXX | E
AMA: 2018,Feb,11; 2018,Jan,8; 2017,Jan,8; 2016,Jan,13; 2015,Jan,16

92371 **spectacle prosthesis for aphakia**
0.33 | 0.33 | FUD XXX | Q1
AMA: 2018,Feb,11; 2018,Jan,8; 2017,Jan,8; 2016,Jan,13; 2015,Jan,16

92499 **Unlisted ophthalmological service or procedure**
0.00 | 0.00 | FUD XXX | Q1 80
AMA: 2020,Aug,14; 2019,Jan,12; 2018,Jul,3; 2018,Feb,11; 2018,Jan,8; 2017,Jan,8; 2016,Jan,13; 2015,Jan,16

92502-92526 [92517, 92518, 92519] Special Procedures of the Ears/Nose/Throat

INCLUDES Anterior rhinoscopy, tuning fork testing, otoscopy, or removal non-impacted cerumen
Diagnostic/treatment services not generally included in E/M service

EXCLUDES *Laryngoscopy with stroboscopy (31579)*

92502 **Otolaryngologic examination under general anesthesia**
2.73 | 2.73 | FUD 000 | T 80
AMA: 2018,Feb,11; 2018,Jan,8; 2017,Jan,8; 2016,Sep,6

92504 **Binocular microscopy (separate diagnostic procedure)**
0.27 | 0.83 | FUD XXX | N 80
AMA: 2018,Feb,11; 2018,Jan,8; 2017,Jan,8; 2016,Sep,6; 2016,Jan,13; 2015,Jan,16

92507 Treatment of speech, language, voice, communication, and/or auditory processing disorder; individual

EXCLUDES *Adaptive behavior treatment ([97153], [97155])*
Auditory rehabilitation:
Postlingual hearing loss (92633)
Prelingual hearing loss (92630)
Programming cochlear implant (92601-92604)

2.25 2.25 FUD XXX A 80

AMA: 2018,Dec,7; 2018,Dec,7; 2018,Nov,3; 2018,Feb,11; 2018,Jan,8; 2017,Jan,8; 2016,Sep,6; 2016,Jan,13; 2015,Jan,16

92508 group, 2 or more individuals

EXCLUDES *Adaptive behavior treatment ([97154], [97158])*
Auditory rehabilitation:
Postlingual hearing loss (92633)
Prelingual hearing loss (92630)
Programming cochlear implant (92601-92604)

0.67 0.67 FUD XXX A 80

AMA: 2018,Nov,3; 2018,Feb,11; 2018,Jan,8; 2017,Jan,8; 2016,Sep,6; 2016,Jan,13; 2015,Jan,16

92511 Nasopharyngoscopy with endoscope (separate procedure)

EXCLUDES *Diagnostic flexible laryngoscopy (31575)*
Nasopharyngoscopic dilation eustachian tube (69705-69706)
Transnasal esophagoscopy (43197-43198)

1.08 3.15 FUD 000 T 80

AMA: 2018,Feb,11; 2018,Jan,8; 2017,Jul,7; 2017,Jan,8; 2016,Dec,13; 2016,Sep,6

92512 Nasal function studies (eg, rhinomanometry)

0.80 1.68 FUD XXX S 80

AMA: 2018,Feb,11; 2018,Jan,8; 2017,Jan,8; 2016,Sep,6

92516 Facial nerve function studies (eg, electroneuronography)

0.65 1.94 FUD XXX S 80

AMA: 2018,Feb,11; 2018,Jan,8; 2017,Jan,8; 2016,Sep,6

92517 **Resequenced code. See code following 92549.**

92518 **Resequenced code. See code following 92549.**

92519 **Resequenced code. See code following 92549.**

92520 Laryngeal function studies (ie, aerodynamic testing and acoustic testing)

EXCLUDES *Other laryngeal function testing (92700)*
Swallowing/laryngeal sensory testing with flexible fiberoptic endoscope (92611-92617)

Code also modifier 52 for single test

1.17 2.28 FUD XXX Q1 80

AMA: 2018,Feb,11; 2018,Jan,8; 2017,Jan,8; 2016,Sep,6; 2016,Jan,13; 2015,Jan,16

92521 Evaluation of speech fluency (eg, stuttering, cluttering)

INCLUDES Ability to execute motor movements needed for speech
Comprehension written and verbal expression
Determination patient's ability to create and communicate expressive thought
Evaluation ability to produce speech sound

3.21 3.21 FUD XXX A 80

AMA: 2018,Feb,11; 2018,Jan,8; 2017,Jan,8; 2016,Sep,6; 2016,Jan,13; 2015,Jan,16

92522 Evaluation of speech sound production (eg, articulation, phonological process, apraxia, dysarthria);

INCLUDES Ability to execute motor movements needed for speech
Comprehension written and verbal expression
Determination patient's ability to create and communicate expressive thought
Evaluation ability to produce speech sound

2.60 2.60 FUD XXX A 80

AMA: 2018,Feb,11; 2018,Jan,8; 2017,Jan,8; 2016,Sep,6; 2016,Jan,13; 2015,Jan,16

92523 with evaluation of language comprehension and expression (eg, receptive and expressive language)

INCLUDES Ability to execute motor movements needed for speech
Comprehension written and verbal expression
Determination patient's ability to create and communicate expressive thought
Evaluation ability to produce speech sound

5.54 5.54 FUD XXX A 80

AMA: 2018,Feb,11; 2018,Jan,8; 2017,Jan,8; 2016,Sep,6; 2016,Jan,13; 2015,Jan,16

92524 Behavioral and qualitative analysis of voice and resonance

INCLUDES Ability to execute motor movements needed for speech
Comprehension written and verbal expression
Determination patient's ability to create and communicate expressive thought
Evaluation ability to produce speech sound

2.51 2.51 FUD XXX A 80

AMA: 2018,Feb,11; 2018,Jan,8; 2017,Jan,8; 2016,Sep,6; 2016,Jan,13; 2015,Jan,16

92526 Treatment of swallowing dysfunction and/or oral function for feeding

2.48 2.48 FUD XXX A 80

AMA: 2018,Feb,11; 2018,Jan,8; 2017,Jan,8; 2016,Sep,6

92531-92519 [92517, 92518, 92519] Vestibular Function Tests

92531 Spontaneous nystagmus, including gaze

EXCLUDES *When performed with E/M services (99202-99215, 99218-99223 [99224, 99225, 99226], 99231-99236, 99241-99245, 99304-99318, 99324-99337)*

0.00 0.00 FUD XXX N

AMA: 2020,Aug,14; 2018,Feb,11

92532 Positional nystagmus test

EXCLUDES *When performed with E/M services (99202-99215, 99218-99223 [99224, 99225, 99226], 99231-99236, 99241-99245, 99304-99318, 99324-99337)*

0.00 0.00 FUD XXX N

AMA: 2020,Aug,14; 2018,Feb,11

92533 Caloric vestibular test, each irrigation (binaural, bithermal stimulation constitutes 4 tests)

INCLUDES Barany caloric test

0.00 0.00 FUD XXX N

AMA: 2020,Aug,14; 2018,Feb,11; 2018,Jan,8; 2017,Jan,8; 2016,Jan,13; 2015,Jan,16

92534 Optokinetic nystagmus test

0.00 0.00 FUD XXX N

AMA: 2020,Aug,14; 2018,Feb,11

92537 Caloric vestibular test with recording, bilateral; bithermal (ie, one warm and one cool irrigation in each ear for a total of four irrigations)

EXCLUDES *Electro-oculography (92270)*
Monothermal caloric vestibular test (92538)

Code also modifier 52 when only three irrigations performed

1.18 1.18 FUD XXX S 80

AMA: 2020,Aug,14; 2018,Feb,11; 2015,Sep,7

92538 monothermal (ie, one irrigation in each ear for a total of two irrigations)

EXCLUDES *Bithermal caloric vestibular test (92537)*
Electro-oculography (92270)

Code also modifier 52 only one irrigation performed

0.64 0.64 FUD XXX S 80

AMA: 2020,Aug,14; 2018,Feb,11; 2015,Sep,7

92540 **Basic vestibular evaluation, includes spontaneous nystagmus test with eccentric gaze fixation nystagmus, with recording, positional nystagmus test, minimum of 4 positions, with recording, optokinetic nystagmus test, bidirectional foveal and peripheral stimulation, with recording, and oscillating tracking test, with recording**

EXCLUDES *Vestibular function tests (92270, 92541-92542, 92544-92545)*

Facility RVU 3.04 Non-Facility RVU 3.04 FUD XXX S 80

AMA: 2020,Aug,14; 2018,Feb,11; 2018,Jan,8; 2017,Jan,8; 2016,Jan,13; 2015,Sep,7

92541 **Spontaneous nystagmus test, including gaze and fixation nystagmus, with recording**

EXCLUDES *Vestibular function tests (92270, 92540, 92542, 92544-92545)*

Facility RVU 0.71 Non-Facility RVU 0.71 FUD XXX Q1 80

AMA: 2020,Aug,14; 2019,Jan,12; 2018,Feb,11; 2018,Jan,8; 2017,Jan,8; 2016,Jan,13; 2015,Sep,7; 2015,Jan,16

92542 **Positional nystagmus test, minimum of 4 positions, with recording**

EXCLUDES *Vestibular function tests (92270, 92540-92541, 92544-92545)*

Facility RVU 0.84 Non-Facility RVU 0.84 FUD XXX Q1 80

AMA: 2020,Aug,14; 2018,Feb,11; 2018,Jan,8; 2017,Jan,8; 2016,Jan,13; 2015,Sep,7; 2015,Jan,16

92544 **Optokinetic nystagmus test, bidirectional, foveal or peripheral stimulation, with recording**

EXCLUDES *Vestibular function tests (92270, 92540-92542, 92545)*

Facility RVU 0.49 Non-Facility RVU 0.49 FUD XXX S 80

AMA: 2020,Aug,14; 2018,Feb,11; 2018,Jan,8; 2017,Jan,8; 2016,Jan,13; 2015,Sep,7; 2015,Jan,16

92545 **Oscillating tracking test, with recording**

EXCLUDES *Vestibular function tests (92270, 92540-92542, 92544)*

Facility RVU 0.47 Non-Facility RVU 0.47 FUD XXX S 80

AMA: 2020,Aug,14; 2018,Feb,11; 2018,Jan,8; 2017,Jan,8; 2016,Jan,13; 2015,Sep,7; 2015,Jan,16

92546 **Sinusoidal vertical axis rotational testing**

EXCLUDES *Electro-oculography (92270)*

Facility RVU 2.95 Non-Facility RVU 2.95 FUD XXX S 80

AMA: 2020,Aug,14; 2018,Feb,11; 2018,Jan,8; 2017,Jan,8; 2016,Jan,13; 2015,Sep,7; 2015,Jan,16

+ **92547** **Use of vertical electrodes (List separately in addition to code for primary procedure)**

EXCLUDES *Electro-oculography (92270)*
Unlisted vestibular tests (92700)

Code first (92540-92546)

Facility RVU 0.21 Non-Facility RVU 0.21 FUD ZZZ N 80 TC

AMA: 2020,Aug,14; 2018,Feb,11; 2018,Jan,8; 2017,Jan,8; 2016,Jan,13; 2015,Sep,7; 2015,Jan,16

92548 **Computerized dynamic posturography sensory organization test (CDP-SOT), 6 conditions (ie, eyes open, eyes closed, visual sway, platform sway, eyes closed platform sway, platform and visual sway), including interpretation and report;**

EXCLUDES *Electro-oculography (92270)*

Facility RVU 1.41 Non-Facility RVU 1.41 FUD XXX Q1 80

AMA: 2020,Aug,14; 2020,Apr,7; 2018,Feb,11; 2018,Jan,8; 2017,Jan,8; 2016,Jan,13; 2015,Sep,7; 2015,Jan,16

92549 **with motor control test (MCT) and adaptation test (ADT)**

EXCLUDES *Electro-oculography (92270)*

Facility RVU 1.80 Non-Facility RVU 1.80 FUD XXX 80

AMA: 2020,Aug,14; 2020,Apr,7

● # **92517** **Vestibular evoked myogenic potential (VEMP) testing, with interpretation and report; cervical (cVEMP)**

EXCLUDES *Electro-oculography (92270)*
Vestibular evoked myogenic potential testing:
Cervical and ocular ([92519])
Ocular ([92518])

Facility RVU 0.00 Non-Facility RVU 0.00 FUD 000

● # **92518** **ocular (oVEMP)**

EXCLUDES *Electro-oculography (92270)*
Vestibular evoked myogenic potential testing:
Cervical ([92517])
Cervical and ocular ([92519])

Facility RVU 0.00 Non-Facility RVU 0.00 FUD 000

● # **92519** **cervical (cVEMP) and ocular (oVEMP)**

EXCLUDES *Electro-oculography (92270)*
Vestibular evoked myogenic potential testing:
Cervical only ([92517])
Ocular only ([92518])

Facility RVU 0.00 Non-Facility RVU 0.00 FUD 000

92550-92597 [92558, 92597, 92650, 92651, 92652, 92653] Hearing and Speech Tests

INCLUDES Calibrated electronic equipment, recording results, and report with interpretation
Diagnostic/treatment services not generally included in comprehensive otorhinolaryngologic evaluation or office visit
Testing both ears
Tuning fork and whisper tests

EXCLUDES *Evaluation speech/language/hearing problems using performance observation/assessment (92521-92524)*

Code also modifier 52 for unilateral testing

92550 **Tympanometry and reflex threshold measurements**

INCLUDES Tympanometry, acoustic reflex testing individual codes (92567-92568)

Facility RVU 0.62 Non-Facility RVU 0.62 FUD XXX Q1 80

AMA: 2018,Feb,11; 2018,Jan,8; 2017,Jan,8; 2016,Jan,13; 2015,Jan,16

92551 **Screening test, pure tone, air only**

Facility RVU 0.33 Non-Facility RVU 0.33 FUD XXX E

AMA: 2018,Feb,11; 2018,Jan,8; 2017,Jan,8; 2016,Jan,13; 2015,Jan,16

92552 **Pure tone audiometry (threshold); air only**

EXCLUDES *Automated test (0208T)*

Facility RVU 0.89 Non-Facility RVU 0.89 FUD XXX Q1 80 TC

AMA: 2018,Feb,11; 2018,Jan,8; 2017,Jan,8; 2016,Jan,13; 2015,Jan,16

92553 **air and bone**

EXCLUDES *Automated test (0209T)*

Facility RVU 1.08 Non-Facility RVU 1.08 FUD XXX Q1 80 TC

AMA: 2018,Feb,11; 2018,Jan,8; 2017,Jan,8; 2016,Jan,13; 2015,Jan,16

92555 **Speech audiometry threshold;**

EXCLUDES *Automated test (0210T)*

Facility RVU 0.68 Non-Facility RVU 0.68 FUD XXX Q1 80 TC

AMA: 2018,Feb,11; 2018,Jan,8; 2017,Jan,8; 2016,Jan,13; 2015,Jan,16

92556 **with speech recognition**

EXCLUDES *Automated test (0211T)*

Facility RVU 1.07 Non-Facility RVU 1.07 FUD XXX Q1 80 TC

AMA: 2018,Feb,11; 2018,Jan,8; 2017,Jan,8; 2016,Jan,13; 2015,Jan,16

92557 **Comprehensive audiometry threshold evaluation and speech recognition (92553 and 92556 combined)**

EXCLUDES *Automated test (0208T-0212T)*
Evaluation/selection hearing aid (92590-92595)

Facility RVU 0.93 Non-Facility RVU 1.08 FUD XXX Q1 80

AMA: 2018,Feb,11; 2018,Jan,8; 2017,Jan,8; 2016,Jan,13; 2015,Jan,16

92558 **Resequenced code. See code before 92587.**

92559 **Audiometric testing of groups**

INCLUDES For group testing, indicate tests performed

Facility RVU 0.00 Non-Facility RVU 0.00 FUD XXX E

AMA: 2018,Feb,11; 2018,Jan,8; 2017,Jan,8; 2016,Jan,13; 2015,Jan,16

92560 Bekesy audiometry; screening
0.00 0.00 FUD XXX E
AMA: 2018,Feb,11; 2018,Jan,8; 2017,Jan,8; 2016,Jan,13; 2015,Jan,16

92561 diagnostic
1.10 1.10 FUD XXX Q1 80 TC
AMA: 2018,Feb,11; 2018,Jan,8; 2017,Jan,8; 2016,Jan,13; 2015,Jan,16

92562 Loudness balance test, alternate binaural or monaural
INCLUDES ABLB test
1.28 1.28 FUD XXX Q1 80 TC
AMA: 2018,Feb,11; 2018,Jan,8; 2017,Jan,8; 2016,Jan,13; 2015,Jan,16

92563 Tone decay test
0.87 0.87 FUD XXX Q1 80 TC
AMA: 2018,Feb,11; 2018,Jan,8; 2017,Jan,8; 2016,Jan,13; 2015,Jan,16

92564 Short increment sensitivity index (SISI)
0.71 0.71 FUD XXX Q1 80 TC
AMA: 2018,Feb,11; 2018,Jan,8; 2017,Jan,8; 2016,Jan,13; 2015,Jan,16

92565 Stenger test, pure tone
0.44 0.44 FUD XXX Q1 80 TC
AMA: 2018,Feb,11; 2018,Jan,8; 2017,Jan,8; 2016,Jan,13; 2015,Jan,16

92567 Tympanometry (impedance testing)
0.31 0.43 FUD XXX Q1 80
AMA: 2018,Feb,11; 2018,Jan,8; 2017,Jan,8; 2016,Jan,13; 2015,Jan,16

92568 Acoustic reflex testing, threshold
0.44 0.45 FUD XXX Q1 80
AMA: 2018,Feb,11; 2018,Jan,8; 2017,Jan,8; 2016,Jan,13; 2015,Jan,16

92570 Acoustic immittance testing, includes tympanometry (impedance testing), acoustic reflex threshold testing, and acoustic reflex decay testing
INCLUDES Tympanometry, acoustic reflex testing individual codes (92567-92568)
0.85 0.94 FUD XXX Q1 80
AMA: 2018,Feb,11; 2018,Jan,8; 2017,Jan,8; 2016,Jan,13; 2015,Jan,16

92571 Filtered speech test
0.76 0.76 FUD XXX Q1 80 TC
AMA: 2018,Feb,11; 2018,Jan,8; 2017,Jan,8; 2016,Jan,13; 2015,Jan,16

92572 Staggered spondaic word test
1.21 1.21 FUD XXX Q1 80 TC
AMA: 2018,Feb,11; 2018,Jan,8; 2017,Jan,8; 2016,Jan,13; 2015,Jan,16

92575 Sensorineural acuity level test
1.79 1.79 FUD XXX Q1 80 TC
AMA: 2018,Feb,11; 2018,Jan,8; 2017,Jan,8; 2016,Jan,13; 2015,Jan,16

92576 Synthetic sentence identification test
1.02 1.02 FUD XXX Q1 80 TC
AMA: 2018,Feb,11; 2018,Jan,8; 2017,Jan,8; 2016,Jan,13; 2015,Jan,16

92577 Stenger test, speech
0.39 0.39 FUD XXX Q1 80 TC
AMA: 2018,Feb,11; 2018,Jan,8; 2017,Jan,8; 2016,Jan,13; 2015,Jan,16

92579 Visual reinforcement audiometry (VRA)
1.09 1.31 FUD XXX Q1 80
AMA: 2018,Feb,11; 2018,Jan,8; 2017,Jan,8; 2016,Jan,13; 2015,Jan,16

92582 Conditioning play audiometry
2.06 2.06 FUD XXX Q1 80 TC
AMA: 2018,Feb,11; 2018,Jan,8; 2017,Jan,8; 2016,Jan,13; 2015,Jan,16

92583 Select picture audiometry
1.35 1.35 FUD XXX Q1 80 TC
AMA: 2018,Feb,11; 2018,Jan,8; 2017,Jan,8; 2016,Jan,13; 2015,Jan,16

92584 Electrocochleography
2.09 2.09 FUD XXX S 80 TC
AMA: 2018,Feb,11; 2018,Jan,8; 2017,Jan,8; 2016,Jan,13; 2015,Jan,16

92585 ~~Auditory evoked potentials for evoked response audiometry and/or testing of the central nervous system; comprehensive~~
To report, see ([92652], [92653])

92586 ~~limited~~
To report, see ([92650], [92651])

● # **92650 Auditory evoked potentials; screening of auditory potential with broadband stimuli, automated analysis**
0.00 0.00 FUD 000

● # **92651 for hearing status determination, broadband stimuli, with interpretation and report**
0.00 0.00 FUD 000

● # **92652 for threshold estimation at multiple frequencies, with interpretation and report**
EXCLUDES *Hearing status determination ([92651])*
0.00 0.00 FUD 000

● # **92653 neurodiagnostic, with interpretation and report**
0.00 0.00 FUD 000

92558 Evoked otoacoustic emissions, screening (qualitative measurement of distortion product or transient evoked otoacoustic emissions), automated analysis
0.25 0.28 FUD XXX E
AMA: 2018,Feb,11; 2018,Jan,8; 2017,Jan,8; 2016,Jan,13; 2015,Jan,16

92587 Distortion product evoked otoacoustic emissions; limited evaluation (to confirm the presence or absence of hearing disorder, 3-6 frequencies) or transient evoked otoacoustic emissions, with interpretation and report
0.63 0.63 FUD XXX S 80
AMA: 2018,Feb,11; 2018,Jan,8; 2017,Jan,8; 2016,Jan,13; 2015,Jan,16

92588 comprehensive diagnostic evaluation (quantitative analysis of outer hair cell function by cochlear mapping, minimum of 12 frequencies), with interpretation and report
EXCLUDES *Evaluation central auditory function (92620-92621)*
0.96 0.96 FUD XXX S 80
AMA: 2018,Feb,11; 2018,Jan,8; 2017,Jan,8; 2016,Jan,13; 2015,Jan,16

92590 Hearing aid examination and selection; monaural
0.00 0.00 FUD XXX E
AMA: 2020,Jul,3; 2018,Feb,11; 2018,Jan,8; 2017,Jan,8; 2016,Jan,13; 2015,Jan,16

92591 binaural
0.00 0.00 FUD XXX E
AMA: 2020,Jul,3; 2018,Feb,11; 2018,Jan,8; 2017,Jan,8; 2016,Jan,13; 2015,Jan,16

92592 Hearing aid check; monaural
0.00 0.00 FUD XXX E
AMA: 2020,Jul,3; 2018,Feb,11; 2018,Jan,8; 2017,Jan,8; 2016,Jan,13; 2015,Jan,16

92593 binaural
0.00 0.00 FUD XXX E
AMA: 2020,Jul,3; 2018,Feb,11; 2018,Jan,8; 2017,Jan,8; 2016,Jan,13; 2015,Jan,16

92594 **Electroacoustic evaluation for hearing aid; monaural**
0.00 0.00 **FUD** XXX E
AMA: 2020,Jul,3; 2018,Feb,11; 2018,Jan,8; 2017,Jan,8; 2016,Jan,13; 2015,Jan,16

92595 **binaural**
0.00 0.00 **FUD** XXX E
AMA: 2020,Jul,3; 2018,Feb,11; 2018,Jan,8; 2017,Jan,8; 2016,Jan,13; 2015,Jan,16

92596 **Ear protector attenuation measurements**
1.89 1.89 **FUD** XXX Q1 80 TC
AMA: 2018,Feb,11; 2018,Jan,8; 2017,Jan,8; 2016,Jan,13; 2015,Jan,16

92597 **Resequenced code. See code following 92604.**

92601-92609 [92597, 92618] Services Related to Hearing and Speech Devices

INCLUDES Diagnostic/treatment services not generally included in comprehensive otorhinolaryngologic evaluation or office visit

92601 **Diagnostic analysis of cochlear implant, patient younger than 7 years of age; with programming** A
INCLUDES Connection to cochlear implant
Postoperative analysis/fitting previously placed external devices
Stimulator programming
EXCLUDES *Cochlear implant placement (69930)*
3.57 4.68 **FUD** XXX S 80
AMA: 2020,Jul,3; 2018,Feb,11; 2018,Jan,8; 2017,Jan,8; 2016,Sep,6; 2016,Jan,13; 2015,Jan,16

92602 **subsequent reprogramming** A
INCLUDES Internal stimulator re-programming
Subsequent sessions for external transmitter measurements/adjustment
EXCLUDES *Analysis with programming (92601)*
Aural rehabilitation services after cochlear implant (92626-92627, 92630-92633)
Cochlear implant placement (69930)
2.02 2.92 **FUD** XXX S 80
AMA: 2020,Jul,3; 2018,Feb,11; 2018,Jan,8; 2017,Jan,8; 2016,Sep,6; 2016,Jan,13; 2015,Jan,16

92603 **Diagnostic analysis of cochlear implant, age 7 years or older; with programming** A
INCLUDES Connection to cochlear implant
Postoperative analysis/fitting previously placed external devices
Stimulator programming
EXCLUDES *Cochlear implant placement (69930)*
3.47 4.37 **FUD** XXX S 80
AMA: 2020,Jul,3; 2018,Feb,11; 2018,Jan,8; 2017,Jan,8; 2016,Sep,6; 2016,Jan,13; 2015,Jan,16

92604 **subsequent reprogramming** A
INCLUDES Internal stimulator reprogramming
Subsequent sessions for external transmitter measurements/adjustment
EXCLUDES *Analysis with programming (92603)*
Cochlear implant placement (69930)
1.94 2.60 **FUD** XXX S 80
AMA: 2020,Jul,3; 2018,Feb,11; 2018,Jan,8; 2017,Jan,8; 2016,Sep,6; 2016,Jan,13; 2015,Jan,16

92597 **Evaluation for use and/or fitting of voice prosthetic device to supplement oral speech**
EXCLUDES *Augmentative or alternative communication device services (92605, [92618], 92607-92608)*
2.06 2.06 **FUD** XXX A 80
AMA: 2018,Feb,11; 2018,Jan,8; 2017,Jan,8; 2016,Jan,13; 2015,Jan,16

92605 **Evaluation for prescription of non-speech-generating augmentative and alternative communication device, face-to-face with the patient; first hour**
EXCLUDES *Prosthetic voice device fitting or use evaluation (92597)*
2.53 2.65 **FUD** XXX A
AMA: 2018,Feb,11; 2018,Jan,8; 2017,Jan,8; 2016,Jan,13; 2015,Jan,16

+ # **92618** **each additional 30 minutes (List separately in addition to code for primary procedure)**
Code first (92605)
0.94 0.96 **FUD** ZZZ A
AMA: 2018,Feb,11

92606 **Therapeutic service(s) for the use of non-speech-generating device, including programming and modification**
2.02 2.35 **FUD** XXX A
AMA: 2018,Feb,11; 2018,Jan,8; 2017,Jan,8; 2016,Jan,13; 2015,Jan,16

92607 **Evaluation for prescription for speech-generating augmentative and alternative communication device, face-to-face with the patient; first hour**
EXCLUDES *Evaluation for prescription non-speech generating device (92605)*
Evaluation for use/fitting voice prosthetic (92597)
3.69 3.69 **FUD** XXX A 80
AMA: 2018,Feb,11; 2018,Jan,8; 2017,Jan,8; 2016,Jan,13; 2015,Jan,16

+ **92608** **each additional 30 minutes (List separately in addition to code for primary procedure)**
Code first initial hour (92607)
1.47 1.47 **FUD** ZZZ A 80
AMA: 2018,Feb,11; 2018,Jan,8; 2017,Jan,8; 2016,Jan,13; 2015,Jan,16

92609 **Therapeutic services for the use of speech-generating device, including programming and modification**
EXCLUDES *Therapeutic services for use non-speech generating device (92606)*
3.08 3.08 **FUD** XXX A 80
AMA: 2018,Feb,11; 2018,Jan,8; 2017,Jan,8; 2016,Jan,13; 2015,Jan,16

92610-92618 [92618] Swallowing Evaluations

92610 **Evaluation of oral and pharyngeal swallowing function**
EXCLUDES *Evaluation with flexible endoscope (92612-92617)*
Motion fluoroscopic evaluation swallowing function (92611)
2.06 2.45 **FUD** XXX A 80
AMA: 2018,Feb,11; 2018,Jan,8; 2017,Apr,8; 2017,Jan,8; 2016,Jan,13; 2015,Jan,16

92611 **Motion fluoroscopic evaluation of swallowing function by cine or video recording**
EXCLUDES *Diagnostic flexible laryngoscopy (31575)*
Evaluation oral/pharyngeal swallowing function (92610)
(74230)
2.55 2.55 **FUD** XXX A 80
AMA: 2020,Aug,9; 2018,Feb,11; 2018,Jan,8; 2017,Apr,8; 2017,Jan,8; 2016,Sep,6; 2016,Jan,13; 2015,Jan,16

92612 **Flexible endoscopic evaluation of swallowing by cine or video recording;**
EXCLUDES *Diagnostic flexible fiberoptic laryngoscopy (31575)*
Flexible endoscopic examination/testing without cine or video recording (92700)
1.94 5.42 **FUD** XXX A 80
AMA: 2018,Feb,11; 2018,Jan,8; 2017,Jul,7; 2017,Apr,8; 2017,Jan,8; 2016,Dec,13; 2016,Sep,6; 2016,Jan,13; 2015,Jan,16

92613 **interpretation and report only**

EXCLUDES *Diagnostic flexible laryngoscopy (31575)*
Oral/pharyngeal swallowing function examination (92610)
Swallowing function motion fluoroscopic examination (92611)

1.07 1.07 FUD XXX B 80

AMA: 2018,Feb,11; 2018,Jan,8; 2017,Jul,7; 2017,Apr,8; 2017,Jan,8; 2016,Dec,13; 2016,Sep,6; 2016,Jan,13; 2015,Jan,16

92614 **Flexible endoscopic evaluation, laryngeal sensory testing by cine or video recording;**

EXCLUDES *Diagnostic flexible laryngoscopy (31575)*
Flexible endoscopic examination/testing without cine or video recording (92700)

1.90 4.03 FUD XXX A 80

AMA: 2018,Feb,11; 2018,Jan,8; 2017,Jul,7; 2017,Apr,8; 2017,Jan,8; 2016,Dec,13; 2016,Sep,6; 2016,Jan,13; 2015,Jan,16

92615 **interpretation and report only**

EXCLUDES *Diagnostic flexible laryngoscopy (31575)*

0.94 0.94 FUD XXX E 80

AMA: 2018,Feb,11; 2018,Jan,8; 2017,Jul,7; 2017,Apr,8; 2017,Jan,8; 2016,Dec,13; 2016,Sep,6; 2016,Jan,13; 2015,Jan,16

92616 **Flexible endoscopic evaluation of swallowing and laryngeal sensory testing by cine or video recording;**

EXCLUDES *Diagnostic flexible fiberoptic laryngoscopy (31575)*
Flexible endoscopic examination/testing without cine or video recording (92700)

2.84 5.85 FUD XXX A 80

AMA: 2018,Feb,11; 2018,Jan,8; 2017,Jul,7; 2017,Apr,8; 2017,Jan,8; 2016,Dec,13; 2016,Sep,6; 2016,Jan,13; 2015,Jan,16

92617 **interpretation and report only**

EXCLUDES *Diagnostic flexible laryngoscopy (31575)*

1.18 1.18 FUD XXX E 80

AMA: 2018,Feb,11; 2018,Jan,8; 2017,Jul,7; 2017,Apr,8; 2017,Jan,8; 2016,Dec,13; 2016,Sep,6; 2016,Jan,13; 2015,Jan,16

92618 **Resequenced code. See code following 92605.**

92620-92700 [92650, 92651, 92652, 92653] Diagnostic Hearing Evaluations and Rehabilitation

INCLUDES Diagnostic/treatment services not generally included in comprehensive otorhinolaryngologic evaluation or office visit

92620 **Evaluation of central auditory function, with report; initial 60 minutes**

EXCLUDES *Voice analysis (92521-92524)*

2.32 2.67 FUD XXX Q1 80

AMA: 2018,Feb,11; 2018,Jan,8; 2017,Jan,8; 2016,Jan,13; 2015,Jan,16

+ **92621** **each additional 15 minutes (List separately in addition to code for primary procedure)**

EXCLUDES *Voice analysis (92521-92524)*.
Code first (92620)

0.54 0.64 FUD ZZZ N 80

AMA: 2018,Feb,11; 2018,Jan,8; 2017,Jan,8; 2016,Jan,13; 2015,Jan,16

92625 **Assessment of tinnitus (includes pitch, loudness matching, and masking)**

EXCLUDES *Loudness test (92562)*
Code also modifier 52 for unilateral procedure

1.78 1.99 FUD XXX Q1 80

AMA: 2018,Feb,11; 2018,Jan,8; 2017,Jan,8; 2016,Jan,13; 2015,Jan,16

92626 **Evaluation of auditory function for surgically implanted device(s) candidacy or postoperative status of a surgically implanted device(s); first hour**

INCLUDES Assessment to determine patient's proficiency in remaining hearing to identify speech
Face-to-face time spent with patient or family

EXCLUDES *Hearing aid evaluation, fitting, follow-up, or selection (92590-92591, 92592-92593, 92594-92595)*

2.16 2.55 FUD XXX Q1 80

AMA: 2020,Jul,3; 2018,Feb,11; 2018,Jan,8; 2017,Jan,8; 2016,Sep,6; 2016,Jan,13; 2015,Jan,16

+ **92627** **each additional 15 minutes (List separately in addition to code for primary procedure)**

INCLUDES Assessment to determine patient's proficiency in remaining hearing to identify speech
Face-to-face time spent with patient or family

EXCLUDES *Hearing aid evaluation, fitting, follow-up, or selection (92590-92591, 92592-92593, 92594-92595)*
Code first initial hour (92626)

0.51 0.64 FUD ZZZ N 80

AMA: 2020,Jul,3; 2018,Feb,11; 2018,Jan,8; 2017,Jan,8; 2016,Sep,6; 2016,Jan,13; 2015,Jan,16

92630 **Auditory rehabilitation; prelingual hearing loss**

0.00 0.00 FUD XXX E

AMA: 2018,Feb,11; 2018,Jan,8; 2017,Jan,8; 2016,Sep,6; 2016,Jan,13; 2015,Jan,16

92633 **postlingual hearing loss**

0.00 0.00 FUD XXX E

AMA: 2018,Feb,11; 2018,Jan,8; 2017,Jan,8; 2016,Sep,6; 2016,Jan,13; 2015,Jan,16

92640 **Diagnostic analysis with programming of auditory brainstem implant, per hour**

EXCLUDES *Nonprogramming services (cardiac monitoring)*

2.73 3.25 FUD XXX S 80

AMA: 2018,Feb,11

92650 **Resequenced code. See code following 92584.**

92651 **Resequenced code. See code following 92584.**

92652 **Resequenced code. See code following 92584.**

92653 **Resequenced code. See code following 92584.**

92700 **Unlisted otorhinolaryngological service or procedure**

INCLUDES Lombard test

0.00 0.00 FUD XXX Q1 80

AMA: 2018,Feb,11; 2018,Jan,8; 2017,Apr,8; 2017,Jan,8; 2016,Sep,6; 2016,Jan,13; 2015,Sep,7; 2015,Sep,12; 2015,Jan,16

92920-92953 [92920, 92921, 92924, 92925, 92928, 92929, 92933, 92934, 92937, 92938, 92941, 92943, 92944] Emergency Cardiac Procedures

92920 **Resequenced code. See code following 92998.**

92921 **Resequenced code. See code following 92998.**

92924 **Resequenced code. See code following 92998.**

92925 **Resequenced code. See code following 92998.**

92928 **Resequenced code. See code following 92998.**

92929 **Resequenced code. See code following 92998.**

92933 **Resequenced code. See code following 92998.**

92934 **Resequenced code. See code following 92998.**

92937 **Resequenced code. See code following 92998.**

92938 **Resequenced code. See code following 92998.**

92941 **Resequenced code. See code following 92998.**

92943 **Resequenced code. See code following 92998.**

92944 **Resequenced code. See code following 92998.**

92950 **Cardiopulmonary resuscitation (eg, in cardiac arrest)**

INCLUDES Cardiac defibrillation

EXCLUDES *Critical care services (99291-99292)*

5.35 8.92 **FUD** 000 S 80

AMA: 2018,Feb,11; 2018,Jan,8; 2017,Jan,8; 2016,Jan,13; 2015,Jan,16

92953 **Temporary transcutaneous pacing**

EXCLUDES *Direction ambulance/rescue personnel by physician or other qualified health care professional (99288)*

0.03 0.03 **FUD** 000 Q3 80

AMA: 2019,Aug,8; 2018,Feb,11; 2018,Jan,8; 2017,Jan,8; 2016,Jan,13; 2015,Jan,16

92960-92961 Cardioversion

92960 **Cardioversion, elective, electrical conversion of arrhythmia; external**

3.13 4.51 **FUD** 000 S 80

AMA: 2018,Feb,11; 2018,Jan,8; 2017,Jan,8; 2016,Jan,13; 2015,Jan,16

92961 **internal (separate procedure)**

EXCLUDES *Device evaluation for implantable defibrillator/multi-lead pacemaker system (93282-93284, 93287, 93289, 93295-93296)*
Electrophysiological studies (93618-93624, 93631, 93640-93642)
Intracardiac ablation (93650-93657, 93662)

7.23 7.23 **FUD** 000 S

AMA: 2018,Feb,11; 2018,Jan,8; 2017,Jan,8; 2016,Jan,13; 2015,Feb,3; 2015,Jan,16

92970-92979 [92973, 92974, 92975, 92977, 92978, 92979] Circulatory Assist: External/Internal

EXCLUDES *Atrial septostomy, any method (33741)*
Catheter placement for use in circulatory assist devices (intra-aortic balloon pump) (33970)

92970 **Cardioassist-method of circulatory assist; internal**

5.52 5.52 **FUD** 000 C 80

AMA: 2018,Feb,11

92971 **external**

2.91 2.91 **FUD** 000 C 80

AMA: 2018,Feb,11

92973 **Resequenced code. See code following 92998.**

92974 **Resequenced code. See code following 92998.**

92975 **Resequenced code. See code following 92998.**

92977 **Resequenced code. See code following 92998.**

92978 **Resequenced code. See code following 92998.**

92979 **Resequenced code. See code following 92998.**

92986-92993 Percutaneous Procedures of Heart Valves and Septum

EXCLUDES *Atrial septostomy, any method (33741)*

92986 **Percutaneous balloon valvuloplasty; aortic valve**

38.3 38.3 **FUD** 090 J 80

AMA: 2018,Feb,11; 2018,Jan,8; 2017,Jan,8; 2016,Jan,13; 2015,Feb,3; 2015,Jan,16

92987 **mitral valve**

39.3 39.3 **FUD** 090 J 80

AMA: 2018,Feb,11; 2018,Jan,8; 2017,Jan,8; 2016,Jan,13; 2015,Feb,3

92990 **pulmonary valve**

31.4 31.4 **FUD** 090 J 80

AMA: 2018,Feb,11; 2018,Jan,8; 2017,Jan,8; 2016,Jan,13; 2015,Jul,10; 2015,Feb,3

92992 ~~**Atrial septectomy or septostomy; transvenous method, balloon (eg, Rashkind type) (includes cardiac catheterization)**~~

92993 ~~**blade method (Park septostomy) (includes cardiac catheterization)**~~

92997-92998 Percutaneous Angioplasty: Pulmonary Artery

92997 **Percutaneous transluminal pulmonary artery balloon angioplasty; single vessel**

18.4 18.4 **FUD** 000 J 80

AMA: 2018,Feb,11; 2018,Jan,8; 2017,Jul,3; 2017,Jan,8; 2016,Mar,5; 2016,Jan,13; 2015,Feb,3

\+ **92998** **each additional vessel (List separately in addition to code for primary procedure)**

Code first single vessel (92997)

9.44 9.44 **FUD** ZZZ N 80

AMA: 2018,Feb,11; 2018,Jan,8; 2017,Jul,3; 2017,Jan,8; 2016,Mar,5; 2016,Jan,13; 2015,Feb,3

92920-92944 [92920, 92921, 92924, 92925, 92928, 92929, 92933, 92934, 92937, 92938, 92941, 92943, 92944]

Intravascular Coronary Procedures

INCLUDES Accessing vessel
- Additional procedures performed in third branch, major coronary artery
- All procedures performed in all branch segments, coronary arteries
  - Branches left anterior descending (diagonals), left circumflex (marginals), and right (posterior descending, posterolaterals)
  - Distal, proximal, and mid segments
- All procedures performed in all segments, major coronary arteries through native vessels:
  - Distal, proximal, and mid segments
  - Left main, left anterior descending, left circumflex, right, and ramus intermedius arteries
- All procedures performed in major coronary arteries or recognized coronary artery branches through coronary artery bypass graft
  - Sequential bypass graft with more than single distal anastomosis as one graft
  - Branching bypass grafts (e.g., "Y" grafts) include coronary vessel for primary graft, with each branch off primary graft making up an additional coronary vessel
  - Each coronary artery bypass graft denotes single coronary vessel
  - Embolic protection devices when used
- Arteriotomy closure through access sheath
- Atherectomy (e.g., directional, laser, rotational)
- Balloon angioplasty (e.g., cryoplasty, cutting balloon, wired balloons)
- Cardiac catheterization and related procedures when included in coronary revascularization service (93454-93461, 93563-93564)
- Imaging once procedure complete
- Percutaneous coronary interventions (PCI) for coronary vessel disease, native and bypass grafts
- Procedures in left main and ramus intermedius coronary artery branches as they are unrecognized for individual code assignment
- Radiological supervision and interpretation intervention(s)
- Reporting most comprehensive treatment in given vessel according to intensity hierarchy for base and add-on codes:
  - Add-on codes: 92944 = 92938 > 92934 > 92925 > 92929 > 92921
  - Base codes (report only one): 92943 = 92941 = 92933 > 92924 > 92937 = 92928 > 92920
- Revascularization achieved with single procedure when single lesion continues from one target vessel (major artery, branch, or bypass graft) to another target vessel
- Selective vessel catheterization
- Stenting (e.g., balloon expandable, bare metal, covered, drug eluting, self-expanding)
- Traversing lesion

EXCLUDES *Application intravascular radioelements (77770-77772)*
- *Insertion device for coronary intravascular brachytherapy (92974)*
- *Reduction septum (e.g., alcohol ablation) (93799)*

Code also add-on codes for procedures performed during same session in additional recognized target vessel branches

Code also diagnostic angiography during interventional procedure when:
- No previous catheter-based coronary angiography study available, and full diagnostic study performed, with decision to perform intervention based on that study
- Previous study available, but documentation states patient's condition changed since previous study or target area visualization inadequate, or change occurs during procedure warranting additional evaluation outside current target area

Code also diagnostic angiography performed at session separate from interventional procedure

Code also individual base codes for treatment major native coronary artery segment and another segment same artery requiring treatment through bypass graft when performed at same time

Code also procedures for both vessels for bifurcation lesion

Code also procedures performed in second branch major coronary artery

Code also treatment arterial segment requiring access through bypass graft

92920 **Percutaneous transluminal coronary angioplasty; single major coronary artery or branch**

15.4 15.4 FUD 000 J J8 80

AMA: 2018,Feb,11; 2018,Jan,8; 2017,Jul,3; 2017,Jan,8; 2016,Jan,13; 2015,Jan,16

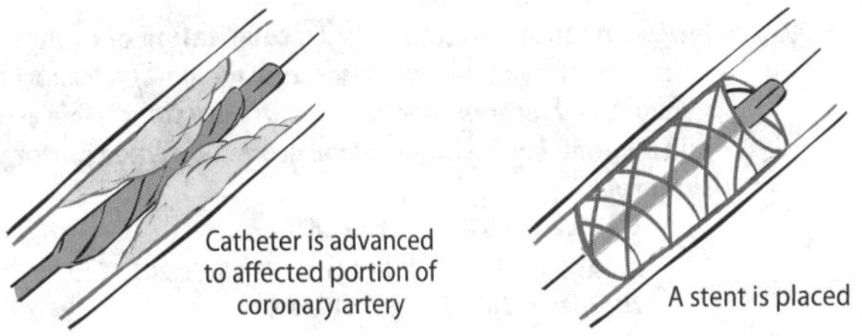

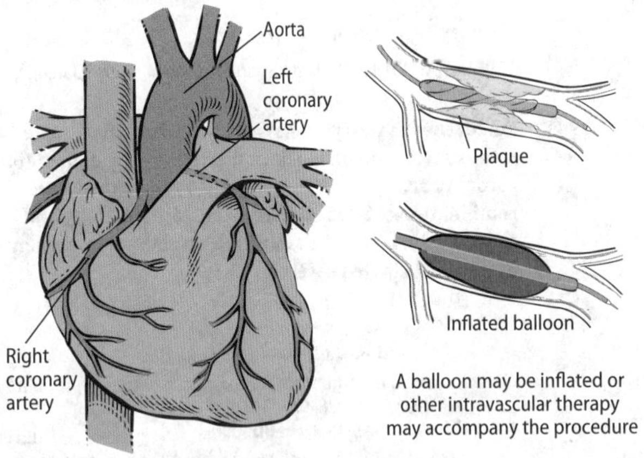

+ # **92921** **each additional branch of a major coronary artery (List separately in addition to code for primary procedure)**

Code first (92920, 92924, 92928, 92933, 92937, 92941, 92943)

0.00 0.00 FUD ZZZ N N1

AMA: 2018,Feb,11; 2018,Jan,8; 2017,Jul,3; 2017,Jan,8; 2016,Jan,13; 2015,Jan,16

92924 **Percutaneous transluminal coronary atherectomy, with coronary angioplasty when performed; single major coronary artery or branch**

18.4 18.4 FUD 000 J 80

AMA: 2018,Feb,11; 2018,Jan,8; 2017,Jul,3; 2017,Jan,8; 2016,Jan,13; 2015,Jan,16

+ # **92925** **each additional branch of a major coronary artery (List separately in addition to code for primary procedure)**

Code first (92924, 92928, 92933, 92937, 92941, 92943)

0.00 0.00 FUD ZZZ N

AMA: 2018,Feb,11; 2018,Jan,8; 2017,Jul,3; 2017,Jan,8; 2016,Jan,13; 2015,Jan,16

92928 **Percutaneous transcatheter placement of intracoronary stent(s), with coronary angioplasty when performed; single major coronary artery or branch**

17.2 17.2 FUD 000 J J8 80

AMA: 2018,Feb,11; 2018,Jan,8; 2017,Jul,3; 2017,Feb,14; 2017,Jan,8; 2017,Jan,6; 2016,Jan,13; 2015,Jan,16

+ # **92929** **each additional branch of a major coronary artery (List separately in addition to code for primary procedure)**

Code first (92928, 92933, 92937, 92941, 92943)

0.00 0.00 FUD ZZZ N N1

AMA: 2018,Feb,11; 2018,Jan,8; 2017,Jul,3; 2017,Jan,8; 2017,Jan,6; 2016,Jan,13; 2015,Jan,16

92933 **Percutaneous transluminal coronary atherectomy, with intracoronary stent, with coronary angioplasty when performed; single major coronary artery or branch**

19.3 19.3 FUD 000 J 80

AMA: 2018,Feb,11; 2018,Jan,8; 2017,Jul,3; 2017,Jan,8; 2016,Jan,13; 2015,Jan,16

+ # **92934** **each additional branch of a major coronary artery (List separately in addition to code for primary procedure)**

Code first (92933, 92937, 92941, 92943)

0.00 0.00 **FUD** ZZZ N

AMA: 2018,Feb,11; 2018,Jan,8; 2017,Jul,3; 2017,Jan,8; 2016,Jan,13; 2015,Jan,16

92937 **Percutaneous transluminal revascularization of or through coronary artery bypass graft (internal mammary, free arterial, venous), any combination of intracoronary stent, atherectomy and angioplasty, including distal protection when performed; single vessel**

17.2 17.2 **FUD** 000 J 80

AMA: 2018,Feb,11; 2018,Jan,8; 2017,Jul,3; 2017,Feb,14; 2017,Jan,8; 2016,Jan,13; 2015,Jan,16

+ # **92938** **each additional branch subtended by the bypass graft (List separately in addition to code for primary procedure)**

Code first (92937)

0.00 0.00 **FUD** ZZZ N

AMA: 2018,Feb,11; 2018,Jan,8; 2017,Jul,3; 2017,Jan,8; 2016,Jan,13; 2015,Jan,16

92941 **Percutaneous transluminal revascularization of acute total/subtotal occlusion during acute myocardial infarction, coronary artery or coronary artery bypass graft, any combination of intracoronary stent, atherectomy and angioplasty, including aspiration thrombectomy when performed, single vessel**

INCLUDES Aspiration thrombectomy, when performed
Embolic protection
Rheolytic thrombectomy

Code also treatment additional vessels, when appropriate (92920-92938, 92943-92944)

19.3 19.3 **FUD** 000 C 80

AMA: 2020,Jul,13; 2018,Feb,11; 2018,Jan,8; 2017,Jul,3; 2017,Feb,14; 2017,Jan,8; 2016,Jan,13; 2015,Jan,16

92943 **Percutaneous transluminal revascularization of chronic total occlusion, coronary artery, coronary artery branch, or coronary artery bypass graft, any combination of intracoronary stent, atherectomy and angioplasty; single vessel**

INCLUDES Antegrade flow deficiency with angiography and clinical criteria indicating chronic total occlusion

19.3 19.3 **FUD** 000 J 80

AMA: 2018,Feb,11; 2018,Jan,8; 2017,Jul,3; 2017,Jan,8; 2016,Jan,13; 2015,Jan,16

+ # **92944** **each additional coronary artery, coronary artery branch, or bypass graft (List separately in addition to code for primary procedure)**

EXCLUDES *Application intravascular radioelements (77770-77772)*

Code first (92924, 92928, 92933, 92937, 92941, 92943)

0.00 0.00 **FUD** ZZZ N

AMA: 2018,Feb,11; 2018,Jan,8; 2017,Jul,3; 2017,Jan,8; 2016,Jan,13; 2015,Jan,16

92973-92979 [92973, 92974, 92975, 92977, 92978, 92979] Additional Coronary Artery Procedures

+ # **92973** **Percutaneous transluminal coronary thrombectomy mechanical (List separately in addition to code for primary procedure)**

EXCLUDES *Aspiration thrombectomy*

Code first (92920, 92924, 92928, 92933, 92937, 92941, 92943, 92975, 93454-93461, 93563-93564)

5.15 5.15 **FUD** ZZZ N 80

AMA: 2020,Jul,13; 2018,Feb,11; 2018,Jan,8; 2017,Feb,14; 2017,Jan,8; 2016,Jan,13; 2015,Jan,16

+ # **92974** **Transcatheter placement of radiation delivery device for subsequent coronary intravascular brachytherapy (List separately in addition to code for primary procedure)**

EXCLUDES *Application intravascular radioelements (77770-77772)*

Code first (92920, 92924, 92928, 92933, 92937, 92941, 92943, 93454-93461)

4.68 4.68 **FUD** ZZZ N 80

AMA: 2018,Feb,11; 2018,Jan,8; 2017,Feb,14; 2017,Jan,8; 2016,Jan,13; 2015,Jan,16

92975 **Thrombolysis, coronary; by intracoronary infusion, including selective coronary angiography**

EXCLUDES *Thrombolysis, cerebral (37195)*
Thrombolysis other than coronary ([37211, 37212, 37213, 37214])

10.9 10.9 **FUD** 000 C 80

AMA: 2018,Feb,11

92977 **by intravenous infusion**

EXCLUDES *Thrombolysis, cerebral (37195)*
Thrombolysis other than coronary ([37211, 37212, 37213, 37214])

1.51 1.51 **FUD** XXX T 80

AMA: 2018,Feb,11

+ # **92978** **Endoluminal imaging of coronary vessel or graft using intravascular ultrasound (IVUS) or optical coherence tomography (OCT) during diagnostic evaluation and/or therapeutic intervention including imaging supervision, interpretation and report; initial vessel (List separately in addition to code for primary procedure)**

Code first primary procedure (92920, 92924, 92928, 92933, 92937, 92941, 92943, 92975, 93454-93461, 93563-93564)

0.00 0.00 **FUD** ZZZ N 80

AMA: 2018,Feb,11; 2018,Jan,8; 2017,Jan,8; 2016,Jan,13; 2015,Jan,16

+ # **92979** **each additional vessel (List separately in addition to code for primary procedure)**

INCLUDES Transducer manipulations/repositioning in vessel examined, before and after therapeutic intervention

EXCLUDES *Intravascular spectroscopy (93799)*

Code first initial vessel (92978)

0.00 0.00 **FUD** ZZZ N 80

AMA: 2018,Feb,11; 2018,Jan,8; 2017,Jan,8; 2016,Jan,13; 2015,Jan,16

93000-93010 Electrocardiographic Services

INCLUDES Specific order for service, separate written and signed report, and documentation medical necessity

EXCLUDES *Acoustic cardiography (93799)*
Echocardiography (93303-93350)
Intracardiac ischemia monitoring system (0525T-0532T)
Reporting codes for telemetry monitoring strip review

93000 **Electrocardiogram, routine ECG with at least 12 leads; with interpretation and report**

0.48 0.48 **FUD** XXX M 80

AMA: 2018,Feb,11; 2018,Jan,8; 2017,Oct,3; 2017,Jan,8; 2016,Jan,13; 2015,Jan,16

93005 **tracing only, without interpretation and report**

0.24 0.24 **FUD** XXX Q1 80 TC

AMA: 2018,Feb,11; 2018,Jan,8; 2017,Oct,3; 2017,Jan,8; 2016,Apr,8; 2016,Jan,13; 2015,Jan,16

93010 **interpretation and report only**
0.24 0.24 FUD XXX B 80 26
AMA: 2018,Feb,11; 2018,Jan,8; 2017,Oct,3; 2017,Jan,8; 2016,Apr,8; 2016,Jan,13; 2015,Jan,16

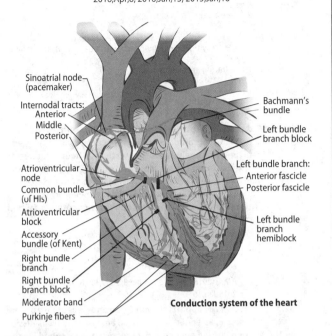

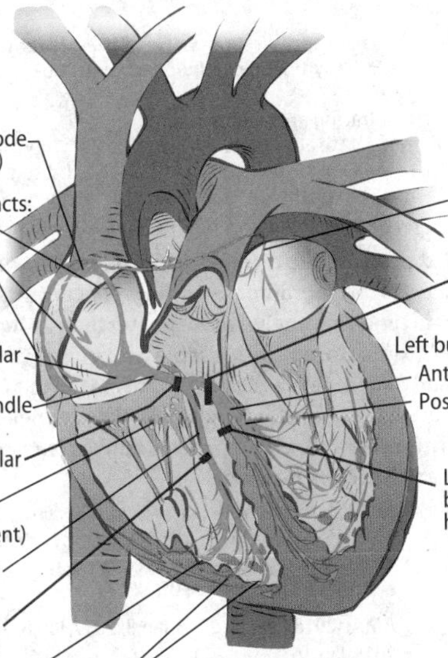

Conduction system of the heart

93015-93018 Stress Test

93015 **Cardiovascular stress test using maximal or submaximal treadmill or bicycle exercise, continuous electrocardiographic monitoring, and/or pharmacological stress; with supervision, interpretation and report**
2.01 2.01 FUD XXX B 80
AMA: 2020,Jul,5; 2018,Feb,11; 2018,Jan,8; 2017,Oct,3; 2017,Jan,8; 2016,Jan,13; 2015,Jan,16

93016 **supervision only, without interpretation and report**
0.63 0.63 FUD XXX B 80 26
AMA: 2020,Jul,5; 2018,Feb,11; 2018,Jan,8; 2017,Oct,3; 2017,Jan,8; 2016,Jan,13; 2015,Jan,16

93017 **tracing only, without interpretation and report**
0.95 0.95 FUD XXX Q1 80 TC
AMA: 2020,Jul,5; 2018,Feb,11; 2018,Jan,8; 2017,Oct,3; 2017,Jan,8; 2016,Jan,13; 2015,Jan,16

93018 **interpretation and report only**
0.42 0.42 FUD XXX B 80 26
AMA: 2020,Jul,5; 2018,Feb,11; 2018,Jan,8; 2017,Oct,3; 2017,Jan,8; 2016,Jan,13; 2015,Jan,16

93024 Provocation Test for Coronary Vasospasm

93024 **Ergonovine provocation test**
3.10 3.10 FUD XXX Q1 80
AMA: 2018,Feb,11

93025 Microvolt T-Wave Alternans

CMS: 100-03,20.30 Microvolt T-Wave Alternans (MTWA); 100-04,32,370 Microvolt T-wave Alternans; 100-04,32,370.1 Coding and Claims Processing for MTWA; 100-04,32,370.2 Messaging for MTWA

INCLUDES Specific order for service, separate written and signed report, and documentation medical necessity

EXCLUDES *Echocardiography (93303-93350)*
Reporting codes for telemetry monitoring strip review

93025 **Microvolt T-wave alternans for assessment of ventricular arrhythmias**
4.23 4.23 FUD XXX S 80
AMA: 2018,Feb,11; 2018,Jan,8; 2017,Jan,8; 2016,Jan,13; 2015,Jan,16

93040-93042 Rhythm Strips

INCLUDES Specific order for service, separate written and signed report, and documentation medical necessity

EXCLUDES *Device evaluation ([93261], 93279-93289 [93260], 93291-93296, 93298)*
Echocardiography (93303-93350)
Reporting codes for telemetry monitoring strip review

93040 **Rhythm ECG, 1-3 leads; with interpretation and report**
0.36 0.36 FUD XXX B 80
AMA: 2020,Sep,7; 2018,Feb,11; 2018,Jan,8; 2017,Oct,3; 2017,Jan,8; 2016,Jan,13; 2015,Jan,16

93041 **tracing only without interpretation and report**
0.16 0.16 FUD XXX Q1 80 TC
AMA: 2018,Feb,11; 2018,Jan,8; 2017,Oct,3; 2017,Jan,8; 2016,Jan,13; 2015,Jan,16

93042 **interpretation and report only**
0.20 0.20 FUD XXX B 80 26
AMA: 2018,Feb,11; 2018,Jan,8; 2017,Oct,3; 2017,Jan,8; 2016,Jan,13; 2015,Jan,16

93050 Arterial Waveform Analysis

EXCLUDES *Reporting code with any intra-arterial diagnostic or interventional procedure*

93050 **Arterial pressure waveform analysis for assessment of central arterial pressures, includes obtaining waveform(s), digitization and application of nonlinear mathematical transformations to determine central arterial pressures and augmentation index, with interpretation and report, upper extremity artery, non-invasive**
0.46 0.46 FUD XXX Q1 80
AMA: 2018,Feb,11

93224-93227 Holter Monitor

INCLUDES Cardiac monitoring using in-person as well as remote technology for electrocardiographic data assessment
Up to 48 hours recording on continuous basis

EXCLUDES *Echocardiography (93303-93355 [93356])*
Implantable patient activated cardiac event recorders (93285, 93291, 93297-93298)
More than 48 hours monitoring ([93241, 93242, 93243, 93244, 93245, 93246, 93247, 93248])

Code also modifier 52 when less than 12 hours continuous recording provided

93224 **External electrocardiographic recording up to 48 hours by continuous rhythm recording and storage; includes recording, scanning analysis with report, review and interpretation by a physician or other qualified health care professional**
2.51 2.51 FUD XXX M 80
AMA: 2018,Feb,11; 2018,Jan,8; 2017,Jan,8; 2016,Jan,13; 2015,Jan,16

93225 **recording (includes connection, recording, and disconnection)**
0.72 0.72 FUD XXX Q1 80 TC
AMA: 2018,Feb,11; 2018,Jan,8; 2017,Jan,8; 2016,Jan,13; 2015,Jan,16

93226 **scanning analysis with report**
1.03 1.03 FUD XXX Q1 80 TC
AMA: 2018,Feb,11; 2018,Jan,8; 2017,Jan,8; 2016,Jan,13; 2015,Jan,16

93227 **review and interpretation by a physician or other qualified health care professional**
0.75 0.75 FUD XXX M 80 26
AMA: 2018,Mar,5; 2018,Feb,11; 2018,Jan,8; 2017,Jan,8; 2016,Jan,13; 2015,Jan,16

93241-93248 [93241, 93242, 93243, 93244, 93245, 93246, 93247, 93248] External Electrocardiographic Recording

INCLUDES Cardiac monitoring using in-person as well as remote technology for electrocardiographic data assessment

EXCLUDES *During same monitoring period:*
- *External ECG event recording up to 30 days (93268-93272)*
- *External ECG event recording without 24 hour attended monitoring (0497T-0498T)*
- *Remote physiological monitoring, collection and interpretation ([99453, 99454], [99091])*

Echocardiography (93303-93355 [93356])

Implantable patient activated cardiac event recorders (93285, 93291, 93297-93298)

Less than 48 hours monitoring (93224-93227)

● # **93241** **External electrocardiographic recording for more than 48 hours up to 7 days by continuous rhythm recording and storage; includes recording, scanning analysis with report, review and interpretation**

EXCLUDES *More than 7 days and up to 15 days monitoring ([93245, 93246, 93247, 93248])*

Facility RVU 0.00 Non-Facility RVU 0.00 **FUD** 000

● # **93242** **recording (includes connection and initial recording)**

EXCLUDES *More than 7 days and up to 15 days monitoring ([93245, 93246, 93247, 93248])*

Facility RVU 0.00 Non-Facility RVU 0.00 **FUD** 000

● # **93243** **scanning analysis with report**

EXCLUDES *More than 7 days and up to 15 days monitoring ([93245, 93246, 93247, 93248])*

Facility RVU 0.00 Non-Facility RVU 0.00 **FUD** 000

● # **93244** **review and interpretation**

EXCLUDES *More than 7 days and up to 15 days monitoring ([93245, 93246, 93247, 93248])*

Facility RVU 0.00 Non-Facility RVU 0.00 **FUD** 000

● # **93245** **External electrocardiographic recording for more than 7 days up to 15 days by continuous rhythm recording and storage; includes recording, scanning analysis with report, review and interpretation**

EXCLUDES *More than 48 hours up to 7 days monitoring ([93241, 93242, 93243, 93244])*

Facility RVU 0.00 Non-Facility RVU 0.00 **FUD** 000

● # **93246** **recording (includes connection and initial recording)**

EXCLUDES *More than 48 hours up to 7 days monitoring ([93241, 93242, 93243, 93244])*

Facility RVU 0.00 Non-Facility RVU 0.00 **FUD** 000

● # **93247** **scanning analysis with report**

EXCLUDES *More than 48 hours up to 7 days monitoring ([93241, 93242, 93243, 93244])*

Facility RVU 0.00 Non-Facility RVU 0.00 **FUD** 000

● # **93248** **review and interpretation**

EXCLUDES *More than 48 hours up to 7 days monitoring ([93241, 93242, 93243, 93244])*

Facility RVU 0.00 Non-Facility RVU 0.00 **FUD** 000

93228-93248 [93241, 93242, 93243, 93244, 93245, 93246, 93247, 93248] Remote Cardiovascular Telemetry

INCLUDES Cardiac monitoring using in-person as well as remote technology for electrocardiographic data assessment

Mobile telemetry monitors with capacity to:
- Detect arrhythmias
- Real-time data analysis for signal quality evaluation quality
- Records ECG rhythm on continuous basis using external electrodes on patient
- Transmit tracing at any time
- Transmit data to attended surveillance center where technician available to respond to device or rhythm alerts and contact physician or qualified health care professional when needed

EXCLUDES *Reporting code more than one time in 30-day period*

93228 **External mobile cardiovascular telemetry with electrocardiographic recording, concurrent computerized real time data analysis and greater than 24 hours of accessible ECG data storage (retrievable with query) with ECG triggered and patient selected events transmitted to a remote attended surveillance center for up to 30 days; review and interpretation with report by a physician or other qualified health care professional**

EXCLUDES *Cardiovascular monitors that do not perform automatic ECG triggered transmissions to attended surveillance center (93224-93227, 93268-93272)*

Facility RVU 0.74 Non-Facility RVU 0.74 **FUD** XXX ★ M 80 26

AMA: 2018,Feb,11; 2018,Jan,8; 2017,Jan,8; 2016,Jan,13; 2015,Jan,16

93229 **technical support for connection and patient instructions for use, attended surveillance, analysis and transmission of daily and emergent data reports as prescribed by a physician or other qualified health care professional**

Facility RVU 19.9 Non-Facility RVU 19.9 **FUD** XXX ★ S 80 TC

AMA: 2018,Feb,11; 2018,Jan,8; 2017,Jan,8; 2016,Jan,13; 2015,Jan,16

93241 **Resequenced code. See code following 93227.**

93242 **Resequenced code. See code following 93227.**

93243 **Resequenced code. See code following 93227.**

93244 **Resequenced code. See code following 93227.**

93245 **Resequenced code. See code following 93227.**

93246 **Resequenced code. See code following 93227.**

93247 **Resequenced code. See code following 93227.**

93248 **Resequenced code. See code following 93227.**

93260-93272 [93260, 93261, 93264] Event Monitors

INCLUDES ECG rhythm derived elements, which differ from physiologic data and include heart rhythm, rate, ST analysis, heart rate variability, T-wave alternans, among others

Event monitors that:
- Record ECGs in response to patient activation or automatic detection algorithm (or both)
- Require attended surveillance
- Transmit data upon request (although not immediately when activated)

EXCLUDES *Monitoring cardiovascular devices (93279-93289 [93260], 93291-93296, 93298)*

93260 **Resequenced code. See code following 93284.**

93261 **Resequenced code. See code following 93289.**

93264 **Resequenced code. See code before 93278.**

93268 **External patient and, when performed, auto activated electrocardiographic rhythm derived event recording with symptom-related memory loop with remote download capability up to 30 days, 24-hour attended monitoring; includes transmission, review and interpretation by a physician or other qualified health care professional**

EXCLUDES *Implantable patient activated cardiac event recorders (93285, 93291, 93298)*

Subcutaneous cardiac rhythm monitor (33285)

Facility RVU 5.70 Non-Facility RVU 5.70 **FUD** XXX ★ M 80

AMA: 2018,Feb,11; 2018,Jan,8; 2017,Jan,8; 2016,Jan,13; 2015,Jan,16

93270 **recording (includes connection, recording, and disconnection)**

0.26 0.26 FUD XXX ★ Q1 80 TC

AMA: 2018,Feb,11; 2018,Jan,8; 2017,Jan,8; 2016,Jan,13; 2015,Jan,16

93271 **transmission and analysis**

4.72 4.72 FUD XXX ★ S 80 TC

AMA: 2018,Feb,11; 2018,Jan,8; 2017,Jan,8; 2016,Jan,13; 2015,Jan,16

93272 **review and interpretation by a physician or other qualified health care professional**

EXCLUDES *Implantable patient activated cardiac event recorders (93285, 93291, 93298)*
Subcutaneous cardiac rhythm monitor (33285)

0.72 0.72 FUD XXX ★ M 80 26

AMA: 2018,Mar,5; 2018,Feb,11; 2018,Jan,8; 2017,Jan,8; 2016,Jan,13; 2015,Jan,16

93278 Signal-averaged Electrocardiography

EXCLUDES *Echocardiography (93303-93355)*

Code also modifier 26 for interpretation and report only

93278 **Signal-averaged electrocardiography (SAECG), with or without ECG**

0.87 0.87 FUD XXX Q1 80

AMA: 2018,Feb,11; 2018,Jan,8; 2017,Jan,8; 2016,Jan,13; 2015,Jan,16

93264 [93264] Wireless Pulmonary Artery Pressure Sensor Monitoring

INCLUDES Data collection from internal sensor in pulmonary artery
Downloads, interpretation, analysis, and report that must occur at least one time per week
Transmission and storage of data

EXCLUDES *Reporting code wehn monitoring for less than 30-day period*
Reporting code more than one time in 30 days

93264 **Remote monitoring of a wireless pulmonary artery pressure sensor for up to 30 days, including at least weekly downloads of pulmonary artery pressure recordings, interpretation(s), trend analysis, and report(s) by a physician or other qualified health care professional**

1.03 1.43 FUD XXX 80

AMA: 2020,Feb,7; 2019,Oct,3; 2019,Jun,3

93279-93298 [93260, 93261] Monitoring of Cardiovascular Devices

INCLUDES Implantable cardiovascular monitor (ICM) interrogation:
- Analysis at least one recorded physiologic cardiovascular data element from either internal or external sensors
- Programmed parameters

Implantable defibrillator interrogation:
- Battery
- Capture and sensing functions
- Leads
- Presence or absence therapy for ventricular tachyarrhythmias
- Programmed parameters
- Underlying heart rhythm

Implantable loop recorder (ILR) interrogation:
- Heart rate and rhythm during recorded episodes from both patient-initiated and device detected events
- Programmed parameters

In-person interrogation/device evaluation (93288)
In-person periprocedural device evaluation/programming device system parameters (93286)
Interrogation evaluation device
Pacemaker interrogation:
- Battery
- Capture and sensing functions
- Heart rhythm
- Leads
- Programmed parameters

Time period established by initiation remote monitoring or 91st day implantable defibrillator/pacemaker monitoring or 31st day ILR monitoring and extending for succeeding 30- or 90-day period

EXCLUDES *Wearable device monitoring (93224-93272)*

93279 **Programming device evaluation (in person) with iterative adjustment of the implantable device to test the function of the device and select optimal permanent programmed values with analysis, review and report by a physician or other qualified health care professional; single lead pacemaker system or leadless pacemaker system in one cardiac chamber**

EXCLUDES *External ECG event recording up to 30 days (93268-93272)*
Peri-procedural and interrogation device evaluation (93286, 93288)
Rhythm strips (93040-93042)

1.72 1.72 FUD XXX Q1 80

AMA: 2019,Oct,3; 2019,Mar,6; 2018,Feb,11; 2018,Jan,8; 2017,Jan,8; 2016,Aug,5; 2016,May,5; 2016,Jan,13; 2015,Jan,16

93280 **dual lead pacemaker system**

EXCLUDES *External ECG event recording up to 30 days (93268-93272)*
Peri-procedural and interrogation device evaluation (93286, 93288)
Rhythm strips (93040-93042)

1.83 1.83 FUD XXX Q1 80

AMA: 2019,Oct,3; 2018,Feb,11; 2018,Jan,8; 2017,Jan,8; 2016,Aug,5; 2016,May,5; 2016,Jan,13; 2015,Jan,16

93281 **multiple lead pacemaker system**

EXCLUDES *External ECG event recording up to 30 days (93268-93272)*
Peri-procedural and interrogation device evaluation (93286, 93288)
Rhythm strips (93040-93042)

2.17 2.17 FUD XXX Q1 80

AMA: 2019,Oct,3; 2018,Feb,11; 2018,Jan,8; 2017,Jan,8; 2016,Aug,5; 2016,May,5; 2016,Jan,13; 2015,Jan,16

93282 **single lead transvenous implantable defibrillator system**

EXCLUDES *Device evaluation subcutaneous lead defibrillator system (93260)*
External ECG event recording up to 30 days (93268-93272)
Peri-procedural and interrogation device evaluation (93287, 93289)
Rhythm strips (93040-93042)
Wearable cardio-defibrillator system services (93745)

2.08 2.08 **FUD** XXX Q1 80

AMA: 2019,Oct,3; 2018,Feb,11; 2018,Jan,8; 2017,Jan,8; 2016,Aug,5; 2016,Jan,13; 2015,Jan,16

93283 **dual lead transvenous implantable defibrillator system**

EXCLUDES *External ECG event recording up to 30 days (93268-93272)*
Peri-procedural and interrogation device evaluation (93287, 93289)
Rhythm strips (93040-93042)

2.60 2.60 **FUD** XXX Q1 80

AMA: 2019,Oct,3; 2018,Feb,11; 2018,Jan,8; 2017,Jan,8; 2016,Aug,5; 2016,'an,13; 2015,Jan,16

93284 **multiple lead transvenous implantable defibrillator system**

EXCLUDES *External ECG event recording up to 30 days (93268-93272)*
Peri-procedural and interrogation device evaluation (93287, 93289)
Rhythm strips (93040-93042)

2.81 2.81 **FUD** XXX Q1 80

AMA: 2019,Oct,3; 2018,Feb,11; 2018,Jan,8; 2017,Jan,8; 2016,Aug,5; 2016,Jan,13; 2015,Jan,16

\# **93260** **implantable subcutaneous lead defibrillator system**

EXCLUDES *Device evaluation (93261, 93282, 93287)*
External ECG event recording up to 30 days (93268-93272)
Insertion/removal/replacement implantable defibrillator (33240, 33241, [33262], [33270, 33271, 33272, 33273])
Rhythm strips (93040-93042)

2.04 2.04 **FUD** XXX Q1 80

AMA: 2019,Oct,3; 2018,Feb,11; 2018,Jan,8; 2017,Jan,8; 2016,Aug,5; 2016,Jan,13; 2015,Jan,16

93285 **subcutaneous cardiac rhythm monitor system**

EXCLUDES *Device evaluation (93279-93284, 93291)*
External ECG event recording up to 30 days (93268-93272)
Insertion subcutaneous cardiac rhythm monitor (33285)
Rhythm strips (93040-93042)

1.52 1.52 **FUD** XXX Q1 80

AMA: 2019,Oct,3; 2019,Apr,3; 2018,Feb,11; 2018,Jan,8; 2017,Jan,8; 2016,Aug,5; 2016,Jan,13; 2015,Jan,16

93286 **Peri-procedural device evaluation (in person) and programming of device system parameters before or after a surgery, procedure, or test with analysis, review and report by a physician or other qualified health care professional; single, dual, or multiple lead pacemaker system, or leadless pacemaker system**

INCLUDES One evaluation and programming (if performed once before and once after, report as two units)

EXCLUDES *Device evaluation (93279-93281, 93288)*
External ECG event recording up to 30 days (93268-93272)
Rhythm strips (93040-93042)
Services related to cardiac contractility modulation systems (0408T-0411T, 0414T-0415T)
Subcutaneous implantable defibrillator peri-procedural device evaluation and programming (93260, 93261)

0.99 0.99 **FUD** XXX N 80

AMA: 2019,Oct,3; 2019,Mar,6; 2018,Feb,11; 2018,Jan,8; 2017,Jan,8; 2016,Aug,5; 2016,May,5; 2016,Jan,13; 2015,Jan,16

93287 **single, dual, or multiple lead implantable defibrillator system**

INCLUDES One evaluation and programming (if performed once before and once after, report as two units)

EXCLUDES *Device evaluation (93282-93284, 93289)*
External ECG event recording up to 30 days (93268-93272)
Rhythm strips (93040-93042)
Services related to cardiac contractility modulation systems (0408T-0411T, 0414T-0415T)
Subcutaneous implantable defibrillator peri-procedural device evaluation and programming (93260, 93261)

1.36 1.36 **FUD** XXX N 80

AMA: 2019,Oct,3; 2018,Feb,11; 2018,Jan,8; 2017,Jan,8; 2016,Aug,5; 2016,May,5; 2016,Jan,13; 2015,Jan,16

93288 **Interrogation device evaluation (in person) with analysis, review and report by a physician or other qualified health care professional, includes connection, recording and disconnection per patient encounter; single, dual, or multiple lead pacemaker system, or leadless pacemaker system**

EXCLUDES *Device evaluation (93279-93281, 93286, 93294-93295)*
External ECG event recording up to 30 days (93268-93272)
Rhythm strips (93040-93042)

1.25 1.25 **FUD** XXX Q1 80

AMA: 2019,Oct,3; 2019,Mar,6; 2018,Feb,11; 2018,Jan,8; 2017,Jan,8; 2016,Aug,5; 2016,May,5; 2016,Jan,13; 2015,Jan,16

93289 **single, dual, or multiple lead transvenous implantable defibrillator system, including analysis of heart rhythm derived data elements**

EXCLUDES *Monitoring physiologic cardiovascular data elements derived from implantable defibrillator (93290)*
Device evaluation (93261, 93282-93284, 93287, 93295-93296)
External ECG event recording up to 30 days (93268-93272)
Rhythm strips (93040-93042)

1.70 1.70 **FUD** XXX Q1 80

AMA: 2019,Oct,3; 2018,Feb,11; 2018,Jan,8; 2017,Jan,8; 2016,Aug,5; 2016,May,5; 2016,Jan,13; 2015,Jan,16

\# **93261** **implantable subcutaneous lead defibrillator system**

EXCLUDES *Device evaluation (93260, 93287, 93289)*
External ECG event recording up to 30 days (93268-93272)
Insertion/removal/replacement implantable defibrillator (33240, 33241, [33262], [33270, 33271, 33272, 33273])
Rhythm strips (93040-93042)

1.87 1.87 **FUD** XXX Q1 80

AMA: 2019,Oct,3; 2018,Feb,11; 2018,Jan,8; 2017,Jan,8; 2016,Aug,5; 2016,Jan,13; 2015,Jan,16

93290 **implantable cardiovascular physiologic monitor system, including analysis of 1 or more recorded physiologic cardiovascular data elements from all internal and external sensors**

EXCLUDES *Device evaluation (93297)*
Heart rhythm derived data (93289)

1.19 1.19 **FUD** XXX Q1 80

AMA: 2020,Feb,7; 2019,Oct,3; 2018,Feb,11; 2018,Jan,8; 2017,Jan,8; 2016,Aug,5; 2016,Jan,13; 2015,Jan,16

93291 **subcutaneous cardiac rhythm monitor system, including heart rhythm derived data analysis**

EXCLUDES *Device evaluation (93288-93290 [93261], 93298)*
External ECG event recording up to 30 days (93268-93272)
Insertion subcutaneous cardiac rhythm monitor (33285)
Rhythm strips (93040-93042)

1.22 1.22 **FUD** XXX Q1 80

AMA: 2019,Oct,3; 2019,Apr,3; 2018,Feb,11; 2018,Jan,8; 2017,Jan,8; 2016,Aug,5; 2016,Jan,13; 2015,Jan,16

93292 **wearable defibrillator system**

EXCLUDES *External ECG event recording up to 30 days (93268-93272)*
Rhythm strips (93040-93042)
Wearable cardioverter-defibrillator system (93745)

1.27 1.27 **FUD** XXX Q1 80

AMA: 2019,Oct,3; 2018,Feb,11; 2018,Jan,8; 2017,Jan,8; 2016,Aug,5; 2016,Jan,13; 2015,Jan,16

93293 **Transtelephonic rhythm strip pacemaker evaluation(s) single, dual, or multiple lead pacemaker system, includes recording with and without magnet application with analysis, review and report(s) by a physician or other qualified health care professional, up to 90 days**

EXCLUDES *Device evaluation (93294)*
External ECG event recording up to 30 days (93268-93272)
Rhythm strips (93040-93042)
Reporting code more than one time in 90-day period
Reporting code when monitoring period less than 30 days

1.48 1.48 **FUD** XXX Q1 80

AMA: 2019,Oct,3; 2018,Feb,11; 2018,Jan,8; 2017,Jan,8; 2016,Aug,5; 2016,Jan,13; 2015,Jan,16

93294 **Interrogation device evaluation(s) (remote), up to 90 days; single, dual, or multiple lead pacemaker system, or leadless pacemaker system with interim analysis, review(s) and report(s) by a physician or other qualified health care professional**

EXCLUDES *Device evaluation (93288, 93293)*
External ECG event recording up to 30 days (93268-93272)
Rhythm strips (93040-93042)
Reporting code more than one time in 90-day period
Reporting code when monitoring period less than 30 days

0.87 0.87 **FUD** XXX M 80 26

AMA: 2019,Oct,3; 2019,Mar,6; 2018,Feb,11; 2018,Jan,8; 2017,Jan,8; 2016,Aug,5; 2016,Jan,13; 2015,Jan,16

93295 **single, dual, or multiple lead implantable defibrillator system with interim analysis, review(s) and report(s) by a physician or other qualified health care professional**

EXCLUDES *Device evaluation (93289)*
External ECG event recording up to 30 days (93268-93272)
Remote interrogation device evaluation implantable cardioverter-defibrillator with substernal lead (0578T, 0579T)
Remote monitoring physiological cardiovascular data (93297)
Rhythm strips (93040-93042)
Reporting code more than one time in 90-day period
Reporting code when monitoring period less than 30 days

1.09 1.09 **FUD** XXX M 80 26

AMA: 2019,Oct,3; 2018,Feb,11; 2018,Jan,8; 2017,Jan,8; 2016,Aug,5; 2016,Jan,13; 2015,Jan,16

93296 **single, dual, or multiple lead pacemaker system, leadless pacemaker system, or implantable defibrillator system, remote data acquisition(s), receipt of transmissions and technician review, technical support and distribution of results**

EXCLUDES *Device evaluation (93288-93289)*
External ECG event recording up to 30 days (93268-93272)
Remote interrogation device evaluation implantable cardioverter-defibrillator with substernal lead (0578T, 0579T)
Rhythm strips (93040-93042)
Reporting code more than one time in 90-day period
Reporting code when monitoring period less than 30 days

0.72 0.72 **FUD** XXX Q1 80 TC

AMA: 2019,Oct,3; 2019,Mar,6; 2019,Jan,6; 2018,Feb,11; 2018,Jan,8; 2017,Jan,8; 2016,Aug,5; 2016,Jan,13; 2015,Jan,16

93297 **Interrogation device evaluation(s), (remote) up to 30 days; implantable cardiovascular physiologic monitor system, including analysis of 1 or more recorded physiologic cardiovascular data elements from all internal and external sensors, analysis, review(s) and report(s) by a physician or other qualified health care professional**

EXCLUDES *Collection and interpretation physiologic data digitally stored and/or transmitted ([99091])*
Device evaluation (93290, 93298)
Heart rhythm derived data (93295)
Remote monitoring physiologic parameter(s) with daily recording(s) or programmed alert(s) ([99454])
Remote monitoring wireless pulmonary artery pressure sensor (93264)
Reporting code more than one time in 30-day period
Reporting code when monitoring period less than 10 days

0.75 0.75 **FUD** XXX M 80 26

AMA: 2020,Feb,12; 2019,Oct,3; 2018,Feb,11; 2018,Jan,8; 2017,Jan,8; 2016,Aug,5; 2016,Jan,13; 2015,Jan,16

93298 **subcutaneous cardiac rhythm monitor system, including analysis of recorded heart rhythm data, analysis, review(s) and report(s) by a physician or other qualified health care professional**

EXCLUDES *Collection and interpretation physiologic data digitally stored and/or transmitted ([99091])*
Device evaluation (93291, 93297)
External ECG event recording up to 30 days (93268-93272)
Implantation patient-activated cardiac event recorder (33285)
Remote monitoring physiologic parameter(s) with daily recording(s) or programmed alert(s) ([99454])
Reporting code more than one time in 30-day period
Reporting code when monitoring period less than 10 days
Rhythm strips (93040-93042)

0.75 0.75 **FUD** XXX M 80 26

AMA: 2020,Feb,12; 2019,Oct,3; 2019,Apr,3; 2018,Feb,11; 2018,Jan,8; 2017,Jan,8; 2016,Aug,5; 2016,Jan,13; 2015,Jan,16

Medicine

93303 — 93321

93303-93356 [93356] Echocardiography

INCLUDES Interpretation and report
Obtaining ultrasonic signals from heart/great arteries
Report study including:
Description recognized abnormalities
Documentation all clinically relevant findings including obtained quantitative measurements
Interpretation all information obtained
Two-dimensional image/doppler ultrasonic signal documentation
Ultrasound exam:
Adjacent great vessels
Cardiac chambers/valves
Pericardium

EXCLUDES *Contrast agents and/or drugs used for pharmacological stress*
Echocardiography, fetal (76825-76828)
Ultrasound with thorough examination organ(s) or anatomic region/documentation image/final written report

93303 **Transthoracic echocardiography for congenital cardiac anomalies; complete**
6.65 6.65 **FUD** XXX S 80
AMA: 2020,Jul,12; 2020,Apr,10; 2020,Jan,7; 2018,Feb,11; 2018,Jan,8; 2017,Jan,8; 2016,Jan,13; 2015,May,10; 2015,Jan,16

93304 **follow-up or limited study**
4.53 4.53 **FUD** XXX S 80
AMA: 2020,Jul,12; 2020,Jan,7; 2018,Feb,11; 2018,Jan,8; 2017,Jan,8; 2016,Jan,13; 2015,May,10; 2015,Jan,16

93306 **Echocardiography, transthoracic, real-time with image documentation (2D), includes M-mode recording, when performed, complete, with spectral Doppler echocardiography, and with color flow Doppler echocardiography**
INCLUDES Doppler and color flow
Two-dimensional and M-mode
EXCLUDES *Transthoracic without spectral and color doppler (93307)*
5.84 5.84 **FUD** XXX S 80
AMA: 2020,Jul,12; 2020,May,12; 2020,Jan,7; 2018,Dec,10; 2018,Dec,10; 2018,Feb,11; 2018,Jan,8; 2017,Jan,8; 2016,Apr,8; 2016,Jan,13; 2015,May,10; 2015,Jan,16

93307 **Echocardiography, transthoracic, real-time with image documentation (2D), includes M-mode recording, when performed, complete, without spectral or color Doppler echocardiography**
INCLUDES Additional structures that may be viewed such as pulmonary vein or artery, pulmonic valve, inferior vena cava
Obtaining/recording appropriate measurements
Two-dimensional/selected M-mode exam:
Adjacent portions aorta
Aortic/mitral/tricuspid valves
Left/right atria
Left/right ventricles
Pericardium
Using multiple views as required to obtain complete functional/anatomic evaluation
EXCLUDES *Doppler echocardiography (93320-93321, 93325)*
3.97 3.97 **FUD** XXX S 80
AMA: 2020,Jul,12; 2020,May,12; 2020,Jan,7; 2018,Feb,11; 2018,Jan,8; 2017,Jan,8; 2016,Apr,8; 2016,Jan,13; 2015,May,10; 2015,Jan,16

93308 **Echocardiography, transthoracic, real-time with image documentation (2D), includes M-mode recording, when performed, follow-up or limited study**
INCLUDES Exam that does not evaluate/document attempt to evaluate all structures comprising complete echocardiographic exam
2.79 2.79 **FUD** XXX S 80
AMA: 2020,Jul,12; 2020,May,12; 2020,Jan,7; 2018,Dec,10; 2018,Dec,10; 2018,Feb,11; 2018,Jan,8; 2017,Jan,8; 2016,Apr,8; 2016,Jan,13; 2015,May,10; 2015,Jan,16

93312 **Echocardiography, transesophageal, real-time with image documentation (2D) (with or without M-mode recording); including probe placement, image acquisition, interpretation and report**
EXCLUDES *Transesophageal echocardiography (93355)*
6.97 6.97 **FUD** XXX S 80
AMA: 2020,Jan,7; 2018,Feb,11; 2018,Jan,8; 2017,Jan,8; 2016,Jan,13; 2015,Jan,16

93313 **placement of transesophageal probe only**
EXCLUDES *Procedure when performed by same person performing transesophageal echocardiography (93355)*
0.33 0.33 **FUD** XXX S 80
AMA: 2020,Jan,7; 2018,Feb,11; 2018,Jan,8; 2017,Jan,8; 2016,Jan,13; 2015,Jan,16

93314 **image acquisition, interpretation and report only**
EXCLUDES *Transesophageal echocardiography (93355)*
6.73 6.73 **FUD** XXX N 80
AMA: 2020,Jan,7; 2018,Feb,11; 2018,Jan,8; 2017,Jan,8; 2016,Jan,13; 2015,Jan,16

93315 **Transesophageal echocardiography for congenital cardiac anomalies; including probe placement, image acquisition, interpretation and report**
EXCLUDES *Transesophageal echocardiography (93355)*
0.00 0.00 **FUD** XXX S 80
AMA: 2020,Jan,7; 2018,Feb,11; 2018,Jan,8; 2017,Jan,8; 2016,Jan,13; 2015,Jan,16

93316 **placement of transesophageal probe only**
EXCLUDES *Transesophageal echocardiography (93355)*
0.79 0.79 **FUD** XXX S 80
AMA: 2020,Jan,7; 2018,Feb,11; 2018,Jan,8; 2017,Jan,8; 2016,Jan,13; 2015,Jan,16

93317 **image acquisition, interpretation and report only**
EXCLUDES *Transesophageal echocardiography (93355)*
0.00 0.00 **FUD** XXX N 80
AMA: 2020,Jan,7; 2018,Feb,11; 2018,Jan,8; 2017,Jan,8; 2016,Jan,13; 2015,Jan,16

93318 **Echocardiography, transesophageal (TEE) for monitoring purposes, including probe placement, real time 2-dimensional image acquisition and interpretation leading to ongoing (continuous) assessment of (dynamically changing) cardiac pumping function and to therapeutic measures on an immediate time basis**
EXCLUDES *Transesophageal echocardiography (93355)*
0.00 0.00 **FUD** XXX S 80
AMA: 2020,Jan,7; 2018,Feb,11; 2018,Jan,8; 2017,Jan,8; 2016,Jan,13; 2015,Jan,16

+ **93320** **Doppler echocardiography, pulsed wave and/or continuous wave with spectral display (List separately in addition to codes for echocardiographic imaging); complete**
EXCLUDES *Transesophageal echocardiography (93355)*
Code first (93303-93304, 93312, 93314-93315, 93317, 93350-93351)
1.51 1.51 **FUD** ZZZ N 80
AMA: 2020,May,12; 2020,Jan,7; 2018,Feb,11; 2018,Jan,8; 2017,Jan,8; 2016,Jan,13; 2015,Jan,16

+ **93321** **follow-up or limited study (List separately in addition to codes for echocardiographic imaging)**
EXCLUDES *Transesophageal echocardiography (93355)*
Code first (93303-93304, 93308, 93312, 93314-93315, 93317, 93350-93351)
0.76 0.76 **FUD** ZZZ N 80
AMA: 2020,Jan,7; 2018,Feb,11; 2018,Jan,8; 2017,Jan,8; 2016,Jan,13; 2015,Jan,16

+ **93325** **Doppler echocardiography color flow velocity mapping (List separately in addition to codes for echocardiography)**

EXCLUDES *Transesophageal echocardiography (93355)*

Code first (76825-76828, 93303-93304, 93308, 93312, 93314-93315, 93317, 93350-93351)

0.70 0.70 FUD ZZZ N 80

AMA: 2020,May,12; 2020,Jan,7; 2018,Feb,11; 2018,Jan,8; 2017,Jan,8; 2016,Jul,8; 2016,Jan,13; 2015,Jan,16

93350 **Echocardiography, transthoracic, real-time with image documentation (2D), includes M-mode recording, when performed, during rest and cardiovascular stress test using treadmill, bicycle exercise and/or pharmacologically induced stress, with interpretation and report;**

EXCLUDES *Cardiovascular stress test, complete procedure (93015)*

Code also exercise stress testing (93016-93018)

5.31 5.31 FUD XXX S 80

AMA: 2020,Jul,12; 2018,Feb,11; 2018,Jan,8; 2017,Jan,8; 2016,Apr,8; 2016,Jan,13; 2015,Jan,16

93351 **including performance of continuous electrocardiographic monitoring, with supervision by a physician or other qualified health care professional**

INCLUDES Stress echocardiogram performed with complete cardiovascular stress test

EXCLUDES *Cardiovascular stress test (93015-93018)*
Echocardiography (93350)
Professional only components complete stress test and stress echocardiogram performed in facility by same physician, append modifier 26
Reporting code for professional component (modifier 26 appended) with (93016, 93018, 93350)

Code also components cardiovascular stress test when professional services not performed by same physician performing stress echocardiogram (93016-93018)

6.63 6.63 FUD XXX S

AMA: 2020,Jul,12; 2018,Feb,11; 2018,Jan,8; 2017,Jan,8; 2016,Apr,8; 2016,Jan,13; 2015,Jan,16

+ # **93356** **Myocardial strain imaging using speckle tracking-derived assessment of myocardial mechanics (List separately in addition to codes for echocardiography imaging)**

EXCLUDES *Reporting code more than one time for each session*

Code first (93303-93304, 93306, 93307, 93308, 93350-93351)

0.34 1.13 FUD ZZZ 80

AMA: 2020,Jul,12; 2020,Apr,10

+ **93352** **Use of echocardiographic contrast agent during stress echocardiography (List separately in addition to code for primary procedure)**

EXCLUDES *Reporting code more than one time for each stress echocardiogram*

Code first (93350, 93351)

0.95 0.95 FUD ZZZ M 80

AMA: 2018,Feb,11; 2018,Jan,8; 2017,Jan,8; 2016,Jan,13; 2015,Jan,16

93355 **Echocardiography, transesophageal (TEE) for guidance of a transcatheter intracardiac or great vessel(s) structural intervention(s) (eg,TAVR, transcatheter pulmonary valve replacement, mitral valve repair, paravalvular regurgitation repair, left atrial appendage occlusion/closure, ventricular septal defect closure) (peri-and intra-procedural), real-time image acquisition and documentation, guidance with quantitative measurements, probe manipulation, interpretation, and report, including diagnostic transesophageal echocardiography and, when performed, administration of ultrasound contrast, Doppler, color flow, and 3D**

EXCLUDES *3D rendering (76376-76377)*
Doppler echocardiography (93320-93321, 93325)
Transesophageal echocardiography (93312-93318)
Transesophageal probe positioning by different provider (93313)

6.57 6.57 FUD XXX N 80

AMA: 2018,Feb,11

93356 **Resequenced code. See code following 93351.**

93451-93505 Heart Catheterization

INCLUDES Access site imaging and placement closure device
Catheter insertion and positioning
Contrast injection (except as listed below)
Imaging and insertion closure device
Radiology supervision and interpretation
Roadmapping angiography

EXCLUDES *Congenital cardiac cath procedures (93530-93533)*

Code also separately identifiable:
Aortography (93567)
Noncardiac angiography (see radiology and vascular codes)
Pulmonary angiography (93568)
Right ventricular or atrial injection (93566)

93451 **Right heart catheterization including measurement(s) of oxygen saturation and cardiac output, when performed**

INCLUDES Cardiac output review
Insertion catheter into one or more right cardiac chambers or areas
Obtaining samples for blood gas

EXCLUDES *Catheterization procedures including right side heart (93453, 93456-93457, 93460-93461)*
Implantation wireless pulmonary artery pressure sensor (33289)
Indicator dilution studies (93561-93562)
Percutaneous repair congenital interatrial defect (93580)
Swan-Ganz catheter insertion (93503)
Transcatheter implantation interatrial septal shunt device, percutaneous approach (0613T)
Transcatheter ultrasound ablation nerves innervating pulmonary arteries, percutaneous approach (0632T)
Valve repair or annulus reconstruction (33418, 0345T, 0483T, 0484T, 0544T, 0545T)

Code also administration medication or exercise to repeat assessment hemodynamic measurement (93463-93464)

22.1 22.1 FUD 000 J 62 80

AMA: 2019,Jun,3; 2019,Mar,6; 2018,Dec,10; 2018,Dec,10; 2018,Feb,11; 2018,Jan,8; 2017,Dec,13; 2017,Jul,3; 2017,Jan,8; 2016,Mar,5; 2016,Jan,13; 2015,Sep,3; 2015,Jan,16

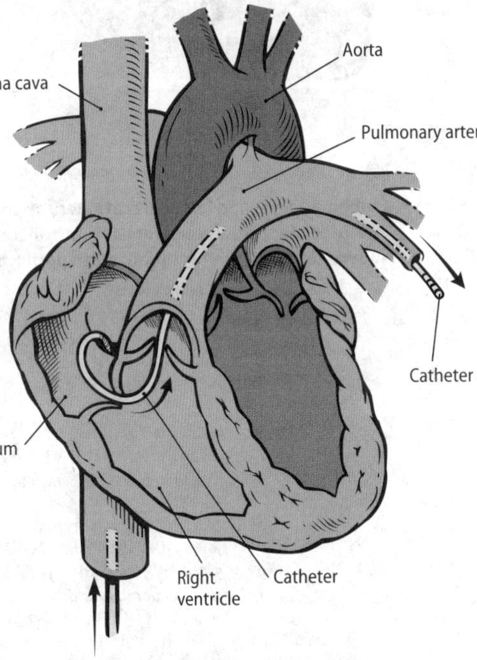

93452 Left heart catheterization including intraprocedural injection(s) for left ventriculography, imaging supervision and interpretation, when performed

INCLUDES Insertion catheter into left cardiac chambers

EXCLUDES *Catheterization procedures including injections for left ventriculography (93453, 93458-93461)*
Injection procedures (93561-93565)
Percutaneous repair congenital interatrial defect (93580)
Services related to cardiac contractility modulation systems (0408T-0411T, 0414T-0415T)
Swan-Ganz catheter insertion (93503)
Valve repair or annulus reconstruction (33418, 0345T, 0483T, 0484T, 0544T, 0545T)

Code also administration medication or exercise to repeat assessment hemodynamic measurement (93463-93464)
Code also transapical or transseptal puncture (93462)

25.9 25.9 **FUD** 000 J G2 80

AMA: 2018,Feb,11; 2018,Jan,8; 2017,Jul,3; 2017,Jan,8; 2016,Jan,13; 2015,Jan,16

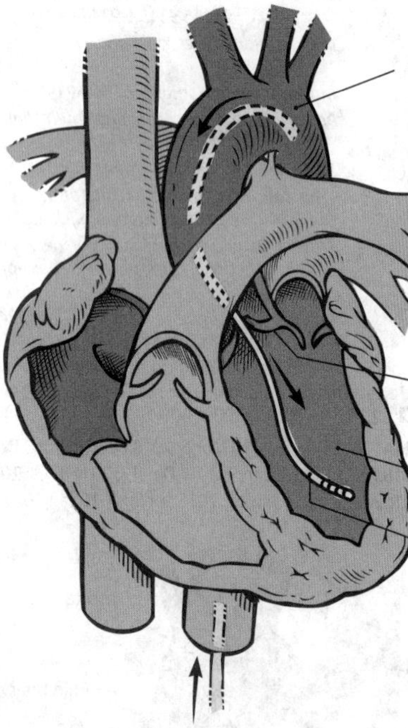

93453 Combined right and left heart catheterization including intraprocedural injection(s) for left ventriculography, imaging supervision and interpretation, when performed

INCLUDES Cardiac output review
Insertion catheter into left cardiac chambers
Insertion catheter into one or more right cardiac chambers or areas
Obtaining samples for blood gas

EXCLUDES *Catheterization procedures (93451-93452, 93456-93461)*
Injection procedures (93561-93565)
Percutaneous repair congenital interatrial defect (93580)
Services related to cardiac contractility modulation systems (0408T-0411T, 0414T-0415T)
Swan-Ganz catheter insertion (93503)
Valve repair or annulus reconstruction (33418, 0345T, 0483T, 0484T, 0544T, 0545T)

Code also administration medication or exercise to repeat assessment hemodynamic measurement (93463-93464)
Code also transapical or transseptal puncture (93462)

33.3 33.3 **FUD** 000 J G2 80

AMA: 2019,Jun,3; 2019,Mar,6; 2018,Feb,11; 2018,Jan,8; 2017,Jul,3; 2017,Jan,8; 2016,Mar,5; 2016,Jan,13; 2015,Sep,3; 2015,Jan,16

93454 Catheter placement in coronary artery(s) for coronary angiography, including intraprocedural injection(s) for coronary angiography, imaging supervision and interpretation;

EXCLUDES *Injection procedures (93561-93565)*
Swan-Ganz catheter insertion (93503)
Valve repair or annulus reconstruction (33418, 0345T, 0483T, 0484T, 0544T, 0545T)

25.9 25.9 **FUD** 000 J G2 80

AMA: 2018,Feb,11; 2018,Jan,8; 2017,Feb,14; 2017,Jan,8; 2016,Mar,5; 2016,Jan,13; 2015,Jan,16

93455 with catheter placement(s) in bypass graft(s) (internal mammary, free arterial, venous grafts) including intraprocedural injection(s) for bypass graft angiography

EXCLUDES *Injection procedures (93561-93565)*
Percutaneous repair congenital interatrial defect (93580)
Swan-Ganz catheter insertion (93503)
Valve repair or annulus reconstruction (33418, 0345T, 0483T, 0484T, 0544T, 0545T)

29.5 29.5 **FUD** 000 J G2 80

AMA: 2018,Feb,11; 2018,Jan,8; 2017,Jan,8; 2016,Mar,5; 2016,Jan,13; 2015,Jan,16

93456 with right heart catheterization

INCLUDES Cardiac output review
Insertion catheter into one or more right cardiac chambers or areas
Obtaining samples for blood gas

EXCLUDES *Injection procedures (93561-93565)*
Percutaneous repair congenital interatrial defect (93580)
Swan-Ganz catheter insertion (93503)
Valve repair or annulus reconstruction (33418, 0345T, 0483T, 0484T, 0544T, 0545T)

Code also administration medication or exercise to repeat assessment hemodynamic measurement (93463-93464)

31.4 31.4 **FUD** 000 J G2 80

AMA: 2019,Jun,3; 2019,Mar,6; 2018,Feb,11; 2018,Jan,8; 2017,Jul,3; 2017,Jan,8; 2016,Mar,5; 2016,Jan,13; 2015,Sep,3; 2015,Jan,16

93457 with catheter placement(s) in bypass graft(s) (internal mammary, free arterial, venous grafts) including intraprocedural injection(s) for bypass graft angiography and right heart catheterization

INCLUDES Cardiac output review
Insertion catheter into one more right cardiac chambers or areas
Obtaining samples for blood gas

EXCLUDES *Injection procedures (93561-93565)*
Percutaneous repair congenital interatrial defect (93580)
Swan-Ganz catheter insertion (93503)
Valve repair or annulus reconstruction (33418, 0345T, 0483T, 0484T, 0544T, 0545T)

Code also administration medication or exercise to repeat assessment hemodynamic measurement (93463-93464)

36.4 36.4 **FUD** 000 J G2 80

AMA: 2019,Jun,3; 2019,Mar,6; 2018,Feb,11; 2018,Jan,8; 2017,Jan,8; 2016,Mar,5; 2016,Jan,13; 2015,Sep,3; 2015,Jan,16

93458 **with left heart catheterization including intraprocedural injection(s) for left ventriculography, when performed**

INCLUDES Insertion catheter into left cardiac chambers

EXCLUDES *Injection procedures (93561-93565)*
Percutaneous repair congenital interatrial defect (93580)
Services related to cardiac contractility modulation systems (0408T-0411T, 0414T-0415T)
Swan-Ganz catheter insertion (93503)
Valve repair or annulus reconstruction (33418, 0345T, 0483T, 0484T, 0544T, 0545T)

Code also administration medication or exercise to repeat assessment hemodynamic measurement (93463-93464)
Code also transapical or transseptal puncture (93462)

30.4 30.4 **FUD** 000 J 62 80

AMA: 2018,Feb,11; 2018,Jan,8; 2017,Jul,3; 2017,Jan,8; 2016,Mar,5; 2016,Jan,13; 2015,Sep,3; 2015,Jan,16

93459 **with left heart catheterization including intraprocedural injection(s) for left ventriculography, when performed, catheter placement(s) in bypass graft(s) (internal mammary, free arterial, venous grafts) with bypass graft angiography**

INCLUDES Insertion catheter into left cardiac chambers

EXCLUDES *Injection procedures (93561-93565)*
Percutaneous repair congenital interatrial defect (93580)
Services related to cardiac contractility modulation systems (0408T-0411T, 0414T-0415T)
Swan-Ganz catheter insertion (93503)
Valve repair or annulus reconstruction (33418, 0345T, 0483T, 0484T, 0544T, 0545T)

Code also administration medication or exercise to repeat assessment hemodynamic measurement (93463-93464)
Code also transapical or transseptal puncture (93462)

32.4 32.4 **FUD** 000 J 62 80

AMA: 2018,Feb,11; 2018,Jan,8; 2017,Jul,3; 2017,Jan,8; 2016,Mar,5; 2016,Jan,13; 2015,Sep,3; 2015,Jan,16

93460 **with right and left heart catheterization including intraprocedural injection(s) for left ventriculography, when performed**

INCLUDES Cardiac output review
Insertion catheter into left cardiac chambers
Insertion catheter into one or more right cardiac chambers or areas
Obtaining samples for blood gas

EXCLUDES *Injection procedures (93561-93565)*
Percutaneous repair congenital interatrial defect (93580)
Services related to cardiac contractility modulation systems (0408T-0411T, 0414T-0415T)
Swan-Ganz catheter insertion (93503)
Valve repair or annulus reconstruction (33418, 0345T, 0483T, 0484T, 0544T, 0545T)

Code also administration medication or exercise to repeat assessment hemodynamic measurement (93463-93464)
Code also transapical or transseptal puncture (93462)

35.4 35.4 **FUD** 000 J 62 80

AMA: 2019,Jun,3; 2019,Mar,6; 2018,Feb,11; 2018,Jan,8; 2017,Jul,3; 2017,Jan,8; 2016,Mar,5; 2016,Jan,13; 2015,Sep,3; 2015,Jan,16

93461 **with right and left heart catheterization including intraprocedural injection(s) for left ventriculography, when performed, catheter placement(s) in bypass graft(s) (internal mammary, free arterial, venous grafts) with bypass graft angiography**

INCLUDES Cardiac output review
Insertion catheter into left cardiac chambers
Insertion catheter into one or more right cardiac chambers or areas
Obtaining samples for blood gas

EXCLUDES *Injection procedures (93561-93565)*
Percutaneous repair congenital interatrial defect (93580)
Services related to cardiac contractility modulation systems (0408T-0411T, 0414T-0415T)
Swan-Ganz catheter insertion (93503)
Valve repair or annulus reconstruction (33418, 0345T, 0483T, 0484T, 0544T, 0545T)

Code also administration medication or exercise to repeat assessment hemodynamic measurement (93463-93464)
Code also transapical or transseptal puncture (93462)

40.0 40.0 **FUD** 000 J 62 80

AMA: 2019,Jun,3; 2019,Mar,6; 2018,Feb,11; 2018,Jan,8; 2017,Jul,3; 2017,Jan,8; 2016,Mar,5; 2016,Jan,13; 2015,Sep,3; 2015,Jan,16

+ **93462** **Left heart catheterization by transseptal puncture through intact septum or by transapical puncture (List separately in addition to code for primary procedure)**

INCLUDES Insertion catheter into left cardiac chambers

EXCLUDES *Comprehensive electrophysiologic evaluation (93656)*
Transseptal approach for percutaneous closure paravalvular leak (93590)
Valve repair or annulus reconstruction unless performed with transapical puncture (0345T, 0544T)

Code also percutaneous closure paravalvular leak when transapical puncture performed (93590-93591)
Code first (33477, 93452-93453, 93458-93461, 93582, 93653-93654)

6.11 6.11 **FUD** ZZZ N N1 80

AMA: 2018,Feb,11; 2018,Jan,8; 2017,Sep,3; 2017,Jul,3; 2017,Jan,8; 2016,Jan,13; 2015,Sep,3; 2015,Jan,16

+ **93463** **Pharmacologic agent administration (eg, inhaled nitric oxide, intravenous infusion of nitroprusside, dobutamine, milrinone, or other agent) including assessing hemodynamic measurements before, during, after and repeat pharmacologic agent administration, when performed (List separately in addition to code for primary procedure)**

EXCLUDES *Coronary interventional procedures (92920-92944, 92975, 92977)*
Reporting code more than one time per catheterization

Code first (33477, 93451-93453, 93456-93461, 93530-93533, 93580-93581)

2.82 2.82 **FUD** ZZZ N 80

AMA: 2018,Feb,11; 2018,Jan,8; 2017,Jan,8; 2016,Jan,13; 2015,Jan,16

+ **93464** **Physiologic exercise study (eg, bicycle or arm ergometry) including assessing hemodynamic measurements before and after (List separately in addition to code for primary procedure)**

EXCLUDES *Administration of pharmacologic agent (93463)*
Bundle of His recording (93600)
Reporting code more than one time per catheterization

Code first (33477, 93451-93453, 93456-93461, 93530-93533)

7.04 7.04 **FUD** ZZZ N 80

AMA: 2018,Feb,11; 2018,Jan,8; 2017,Jan,8; 2016,Jan,13; 2015,Jan,16

93503 **Insertion and placement of flow directed catheter (eg, Swan-Ganz) for monitoring purposes**

EXCLUDES *Diagnostic cardiac catheterization (93451-93461, 93530-93533)*
Subsequent monitoring (99356-99357)
Transcatheter ultrasound ablation nerves innervating pulmonary arteries, percutaneous approach (0632T)

2.55 2.55 **FUD** 000 T 80

AMA: 2018,Feb,11; 2018,Jan,8; 2017,Jan,8; 2016,Jan,13; 2015,Jan,16

93505 **Endomyocardial biopsy**

EXCLUDES *Intravascular brachytherapy radionuclide insertion (77770-77772)*
Transcatheter insertion brachytherapy delivery device (92974)

20.1 20.1 **FUD** 000 T 80

AMA: 2018,Feb,11; 2018,Jan,8; 2017,Dec,13; 2017,Jan,8; 2016,Jan,13; 2015,Jan,16

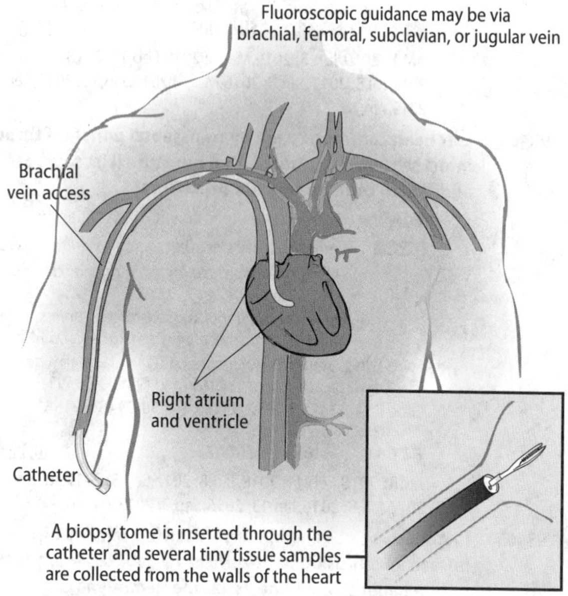
Fluoroscopic guidance may be via brachial, femoral, subclavian, or jugular vein
Brachial vein access
Right atrium and ventricle
Catheter
A biopsy tome is inserted through the catheter and several tiny tissue samples are collected from the walls of the heart

93530-93533 Congenital Heart Defect Catheterization

INCLUDES Access site imaging and placement closure device
Cardiac output review
Insertion catheter into one or more right cardiac chambers or areas
Obtaining samples for blood gas
Radiology supervision and interpretation
Roadmapping angiography

EXCLUDES *Cardiac cath on noncongenital heart (93451-93453, 93456-93461)*
Percutaneous repair congenital interatrial defect (93580)
Swan-Ganz catheter insertion (93503)

Code also (93563-93568)

93530 **Right heart catheterization, for congenital cardiac anomalies**

0.00 0.00 **FUD** 000 J 80

AMA: 2019,Jun,3; 2019,Mar,6; 2018,Feb,11; 2018,Jan,8; 2017,Jul,3; 2017,Jan,8; 2016,Mar,5; 2016,Jan,13; 2015,Sep,3; 2015,Jan,16

93531 **Combined right heart catheterization and retrograde left heart catheterization, for congenital cardiac anomalies**

0.00 0.00 **FUD** 000 J 80

AMA: 2019,Jun,3; 2019,Mar,6; 2018,Feb,11; 2018,Jan,8; 2017,Jul,3; 2017,Jan,8; 2016,Mar,5; 2016,Jan,13; 2015,Sep,3; 2015,Jan,16

93532 **Combined right heart catheterization and transseptal left heart catheterization through intact septum with or without retrograde left heart catheterization, for congenital cardiac anomalies**

0.00 0.00 **FUD** 000 J 80

AMA: 2019,Jun,3; 2019,Mar,6; 2018,Feb,11; 2018,Jan,8; 2017,Jul,3; 2017,Jan,8; 2016,Mar,5; 2016,Jan,13; 2015,Sep,3; 2015,Jan,16

93533 **Combined right heart catheterization and transseptal left heart catheterization through existing septal opening, with or without retrograde left heart catheterization, for congenital cardiac anomalies**

0.00 0.00 **FUD** 000 J 80

AMA: 2019,Jun,3; 2019,Mar,6; 2018,Feb,11; 2018,Jan,8; 2017,Jul,3; 2017,Jan,8; 2016,Mar,5; 2016,Jan,13; 2015,Sep,3; 2015,Jan,16

93561-93568 Injection Procedures

INCLUDES Automatic power injector
Catheter repositioning
Radiology supervision and interpretation

93561 **Indicator dilution studies such as dye or thermodilution, including arterial and/or venous catheterization; with cardiac output measurement (separate procedure)**

EXCLUDES *Cardiac output, radioisotope method (78472-78473, 78481)*
Catheterization procedures (93451-93462)
Percutaneous closure patent ductus arteriosus (93582)

0.00 0.00 **FUD** ZZZ N 80

AMA: 2019,Aug,8; 2018,Feb,11; 2018,Jan,8; 2017,Jan,8; 2016,Jan,13; 2015,Jan,16

93562 **subsequent measurement of cardiac output**

EXCLUDES *Cardiac output, radioisotope method (78472-78473, 78481)*
Catheterization procedures (93451-93462)
Percutaneous closure patent ductus arteriosus (93582)

0.00 0.00 **FUD** ZZZ N 80

AMA: 2019,Aug,8; 2018,Feb,11; 2018,Jan,8; 2017,Jan,8; 2016,Jan,13; 2015,Jan,16

\+ **93563** **Injection procedure during cardiac catheterization including imaging supervision, interpretation, and report; for selective coronary angiography during congenital heart catheterization (List separately in addition to code for primary procedure)**

EXCLUDES *Catheterization procedures (93452-93461)*
Valve repair or annulus reconstruction (33418, 0345T, 0483T, 0484T, 0544T, 0545T)

Code first (93530-93533)

1.69 1.69 **FUD** ZZZ N 80

AMA: 2018,Feb,11; 2018,Jan,8; 2017,Jan,8; 2016,Mar,5; 2016,Jan,13; 2015,Jan,16

\+ **93564** **for selective opacification of aortocoronary venous or arterial bypass graft(s) (eg, aortocoronary saphenous vein, free radial artery, or free mammary artery graft) to one or more coronary arteries and in situ arterial conduits (eg, internal mammary), whether native or used for bypass to one or more coronary arteries during congenital heart catheterization, when performed (List separately in addition to code for primary procedure)**

EXCLUDES *Catheterization procedures (93452-93461)*
Percutaneous repair congenital interatrial defect (93580)
Valve repair or annulus reconstruction (33418, 0345T, 0483T, 0484T, 0544T, 0545T)

Code first (93530-93533)

1.79 1.79 **FUD** ZZZ N 80

AMA: 2018,Feb,11; 2018,Jan,8; 2017,Jan,8; 2016,Mar,5; 2016,Jan,13; 2015,Jan,16

\+ 93565 **for selective left ventricular or left atrial angiography (List separately in addition to code for primary procedure)**

EXCLUDES *Catheterization procedures (93452-93461)*
Percutaneous repair congenital interatrial defect (93580)
Code first (93530-93533)
1.31 1.31 FUD ZZZ N 80
AMA: 2018,Feb,11; 2018,Jan,8; 2017,Jan,8; 2016,Jan,13; 2015,Jan,16

\+ 93566 **for selective right ventricular or right atrial angiography (List separately in addition to code for primary procedure)**

EXCLUDES *Annulus reconstruction (0545T)*
Percutaneous repair congenital interatrial defect (93580)
Right ventriculography when performed during insertion leadless pacemaker ([33274])
Code first (93451, 93453, 93456-93457, 93460-93461, 93530-93533)
1.35 4.38 FUD ZZZ N N1 80
AMA: 2019,Mar,6; 2018,Feb,11; 2018,Jan,8; 2017,Jan,8; 2016,Aug,5; 2016,May,5; 2016,Mar,5; 2016,Jan,13; 2015,May,3; 2015,Jan,16

\+ 93567 **for supravalvular aortography (List separately in addition to code for primary procedure)**

EXCLUDES *Abdominal aortography or non-supravalvular thoracic aortography at same time as cardiac catheterization (36221, 75600-75630)*
Code first (93451-93461, 93530-93533)
1.53 3.71 FUD ZZZ N N1 80
AMA: 2018,Feb,11; 2018,Jan,8; 2017,Jan,8; 2016,Mar,5; 2016,Jan,13; 2015,Jan,16

\+ 93568 **for pulmonary angiography (List separately in addition to code for primary procedure)**

EXCLUDES *Transcatheter ultrasound ablation nerves innervating pulmonary arteries, percutaneous approach (0632T)*
Code first (93451, 93453, 93456-93457, 93460-93461, 93530-93533, 93582-93583)
1.38 3.97 FUD ZZZ N N1 80
AMA: 2019,Jun,3; 2019,Apr,10; 2018,Feb,11; 2018,Jan,8; 2017,Jan,8; 2016,Mar,5; 2016,Jan,13; 2015,Jan,16

93571-93572 Coronary Artery Doppler Studies

INCLUDES Doppler transducer manipulations/repositioning within vessel examined, during coronary angiography/therapeutic intervention (angioplasty)
EXCLUDES *Intraprocedural coronary fractional flow reserve (FFR) ([0523T])*

\+ 93571 **Intravascular Doppler velocity and/or pressure derived coronary flow reserve measurement (coronary vessel or graft) during coronary angiography including pharmacologically induced stress; initial vessel (List separately in addition to code for primary procedure)**

Code first (92920, 92924, 92928, 92933, 92937, 92941, 92943, 92975, 93454-93461, 93563-93564)
0.00 0.00 FUD ZZZ N N1 80
AMA: 2018,Feb,11; 2018,Jan,8; 2017,Jan,8; 2016,Jan,13; 2015,Dec,18; 2015,May,10; 2015,Jan,16

\+ 93572 **each additional vessel (List separately in addition to code for primary procedure)**

Code first initial vessel (93571)
0.00 0.00 FUD ZZZ N N1 80
AMA: 2018,Feb,11; 2018,Jan,8; 2017,Jan,8; 2016,Jan,13; 2015,Dec,18; 2015,May,10; 2015,Jan,16

93580-93583 Percutaneous Repair of Congenital Heart Defects

93580 **Percutaneous transcatheter closure of congenital interatrial communication (ie, Fontan fenestration, atrial septal defect) with implant**

INCLUDES Injection contrast for right heart atrial/ventricular angiograms (93564-93566)
Right heart catheterization (93451, 93453, 93456-93457, 93460-93461, 93530-93533)
EXCLUDES *Bypass graft angiography (93455)*
Injection contrast for left heart atrial/ventricular angiograms (93458-93459)
Left heart catheterization (93452, 93458-93459)
Code also echocardiography, when performed (93303-93317, 93662)
28.2 28.2 FUD 000 J 80
AMA: 2018,Feb,11; 2018,Jan,8; 2017,Jan,8; 2016,Jan,13; 2015,Jan,16

93581 **Percutaneous transcatheter closure of a congenital ventricular septal defect with implant**

INCLUDES Injection contrast for right heart atrial/ventricular angiograms (93564-93566)
Right heart catheterization (93451, 93453, 93456-93457, 93460-93461, 93530-93533)
EXCLUDES *Bypass graft angiography (93455)*
Injection contrast for left heart atrial/ventricular angiograms (93458-93459)
Left heart catheterization (93452, 93458-93459)
Code also echocardiography, when performed (93303-93317, 93662)
38.7 38.7 FUD 000 J 80
AMA: 2018,Feb,11; 2018,Jan,8; 2017,Jan,8; 2016,Jan,13; 2015,Jan,16

93582 **Percutaneous transcatheter closure of patent ductus arteriosus**

INCLUDES Aorta catheter placement (36200)
Aortography (75600-75605, 93567)
Heart catheterization (93451-93461, 93530-93533)
EXCLUDES *Catheterization pulmonary artery (36013-36014)*
Intracardiac echocardiographic services (93662)
Left heart catheterization performed via transapical puncture or transseptal puncture through intact septum (93462)
Ligation repair (33820, 33822, 33824)
Other cardiac angiographic procedures (93563-93566, 93568)
Other echocardiographic services by different provider (93315-93317)
19.4 19.4 FUD 000 J 80
AMA: 2019,Apr,10; 2018,Feb,11; 2018,Jan,8; 2017,Jan,8; 2016,Jan,13; 2015,Jan,16

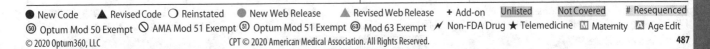

93583 Percutaneous transcatheter septal reduction therapy (eg, alcohol septal ablation) including temporary pacemaker insertion when performed

INCLUDES Alcohol injection (93463)
Coronary angiography during procedure to roadmap, guide intervention, measure vessel, and complete angiography (93454-93461, 93531-93533, 93563, 93563, 93565)
Left heart catheterization (93452-93453, 93458-93461, 93531-93533)
Temporary pacemaker insertion (33210)

EXCLUDES *Intracardiac echocardiographic services when performed (93662)*
Myectomy (surgical ventriculomyotomy) to treat idiopathic hypertrophic subaortic stenosis (33416)
Other echocardiographic services rendered by different provider (93312-93317)

Code also diagnostic cardiac catheterization procedures if patient's condition (clinical indication) changed since intervention or prior study, no available prior catheter-based diagnostic study in treatment zone, or prior study not adequate (93451, 93454-93457, 93530, 93563-93564, 93566-93568)

21.6 21.6 FUD 000 C 80

AMA: 2018,Feb,11

93590-93592 Percutaneous Repair Paravalvular Leak

INCLUDES Access with insertion and positioning of device
Angiography
Fluoroscopy (76000)
Imaging guidance
Left heart catheterization (93452-93453, 93459-93461, 93531-93533)

Code also diagnostic right heart catheterization and angiography performed:
Previous study available but documentation states patient's condition changed since previous study; visualization insufficient; or change necessitates re-evaluation; append modifier 59
When no previous study available and complete diagnostic study performed; append modifier 59

93590 Percutaneous transcatheter closure of paravalvular leak; initial occlusion device, mitral valve

INCLUDES Transseptal puncture (93462)
Code also for transapical puncture (93462)

31.0 31.0 FUD 000 J 80

AMA: 2018,Feb,11; 2018,Jan,8; 2017,Sep,3

93591 initial occlusion device, aortic valve

EXCLUDES *Transapical or transseptal puncture (93462)*

25.8 25.8 FUD 000 J 80

AMA: 2018,Feb,11; 2018,Jan,8; 2017,Sep,3

\+ **93592 each additional occlusion device (List separately in addition to code for primary procedure)**

Code first (93590-93591)

11.3 11.3 FUD ZZZ N 80

AMA: 2018,Feb,11; 2018,Jan,8; 2017,Sep,3

93600-93603 Recording of Intracardiac Electrograms

INCLUDES Unusual situations in which there may be recording/pacing/attempt at arrhythmia induction from only one side heart

EXCLUDES *Comprehensive electrophysiological studies (93619-93620, 93653-93654, 93656)*

93600 Bundle of His recording

0.00 0.00 FUD 000 J 80

AMA: 2018,Feb,11; 2018,Jan,8; 2017,Jan,8; 2016,Jan,13; 2015,Jan,16

93602 Intra-atrial recording

0.00 0.00 FUD 000 J 80

AMA: 2018,Feb,11; 2018,Jan,8; 2017,Jan,8; 2016,Jan,13; 2015,Jan,16

93603 Right ventricular recording

0.00 0.00 FUD 000 J 80

AMA: 2018,Feb,11; 2018,Jan,8; 2017,Jan,8; 2016,Jan,13; 2015,Jan,16

93609-93613 Intracardiac Mapping and Pacing

\+ **93609 Intraventricular and/or intra-atrial mapping of tachycardia site(s) with catheter manipulation to record from multiple sites to identify origin of tachycardia (List separately in addition to code for primary procedure)**

EXCLUDES *Intracardiac 3D mapping (93613)*
Intracardiac ablation with 3D mapping (93654)

Code first (93620, 93653, 93656)

0.00 0.00 FUD ZZZ N 80

AMA: 2018,Feb,11; 2018,Jan,8; 2017,Jan,8; 2016,Jan,13; 2015,Jan,16

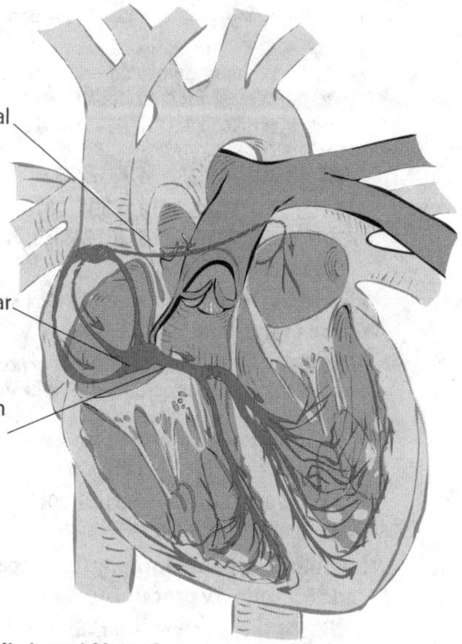

Tachycardia is rapid heartbeat

93610 Intra-atrial pacing

INCLUDES Unusual situations in which there may be recording/pacing/attempt at arrhythmia induction from only one side heart

EXCLUDES *Comprehensive electrophysiological studies (93619-93620)*
Intracardiac ablation (93653-93654, 93656)

0.00 0.00 FUD 000 J 80

AMA: 2018,Feb,11; 2018,Jan,8; 2017,Jan,8; 2016,Jan,13; 2015,Jan,16

93612 Intraventricular pacing

INCLUDES Unusual situations in which there may be recording/pacing/attempt at arrhythmia induction from only one side heart

EXCLUDES *Comprehensive electrophysiological studies (93619-93622)*
Intracardiac ablation (93653-93654, 93656)

0.00 0.00 FUD 000 J 80

AMA: 2018,Feb,11; 2018,Jan,8; 2017,Jan,8; 2016,Jan,13; 2015,Jan,16

\+ **93613 Intracardiac electrophysiologic 3-dimensional mapping (List separately in addition to code for primary procedure)**

EXCLUDES *Intracardiac ablation with 3D mapping (93654)*
Mapping tachycardia site (93609)

Code first (93620, 93653, 93656)

8.63 8.63 FUD ZZZ N 80

AMA: 2018,Feb,11; 2018,Jan,8; 2017,Jan,8; 2016,Jan,13; 2015,Jan,16

93615-93616 Recording and Pacing via Esophagus

93615 **Esophageal recording of atrial electrogram with or without ventricular electrogram(s);**
0.00 0.00 FUD 000
AMA: 2018,Feb,11; 2018,Jan,8; 2017,Jan,8; 2016,Jan,13; 2015,Jan,16

93616 **with pacing**
0.00 0.00 FUD 000
AMA: 2018,Feb,11; 2018,Jan,8; 2017,Jan,8; 2016,Jan,13; 2015,Jan,16

93618 Pacing to Produce an Arrhythmia

CMS: 100-03,20.12 Diagnostic Endocardial Electrical Stimulation (Pacing)

INCLUDES Unusual situations in which there may be recording/pacing/attempt at arrhythmia induction from only one side heart

EXCLUDES *Comprehensive electrophysiological studies (93619-93622)*
Intracardiac ablation (93653-93654, 93656)
Intracardiac phonocardiogram (93799)

93618 **Induction of arrhythmia by electrical pacing**
0.00 0.00 FUD 000
AMA: 2018,Feb,11; 2018,Jan,8; 2017,Jan,8; 2016,Jan,13; 2015,Jan,16

93619-93623 Comprehensive Electrophysiological Studies

CMS: 100-03,20.12 Diagnostic Endocardial Electrical Stimulation (Pacing)

93619 **Comprehensive electrophysiologic evaluation with right atrial pacing and recording, right ventricular pacing and recording, His bundle recording, including insertion and repositioning of multiple electrode catheters, without induction or attempted induction of arrhythmia**

INCLUDES Evaluation sinus node/atrioventricular node/His-Purkinje conduction system without arrhythmia induction

EXCLUDES *Comprehensive electrophysiological studies (93620-93622)*
Intracardiac ablation (93653-93657)
Intracardiac pacing (93610, 93612, 93618)
Recording intracardiac electrograms (93600-93603)

0.00 0.00 FUD 000
AMA: 2018,Feb,11; 2018,Jan,8; 2017,Jan,8; 2016,Jan,13; 2015,Jan,16

93620 **Comprehensive electrophysiologic evaluation including insertion and repositioning of multiple electrode catheters with induction or attempted induction of arrhythmia; with right atrial pacing and recording, right ventricular pacing and recording, His bundle recording**

INCLUDES Recording/pacing/attempted arrhythmia induction from one or more site(s) in heart

EXCLUDES *Comprehensive electrophysiological study without induction/attempted induction arrhythmia (93619)*
Intracardiac ablation (93653-93657)
Intracardiac pacing (93610, 93612, 93618)
Recording intracardiac electrograms (93600-93603)

0.00 0.00 FUD 000
AMA: 2018,Feb,11; 2018,Jan,8; 2017,Jan,8; 2016,Jan,13; 2015,Jan,16

\+ **93621** **with left atrial pacing and recording from coronary sinus or left atrium (List separately in addition to code for primary procedure)**

INCLUDES Recording/pacing/attempted arrhythmia induction from one or more site(s) in heart

EXCLUDES *Intracardiac ablation (93656)*

Code first (93620, 93653-93654)
0.00 0.00 FUD ZZZ
AMA: 2018,Feb,11; 2018,Jan,8; 2017,Jan,8; 2016,Jan,13; 2015,Jan,16

\+ **93622** **with left ventricular pacing and recording (List separately in addition to code for primary procedure)**

EXCLUDES *Intracardiac ablation (93654)*

Code first (93620, 93653, 93656)
0.00 0.00 FUD ZZZ
AMA: 2018,Feb,11; 2018,Jan,8; 2017,Jan,8; 2016,Jan,13; 2015,Jan,16

\+ **93623** **Programmed stimulation and pacing after intravenous drug infusion (List separately in addition to code for primary procedure)**

INCLUDES Recording/pacing/attempted arrhythmia induction from one or more site(s) in heart

EXCLUDES *Reporting code more than one time per day*

Code first comprehensive electrophysiologic evaluation (93610, 93612, 93619-93620, 93653-93654, 93656)
0.00 0.00 FUD ZZZ
AMA: 2018,Feb,11; 2018,Jan,8; 2017,Jan,8; 2016,Jan,13; 2015,Jan,16

93624-93631 Followup and Intraoperative Electrophysiologic Studies

CMS: 100-03,20.12 Diagnostic Endocardial Electrical Stimulation (Pacing)

93624 **Electrophysiologic follow-up study with pacing and recording to test effectiveness of therapy, including induction or attempted induction of arrhythmia**

INCLUDES Recording/pacing/attempted arrhythmia induction from one or more site(s) in heart

0.00 0.00 FUD 000
AMA: 2018,Feb,11; 2018,Jan,8; 2017,Jan,8; 2016,Jan,13; 2015,Jan,16

93631 **Intra-operative epicardial and endocardial pacing and mapping to localize the site of tachycardia or zone of slow conduction for surgical correction**

EXCLUDES *Operative ablation arrhythmogenic focus or pathway by separate provider (33250-33261)*

0.00 0.00 FUD 000
AMA: 2018,Feb,11; 2018,Jan,8; 2017,Jan,8; 2016,Jan,13; 2015,Jan,16

93640-93644 Electrophysiologic Studies of Cardioverter-Defibrillators

INCLUDES Recording/pacing/attempted arrhythmia induction from one or more site(s) in heart

93640 **Electrophysiologic evaluation of single or dual chamber pacing cardioverter-defibrillator leads including defibrillation threshold evaluation (induction of arrhythmia, evaluation of sensing and pacing for arrhythmia termination) at time of initial implantation or replacement;**
0.00 0.00 FUD 000
AMA: 2018,Feb,11; 2018,Jan,8; 2017,Jan,8; 2016,Jan,13; 2015,Jan,16

93641 **with testing of single or dual chamber pacing cardioverter-defibrillator pulse generator**

EXCLUDES *Single/dual chamber pacing cardioverter-defibrillators reprogramming/electronic analysis, subsequent/periodic (93282-93283, 93289, 93292, 93295, 93642)*

0.00 0.00 FUD 000
AMA: 2018,Feb,11; 2018,Jan,8; 2017,Jan,8; 2016,Jan,13; 2015,Jan,16

93642 **Electrophysiologic evaluation of single or dual chamber transvenous pacing cardioverter-defibrillator (includes defibrillation threshold evaluation, induction of arrhythmia, evaluation of sensing and pacing for arrhythmia termination, and programming or reprogramming of sensing or therapeutic parameters)**
9.71 9.71 FUD 000
AMA: 2018,Feb,11; 2018,Jan,8; 2017,Jan,8; 2016,Jan,13; 2015,Jan,16

93644 Electrophysiologic evaluation of subcutaneous implantable defibrillator (includes defibrillation threshold evaluation, induction of arrhythmia, evaluation of sensing for arrhythmia termination, and programming or reprogramming of sensing or therapeutic parameters)

EXCLUDES *Electrophysiological evaluation subcutaneous implantable defibrillator system with substernal electrode (0577T)*
Insertion/replacement subcutaneous implantable defibrillator ([33270])
Subcutaneous cardioverter-defibrillator electrophysiologic evaluation, subsequent/periodic (93260-93261)

5.65 | 5.65 | FUD 000 | N 80

AMA: 2018,Feb,11

93650-93657 Intracardiac Ablation

INCLUDES Ablation services include selective delivery cryo-energy or radiofrequency to targeted tissue
Electrophysiologic studies performed in same session with ablation

93650 Intracardiac catheter ablation of atrioventricular node function, atrioventricular conduction for creation of complete heart block, with or without temporary pacemaker placement

17.2 | 17.2 | FUD 000 | J 80

AMA: 2018,Feb,11; 2018,Jan,8; 2017,Jan,8; 2016,Jan,13; 2015,Jan,16

93653 Comprehensive electrophysiologic evaluation including insertion and repositioning of multiple electrode catheters with induction or attempted induction of an arrhythmia with right atrial pacing and recording, right ventricular pacing and recording (when necessary), and His bundle recording (when necessary) with intracardiac catheter ablation of arrhythmogenic focus; with treatment of supraventricular tachycardia by ablation of fast or slow atrioventricular pathway, accessory atrioventricular connection, cavo-tricuspid isthmus or other single atrial focus or source of atrial re-entry

EXCLUDES *Comprehensive electrophysiological studies (93619-93620)*
Electrophysiologic evaluation pacing cardioverter defibrillator (93642)
Intracardiac ablation with transseptal catheterization (93656)
Intracardiac ablation with treatment ventricular arrhythmia (93654)
Intracardiac pacing (93610, 93612, 93618)
Recording intracardiac electrograms (93600-93603)

24.3 | 24.3 | FUD 000 | J 80

AMA: 2018,Feb,11; 2018,Jan,8; 2017,Jan,8; 2016,Jan,13; 2015,Jan,16

93654 with treatment of ventricular tachycardia or focus of ventricular ectopy including intracardiac electrophysiologic 3D mapping, when performed, and left ventricular pacing and recording, when performed

EXCLUDES *Comprehensive electrophysiological studies (93619-93620, 93622)*
Device evaluation (93279-93284, 93286-93289)
Electrophysiologic evaluation pacing cardioverter defibrillator (93642)
Intracardiac ablation with transseptal catheterization (93656)
Intracardiac ablation with treatment supraventricular tachycardia (93653)
Intracardiac pacing (93609-93613, 93618)
Recording intracardiac electrograms (93600-93603)

32.6 | 32.6 | FUD 000 | J 80

AMA: 2018,Feb,11; 2018,Jan,8; 2017,Jan,8; 2016,Jan,13; 2015,Jan,16

\+ **93655 Intracardiac catheter ablation of a discrete mechanism of arrhythmia which is distinct from the primary ablated mechanism, including repeat diagnostic maneuvers, to treat a spontaneous or induced arrhythmia (List separately in addition to code for primary procedure)**

Code first (93653-93654, 93656)

12.4 | 12.4 | FUD ZZZ | N 80

AMA: 2018,Feb,11; 2018,Jan,8; 2017,Jan,8; 2016,Jan,13; 2015,Jan,16

93656 Comprehensive electrophysiologic evaluation including transseptal catheterizations, insertion and repositioning of multiple electrode catheters with induction or attempted induction of an arrhythmia including left or right atrial pacing/recording when necessary, right ventricular pacing/recording when necessary, and His bundle recording when necessary with intracardiac catheter ablation of atrial fibrillation by pulmonary vein isolation

INCLUDES His bundle recording when indicated
Left atrial pacing/recording
Right ventricular pacing/recording

EXCLUDES *Comprehensive electrophysiological studies (93619-93621)*
Device evaluation (93279-93284, 93286-93289)
Electrophysiologic evaluation with treatment ventricular tachycardia (93654)
Intracardiac ablation with treatment supraventricular tachycardia (93653)
Intracardiac pacing (93610, 93612, 93618)
Left heart catheterization by transseptal puncture (93462)
Recording intracardiac electrograms (93600-93603)

32.7 | 32.7 | FUD 000 | J 80

AMA: 2019,Sep,10; 2018,Feb,11; 2018,Jan,8; 2017,Jan,8; 2016,Jan,13; 2015,Jan,16

\+ **93657 Additional linear or focal intracardiac catheter ablation of the left or right atrium for treatment of atrial fibrillation remaining after completion of pulmonary vein isolation (List separately in addition to code for primary procedure)**

Code first (93656)

12.3 | 12.3 | FUD ZZZ | N 80

AMA: 2019,Sep,10; 2018,Feb,11; 2018,Jan,8; 2017,Jan,8; 2016,Jan,13; 2015,Jan,16

93660-93662 Other Tests for Cardiac Function

93660 Evaluation of cardiovascular function with tilt table evaluation, with continuous ECG monitoring and intermittent blood pressure monitoring, with or without pharmacological intervention

EXCLUDES *Autonomic nervous system function testing (95921, 95924, [95943])*

4.50 | 4.50 | FUD 000 | S 80

AMA: 2018,Feb,11; 2018,Jan,8; 2017,Jan,8; 2016,Jan,13; 2015,Jan,16

\+ **93662 Intracardiac echocardiography during therapeutic/diagnostic intervention, including imaging supervision and interpretation (List separately in addition to code for primary procedure)**

EXCLUDES *Internal cardioversion (92961)*
Transcatheter implantation interatrial septal shunt device, percutaneous approach (0613T)
Transcatheter tricuspid valve repair with prosthesis, percutaneous approach (0569T-0570T)

Code first (as appropriate) (92987, 93453, 93460-93462, 93532, 93580-93583, 93620-93622, 93653-93654, 93656)

0.00 | 0.00 | FUD ZZZ | N 80

AMA: 2018,Feb,11; 2018,Jan,8; 2017,Jan,8; 2016,Jan,13; 2015,Jan,16

93668 Rehabilitation Services: Peripheral Arterial Disease

CMS: 100-03,1,20.35 Supervised Exercise Therapy (SET) for Symptomatic Peripheral Artery Disease (PAD)(Effective May 25, 2017; 100-04,32,390 Supervised exercise therapy (SET) Symptomatic Peripheral Artery Disease; 100-04,32,390.1 General Billing Requirements for Supervised exercise therapy (SET) for PAD; 100-04,32,390.2 Coding Requirements for SET for PAD; 100-04,32,390.3 Special Billing Requirements for Professional Claims; 100-04,32,390.4 Special Billing Requirements for Institutional Claims; 100-04,32,390.5 Common Working File (CWF) Requirements; 100-04,32,390.6 Applicable Medicare Summary Notice (MSN), Remittance Advice Remark Codes (RARCs), and Claim Adjustment Reason Code (CARC) Messaging

INCLUDES Monitoring:
- Other cardiovascular limitations for workload adjustment
- Patient's claudication threshold

Motorized treadmill or track
Sessions lasting 45-60 minutes
Supervision by exercise physiologist/nurse

Code also appropriate E/M service, when performed

93668 **Peripheral arterial disease (PAD) rehabilitation, per session**
0.50 0.50 **FUD** XXX S 80 TC
AMA: 2018,Feb,11

93701-93702 Thoracic Electrical Bioimpedance

EXCLUDES *Bioelectrical impedance analysis whole body (0358T)*
Indirect measurement left ventricular filling pressure by computerized calibration arterial waveform response to Valsalva (93799)

93701 **Bioimpedance-derived physiologic cardiovascular analysis**
0.71 0.71 **FUD** XXX Q1 80 TC
AMA: 2018,Feb,11; 2018,Jan,8; 2017,Jan,8; 2016,Jan,13; 2015,Jan,16

93702 **Bioimpedance spectroscopy (BIS), extracellular fluid analysis for lymphedema assessment(s)**
3.57 3.57 **FUD** XXX S 80 TC
AMA: 2018,Feb,11

93724 Electronic Analysis of Pacemaker Function

93724 **Electronic analysis of antitachycardia pacemaker system (includes electrocardiographic recording, programming of device, induction and termination of tachycardia via implanted pacemaker, and interpretation of recordings)**
8.04 8.04 **FUD** 000 S 80
AMA: 2018,Feb,11; 2018,Jan,8; 2017,Jan,8; 2016,Jan,13; 2015,Jan,16

93740 Temperature Gradient Assessment

93740 **Temperature gradient studies**
0.23 0.23 **FUD** XXX Q1
AMA: 2018,Feb,11

93745 Wearable Cardioverter-Defibrillator System Services

EXCLUDES *Device evaluation (93282, 93292)*

93745 **Initial set-up and programming by a physician or other qualified health care professional of wearable cardioverter-defibrillator includes initial programming of system, establishing baseline electronic ECG, transmission of data to data repository, patient instruction in wearing system and patient reporting of problems or events**
0.00 0.00 **FUD** XXX S 80
AMA: 2018,Feb,11

93750 Ventricular Assist Device (VAD) Interrogation

CMS: 100-03,20.9 Artificial Hearts and Related Devices; 100-03,20.9.1 Ventricular Assist Devices; 100-04,32,320.1 Artificial Hearts Prior to May 1, 2008; 100-04,32,320.2 Coding for Artificial Hearts After May 1, 2008; 100-04,32,320.3 Ventricular Assist Devices; 100-04,32,320.3.1 Post-cardiotomy; 100-04,32,320.3.2 Bridge- to -Transplantation

EXCLUDES *Insertion ventricular assist device (33975-33976, 33979)*
Removal/replacement ventricular assist device (33981-33983)

93750 **Interrogation of ventricular assist device (VAD), in person, with physician or other qualified health care professional analysis of device parameters (eg, drivelines, alarms, power surges), review of device function (eg, flow and volume status, septum status, recovery), with programming, if performed, and report**
1.32 1.58 **FUD** XXX S 80
AMA: 2018,Dec,10; 2018,Dec,10; 2018,Feb,11; 2018,Jan,8; 2017,Jan,8; 2016,Jan,13; 2015,Jan,16

93770 Peripheral Venous Blood Pressure Assessment

CMS: 100-03,20.19 Ambulatory Blood Pressure Monitoring (20.19)

EXCLUDES *Cannulization, central venous (36500, 36555-36556)*

93770 **Determination of venous pressure**
0.23 0.23 **FUD** XXX N
AMA: 2018,Feb,11

93784-93790 Ambulatory Blood Pressure Monitoring

CMS: 100-03,20.19 Ambulatory Blood Pressure Monitoring (20.19); 100-04,32,10.1 Ambulatory Blood Pressure Monitoring Billing Requirements

EXCLUDES *Self-measured blood pressure monitoring ([99473, 99474])*

93784 **Ambulatory blood pressure monitoring, utilizing report-generating software, automated, worn continuously for 24 hours or longer; including recording, scanning analysis, interpretation and report**
1.51 1.51 **FUD** XXX B 80
AMA: 2020,Apr,5; 2018,Feb,11

93786 **recording only**
0.83 0.83 **FUD** XXX Q1 80 TC
AMA: 2020,Apr,5; 2018,Feb,11

93788 **scanning analysis with report**
0.14 0.14 **FUD** XXX Q1 80 TC
AMA: 2020,Apr,5; 2018,Feb,11

93790 **review with interpretation and report**
0.53 0.53 **FUD** XXX M 80 26
AMA: 2020,Apr,5; 2018,Feb,11

93792-93793 INR Monitoring

CMS: 100-03,190.11 Home PT/INR Monitoring for Anticoagulation Management; 100-04,32,60.4.1 Anticoagulation Management: Covered Diagnosis Codes

EXCLUDES *Chronic care management services provided during same month ([99439, 99490, 99491])*
Complex chronic care management services provided during same month (99487-99489)
Online digital assessment and management services by nonphysician healthcare professional (98970-98972)
Online digital evaluation and management services by physician or other qualified health care professional ([99421, 99422, 99423])
Telephone assessment and management service by nonphysician healthcare professional (98966-98968)
Telephone evaluation and management service by physician or other qualified healthcare professional (99441-99443)

93792 **Patient/caregiver training for initiation of home international normalized ratio (INR) monitoring under the direction of a physician or other qualified health care professional, face-to-face, including use and care of the INR monitor, obtaining blood sample, instructions for reporting home INR test results, and documentation of patient's/caregiver's ability to perform testing and report results**

Code also INR home monitoring equipment with appropriate supply code or (99070)
Code also significantly separately identifiable E/M service on same date service using modifier 25

1.84 1.84 **FUD** XXX B 80 TC
AMA: 2018,Mar,7; 2018,Feb,11

93793 **Anticoagulant management for a patient taking warfarin, must include review and interpretation of a new home, office, or lab international normalized ratio (INR) test result, patient instructions, dosage adjustment (as needed), and scheduling of additional test(s), when performed**

EXCLUDES *E/M services performed same date (99202-99215, 99241-99245)*
Reporting code more than one time per day

0.33 0.33 **FUD** XXX B 80 26

AMA: 2020,Feb,7; 2018,Mar,7; 2018,Feb,11; 2018,Jan,8; 2017,Nov,10

93797-93799 Cardiac Rehabilitation

CMS: 100-02,15,232 Cardiac Rehabilitation (CR) and Intensive Cardiac Rehabilitation (ICR) Services Furnished On or After January 1, 2010; 100-04,32,140.2 Cardiac Rehabilitation On or After January 1, 2010; 100-04,32,140.2.1 Coding Cardiac Rehabilitation Services On or After January 1, 2010; 100-04,32,140.2.2 Institutional Claims for CR and ICR Services; 100-04,32,140.2.2.4 CR Services Exceeding 36 Sessions; 100-04,32,140.3 Intensive Cardiac Rehabilitation Program Services Furnished On or After January 1, 2010; 100-08,15,4.2.8 Cardiac Rehabilitation (CR) and Intensive Cardiac Rehabilitation (ICR)

93797 **Physician or other qualified health care professional services for outpatient cardiac rehabilitation; without continuous ECG monitoring (per session)**

0.25 0.46 **FUD** 000 S 80

AMA: 2018,Feb,11

93798 **with continuous ECG monitoring (per session)**

0.40 0.72 **FUD** 000 S 80

AMA: 2018,Feb,11

93799 **Unlisted cardiovascular service or procedure**

0.00 0.00 **FUD** XXX S 80

AMA: 2018,Dec,10; 2018,Dec,10; 2018,Sep,10; 2018,Aug,10; 2018,Feb,11; 2018,Jan,8; 2017,Jan,8; 2016,May,5; 2016,Jan,13; 2015,Jan,16

93880-93895 Noninvasive Tests Extracranial/Intracranial Arteries

INCLUDES Patient care required to perform/supervise studies and interpret results
EXCLUDES *Hand-held Dopplers that do not provide hard copy or vascular flow bidirectional analysis (see E/M codes)*

93880 **Duplex scan of extracranial arteries; complete bilateral study**

EXCLUDES *Common carotid intima-media thickness (IMT) studies (93895)*

5.64 5.64 **FUD** XXX S 80

AMA: 2018,Feb,11; 2018,Jan,8; 2017,Jan,8; 2016,Jan,13; 2015,Jan,16

93882 **unilateral or limited study**

EXCLUDES *Common carotid intima-media thickness (IMT) studies (93895)*

3.64 3.64 **FUD** XXX S 80

AMA: 2018,Feb,11; 2018,Jan,8; 2017,Jan,8; 2016,Jan,13; 2015,Jan,16

93886 **Transcranial Doppler study of the intracranial arteries; complete study**

INCLUDES Complete transcranial doppler (TCD) study
Ultrasound evaluation right/left anterior circulation territories and posterior circulation territory

7.70 7.70 **FUD** XXX S 80

AMA: 2018,Feb,11; 2018,Jan,8; 2017,Jan,8; 2016,Jan,13; 2015,Jan,16

93888 **limited study**

INCLUDES Limited TCD study
Ultrasound examination two or fewer territories (right/left anterior circulation, posterior circulation)

4.47 4.47 **FUD** XXX S 80

AMA: 2018,Feb,11; 2018,Jan,8; 2017,Jan,8; 2016,Jan,13; 2015,Jan,16

93890 **vasoreactivity study**

EXCLUDES *Limited TCD study (93888)*

7.82 7.82 **FUD** XXX Q1 80

AMA: 2018,Feb,11; 2018,Jan,8; 2017,Jan,8; 2016,Jan,13; 2015,Jan,16

93892 **emboli detection without intravenous microbubble injection**

EXCLUDES *Limited TCD study (93888)*

8.81 8.81 **FUD** XXX Q1 80

AMA: 2018,Feb,11; 2018,Jan,8; 2017,Jan,8; 2016,Jan,13; 2015,Jan,16

93893 **emboli detection with intravenous microbubble injection**

EXCLUDES *Limited TCD study (93888)*

9.81 9.81 **FUD** XXX Q1 80

AMA: 2018,Feb,11; 2018,Jan,8; 2017,Jan,8; 2016,Jan,13; 2015,Jan,16

93895 **Quantitative carotid intima media thickness and carotid atheroma evaluation, bilateral**

EXCLUDES *Complete and limited duplex studies (93880, 93882)*

0.00 0.00 **FUD** XXX E 80

AMA: 2018,Feb,11

93922-93971 Noninvasive Vascular Studies: Extremities

CMS: 100-04,8,180 Noninvasive Studies for ESRD Patients

INCLUDES Patient care required to perform/supervise studies and interpret results

EXCLUDES *Hand-held dopplers that do not provide hard copy or vascular flow bidirectional analysis (see E/M codes)*

93922 Limited bilateral noninvasive physiologic studies of upper or lower extremity arteries, (eg, for lower extremity: ankle/brachial indices at distal posterior tibial and anterior tibial/dorsalis pedis arteries plus bidirectional, Doppler waveform recording and analysis at 1-2 levels, or ankle/brachial indices at distal posterior tibial and anterior tibial/dorsalis pedis arteries plus volume plethysmography at 1-2 levels, or ankle/brachial indices at distal posterior tibial and anterior tibial/dorsalis pedis arteries with, transcutaneous oxygen tension measurement at 1-2 levels)

INCLUDES Evaluation:
- Doppler analysis bidirectional blood flow
- Nonimaging physiologic recordings pressure
- Oxygen tension measurements and/or plethysmography

Lower extremity (potential levels include high thigh, low thigh, calf, ankle, metatarsal and toes) limited study includes either:
- Ankle/brachial indices distal posterior tibial and anterior tibial/dorsalis pedis arteries plus bidirectional Doppler waveform recording and analysis 1-2 levels; OR
- Ankle/brachial indices distal posterior tibial and anterior tibial/dorsalis pedis arteries plus volume plethysmography 1-2 levels; OR
- Ankle/brachial indices distal posterior tibial and anterior tibial/dorsalis pedis arteries with transcutaneous oxygen tension measurements 1-2 levels

Unilateral provocative functional measurement

Unilateral study 3 or move levels

Upper extremity (potential levels include arm, forearm, wrist, and digits) limited study includes:
- Doppler-determined systolic pressures and bidirectional waveform recording with analysis 1-2 levels; OR
- Doppler-determined systolic pressures and transcutaneous oxygen tension measurements 1-2 levels; OR
- Doppler-determined systolic pressures and volume plethysmography 1-2 levels

EXCLUDES *Reporting code more than one time for lower extremity(ies)*

Reporting code more than one time for upper extremity(ies)

Transcutaneous oxyhemoglobin, deoxyhemoglobin and tissue oxygenation measurement (0631T)

Transcutaneous oxyhemoglobin measurement (0493T)

Code also modifier 52 for unilateral study 1-2 levels

Code also twice for upper and lower extremity study and append modifier 59

2.40 2.40 **FUD** XXX Q1 80

AMA: 2019,Oct,8; 2018,Feb,11; 2018,Jan,8; 2017,Jan,8; 2016,Jan,13; 2015,Jan,16

93923 Complete bilateral noninvasive physiologic studies of upper or lower extremity arteries, 3 or more levels (eg, for lower extremity: ankle/brachial indices at distal posterior tibial and anterior tibial/dorsalis pedis arteries plus segmental blood pressure measurements with bidirectional Doppler waveform recording and analysis, at 3 or more levels, or ankle/brachial indices at distal posterior tibial and anterior tibial/dorsalis pedis arteries plus segmental volume plethysmography at 3 or more levels, or ankle/brachial indices at distal posterior tibial and anterior tibial/dorsalis pedis arteries plus segmental transcutaneous oxygen tension measurements at 3 or more levels), or single level study with provocative functional maneuvers (eg, measurements with postural provocative tests, or measurements with reactive hyperemia)

INCLUDES Evaluation:
- Doppler analysis bidirectional blood flow
- Nonimaging physiologic recordings pressures
- Oxygen tension measurements

Lower extremity:
- Ankle/brachial indices distal posterior tibial and anterior tibial/dorsalis pedis arteries plus bidirectional Doppler waveform recording and analysis 3 or more levels; OR
- Ankle/brachial indices distal posterior tibial and anterior tibial/dorsalis pedis arteries with transcutaneous oxygen tension measurements 3 or more levels; OR
- Ankle/brachial indices distal posterior tibial and anterior tibial/dorsalis pedis arteries plus volume plethysmography 3 or more levels; OR

Provocative functional maneuvers and measurement single level

Upper extremity complete study:
- Doppler-determined systolic pressures and bidirectional waveform recording with analysis 3 or more levels; OR
- Doppler-determined systolic pressures and transcutaneous oxygen tension measurements 3 or more levels; OR
- Doppler-determined systolic pressures and volume plethysmography 3 or more levels; OR

EXCLUDES *Reporting code more than one time for lower extremity(ies)*

Reporting coe more than one time for upper extremity(ies)

Transcutaneous oxyhemoglobin, deoxyhemoglobin and tissue oxygenation measurement (0631T)

Unilateral study 3 or more levels (93922)

Code also twice for upper and lower extremity study and append modifier 59

3.78 3.78 **FUD** XXX S 80

AMA: 2020,Sep,14; 2019,Oct,8; 2018,Feb,11; 2018,Jan,8; 2017,Jan,8; 2016,Jan,13; 2015,Jan,16

93924 Noninvasive physiologic studies of lower extremity arteries, at rest and following treadmill stress testing, (ie, bidirectional Doppler waveform or volume plethysmography recording and analysis at rest with ankle/brachial indices immediately after and at timed intervals following performance of a standardized protocol on a motorized treadmill plus recording of time of onset of claudication or other symptoms, maximal walking time, and time to recovery) complete bilateral study

INCLUDES Evaluation:
- Doppler analysis bidirectional blood flow
- Nonimaging physiologic recordings pressures
- Oxygen tension measurements
- Plethysmography

EXCLUDES *Noninvasive vascular studies extremities (93922-93923)*

Other types exercise

4.62 4.62 **FUD** XXX S 80

AMA: 2019,Oct,8; 2018,Feb,11; 2018,Jan,8; 2017,Jan,8; 2016,Jan,13; 2015,Jan,16

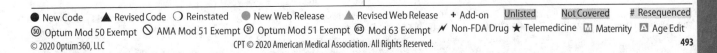

Medicine
93925 — 94004

93925 **Duplex scan of lower extremity arteries or arterial bypass grafts; complete bilateral study**
EXCLUDES *Preoperative arterial inflow and venous outflow duplex scan for creation hemodialysis access, same extremities (93985)*
7.25 7.25 FUD XXX S 80
AMA: 2019,Oct,8; 2018,Feb,11; 2018,Jan,8; 2017,Jan,8; 2016,Sep,9; 2016,Jan,13; 2015,Jan,16

93926 **unilateral or limited study**
EXCLUDES *Preoperative arterial inflow and venous outflow duplex scan for creation hemodialysis access, same extremity (93986)*
4.24 4.24 FUD XXX S 80
AMA: 2019,Oct,8; 2018,Feb,11; 2018,Jan,8; 2017,Jan,8; 2016,Sep,9; 2016,Jan,13; 2015,Jan,16

93930 **Duplex scan of upper extremity arteries or arterial bypass grafts; complete bilateral study**
EXCLUDES *Preoperative arterial inflow and venous outflow duplex scan for creation hemodialysis access, same extremity(ies) (93985-93986)*
5.83 5.83 FUD XXX S 80
AMA: 2019,Oct,8; 2018,Feb,11; 2018,Jan,8; 2017,Jan,8; 2016,Sep,9; 2016,Jan,13; 2015,Jan,16

93931 **unilateral or limited study**
EXCLUDES *Preoperative arterial inflow and venous outflow duplex scan for creation hemodialysis access, same extremity (93985-93986)*
3.63 3.63 FUD XXX S 80
AMA: 2019,Oct,8; 2018,Feb,11; 2018,Jan,8; 2017,Jan,8; 2016,Sep,9; 2016,Jan,13; 2015,Jan,16

93970 **Duplex scan of extremity veins including responses to compression and other maneuvers; complete bilateral study**
EXCLUDES *Endovenous ablation (36475-36476, 36478-36479)*
Preoperative arterial inflow and venous outflow duplex scan for creation hemodialysis access, same extremity(ies) (93985-93986)
5.52 5.52 FUD XXX S 80
AMA: 2019,Oct,8; 2018,Mar,3; 2018,Feb,11; 2018,Jan,8; 2017,Jan,8; 2016,Nov,3; 2016,Sep,9; 2016,Jan,13; 2015,Jan,16

93971 **unilateral or limited study**
EXCLUDES *Endovenous ablation (36475-36476, 36478-36479)*
Preoperative arterial inflow and venous outflow duplex scan for creation hemodialysis access, same extremity (93985-93986)
3.44 3.44 FUD XXX S 80
AMA: 2019,Oct,8; 2018,Mar,3; 2018,Feb,11; 2018,Jan,8; 2017,Jan,8; 2016,Nov,3; 2016,Sep,9; 2016,Jan,13; 2015,Aug,8; 2015,Jan,16

93975-93981 Noninvasive Vascular Studies: Abdomen/Chest/Pelvis

93975 **Duplex scan of arterial inflow and venous outflow of abdominal, pelvic, scrotal contents and/or retroperitoneal organs; complete study**
7.83 7.83 FUD XXX S 80
AMA: 2018,Feb,11; 2018,Jan,8; 2017,Jan,8; 2016,Aug,9; 2016,Jan,13; 2015,Mar,9; 2015,Jan,16

93976 **limited study**
4.64 4.64 FUD XXX S 80
AMA: 2018,Feb,11; 2018,Jan,8; 2017,Jan,8; 2016,Aug,9; 2016,Jan,13; 2015,Mar,9; 2015,Jan,16

93978 **Duplex scan of aorta, inferior vena cava, iliac vasculature, or bypass grafts; complete study**
EXCLUDES *Ultrasound screening for abdominal aortic aneurysm (76706)*
5.34 5.34 FUD XXX S 80
AMA: 2018,Feb,11; 2018,Jan,8; 2017,Jan,8; 2016,Jan,13; 2015,Jan,16

93979 **unilateral or limited study**
EXCLUDES *Ultrasound screening for abdominal aortic aneurysm (76706)*
3.40 3.40 FUD XXX Q1 80
AMA: 2018,Feb,11; 2018,Jan,8; 2017,Jan,8; 2016,Jan,13; 2015,Jan,16

93980 **Duplex scan of arterial inflow and venous outflow of penile vessels; complete study**
3.53 3.53 FUD XXX S 80
AMA: 2018,Feb,11; 2018,Jan,8; 2017,Jan,8; 2016,Jan,13; 2015,Jan,16

93981 **follow-up or limited study**
2.15 2.15 FUD XXX S 80
AMA: 2018,Feb,11; 2018,Jan,8; 2017,Jan,8; 2016,Jan,13; 2015,Jan,16

93985-93998 Noninvasive Vascular Studies: Hemodialysis Access

93985 **Duplex scan of arterial inflow and venous outflow for preoperative vessel assessment prior to creation of hemodialysis access; complete bilateral study**
EXCLUDES *Duplex scan extremity arteries only, same extremity(ies) (93925, 93930)*
Duplex scan extremity veins only, same extremity(ies) (93970)
Duplex scan hemodialysis access, arterial inflow, and venous outflow, same extremity(ies) (93990)
Physiologic arterial evaluation extremities (93922-93924)
7.53 7.53 FUD XXX P2 80

93986 **complete unilateral study**
EXCLUDES *Duplex scan extremity arteries only, same extremity (93926, 93931)*
Duplex scan extremity veins only, same extremity (93971)
Duplex scan hemodialysis access, arterial inflow and venous outflow, same extremity (93990)
Physiologic arterial evaluation extremities (93922-93924)
4.37 4.37 FUD XXX P2 80

93990 **Duplex scan of hemodialysis access (including arterial inflow, body of access and venous outflow)**
EXCLUDES *Hemodialysis access flow measurement by indicator method (90940)*
4.39 4.39 FUD XXX Q1 80
AMA: 2019,Oct,8; 2018,Feb,11; 2018,Jan,8; 2017,Jan,8; 2016,Jan,13; 2015,Jan,16

93998 **Unlisted noninvasive vascular diagnostic study**
0.00 0.00 FUD XXX Q1 80
AMA: 2018,Feb,11; 2018,Jan,8; 2017,Jan,8; 2016,Jan,13; 2015,Jan,16

94002-94005 Ventilator Management Services

94002 **Ventilation assist and management, initiation of pressure or volume preset ventilators for assisted or controlled breathing; hospital inpatient/observation, initial day**
EXCLUDES *E/M services*
2.63 2.63 FUD XXX Q3 80
AMA: 2019,Aug,8; 2018,Feb,11; 2018,Jan,8; 2017,Jan,8; 2016,Jan,13; 2015,Jan,16

94003 **hospital inpatient/observation, each subsequent day**
EXCLUDES *E/M services*
1.90 1.90 FUD XXX Q3 80
AMA: 2019,Aug,8; 2018,Feb,11; 2018,Jan,8; 2017,Jan,8; 2016,Jan,13; 2015,Jan,16

94004 **nursing facility, per day**
EXCLUDES *E/M services*
1.40 1.40 FUD XXX B 80
AMA: 2019,Aug,8; 2018,Feb,11; 2018,Jan,8; 2017,Jan,8; 2016,Jan,13; 2015,Jan,16

94005 Home ventilator management care plan oversight of a patient (patient not present) in home, domiciliary or rest home (eg, assisted living) requiring review of status, review of laboratories and other studies and revision of orders and respiratory care plan (as appropriate), within a calendar month, 30 minutes or more

Code also when different provider reports care plan oversight in same 30 days (99339-99340, 99374-99378)

2.61 2.61 FUD XXX M

AMA: 2018,Feb,11; 2018,Jan,8; 2017,Jan,8; 2016,Jan,13; 2015,Jan,16

94010-94799 [94619] Respiratory Services: Diagnostic and Therapeutic

INCLUDES Laboratory procedure(s)
Test results interpretation

EXCLUDES *Separately identifiable E/M service*

94010 Spirometry, including graphic record, total and timed vital capacity, expiratory flow rate measurement(s), with or without maximal voluntary ventilation

INCLUDES Measurement expiratory airflow and volumes

EXCLUDES *Diffusing capacity (94729)*
Other respiratory function services (94150, 94200, 94375, 94728)

1.00 1.00 FUD XXX Q1 80

AMA: 2019,May,10; 2019,Mar,10; 2019,Apr,10; 2018,Feb,11; 2018,Jan,8; 2017,Jan,8; 2016,Jan,13; 2015,Sep,9; 2015,Jan,16

94011 Measurement of spirometric forced expiratory flows in an infant or child through 2 years of age

2.46 2.46 FUD XXX Q1 80

AMA: 2019,Mar,10; 2018,Feb,11; 2018,Jan,8; 2017,Jan,8; 2016,Jan,13; 2015,Jan,16

94012 Measurement of spirometric forced expiratory flows, before and after bronchodilator, in an infant or child through 2 years of age

4.02 4.02 FUD XXX Q1 80

AMA: 2019,Mar,10; 2018,Feb,11; 2018,Jan,8; 2017,Jan,8; 2016,Jan,13; 2015,Jan,16

94013 Measurement of lung volumes (ie, functional residual capacity [FRC], forced vital capacity [FVC], and expiratory reserve volume [ERV]) in an infant or child through 2 years of age

0.55 0.55 FUD XXX S 80

AMA: 2019,Mar,10; 2018,Feb,11; 2018,Jan,8; 2017,Jan,8; 2016,Jan,13; 2015,Jan,16

94014 Patient-initiated spirometric recording per 30-day period of time; includes reinforced education, transmission of spirometric tracing, data capture, analysis of transmitted data, periodic recalibration and review and interpretation by a physician or other qualified health care professional

1.58 1.58 FUD XXX Q1 80

AMA: 2019,Mar,10; 2018,Feb,11; 2018,Jan,8; 2017,Jan,8; 2016,Jan,13; 2015,Jan,16

94015 recording (includes hook-up, reinforced education, data transmission, data capture, trend analysis, and periodic recalibration)

0.86 0.86 FUD XXX Q1 80 TC

AMA: 2019,Mar,10; 2018,Feb,11; 2018,Jan,8; 2017,Jan,8; 2016,Jan,13; 2015,Jan,16

94016 review and interpretation only by a physician or other qualified health care professional

0.72 0.72 FUD XXX A 80 26

AMA: 2019,Mar,10; 2018,Feb,11; 2018,Jan,8; 2017,Jan,8; 2016,Jan,13; 2015,Jan,16

94060 Bronchodilation responsiveness, spirometry as in 94010, pre- and post-bronchodilator administration

INCLUDES Spirometry performed prior to and after bronchodilator has been administered

EXCLUDES *Bronchospasm prolonged exercise test with pre- and post-spirometry (94617, [94619])*
Diffusing capacity (94729)
Other respiratory function services (94150, 94200, 94375, 94640, 94728)

Code also bronchodilator supply with appropriate supply code or (99070)

1.68 1.68 FUD XXX S 80

AMA: 2019,Mar,10; 2019,Apr,10; 2018,Feb,11; 2018,Jan,8; 2017,Jan,8; 2016,Jan,13; 2015,Sep,9; 2015,Jan,16

94070 Bronchospasm provocation evaluation, multiple spirometric determinations as in 94010, with administered agents (eg, antigen[s], cold air, methacholine)

EXCLUDES *Diffusing capacity (94729)*
Inhalation treatment (diagnostic or therapeutic) (94640)

Code also antigen(s) administration with appropriate supply code or (99070)

1.67 1.67 FUD XXX S 80

AMA: 2019,Mar,10; 2018,Feb,11; 2018,Jan,8; 2017,Jan,8; 2016,Jan,13; 2015,Sep,9; 2015,Jan,16

94150 Vital capacity, total (separate procedure)

EXCLUDES *Other respiratory function services (94010, 94060, 94728)*
Thoracic gas volumes (94726-94727)

0.71 0.71 FUD XXX Q1

AMA: 2019,Mar,10; 2018,Sep,14; 2018,Feb,11; 2018,Jan,8; 2017,Jan,8; 2016,Jan,13; 2015,Jan,16

94200 Maximum breathing capacity, maximal voluntary ventilation

EXCLUDES *Other respiratory function services (94010, 94060)*

0.78 0.78 FUD XXX Q1 80

AMA: 2019,Mar,10; 2018,Feb,11; 2018,Jan,8; 2017,Jan,8; 2016,Jan,13; 2015,Jan,16

94250 ~~Expired gas collection, quantitative, single procedure (separate procedure)~~

94375 Respiratory flow volume loop

INCLUDES Obstruction pattern identification in central or peripheral airways (inspiratory and/or expiratory)

EXCLUDES *Diffusing capacity (94729)*
Other respiratory function services (94010, 94060, 94728)

1.10 1.10 FUD XXX Q1 80

AMA: 2019,Mar,10; 2018,Feb,11; 2018,Jan,8; 2017,Jan,8; 2016,Jan,13; 2015,Jan,16

94400 ~~Breathing response to CO2 (CO2 response curve)~~

94450 Breathing response to hypoxia (hypoxia response curve)

EXCLUDES *HAST - high altitude simulation test (94452, 94453)*

1.88 1.88 FUD XXX Q1 80

AMA: 2019,Mar,10; 2018,Feb,11; 2018,Jan,8; 2017,Jan,8; 2016,Jan,13; 2015,Jan,16

94452 High altitude simulation test (HAST), with interpretation and report by a physician or other qualified health care professional;

EXCLUDES *HAST test with supplemental oxygen titration (94453)*
Noninvasive pulse oximetry (94760-94761)
Obtaining arterial blood gases (36600)

1.48 1.48 FUD XXX Q1 80

AMA: 2019,Mar,10; 2018,Feb,11; 2018,Jan,8; 2017,Jan,8; 2016,Jan,13; 2015,Jan,16

94453 **with supplemental oxygen titration**

EXCLUDES *HAST test without supplemental oxygen titration (94452)*
Noninvasive pulse oximetry (94760-94761)
Obtaining arterial blood gases (36600)

2.03 2.03 FUD XXX Q1 80

AMA: 2019,Mar,10; 2018,Feb,11; 2018,Jan,8; 2017,Jan,8; 2016,Jan,13; 2015,Jan,16

94610 **Intrapulmonary surfactant administration by a physician or other qualified health care professional through endotracheal tube**

INCLUDES Reporting once per dosing episode

EXCLUDES *Intubation, endotracheal (31500)*
Neonatal critical care (99468-99472)

1.59 1.59 FUD XXX Q1 80

AMA: 2019,Mar,10; 2018,Feb,11; 2018,Jan,8; 2017,Jan,8; 2016,Jan,13; 2015,Jan,16

▲ **94617** **Exercise test for bronchospasm, including pre- and post-spirometry and pulse oximetry; with electrocardiographic recording(s)**

EXCLUDES *Cardiovascular stress test (93015-93018)*
ECG monitoring (93000-93010, 93040-93042)
Pulse oximetry (94760-94761)

2.66 2.66 FUD XXX Q1 80

AMA: 2019,May,10; 2019,Mar,10; 2018,Feb,11; 2018,Jan,8; 2017,Oct,3

● # **94619** **without electrocardiographic recording(s)**

EXCLUDES *Cardiovascular stress test (93015-93018)*
ECG monitoring (93000-93010, 93040-93042)
Pulse oximetry (94760-94761)

0.00 0.00 FUD 000

94618 **Pulmonary stress testing (eg, 6-minute walk test), including measurement of heart rate, oximetry, and oxygen titration, when performed**

EXCLUDES *Pulse oximetry (94760-94761)*

0.95 0.95 FUD XXX Q1 80

AMA: 2019,May,10; 2019,Mar,10; 2018,Feb,11; 2018,Jan,8; 2017,Oct,3

94619 **Resequenced code. See code following 94617.**

94621 **Cardiopulmonary exercise testing, including measurements of minute ventilation, CO2 production, O2 uptake, and electrocardiographic recordings**

EXCLUDES *Cardiovascular stress test (93015-93018)*
ECG monitoring (93000-93010, 93040-93042)
Oxygen uptake expired gas analysis (94680-94690)
Pulse oximetry (94760-94761)

4.50 4.50 FUD XXX S 80

AMA: 2019,May,10; 2019,Mar,10; 2018,Feb,11; 2018,Jan,8; 2017,Oct,3; 2017,Jan,8; 2016,Jan,13; 2015,Jan,16

94640 **Pressurized or nonpressurized inhalation treatment for acute airway obstruction for therapeutic purposes and/or for diagnostic purposes such as sputum induction with an aerosol generator, nebulizer, metered dose inhaler or intermittent positive pressure breathing (IPPB) device**

EXCLUDES *One hour or more continuous inhalation treatment (94644, 94645)*
Other respiratory function services (94060, 94070)

Code also modifier 76 when more than one inhalation treatment performed on same date

0.51 0.51 FUD XXX Q1 80

AMA: 2019,Mar,10; 2018,Feb,11; 2018,Jan,8; 2017,Jan,8; 2016,Jan,13; 2015,Sep,9; 2015,Jan,16

94642 **Aerosol inhalation of pentamidine for pneumocystis carinii pneumonia treatment or prophylaxis**

0.00 0.00 FUD XXX Q1 80

AMA: 2019,Mar,10; 2018,Feb,11; 2018,Jan,8; 2017,Jan,8; 2016,Jan,13; 2015,Jan,16

94644 **Continuous inhalation treatment with aerosol medication for acute airway obstruction; first hour**

EXCLUDES *Services less than one hour (94640)*

1.51 1.51 FUD XXX Q1 80

AMA: 2019,Mar,10; 2018,Feb,11; 2018,Jan,8; 2017,Jan,8; 2016,Jan,13; 2015,Sep,9; 2015,Jan,16

\+ **94645** **each additional hour (List separately in addition to code for primary procedure)**

Code first initial hour (94644)

0.47 0.47 FUD XXX N 80

AMA: 2019,Mar,10; 2018,Feb,11; 2018,Jan,8; 2017,Jan,8; 2016,Jan,13; 2015,Sep,9; 2015,Jan,16

94660 **Continuous positive airway pressure ventilation (CPAP), initiation and management**

1.09 1.81 FUD XXX Q1 80

AMA: 2019,Aug,8; 2019,Mar,10; 2018,Feb,11; 2018,Jan,8; 2017,Jan,8; 2016,Jan,13; 2015,Jan,16

94662 **Continuous negative pressure ventilation (CNP), initiation and management**

1.03 1.03 FUD XXX Q3 80

AMA: 2019,Aug,8; 2019,Mar,10; 2018,Feb,11; 2018,Jan,8; 2017,Jan,8; 2016,Jan,13; 2015,Jan,16

94664 **Demonstration and/or evaluation of patient utilization of an aerosol generator, nebulizer, metered dose inhaler or IPPB device**

INCLUDES Reporting only one time per day

0.48 0.48 FUD XXX Q1 80

AMA: 2019,Mar,10; 2018,Feb,11; 2018,Jan,8; 2017,Jan,8; 2016,Jan,13; 2015,Jan,16

94667 **Manipulation chest wall, such as cupping, percussing, and vibration to facilitate lung function; initial demonstration and/or evaluation**

0.71 0.71 FUD XXX Q1 80

AMA: 2019,Mar,10; 2018,Feb,11; 2018,Jan,8; 2017,Jan,8; 2016,Jan,13; 2015,Sep,9; 2015,Jan,16

94668 **subsequent**

0.92 0.92 FUD XXX Q1 80

AMA: 2019,Mar,10; 2018,Feb,11; 2018,Jan,8; 2017,Jan,8; 2016,Jan,13; 2015,Sep,9; 2015,Jan,16

94669 **Mechanical chest wall oscillation to facilitate lung function, per session**

INCLUDES Application external wrap or vest to provide mechanical oscillation

0.90 0.90 FUD XXX Q1 80

AMA: 2019,Mar,10; 2018,Feb,11; 2018,Jan,8; 2017,Jan,8; 2016,Jan,13; 2015,Jan,16

94680 **Oxygen uptake, expired gas analysis; rest and exercise, direct, simple**

EXCLUDES *Cardiopulmonary stress testing (94621)*

1.51 1.51 FUD XXX Q1 80

AMA: 2019,Mar,10; 2018,Feb,11; 2018,Jan,8; 2017,Oct,3; 2017,Jan,8; 2016,Jan,13; 2015,Jan,16

94681 **including CO2 output, percentage oxygen extracted**

EXCLUDES *Cardiopulmonary stress testing (94621)*

1.49 1.49 FUD XXX Q1 80

AMA: 2019,Mar,10; 2018,Feb,11; 2018,Jan,8; 2017,Oct,3; 2017,Jan,8; 2016,Jan,13; 2015,Jan,16

94690 **rest, indirect (separate procedure)**

EXCLUDES *Arterial puncture (36600)*
Cardiopulmonary stress testing (94621)

1.49 1.49 FUD XXX Q1 80

AMA: 2019,Mar,10; 2018,Feb,11; 2018,Jan,8; 2017,Oct,3; 2017,Jan,8; 2016,Jan,13; 2015,Jan,16

94726 **Plethysmography for determination of lung volumes and, when performed, airway resistance**

INCLUDES Airway resistance
Determination:
Functional residual capacity
Residual volume
Total lung capacity

EXCLUDES *Airway resistance by oscillometry (94728)*
Bronchial provocation (94070)
Diffusing capacity (94729)
Gas dilution or washout (94727)
Spirometry (94010, 94060)

1.52 1.52 **FUD** XXX Q1 80

AMA: 2019,Mar,10; 2018,Feb,11; 2018,Jan,8; 2017,Jan,8; 2016,Jan,13; 2015,Jan,16

94727 **Gas dilution or washout for determination of lung volumes and, when performed, distribution of ventilation and closing volumes**

INCLUDES Closing volume
Lung volume measurement
Ventilation distribution

EXCLUDES *Bronchial provocation (94070)*
Diffusing capacity (94729)
Plethysmography for lung volume/airway resistance (94726)
Spirometry (94010, 94060)

1.23 1.23 **FUD** XXX Q1 80

AMA: 2019,Mar,10; 2018,Feb,11; 2018,Jan,8; 2017,Jan,8; 2016,Jan,13; 2015,Jan,16

94728 **Airway resistance by oscillometry**

EXCLUDES *Diffusing capacity (94729)*
Gas dilution techniques
Other respiratory function services (94010, 94060, 94070, 94375, 94726)

1.15 1.15 **FUD** XXX Q1 80

AMA: 2019,Mar,10; 2018,Feb,11; 2018,Jan,8; 2017,Jan,8; 2016,Jan,13; 2015,Jan,16

+ 94729 **Diffusing capacity (eg, carbon monoxide, membrane) (List separately in addition to code for primary procedure)**

Code first (94010, 94060, 94070, 94375, 94726-94728)

1.56 1.56 **FUD** ZZZ N 80

AMA: 2019,Mar,10; 2018,Feb,11; 2018,Jan,8; 2017,Jan,8; 2016,Jan,13; 2015,Jan,16

~~94750 **Pulmonary compliance study (eg, plethysmography, volume and pressure measurements)**~~

94760 **Noninvasive ear or pulse oximetry for oxygen saturation; single determination**

EXCLUDES *Blood gases (82803-82810)*
Cardiopulmonary stress testing (94621)
Exercise test for bronchospasm (94617)
Pulmonary stress testing (94618)

0.07 0.07 **FUD** XXX N 80 TC

AMA: 2019,Aug,8; 2019,Mar,10; 2019,Jan,6; 2018,Feb,11; 2018,Jan,8; 2017,Oct,3; 2017,Jan,8; 2016,Jan,13; 2015,Jan,16

94761 **multiple determinations (eg, during exercise)**

EXCLUDES *Cardiopulmonary stress testing (94621)*
Exercise test for bronchospasm (94617, [94619])
Pulmonary stress testing (94618)

0.11 0.11 **FUD** XXX N 80 TC

AMA: 2019,Aug,8; 2019,Mar,10; 2018,Feb,11; 2018,Jan,8; 2017,Oct,3; 2017,Jan,8; 2016,Jan,13; 2015,Jan,16

94762 **by continuous overnight monitoring (separate procedure)**

0.71 0.71 **FUD** XXX Q3 80 TC

AMA: 2019,Aug,8; 2019,Mar,10; 2018,Feb,11; 2018,Jan,8; 2017,Jan,8; 2016,Jan,13; 2015,Jan,16

~~94770 **Carbon dioxide, expired gas determination by infrared analyzer**~~

94772 **Circadian respiratory pattern recording (pediatric pneumogram), 12-24 hour continuous recording, infant** A

EXCLUDES *Electromyograms/EEG/ECG/respiration recordings*

0.00 0.00 **FUD** XXX S 80

AMA: 2019,Mar,10; 2018,Feb,11; 2018,Jan,8; 2017,Jan,8; 2016,Jan,13; 2015,Jan,16

94774 **Pediatric home apnea monitoring event recording including respiratory rate, pattern and heart rate per 30-day period of time; includes monitor attachment, download of data, review, interpretation, and preparation of a report by a physician or other qualified health care professional** A

INCLUDES Oxygen saturation monitoring

EXCLUDES *Event monitors (93268-93272)*
Holter monitor (93224-93227)
Pediatric home apnea services (94775-94777)
Remote cardiovascular telemetry (93228-93229)
Sleep testing (95805-95811 [95800, 95801])

0.00 0.00 **FUD** YYY B 80

AMA: 2019,Mar,10; 2018,Feb,11; 2018,Jan,8; 2017,Jan,8; 2016,Jan,13; 2015,Jan,16

94775 **monitor attachment only (includes hook-up, initiation of recording and disconnection)** A

INCLUDES Oxygen saturation monitoring

EXCLUDES *Event monitors (93268-93272)*
Holter monitor (93224-93227)
Remote cardiovascular telemetry (93228-93229)
Sleep testing (95805-95811 [95800, 95801])

0.00 0.00 **FUD** YYY S 80 TC

AMA: 2019,Mar,10; 2018,Feb,11; 2018,Jan,8; 2017,Jan,8; 2016,Jan,13; 2015,Jan,16

94776 **monitoring, download of information, receipt of transmission(s) and analyses by computer only** A

INCLUDES Oxygen saturation monitoring

EXCLUDES *Event monitors (93268-93272)*
Holter monitor (93224-93227)
Remote cardiovascular telemetry (93228-93229)
Sleep testing (95805-95811 [95800, 95801])

0.00 0.00 **FUD** YYY S 80 TC

AMA: 2019,Mar,10; 2018,Feb,11; 2018,Jan,8; 2017,Jan,8; 2016,Jan,13; 2015,Jan,16

94777 **review, interpretation and preparation of report only by a physician or other qualified health care professional** A

INCLUDES Oxygen saturation monitoring

EXCLUDES *Event monitors (93268-93272)*
Holter monitor (93224-93227)
Remote cardiovascular telemetry (93228-93229)
Sleep testing (95805-95811 [95800, 95801])

0.00 0.00 **FUD** YYY B 80 26

AMA: 2019,Mar,10; 2018,Feb,11; 2018,Jan,8; 2017,Jan,8; 2016,Jan,13; 2015,Jan,16

94780 **Car seat/bed testing for airway integrity, for infants through 12 months of age, with continual clinical staff observation and continuous recording of pulse oximetry, heart rate and respiratory rate, with interpretation and report; 60 minutes** A

EXCLUDES *Pediatric and neonatal critical care services (99468-99476, 99477-99480)*
Pulse oximetry (94760-94761)
Reporting code for service less than 60 minutes
Rhythm strips (93040-93042)

0.68 1.45 **FUD** XXX Q1

AMA: 2019,Mar,10; 2018,Feb,11; 2018,Jan,8; 2017,Jan,8; 2016,Jan,13; 2015,May,10; 2015,Jan,16

+ **94781** **each additional full 30 minutes (List separately in addition to code for primary procedure)** A

Code first (94780)

0.24 0.57 FUD ZZZ N

AMA: 2019,Mar,10; 2018,Feb,11; 2018,Jan,8; 2017,Jan,8; 2016,Jan,13; 2015,May,10; 2015,Jan,16

94799 **Unlisted pulmonary service or procedure**

0.00 0.00 FUD XXX Q1 80

AMA: 2019,Mar,10; 2018,Sep,14; 2018,Feb,11; 2018,Jan,8; 2017,Jan,8; 2016,Jan,13; 2015,Dec,16; 2015,May,10; 2015,Jan,16

95004-95071 Allergy Tests

EXCLUDES *Drugs administered for intractable/severe allergic reaction (eg, antihistamines, epinephrine, steroids) (96372)*

E/M services when reporting test interpretation/report

Laboratory tests for allergies (86000-86999 [86152, 86153])

Code also medical conferences regarding equipment use (eg, air filters, humidifiers, dehumidifiers), climate therapy, physical, occupational, and recreation therapy using appropriate E/M codes

Code also significant, separately identifiable E/M services using modifier 25, when performed (99202-99215, 99217-99223 [99224, 99225, 99226], 99231-99233, 99241-99255, 99281-99285, 99304-99318, 99324-99337, 99341-99350, 99381-99429 [99415, 99416, 99417, 99421, 99422, 99423])

95004 **Percutaneous tests (scratch, puncture, prick) with allergenic extracts, immediate type reaction, including test interpretation and report, specify number of tests**

0.12 0.12 FUD XXX Q1 80

AMA: 2018,Feb,11; 2018,Jan,8; 2017,Jan,8; 2016,Jan,13; 2015,Jan,16

95012 **Nitric oxide expired gas determination**

0.56 0.56 FUD XXX Q1 80

AMA: 2018,Feb,11; 2018,Jan,8; 2017,Jan,8; 2016,Jan,13; 2015,Jan,16

95017 **Allergy testing, any combination of percutaneous (scratch, puncture, prick) and intracutaneous (intradermal), sequential and incremental, with venoms, immediate type reaction, including test interpretation and report, specify number of tests**

0.11 0.23 FUD XXX Q1 80

AMA: 2018,Feb,11; 2018,Jan,8; 2017,Jan,8; 2016,Jan,13; 2015,Jul,9; 2015,Jan,16

95018 **Allergy testing, any combination of percutaneous (scratch, puncture, prick) and intracutaneous (intradermal), sequential and incremental, with drugs or biologicals, immediate type reaction, including test interpretation and report, specify number of tests**

0.21 0.61 FUD XXX Q1 80

AMA: 2018,Feb,11; 2018,Jan,8; 2017,Jan,8; 2016,Jan,13; 2015,Jul,9; 2015,Jan,16

95024 **Intracutaneous (intradermal) tests with allergenic extracts, immediate type reaction, including test interpretation and report, specify number of tests**

0.03 0.23 FUD XXX Q1 80

AMA: 2018,Feb,11; 2018,Jan,8; 2017,Jan,8; 2016,Jan,13; 2015,Jan,16

95027 **Intracutaneous (intradermal) tests, sequential and incremental, with allergenic extracts for airborne allergens, immediate type reaction, including test interpretation and report, specify number of tests**

0.14 0.14 FUD XXX Q1 80

AMA: 2018,Feb,11; 2018,Jan,8; 2017,Jan,8; 2016,Jan,13; 2015,Jan,16

95028 **Intracutaneous (intradermal) tests with allergenic extracts, delayed type reaction, including reading, specify number of tests**

0.37 0.37 FUD XXX Q1 80 TC

AMA: 2018,Feb,11; 2018,Jan,8; 2017,Jan,8; 2016,Jan,13; 2015,Jan,16

95044 **Patch or application test(s) (specify number of tests)**

0.16 0.16 FUD XXX Q1 80

AMA: 2018,Feb,11; 2018,Jan,8; 2017,Jan,8; 2016,Jan,13; 2015,Jan,16

95052 **Photo patch test(s) (specify number of tests)**

0.18 0.18 FUD XXX Q1 80

AMA: 2018,Feb,11; 2018,Jan,8; 2017,Jan,8; 2016,Jan,13; 2015,Jan,16

95056 **Photo tests**

1.31 1.31 FUD XXX Q1 80

AMA: 2018,Feb,11; 2018,Jan,8; 2017,Jan,8; 2016,Jan,13; 2015,Jan,16

95060 **Ophthalmic mucous membrane tests**

0.99 0.99 FUD XXX Q1 80 TC

AMA: 2018,Feb,11; 2018,Jan,8; 2017,Jan,8; 2016,Jan,13; 2015,Jan,16

95065 **Direct nasal mucous membrane test**

0.73 0.73 FUD XXX Q1 80 TC

AMA: 2018,Feb,11; 2018,Jan,8; 2017,Jan,8; 2016,Jan,13; 2015,Jan,16

▲ **95070** **Inhalation bronchial challenge testing (not including necessary pulmonary function tests), with histamine, methacholine, or similar compounds**

EXCLUDES *Pulmonary function tests (94060, 94070)*

0.90 0.90 FUD XXX S 80 TC

AMA: 2018,Feb,11; 2018,Jan,8; 2017,Jan,8; 2016,Jan,13; 2015,Jan,16

~~**95071** **with antigens or gases, specify**~~

95076-95079 Challenge Ingestion Testing

CMS: 100-03,110.12 Challenge Ingestion Food Testing

INCLUDES Assessment and monitoring for allergic reactions (eg, blood pressure, peak flow meter)

Testing time until test ends or to point E/M service needed

EXCLUDES *Reporting code for testing time less than 61 minutes, such as positive challenge resulting in ending test (report E/M codes as appropriate)*

Code also interventions when appropriate (eg, injection of epinephrine or steroid)

95076 **Ingestion challenge test (sequential and incremental ingestion of test items, eg, food, drug or other substance); initial 120 minutes of testing**

INCLUDES First 120 minutes testing time (not face-to-face time with physician)

2.15 3.43 FUD XXX S 80

AMA: 2018,Feb,11; 2018,Jan,8; 2017,Jan,8; 2016,Jan,13; 2015,Jan,16

+ **95079** **each additional 60 minutes of testing (List separately in addition to code for primary procedure)**

INCLUDES Includes each 60 minutes additional testing time (not face-to-face time with physician)

Code first (95076)

1.97 2.42 FUD ZZZ N 80

AMA: 2018,Feb,11; 2018,Jan,8; 2017,Jan,8; 2016,Jan,13; 2015,Jan,16

95115-95199 Allergy Immunotherapy

CMS: 100-03,110.9 Antigens Prepared for Sublingual Administration

INCLUDES Allergen immunotherapy professional services

EXCLUDES *Bacterial/viral/fungal extracts skin testing (86485-86580, 95028)*
Procedures for testing: (see Pathology/Immunology section or code:) (95199)
Leukocyte histamine release (LHR)
Lymphocytic transformation test (LTT)
Mast cell degranulation test (MCDT)
Migration inhibitory factor test (MIF)
Nitroblue tetrazolium dye test (NTD)
Radioallergosorbent testing (RAST)
Rat mast cell technique (RMCT)
Transfer factor test (TFT)
Special reports for allergy patients (99080)

Code also significant separately identifiable E/M services, when performed

95115 **Professional services for allergen immunotherapy not including provision of allergenic extracts; single injection**
0.26 0.26 FUD XXX Q1 80
AMA: 2020,Sep,14; 2019,Jun,14; 2018,Feb,11; 2018,Jan,8; 2017,Jan,8; 2016,Jan,13; 2015,Jan,16

95117 **2 or more injections**
0.30 0.30 FUD XXX Q1 80
AMA: 2020,Sep,14; 2019,Jun,14; 2018,Feb,11; 2018,Jan,8; 2017,Jan,8; 2016,Jan,13; 2015,Jan,16

95120 **Professional services for allergen immunotherapy in the office or institution of the prescribing physician or other qualified health care professional, including provision of allergenic extract; single injection**
0.00 0.00 FUD XXX E
AMA: 2018,Feb,11; 2018,Jan,8; 2017,Jan,8; 2016,Jan,13; 2015,Jan,16

95125 **2 or more injections**
0.00 0.00 FUD XXX E
AMA: 2018,Feb,11; 2018,Jan,8; 2017,Jan,8; 2016,Jan,13; 2015,Jan,16

95130 **single stinging insect venom**
0.00 0.00 FUD XXX E
AMA: 2018,Feb,11; 2018,Jan,8; 2017,Jan,8; 2016,Jan,13; 2015,Jan,16

95131 **2 stinging insect venoms**
0.00 0.00 FUD XXX E
AMA: 2018,Feb,11; 2018,Jan,8; 2017,Jan,8; 2016,Jan,13; 2015,Jan,16

95132 **3 stinging insect venoms**
0.00 0.00 FUD XXX E
AMA: 2018,Feb,11; 2018,Jan,8; 2017,Jan,8; 2016,Jan,13; 2015,Jan,16

95133 **4 stinging insect venoms**
0.00 0.00 FUD XXX E
AMA: 2018,Feb,11; 2018,Jan,8; 2017,Jan,8; 2016,Jan,13; 2015,Jan,16

95134 **5 stinging insect venoms**
0.00 0.00 FUD XXX E
AMA: 2018,Feb,11; 2018,Jan,8; 2017,Jan,8; 2016,Jan,13; 2015,Jan,16

95144 **Professional services for the supervision of preparation and provision of antigens for allergen immunotherapy, single dose vial(s) (specify number of vials)**
INCLUDES Single dose vial/single dose of antigen administered in one injection
0.09 0.41 FUD XXX Q1 80
AMA: 2018,Feb,11; 2018,Jan,8; 2017,Jan,8; 2016,Jan,13; 2015,Jan,16

95145 **Professional services for the supervision of preparation and provision of antigens for allergen immunotherapy (specify number of doses); single stinging insect venom**
0.09 0.81 FUD XXX Q1 80
AMA: 2018,Feb,11; 2018,Jan,8; 2017,Jan,8; 2016,Jan,13; 2015,Jan,16

95146 **2 single stinging insect venoms**
0.09 1.50 FUD XXX Q1 80
AMA: 2018,Feb,11; 2018,Jan,8; 2017,Jan,8; 2016,Jan,13; 2015,Jan,16

95147 **3 single stinging insect venoms**
0.09 1.55 FUD XXX Q1 80
AMA: 2018,Feb,11; 2018,Jan,8; 2017,Jan,8; 2016,Jan,13; 2015,Jan,16

95148 **4 single stinging insect venoms**
0.09 2.23 FUD XXX Q1 80
AMA: 2018,Feb,11; 2018,Jan,8; 2017,Jan,8; 2016,Jan,13; 2015,Jan,16

95149 **5 single stinging insect venoms**
0.09 3.12 FUD XXX Q1 80
AMA: 2018,Feb,11; 2018,Jan,8; 2017,Jan,8; 2016,Jan,13; 2015,Jan,16

95165 **Professional services for the supervision of preparation and provision of antigens for allergen immunotherapy; single or multiple antigens (specify number of doses)**
0.09 0.40 FUD XXX Q1 80
AMA: 2018,Feb,11; 2018,Jan,8; 2017,Jan,8; 2016,Jan,13; 2015,Jan,16

95170 **whole body extract of biting insect or other arthropod (specify number of doses)**
INCLUDES Dose which is amount of antigen(s) administered in single injection from multiple dose vial
0.09 0.31 FUD XXX Q1 80
AMA: 2018,Feb,11; 2018,Jan,8; 2017,Jan,8; 2016,Jan,13; 2015,Jan,16

95180 **Rapid desensitization procedure, each hour (eg, insulin, penicillin, equine serum)**
2.96 3.92 FUD XXX Q1 80
AMA: 2019,Jun,14; 2018,Feb,11; 2018,Jan,8; 2017,Jan,8; 2016,Jan,13; 2015,Jan,16

95199 **Unlisted allergy/clinical immunologic service or procedure**
0.00 0.00 FUD XXX Q1 80
AMA: 2018,Feb,11; 2018,Jan,8; 2017,Jan,8; 2016,Jan,13; 2015,Jan,16

95249-95251 [95249] Glucose Monitoring By Subcutaneous Device

EXCLUDES *Physiologic data collection/interpretation (99091)*

Code also when data receiver owned by patient for sensor placement, hook-up, monitor calibration, training, and printout (95999)

95249 **Resequenced code. See code following 95250.**

95250 **Ambulatory continuous glucose monitoring of interstitial tissue fluid via a subcutaneous sensor for a minimum of 72 hours; physician or other qualified health care professional (office) provided equipment, sensor placement, hook-up, calibration of monitor, patient training, removal of sensor, and printout of recording**
EXCLUDES *Reporting code more than one time per month*
Subcutaneous pocket with insertion interstitial glucose monitor (0446T)
4.23 4.23 FUD XXX V 80 TC
AMA: 2019,Jan,6; 2018,Jun,6; 2018,Mar,5; 2018,Feb,11; 2018,Jan,8; 2017,Jan,8; 2016,Jan,13; 2015,Jan,16

\# **95249** **patient-provided equipment, sensor placement, hook-up, calibration of monitor, patient training, and printout of recording**
INCLUDES Performing complete collection initial data in provider's office
EXCLUDES *Reporting code more than one time during period patient owns data receiver*
Subcutaneous pocket with insertion interstitial glucose monitor (0446T)
1.54 1.54 FUD XXX S 80 TC
AMA: 2018,Jun,6; 2018,Feb,11

95251 **analysis, interpretation and report**

EXCLUDES *Reporting code more than one time per month*

1.02 1.02 **FUD** XXX B 80 26

AMA: 2018,Jun,6; 2018,Mar,5; 2018,Feb,11; 2018,Jan,8; 2017,Jan,8; 2016,Jan,13; 2015,Jan,16

95700-95783 [95700, 95705, 95706, 95707, 95708, 95709, 95710, 95711, 95712, 95713, 95714, 95715, 95716, 95717, 95718, 95719, 95720, 95721, 95722, 95723, 95724, 95725, 95726, 95782, 95783, 95800, 95801] Sleep Studies

INCLUDES Assessment sleep disorders in adults and children
Continuous and simultaneous monitoring and recording physiological sleep parameters six hours or more
Evaluation patient's response to therapies
Physician:
- Interpretation
- Recording
- Report

Portable and in-laboratory technology
Recording sessions may be:
- Attended studies that include technologist or qualified health care professional presence to respond to patient needs or technical issues at bedside
- Remote without technologist or qualified health professional presence
- Unattended without technologist or qualified health care professional presence

Testing parameters include:
- Actigraphy: Noninvasive portable device to record gross motor movements to approximate sleep and wakeful periods
- Electrooculogram (EOG): Records electrical activity associated with eye movements
- Maintenance of wakefulness test (MWT): Attended study to determine patient's ability to stay awake
- Multiple sleep latency test (MSLT): Attended study to determine patient tendency to fall asleep
- Peripheral arterial tonometry (PAT): Pulsatile volume changes in digit measured to determine activity in sympathetic nervous system for respiratory analysis
- Polysomnography: Attended continuous, simultaneous recording physiological sleep parameters for at least six hours in sleep laboratory setting that also includes four or more:
  1. Airflow-oral and/or nasal
  2. Bilateral anterior tibialis EMG
  3. Electrocardiogram (ECG)
  4. Oxyhemoglobin saturation, SpO2
  5. Respiratory effort
- Positive airway pressure (PAP): Noninvasive devices to treat sleep-related disorders
- Respiratory airflow (ventilation): Assessment air movement during inhalation and exhalation as measured by nasal pressure sensors and thermistor
- Respiratory analysis: Assessment respiration components obtained by other methods such as airflow or peripheral arterial tone
- Respiratory effort: Diaphragm and/or intercostal muscle contraction for airflow measured using transducers to estimate thoracic and abdominal motion
- Respiratory movement: Measures chest and abdomen movement during respiration
- Sleep latency: Pertains to time it takes to get to sleep
- Sleep staging: Determining separate sleep levels according to physiological measurements

Total sleep time: Determined by actigraphy and other methods

EXCLUDES *E/M services*

95700 **Resequenced code. See code following 95967.**

95705 **Resequenced code. See code following 95967.**

95706 **Resequenced code. See code following 95967.**

95707 **Resequenced code. See code following 95967.**

95708 **Resequenced code. See code following 95967.**

95709 **Resequenced code. See code following 95967.**

95710 **Resequenced code. See code following 95967.**

95711 **Resequenced code. See code following 95967.**

95712 **Resequenced code. See code following 95967.**

95713 **Resequenced code. See code following 95967.**

95714 **Resequenced code. See code following 95967.**

95715 **Resequenced code. See code following 95967.**

95716 **Resequenced code. See code following 95967.**

95717 **Resequenced code. See code following 95967.**

95718 **Resequenced code. See code following 95967.**

95719 **Resequenced code. See code following 95967.**

95720 **Resequenced code. See code following 95967.**

95721 **Resequenced code. See code following 95967.**

95722 **Resequenced code. See code following 95967.**

95723 **Resequenced code. See code following 95967.**

95724 **Resequenced code. See code following 95967.**

95725 **Resequenced code. See code following 95967.**

95726 **Resequenced code. See code following 95967.**

95782 **Resequenced code. See code following 95811.**

95783 **Resequenced code. See code following 95811.**

95800 **Resequenced code. See code following 95806.**

95801 **Resequenced code. See code following 95806.**

95803 **Actigraphy testing, recording, analysis, interpretation, and report (minimum of 72 hours to 14 consecutive days of recording)**

EXCLUDES *Reporting code more than one time in 14-day period*
Sleep studies (95806-95811 [95800, 95801])

4.22 4.22 **FUD** XXX Q1 80

AMA: 2018,Feb,11; 2018,Jan,8; 2017,Jan,8; 2016,Jan,13; 2015,Jan,16

95805 **Multiple sleep latency or maintenance of wakefulness testing, recording, analysis and interpretation of physiological measurements of sleep during multiple trials to assess sleepiness**

INCLUDES Physiological sleep parameters as measured by:
- Frontal, central, and occipital EEG leads (three leads)
- Left and right EOG
- Submental EMG lead

EXCLUDES *Polysomnography (95808-95811)*
Sleep study, not attended (95806)

Code also modifier 52 when less than four nap opportunities recorded

11.7 11.7 **FUD** XXX S 80

AMA: 2018,Feb,11; 2018,Jan,8; 2017,Jan,8; 2016,Jan,13; 2015,Jan,16

95806 **Sleep study, unattended, simultaneous recording of, heart rate, oxygen saturation, respiratory airflow, and respiratory effort (eg, thoracoabdominal movement)**

EXCLUDES *Arterial waveform analysis (93050)*
Event monitors (93268-93272)
Holter monitor (93224-93227)
Remote cardiovascular telemetry (93228-93229)
Rhythm strips (93041-93042)
Unattended sleep study with minimum heart rate, oxygen saturation, and respiratory analysis measurement ([95801])
Unattended sleep study with heart rate, oxygen saturation, respiratory analysis, and sleep time measurement ([95800])

Code also modifier 52 for fewer than six hours recording

3.90 3.90 **FUD** XXX S 80

AMA: 2018,Feb,11; 2018,Jan,8; 2017,Jan,8; 2016,Jan,13; 2015,Jan,16

\# **95800** **Sleep study, unattended, simultaneous recording; heart rate, oxygen saturation, respiratory analysis (eg, by airflow or peripheral arterial tone), and sleep time**

EXCLUDES *Actigraphy testing (95803)*
Arterial waveform analysis (93050)
Event monitors (93268-93272)
Holter monitor (93224-93227)
Remote cardiovascular telemetry (93228-93229)
Rhythm strips (93041-93042)
Unattended sleep study with heart rate, oxygen saturation, respiratory airflow and respiratory effort measurement (95806)
Unattended sleep study with minimum heart rate, oxygen saturation, and respiratory analysis measurement ([95801])

Code also modifier 52 for fewer than 6 hours recording
4.68 4.68 **FUD** XXX S 80
AMA: 2018,Feb,11; 2018,Jan,8; 2017,Jan,8; 2016,Jan,13; 2015,Jan,16

\# **95801** **minimum of heart rate, oxygen saturation, and respiratory analysis (eg, by airflow or peripheral arterial tone)**

EXCLUDES *Arterial waveform analysis (93050)*
Event monitors (93268-93272)
Holter monitor (93224-93227)
Remote cardiovascular telemetry (93228-93229)
Rhythm strips (93041-93042)
Unattended sleep study with heart rate, oxygen saturation, respiratory airflow and respiratory effort measurement (95806)
Unattended sleep study with heart rate, oxygen saturation, respiratory analysis, and sleep time measurement ([95800])

Code also modifier 52 for fewer than 6 hours recording
2.57 2.57 **FUD** XXX Q1 80
AMA: 2018,Feb,11; 2018,Jan,8; 2017,Jan,8; 2016,Jan,13; 2015,Jan,16

95807 **Sleep study, simultaneous recording of ventilation, respiratory effort, ECG or heart rate, and oxygen saturation, attended by a technologist**

EXCLUDES *Polysomnography (95808-95811)*
Sleep study, not attended (95806)

Code also modifier 52 for fewer than six hours recording
11.4 11.4 **FUD** XXX S 80
AMA: 2018,Feb,11; 2018,Jan,8; 2017,Jan,8; 2016,Jan,13; 2015,Jan,16

95808 **Polysomnography; any age, sleep staging with 1-3 additional parameters of sleep, attended by a technologist**

EXCLUDES *Sleep study, not attended (95806)*

18.4 18.4 **FUD** XXX S 80
AMA: 2018,Feb,11; 2018,Jan,8; 2017,Jan,8; 2016,Jan,13; 2015,Jan,16

95810 **age 6 years or older, sleep staging with 4 or more additional parameters of sleep, attended by a technologist** A

EXCLUDES *Sleep study, not attended (95806)*

Code also modifier 52 for fewer than six hours recording
17.2 17.2 **FUD** XXX S 80
AMA: 2018,Feb,11; 2018,Jan,8; 2017,Jan,8; 2016,Jan,13; 2015,Jan,16

95811 **age 6 years or older, sleep staging with 4 or more additional parameters of sleep, with initiation of continuous positive airway pressure therapy or bilevel ventilation, attended by a technologist** A

EXCLUDES *Sleep study, not attended (95806)*

Code also modifier 52 for fewer than six hours recording
17.9 17.9 **FUD** XXX S 80
AMA: 2018,Feb,11; 2018,Jan,8; 2017,Jan,8; 2016,Jan,13; 2015,Jan,16

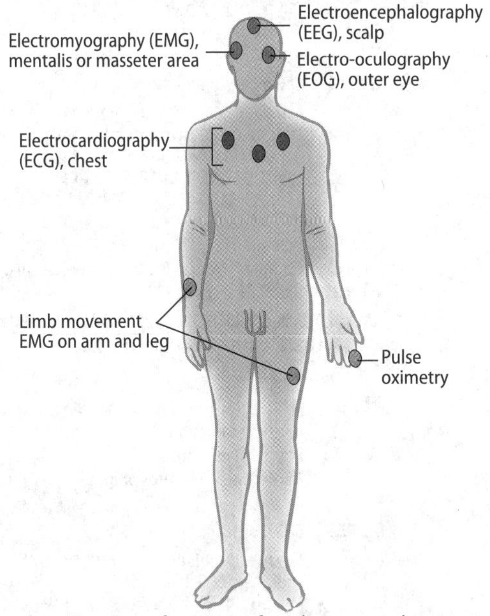

Core areas of monitoring for polysomnography

\# **95782** **younger than 6 years, sleep staging with 4 or more additional parameters of sleep, attended by a technologist** A

Code also modifier 52 for fewer than 7 hours recording
25.4 25.4 **FUD** XXX S 80
AMA: 2018,Feb,11; 2018,Jan,8; 2017,Jan,8; 2016,Jan,13; 2015,Jan,16

\# **95783** **younger than 6 years, sleep staging with 4 or more additional parameters of sleep, with initiation of continuous positive airway pressure therapy or bi-level ventilation, attended by a technologist** A

Code also modifier 52 for fewer than seven hours recording
27.1 27.1 **FUD** XXX S 80
AMA: 2018,Feb,11; 2018,Jan,8; 2017,Jan,8; 2016,Jan,13; 2015,Jan,16

95812-95830 [95829] Evaluation of Brain Activity by Electroencephalogram

INCLUDES Only time when time is recorded, data collected, and does not include set-up and take-down

EXCLUDES *E/M services*

95812 Electroencephalogram (EEG) extended monitoring; 41-60 minutes

INCLUDES Hyperventilation
Photic stimulation
Physician interpretation
Recording 41-60 minutes
Report

EXCLUDES *EEG digital analysis (95957)*
EEG during nonintracranial surgery (95955)
Long-term EEG (two hours or more) ([95700, 95705, 95706, 95707, 95708, 95709, 95710, 95711, 95712, 95713, 95714, 95715, 95716, 95717, 95718, 95719, 95720, 95721, 95722, 95723, 95724, 95725, 95726])
Wada test (95958)

Code also modifier 26 for physician interpretation only

Facility RVU 9.29 Non-Facility RVU 9.29 **FUD** XXX S 80 CCI

AMA: 2018,Dec,3; 2018,Dec,3; 2018,Feb,11; 2018,Jan,8; 2017,Jan,8; 2016,Jan,13; 2015,Jan,16

95813 61-119 minutes

INCLUDES Hyperventilation
Photic stimulation
Physician interpretation
Recording 61 minutes or more
Report

EXCLUDES *EEG digital analysis (95957)*
EEG during nonintracranial surgery (95955)
Long-term EEG (two hours or more) ([95700, 95705, 95706, 95707, 95708, 95709, 95710, 95711, 95712, 95713, 95714, 95715, 95716, 95717, 95718, 95719, 95720, 95721, 95722, 95723, 95724, 95725, 95726])
Wada test (95958)

Code also modifier 26 for physician interpretation only

Facility RVU 11.4 Non-Facility RVU 11.4 **FUD** XXX S 80 CCI

AMA: 2018,Dec,3; 2018,Dec,3; 2018,Feb,11; 2018,Jan,8; 2017,Jan,8; 2016,Jan,13; 2015,Jan,16

95816 Electroencephalogram (EEG); including recording awake and drowsy

INCLUDES Photic stimulation
Physician interpretation
Recording 20-40 minutes
Report

EXCLUDES *EEG digital analysis (95957)*
EEG during nonintracranial surgery (95955)
Long-term EEG (two hours or more) ([95700, 95705, 95706, 95707, 95708, 95709, 95710, 95711, 95712, 95713, 95714, 95715, 95716, 95717, 95718, 95719, 95720, 95721, 95722, 95723, 95724, 95725, 95726])
Wada test (95958)

Code also modifier 26 for physician interpretation only

Facility RVU 10.2 Non-Facility RVU 10.2 **FUD** XXX S 80 CCI

AMA: 2018,Dec,3; 2018,Dec,3; 2018,Feb,11; 2018,Jan,8; 2017,Jan,8; 2016,Jan,13; 2015,Dec,16; 2015,Jan,16

95819 including recording awake and asleep

INCLUDES Hyperventilation
Photic stimulation
Physician interpretation
Recording 20-40 minutes
Report

EXCLUDES *EEG digital analysis (95957)*
EEG during nonintracranial surgery (95955)
Long-term EEG (two hours or more) ([95700, 95705, 95706, 95707, 95708, 95709, 95710, 95711, 95712, 95713, 95714, 95715, 95716, 95717, 95718, 95719, 95720, 95721, 95722, 95723, 95724, 95725, 95726])
Wada test (95958)

Code also modifier 26 for interpretation only

Facility RVU 12.0 Non-Facility RVU 12.0 **FUD** XXX S 80 CCI

AMA: 2018,Dec,3; 2018,Dec,3; 2018,Feb,11; 2018,Jan,8; 2017,Jan,8; 2016,Jan,13; 2015,Dec,16; 2015,Jan,16

95822 recording in coma or sleep only

INCLUDES Hyperventilation
Photic stimulation
Physician interpretation
Recording 20-40 minutes
Report

EXCLUDES *EEG digital analysis (95957)*
EEG during nonintracranial surgery (95955)
Long-term EEG (two hours or more) ([95700, 95705, 95706, 95707, 95708, 95709, 95710, 95711, 95712, 95713, 95714, 95715, 95716, 95717, 95718, 95719, 95720, 95721, 95722, 95723, 95724, 95725, 95726])
Wada test (95958)

Code also modifier 26 for interpretation only

Facility RVU 10.9 Non-Facility RVU 10.9 **FUD** XXX S 80 CCI

AMA: 2018,Dec,3; 2018,Dec,3; 2018,Feb,11; 2018,Jan,8; 2017,Jan,8; 2016,Jan,13; 2015,Jan,16

95824 cerebral death evaluation only

INCLUDES Physician interpretation
Recording
Report

EXCLUDES *EEG digital analysis (95957)*
EEG during nonintracranial surgery (95955)
Long-term EEG (two hours or more) ([95700, 95705, 95706, 95707, 95708, 95709, 95710, 95711, 95712, 95713, 95714, 95715, 95716, 95717, 95718, 95719, 95720, 95721, 95722, 95723, 95724, 95725, 95726])
Wada test (95958)

Code also modifier 26 for physician interpretation only

Facility RVU 0.00 Non-Facility RVU 0.00 **FUD** XXX S 80 CCI

AMA: 2018,Feb,11

95829 **Resequenced code. See code following 95830.**

95830 Insertion by physician or other qualified health care professional of sphenoidal electrodes for electroencephalographic (EEG) recording

Facility RVU 2.64 Non-Facility RVU 10.9 **FUD** XXX B 80 CCI

AMA: 2018,Feb,11

95829-95836 [95829, 95836] Evaluation of Brain Activity by Electrocorticography

\# **95829 Electrocorticogram at surgery (separate procedure)**

INCLUDES EEG recording from electrodes placed in or on brain
Interpretation and review during surgical procedure

Code also modifier 26 for interpretation only

Facility RVU 52.9 Non-Facility RVU 52.9 **FUD** XXX N 80 CCI

AMA: 2018,Dec,3; 2018,Dec,3; 2018,Feb,11

95836 **Electrocorticogram from an implanted brain neurostimulator pulse generator/transmitter, including recording, with interpretation and written report, up to 30 days**

INCLUDES Intracranial recordings up to 30 days (unattended) with storage for later review

EXCLUDES *EEG digital analysis (95957)*

Programming neurostimulator during 30-day period ([95983, 95984])

Reporting code more than one time for documented 30-day period

3.19 3.19 FUD XXX 80

AMA: 2018,Dec,3; 2018,Dec,3

95836-95857 [95836] Evaluation of Muscles and Range of Motion

95836 **Resequenced code. See code following 95830.**

95851 **Range of motion measurements and report (separate procedure); each extremity (excluding hand) or each trunk section (spine)**

0.22 0.59 FUD XXX A 80

AMA: 2018,Feb,11; 2018,Jan,8; 2017,Jan,8; 2016,Dec,16; 2016,Jan,13; 2015,Jan,16

95852 **hand, with or without comparison with normal side**

0.17 0.53 FUD XXX A 80

AMA: 2018,Feb,11; 2018,Jan,8; 2017,Jan,8; 2016,Jan,13; 2015,Jan,16

95857 **Cholinesterase inhibitor challenge test for myasthenia gravis**

0.85 1.54 FUD XXX S 80

AMA: 2018,Feb,11; 2018,Jan,8; 2017,Jan,8; 2016,Jan,13; 2015,Jan,16

95860-95887 [95885, 95886, 95887] Evaluation of Nerve and Muscle Function: EMGs with/without Nerve Conduction Studies

INCLUDES Physician interpretation
Recording
Report

EXCLUDES *E/M services*

95860 **Needle electromyography; 1 extremity with or without related paraspinal areas**

INCLUDES Testing five or more muscles per extremity

EXCLUDES *Dynamic electromyography during motion analysis studies (96002-96003)*

Guidance for chemodenervation (95873-95874)

Code also modifier 26 for interpretation only

3.43 3.43 FUD XXX Q1 80

AMA: 2018,Feb,11; 2018,Jan,8; 2017,Jan,8; 2016,Jan,13; 2015,Mar,6; 2015,Jan,16

95861 **2 extremities with or without related paraspinal areas**

INCLUDES Testing five or more muscles per extremity

EXCLUDES *Dynamic electromyography during motion analysis studies (96002-96003)*

Guidance for chemodenervation (95873-95874)

Code also modifier 26 for interpretation only

4.90 4.90 FUD XXX Q1 80

AMA: 2018,Feb,11; 2018,Jan,8; 2017,Jan,8; 2016,Jan,13; 2015,Mar,6; 2015,Jan,16

95863 **3 extremities with or without related paraspinal areas**

INCLUDES Testing five or more muscles per extremity

EXCLUDES *Dynamic electromyography during motion analysis studies (96002-96003)*

Guidance for chemodenervation (95873-95874)

Code also modifier 26 for interpretation only

6.15 6.15 FUD XXX S 80

AMA: 2018,Feb,11; 2018,Jan,8; 2017,Jan,8; 2016,Jan,13; 2015,Mar,6; 2015,Jan,16

95864 **4 extremities with or without related paraspinal areas**

INCLUDES Testing five or more muscles per extremity

EXCLUDES *Dynamic electromyography during motion analysis studies (96002-96003)*

Guidance for chemodenervation (95873-95874)

Code also modifier 26 for interpretation only

7.07 7.07 FUD XXX S 80

AMA: 2018,Feb,11; 2018,Jan,8; 2017,Jan,8; 2016,Jan,13; 2015,Mar,6; 2015,Jan,16

95865 **larynx**

EXCLUDES *Dynamic electromyography during motion analysis studies (96002-96003)*

Guidance for chemodenervation (95873-95874)

Code also modifier 26 for interpretation only

Code also modifier 52 for unilateral procedure

4.34 4.34 FUD XXX Q1 80

AMA: 2018,Feb,11; 2018,Jan,8; 2017,Jan,8; 2016,Jan,13; 2015,Mar,6; 2015,Jan,16

95866 **hemidiaphragm**

EXCLUDES *Dynamic electromyography during motion analysis studies (96002-96003)*

Guidance for chemodenervation (95873-95874)

Code also modifier 26 for interpretation only

3.90 3.90 FUD XXX Q1 80

AMA: 2018,Feb,11; 2018,Jan,8; 2017,Jan,8; 2016,Jan,13; 2015,Mar,6; 2015,Jan,16

95867 **cranial nerve supplied muscle(s), unilateral**

EXCLUDES *Guidance for chemodenervation (95873-95874)*

Code also modifier 26 for interpretation only

3.05 3.05 FUD XXX S 80

AMA: 2018,Feb,11; 2018,Jan,8; 2017,Jan,8; 2016,Jan,13; 2015,Mar,6; 2015,Jan,16

95868 **cranial nerve supplied muscles, bilateral**

EXCLUDES *Guidance for chemodenervation (95873-95874)*

3.93 3.93 FUD XXX S 80

AMA: 2018,Feb,11; 2018,Jan,8; 2017,Jan,8; 2016,Jan,13; 2015,Mar,6; 2015,Jan,16

95869 **thoracic paraspinal muscles (excluding T1 or T12)**

EXCLUDES *Dynamic electromyography during motion analysis studies (96002-96003)*

Guidance for chemodenervation (95873-95874)

2.67 2.67 FUD XXX Q1 80

AMA: 2018,Feb,11; 2018,Jan,8; 2017,Jan,8; 2016,Jan,13; 2015,Mar,6; 2015,Jan,16

95870 **limited study of muscles in 1 extremity or non-limb (axial) muscles (unilateral or bilateral), other than thoracic paraspinal, cranial nerve supplied muscles, or sphincters**

INCLUDES Adson test

Testing four or less muscles per extremity

EXCLUDES *Anal/urethral sphincter/detrusor/urethra/perineum musculature (51785-51792)*

Complete study extremities (95860-95864)

Dynamic electromyography during motion analysis studies (96002-96003)

Eye muscles (92265)

Guidance for chemodenervation (95873-95874)

2.56 2.56 FUD XXX Q1 80

AMA: 2018,Feb,11; 2018,Jan,8; 2017,Jan,8; 2016,Jan,13; 2015,Mar,6; 2015,Jan,16

95872 **Needle electromyography using single fiber electrode, with quantitative measurement of jitter, blocking and/or fiber density, any/all sites of each muscle studied**

EXCLUDES *Dynamic electromyography during motion analysis studies (96002-96003)*

5.66 5.66 FUD XXX S 80

AMA: 2018,Feb,11; 2018,Jan,8; 2017,Jan,8; 2016,Jan,13; 2015,Mar,6; 2015,Jan,16

+ # **95885** **Needle electromyography, each extremity, with related paraspinal areas, when performed, done with nerve conduction, amplitude and latency/velocity study; limited (List separately in addition to code for primary procedure)**

INCLUDES Testing four or less muscles per extremity

EXCLUDES *Dynamic electromyography during motion analysis studies (96002-96003)*
Motor and sensory nerve conduction (95905)
Needle electromyography extremities (95860-95864, 95870)
Reporting code more than one time per extremity

Code also, when applicable, for combined maximum total four units per patient when all four extremities tested ([95886])

Code first nerve conduction tests (95907-95913)

1.77 1.77 **FUD** ZZZ N 80

AMA: 2018,Feb,11; 2018,Jan,8; 2017,Jul,10; 2017,Jan,8; 2016,Jan,13; 2015,Mar,6; 2015,Jan,16

+ # **95886** **complete, five or more muscles studied, innervated by three or more nerves or four or more spinal levels (List separately in addition to code for primary procedure)**

INCLUDES Testing five or more muscles per extremity

EXCLUDES *Dynamic electromyography during motion analysis studies (96002-96003)*
Motor and sensory nerve conduction (95905)
Needle electromyography extremities (95860-95864, 95870)
Reporting code more than one time per extremity

Code also, when applicable, for combined maximum total four units per patient when all four extremities tested ([95885])

Code first nerve conduction tests (95907-95913)

2.68 2.68 **FUD** ZZZ N 80

AMA: 2018,Feb,11; 2018,Jan,8; 2017,Jul,10; 2017,Jan,8; 2016,Jan,13; 2015,Mar,6; 2015,Jan,16

+ # **95887** **Needle electromyography, non-extremity (cranial nerve supplied or axial) muscle(s) done with nerve conduction, amplitude and latency/velocity study (List separately in addition to code for primary procedure)**

INCLUDES Nerve study unilateral cranial nerve innervated muscles

EXCLUDES *Dynamic electromyography during motion analysis studies (96002-96003)*
Guidance for chemodenervation (95874)
Motor and sensory nerve conduction (95905)
Needle electromyography cranial nerve supplied muscles (95867-95868)
Needle electromyography except for thoracic paraspinal, cranial nerve supplied muscles, or sphincters (95870)
Nerve study extra-ocular or laryngeal nerves
Reporting code more than once per anatomic site

Code also twice when performed bilaterally

Code first nerve conduction tests (95907-95913)

2.40 2.40 **FUD** ZZZ N 80

AMA: 2018,Feb,11; 2018,Jan,8; 2017,Jul,10; 2017,Jan,8; 2016,Jan,13; 2015,Mar,6; 2015,Jan,16

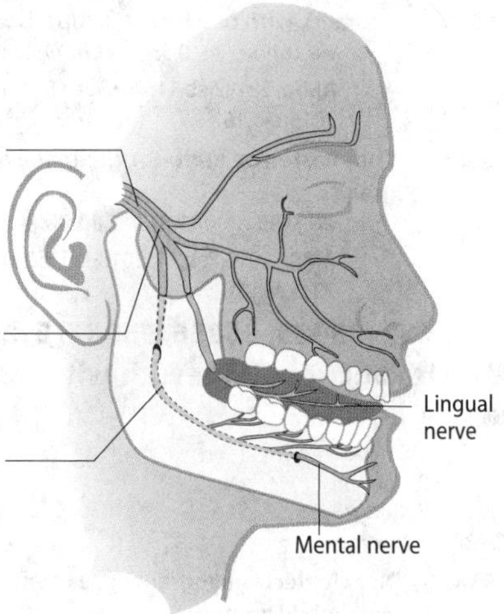

Cranial nerves: trigeminal branches of lower face and select facial nerves

Needle EMG is performed to determine conduction, amplitude, and latency/velocity

+ **95873** **Electrical stimulation for guidance in conjunction with chemodenervation (List separately in addition to code for primary procedure)**

EXCLUDES *Chemodenervation larynx (64617)*
Injection anesthetic or steroid, sacroiliac joint (64451)
Needle electromyography (95860-95870)
Needle electromyography guidance for chemodenervation (95874)
Radiofrequency ablation, sacroiliac joint ([64625])
Reporting more than one guidance code for each chemodenervation code

Code first chemodenervation (64612, 64615-64616, 64642-64647)

2.17 2.17 **FUD** ZZZ N 80

AMA: 2019,Dec,8; 2019,Apr,9; 2018,Feb,11; 2018,Jan,8; 2017,Jan,8; 2016,Jan,13; 2015,Mar,6; 2015,Jan,16

+ **95874** **Needle electromyography for guidance in conjunction with chemodenervation (List separately in addition to code for primary procedure)**

EXCLUDES *Chemodenervation larynx (64617)*
Injection anesthetic or steroid, sacroiliac joint (64451)
Needle electromyography (95860-95870)
Needle electromyography guidance for chemodenervation (95873)
Radiofrequency ablation, sacroiliac joint ([64625])
Reporting more than one guidance code for each chemodenervation code

Code first chemodenervation (64612, 64615-64616, 64642-64647)

2.23 2.23 **FUD** ZZZ N 80

AMA: 2019,Dec,8; 2019,Apr,9; 2018,Feb,11; 2018,Jan,8; 2017,Jan,8; 2016,Jan,13; 2015,Mar,6; 2015,Jan,16

95875 **Ischemic limb exercise test with serial specimen(s) acquisition for muscle(s) metabolite(s)**

3.75 3.75 **FUD** XXX S 80

AMA: 2018,Feb,11; 2018,Jan,8; 2017,Jan,8; 2016,Jan,13; 2015,Mar,6; 2015,Jan,16

95885 **Resequenced code. See code following 95872.**

95886 **Resequenced code. See code following 95872.**

95887 **Resequenced code. See code before 95873.**

95905-95913 Evaluation of Nerve Function: Nerve Conduction Studies

INCLUDES Conduction studies motor and sensory nerves
Reports from on-site examiner including interpretation results using established methodologies, calculations, comparisons to normal studies, and interpretation by physician or other qualified health care professional
Single conduction study comprising sensory and motor conduction test with/without F or H wave testing, and all orthodromic and antidromic impulses
Total number tests performed indicate appropriate code

EXCLUDES *Reporting code for more than one study when multiple sites on same nerve tested*

Code also electromyography performed with nerve conduction studies, as appropriate ([95885, 95886, 95887])

95905 **Motor and/or sensory nerve conduction, using preconfigured electrode array(s), amplitude and latency/velocity study, each limb, includes F-wave study when performed, with interpretation and report**

INCLUDES Study with preconfigured electrodes that are customized to a specific body location

EXCLUDES *Needle electromyography ([95885, 95886])*
Nerve conduction studies (95907-95913)
Reporting code more than one time for each limb studied

1.80 1.80 **FUD** XXX ⊘ 01 80

AMA: 2018,Feb,11; 2018,Jan,8; 2017,Jan,8; 2016,Jan,13; 2015,Jan,16

95907 **Nerve conduction studies; 1-2 studies**

2.71 2.71 **FUD** XXX S 80

AMA: 2018,Aug,10; 2018,Feb,11; 2018,Jan,8; 2017,Dec,14; 2017,Jan,8; 2016,Jan,13; 2015,Jan,16

95908 **3-4 studies**

3.44 3.44 **FUD** XXX S 80

AMA: 2018,Aug,10; 2018,Feb,11; 2018,Jan,8; 2017,Jan,8; 2016,Jan,13; 2015,Mar,6; 2015,Jan,16

95909 **5-6 studies**

4.20 4.20 **FUD** XXX S 80

AMA: 2018,Aug,10; 2018,Feb,11; 2018,Jan,8; 2017,Jan,8; 2016,Jan,13; 2015,Jan,16

95910 **7-8 studies**

5.42 5.42 **FUD** XXX S 80

AMA: 2018,Aug,10; 2018,Feb,11; 2018,Jan,8; 2017,Jan,8; 2016,Jan,13; 2015,Jan,16

95911 **9-10 studies**

6.49 6.49 **FUD** XXX S 80

AMA: 2018,Aug,10; 2018,Feb,11; 2018,Jan,8; 2017,Jan,8; 2016,Jan,13; 2015,Jan,16

95912 **11-12 studies**

7.43 7.43 **FUD** XXX S 80

AMA: 2018,Aug,10; 2018,Feb,11; 2018,Jan,8; 2017,Jan,8; 2016,Jan,13; 2015,Jan,16

95913 **13 or more studies**

8.60 8.60 **FUD** XXX S 80

AMA: 2018,Aug,10; 2018,Feb,11; 2018,Jan,8; 2017,Jan,8; 2016,Jan,13; 2015,Jan,16

95940-95941 [95940, 95941] Intraoperative Neurophysiological Monitoring

INCLUDES Monitoring, testing, and data evaluation during surgical procedures by monitoring professional dedicated only to performing necessary testing and monitoring
Monitoring services provided by anesthesiologist or surgeon separately

EXCLUDES *Baseline neurophysiologic monitoring*
EEG during nonintracranial surgery (95955)
Electrocorticography ([95829])
Intraoperative cortical and subcortical mapping (95961-95962)
Neurostimulator programming/analysis (95971-95972, 95976-95977, [95983, 95984])
Time required for set-up, recording, interpretation, and electrode removal

Code also baseline studies (eg, EMGs, NCVs), no more than one time per operative session
Code also services provided after midnight using date when monitoring started and total monitoring time
Code also standby time prior to procedure (99360)
Code first ([92653], 95822, 95860-95870, 95907-95913, 95925-95937 [95938, 95939])

+ # **95940** **Continuous intraoperative neurophysiology monitoring in the operating room, one on one monitoring requiring personal attendance, each 15 minutes (List separately in addition to code for primary procedure)**

INCLUDES 15 minute increments monitoring service
Based on time spent monitoring, despite number tests or parameters monitored
Continuous intraoperative neurophysiologic monitoring by dedicated monitoring professional in operating room providing one-on-one patient care
Monitoring time distinct from baseline neurophysiologic study time(s) or other services (e.g., mapping)
Monitoring time may begin prior to incision
Total all monitoring time for procedures overlapping midnight

EXCLUDES *Time spent in executing or interpreting baseline neurophysiologic study or studies*

Code also monitoring from outside operative room, when applicable ([95941])

0.93 0.93 **FUD** XXX N 80

AMA: 2018,Feb,11; 2018,Jan,8; 2017,Aug,8; 2017,Jan,8; 2016,Jan,13; 2015,Jan,16

+ # **95941** **Continuous intraoperative neurophysiology monitoring, from outside the operating room (remote or nearby) or for monitoring of more than one case while in the operating room, per hour (List separately in addition to code for primary procedure)**

INCLUDES Based on time spent monitoring, despite number tests or parameters monitored
Monitoring time distinct from baseline neurophysiologic study time(s) or other services (e.g., mapping)
One hour increments monitoring service

0.00 0.00 **FUD** XXX N

AMA: 2018,Feb,11; 2018,Jan,8; 2017,Aug,8; 2017,Jan,8; 2016,Jan,13; 2015,Jan,16

95921-95943 [95943] Evaluation of Autonomic Nervous System

INCLUDES Physician interpretation
Recording
Report
Testing for autonomic dysfunction including site and autonomic subsystems

95921 Testing of autonomic nervous system function; cardiovagal innervation (parasympathetic function), including 2 or more of the following: heart rate response to deep breathing with recorded R-R interval, Valsalva ratio, and 30:15 ratio

INCLUDES Data storage for waveform analysis
Display on monitor
Minimum two elements performed:
- Cardiovascular function indicated by 30:15 ration (R/R interval at beat 30)/(R-R interval at beat 15)
- Heart rate response to deep breathing obtained by visual quantitative recording analysis with patient taking five to six breaths per minute
- Valsalva ratio (at least two) obtained by dividing highest heart rate by lowest

Monitoring heart rate by electrocardiography; rate obtained from time between two successive R waves (R-R interval)
Testing most usually in prone position
Tilt table testing, when performed

EXCLUDES *Autonomic nervous system testing with sympathetic adrenergic function testing (95922, 95924)*
Simultaneous measures parasympathetic and sympathetic function ([95943])

2.36 2.36 **FUD** XXX S 80

AMA: 2020,Sep,7; 2018,Feb,11; 2018,Jan,8; 2017,Jan,8; 2016,Jan,13; 2015,Jan,16

95922 vasomotor adrenergic innervation (sympathetic adrenergic function), including beat-to-beat blood pressure and R-R interval changes during Valsalva maneuver and at least 5 minutes of passive tilt

EXCLUDES *Autonomic nervous system testing with parasympathetic function (95921, 95924)*
Simultaneous measures parasympathetic and sympathetic function ([95943])

2.79 2.79 **FUD** XXX Q1 80

AMA: 2020,Sep,7; 2018,Feb,11; 2018,Jan,8; 2017,Jan,8; 2016,Jan,13; 2015,Jan,16

95923 sudomotor, including 1 or more of the following: quantitative sudomotor axon reflex test (QSART), silastic sweat imprint, thermoregulatory sweat test, and changes in sympathetic skin potential

3.64 3.64 **FUD** XXX Q1 80

AMA: 2020,Sep,7; 2018,Feb,11; 2018,Jan,8; 2017,Jan,8; 2016,Jan,13; 2015,Jan,16

95924 combined parasympathetic and sympathetic adrenergic function testing with at least 5 minutes of passive tilt

INCLUDES Tilt table testing adrenergic and parasympathetic function

EXCLUDES *Autonomic nervous system testing with parasympathetic function (95921-95922)*
Simultaneous measures parasympathetic and sympathetic function ([95943])

4.25 4.25 **FUD** XXX S 80

AMA: 2020,Sep,7; 2018,Feb,11; 2018,Jan,8; 2017,Jan,8; 2016,Jan,13; 2015,Jan,16

95943 Simultaneous, independent, quantitative measures of both parasympathetic function and sympathetic function, based on time-frequency analysis of heart rate variability concurrent with time-frequency analysis of continuous respiratory activity, with mean heart rate and blood pressure measures, during rest, paced (deep) breathing, Valsalva maneuvers, and head-up postural change

EXCLUDES *Autonomic nervous system testing (95921-95922, 95924)*
Rhythm ECG (93040)

0.00 0.00 **FUD** XXX S 80

AMA: 2020,Sep,7; 2018,Feb,11; 2018,Jan,8; 2017,Jan,8; 2016,Jan,13; 2015,Jan,16

95925-95943 [95938, 95939, 95940, 95941, 95943] Neurotransmission Studies

95925 Short-latency somatosensory evoked potential study, stimulation of any/all peripheral nerves or skin sites, recording from the central nervous system; in upper limbs

EXCLUDES *Auditory evoked potentials ([92653])*
Evoked potential study both upper and lower limbs ([95938])
Evoked potential study lower limbs (95926)

3.95 3.95 **FUD** XXX S 80

AMA: 2018,Feb,11; 2018,Jan,8; 2017,Jan,8; 2016,Jan,13; 2015,Jan,16

95926 in lower limbs

EXCLUDES *Auditory evoked potentials ([92653])*
Evoked potential study both upper and lower limbs ([95938])
Evoked potential study upper limbs (95925)

3.76 3.76 **FUD** XXX S 80

AMA: 2018,Feb,11; 2018,Jan,8; 2017,Jan,8; 2016,Jan,13; 2015,Jan,16

95938 in upper and lower limbs

9.79 9.79 **FUD** XXX S 80

AMA: 2018,Feb,11; 2018,Jan,8; 2017,Jan,8; 2016,Jan,13; 2015,Jan,16

95927 in the trunk or head

EXCLUDES *Auditory evoked potentials ([92653])*

Code also modifier 52 for unilateral test

3.74 3.74 **FUD** XXX S 80

AMA: 2018,Feb,11; 2018,Jan,8; 2017,Jan,8; 2016,Jan,13; 2015,Jan,16

95928 Central motor evoked potential study (transcranial motor stimulation); upper limbs

EXCLUDES *Central motor evoked potential study lower limbs (95929)*

6.38 6.38 **FUD** XXX S 80

AMA: 2018,Feb,11; 2018,Jan,8; 2017,Jan,8; 2016,Jan,13; 2015,Jan,16

95929 lower limbs

EXCLUDES *Central motor evoked potential study upper limbs (95928)*

6.57 6.57 **FUD** XXX S 80

AMA: 2018,Feb,11; 2018,Jan,8; 2017,Jan,8; 2016,Jan,13; 2015,Jan,16

95939 in upper and lower limbs

EXCLUDES *Central motor evoked potential study either lower or upper limbs (95928-95929)*

14.5 14.5 **FUD** XXX S 80

AMA: 2018,Feb,11; 2018,Jan,8; 2017,Jan,8; 2016,Jan,13; 2015,Jan,16

95930 **Visual evoked potential (VEP) checkerboard or flash testing, central nervous system except glaucoma, with interpretation and report**

EXCLUDES *Visual acuity screening using automated visual evoked potential devices (0333T)*
Visual evoked glaucoma testing ([0464T])

1.88 1.88 FUD XXX S 80

AMA: 2018,Feb,11; 2018,Feb,3; 2018,Jan,8; 2017,Jan,8; 2016,Jan,13; 2015,Jan,16

95933 **Orbicularis oculi (blink) reflex, by electrodiagnostic testing**

2.30 2.30 FUD XXX 01 80

AMA: 2018,Feb,11; 2018,Jan,8; 2017,Jul,10; 2017,Jan,8; 2016,Jan,13; 2015,Jan,16

95937 **Neuromuscular junction testing (repetitive stimulation, paired stimuli), each nerve, any 1 method**

2.48 2.48 FUD XXX S 80

AMA: 2020,Aug,14; 2018,Feb,11; 2018,Jan,8; 2017,Jan,8; 2016,Feb,13; 2016,Jan,13; 2015,Jan,16

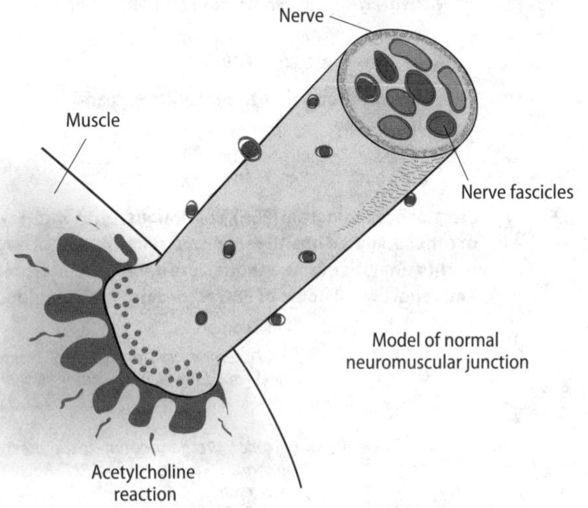

A selected neuromusular junction is repeatedly stimulated. The test is useful to demonstrate reduced muscle action potential from fatigue

95938 **Resequenced code. See code following 95926.**

95939 **Resequenced code. See code following 95929.**

95940 **Resequenced code. See code following 95913.**

95941 **Resequenced code. See code following 95913.**

95943 **Resequenced code. See code following 95924.**

95954-95962 Electroencephalography For Seizure Monitoring/Intraoperative Use

EXCLUDES *E/M services*

95954 **Pharmacological or physical activation requiring physician or other qualified health care professional attendance during EEG recording of activation phase (eg, thiopental activation test)**

11.0 11.0 FUD XXX S 80

AMA: 2018,Feb,11; 2018,Jan,8; 2017,Jan,8; 2016,Jan,13; 2015,Jan,16

95955 **Electroencephalogram (EEG) during nonintracranial surgery (eg, carotid surgery)**

5.94 5.94 FUD XXX N 80

AMA: 2018,Feb,11; 2018,Jan,8; 2017,Jan,8; 2016,Jan,13; 2015,Jan,16

95957 **Digital analysis of electroencephalogram (EEG) (eg, for epileptic spike analysis)**

EXCLUDES *Use of automated spike and seizure detection/trending software, when performed ([95700, 95705, 95706, 95707, 95708, 95709, 95710, 95711, 95712, 95713, 95714, 95715, 95716, 95717, 95718, 95719, 95720, 95721, 95722, 95723, 95724, 95725, 95726])*

7.62 7.62 FUD XXX N 80

AMA: 2018,Dec,3; 2018,Dec,3; 2018,Feb,11; 2018,Jan,8; 2017,Jan,8; 2016,Jan,13; 2015,Jan,16

95958 **Wada activation test for hemispheric function, including electroencephalographic (EEG) monitoring**

16.3 16.3 FUD XXX S 80

AMA: 2018,Feb,11

95961 **Functional cortical and subcortical mapping by stimulation and/or recording of electrodes on brain surface, or of depth electrodes, to provoke seizures or identify vital brain structures; initial hour of attendance by a physician or other qualified health care professional**

INCLUDES One hour attendance by physician or other qualified health care professional

Code also each additional hour attendance by physician or other qualified health care professional, when appropriate (95962)

Code also long-term EEG (two hours or more), when performed ([95700, 95705, 95706, 95707, 95708, 95709, 95710, 95711, 95712, 95713, 95714, 95715, 95716, 95717, 95718, 95719, 95720, 95721, 95722, 95723, 95724, 95725, 95726])

Code also modifier 52 for 30 minutes or less attendance by physician or other qualified health care professional

8.79 8.79 FUD XXX S 80

AMA: 2018,Dec,3; 2018,Dec,3; 2018,Feb,11; 2018,Jan,8; 2017,Jan,8; 2016,Jan,13; 2015,Jan,16

+ **95962** **each additional hour of attendance by a physician or other qualified health care professional (List separately in addition to code for primary procedure)**

INCLUDES One hour attendance by physician or other qualified health care professional

Code also long-term EEG (two hours or more), when performed ([95700, 95705, 95706, 95707, 95708, 95709, 95710, 95711, 95712, 95713, 95714, 95715, 95716, 95717, 95718, 95719, 95720, 95721, 95722, 95723, 95724, 95725, 95726])

Code first initial hour (95961)

7.46 7.46 FUD ZZZ N 80

AMA: 2018,Feb,11; 2018,Jan,8; 2017,Jan,8; 2016,Jan,13; 2015,Jan,16

95965-95967 Magnetoencephalography

INCLUDES Physician interpretation
Recording
Report

EXCLUDES *CT provided with magnetoencephalography (70450-70470, 70496)*
Electroencephalography provided with magnetoencephalography (95812-95824)
E/M services
MRI provided with magnetoencephalography (70551-70553)
Somatosensory evoked potentials/auditory evoked potentials/visual evoked potentials provided with magnetic evoked field responses ([92653], 95925, 95926, 95930)

95965 **Magnetoencephalography (MEG), recording and analysis; for spontaneous brain magnetic activity (eg, epileptic cerebral cortex localization)**

0.00 0.00 FUD XXX S 80

AMA: 2018,Feb,11

95966 **for evoked magnetic fields, single modality (eg, sensory, motor, language, or visual cortex localization)**

0.00 0.00 FUD XXX S 80

AMA: 2018,Feb,11

+ **95967** **for evoked magnetic fields, each additional modality (eg, sensory, motor, language, or visual cortex localization) (List separately in addition to code for primary procedure)**

Code first single modality (95966)

0.00 0.00 FUD ZZZ N 80

AMA: 2018,Feb,11

95700-95726 [95700, 95705, 95706, 95707, 95708, 95709, 95710, 95711, 95712, 95713, 95714, 95715, 95716, 95717, 95718, 95719, 95720, 95721, 95722, 95723, 95724, 95725, 95726] Electronencephalogram (EEG)

INCLUDES Automated spike and seizure detection/trending software, when performed
Determination:
Eligibility for epilepsy surgery
Location and type seizures
Differentiation seizures from other conditions
Monitoring:
Seizure treatment
Status epilepticus

EXCLUDES *Diagnostic EEG recording time less than two hours*
Routine EEG (95812-95813, 95816, 95819, 95822)

Code also cortical or subcortical mapping, when performed (95961-95962)

\# **95700** **Electroencephalogram (EEG) continuous recording, with video when performed, setup, patient education, and takedown when performed, administered in person by EEG technologist, minimum of 8 channels**

INCLUDES Technical component
EXCLUDES *EEG performed using patient-placed electrodes, performed by non-EEG technologist, or remote supervision by EEG technologist (95999)*
Reporting code more than one time each session

0.00 0.00 FUD XXX 80

\# **95705** **Electroencephalogram (EEG), without video, review of data, technical description by EEG technologist, 2-12 hours; unmonitored**

INCLUDES Technical component
EXCLUDES *Reporting code more than one time to capture complete long-term EEG session or final 2-12 hour segment past 26 hours*

0.00 0.00 FUD XXX 80

\# **95706** **with intermittent monitoring and maintenance**

INCLUDES Technical component
EXCLUDES *Reporting code more than one time to capture complete long-term EEG session or final 2-12 hour segment past 26 hours*

0.00 0.00 FUD XXX 80

\# **95707** **with continuous, real-time monitoring and maintenance**

INCLUDES Technical component
EXCLUDES *Reporting code more than one time to capture complete long-term EEG session or final 2-12 hour segment past 26 hours*

0.00 0.00 FUD XXX 80

\# **95708** **Electroencephalogram (EEG), without video, review of data, technical description by EEG technologist, each increment of 12-26 hours; unmonitored**

INCLUDES Technical component

0.00 0.00 FUD XXX 80

\# **95709** **with intermittent monitoring and maintenance**

INCLUDES Technical component

0.00 0.00 FUD XXX 80

\# **95710** **with continuous, real-time monitoring and maintenance**

INCLUDES Technical component

0.00 0.00 FUD XXX 80

\# **95711** **Electroencephalogram with video (VEEG), review of data, technical description by EEG technologist, 2-12 hours; unmonitored**

INCLUDES Technical component
EXCLUDES *Reporting code more than one time to capture complete long-term EEG session or final 2-12 hour segment past 26 hours*

0.00 0.00 FUD XXX 80

\# **95712** **with intermittent monitoring and maintenance**

INCLUDES Technical component
EXCLUDES *Reporting code more than one time to capture complete long-term EEG session or final 2-12 hour segment past 26 hours*

0.00 0.00 FUD XXX 80

\# **95713** **with continuous, real-time monitoring and maintenance**

INCLUDES Technical component
EXCLUDES *Reporting code more than one time to capture complete long-term EEG session or final 2-12 hour segment past 26 hours*

0.00 0.00 FUD XXX 80

\# **95714** **Electroencephalogram with video (VEEG), review of data, technical description by EEG technologist, each increment of 12-26 hours; unmonitored**

INCLUDES Technical component

0.00 0.00 FUD XXX 80

\# **95715** **with intermittent monitoring and maintenance**

INCLUDES Technical component

0.00 0.00 FUD XXX 80

\# **95716** **with continuous, real-time monitoring and maintenance**

INCLUDES Technical component

0.00 0.00 FUD XXX 80

\# **95717** **Electroencephalogram (EEG), continuous recording, physician or other qualified health care professional review of recorded events, analysis of spike and seizure detection, interpretation and report, 2-12 hours of EEG recording; without video**

INCLUDES Professional component
EXCLUDES *Professional interpretation for recordings greater than 36 hours and for which entire professional report generated retroactively ([95721, 95722, 95723, 95724, 95725, 95726])*
Reporting code more than one time to capture complete long-term EEG session or final 2-12 hour segment past 24 hours

2.90 2.94 FUD XXX 80

\# **95718** **with video (VEEG)**

INCLUDES Professional component
EXCLUDES *Professional interpretation for recordings greater than 36 hours and for which entire professional report generated retroactively ([95721, 95722, 95723, 95724, 95725, 95726])*
Reporting code more than one time to capture complete long-term EEG session or final 2-12 hour segment past 24 hours

3.81 3.87 FUD XXX 80

\# **95719** **Electroencephalogram (EEG), continuous recording, physician or other qualified health care professional review of recorded events, analysis of spike and seizure detection, each increment of greater than 12 hours, up to 26 hours of EEG recording, interpretation and report after each 24-hour period; without video**

INCLUDES Professional component
Single report or multiple reports during 26-hour reporting period
EXCLUDES *Professional interpretation for recordings greater than 36 hours and for which entire professional report generated retroactively ([95721, 95722, 95723, 95724, 95725, 95726])*
Reporting code more than once for multiple day studies after each 24-hour period during extended EEG recording time ([95719, 95720])
Reporting code more than one time to capture between12-26 hours

Code also EEG, 2-12 hours for studies longer than 26 hours ([95717, 95718])

4.50 4.55 FUD XXX 80

95720 with video (VEEG)

INCLUDES Professional component
Single report or multiple reports during 26-hour reporting period

EXCLUDES *Professional interpretation for recordings greater than 36 hours and for which entire professional report generated retroactively ([95721, 95722, 95723, 95724, 95725, 95726])*
Reporting code more than one time to capture between 12-26 hours
Reporting code more than once for multiple day studies after each 24-hour period during extended EEG recording time ([95719, 95720])

Code also EEG, 2-12 hours for studies longer than 26 hours ([95717, 95718])

5.90 5.99 FUD XXX 80

95721 **Electroencephalogram (EEG), continuous recording, physician or other qualified health care professional review of recorded events, analysis of spike and seizure detection, interpretation, and summary report, complete study; greater than 36 hours, up to 60 hours of EEG recording, without video**

INCLUDES Professional interpretation for recordings greater than 36 hours and for which entire professional report generated retroactively

EXCLUDES *EEG, continuous recording, less than 36 hours ([95717, 95718, 95719, 95720])*

5.92 6.04 FUD XXX 80

95722 **greater than 36 hours, up to 60 hours of EEG recording, with video (VEEG)**

INCLUDES Professional interpretation for recordings greater than 36 hours and for which entire professional report generated retroactively

EXCLUDES *EEG, continuous recording, less than 36 hours ([95717, 95718, 95719, 95720])*

7.20 7.33 FUD XXX 80

95723 **greater than 60 hours, up to 84 hours of EEG recording, without video**

INCLUDES Professional interpretation for recordings greater than 36 hours and for which entire professional report generated retroactively

EXCLUDES *EEG, continuous recording, less than 36 hours ([95717, 95718, 95719, 95720])*

7.33 7.49 FUD XXX 80

95724 **greater than 60 hours, up to 84 hours of EEG recording, with video (VEEG)**

INCLUDES Professional interpretation for recordings greater than 36 hours and for which entire professional report generated retroactively

EXCLUDES *EEG, continuous recording, less than 36 hours ([95717, 95718, 95719, 95720])*

9.18 9.36 FUD XXX 80

95725 **greater than 84 hours of EEG recording, without video**

INCLUDES Professional interpretation for recordings greater than 36 hours and for which entire professional report generated retroactively

EXCLUDES *EEG, continuous recording, less than 36 hours ([95717, 95718, 95719, 95720])*

8.34 8.55 FUD XXX 80

AMA: 2011,Jan,11; 2009,Jan,11-31

95726 **greater than 84 hours of EEG recording, with video (VEEG)**

INCLUDES Professional interpretation for recordings greater than 36 hours and for which entire professional report generated retroactively

EXCLUDES *EEG, continuous recording, less than 36 hours ([95717, 95718, 95719, 95720])*

11.6 11.8 FUD XXX 80

95970-95984 [95983, 95984] Evaluation of Implanted Neurostimulator with/without Programming

INCLUDES Documentation settings, electrode impedances system parameters before programming
Insertion electrode array(s) into target area (permanent or trial)
Multiple adjustments to parameters necessary during programming session
Neurostimulators distinguished by nervous system area stimulated:
- Brain: Deep brain stimulation or cortical stimulation (brain surface)
- Cranial nerves: Includes12 pairs cranial nerves, branches, divisions, intracranial and extracranial segments
- Spinal cord and peripheral nerves: Nerves originating in spinal cord and nerves and ganglia outside spinal cord

Parameters (vary by system) include:
- Amplitude
- Burst
- Cycling on/off
- Detection algorithms
- Dose lockout
- Frequency
- Pulse width
- Responsive neurostimulation

EXCLUDES *Implantation/replacement neurostimulator electrodes (43647, 43881, 61850-61868, 63650-63655, 64553-64581)*
Neurostimulation system, posterior tibial nerve (0587T-0590T)
Neurostimulator pulse generator/receiver:
Insertion (61885-61886, 63685, 64568, 64590)
Revision/removal (61888, 63688, 64569, 64570, 64595)
Revision/removal neurostimulator electrodes (43648, 43882, 61880, 63661-63664, 64569-64570, 64585)

95970 **Electronic analysis of implanted neurostimulator pulse generator/transmitter (eg, contact group[s], interleaving, amplitude, pulse width, frequency [Hz], on/off cycling, burst, magnet mode, dose lockout, patient selectable parameters, responsive neurostimulation, detection algorithms, closed loop parameters, and passive parameters) by physician or other qualified health care professional; with brain, cranial nerve, spinal cord, peripheral nerve, or sacral nerve, neurostimulator pulse generator/transmitter, without programming**

INCLUDES Analysis implanted neurostimulator without programming

EXCLUDES *Programming with analysis (95971-95972, 95976-95977, [95983, 95984])*

0.54 0.55 FUD XXX Q1 80

AMA: 2019,Feb,6; 2018,Oct,8; 2018,Feb,11; 2018,Jan,8; 2017,Jan,8; 2016,Jul,7; 2016,Jan,13; 2015,Jan,16

95971 **with simple spinal cord or peripheral nerve (eg, sacral nerve) neurostimulator pulse generator/transmitter programming by physician or other qualified health care professional**

EXCLUDES *Programming neurostimulator for complex spinal cord or peripheral nerve (95972)*

1.17 1.44 FUD XXX S 80

AMA: 2019,Feb,6; 2018,Oct,8; 2018,Feb,11; 2018,Jan,8; 2017,Jan,8; 2016,Jul,7; 2016,Jan,13; 2015,Jan,16

95972 **with complex spinal cord or peripheral nerve (eg, sacral nerve) neurostimulator pulse generator/transmitter programming by physician or other qualified health care professional**

1.19 1.62 FUD XXX S 80

AMA: 2019,Feb,6; 2018,Oct,8; 2018,Feb,11; 2018,Jan,8; 2017,Jan,8; 2016,Jul,7; 2016,Jan,13; 2015,Jan,16

95976 **with simple cranial nerve neurostimulator pulse generator/transmitter programming by physician or other qualified health care professional**

EXCLUDES *Programming neurostimulator for complex cranial nerve (95977)*

1.16 1.18 FUD XXX 80

AMA: 2019,Feb,6

95977 with complex cranial nerve neurostimulator pulse generator/transmitter programming by physician or other qualified health care professional
1.52 1.54 FUD XXX 80
AMA: 2019,Feb,6

95983 with brain neurostimulator pulse generator/transmitter programming, first 15 minutes face-to-face time with physician or other qualified health care professional
1.44 1.46 FUD XXX 80
AMA: 2019,Feb,6; 2018,Dec,3; 2018,Dec,3

+ # 95984 with brain neurostimulator pulse generator/transmitter programming, each additional 15 minutes face-to-face time with physician or other qualified health care professional (List separately in addition to code for primary procedure)
Code first ([95983])
1.26 1.27 FUD ZZZ 80
AMA: 2019,Feb,6; 2018,Dec,3; 2018,Dec,3

95980 Electronic analysis of implanted neurostimulator pulse generator system (eg, rate, pulse amplitude and duration, configuration of wave form, battery status, electrode selectability, output modulation, cycling, impedance and patient measurements) gastric neurostimulator pulse generator/transmitter; intraoperative, with programming
INCLUDES Gastric neurostimulator lesser curvature
EXCLUDES *Analysis, with programming when performed, vagus nerve trunk stimulator for morbid obesity (0312T, 0317T)*
1.32 1.32 FUD XXX N 80
AMA: 2018,Feb,11; 2018,Jan,8; 2017,Jan,8; 2016,Jul,7; 2016,Jan,13; 2015,Jan,16

95981 subsequent, without reprogramming
EXCLUDES *Analysis, with programming when performed, vagus nerve trunk stimulator for morbid obesity (0312T, 0317T)*
0.51 1.01 FUD XXX Q1 80
AMA: 2018,Feb,11; 2018,Jan,8; 2017,Jan,8; 2016,Jul,7; 2016,Jan,13; 2015,Jan,16

95982 subsequent, with reprogramming
EXCLUDES *Analysis, with programming when performed, vagus nerve trunk stimulator for morbid obesity (0312T, 0317T)*
1.06 1.61 FUD XXX Q1 80
AMA: 2018,Feb,11; 2018,Jan,8; 2017,Jan,8; 2016,Jul,7; 2016,Jan,13; 2015,Jan,16

95983 Resequenced code. See code following 95977.

95984 Resequenced code. See code following 95977.

95990-95991 Refill/Upkeep of Implanted Drug Delivery Pump to Central Nervous System

EXCLUDES *Analysis/reprogramming implanted pump for infusion (62367-62370)*
E/M services

95990 Refilling and maintenance of implantable pump or reservoir for drug delivery, spinal (intrathecal, epidural) or brain (intraventricular), includes electronic analysis of pump, when performed;
2.55 2.55 FUD XXX S 80
AMA: 2018,Feb,11; 2018,Jan,8; 2017,Jan,8; 2016,Jan,13; 2015,Jan,16

95991 requiring skill of a physician or other qualified health care professional
1.14 3.30 FUD XXX T 80
AMA: 2018,Feb,11; 2018,Jan,8; 2017,Jan,8; 2016,Jan,13; 2015,Jan,16

95992-95999 Other and Unlisted Neurological Procedures

95992 Canalith repositioning procedure(s) (eg, Epley maneuver, Semont maneuver), per day
EXCLUDES *Nystagmus testing (92531-92532)*
1.08 1.27 FUD XXX A 80
AMA: 2018,Feb,11; 2018,Jan,8; 2017,Jan,8; 2016,Jan,13; 2015,Jan,16

95999 Unlisted neurological or neuromuscular diagnostic procedure
0.00 0.00 FUD XXX Q1 80
AMA: 2018,Aug,10; 2018,Feb,11; 2018,Jan,8; 2017,Jan,8; 2016,Jan,13; 2015,Aug,8; 2015,Jan,16

96000-96004 Motion Analysis Studies

CMS: 100-02,15,230.4 Services By a Physical/Occupational Therapist in Private Practice

INCLUDES Services provided as part major therapeutic/diagnostic decision making
Services provided in dedicated motion analysis department with these capabilities:
3D kinetics/dynamic electromyography
Computerized 3D kinematics
Videotaping from front/back/both sides
EXCLUDES *E/M services*
Gait training (97116)
Needle electromyography (95860-95872 [95885, 95886, 95887])

96000 Comprehensive computer-based motion analysis by video-taping and 3D kinematics;
2.72 2.72 FUD XXX S 80
AMA: 2018,Feb,11; 2018,Jan,8; 2017,Jan,8; 2016,Jan,13; 2015,Jan,16

96001 with dynamic plantar pressure measurements during walking
3.65 3.65 FUD XXX S 80
AMA: 2018,Feb,11; 2018,Jan,8; 2017,Jan,8; 2016,Jan,13; 2015,Jan,16

96002 Dynamic surface electromyography, during walking or other functional activities, 1-12 muscles
0.63 0.63 FUD XXX S 80
AMA: 2018,Feb,11; 2018,Jan,8; 2017,Jan,8; 2016,Jan,13; 2015,Aug,8; 2015,Jan,16

96003 Dynamic fine wire electromyography, during walking or other functional activities, 1 muscle
0.49 0.49 FUD XXX Q1 80
AMA: 2018,Feb,11; 2018,Jan,8; 2017,Jan,8; 2016,Jan,13; 2015,Jan,16

96004 Review and interpretation by physician or other qualified health care professional of comprehensive computer-based motion analysis, dynamic plantar pressure measurements, dynamic surface electromyography during walking or other functional activities, and dynamic fine wire electromyography, with written report
3.24 3.24 FUD XXX B 80 26
AMA: 2018,Feb,11; 2018,Jan,8; 2017,Jan,8; 2016,Jan,13; 2015,Aug,8; 2015,Jan,16

96020 Neurofunctional Brain Testing

INCLUDES Selection/administration, testing:
- Cognition
- Determining validity neurofunctional testing relative to separately interpreted functional magnetic resonance images
- Functional neuroimaging
- Language
- Memory
- Monitoring performance of testing
- Movement
- Other neurological functions
- Sensation

EXCLUDES *Clinical depression treatment by repetitive transcranial magnetic stimulation (90867-90868)*
Developmental test administration (96112-96113)
E/M services on same date
MRI brain (70554-70555)
Neurobehavioral status examination (96116, 96121)
Neuropsychological testing (96132-96133)
Psychological testing (96130-96131)

96020 Neurofunctional testing selection and administration during noninvasive imaging functional brain mapping, with test administered entirely by a physician or other qualified health care professional (ie, psychologist), with review of test results and report

0.00 0.00 **FUD** XXX N 80

AMA: 2018,Feb,11; 2018,Jan,8; 2017,Jan,8; 2016,Jan,13; 2015,Jan,16

96040 Genetic Counseling Services

INCLUDES Analysis for genetic risk assessment
Counseling patient/family
Counseling services
Face-to-face interviews
Obtaining structured family genetic history
Pedigree construction
Review medical data/family information
Services provided by trained genetic counselor
Services provided during one or more sessions
Thirty minutes face-to-face time, reported one time for each 16-30 minutes service

EXCLUDES *Education/genetic counseling by physician or other qualified health care provider to group (99078)*
Education/genetic counseling by physician or other qualified health care provider to individual; report appropriate E/M code
Education regarding genetic risks by nonphysician to group (98961, 98962)
Genetic counseling and/or risk factor reduction intervention from physician or other qualified health care provider provided to patients without symptoms/diagnosis (99401-99412)
Reporting code when 15 minutes or less face-to-face time provided

96040 Medical genetics and genetic counseling services, each 30 minutes face-to-face with patient/family

1.30 1.30 **FUD** XXX ★ B

AMA: 2018,Feb,11; 2018,Jan,8; 2017,Jan,8; 2016,Jan,13; 2015,Jan,16

97151-97158 [97151, 97152, 97153, 97154, 97155, 97156, 97157, 97158] Adaptive Behavior Assessments and Treatments

INCLUDES Adaptive behavior deficits (e.g., impairment in social, communication, self care skills)
Assessment and treatment that focuses on:
- Maladaptive behaviors (e.g., repetitive movements, risk harm to self, others, property)
- Secondary functional impairment due to consequences deficient adaptive and maladaptive behaviors (e.g., communication, play, leisure, social interactions)
- Treatment determined based on goals and targets identified in assessments

\# **97151 Behavior identification assessment, administered by a physician or other qualified health care professional, each 15 minutes of the physician's or other qualified health care professional's time face-to-face with patient and/or guardian(s)/caregiver(s) administering assessments and discussing findings and recommendations, and non-face-to-face analyzing past data, scoring/interpreting the assessment, and preparing the report/treatment plan**

EXCLUDES *Health and behavior assessment and intervention (96156, 96158-96159, [96164, 96165], [96167, 96168], [96170, 96171])*
Medical team conference (99366-99368)
Neurobehavioral status examination (96116, 96121)
Neuropsychological testing (96132-96133, 96136-96139, 96146)
Psychiatric diagnostic evaluation (90791-90792)
Speech evaluations (92521-92524)

Code also more than one time on same or different days until assessment complete
Code also supporting assessment depending on time patient spends face-to-face with one or more technicians (counting only time spent by one technician) ([97152], 0362T)

0.00 0.00 **FUD** XXX 80

AMA: 2018,Nov,3

\# **97152 Behavior identification-supporting assessment, administered by one technician under the direction of a physician or other qualified health care professional, face-to-face with the patient, each 15 minutes**

EXCLUDES *Health and behavior assessment and intervention (96156, 96158-96159, [96164, 96165], [96167, 96168], [96170, 96171])*
Medical team conference (99366-99368)
Neurobehavioral status examination (96116, 96121)
Neuropsychological testing (96132-96133, 96136-96139, 96146)
Psychiatric diagnostic evaluation (90791-90792)
Speech evaluations (92521-92524)

Code also more than one time on same or different days until assessment complete
Code also supporting assessment depending on time patient spends face-to-face with one or more technicians (counting only time spent by one technician) ([97152], 0362T)

0.00 0.00 **FUD** XXX 80

AMA: 2018,Nov,3

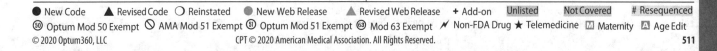

97153 Adaptive behavior treatment by protocol, administered by technician under the direction of a physician or other qualified health care professional, face-to-face with one patient, each 15 minutes

INCLUDES Face-to-face service with one patient only
Provided by technician under physician/other qualified healthcare professional direction

EXCLUDES *Aphasia and cognitive performance testing (96105, [96125])*
Behavioral/developmental screening/testing (96110-96113 [96127])
Health and behavior assessment and intervention (96156, 96158-96159, [96164, 96165], [96167, 96168], [96170, 96171])
Health risk assessment (96160-96161)
Neurobehavioral status examination (96116, 96121)
Psychiatric services (90785-90899)
Testing administration with scoring (96136-96139, 96146)
Testing evaluation (96130-96133)
Therapeutic procedure(s), individual patient (97129)
Treatment speech disorders (individual) (92507)

0.00 0.00 **FUD** XXX 80

AMA: 2020,Jul,10; 2018,Nov,3

97154 Group adaptive behavior treatment by protocol, administered by technician under the direction of a physician or other qualified health care professional, face-to-face with two or more patients, each 15 minutes

INCLUDES Face-to-face service with one patient only
Provided by technician under physician/other qualified healthcare professional direction

EXCLUDES *Aphasia and cognitive performance testing (96105, [96125])*
Behavioral/developmental screening/testing (96110-96113, [96127])
Health and behavior assessment and intervention (96156, 96158-96159, [96164, 96165], [96167, 96168], [96170, 96171])
Neurobehavioral status examination (96116, 96121)
Psychiatric services (90785-90899)
Testing administration with scoring (96136-96139, 96146)
Testing evaluation (96130-96133)
Therapeutic procedure(s) group, two or more patients (97150)
Treatment speech disorders (group) (92508)

0.00 0.00 **FUD** XXX 80

AMA: 2018,Nov,3

97155 Adaptive behavior treatment with protocol modification, administered by physician or other qualified health care professional, which may include simultaneous direction of technician, face-to-face with one patient, each 15 minutes

INCLUDES Face-to-face service with one patient only
Provided by technician under physician/other qualified healthcare professional direction

EXCLUDES *Aphasia and cognitive performance testing (96105, [96125])*
Behavioral/developmental screening/testing (96110-96113, [96127])
Health and behavior assessment and intervention (96156, 96158-96159, [96164, 96165], [96167, 96168], [96170, 96171])
Neurobehavioral status examination (96116, 96121)
Psychiatric services (90785-90899)
Testing administration with scoring (96136-96139, 96146)
Testing evaluation (96130-96133)
Therapeutic procedure(s), individual patient (97129)
Treatment speech disorders (individual) (92507)

0.00 0.00 **FUD** XXX 80

AMA: 2020,Jul,10; 2018,Nov,3

97156 Family adaptive behavior treatment guidance, administered by physician or other qualified health care professional (with or without the patient present), face-to-face with guardian(s)/caregiver(s), each 15 minutes

INCLUDES Provided by physician/other qualified healthcare professional
Without patient presence

EXCLUDES *Aphasia and cognitive performance testing (96105, [96125])*
Behavioral/developmental screening/testing (96110-96113 [96127])
Health and behavior assessment and intervention (96156, 96158-96159, [96164, 96165], [96167, 96168], [96170, 96171])
Neurobehavioral status examination (96116, 96121)
Psychiatric services (90785-90899)
Testing administration with scoring (96136-96139, 96146)
Testing evaluation (96130-96133)

0.00 0.00 **FUD** XXX 80

AMA: 2018,Nov,3

97157 Multiple-family group adaptive behavior treatment guidance, administered by physician or other qualified health care professional (without the patient present), face-to-face with multiple sets of guardians/caregivers, each 15 minutes

INCLUDES Provided by physician/other qualified healthcare professional
Without patient presence

EXCLUDES *Aphasia and cognitive performance testing (96105, [96125])*
Behavioral/developmental screening/testing (96110-96113 [96127])
Groups more than eight families
Health and behavior assessment and intervention (96156, 96158-96159, [96164, 96165], [96167, 96168], [96170, 96171])
Neurobehavioral status examination (96116, 96121)
Psychiatric services (90785-90899)
Testing administration with scoring (96136-96139, 96146)
Testing evaluation (96130-96133)

0.00 0.00 **FUD** XXX 80

AMA: 2018,Nov,3

97158 Group adaptive behavior treatment with protocol modification, administered by physician or other qualified health care professional, face-to-face with multiple patients, each 15 minutes

INCLUDES Face-to-face service with one patient only
Provided by technician under physician/other qualified healthcare professional direction

EXCLUDES *Aphasia and cognitive performance testing (96105, [96125])*
Behavioral/developmental screening/testing (96110-96113 [96127])
Groups more than eight families
Health and behavior assessment and intervention (96156, 96158-96159, [96164, 96165], [96167, 96168], [96170, 96171])
Neurobehavioral status examination (96116, 96121)
Psychiatric services (90785-90899)
Testing administration with scoring (96136-96139, 96146)
Testing evaluation (96130-96133)
Therapeutic procedure(s) group of two or more patients (97150)
Treatment speech disorders (group) (92508)

0.00 0.00 **FUD** XXX 80

AMA: 2018,Nov,3

96105-96146 [96125, 96127] Testing Services

INCLUDES Interpretation and report when performed by qualified healthcare professional
Results when automatically generated

EXCLUDES *Adaptive behavior assessments and treatments ([97151, 97152, 97153, 97154, 97155, 97156, 97157, 97158], 0362T, 0373T)*
Cognitive skills development (97129, 97533)

96105 **Assessment of aphasia (includes assessment of expressive and receptive speech and language function, language comprehension, speech production ability, reading, spelling, writing, eg, by Boston Diagnostic Aphasia Examination) with interpretation and report, per hour**

EXCLUDES *Reporting code for less than 31 minutes*
2.96 2.96 FUD XXX A 80
AMA: 2018,Nov,3; 2018,Oct,5; 2018,Feb,11; 2018,Jan,8; 2017,Jan,8; 2016,Jan,13; 2015,Aug,5; 2015,Jan,16

\# **96125** **Standardized cognitive performance testing (eg, Ross Information Processing Assessment) per hour of a qualified health care professional's time, both face-to-face time administering tests to the patient and time interpreting these test results and preparing the report**

EXCLUDES *Neuropsychological testing (96132-96139, 96146)*
3.10 3.10 FUD XXX A 80
AMA: 2018,Nov,3; 2018,Oct,5; 2018,Feb,11; 2018,Jan,8; 2017,Jan,8; 2016,Jan,13; 2015,Aug,5; 2015,Jan,16

96110 **Developmental screening (eg, developmental milestone survey, speech and language delay screen), with scoring and documentation, per standardized instrument**

EXCLUDES *Emotional/behavioral assessment ([96127])*
0.28 0.28 FUD XXX E
AMA: 2018,Nov,3; 2018,Feb,11; 2018,Jan,8; 2017,Feb,14; 2017,Jan,8; 2016,Jan,13; 2015,Aug,5; 2015,Jan,16

96112 **Developmental test administration (including assessment of fine and/or gross motor, language, cognitive level, social, memory and/or executive functions by standardized developmental instruments when performed), by physician or other qualified health care professional, with interpretation and report; first hour**

EXCLUDES *Reporting code for less than 31 minutes*
3.61 3.83 FUD XXX 80
AMA: 2018,Nov,3

\+ **96113** **each additional 30 minutes (List separately in addition to code for primary procedure)**

EXCLUDES *Reporting code for less than 16 minutes*
1.65 1.74 FUD ZZZ 80
AMA: 2018,Nov,3

\# **96127** **Brief emotional/behavioral assessment (eg, depression inventory, attention-deficit/hyperactivity disorder [ADHD] scale), with scoring and documentation, per standardized instrument**

0.15 0.15 FUD XXX Q1 80 TC
AMA: 2018,Nov,3; 2018,Oct,5; 2018,Apr,9; 2018,Feb,11; 2018,Jan,8; 2017,Feb,14; 2017,Jan,8; 2016,Jan,13; 2015,Aug,5

96116 **Neurobehavioral status exam (clinical assessment of thinking, reasoning and judgment, [eg, acquired knowledge, attention, language, memory, planning and problem solving, and visual spatial abilities]), by physician or other qualified health care professional, both face-to-face time with the patient and time interpreting test results and preparing the report; first hour**

EXCLUDES *Neuropsychological testing (96132-96139, 96146)*
Reporting code for less than 31 minutes
2.41 2.70 FUD XXX ★ 03 80
AMA: 2018,Nov,3; 2018,Oct,5; 2018,Feb,11; 2018,Jan,8; 2017,Jan,8; 2016,Jan,13; 2015,Aug,5; 2015,Jan,16

\+ **96121** **each additional hour (List separately in addition to code for primary procedure)**

EXCLUDES *Reporting code for less than 31 minutes*
Code first (96116)
2.22 2.39 FUD ZZZ 80
AMA: 2018,Nov,3

96125 **Resequenced code. See code following 96105.**

96127 **Resequenced code. See code following 96113.**

96130 **Psychological testing evaluation services by physician or other qualified health care professional, including integration of patient data, interpretation of standardized test results and clinical data, clinical decision making, treatment planning and report, and interactive feedback to the patient, family member(s) or caregiver(s), when performed; first hour**

EXCLUDES *Reporting code for less than 31 minutes*
3.08 3.38 FUD XXX 80
AMA: 2019,Dec,14; 2019,Sep,10; 2018,Nov,3

\+ **96131** **each additional hour (List separately in addition to code for primary procedure)**

EXCLUDES *Reporting code for less than 31 minutes*
2.37 2.60 FUD ZZZ 80
AMA: 2019,Dec,14; 2019,Sep,10; 2018,Nov,3

96132 **Neuropsychological testing evaluation services by physician or other qualified health care professional, including integration of patient data, interpretation of standardized test results and clinical data, clinical decision making, treatment planning and report, and interactive feedback to the patient, family member(s) or caregiver(s), when performed; first hour**

EXCLUDES *Reporting code for less than 31 minutes*
3.04 3.78 FUD XXX 80
AMA: 2019,Dec,14; 2019,Sep,10; 2018,Nov,3

\+ **96133** **each additional hour (List separately in addition to code for primary procedure)**

EXCLUDES *Reporting code for less than 16 minutes*
2.34 2.84 FUD ZZZ 80
AMA: 2019,Dec,14; 2019,Sep,10; 2018,Nov,3

96136 **Psychological or neuropsychological test administration and scoring by physician or other qualified health care professional, two or more tests, any method; first 30 minutes**

EXCLUDES *Reporting code for less than 16 minutes*
Code also testing evaluation on same or different days (96130-96133)
0.70 1.33 FUD XXX 80
AMA: 2020,Aug,3; 2019,Dec,14; 2019,Sep,10; 2018,Nov,3

\+ **96137** **each additional 30 minutes (List separately in addition to code for primary procedure)**

EXCLUDES *Reporting code for less than 16 minutes*
Code also testing evaluation on same or different days (96130-96133)
0.55 1.22 FUD ZZZ 80
AMA: 2020,Aug,3; 2019,Dec,14; 2019,Sep,10; 2018,Nov,3

96138 **Psychological or neuropsychological test administration and scoring by technician, two or more tests, any method; first 30 minutes**

EXCLUDES *Reporting code for less than 16 minutes*
Code also testing evaluation on same or different days (96130-96133)
1.07 1.07 FUD XXX 80
AMA: 2018,Nov,3

\+ **96139** **each additional 30 minutes (List separately in addition to code for primary procedure)**

EXCLUDES *Reporting code for less than 16 minutes*
Code also testing evaluation on same or different days (96130-96133)
1.07 1.07 FUD ZZZ 80
AMA: 2018,Nov,3

96146 **Psychological or neuropsychological test administration, with single automated, standardized instrument via electronic platform, with automated result only**

EXCLUDES *Testing provided by physician, other qualified healthcare professional, or technician ([96127], 96136-96139)*

0.06 0.06 FUD XXX 80

AMA: 2018,Nov,3

96156-96171 [96164, 96165, 96167, 96168, 96170, 96171] Biopsychosocial Assessment/Intervention

INCLUDES Services for patients that have primary physical illnesses/diagnoses/symptoms who may benefit from assessments/interventions that focus on biopsychosocial factors related to patient's health status

Services used to identify factors important to prevention/treatment/management physical health problems:

- Behavioral
- Cognitive
- Emotional
- Psychological
- Social

EXCLUDES *Adaptive behavior services ([97151, 97152, 97153, 97154, 97155, 97156, 97157, 97158], 0362T, 0373T)*

E/M services same date

Health and behavior assessment and intervention (96156, 96158-96159)

Preventive medicine counseling services (99401-99412)

96156 **Health behavior assessment, or re-assessment (ie, health-focused clinical interview, behavioral observations, clinical decision making)**

EXCLUDES *Psychotherapy services (90785-90899)*

2.51 2.77 FUD XXX 80

AMA: 2020,Aug,3; 2020,Jul,7

96158 **Health behavior intervention, individual, face-to-face; initial 30 minutes**

EXCLUDES *Psychotherapy services (90785-90899)*

1.71 1.89 FUD XXX 80

AMA: 2020,Aug,3; 2020,Jul,7

+ 96159 **each additional 15 minutes (List separately in addition to code for primary service)**

EXCLUDES *Psychotherapy services (90785-90899)*

Code first (96158)

0.59 0.66 FUD ZZZ 80

AMA: 2020,Aug,3; 2020,Jul,7

96164 **Health behavior intervention, group (2 or more patients), face-to-face; initial 30 minutes**

EXCLUDES *Psychotherapy services (90785-90899)*

0.25 0.28 FUD XXX 80

AMA: 2020,Aug,3; 2020,Jul,7

+ # 96165 **each additional 15 minutes (List separately in addition to code for primary service)**

EXCLUDES *Psychotherapy services (90785-90899)*

Code first ([96164])

0.11 0.13 FUD ZZZ 80

AMA: 2020,Aug,3; 2020,Jul,7

96167 **Health behavior intervention, family (with the patient present), face-to-face; initial 30 minutes**

EXCLUDES *Psychotherapy services (90785-90899)*

1.83 2.03 FUD XXX 80

AMA: 2020,Aug,3

+ # 96168 **each additional 15 minutes (List separately in addition to code for primary service)**

EXCLUDES *Psychotherapy services (90785-90899)*

Code first ([96167])

0.65 0.72 FUD ZZZ 80

AMA: 2020,Aug,3

96170 **Health behavior intervention, family (without the patient present), face-to-face; initial 30 minutes**

EXCLUDES *Psychotherapy services (90785-90899)*

2.19 2.30 FUD XXX

AMA: 2020,Aug,3

+ # 96171 **each additional 15 minutes (List separately in addition to code for primary service)**

EXCLUDES *Psychotherapy services (90785-90899)*

Code first ([96170])

0.80 0.84 FUD ZZZ

AMA: 2020,Aug,3

96160-96171 [96164, 96165, 96167, 96168, 96170, 96171] Health Risk Assessments

96160 **Administration of patient-focused health risk assessment instrument (eg, health hazard appraisal) with scoring and documentation, per standardized instrument**

0.11 0.11 FUD ZZZ S

AMA: 2020,Aug,3; 2018,Feb,11; 2018,Jan,8; 2017,Feb,14; 2017,Jan,8; 2016,Nov,5

96161 **Administration of caregiver-focused health risk assessment instrument (eg, depression inventory) for the benefit of the patient, with scoring and documentation, per standardized instrument**

0.09 0.09 FUD ZZZ S

AMA: 2020,Aug,3; 2018,Feb,11; 2018,Jan,8; 2017,Feb,14; 2017,Jan,8; 2016,Nov,5

96164 **Resequenced code. See code following 96159.**

96165 **Resequenced code. See code following 96159.**

96167 **Resequenced code. See code following 96159.**

96168 **Resequenced code. See code following 96159.**

96170 **Resequenced code. See code following 96159.**

96171 **Resequenced code. See code following 96159.**

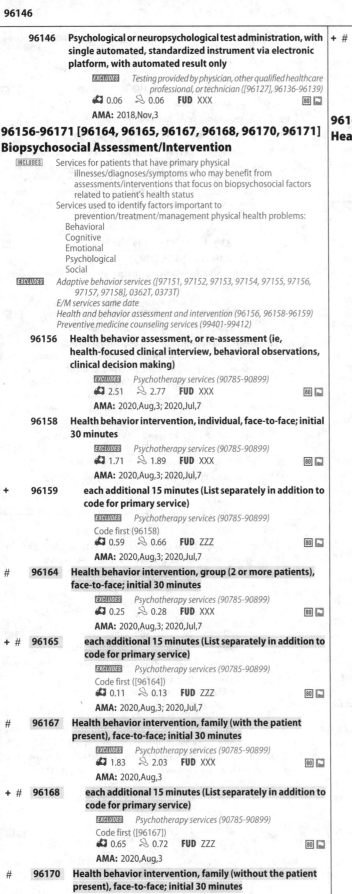

96360-96361 Intravenous Fluid Infusion for Hydration (Nonchemotherapy)

CMS: 100-04,4,230.2 OPPS Drug Administration

INCLUDES Administration prepackaged fluids and electrolytes
Coding hierarchy rules for facility reporting only:
Chemotherapy services primary to diagnostic, prophylactic, and therapeutic services
Diagnostic, prophylactic, and therapeutic services primary to hydration services
Infusions primary to pushes
Pushes primary to injections
Constant observance/attendance by person administering drug or substance
Infusion 15 minutes or less
Direct supervision by physician or other qualified health care provider:
Direction personnel
Minimal supervision for:
Consent
Safety oversight
Supervision personnel
If done to facilitate injection/infusion:
Flush at infusion end
Indwelling IV, subcutaneous catheter/port access
Local anesthesia
Start IV
Supplies/tubing/syringes
Report initial code for primary reason for visit despite order infusions or injections given
Treatment plan verification

EXCLUDES *Catheter/port declotting (36593)*
Drugs/other substances
Minimal infusion to keep vein open or during other therapeutic infusions
Reporting code for hydration infusion 31 minutes or less
Reporting code for second initial service on same date for accessing multilumen catheter, restarting IV, or when two IV lines are needed to meet infusion rate
Services provided by physicians or other qualified health care providers in facility settings
Significant separately identifiable E/M service, when performed

96360 Intravenous infusion, hydration; initial, 31 minutes to 1 hour

EXCLUDES *Reporting code when service performed as concurrent infusion*

1.07 1.07 **FUD** XXX S 80

AMA: 2019,Jun,5; 2018,Feb,11; 2018,Jan,8; 2017,Jan,8; 2016,Jan,13; 2015,Jan,16

\+ **96361 each additional hour (List separately in addition to code for primary procedure)**

INCLUDES Hydration infusion of more than 30 minutes beyond 1 hour
Hydration provided as secondary or subsequent service after different initial service via same IV access site

Code first (96360)

0.38 0.38 **FUD** ZZZ S 80

AMA: 2019,Jun,5; 2018,Feb,11; 2018,Jan,8; 2017,Jan,8; 2016,Jan,13; 2015,Jan,16

96365-96371 Infusions: Diagnostic/Preventive/Therapeutic

CMS: 100-04,4,230.2 OPPS Drug Administration

INCLUDES Administration fluid
Administration substances/drugs
Coding hierarchy rules for facility reporting:
Chemotherapy services primary to diagnostic, prophylactic, and therapeutic services
Diagnostic, prophylactic, and therapeutic services primary to hydration services
Infusions primary to pushes
Pushes primary to injections
Constant presence by health care professional administering substance/drug
Direct supervision by physician or other qualified health care provider:
Consent
Direction personnel
Patient assessment
Safety oversight
Supervision personnel
If done to facilitate injection/infusion:
Flush at infusion end
Indwelling IV, subcutaneous catheter/port access
Local anesthesia
Start IV
Supplies/tubing/syringes
Infusion 16 minutes or more
Training to assess patient and monitor vital signs
Training to prepare/dose/dispose
Treatment plan verification

EXCLUDES *Catheter/port declotting (36593)*
Services provided by physicians or other qualified health care providers in facility settings
Significant separately identifiable E/M service, when performed
Reporting code for second initial service on same date for accessing multilumen catheter, restarting IV, or when two IV lines needed to meet infusion rate
Reporting code with other procedures where IV push or infusion is integral to procedure

Code also drugs/materials

96365 Intravenous infusion, for therapy, prophylaxis, or diagnosis (specify substance or drug); initial, up to 1 hour

Code also second initial service with modifier 59 when patient's condition or drug protocol mandates use of two IV lines

2.00 2.00 **FUD** XXX S 80

AMA: 2020,Jan,11; 2018,Dec,8; 2018,Dec,8; 2018,Sep,14; 2018,May,10; 2018,Feb,11; 2018,Jan,8; 2017,Jan,8; 2016,Jan,13; 2015,Jan,16

\+ **96366 each additional hour (List separately in addition to code for primary procedure)**

INCLUDES Additional hours sequential infusion
Infusion intervals more than 30 minutes beyond one hour
Second and subsequent infusions same drug or substance

Code also additional infusion, when appropriate (96367)
Code first (96365)

0.61 0.61 **FUD** ZZZ S 80

AMA: 2020,Jan,11; 2018,Sep,14; 2018,Feb,11; 2018,Jan,8; 2017,Jan,8; 2016,Jan,13; 2015,Jan,16

\+ **96367 additional sequential infusion of a new drug/substance, up to 1 hour (List separately in addition to code for primary procedure)**

INCLUDES Secondary or subsequent service with new drug or substance after different initial service via same IV access

EXCLUDES *Reporting code more than one time per sequential infusion same mix*

Code first (96365, 96374, 96409, 96413)

0.87 0.87 **FUD** ZZZ S 80

AMA: 2020,Jan,11; 2018,Feb,11; 2018,Jan,8; 2017,Jan,8; 2016,Jan,13; 2015,Jan,16

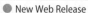

+ **96368** **concurrent infusion (List separately in addition to code for primary procedure)**

EXCLUDES *Reporting code more than one time per service date*

Code first (96365, 96366, 96413, 96415, 96416)

0.59 0.59 FUD ZZZ N 80

AMA: 2020,Jan,11; 2018,Feb,11; 2018,Jan,8; 2017,Jan,8; 2016,Jan,13; 2015,Jan,16

96369 **Subcutaneous infusion for therapy or prophylaxis (specify substance or drug); initial, up to 1 hour, including pump set-up and establishment of subcutaneous infusion site(s)**

EXCLUDES *Infusions 15 minutes or less (96372)*
Reporting code more than one time per encounter

4.69 4.69 FUD XXX S 80

AMA: 2020,Jan,11; 2018,Feb,11; 2018,Jan,8; 2017,Jan,8; 2016,Jan,13; 2015,Jan,16

+ **96370** **each additional hour (List separately in addition to code for primary procedure)**

INCLUDES Infusions more than 30 minutes beyond one hour

Code first (96369)

0.44 0.44 FUD ZZZ S 80

AMA: 2020,Jan,11; 2018,Feb,11; 2018,Jan,8; 2017,Jan,8; 2016,Jan,13; 2015,Jan,16

+ **96371** **additional pump set-up with establishment of new subcutaneous infusion site(s) (List separately in addition to code for primary procedure)**

EXCLUDES *Reporting code more than one time per encounter*

Code first (96369)

1.84 1.84 FUD ZZZ Q1 80

AMA: 2020,Jan,11; 2018,Feb,11; 2018,Jan,8; 2017,Jan,8; 2016,Jan,13; 2015,Jan,16

96372-96379 Injections: Diagnostic/Preventive/Therapeutic

CMS: 100-04,4,230.2 OPPS Drug Administration

INCLUDES Administration fluid
Administration substances/drugs
Coding hierarchy rules for facility reporting:
  Chemotherapy services primary to diagnostic, prophylactic, and therapeutic services
  Diagnostic, prophylactic, and therapeutic services primary to hydration services
  Infusions primary to pushes
  Pushes primary to injections
Constant presence by health care professional administering substance/drug
Direct supervision by physician or other qualified health care provider:
  Consent
  Direction personnel
  Patient assessment
  Safety oversight
  Supervision personnel
If done to facilitate injection/infusion:
  Flush at infusion end
  Indwelling IV, subcutaneous catheter/port access
  Local anesthesia
  Start IV
  Supplies/tubing/syringes
Infusion 15 minutes or less
Training to assess patient and monitor vital signs
Training to prepare/dose/dispose
Treatment plan verification

EXCLUDES *Catheter/port declotting (36593)*
Reporting code for second initial service on same date for accessing multilumen catheter, restarting IV, or when two IV lines needed to meet infusion rate
Reporting code with other procedures where IV push or infusion is integral to procedure
Services provided by physicians or other qualified health care providers in facility settings
Significant separately identifiable E/M service, when performed

Code also drugs/materials

96372 **Therapeutic, prophylactic, or diagnostic injection (specify substance or drug); subcutaneous or intramuscular**

INCLUDES Direct supervision by physician or other qualified health care provider when reported by physician/other qualified health care provider. When reported by hospital, physician/other qualified health care provider need not be present
Hormonal therapy injections (non-antineoplastic) (96372)

EXCLUDES *Administration vaccines/toxoids (90460-90474)*
Allergen immunotherapy injections (95115-95117)
Antineoplastic hormonal injections (96402)
Antineoplastic nonhormonal injections (96401)
Injections administered without direct supervision by physician or other qualified health care provider (99211)

0.40 0.40 FUD XXX Q1 80

AMA: 2018,Dec,10; 2018,Dec,10; 2018,Feb,11; 2018,Jan,8; 2017,Jan,8; 2016,Oct,9; 2016,Jan,13; 2015,Jan,16

96373 **intra-arterial**

0.53 0.53 FUD XXX S 80

AMA: 2018,Feb,11; 2018,Jan,8; 2017,Jan,8; 2016,Jan,13; 2015,Jan,16

96374 **intravenous push, single or initial substance/drug**

1.10 1.10 FUD XXX S 80

AMA: 2020,Jan,11; 2019,Sep,5; 2019,Jun,9; 2018,Feb,11; 2018,Jan,8; 2017,Jan,8; 2016,Jan,13; 2015,Nov,3; 2015,Jan,16

+ **96375** **each additional sequential intravenous push of a new substance/drug (List separately in addition to code for primary procedure)**

INCLUDES IV push new substance/drug provided as secondary or subsequent service after different initial service via same IV access site

Code first (96365, 96374, 96409, 96413)

0.47 0.47 FUD ZZZ S 80

AMA: 2019,Sep,5; 2018,Feb,11; 2018,Jan,8; 2017,Jan,8; 2016,Jan,13; 2015,Nov,3; 2015,Jan,16

\+ **96376** **each additional sequential intravenous push of the same substance/drug provided in a facility (List separately in addition to code for primary procedure)**

INCLUDES Facilities only

EXCLUDES *IV push performed within 30 minutes push same substance or drug*

Services performed by any nonfacilty provider

Code first (96365, 96374, 96409, 96413)

0.00 0.00 **FUD** ZZZ N

AMA: 2018,Dec,8; 2018,Dec,8; 2018,Feb,11; 2018,Jan,8; 2017,Jan,8; 2016,Jan,13; 2015,Jan,16

96377 **Application of on-body injector (includes cannula insertion) for timed subcutaneous injection**

0.56 0.56 **FUD** XXX Q1 80

AMA: 2018,Feb,11; 2018,Jan,8; 2017,Jan,8; 2016,Oct,9

96379 **Unlisted therapeutic, prophylactic, or diagnostic intravenous or intra-arterial injection or infusion**

0.00 0.00 **FUD** XXX Q1 80

AMA: 2018,Feb,11; 2018,Jan,8; 2017,Jan,8; 2016,Jan,13; 2015,Jan,16

96401-96411 Chemotherapy and Other Complex Drugs, Biologicals: Injection and IV Push

CMS: 100-03,110.2 Certain Drugs Distributed by the National Cancer Institute; 100-03,110.6 Scalp Hypothermia During Chemotherapy, to Prevent Hair Loss; 100-04,4,230.2 OPPS Drug Administration

INCLUDES Highly complex services that require direct supervision for:
- Consent
- Patient assessment
- Safety oversight
- Supervision

More intense work and monitoring clinical staff by physician or other qualified health care provider due to greater risk severe patient reactions

Parenteral administration:
- Anti-neoplastic agents for noncancer diagnoses
- Monoclonal antibody agents
- Nonradionuclide antineoplastic drugs
- Other biologic response modifiers

EXCLUDES *Reporting code for second initial service on same date for accessing multilumen catheter, restarting IV, or when two IV lines needed to meet infusion rate*

96401 **Chemotherapy administration, subcutaneous or intramuscular; non-hormonal anti-neoplastic**

EXCLUDES *Services performed by physicians or other qualified health care providers in facility settings*

2.22 2.22 **FUD** XXX Q1 80

AMA: 2018,Feb,11; 2018,Jan,8; 2017,Jan,8; 2016,Jan,13; 2015,Jan,16

96402 **hormonal anti-neoplastic**

EXCLUDES *Services performed by physicians or other qualified health care providers in facility settings*

0.87 0.87 **FUD** XXX Q1 80

AMA: 2018,Feb,11; 2018,Jan,8; 2017,Jan,8; 2016,Jan,13; 2015,Jan,16

96405 **Chemotherapy administration; intralesional, up to and including 7 lesions**

0.84 2.31 **FUD** 000 Q1

AMA: 2018,Feb,11; 2018,Jan,8; 2017,Jan,8; 2016,Jan,13; 2015,Jan,16

96406 **intralesional, more than 7 lesions**

1.31 3.46 **FUD** 000 S

AMA: 2018,Feb,11; 2018,Jan,8; 2017,Jan,8; 2016,Jan,13; 2015,Jan,16

96409 **intravenous, push technique, single or initial substance/drug**

INCLUDES Push technique includes:
- Administration injection directly into vessel or access line by health care professional; or
- Infusion less than or equal to 15 minutes

EXCLUDES *Insertion arterial and venous cannula(s) for extracorpororeal circulation (36823)*

Services performed by physicians or other qualified health care providers in facility settings

3.05 3.05 **FUD** XXX S 80

AMA: 2018,Feb,11; 2018,Jan,8; 2017,Jan,8; 2016,Jan,13; 2015,Jan,16

\+ **96411** **intravenous, push technique, each additional substance/drug (List separately in addition to code for primary procedure)**

INCLUDES Push technique includes:
- Administration injection directly into vessel or access line by health care professional; or
- Infusion less than or equal to 15 minutes

EXCLUDES *Insertion arterial and venous cannula(s) for extracorpororeal circulation (36823)*

Services performed by physicians or other qualified health care providers in facility settings

Code first initial substance/drug (96409, 96413)

1.65 1.65 **FUD** ZZZ S 80

AMA: 2018,Feb,11; 2018,Jan,8; 2017,Jan,8; 2016,Jan,13; 2015,Jan,16

96413-96417 Chemotherapy and Complex Drugs, Biologicals: Intravenous Infusion

CMS: 100-03,110.2 Certain Drugs Distributed by the National Cancer Institute; 100-03,110.6 Scalp Hypothermia During Chemotherapy, to Prevent Hair Loss; 100-04,4,230.2 OPPS Drug Administration

INCLUDES Administration:
- Access to IV/catheter/port
- Drug preparation
- Flushing at infusion completion
- Hydration fluid
- Local anesthesia
- Routine tubing/syringe/supplies
- Starting IV

Highly complex services that require direct supervision for:
- Consent
- Patient assessment
- Safety oversight
- Supervision

More intense work and monitoring clinical staff by physician or other qualified health care provider due to greater risk severe patient reactions

Parenteral administration:
- Antineoplastic agents for noncancer diagnoses
- Monoclonal antibody agents
- Nonradionuclide antineoplastic drugs
- Other biologic response modifiers

EXCLUDES *Administration nonchemotherapy agents such as antibiotics/steroids/analgesics*
Declotting catheter/port (36593)
Home infusion (99601-99602)
Insertion arterial and venous cannula(s) for extracorpororeal circulation (36823)
Reporting code for second initial service on same date for accessing multilumen catheter, restarting IV, or when two IV lines needed to meet infusion rate
Services provided by physicians or other qualified health care providers in facility settings

Code also drug or substance
Code also significant separately identifiable E/M service, when performed

96413 Chemotherapy administration, intravenous infusion technique; up to 1 hour, single or initial substance/drug

INCLUDES Push technique includes:
- Administration injection directly into vessel or access line by health care professional; or
- Infusion less than or equal to 15 minutes

EXCLUDES *Hydration administered as secondary or subsequent service via same IV access site (96361)*
Therapeutic/prophylactic/diagnostic drug infusion/injection through the same intravenous access (96366, 96367, 96375)

Code also second initial service with modifier 59 when patient's condition or drug protocol mandates use of two IV lines

3.97 3.97 **FUD** XXX S 80

AMA: 2018,Feb,11; 2018,Jan,8; 2017,Jan,8; 2016,Jan,13; 2015,Jan,16

\+ **96415 each additional hour (List separately in addition to code for primary procedure)**

INCLUDES Infusion intervals more than 30 minutes past 1-hour increments

Code first initial hour (96413)

0.86 0.86 **FUD** ZZZ S 80

AMA: 2018,Feb,11; 2018,Jan,8; 2017,Jan,8; 2016,Jan,13; 2015,Jan,16

96416 initiation of prolonged chemotherapy infusion (more than 8 hours), requiring use of a portable or implantable pump

EXCLUDES *Portable or implantable infusion pump/reservoir refilling/maintenance for drug delivery (96521-96523)*

3.98 3.98 **FUD** XXX S 80

AMA: 2018,Feb,11; 2018,Jan,8; 2017,Jan,8; 2016,Jan,13; 2015,Jan,16

\+ **96417 each additional sequential infusion (different substance/drug), up to 1 hour (List separately in addition to code for primary procedure)**

INCLUDES Push technique includes:
- Administration injection directly into vessel or access line by health care professional; or
- Infusion less than or equal to 15 minutes

EXCLUDES *Additional hour(s) sequential infusion (96415)*
Reporting code more than one time per sequential infusion

Code first initial substance/drug (96413)

1.92 1.92 **FUD** ZZZ S 80

AMA: 2018,Feb,11; 2018,Jan,8; 2017,Jan,8; 2016,Jan,13; 2015,Jan,16

96420-96425 Chemotherapy and Complex Drugs, Biologicals: Intra-arterial

CMS: 100-03,110.2 Certain Drugs Distributed by the National Cancer Institute; 100-03,110.6 Scalp Hypothermia During Chemotherapy, to Prevent Hair Loss; 100-04,4,230.2 OPPS Drug Administration

INCLUDES Administration:
- Access to IV/catheter/port
- Drug preparation
- Flushing at infusion completion
- Hydration fluid
- Local anesthesia
- Routine tubing/syringe/supplies
- Starting IV

Highly complex services that require direct supervision for:
- Consent
- Patient assessment
- Safety oversight
- Supervision

More intense work and monitoring clinical staff by physician or other qualified health care provider due to greater risk severe patient reactions

Parenteral administration:
- Antineoplastic agents for noncancer diagnoses
- Monoclonal antibody agents
- Nonradionuclide antineoplastic drugs
- Other biologic response modifiers

EXCLUDES *Administration nonchemotherapy agents such as antibiotics/steroids/analgesics*
Declotting catheter/port (36593)
Home infusion (99601-99602)
Reporting code for second initial service on same date for accessing multilumen catheter, restarting IV, or when two IV lines needed to meet an infusion rate
Services provided by physicians or other qualified health care providers in facility settings

Code also drug or substance
Code also significant separately identifiable E/M service, when performed

96420 Chemotherapy administration, intra-arterial; push technique

INCLUDES Push technique includes:
- Administration injection directly into vessel or access line by health care professional; or
- Infusion less than or equal to 15 minutes

Regional chemotherapy perfusion

EXCLUDES *Insertion arterial and venous cannula(s) for extracorpororeal circulation (36823)*
Placement intra-arterial catheter

2.95 2.95 **FUD** XXX S 80

AMA: 2018,Feb,11; 2018,Jan,8; 2017,Jan,8; 2016,Mar,3; 2016,Jan,13; 2015,Nov,3; 2015,Jan,16

96422 infusion technique, up to 1 hour

INCLUDES Push technique includes:
- Administration injection directly into vessel or access line by health care professional; or
- Infusion less than or equal to 15 minutes

Regional chemotherapy perfusion

EXCLUDES *Insertion arterial and venous cannula(s) for extracorpororeal circulation (36823)*
Placement intra-arterial catheter

4.85 4.85 **FUD** XXX S 80

AMA: 2018,Feb,11; 2018,Jan,8; 2017,Jan,8; 2016,Mar,3; 2016,Jan,13; 2015,Nov,3; 2015,Jan,16

+ **96423** **infusion technique, each additional hour (List separately in addition to code for primary procedure)**

INCLUDES Infusion intervals more than 30 minutes past 1-hour increments
Regional chemotherapy perfusion

EXCLUDES *Insertion arterial and venous cannula(s) for extracorpororeal circulation (36823)*
Placement intra-arterial catheter

Code first initial hour (96422)

2.24 2.24 **FUD** ZZZ S 80

AMA: 2018,Feb,11; 2018,Jan,8; 2017,Jan,8; 2016,Mar,3; 2016,Jan,13; 2015,Nov,3; 2015,Jan,16

96425 **infusion technique, initiation of prolonged infusion (more than 8 hours), requiring the use of a portable or implantable pump**

INCLUDES Regional chemotherapy perfusion

EXCLUDES *Insertion arterial and venous cannula(s) for extracorpororeal circulation (36823)*
Placement intra-arterial catheter
Portable or implantable infusion pump/reservoir refilling/maintenance for drug delivery (96521-96523)

5.14 5.14 **FUD** XXX S 80

AMA: 2018,Feb,11; 2018,Jan,8; 2017,Jan,8; 2016,Mar,3; 2016,Jan,13; 2015,Nov,3; 2015,Jan,16

96440-96450 Chemotherapy Administration: Intrathecal/Peritoneal Cavity/Pleural Cavity

CMS: 100-03,110.2 Certain Drugs Distributed by the National Cancer Institute; 100-04,4,230.2 OPPS Drug Administration

96440 **Chemotherapy administration into pleural cavity, requiring and including thoracentesis**

3.57 23.6 **FUD** 000 S 80

AMA: 2018,Feb,11; 2018,Jan,8; 2017,Jan,8; 2016,Jan,13; 2015,Jan,16

96446 **Chemotherapy administration into the peritoneal cavity via indwelling port or catheter**

0.79 5.78 **FUD** XXX S 80

AMA: 2018,Feb,11; 2018,Jan,8; 2017,Jan,8; 2016,Jan,13; 2015,Jan,16

96450 **Chemotherapy administration, into CNS (eg, intrathecal), requiring and including spinal puncture**

EXCLUDES *Chemotherapy administration, intravesical/bladder (51720)*
Fluoroscopy (77003)
Insertion catheter/reservoir:
Intraventricular (61210, 61215)
Subarachnoid (62350-62351, 62360-62362)

2.27 5.13 **FUD** 000 S 80

AMA: 2018,Feb,11; 2018,Jan,8; 2017,Jan,8; 2016,Jan,13; 2015,Jan,16

96521-96523 Refill/Upkeep of Drug Delivery Device

CMS: 100-04,4,230.2 OPPS Drug Administration

INCLUDES Administration:
- Access to IV/catheter/port
- Drug preparation
- Flushing at infusion completion
- Hydration fluid
- Local anesthesia
- Routine tubing/syringe/supplies
- Starting IV

Highly complex services that require direct supervision for:
- Consent
- Patient assessment
- Safety oversight
- Supervision

Parenteral administration:
- Antineoplastic agents for noncancer diagnoses
- Monoclonal antibody agents
- Nonradionuclide antineoplastic drugs
- Other biologic response modifiers

Therapeutic drugs other than chemotherapy

EXCLUDES *Administration nonchemotherapy agents such as antibiotics/steroids/analgesics*
Blood specimen collection from completely implantable venous access device (36591)
Declotting catheter/port (36593)
Home infusion (99601-99602)
Services provided by physicians or other qualified health care providers in facility settings

Code also drug or substance
Code also significant separately identifiable E/M service, when performed

96521 **Refilling and maintenance of portable pump**

4.13 4.13 **FUD** XXX S 80

AMA: 2018,Feb,11; 2018,Jan,8; 2017,Jan,8; 2016,Jan,13; 2015,Jan,16

96522 **Refilling and maintenance of implantable pump or reservoir for drug delivery, systemic (eg, intravenous, intra-arterial)**

EXCLUDES *Implantable infusion pump refilling/maintenance for spinal/brain drug delivery (95990-95991)*

3.45 3.45 **FUD** XXX S 80

AMA: 2018,Feb,11; 2018,Jan,8; 2017,Jan,8; 2016,Jan,13; 2015,Jan,16

96523 **Irrigation of implanted venous access device for drug delivery systems**

EXCLUDES *Direct supervision by physician or other qualified health care provider in facility settings*
Reporting code with any other services on same service date

0.77 0.77 **FUD** XXX Q1 80

AMA: 2018,Feb,11; 2018,Jan,8; 2017,Jan,8; 2016,Jan,13; 2015,Jan,16

96542-96549 Chemotherapy Injection Into Brain

CMS: 100-04,4,230.2 OPPS Drug Administration

INCLUDES Administration:
- Access to IV/catheter/port
- Drug preparation
- Flushing at infusion completion
- Hydration fluid
- Local anesthesia
- Routine tubing/syringe/supplies
- Starting IV

Highly complex services that require direct supervision for:
- Consent
- Patient assessment
- Safety oversight
- Supervision

Parenteral administration:
- Antineoplastic agents for noncancer diagnoses
- Monoclonal antibody agents
- Nonradionuclide antineoplastic drugs
- Other biologic response modifiers

EXCLUDES *Administration nonchemotherapy agents such as antibiotics/steroids/analgesics*
Blood specimen collection from completely implantable venous access device (36591)
Declotting catheter/port (36593)
Home infusion (99601-99602)

Code also drug or substance
Code also significant separately identifiable E/M service, when performed

96542 Chemotherapy injection, subarachnoid or intraventricular via subcutaneous reservoir, single or multiple agents

EXCLUDES *Oral radioactive isotope therapy (79005)*

1.19 3.77 **FUD** XXX S 80

AMA: 2018,Feb,11; 2018,Jan,8; 2017,Jan,8; 2016,Jan,13; 2015,Jan,16

96549 Unlisted chemotherapy procedure

0.00 0.00 **FUD** XXX Q1 80

AMA: 2018,Feb,11; 2018,Jan,8; 2017,Jan,8; 2016,Jan,13; 2015,Jan,16

96567-96574 Destruction of Lesions: Photodynamic Therapy

EXCLUDES *Ocular photodynamic therapy (67221)*

96567 Photodynamic therapy by external application of light to destroy premalignant lesions of the skin and adjacent mucosa with application and illumination/activation of photosensitive drug(s), per day

INCLUDES Services provided without direct participation by physician or other qualified healthcare professional

3.50 3.50 **FUD** XXX Q1 80

AMA: 2018,Jul,14; 2018,Feb,10; 2018,Feb,11; 2018,Jan,8; 2017,Jan,8; 2016,Jan,13; 2015,Jan,16

\+ **96570 Photodynamic therapy by endoscopic application of light to ablate abnormal tissue via activation of photosensitive drug(s); first 30 minutes (List separately in addition to code for endoscopy or bronchoscopy procedures of lung and gastrointestinal tract)**

Code also for 38-52 minutes (96571)
Code also modifier 52 when services with report less than 23 minutes
Code first (31641, 43229)

1.48 1.48 **FUD** ZZZ N

AMA: 2018,Feb,11; 2018,Jan,8; 2017,Jan,8; 2016,Jan,13; 2015,Jan,16

\+ **96571 each additional 15 minutes (List separately in addition to code for endoscopy or bronchoscopy procedures of lung and gastrointestinal tract)**

EXCLUDES *23-37 minutes service (96570)*

Code first (96570)
Code first when appropriate (31641, 43229)

0.83 0.83 **FUD** ZZZ N

AMA: 2018,Feb,11; 2018,Jan,8; 2017,Jan,8; 2016,Jan,13; 2015,Jan,16

96573 Photodynamic therapy by external application of light to destroy premalignant lesions of the skin and adjacent mucosa with application and illumination/activation of photosensitizing drug(s) provided by a physician or other qualified health care professional, per day

INCLUDES Application photosensitizer to lesions at anatomical site
Debridement, when performed
Light to activate photosensitizer for destruction premalignant lesions

EXCLUDES *Debridement lesion with photodynamic therapy provided by physician or other qualified healthcare professional (96574)*
Photodynamic therapy by external application light to same anatomical site (96567)
Services provided to same area on same date as photodynamic therapy:
- *Biopsy (11102-11107)*
- *Debridement (11000-11001, 11004-11005)*
- *Excision lesion (11400-11471)*
- *Shaving lesion (11300-11313)*

6.03 6.03 **FUD** 000 Q1 80

AMA: 2018,Jul,14; 2018,Feb,11; 2018,Feb,10

96574 Debridement of premalignant hyperkeratotic lesion(s) (ie, targeted curettage, abrasion) followed with photodynamic therapy by external application of light to destroy premalignant lesions of the skin and adjacent mucosa with application and illumination/activation of photosensitizing drug(s) provided by a physician or other qualified health care professional, per day

INCLUDES Application photosensitizer to lesions at anatomical site
Debridement, when performed
Light to activate photosensitizer for destruction premalignant lesions

EXCLUDES *Photodynamic therapy by external application light for destruction premalignant lesions (96573)*
Photodynamic therapy by external application light to same anatomical site (96567)
Services provided to same area on same as photodynamic therapy:
- *Biopsy (11102-11107)*
- *Debridement (11000-11001, 11004-11005)*
- *Excision lesion (11400-11471)*
- *Shaving lesion (11300-11313)*

7.25 7.25 **FUD** 000 Q1 80

AMA: 2018,Feb,10; 2018,Feb,11

96900-96999 Diagnostic/Therapeutic Skin Procedures

EXCLUDES *E/M services*
Injection, intralesional (11900-11901)

96900 Actinotherapy (ultraviolet light)

EXCLUDES *Rhinophototherapy (30999)*

(88160-88161)

0.61 0.61 **FUD** XXX Q1 80

AMA: 2018,Feb,11; 2018,Jan,8; 2017,Jan,8; 2016,Nov,9; 2016,Sep,3; 2016,Jan,13; 2015,Jan,16

96902 Microscopic examination of hairs plucked or clipped by the examiner (excluding hair collected by the patient) to determine telogen and anagen counts, or structural hair shaft abnormality

(88160-88161)

0.59 0.62 **FUD** XXX N

AMA: 2018,Feb,11

96904 Whole body integumentary photography, for monitoring of high risk patients with dysplastic nevus syndrome or a history of dysplastic nevi, or patients with a personal or familial history of melanoma

(88160-88161)

1.82 1.82 **FUD** XXX N 80

AMA: 2018,Feb,11

96910 **Photochemotherapy; tar and ultraviolet B (Goeckerman treatment) or petrolatum and ultraviolet B**
(88160-88161)
3.28 3.28 FUD XXX Q1 80
AMA: 2018,Feb,11; 2018,Jan,8; 2017,Jan,8; 2016,Sep,3; 2016,Jan,13; 2015,Jan,16

96912 **psoralens and ultraviolet A (PUVA)**
(88160-88161)
2.80 2.80 FUD XXX Q1 80
AMA: 2018,Feb,11; 2018,Jan,8; 2017,Jan,8; 2016,Sep,3; 2016,Jan,13; 2015,Jan,16

96913 **Photochemotherapy (Goeckerman and/or PUVA) for severe photoresponsive dermatoses requiring at least 4-8 hours of care under direct supervision of the physician (includes application of medication and dressings)**
(88160-88161)
4.06 4.06 FUD XXX T 80
AMA: 2018,Feb,11; 2018,Jan,8; 2017,Jan,8; 2016,Sep,3

96920 **Laser treatment for inflammatory skin disease (psoriasis); total area less than 250 sq cm**
EXCLUDES *Destruction by laser:*
Benign lesions (17110-17111)
Cutaneous vascular proliferative lesions (17106-17108)
Malignant lesions (17260-17286)
Premalignant lesions (17000-17004)
(88160-88161)
1.90 4.64 FUD 000 Q1
AMA: 2020,Jul,13; 2018,Feb,11; 2018,Jan,8; 2017,Jan,8; 2016,Sep,3; 2016,Jan,13; 2015,Jan,16

96921 **250 sq cm to 500 sq cm**
EXCLUDES *Destruction by laser:*
Benign lesions (17110-17111)
Cutaneous vascular proliferative lesions (17106-17108)
Malignant lesions (17260-17286)
Premalignant lesions (17000-17004)
(88160-88161)
2.14 5.09 FUD 000 Q1
AMA: 2020,Jul,13; 2018,Feb,11; 2018,Jan,8; 2017,Jan,8; 2016,Sep,3; 2016,Jan,13; 2015,Jan,16

96922 **over 500 sq cm**
EXCLUDES *Destruction by laser:*
Benign lesions (17110-17111)
Cutaneous vascular proliferative lesions (17106-17108)
Malignant lesions (17260-17286)
Premalignant lesions (17000-17004)
(88160-88161)
3.43 6.91 FUD 000 Q1
AMA: 2020,Jul,13; 2018,Feb,11; 2018,Jan,8; 2017,Jan,8; 2016,Sep,3; 2016,Jan,13; 2015,Jan,16

96931 **Reflectance confocal microscopy (RCM) for cellular and sub-cellular imaging of skin; image acquisition and interpretation and report, first lesion**
EXCLUDES *Optical coherence tomography for skin imaging (0470T-0471T)*
Reflectance confocal microscopy examination without generated mosaic images (96999)
4.78 4.78 FUD XXX M 80
AMA: 2018,Feb,11; 2018,Jan,8; 2017,Sep,9

96932 **image acquisition only, first lesion**
EXCLUDES *Optical coherence tomography for skin imaging (0470T-0471T)*
Reflectance confocal microscopy examination without generated mosaic images (96999)
3.47 3.47 FUD XXX Q1 80 TC
AMA: 2018,Feb,11; 2018,Jan,8; 2017,Sep,9

96933 **interpretation and report only, first lesion**
EXCLUDES *Optical coherence tomography for skin imaging (0470T-0471T)*
Reflectance confocal microscopy examination without generated mosaic images (96999)
1.32 1.32 FUD XXX B 80 26
AMA: 2018,Feb,11; 2018,Jan,8; 2017,Sep,9

\+ **96934** **image acquisition and interpretation and report, each additional lesion (List separately in addition to code for primary procedure)**
EXCLUDES *Optical coherence tomography for skin imaging (0470T-0471T)*
Reflectance confocal microscopy examination without generated mosaic images (96999)
Code first (96931)
2.10 2.10 FUD ZZZ N 80
AMA: 2018,Feb,11; 2018,Jan,8; 2017,Sep,9

\+ **96935** **image acquisition only, each additional lesion (List separately in addition to code for primary procedure)**
EXCLUDES *Optical coherence tomography for skin imaging (0470T-0471T)*
Reflectance confocal microscopy examination without generated mosaic images (96999)
Code first (96932)
0.99 0.99 FUD ZZZ N 80 TC
AMA: 2018,Feb,11; 2018,Jan,8; 2017,Sep,9

\+ **96936** **interpretation and report only, each additional lesion (List separately in addition to code for primary procedure)**
EXCLUDES *Optical coherence tomography for skin imaging (0470T-0471T)*
Reflectance confocal microscopy examination without generated mosaic images (96999)
Code first (96933)
1.11 1.11 FUD ZZZ N 80 26
AMA: 2018,Feb,11; 2018,Jan,8; 2017,Sep,9

96999 **Unlisted special dermatological service or procedure**
0.00 0.00 FUD XXX Q1 80
AMA: 2020,Jul,13; 2018,Feb,11; 2018,Jan,8; 2017,Sep,9; 2017,Jan,8; 2016,Sep,3; 2016,Jan,13; 2015,Jan,16

97161-97164 [97161, 97162, 97163, 97164] Assessment: Physical Therapy

CMS: 100-02,15,220 Coverage of Outpatient Rehabilitation Therapy Services; 100-02,15,220.4 Functional Reporting; 100-02,15,230 Practice of Physical Therapy, Occupational Therapy, and Speech-Language Pathology; 100-02,15,230.1 Practice of Physical Therapy; 100-02,15,230.4 Services By a Physical/Occupational Therapist in Private Practice; 100-04,5,10.3.2 Therapy Cap Exceptions; 100-04,5,10.3.3 Use of the KX Modifier; 100-04,5,10.6 Functional Reporting; 100-04,5,20.2 Reporting Units of Service

INCLUDES Care plan creation
Evaluation body systems as defined in 1997 E/M documentation guidelines:
Cardiovascular system: Vital signs, edema extremities
Integumentary system: Inspection for skin abnormalities
Mental status: Orientation, judgment, thought processes
Musculoskeletal system: Evaluation gait and station, motion range, muscle strength, height, and weight
Neuromuscular evaluation: Balance, abnormal movements

EXCLUDES *Biofeedback traning via EMG (90901)*
Joint motion range (95851-95852)
Transcutaneous nerve stimulation (TENS) (97014, 97032)

\# **97161** **Physical therapy evaluation: low complexity, requiring these components: A history with no personal factors and/or comorbidities that impact the plan of care; An examination of body system(s) using standardized tests and measures addressing 1-2 elements from any of the following: body structures and functions, activity limitations, and/or participation restrictions; A clinical presentation with stable and/or uncomplicated characteristics; and Clinical decision making of low complexity using standardized patient assessment instrument and/or measurable assessment of functional outcome. Typically, 20 minutes are spent face-to-face with the patient and/or family.**
2.38 2.38 FUD XXX 51 A 80
AMA: 2018,May,5; 2018,Feb,11; 2018,Jan,8; 2017,Aug,3; 2017,Jun,6; 2017,Jan,8

\# **97162** **Physical therapy evaluation: moderate complexity, requiring these components: A history of present problem with 1-2 personal factors and/or comorbidities that impact the plan of care; An examination of body systems using standardized tests and measures in addressing a total of 3 or more elements from any of the following: body structures and functions, activity limitations, and/or participation restrictions; An evolving clinical presentation with changing characteristics; and Clinical decision making of moderate complexity using standardized patient assessment instrument and/or measurable assessment of functional outcome. Typically, 30 minutes are spent face-to-face with the patient and/or family.**

2.38 2.38 **FUD** XXX (51) A 80

AMA: 2018,May,5; 2018,Feb,11; 2018,Jan,8; 2017,Aug,3; 2017,Jun,6; 2017,Jan,8

\# **97163** **Physical therapy evaluation: high complexity, requiring these components: A history of present problem with 3 or more personal factors and/or comorbidities that impact the plan of care; An examination of body systems using standardized tests and measures addressing a total of 4 or more elements from any of the following: body structures and functions, activity limitations, and/or participation restrictions; A clinical presentation with unstable and unpredictable characteristics; and Clinical decision making of high complexity using standardized patient assessment instrument and/or measurable assessment of functional outcome. Typically, 45 minutes are spent face-to-face with the patient and/or family.**

2.40 2.40 **FUD** XXX (51) A 80

AMA: 2018,May,5; 2018,Feb,11; 2018,Jan,8; 2017,Aug,3; 2017,Jun,6; 2017,Jan,8

\# **97164** **Re-evaluation of physical therapy established plan of care, requiring these components: An examination including a review of history and use of standardized tests and measures is required; and Revised plan of care using a standardized patient assessment instrument and/or measurable assessment of functional outcome Typically, 20 minutes are spent face-to-face with the patient and/or family.**

1.63 1.63 **FUD** XXX (51) A 80

AMA: 2018,May,5; 2018,Feb,11; 2018,Jan,8; 2017,Aug,3; 2017,Jun,6; 2017,Jan,8

97165-97168 [97165, 97166, 97167, 97168] Assessment: Occupational Therapy

CMS: 100-02,15,220 Coverage of Outpatient Rehabilitation Therapy Services; 100-02,15,220.4 Functional Reporting; 100-02,15,230 Practice of Physical Therapy, Occupational Therapy, and Speech-Language Pathology; 100-02,15,230.1 Practice of Physical Therapy; 100-02,15,230.2 Practice of Occupational Therapy; 100-02,15,230.4 Services By a Physical/Occupational Therapist in Private Practice; 100-04,5,10.3.2 Exceptions Process; 100-04,5,10.3.3 Use of the KX Modifier; 100-04,5,10.6 Functional Reporting; 100-04,5,20.2 Reporting Units of Service

INCLUDES Care plan creation
Evaluations as appropriate
Medical history
Occupational status
Past therapy history

\# **97165** **Occupational therapy evaluation, low complexity, requiring these components: An occupational profile and medical and therapy history, which includes a brief history including review of medical and/or therapy records relating to the presenting problem; An assessment(s) that identifies 1-3 performance deficits (ie, relating to physical, cognitive, or psychosocial skills) that result in activity limitations and/or participation restrictions; and Clinical decision making of low complexity, which includes an analysis of the occupational profile, analysis of data from problem-focused assessment(s), and consideration of a limited number of treatment options. Patient presents with no comorbidities that affect occupational performance. Modification of tasks or assistance (eg, physical or verbal) with assessment(s) is not necessary to enable completion of evaluation component. Typically, 30 minutes are spent face-to-face with the patient and/or family.**

2.57 2.57 **FUD** XXX (51) A 80

AMA: 2018,May,5; 2018,Feb,11; 2018,Jan,8; 2017,Jun,6; 2017,Feb,3; 2017,Jan,8

\# **97166** **Occupational therapy evaluation, moderate complexity, requiring these components: An occupational profile and medical and therapy history, which includes an expanded review of medical and/or therapy records and additional review of physical, cognitive, or psychosocial history related to current functional performance; An assessment(s) that identifies 3-5 performance deficits (ie, relating to physical, cognitive, or psychosocial skills) that result in activity limitations and/or participation restrictions; and Clinical decision making of moderate analytic complexity, which includes an analysis of the occupational profile, analysis of data from detailed assessment(s), and consideration of several treatment options. Patient may present with comorbidities that affect occupational performance. Minimal to moderate modification of tasks or assistance (eg, physical or verbal) with assessment(s) is necessary to enable patient to complete evaluation component. Typically, 45 minutes are spent face-to-face with the patient and/or family.**

2.58 2.58 **FUD** XXX (51) A 80

AMA: 2018,May,5; 2018,Feb,11; 2018,Jan,8; 2017,Jun,6; 2017,Feb,3; 2017,Jan,8

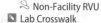

97167 Occupational therapy evaluation, high complexity, requiring these components: An occupational profile and medical and therapy history, which includes review of medical and/or therapy records and extensive additional review of physical, cognitive, or psychosocial history related to current functional performance; An assessment(s) that identifies 5 or more performance deficits (ie, relating to physical, cognitive, or psychosocial skills) that result in activity limitations and/or participation restrictions; and Clinical decision making of high analytic complexity, which includes an analysis of the patient profile, analysis of data from comprehensive assessment(s), and consideration of multiple treatment options. Patient presents with comorbidities that affect occupational performance. Significant modification of tasks or assistance (eg, physical or verbal) with assessment(s) is necessary to enable patient to complete evaluation component. Typically, 60 minutes are spent face-to-face with the patient and/or family.

2.57 2.57 FUD XXX ⑤① A 80

AMA: 2018,May,5; 2018,Feb,11; 2018,Jan,8; 2017,Jun,6; 2017,Feb,3; 2017,Jan,8

97168 Re-evaluation of occupational therapy established plan of care, requiring these components: An assessment of changes in patient functional or medical status with revised plan of care; An update to the initial occupational profile to reflect changes in condition or environment that affect future interventions and/or goals; and A revised plan of care. A formal reevaluation is performed when there is a documented change in functional status or a significant change to the plan of care is required. Typically, 30 minutes are spent face-to-face with the patient and/or family.

1.75 1.75 FUD XXX ⑤① A 80

AMA: 2018,May,5; 2018,Feb,11; 2018,Jan,8; 2017,Jun,6; 2017,Feb,3; 2017,Jan,8

97169-97172 [97169, 97170, 97171, 97172] Assessment: Athletic Training

CMS: 100-02,15,220 Coverage of Outpatient Rehabilitation Therapy Services; 100-02,15,230 Practice of Physical Therapy, Occupational Therapy, and Speech-Language Pathology; 100-02,15,230.1 Practice of Physical Therapy

INCLUDES Care plan creation
Evaluation body systems as defined in 1997 E/M documentation guidelines:
Cardiovascular system: Vital signs, edema extremities
Integumentary system: Inspection for skin abnormalities
Musculoskeletal system: Evaluation gait and station, motion range, muscle strength, height, and weight
Neuromuscular evaluation: Balance, abnormal movements

97169 Athletic training evaluation, low complexity, requiring these components: A history and physical activity profile with no comorbidities that affect physical activity; An examination of affected body area and other symptomatic or related systems addressing 1-2 elements from any of the following: body structures, physical activity, and/or participation deficiencies; and Clinical decision making of low complexity using standardized patient assessment instrument and/or measurable assessment of functional outcome. Typically, 15 minutes are spent face-to-face with the patient and/or family.

0.00 0.00 FUD XXX ⑤① E

AMA: 2018,May,5; 2018,Feb,11; 2018,Jan,8; 2017,Jun,6; 2017,Jan,8

97170 Athletic training evaluation, moderate complexity, requiring these components: A medical history and physical activity profile with 1-2 comorbidities that affect physical activity; An examination of affected body area and other symptomatic or related systems addressing a total of 3 or more elements from any of the following: body structures, physical activity, and/or participation deficiencies; and Clinical decision making of moderate complexity using standardized patient assessment instrument and/or measurable assessment of functional outcome. Typically, 30 minutes are spent face-to-face with the patient and/or family.

0.00 0.00 FUD XXX ⑤① E

AMA: 2018,May,5; 2018,Feb,11; 2018,Jan,8; 2017,Jun,6; 2017,Jan,8

97171 Athletic training evaluation, high complexity, requiring these components: A medical history and physical activity profile, with 3 or more comorbidities that affect physical activity; A comprehensive examination of body systems using standardized tests and measures addressing a total of 4 or more elements from any of the following: body structures, physical activity, and/or participation deficiencies; Clinical presentation with unstable and unpredictable characteristics; and Clinical decision making of high complexity using standardized patient assessment instrument and/or measurable assessment of functional outcome. Typically, 45 minutes are spent face-to-face with the patient and/or family.

0.00 0.00 FUD XXX ⑤① E

AMA: 2018,May,5; 2018,Feb,11; 2018,Jan,8; 2017,Jun,6; 2017,Jan,8

97172 Re-evaluation of athletic training established plan of care requiring these components: An assessment of patient's current functional status when there is a documented change; and A revised plan of care using a standardized patient assessment instrument and/or measurable assessment of functional outcome with an update in management options, goals, and interventions. Typically, 20 minutes are spent face-to-face with the patient and/or family.

0.00 0.00 FUD XXX ⑤① E

AMA: 2018,May,5; 2018,Feb,11; 2018,Jan,8; 2017,Jun,6; 2017,Jan,8

97010-97028 Physical Therapy Treatment Modalities: Supervised

CMS: 100-02,15,220 Coverage of Outpatient Rehabilitation Therapy Services; 100-02,15,220.4 Functional Reporting; 100-02,15,230 Practice of Physical Therapy, Occupational Therapy, and Speech-Language Pathology; 100-02,15,230.1 Practice of Physical Therapy; 100-02,15,230.2 Practice of Occupational Therapy; 100-02,15,230.4 Services By a Physical/Occupational Therapist in Private Practice; 100-03,10.3 Inpatient Pain Rehabilitation Programs; 100-03,10.4 Outpatient Hospital Pain Rehabilitation Programs; 100-03,160.17 Payment for L-Dopa /Associated Inpatient Hospital Services; 100-04,5,10 Part B Outpatient Rehabilitation and Comprehensive Outpatient Rehabilitation Facility (CORF) Services - General; 100-04,5,10.3.2 Exceptions Process; 100-04,5,10.3.3 Use of the KX Modifier; 100-04,5,20.2 Reporting Units of Service

INCLUDES Adding incremental treatment time intervals for same visit to calculate total service time

EXCLUDES *Direct patient contact by provider*
Electromyography (95860-95872 [95885, 95886, 95887])
EMG biofeedback training (90901)
Muscle and motion range tests ([97161, 97162, 97163, 97164, 97165, 97166, 97167, 97168, 97169, 97170, 97171, 97172])
Nerve conduction studies (95905-95913)

97010 **Application of a modality to 1 or more areas; hot or cold packs**

0.18 0.18 FUD XXX ⑤① A

AMA: 2018,May,5; 2018,Feb,11; 2018,Jan,8; 2017,Jan,8; 2016,Jun,8; 2016,Jan,13; 2015,Jan,16

97012 **traction, mechanical**

0.42 0.42 FUD XXX ⑤① A 80

AMA: 2020,Jul,13; 2018,May,5; 2018,Feb,11; 2018,Jan,8; 2017,Jan,8; 2016,Jun,8; 2016,Jan,13; 2015,Jan,16

97014 **electrical stimulation (unattended)**

[EXCLUDES] *Acupuncture with electrical stimulation (97813, 97814)*

🏥 0.42 ⚕ 0.42 **FUD** XXX [51] [E] ⚑

AMA: 2019,Jul,10; 2018,Oct,11; 2018,Oct,8; 2018,May,5; 2018,Feb,11; 2018,Jan,8; 2017,Jan,8; 2016,Jan,13; 2015,Jan,16

97016 **vasopneumatic devices**

🏥 0.36 ⚕ 0.36 **FUD** XXX [51] [A] [80] ⚑

AMA: 2018,May,5; 2018,Feb,11; 2018,Jan,8; 2017,Jan,8; 2016,Jan,13; 2015,Jan,16

97018 **paraffin bath**

🏥 0.20 ⚕ 0.20 **FUD** XXX [51] [A] [80] ⚑

AMA: 2018,May,5; 2018,Feb,11; 2018,Jan,8; 2017,Jan,8; 2016,Jan,13; 2015,Jan,16

97022 **whirlpool**

🏥 0.51 ⚕ 0.51 **FUD** XXX [51] [A] [80] ⚑

AMA: 2018,May,5; 2018,Feb,11; 2018,Jan,8; 2017,Jan,8; 2016,Jan,13; 2015,Jan,16

97024 **diathermy (eg, microwave)**

🏥 0.20 ⚕ 0.20 **FUD** XXX [51] [A] [80] ⚑

AMA: 2018,May,5; 2018,Feb,11; 2018,Jan,8; 2017,Jan,8; 2016,Jan,13; 2015,Jan,16

97026 **infrared**

🏥 0.18 ⚕ 0.18 **FUD** XXX [51] [A] [80] ⚑

AMA: 2018,May,5; 2018,Feb,11; 2018,Jan,8; 2017,Jan,8; 2016,Jan,13; 2015,Jan,16

97028 **ultraviolet**

🏥 0.23 ⚕ 0.23 **FUD** XXX [51] [A] [80] ⚑

AMA: 2018,May,5; 2018,Feb,11; 2018,Jan,8; 2017,Jan,8; 2016,Jan,13; 2015,Jan,16

97032-97039 Physical Therapy Treatment Modalities: Constant Attendance

CMS: 100-02,15,220 Coverage of Outpatient Rehabilitation Therapy Services; 100-02,15,220.4 Functional Reporting; 100-02,15,230 Practice of Physical Therapy, Occupational Therapy, and Speech-Language Pathology; 100-02,15,230.1 Practice of Physical Therapy; 100-02,15,230.2 Practice of Occupational Therapy; 100-02,15,230.4 Services By a Physical/Occupational Therapist in Private Practice; 100-03,10.3 Inpatient Pain Rehabilitation Programs; 100-03,10.4 Outpatient Hospital Pain Rehabilitation Programs; 100-03,160.17 Payment for L-Dopa /Associated Inpatient Hospital Services; 100-04,5,10 Part B Outpatient Rehabilitation and Comprehensive Outpatient Rehabilitation Facility (CORF) Services - General; 100-04,5,10.3.2 Exceptions Process; 100-04,5,10.3.3 Use of the KX Modifier; 100-04,5,20.2 Reporting Units of Service

[INCLUDES] Adding incremental treatment time intervals for same visit to calculate total service time
Direct patient contact by provider

[EXCLUDES] *Electromyography (95860-95872 [95885, 95886, 95887])*
EMG biofeedback training (90901)
Muscle and motion range tests ([97161, 97162, 97163, 97164, 97165, 97166, 97167, 97168, 97169, 97170, 97171, 97172])
Nerve conduction studies (95905-95913)

97032 **Application of a modality to 1 or more areas; electrical stimulation (manual), each 15 minutes**

[EXCLUDES] *Transcutaneous electrical modulation pain reprocessing (TEMPR) (scrambler therapy) (0278T)*

🏥 0.42 ⚕ 0.42 **FUD** XXX [51] [A] [80] ⚑

AMA: 2019,Jul,10; 2018,Oct,11; 2018,Oct,8; 2018,May,5; 2018,Feb,11; 2018,Jan,8; 2017,Jan,8; 2016,Jan,13; 2015,Jan,16

97033 **iontophoresis, each 15 minutes**

🏥 0.59 ⚕ 0.59 **FUD** XXX [51] [A] [80] ⚑

AMA: 2018,May,5; 2018,Feb,11; 2018,Jan,8; 2017,Jan,8; 2016,Jan,13; 2015,Jan,16

97034 **contrast baths, each 15 minutes**

🏥 0.43 ⚕ 0.43 **FUD** XXX [51] [A] [80] ⚑

AMA: 2018,May,5; 2018,Feb,11; 2018,Jan,8; 2017,Jan,8; 2016,Jan,13; 2015,Jan,16

97035 **ultrasound, each 15 minutes**

🏥 0.39 ⚕ 0.39 **FUD** XXX [51] [A] [80] ⚑

AMA: 2018,May,5; 2018,Feb,11; 2018,Jan,8; 2017,Jan,8; 2016,Jan,13; 2015,Jan,16

97036 **Hubbard tank, each 15 minutes**

🏥 0.99 ⚕ 0.99 **FUD** XXX [51] [A] [80] ⚑

AMA: 2018,May,5; 2018,Feb,11; 2018,Jan,8; 2017,Jan,8; 2016,Jan,13; 2015,Jan,16

97039 **Unlisted modality (specify type and time if constant attendance)**

🏥 0.00 ⚕ 0.00 **FUD** XXX [A] [80] ⚑

AMA: 2020,Jul,13; 2018,May,5; 2018,Feb,11; 2018,Jan,8; 2017,Jan,8; 2016,Nov,9; 2016,Jun,8; 2016,Jan,13; 2015,Jan,16

97110-97546 [97151, 97152, 97153, 97154, 97155, 97156, 97157, 97158, 97161, 97162, 97163, 97164, 97165, 97166, 97167, 97168, 97169, 97170, 97171, 97172] Other Therapeutic Techniques With Direct Patient Contact

CMS: 100-02,15,220 Coverage of Outpatient Rehabilitation Therapy Services; 100-02,15,230 Practice of Physical Therapy, Occupational Therapy, and Speech-Language Pathology; 100-02,15,230.1 Practice of Physical Therapy; 100-02,15,230.2 Practice of Occupational Therapy; 100-02,15,230.4 Services By a Physical/Occupational Therapist in Private Practice; 100-03,10.3 Inpatient Pain Rehabilitation Programs; 100-03,10.4 Outpatient Hospital Pain Rehabilitation Programs; 100-04,5,10 Part B Outpatient Rehabilitation and Comprehensive Outpatient Rehabilitation Facility (CORF) Services - General; 100-04,5,20.2 Reporting Units of Service

[INCLUDES] Application clinical skills/services to improve function
Direct patient contact by provider

[EXCLUDES] *Electromyography (95860-95872 [95885, 95886, 95887])*
EMG biofeedback training (90901)
Muscle and motion range tests ([97161, 97162, 97163, 97164, 97165, 97166, 97167, 97168, 97169, 97170, 97171, 97172])
Nerve conduction studies (95905-95913)

97110 **Therapeutic procedure, 1 or more areas, each 15 minutes; therapeutic exercises to develop strength and endurance, range of motion and flexibility**

🏥 0.87 ⚕ 0.87 **FUD** XXX [51] [A] [80] ⚑

AMA: 2019,Jun,14; 2018,Dec,7; 2018,Dec,7; 2018,May,5; 2018,Feb,11; 2018,Jan,8; 2017,Dec,14; 2017,Jan,8; 2016,Jun,8; 2016,Jan,13; 2015,Jan,16

97112 **neuromuscular reeducation of movement, balance, coordination, kinesthetic sense, posture, and/or proprioception for sitting and/or standing activities**

🏥 0.99 ⚕ 0.99 **FUD** XXX [51] [A] [80] ⚑

AMA: 2018,May,5; 2018,Feb,11; 2018,Jan,8; 2017,Jan,8; 2016,Jan,13; 2015,Jan,16

97113 **aquatic therapy with therapeutic exercises**

🏥 1.10 ⚕ 1.10 **FUD** XXX [51] [A] [80] ⚑

AMA: 2018,May,5; 2018,Feb,11; 2018,Jan,8; 2017,Jan,8; 2016,Jan,13; 2015,Jan,16

97116 **gait training (includes stair climbing)**

[EXCLUDES] *Comprehensive gait/motion analysis (96000-96003)*

🏥 0.86 ⚕ 0.86 **FUD** XXX [51] [A] [80] ⚑

AMA: 2018,May,5; 2018,Feb,11; 2018,Jan,8; 2017,Jan,8; 2016,Jan,13; 2015,Jan,16

97124 **massage, including effleurage, petrissage and/or tapotement (stroking, compression, percussion)**

[EXCLUDES] *Myofascial release (97140)*

🏥 0.81 ⚕ 0.81 **FUD** XXX [51] [A] [80] ⚑

AMA: 2020,Jul,10; 2019,Jun,14; 2018,May,5; 2018,Feb,11; 2018,Jan,8; 2017,Jan,8; 2016,Jun,8; 2016,Jan,13; 2015,Jan,16

97129 **Therapeutic interventions that focus on cognitive function (eg, attention, memory, reasoning, executive function, problem solving, and/or pragmatic functioning) and compensatory strategies to manage the performance of an activity (eg, managing time or schedules, initiating, organizing, and sequencing tasks), direct (one-on-one) patient contact; initial 15 minutes**

[EXCLUDES] *Adaptive behavior treatment ([97153], [97155])*
Reporting code more than one time per day

🏥 0.67 ⚕ 0.68 **FUD** XXX [51] [80] ⚑

AMA: 2020,Jul,10

+ **97130** **each additional 15 minutes (List separately in addition to code for primary procedure)**

[EXCLUDES] *Adaptive behavior treatment ([97153], [97155])*

Code first (97129)

🏢 0.65 🩺 0.65 **FUD** ZZZ [51] [80] ⚑

AMA: 2020,Jul,10

97139 **Unlisted therapeutic procedure (specify)**

🏢 0.00 🩺 0.00 **FUD** XXX [A] [80] ⚑

AMA: 2018,May,5; 2018,Feb,11; 2018,Jan,8; 2017,Jan,8; 2016,Jan,13; 2015,Jan,16

97140 **Manual therapy techniques (eg, mobilization/ manipulation, manual lymphatic drainage, manual traction), 1 or more regions, each 15 minutes**

[EXCLUDES] *Insertion needle without injection ([20560, 20561])*

🏢 0.80 🩺 0.80 **FUD** XXX [51] [A] [80] ⚑

AMA: 2020,Jul,10; 2020,Feb,9; 2019,Jun,14; 2018,May,5; 2018,Feb,11; 2018,Jan,8; 2017,Jan,8; 2016,Nov,9; 2016,Sep,9; 2016,Aug,3; 2016,Jan,13; 2015,Mar,9; 2015,Jan,16

97150 **Therapeutic procedure(s), group (2 or more individuals)**

[INCLUDES] Constant attendance by physician/therapist

Reporting this procedure for each group member

[EXCLUDES] *Adaptive behavior services ([97154], [97158])*

Osteopathic manipulative treatment (98925-98929)

🏢 0.52 🩺 0.52 **FUD** XXX [51] [A] [80] ⚑

AMA: 2020,Jul,7; 2018,Nov,3; 2018,May,5; 2018,Feb,11; 2018,Jan,8; 2017,Jan,8; 2016,Jan,13; 2015,Jan,16

97151 **Resequenced code. See code following 96040.**

97152 **Resequenced code. See code following 96040.**

97153 **Resequenced code. See code following 96040.**

97154 **Resequenced code. See code following 96040.**

97155 **Resequenced code. See code following 96040.**

97156 **Resequenced code. See code following 96040.**

97157 **Resequenced code. See code following 96040.**

97158 **Resequenced code. See code following 96040.**

97161 **Resequenced code. See code before 97010.**

97162 **Resequenced code. See code before 97010.**

97163 **Resequenced code. See code before 97010.**

97164 **Resequenced code. See code before 97010.**

97165 **Resequenced code. See code before 97010.**

97166 **Resequenced code. See code before 97010.**

97167 **Resequenced code. See code before 97010.**

97168 **Resequenced code. See code before 97010.**

97169 **Resequenced code. See code before 97010.**

97170 **Resequenced code. See code before 97010.**

97171 **Resequenced code. See code before 97010.**

97172 **Resequenced code. See code before 97010.**

97530 **Therapeutic activities, direct (one-on-one) patient contact (use of dynamic activities to improve functional performance), each 15 minutes**

🏢 1.13 🩺 1.13 **FUD** XXX [51] [A] [80] ⚑

AMA: 2018,Dec,7; 2018,Dec,7; 2018,May,5; 2018,Feb,11; 2018,Jan,8; 2017,Jan,8; 2016,Jan,13; 2015,Jan,16

97533 **Sensory integrative techniques to enhance sensory processing and promote adaptive responses to environmental demands, direct (one-on-one) patient contact, each 15 minutes**

🏢 1.47 🩺 1.47 **FUD** XXX [51] [A] [80] ⚑

AMA: 2018,May,5; 2018,Feb,11; 2018,Jan,8; 2017,Jan,8; 2016,Jan,13; 2015,Jan,16

97535 **Self-care/home management training (eg, activities of daily living (ADL) and compensatory training, meal preparation, safety procedures, and instructions in use of assistive technology devices/adaptive equipment) direct one-on-one contact, each 15 minutes**

🏢 0.97 🩺 0.97 **FUD** XXX [51] [A] [80] ⚑

AMA: 2018,May,5; 2018,Feb,11; 2018,Jan,8; 2017,Jan,8; 2016,Aug,3; 2016,Jan,13; 2015,Jun,10; 2015,Mar,9; 2015,Jan,16

97537 **Community/work reintegration training (eg, shopping, transportation, money management, avocational activities and/or work environment/modification analysis, work task analysis, use of assistive technology device/adaptive equipment), direct one-on-one contact, each 15 minutes**

[EXCLUDES] *Wheelchair management/propulsion training (97542)*

🏢 0.93 🩺 0.93 **FUD** XXX [51] [A] [80] ⚑

AMA: 2018,May,5; 2018,Feb,11; 2018,Jan,8; 2017,Jan,8; 2016,Jan,13; 2015,Jan,16

97542 **Wheelchair management (eg, assessment, fitting, training), each 15 minutes**

🏢 0.94 🩺 0.94 **FUD** XXX [51] [A] [80] ⚑

AMA: 2018,May,5; 2018,Feb,11; 2018,Jan,8; 2017,Jan,8; 2016,Jan,13; 2015,Jun,10; 2015,Jan,16

97545 **Work hardening/conditioning; initial 2 hours**

🏢 0.00 🩺 0.00 **FUD** XXX [51] [A] [80] ⚑

AMA: 2018,May,5; 2018,Feb,11; 2018,Jan,8; 2017,Jan,8; 2016,Jan,13; 2015,Jan,16

+ **97546** **each additional hour (List separately in addition to code for primary procedure)**

Code first initial two hours (97545)

🏢 0.00 🩺 0.00 **FUD** ZZZ [51] [A] [80] ⚑

AMA: 2018,May,5; 2018,Feb,11; 2018,Jan,8; 2017,Jan,8; 2016,Jan,13; 2015,Jan,16

97597-97610 Treatment of Wounds

CMS: 100-02,15,220.4 Functional Reporting; 100-02,15,230.4 Services By a Physical/Occupational Therapist in Private Practice; 100-03,270.3 Blood-derived Products for Chronic Nonhealing Wounds; 100-04,4,200.9 Billing for "Sometimes Therapy" Services that May be Paid as Non-Therapy Services; 100-04,5,10 Part B Outpatient Rehabilitation and Comprehensive Outpatient Rehabilitation Facility (CORF) Services - General; 100-04,5,10.3.2 Exceptions Process; 100-04,5,10.3.3 Use of the KX Modifier

INCLUDES Direct patient contact
Removing devitalized/necrotic tissue and promoting healing

EXCLUDES *Burn wound debridement (16020-16030)*

97597 **Debridement (eg, high pressure waterjet with/without suction, sharp selective debridement with scissors, scalpel and forceps), open wound, (eg, fibrin, devitalized epidermis and/or dermis, exudate, debris, biofilm), including topical application(s), wound assessment, use of a whirlpool, when performed and instruction(s) for ongoing care, per session, total wound(s) surface area; first 20 sq cm or less**

INCLUDES Chemical cauterization (17250)

0.68 2.52 **FUD** 000 51 T 80

AMA: 2018,May,5; 2018,Feb,11; 2018,Jan,8; 2017,Jan,8; 2016,Oct,3; 2016,Aug,9; 2016,Jan,13; 2015,Jan,16

Wound may be washed, addressed with scissors, and/or tweezers and scalpel

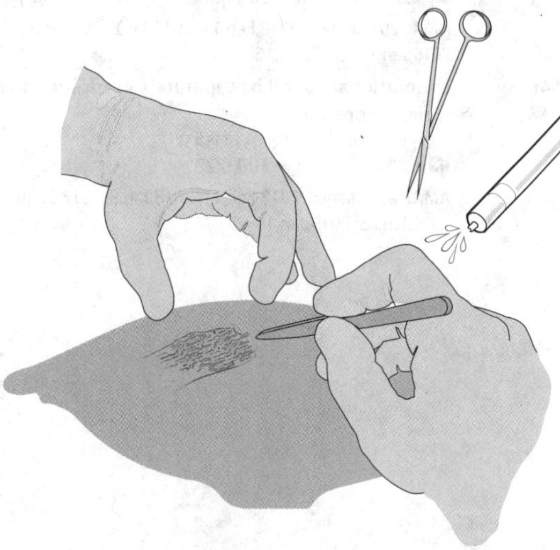

\+ **97598** **each additional 20 sq cm, or part thereof (List separately in addition to code for primary procedure)**

INCLUDES Chemical cauterization (17250)

Code first (97597)

0.74 1.31 **FUD** ZZZ 51 N 80

AMA: 2018,May,5; 2018,Feb,11; 2018,Jan,8; 2017,Jan,8; 2016,Oct,3; 2016,Aug,9; 2016,Jan,13; 2015,Jan,16

97602 **Removal of devitalized tissue from wound(s), non-selective debridement, without anesthesia (eg, wet-to-moist dressings, enzymatic, abrasion, larval therapy), including topical application(s), wound assessment, and instruction(s) for ongoing care, per session**

INCLUDES Chemical cauterization (17250)

0.00 0.00 **FUD** XXX 51 Q1

AMA: 2018,May,5; 2018,Feb,11; 2018,Jan,8; 2017,Jan,8; 2016,Oct,3; 2016,Jan,13; 2015,Jan,16

97605 **Negative pressure wound therapy (eg, vacuum assisted drainage collection), utilizing durable medical equipment (DME), including topical application(s), wound assessment, and instruction(s) for ongoing care, per session; total wound(s) surface area less than or equal to 50 square centimeters**

EXCLUDES *Negative pressure wound therapy using disposable medical equipment (97607-97608)*

0.74 1.24 **FUD** XXX 51 Q1 80

AMA: 2018,May,5; 2018,Feb,11; 2018,Jan,8; 2017,Jan,8; 2016,Feb,13; 2016,Jan,13; 2015,Jan,16

97606 **total wound(s) surface area greater than 50 square centimeters**

EXCLUDES *Negative pressure wound therapy using disposable medical equipment (97607-97608)*

0.80 1.46 **FUD** XXX 51 Q1 80

AMA: 2018,May,5; 2018,Feb,11; 2018,Jan,8; 2017,Jan,8; 2016,Feb,13; 2016,Jan,13; 2015,Jan,16

97607 **Negative pressure wound therapy, (eg, vacuum assisted drainage collection), utilizing disposable, non-durable medical equipment including provision of exudate management collection system, topical application(s), wound assessment, and instructions for ongoing care, per session; total wound(s) surface area less than or equal to 50 square centimeters**

EXCLUDES *Negative pressure wound therapy using durable medical equipment (97605-97606)*

0.00 0.00 **FUD** XXX 51 T 80

AMA: 2018,May,5; 2018,Feb,11; 2018,Jan,8; 2017,Jan,8; 2016,Jan,13; 2015,Jan,16

97608 **total wound(s) surface area greater than 50 square centimeters**

EXCLUDES *Negative pressure wound therapy using durable medical equipment (97605-97606)*

0.00 0.00 **FUD** XXX 51 T 80

AMA: 2018,May,5; 2018,Feb,11; 2018,Jan,8; 2017,Jan,8; 2016,Jan,13; 2015,Jan,16

97610 **Low frequency, non-contact, non-thermal ultrasound, including topical application(s), when performed, wound assessment, and instruction(s) for ongoing care, per day**

0.48 6.39 **FUD** XXX 51 Q1 80

AMA: 2018,May,5; 2018,Feb,11; 2018,Jan,8; 2017,Jan,8; 2016,Jan,13; 2015,Jan,16

97750-97799 Assessments and Training

CMS: 100-02,15,220 Coverage of Outpatient Rehabilitation Therapy Services; 100-02,15,220.4 Functional Reporting; 100-02,15,230 Practice of Physical Therapy, Occupational Therapy, and Speech-Language Pathology; 100-02,15,230.1 Practice of Physical Therapy; 100-02,15,230.2 Practice of Occupational Therapy; 100-02,15,230.4 Services By a Physical/Occupational Therapist in Private Practice; 100-04,5,10 Part B Outpatient Rehabilitation and Comprehensive Outpatient Rehabilitation Facility (CORF) Services - General; 100-04,5,10.3.2 Therapy Cap Exceptions; 100-04,5,10.3.3 Use of the KX Modifier

97750 **Physical performance test or measurement (eg, musculoskeletal, functional capacity), with written report, each 15 minutes**

INCLUDES Direct patient contact

EXCLUDES *Electromyography (95860-95872, [95885, 95886, 95887])*
Joint motion range (95851-95852)
Nerve velocity determination (95905, 95907-95913)

0.99 0.99 **FUD** XXX 51 A 80

AMA: 2018,May,5; 2018,Feb,11; 2018,Jan,8; 2017,Jan,8; 2016,Jan,13; 2015,Jan,16

97755 Assistive technology assessment (eg, to restore, augment or compensate for existing function, optimize functional tasks and/or maximize environmental accessibility), direct one-on-one contact, with written report, each 15 minutes

INCLUDES Direct patient contact

EXCLUDES *Augmentative/alternative communication device (92605, 92607)*
Electromyography (95860-95872, [95885, 95886, 95887])
Joint motion range (95851-95852)
Nerve velocity determination (95905, 95907-95913)

1.09 1.09 **FUD** XXX

AMA: 2018,May,5; 2018,Feb,11

97760 Orthotic(s) management and training (including assessment and fitting when not otherwise reported), upper extremity(ies), lower extremity(ies) and/or trunk, initial orthotic(s) encounter, each 15 minutes

EXCLUDES *Gait training, when performed on same extremity (97116)*

1.40 1.40 **FUD** XXX

AMA: 2018,May,5; 2018,Feb,11; 2018,Jan,8; 2017,Jan,8; 2016,Jan,13; 2015,Jan,16

97761 Prosthetic(s) training, upper and/or lower extremity(ies), initial prosthetic(s) encounter, each 15 minutes

1.16 1.16 **FUD** XXX

AMA: 2018,May,5; 2018,Feb,11; 2018,Jan,8; 2017,Jan,8; 2016,Jan,13; 2015,Jan,16

97763 Orthotic(s)/prosthetic(s) management and/or training, upper extremity(ies), lower extremity(ies), and/or trunk, subsequent orthotic(s)/prosthetic(s) encounter, each 15 minutes

EXCLUDES *Initial encounter for orthotics and prosthetics management and training (97760-97761)*

1.50 1.50 **FUD** XXX

AMA: 2018,May,5; 2018,Feb,11

97799 Unlisted physical medicine/rehabilitation service or procedure

0.00 0.00 **FUD** XXX

AMA: 2018,May,5; 2018,Feb,11; 2018,Jan,8; 2017,Jan,8; 2016,Nov,9; 2016,Jan,13; 2015,Jan,16

97802-97804 Medical Nutrition Therapy Services

CMS: 100-02,13,220 Preventive Health Services; 100-03,180.1 Medical Nutrition Therapy; 100-04,12,190.3 List of Telehealth Services; 100-04,12,190.6 Payment Methodology for Physician/Practitioner at the Distant Site ; 100-04,12,190.6.1 Submission of Telehealth Claims for Distant Site Practitioners; 100-04,12,190.7 Contractor Editing of Telehealth Claims; 100-04,4,300 Medical Nutrition Therapy Services; 100-04,4,300.6 CWF Edits for MNT/DSMT

EXCLUDES *Medical nutrition therapy assessment/intervention provided by physician or other qualified health care provider; report appropriate E/M codes*

97802 Medical nutrition therapy; initial assessment and intervention, individual, face-to-face with the patient, each 15 minutes

0.96 1.05 **FUD** XXX ★

AMA: 2020,Jul,7; 2018,Feb,11; 2018,Jan,8; 2017,Jan,8; 2016,Jan,13; 2015,Jan,16

97803 re-assessment and intervention, individual, face-to-face with the patient, each 15 minutes

0.81 0.92 **FUD** XXX ★

AMA: 2020,Jul,7; 2018,Feb,11; 2018,Jan,8; 2017,Jan,8; 2016,Jan,13; 2015,Jan,16

97804 group (2 or more individual(s)), each 30 minutes

0.45 0.48 **FUD** XXX ★

AMA: 2020,Jul,7; 2018,Feb,11; 2018,Jan,8; 2017,Jan,8; 2016,Jan,13; 2015,Jan,16

97810-97814 Acupuncture

CMS: 100-03,10.3 Inpatient Pain Rehabilitation Programs; 100-03,10.4 Outpatient Hospital Pain Rehabilitation Programs; 100-03,30.3 Acupuncture; 100-03,30.3.1 Acupuncture for Fibromyalgia; 100-03,30.3.2 Acupuncture for Osteoarthritis

INCLUDES 15 minute increments face-to-face contact with patient
Reporting only one code for each 15 minute increment

EXCLUDES *Insertion needle without injection ([20560, 20561])*

Code also significant separately identifiable E/M service with modifier 25, when performed

97810 Acupuncture, 1 or more needles; without electrical stimulation, initial 15 minutes of personal one-on-one contact with the patient

EXCLUDES *Treatment with electrical stimulation (97813-97814)*

0.87 1.03 **FUD** XXX

AMA: 2020,Feb,9; 2018,Feb,11; 2018,Jan,8; 2017,Jan,8; 2016,Jan,13; 2015,Jan,16

+ **97811 without electrical stimulation, each additional 15 minutes of personal one-on-one contact with the patient, with re-insertion of needle(s) (List separately in addition to code for primary procedure)**

EXCLUDES *Treatment with electrical stimulation (97813-97814)*

Code first initial 15 minutes (97810)

0.72 0.78 **FUD** ZZZ

AMA: 2020,Feb,9; 2018,Feb,11; 2018,Jan,8; 2017,Jan,8; 2016,Jan,13; 2015,Jan,16

97813 with electrical stimulation, initial 15 minutes of personal one-on-one contact with the patient

EXCLUDES *Treatment without electrical stimulation (97813-97814)*

0.94 1.13 **FUD** XXX

AMA: 2020,Feb,9; 2018,Feb,11; 2018,Jan,8; 2017,Jan,8; 2016,Jan,13; 2015,Jan,16

+ **97814 with electrical stimulation, each additional 15 minutes of personal one-on-one contact with the patient, with re-insertion of needle(s) (List separately in addition to code for primary procedure)**

EXCLUDES *Treatment without electrical stimulation (97813-97814)*

Code first initial 15 minutes (97813)

0.79 0.91 **FUD** ZZZ

AMA: 2020,Feb,9; 2018,Feb,11; 2018,Jan,8; 2017,Jan,8; 2016,Jan,13; 2015,Jan,16

98925-98929 Osteopathic Manipulation

CMS: 100-03,150.1 Manipulation

INCLUDES Body regions:
Abdomen/visceral region
Cervical region
Head region
Lower extremities
Lumbar region
Pelvic region
Rib cage region
Sacral region
Thoracic region
Upper extremities
Physician applied manual treatment done to eliminate/alleviate somatic dysfunction and related disorders with multiple techniques

Code also significant separately identifiable E/M service with modifier 25, when performed

98925 Osteopathic manipulative treatment (OMT); 1-2 body regions involved

0.68 0.89 **FUD** 000

AMA: 2018,Aug,9; 2018,Feb,11; 2018,Jan,8; 2017,Dec,14; 2017,Jan,8; 2016,Jan,13; 2015,Jan,16

98926 3-4 body regions involved

1.03 1.29 **FUD** 000

AMA: 2018,Aug,9; 2018,Feb,11; 2018,Jan,8; 2017,Jan,8; 2016,Jan,13; 2015,Jan,16

98927 5-6 body regions involved

1.35 1.68 **FUD** 000

AMA: 2018,Aug,9; 2018,Feb,11; 2018,Jan,8; 2017,Jan,8; 2016,Jan,13; 2015,Jan,16

98928 **7-8 body regions involved**
Facility RVU 1.69 Non-Facility RVU 2.05 **FUD** 000 Q1 80 CCI
AMA: 2018,Aug,9; 2018,Feb,11; 2018,Jan,8; 2017,Jan,8; 2016,Jan,13; 2015,Jan,16

98929 **9-10 body regions involved**
Facility RVU 2.07 Non-Facility RVU 2.45 **FUD** 000 Q1 80 CCI
AMA: 2018,Aug,9; 2018,Feb,11; 2018,Jan,8; 2017,Jan,8; 2016,Jan,13; 2015,Jan,16

98940-98943 Chiropractic Manipulation

CMS: 100-01,5,70.6 Chiropractors; 100-02,15,240 Chiropractic Services - General; 100-02,15,240.1.3 Necessity for Treatment; 100-02,15,30.5 Chiropractor's Services; 100-03,150.1 Manipulation

INCLUDES Five extraspinal regions:
- Abdomen
- Head, including temporomandibular joint, excluding atlanto-occipital region
- Lower extremities
- Rib cage, not including costotransverse/costovertebral joints
- Upper extremities

Five spinal regions:
- Cervical region (atlanto-occipital joint)
- Lumbar region
- Pelvic region (sacro-iliac joint)
- Sacral region
- Thoracic region (costovertebral/costotransverse joints)

Manual treatment performed to influence joint/neurophysical function

Code also significant separately identifiable E/M service with modifier 25, when performed

98940 **Chiropractic manipulative treatment (CMT); spinal, 1-2 regions**
Facility RVU 0.64 Non-Facility RVU 0.80 **FUD** 000 Q1 80 CCI
AMA: 2018,Nov,11; 2018,Feb,11; 2018,Jan,8; 2017,Jan,8; 2016,Jan,13; 2015,Jan,16

98941 **spinal, 3-4 regions**
Facility RVU 0.98 Non-Facility RVU 1.15 **FUD** 000 Q1 80 CCI
AMA: 2018,Nov,11; 2018,Feb,11; 2018,Jan,8; 2017,Jan,8; 2016,Jan,13; 2015,Jan,16

98942 **spinal, 5 regions**
Facility RVU 1.33 Non-Facility RVU 1.50 **FUD** 000 Q1 80 CCI
AMA: 2018,Nov,11; 2018,Feb,11; 2018,Jan,8; 2017,Jan,8; 2016,Jan,13; 2015,Jan,16

98943 **extraspinal, 1 or more regions**
Facility RVU 0.67 Non-Facility RVU 0.77 **FUD** XXX E CCI
AMA: 2018,Nov,11; 2018,Feb,11; 2018,Jan,8; 2017,Jan,8; 2016,Jan,13; 2015,Jan,16

98960-98962 Self-Management Training

INCLUDES Education/training services:
- Prescribed by physician or other qualified health care professional
- Provided by qualified nonphysician health care provider

Standardized curriculum that may be modified as necessary for:
- Clinical needs
- Cultural norms
- Health literacy

Teaching patient how to manage illness/delay comorbidity(s)

EXCLUDES *Collection/interpretation physiologic data ([99091])*
Complex chronic care management (99487, 99489)
Counseling/education to group (99078)
Counseling/risk factor reduction without symptoms/established disease (99401-99412)
Genetic counseling education services (96040, 98961-98962)
Health and behavior assessment and intervention (96156, 96158-96159, [96164, 96165], [96167, 96168], [96170, 96171])
Medical nutrition therapy (97802-97804)
Physician supervision in home, domiciliary, or rest home (99339, 99340, 99374-99375, 99379-99380)
Services provided in which time would be reported with other services
Services provided with cumulative time of less than 5 minutes
Supervision hospice patient (99377-99378)
Transitional care management (99495, 99496)

98960 **Education and training for patient self-management by a qualified, nonphysician health care professional using a standardized curriculum, face-to-face with the patient (could include caregiver/family) each 30 minutes; individual patient**
Facility RVU 0.77 Non-Facility RVU 0.77 **FUD** XXX ★ E CCI
AMA: 2020,Jul,7; 2018,Aug,6; 2018,Feb,11; 2018,Jan,8; 2017,Jan,8; 2016,Jan,13; 2015,Jan,16

98961 **2-4 patients**
INCLUDES Group education regarding genetic risks
Facility RVU 0.37 Non-Facility RVU 0.37 **FUD** XXX ★ E CCI
AMA: 2020,Jul,7; 2018,Aug,6; 2018,Feb,11; 2018,Jan,8; 2017,Jan,8; 2016,Jan,13; 2015,Jan,16

98962 **5-8 patients**
INCLUDES Group education regarding genetic risks
Facility RVU 0.27 Non-Facility RVU 0.27 **FUD** XXX ★ E CCI
AMA: 2020,Jul,7; 2018,Aug,6; 2018,Feb,11; 2018,Jan,8; 2017,Jan,8; 2016,Jan,13; 2015,Jan,16

98966-98968 Nonphysician Telephone Services

INCLUDES Assessment and management services provided by telephone by qualified health care professional
Care episodes initiated by established patient or his/her guardian

EXCLUDES *Call initiated by qualified health care professional*
Calls during postoperative period
Decision to see patient at next available urgent care appointment
Decision to see patient within 24 hours from patient call
Monitoring INR (93792-93793)
Patient management services during same time frame as ([99439, 99490, 99491], 99487-99489)
Reporting codes when same codes billed within past seven days
Telephone services considered previous or subsequent service component
Telephone services provided by physician (99441-99443)

98966 **Telephone assessment and management service provided by a qualified nonphysician health care professional to an established patient, parent, or guardian not originating from a related assessment and management service provided within the previous 7 days nor leading to an assessment and management service or procedure within the next 24 hours or soonest available appointment; 5-10 minutes of medical discussion**
Facility RVU 0.36 Non-Facility RVU 0.39 **FUD** XXX E 80 CCI
AMA: 2018,Mar,7; 2018,Feb,11; 2018,Jan,8; 2017,Jan,8; 2016,Jan,13; 2015,Jan,16

98967 **11-20 minutes of medical discussion**
Facility RVU 0.72 Non-Facility RVU 0.76 **FUD** XXX E 80 CCI
AMA: 2018,Mar,7; 2018,Feb,11; 2018,Jan,8; 2017,Jan,8; 2016,Jan,13; 2015,Jan,16

98968 **21-30 minutes of medical discussion**
1.08 1.12 FUD XXX E 80
AMA: 2018,Mar,7; 2018,Feb,11; 2018,Jan,8; 2017,Jan,8; 2016,Jan,13; 2015,Jan,16

98970-98972 Nonphysician Online Service

Timely reply to patient as well as:
Ordering laboratory services
Permanent service record; either hard copy or electronic
Providing prescription
Related telephone calls

EXCLUDES *Monitoring INR (93792-93793)*
Online digital assessment and management service provided by qualified health care professional ([99421, 99422, 99423])
Online evaluation service:
Provided during postoperative period
Provided more than once in seven day period
Related to service provided in previous seven days
Provided with cumulative time less than 5 minutes
Where time would be reported as another service
Patient management services during same time frame as:
Chronic care management ([99439, 99490, 99491])
Collection/interpretation physiologic data ([99091])
Complex chronic care management (99487-99489)
Physician supervision in home, domiciliary, or rest home (99339-99340, 99374-99375, 99379-99380)
Supervision hospice patient (99377-99378)

98970 **Qualified nonphysician health care professional online digital assessment and management, for an established patient, for up to 7 days, cumulative time during the 7 days; 5-10 minutes**
0.00 0.00 FUD XXX
AMA: 2020,Jan,3

98971 **11-20 minutes**
0.00 0.00 FUD XXX
AMA: 2020,Jan,3

98972 **21 or more minutes**
0.00 0.00 FUD XXX
AMA: 2020,Jan,3

99000-99091 [99091] Supplemental Services and Supplies

INCLUDES Supplemental reporting for services adjunct to basic service provided

99000 **Handling and/or conveyance of specimen for transfer from the office to a laboratory**
0.00 0.00 FUD XXX E
AMA: 2018,Dec,10; 2018,Dec,10; 2018,Feb,11; 2018,Jan,8; 2017,Jan,8; 2016,Jan,13; 2015,Jan,16

99001 **Handling and/or conveyance of specimen for transfer from the patient in other than an office to a laboratory (distance may be indicated)**
0.00 0.00 FUD XXX E
AMA: 2018,Dec,10; 2018,Dec,10; 2018,Feb,11; 2018,Jan,8; 2017,Jan,8; 2016,Jan,13; 2015,Jan,16

99002 **Handling, conveyance, and/or any other service in connection with the implementation of an order involving devices (eg, designing, fitting, packaging, handling, delivery or mailing) when devices such as orthotics, protectives, prosthetics are fabricated by an outside laboratory or shop but which items have been designed, and are to be fitted and adjusted by the attending physician or other qualified health care professional**
EXCLUDES *Venous blood routine collection (36415)*
0.00 0.00 FUD XXX B
AMA: 2018,Dec,10; 2018,Dec,10; 2018,Feb,11; 2018,Jan,8; 2017,Jan,8; 2016,Jan,13; 2015,Jan,16

99024 **Postoperative follow-up visit, normally included in the surgical package, to indicate that an evaluation and management service was performed during a postoperative period for a reason(s) related to the original procedure**
0.00 0.00 FUD XXX B
AMA: 2018,Dec,10; 2018,Dec,10; 2018,Feb,11; 2018,Jan,8; 2017,Jul,9; 2017,Jan,3; 2017,Jan,8; 2016,Jan,13; 2015,Mar,3; 2015,Jan,16

99026 **Hospital mandated on call service; in-hospital, each hour**
EXCLUDES *Physician stand-by services with prolonged physician attendance (99360)*
Time spent providing procedures or services that may be separately reported
0.00 0.00 FUD XXX E
AMA: 2018,Dec,10; 2018,Dec,10; 2018,Feb,11; 2018,Jan,8; 2017,Jan,8; 2016,Jan,13; 2015,Jan,16

99027 **out-of-hospital, each hour**
EXCLUDES *Physician stand-by services with prolonged physician attendance (99360)*
Time spent providing procedures or services that may be separately reported
0.00 0.00 FUD XXX E
AMA: 2018,Dec,10; 2018,Dec,10; 2018,Feb,11; 2018,Jan,8; 2017,Jan,8; 2016,Jan,13; 2015,Jan,16

99050 **Services provided in the office at times other than regularly scheduled office hours, or days when the office is normally closed (eg, holidays, Saturday or Sunday), in addition to basic service**
Code also more than one adjunct code per encounter when appropriate
Code first basic service provided
0.00 0.00 FUD XXX ⑤ B
AMA: 2018,Dec,10; 2018,Dec,10; 2018,Feb,11; 2018,Jan,8; 2017,Jan,8; 2016,Jan,13; 2015,Jan,16

99051 **Service(s) provided in the office during regularly scheduled evening, weekend, or holiday office hours, in addition to basic service**
Code also more than one adjunct code per encounter when appropriate
Code first basic service provided
0.00 0.00 FUD XXX ⑤ B
AMA: 2018,Dec,10; 2018,Dec,10; 2018,Feb,11; 2018,Jan,8; 2017,Jan,8; 2016,Jan,13; 2015,Jan,16

99053 **Service(s) provided between 10:00 PM and 8:00 AM at 24-hour facility, in addition to basic service**
Code also more than one adjunct code per encounter when appropriate
Code first basic service provided
0.00 0.00 FUD XXX ⑤ B
AMA: 2018,Dec,10; 2018,Dec,10; 2018,Feb,11; 2018,Jan,8; 2017,Jan,8; 2016,Jan,13; 2015,Jan,16

99056 **Service(s) typically provided in the office, provided out of the office at request of patient, in addition to basic service**
Code also more than one adjunct code per encounter when appropriate
Code first basic service provided
0.00 0.00 FUD XXX ⑤ B
AMA: 2018,Dec,10; 2018,Dec,10; 2018,Feb,11; 2018,Jan,8; 2017,Jan,8; 2016,Jan,13; 2015,Jan,16

99058 **Service(s) provided on an emergency basis in the office, which disrupts other scheduled office services, in addition to basic service**
Code also more than one adjunct code per encounter when appropriate
Code first basic service provided
0.00 0.00 FUD XXX ⑤ B
AMA: 2018,Dec,10; 2018,Dec,10; 2018,Feb,11; 2018,Jan,8; 2017,Jan,8; 2016,Jan,13; 2015,Jan,16

99060 **Service(s) provided on an emergency basis, out of the office, which disrupts other scheduled office services, in addition to basic service**
Code also more than one adjunct code per encounter when appropriate
Code first basic service provided
0.00 0.00 FUD XXX ⑤ B
AMA: 2018,Dec,10; 2018,Dec,10; 2018,Feb,11; 2018,Jan,8; 2017,Jan,8; 2016,Jan,13; 2015,Jan,16

99070 **Supplies and materials (except spectacles), provided by the physician or other qualified health care professional over and above those usually included with the office visit or other services rendered (list drugs, trays, supplies, or materials provided)**

EXCLUDES *Additional supplies, materials, and clinical staff time required for patient symptom review, personal protective equipment (PPE) use, and heightened cleaning processes due to respiratory-transmitted infectious disease during a declared public health emergency (PHE), as defined by law (99072)*

Spectacles supply

0.00 0.00 FUD XXX B

AMA: 2020,SepSE,1; 2020,SepSE,1; 2019,Apr,10; 2019,Feb,10; 2018,Dec,10; 2018,Dec,10; 2018,Jun,11; 2018,Mar,7; 2018,Jan,3; 2018,Jan,8; 2017,Sep,14; 2017,Jan,8; 2017,Jan,6; 2016,Jan,13; 2015,Jan,16

99071 **Educational supplies, such as books, tapes, and pamphlets, for the patient's education at cost to physician or other qualified health care professional**

0.00 0.00 FUD XXX B

AMA: 2018,Dec,10; 2018,Dec,10; 2018,Jan,8; 2017,Jan,8; 2016,Jan,13; 2015,Jan,16

● **99072** **Additional supplies, materials, and clinical staff time over and above those usually included in an office visit or other nonfacility service(s), when performed during a Public Health Emergency, as defined by law, due to respiratory-transmitted infectious disease**

INCLUDES Additional supplies, materials, and clinical staff time required for patient symptom review, personal protective equipment (PPE) use, and heightened cleaning processes due to respiratory-transmitted infectious disease during a declared public health emergency (PHE), as defined by law

EXCLUDES *Reporting more than one time per encounter, despite number services provided during encounter*

Supplies and materials provided, above those normally included in the encounter, unrelated to a declared PHE (99070)

AMA: 2020,SepSE,1

99075 **Medical testimony**

0.00 0.00 FUD XXX E

AMA: 2018,Dec,10; 2018,Dec,10; 2018,Jan,8; 2017,Jan,8; 2016,Jan,13; 2015,Jan,16

99078 **Physician or other qualified health care professional qualified by education, training, licensure/regulation (when applicable) educational services rendered to patients in a group setting (eg, prenatal, obesity, or diabetic instructions)**

0.00 0.00 FUD XXX N

AMA: 2018,Dec,10; 2018,Dec,10; 2018,Jan,8; 2017,Jan,8; 2016,Jan,13; 2015,Jan,16

99080 **Special reports such as insurance forms, more than the information conveyed in the usual medical communications or standard reporting form**

EXCLUDES *Completion workmen's compensation forms (99455-99456)*

0.00 0.00 FUD XXX B

AMA: 2018,Dec,10; 2018,Dec,10; 2018,Jan,8; 2017,Jan,8; 2016,Jan,13; 2015,Jan,16

99082 **Unusual travel (eg, transportation and escort of patient)**

0.00 0.00 FUD XXX B 80

AMA: 2018,Dec,10; 2018,Dec,10; 2018,Jan,8; 2017,Jan,8; 2016,Jan,13; 2015,Jan,16

99091 **Resequenced code. See code following resequenced code 99454.**

99100-99140 Modifying Factors for Anesthesia Services

CMS: 100-04,12,140.3 Payment for Qualified Nonphysician Anesthetists; 100-04,12,140.3.3 Billing Modifiers; 100-04,12,140.3.4 General Billing Instructions; 100-04,12,140.4.1 Anesthesiologist/Qualified Nonphysican Anesthetist; 100-04,12,140.4.2 Anesthetist and Anesthesiologist in a Single Procedure; 100-04,12,140.4.4 Conversion Factors for Anesthesia Services; 100-04,4,250.3.2 Anesthesia in a Hospital Outpatient Setting

Code first primary anesthesia procedure

\+ **99100** **Anesthesia for patient of extreme age, younger than 1 year and older than 70 (List separately in addition to code for primary anesthesia procedure)** A

EXCLUDES *Anesthesia services for infants one year old or less (00326, 00561, 00834, 00836)*

0.00 0.00 FUD ZZZ B

AMA: 2019,Oct,10; 2018,Jan,8; 2017,Dec,8; 2017,Jan,8; 2016,Jan,13; 2015,Jan,16

\+ **99116** **Anesthesia complicated by utilization of total body hypothermia (List separately in addition to code for primary anesthesia procedure)**

EXCLUDES *Anesthesia for procedures on heart/pericardial sac/great vessels chest with pump oxygenator (00561)*

0.00 0.00 FUD ZZZ B

AMA: 2019,Oct,10; 2018,Jan,8; 2017,Dec,8; 2017,Jan,8; 2016,Jan,13; 2015,Jan,16

\+ **99135** **Anesthesia complicated by utilization of controlled hypotension (List separately in addition to code for primary anesthesia procedure)**

EXCLUDES *Anesthesia for procedures on heart/pericardial sac/great vessels chest with pump oxygenator (00561)*

0.00 0.00 FUD ZZZ B

AMA: 2019,Oct,10; 2018,Jan,8; 2017,Dec,8; 2017,Jan,8; 2016,Jan,13; 2015,Jan,16

\+ **99140** **Anesthesia complicated by emergency conditions (specify) (List separately in addition to code for primary anesthesia procedure)**

INCLUDES Conditions where treatment delay could be dangerous to life or health

0.00 0.00 FUD ZZZ B

AMA: 2019,Oct,10; 2018,Jan,8; 2017,Dec,8; 2017,Jan,8; 2016,Jan,13; 2015,Jan,16

99151-99157 Moderate Sedation Services

INCLUDES Intraservice work that begins with sedation administration and ends when procedure complete

Monitoring:

- Patient response to drugs
- Vital signs

Ordering and providing drug to patient (first and subsequent)

Pre- and postservice procedures

99151 **Moderate sedation services provided by the same physician or other qualified health care professional performing the diagnostic or therapeutic service that the sedation supports, requiring the presence of an independent trained observer to assist in the monitoring of the patient's level of consciousness and physiological status; initial 15 minutes of intraservice time, patient younger than 5 years of age**

INCLUDES First 15 minutes intraservice time for patients under age 5

Services provided to patients by same service provider for which moderate sedation necessary with monitoring by trained observer

0.70 2.20 FUD XXX N

AMA: 2019,Feb,10; 2018,Jan,8; 2017,Sep,11; 2017,Jun,3; 2017,Jan,3

99152 **initial 15 minutes of intraservice time, patient age 5 years or older**

INCLUDES First 15 minutes intraservice time for patients age 5 and over

Services provided to patients by same service provider for which moderate sedation necessary with monitoring by trained observer

0.35 1.44 FUD XXX N

AMA: 2019,May,10; 2019,Feb,10; 2018,Jan,8; 2017,Sep,11; 2017,Jun,3; 2017,Jan,3

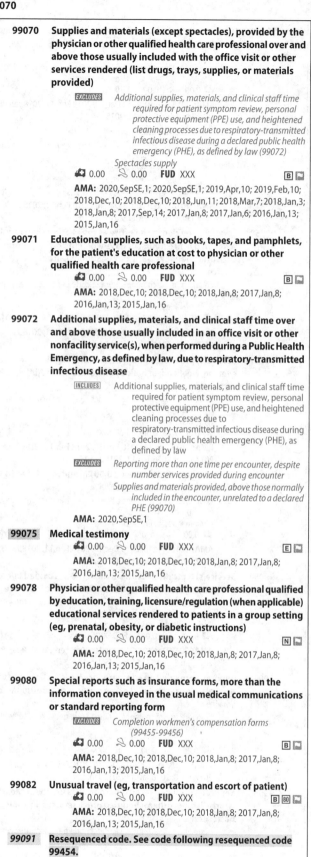

+ 99153 **each additional 15 minutes intraservice time (List separately in addition to code for primary service)**

INCLUDES Services provided to patients by same service provider for which moderate sedation necessary with monitoring by trained observer (99155-99157)

EXCLUDES *Services provided to patients by physician/other qualified health care professional other than provider rendering service*

Code first (99151-99152)

0.31 0.31 FUD ZZZ N TC

AMA: 2019,May,10; 2019,Feb,10; 2018,Jan,8; 2017,Sep,11; 2017,Jun,3; 2017,Jan,3

99155 **Moderate sedation services provided by a physician or other qualified health care professional other than the physician or other qualified health care professional performing the diagnostic or therapeutic service that the sedation supports; initial 15 minutes of intraservice time, patient younger than 5 years of age**

INCLUDES First 15 minutes intraservice time for patients under age 5

Services provided to patients by physician/other qualified health care professional other than provider rendering service for which moderate sedation necessary

2.54 2.54 FUD XXX N

AMA: 2019,Feb,10; 2018,Jan,8; 2017,Sep,11; 2017,Jun,3; 2017,Jan,3

99156 **initial 15 minutes of intraservice time, patient age 5 years or older**

INCLUDES First 15 minutes intraservice time for patients age 5 and over

Services provided to patients by physician/other qualified health care professional other than provider rendering service for which moderate sedation necessary

2.24 2.24 FUD XXX N

AMA: 2019,Feb,10; 2018,Jan,8; 2017,Sep,11; 2017,Jun,3; 2017,Jan,3

+ 99157 **each additional 15 minutes intraservice time (List separately in addition to code for primary service)**

INCLUDES Each subsequent 15 minutes services

Services provided to patients by physician/other qualified health care professional other than provider rendering service for which moderate sedation necessary (99151-99152)

EXCLUDES *Services provided to patients by same service provider for which moderate sedation necessary with monitoring by trained observer (99151-99152)*

Code first (99155-99156)

1.64 1.64 FUD ZZZ N

AMA: 2019,Feb,10; 2018,Jan,8; 2017,Sep,11; 2017,Jun,3; 2017,Jan,3

99170 Specialized Examination of Child

EXCLUDES *Moderate sedation (99151-99157)*

99170 **Anogenital examination, magnified, in childhood for suspected trauma, including image recording when performed** A

2.47 4.48 FUD 000 T

AMA: 2018,Jan,8; 2017,Jan,8; 2016,Jan,13; 2015,Jan,16

99172-99173 Visual Acuity Screening Tests

INCLUDES Graduated visual acuity stimuli that allow quantitative determination/estimation visual acuity

EXCLUDES *General ophthalmological or E/M services*

99172 **Visual function screening, automated or semi-automated bilateral quantitative determination of visual acuity, ocular alignment, color vision by pseudoisochromatic plates, and field of vision (may include all or some screening of the determination[s] for contrast sensitivity, vision under glare)**

EXCLUDES *Screening for visual acuity, amblyogenic factors, retinal polarization scan (99173, 99174 [99177], 0469T)*

0.00 0.00 FUD XXX E

AMA: 2018,Jan,8; 2017,Jan,8; 2016,Jan,13; 2015,Jan,16

99173 **Screening test of visual acuity, quantitative, bilateral**

EXCLUDES *Screening for visual function, amblyogenic factors (99172, 99174, [99177])*

0.08 0.08 FUD XXX E

AMA: 2018,Jan,8; 2017,Jan,8; 2016,Jan,13; 2015,Jan,16

99174-99177 [99177] Screening For Amblyogenic Factors

EXCLUDES *General ophthalmological services (92002-92014)*

Screening for visual acuity (99172-99173, [99177])

99174 **Instrument-based ocular screening (eg, photoscreening, automated-refraction), bilateral; with remote analysis and report**

EXCLUDES *Ocular screening on-site analysis ([99177])*

0.16 0.16 FUD XXX E

AMA: 2018,Feb,3; 2018,Jan,8; 2017,Jan,8; 2016,Mar,10; 2016,Jan,13; 2015,Jan,16

99177 **with on-site analysis**

EXCLUDES *Remote ocular screening (99174)*

Retinal polarization scan (0469T)

0.14 0.14 FUD XXX E

AMA: 2018,Feb,3; 2018,Jan,8; 2017,Jan,8; 2016,Mar,10

99175-99177 [99177] Drug Administration to Induce Vomiting

EXCLUDES *Diagnostic gastric lavage (43754-43755)*

Diagnostic gastric intubation (43754-43755)

99175 **Ipecac or similar administration for individual emesis and continued observation until stomach adequately emptied of poison**

0.73 0.73 FUD XXX N 80

AMA: 1997,Nov,1

99177 **Resequenced code. See code following 99174.**

99183-99184 Hyperbaric Oxygen Therapy

CMS: 100-03,20.29 Hyperbaric Oxygen Therapy; 100-04,32,30.1 HBO Therapy for Lower Extremity Diabetic Wounds

EXCLUDES *E/M services, when performed*

Other procedures such as wound debridement, when performed

99183 **Physician or other qualified health care professional attendance and supervision of hyperbaric oxygen therapy, per session**

3.12 3.12 FUD XXX B 80 26

AMA: 2018,Jan,8; 2017,Jan,8; 2016,Jan,13; 2015,Jan,16

99184 **Initiation of selective head or total body hypothermia in the critically ill neonate, includes appropriate patient selection by review of clinical, imaging and laboratory data, confirmation of esophageal temperature probe location, evaluation of amplitude EEG, supervision of controlled hypothermia, and assessment of patient tolerance of cooling** A

EXCLUDES *Reporting code more than one time per hospitalization*

6.33 6.33 FUD XXX C 80

AMA: 2018,Jan,8; 2017,Jan,8; 2016,Jan,13; 2015,Oct,8

Medicine

99153 — 99184

99188 Topical Fluoride Application

99188 **Application of topical fluoride varnish by a physician or other qualified health care professional**
Facility RVU 0.29 Non-Facility RVU 0.35 FUD XXX E 80 CCI

99190-99192 Assemble and Manage Pump with Oxygenator/Heat Exchange

99190 **Assembly and operation of pump with oxygenator or heat exchanger (with or without ECG and/or pressure monitoring); each hour**
Facility RVU 0.00 Non-Facility RVU 0.00 FUD XXX C CCI
AMA: 1997,Nov,1

99191 **45 minutes**
Facility RVU 0.00 Non-Facility RVU 0.00 FUD XXX C CCI
AMA: 1997,Nov,1

99192 **30 minutes**
Facility RVU 0.00 Non-Facility RVU 0.00 FUD XXX C CCI
AMA: 1997,Nov,1

99195-99199 Therapeutic Phlebotomy and Unlisted Procedures

99195 **Phlebotomy, therapeutic (separate procedure)**
Facility RVU 2.86 Non-Facility RVU 2.86 FUD XXX Q1 80 CCI
AMA: 2018,Jan,8; 2017,Jan,8; 2016,Jan,13; 2015,Jan,16

99199 **Unlisted special service, procedure or report**
Facility RVU 0.00 Non-Facility RVU 0.00 FUD XXX B 80 CCI
AMA: 2018,Jan,8; 2017,Jan,8; 2016,Jan,13; 2015,Jan,16

99500-99602 Home Visit By Non-Physician Professionals

INCLUDES Services performed by non-physician providers
Services provided in patient's:
- Assisted living apartment
- Custodial care facility
- Group home
- Nontraditional private home
- Residence
- School

EXCLUDES *Home visits performed by physicians (99341-99350)*
Other services/procedures provided by physicians to patients at home

Code also home visit E/M codes when health care provider authorized to report (99341-99350)

Code also significant separately identifiable E/M service, when performed

99500 **Home visit for prenatal monitoring and assessment to include fetal heart rate, non-stress test, uterine monitoring, and gestational diabetes monitoring** M ♀
Facility RVU 0.00 Non-Facility RVU 0.00 FUD XXX E CCI
AMA: 2018,Jan,8; 2017,Jan,8; 2016,Jan,13; 2015,Jan,16

99501 **Home visit for postnatal assessment and follow-up care** M ♀
Facility RVU 0.00 Non-Facility RVU 0.00 FUD XXX E CCI
AMA: 2018,Jan,8; 2017,Jan,8; 2016,Jan,13; 2015,Jan,16

99502 **Home visit for newborn care and assessment** A
Facility RVU 0.00 Non-Facility RVU 0.00 FUD XXX E CCI
AMA: 2018,Jan,8; 2017,Jan,8; 2016,Jan,13; 2015,Jan,16

99503 **Home visit for respiratory therapy care (eg, bronchodilator, oxygen therapy, respiratory assessment, apnea evaluation)**
Facility RVU 0.00 Non-Facility RVU 0.00 FUD XXX E CCI
AMA: 2018,Jan,8; 2017,Jan,8; 2016,Jan,13; 2015,Jan,16

99504 **Home visit for mechanical ventilation care**
Facility RVU 0.00 Non-Facility RVU 0.00 FUD XXX E CCI
AMA: 2018,Jan,8; 2017,Jan,8; 2016,Jan,13; 2015,Jan,16

99505 **Home visit for stoma care and maintenance including colostomy and cystostomy**
Facility RVU 0.00 Non-Facility RVU 0.00 FUD XXX E CCI
AMA: 2018,Jan,8; 2017,Jan,8; 2016,Jan,13; 2015,Jan,16

99506 **Home visit for intramuscular injections**
Facility RVU 0.00 Non-Facility RVU 0.00 FUD XXX E CCI
AMA: 2018,Jan,8; 2017,Jan,8; 2016,Jan,13; 2015,Jan,16

99507 **Home visit for care and maintenance of catheter(s) (eg, urinary, drainage, and enteral)**
Facility RVU 0.00 Non-Facility RVU 0.00 FUD XXX E CCI
AMA: 2018,Jan,8; 2017,Jan,8; 2016,Jan,13; 2015,Jan,16

99509 **Home visit for assistance with activities of daily living and personal care**
EXCLUDES *Medical nutrition therapy/assessment home services (97802-97804)*
Self-care/home management training (97535)
Speech therapy home services (92507-92508)
Facility RVU 0.00 Non-Facility RVU 0.00 FUD XXX E CCI
AMA: 2018,Jan,8; 2017,Jan,8; 2016,Jan,13; 2015,Jan,16

99510 **Home visit for individual, family, or marriage counseling**
Facility RVU 0.00 Non-Facility RVU 0.00 FUD XXX E CCI
AMA: 2018,Jan,8; 2017,Jan,8; 2016,Jan,13; 2015,Jan,16

99511 **Home visit for fecal impaction management and enema administration**
Facility RVU 0.00 Non-Facility RVU 0.00 FUD XXX E CCI
AMA: 2018,Jan,8; 2017,Jan,8; 2016,Jan,13; 2015,Jan,16

99512 **Home visit for hemodialysis**
EXCLUDES *Peritoneal dialysis home infusion (99601-99602)*
Facility RVU 0.00 Non-Facility RVU 0.00 FUD XXX E CCI
AMA: 2018,Jan,8; 2017,Jan,8; 2016,Jan,13; 2015,Jan,16

99600 **Unlisted home visit service or procedure**
Facility RVU 0.00 Non-Facility RVU 0.00 FUD XXX E CCI
AMA: 2018,Jan,8; 2017,Jan,8; 2016,Jan,13; 2015,Jan,16

99601 **Home infusion/specialty drug administration, per visit (up to 2 hours);**
Facility RVU 0.00 Non-Facility RVU 0.00 FUD XXX E CCI
AMA: 2005,Nov,1-9; 2003,Oct,7

\+ **99602** **each additional hour (List separately in addition to code for primary procedure)**
Code first (99601)
Facility RVU 0.00 Non-Facility RVU 0.00 FUD XXX E CCI
AMA: 2005,Nov,1-9; 2003,Oct,7

99605-99607 Medication Management By Pharmacist

INCLUDES Direct (face-to-face) assessment and intervention by pharmacist:
- Managing medication complications and/or interactions
- Maximizing patient's response to drug therapy

Documenting required elements:
- Advice given regarding improvement treatment compliance and outcomes
- Medication profile (prescription and nonprescription)
- Review applicable patient history

EXCLUDES *Routine tasks associated with dispensing and related activities (e.g., providing product information)*

99605 **Medication therapy management service(s) provided by a pharmacist, individual, face-to-face with patient, with assessment and intervention if provided; initial 15 minutes, new patient**
Facility RVU 0.00 Non-Facility RVU 0.00 FUD XXX E CCI
AMA: 2018,Apr,9; 2018,Jan,8; 2017,Jan,8; 2016,Jan,13; 2015,Jan,16

99606 **initial 15 minutes, established patient**
Facility RVU 0.00 Non-Facility RVU 0.00 FUD XXX E CCI
AMA: 2018,Apr,9; 2018,Jan,8; 2017,Jan,8; 2016,Jan,13; 2015,Jan,16

\+ **99607** **each additional 15 minutes (List separately in addition to code for primary service)**
Code first (99605, 99606)
Facility RVU 0.00 Non-Facility RVU 0.00 FUD XXX E CCI
AMA: 2018,Apr,9; 2018,Jan,8; 2017,Jan,8; 2016,Jan,13; 2015,Jan,16

Evaluation and Management (E/M) Services Guidelines

Information unique to this section is defined or identified below.

For additional information about evaluation and management services, see Appendix C: Evaluation and Management Extended Guidelines. This appendix includes comprehensive explanations and instructions for the correct selection of an E&M service code based on federal documentation standards.

Classification of Evaluation and Management (E/M) Services

The E/M section is divided into broad categories such as office visits, hospital visits, and consultations. Most of the categories are further divided into two or more subcategories of E/M services. For example, there are two subcategories of office visits (new patient and established patient) and there are two subcategories of hospital visits (initial and subsequent). The subcategories of E/M services are further classified into levels of E/M services that are identified by specific codes.

The basic format of the levels of E/M services is the same for most categories. First, a unique code number is listed. Second, the place and/or type of service is specified, eg, office consultation. Third, the content of the service is defined. Fourth, time is specified. (A detailed discussion of time is provided following the Decision Tree for New vs Established Patients.)

Definitions of Commonly Used Terms

Certain key words and phrases are used throughout the E/M section. The following definitions are intended to reduce the potential for differing interpretations and to increase the consistency of reporting by physicians and other qualified health care professionals. The definitions in the E/M section are provided solely for the basis of code selection.

Some definitions are common to all categories of services, and others are specific to one or more categories only.

New and Established Patient

Solely for the purposes of distinguishing between new and established patients, professional services are those face-to-face services rendered by physicians and other qualified health care professionals who may report E/M services with a specific CPT® code or codes. A new patient is one who has not received any professional services from the physician/qualified health care professional or another physician/qualified health care professional of the exact same specialty and subspecialty who belongs to the same group practice, within the past three years.

An established patient is one who has received professional services from the physician/qualified health care professional or another physician/qualified health care professional of the exact same specialty and subspecialty who belongs to the same group practice, within the past three years. See the decision tree at right.

When a physician/qualified health care professional is on call or covering for another physician/qualified health care professional, the patient's encounter is classified as it would have been by the physician/qualified health care professional who is not available. When advanced practice nurses and physician assistants are working with physicians, they are considered as working in the exact same specialty and exact same subspecialties as the physician.

No distinction is made between new and established patients in the emergency department. E/M services in the emergency department category may be reported for any new or established patient who presents for treatment in the emergency department.

The decision tree in the next column is provided to aid in determining whether to report the E/M service provided as a new or an established patient encounter.

Time

The inclusion of time in the definitions of levels of E/M services has been implicit in prior editions of the CPT codebook. The inclusion of time as an explicit factor beginning in CPT 1992 was done to assist in selecting the most appropriate level of E/M services. Beginning with CPT 2021, except for 99211, time alone may be used to select the appropriate code level for the office or other outpatient E/M services codes (99202, 99203, 99204, 99205, 99212, 99213, 99214, 99215). Different categories of services use time differently. It is important to review the instructions for each category.

Time is **not** a descriptive component for the emergency department levels of E/M services because emergency department services are typically provided on a variable intensity basis, often involving multiple encounters with several patients over an extended period of time. Therefore, it is often difficult to provide accurate estimates of the time spent face-to-face with the patient.

Time may be used to select a code level in office or other outpatient services whether or not counseling and/or coordination of care dominates the service. Time may only be used for selecting the level of the ***other*** E/M services when counseling and/or coordination of care dominates the service.

When time is used for reporting E/M services codes, the time defined in the service descriptors is used for selecting the appropriate level of services. The E/M services for which these guidelines apply require a face-to-face encounter with the physician or other qualified health care professional. For office or other outpatient services, if the physician's or other qualified health care professional's time is spent in the supervision of clinical staff who perform the face-to-face services of the encounter, use 99211.

A shared or split visit is defined as a visit in which a physician and other qualified health care professional(s) jointly provide the face-to-face and non-face-to-face work related to the visit. When time is being used to select the appropriate level of services for which time-based reporting of shared or split visits is allowed, the time personally spent by the physician and other qualified health care professional(s) assessing and managing the patient on the date of the encounter is summed to define total time. Only distinct time should be summed for shared or split visits (ie, when two or more individuals jointly meet with or discuss the patient, only the time of one individual should be counted).

When prolonged time occurs, the appropriate prolonged services code may be reported. The appropriate time should be documented in the medical record when it is used as the basis for code selection.

Face-to-face time (outpatient consultations [99241, 99242, 99243, 99244, 99245], domiciliary, rest home, or custodial services [99324, 99325, 99326, 99327, 99328, 99334, 99335, 99336, 99337], home services [99341, 99342, 99343, 99344, 99345, 99347, 99348, 99349, 99350], cognitive assessment and care plan services [99483]): For coding purposes, face-to-face time for these services is defined as only that time spent face-to-face with the patient and/or family. This includes the time spent performing such tasks as obtaining a history, examination, and counseling the patient.

Unit/floor time (hospital observation services [99218, 99219, 99220, 99224, 99225, 99226, 99234, 99235, 99236], hospital inpatient services [99221, 99222, 99223, 99231, 99232, 99233], inpatient consultations [99251, 99252, 99253, 99254, 99255], nursing facility services [99304, 99305, 99306, 99307, 99308, 99309, 99310, 99315, 99316, 99318]): For coding purposes, time for these services is defined as unit/floor time, which includes the time present on the patient's hospital unit and at the bedside rendering services for that patient. This includes the time to establish and/or review the patient's chart, examine the patient, write notes, and communicate with other professionals and the patient's family.

Total time on the date of the encounter (office or other outpatient services [99202, 99203, 99204, 99205, 99212, 99213, 99214, 99215]): For coding purposes, time for these services is the total time on the date of the encounter. It includes both the face-to-face and non-face-to-face time personally spent by the physician and/or other qualified health care professional(s) on the day of the encounter (includes time in activities that require the physician or other qualified health care professional and does not include time in activities normally performed by clinical staff).

Physician/other qualified health care professional time includes the following activities, when performed:

- Preparing to see the patient (e.g., review of tests)

- Obtaining and/or reviewing separately obtained history
- Performing a medically appropriate examination and/or evaluation
- Counseling and educating the patient/family/caregiver
- Ordering medications, tests, or procedures
- Referring and communicating with other health care professionals (when not separately reported)
- Documenting clinical information in the electronic or other health record
- Independently interpreting results (not separately reported) and communicating results to the patient/family/caregiver
- Care coordination (not separately reported)

Concurrent Care and Transfer of Care

Concurrent care is the provision of similar services (e.g., hospital visits) to the same patient by more than one physician or other qualified health care professional on the same day. When concurrent care is provided, no special reporting is required. Transfer of care is the process whereby a physician or other qualified health care professional who is managing some or all of a patient's problems relinquishes this responsibility to another physician or other qualified health care professional who explicitly agrees to accept this responsibility and who, from the initial encounter, is not providing consultative services. The physician or other qualified health care professional transferring care is then no longer providing care for these problems though he or she may continue providing care for other conditions when appropriate. Consultation codes should not be reported by the physician or other qualified health care professional who has agreed to accept transfer of care before an initial evaluation, but they are appropriate to report if the decision to accept transfer of care cannot be made until after the initial consultation evaluation, regardless of site of service.

Decision Tree for New vs Established Patients

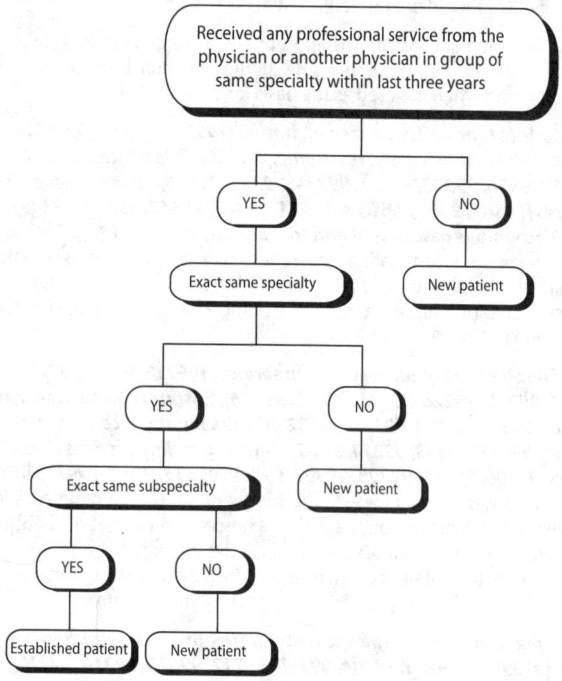

Counseling

Counseling is a discussion with a patient and/or family concerning one or more of the following areas:

- Diagnostic results, impressions, and/or recommended diagnostic studies
- Prognosis
- Risks and benefits of management (treatment) options
- Instructions for management (treatment) and/or follow-up
- Importance of compliance with chosen management (treatment) options
- Risk factor reduction
- Patient and family education
  (For psychotherapy, see 90832–90834, 90836–90840)

Services Reported Separately

Any specifically identifiable procedure or service (ie, identified with a specific CPT code) performed on the date of E/M services may be reported separately.

The actual performance and/or interpretation of diagnostic tests/studies during a patient encounter are not included in determining the levels of E/M services when reported separately. Physician performance of diagnostic tests/studies for which specific CPT codes are available may be reported separately, in addition to the appropriate E/M code. The physician's interpretation of the results of diagnostic tests/studies (ie, professional component) with preparation of a separation distinctly identifiable signed written report may also be reported separately, using the appropriate CPT code and, if required, with modifier 26 appended. If a test/study is independently interpreted in order to manage the patient as part of the E/M service, but is not separately reported, it is part of MDM.

The physician or other qualified health care professional may need to indicate that on the day a procedure or service identified by a CPT code was performed, the patient's condition required a significant separately identifiable E/M service. The E/M service may be caused or prompted by the symptoms or condition for which the procedure and/or service was provided. This circumstance may be reported by adding modifier 25 to the appropriate level of E/M service. As such, different diagnoses are not required for reporting of the procedure and the E/M services on the same date.

Levels of E/M Services

Within each category or subcategory of E/M service, there are three to five levels of E/M services available for reporting purposes. Levels of E/M services are **not** interchangeable among the different categories or subcategories of service. For example, the first level of E/M services in the subcategory of office visit, new patient, does not have the same definition as the first level of E/M services in the subcategory of office visit, established patient. Each level of E/M services may be used by all physicians or other qualified health care professionals.

The levels of E/M services include examinations, evaluations, treatments, conferences with or concerning patients, preventive pediatric and adult health supervision, and similar medical services, such as the determination of the need and/or location for appropriate care. Medical screening includes the history, examination, and medical decision-making required to determine the need and/or location for appropriate care and treatment of the patient (eg, office and other outpatient setting, emergency department, nursing facility). The levels of E/M services encompass the wide variations in skill, effort, time, responsibility, and medical knowledge required for the prevention or diagnosis and treatment of illness or injury and the promotion of optimal health. Each level of E/M services may be used by all physicians or other qualified health care professionals.

The descriptors for the levels of E/M services recognize seven components, six of which are used in defining the levels of E/M services. These components are:

- History
- Examination
- Medical decision making
- Counseling
- Coordination of care
- Nature of presenting problem
- Time

The first three of these components (history, examination, and medical decision making) are considered the **key** components in selecting a level of E/M services. (See "Determine the Extent of History Obtained.")

The next three components (counseling, coordination of care, and the nature of the presenting problem) are considered **contributory** factors in the majority of encounters. Although the first two of these contributory factors are important E/M services, it is not required that these services be provided at every patient encounter.

Coordination of care with other physicians, other qualified health care professionals, or agencies without a patient encounter on that day is reported using the case management codes.

The final component, time, is discussed in detail before the Decision Tree for New vs Established Patients.

Chief Complaint

A chief complaint is a concise statement describing the symptom, problem, condition, diagnosis, or other factor that is the reason for the encounter, usually stated in the patient's words.

History of Present Illness

A chronological description of the development of the patient's present illness from the first sign and/or symptom to the present. This includes a description of location, quality, severity, timing, context, modifying factors, and associated signs and symptoms significantly related to the presenting problem.

Nature of Presenting Problem

A presenting problem is a disease, condition, illness, injury, symptom, sign, finding, complaint, or other reason for encounter, with or without a diagnosis being established at the time of the encounter. The E/M codes recognize five types of presenting problems that are defined as follows:

Minimal: A problem that may not require the presence of the physician or other qualified health care professional, but service is provided under the physician's or other qualified health care professional's supervision.

Self-limited or minor: A problem that runs a definite and prescribed course, is transient in nature, and is not likely to permanently alter health status.

Low severity: A problem where the risk of morbidity without treatment is low; there is little to no risk of mortality without treatment; full recovery without functional impairment is expected.

Moderate severity: A problem where the risk of morbidity without treatment is moderate; there is moderate risk of mortality without treatment; uncertain prognosis OR increased probability of prolonged functional impairment.

High severity: A problem where the risk of morbidity without treatment is high to extreme; there is a moderate to high risk of mortality without treatment OR high probability of severe, prolonged functional impairment.

Past History

A review of the patient's past experiences with illnesses, injuries, and treatments that includes significant information about:

- Prior major illnesses and injuries
- Prior operations
- Prior hospitalizations
- Current medications
- Allergies (eg, drug, food)
- Age appropriate immunization status
- Age appropriate feeding/dietary status

Family History

A review of medical events in the patient's family that includes significant information about:

- The health status of cause of death of parents, siblings, and children
- Specific diseases related to problems identified in the Chief Complaint or History of the Present Illness, and/or System Review
- Diseases of family members that may be hereditary or place the patient at risk

Social History

An age appropriate review of past and current activities that includes significant information about:

- Marital status and/or living arrangements
- Current employment
- Occupational history
- Military history
- Use of drugs, alcohol, and tobacco
- Level of education
- Sexual history
- Other relevant social factors

System Review (Review of Systems)

An inventory of body systems obtained through a series of questions seeking to identify signs and/or symptoms that the patient may be experiencing or has experienced. For the purposes of the CPT codebook the following elements of a system review have been identified:

- Constitutional symptoms (fever, weight loss, etc)
- Eyes
- Ears, nose, mouth, throat
- Cardiovascular
- Respiratory
- Gastrointestinal
- Genitourinary
- Musculoskeletal
- Integumentary (skin and/or breast)
- Neurological
- Psychiatric
- Endocrine
- Hematologic/lymphatic
- Allergic/immunologic

The review of systems helps define the problem, clarify the differential diagnosis, identify needed testing, or serves as baseline data on other systems that might be affected by any possible management options.

Instructions for Selecting a Level of E/M Service

Review the Reporting Instructions for the Selected Category or Subcategory

Most of the categories and many of the subcategories of service have special guidelines or instructions unique to that category or subcategory. Where these are indicated, eg, "Inpatient Hospital Care," special instructions will be presented preceding the levels of E/M services.

Review the Level of E/M Service Descriptors and Examples in the Selected Category or Subcategory

The descriptors for the levels of E/M services recognize seven components, six of which are used in defining the levels of E/M services. These components are:

- History
- Examination
- Medical decision making
- Counseling
- Coordination of care
- Nature of presenting problem
- Time

The first three of these components (ie, history, examination, and medical decision making) should be considered the **key** components in selecting the level of E/M services. An exception to this rule is in the case of visits that consist predominantly of counseling or coordination of care.

The nature of the presenting problem and time are provided in some levels to assist the physician in determining the appropriate level of E/M service.

Determine the Extent of History Obtained

The extent of the history is dependent upon clinical judgment and on the nature of the presenting problem(s). The levels of E/M services recognize four types of history that are defined as follows:

Problem focused: Chief complaint; brief history of present illness or problem.

Expanded problem focused: Chief complaint; brief history of present illness; problem pertinent system review.

Detailed: Chief complaint; extended history of present illness; problem pertinent system review extended to include a review of a limited number of additional systems; pertinent past, family, and/or social history directly related to the patient's problems.

Comprehensive: Chief complaint; extended history of present illness; review of systems that is directly related to the problem(s) identified in the history of the present illness plus a review of all additional body systems; **complete** past, family, and social history.

The comprehensive history obtained as part of the preventive medicine E/M service is not problem-oriented and does not involve a chief complaint or present illness. It does, however, include a comprehensive system review and comprehensive or interval past, family, and social history as well as a comprehensive assessment/history of pertinent risk factors.

Determine the Extent of Examination Performed

The extent of the examination performed is dependent on clinical judgment and on the nature of the presenting problem(s). The levels of E/M services recognize four types of examination that are defined as follows:

Problem focused: A limited examination of the affected body area or organ system.

Expanded problem focused: A limited examination of the affected body area or organ system and other symptomatic or related organ system(s).

Detailed: An extended examination of the affected body area(s) and other symptomatic or related organ system(s).

Comprehensive: A general multisystem examination or a complete examination of a single organ system. **Note:** The comprehensive examination performed as part of the preventive medicine E/M service is multisystem, but its extent is based on age and risk factors identified.

For the purposes of these CPT definitions, the following body areas are recognized:

- Head, including the face
- Neck
- Chest, including breasts and axilla
- Abdomen
- Genitalia, groin, buttocks
- Back
- Each extremity

For the purposes of these CPT definitions, the following organ systems are recognized:

- Eyes
- Ears, nose, mouth, and throat
- Cardiovascular
- Respiratory
- Gastrointestinal
- Genitourinary
- Musculoskeletal
- Skin
- Neurologic
- Psychiatric
- Hematologic/lymphatic/immunologic

Determine the Complexity of Medical Decision Making

Medical decision making refers to the complexity of establishing a diagnosis and/or selecting a management option as measured by:

- The number of possible diagnoses and/or the number of management options that must be considered
- The amount and/or complexity of medical records, diagnostic tests, and/or other information that must be obtained, reviewed, and analyzed
- The risk of significant complications, morbidity, and/or mortality, as well as comorbidities associated with the patient's presenting problem(s), the diagnostic procedure(s), and/or the possible management options

Four types of medical decision making are recognized: straightforward, low complexity, moderate complexity, and high complexity. To qualify for a given type of decision making, two of the three elements in Table 1 must be met or exceeded.

Comorbidities and underlying diseases, in and of themselves, are not considered in selecting a level of E/M services unless their presence significantly increases the complexity of the medical decision making.

Select the Appropriate Level of E/M Services Based on the Following

For the following categories/subcategories, **all of the key components**, ie, history, examination, and medical decision making, must meet or exceed the stated requirements to qualify for a particular level of E/M service: initial observation care; initial hospital care; observation or inpatient hospital care (including admission and discharge services); office or other outpatient consultations; inpatient consultations; emergency department services; initial nursing facility care; other nursing facility services; domiciliary care, new patient; and home services, new patient.

For the following categories/subcategories, **two of the three key components** (ie, history, examination, and medical decision making) must meet or exceed the stated requirements to qualify for a particular level of E/M services: subsequent observation care; subsequent hospital care; subsequent nursing facility care; domiciliary care, established patient; and home services, established patient.

When counseling and/or coordination of care dominates (more than 50 percent) the encounter with the patient and/or family (face-to-face time in the office or other outpatient setting or floor/unit time in the hospital or nursing facility), then **time** shall be considered the key or controlling factor to qualify for a particular level of E/M services. This includes time spent with parties who have assumed responsibility for the care of the patient or decision making whether or not they are family members (e.g., foster parents, person acting in loco parentis, legal guardian). The extent of counseling and/or coordination of care must be documented in the medical record.

CONSULTATION CODES AND MEDICARE REIMBURSEMENT

The Centers for Medicare and Medicaid Services (CMS) no longer provides benefits for CPT consultation codes. CMS has, however, redistributed the value of the consultation codes across the other E/M codes for services which are covered by Medicare. CMS has retained codes 99241 - 99251 in the Medicare Physician Fee Schedule for those private payers that use this data for reimbursement. Note that private payers may choose to follow CMS or CPT guidelines, and the use of consultation codes should be verified with individual payers.

Table 1

Complexity of Medical Decision Making

Number of Diagnoses or Management Options	*Amount and/or Complexity of Data to Be Reviewed*	*Risk of Complications and/or Morbidity or Mortality*	*Type of Decision Making*
minimal	minimal or none	minimal	**straightforward**
limited	limited	low	**low complexity**
multiple	moderate	moderate	**moderate complexity**
extensive	extensive	high	**high complexity**

Guidelines for Office or Other Outpatient E/M Services

History and/or Examination

Office or other outpatient services include a medically appropriate history and/or physical examination, when performed. The nature and extent of the history and/or physical examination are determined by the treating physician or other qualified health care professional reporting the service. The care team may collect information and the patient or caregiver may supply information directly (eg, by electronic health record [EHR] portal or questionnaire) that is reviewed by the reporting physician or other qualified health care professional. The extent of history and physical examination is not an element in selection of the level of office or other outpatient code.

Number and Complexity of Problems Addressed at the Encounter

One element used in selecting the level of office or other outpatient services is the number and complexity of the problems that are addressed at an encounter. Multiple new or established conditions may be addressed at the same time and may affect MDM. Symptoms may cluster around a specific diagnosis and each symptom is not necessarily a unique condition. Comorbidities/underlying diseases, in and of themselves, are not considered in selecting a level of E/M services **unless** they are addressed, and their presence increases the amount and/or complexity of data to be reviewed and analyzed or the risk of complications and/or morbidity or mortality of patient management. The final diagnosis for a condition does not, in and of itself, determine the complexity or risk, as extensive evaluation may be required to reach the conclusion that the signs or symptoms do not represent a highly morbid condition. Multiple problems of a lower severity may, in the aggregate, create higher risk due to interaction. Definitions for the elements of MDM (see Table 2, Levels of Medical Decision Making) for other office or other outpatient services are:

Problem: A problem is a disease, condition, illness, injury, symptom, sign, finding, complaint, or other matter addressed at the encounter, with or without a diagnosis being established at the time of the encounter.

Problem addressed: A problem is addressed or managed when it is evaluated or treated at the encounter by the physician or other qualified health care professional reporting the service. This includes consideration of further testing or treatment that may not be elected by virtue of risk/benefit analysis or patient/parent/guardian/surrogate choice. Notation in the patient's medical record that another professional is managing the problem without additional assessment or care coordination documented does not qualify as being addressed or managed by the physician or other qualified health care professional reporting the service. Referral without evaluation (by history, examination, or diagnostic study[ies]) or consideration of treatment does not qualify as being addressed or managed by the physician or other qualified health care professional reporting the service.

Minimal problem: A problem that may not require the presence of the physician or other qualified health care professional, but the service is provided under the physician's or other qualified health care professional's supervision (see 99211).

Self-limited or minor problem: A problem that runs a definite and prescribed course, is transient in nature, and is not likely to permanently alter health status.

Stable, chronic illness: A problem with an expected duration of at least one year or until the death of the patient. For the purpose of defining chronicity, conditions are treated as chronic whether or not stage or severity changes (eg, uncontrolled diabetes and controlled diabetes are a single chronic condition). "Stable" for the purposes of categorizing MDM is defined by the specific treatment goals for an individual patient. A patient who is not at his or her treatment goal is not stable, even if the condition has not changed and there is no short\term threat to life or function. For example, in a patient with persistently poorly controlled blood pressure for whom better control is a goal is not stable, even if the pressures are not changing and the patient is asymptomatic, the risk of morbidity **without** treatment is significant. Examples may include well-controlled hypertension, non-insulin dependent diabetes, cataract, or benign prostatic hyperplasia.

Acute, uncomplicated illness or injury: A recent or new short-term problem with low risk of morbidity for which treatment is considered. There is little to no risk of mortality with treatment, and full recovery without functional impairment is expected. A problem that is normally self-limited or minor but is not resolving consistent with a definite and prescribed course is an acute, uncomplicated illness. Examples may include cystitis, allergic rhinitis, or a simple sprain.

Chronic illness with exacerbation, progression, or side effects of treatment: A chronic illness that is acutely worsening, poorly controlled, or progressing with an intent to control progression and requiring additional supportive care or requiring attention to treatment for side effects but that does not require consideration of hospital level of care.

Undiagnosed new problem with uncertain prognosis: A problem in the differential diagnosis that represents a condition likely to result in a high risk of morbidity without treatment. An example may be a lump in the breast.

Acute illness with systemic symptoms: An illness that causes systemic symptoms and has a high risk of morbidity without treatment. For systemic general symptoms, such as fever, body aches, or fatigue in a minor illness that may be treated to alleviate symptoms, shorten the course of illness, or to prevent complications, see the definitions for self-limited or minor problem or acute, uncomplicated illness or injury. Systemic symptoms may not be general but may be single system. Examples may include pyelonephritis, pneumonitis, or colitis.

Acute, complicated injury: An injury which requires treatment that includes evaluation of body systems that are not directly part of the injured organ, the injury is extensive, or the treatment options are multiple and/or associated with risk of morbidity. An example may be a head injury with brief loss of consciousness.

Chronic illness with severe exacerbation, progression, or side effects of treatment: The severe exacerbation or progression of a chronic illness or severe side effects of treatment that have significant risk of morbidity and may require hospital level of care.

Acute or chronic illness or injury that poses a threat to life or bodily function: An acute illness with systemic symptoms, an acute complicated injury, or a chronic illness or injury with exacerbation and/or progression or side effects of treatment, that poses a threat to life or bodily function in the near term without treatment. Examples may include acute myocardial infarction, pulmonary embolus, severe respiratory distress, progressive severe rheumatoid arthritis, psychiatric illness with potential threat to self or others, peritonitis, acute renal failure, or an abrupt change in neurologic status.

Test: Tests are imaging, laboratory, psychometric, or physiologic data. A clinical laboratory panel (eg, basic metabolic panel [80047]) is a single test. The differentiation between single or multiple unique tests is defined in accordance with the CPT code set.

External: External records, communications and/or test results are from an external physician, other qualified health care professional, facility, or health care organization.

External physician or other qualified health care professional: An external physician or other qualified health care professional who is not in the same group practice or is of a different specialty or subspecialty. This includes licensed professionals who are practicing independently. The individual may also be a facility or organizational provider such as from a hospital, nursing facility, or home health care agency.

Independent historian(s): An individual (eg, parent, guardian, surrogate, spouse, witness) who provides a history in addition to a history provided by the patient who is unable to provide a complete or reliable history (eg, due to developmental stage, dementia, or psychosis) or because a confirmatory history is judged to be necessary. In the case where there may be conflict or poor communication between multiple historians and more than one historian is needed, the independent historian requirement is met.

Independent interpretation: The interpretation of a test for which there is a CPT code and an interpretation or report is customary. This does not apply when the physician or other qualified health care professional is reporting the service or has previously report the service for the patient. A form of interpretation should be documented but need not conform to the usual standards of a complete report for the test.

Appropriate source: For the purpose of the **discussion of management** data element (see Table 2, Levels of Medical Decision Making), an appropriate source includes professionals who are not health care professionals but may be involved in the management of the patient (eg, lawyer, parole officer, case manager, teacher). It does not include discussion with family or informal caregivers.

Risk: The probability and/or consequences of an event. The assessment of the level of risk is affected by the nature of the event under consideration. For example, a low probability of death may be high risk, whereas a high chance of a minor, self-limited adverse effect of treatment may be low risk. Definitions of risk are based upon the usual behavior and thought processes of a physician or other qualified health care professional in the same specialty. Trained clinicians apply common language usage meanings to terms such as high, medium, low, or minimal risk and do not require quantification for these definitions (though quantification may be provided when evidence-based medicine has established probabilities). For the purposes of MDM, level of risk is based upon consequences of the problem(s) addressed at the encounter when appropriately treated. Risk also includes MDM related to the need to initiate or forego further testing, treatment, and/or hospitalization.

Morbidity: A state of illness or functional impairment that is expected to be of substantial duration during which function is limited, quality of life is impaired, or there is organ damage that may not be transient despite treatment.

Social determinants of health: Economic and social conditions that influence the health of people and communities. Examples may include food and housing insecurity.

Drug therapy requiring intensive monitoring for toxicity: A drug that requires intensive monitoring is a therapeutic agent that has the potential to cause serious morbidity or death., The monitoring is performed for assessment of these adverse effects and not primarily for assessment of therapeutic efficacy. The monitoring should be that which is generally accepted practice for the agent but may be patient-specific in some cases. Intensive monitoring may be long-term or short-term. Long-term intensive monitoring is not performed less than quarterly. The monitoring may be performed with a laboratory test, a physiologic test, or imaging. Monitoring by history or examination does not qualify. The monitoring affects the level of MDM in an encounter in which it is considered in the management of the patient. Examples may include monitoring for cytopenia in the use of an antineoplastic agent between dose cycles or the short-term intensive monitoring of electrolytes and renal function in a patient who is undergoing diuresis. Examples of monitoring that do not qualify include monitoring glucose levels during insulin therapy, as the primary reason is the therapeutic effect (even if hypoglycemia is a concern) or annual electrolytes and renal function for a patient on a diuretic, as the frequency does not meet the threshold.

Instructions for Selecting a Level of Office or Other Outpatient E/M Services

Select the appropriate level of E/M services based on the following:

1. The level of the MDM as defined for each service, or
2. The total time for E/M services performed on the date of the encounter.

Medical Decision Making

MDM includes establishing diagnoses, assessing the status of a condition, and/or selecting a management option. MDM in the office or other outpatient services codes is defined by three elements:

- The number and complexity of problem(s) that are addressed during the encounter.
- The amount and/or complexity of data to be reviewed and analyzed. These data include medical records, tests, and/or other information that must be obtained, ordered, reviewed, and analyzed for the encounter. This includes information obtained from multiple sources or interprofessional communications that are not reported separately and interpretation of tests that are not reported separately. Ordering a test is included in the category of test result(s) and the review of the test result is part of the encounter and not a subsequent encounter. Data are divided into three categories:
    - — Tests, documents, orders, or independent historian(s). (Each unique test, order, or document is counted to meet a threshold number.)
    - — Independent interpretation of tests.
    - — Discussion of management or test interpretation with external physician or other qualified health care professional or appropriate source.
- The risk of complications and/or morbidity or mortality of patient management decisions made at the visit, associated with the patient's problem(s), the diagnostic procedure(s), treatment(s). This includes the possible management options selected and those considered but not selected, after shared MDM with the patient and/or family. For example, a decision about hospitalization includes consideration of alternative levels of care. Examples may include a psychiatric patient with a sufficient degree of support in the outpatient setting or the decision to not hospitalize a patient with advanced dementia with an acute condition that would generally warrant in patient care, but for whom the goal is palliative treatment.

Four types of MDM are recognized: straightforward, low, moderate, and high. The concept of the level of MDM does not apply to 99211. Shared MDM involves eliciting patient and/or family preferences, patient and/or family education, and explaining risks and benefits of management options. MDM may be impacted by role and management responsibility.

When the physician or other qualified health care professional is reporting a separate CPT code that includes interpretation and/or report, the interpretation and/or report should not count toward the MDM when selecting a level of office or other outpatient services. When the physician or other qualified health care professional is reporting a separate service for discussion of management with a physician or another qualified health care professional, the discussion is not counted toward the MDM when selecting a level of office or other outpatient services.

The Levels of Medical Decision Making (MDM) table (Table2) is a guide to assist in selecting the level of MDM for reporting an office or other outpatient E/M services code. The table includes the four levels of MDM (ie, straightforward, low, moderate, high) and the three elements of MDM (ie, number and complexity of problems addressed at the encounter, amount and/or complexity of data reviewed and analyzed, and risk of complications and/or morbidity or mortality of patient management). To qualify for a particular level of MDM, two of the three elements for that level of MDM must be met or exceeded. See Table 2: Levels of Medical Decision Making (MDM) below.

Table 2: Levels of Medical Decision Making (MDM)

		Elements of Medical Decision Making		
Code	**Level of MDM (Based on 2 out of 3 Elements of MDM)**	**Number and Complexity of Problems Addressed**	**Amount and/or Complexity of Data to be Reviewed and Analyzed**	**Risk of Complications and/or Morbidity or Mortality of Patient Management**
99211	N/A	N/A	N/A	N/A
99202 **99212**	**Straightforward**	**Minimal** • **1** self-limited or minor problem	**Minimal or none**	**Minimal risk of morbidity from additional diagnostic testing or treatment**
99203 **99213**	**Low**	**Low** • **2** or more self-limited or minor problems; **or** • stable chronic illness; **or** • **1** acute, uncomplicated illness or injury	**Limited** *(Must meet the requirements of at least 1 of the 2 categories)* **Category 1: Tests and documents** • Any combination of 2 from the following: - Review of prior external note(s) from each unique source*; - review of the result(s) of each unique test*; - ordering of each unique test* **or** **Category 2: Assessment requiring an independent historian(s)** *(For the categories of independent interpretation of tests and discussion of management or test interpretation, see moderate or high)*	**Low risk of morbidity from additional diagnostic testing or treatment**

**Each unique test, order, or document contributes to the combination of 2 or combination of 3 in Category 1 below.*

Code	Level of MDM (Based on 2 out of 3 Elements of MDM)	Elements of Medical Decision Making: Number and Complexity of Problems Addressed	Amount and/or Complexity of Data to be Reviewed and Analyzed	Risk of Complications and/or Morbidity or Mortality of Patient Management
99204 99214	**Moderate**	**Moderate** • **1** or more chronic illnesses with exacerbation, progression, or side effects of treatment; **or** • **2** or more stable chronic illnesses; **or** • **1** undiagnosed new problem with uncertain prognosis; **or** • **1** acute illness with systemic symptoms; **or** • **1** acute complicated injury	**Moderate** *(Must meet the requirements of at least 1 out of 3 categories)* **Category 1: Tests, documents, or independent historian(s)** • Any combination of 3 from the following: - Review of prior external note(s) from each unique source*; - Review of the result(s) of each unique test*; - Ordering of each unique test*; - Assessment requiring an independent historian(s) **or** **Category 2: Independent interpretation of tests** • Independent interpretation of a test performed by another physician/other qualified health care professional (not separately reported); **or** **Category 3: Discussion of management or test interpretation** Discussion of management or test interpretation with external physician/other qualified health care professional\appropriate source (not separately reported)	**Moderate risk of morbidity from additional diagnostic testing or treatment** *Examples only:* • Prescription drug management • Decision regarding minor surgery with identified patient or procedure risk factors • Decision regarding elective major surgery without identified patient or procedure risk factors Diagnosis or treatment significantly limited by social determinants of health
99205 99215	**High**	**High** • **1** or more chronic illnesses with severe exacerbation, progression, or side effects of treatment; **or** • **1** acute or chronic illness or injury that poses a threat to life or bodily function	**Extensive** *(Must meet the requirements of at least 2 out of 3 categories)* **Category 1: Tests, documents, or independent historian(s)** • **Any combination of 3 from the following:** - Review of prior external note(s) from each unique source*; - Review of the result(s) of each unique test*; - Ordering of each unique test*; - Assessment requiring an independent historian(s) **or** **Category 2: Independent interpretation of tests** • **Independent interpretation of a test performed by another physician/other qualified health care professional (not separately reported);** **or** **Category 3: Discussion of management or test interpretation** • Discussion of management or test interpretation with external physician/other qualified health care professional/appropriate source (not separately reported)	**High risk of morbidity from additional diagnostic testing or treatment** *Examples only:* • Drug therapy requiring intensive monitoring for toxicity • Decision regarding elective major surgery with identified patient or procedure risk factors • Decision regarding emergency major surgery • Decision regarding hospitalization • Decision not to resuscitate or to de-escalate care because of poor prognosis

**Each unique test, order, or document contributes to the combination of 2 or combination of 3 in Category 1 below.*

Time

For instructions on using time to select the level of office or other outpatient E/M services code, see the ***Time*** subsection in the ***Guidelines Common to All E/M Services.***

Unlisted Service

An E/M service may be provided that is not listed in this section of the CPT codebook. When reporting such a service, the appropriate unlisted code may be used to indicate the service, identifying it by "Special Report," as discussed in the following paragraph. The "Unlisted Services" and accompanying codes for the E/M section are as follows:

99429 **Unlisted preventive** medicine service

99499 **Unlisted evaluation and management** service

Special Report

An unlisted service or one that is unusual, variable, or new may require a special report demonstrating the medical appropriateness of the service. Pertinent information should include an adequate definition or description of the nature, extent, and need for the procedure and the time, effort, and equipment necessary to provide the service. Additional items that may be included are complexity of symptoms, final diagnosis, pertinent physical findings, diagnostic and therapeutic procedures, concurrent problems, and follow-up care.

Clinical Examples

Clinical examples of the codes for E/M services are provided to assist in understanding the meaning of the descriptors and selecting the correct code. The clinical examples are listed in Appendix C. Each example was developed by the specialties shown. The same problem, when seen by different specialties, may involve different amounts of work. Therefore, the appropriate level of encounter should be reported using the descriptors rather than the examples.

99201-99215 Outpatient and Other Visits

CMS: 100-04,11,40.1.3 Independent Attending Physician Services; 100-04,12,190.3 List of Telehealth Services; 100-04,12,190.6 Payment Methodology for Physician/Practitioner at the Distant Site ; 100-04,12,190.6.1 Submission of Telehealth Claims for Distant Site Practitioners; 100-04,12,190.7 Contractor Editing of Telehealth Claims; 100-04,12,230 Primary Care Incentive Payment Program; 100-04,12,230.1 Definition of Primary Care Practitioners and Services; 100-04,12,230.2 Coordination with Other Payments; 100-04,12,230.3 Claims Processing and Payment; 100-04,12,30.6.10 Consultation Services; 100-04,12,30.6.15.1 Prolonged Services With Direct Face-to-Face Patient Contact; 100-04,12,30.6.4 Services Furnished Incident to Physician's Service; 100-04,12,30.6.7 Payment for Office or Other Outpatient E&M Visits; 100-04,12,40.3 Global Surgery Review; 100-04,18,80.2 Contractor Billing Requirements; 100-04,32,12.1 Counseling to Prevent Tobacco Use HCPCS and Diagnosis Coding; 100-04,32,130.1 Billing and Payment of External counterpulsation (ECP)

INCLUDES Established patients: received prior professional services from physician or qualified health care professional or another physician or qualified health care professional in exact same specialty practice and subspecialty in previous three years (99211-99215)

New patients: have not received professional services from physician or qualified health care professional or any other physician or qualified health care professional in same practice in exact same specialty and subspecialty in previous three years (99202-99205)

Office visits

Outpatient services (including services prior to formal admission to facility)

EXCLUDES *Services provided in:*

Emergency department (99281-99285)

Hospital observation (99217-99220 [99224, 99225, 99226])

Hospital observation or inpatient with same day admission and discharge (99234-99236)

~~99201~~ ~~**Office or other outpatient visit for the evaluation and management of a new patient, which requires these 3 key components: A problem focused history; A problem focused examination; Straightforward medical decision making. Counseling and/or coordination of care with other physicians, other qualified health care professionals, or agencies are provided consistent with the nature of the problem(s) and the patient's and/or family's needs. Usually, the presenting problem(s) are self limited or minor. Typically, 10 minutes are spent face-to-face with the patient and/or family.**~~

To report, see (99202)

▲ **99202** **Office or other outpatient visit for the evaluation and management of a new patient, which requires a medically appropriate history and/or examination and straightforward medical decision making. When using time for code selection, 15-29 minutes of total time is spent on the date of the encounter.**

1.43 2.15 **FUD** XXX ★ B 80

AMA: 2020,Sep,14; 2020,Sep,3; 2020,Jun,3; 2020,May,3; 2020,Feb,3; 2020,Jan,3; 2019,Oct,10; 2019,Feb,3; 2019,Jan,3; 2018,Sep,14; 2018,Apr,10; 2018,Apr,9; 2018,Mar,7; 2018,Jan,8; 2017,Aug,3; 2017,Jun,6; 2017,Jan,8; 2016,Dec,11; 2016,Sep,6; 2016,Mar,10; 2016,Jan,13; 2016,Jan,7; 2015,Dec,3; 2015,Oct,3; 2015,Jan,16; 2015,Jan,12

▲ **99203** **Office or other outpatient visit for the evaluation and management of a new patient, which requires a medically appropriate history and/or examination and low level of medical decision making. When using time for code selection, 30-44 minutes of total time is spent on the date of the encounter.**

2.15 3.05 **FUD** XXX ★ B 80

AMA: 2020,Sep,3; 2020,Sep,14; 2020,Jun,3; 2020,May,3; 2020,Feb,3; 2020,Jan,3; 2019,Oct,10; 2019,Feb,3; 2019,Jan,3; 2018,Sep,14; 2018,Apr,9; 2018,Apr,10; 2018,Mar,7; 2018,Jan,8; 2017,Aug,3; 2017,Jun,6; 2017,Jan,8; 2016,Dec,11; 2016,Sep,6; 2016,Mar,10; 2016,Jan,7; 2016,Jan,13; 2015,Dec,3; 2015,Oct,3; 2015,Jan,12; 2015,Jan,16

▲ **99204** **Office or other outpatient visit for the evaluation and management of a new patient, which requires a medically appropriate history and/or examination and moderate level of medical decision making. When using time for code selection, 45-59 minutes of total time is spent on the date of the encounter.**

3.64 4.63 **FUD** XXX ★ B 80

AMA: 2020,Sep,3; 2020,Sep,14; 2020,Jun,3; 2020,May,3; 2020,Feb,3; 2020,Jan,3; 2019,Oct,10; 2019,Feb,3; 2019,Jan,3; 2018,Sep,14; 2018,Apr,9; 2018,Apr,10; 2018,Mar,7; 2018,Jan,8; 2017,Aug,3; 2017,Jun,6; 2017,Jan,8; 2016,Dec,11; 2016,Sep,6; 2016,Mar,10; 2016,Jan,7; 2016,Jan,13; 2015,Dec,3; 2015,Oct,3; 2015,Jan,12; 2015,Jan,16

▲ **99205** **Office or other outpatient visit for the evaluation and management of a new patient, which requires a medically appropriate history and/or examination and high level of medical decision making. When using time for code selection, 60-74 minutes of total time is spent on the date of the encounter.**

Prolonged services (lasting 75 minutes or more) ([99417])

4.75 5.82 **FUD** XXX ★ B 80

AMA: 2020,Sep,3; 2020,Sep,14; 2020,Jun,3; 2020,May,3; 2020,Feb,3; 2020,Jan,3; 2019,Oct,10; 2019,Feb,3; 2019,Jan,3; 2018,Sep,14; 2018,Apr,9; 2018,Apr,10; 2018,Mar,7; 2018,Jan,8; 2017,Aug,3; 2017,Jun,6; 2017,Jan,8; 2016,Dec,11; 2016,Sep,6; 2016,Mar,10; 2016,Jan,7; 2016,Jan,13; 2015,Dec,3; 2015,Oct,3; 2015,Jan,12; 2015,Jan,16

▲ **99211** **Office or other outpatient visit for the evaluation and management of an established patient, that may not require the presence of a physician or other qualified health care professional. Usually, the presenting problem(s) are minimal.**

0.26 0.65 **FUD** XXX B 80

AMA: 2020,Sep,3; 2020,Sep,14; 2020,Jun,3; 2020,May,3; 2020,Feb,3; 2020,Jan,3; 2019,Oct,10; 2019,Feb,3; 2019,Jan,3; 2018,Sep,14; 2018,Apr,10; 2018,Apr,9; 2018,Mar,7; 2018,Jan,8; 2017,Aug,3; 2017,Jun,6; 2017,Mar,10; 2017,Jan,8; 2016,Dec,11; 2016,Sep,6; 2016,Mar,10; 2016,Jan,13; 2016,Jan,7; 2015,Dec,3; 2015,Oct,3; 2015,Jan,16; 2015,Jan,12

▲ **99212** **Office or other outpatient visit for the evaluation and management of an established patient, which requires a medically appropriate history and/or examination and straightforward medical decision making. When using time for code selection, 10-19 minutes of total time is spent on the date of the encounter.**

0.73 1.28 **FUD** XXX ★ B 80

AMA: 2020,Sep,3; 2020,Sep,14; 2020,Jun,3; 2020,May,3; 2020,Feb,3; 2020,Jan,3; 2019,Oct,10; 2019,Feb,3; 2019,Jan,3; 2018,Sep,14; 2018,Apr,9; 2018,Apr,10; 2018,Mar,7; 2018,Jan,8; 2017,Oct,5; 2017,Aug,3; 2017,Jun,6; 2017,Jan,8; 2016,Dec,11; 2016,Sep,6; 2016,Mar,10; 2016,Jan,7; 2016,Jan,13; 2015,Dec,3; 2015,Oct,3; 2015,Jan,12; 2015,Jan,16

▲ **99213** **Office or other outpatient visit for the evaluation and management of an established patient, which requires a medically appropriate history and/or examination and low level of medical decision making. When using time for code selection, 20-29 minutes of total time is spent on the date of the encounter.**

1.45 2.11 **FUD** XXX ★ B 80

AMA: 2020,Sep,3; 2020,Sep,14; 2020,Jun,3; 2020,May,3; 2020,Feb,3; 2020,Jan,3; 2019,Oct,10; 2019,Feb,3; 2019,Jan,3; 2018,Sep,14; 2018,Apr,9; 2018,Apr,10; 2018,Mar,7; 2018,Jan,8; 2017,Aug,3; 2017,Jun,6; 2017,Jan,8; 2016,Dec,11; 2016,Sep,6; 2016,Mar,10; 2016,Jan,13; 2016,Jan,7; 2015,Dec,3; 2015,Oct,3; 2015,Jan,12; 2015,Jan,16

▲ **99214 Office or other outpatient visit for the evaluation and management of an established patient, which requires a medically appropriate history and/or examination and moderate level of medical decision making. When using time for code selection, 30-39 minutes of total time is spent on the date of the encounter.**

2.22 3.06 **FUD** XXX ★ B 80

AMA: 2020,Sep,3; 2020,Sep,14; 2020,Jun,3; 2020,May,3; 2020,Feb,3; 2020,Jan,3; 2019,Oct,10; 2019,Feb,3; 2019,Jan,3; 2018,Sep,14; 2018,Apr,9; 2018,Apr,10; 2018,Mar,7; 2018,Jan,8; 2017,Aug,3; 2017,Jun,6; 2017,Jan,8; 2016,Dec,11; 2016,Sep,6; 2016,Mar,10; 2016,Jan,13; 2016,Jan,7; 2015,Dec,3; 2015,Oct,3; 2015,Jan,16; 2015,Jan,12

▲ **99215 Office or other outpatient visit for the evaluation and management of an established patient, which requires a medically appropriate history and/or examination and high level of medical decision making. When using time for code selection, 40-54 minutes of total time is spent on the date of the encounter.**

EXCLUDES *Prolonged services (lasting 55 minutes or more) ([99417])*

3.13 4.10 **FUD** XXX ★ B 80

AMA: 2020,Sep,3; 2020,Sep,14; 2020,Jun,3; 2020,May,3; 2020,Feb,3; 2020,Jan,3; 2019,Oct,10; 2019,Feb,3; 2019,Jan,3; 2018,Sep,14; 2018,Apr,9; 2018,Apr,10; 2018,Mar,7; 2018,Jan,8; 2017,Aug,3; 2017,Jun,6; 2017,Jan,8; 2016,Dec,11; 2016,Sep,6; 2016,Mar,10; 2016,Jan,13; 2016,Jan,7; 2015,Dec,3; 2015,Oct,3; 2015,Jan,16; 2015,Jan,12

99217-99220 Facility Observation Visits: Initial and Discharge

CMS: 100-04,11,40.1.3 Independent Attending Physician Services; 100-04,12,30.6.4 Services Furnished Incident to Physician's Service; 100-04,12,30.6.8 Payment for Hospital Observation Services; 100-04,12,40.3 Global Surgery Review; 100-04,32,130.1 Billing and Payment of External counterpulsation (ECP)

INCLUDES Services provided on same date in other settings or departments associated with observation status admission (99202-99215, 99281-99285, 99304-99318, 99324-99337, 99341-99350, 99381-99429 [99415, 99416, 99417, 99421, 99422, 99423])
Services provided to new and established patients admitted to hospital specifically for observation (not required to be designated hospital area)

EXCLUDES *Services provided by physicians or another qualified health care professional other than admitting physician ([99224, 99225, 99226], 99241-99245)*
Services provided to patient admitted and discharged from observation status on same date (99234-99236)
Services provided to patient admitted to hospital following observation status (99221-99223)
Services provided to patient discharged from inpatient care (99238-99239)

99217 Observation care discharge day management (This code is to be utilized to report all services provided to a patient on discharge from outpatient hospital "observation status" if the discharge is on other than the initial date of "observation status." To report services to a patient designated as "observation status" or "inpatient status" and discharged on the same date, use the codes for Observation or Inpatient Care Services [including Admission and Discharge Services, 99234-99236 as appropriate.])

INCLUDES Discussing observation admission with patient
Final patient evaluation:
Discharge instructions
Sign off on discharge medical records

2.06 2.06 **FUD** XXX B 80

AMA: 2019,Jul,10; 2018,Jan,8; 2017,Aug,3; 2017,Jun,6; 2017,Jan,8; 2016,Dec,11; 2016,Jan,13; 2016,Jan,7; 2015,Dec,3; 2015,Jan,16

99218 Initial observation care, per day, for the evaluation and management of a patient which requires these 3 key components: A detailed or comprehensive history; A detailed or comprehensive examination; and Medical decision making that is straightforward or of low complexity. Counseling and/or coordination of care with other physicians, other qualified health care professionals, or agencies are provided consistent with the nature of the problem(s) and the patient's and/or family's needs. Usually, the problem(s) requiring admission to outpatient hospital "observation status" are of low severity. Typically, 30 minutes are spent at the bedside and on the patient's hospital floor or unit.

2.81 2.81 **FUD** XXX B 80

AMA: 2020,Sep,3; 2019,Jul,10; 2018,Dec,8; 2018,Dec,8; 2018,Jan,8; 2017,Aug,3; 2017,Jun,6; 2017,Jan,8; 2016,Dec,11; 2016,Jan,7; 2016,Jan,13; 2015,Dec,3; 2015,Jul,3; 2015,Mar,3; 2015,Jan,16

99219 Initial observation care, per day, for the evaluation and management of a patient, which requires these 3 key components: A comprehensive history; A comprehensive examination; and Medical decision making of moderate complexity. Counseling and/or coordination of care with other physicians, other qualified health care professionals, or agencies are provided consistent with the nature of the problem(s) and the patient's and/or family's needs. Usually, the problem(s) requiring admission to outpatient hospital "observation status" are of moderate severity. Typically, 50 minutes are spent at the bedside and on the patient's hospital floor or unit.

3.83 3.83 **FUD** XXX B 80

AMA: 2020,Sep,3; 2019,Jul,10; 2018,Dec,8; 2018,Dec,8; 2018,Jan,8; 2017,Aug,3; 2017,Jun,6; 2017,Jan,8; 2016,Dec,11; 2016,Jan,13; 2016,Jan,7; 2015,Dec,3; 2015,Jul,3; 2015,Jan,16

99220 Initial observation care, per day, for the evaluation and management of a patient, which requires these 3 key components: A comprehensive history; A comprehensive examination; and Medical decision making of high complexity. Counseling and/or coordination of care with other physicians, other qualified health care professionals, or agencies are provided consistent with the nature of the problem(s) and the patient's and/or family's needs. Usually, the problem(s) requiring admission to outpatient hospital "observation status" are of high severity. Typically, 70 minutes are spent at the bedside and on the patient's hospital floor or unit.

5.22 5.22 **FUD** XXX B 80

AMA: 2020,Sep,3; 2019,Jul,10; 2018,Dec,8; 2018,Dec,8; 2018,Jan,8; 2017,Aug,3; 2017,Jun,6; 2017,Jan,8; 2016,Dec,11; 2016,Jan,13; 2016,Jan,7; 2015,Dec,3; 2015,Jul,3; 2015,Jan,16

99224-99226 [99224, 99225, 99226] Facility Observation Visits: Subsequent

CMS: 100-04,11,40.1.3 Independent Attending Physician Services; 100-04,12,30.6.4 Services Furnished Incident to Physician's Service; 100-04,12,30.6.8 Payment for Hospital Observation Services; 100-04,12,30.6.9.1 Initial Hospital Care and Observation or Inpatient Care Services

INCLUDES Changes in patient's status (e.g., physical condition, history; response to medical management)
Medical record review
Review diagnostic test results
Services provided on same date in other settings or departments associated with observation status admission (99202-99215, 99281-99285, 99304-99318, 99324-99337, 99341-99350, 99381-99429 [99415, 99416, 99417, 99421, 99422, 99423])

EXCLUDES *Observation admission and discharge on same day (99234-99236)*

\# **99224** **Subsequent observation care, per day, for the evaluation and management of a patient, which requires at least 2 of these 3 key components: Problem focused interval history; Problem focused examination; Medical decision making that is straightforward or of low complexity. Counseling and/or coordination of care with other physicians, other qualified health care professionals, or agencies are provided consistent with the nature of the problem(s) and the patient's and/or family's needs. Usually, the patient is stable, recovering, or improving. Typically, 15 minutes are spent at the bedside and on the patient's hospital floor or unit.**

1.12 1.12 **FUD** XXX B 80

AMA: 2020,Sep,3; 2019,Jul,10; 2018,Jan,8; 2017,Aug,3; 2017,Jun,6; 2017,Jan,8; 2016,Dec,11; 2016,Jan,7; 2016,Jan,13; 2015,Dec,3; 2015,Jan,16

\# **99225** **Subsequent observation care, per day, for the evaluation and management of a patient, which requires at least 2 of these 3 key components: An expanded problem focused interval history; An expanded problem focused examination; Medical decision making of moderate complexity. Counseling and/or coordination of care with other physicians, other qualified health care professionals, or agencies are provided consistent with the nature of the problem(s) and the patient's and/or family's needs. Usually, the patient is responding inadequately to therapy or has developed a minor complication. Typically, 25 minutes are spent at the bedside and on the patient's hospital floor or unit.**

2.06 2.06 **FUD** XXX B 80

AMA: 2020,Sep,3; 2019,Jul,10; 2018,Jan,8; 2017,Aug,3; 2017,Jun,6; 2017,Jan,8; 2016,Dec,11; 2016,Jan,7; 2016,Jan,13; 2015,Dec,3; 2015,Jan,16

\# **99226** **Subsequent observation care, per day, for the evaluation and management of a patient, which requires at least 2 of these 3 key components: A detailed interval history; A detailed examination; Medical decision making of high complexity. Counseling and/or coordination of care with other physicians, other qualified health care professionals, or agencies are provided consistent with the nature of the problem(s) and the patient's and/or family's needs. Usually, the patient is unstable or has developed a significant complication or a significant new problem. Typically, 35 minutes are spent at the bedside and on the patient's hospital floor or unit.**

2.95 2.95 **FUD** XXX B 80

AMA: 2020,Sep,3; 2019,Jul,10; 2018,Jan,8; 2017,Aug,3; 2017,Jun,6; 2017,Jan,8; 2016,Dec,11; 2016,Jan,7; 2016,Jan,13; 2015,Dec,3; 2015,Jan,16

99221-99233 [99224, 99225, 99226] Inpatient Hospital Visits: Initial and Subsequent

CMS: 100-04,11,40.1.3 Independent Attending Physician Services; 100-04,12,30.6.10 Consultation Services; 100-04,12,30.6.15.1 Prolonged Services With Direct Face-to-Face Patient Contact; 100-04,12,30.6.4 Services Furnished Incident to Physician's Service; 100-04,12,30.6.9 Hospital Visit and Critical Care on Same Day

INCLUDES Initial physician services provided to patient in hospital or "partial" hospital settings (99221-99223)
Services provided on admission date in other settings or departments associated with observation status admission (99202-99215, 99281-99285, 99304-99318, 99324-99337, 99341-99350, 99381-99397)
Services provided to new or established patient

EXCLUDES *Inpatient admission and discharge on same date (99234-99236)*
Inpatient E/M services provided by other than admitting physician

99221 **Initial hospital care, per day, for the evaluation and management of a patient, which requires these 3 key components: A detailed or comprehensive history; A detailed or comprehensive examination; and Medical decision making that is straightforward or of low complexity. Counseling and/or coordination of care with other physicians, other qualified health care professionals, or agencies are provided consistent with the nature of the problem(s) and the patient's and/or family's needs. Usually, the problem(s) requiring admission are of low severity. Typically, 30 minutes are spent at the bedside and on the patient's hospital floor or unit.**

2.86 2.86 **FUD** XXX B 80

AMA: 2020,Sep,3; 2018,Dec,8; 2018,Dec,8; 2018,Jan,8; 2017,Aug,3; 2017,Jun,6; 2017,Jan,8; 2016,Dec,11; 2016,Mar,10; 2016,Jan,13; 2016,Jan,7; 2015,Dec,3; 2015,Dec,18; 2015,Jul,3; 2015,Jan,16

99222 **Initial hospital care, per day, for the evaluation and management of a patient, which requires these 3 key components: A comprehensive history; A comprehensive examination; and Medical decision making of moderate complexity. Counseling and/or coordination of care with other physicians, other qualified health care professionals, or agencies are provided consistent with the nature of the problem(s) and the patient's and/or family's needs. Usually, the problem(s) requiring admission are of moderate severity. Typically, 50 minutes are spent at the bedside and on the patient's hospital floor or unit.**

3.86 3.86 **FUD** XXX B 80

AMA: 2020,Sep,3; 2018,Dec,8; 2018,Dec,8; 2018,Jan,8; 2017,Aug,3; 2017,Jun,6; 2017,Jan,8; 2016,Dec,11; 2016,Mar,10; 2016,Jan,13; 2016,Jan,7; 2015,Dec,3; 2015,Dec,18; 2015,Jul,3; 2015,Mar,3; 2015,Jan,16

99223 **Initial hospital care, per day, for the evaluation and management of a patient, which requires these 3 key components: A comprehensive history; A comprehensive examination; and Medical decision making of high complexity. Counseling and/or coordination of care with other physicians, other qualified health care professionals, or agencies are provided consistent with the nature of the problem(s) and the patient's and/or family's needs. Usually, the problem(s) requiring admission are of high severity. Typically, 70 minutes are spent at the bedside and on the patient's hospital floor or unit.**

5.71 5.71 **FUD** XXX B 80

AMA: 2020,Sep,3; 2018,Dec,8; 2018,Dec,8; 2018,Jan,8; 2017,Aug,3; 2017,Jun,6; 2017,Jan,8; 2016,Dec,11; 2016,Mar,10; 2016,Jan,13; 2016,Jan,7; 2015,Dec,3; 2015,Dec,18; 2015,Jul,3; 2015,Jan,16

99224 **Resequenced code. See code following 99220.**

99225 **Resequenced code. See code following 99220.**

99226 **Resequenced code. See code following 99220.**

99231 **Subsequent hospital care, per day, for the evaluation and management of a patient, which requires at least 2 of these 3 key components: A problem focused interval history; A problem focused examination; Medical decision making that is straightforward or of low complexity. Counseling and/or coordination of care with other physicians, other qualified health care professionals, or agencies are provided consistent with the nature of the problem(s) and the patient's and/or family's needs. Usually, the patient is stable, recovering or improving. Typically, 15 minutes are spent at the bedside and on the patient's hospital floor or unit.**

1.11 1.11 **FUD** XXX ★ B 80

AMA: 2020,Sep,3; 2018,Dec,8; 2018,Dec,8; 2018,Jan,8; 2017,Aug,3; 2017,Jun,6; 2017,Jan,8; 2016,Dec,11; 2016,Jan,13; 2016,Jan,7; 2015,Dec,3; 2015,Jul,3; 2015,Jan,16

99232 **Subsequent hospital care, per day, for the evaluation and management of a patient, which requires at least 2 of these 3 key components: An expanded problem focused interval history; An expanded problem focused examination; Medical decision making of moderate complexity. Counseling and/or coordination of care with other physicians, other qualified health care professionals, or agencies are provided consistent with the nature of the problem(s) and the patient's and/or family's needs. Usually, the patient is responding inadequately to therapy or has developed a minor complication. Typically, 25 minutes are spent at the bedside and on the patient's hospital floor or unit.**

2.05 2.05 **FUD** XXX ★ B 80

AMA: 2020,Sep,3; 2018,Dec,8; 2018,Dec,8; 2018,Jan,8; 2017,Aug,3; 2017,Jun,6; 2017,Jan,8; 2016,Dec,11; 2016,Oct,8; 2016,Jan,13; 2016,Jan,7; 2015,Dec,3; 2015,Jul,3; 2015,Jan,16

99233 **Subsequent hospital care, per day, for the evaluation and management of a patient, which requires at least 2 of these 3 key components: A detailed interval history; A detailed examination; Medical decision making of high complexity. Counseling and/or coordination of care with other physicians, other qualified health care professionals, or agencies are provided consistent with the nature of the problem(s) and the patient's and/or family's needs. Usually, the patient is unstable or has developed a significant complication or a significant new problem. Typically, 35 minutes are spent at the bedside and on the patient's hospital floor or unit.**

2.93 2.93 **FUD** XXX ★ B 80

AMA: 2020,Sep,3; 2018,Dec,8; 2018,Dec,8; 2018,Jan,8; 2017,Aug,3; 2017,Jun,6; 2017,Jan,8; 2016,Dec,11; 2016,Oct,8; 2016,Jan,13; 2016,Jan,7; 2015,Dec,3; 2015,Jul,3; 2015,Jan,16

99234-99236 Observation/Inpatient Visits: Admitted/Discharged on Same Date

CMS: 100-04,11,40.1.3 Independent Attending Physician Services; 100-04,12,30.6.4 Services Furnished Incident to Physician's Service; 100-04,12,30.6.8 Payment for Hospital Observation Services; 100-04,12,30.6.9 Payment for Inpatient Hospital Visits - General; 100-04,12,30.6.9.1 Initial Hospital Care and Observation or Inpatient Care Services; 100-04,12,30.6.9.2 Subsequent Hospital Visit and Discharge Management; 100-04,12,40.3 Global Surgery Review

INCLUDES Admission and discharge services on same date in observation or inpatient setting

All services provided by admitting physician or other qualified health care professional on same date, even when initiated in another setting (e.g., emergency department, nursing facility, office)

EXCLUDES *Services provided to patients admitted to observation and discharged on different date (99217-99220, [99224, 99225, 99226])*

99234 **Observation or inpatient hospital care, for the evaluation and management of a patient including admission and discharge on the same date, which requires these 3 key components: A detailed or comprehensive history; A detailed or comprehensive examination; and Medical decision making that is straightforward or of low complexity. Counseling and/or coordination of care with other physicians, other qualified health care professionals, or agencies are provided consistent with the nature of the problem(s) and the patient's and/or family's needs. Usually the presenting problem(s) requiring admission are of low severity. Typically, 40 minutes are spent at the bedside and on the patient's hospital floor or unit.**

3.75 3.75 **FUD** XXX B 80

AMA: 2020,Sep,3; 2018,Dec,8; 2018,Dec,8; 2018,Apr,10; 2018,Jan,8; 2017,Aug,3; 2017,Jun,6; 2017,Jan,8; 2016,Dec,11; 2016,Jan,13; 2015,Jul,3; 2015,Jan,16

99235 **Observation or inpatient hospital care, for the evaluation and management of a patient including admission and discharge on the same date, which requires these 3 key components: A comprehensive history; A comprehensive examination; and Medical decision making of moderate complexity. Counseling and/or coordination of care with other physicians, other qualified health care professionals, or agencies are provided consistent with the nature of the problem(s) and the patient's and/or family's needs. Usually the presenting problem(s) requiring admission are of moderate severity. Typically, 50 minutes are spent at the bedside and on the patient's hospital floor or unit.**

4.77 4.77 **FUD** XXX B 80

AMA: 2020,Sep,3; 2018,Dec,8; 2018,Dec,8; 2018,Apr,10; 2018,Jan,8; 2017,Aug,3; 2017,Jun,6; 2017,Jan,8; 2016,Dec,11; 2016,Jan,13; 2015,Jul,3; 2015,Jan,16

99236 **Observation or inpatient hospital care, for the evaluation and management of a patient including admission and discharge on the same date, which requires these 3 key components: A comprehensive history; A comprehensive examination; and Medical decision making of high complexity. Counseling and/or coordination of care with other physicians, other qualified health care professionals, or agencies are provided consistent with the nature of the problem(s) and the patient's and/or family's needs. Usually the presenting problem(s) requiring admission are of high severity. Typically, 55 minutes are spent at the bedside and on the patient's hospital floor or unit.**

6.14 6.14 **FUD** XXX B 80

AMA: 2020,Sep,3; 2018,Dec,8; 2018,Dec,8; 2018,Apr,10; 2018,Jan,8; 2017,Aug,3; 2017,Jun,6; 2017,Jan,8; 2016,Dec,11; 2016,Jan,13; 2015,Jul,3; 2015,Jan,16

99238-99239 Inpatient Hospital Discharge Services

CMS: 100-04,11,40.1.3 Independent Attending Physician Services; 100-04,12,30.6.4 Services Furnished Incident to Physician's Service; 100-04,12,30.6.9 Swing Bed Visits; 100-04,12,30.6.9.1 Initial Hospital Care and Observation or Inpatient Care Services; 100-04,12,30.6.9.2 Subsequent Hospital Visit and Discharge Management; 100-04,12,40.3 Global Surgery Review

INCLUDES All services on discharge day when discharge and admission are not on same day
Discharge instructions
Final patient evaluation
Final preparation patient's medical records
Provision prescriptions/referrals, as needed
Review inpatient admission

EXCLUDES *Admission/discharge on same date (99234-99236)*
Discharge from observation (99217)
Discharge from nursing facility (99315-99316)
Healthy newborn evaluated and discharged on same date (99463)
Services provided by other than attending physician or other qualified health care professional on discharge date (99231-99233)

99238 **Hospital discharge day management; 30 minutes or less**
2.06 2.06 FUD XXX B 80
AMA: 2018,Dec,8; 2018,Dec,8; 2018,Jan,8; 2017,Aug,3; 2017,Jun,6; 2017,Jan,8; 2016,Dec,11; 2016,Jan,13; 2015,Jan,16

99239 **more than 30 minutes**
3.02 3.02 FUD XXX B 80
AMA: 2018,Dec,8; 2018,Dec,8; 2018,Jan,8; 2017,Aug,3; 2017,Jun,6; 2017,Jan,8; 2016,Dec,11; 2016,Jan,13; 2015,Jan,16

99241-99245 Consultations: Office and Outpatient

CMS: 100-04,11,40.1.3 Independent Attending Physician Services; 100-04,12,190.6 Payment Methodology for Physician/Practitioner at the Distant Site ; 100-04,12,190.6.1 Submission of Telehealth Claims for Distant Site Practitioners; 100-04,12,190.7 Contractor Editing of Telehealth Claims; 100-04,12,30.6.10 Consultation Services; 100-04,12,30.6.15.1 Prolonged Services With Direct Face-to-Face Patient Contact; 100-04,12,30.6.4 Services Furnished Incident to Physician's Service; 100-04,12,30.6.9.1 Initial Hospital Care and Observation or Inpatient Care Services; 100-04,12,40.3 Global Surgery Review; 100-04,32,130.1 Billing and Payment of External counterpulsation (ECP); 100-04,4,160 Clinic and Emergency Visits Under OPPS

INCLUDES All outpatient consultations provided in office, outpatient or other ambulatory facility, domiciliary/rest home, emergency department, patient's home, and hospital observation
Documentation consultation request from appropriate source
Documentation need for consultation in patient's medical record
One consultation per consultant
Provision by physician or qualified nonphysician practitioner whose advice, opinion, recommendation, suggestion, direction, or counsel, etc., requested for evaluating/treating patient since that individual's specific medical expertise beyond requesting physician knowledge
Provision written report, findings/recommendations from consultant to referring physician
Third-party mandated consultation; append modifier 32

EXCLUDES *Another appropriately requested and documented consultation pertaining to same/new problem; repeat consultation code reporting*
Any distinctly recognizable procedure/service provided on or following consultation
Care assumption (all or partial); report subsequent codes as appropriate for place of service (99211-99215, 99334-99337, 99347-99350)
Consultation prompted by patient/family; report codes for office, domiciliary/rest home, or home visits instead (99202-99215, 99324-99337, 99341-99350)
Services provided to Medicare patients; E/M code as appropriate for place of service or HCPCS code (99202-99215, 99221-99223, 99231-99233, G0406-G0408, G0425-G0427)

99241 **Office consultation for a new or established patient, which requires these 3 key components: A problem focused history; A problem focused examination; and Straightforward medical decision making. Counseling and/or coordination of care with other physicians, other qualified health care professionals, or agencies are provided consistent with the nature of the problem(s) and the patient's and/or family's needs. Usually, the presenting problem(s) are self limited or minor. Typically, 15 minutes are spent face-to-face with the patient and/or family.**
0.92 1.34 FUD XXX ★ E
AMA: 2020,Sep,3; 2018,Apr,9; 2018,Apr,10; 2018,Mar,7; 2018,Jan,8; 2017,Aug,3; 2017,Jun,6; 2017,Jan,8; 2016,Dec,11; 2016,Sep,6; 2016,Jan,13; 2016,Jan,7; 2015,Jan,12; 2015,Jan,16

99242 **Office consultation for a new or established patient, which requires these 3 key components: An expanded problem focused history; An expanded problem focused examination; and Straightforward medical decision making. Counseling and/or coordination of care with other physicians, other qualified health care professionals, or agencies are provided consistent with the nature of the problem(s) and the patient's and/or family's needs. Usually, the presenting problem(s) are of low severity. Typically, 30 minutes are spent face-to-face with the patient and/or family.**
1.93 2.52 FUD XXX ★ E
AMA: 2020,Sep,3; 2018,Apr,9; 2018,Apr,10; 2018,Mar,7; 2018,Jan,8; 2017,Aug,3; 2017,Jun,6; 2017,Jun,8; 2017,Jan,8; 2016,Dec,11; 2016,Sep,6; 2016,Jan,7; 2016,Jan,13; 2015,Jan,12; 2015,Jan,16

99243 **Office consultation for a new or established patient, which requires these 3 key components: A detailed history; A detailed examination; and Medical decision making of low complexity. Counseling and/or coordination of care with other physicians, other qualified health care professionals, or agencies are provided consistent with the nature of the problem(s) and the patient's and/or family's needs. Usually, the presenting problem(s) are of moderate severity. Typically, 40 minutes are spent face-to-face with the patient and/or family.**
2.74 3.49 FUD XXX ★ E
AMA: 2020,Sep,3; 2018,Apr,9; 2018,Apr,10; 2018,Mar,7; 2018,Jan,8; 2017,Aug,3; 2017,Jun,6; 2017,Jan,8; 2016,Dec,11; 2016,Sep,6; 2016,Jan,7; 2016,Jan,13; 2015,Jan,12; 2015,Jan,16

99244 **Office consultation for a new or established patient, which requires these 3 key components: A comprehensive history; A comprehensive examination; and Medical decision making of moderate complexity. Counseling and/or coordination of care with other physicians, other qualified health care professionals, or agencies are provided consistent with the nature of the problem(s) and the patient's and/or family's needs. Usually, the presenting problem(s) are of moderate to high severity. Typically, 60 minutes are spent face-to-face with the patient and/or family.**
4.41 5.23 FUD XXX ★ E
AMA: 2020,Sep,3; 2018,Apr,9; 2018,Apr,10; 2018,Mar,7; 2018,Jan,8; 2017,Aug,3; 2017,Jun,6; 2017,Jan,8; 2016,Dec,11; 2016,Sep,6; 2016,Jan,7; 2016,Jan,13; 2015,Jan,16; 2015,Jan,12

99245 **Office consultation for a new or established patient, which requires these 3 key components: A comprehensive history; A comprehensive examination; and Medical decision making of high complexity. Counseling and/or coordination of care with other physicians, other qualified health care professionals, or agencies are provided consistent with the nature of the problem(s) and the patient's and/or family's needs. Usually, the presenting problem(s) are of moderate to high severity. Typically, 80 minutes are spent face-to-face with the patient and/or family.**
5.37 6.29 FUD XXX ★ E
AMA: 2020,Sep,3; 2018,Apr,9; 2018,Apr,10; 2018,Mar,7; 2018,Jan,8; 2017,Aug,3; 2017,Jun,6; 2017,Jan,8; 2016,Dec,11; 2016,Sep,6; 2016,Jan,7; 2016,Jan,13; 2015,Jan,12; 2015,Jan,16

99251-99255 Consultations: Inpatient

CMS: 100-04,11,40.1.3 Independent Attending Physician Services; 100-04,12,190.6 Payment Methodology for Physician/Practitioner at the Distant Site ; 100-04,12,190.6.1 Submission of Telehealth Claims for Distant Site Practitioners; 100-04,12,190.7 Contractor Editing of Telehealth Claims; 100-04,12,30.6.10 Consultation Services; 100-04,12,30.6.15.1 Prolonged Services With Direct Face-to-Face Patient Contact; 100-04,12,30.6.4 Services Furnished Incident to Physician's Service; 100-04,12,30.6.9.1 Initial Hospital Care and Observation or Inpatient Care Services; 100-04,12,40.3 Global Surgery Review

INCLUDES All outpatient consultations provided in office, outpatient or other ambulatory facility, domiciliary/rest home, emergency department, patient's home, and hospital observation
Documentation consultation request from appropriate source
Documentation need for consultation in patient's medical record
One consultation per consultant
Provision by physician or qualified nonphysician practitioner whose advice, opinion, recommendation, suggestion, direction, or counsel, etc., requested for evaluating/treating patient since that individual's specific medical expertise beyond requesting physician knowledge
Provision written report, findings/recommendations from consultant to referring physician
Third-party mandated consultation; append modifier 32

EXCLUDES *Another appropriately requested and documented consultation pertaining to same/new problem; repeat consultation code reporting*
Any distinctly recognizable procedure/service provided on or following consultation
Care assumption (all or partial); report subsequent codes as appropriate for place of service (99231-99233, 99307-99310)
Consultation prompted by patient/family; report codes for office, domiciliary/rest home, or home visits instead (99202-99215, 99234-99337, 99341-99350)
Services provided to Medicare patients; E/M code as appropriate for place of service or HCPCS code (99202-99215, 99324-99337, 99341-99350)

99251 **Inpatient consultation for a new or established patient, which requires these 3 key components: A problem focused history; A problem focused examination; and Straightforward medical decision making. Counseling and/or coordination of care with other physicians, other qualified health care professionals, or agencies are provided consistent with the nature of the problem(s) and the patient's and/or family's needs. Usually, the presenting problem(s) are self limited or minor. Typically, 20 minutes are spent at the bedside and on the patient's hospital floor or unit.**

1.38 1.38 FUD XXX ★ E

AMA: 2020,Sep,3; 2018,Jan,8; 2017,Aug,3; 2017,Jun,6; 2017,Jan,8; 2016,Dec,11; 2016,Jan,7; 2016,Jan,13; 2015,Jan,16

99252 **Inpatient consultation for a new or established patient, which requires these 3 key components: An expanded problem focused history; An expanded problem focused examination; and Straightforward medical decision making. Counseling and/or coordination of care with other physicians, other qualified health care professionals, or agencies are provided consistent with the nature of the problem(s) and the patient's and/or family's needs. Usually, the presenting problem(s) are of low severity. Typically, 40 minutes are spent at the bedside and on the patient's hospital floor or unit.**

2.13 2.13 FUD XXX ★ E

AMA: 2020,Sep,3; 2018,Jan,8; 2017,Aug,3; 2017,Jun,6; 2017,Jan,8; 2016,Dec,11; 2016,Jan,13; 2016,Jan,7; 2015,Jan,16

99253 **Inpatient consultation for a new or established patient, which requires these 3 key components: A detailed history; A detailed examination; and Medical decision making of low complexity. Counseling and/or coordination of care with other physicians, other qualified health care professionals, or agencies are provided consistent with the nature of the problem(s) and the patient's and/or family's needs. Usually, the presenting problem(s) are of moderate severity. Typically, 55 minutes are spent at the bedside and on the patient's hospital floor or unit.**

3.25 3.25 FUD XXX ★ E

AMA: 2020,Sep,3; 2018,Jan,8; 2017,Aug,3; 2017,Jun,6; 2017,Jan,8; 2016,Dec,11; 2016,Jan,13; 2016,Jan,7; 2015,Jan,16

99254 **Inpatient consultation for a new or established patient, which requires these 3 key components: A comprehensive history; A comprehensive examination; and Medical decision making of moderate complexity. Counseling and/or coordination of care with other physicians, other qualified health care professionals, or agencies are provided consistent with the nature of the problem(s) and the patient's and/or family's needs. Usually, the presenting problem(s) are of moderate to high severity. Typically, 80 minutes are spent at the bedside and on the patient's hospital floor or unit.**

4.72 4.72 FUD XXX ★ E

AMA: 2020,Sep,3; 2018,Jan,8; 2017,Aug,3; 2017,Jun,6; 2017,Jan,8; 2016,Dec,11; 2016,Jan,7; 2016,Jan,13; 2015,Jan,16

99255 **Inpatient consultation for a new or established patient, which requires these 3 key components: A comprehensive history; A comprehensive examination; and Medical decision making of high complexity. Counseling and/or coordination of care with other physicians, other qualified health care professionals, or agencies are provided consistent with the nature of the problem(s) and the patient's and/or family's needs. Usually, the presenting problem(s) are of moderate to high severity. Typically, 110 minutes are spent at the bedside and on the patient's hospital floor or unit.**

5.76 5.76 FUD XXX ★ E

AMA: 2020,Sep,3; 2018,Jan,8; 2017,Aug,3; 2017,Jun,6; 2017,Jan,8; 2016,Dec,11; 2016,Jan,7; 2016,Jan,13; 2015,Jan,16

99281-99288 Emergency Department Visits

CMS: 100-04,11,40.1.3 Independent Attending Physician Services; 100-04,12,30.6.11 Emergency Department Visits; 100-04,4,160 Clinic and Emergency Visits Under OPPS

INCLUDES Any time spent with patient, which usually involves multiple encounters while patient in emergency department
Care provided to new and established patients

EXCLUDES *Critical care services (99291-99292)*
Observation services (99217-99220, 99234-99236)

99281 **Emergency department visit for the evaluation and management of a patient, which requires these 3 key components: A problem focused history; A problem focused examination; and Straightforward medical decision making. Counseling and/or coordination of care with other physicians, other qualified health care professionals, or agencies are provided consistent with the nature of the problem(s) and the patient's and/or family's needs. Usually, the presenting problem(s) are self limited or minor.**

0.60 0.60 FUD XXX J 80

AMA: 2020,Jul,13; 2019,Jul,10; 2018,Jan,8; 2017,Aug,3; 2017,Jun,6; 2017,Jan,8; 2016,Jan,13; 2016,Jan,7; 2015,Jan,16; 2015,Jan,12

99282 **Emergency department visit for the evaluation and management of a patient, which requires these 3 key components: An expanded problem focused history; An expanded problem focused examination; and Medical decision making of low complexity. Counseling and/or coordination of care with other physicians, other qualified health care professionals, or agencies are provided consistent with the nature of the problem(s) and the patient's and/or family's needs. Usually, the presenting problem(s) are of low to moderate severity.**

1.17 1.17 FUD XXX J 80

AMA: 2020,Jul,13; 2019,Jul,10; 2018,Jan,8; 2017,Aug,3; 2017,Jun,6; 2017,Jan,8; 2016,Jan,7; 2016,Jan,13; 2015,Jan,12; 2015,Jan,16

99283 **Emergency department visit for the evaluation and management of a patient, which requires these 3 key components: An expanded problem focused history; An expanded problem focused examination; and Medical decision making of moderate complexity. Counseling and/or coordination of care with other physicians, other qualified health care professionals, or agencies are provided consistent with the nature of the problem(s) and the patient's and/or family's needs. Usually, the presenting problem(s) are of moderate severity.**

1.84 1.84 **FUD** XXX J 80

AMA: 2020,Jul,13; 2019,Jul,10; 2018,Jan,8; 2017,Aug,3; 2017,Jun,6; 2017,Jan,8; 2016,Jan,7; 2016,Jan,13; 2015,Jan,16; 2015,Jan,12

99284 **Emergency department visit for the evaluation and management of a patient, which requires these 3 key components: A detailed history; A detailed examination; and Medical decision making of moderate complexity. Counseling and/or coordination of care with other physicians, other qualified health care professionals, or agencies are provided consistent with the nature of the problem(s) and the patient's and/or family's needs. Usually, the presenting problem(s) are of high severity, and require urgent evaluation by the physician, or other qualified health care professionals but do not pose an immediate significant threat to life or physiologic function.**

3.38 3.38 **FUD** XXX J 80

AMA: 2020,Jul,13; 2019,Jul,10; 2018,Jan,8; 2017,Aug,3; 2017,Jun,6; 2017,Jan,8; 2016,Jan,13; 2016,Jan,7; 2015,Jan,16; 2015,Jan,12

99285 **Emergency department visit for the evaluation and management of a patient, which requires these 3 key components within the constraints imposed by the urgency of the patient's clinical condition and/or mental status: A comprehensive history; A comprehensive examination; and Medical decision making of high complexity. Counseling and/or coordination of care with other physicians, other qualified health care professionals, or agencies are provided consistent with the nature of the problem(s) and the patient's and/or family's needs. Usually, the presenting problem(s) are of high severity and pose an immediate significant threat to life or physiologic function.**

4.89 4.89 **FUD** XXX J 80

AMA: 2020,Jul,13; 2020,Jan,12; 2019,Jul,10; 2018,Jan,8; 2017,Aug,3; 2017,Jun,6; 2017,Jan,8; 2016,Jan,7; 2016,Jan,13; 2015,Jan,12; 2015,Jan,16

99288 **Physician or other qualified health care professional direction of emergency medical systems (EMS) emergency care, advanced life support**

INCLUDES Management provided by emergency/intensive care based physician or other qualified health care professional via voice contact to ambulance/rescue staff for services such as heart monitoring and drug administration

0.00 0.00 **FUD** XXX B

AMA: 2018,Jan,8; 2017,Aug,3; 2017,Jun,6; 2017,Jan,8; 2016,Jan,13; 2015,Jan,16

99291-99292 Critical Care Visits: Patients 72 Months of Age and Older

CMS: 100-04,11,40.1.3 Independent Attending Physician Services; 100-04,12,30.6.4 Services Furnished Incident to Physician's Service; 100-04,12,30.6.9 Swing Bed Visits; 100-04,12,40.3 Global Surgery Review; 100-04,4,160 Clinic and Emergency Visits Under OPPS; 100-04,4,160.1 Critical Care Services

INCLUDES 30 minutes or more direct care provided by physician or other qualified health care professional to critically ill or injured patient, any location
All activities performed outside unit or off floor
All time spent exclusively with patient/family/caregivers on nursing unit or elsewhere
Outpatient critical care provided to neonates and pediatric patients age 71 months or younger
Physician or other qualified health care professional presence during interfacility transfer for critically ill/injured patients age 24 months or older
Professional services for interpretation:
Blood gases
Chest films (71045-71046)
Measurement cardiac output (93561-93562)
Other computer stored information
Pulse oximetry (94760-94762)
Professional services:
Gastric intubation (43752-43753)
Transcutaneous pacing, temporary (92953)
Venous access, arterial puncture (36000, 36410, 36415, 36591, 36600)
Ventilation assistance and management, includes CPAP, CNP (94002-94004, 94660, 94662)

EXCLUDES *All services less than 30 minutes; report appropriate E/M code*
Inpatient critical care services provided to child age 2 through 5 years old (99475-99476)
Inpatient critical care services provided to infants age 29 days through 24 months old (99471-99472)
Inpatient critical care services provided to neonates age 28 days or younger (99468-99469)
Other procedures not listed as included performed by physician or other qualified health care professional rendering critical care
Patients not critically ill but in critical care department (report appropriate E/M code)
Physician or other qualified health care professional presence during interfacility transfer for critically ill/injured patients age 24 months or younger (99466-99467)
Supervisory services control physician during interfacility transfer for critically ill/injured patients age 24 months or younger ([99485, 99486])

99291 **Critical care, evaluation and management of the critically ill or critically injured patient; first 30-74 minutes**

6.28 7.89 **FUD** XXX J 80

AMA: 2020,Feb,7; 2020,Jan,12; 2019,Dec,14; 2019,Aug,8; 2019,Jul,10; 2018,Dec,8; 2018,Dec,8; 2018,Jun,9; 2018,Jan,8; 2017,Aug,3; 2017,Jun,6; 2017,Jan,8; 2016,Oct,8; 2016,Aug,9; 2016,May,3; 2016,Jan,13; 2015,Jul,3; 2015,Feb,10; 2015,Jan,16

\+ 99292 **each additional 30 minutes (List separately in addition to code for primary service)**

Code first (99291)

3.16 3.49 **FUD** ZZZ N 80

AMA: 2020,Feb,7; 2019,Dec,14; 2019,Aug,8; 2019,Jul,10; 2018,Dec,8; 2018,Dec,8; 2018,Jun,9; 2018,Jan,8; 2017,Aug,3; 2017,Jun,6; 2017,Jan,8; 2016,Aug,9; 2016,May,3; 2016,Jan,13; 2015,Jul,3; 2015,Feb,10; 2015,Jan,16

99304-99310 Nursing Facility Visits

CMS: 100-04,11,40.1.3 Independent Attending Physician Services; 100-04,12,230 Primary Care Incentive Payment Program; 100-04,12,230.1 Definition of Primary Care Practitioners and Services; 100-04,12,230.2 Coordination with Other Payments; 100-04,12,230.3 Claims Processing and Payment; 100-04,12,30.6.10 Consultation Services; 100-04,12,30.6.13 Nursing Facility Visits; 100-04,12,30.6.15.1 Prolonged Services With Direct Face-to-Face Patient Contact; 100-04,12,30.6.4 Services Furnished Incident to Physician's Service; 100-04,12,30.6.9 Swing Bed Visits

INCLUDES All E/M services provided by admitting physician on nursing facility admission date in other locations (e.g., office, emergency department)
Initial care, subsequent care, discharge, and yearly assessments
Initial services include patient assessment and physician participation in developing plan of care (99304-99306)
Services provided in psychiatric residential treatment center
Services provided to new and established patients in nursing facility (skilled, intermediate, and long-term care facilities)
Subsequent services include physician review medical records, reassessment, and review test results (99307-99310)

EXCLUDES *Care plan oversight services (99379-99380)*

Code also hospital discharge services on same admission or readmission date to nursing home (99217, 99234-99236, 99238-99239)

99304 **Initial nursing facility care, per day, for the evaluation and management of a patient, which requires these 3 key components: A detailed or comprehensive history; A detailed or comprehensive examination; and Medical decision making that is straightforward or of low complexity. Counseling and/or coordination of care with other physicians, other qualified health care professionals, or agencies are provided consistent with the nature of the problem(s) and the patient's and/or family's needs. Usually, the problem(s) requiring admission are of low severity. Typically, 25 minutes are spent at the bedside and on the patient's facility floor or unit.**

2.55 2.55 **FUD** XXX B 80

AMA: 2020,Sep,3; 2018,Jan,8; 2017,Aug,3; 2017,Jun,6; 2017,Jan,8; 2016,Dec,11; 2016,Jan,13; 2016,Jan,7; 2015,Jan,16

99305 **Initial nursing facility care, per day, for the evaluation and management of a patient, which requires these 3 key components: A comprehensive history; A comprehensive examination; and Medical decision making of moderate complexity. Counseling and/or coordination of care with other physicians, other qualified health care professionals, or agencies are provided consistent with the nature of the problem(s) and the patient's and/or family's needs. Usually, the problem(s) requiring admission are of moderate severity. Typically, 35 minutes are spent at the bedside and on the patient's facility floor or unit.**

3.65 3.65 **FUD** XXX B 80

AMA: 2020,Sep,3; 2018,Jan,8; 2017,Aug,3; 2017,Jun,6; 2017,Jan,8; 2016,Dec,11; 2016,Jan,13; 2016,Jan,7; 2015,Jan,16

99306 **Initial nursing facility care, per day, for the evaluation and management of a patient, which requires these 3 key components: A comprehensive history; A comprehensive examination; and Medical decision making of high complexity. Counseling and/or coordination of care with other physicians, other qualified health care professionals, or agencies are provided consistent with the nature of the problem(s) and the patient's and/or family's needs. Usually, the problem(s) requiring admission are of high severity. Typically, 45 minutes are spent at the bedside and on the patient's facility floor or unit.**

4.71 4.71 **FUD** XXX B 80

AMA: 2020,Sep,3; 2018,Jan,8; 2017,Aug,3; 2017,Jun,6; 2017,Jan,8; 2016,Dec,11; 2016,Jan,13; 2016,Jan,7; 2015,Jan,16

99307 **Subsequent nursing facility care, per day, for the evaluation and management of a patient, which requires at least 2 of these 3 key components: A problem focused interval history; A problem focused examination; Straightforward medical decision making. Counseling and/or coordination of care with other physicians, other qualified health care professionals, or agencies are provided consistent with the nature of the problem(s) and the patient's and/or family's needs. Usually, the patient is stable, recovering, or improving. Typically, 10 minutes are spent at the bedside and on the patient's facility floor or unit.**

1.24 1.24 **FUD** XXX ★ B 80

AMA: 2020,Sep,3; 2018,Jan,8; 2017,Aug,3; 2017,Jun,6; 2017,Jan,8; 2016,Dec,11; 2016,Jan,13; 2016,Jan,7; 2015,Jan,16

99308 **Subsequent nursing facility care, per day, for the evaluation and management of a patient, which requires at least 2 of these 3 key components: An expanded problem focused interval history; An expanded problem focused examination; Medical decision making of low complexity. Counseling and/or coordination of care with other physicians, other qualified health care professionals, or agencies are provided consistent with the nature of the problem(s) and the patient's and/or family's needs. Usually, the patient is responding inadequately to therapy or has developed a minor complication. Typically, 15 minutes are spent at the bedside and on the patient's facility floor or unit.**

1.94 1.94 **FUD** XXX ★ B 80

AMA: 2020,Sep,3; 2018,Jan,8; 2017,Aug,3; 2017,Jun,6; 2017,Jan,8; 2016,Dec,11; 2016,Jan,13; 2016,Jan,7; 2015,Jan,16

99309 **Subsequent nursing facility care, per day, for the evaluation and management of a patient, which requires at least 2 of these 3 key components: A detailed interval history; A detailed examination; Medical decision making of moderate complexity. Counseling and/or coordination of care with other physicians, other qualified health care professionals, or agencies are provided consistent with the nature of the problem(s) and the patient's and/or family's needs. Usually, the patient has developed a significant complication or a significant new problem. Typically, 25 minutes are spent at the bedside and on the patient's facility floor or unit.**

2.57 2.57 **FUD** XXX ★ B 80

AMA: 2020,Sep,3; 2018,Jan,8; 2017,Aug,3; 2017,Jun,6; 2017,Jan,8; 2016,Dec,11; 2016,Jan,13; 2016,Jan,7; 2015,Jan,16

99310 **Subsequent nursing facility care, per day, for the evaluation and management of a patient, which requires at least 2 of these 3 key components: A comprehensive interval history; A comprehensive examination; Medical decision making of high complexity. Counseling and/or coordination of care with other physicians, other qualified health care professionals, or agencies are provided consistent with the nature of the problem(s) and the patient's and/or family's needs. The patient may be unstable or may have developed a significant new problem requiring immediate physician attention. Typically, 35 minutes are spent at the bedside and on the patient's facility floor or unit.**

3.79 3.79 **FUD** XXX ★ B 80

AMA: 2020,Sep,3; 2018,Jan,8; 2017,Aug,3; 2017,Jun,6; 2017,Jan,8; 2016,Dec,11; 2016,Jan,13; 2016,Jan,7; 2015,Jan,16

99315-99316 Nursing Home Discharge

CMS: 100-04,11,40.1.3 Independent Attending Physician Services; 100-04,12,230 Primary Care Incentive Payment Program; 100-04,12,230.1 Definition of Primary Care Practitioners and Services; 100-04,12,230.2 Coordination with Other Payments; 100-04,12,230.3 Claims Processing and Payment; 100-04,12,30.6.13 Nursing Facility Visits; 100-04,12,30.6.4 Services Furnished Incident to Physician's Service; 100-04,12,40.3 Global Surgery Review

INCLUDES Discharge services include all time spent by physician or other qualified health care professional:
- Completion discharge records
- Discharge instructions for patient and caregivers
- Discussion regarding stay in facility
- Final patient examination
- Provide prescriptions and referrals as appropriate

99315 **Nursing facility discharge day management; 30 minutes or less**

2.07 2.07 FUD XXX B 80

AMA: 2018,Jan,8; 2017,Aug,3; 2017,Jun,6; 2017,Jan,8; 2016,Dec,11; 2016,Jan,13; 2016,Jan,7; 2015,Jan,16

99316 **more than 30 minutes**

2.97 2.97 FUD XXX B 80

AMA: 2018,Jan,8; 2017,Aug,3; 2017,Jun,6; 2017,Jan,8; 2016,Dec,11; 2016,Jan,13; 2016,Jan,7; 2015,Jan,16

99318 Annual Nursing Home Assessment

CMS: 100-04,11,40.1.3 Independent Attending Physician Services; 100-04,12,230 Primary Care Incentive Payment Program; 100-04,12,230.1 Definition of Primary Care Practitioners and Services; 100-04,12,230.2 Coordination with Other Payments; 100-04,12,230.3 Claims Processing and Payment; 100-04,12,30.6.13 Nursing Facility Visits; 100-04,12,30.6.15.1 Prolonged Services With Direct Face-to-Face Patient Contact; 100-04,12,30.6.4 Services Furnished Incident to Physician's Service; 100-04,12,30.6.9 Swing Bed Visits

INCLUDES Includes nursing facility visits on same date as (99304-99316)

99318 **Evaluation and management of a patient involving an annual nursing facility assessment, which requires these 3 key components: A detailed interval history; A comprehensive examination; and Medical decision making that is of low to moderate complexity. Counseling and/or coordination of care with other physicians, other qualified health care professionals, or agencies are provided consistent with the nature of the problem(s) and the patient's and/or family's needs. Usually, the patient is stable, recovering, or improving. Typically, 30 minutes are spent at the bedside and on the patient's facility floor or unit.**

2.70 2.70 FUD XXX B 80

AMA: 2018,Jan,8; 2017,Aug,3; 2017,Jun,6; 2017,Jan,8; 2016,Dec,11; 2016,Jan,7; 2016,Jan,13; 2015,Jan,16

99324-99337 Domiciliary Care, Rest Home, Assisted Living Visits

CMS: 100-04,12,230 Primary Care Incentive Payment Program; 100-04,12,230.1 Definition of Primary Care Practitioners and Services; 100-04,12,230.2 Coordination with Other Payments; 100-04,12,230.3 Claims Processing and Payment; 100-04,12,30.6.14 Domiciliary Care, Rest Home, Assisted Living Visits; 100-04,12,30.6.15.1 Prolonged Services With Direct Face-to-Face Patient Contact; 100-04,12,30.6.4 Services Furnished Incident to Physician's Service

INCLUDES E/M services for patients residing in assisted living, domiciliary care, and rest homes where medical care not included
Services provided to new patients or established patients (99324-99328, 99334-99337)

EXCLUDES *Care plan oversight services provided to patient in rest home under home health agency care (99374-99375)*
Care plan oversight services provided to patient under hospice agency care (99377-99378)

99324 **Domiciliary or rest home visit for the evaluation and management of a new patient, which requires these 3 key components: A problem focused history; A problem focused examination; and Straightforward medical decision making. Counseling and/or coordination of care with other physicians, other qualified health care professionals, or agencies are provided consistent with the nature of the problem(s) and the patient's and/or family's needs. Usually, the presenting problem(s) are of low severity. Typically, 20 minutes are spent with the patient and/or family or caregiver.**

1.54 1.54 FUD XXX B 80

AMA: 2020,Sep,3; 2018,Apr,9; 2018,Jan,8; 2017,Aug,3; 2017,Jun,6; 2017,Jan,8; 2016,Dec,11; 2016,Jan,7; 2016,Jan,13; 2015,Jan,16

99325 **Domiciliary or rest home visit for the evaluation and management of a new patient, which requires these 3 key components: An expanded problem focused history; An expanded problem focused examination; and Medical decision making of low complexity. Counseling and/or coordination of care with other physicians, other qualified health care professionals, or agencies are provided consistent with the nature of the problem(s) and the patient's and/or family's needs. Usually, the presenting problem(s) are of moderate severity. Typically, 30 minutes are spent with the patient and/or family or caregiver.**

2.26 2.26 FUD XXX B 80

AMA: 2020,Sep,3; 2018,Apr,9; 2018,Jan,8; 2017,Aug,3; 2017,Jun,6; 2017,Jan,8; 2016,Dec,11; 2016,Jan,7; 2016,Jan,13; 2015,Jan,16

99326 **Domiciliary or rest home visit for the evaluation and management of a new patient, which requires these 3 key components: A detailed history; A detailed examination; and Medical decision making of moderate complexity. Counseling and/or coordination of care with other physicians, other qualified health care professionals, or agencies are provided consistent with the nature of the problem(s) and the patient's and/or family's needs. Usually, the presenting problem(s) are of moderate to high severity. Typically, 45 minutes are spent with the patient and/or family or caregiver.**

3.92 3.92 FUD XXX B 80

AMA: 2020,Sep,3; 2018,Apr,9; 2018,Jan,8; 2017,Aug,3; 2017,Jun,6; 2017,Jan,8; 2016,Dec,11; 2016,Jan,7; 2016,Jan,13; 2015,Jan,16

99327 **Domiciliary or rest home visit for the evaluation and management of a new patient, which requires these 3 key components: A comprehensive history; A comprehensive examination; and Medical decision making of moderate complexity. Counseling and/or coordination of care with other physicians, other qualified health care professionals, or agencies are provided consistent with the nature of the problem(s) and the patient's and/or family's needs. Usually, the presenting problem(s) are of high severity. Typically, 60 minutes are spent with the patient and/or family or caregiver.**

5.26 5.26 **FUD** XXX B 80

AMA: 2020,Sep,3; 2018,Apr,9; 2018,Jan,8; 2017,Aug,3; 2017,Jun,6; 2017,Jan,8; 2016,Dec,11; 2016,Jan,7; 2016,Jan,13; 2015,Jan,16

99328 **Domiciliary or rest home visit for the evaluation and management of a new patient, which requires these 3 key components: A comprehensive history; A comprehensive examination; and Medical decision making of high complexity. Counseling and/or coordination of care with other physicians, other qualified health care professionals, or agencies are provided consistent with the nature of the problem(s) and the patient's and/or family's needs. Usually, the patient is unstable or has developed a significant new problem requiring immediate physician attention. Typically, 75 minutes are spent with the patient and/or family or caregiver.**

6.20 6.20 **FUD** XXX B 80

AMA: 2020,Sep,3; 2018,Apr,9; 2018,Jan,8; 2017,Aug,3; 2017,Jun,6; 2017,Jan,8; 2016,Dec,11; 2016,Jan,7; 2016,Jan,13; 2015,Jan,16

99334 **Domiciliary or rest home visit for the evaluation and management of an established patient, which requires at least 2 of these 3 key components: A problem focused interval history; A problem focused examination; Straightforward medical decision making. Counseling and/or coordination of care with other physicians, other qualified health care professionals, or agencies are provided consistent with the nature of the problem(s) and the patient's and/or family's needs. Usually, the presenting problem(s) are self-limited or minor. Typically, 15 minutes are spent with the patient and/or family or caregiver.**

1.70 1.70 **FUD** XXX B 80

AMA: 2020,Sep,3; 2018,Apr,9; 2018,Jan,8; 2017,Aug,3; 2017,Jun,6; 2017,Jan,8; 2016,Dec,11; 2016,Jan,7; 2016,Jan,13; 2015,Jan,16

99335 **Domiciliary or rest home visit for the evaluation and management of an established patient, which requires at least 2 of these 3 key components: An expanded problem focused interval history; An expanded problem focused examination; Medical decision making of low complexity. Counseling and/or coordination of care with other physicians, other qualified health care professionals, or agencies are provided consistent with the nature of the problem(s) and the patient's and/or family's needs. Usually, the presenting problem(s) are of low to moderate severity. Typically, 25 minutes are spent with the patient and/or family or caregiver.**

2.68 2.68 **FUD** XXX B 80

AMA: 2020,Sep,3; 2018,Apr,9; 2018,Jan,8; 2017,Aug,3; 2017,Jun,6; 2017,Jan,8; 2016,Dec,11; 2016,Jan,7; 2016,Jan,13; 2015,Jan,16

99336 **Domiciliary or rest home visit for the evaluation and management of an established patient, which requires at least 2 of these 3 key components: A detailed interval history; A detailed examination; Medical decision making of moderate complexity. Counseling and/or coordination of care with other physicians, other qualified health care professionals, or agencies are provided consistent with the nature of the problem(s) and the patient's and/or family's needs. Usually, the presenting problem(s) are of moderate to high severity. Typically, 40 minutes are spent with the patient and/or family or caregiver.**

3.80 3.80 **FUD** XXX B 80

AMA: 2020,Sep,3; 2018,Apr,9; 2018,Jan,8; 2017,Aug,3; 2017,Jun,6; 2017,Jan,8; 2016,Dec,11; 2016,Jan,7; 2016,Jan,13; 2015,Jan,16

99337 **Domiciliary or rest home visit for the evaluation and management of an established patient, which requires at least 2 of these 3 key components: A comprehensive interval history; A comprehensive examination; Medical decision making of moderate to high complexity. Counseling and/or coordination of care with other physicians, other qualified health care professionals, or agencies are provided consistent with the nature of the problem(s) and the patient's and/or family's needs. Usually, the presenting problem(s) are of moderate to high severity. The patient may be unstable or may have developed a significant new problem requiring immediate physician attention. Typically, 60 minutes are spent with the patient and/or family or caregiver.**

5.47 5.47 **FUD** XXX B 80

AMA: 2020,Sep,3; 2018,Apr,9; 2018,Jan,8; 2017,Aug,3; 2017,Jun,6; 2017,Jan,8; 2016,Dec,11; 2016,Jan,7; 2016,Jan,13; 2015,Jan,16

99339-99340 Care Plan Oversight: Rest Home, Domiciliary Care, Assisted Living, and Home

CMS: 100-04,12,180 Payment of Care Plan Oversight (CPO); 100-04,12,180.1 Billing for Care Plan Oversight (CPO); 100-04,12,230 Primary Care Incentive Payment Program; 100-04,12,230.1 Definition of Primary Care Practitioners and Services; 100-04,12,230.2 Coordination with Other Payments; 100-04,12,230.3 Claims Processing and Payment; 100-04,12,30.6.14 Domiciliary Care, Rest Home, Assisted Living Visits; 100-04,12,30.6.4 Services Furnished Incident to Physician's Service

INCLUDES Care plan oversight for patients residing in assisted living, domiciliary care, private residences, and rest homes

Patient management services during same time frame as ([99421, 99422, 99423], 99441-99443, 98966-98968)

EXCLUDES *Care plan oversight services furnished under home health agency, nursing facility, or hospice (99374-99380)*

99339 **Individual physician supervision of a patient (patient not present) in home, domiciliary or rest home (eg, assisted living facility) requiring complex and multidisciplinary care modalities involving regular physician development and/or revision of care plans, review of subsequent reports of patient status, review of related laboratory and other studies, communication (including telephone calls) for purposes of assessment or care decisions with health care professional(s), family member(s), surrogate decision maker(s) (eg, legal guardian) and/or key caregiver(s) involved in patient's care, integration of new information into the medical treatment plan and/or adjustment of medical therapy, within a calendar month; 15-29 minutes**

2.17 2.17 **FUD** XXX B

AMA: 2019,Jan,6; 2018,Oct,9; 2018,Jan,8; 2017,Aug,3; 2017,Jun,6; 2017,Jan,8; 2016,Jan,13; 2015,Jan,16

99340 **30 minutes or more**

3.05 3.05 **FUD** XXX B

AMA: 2019,Jan,6; 2018,Oct,9; 2018,Jan,8; 2017,Aug,3; 2017,Jun,6; 2017,Jan,8; 2016,Jan,13; 2015,Jan,16

99341-99350 Home Visits

CMS: 100-04,11,40.1.3 Independent Attending Physician Services; 100-04,12,230 Primary Care Incentive Payment Program; 100-04,12,230.1 Definition of Primary Care Practitioners and Services; 100-04,12,230.2 Coordination with Other Payments; 100-04,12,230.3 Claims Processing and Payment; 100-04,12,30.6.14 Domiciliary Care, Rest Home, Assisted Living Visits; 100-04,12,30.6.14.1 Home Visits; 100-04,12,30.6.15.1 Prolonged Services With Direct Face-to-Face Patient Contact; 100-04,12,30.6.4 Services Furnished Incident to Physician's Service; 100-04,12,40.3 Global Surgery Review; 100-04,30.6.14.1 Home Services (Codes 99341 - 99350)

INCLUDES Services for new or established patient (99341-99345, 99347-99350)
Services provided to patient in private home (e.g., private residence, temporary or short-term housing such as campground, cruise ship, hostel, or hotel)

EXCLUDES *Services provided to patients under home health agency or hospice care (99374-99378)*

99341 **Home visit for the evaluation and management of a new patient, which requires these 3 key components: A problem focused history; A problem focused examination; and Straightforward medical decision making. Counseling and/or coordination of care with other physicians, other qualified health care professionals, or agencies are provided consistent with the nature of the problem(s) and the patient's and/or family's needs. Usually, the presenting problem(s) are of low severity. Typically, 20 minutes are spent face-to-face with the patient and/or family.**

1.56 1.56 **FUD** XXX B 80

AMA: 2020,Sep,3; 2018,Apr,9; 2018,Jan,8; 2017,Aug,3; 2017,Jun,6; 2017,Jan,8; 2016,Dec,11; 2016,Jan,7; 2016,Jan,13; 2015,Jan,16

99342 **Home visit for the evaluation and management of a new patient, which requires these 3 key components: An expanded problem focused history; An expanded problem focused examination; and Medical decision making of low complexity. Counseling and/or coordination of care with other physicians, other qualified health care professionals, or agencies are provided consistent with the nature of the problem(s) and the patient's and/or family's needs. Usually, the presenting problem(s) are of moderate severity. Typically, 30 minutes are spent face-to-face with the patient and/or family.**

2.25 2.25 **FUD** XXX B 80

AMA: 2020,Sep,3; 2018,Apr,9; 2018,Jan,8; 2017,Aug,3; 2017,Jun,6; 2017,Jan,8; 2016,Dec,11; 2016,Jan,7; 2016,Jan,13; 2015,Jan,16

99343 **Home visit for the evaluation and management of a new patient, which requires these 3 key components: A detailed history; A detailed examination; and Medical decision making of moderate complexity. Counseling and/or coordination of care with other physicians, other qualified health care professionals, or agencies are provided consistent with the nature of the problem(s) and the patient's and/or family's needs. Usually, the presenting problem(s) are of moderate to high severity. Typically, 45 minutes are spent face-to-face with the patient and/or family.**

3.67 3.67 **FUD** XXX B 80

AMA: 2020,Sep,3; 2018,Apr,9; 2018,Jan,8; 2017,Aug,3; 2017,Jun,6; 2017,Jan,8; 2016,Dec,11; 2016,Jan,7; 2016,Jan,13; 2015,Jan,16

99344 **Home visit for the evaluation and management of a new patient, which requires these 3 key components: A comprehensive history; A comprehensive examination; and Medical decision making of moderate complexity. Counseling and/or coordination of care with other physicians, other qualified health care professionals, or agencies are provided consistent with the nature of the problem(s) and the patient's and/or family's needs. Usually, the presenting problem(s) are of high severity. Typically, 60 minutes are spent face-to-face with the patient and/or family.**

5.14 5.14 **FUD** XXX B 80

AMA: 2020,Sep,3; 2018,Apr,9; 2018,Jan,8; 2017,Aug,3; 2017,Jun,6; 2017,Jan,8; 2016,Dec,11; 2016,Jan,7; 2016,Jan,13; 2015,Jan,16

99345 **Home visit for the evaluation and management of a new patient, which requires these 3 key components: A comprehensive history; A comprehensive examination; and Medical decision making of high complexity. Counseling and/or coordination of care with other physicians, other qualified health care professionals, or agencies are provided consistent with the nature of the problem(s) and the patient's and/or family's needs. Usually, the patient is unstable or has developed a significant new problem requiring immediate physician attention. Typically, 75 minutes are spent face-to-face with the patient and/or family.**

6.27 6.27 **FUD** XXX B 80

AMA: 2020,Sep,3; 2018,Apr,9; 2018,Jan,8; 2017,Aug,3; 2017,Jun,6; 2017,Jan,8; 2016,Dec,11; 2016,Jan,7; 2016,Jan,13; 2015,Jan,16

99347 **Home visit for the evaluation and management of an established patient, which requires at least 2 of these 3 key components: A problem focused interval history; A problem focused examination; Straightforward medical decision making. Counseling and/or coordination of care with other physicians, other qualified health care professionals, or agencies are provided consistent with the nature of the problem(s) and the patient's and/or family's needs. Usually, the presenting problem(s) are self limited or minor. Typically, 15 minutes are spent face-to-face with the patient and/or family.**

1.56 1.56 **FUD** XXX B 80

AMA: 2020,Sep,3; 2018,Apr,9; 2018,Jan,8; 2017,Aug,3; 2017,Jun,6; 2017,Jan,8; 2016,Dec,11; 2016,Jan,7; 2016,Jan,13; 2015,Jan,16

99348 **Home visit for the evaluation and management of an established patient, which requires at least 2 of these 3 key components: An expanded problem focused interval history; An expanded problem focused examination; Medical decision making of low complexity. Counseling and/or coordination of care with other physicians, other qualified health care professionals, or agencies are provided consistent with the nature of the problem(s) and the patient's and/or family's needs. Usually, the presenting problem(s) are of low to moderate severity. Typically, 25 minutes are spent face-to-face with the patient and/or family.**

2.37 2.37 **FUD** XXX B 80

AMA: 2020,Sep,3; 2018,Apr,9; 2018,Jan,8; 2017,Aug,3; 2017,Jun,6; 2017,Jan,8; 2016,Dec,11; 2016,Jan,7; 2016,Jan,13; 2015,Jan,16

99349 **Home visit for the evaluation and management of an established patient, which requires at least 2 of these 3 key components: A detailed interval history; A detailed examination; Medical decision making of moderate complexity. Counseling and/or coordination of care with other physicians, other qualified health care professionals, or agencies are provided consistent with the nature of the problem(s) and the patient's and/or family's needs. Usually, the presenting problem(s) are moderate to high severity. Typically, 40 minutes are spent face-to-face with the patient and/or family.**

3.64 3.64 **FUD** XXX B 80

AMA: 2020,Sep,3; 2018,Apr,9; 2018,Jan,8; 2017,Aug,3; 2017,Jun,6; 2017,Jan,8; 2016,Dec,11; 2016,Jan,7; 2016,Jan,13; 2015,Jan,16

99350 **Home visit for the evaluation and management of an established patient, which requires at least 2 of these 3 key components: A comprehensive interval history; A comprehensive examination; Medical decision making of moderate to high complexity. Counseling and/or coordination of care with other physicians, other qualified health care professionals, or agencies are provided consistent with the nature of the problem(s) and the patient's and/or family's needs. Usually, the presenting problem(s) are of moderate to high severity. The patient may be unstable or may have developed a significant new problem requiring immediate physician attention. Typically, 60 minutes are spent face-to-face with the patient and/or family.**

5.05 5.05 **FUD** XXX B 80

AMA: 2020,Sep,3; 2018,Apr,9; 2018,Jan,8; 2017,Aug,3; 2017,Jun,6; 2017,Jan,8; 2016,Dec,11; 2016,Jan,7; 2016,Jan,13; 2015,Jan,16

99354-99357 Prolonged Services Direct Contact

CMS: 100-04,11,40.1.3 Independent Attending Physician Services; 100-04,12,30.6.15.1 Prolonged Services With Direct Face-to-Face Patient Contact; 100-04,12,30.6.4 Services Furnished Incident to Physician's Service

INCLUDES Personal contact with patient by physician or other qualified health professional
Services extending beyond customary service provided in inpatient, observation, or outpatient setting
Time spent providing additional indirect contact services on floor, hospital unit, or nursing facility during same session as direct contact
Time spent providing prolonged services on service date, even when time not continuous

EXCLUDES *Services less than 30 minutes, less than15 minutes after first hour, or after final 30 minutes*
Services provided independent from personal contact date with patient (99358-99359)

Code first E/M service code, as appropriate

▲ + 99354 **Prolonged service(s) in the outpatient setting requiring direct patient contact beyond the time of the usual service; first hour (List separately in addition to code for outpatient Evaluation and Management or psychotherapy service, except with office or other outpatient services [99202, 99203, 99204, 99205, 99212, 99213, 99214, 99215])**

EXCLUDES *Office or other outpatient visit (99202-99205, 99212-99215)*
Prolonged office/outpatient services ([99417])
Prolonged service provided by clinical staff under supervision ([99415, 99416])
Reporting code more than one time per service date

Code first (99241-99245, 99324-99337, 99341-99350, 90837, 90847)

3.44 3.67 **FUD** ZZZ ★ N 80

AMA: 2020,Sep,3; 2020,Feb,3; 2019,Oct,10; 2019,Jun,7; 2018,Jan,8; 2017,Jan,8; 2016,Dec,11; 2016,Jan,13; 2015,Oct,9; 2015,Oct,3; 2015,Jan,16

▲ + 99355 **each additional 30 minutes (List separately in addition to code for prolonged service)**

EXCLUDES *Office or other outpatient visit (99202-99205, 99212-99215)*
Prolonged office/outpatient services ([99417])
Prolonged service provided by clinical staff under supervision ([99415, 99416])

Code first (99354)

2.60 2.80 **FUD** ZZZ ★ N 80

AMA: 2020,Sep,3; 2020,Feb,3; 2019,Oct,10; 2019,Jun,7; 2018,Jan,8; 2017,Jan,8; 2016,Dec,11; 2016,Jan,13; 2015,Oct,9; 2015,Oct,3; 2015,Jan,16

▲ + 99356 **Prolonged service in the inpatient or observation setting, requiring unit/floor time beyond the usual service; first hour (List separately in addition to code for inpatient or observation Evaluation and Management service)**

EXCLUDES *Reporting code more than one time per service date*

Code first (99218-99223 [99224, 99225, 99226], 99231-99236, 99251-99255, 99304-99310, 90837, 90847)

2.60 2.60 **FUD** ZZZ C 80

AMA: 2020,Sep,3; 2019,Jun,7; 2018,Jan,8; 2017,Jan,8; 2016,Dec,11; 2016,Jan,13; 2015,Oct,3; 2015,Oct,9; 2015,Jan,16

+ 99357 **each additional 30 minutes (List separately in addition to code for prolonged service)**

Code first (99356)

2.61 2.61 **FUD** ZZZ C 80

AMA: 2020,Sep,3; 2019,Jun,7; 2018,Jan,8; 2017,Jan,8; 2016,Dec,11; 2016,Jan,13; 2015,Oct,3; 2015,Oct,9; 2015,Jan,16

99358-99359 Prolonged Services Indirect Contact

CMS: 100-04,11,40.1.3 Independent Attending Physician Services; 100-04,12,30.6.15.2 Prolonged Services Without Face to Face Service; 100-04,12,30.6.4 Services Furnished Incident to Physician's Service

INCLUDES Services extending beyond customary service
Time spent providing indirect contact services by physician or other qualified health care professional in relation to patient management where face-to-face services have or will occur on different date
Time spent providing prolonged services on service date, even when time not continuous

EXCLUDES *Any additional unit or floor time in hospital or nursing facility during same evaluation and management session*
Behavioral health integration care management services (99484)
Time without direct patient contact for other services:
Care plan oversight (99339-99340, 99374-99380)
Chronic care management services provided during same month ([99491])
INR monitoring services (93792-93793)
Medical team conference (99366-99368)
Online and telephone consultative services (99446-99452 [99451, 99452])
Online medical services ([99421, 99422, 99423])
Patient management services during same time frame as (99487-99489, 99495-99496)
Psychiatric collaborative care management services during same month (99492-99494)
Reporting code more than one time per service date
Services less than 30 minutes, less than15 minutes after first hour, or after final 30 minutes

Code also E/M or other services provided, excluding (99202-99205, 99212-99215, 99217)

99358 **Prolonged evaluation and management service before and/or after direct patient care; first hour**

EXCLUDES *Use of code more than one time per date of service*

3.15 3.15 **FUD** XXX N 80

AMA: 2020,Sep,3; 2020,Feb,3; 2019,Jun,7; 2019,Jan,13; 2018,Oct,9; 2018,Jan,8; 2017,Jan,8; 2016,Jan,13; 2015,Jan,16

+ 99359 **each additional 30 minutes (List separately in addition to code for prolonged service)**

Code first (99358)

1.52 1.52 **FUD** ZZZ N 80

AMA: 2020,Sep,3; 2020,Feb,3; 2019,Jun,7; 2019,Jan,13; 2018,Oct,9; 2018,Jan,8; 2017,Jan,8; 2016,Jan,13; 2015,Jan,16

99415-99417 [99415, 99416, 99417] Prolonged Clinical Staff Services Under Supervision

INCLUDES Time spent by clinical staff providing prolonged face-to-face services extending beyond customary service under physician or other qualified health professional supervision
Time spent by clinical staff providing prolonged services on service date, even when time not continuous

EXCLUDES *Prolonged service provided by physician or other qualified health care professional (99354-99355, [99417])*

▲ + # 99415 **Prolonged clinical staff service (the service beyond the highest time in the range of total time of the service) during an evaluation and management service in the office or outpatient setting, direct patient contact with physician supervision; first hour (List separately in addition to code for outpatient Evaluation and Management service)**

EXCLUDES *Reporting code more than one time per service date*
Reporting code with ([99417])
Services less than 30 minutes
Services provided to more than two patients at same time

Code first (99202-99205, 99212-99215)

0.28 0.28 **FUD** ZZZ N 80 TC

AMA: 2020,Sep,3; 2020,Feb,3; 2019,Oct,10; 2018,Jan,8; 2017,Jan,8; 2016,Mar,8; 2016,Feb,13; 2016,Jan,13; 2015,Oct,3

▲+ #99416 **each additional 30 minutes (List separately in addition to code for prolonged service)**

EXCLUDES *Reporting code with ([99417])*
Services less than 30 minutes, less than 15 minutes after first hour, or after final 30 minutes
Services provided to more than two patients at same time

Code first ([99415])

Facility RVU 0.13 Non-Facility RVU 0.13 **FUD** ZZZ N 80 TC CCI

AMA: 2020,Sep,3; 2020,Feb,3; 2019,Oct,10; 2018,Jan,8; 2017,Jan,8; 2016,Mar,8; 2016,Feb,13; 2016,Jan,13; 2015,Oct,3

●+ #99417 **Prolonged office or other outpatient evaluation and management service(s) beyond the minimum required time of the primary procedure which has been selected using total time, requiring total time with or without direct patient contact beyond the usual service, on the date of the primary service, each 15 minutes of total time (List separately in addition to codes 99205, 99215 for office or other outpatient Evaluation and Management services)**

INCLUDES Total time prolonged services provided same date with both direct and indirect patient contact by physician or QHCP

EXCLUDES *Services less than 15 minutes*

Code first (99205 or 99215)

Facility RVU 0.00 Non-Facility RVU 0.00 **FUD** 000 ★

99360 Standby Services

CMS: 100-04,11,40.1.3 Independent Attending Physician Services; 100-04,12,30.6.15.3 Standby Services; 100-04,12,30.6.4 Services Furnished Incident to Physician's Service

INCLUDES Services requested by physician or qualified health care professional that involve no direct patient contact
Total standby time for day

EXCLUDES *Delivery attendance (99464)*
Less than 30 minutes standby time
On-call services mandated by hospital (99026-99027)

Code also as appropriate (99460, 99465)

99360 **Standby service, requiring prolonged attendance, each 30 minutes (eg, operative standby, standby for frozen section, for cesarean/high risk delivery, for monitoring EEG)**

Facility RVU 1.75 Non-Facility RVU 1.75 **FUD** XXX B CCI

AMA: 2018,Jan,8; 2017,Jan,8; 2016,Jan,13; 2015,Jan,16

99366-99368 Interdisciplinary Conferences

CMS: 100-04,11,40.1.3 Independent Attending Physician Services

INCLUDES Documentation conference participation, contribution, and recommendations
Face-to-face participation by minimum of three qualified people from different specialties or disciplines
Individual patient review from start to conclusion
Only participants who have performed face-to-face evaluations or direct treatment to patient within previous 60 days
Team conferences 30 minutes or more

EXCLUDES *Conferences less than 30 minutes (not reportable)*
More than one individual from same specialty at same encounter
Patient management services during same month as ([99439, 99490, 99491], 99487-99489)
Time spent record keeping or writing report

99366 **Medical team conference with interdisciplinary team of health care professionals, face-to-face with patient and/or family, 30 minutes or more, participation by nonphysician qualified health care professional**

EXCLUDES *Team conferences by physician with patient or family present, see appropriate E/M service code*

Facility RVU 1.19 Non-Facility RVU 1.21 **FUD** XXX N CCI

AMA: 2018,Apr,9; 2018,Jan,8; 2017,Jan,8; 2016,Jan,13; 2015,Jan,16

99367 **Medical team conference with interdisciplinary team of health care professionals, patient and/or family not present, 30 minutes or more; participation by physician**

Facility RVU 1.60 Non-Facility RVU 1.60 **FUD** XXX N CCI

AMA: 2019,Dec,14; 2018,Apr,9; 2018,Jan,8; 2017,Jan,8; 2016,Jan,13; 2015,Jan,16

99368 **participation by nonphysician qualified health care professional**

Facility RVU 1.04 Non-Facility RVU 1.04 **FUD** XXX N CCI

AMA: 2018,Apr,9; 2018,Jan,8; 2017,Jan,8; 2016,Jan,13; 2015,Jan,16

99374-99380 Care Plan Oversight: Patient Under Care of HHA, Hospice, or Nursing Facility

CMS: 100-04,11,40.1.3 Independent Attending Physician Services; 100-04,12,180 Payment of Care Plan Oversight (CPO); 100-04,12,180.1 Billing for Care Plan Oversight (CPO); 100-04,12,30.6.4 Services Furnished Incident to Physician's Service

INCLUDES Analysis reports, diagnostic tests, treatment plans
Discussions with other health care providers, outside practice, involved in patient's care
Establishment and revisions to care plans within 30-day period
Payment to one physician per month for covered care plan oversight services (must be same one who signed plan of care)

EXCLUDES *Care plan oversight services provided in hospice agency (99377-99378)*
Care plan oversight services provided in assisted living, domiciliary care, or private residence, not under home health agency or hospice care (99339-99340)
Patient management services during same time frame as ([99421, 99422, 99423], 99441-99443, 98966-98968)
Routine postoperative care provided during global surgery period
Time discussing treatment with patient and/or caregivers

Code also office/outpatient visits, hospital, home, nursing facility, domiciliary, or non-face-to-face services

99374 **Supervision of a patient under care of home health agency (patient not present) in home, domiciliary or equivalent environment (eg, Alzheimer's facility) requiring complex and multidisciplinary care modalities involving regular development and/or revision of care plans by that individual, review of subsequent reports of patient status, review of related laboratory and other studies, communication (including telephone calls) for purposes of assessment or care decisions with health care professional(s), family member(s), surrogate decision maker(s) (eg, legal guardian) and/or key caregiver(s) involved in patient's care, integration of new information into the medical treatment plan and/or adjustment of medical therapy, within a calendar month; 15-29 minutes**

Facility RVU 1.60 Non-Facility RVU 1.96 **FUD** XXX B CCI

AMA: 2019,Jan,6; 2018,Jan,8; 2017,Jan,8; 2016,Jan,13; 2015,Jan,16

99375 **30 minutes or more**

Facility RVU 2.53 Non-Facility RVU 2.96 **FUD** XXX E CCI

AMA: 2019,Jan,6; 2018,Jan,8; 2017,Jan,8; 2016,Jan,13; 2015,Jan,16

99377 **Supervision of a hospice patient (patient not present) requiring complex and multidisciplinary care modalities involving regular development and/or revision of care plans by that individual, review of subsequent reports of patient status, review of related laboratory and other studies, communication (including telephone calls) for purposes of assessment or care decisions with health care professional(s), family member(s), surrogate decision maker(s) (eg, legal guardian) and/or key caregiver(s) involved in patient's care, integration of new information into the medical treatment plan and/or adjustment of medical therapy, within a calendar month; 15-29 minutes**

Facility RVU 1.60 Non-Facility RVU 1.96 **FUD** XXX B CCI

AMA: 2019,Jan,6; 2018,Jan,8; 2017,Jan,8; 2016,Jan,13; 2015,Jan,16

99378 **30 minutes or more**

Facility RVU 2.50 Non-Facility RVU 2.94 **FUD** XXX E CCI

AMA: 2019,Jan,6; 2018,Jan,8; 2017,Jan,8; 2016,Jan,13; 2015,Jan,16

99379 **Supervision of a nursing facility patient (patient not present) requiring complex and multidisciplinary care modalities involving regular development and/or revision of care plans by that individual, review of subsequent reports of patient status, review of related laboratory and other studies, communication (including telephone calls) for purposes of assessment or care decisions with health care professional(s), family member(s), surrogate decision maker(s) (eg, legal guardian) and/or key caregiver(s) involved in patient's care, integration of new information into the medical treatment plan and/or adjustment of medical therapy, within a calendar month; 15-29 minutes**
1.60 1.96 **FUD** XXX B
AMA: 2019,Jan,6; 2018,Jan,8; 2017,Jan,8; 2016,Jan,13; 2015,Jan,16

99380 **30 minutes or more**
2.53 2.96 **FUD** XXX B
AMA: 2019,Jan,6; 2018,Jan,8; 2017,Jan,8; 2016,Jan,13; 2015,Jan,16

99381-99397 Preventive Medicine Visits

CMS: 100-04,11,40.1.3 Independent Attending Physician Services; 100-04,12,30.6.2 Medically Necessary and Preventive Medicine Service on Same Date; 100-04,12,30.6.4 Services Furnished Incident to Physician's Service

INCLUDES Care for small problem or pre-existing condition that requires no extra work
New patients or established patients (99381-99387, 99391-99397)
Regular preventive care (e.g., well-child exams) for all age groups

EXCLUDES *Behavioral change interventions (99406-99409)*
Counseling/risk factor reduction interventions not provided with preventive medical examination (99401-99412)
Diagnostic tests and other procedures

Code also immunization counseling, administration, and product (90460-90461, 90471-90474, 90476-90749 [90620, 90621, 90625, 90630, 90644, 90672, 90673, 90674, 90750, 90756])
Code also significant, separately identifiable E/M service on same date for substantial problems requiring additional work using modifier 25 and (99202-99215)

99381 **Initial comprehensive preventive medicine evaluation and management of an individual including an age and gender appropriate history, examination, counseling/anticipatory guidance/risk factor reduction interventions, and the ordering of laboratory/diagnostic procedures, new patient; infant (age younger than 1 year)** A
2.19 3.13 **FUD** XXX E
AMA: 2018,Jan,8; 2017,Jan,8; 2016,Mar,8; 2016,Jan,13; 2015,Jan,16

99382 **early childhood (age 1 through 4 years)** A
2.32 3.28 **FUD** XXX E
AMA: 2018,Jan,8; 2017,Jan,8; 2016,Mar,8; 2016,Jan,13; 2015,Jan,16

99383 **late childhood (age 5 through 11 years)** A
2.46 3.41 **FUD** XXX E
AMA: 2018,Jan,8; 2017,Jan,8; 2016,Mar,8; 2016,Jan,13; 2015,Jan,16

99384 **adolescent (age 12 through 17 years)** A
2.88 3.85 **FUD** XXX E
AMA: 2018,Jan,8; 2017,Jan,8; 2016,Mar,8; 2016,Jan,13; 2015,Jan,12; 2015,Jan,16

99385 **18-39 years** A
2.76 3.72 **FUD** XXX E
AMA: 2018,Jan,8; 2017,Jan,8; 2016,Mar,8; 2016,Jan,13; 2015,Jan,12; 2015,Jan,16

99386 **40-64 years** A
3.36 4.32 **FUD** XXX E
AMA: 2018,Jan,8; 2017,Jan,8; 2016,Mar,8; 2016,Jan,13; 2015,Jan,12; 2015,Jan,16

99387 **65 years and older** A
3.67 4.72 **FUD** XXX E
AMA: 2018,Jan,8; 2017,Jan,8; 2016,Mar,8; 2016,Jan,13; 2015,Jan,16

99391 **Periodic comprehensive preventive medicine reevaluation and management of an individual including an age and gender appropriate history, examination, counseling/anticipatory guidance/risk factor reduction interventions, and the ordering of laboratory/diagnostic procedures, established patient; infant (age younger than 1 year)** A
1.98 2.82 **FUD** XXX E
AMA: 2018,Jan,8; 2017,Jan,8; 2016,Mar,8; 2016,Jan,13; 2015,Jan,16

99392 **early childhood (age 1 through 4 years)** A
2.17 3.01 **FUD** XXX E
AMA: 2018,Jan,8; 2017,Jan,8; 2016,Mar,8; 2016,Jan,13; 2015,Jan,16

99393 **late childhood (age 5 through 11 years)** A
2.17 3.00 **FUD** XXX E
AMA: 2018,Jan,8; 2017,Jan,8; 2016,Mar,8; 2016,Jan,13; 2015,Jan,16

99394 **adolescent (age 12 through 17 years)** A
2.46 3.29 **FUD** XXX E
AMA: 2018,Jan,8; 2017,Jan,8; 2016,Mar,8; 2016,Jan,13; 2015,Jan,12; 2015,Jan,16

99395 **18-39 years** A
2.53 3.36 **FUD** XXX E
AMA: 2018,Jan,8; 2017,Jan,8; 2016,Mar,8; 2016,Jan,13; 2015,Jan,16; 2015,Jan,12

99396 **40-64 years** A
2.74 3.58 **FUD** XXX E
AMA: 2018,Jan,8; 2017,Sep,11; 2017,Jan,8; 2016,Mar,8; 2016,Jan,13; 2015,Jan,12; 2015,Jan,16

99397 **65 years and older** A
2.93 3.87 **FUD** XXX E
AMA: 2018,Jan,8; 2017,Jan,8; 2016,Mar,8; 2016,Jan,13; 2015,Jan,16

99401-99423 [99415, 99416, 99417, 99421, 99422, 99423] Counseling Services: Risk Factor and Behavioral Change Modification

INCLUDES Face-to-face services for new and established patients based on 15- to 60-minute time increments
Health and behavioral services provided on same day (96156-96159 [96164, 96165, 96167, 96168, 96170, 96171])
Issues such as healthy diet, exercise, alcohol, and drug abuse
Services provided by physician or other qualified healthcare professional for promoting health and reducing illness and injury

EXCLUDES *Counseling and risk factor reduction interventions included in preventive medicine services (99381-99397)*
Counseling services provided to patient groups with existing symptoms or illness (99078)

Code also significant, separately identifiable E/M services when performed and append modifier 25 to service

99401 **Preventive medicine counseling and/or risk factor reduction intervention(s) provided to an individual (separate procedure); approximately 15 minutes**
0.70 1.10 **FUD** XXX E
AMA: 2020,Aug,3; 2018,Jan,8; 2017,Jan,8; 2016,Mar,8; 2016,Jan,13; 2015,Jan,16

99402 **approximately 30 minutes**
1.42 1.81 **FUD** XXX E
AMA: 2020,Aug,3; 2018,Jan,8; 2017,Jan,8; 2016,Mar,8; 2016,Jan,13; 2015,Jan,16

99403 **approximately 45 minutes**
2.12 2.51 **FUD** XXX E
AMA: 2020,Aug,3; 2018,Jan,8; 2017,Jan,8; 2016,Mar,8; 2016,Jan,13; 2015,Jan,16

99404 **approximately 60 minutes**
2.81 3.21 **FUD** XXX E
AMA: 2020,Aug,3; 2018,Jan,8; 2017,Jan,8; 2016,Mar,8; 2016,Jan,13; 2015,Jan,16

99406 **Smoking and tobacco use cessation counseling visit; intermediate, greater than 3 minutes up to 10 minutes**
0.35 0.43 FUD XXX ★ S 80
AMA: 2020,Sep,14; 2020,Aug,3; 2018,Jan,8; 2017,Nov,3; 2017,Jan,8; 2016,Mar,8; 2016,Jan,13; 2015,Jan,16

99407 **intensive, greater than 10 minutes**
INCLUDES Services 11-14 minutes
0.73 0.80 FUD XXX ★ S 80
AMA: 2020,Aug,3; 2018,Jan,8; 2017,Nov,3; 2017,Jan,8; 2016,Mar,8; 2016,Jan,13; 2015,Jan,16

99408 **Alcohol and/or substance (other than tobacco) abuse structured screening (eg, AUDIT, DAST), and brief intervention (SBI) services; 15 to 30 minutes**
INCLUDES Health risk assessment (96160-96161)
Services 15 minutes or more
Only initial screening and brief intervention
0.94 1.01 FUD XXX ★ E
AMA: 2020,Aug,3; 2018,Jan,8; 2017,Nov,3; 2017,Jan,8; 2016,Nov,5; 2016,Mar,8; 2016,Jan,13; 2015,Jan,16

99409 **greater than 30 minutes**
INCLUDES Health risk assessment (96160-96161)
Only initial screening and brief intervention
Services 31 minutes or more
1.88 1.95 FUD XXX ★ E
AMA: 2020,Aug,3; 2018,Jan,8; 2017,Nov,3; 2017,Jan,8; 2016,Nov,5; 2016,Mar,8; 2016,Jan,13; 2015,Jan,16

99411 **Preventive medicine counseling and/or risk factor reduction intervention(s) provided to individuals in a group setting (separate procedure); approximately 30 minutes**
0.22 0.55 FUD XXX E
AMA: 2020,Aug,3; 2018,Jan,8; 2017,Jan,8; 2016,Mar,8; 2016,Jan,13; 2015,Jan,16

99412 **approximately 60 minutes**
0.36 0.69 FUD XXX E
AMA: 2020,Aug,3; 2018,Jan,8; 2017,Jan,8; 2016,Mar,8; 2016,Jan,13; 2015,Jan,16

99415 **Resequenced code. See code following 99359.**

99416 **Resequenced code. See code following 99359.**

99421 **Resequenced code. See code following 99443.**

99422 **Resequenced code. See code following 99443.**

99423 **Resequenced code. See code following 99443.**

99429-99439 [99439] Other Preventive Medicine

99429 **Unlisted preventive medicine service**
0.00 0.00 FUD XXX E
AMA: 2018,Jan,8; 2017,Jan,8; 2016,Mar,8; 2016,Jan,13; 2015,Jan,16

99439 **Resequenced code. See code following resequenced code 99490.**

99441-99443 Telephone Calls for Patient Management

CMS: 100-04,11,40.1.3 Independent Attending Physician Services

INCLUDES Care initiated by established patient or patient's guardian
Non-face-to-face E/M services provided by physician or other health care provider qualified to report E/M services
Related E/M services provided within:
Postoperative period
Seven days prior to service

EXCLUDES *Patient management services during same time frame as (99339-99340, 99374-99380, 99487-99489, 99495-99496, 93792-93793)*
Reporting codes more than one time for telephone and online services when reported within 7-day time period by same provider
Services provided by qualified nonphysician health care professional unable to report E/M codes (98966-98968)

99441 **Telephone evaluation and management service by a physician or other qualified health care professional who may report evaluation and management services provided to an established patient, parent, or guardian not originating from a related E/M service provided within the previous 7 days nor leading to an E/M service or procedure within the next 24 hours or soonest available appointment; 5-10 minutes of medical discussion**
0.36 0.39 FUD XXX E 80
AMA: 2020,JulBULL,1; 2019,Mar,8; 2018,Mar,7; 2018,Jan,8; 2017,Jan,8; 2016,Jan,13; 2015,Jan,16

99442 **11-20 minutes of medical discussion**
0.72 0.76 FUD XXX E 80
AMA: 2020,JulBULL,1; 2019,Mar,8; 2018,Mar,7; 2018,Jan,8; 2017,Jan,8; 2016,Jan,13; 2015,Jan,16

99443 **21-30 minutes of medical discussion**
1.08 1.12 FUD XXX E 80
AMA: 2020,JulBULL,1; 2019,Mar,8; 2018,Mar,7; 2018,Jan,8; 2017,Jan,8; 2016,Jan,13; 2015,Jan,16

99421-99423 [99421, 99422, 99423] Digital Evaluation and Management Services

CMS: 100-04,11,40.1.3 Independent Attending Physician Services

INCLUDES Cumulative service time within seven-day time frame needed to evaluate, assess, and manage the patient:
Ordering tests
Prescription generation
Separate digital inquiry for new and unrelated problem
Subsequent communication digitally supported (i.e., email, online, telephone)
Digital service initiated by established patient

EXCLUDES *Clinical staff time*
Digital evaluation by qualified nonphysician health care professional (98970-98972)
Digital evaluation peformed with separately reportable E/M services during same time frame for new or established patient:
Inquiries related to previously completed procedure and within postoperative period
INR monitoring (93792-93793)
Office consultation (99241-99245)
Office or other outpatient visit (99202-99205, 99212-99215)
Patient management services (99339-99340, 99374-99380, [99091], 99487-99489)
Digital service less than 5 minutes
Reporting code more than one time in 7 days

\# **99421** **Online digital evaluation and management service, for an established patient, for up to 7 days, cumulative time during the 7 days; 5-10 minutes**
0.37 0.43 FUD XXX 80
AMA: 2020,Jan,3

\# **99422** **11-20 minutes**
0.76 0.86 FUD XXX 80
AMA: 2020,Jan,3

\# **99423** **21 or more minutes**
1.21 1.39 FUD XXX 80
AMA: 2020,Jan,3

99446-99452 [99451, 99452] Online and Telephone Consultative Services

INCLUDES Multiple telephone and/or internet contact needed to complete consultation (e.g., test result(s) follow-up)
New or established patient with new problem or exacerbation existing problem and not seen within last 14 days
Review pertinent lab, imaging and/or pathology studies, medical records, medications

EXCLUDES *Any service less than 5 minutes*
Communication with family with or without patient present ([99421, 99422, 99423], 99441-99443, 98966-98967)
Transfer care only

99446 Interprofessional telephone/Internet/electronic health record assessment and management service provided by a consultative physician, including a verbal and written report to the patient's treating/requesting physician or other qualified health care professional; 5-10 minutes of medical consultative discussion and review

INCLUDES Verbal and written reports from consultant to requesting provider

EXCLUDES *Prolonged services without direct patient contact (99358-99359)*
Reporting code more than one time in 7 days

0.51 0.51 **FUD** XXX E 80

AMA: 2019,Jun,7; 2019,Jan,3; 2018,Jan,8; 2017,Jan,8; 2016,Jan,13; 2015,Jan,16

99447 11-20 minutes of medical consultative discussion and review

INCLUDES Verbal and written reports from consultant to requesting provider

EXCLUDES *Prolonged services without direct patient contact (99358-99359)*
Reporting code more than one time in 7 days

1.01 1.01 **FUD** XXX E 80

AMA: 2019,Jun,7; 2019,Jan,3; 2018,Jan,8; 2017,Jan,8; 2016,Jan,13; 2015,Jan,16

99448 21-30 minutes of medical consultative discussion and review

INCLUDES Verbal and written reports from consultant to requesting provider

EXCLUDES *Prolonged services without direct patient contact (99358-99359)*
Reporting code more than one time in 7 days

1.52 1.52 **FUD** XXX E 80

AMA: 2019,Jun,7; 2019,Jan,3; 2018,Jan,8; 2017,Jan,8; 2016,Jan,13; 2015,Jan,16

99449 31 minutes or more of medical consultative discussion and review

INCLUDES Verbal and written reports from consultant to requesting provider

EXCLUDES *Prolonged services without direct patient contact (99358-99359)*
Reporting code more than one time in 7 days

2.02 2.02 **FUD** XXX E 80

AMA: 2019,Jun,7; 2019,Jan,3; 2018,Jan,8; 2017,Jan,8; 2016,Jan,13; 2015,Jan,16

\# **99451 Interprofessional telephone/Internet/electronic health record assessment and management service provided by a consultative physician, including a written report to the patient's treating/requesting physician or other qualified health care professional, 5 minutes or more of medical consultative time**

INCLUDES Verbal and written reports from consultant to requesting provider

EXCLUDES *Prolonged services without direct patient contact (99358-99359)*
Reporting code more than one time in 7 days

1.04 1.04 **FUD** XXX 80

AMA: 2019,Jun,7; 2019,Jan,3

\# **99452 Interprofessional telephone/Internet/electronic health record referral service(s) provided by a treating/requesting physician or other qualified health care professional, 30 minutes**

INCLUDES Time preparing for referral, 16 to 30 minutes

EXCLUDES *Requesting physician's time 30 minutes over typical E/M service, patient not on site (99358-99359)*
Requesting physician's time 30 minutes over typical E/M service, patient on site (99354-99357)
Reporting code more than one time every 14 days

1.04 1.04 **FUD** XXX 80

AMA: 2020,Jun,3; 2019,Jun,7; 2019,Jan,3

99453-99474 [99091, 99453, 99454, 99473, 99474] Remote Monitoring/Collection Biological Data

\# **99453 Remote monitoring of physiologic parameter(s) (eg, weight, blood pressure, pulse oximetry, respiratory flow rate), initial; set-up and patient education on use of equipment**

INCLUDES 30-day period physiologic monitoring parameters such as weight, blood pressure, pulse oximetry
Services ordered by physician or other qualified healthcare professional
Services provided for each care episode (starts when monitoring begins and ends when treatment goals achieved)
Set-up and instructions for use
Treatment with device approved by FDA

EXCLUDES *Monitoring less than 16 days*
Reporting codes when services included in other monitoring services (e.g., 93296, 94760, 95250)

0.52 0.52 **FUD** XXX 80

AMA: 2020,Apr,5; 2019,Mar,10; 2019,Jan,3; 2019,Jan,6

\# **99454 device(s) supply with daily recording(s) or programmed alert(s) transmission, each 30 days**

INCLUDES 30-day period physiologic monitoring parameters such as weight, blood pressure, pulse oximetry
Service ordered by physician or other qualified healthcare professional
Supplying device
Treatment with device approved by FDA

EXCLUDES *Monitoring less than 16 days*
Remote monitoring treatment management
Reporting codes when services included in other monitoring services (e.g., 93296, 94760, 95250)
Self-measured blood pressure monitoring ([99473, 99474])

1.73 1.73 **FUD** XXX 80

AMA: 2020,Apr,5; 2019,Oct,3; 2019,Mar,10; 2019,Jan,3; 2019,Jan,6

\# **99091 Collection and interpretation of physiologic data (eg, ECG, blood pressure, glucose monitoring) digitally stored and/or transmitted by the patient and/or caregiver to the physician or other qualified health care professional, qualified by education, training, licensure/regulation (when applicable) requiring a minimum of 30 minutes of time, each 30 days**

INCLUDES E/M services provided on same service date

EXCLUDES *Care plan oversight services within same calendar month (99339-99340, 99374-99380)*
Chronic care management services within same calendar month ([99491])
Data transfer/interpretation from clinical lab or hospital computers
Remote physiologic monitoring treatment management within same calendar month ([99457])
Reporting code more than one time in 30 days
Reporting codes when services included in other monitoring services such as (93227, 93272, 95250)
Services for which more specific codes exist, such as:
Ambulatory continuous glucose monitoring (95250)
Electrocardiographic services (93227, 93272)

1.62 1.62 **FUD** XXX N 80

AMA: 2020,Apr,5; 2020,Feb,7; 2019,Oct,3; 2019,Jun,3; 2019,Jan,6; 2018,Dec,10; 2018,Dec,10; 2018,Jun,6; 2018,Mar,5; 2018,Feb,7; 2018,Jan,8; 2017,Jan,8; 2016,Jan,13; 2015,Jan,16

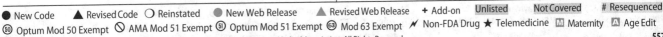

\# **99473** **Self-measured blood pressure using a device validated for clinical accuracy; patient education/training and device calibration**

EXCLUDES *Reporting code more than once per device*
Reporting codes when services included in same calendar month as:
Ambulatory blood pressure monitoring (93784-93790)
Chronic care management service ([99439, 99490, 99491], 99487-99489)
Remote physiologic monitoring, collection and interpretation ([99453, 99454], [99091], [99457])

Facility RVU 0.31 Non-Facility RVU 0.31 **FUD** XXX 80

AMA: 2020,Apr,5; 2020,Feb,7; 2020,Jan,3

\# **99474** **separate self-measurements of two readings one minute apart, twice daily over a 30-day period (minimum of 12 readings), collection of data reported by the patient and/or caregiver to the physician or other qualified health care professional, with report of average systolic and diastolic pressures and subsequent communication of a treatment plan to the patient**

EXCLUDES *Reporting code more than once per device*
Reporting codes when services included in same calendar month as:
Ambulatory blood pressure monitoring (93784-93790)
Chronic care management services ([99439, 99490, 99491], 99487-99489)
Remote physiologic monitoring, collection and interpretation services ([99453, 99454], [99091], [99457])

Facility RVU 0.25 Non-Facility RVU 0.42 **FUD** XXX 80

AMA: 2020,Apr,5; 2020,Feb,7; 2020,Jan,3

99457-99458 [99457, 99458] Remote Monitoring Management

CMS: 100-04,11,40.1.3 Independent Attending Physician Services

INCLUDES Interactive live communication with patient at least 20 minutes per month
Remote monitoring results used for patient management
Reporting code each 30 days no matter number parameters monitored
Service ordered by physician or other qualified healthcare professional
Time managing care when more specific service codes not available
Treatment with device approved by FDA

EXCLUDES *Reporting code for services lasting less than 20 mintues*
Reporting code on same service date as E/M services (99202-99215, 99221-99223, 99231-99233, 99251-99255, 99324-99328, 99334-99337, 99341-99350)

Code also, when appropriate:
Behavioral health integration services ([99484], 99492-99494)
Chronic care management services ([99439], [99490], [99491], 99487, 99489)
Transitional care management services (99495-99496)

\# **99457** **Remote physiologic monitoring treatment management services, clinical staff/physician/other qualified health care professional time in a calendar month requiring interactive communication with the patient/caregiver during the month; first 20 minutes**

EXCLUDES *Collection and interpretation physiologic data ([99091])*

Facility RVU 0.90 Non-Facility RVU 1.43 **FUD** XXX 80

AMA: 2020,Apr,5; 2020,Feb,7; 2019,Jun,3; 2019,Jan,3; 2019,Jan,6

\+ # **99458** **each additional 20 minutes (List separately in addition to code for primary procedure)**

EXCLUDES *Reporting code when 20 minutes additional treatment time not obtained ([99457])*

Code first ([99457])

Facility RVU 0.91 Non-Facility RVU 1.17 **FUD** ZZZ 80

AMA: 2020,Feb,7

99450-99458 [99451, 99452, 99453, 99454, 99457, 99458] Life/Disability Insurance Eligibility Visits

INCLUDES Assessment services for insurance eligibility and work-related disability without medical management of the patient's illness/injury
Services provided to new/established patients at any site of service

EXCLUDES *Any additional E&M services or procedures performed on the same date of service: report with appropriate code*

99450 **Basic life and/or disability examination that includes: Measurement of height, weight, and blood pressure; Completion of a medical history following a life insurance pro forma; Collection of blood sample and/or urinalysis complying with "chain of custody" protocols; and Completion of necessary documentation/certificates.**

Facility RVU 0.00 Non-Facility RVU 0.00 **FUD** XXX E

AMA: 2019,Jun,7; 2018,Jan,8; 2017,Jan,8; 2016,Jan,13; 2015,Jan,16

99451 **Resequenced code. See code following 99449.**

99452 **Resequenced code. See code following 99449.**

99453 **Resequenced code. See code following 99449.**

99454 **Resequenced code. See code following 99449.**

99455 **Work related or medical disability examination by the treating physician that includes: Completion of a medical history commensurate with the patient's condition; Performance of an examination commensurate with the patient's condition; Formulation of a diagnosis, assessment of capabilities and stability, and calculation of impairment; Development of future medical treatment plan; and Completion of necessary documentation/certificates and report.**

INCLUDES Special reports (99080)

Facility RVU 0.00 Non-Facility RVU 0.00 **FUD** XXX B 80

AMA: 2018,Jan,8; 2017,Jan,8; 2016,Jan,13; 2015,Jan,16

99456 **Work related or medical disability examination by other than the treating physician that includes: Completion of a medical history commensurate with the patient's condition; Performance of an examination commensurate with the patient's condition; Formulation of a diagnosis, assessment of capabilities and stability, and calculation of impairment; Development of future medical treatment plan; and Completion of necessary documentation/certificates and report.**

INCLUDES Special reports (99080)

Facility RVU 0.00 Non-Facility RVU 0.00 **FUD** XXX B 80

AMA: 2018,Jan,8; 2017,Jan,8; 2016,Jan,13; 2015,Jan,16

99457 **Resequenced code. See code before resequenced code 99474.**

99458 **Resequenced code. See code before 99450.**

99460-99463 Evaluation and Management Services for Age 28 Days or Less

CMS: 100-04,12,30.6.4 Services Furnished Incident to Physician's Service

INCLUDES Family consultation
Healthy newborn history and physical
Medical record documentation
Ordering diagnostic test and treatments
Services provided to healthy newborns age 28 days or younger

EXCLUDES *Neonatal intensive and critical care services (99466-99469 [99485, 99486], 99477-99480)*
Newborn follow-up services in office or outpatient setting (99202-99215, 99381, 99391)
Newborn hospital discharge services when provided on date subsequent to admission (99238-99239)
Nonroutine neonatal inpatient evaluation and management services (99221-99233)

Code also attendance at delivery (99464)
Code also circumcision (54150)
Code also emergency resuscitation services (99465)

99460 **Initial hospital or birthing center care, per day, for evaluation and management of normal newborn infant** A

Facility RVU 2.70 Non-Facility RVU 2.70 **FUD** XXX V 80

AMA: 2018,Jan,8; 2017,Jan,8; 2016,Jan,13; 2015,Jan,16

99461 Initial care, per day, for evaluation and management of normal newborn infant seen in other than hospital or birthing center A
1.78 2.57 FUD XXX M 80
AMA: 2018,Jan,8; 2017,Jan,8; 2016,Jan,13; 2015,Jan,16

99462 Subsequent hospital care, per day, for evaluation and management of normal newborn A
1.19 1.19 FUD XXX C 80
AMA: 2018,Jan,8; 2017,Jan,8; 2016,Jan,13; 2015,Jan,16

99463 Initial hospital or birthing center care, per day, for evaluation and management of normal newborn infant admitted and discharged on the same date A
3.13 3.13 FUD XXX V 80
AMA: 2018,Jan,8; 2017,Jan,8; 2016,Jan,13; 2015,Jan,16

99464-99465 Newborn Delivery Attendance/Resuscitation

CMS: 100-04,12,30.6.4 Services Furnished Incident to Physician's Service

99464 Attendance at delivery (when requested by the delivering physician or other qualified health care professional) and initial stabilization of newborn A
EXCLUDES *Resuscitation at delivery (99465)*
2.12 2.12 FUD XXX N 80
AMA: 2018,Jan,8; 2017,Jan,8; 2016,Jan,13; 2015,Jan,16

99465 Delivery/birthing room resuscitation, provision of positive pressure ventilation and/or chest compressions in the presence of acute inadequate ventilation and/or cardiac output A
EXCLUDES *Attendance at delivery (99464)*
Code also any necessary procedures performed as resuscitation component
4.13 4.13 FUD XXX S 80
AMA: 2018,Jan,8; 2017,Jan,8; 2016,Jan,13; 2015,Jan,16

99466-99467 Critical Care Transport Age 24 Months or Younger

CMS: 100-04,12,30.6.4 Services Furnished Incident to Physician's Service

INCLUDES Face-to-face care starting when physician assumes patient responsibility at referring facility until receiving facility accepts patient
Physician presence during interfacility transfer critically ill/injured patient age 24 months or younger
Services provided by physician during transport:
- Blood gases
- Chest x-rays (71045-71046)
- Data stored in computers (e.g., ECGs, blood pressures, hematologic data)
- Gastric intubation (43752-43753)
- Interpretation cardiac output measurements (93562)
- Pulse oximetry (94760-94762)
- Routine monitoring:
  - Heart rate
  - Respiratory rate
- Temporary transcutaneous pacing (92953)
- Vascular access procedures (36000, 36400, 36405-36406, 36415, 36591, 36600)
- Ventilatory management (94002-94003, 94660, 94662)

EXCLUDES *Neonatal hypothermia (99184)*
Patient critical care transport services with personal patient contact less than 30 minutes
Physician directed emergency care via two-way voice communication with transporting staff (99288, [99485, 99486])
Physician services directing transport (control physician) ([99485, 99486])
Services less than 30 minutes in duration (see E/M codes)

Code also any services not designated as included in critical care transport service

99466 Critical care face-to-face services, during an interfacility transport of critically ill or critically injured pediatric patient, 24 months of age or younger; first 30-74 minutes of hands-on care during transport A
6.75 6.75 FUD XXX N 80
AMA: 2018,Jun,9; 2018,Jan,8; 2017,Jan,8; 2016,Jan,13; 2015,Jan,16

\+ **99467 each additional 30 minutes (List separately in addition to code for primary service)** A
Code first (99466)
3.38 3.38 FUD ZZZ N 80
AMA: 2018,Jun,9; 2018,Jan,8; 2017,Jan,8; 2016,Jan,13; 2015,Jan,16

99485-99486 [99485, 99486] Critical Care Transport Supervision Age 24 Months or Younger

INCLUDES Advice for treatment to transport team from control physician
Non face-to-face care starts with first contact by control physician with transport team and ends when patient responsibility assumed by receiving facility

EXCLUDES *Emergency systems physician direction for pediatric patient older than 24 months (99288)*
Services less than 15 minutes
Services performed by control physician for same time period
Services performed by same physician providing critical care transport (99466-99467)
Services provided by transport team

\# **99485 Supervision by a control physician of interfacility transport care of the critically ill or critically injured pediatric patient, 24 months of age or younger, includes two-way communication with transport team before transport, at the referring facility and during the transport, including data interpretation and report; first 30 minutes** A
2.17 2.17 FUD XXX B
AMA: 2018,Jun,9; 2018,Jan,8; 2017,Jan,8; 2016,Jan,13; 2015,Jan,16

\+ # **99486 each additional 30 minutes (List separately in addition to code for primary procedure)** A
Code first ([99485])
1.88 1.88 FUD XXX B
AMA: 2018,Jun,9; 2018,Jan,8; 2017,Jan,8; 2016,Jan,13; 2015,Jan,16

99468-99476 [99473, 99474] Critical Care Age 5 Years or Younger

CMS: 100-04,12,30.6.4 Services Furnished Incident to Physician's Service

INCLUDES All services included in codes 99291-99292 as well as (which may be reported by facilities only):
- Administration blood/blood components (36430, 36440)
- Administration intravenous fluids (96360-96361)
- Administration surfactant (94610)
- Bladder aspiration, suprapubic (51100)
- Bladder catheterization (51701, 51702)
- Car seat evaluation (94780-94781)
- Catheterization umbilical artery (36660)
- Catheterization umbilical vein (36510)
- Central venous catheter, centrally inserted (36555)
- Endotracheal intubation (31500)
- Lumbar puncture (62270)
- Oral or nasogastric tube placement (43752)
- Pulmonary function testing, performed at bedside (94375)
- Pulse or ear oximetry (94760-94762)
- Vascular access, arteries (36140, 36620)
- Vascular access, venous (36400-36406, 36420, 36600)
- Ventilatory management (94002-94004, 94660)

Initial and subsequent care provided to critically ill infant or child

Other hospital care or intensive care services by same group or individual done on same day patient transferred to initial neonatal/pediatric critical care

Readmission to critical unit on same day or during same stay (subsequent care)

EXCLUDES *Critical care services for patients age six years or older (99291-99292)*

Critical care services provided by second physician or different physician specialty (99291-99292)

Interfacility transport services by same or different individual, same or different specialty or group, on same service date (99466-99467, [99485, 99486])

Neonatal hypothermia (99184)

Services performed by individual in another group receiving patient transferred to lower care level (99231-99233, 99478-99480)

Services performed by individual transferring patient to lower care level (99231-99233, 99291-99292)

Services performed by same or different individual in same group on same day (99291-99292)

Services performed by transferring individual prior to patient transfer to individual in different group (99221-99233, 99291-99292, 99460-99462, 99477-99480)

Code also normal newborn care when done on same day by same group or individual providing critical care. Report modifier 25 with initial critical care code (99460-99462)

99468 Initial inpatient neonatal critical care, per day, for the evaluation and management of a critically ill neonate, 28 days of age or younger A

26.0 | 26.0 | **FUD** XXX | C 80

AMA: 2018,Dec,8; 2018,Dec,8; 2018,Jun,9; 2018,Jan,8; 2017,Jan,8; 2016,May,3; 2016,Jan,13; 2015,Oct,8; 2015,Jul,3; 2015,Feb,10; 2015,Jan,16

99469 Subsequent inpatient neonatal critical care, per day, for the evaluation and management of a critically ill neonate, 28 days of age or younger A

11.2 | 11.2 | **FUD** XXX | C 80

AMA: 2018,Dec,8; 2018,Dec,8; 2018,Jun,9; 2018,Jan,8; 2017,Jan,8; 2016,May,3; 2016,Jan,13; 2015,Oct,8; 2015,Jul,3; 2015,Feb,10; 2015,Jan,16

99471 Initial inpatient pediatric critical care, per day, for the evaluation and management of a critically ill infant or young child, 29 days through 24 months of age A

22.5 | 22.5 | **FUD** XXX | C 80

AMA: 2018,Dec,8; 2018,Dec,8; 2018,Jun,9; 2018,Jan,8; 2017,Jan,8; 2016,May,3; 2016,Jan,13; 2015,Jul,3; 2015,Feb,10; 2015,Jan,16

99472 Subsequent inpatient pediatric critical care, per day, for the evaluation and management of a critically ill infant or young child, 29 days through 24 months of age A

11.5 | 11.5 | **FUD** XXX | C 80

AMA: 2018,Dec,8; 2018,Dec,8; 2018,Jun,9; 2018,Jan,8; 2017,Jan,8; 2016,May,3; 2016,Jan,13; 2015,Jul,3; 2015,Feb,10; 2015,Jan,16

99473 **Resequenced code. See code before 99450.**

99474 **Resequenced code. See code before 99450.**

99475 Initial inpatient pediatric critical care, per day, for the evaluation and management of a critically ill infant or young child, 2 through 5 years of age A

15.8 | 15.8 | **FUD** XXX | C 80

AMA: 2018,Dec,8; 2018,Dec,8; 2018,Jun,9; 2018,Jan,8; 2017,Jan,8; 2016,May,3; 2016,Jan,13; 2015,Jul,3; 2015,Feb,10; 2015,Jan,16

99476 Subsequent inpatient pediatric critical care, per day, for the evaluation and management of a critically ill infant or young child, 2 through 5 years of age A

9.86 | 9.86 | **FUD** XXX | C 80

AMA: 2018,Dec,8; 2018,Dec,8; 2018,Jun,9; 2018,Jan,8; 2017,Jan,8; 2016,May,3; 2016,Jan,13; 2015,Jul,3; 2015,Feb,10; 2015,Jan,16

99477-99480 Initial Inpatient Neonatal Intensive Care and Other Services

CMS: 100-04,12,30.6.4 Services Furnished Incident to Physician's Service

INCLUDES All services included in codes 99291-99292 as well as (which may be reported by facilities only):
- Adjustments to enteral and/or parenteral nutrition
- Airway and ventilator management (31500, 94002-94004, 94375, 94610, 94660)
- Bladder catheterization (51701-51702)
- Blood transfusion (36430, 36440)
- Car seat evaluation (94780-94781)
- Constant and/or frequent monitoring vital signs
- Continuous observation by the healthcare team
- Heat maintenance
- Intensive cardiac or respiratory monitoring
- Oral or nasogastric tube insertion (43752)
- Oxygen saturation (94760-94762)
- Spinal puncture (62270)
- Suprapubic catheterization (51100)
- Vascular access procedures (36000, 36140, 36400, 36405-36406, 36420, 36510, 36555, 36600, 36620, 36660)

EXCLUDES *Critical care services for patient transferred after initial or subsequent intensive care provided (99291-99292)*

Initial day intensive care provided by transferring individual same day neonate/infant transferred to lower care level (99477)

Inpatient neonatal/pediatric critical care services received on same day (99468-99476)

Necessary resuscitation services done as delivery care component prior to admission

Neonatal hypothermia (99184)

Services provided by receiving individual when patient transferred for critical care (99468-99476)

Services for receiving provider when patient improves after initial day and transferred to lower care level (99231-99233, 99478-99480)

Subsequent care sick neonate, under age 28 days, more than 5000 grams, not requiring critical or intensive care services (99231-99233)

Code also care provided by receiving individual when patient transferred to individual in different group (99231-99233, 99462)

Code also initial neonatal intensive care service when physician or other qualified health care professional present for delivery and/or neonate requires resuscitation (99464-99465); append modifier 25 to (99477)

99477 Initial hospital care, per day, for the evaluation and management of the neonate, 28 days of age or younger, who requires intensive observation, frequent interventions, and other intensive care services A

EXCLUDES *Initiation care critically ill neonate (99468)*

Initiation inpatient care normal newborn (99460)

9.85 | 9.85 | **FUD** XXX | C 80

AMA: 2018,Dec,8; 2018,Dec,8; 2018,Jan,8; 2017,Jan,8; 2016,Jan,13; 2015,Jul,3; 2015,Jan,16

99478 Subsequent intensive care, per day, for the evaluation and management of the recovering very low birth weight infant (present body weight less than 1500 grams) A

3.87 | 3.87 | **FUD** XXX | C 80

AMA: 2018,Dec,8; 2018,Dec,8; 2018,Jun,11; 2018,Jan,8; 2017,Jan,8; 2016,Jan,13; 2015,Jul,3; 2015,Jan,16

99479 **Subsequent intensive care, per day, for the evaluation and management of the recovering low birth weight infant (present body weight of 1500-2500 grams)** A
3.52 3.52 FUD XXX C 80
AMA: 2018,Dec,8; 2018,Dec,8; 2018,Jun,11; 2018,Jan,8; 2017,Jan,8; 2016,Jan,13; 2015,Jul,3; 2015,Jan,16

99480 **Subsequent intensive care, per day, for the evaluation and management of the recovering infant (present body weight of 2501-5000 grams)** A
3.37 3.37 FUD XXX C 80
AMA: 2018,Dec,8; 2018,Dec,8; 2018,Jun,11; 2018,Jan,8; 2017,Jan,8; 2016,Jan,13; 2015,Jul,3; 2015,Jan,16

99483-99486 [99484, 99485, 99486] Cognitive Impairment Services

INCLUDES Assessment and care plan services during same time frame as:
- E/M services (99202-99215, 99241-99245, 99324-99337, 99341-99350, 99366-99368, 99497-99498)
- Medication management (99605-99607)
- Need for services evaluation (e.g., legal, financial, meals, personal care)
- Patient and caregiver focused risk assessment (96160-96161)
- Psychiatric and psychological services (90785, 90791-90792, [96127])
- Psychological or neuropsychological tests (96146)

Consideration other conditions that may cause cognitive impairment (e.g., infection, hydrocephalus, stroke, medications)
Evaluation and care plans for new or existing patients with cognitive impairment symptoms

EXCLUDES *Reporting code more than one time per 180-day period*

99483 **Assessment of and care planning for a patient with cognitive impairment, requiring an independent historian, in the office or other outpatient, home or domiciliary or rest home, with all of the following required elements: Cognition-focused evaluation including a pertinent history and examination; Medical decision making of moderate or high complexity; Functional assessment (eg, basic and instrumental activities of daily living), including decision-making capacity; Use of standardized instruments for staging of dementia (eg, functional assessment staging test [FAST], clinical dementia rating [CDR]); Medication reconciliation and review for high-risk medications; Evaluation for neuropsychiatric and behavioral symptoms, including depression, including use of standardized screening instrument(s); Evaluation of safety (eg, home), including motor vehicle operation; Identification of caregiver(s), caregiver knowledge, caregiver needs, social supports, and the willingness of caregiver to take on caregiving tasks; Development, updating or revision, or review of an Advance Care Plan; Creation of a written care plan, including initial plans to address any neuropsychiatric symptoms, neuro-cognitive symptoms, functional limitations, and referral to community resources as needed (eg, rehabilitation services, adult day programs, support groups) shared with the patient and/or caregiver with initial education and support. Typically, 50 minutes are spent face-to-face with the patient and/or family or caregiver.**
5.12 7.35 FUD XXX S 80
AMA: 2020,Sep,3; 2018,Jul,12; 2018,Apr,9; 2018,Jan,8

99484 **Resequenced code. See code before 99450.**

99485 **Resequenced code. See code following 99467.**

99486 **Resequenced code. See code following 99467.**

99490-99491 [99439, 99490, 99491] Coordination of Services for Chronic Care

CMS: 100-02,13,230.2 Chronic Care Management and General Behavioral Health Integration Services; 100-04,11,40.1.3 Independent Attending Physician Services

INCLUDES Case management services provided to patients that:
- Have two or more conditions anticipated to endure more than 12 months or until patient's death
- High risk that conditions will result in decompensation, deterioration, or death
- Require at least 20 minutes staff time monthly

EXCLUDES *Patient management services during same time frame as (99339-99340, 99374-99380, 99487-99489, 90951-90970, 99605-99607)*
Service time reported with (99358-99359, 99366-99368, [99421, 99422, 99423], 99441-99443, [99091], [99484], 99492-99494, 93792-93793, 98960-98962, 98966-98968, 99071, 99078, 99080)

▲ # **99490** **Chronic care management services with the following required elements: multiple (two or more) chronic conditions expected to last at least 12 months, or until the death of the patient, chronic conditions place the patient at significant risk of death, acute exacerbation/decompensation, or functional decline, comprehensive care plan established, implemented, revised, or monitored; first 20 minutes of clinical staff time directed by a physician or other qualified health care professional, per calendar month.**
EXCLUDES *Chronic care management provided personally by physician or other qualified health care professional ([99491])*
Reporting code more than once per calendar month
Qualified nonphysician health care professional online digital assessment and management (98970-98972)
0.90 1.17 FUD XXX S 80
AMA: 2020,Apr,5; 2020,Feb,7; 2019,Jan,6; 2018,Oct,9; 2018,Jul,12; 2018,Apr,9; 2018,Mar,7; 2018,Mar,5; 2018,Feb,7; 2018,Jan,8; 2017,Jan,8; 2016,Jan,13; 2015,Feb,3; 2015,Jan,16

● + # **99439** **Chronic care management services with the following required elements: multiple (two or more) chronic conditions expected to last at least 12 months, or until the death of the patient, chronic conditions place the patient at significant risk of death, acute exacerbation/decompensation, or functional decline, comprehensive care plan established, implemented, revised, or monitored; each additional 20 minutes of clinical staff time directed by a physician or other qualified health care professional, per calendar month (List separately in addition to code for primary procedure)**
EXCLUDES *Reporting code more than twice per calendar month*
Qualified nonphysician health care professional online digital assessment and management (98970-98972)
Code first ([99490])
0.00 0.00 FUD 000

99491 **Chronic care management services, provided personally by a physician or other qualified health care professional, at least 30 minutes of physician or other qualified health care professional time, per calendar month, with the following required elements: multiple (two or more) chronic conditions expected to last at least 12 months, or until the death of the patient; chronic conditions place the patient at significant risk of death, acute exacerbation/decompensation, or functional decline; comprehensive care plan established, implemented, revised, or monitored**
EXCLUDES *Chronic care management provided by medically directed clinical staff only ([99439], [99490])*
Reporting code more than once per calendar month
Transitional care management services (99495-99496)
2.33 2.33 FUD XXX 80
AMA: 2020,Apr,5

99487-99491 [99490, 99491] Coordination of Complex Services for Chronic Care

INCLUDES All clinical non-face-to-face time with patient, family, and caregivers
Only services given by physician or other qualified health caregiver who has care coordination role for patient for month
Patient management services during same time frame as (99339-99340, 99374-99380, [99439, 99490, 99491], 90951-90970, 99605-99607)
Service time reported with (99358-99359, 99366-99368, [99421, 99422, 99423], 99441-99443, [99091], 93792-93793, 98960-98962, 98966-98972, 99071, 99078, 99080, 99605-99607)
Services provided to patients in rest home, domiciliary, assisted living facility, or at home including:
Caregiver education to family or patient, addressing independent living and self-management
Communication with patient and all caregivers and professionals regarding care
Determining which community and health resources benefit patient
Developing and maintaining care plan
Facilitation services and care
Health outcomes data and registry documentation
Providing communication with home health and other patient utilized services
Support for treatment and medication adherence
Services that address activities daily living, psychosocial, and medical needs

EXCLUDES *E/M services by same/different individual during care management services time frame*
Psychiatric collaborative care management (99484, 99492-99494)

▲ **99487** **Complex chronic care management services with the following required elements: multiple (two or more) chronic conditions expected to last at least 12 months, or until the death of the patient, chronic conditions place the patient at significant risk of death, acute exacerbation/decompensation, or functional decline, comprehensive care plan established, implemented, revised, or monitored, moderate or high complexity medical decision making; first 60 minutes of clinical staff time directed by a physician or other qualified health care professional, per calendar month.**

INCLUDES Clinical services, 60 to 74 minutes, during calendar month

1.47 2.58 **FUD** XXX S 80

AMA: 2020,Apr,5; 2020,Feb,7; 2019,Jan,6; 2018,Oct,9; 2018,Jul,12; 2018,Apr,9; 2018,Mar,7; 2018,Mar,5; 2018,Feb,7; 2018,Jan,8; 2017,Apr,9; 2017,Jan,8; 2016,Jan,13; 2015,Jan,16

▲ + **99489** **each additional 30 minutes of clinical staff time directed by a physician or other qualified health care professional, per calendar month (List separately in addition to code for primary procedure)**

EXCLUDES *Clinical services less than 30 minutes beyond initial 60 minutes, per calendar month*

Code first (99487)

0.74 1.29 **FUD** ZZZ N 80

AMA: 2020,Apr,5; 2020,Feb,7; 2019,Jan,6; 2018,Oct,9; 2018,Jul,12; 2018,Apr,9; 2018,Mar,7; 2018,Mar,5; 2018,Feb,7; 2018,Jan,8; 2017,Apr,9; 2017,Jan,8; 2016,Jan,13; 2015,Jan,16

99490 **Resequenced code. See code before 99487.**

99491 **Resequenced code. See code before 99487.**

99492-99494 Psychiatric Collaborative Care

CMS: 100-02,13,230.2 Chronic Care Management and General Behavioral Health Integration Services

INCLUDES Services provided during calendar month by physician or other qualified healthcare profession for patients with psychiatric diagnosis
Assessment behavioral health status
Creation and care plan revision
Treatment provided during care episode during which goals may be met, not achieved, or lack of services during six-month period

EXCLUDES *Additional services provided by behavioral health care manager during same calendar month period (do not count as time for 99492-99494):*
Psychiatric evaluation (90791-90792)
Psychotherapy (99406-99407, 99408-99409, 90832-90834, 90836-90838, 90839-90840, 90846-90847, 90849, 90853)
Services provided by psychiatric consultant (do not count as time for 99492-99494): (E/M services) and psychiatric evaluation (90791-90792)

99492 **Initial psychiatric collaborative care management, first 70 minutes in the first calendar month of behavioral health care manager activities, in consultation with a psychiatric consultant, and directed by the treating physician or other qualified health care professional, with the following required elements: outreach to and engagement in treatment of a patient directed by the treating physician or other qualified health care professional; initial assessment of the patient, including administration of validated rating scales, with the development of an individualized treatment plan; review by the psychiatric consultant with modifications of the plan if recommended; entering patient in a registry and tracking patient follow-up and progress using the registry, with appropriate documentation, and participation in weekly caseload consultation with the psychiatric consultant; and provision of brief interventions using evidence-based techniques such as behavioral activation, motivational interviewing, and other focused treatment strategies.**

EXCLUDES *Services less than 36 minutes*
Subsequent collaborative care managment in same calendar month (99493)

2.50 4.35 **FUD** XXX S 80

AMA: 2020,Feb,7; 2019,Jan,6; 2018,Jul,12; 2018,Mar,5; 2018,Feb,7; 2018,Jan,8; 2017,Nov,3

99493 **Subsequent psychiatric collaborative care management, first 60 minutes in a subsequent month of behavioral health care manager activities, in consultation with a psychiatric consultant, and directed by the treating physician or other qualified health care professional, with the following required elements: tracking patient follow-up and progress using the registry, with appropriate documentation; participation in weekly caseload consultation with the psychiatric consultant; ongoing collaboration with and coordination of the patient's mental health care with the treating physician or other qualified health care professional and any other treating mental health providers; additional review of progress and recommendations for changes in treatment, as indicated, including medications, based on recommendations provided by the psychiatric consultant; provision of brief interventions using evidence-based techniques such as behavioral activation, motivational interviewing, and other focused treatment strategies; monitoring of patient outcomes using validated rating scales; and relapse prevention planning with patients as they achieve remission of symptoms and/or other treatment goals and are prepared for discharge from active treatment.**

EXCLUDES *Initial collaborative care managment in same calendar month (99492)*

2.25 3.50 **FUD** XXX S 80

AMA: 2020,Feb,7; 2019,Jan,6; 2018,Jul,12; 2018,Mar,5; 2018,Feb,7; 2018,Jan,8; 2017,Nov,3

+ 99494 **Initial or subsequent psychiatric collaborative care management, each additional 30 minutes in a calendar month of behavioral health care manager activities, in consultation with a psychiatric consultant, and directed by the treating physician or other qualified health care professional (List separately in addition to code for primary procedure)**

INCLUDES Coordination care with emergency department staff

Code first (99492, 99493)

1.20 1.77 FUD ZZZ N 80

AMA: 2020,Feb,7; 2019,Jan,6; 2018,Jul,12; 2018,Mar,5; 2018,Feb,7; 2018,Jan,8; 2017,Nov,3

99495-99496 Management of Transitional Care Services

CMS: 100-02,13,230.1 Transitional Care Management Services; 100-04,11,40.1.3 Independent Attending Physician Services; 100-04,12,190.3 List of Telehealth Services

INCLUDES First interaction (face-to-face, by telephone, or electronic) with patient or his/her caregiver and must be done within two working days from discharge
- Initial face-to-face; must be done within code time frame and include medication management
- New or established patient with moderate to high complexity medical decision making needs during care transitions
- Patient management services during same time frame as (99339-99340, 99358-99359, 99366-99368, 99374-99380, 99441-99443, [99091], 99487-99489, 90951-90970, 93792-93793, 98960-98962, 98966-98968, 99071, 99078, 99080, 99605-99607)
- Services from discharge day up to 29 days post discharge
- Subsequent discharge within 30 days
- Without face-to-face patient care given by physician or other qualified health care professional includes:
  - Contacting qualified health care professionals for specific patient problems
  - Discharge information review
  - Follow-up and referral arrangements with community resources and providers
  - Need for follow-up care review based on tests and treatments
  - Patient, family, and caregiver education
- Without face-to-face patient care given by staff under physician guidance or other qualified health care professional includes:
  - Caregiver education to family or patient, addressing independent living and self-management
  - Communication with patient and all caregivers and professionals regarding care
  - Determining which community and health resources benefit patient
  - Facilitation services and care
  - Providing communication with home health and other patient utilized services
  - Support for treatment and medication adherence

EXCLUDES *E/M services after first face-to-face visit*

99495 **Transitional Care Management Services with the following required elements: Communication (direct contact, telephone, electronic) with the patient and/or caregiver within 2 business days of discharge Medical decision making of at least moderate complexity during the service period Face-to-face visit, within 14 calendar days of discharge**

3.11 4.62 FUD XXX ★ V 80

AMA: 2020,Feb,7; 2020,Jan,3; 2019,Jan,6; 2018,Jul,12; 2018,Apr,9; 2018,Mar,5; 2018,Mar,7; 2018,Feb,7; 2018,Jan,8; 2017,Jan,8; 2016,Jan,13; 2015,Jan,16

99496 **Transitional Care Management Services with the following required elements: Communication (direct contact, telephone, electronic) with the patient and/or caregiver within 2 business days of discharge Medical decision making of high complexity during the service period Face-to-face visit, within 7 calendar days of discharge**

4.51 6.52 FUD XXX ★ V 80

AMA: 2020,Feb,7; 2020,Jan,3; 2019,Jan,6; 2018,Jul,12; 2018,Apr,9; 2018,Mar,5; 2018,Mar,7; 2018,Feb,7; 2018,Jan,8; 2017,Jan,8; 2016,Jan,13; 2015,Jan,16

99497-99498 Advance Directive Guidance

CMS: 100-02,15,280.5.1 Advance Care Planning with an Annual Wellness Visit; 100-04,11,40.1.3 Independent Attending Physician Services; 100-04,18,140.8 Advance Care Planning with an Annual Wellness Visit (AWV); 100-04,4,200.11 Advance Care Planning as an Optional Element of an Annual Wellness Visit

EXCLUDES *Critical care services (99291-99292, 99468-99469, 99471-99472, 99475-99476, 99477-99480)*
- *Services for cognitive care (99483)*
- *Treatment/management for active problem (see appropriate E/M service)*

99497 **Advance care planning including the explanation and discussion of advance directives such as standard forms (with completion of such forms, when performed), by the physician or other qualified health care professional; first 30 minutes, face-to-face with the patient, family member(s), and/or surrogate**

2.23 2.40 FUD XXX Q1 80

AMA: 2018,Apr,9; 2018,Jan,8; 2017,Jan,8; 2016,Feb,7; 2016,Jan,13; 2015,Jan,16

+ 99498 **each additional 30 minutes (List separately in addition to code for primary procedure)**

Code first (99497)

2.10 2.11 FUD ZZZ N 80

AMA: 2018,Apr,9; 2018,Jan,8; 2017,Jan,8; 2016,Feb,7; 2016,Jan,13; 2015,Jan,16

99484 [99484] Behavioral Health Integration Care

CMS: 100-02,13,230.2 Chronic Care Management and General Behavioral Health Integration Services

INCLUDES Care management services requiring 20 minutes or more per calendar month
- Coordination of care with emergency department staff
- Face to face services when necessary
- Provided as outpatient service
- Provision services by clinical staff and reported by supervising physician or other qualified healthcare professional
- Provision services to patients with ongoing relationship
- Treatment plan and specific service components

EXCLUDES *Other services for which time or activities associated with service not used to meet requirements for 99484:*
- *Behavioral health integration care in same month ([99484])*
- *Chronic care management ([99439], [99490], 99487-99489)*
- *Psychiatric collaborative care in same calendar month (99492-99494)*
- *Psychotherapy services (90785-90899)*
- *Transitional care management (99495-99496)*

99484 **Care management services for behavioral health conditions, at least 20 minutes of clinical staff time, directed by a physician or other qualified health care professional, per calendar month, with the following required elements: initial assessment or follow-up monitoring, including the use of applicable validated rating scales; behavioral health care planning in relation to behavioral/psychiatric health problems, including revision for patients who are not progressing or whose status changes; facilitating and coordinating treatment such as psychotherapy, pharmacotherapy, counseling and/or psychiatric consultation; and continuity of care with a designated member of the care team.**

0.91 1.33 FUD XXX S 80

AMA: 2020,Feb,7; 2019,Jan,6; 2018,Jul,12; 2018,Mar,5; 2018,Feb,7; 2018,Jan,8

99499 Unlisted Evaluation and Management Services

CMS: 100-04,12,30.6.10 Consultation Services; 100-04,12,30.6.4 Services Furnished Incident to Physician's Service; 100-04,12,30.6.9.1 Initial Hospital Care and Observation or Inpatient Care Services

99499 **Unlisted evaluation and management service**

0.00 0.00 FUD XXX B 80

AMA: 2019,Aug,8; 2018,Jan,8; 2017,Jan,8; 2016,Jan,13; 2015,Jan,16

0001F-0015F Quality Measures with Multiple Components

INCLUDES Several measures grouped within single code descriptor to make possible reporting for clinical conditions when all components have been met

0001F **Heart failure assessed (includes assessment of all the following components) (CAD): Blood pressure measured (2000F) Level of activity assessed (1003F) Clinical symptoms of volume overload (excess) assessed (1004F) Weight, recorded (2001F) Clinical signs of volume overload (excess) assessed (2002F)**

INCLUDES Blood pressure measured (2000F)
Clinical signs volume overload (excess) assessed (2002F)
Clinical symptoms volume overload (excess) assessed (1004F)
Level activity assessed (1003F)
Weight recorded (2001F)

0.00 0.00 **FUD** XXX E

AMA: 2018,Jan,8; 2017,Jan,8; 2016,Jan,13; 2015,Jan,16

0005F **Osteoarthritis assessed (OA) Includes assessment of all the following components: Osteoarthritis symptoms and functional status assessed (1006F) Use of anti-inflammatory or over-the-counter (OTC) analgesic medications assessed (1007F) Initial examination of the involved joint(s) (includes visual inspection, palpation, range of motion) (2004F)**

INCLUDES Anti-inflammatory or over-the-counter (OTC) analgesic medication usage assessed (1007F)
Initial examination involved joint(s) (includes visual inspection/palpation/range) (2004F)
Osteoarthritis symptoms and functional status assessed (1006F)

0.00 0.00 **FUD** XXX E

AMA: 2005,Oct,1-5

0012F **Community-acquired bacterial pneumonia assessment (includes all of the following components) (CAP): Co-morbid conditions assessed (1026F) Vital signs recorded (2010F) Mental status assessed (2014F) Hydration status assessed (2018F)**

INCLUDES Co-morbid conditions assessed (1026F)
Hydration status assessed (2018F)
Mental status assessed (2014F)
Vital signs recorded (2010F)

0.00 0.00 **FUD** XXX E

0014F **Comprehensive preoperative assessment performed for cataract surgery with intraocular lens (IOL) placement (includes assessment of all of the following components) (EC): Dilated fundus evaluation performed within 12 months prior to cataract surgery (2020F) Pre-surgical (cataract) axial length, corneal power measurement and method of intraocular lens power calculation documented (must be performed within 12 months prior to surgery) (3073F) Preoperative assessment of functional or medical indication(s) for surgery prior to the cataract surgery with intraocular lens placement (must be performed within 12 months prior to cataract surgery) (3325F)**

INCLUDES Evaluation dilated fundus done within 12 months prior to surgery (2020F)
Preoperative assessment functional or medical indications done within 12 months prior to surgery (3325F)
Presurgical measurement axial length, corneal power, and IOL power calculation performed within 12 months prior to surgery (3073F)

0.00 0.00 **FUD** XXX E

AMA: 2008,Mar,8-12

0015F **Melanoma follow up completed (includes assessment of all of the following components) (ML): History obtained regarding new or changing moles (1050F) Complete physical skin exam performed (2029F) Patient counseled to perform a monthly self skin examination (5005F)**

INCLUDES Complete physical skin exam (2029F)
Counseling to perform monthly skin self-examination (5005F)
History obtained new or changing moles (1050F)

0.00 0.00 **FUD** XXX E

AMA: 2008,Mar,8-12

0500F-0584F Care Provided According to Prevailing Guidelines

INCLUDES Utilization measures or patient care provided for certain clinical purposes

0500F **Initial prenatal care visit (report at first prenatal encounter with health care professional providing obstetrical care. Report also date of visit and, in a separate field, the date of the last menstrual period [LMP]) (Prenatal)** M ♀

0.00 0.00 **FUD** XXX E

AMA: 2018,Jan,8; 2017,Jan,8; 2016,Jan,13; 2015,Jan,16

0501F **Prenatal flow sheet documented in medical record by first prenatal visit (documentation includes at minimum blood pressure, weight, urine protein, uterine size, fetal heart tones, and estimated date of delivery). Report also: date of visit and, in a separate field, the date of the last menstrual period [LMP] (Note: If reporting 0501F Prenatal flow sheet, it is not necessary to report 0500F Initial prenatal care visit) (Prenatal)** M ♀

0.00 0.00 **FUD** XXX E

AMA: 2004,Nov,1

0502F **Subsequent prenatal care visit (Prenatal) [Excludes: patients who are seen for a condition unrelated to pregnancy or prenatal care (eg, an upper respiratory infection; patients seen for consultation only, not for continuing care)]** M ♀

EXCLUDES *Patients seen for unrelated pregnancy/prenatal care condition (e.g., upper respiratory infection; patients seen for consultation only, not for continuing care)*

0.00 0.00 **FUD** XXX E

AMA: 2004,Nov,1

0503F **Postpartum care visit (Prenatal)** M ♀

0.00 0.00 **FUD** XXX E

AMA: 2004,Nov,1

0505F **Hemodialysis plan of care documented (ESRD, P-ESRD)**

0.00 0.00 **FUD** XXX E

AMA: 2008,Mar,8-12

0507F **Peritoneal dialysis plan of care documented (ESRD)**

0.00 0.00 **FUD** XXX E

AMA: 2008,Mar,8-12

0509F **Urinary incontinence plan of care documented (GER)**

0.00 0.00 **FUD** XXX M

0513F **Elevated blood pressure plan of care documented (CKD)**

0.00 0.00 **FUD** XXX M

AMA: 2008,Mar,8-12

0514F **Plan of care for elevated hemoglobin level documented for patient receiving Erythropoiesis-Stimulating Agent therapy (ESA) (CKD)**

0.00 0.00 **FUD** XXX E

AMA: 2008,Mar,8-12

0516F **Anemia plan of care documented (ESRD)**

0.00 0.00 **FUD** XXX E

AMA: 2008,Mar,8-12

0517F **Glaucoma plan of care documented (EC)**

0.00 0.00 **FUD** XXX M

AMA: 2008,Mar,8-12

0518F **Falls plan of care documented (GER)**
0.00 0.00 FUD XXX M
AMA: 2008,Mar,8-12

0519F **Planned chemotherapy regimen, including at a minimum: drug(s) prescribed, dose, and duration, documented prior to initiation of a new treatment regimen (ONC)**
0.00 0.00 FUD XXX E
AMA: 2008,Mar,8-12

0520F **Radiation dose limits to normal tissues established prior to the initiation of a course of 3D conformal radiation for a minimum of 2 tissue/organ (ONC)**
0.00 0.00 FUD XXX M
AMA: 2008,Mar,8-12

0521F **Plan of care to address pain documented (COA) (ONC)**
0.00 0.00 FUD XXX M
AMA: 2008,Mar,8-12

0525F **Initial visit for episode (BkP)**
0.00 0.00 FUD XXX E
AMA: 2008,Mar,8-12

0526F **Subsequent visit for episode (BkP)**
0.00 0.00 FUD XXX M
AMA: 2008,Mar,8-12

0528F **Recommended follow-up interval for repeat colonoscopy of at least 10 years documented in colonoscopy report (End/Polyp)**
0.00 0.00 FUD XXX M

0529F **Interval of 3 or more years since patient's last colonoscopy, documented (End/Polyp)**
0.00 0.00 FUD XXX M

0535F **Dyspnea management plan of care, documented (Pall Cr)**
0.00 0.00 FUD XXX E

0540F **Glucorticoid Management Plan Documented (RA)**
0.00 0.00 FUD XXX M

0545F **Plan for follow-up care for major depressive disorder, documented (MDD ADOL)**
0.00 0.00 FUD XXX E

0550F **Cytopathology report on routine nongynecologic specimen finalized within two working days of accession date (PATH)**
0.00 0.00 FUD XXX E

0551F **Cytopathology report on nongynecologic specimen with documentation that the specimen was non-routine (PATH)**
0.00 0.00 FUD XXX E

0555F **Symptom management plan of care documented (HF)**
0.00 0.00 FUD XXX E

0556F **Plan of care to achieve lipid control documented (CAD)**
0.00 0.00 FUD XXX E

0557F **Plan of care to manage anginal symptoms documented (CAD)**
0.00 0.00 FUD XXX E

0575F **HIV RNA control plan of care, documented (HIV)**
0.00 0.00 FUD XXX E

0580F **Multidisciplinary care plan developed or updated (ALS)**
0.00 0.00 FUD XXX E

0581F **Patient transferred directly from anesthetizing location to critical care unit (Peri2)**
0.00 0.00 FUD XXX M

0582F **Patient not transferred directly from anesthetizing location to critical care unit (Peri2)**
0.00 0.00 FUD XXX E

0583F **Transfer of care checklist used (Peri2)**
0.00 0.00 FUD XXX M

0584F **Transfer of care checklist not used (Peri2)**
0.00 0.00 FUD XXX E

1000F-1505F Elements of History/Review of Systems

INCLUDES Measures for specific aspects patient history or systems review

1000F **Tobacco use assessed (CAD, CAP, COPD, PV) (DM)**
0.00 0.00 FUD XXX E
AMA: 2018,Jan,8; 2017,Jan,8; 2016,Jan,13; 2015,Jan,16

1002F **Anginal symptoms and level of activity assessed (NMA-No Measure Associated)**
0.00 0.00 FUD XXX E
AMA: 2004,Nov,1

1003F **Level of activity assessed (NMA-No Measure Associated)**
0.00 0.00 FUD XXX E
AMA: 2006,Dec,10-12

1004F **Clinical symptoms of volume overload (excess) assessed (NMA-No Measure Associated)**
0.00 0.00 FUD XXX E
AMA: 2006,Dec,10-12

1005F **Asthma symptoms evaluated (includes documentation of numeric frequency of symptoms or patient completion of an asthma assessment tool/survey/questionnaire) (NMA-No Measure Associated)**
0.00 0.00 FUD XXX E

1006F **Osteoarthritis symptoms and functional status assessed (may include the use of a standardized scale or the completion of an assessment questionnaire, such as the SF-36, AAOS Hip & Knee Questionnaire) (OA) [Instructions: Report when osteoarthritis is addressed during the patient encounter]**
INCLUDES Osteoarthritis when addressed during patient encounter
0.00 0.00 FUD XXX M

1007F **Use of anti-inflammatory or analgesic over-the-counter (OTC) medications for symptom relief assessed (OA)**
0.00 0.00 FUD XXX E

1008F **Gastrointestinal and renal risk factors assessed for patients on prescribed or OTC non-steroidal anti-inflammatory drug (NSAID) (OA)**
0.00 0.00 FUD XXX E

1010F **Severity of angina assessed by level of activity (CAD)**
0.00 0.00 FUD XXX E

1011F **Angina present (CAD)**
0.00 0.00 FUD XXX E

1012F **Angina absent (CAD)**
0.00 0.00 FUD XXX E

1015F **Chronic obstructive pulmonary disease (COPD) symptoms assessed (Includes assessment of at least 1 of the following: dyspnea, cough/sputum, wheezing), or respiratory symptom assessment tool completed (COPD)**
0.00 0.00 FUD XXX E

1018F **Dyspnea assessed, not present (COPD)**
0.00 0.00 FUD XXX E

1019F **Dyspnea assessed, present (COPD)**
0.00 0.00 FUD XXX E

1022F **Pneumococcus immunization status assessed (CAP, COPD)**
0.00 0.00 FUD XXX E
AMA: 2010,Jul,3-5; 2008,Mar,8-12

1026F **Co-morbid conditions assessed (eg, includes assessment for presence or absence of: malignancy, liver disease, congestive heart failure, cerebrovascular disease, renal disease, chronic obstructive pulmonary disease, asthma, diabetes, other co-morbid conditions) (CAP)**
0.00 0.00 FUD XXX E

1030F **Influenza immunization status assessed (CAP)**
0.00 0.00 FUD XXX E
AMA: 2008,Mar,8-12

1031F **Smoking status and exposure to second hand smoke in the home assessed (Asthma)**
0.00 0.00 FUD XXX E

1032F **Current tobacco smoker or currently exposed to secondhand smoke (Asthma)**
0.00 0.00 FUD XXX E

1033F **Current tobacco non-smoker and not currently exposed to secondhand smoke (Asthma)**
0.00 0.00 FUD XXX E

1034F **Current tobacco smoker (CAD, CAP, COPD, PV) (DM)**
0.00 0.00 FUD XXX E
AMA: 2008,Mar,8-12

1035F **Current smokeless tobacco user (eg, chew, snuff) (PV)**
0.00 0.00 FUD XXX E
AMA: 2008,Mar,8-12

1036F **Current tobacco non-user (CAD, CAP, COPD, PV) (DM) (IBD)**
0.00 0.00 FUD XXX M
AMA: 2008,Mar,8-12

1038F **Persistent asthma (mild, moderate or severe) (Asthma)**
0.00 0.00 FUD XXX M
AMA: 2018,Jan,8; 2017,Jan,8; 2016,Jan,13; 2015,Jan,16

1039F **Intermittent asthma (Asthma)**
0.00 0.00 FUD XXX M
AMA: 2018,Jan,8; 2017,Jan,8; 2016,Jan,13; 2015,Jan,16

1040F **DSM-5 criteria for major depressive disorder documented at the initial evaluation (MDD, MDD ADOL)**
0.00 0.00 FUD XXX E
AMA: 2008,Mar,8-12

1050F **History obtained regarding new or changing moles (ML)**
0.00 0.00 FUD XXX E
AMA: 2008,Mar,8-12

1052F **Type, anatomic location, and activity all assessed (IBD)**
0.00 0.00 FUD XXX E

1055F **Visual functional status assessed (EC)**
0.00 0.00 FUD XXX E

1060F **Documentation of permanent or persistent or paroxysmal atrial fibrillation (STR)**
0.00 0.00 FUD XXX E

1061F **Documentation of absence of permanent and persistent and paroxysmal atrial fibrillation (STR)**
0.00 0.00 FUD XXX E

1065F **Ischemic stroke symptom onset of less than 3 hours prior to arrival (STR)**
0.00 0.00 FUD XXX E

1066F **Ischemic stroke symptom onset greater than or equal to 3 hours prior to arrival (STR)**
0.00 0.00 FUD XXX E

1070F **Alarm symptoms (involuntary weight loss, dysphagia, or gastrointestinal bleeding) assessed; none present (GERD)**
0.00 0.00 FUD XXX E

1071F **1 or more present (GERD)**
0.00 0.00 FUD XXX E

1090F **Presence or absence of urinary incontinence assessed (GER)**
0.00 0.00 FUD XXX M

1091F **Urinary incontinence characterized (eg, frequency, volume, timing, type of symptoms, how bothersome) (GER)**
0.00 0.00 FUD XXX E

1100F **Patient screened for future fall risk; documentation of 2 or more falls in the past year or any fall with injury in the past year (GER)**
0.00 0.00 FUD XXX M
AMA: 2008,Mar,8-12

1101F **documentation of no falls in the past year or only 1 fall without injury in the past year (GER)**
0.00 0.00 FUD XXX M
AMA: 2008,Mar,8-12

1110F **Patient discharged from an inpatient facility (eg, hospital, skilled nursing facility, or rehabilitation facility) within the last 60 days (GER)**
0.00 0.00 FUD XXX E

1111F **Discharge medications reconciled with the current medication list in outpatient medical record (COA) (GER)**
0.00 0.00 FUD XXX M

1116F **Auricular or periauricular pain assessed (AOE)**
0.00 0.00 FUD XXX E
AMA: 2008,Mar,8-12

1118F **GERD symptoms assessed after 12 months of therapy (GERD)**
0.00 0.00 FUD XXX E
AMA: 2008,Mar,8-12

1119F **Initial evaluation for condition (HEP C)(EPI, DSP)**
0.00 0.00 FUD XXX E
AMA: 2008,Mar,8-12

1121F **Subsequent evaluation for condition (HEP C)(EPI)**
0.00 0.00 FUD XXX E
AMA: 2008,Mar,8-12

1123F **Advance Care Planning discussed and documented advance care plan or surrogate decision maker documented in the medical record (DEM) (GER, Pall Cr)**
0.00 0.00 FUD XXX M
AMA: 2008,Mar,8-12

1124F **Advance Care Planning discussed and documented in the medical record, patient did not wish or was not able to name a surrogate decision maker or provide an advance care plan (DEM) (GER, Pall Cr)**
0.00 0.00 FUD XXX M
AMA: 2008,Mar,8-12

1125F **Pain severity quantified; pain present (COA) (ONC)**
0.00 0.00 FUD XXX M
AMA: 2008,Mar,8-12

1126F **no pain present (COA) (ONC)**
0.00 0.00 FUD XXX M
AMA: 2008,Mar,8-12

1127F **New episode for condition (NMA-No Measure Associated)**
0.00 0.00 FUD XXX E
AMA: 2008,Mar,8-12

1128F **Subsequent episode for condition (NMA-No Measure Associated)**
0.00 0.00 FUD XXX E
AMA: 2008,Mar,8-12

1130F **Back pain and function assessed, including all of the following: Pain assessment and functional status and patient history, including notation of presence or absence of "red flags" (warning signs) and assessment of prior treatment and response, and employment status (BkP)**
0.00 0.00 FUD XXX E
AMA: 2008,Mar,8-12

1134F **Episode of back pain lasting 6 weeks or less (BkP)**
0.00 0.00 FUD XXX E
AMA: 2008,Mar,8-12

1135F **Episode of back pain lasting longer than 6 weeks (BkP)**
0.00 0.00 FUD XXX E
AMA: 2008,Mar,8-12

1136F **Episode of back pain lasting 12 weeks or less (BkP)**
0.00 0.00 FUD XXX E
AMA: 2008,Mar,8-12

1137F **Episode of back pain lasting longer than 12 weeks (BkP)**
0.00 0.00 FUD XXX E
AMA: 2008,Mar,8-12

1150F **Documentation that a patient has a substantial risk of death within 1 year (Pall Cr)**
0.00 0.00 FUD XXX E

1151F **Documentation that a patient does not have a substantial risk of death within one year (Pall Cr)**
0.00 0.00 FUD XXX E

1152F **Documentation of advanced disease diagnosis, goals of care prioritize comfort (Pall Cr)**
0.00 0.00 FUD XXX E

1153F **Documentation of advanced disease diagnosis, goals of care do not prioritize comfort (Pall Cr)**
0.00 0.00 FUD XXX E

1157F **Advance care plan or similar legal document present in the medical record (COA)**
0.00 0.00 FUD XXX E

1158F **Advance care planning discussion documented in the medical record (COA)**
0.00 0.00 FUD XXX M

1159F **Medication list documented in medical record (COA)**
0.00 0.00 FUD XXX E

1160F **Review of all medications by a prescribing practitioner or clinical pharmacist (such as, prescriptions, OTCs, herbal therapies and supplements) documented in the medical record (COA)**
0.00 0.00 FUD XXX E

1170F **Functional status assessed (COA) (RA)**
0.00 0.00 FUD XXX M

1175F **Functional status for dementia assessed and results reviewed (DEM)**
0.00 0.00 FUD XXX E

1180F **All specified thromboembolic risk factors assessed (AFIB)**
0.00 0.00 FUD XXX E

1181F **Neuropsychiatric symptoms assessed and results reviewed (DEM)**
0.00 0.00 FUD XXX E

1182F **Neuropsychiatric symptoms, one or more present (DEM)**
0.00 0.00 FUD XXX E

1183F **Neuropsychiatric symptoms, absent (DEM)**
0.00 0.00 FUD XXX E

1200F **Seizure type(s) and current seizure frequency(ies) documented (EPI)**
0.00 0.00 FUD XXX E

1205F **Etiology of epilepsy or epilepsy syndrome(s) reviewed and documented (EPI)**
0.00 0.00 FUD XXX E

1220F **Patient screened for depression (SUD)**
0.00 0.00 FUD XXX E

1400F **Parkinson's disease diagnosis reviewed (Prkns)**
0.00 0.00 FUD XXX E

1450F **Symptoms improved or remained consistent with treatment goals since last assessment (HF)**
0.00 0.00 FUD XXX E

1451F **Symptoms demonstrated clinically important deterioration since last assessment (HF)**
0.00 0.00 FUD XXX E

1460F **Qualifying cardiac event/diagnosis in previous 12 months (CAD)**
0.00 0.00 FUD XXX M

1461F **No qualifying cardiac event/diagnosis in previous 12 months (CAD)**
0.00 0.00 FUD XXX M

1490F **Dementia severity classified, mild (DEM)**
0.00 0.00 FUD XXX E

1491F **Dementia severity classified, moderate (DEM)**
0.00 0.00 FUD XXX E

1493F **Dementia severity classified, severe (DEM)**
0.00 0.00 FUD XXX E

1494F **Cognition assessed and reviewed (DEM)**
0.00 0.00 FUD XXX E

1500F **Symptoms and signs of distal symmetric polyneuropathy reviewed and documented (DSP)**
0.00 0.00 FUD XXX E

1501F **Not initial evaluation for condition (DSP)**
0.00 0.00 FUD XXX E

1502F **Patient queried about pain and pain interference with function using a valid and reliable instrument (DSP)**
0.00 0.00 FUD XXX E

1503F **Patient queried about symptoms of respiratory insufficiency (ALS)**
0.00 0.00 FUD XXX E

1504F **Patient has respiratory insufficiency (ALS)**
0.00 0.00 FUD XXX E

1505F **Patient does not have respiratory insufficiency (ALS)**
0.00 0.00 FUD XXX E

2000F-2060F [2033F] Elements of Examination

INCLUDES Components clinical assessment or physical exam

2000F **Blood pressure measured (CKD)(DM)**
0.00 0.00 FUD XXX M
AMA: 2018,Jan,8; 2017,Jan,8; 2016,Jan,13; 2015,Jan,16

2001F **Weight recorded (PAG)**
0.00 0.00 FUD XXX E
AMA: 2006,Dec,10-12

2002F **Clinical signs of volume overload (excess) assessed (NMA-No Measure Associated)**
0.00 0.00 FUD XXX E
AMA: 2006,Dec,10-12

2004F **Initial examination of the involved joint(s) (includes visual inspection, palpation, range of motion) (OA) [Instructions: Report only for initial osteoarthritis visit or for visits for new joint involvement]**
INCLUDES Visits for initial osteoarthritis examination or new joint involvement
0.00 0.00 FUD XXX E
AMA: 2004,Feb,3; 2003,Aug,1

2010F **Vital signs (temperature, pulse, respiratory rate, and blood pressure) documented and reviewed (CAP) (EM)**
0.00 0.00 FUD XXX E

2014F **Mental status assessed (CAP) (EM)**
0.00 0.00 FUD XXX E

2015F **Asthma impairment assessed (Asthma)**
0.00 0.00 FUD XXX E

2016F **Asthma risk assessed (Asthma)**
0.00 0.00 FUD XXX E

2018F **Hydration status assessed (normal/mildly dehydrated/severely dehydrated) (CAP)**
0.00 0.00 FUD XXX E

2019F **Dilated macular exam performed, including documentation of the presence or absence of macular thickening or hemorrhage and the level of macular degeneration severity (EC)**
0.00 0.00 FUD XXX E

2020F **Dilated fundus evaluation performed within 12 months prior to cataract surgery (EC)**
0.00 0.00 FUD XXX E
AMA: 2008,Mar,8-12

2021F **Dilated macular or fundus exam performed, including documentation of the presence or absence of macular edema and level of severity of retinopathy (EC)**
0.00 0.00 FUD XXX E

2022F **Dilated retinal eye exam with interpretation by an ophthalmologist or optometrist documented and reviewed; with evidence of retinopathy (DM)**
0.00 0.00 FUD XXX M
AMA: 2008,Mar,8-12

2023F **without evidence of retinopathy (DM)**
0.00 0.00 FUD XXX

2024F **7 standard field stereoscopic retinal photos with interpretation by an ophthalmologist or optometrist documented and reviewed; with evidence of retinopathy (DM)**
0.00 0.00 FUD XXX M
AMA: 2008,Mar,8-12

2025F **without evidence of retinopathy (DM)**
0.00 0.00 FUD XXX

2026F **Eye imaging validated to match diagnosis from 7 standard field stereoscopic retinal photos results documented and reviewed; with evidence of retinopathy (DM)**
0.00 0.00 FUD XXX M
AMA: 2008,Mar,8-12

\# 2033F **without evidence of retinopathy (DM)**
0.00 0.00 FUD XXX

2027F **Optic nerve head evaluation performed (EC)**
0.00 0.00 FUD XXX M

2028F **Foot examination performed (includes examination through visual inspection, sensory exam with monofilament, and pulse exam - report when any of the 3 components are completed) (DM)**
0.00 0.00 FUD XXX E

2029F **Complete physical skin exam performed (ML)**
0.00 0.00 FUD XXX E
AMA: 2008,Mar,8-12

2030F **Hydration status documented, normally hydrated (PAG)**
0.00 0.00 FUD XXX E

2031F **Hydration status documented, dehydrated (PAG)**
0.00 0.00 FUD XXX E

2033F **Resequenced code. See code following 2026F.**

2035F **Tympanic membrane mobility assessed with pneumatic otoscopy or tympanometry (OME)**
0.00 0.00 FUD XXX E
AMA: 2008,Mar,8-12

2040F **Physical examination on the date of the initial visit for low back pain performed, in accordance with specifications (BkP)**
0.00 0.00 FUD XXX E
AMA: 2008,Mar,8-12

2044F **Documentation of mental health assessment prior to intervention (back surgery or epidural steroid injection) or for back pain episode lasting longer than 6 weeks (BkP)**
0.00 0.00 FUD XXX E
AMA: 2008,Mar,8-12

2050F **Wound characteristics including size and nature of wound base tissue and amount of drainage prior to debridement documented (CWC)**
0.00 0.00 FUD XXX E

2060F **Patient interviewed directly on or before date of diagnosis of major depressive disorder (MDD ADOL)**
0.00 0.00 FUD XXX E

3006F-3776F [3051F, 3052F] Findings from Diagnostic or Screening Tests

INCLUDES Results and medical decision making with regards to ordered tests:
Clinical laboratory tests
Other examination procedures
Radiological examinations

3006F **Chest X-ray results documented and reviewed (CAP)**
0.00 0.00 FUD XXX E
AMA: 2018,Jan,8; 2017,Jan,8; 2016,Jan,13; 2015,Jan,16

3008F **Body Mass Index (BMI), documented (PV)**
0.00 0.00 FUD XXX E

3011F **Lipid panel results documented and reviewed (must include total cholesterol, HDL-C, triglycerides and calculated LDL-C) (CAD)**
0.00 0.00 FUD XXX E

3014F **Screening mammography results documented and reviewed (PV)**
0.00 0.00 FUD XXX E
AMA: 2008,Mar,8-12

3015F **Cervical cancer screening results documented and reviewed (PV)** ♀
0.00 0.00 FUD XXX E

3016F **Patient screened for unhealthy alcohol use using a systematic screening method (PV) (DSP)**
0.00 0.00 FUD XXX E

3017F **Colorectal cancer screening results documented and reviewed (PV)**
0.00 0.00 FUD XXX M
AMA: 2008,Mar,8-12

3018F **Pre-procedure risk assessment and depth of insertion and quality of the bowel prep and complete description of polyp(s) found, including location of each polyp, size, number and gross morphology and recommendations for follow-up in final colonoscopy report documented (End/Polyp)**
0.00 0.00 FUD XXX E

3019F **Left ventricular ejection fraction (LVEF) assessment planned post discharge (HF)**
0.00 0.00 FUD XXX E

3020F **Left ventricular function (LVF) assessment (eg, echocardiography, nuclear test, or ventriculography) documented in the medical record (Includes quantitative or qualitative assessment results) (NMA-No Measure Associated)**
0.00 0.00 FUD XXX E
AMA: 2006,Dec,10-12

3021F **Left ventricular ejection fraction (LVEF) less than 40% or documentation of moderately or severely depressed left ventricular systolic function (CAD, HF)**
0.00 0.00 FUD XXX M

3022F **Left ventricular ejection fraction (LVEF) greater than or equal to 40% or documentation as normal or mildly depressed left ventricular systolic function (CAD, HF)**
0.00 0.00 FUD XXX M

3023F **Spirometry results documented and reviewed (COPD)**
0.00 0.00 FUD XXX M

3025F **Spirometry test results demonstrate FEV1/FVC less than 70% with COPD symptoms (eg, dyspnea, cough/sputum, wheezing) (CAP, COPD)**
0.00 0.00 FUD XXX E

3027F **Spirometry test results demonstrate FEV1/FVC greater than or equal to 70% or patient does not have COPD symptoms (COPD)**
0.00 0.00 FUD XXX E

3028F **Oxygen saturation results documented and reviewed (includes assessment through pulse oximetry or arterial blood gas measurement) (CAP, COPD) (EM)**
0.00 0.00 FUD XXX E

3035F **Oxygen saturation less than or equal to 88% or a PaO2 less than or equal to 55 mm Hg (COPD)**
0.00 0.00 FUD XXX E

3037F **Oxygen saturation greater than 88% or PaO2 greater than 55 mm Hg (COPD)**
0.00 0.00 FUD XXX E

3038F **Pulmonary function test performed within 12 months prior to surgery (Lung/Esop Cx)**
0.00 0.00 FUD XXX E

3040F **Functional expiratory volume (FEV1) less than 40% of predicted value (COPD)**
0.00 0.00 FUD XXX E

3042F **Functional expiratory volume (FEV1) greater than or equal to 40% of predicted value (COPD)**
0.00 0.00 FUD XXX E

3044F **Most recent hemoglobin A1c (HbA1c) level less than 7.0% (DM)**
0.00 0.00 FUD XXX M

\# **3051F** **Most recent hemoglobin A1c (HbA1c) level greater than or equal to 7.0% and less than 8.0% (DM)**
0.00 0.00 FUD XXX

\# **3052F** **Most recent hemoglobin A1c (HbA1c) level greater than or equal to 8.0% and less than or equal to 9.0% (DM)**
0.00 0.00 FUD XXX

3046F **Most recent hemoglobin A1c level greater than 9.0% (DM)**
EXCLUDES *Hemoglobin A1c less than or equal to 9.0% (3044F, [3051F], [3052F])*
0.00 0.00 FUD XXX M

3048F **Most recent LDL-C less than 100 mg/dL (CAD) (DM)**
0.00 0.00 FUD XXX E

3049F **Most recent LDL-C 100-129 mg/dL (CAD) (DM)**
0.00 0.00 FUD XXX E

3050F **Most recent LDL-C greater than or equal to 130 mg/dL (CAD) (DM)**
0.00 0.00 FUD XXX E

3051F **Resequenced code. See code following 3044F.**

3052F **Resequenced code. See code before 3046F.**

3055F **Left ventricular ejection fraction (LVEF) less than or equal to 35% (HF)**
0.00 0.00 FUD XXX E

3056F **Left ventricular ejection fraction (LVEF) greater than 35% or no LVEF result available (HF)**
0.00 0.00 FUD XXX E

3060F **Positive microalbuminuria test result documented and reviewed (DM)**
0.00 0.00 FUD XXX M

3061F **Negative microalbuminuria test result documented and reviewed (DM)**
0.00 0.00 FUD XXX M

3062F **Positive macroalbuminuria test result documented and reviewed (DM)**
0.00 0.00 FUD XXX M

3066F **Documentation of treatment for nephropathy (eg, patient receiving dialysis, patient being treated for ESRD, CRF, ARF, or renal insufficiency, any visit to a nephrologist) (DM)**
0.00 0.00 FUD XXX M

3072F **Low risk for retinopathy (no evidence of retinopathy in the prior year) (DM)**
0.00 0.00 FUD XXX M
AMA: 2008,Mar,8-12

3073F **Pre-surgical (cataract) axial length, corneal power measurement and method of intraocular lens power calculation documented within 12 months prior to surgery (EC)**
0.00 0.00 FUD XXX E
AMA: 2008,Mar,8-12

3074F **Most recent systolic blood pressure less than 130 mm Hg (DM), (HTN, CKD, CAD)**
0.00 0.00 FUD XXX E
AMA: 2008,Mar,8-12

3075F **Most recent systolic blood pressure 130-139 mm Hg (DM) (HTN, CKD, CAD)**
0.00 0.00 FUD XXX E
AMA: 2008,Mar,8-12

3077F **Most recent systolic blood pressure greater than or equal to 140 mm Hg (HTN, CKD, CAD) (DM)**
0.00 0.00 FUD XXX E
AMA: 2008,Mar,8-12

3078F **Most recent diastolic blood pressure less than 80 mm Hg (HTN, CKD, CAD) (DM)**
0.00 0.00 FUD XXX E
AMA: 2008,Mar,8-12

3079F **Most recent diastolic blood pressure 80-89 mm Hg (HTN, CKD, CAD) (DM)**
0.00 0.00 FUD XXX E
AMA: 2008,Mar,8-12

3080F **Most recent diastolic blood pressure greater than or equal to 90 mm Hg (HTN, CKD, CAD) (DM)**
0.00 0.00 FUD XXX E
AMA: 2008,Mar,8-12

3082F **Kt/V less than 1.2 (Clearance of urea [Kt]/volume [V]) (ESRD, P-ESRD)**
0.00 0.00 FUD XXX E
AMA: 2008,Mar,8-12

3083F **Kt/V equal to or greater than 1.2 and less than 1.7 (Clearance of urea [Kt]/volume [V]) (ESRD, P-ESRD)**
0.00 0.00 FUD XXX E
AMA: 2008,Mar,8-12

3084F **Kt/V greater than or equal to 1.7 (Clearance of urea [Kt]/volume [V]) (ESRD, P-ESRD)**
0.00 0.00 FUD XXX E
AMA: 2008,Mar,8-12

3085F **Suicide risk assessed (MDD, MDD ADOL)**
0.00 0.00 FUD XXX E

3088F **Major depressive disorder, mild (MDD)**
0.00 0.00 FUD XXX E

3089F **Major depressive disorder, moderate (MDD)**
0.00 0.00 FUD XXX E

3090F **Major depressive disorder, severe without psychotic features (MDD)**
0.00 0.00 FUD XXX E

3091F **Major depressive disorder, severe with psychotic features (MDD)**
0.00 0.00 FUD XXX E

3092F **Major depressive disorder, in remission (MDD)**
0.00 0.00 FUD XXX E

3093F **Documentation of new diagnosis of initial or recurrent episode of major depressive disorder (MDD)**
0.00 0.00 FUD XXX E
AMA: 2008,Mar,8-12

3095F **Central dual-energy X-ray absorptiometry (DXA) results documented (OP)(IBD)**
0.00 0.00 FUD XXX M

3096F **Central dual-energy X-ray absorptiometry (DXA) ordered (OP)(IBD)**
0.00 0.00 FUD XXX E

3100F **Carotid imaging study report (includes direct or indirect reference to measurements of distal internal carotid diameter as the denominator for stenosis measurement) (STR, RAD)**
0.00 0.00 FUD XXX M
AMA: 2008,Mar,8-12

3110F **Documentation in final CT or MRI report of presence or absence of hemorrhage and mass lesion and acute infarction (STR)**
0.00 0.00 FUD XXX E

3111F **CT or MRI of the brain performed in the hospital within 24 hours of arrival or performed in an outpatient imaging center, to confirm initial diagnosis of stroke, TIA or intracranial hemorrhage (STR)**
0.00 0.00 FUD XXX E

3112F **CT or MRI of the brain performed greater than 24 hours after arrival to the hospital or performed in an outpatient imaging center for purpose other than confirmation of initial diagnosis of stroke, TIA, or intracranial hemorrhage (STR)**
0.00 0.00 FUD XXX E

3115F **Quantitative results of an evaluation of current level of activity and clinical symptoms (HF)**
0.00 0.00 FUD XXX E

3117F **Heart failure disease specific structured assessment tool completed (HF)**
0.00 0.00 FUD XXX E

3118F **New York Heart Association (NYHA) Class documented (HF)**
0.00 0.00 FUD XXX E

3119F **No evaluation of level of activity or clinical symptoms (HF)**
0.00 0.00 FUD XXX E

3120F **12-Lead ECG Performed (EM)**
0.00 0.00 FUD XXX E

3126F **Esophageal biopsy report with a statement about dysplasia (present, absent, or indefinite, and if present, contains appropriate grading) (PATH)**
0.00 0.00 FUD XXX M

3130F **Upper gastrointestinal endoscopy performed (GERD)**
0.00 0.00 FUD XXX E

3132F **Documentation of referral for upper gastrointestinal endoscopy (GERD)**
0.00 0.00 FUD XXX E

3140F **Upper gastrointestinal endoscopy report indicates suspicion of Barrett's esophagus (GERD)**
0.00 0.00 FUD XXX E

3141F **Upper gastrointestinal endoscopy report indicates no suspicion of Barrett's esophagus (GERD)**
0.00 0.00 FUD XXX E

3142F **Barium swallow test ordered (GERD)**
INCLUDES Documentation barium swallow test
0.00 0.00 FUD XXX E

3150F **Forceps esophageal biopsy performed (GERD)**
0.00 0.00 FUD XXX E

3155F **Cytogenetic testing performed on bone marrow at time of diagnosis or prior to initiating treatment (HEM)**
0.00 0.00 FUD XXX M
AMA: 2008,Mar,8-12

3160F **Documentation of iron stores prior to initiating erythropoietin therapy (HEM)**
0.00 0.00 FUD XXX M
AMA: 2008,Mar,8-12

▲ 3170F **Baseline flow cytometry studies performed at time of diagnosis or prior to initiating treatment (HEM)**
0.00 0.00 FUD XXX M
AMA: 2008,Mar,8-12

3200F **Barium swallow test not ordered (GERD)**
0.00 0.00 FUD XXX E

3210F **Group A Strep Test Performed (PHAR)**
0.00 0.00 FUD XXX M
AMA: 2008,Mar,8-12

3215F **Patient has documented immunity to Hepatitis A (HEP-C)**
0.00 0.00 FUD XXX E
AMA: 2008,Mar,8-12

3216F **Patient has documented immunity to Hepatitis B (HEP-C)(IBD)**
0.00 0.00 FUD XXX E
AMA: 2008,Mar,8-12

3218F **RNA testing for Hepatitis C documented as performed within 6 months prior to initiation of antiviral treatment for Hepatitis C (HEP-C)**
0.00 0.00 FUD XXX E
AMA: 2008,Mar,8-12

3220F **Hepatitis C quantitative RNA testing documented as performed at 12 weeks from initiation of antiviral treatment (HEP-C)**
0.00 0.00 FUD XXX E
AMA: 2008,Mar,8-12

3230F **Documentation that hearing test was performed within 6 months prior to tympanostomy tube insertion (OME)**
0.00 0.00 FUD XXX E
AMA: 2008,Mar,8-12

3250F **Specimen site other than anatomic location of primary tumor (PATH)**
0.00 0.00 FUD XXX M

3260F **pT category (primary tumor), pN category (regional lymph nodes), and histologic grade documented in pathology report (PATH)**
0.00 0.00 FUD XXX M
AMA: 2008,Mar,8-12

3265F **Ribonucleic acid (RNA) testing for Hepatitis C viremia ordered or results documented (HEP C)**
0.00 0.00 FUD XXX E
AMA: 2008,Mar,8-12

3266F **Hepatitis C genotype testing documented as performed prior to initiation of antiviral treatment for Hepatitis C (HEP C)**
0.00 0.00 FUD XXX E
AMA: 2008,Mar,8-12

3267F **Pathology report includes pT category, pN category, Gleason score, and statement about margin status (PATH)**
0.00 0.00 FUD XXX M

3268F **Prostate-specific antigen (PSA), and primary tumor (T) stage, and Gleason score documented prior to initiation of treatment (PRCA)**
0.00 0.00 FUD XXX E
AMA: 2008,Mar,8-12

3269F **Bone scan performed prior to initiation of treatment or at any time since diagnosis of prostate cancer (PRCA)**
0.00 0.00 FUD XXX M
AMA: 2008,Mar,8-12

3270F **Bone scan not performed prior to initiation of treatment nor at any time since diagnosis of prostate cancer (PRCA)**
0.00 0.00 FUD XXX M
AMA: 2008,Mar,8-12

3271F **Low risk of recurrence, prostate cancer (PRCA)**
0.00 0.00 FUD XXX E
AMA: 2008,Mar,8-12

3272F **Intermediate risk of recurrence, prostate cancer (PRCA)**
0.00 0.00 FUD XXX E
AMA: 2008,Mar,8-12

3273F **High risk of recurrence, prostate cancer (PRCA)**
0.00 0.00 FUD XXX E
AMA: 2008,Mar,8-12

3274F **Prostate cancer risk of recurrence not determined or neither low, intermediate nor high (PRCA)**
0.00 0.00 FUD XXX E
AMA: 2008,Mar,8-12

3278F **Serum levels of calcium, phosphorus, intact Parathyroid Hormone (PTH) and lipid profile ordered (CKD)**
0.00 0.00 FUD XXX E
AMA: 2008,Mar,8-12

3279F **Hemoglobin level greater than or equal to 13 g/dL (CKD, ESRD)**
0.00 0.00 FUD XXX E
AMA: 2008,Mar,8-12

3280F **Hemoglobin level 11 g/dL to 12.9 g/dL (CKD, ESRD)**
0.00 0.00 FUD XXX E
AMA: 2008,Mar,8-12

3281F **Hemoglobin level less than 11 g/dL (CKD, ESRD)**
0.00 0.00 FUD XXX E
AMA: 2008,Mar,8-12

3284F **Intraocular pressure (IOP) reduced by a value of greater than or equal to 15% from the pre-intervention level (EC)**
0.00 0.00 FUD XXX M
AMA: 2008,Mar,8-12

3285F **Intraocular pressure (IOP) reduced by a value less than 15% from the pre-intervention level (EC)**
0.00 0.00 FUD XXX M
AMA: 2008,Mar,8-12

3288F **Falls risk assessment documented (GER)**
0.00 0.00 FUD XXX M
AMA: 2008,Mar,8-12

3290F **Patient is D (Rh) negative and unsensitized (Pre-Cr)**
0.00 0.00 FUD XXX E
AMA: 2008,Mar,8-12

3291F **Patient is D (Rh) positive or sensitized (Pre-Cr)**
0.00 0.00 FUD XXX E
AMA: 2008,Mar,8-12

3292F **HIV testing ordered or documented and reviewed during the first or second prenatal visit (Pre-Cr)**
0.00 0.00 FUD XXX E

3293F **ABO and Rh blood typing documented as performed (Pre-Cr)**
0.00 0.00 FUD XXX E

3294F **Group B Streptococcus (GBS) screening documented as performed during week 35-37 gestation (Pre-Cr)**
0.00 0.00 FUD XXX E

3300F **American Joint Committee on Cancer (AJCC) stage documented and reviewed (ONC)**
0.00 0.00 FUD XXX M
AMA: 2008,Mar,8-12

3301F **Cancer stage documented in medical record as metastatic and reviewed (ONC)**
EXCLUDES *Cancer staging measures (3321F-3390F)*
0.00 0.00 FUD XXX M
AMA: 2008,Mar,8-12

3315F **Estrogen receptor (ER) or progesterone receptor (PR) positive breast cancer (ONC)**
0.00 0.00 FUD XXX E
AMA: 2008,Mar,8-12

3316F **Estrogen receptor (ER) and progesterone receptor (PR) negative breast cancer (ONC)**
0.00 0.00 FUD XXX E
AMA: 2008,Mar,8-12

3317F **Pathology report confirming malignancy documented in the medical record and reviewed prior to the initiation of chemotherapy (ONC)**
0.00 0.00 FUD XXX E
AMA: 2008,Mar,8-12

3318F **Pathology report confirming malignancy documented in the medical record and reviewed prior to the initiation of radiation therapy (ONC)**
0.00 0.00 FUD XXX E
AMA: 2008,Mar,8-12

3319F **1 of the following diagnostic imaging studies ordered: chest x-ray, CT, Ultrasound, MRI, PET, or nuclear medicine scans (ML)**
0.00 0.00 FUD XXX M
AMA: 2008,Mar,8-12

3320F **None of the following diagnostic imaging studies ordered: chest X-ray, CT, Ultrasound, MRI, PET, or nuclear medicine scans (ML)**
0.00 0.00 FUD XXX M
AMA: 2008,Mar,8-12

3321F **AJCC Cancer Stage 0 or IA Melanoma, documented (ML)**
0.00 0.00 FUD XXX M

3322F **Melanoma greater than AJCC Stage 0 or IA (ML)**
0.00 0.00 FUD XXX M

3323F **Clinical tumor, node and metastases (TNM) staging documented and reviewed prior to surgery (Lung/Esop Cx)**
0.00 0.00 FUD XXX E

3324F **MRI or CT scan ordered, reviewed or requested (EPI)**
0.00 0.00 FUD XXX E

3325F **Preoperative assessment of functional or medical indication(s) for surgery prior to the cataract surgery with intraocular lens placement (must be performed within 12 months prior to cataract surgery) (EC)**
0.00 0.00 FUD XXX E
AMA: 2008,Mar,8-12

3328F **Performance status documented and reviewed within 2 weeks prior to surgery (Lung/Esop Cx)**
0.00 0.00 FUD XXX E

3330F **Imaging study ordered (BkP)**
0.00 0.00 FUD XXX E
AMA: 2008,Mar,8-12

3331F **Imaging study not ordered (BkP)**
0.00 0.00 FUD XXX E
AMA: 2008,Mar,8-12

3340F **Mammogram assessment category of "incomplete: need additional imaging evaluation" documented (RAD)**
0.00 0.00 FUD XXX M
AMA: 2008,Mar,8-12

3341F **Mammogram assessment category of "negative," documented (RAD)**
0.00 0.00 FUD XXX M
AMA: 2008,Mar,8-12

3342F **Mammogram assessment category of "benign," documented (RAD)**
0.00 0.00 FUD XXX M
AMA: 2008,Mar,8-12

3343F **Mammogram assessment category of "probably benign," documented (RAD)**
0.00 0.00 FUD XXX M
AMA: 2008,Mar,8-12

3344F **Mammogram assessment category of "suspicious," documented (RAD)**
0.00 0.00 FUD XXX M
AMA: 2008,Mar,8-12

3345F **Mammogram assessment category of "highly suggestive of malignancy," documented (RAD)**
0.00 0.00 FUD XXX M
AMA: 2008,Mar,8-12

3350F **Mammogram assessment category of "known biopsy proven malignancy," documented (RAD)**
0.00 0.00 FUD XXX M
AMA: 2008,Mar,8-12

3351F **Negative screen for depressive symptoms as categorized by using a standardized depression screening/assessment tool (MDD)**
0.00 0.00 FUD XXX E

3352F **No significant depressive symptoms as categorized by using a standardized depression assessment tool (MDD)**
0.00 0.00 FUD XXX E

3353F **Mild to moderate depressive symptoms as categorized by using a standardized depression screening/assessment tool (MDD)**
0.00 0.00 FUD XXX E

3354F **Clinically significant depressive symptoms as categorized by using a standardized depression screening/assessment tool (MDD)**
0.00 0.00 FUD XXX E

3370F **AJCC Breast Cancer Stage 0 documented (ONC)**
0.00 0.00 FUD XXX E

3372F **AJCC Breast Cancer Stage I: T1mic, T1a or T1b (tumor size ≤ 1 cm) documented (ONC)**
0.00 0.00 FUD XXX E

3374F **AJCC Breast Cancer Stage I: T1c (tumor size > 1 cm to 2 cm) documented (ONC)**
0.00 0.00 FUD XXX E

3376F **AJCC Breast Cancer Stage II documented (ONC)**
0.00 0.00 FUD XXX E

3378F **AJCC Breast Cancer Stage III documented (ONC)**
0.00 0.00 FUD XXX E

3380F **AJCC Breast Cancer Stage IV documented (ONC)**
0.00 0.00 FUD XXX E

3382F **AJCC colon cancer, Stage 0 documented (ONC)**
0.00 0.00 FUD XXX E

3384F **AJCC colon cancer, Stage I documented (ONC)**
0.00 0.00 FUD XXX E

3386F **AJCC colon cancer, Stage II documented (ONC)**
0.00 0.00 FUD XXX E

3388F **AJCC colon cancer, Stage III documented (ONC)**
0.00 0.00 FUD XXX E

3390F **AJCC colon cancer, Stage IV documented (ONC)**
0.00 0.00 FUD XXX E

3394F **Quantitative HER2 immunohistochemistry (IHC) evaluation of breast cancer consistent with the scoring system defined in the ASCO/CAP guidelines (PATH)**
0.00 0.00 FUD XXX M

3395F **Quantitative non-HER2 immunohistochemistry (IHC) evaluation of breast cancer (eg, testing for estrogen or progesterone receptors [ER/PR]) performed (PATH)**
0.00 0.00 FUD XXX M

3450F **Dyspnea screened, no dyspnea or mild dyspnea (Pall Cr)**
0.00 0.00 FUD XXX E

3451F **Dyspnea screened, moderate or severe dyspnea (Pall Cr)**
0.00 0.00 FUD XXX E

3452F **Dyspnea not screened (Pall Cr)**
0.00 0.00 FUD XXX E

3455F **TB screening performed and results interpreted within six months prior to initiation of first-time biologic disease modifying anti-rheumatic drug therapy for RA (RA)**
0.00 0.00 FUD XXX M

3470F **Rheumatoid arthritis (RA) disease activity, low (RA)**
0.00 0.00 FUD XXX M

3471F **Rheumatoid arthritis (RA) disease activity, moderate (RA)**
0.00 0.00 FUD XXX M

3472F **Rheumatoid arthritis (RA) disease activity, high (RA)**
0.00 0.00 FUD XXX M

3475F **Disease prognosis for rheumatoid arthritis assessed, poor prognosis documented (RA)**
0.00 0.00 FUD XXX M

3476F **Disease prognosis for rheumatoid arthritis assessed, good prognosis documented (RA)**
0.00 0.00 FUD XXX M

3490F **History of AIDS-defining condition (HIV)**
0.00 0.00 FUD XXX E

3491F **HIV indeterminate (infants of undetermined HIV status born of HIV-infected mothers) (HIV)**
0.00 0.00 FUD XXX E

3492F **History of nadir CD4+ cell count <350 cells/mm3 (HIV)**
0.00 0.00 FUD XXX E

3493F **No history of nadir CD4+ cell count <350 cells/mm3 and no history of AIDS-defining condition (HIV)**
0.00 0.00 FUD XXX E

3494F **CD4+ cell count <200 cells/mm3 (HIV)**
0.00 0.00 FUD XXX E

3495F **CD4+ cell count 200 - 499 cells/mm3 (HIV)**
0.00 0.00 FUD XXX E

3496F **CD4+ cell count ≥ 500 cells/mm3 (HIV)**
0.00 0.00 FUD XXX E

3497F **CD4+ cell percentage <15% (HIV)**
0.00 0.00 FUD XXX E

3498F **CD4+ cell percentage ≥ 15% (HIV)**
0.00 0.00 FUD XXX E

3500F **CD4+ cell count or CD4+ cell percentage documented as performed (HIV)**
0.00 0.00 FUD XXX E

3502F **HIV RNA viral load below limits of quantification (HIV)**
0.00 0.00 FUD XXX E

3503F **HIV RNA viral load not below limits of quantification (HIV)**
0.00 0.00 FUD XXX E

3510F **Documentation that tuberculosis (TB) screening test performed and results interpreted (HIV) (IBD)**
0.00 0.00 FUD XXX E

3511F **Chlamydia and gonorrhea screenings documented as performed (HIV)**
0.00 0.00 FUD XXX E

3512F **Syphilis screening documented as performed (HIV)**
0.00 0.00 FUD XXX E

3513F **Hepatitis B screening documented as performed (HIV)**
0.00 0.00 FUD XXX E

3514F **Hepatitis C screening documented as performed (HIV)**
0.00 0.00 FUD XXX E

3515F **Patient has documented immunity to Hepatitis C (HIV)**
0.00 0.00 FUD XXX E

3517F **Hepatitis B Virus (HBV) status assessed and results interpreted within one year prior to receiving a first course of anti-TNF (tumor necrosis factor) therapy (IBD)**
0.00 0.00 FUD XXX E

3520F **Clostridium difficile testing performed (IBD)**
0.00 0.00 FUD XXX E

3550F **Low risk for thromboembolism (AFIB)**
0.00 0.00 FUD XXX E

3551F **Intermediate risk for thromboembolism (AFIB)**
0.00 0.00 FUD XXX E

3552F **High risk for thromboembolism (AFIB)**
0.00 0.00 FUD XXX E

3555F **Patient had International Normalized Ratio (INR) measurement performed (AFIB)**
0.00 0.00 FUD XXX E
AMA: 2010,Jul,3-5

3570F **Final report for bone scintigraphy study includes correlation with existing relevant imaging studies (eg, X-ray, MRI, CT) corresponding to the same anatomical region in question (NUC_MED)**
0.00 0.00 FUD XXX M

3572F **Patient considered to be potentially at risk for fracture in a weight-bearing site (NUC_MED)**
0.00 0.00 FUD XXX E

3573F **Patient not considered to be potentially at risk for fracture in a weight-bearing site (NUC_MED)**
0.00 0.00 FUD XXX E

3650F **Electroencephalogram (EEG) ordered, reviewed or requested (EPI)**
0.00 0.00 FUD XXX E

3700F **Psychiatric disorders or disturbances assessed (Prkns)**
0.00 0.00 FUD XXX E

3720F **Cognitive impairment or dysfunction assessed (Prkns)**
0.00 0.00 FUD XXX M

3725F **Screening for depression performed (DEM)**
0.00 0.00 FUD XXX M

3750F **Patient not receiving dose of corticosteroids greater than or equal to 10mg/day for 60 or greater consecutive days (IBD)**
0.00 0.00 FUD XXX E

3751F **Electrodiagnostic studies for distal symmetric polyneuropathy conducted (or requested), documented, and reviewed within 6 months of initial evaluation for condition (DSP)**
0.00 0.00 FUD XXX E

3752F **Electrodiagnostic studies for distal symmetric polyneuropathy not conducted (or requested), documented, or reviewed within 6 months of initial evaluation for condition (DSP)**
0.00 0.00 FUD XXX E

3753F **Patient has clear clinical symptoms and signs that are highly suggestive of neuropathy AND cannot be attributed to another condition, AND has an obvious cause for the neuropathy (DSP)**
0.00 0.00 FUD XXX E

3754F **Screening tests for diabetes mellitus reviewed, requested, or ordered (DSP)**
0.00 0.00 FUD XXX E

3755F **Cognitive and behavioral impairment screening performed (ALS)**
0.00 0.00 FUD XXX E

3756F **Patient has pseudobulbar affect, sialorrhea, or ALS-related symptoms (ALS)**
0.00 0.00 FUD XXX E

3757F **Patient does not have pseudobulbar affect, sialorrhea, or ALS-related symptoms (ALS)**
0.00 0.00 FUD XXX E

3758F **Patient referred for pulmonary function testing or peak cough expiratory flow (ALS)**
0.00 0.00 FUD XXX E

3759F **Patient screened for dysphagia, weight loss, and impaired nutrition, and results documented (ALS)**
0.00 0.00 FUD XXX E

3760F **Patient exhibits dysphagia, weight loss, or impaired nutrition (ALS)**
0.00 0.00 FUD XXX E

3761F **Patient does not exhibit dysphagia, weight loss, or impaired nutrition (ALS)**
0.00 0.00 FUD XXX E

3762F **Patient is dysarthric (ALS)**
0.00 0.00 FUD XXX E

3763F **Patient is not dysarthric (ALS)**
0.00 0.00 FUD XXX E

3775F **Adenoma(s) or other neoplasm detected during screening colonoscopy (SCADR)**
0.00 0.00 FUD XXX E

3776F **Adenoma(s) or other neoplasm not detected during screening colonoscopy (SCADR)**
0.00 0.00 FUD XXX E

4000F-4563F Therapies Provided (Includes Preventive Services)

INCLUDES Behavioral/pharmacologic/procedural therapies
Preventive services including patient education/counseling

4000F **Tobacco use cessation intervention, counseling (COPD, CAP, CAD, Asthma) (DM) (PV)**
0.00 0.00 FUD XXX E
AMA: 2018,Jan,8; 2017,Jan,8; 2016,Jan,13; 2015,Jan,16

4001F **Tobacco use cessation intervention, pharmacologic therapy (COPD, CAD, CAP, PV, Asthma) (DM) (PV)**
0.00 0.00 FUD XXX E
AMA: 2008,Mar,8-12; 2004,Nov,1

4003F **Patient education, written/oral, appropriate for patients with heart failure, performed (NMA-No Measure Associated)**
0.00 0.00 FUD XXX E
AMA: 2004,Nov,1

4004F **Patient screened for tobacco use and received tobacco cessation intervention (counseling, pharmacotherapy, or both), if identified as a tobacco user (PV, CAD)**
0.00 0.00 FUD XXX M

4005F **Pharmacologic therapy (other than minerals/vitamins) for osteoporosis prescribed (OP) (IBD)**
0.00 0.00 FUD XXX E

4008F **Beta-blocker therapy prescribed or currently being taken (CAD,HF)**
0.00 0.00 FUD XXX M

4010F **Angiotensin Converting Enzyme (ACE) Inhibitor or Angiotensin Receptor Blocker (ARB) therapy prescribed or currently being taken (CAD, CKD, HF) (DM)**
0.00 0.00 FUD XXX M

4011F **Oral antiplatelet therapy prescribed (CAD)**
0.00 0.00 FUD XXX E
AMA: 2004,Nov,1

4012F **Warfarin therapy prescribed (NMA-No Measure Associated)**
0.00 0.00 FUD XXX E

4013F **Statin therapy prescribed or currently being taken (CAD)**
0.00 0.00 FUD XXX E

4014F **Written discharge instructions provided to heart failure patients discharged home (Instructions include all of the following components: activity level, diet, discharge medications, follow-up appointment, weight monitoring, what to do if symptoms worsen) (NMA-No Measure Associated)**
0.00 0.00 FUD XXX E

4015F **Persistent asthma, preferred long term control medication or an acceptable alternative treatment, prescribed (NMA-No Measure Associated)**
EXCLUDES *Reporting code with modifier 1P*
Code also modifier 2P for patient reasons for not prescribing
0.00 0.00 FUD XXX E

4016F **Anti-inflammatory/analgesic agent prescribed (OA) (Use for prescribed or continued medication[s], including over-the-counter medication[s])**
INCLUDES Over-the-counter medication(s)
Prescribed/continued medication(s)
0.00 0.00 FUD XXX E

4017F **Gastrointestinal prophylaxis for NSAID use prescribed (OA)**
0.00 0.00 FUD XXX E

4018F **Therapeutic exercise for the involved joint(s) instructed or physical or occupational therapy prescribed (OA)**
0.00 0.00 FUD XXX E

4019F **Documentation of receipt of counseling on exercise and either both calcium and vitamin D use or counseling regarding both calcium and vitamin D use (OP)**
0.00 0.00 FUD XXX E

4025F **Inhaled bronchodilator prescribed (COPD)**
0.00 0.00 FUD XXX E

4030F **Long-term oxygen therapy prescribed (more than 15 hours per day) (COPD)**
0.00 0.00 FUD XXX E

4033F **Pulmonary rehabilitation exercise training recommended (COPD)**
Code also dyspnea assessed, present (1019F)
0.00 0.00 FUD XXX E

4035F **Influenza immunization recommended (COPD) (IBD)**
0.00 0.00 FUD XXX E
AMA: 2008,Mar,8-12

4037F **Influenza immunization ordered or administered (COPD, PV, CKD, ESRD)(IBD)**
0.00 0.00 FUD XXX E
AMA: 2008,Mar,8-12

4040F **Pneumococcal vaccine administered or previously received (COPD) (PV), (IBD)**
0.00 0.00 FUD XXX M
AMA: 2008,Mar,8-12

4041F **Documentation of order for cefazolin OR cefuroxime for antimicrobial prophylaxis (PERI 2)**
0.00 0.00 FUD XXX E

4042F **Documentation that prophylactic antibiotics were neither given within 4 hours prior to surgical incision nor given intraoperatively (PERI 2)**
0.00 0.00 FUD XXX E

4043F **Documentation that an order was given to discontinue prophylactic antibiotics within 48 hours of surgical end time, cardiac procedures (PERI 2)**
0.00 0.00 FUD XXX E

4044F **Documentation that an order was given for venous thromboembolism (VTE) prophylaxis to be given within 24 hours prior to incision time or 24 hours after surgery end time (PERI 2)**
0.00 0.00 FUD XXX M

4045F **Appropriate empiric antibiotic prescribed (CAP), (EM)**
0.00 0.00 FUD XXX E

4046F **Documentation that prophylactic antibiotics were given within 4 hours prior to surgical incision or given intraoperatively (PERI 2)**
0.00 0.00 FUD XXX E

4047F **Documentation of order for prophylactic parenteral antibiotics to be given within 1 hour (if fluoroquinolone or vancomycin, 2 hours) prior to surgical incision (or start of procedure when no incision is required) (PERI 2)**
0.00 0.00 FUD XXX E

4048F **Documentation that administration of prophylactic parenteral antibiotic was initiated within 1 hour (if fluoroquinolone or vancomycin, 2 hours) prior to surgical incision (or start of procedure when no incision is required) as ordered (PERI 2)**
0.00 0.00 FUD XXX E

4049F **Documentation that order was given to discontinue prophylactic antibiotics within 24 hours of surgical end time, non-cardiac procedure (PERI 2)**
0.00 0.00 FUD XXX E

4050F **Hypertension plan of care documented as appropriate (NMA-No Measure Associated)**
0.00 0.00 FUD XXX E

4051F **Referred for an arteriovenous (AV) fistula (ESRD, CKD)**
0.00 0.00 FUD XXX E
AMA: 2008,Mar,8-12

4052F **Hemodialysis via functioning arteriovenous (AV) fistula (ESRD)**
0.00 0.00 FUD XXX E
AMA: 2008,Mar,8-12

4053F **Hemodialysis via functioning arteriovenous (AV) graft (ESRD)**
0.00 0.00 FUD XXX E
AMA: 2008,Mar,8-12

4054F **Hemodialysis via catheter (ESRD)**
0.00 0.00 FUD XXX E
AMA: 2008,Mar,8-12

4055F **Patient receiving peritoneal dialysis (ESRD)**
0.00 0.00 FUD XXX E
AMA: 2008,Mar,8-12

4056F **Appropriate oral rehydration solution recommended (PAG)**
0.00 0.00 FUD XXX E

4058F **Pediatric gastroenteritis education provided to caregiver (PAG)**
0.00 0.00 FUD XXX E

4060F **Psychotherapy services provided (MDD, MDD ADOL)**
0.00 0.00 FUD XXX E

4062F **Patient referral for psychotherapy documented (MDD, MDD ADOL)**
0.00 0.00 FUD XXX E

4063F **Antidepressant pharmacotherapy considered and not prescribed (MDD ADOL)**
0.00 0.00 FUD XXX E

4064F **Antidepressant pharmacotherapy prescribed (MDD, MDD ADOL)**
0.00 0.00 FUD XXX E

4065F **Antipsychotic pharmacotherapy prescribed (MDD)**
0.00 0.00 FUD XXX E

4066F **Electroconvulsive therapy (ECT) provided (MDD)**
0.00 0.00 FUD XXX E

4067F **Patient referral for electroconvulsive therapy (ECT) documented (MDD)**
0.00 0.00 FUD XXX E

4069F **Venous thromboembolism (VTE) prophylaxis received (IBD)**
0.00 0.00 FUD XXX E

4070F **Deep vein thrombosis (DVT) prophylaxis received by end of hospital day 2 (STR)**
0.00 0.00 FUD XXX E

4073F **Oral antiplatelet therapy prescribed at discharge (STR)**
0.00 0.00 FUD XXX E

4075F **Anticoagulant therapy prescribed at discharge (STR)**
0.00 0.00 FUD XXX E

4077F **Documentation that tissue plasminogen activator (t-PA) administration was considered (STR)**
0.00 0.00 FUD XXX E

4079F **Documentation that rehabilitation services were considered (STR)**
0.00 0.00 FUD XXX E

4084F **Aspirin received within 24 hours before emergency department arrival or during emergency department stay (EM)**
0.00 0.00 FUD XXX E

4086F **Aspirin or clopidogrel prescribed or currently being taken (CAD)**
0.00 0.00 FUD XXX M

4090F **Patient receiving erythropoietin therapy (HEM)**
0.00 0.00 FUD XXX M
AMA: 2008,Mar,8-12

4095F **Patient not receiving erythropoietin therapy (HEM)**
0.00 0.00 FUD XXX E
AMA: 2008,Mar,8-12

4100F **Bisphosphonate therapy, intravenous, ordered or received (HEM)**
0.00 0.00 FUD XXX M
AMA: 2008,Mar,8-12

4110F **Internal mammary artery graft performed for primary, isolated coronary artery bypass graft procedure (CABG)**
0.00 0.00 FUD XXX M

4115F **Beta blocker administered within 24 hours prior to surgical incision (CABG)**
0.00 0.00 FUD XXX M

4120F **Antibiotic prescribed or dispensed (URI, PHAR), (A-BRONCH)**
0.00 0.00 FUD XXX M
AMA: 2008,Mar,8-12

4124F **Antibiotic neither prescribed nor dispensed (URI, PHAR), (A-BRONCH)**
0.00 0.00 FUD XXX M
AMA: 2008,Mar,8-12

4130F **Topical preparations (including OTC) prescribed for acute otitis externa (AOE)**
0.00 0.00 FUD XXX M
AMA: 2010,Jan,6-7; 2008,Mar,8-12

4131F **Systemic antimicrobial therapy prescribed (AOE)**
0.00 0.00 FUD XXX M
AMA: 2008,Mar,8-12

4132F **Systemic antimicrobial therapy not prescribed (AOE)**
0.00 0.00 FUD XXX M
AMA: 2008,Mar,8-12

4133F **Antihistamines or decongestants prescribed or recommended (OME)**
0.00 0.00 FUD XXX E
AMA: 2008,Mar,8-12

4134F **Antihistamines or decongestants neither prescribed nor recommended (OME)**
0.00 0.00 FUD XXX E
AMA: 2008,Mar,8-12

4135F **Systemic corticosteroids prescribed (OME)**
0.00 0.00 FUD XXX E
AMA: 2008,Mar,8-12

4136F **Systemic corticosteroids not prescribed (OME)**
0.00 0.00 FUD XXX E
AMA: 2008,Mar,8-12

4140F **Inhaled corticosteroids prescribed (Asthma)**
0.00 0.00 FUD XXX E

4142F **Corticosteroid sparing therapy prescribed (IBD)**
0.00 0.00 FUD XXX E

4144F **Alternative long-term control medication prescribed (Asthma)**
0.00 0.00 FUD XXX E

4145F **Two or more anti-hypertensive agents prescribed or currently being taken (CAD, HTN)**
0.00 0.00 FUD XXX E

4148F **Hepatitis A vaccine injection administered or previously received (HEP-C)**
0.00 0.00 FUD XXX E

4149F **Hepatitis B vaccine injection administered or previously received (HEP-C, HIV) (IBD)**
0.00 0.00 FUD XXX E

4150F **Patient receiving antiviral treatment for Hepatitis C (HEP-C)**
0.00 0.00 FUD XXX E
AMA: 2008,Mar,8-12

4151F **Patient did not start or is not receiving antiviral treatment for Hepatitis C during the measurement period (HEP-C)**
0.00 0.00 FUD XXX E
AMA: 2008,Mar,8-12

4153F **Combination peginterferon and ribavirin therapy prescribed (HEP-C)**
0.00 0.00 FUD XXX E
AMA: 2008,Mar,8-12

4155F **Hepatitis A vaccine series previously received (HEP-C)**
0.00 0.00 FUD XXX E
AMA: 2008,Mar,8-12

4157F **Hepatitis B vaccine series previously received (HEP-C)**
0.00 0.00 FUD XXX E
AMA: 2008,Mar,8-12

4158F **Patient counseled about risks of alcohol use (HEP-C)**
0.00 0.00 FUD XXX E
AMA: 2008,Mar,8-12

4159F **Counseling regarding contraception received prior to initiation of antiviral treatment (HEP-C)**
0.00 0.00 FUD XXX E
AMA: 2008,Mar,8-12

4163F **Patient counseling at a minimum on all of the following treatment options for clinically localized prostate cancer: active surveillance, and interstitial prostate brachytherapy, and external beam radiotherapy, and radical prostatectomy, provided prior to initiation of treatment (PRCA)**
0.00 0.00 FUD XXX E
AMA: 2008,Mar,8-12

4164F **Adjuvant (ie, in combination with external beam radiotherapy to the prostate for prostate cancer) hormonal therapy (gonadotropin-releasing hormone [GnRH] agonist or antagonist) prescribed/administered (PRCA)**
0.00 0.00 FUD XXX E
AMA: 2008,Mar,8-12

4165F **3-dimensional conformal radiotherapy (3D-CRT) or intensity modulated radiation therapy (IMRT) received (PRCA)**
0.00 0.00 FUD XXX E
AMA: 2008,Mar,8-12

4167F **Head of bed elevation (30-45 degrees) on first ventilator day ordered (CRIT)**
0.00 0.00 FUD XXX E
AMA: 2008,Mar,8-12

4168F **Patient receiving care in the intensive care unit (ICU) and receiving mechanical ventilation, 24 hours or less (CRIT)**
0.00 0.00 FUD XXX E
AMA: 2008,Mar,8-12

4169F **Patient either not receiving care in the intensive care unit (ICU) OR not receiving mechanical ventilation OR receiving mechanical ventilation greater than 24 hours (CRIT)**
0.00 0.00 FUD XXX E
AMA: 2008,Mar,8-12

4171F **Patient receiving erythropoiesis-stimulating agents (ESA) therapy (CKD)**
0.00 0.00 FUD XXX E
AMA: 2008,Mar,8-12

4172F **Patient not receiving erythropoiesis-stimulating agents (ESA) therapy (CKD)**
0.00 0.00 FUD XXX E
AMA: 2008,Mar,8-12

4174F **Counseling about the potential impact of glaucoma on visual functioning and quality of life, and importance of treatment adherence provided to patient and/or caregiver(s) (EC)**
0.00 0.00 FUD XXX E
AMA: 2008,Mar,8-12

4175F **Best-corrected visual acuity of 20/40 or better (distance or near) achieved within the 90 days following cataract surgery (EC)**
0.00 0.00 FUD XXX M
AMA: 2008,Mar,8-12

4176F **Counseling about value of protection from UV light and lack of proven efficacy of nutritional supplements in prevention or progression of cataract development provided to patient and/or caregiver(s) (NMA-No Measure Associated)**
0.00 0.00 FUD XXX E

4177F **Counseling about the benefits and/or risks of the Age-Related Eye Disease Study (AREDS) formulation for preventing progression of age-related macular degeneration (AMD) provided to patient and/or caregiver(s) (EC)**
0.00 0.00 FUD XXX M
AMA: 2008,Mar,8-12

4178F **Anti-D immune globulin received between 26 and 30 weeks gestation (Pre-Cr)** M
0.00 0.00 FUD XXX E
AMA: 2008,Mar,8-12

4179F **Tamoxifen or aromatase inhibitor (AI) prescribed (ONC)**
0.00 0.00 FUD XXX E
AMA: 2008,Mar,8-12

4180F **Adjuvant chemotherapy referred, prescribed, or previously received for Stage III colon cancer (ONC)**
0.00 0.00 FUD XXX E
AMA: 2008,Mar,8-12

4181F **Conformal radiation therapy received (NMA-No Measure Associated)**
0.00 0.00 FUD XXX E

4182F **Conformal radiation therapy not received (NMA-No Measure Associated)**
0.00 0.00 FUD XXX E

4185F **Continuous (12-months) therapy with proton pump inhibitor (PPI) or histamine H2 receptor antagonist (H2RA) received (GERD)**
0.00 0.00 FUD XXX E
AMA: 2008,Mar,8-12

4186F **No continuous (12-months) therapy with either proton pump inhibitor (PPI) or histamine H2 receptor antagonist (H2RA) received (GERD)**
0.00 0.00 FUD XXX E
AMA: 2008,Mar,8-12

4187F **Disease modifying anti-rheumatic drug therapy prescribed or dispensed (RA)**
0.00 0.00 FUD XXX E

4188F **Appropriate angiotensin converting enzyme (ACE)/angiotensin receptor blockers (ARB) therapeutic monitoring test ordered or performed (AM)**
0.00 0.00 FUD XXX E
AMA: 2008,Mar,8-12

4189F **Appropriate digoxin therapeutic monitoring test ordered or performed (AM)**
0.00 0.00 FUD XXX E
AMA: 2008,Mar,8-12

4190F **Appropriate diuretic therapeutic monitoring test ordered or performed (AM)**
0.00 0.00 FUD XXX E
AMA: 2008,Mar,8-12

4191F **Appropriate anticonvulsant therapeutic monitoring test ordered or performed (AM)**
0.00 0.00 FUD XXX E
AMA: 2008,Mar,8-12

4192F **Patient not receiving glucocorticoid therapy (RA)**
0.00 0.00 FUD XXX M

4193F **Patient receiving <10 mg daily prednisone (or equivalent), or RA activity is worsening, or glucocorticoid use is for less than 6 months (RA)**
0.00 0.00 FUD XXX M

4194F **Patient receiving ≥10 mg daily prednisone (or equivalent) for longer than 6 months, and improvement or no change in disease activity (RA)**
0.00 0.00 FUD XXX M

4195F **Patient receiving first-time biologic disease modifying anti-rheumatic drug therapy for rheumatoid arthritis (RA)**
0.00 0.00 FUD XXX M

4196F **Patient not receiving first-time biologic disease modifying anti-rheumatic drug therapy for rheumatoid arthritis (RA)**
0.00 0.00 FUD XXX M

4200F **External beam radiotherapy as primary therapy to prostate with or without nodal irradiation (PRCA)**
0.00 0.00 FUD XXX E
AMA: 2008,Mar,8-12

4201F **External beam radiotherapy with or without nodal irradiation as adjuvant or salvage therapy for prostate cancer patient (PRCA)**
0.00 0.00 FUD XXX E
AMA: 2008,Mar,8-12

4210F **Angiotensin converting enzyme (ACE) or angiotensin receptor blockers (ARB) medication therapy for 6 months or more (MM)**
0.00 0.00 FUD XXX E
AMA: 2008,Mar,8-12

4220F **Digoxin medication therapy for 6 months or more (MM)**
0.00 0.00 FUD XXX E
AMA: 2008,Mar,8-12

4221F **Diuretic medication therapy for 6 months or more (MM)**
0.00 0.00 FUD XXX E
AMA: 2008,Mar,8-12

4230F **Anticonvulsant medication therapy for 6 months or more (MM)**
0.00 0.00 FUD XXX E
AMA: 2008,Mar,8-12

4240F **Instruction in therapeutic exercise with follow-up provided to patients during episode of back pain lasting longer than 12 weeks (BkP)**
0.00 0.00 FUD XXX E
AMA: 2008,Mar,8-12

4242F **Counseling for supervised exercise program provided to patients during episode of back pain lasting longer than 12 weeks (BkP)**
0.00 0.00 FUD XXX E
AMA: 2008,Mar,8-12

4245F **Patient counseled during the initial visit to maintain or resume normal activities (BkP)**
0.00 0.00 FUD XXX E
AMA: 2008,Mar,8-12

4248F **Patient counseled during the initial visit for an episode of back pain against bed rest lasting 4 days or longer (BkP)**
0.00 0.00 FUD XXX E
AMA: 2008,Mar,8-12

4250F **Active warming used intraoperatively for the purpose of maintaining normothermia, or at least 1 body temperature equal to or greater than 36 degrees Centigrade (or 96.8 degrees Fahrenheit) recorded within the 30 minutes immediately before or the 15 minutes immediately after anesthesia end time (CRIT)**
0.00 0.00 FUD XXX E
AMA: 2008,Mar,8-12

4255F **Duration of general or neuraxial anesthesia 60 minutes or longer, as documented in the anesthesia record (CRIT) (Peri2)**
0.00 0.00 FUD XXX M

4256F **Duration of general or neuraxial anesthesia less than 60 minutes, as documented in the anesthesia record (CRIT) (Peri2)**
0.00 0.00 FUD XXX E

4260F **Wound surface culture technique used (CWC)**
0.00 0.00 FUD XXX E

4261F **Technique other than surface culture of the wound exudate used (eg, Levine/deep swab technique, semi-quantitative or quantitative swab technique) or wound surface culture technique not used (CWC)**
0.00 0.00 FUD XXX E

4265F **Use of wet to dry dressings prescribed or recommended (CWC)**
0.00 0.00 FUD XXX E

4266F **Use of wet to dry dressings neither prescribed nor recommended (CWC)**
0.00 0.00 FUD XXX E

4267F **Compression therapy prescribed (CWC)**
0.00 0.00 FUD XXX E

4268F **Patient education regarding the need for long term compression therapy including interval replacement of compression stockings received (CWC)**
0.00 0.00 FUD XXX E

4269F **Appropriate method of offloading (pressure relief) prescribed (CWC)**
0.00 0.00 FUD XXX E

4270F **Patient receiving potent antiretroviral therapy for 6 months or longer (HIV)**
0.00 0.00 FUD XXX E

4271F **Patient receiving potent antiretroviral therapy for less than 6 months or not receiving potent antiretroviral therapy (HIV)**
0.00 0.00 FUD XXX E

4274F **Influenza immunization administered or previously received (HIV) (P-ESRD)**
0.00 0.00 FUD XXX E

4276F **Potent antiretroviral therapy prescribed (HIV)**
0.00 0.00 FUD XXX E

4279F **Pneumocystis jiroveci pneumonia prophylaxis prescribed (HIV)**
0.00 0.00 FUD XXX E

4280F **Pneumocystis jiroveci pneumonia prophylaxis prescribed within 3 months of low CD4+ cell count or percentage (HIV)**
0.00 0.00 FUD XXX E

4290F **Patient screened for injection drug use (HIV)**
0.00 0.00 FUD XXX E

4293F **Patient screened for high-risk sexual behavior (HIV)**
0.00 0.00 FUD XXX E

4300F **Patient receiving warfarin therapy for nonvalvular atrial fibrillation or atrial flutter (AFIB)**
0.00 0.00 FUD XXX E

4301F **Patient not receiving warfarin therapy for nonvalvular atrial fibrillation or atrial flutter (AFIB)**
0.00 0.00 FUD XXX E

4305F **Patient education regarding appropriate foot care and daily inspection of the feet received (CWC)**
0.00 0.00 FUD XXX E

4306F **Patient counseled regarding psychosocial and pharmacologic treatment options for opioid addiction (SUD)**
0.00 0.00 FUD XXX E

4320F **Patient counseled regarding psychosocial and pharmacologic treatment options for alcohol dependence (SUD)**
0.00 0.00 FUD XXX E

4322F **Caregiver provided with education and referred to additional resources for support (DEM)**
0.00 0.00 FUD XXX M

4324F **Patient (or caregiver) queried about Parkinson's disease medication related motor complications (Prkns)**
0.00 0.00 FUD XXX E

4325F **Medical and surgical treatment options reviewed with patient (or caregiver) (Prkns)**
0.00 0.00 FUD XXX M

4326F **Patient (or caregiver) queried about symptoms of autonomic dysfunction (Prkns)**
0.00 0.00 FUD XXX E

4328F **Patient (or caregiver) queried about sleep disturbances (Prkns)**
0.00 0.00 FUD XXX E

4330F **Counseling about epilepsy specific safety issues provided to patient (or caregiver(s)) (EPI)**
0.00 0.00 FUD XXX E

4340F **Counseling for women of childbearing potential with epilepsy (EPI)**
0.00 0.00 FUD XXX M

4350F Counseling provided on symptom management, end of life decisions, and palliation (DEM)
0.00 0.00 FUD XXX E

4400F Rehabilitative therapy options discussed with patient (or caregiver) (Prkns)
0.00 0.00 FUD XXX M

4450F Self-care education provided to patient (HF)
0.00 0.00 FUD XXX E

4470F Implantable cardioverter-defibrillator (ICD) counseling provided (HF)
0.00 0.00 FUD XXX E

4480F Patient receiving ACE inhibitor/ARB therapy and beta-blocker therapy for 3 months or longer (HF)
0.00 0.00 FUD XXX E

4481F Patient receiving ACE inhibitor/ARB therapy and beta-blocker therapy for less than 3 months or patient not receiving ACE inhibitor/ARB therapy and beta blocker therapy (HF)
0.00 0.00 FUD XXX E

4500F Referred to an outpatient cardiac rehabilitation program (CAD)
0.00 0.00 FUD XXX M

4510F Previous cardiac rehabilitation for qualifying cardiac event completed (CAD)
0.00 0.00 FUD XXX M

4525F Neuropsychiatric intervention ordered (DEM)
0.00 0.00 FUD XXX E

4526F Neuropsychiatric intervention received (DEM)
0.00 0.00 FUD XXX E

4540F Disease modifying pharmacotherapy discussed (ALS)
0.00 0.00 FUD XXX E

4541F Patient offered treatment for pseudobulbar affect, sialorrhea, or ALS-related symptoms (ALS)
0.00 0.00 FUD XXX E

4550F Options for noninvasive respiratory support discussed with patient (ALS)
0.00 0.00 FUD XXX E

4551F Nutritional support offered (ALS)
0.00 0.00 FUD XXX E

4552F Patient offered referral to a speech language pathologist (ALS)
0.00 0.00 FUD XXX E

4553F Patient offered assistance in planning for end of life issues (ALS)
0.00 0.00 FUD XXX E

4554F Patient received inhalational anesthetic agent (Peri2)
0.00 0.00 FUD XXX M

4555F Patient did not receive inhalational anesthetic agent (Peri2)
0.00 0.00 FUD XXX E

4556F Patient exhibits 3 or more risk factors for post-operative nausea and vomiting (Peri2)
0.00 0.00 FUD XXX M

4557F Patient does not exhibit 3 or more risk factors for post-operative nausea and vomiting (Peri2)
0.00 0.00 FUD XXX E

4558F Patient received at least 2 prophylactic pharmacologic anti-emetic agents of different classes preoperatively and intraoperatively (Peri2)
0.00 0.00 FUD XXX E

4559F At least 1 body temperature measurement equal to or greater than 35.5 degrees Celsius (or 95.9 degrees Fahrenheit) recorded within the 30 minutes immediately before or the 15 minutes immediately after anesthesia end time (Peri2)
0.00 0.00 FUD XXX E

4560F Anesthesia technique did not involve general or neuraxial anesthesia (Peri2)
0.00 0.00 FUD XXX E

4561F Patient has a coronary artery stent (Peri2)
0.00 0.00 FUD XXX E

4562F Patient does not have a coronary artery stent (Peri2)
0.00 0.00 FUD XXX E

4563F Patient received aspirin within 24 hours prior to anesthesia start time (Peri2)
0.00 0.00 FUD XXX E

5005F-5250F Results Conveyed and Documented

INCLUDES Patient's:
- Functional status
- Morbidity/mortality
- Satisfaction/experience with care

Review/communication test results to patients

5005F Patient counseled on self-examination for new or changing moles (ML)
0.00 0.00 FUD XXX E
AMA: 2008,Mar,8-12

5010F Findings of dilated macular or fundus exam communicated to the physician or other qualified health care professional managing the diabetes care (EC)
0.00 0.00 FUD XXX M

5015F Documentation of communication that a fracture occurred and that the patient was or should be tested or treated for osteoporosis (OP)
0.00 0.00 FUD XXX M

5020F Treatment summary report communicated to physician(s) or other qualified health care professional(s) managing continuing care and to the patient within 1 month of completing treatment (ONC)
0.00 0.00 FUD XXX E
AMA: 2008,Mar,8-12

5050F Treatment plan communicated to provider(s) managing continuing care within 1 month of diagnosis (ML)
0.00 0.00 FUD XXX M
AMA: 2008,Mar,8-12

5060F Findings from diagnostic mammogram communicated to practice managing patient's on-going care within 3 business days of exam interpretation (RAD)
0.00 0.00 FUD XXX E
AMA: 2008,Mar,8-12

5062F Findings from diagnostic mammogram communicated to the patient within 5 days of exam interpretation (RAD)
0.00 0.00 FUD XXX E
AMA: 2008,Mar,8-12

5100F Potential risk for fracture communicated to the referring physician or other qualified health care professional within 24 hours of completion of the imaging study (NUC_MED)
0.00 0.00 FUD XXX E

5200F Consideration of referral for a neurological evaluation of appropriateness for surgical therapy for intractable epilepsy within the past 3 years (EPI)
0.00 0.00 FUD XXX E

5250F Asthma discharge plan provided to patient (Asthma)
0.00 0.00 FUD XXX E

6005F-6150F Elements Related to Patient Safety Processes

INCLUDES Patient safety practices

6005F **Rationale (eg, severity of illness and safety) for level of care (eg, home, hospital) documented (CAP)**
0.00 0.00 **FUD** XXX E
AMA: 2018,Jan,8; 2017,Jan,8; 2016,Jan,13; 2015,Jan,16

6010F **Dysphagia screening conducted prior to order for or receipt of any foods, fluids, or medication by mouth (STR)**
0.00 0.00 **FUD** XXX E

6015F **Patient receiving or eligible to receive foods, fluids, or medication by mouth (STR)**
0.00 0.00 **FUD** XXX E

6020F **NPO (nothing by mouth) ordered (STR)**
0.00 0.00 **FUD** XXX E

6030F **All elements of maximal sterile barrier technique, hand hygiene, skin preparation and, if ultrasound is used, sterile ultrasound techniques followed (CRIT)**
0.00 0.00 **FUD** XXX M
AMA: 2008,Mar,8-12

6040F **Use of appropriate radiation dose reduction devices OR manual techniques for appropriate moderation of exposure, documented (RAD)**
0.00 0.00 **FUD** XXX E

6045F **Radiation exposure or exposure time in final report for procedure using fluoroscopy, documented (RAD)**
0.00 0.00 **FUD** XXX E
AMA: 2008,Mar,8-12

6070F **Patient queried and counseled about anti-epileptic drug (AED) side effects (EPI)**
0.00 0.00 **FUD** XXX E

6080F **Patient (or caregiver) queried about falls (Prkns, DSP)**
0.00 0.00 **FUD** XXX E

6090F **Patient (or caregiver) counseled about safety issues appropriate to patient's stage of disease (Prkns)**
0.00 0.00 **FUD** XXX E

6100F **Timeout to verify correct patient, correct site, and correct procedure, documented (PATH)**
0.00 0.00 **FUD** XXX E

6101F **Safety counseling for dementia provided (DEM)**
0.00 0.00 **FUD** XXX E

6102F **Safety counseling for dementia ordered (DEM)**
0.00 0.00 **FUD** XXX E

6110F **Counseling provided regarding risks of driving and the alternatives to driving (DEM)**
0.00 0.00 **FUD** XXX E

6150F **Patient not receiving a first course of anti-TNF (tumor necrosis factor) therapy (IBD)**
0.00 0.00 **FUD** XXX E

7010F-7025F Recall/Reminder System in Place

INCLUDES Provider capabilities
Measures that address setting or care system provided

7010F **Patient information entered into a recall system that includes: target date for the next exam specified and a process to follow up with patients regarding missed or unscheduled appointments (ML)**
0.00 0.00 **FUD** XXX M
AMA: 2008,Mar,8-12

7020F **Mammogram assessment category (eg, Mammography Quality Standards Act [MQSA], Breast Imaging Reporting and Data System [BI-RADS], or FDA approved equivalent categories) entered into an internal database to allow for analysis of abnormal interpretation (recall) rate (RAD)**
0.00 0.00 **FUD** XXX E
AMA: 2008,Mar,8-12

7025F **Patient information entered into a reminder system with a target due date for the next mammogram (RAD)**
0.00 0.00 **FUD** XXX M
AMA: 2008,Mar,8-12

9001F-9007F No Measure Associated

INCLUDES Care aspects not associated with measures at current time

9001F **Aortic aneurysm less than 5.0 cm maximum diameter on centerline formatted CT or minor diameter on axial formatted CT (NMA-No Measure Associated)**
0.00 0.00 **FUD** XXX E

9002F **Aortic aneurysm 5.0 - 5.4 cm maximum diameter on centerline formatted CT or minor diameter on axial formatted CT (NMA-No Measure Associated)**
0.00 0.00 **FUD** XXX E

9003F **Aortic aneurysm 5.5 - 5.9 cm maximum diameter on centerline formatted CT or minor diameter on axial formatted CT (NMA-No Measure Associated)**
0.00 0.00 **FUD** XXX M

9004F **Aortic aneurysm 6.0 cm or greater maximum diameter on centerline formatted CT or minor diameter on axial formatted CT (NMA-No Measure Associated)**
0.00 0.00 **FUD** XXX M

9005F **Asymptomatic carotid stenosis: No history of any transient ischemic attack or stroke in any carotid or vertebrobasilar territory (NMA-No Measure Associated)**
0.00 0.00 **FUD** XXX E

9006F **Symptomatic carotid stenosis: Ipsilateral carotid territory TIA or stroke less than 120 days prior to procedure (NMA-No Measure Associated)**
0.00 0.00 **FUD** XXX M

9007F **Other carotid stenosis: Ipsilateral TIA or stroke 120 days or greater prior to procedure or any prior contralateral carotid territory or vertebrobasilar TIA or stroke (NMA-No Measure Associated)**
0.00 0.00 **FUD** XXX M

0042T

0042T Cerebral perfusion analysis using computed tomography with contrast administration, including post-processing of parametric maps with determination of cerebral blood flow, cerebral blood volume, and mean transit time

0.00 0.00 FUD XXX N 80

AMA: 2003,Nov,5

0054T-0055T

+ **0054T Computer-assisted musculoskeletal surgical navigational orthopedic procedure, with image-guidance based on fluoroscopic images (List separately in addition to code for primary procedure)**

Code first primary procedure

0.00 0.00 FUD XXX N 80

AMA: 2018,Jan,8; 2017,Jan,8; 2016,Jan,13; 2015,Jan,16

+ **0055T Computer-assisted musculoskeletal surgical navigational orthopedic procedure, with image-guidance based on CT/MRI images (List separately in addition to code for primary procedure)**

INCLUDES Performance both CT and MRI in same session (one unit)

Code first primary procedure

0.00 0.00 FUD XXX N 80

AMA: 2018,Jan,8; 2017,Jan,8; 2016,Jan,13; 2015,Jan,16

0058T

EXCLUDES *Cryopreservation:*
- *Embryos (89258)*
- *Oocyte(s), immature (89398)*
- *Oocyte(s), mature (89337)*
- *Sperm (89259)*
- *Testicular reproductive tissue (89335)*

~~0058T~~ **~~Cryopreservation; reproductive tissue, ovarian~~**

To report, see (89398)

0071T-0072T

EXCLUDES *Insertion bladder catheter (51702)*
MRI guidance for parenchymal tissue ablation (77022)

0071T Focused ultrasound ablation of uterine leiomyomata, including MR guidance; total leiomyomata volume less than 200 cc of tissue ♀

0.00 0.00 FUD XXX J 80

AMA: 2005,Mar,1-6; 2005,Dec,3-6

0072T total leiomyomata volume greater or equal to 200 cc of tissue ♀

0.00 0.00 FUD XXX J 80

AMA: 2005,Mar,1-6; 2005,Dec,3-6

0075T-0076T

INCLUDES All diagnostic services for stenting
Ipsilateral extracranial vertebral selective catheterization when confirming need for stenting

EXCLUDES *Selective catheterization and imaging when stenting not required (report only selective catheterization codes)*

0075T Transcatheter placement of extracranial vertebral artery stent(s), including radiologic supervision and interpretation, open or percutaneous; initial vessel

0.00 0.00 FUD XXX C 80

AMA: 2018,Jan,8; 2017,Jan,8; 2016,Jan,13; 2015,Jan,16

+ **0076T each additional vessel (List separately in addition to code for primary procedure)**

Code first (0075T)

0.00 0.00 FUD XXX C 80

AMA: 2018,Jan,8; 2017,Jan,8; 2016,Jan,13; 2015,Jan,16

0085T

~~0085T~~ **~~Breath test for heart transplant rejection~~**

To report, see (84999)

0095T-0098T

INCLUDES Fluoroscopy

+ **0095T Removal of total disc arthroplasty (artificial disc), anterior approach, each additional interspace, cervical (List separately in addition to code for primary procedure)**

EXCLUDES *Lumbar disc (0164T)*
Revision total disc arthroplasty, cervical (22861)
Revision total disc arthroplasty, lumbar (22862)

Code first (22864)

0.00 0.00 FUD XXX C 80

AMA: 2006,Feb,1-6; 2005,Jun,6-8

+ **0098T Revision including replacement of total disc arthroplasty (artificial disc), anterior approach, each additional interspace, cervical (List separately in addition to code for primary procedure)**

EXCLUDES *Application intervertebral biomechanical device(s) at same level (22853-22854, [22859])*
Removal total disc arthroplasty (0095T)
Spinal cord decompression (63001-63048)

Code first (22861)

0.00 0.00 FUD XXX C 80

AMA: 2006,Feb,1-6; 2005,Jun,6-8

0100T

0100T Placement of a subconjunctival retinal prosthesis receiver and pulse generator, and implantation of intra-ocular retinal electrode array, with vitrectomy

EXCLUDES *Evaluation and initial programming implantable retinal electrode array device (0472T)*

0.00 0.00 FUD XXX T J8 80

AMA: 2018,Feb,3; 2018,Jan,8; 2017,Jan,8; 2016,Jan,13; 2015,Jan,16

0101T-0513T [0512T, 0513T]

0101T Extracorporeal shock wave involving musculoskeletal system, not otherwise specified, high energy

EXCLUDES *Extracorporeal shock wave therapy integumentary system not otherwise specified ([0512T, 0513T])*

0.00 0.00 FUD XXX J G2 80

AMA: 2018,Dec,5; 2018,Dec,5; 2018,Jan,8; 2017,Jan,8; 2016,Jan,13; 2015,Jan,16

0102T Extracorporeal shock wave, high energy, performed by a physician, requiring anesthesia other than local, involving lateral humeral epicondyle

0.00 0.00 FUD XXX J G2 80

AMA: 2019,Jun,11; 2018,Dec,5; 2018,Dec,5; 2018,Jan,8; 2017,Jan,8; 2016,Jan,13; 2015,Jan,16

0512T Extracorporeal shock wave for integumentary wound healing, high energy, including topical application and dressing care; initial wound

0.00 0.00 FUD YYY R2 80

AMA: 2018,Dec,5; 2018,Dec,5

+ # **0513T each additional wound (List separately in addition to code for primary procedure)**

Code first ([0512T])

0.00 0.00 FUD ZZZ N1 80

AMA: 2018,Dec,5; 2018,Dec,5

0106T-0110T

0106T Quantitative sensory testing (QST), testing and interpretation per extremity; using touch pressure stimuli to assess large diameter sensation

0.00 0.00 FUD XXX Q1 80

AMA: 2018,Jan,8; 2017,Jan,8; 2016,Jan,13; 2015,Jan,16

0107T using vibration stimuli to assess large diameter fiber sensation

0.00 0.00 FUD XXX Q1 80

AMA: 2018,Jan,8; 2017,Jan,8; 2016,Jan,13; 2015,Jan,16

0108T **using cooling stimuli to assess small nerve fiber sensation and hyperalgesia**
0.00 0.00 FUD XXX Q1 80
AMA: 2018,Jan,8; 2017,Jan,8; 2016,Jan,13; 2015,Jan,16

0109T **using heat-pain stimuli to assess small nerve fiber sensation and hyperalgesia**
0.00 0.00 FUD XXX Q1 80
AMA: 2018,Jan,8; 2017,Jan,8; 2016,Jan,13; 2015,Jan,16

0110T **using other stimuli to assess sensation**
0.00 0.00 FUD XXX Q1 80
AMA: 2018,Jan,8; 2017,Jan,8; 2016,Jan,13; 2015,Jan,16

0111T-0126T

~~0111T~~ ~~**Long-chain (C20-22) omega-3 fatty acids in red blood cell (RBC) membranes**~~
To report, see (82726)

~~0126T~~ ~~**Common carotid intima-media thickness (IMT) study for evaluation of atherosclerotic burden or coronary heart disease risk factor assessment**~~
To report, see (93998)

0163T-0165T

CMS: 100-03,150.10 Lumbar Artificial Disc Replacement (LADR)

INCLUDES Fluoroscopy

EXCLUDES *Application intervertebral biomechanical device(s) at same level (22853-22854, [22859])*
Cervical disc procedures (22856)
Decompression (63001-63048)
Exploration retroperitoneal area at same level (49010)

\+ 0163T **Total disc arthroplasty (artificial disc), anterior approach, including discectomy to prepare interspace (other than for decompression), each additional interspace, lumbar (List separately in addition to code for primary procedure)**
Code first (22857)
0.00 0.00 FUD YYY C 80
AMA: 2018,Jan,8; 2017,Jan,8; 2016,Jan,13; 2015,Jan,16

\+ 0164T **Removal of total disc arthroplasty, (artificial disc), anterior approach, each additional interspace, lumbar (List separately in addition to code for primary procedure)**
Code first (22865)
0.00 0.00 FUD YYY C 80
AMA: 2018,Jan,8; 2017,Jan,8; 2016,Jan,13; 2015,Jan,16

\+ 0165T **Revision including replacement of total disc arthroplasty (artificial disc), anterior approach, each additional interspace, lumbar (List separately in addition to code for primary procedure)**
Code first (22862)
0.00 0.00 FUD YYY C 80
AMA: 2018,Jan,8; 2017,Jan,8; 2016,Jan,13; 2015,Jan,16

0174T-0175T

\+ 0174T **Computer-aided detection (CAD) (computer algorithm analysis of digital image data for lesion detection) with further physician review for interpretation and report, with or without digitization of film radiographic images, chest radiograph(s), performed concurrent with primary interpretation (List separately in addition to code for primary procedure)**
Code first (71045-71048)
0.00 0.00 FUD XXX N 80
AMA: 2018,Apr,7

0175T **Computer-aided detection (CAD) (computer algorithm analysis of digital image data for lesion detection) with further physician review for interpretation and report, with or without digitization of film radiographic images, chest radiograph(s), performed remote from primary interpretation**
INCLUDES Chest x-rays (71045-71048)
0.00 0.00 FUD XXX N 80
AMA: 2018,Apr,7

0184T

0184T **Excision of rectal tumor, transanal endoscopic microsurgical approach (ie, TEMS), including muscularis propria (ie, full thickness)**
INCLUDES Operating microscope (66990)
Proctosigmoidoscopy (45300, 45308-45309, 45315, 45317, 45320)
EXCLUDES *Nonendoscopic excision rectal tumor (45160, 45171-45172)*
0.00 0.00 FUD XXX J 80
AMA: 2018,Feb,11; 2018,Jan,8; 2017,Jan,8; 2016,Feb,12; 2016,Jan,13; 2015,Jan,16

0191T-0253T [0253T, 0376T]

0191T **Insertion of anterior segment aqueous drainage device, without extraocular reservoir, internal approach, into the trabecular meshwork; initial insertion**
0.00 0.00 FUD XXX J J8 80
AMA: 2018,Jul,3; 2018,Feb,3; 2018,Jan,8; 2017,Jan,8; 2016,Jan,13; 2015,Jan,16

\+ # 0376T **each additional device insertion (List separately in addition to code for primary procedure)**
Code first (0191T)
0.00 0.00 FUD XXX N N1 80
AMA: 2018,Jul,3; 2018,Feb,3

\# 0253T **Insertion of anterior segment aqueous drainage device, without extraocular reservoir, internal approach, into the suprachoroidal space**
EXCLUDES *Insertion aqueous drainage device, external approach (66183)*
0.00 0.00 FUD YYY J J8 80
AMA: 2018,Jul,3

0198T

0198T **Measurement of ocular blood flow by repetitive intraocular pressure sampling, with interpretation and report**
0.00 0.00 FUD XXX Q1 80
AMA: 2018,Jan,8; 2017,Jan,8; 2016,Jan,13; 2015,Jan,16

0200T-0201T

INCLUDES Deep bone biopsy (20225)

0200T **Percutaneous sacral augmentation (sacroplasty), unilateral injection(s), including the use of a balloon or mechanical device, when used, 1 or more needles, includes imaging guidance and bone biopsy, when performed**
0.00 0.00 FUD XXX J J8 80 50
AMA: 2018,Jan,8; 2017,Jan,8; 2016,Jan,13; 2015,Dec,18; 2015,Apr,8; 2015,Jan,8

0201T **Percutaneous sacral augmentation (sacroplasty), bilateral injections, including the use of a balloon or mechanical device, when used, 2 or more needles, includes imaging guidance and bone biopsy, when performed**
0.00 0.00 FUD XXX J G2 80
AMA: 2018,Jan,8; 2017,Jan,8; 2016,Jan,13; 2015,Dec,18; 2015,Apr,8; 2015,Jan,8

0202T-0563T [0563T]

0202T **Posterior vertebral joint(s) arthroplasty (eg, facet joint[s] replacement), including facetectomy, laminectomy, foraminotomy, and vertebral column fixation, injection of bone cement, when performed, including fluoroscopy, single level, lumbar spine**
INCLUDES Instrumentation (22840, 22853-22854, [22859])
Laminectomy (63005, 63012, 63017, 63047)
Laminotomy (63030, 63042)
Lumbar arthroplasty (22857)
Percutaneous lumbar vertebral augmentation (22514)
Percutaneous vertebroplasty (22511)
Spinal cord decompression (63056)
0.00 0.00 FUD XXX C 80

0207T **Evacuation of meibomian glands, automated, using heat and intermittent pressure, unilateral**

EXCLUDES *Evacuation using:*
Heat through wearable device ([0563T])
Manual expression only, report appropriate E/M code

0.00 0.00 FUD XXX 01 80

AMA: 2018,Jan,8; 2017,Jan,8; 2016,Jan,13; 2015,Jan,16

0563T **Evacuation of meibomian glands, using heat delivered through wearable, open-eye eyelid treatment devices and manual gland expression, bilateral**

EXCLUDES *Evacuation using:*
Heat and intermittent pressure (0207T)
Manual expression only, report appropriate E/M code

0.00 0.00 FUD YYY 80

0208T-0212T

EXCLUDES *Manual audiometric testing by qualified health care professional, using audiometers (92551-92557)*

0208T **Pure tone audiometry (threshold), automated; air only**

0.00 0.00 FUD XXX 01 80 TC

AMA: 2018,Jan,8; 2017,Jan,8; 2016,Jan,13; 2015,Jan,16

0209T **air and bone**

0.00 0.00 FUD XXX 01 80 TC

AMA: 2018,Jan,8; 2017,Jan,8; 2016,Jan,13; 2015,Jan,16

0210T **Speech audiometry threshold, automated;**

0.00 0.00 FUD XXX 01 80 TC

AMA: 2014,Aug,3

0211T **with speech recognition**

0.00 0.00 FUD XXX 01 80 TC

AMA: 2018,Jan,8; 2017,Jan,8; 2016,Jan,13; 2015,Jan,16

0212T **Comprehensive audiometry threshold evaluation and speech recognition (0209T, 0211T combined), automated**

0.00 0.00 FUD XXX 01 80 TC

AMA: 2018,Jan,8; 2017,Jan,8; 2016,Jan,13; 2015,Jan,16

0213T-0215T

INCLUDES Ultrasound guidance (76942)

0213T **Injection(s), diagnostic or therapeutic agent, paravertebral facet (zygapophyseal) joint (or nerves innervating that joint) with ultrasound guidance, cervical or thoracic; single level**

0.00 0.00 FUD XXX T R2 80 50

AMA: 2018,Jan,8; 2017,Jan,8; 2016,Jan,13; 2015,Jan,16

+ 0214T **second level (List separately in addition to code for primary procedure)**

EXCLUDES *Reporting with modifier 50. Report once for each side when performed bilaterally*

Code first (0213T)

0.00 0.00 FUD ZZZ N N1 80 50

AMA: 2018,Jan,8; 2017,Jan,8; 2016,Jan,13; 2015,Jan,16

+ 0215T **third and any additional level(s) (List separately in addition to code for primary procedure)**

EXCLUDES *Reporting code more than one time per service date*
Reporting with modifier 50. Report once for each side when performed bilaterally

Code first (0213T-0214T)

0.00 0.00 FUD ZZZ N N1 80 50

AMA: 2018,Jan,8; 2017,Jan,8; 2016,Jan,13; 2015,Jan,16

0216T-0218T

INCLUDES Ultrasound guidance (76942)

EXCLUDES *Injection with CT or fluoroscopic guidance (64490-64495)*

0216T **Injection(s), diagnostic or therapeutic agent, paravertebral facet (zygapophyseal) joint (or nerves innervating that joint) with ultrasound guidance, lumbar or sacral; single level**

0.00 0.00 FUD XXX T R2 80 50

AMA: 2018,Jan,8; 2017,Jan,8; 2016,Jan,13; 2015,Jan,16

+ 0217T **second level (List separately in addition to code for primary procedure)**

EXCLUDES *Reporting with modifier 50. Report once for each side when performed bilaterally*

Code first (0216T)

0.00 0.00 FUD ZZZ N N1 80 50

AMA: 2018,Jan,8; 2017,Jan,8; 2016,Jan,13; 2015,Jan,16

+ 0218T **third and any additional level(s) (List separately in addition to code for primary procedure)**

EXCLUDES *Reporting code more than one time per service date*
Reporting with modifier 50. Report once for each side when performed bilaterally

Code first (0216T-0217T)

0.00 0.00 FUD ZZZ N N1 80 50

AMA: 2018,Jan,8; 2017,Jan,8; 2016,Jan,13; 2015,Jan,16

0219T-0222T

INCLUDES Allografts at same level (20930-20931)
Application intervertebral biomechanical device(s) at same level (22853-22854, [22859])
Arthrodesis at same level (22600-22614)
Instrumentation at same level (22840)
Radiologic services

0219T **Placement of a posterior intrafacet implant(s), unilateral or bilateral, including imaging and placement of bone graft(s) or synthetic device(s), single level; cervical**

0.00 0.00 FUD XXX C 80

AMA: 2018,Jan,8; 2017,Jan,8; 2016,Jan,13; 2015,Jan,16

0220T **thoracic**

0.00 0.00 FUD XXX C 80

AMA: 2018,Jan,8; 2017,Jan,8; 2016,Jan,13; 2015,Jan,16

0221T **lumbar**

0.00 0.00 FUD XXX J 80

AMA: 2018,Jan,8; 2017,Jan,8; 2016,Jan,13; 2015,Jan,16

+ 0222T **each additional vertebral segment (List separately in addition to code for primary procedure)**

Code first (0219T-0221T)

0.00 0.00 FUD ZZZ N 80

AMA: 2018,Jan,8; 2017,Jan,8; 2016,Jan,13; 2015,Jan,16

0228T-0231T

~~0228T~~ ~~**Injection(s), anesthetic agent and/or steroid, transforaminal epidural, with ultrasound guidance, cervical or thoracic; single level**~~

To report, see (64999)

~~0229T~~ ~~**each additional level (List separately in addition to code for primary procedure)**~~

To report, see (64999)

~~0230T~~ ~~**Injection(s), anesthetic agent and/or steroid, transforaminal epidural, with ultrasound guidance, lumbar or sacral; single level**~~

To report, see (64999)

~~0231T~~ ~~**each additional level (List separately in addition to code for primary procedure)**~~

To report, see (64999)

0232T

INCLUDES Arthrocentesis (20600-20611)
Blood collection (36415, 36592)
Fat and other soft tissue grafts ([15769], 15771-15774)
Imaging guidance (76942, 77002, 77012, 77021)
Injections (20550-20551)
Platelet/blood product pooling (86965)

EXCLUDES *Aspiration bone marrow for grafting, biopsy, harvesting for transplant (38220-38221, 38230)*
Injections white cell concentrate (0481T)

0232T **Injection(s), platelet rich plasma, any site, including image guidance, harvesting and preparation when performed**

0.00 0.00 FUD XXX 01 N1

AMA: 2019,Oct,5; 2019,Apr,10; 2018,May,3; 2018,Jan,8; 2017,Jan,8; 2016,Jan,13; 2015,Jan,16

0234T-0253T [0253T]

INCLUDES Atherectomy by any technique in arteries above inguinal ligaments
Radiology supervision and interpretation

EXCLUDES *Accessing and catheterization vessel*
Atherectomy performed below inguinal ligaments (37225, 37227, 37229, 37231, 37233, 37235)
Closure arteriotomy by any technique
Negotiating lesion
Other interventions to same or different vessels
Protection from embolism

0234T Transluminal peripheral atherectomy, open or percutaneous, including radiological supervision and interpretation; renal artery
0.00 0.00 FUD YYY J 80
AMA: 2018,Jan,8; 2017,Jan,8; 2016,Jan,13; 2015,Jan,16

0235T visceral artery (except renal), each vessel
0.00 0.00 FUD YYY C 80
AMA: 2018,Jan,8; 2017,Jan,8; 2016,Jan,13; 2015,Jan,16

0236T abdominal aorta
0.00 0.00 FUD YYY J 80
AMA: 2018,Jan,8; 2017,Jan,8; 2016,Jan,13; 2015,Jan,16

0237T brachiocephalic trunk and branches, each vessel
0.00 0.00 FUD YYY J 80
AMA: 2018,Jan,8; 2017,Jan,8; 2016,Jan,13; 2015,Jan,16

0238T iliac artery, each vessel
0.00 0.00 FUD YYY J J8 80
AMA: 2018,Jan,8; 2017,Jan,8; 2016,Jan,13; 2015,Jan,16

0253T **Resequenced code. See code before 0198T.**

0263T-0265T

EXCLUDES *Bone marrow and stem cell services (38204-38242 [38243])*

0263T Intramuscular autologous bone marrow cell therapy, with preparation of harvested cells, multiple injections, one leg, including ultrasound guidance, if performed; complete procedure including unilateral or bilateral bone marrow harvest
INCLUDES Duplex scan (93925-93926)
Ultrasound guidance (76942)
0.00 0.00 FUD XXX S G2 80

0264T complete procedure excluding bone marrow harvest
INCLUDES Bone marrow harvest only (0265T)
Duplex scan (93925-93926)
Ultrasound guidance (76942)
0.00 0.00 FUD XXX S G2 80

0265T unilateral or bilateral bone marrow harvest only for intramuscular autologous bone marrow cell therapy
EXCLUDES *Complete procedure (0263T-0264T)*
0.00 0.00 FUD XXX S G2 80

0266T-0273T

0266T Implantation or replacement of carotid sinus baroreflex activation device; total system (includes generator placement, unilateral or bilateral lead placement, intra-operative interrogation, programming, and repositioning, when performed)
INCLUDES Components complete procedure (0267T-0268T)
0.00 0.00 FUD YYY C 80

0267T lead only, unilateral (includes intra-operative interrogation, programming, and repositioning, when performed)
EXCLUDES *Complete procedure (0266T)*
Device interrogation (0272T-0273T)
Removal/revision device or components (0269T-0271T)
0.00 0.00 FUD YYY T 80

0268T pulse generator only (includes intra-operative interrogation, programming, and repositioning, when performed)
EXCLUDES *Complete procedure (0266T)*
Device interrogation (0272T-0273T)
Removal/revision device or components (0269T-0271T)
0.00 0.00 FUD YYY J 80

0269T Revision or removal of carotid sinus baroreflex activation device; total system (includes generator placement, unilateral or bilateral lead placement, intra-operative interrogation, programming, and repositioning, when performed)
EXCLUDES *Device interrogation (0272T-0273T)*
Implantation/replacement device and/or components (0266T-0268T)
Removal/revision device or components (0270T-0271T)
0.00 0.00 FUD XXX 02 G2 80

0270T lead only, unilateral (includes intra-operative interrogation, programming, and repositioning, when performed)
EXCLUDES *Device interrogation (0272T-0273T)*
Implantation/replacement device and/or components (0266T-0269T)
Removal/revision device or components (0271T)
0.00 0.00 FUD XXX 02 G2 80

0271T pulse generator only (includes intra-operative interrogation, programming, and repositioning, when performed)
EXCLUDES *Device interrogation (0272T-0273T)*
Implantation/replacement device and/or components (0266T-0268T)
Removal/revision device or components (0271T-0273T)
0.00 0.00 FUD XXX 02 G2 80

0272T Interrogation device evaluation (in person), carotid sinus baroreflex activation system, including telemetric iterative communication with the implantable device to monitor device diagnostics and programmed therapy values, with interpretation and report (eg, battery status, lead impedance, pulse amplitude, pulse width, therapy frequency, pathway mode, burst mode, therapy start/stop times each day);
EXCLUDES *Device interrogation (0273T)*
Implantation/replacement device and/or components (0266T-0268T)
Removal/revision device or components (0269T-0271T)
0.00 0.00 FUD XXX S 80

0273T with programming
EXCLUDES *Device interrogation (0272T)*
Implantation/replacement device and/or components (0266T-0268T)
Removal/revision device or components (0269T-0271T)
0.00 0.00 FUD XXX S 80

0274T-0275T

EXCLUDES *Laminotomy/hemilaminectomy by open and endoscopically assisted approach (63020-63035)*
Percutaneous decompression nucleus pulposus intervertebral disc by needle-based technique (62287)

0274T Percutaneous laminotomy/laminectomy (interlaminar approach) for decompression of neural elements, (with or without ligamentous resection, discectomy, facetectomy and/or foraminotomy), any method, under indirect image guidance (eg, fluoroscopic, CT), single or multiple levels, unilateral or bilateral; cervical or thoracic
0.00 0.00 FUD YYY J G2 80
AMA: 2018,Jan,8; 2017,Feb,12; 2017,Jan,8; 2016,Jan,13; 2015,Jan,16

0275T lumbar
0.00 0.00 FUD YYY J G2 80
AMA: 2018,Jan,8; 2017,Feb,12; 2017,Jan,8; 2016,Jan,13; 2015,Jan,16

0278T

0278T Transcutaneous electrical modulation pain reprocessing (eg, scrambler therapy), each treatment session (includes placement of electrodes)
0.00 0.00 **FUD** XXX Q1 N1 80

0290T

\+ **0290T Corneal incisions in the recipient cornea created using a laser, in preparation for penetrating or lamellar keratoplasty (List separately in addition to code for primary procedure)**
Code first (65710, 65730, 65750, 65755)
0.00 0.00 **FUD** ZZZ N N1 80
AMA: 2018,Jan,8; 2017,Jan,8; 2016,Jan,13; 2015,Jan,16

0295T-0298T

~~**0295T External electrocardiographic recording for more than 48 hours up to 21 days by continuous rhythm recording and storage; includes recording, scanning analysis with report, review and interpretation**~~
To report, see ([93241, 93242, 93243, 93244, 93245, 93246, 93247, 93248])

~~**0296T recording (includes connection and initial recording)**~~
To report, see ([93241, 93242, 93243, 93244, 93245, 93246, 93247, 93248])

~~**0297T scanning analysis with report**~~
To report, see ([93241, 93242, 93243, 93244, 93245, 93246, 93247, 93248])

~~**0298T review and interpretation**~~
To report, see ([93241, 93242, 93243, 93244, 93245, 93246, 93247, 93248])

0308T

0308T Insertion of ocular telescope prosthesis including removal of crystalline lens or intraocular lens prosthesis
INCLUDES Injection procedures (66020, 66030)
Iridectomy when performed (66600-66635, 66761)
Operating microscope (69990)
Repositioning intraocular lens (66825)
EXCLUDES *Cataract extraction (66982-66986)*
0.00 0.00 **FUD** YYY J J8 50
AMA: 2019,Dec,6; 2018,Jan,8; 2017,Jan,8; 2016,Jan,13; 2015,Jan,16

0312T-0317T

EXCLUDES *Analysis and/or programming (or reprogramming) vagus nerve stimulator (95970, 95976-95977)*
Implantation, replacement, removal, and/or revision vagus nerve neurostimulator (electrode array and/or pulse generator) for stimulation vagus nerve other than at esophagogastric junction (64568-64570)

0312T Vagus nerve blocking therapy (morbid obesity); laparoscopic implantation of neurostimulator electrode array, anterior and posterior vagal trunks adjacent to esophagogastric junction (EGJ), with implantation of pulse generator, includes programming
0.00 0.00 **FUD** XXX J 80
AMA: 2018,Jan,8; 2017,Jan,8; 2016,Jan,13; 2015,Jan,16

0313T laparoscopic revision or replacement of vagal trunk neurostimulator electrode array, including connection to existing pulse generator
0.00 0.00 **FUD** XXX T J8 80
AMA: 2018,Jan,8; 2017,Jan,8; 2016,Jan,13; 2015,Jan,16

0314T laparoscopic removal of vagal trunk neurostimulator electrode array and pulse generator
0.00 0.00 **FUD** XXX Q2 G2 80
AMA: 2018,Jan,8; 2017,Jan,8; 2016,Jan,13; 2015,Jan,16

0315T removal of pulse generator
EXCLUDES *Removal with replacement pulse generator (0316T)*
0.00 0.00 **FUD** XXX Q2 G2 80
AMA: 2018,Jan,8; 2017,Jan,8; 2016,Jan,13; 2015,Jan,16

0316T replacement of pulse generator
EXCLUDES *Removal without replacement pulse generator (0315T)*
0.00 0.00 **FUD** XXX J J8 80
AMA: 2018,Jan,8; 2017,Jan,8; 2016,Jan,13; 2015,Jan,16

0317T neurostimulator pulse generator electronic analysis, includes reprogramming when performed
EXCLUDES *Analysis and/or programming (or reprogramming) vagus nerve stimulator (95970, 95976-95977)*
0.00 0.00 **FUD** XXX Q1 80
AMA: 2018,Jan,8; 2017,Jan,8; 2016,Jan,13; 2015,Jan,16

0329T-0330T

0329T Monitoring of intraocular pressure for 24 hours or longer, unilateral or bilateral, with interpretation and report
0.00 0.00 **FUD** YYY E
AMA: 2018,Jan,8; 2017,Jan,8; 2016,Jan,13; 2015,Jan,16

0330T Tear film imaging, unilateral or bilateral, with interpretation and report
0.00 0.00 **FUD** YYY Q1 N1
AMA: 2018,Jan,8; 2017,Jan,8; 2016,Jan,13; 2015,Jan,16

0331T-0332T

EXCLUDES *Myocardial infarction avid imaging (78466, 78468, 78469)*

0331T Myocardial sympathetic innervation imaging, planar qualitative and quantitative assessment;
0.00 0.00 **FUD** YYY S Z2
AMA: 2018,Jan,8; 2017,Jan,8; 2016,Jan,13; 2015,Jan,16

0332T with tomographic SPECT
0.00 0.00 **FUD** YYY S Z2
AMA: 2018,Jan,8; 2017,Jan,8; 2016,Jan,13; 2015,Jan,16

0333T-0464T [0464T]

0333T Visual evoked potential, screening of visual acuity, automated, with report
EXCLUDES *Visual evoked potential testing for glaucoma ([0464T])*
0.00 0.00 **FUD** YYY E
AMA: 2018,Feb,3; 2018,Jan,8; 2017,Jan,8; 2016,Jan,13; 2015,Jan,16

\# **0464T Visual evoked potential, testing for glaucoma, with interpretation and report**
EXCLUDES *Visual evoked potential for visual acuity (0333T)*
0.00 0.00 **FUD** YYY S
AMA: 2018,Feb,3

0335T-0511T [0510T, 0511T]

0335T Insertion of sinus tarsi implant
EXCLUDES *Arthroscopic subtalar arthrodesis (29907)*
Open talotarsal joint dislocation repair (28585)
Subtalar arthrodesis (28725)
0.00 0.00 **FUD** YYY J J8

\# **0510T Removal of sinus tarsi implant**
0.00 0.00 **FUD** YYY G2 50

\# **0511T Removal and reinsertion of sinus tarsi implant**
0.00 0.00 **FUD** YYY J8 50

0338T-0339T

INCLUDES Selective catheter placement renal arteries (36251-36254)

0338T Transcatheter renal sympathetic denervation, percutaneous approach including arterial puncture, selective catheter placement(s) renal artery(ies), fluoroscopy, contrast injection(s), intraprocedural roadmapping and radiological supervision and interpretation, including pressure gradient measurements, flush aortogram and diagnostic renal angiography when performed; unilateral
0.00 0.00 **FUD** YYY J G2

0339T bilateral
0.00 0.00 **FUD** YYY J G2

0342T

0342T Therapeutic apheresis with selective HDL delipidation and plasma reinfusion
0.00 0.00 FUD YYY S G2

0345T

0345T Transcatheter mitral valve repair percutaneous approach via the coronary sinus
INCLUDES Coronary angiography (93563-93564)
EXCLUDES *Diagnostic cardiac catheterization procedures integral to valve procedure (93451-93461, 93530-93533, 93563-93564)*
Repair mitral valve including transseptal puncture (33418-33419)
Transcatheter implantation/replacement mitral valve (TMVI) (0483T-0484T)
Transcatheter mitral valve annulus reconstruction (0544T)
Code also transvascular ventricular support, when performed:
Balloon pump insertion (33967, 33970, 33973)
Ventricular assist device ([33995], 33990-33993, [33997])
0.00 0.00 FUD YYY C
AMA: 2018,Jan,8; 2017,Jan,8; 2016,Jan,13; 2015,Sep,3

0347T

0347T Placement of interstitial device(s) in bone for radiostereometric analysis (RSA)
0.00 0.00 FUD YYY Q1 N1
AMA: 2018,Jan,8; 2017,Jan,8; 2016,Jan,13; 2015,Jun,8

0348T-0350T

0348T Radiologic examination, radiostereometric analysis (RSA); spine, (includes cervical, thoracic and lumbosacral, when performed)
0.00 0.00 FUD YYY Q1 N1
AMA: 2018,Jan,8; 2017,Jan,8; 2016,Jan,13; 2015,Jun,8

0349T upper extremity(ies), (includes shoulder, elbow, and wrist, when performed)
0.00 0.00 FUD YYY Q1 N1
AMA: 2018,Jan,8; 2017,Jan,8; 2016,Jan,13; 2015,Jun,8

0350T lower extremity(ies), (includes hip, proximal femur, knee, and ankle, when performed)
0.00 0.00 FUD YYY Q1 N1
AMA: 2018,Jan,8; 2017,Jan,8; 2016,Jan,13; 2015,Jun,8

0351T-0354T

0351T Optical coherence tomography of breast or axillary lymph node, excised tissue, each specimen; real-time intraoperative
INCLUDES Interpretation and report (0352T)
0.00 0.00 FUD YYY N N1
AMA: 2018,Jan,8; 2017,Jan,8; 2016,Jan,13; 2015,Apr,6

0352T interpretation and report, real-time or referred
INCLUDES Interpretation and report (0351T)
0.00 0.00 FUD YYY B
AMA: 2018,Jan,8; 2017,Jan,8; 2016,Jan,13; 2015,Apr,6

0353T Optical coherence tomography of breast, surgical cavity; real-time intraoperative
INCLUDES Interpretation and report (0354T)
EXCLUDES *Reporting code more than one time per session*
0.00 0.00 FUD YYY N N1
AMA: 2018,Jan,8; 2017,Jan,8; 2016,Jan,13; 2015,Apr,6

0354T interpretation and report, real time or referred
0.00 0.00 FUD YYY B
AMA: 2018,Jan,8; 2017,Jan,8; 2016,Jan,13; 2015,Apr,6

0355T-0358T

0355T Gastrointestinal tract imaging, intraluminal (eg, capsule endoscopy), colon, with interpretation and report
INCLUDES Distal ileum imaging when performed
EXCLUDES *Capsule endoscopy esophagus only (91111)*
Capsule endoscopy esophagus through ileum (91110)
0.00 0.00 FUD YYY J

0356T Insertion of drug-eluting implant (including punctal dilation and implant removal when performed) into lacrimal canaliculus, each
EXCLUDES *Drug-eluting ocular insert (0444T-0445T)*
0.00 0.00 FUD YYY Q1 N1
AMA: 2018,Jan,8; 2017,Aug,7

0358T Bioelectrical impedance analysis whole body composition assessment, with interpretation and report
0.00 0.00 FUD YYY Q1

0362T-0376T [0376T]

INCLUDES Only one technician time when more than one technician in attendance
Provided by physician/other qualified healthcare professional while on-site (immediately available during procedure), but does not need to be face-to-face
Provided in environment appropriate for patient
Provided to patients with destructive behaviors
EXCLUDES *Adaptive behavior services ([97153, 97154, 97155, 97156, 97157, 97158])*
Aphasia assessment (96105)
Behavioral/developmental screening/testing (96110-96113, [96127])
Behavior/health assessment (96156-96159 [96164, 96165, 96167, 96168, 96170, 96171])
Cognitive testing ([96125])
Neurobehavioral testing (96116-96121)
Psychiatric evaluations/psychotherapy/interactive complexity (90785-90899)
Psychological/neuropsychological evaluation/testing (96130-96146)

0362T Behavior identification supporting assessment, each 15 minutes of technicians' time face-to-face with a patient, requiring the following components: administration by the physician or other qualified health care professional who is on site; with the assistance of two or more technicians; for a patient who exhibits destructive behavior; completion in an environment that is customized to the patient's behavior.
INCLUDES Comprises:
Functional analysis and behavioral assessment
Procedures and instruments to assess functional impairment and behavior levels
Structured observation with data collection not including direct patient involvement
EXCLUDES *Conferences by medical team (99366-99368)*
Occupational therapy evaluation ([97165, 97166, 97167, 97168])
Speech evaluation (92521-92524)
Code also when performed on different days until behavioral and supporting assessments complete
0.00 0.00 FUD YYY S
AMA: 2018,Nov,3; 2018,Jan,8; 2017,Jan,8; 2016,Jan,13; 2015,Jan,16

0373T Adaptive behavior treatment with protocol modification, each 15 minutes of technicians' time face-to-face with a patient, requiring the following components: administration by the physician or other qualified health care professional who is on site; with the assistance of two or more technicians; for a patient who exhibits destructive behavior; completion in an environment that is customized to the patient's behavior.
0.00 0.00 FUD YYY S
AMA: 2018,Nov,3; 2018,Jan,8; 2017,Jan,8; 2016,Jan,13; 2015,Jan,16

0376T **Resequenced code. See code following 0191T.**

0378T-0379T

0378T **Visual field assessment, with concurrent real time data analysis and accessible data storage with patient initiated data transmitted to a remote surveillance center for up to 30 days; review and interpretation with report by a physician or other qualified health care professional**

0.00 0.00 FUD XXX B 80

AMA: 2018,Jan,8; 2017,Jan,8; 2016,Jan,13; 2015,Jan,10

0379T **technical support and patient instructions, surveillance, analysis and transmission of daily and emergent data reports as prescribed by a physician or other qualified health care professional**

0.00 0.00 FUD XXX Q1 N1 80

AMA: 2018,Jan,8; 2017,Jan,8; 2016,Jan,13; 2015,Jan,10

0381T-0386T

~~0381T~~ **~~External heart rate and 3-axis accelerometer data recording up to 14 days to assess changes in heart rate and to monitor motion analysis for the purposes of diagnosing nocturnal epilepsy seizure events; includes report, scanning analysis with report, review and interpretation by a physician or other qualified health care professional~~**

To report, see (95999)

~~0382T~~ **~~review and interpretation only~~**

To report, see (95999)

~~0383T~~ **~~External heart rate and 3-axis accelerometer data recording from 15 to 30 days to assess changes in heart rate and to monitor motion analysis for the purposes of diagnosing nocturnal epilepsy seizure events; includes report, scanning analysis with report, review and interpretation by a physician or other qualified health care professional~~**

To report, see (95999)

~~0384T~~ **~~review and interpretation only~~**

To report, see (95999)

~~0385T~~ **~~External heart rate and 3-axis accelerometer data recording more than 30 days to assess changes in heart rate and to monitor motion analysis for the purposes of diagnosing nocturnal epilepsy seizure events; includes report, scanning analysis with report, review and interpretation by a physician or other qualified health care professional~~**

To report, see (95999)

~~0386T~~ **~~review and interpretation only~~**

To report, see (95999)

0394T-0395T

EXCLUDES *Radiation oncology procedures (77261-77263, 77300, 77306-77307, 77316-77318, 77332-77334, 77336, 77427-77499, 77761-77772, 77778, 77789)*

0394T **High dose rate electronic brachytherapy, skin surface application, per fraction, includes basic dosimetry, when performed**

EXCLUDES *Superficial non-brachytherapy radiation (77401)*

0.00 0.00 FUD XXX S Z2 80

0395T **High dose rate electronic brachytherapy, interstitial or intracavitary treatment, per fraction, includes basic dosimetry, when performed**

EXCLUDES *High dose rate skin surface application (0394T)*

0.00 0.00 FUD XXX S Z2 80

0396T-0398T

~~0396T~~ **~~Intra-operative use of kinetic balance sensor for implant stability during knee replacement arthroplasty (List separately in addition to code for primary procedure)~~**

To report, see (27599)

+ **0397T** **Endoscopic retrograde cholangiopancreatography (ERCP), with optical endomicroscopy (List separately in addition to code for primary procedure)**

INCLUDES Optical endomicroscopic image(s) (88375)

EXCLUDES *Reporting code more than one time per operative session*

Code first (43260-43265, [43274], [43275], [43276], [43277], [43278])

0.00 0.00 FUD XXX N N1 80

0398T **Magnetic resonance image guided high intensity focused ultrasound (MRgFUS), stereotactic ablation lesion, intracranial for movement disorder including stereotactic navigation and frame placement when performed**

INCLUDES Application stereotactic headframe (61800)
Stereotactic computer-assisted navigation (61781)

0.00 0.00 FUD XXX S 80

0400T-0401T

~~0400T~~ **~~Multi-spectral digital skin lesion analysis of clinically atypical cutaneous pigmented lesions for detection of melanomas and high risk melanocytic atypia; one to five lesions~~**

To report, see (96999)

~~0401T~~ **~~six or more lesions~~**

To report, see (96999)

0402T

0402T **Collagen cross-linking of cornea, including removal of the corneal epithelium and intraoperative pachymetry, when performed (Report medication separately)**

INCLUDES Corneal epithelium removal (65435)
Corneal pachymetry (76514)
Operating microscope (69990)

0.00 0.00 FUD XXX J R2 80

AMA: 2018,Jun,11; 2018,Jan,8; 2017,Jan,8; 2016,Feb,12

0403T-0488T [0488T]

INCLUDES Intensive behavioral counseling by trained lifestyle coach
Standardized course with emphasis on weight, exercise, stress management, and nutrition

0403T **Preventive behavior change, intensive program of prevention of diabetes using a standardized diabetes prevention program curriculum, provided to individuals in a group setting, minimum 60 minutes, per day**

EXCLUDES *Online/electronic diabetes prevention program ([0488T])*
Self-management training and education by nonphysician health care professional (98960-98962)

0.00 0.00 FUD XXX E 80

AMA: 2020,Jul,7; 2018,Aug,6; 2015,Aug,4

0488T **Preventive behavior change, online/electronic structured intensive program for prevention of diabetes using a standardized diabetes prevention program curriculum, provided to an individual, per 30 days**

INCLUDES In person elements when appropriate

EXCLUDES *Group diabetes prevention program (0403T)*
Self-management training and education by nonphysician health care professional (98960-98962)

0.00 0.00 FUD XXX E

AMA: 2020,Jul,7; 2018,Aug,6

0404T-0405T

0404T **Transcervical uterine fibroid(s) ablation with ultrasound guidance, radiofrequency** ♀

0.00 0.00 FUD XXX J 80

~~0405T~~ **~~Oversight of the care of an extracorporeal liver assist system patient requiring review of status, review of laboratories and other studies, and revision of orders and liver assist care plan (as appropriate), within a calendar month, 30 minutes or more of non-face-to-face time~~**

To report, see (99499)

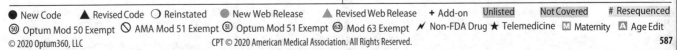

0408T-0418T

0408T Insertion or replacement of permanent cardiac contractility modulation system, including contractility evaluation when performed, and programming of sensing and therapeutic parameters; pulse generator with transvenous electrodes

INCLUDES Device evaluation (93286-93287, 0415T, 0417T-0418T)
Insertion or replacement entire system

EXCLUDES *Cardiac catheterization (93452-93453, 93456-93461)*

Code also removal each electrode when pulse generator and electrodes removed and replaced (0410T-0411T)

0.00 0.00 FUD XXX J J8 80

0409T pulse generator only

INCLUDES Device evaluation (93286-93287, 0415T, 0417T-0418T)

EXCLUDES *Cardiac catheterization (93452-93453, 93456-93461)*

0.00 0.00 FUD XXX J J8 80

0410T atrial electrode only

INCLUDES Device evaluation (93286-93287, 0415T, 0417T-0418T)
Each atrial electrode inserted or replaced

EXCLUDES *Cardiac catheterization (93452-93453, 93456-93461)*

0.00 0.00 FUD XXX J J8 80

0411T ventricular electrode only

INCLUDES Device evaluation (93286-93287, 0415T, 0417T-0418T)
Each ventricular electrode inserted or replaced

EXCLUDES *Cardiac catheterization (93452-93453, 93456-93461)*
Insertion or replacement complete CCM system (0408T)

0.00 0.00 FUD XXX J J8 80

0412T Removal of permanent cardiac contractility modulation system; pulse generator only

EXCLUDES *Device evaluation (0417T-0418T)*
Insertion or replacement complete CCM system (0408T)

0.00 0.00 FUD XXX Q2 G2 80

0413T transvenous electrode (atrial or ventricular)

INCLUDES Each electrode removed

EXCLUDES *Device evaluation (0417T-0418T)*
Insertion or replacement complete CCM system (0408T)

Code also removal and replacement electrode(s), as appropriate (0410T-0411T)

Code also removal pulse generator when leads also removed (0412T)

0.00 0.00 FUD XXX Q2 G2 80

0414T Removal and replacement of permanent cardiac contractility modulation system pulse generator only

INCLUDES Device evaluation (93286-93287, 0417T-0418T)

EXCLUDES *Cardiac catheterization (93452-93453, 93456-93461)*

Code also replacement pulse generator when leads also removed and replaced (0408T, 0412T-0413T)

0.00 0.00 FUD XXX J J8 80

0415T Repositioning of previously implanted cardiac contractility modulation transvenous electrode, (atrial or ventricular lead)

INCLUDES Device evaluation (93286-93287, 0417T-0418T)

EXCLUDES *Cardiac catheterization (93452-93453, 93456-93461)*
Insertion or replacement entire system or components (0408T-0411T)

0.00 0.00 FUD XXX T G2 80

0416T Relocation of skin pocket for implanted cardiac contractility modulation pulse generator

0.00 0.00 FUD XXX T G2 80

0417T Programming device evaluation (in person) with iterative adjustment of the implantable device to test the function of the device and select optimal permanent programmed values with analysis, including review and report, implantable cardiac contractility modulation system

EXCLUDES *Insertion/replacement/removal/repositioning device or components (0408T-0415T, 0418T)*

0.00 0.00 FUD XXX Q1 80

0418T Interrogation device evaluation (in person) with analysis, review and report, includes connection, recording and disconnection per patient encounter, implantable cardiac contractility modulation system

EXCLUDES *Insertion/replacement/removal/repositioning device or components (0408T-0415T, 0417T)*

0.00 0.00 FUD XXX Q1 80

0419T-0420T

EXCLUDES *Neurofibroma excision (64792)*
Reporting code more than one time per session

0419T Destruction of neurofibroma, extensive (cutaneous, dermal extending into subcutaneous); face, head and neck, greater than 50 neurofibromas

0.00 0.00 FUD XXX T R2 80

AMA: 2018,Jan,8; 2017,Jan,8; 2016,Apr,3

0420T trunk and extremities, extensive, greater than 100 neurofibromas

0.00 0.00 FUD XXX T R2 80

AMA: 2018,Jan,8; 2017,Jan,8; 2016,Apr,3

0421T-0423T

0421T Transurethral waterjet ablation of prostate, including control of post-operative bleeding, including ultrasound guidance, complete (vasectomy, meatotomy, cystourethroscopy, urethral calibration and/or dilation, and internal urethrotomy are included when performed) ♂

EXCLUDES *Transrectal ultrasound (76872)*
Transurethral prostate resection (52500, 52630)

0.00 0.00 FUD XXX J G2 80

AMA: 2020,Aug,6

0422T Tactile breast imaging by computer-aided tactile sensors, unilateral or bilateral

0.00 0.00 FUD XXX Q1 Z2 80

0423T Secretory type II phospholipase A2 (sPLA2-IIA)

EXCLUDES *Lipoprotein-associated phospholipase A2 [LpPLA2] (83698)*

0.00 0.00 FUD XXX A

0424T-0436T

INCLUDES Phrenic nerve stimulation system includes:
Pulse generator
Sensing lead (placed in azygos vein)
Stimulation lead (placed into right brachiocephalic vein or left pericardiophrenic vein)

0424T Insertion or replacement of neurostimulator system for treatment of central sleep apnea; complete system (transvenous placement of right or left stimulation lead, sensing lead, implantable pulse generator)

INCLUDES Device evaluation (0434T-0436T)
Insertion or replacement system components (0425T-0427T)
Repositioning leads (0432T-0433T)

Code also when pulse generator and all leads removed and replaced (0428T-0430T)

0.00 0.00 FUD XXX J J8 80

0425T sensing lead only

EXCLUDES *Device evaluation (0434T-0436T)*
Insertion/replacement complete system (0424T)
Repositioning leads (0432T-0433T)

0.00 0.00 FUD XXX J G2 80

0426T stimulation lead only

EXCLUDES *Device evaluation (0434T-0436T)*
Insertion/replacement complete system (0424T)
Repositioning leads (0432T-0433T)

0.00 0.00 FUD XXX J G2 80

0427T pulse generator only

EXCLUDES *Device evaluation (0434T-0436T)*
Insertion/replacement complete system (0424T)
Repositioning leads (0432T-0433T)

0.00 0.00 FUD XXX J G2 80

0428T **Removal of neurostimulator system for treatment of central sleep apnea; pulse generator only**

EXCLUDES *Device evaluation (0434T-0436T)*
Removal with replacement of pulse generator and all leads (0424T, 0429T-0430T)
Repositioning leads (0432T-0433T)

Code also when lead removed (0429T-0430T)

0.00 0.00 FUD XXX Q2 G2 80

0429T **sensing lead only**

INCLUDES Removal one sensing lead

EXCLUDES *Device evaluation (0434T-0436T)*

0.00 0.00 FUD XXX Q2 G2 80

0430T **stimulation lead only**

INCLUDES Removal one stimulation lead

EXCLUDES *Device evaluation (0434T-0436T)*

0.00 0.00 FUD XXX Q2 G2 80

AMA: 2015,Aug,4

0431T **Removal and replacement of neurostimulator system for treatment of central sleep apnea, pulse generator only**

EXCLUDES *Device evaluation (0434T-0436T)*
Removal with replacement generator and all three leads (0424T, 0428T-0430T)

0.00 0.00 FUD XXX J J8 80

0432T **Repositioning of neurostimulator system for treatment of central sleep apnea; stimulation lead only**

EXCLUDES *Device evaluation (0434T-0436T)*
Insertion/replacement complete system or components (0424T-0427T)

0.00 0.00 FUD XXX T G2 80

0433T **sensing lead only**

EXCLUDES *Device evaluation (0434T-0436T)*
Insertion/replacement complete system or components (0424T-0427T)

0.00 0.00 FUD XXX T G2 80

0434T **Interrogation device evaluation implanted neurostimulator pulse generator system for central sleep apnea**

EXCLUDES *Insertion/replacement complete system or components (0424T-0427T)*
Removal system or components (0428T-0431T)
Repositioning leads (0432T-0433T)

0.00 0.00 FUD XXX S G2 80

0435T **Programming device evaluation of implanted neurostimulator pulse generator system for central sleep apnea; single session**

EXCLUDES *Device evaluation (0436T)*
Insertion/replacement complete system or components (0424T-0427T)
Removal system or components (0428T-0431T)
Repositioning leads (0432T-0433T)

0.00 0.00 FUD XXX S 80

0436T **during sleep study**

EXCLUDES *Device evaluation (0435T)*
Insertion/replacement complete system or components (0424T-0427T)
Removal system or components (0428T-0431T)
Reporting code more than one time for each sleep study
Repositioning leads (0432T-0433T)

0.00 0.00 FUD XXX S 80

0437T-0439T

\+ 0437T **Implantation of non-biologic or synthetic implant (eg, polypropylene) for fascial reinforcement of the abdominal wall (List separately in addition to code for primary procedure)**

EXCLUDES *Implantation mesh, other material for repair incisional or ventral hernia (49560-49561, 49565-49566, 49568)*
Insertion mesh, other material for closure wound caused by necrotizing soft tissue infection (11004-11006, 49568)

0.00 0.00 FUD ZZZ N N1 80

\+ 0439T **Myocardial contrast perfusion echocardiography, at rest or with stress, for assessment of myocardial ischemia or viability (List separately in addition to code for primary procedure)**

Code first (93306-93308, 93350-93351)

0.00 0.00 FUD ZZZ N N1 80

AMA: 2018,Jan,8; 2017,Jan,8; 2016,Apr,8

0440T-0442T

0440T **Ablation, percutaneous, cryoablation, includes imaging guidance; upper extremity distal/peripheral nerve**

0.00 0.00 FUD YYY J G2 80

AMA: 2019,Apr,9; 2018,Jan,8

0441T **lower extremity distal/peripheral nerve**

0.00 0.00 FUD YYY J G2 80

AMA: 2019,Apr,9; 2018,Jan,8

0442T **nerve plexus or other truncal nerve (eg, brachial plexus, pudendal nerve)**

0.00 0.00 FUD YYY J J8 80

AMA: 2019,Apr,9; 2018,Jan,8

0443T

\+ 0443T **Real-time spectral analysis of prostate tissue by fluorescence spectroscopy, including imaging guidance (List separately in addition to code for primary procedure)** ♂

EXCLUDES *Reporting code more than one time for each session*

Code also (55700)

0.00 0.00 FUD ZZZ N N1 80

0444T-0445T

EXCLUDES *Insertion/removal drug-eluting stent into canaliculus (0356T)*

0444T **Initial placement of a drug-eluting ocular insert under one or more eyelids, including fitting, training, and insertion, unilateral or bilateral**

0.00 0.00 FUD YYY N N1 80

AMA: 2018,Jan,8; 2017,Aug,7

0445T **Subsequent placement of a drug-eluting ocular insert under one or more eyelids, including re-training, and removal of existing insert, unilateral or bilateral**

0.00 0.00 FUD YYY N N1 80

AMA: 2018,Jan,8; 2017,Aug,7

0446T-0448T

EXCLUDES *Placement non-implantable interstitial glucose sensor without pocket (95250)*

0446T **Creation of subcutaneous pocket with insertion of implantable interstitial glucose sensor, including system activation and patient training**

EXCLUDES *Interpretation/report ambulatory glucose monitoring interstitial tissue (95251)*
Removal interstitial glucose sensor (0447T-0448T)

0.00 0.00 FUD YYY T G2

AMA: 2018,Jun,6

0447T **Removal of implantable interstitial glucose sensor from subcutaneous pocket via incision**

0.00 0.00 FUD YYY Q2 G2

0448T **Removal of implantable interstitial glucose sensor with creation of subcutaneous pocket at different anatomic site and insertion of new implantable sensor, including system activation**

EXCLUDES *Initial insertion sensor (0446T)*
Removal sensor (0447T)

0.00 0.00 FUD YYY T G2

0449T-0450T

EXCLUDES *Removal by internal approach aqueous drainage device without extraocular reservoir in subconjunctival space (92499)*

0449T **Insertion of aqueous drainage device, without extraocular reservoir, internal approach, into the subconjunctival space; initial device**

0.00 0.00 FUD YYY J J8

AMA: 2018,Sep,3; 2018,Jul,3

\+ **0450T** **each additional device (List separately in addition to code for primary procedure)**

Code first (0449T)

0.00 0.00 FUD YYY N N1

AMA: 2018,Jul,3

0451T-0463T

INCLUDES Access procedures (36000-36010)
Catheterization vessel (36200-36228)
Diagnostic angiography (75600-75774)
Imaging guidance (76000, 76936-76937, 77001-77002, 77011-77012, 77021)
Injection procedures (93561-93572)
Radiological supervision and interpretation

EXCLUDES *Cardiac catheterization (93451-93533)*

0451T **Insertion or replacement of a permanently implantable aortic counterpulsation ventricular assist system, endovascular approach, and programming of sensing and therapeutic parameters; complete system (counterpulsation device, vascular graft, implantable vascular hemostatic seal, mechano-electrical skin interface and subcutaneous electrodes)**

EXCLUDES *Aortic counterpulsation ventricular assist system procedures (0452T-0458T)*
Insertion intra-aortic balloon assist device (33967, 33970, 33973)
Insertion/removal percutaneous ventricular assist device ([33995], 33990-33991, [33997])
Insertion/replacement extracorporeal ventricular assist device (33975-33976, 33981)
Insertion/replacement intracorporeal ventricular assist device (33979, 33982-33983)

0.00 0.00 FUD YYY C

AMA: 2017,Dec,3

0452T **aortic counterpulsation device and vascular hemostatic seal**

EXCLUDES *Insertion intra-aortic balloon assist device (33973)*
Insertion intracorporeal ventricular assist device (33979, 33982-33983)
Insertion/removal percutaneous ventricular assist device ([33995], 33990-33991, [33997])
Insertion/replacement counterpulsation ventricular assist system procedures (0451T)
Removal counterpulsation ventricular assist system (0455T-0456T)

0.00 0.00 FUD YYY C

AMA: 2017,Dec,3

0453T **mechano-electrical skin interface**

EXCLUDES *Insertion intra-aortic balloon assist device (33973)*
Insertion intracorporeal ventricular assist device (33979, 33982-33983)
Insertion/removal percutaneous ventricular assist device ([33995], 33990-33991, [33997])
Insertion/replacement counterpulsation ventricular assist system procedures (0451T)
Removal counterpulsation ventricular assist system (0455T, 0457T)

0.00 0.00 FUD YYY J

0454T **subcutaneous electrode**

INCLUDES Each electrode inserted or replaced

EXCLUDES *Insertion intra-aortic balloon assist device (33973, 33982-33983)*
Insertion/removal percutaneous ventricular assist device ([33995], 33990-33991, [33997])
Insertion/replacement counterpulsation ventricular assist system (0451T)
Insertion/replacement intracorporeal ventricular assist device (33979, 33982-33983)
Removal device or component (0455T, 0458T)

0.00 0.00 FUD YYY J

0455T **Removal of permanently implantable aortic counterpulsation ventricular assist system; complete system (aortic counterpulsation device, vascular hemostatic seal, mechano-electrical skin interface and electrodes)**

EXCLUDES *Insertion/replacement system or component (0451T-0454T)*
Removal:
Extracorporeal ventricular assist device (33977-33978)
Intra-aortic balloon assist device (33968, 33971, 33974)
Intracorporeal ventricular assist device (33980)
Percutaneous ventricular assist device (33992)
System or component (0456T-0458T)

0.00 0.00 FUD YYY C

AMA: 2017,Dec,3

0456T **aortic counterpulsation device and vascular hemostatic seal**

EXCLUDES *Insertion/replacement system or component (0451T-0452T)*
Removal:
Aortic counterpulsation ventricular assist system (0455T)
Intra-aortic balloon assist device (33974)
Intracorporeal ventricular assist device (33980)
Percutaneous ventricular assist device (33992)

0.00 0.00 FUD YYY C

AMA: 2017,Dec,3

0457T **mechano-electrical skin interface**

EXCLUDES *Insertion/replacement system or component (0451T, 0453T)*
Removal:
Aortic counterpulsation ventricular assist system (0455T)
Intra-aortic balloon assist device (33974)
Intracorporeal ventricular assist device (33980)
Percutaneous ventricular assist device (33992)

0.00 0.00 FUD YYY Q2

0458T **subcutaneous electrode**

INCLUDES Each electrode removed

EXCLUDES *Insertion/replacement system or component (0451T, 0454T)*
Removal:
Aortic counterpulsation ventricular assist system (0455T)
Intra-aortic balloon assist device (33974)
Intracorporeal ventricular assist device (33980)
Percutaneous ventricular assist device (33992)

0.00 0.00 FUD YYY Q2

0459T **Relocation of skin pocket with replacement of implanted aortic counterpulsation ventricular assist device, mechano-electrical skin interface and electrodes**

EXCLUDES *Repositioning percutaneous ventricular assist device (33993)*

0.00 0.00 FUD YYY C

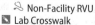

0460T **Repositioning of previously implanted aortic counterpulsation ventricular assist device; subcutaneous electrode**

INCLUDES Repositioning each electrode

EXCLUDES *Insertion/replacement system or component (0451T, 0454T)*

Repositioning percutaneous ventricular assist device (33993)

0.00 0.00 FUD YYY T

0461T **aortic counterpulsation device**

EXCLUDES *Repositioning percutaneous ventricular assist device (33993)*

0.00 0.00 FUD YYY C

0462T **Programming device evaluation (in person) with iterative adjustment of the implantable mechano-electrical skin interface and/or external driver to test the function of the device and select optimal permanent programmed values with analysis, including review and report, implantable aortic counterpulsation ventricular assist system, per day**

EXCLUDES *Device evaluation (0463T)*

Insertion/replacement system or component (0451T-0454T)

Relocation pocket (0459T)

Removal system or component (0455T-0458T)

Repositioning device (0460T-0461T)

0.00 0.00 FUD YYY S

0463T **Interrogation device evaluation (in person) with analysis, review and report, includes connection, recording and disconnection per patient encounter, implantable aortic counterpulsation ventricular assist system, per day**

EXCLUDES *Device evaluation (0462T)*

Insertion/replacement system or component (0451T-0454T)

Relocation pocket (0459T)

Removal system or component (0455T-0458T)

Repositioning device (0460T-0461T)

0.00 0.00 FUD YYY S

0464T [0464T]

0464T **Resequenced code. See code following 0333T.**

0465T-0469T

EXCLUDES *Replacement/revision cranial nerve neurostimulator electrode array (64569)*

0465T **Suprachoroidal injection of a pharmacologic agent (does not include supply of medication)**

EXCLUDES *Intravitreal implantation or injection (67025-67028)*

0.00 0.00 FUD YYY T R2

AMA: 2018,Feb,3

\+ **0466T** **Insertion of chest wall respiratory sensor electrode or electrode array, including connection to pulse generator (List separately in addition to code for primary procedure)**

EXCLUDES *Revision/removal chest wall respiratory sensor electrode or array (0467T-0468T)*

Code first (64568)

0.00 0.00 FUD YYY N N1

AMA: 2018,Mar,9; 2018,Jan,8; 2017,Jan,8; 2016,Nov,6

0467T **Revision or replacement of chest wall respiratory sensor electrode or electrode array, including connection to existing pulse generator**

EXCLUDES *Insertion/removal chest wall respiratory sensor electrode or array (0466T, 0468T)*

Replacement/revision cranial nerve neurostimulator electrode array (64569)

0.00 0.00 FUD YYY Q2 G2

AMA: 2018,Mar,9; 2018,Jan,8; 2017,Jan,8; 2016,Nov,6

0468T **Removal of chest wall respiratory sensor electrode or electrode array**

EXCLUDES *Insertion/removal chest wall respiratory sensor electrode or array (0466T-0467T)*

Removal cranial neurostimulator electrode array (64570)

0.00 0.00 FUD YYY Q2 G2

AMA: 2018,Mar,9; 2018,Jan,8; 2017,Jan,8; 2016,Nov,6

0469T **Retinal polarization scan, ocular screening with on-site automated results, bilateral**

INCLUDES Ophthalmic medical services (92002-92014)

EXCLUDES *Ocular screening (99174, [99177])*

0.00 0.00 FUD XXX E

AMA: 2018,Feb,3

0470T-0471T

EXCLUDES *Optical coherence tomography coronary vessel or graft (92978-92979)*

Reflectance confocal microscopy (RCM) for cellular and subcellular skin imaging (96931-96936)

0470T **Optical coherence tomography (OCT) for microstructural and morphological imaging of skin, image acquisition, interpretation, and report; first lesion**

0.00 0.00 FUD XXX M

\+ **0471T** **each additional lesion (List separately in addition to code for primary procedure)**

Code first (0470T)

0.00 0.00 FUD XXX N N1

0472T-0474T

0472T **Device evaluation, interrogation, and initial programming of intraocular retinal electrode array (eg, retinal prosthesis), in person, with iterative adjustment of the implantable device to test functionality, select optimal permanent programmed values with analysis, including visual training, with review and report by a qualified health care professional**

0.00 0.00 FUD XXX Q1

AMA: 2018,Feb,3

0473T **Device evaluation and interrogation of intraocular retinal electrode array (eg, retinal prosthesis), in person, including reprogramming and visual training, when performed, with review and report by a qualified health care professional**

INCLUDES Reprogramming device (0473T)

EXCLUDES *Placement intraocular retinal electrode display (0100T)*

0.00 0.00 FUD XXX Q1

AMA: 2018,Feb,3

0474T **Insertion of anterior segment aqueous drainage device, with creation of intraocular reservoir, internal approach, into the supraciliary space**

0.00 0.00 FUD XXX J

AMA: 2018,Dec,8; 2018,Dec,8; 2018,Jul,3; 2018,Feb,3

0475T-0478T

0475T **Recording of fetal magnetic cardiac signal using at least 3 channels; patient recording and storage, data scanning with signal extraction, technical analysis and result, as well as supervision, review, and interpretation of report by a physician or other qualified health care professional**

0.00 0.00 FUD XXX M

0476T **patient recording, data scanning, with raw electronic signal transfer of data and storage**

0.00 0.00 FUD XXX Q1

0477T **signal extraction, technical analysis, and result**

0.00 0.00 FUD XXX Q1

0478T **review, interpretation, report by physician or other qualified health care professional**

0.00 0.00 FUD XXX M

0479T-0480T

EXCLUDES *Ablative laser treatment for additional square cm open wound (0492T)*
Cicatricial lesion excision (11400-11446)
Reporting code more than one time per day

0479T Fractional ablative laser fenestration of burn and traumatic scars for functional improvement; first 100 cm2 or part thereof, or 1% of body surface area of infants and children
0.00 0.00 **FUD** 000 T G2
AMA: 2018,Jan,8; 2017,Dec,13

+ **0480T each additional 100 cm2, or each additional 1% of body surface area of infants and children, or part thereof (List separately in addition to code for primary procedure)**
Code first (0479T)
0.00 0.00 **FUD** ZZZ N N1
AMA: 2018,Jan,8; 2017,Dec,13

0481T

0481T Injection(s), autologous white blood cell concentrate (autologous protein solution), any site, including image guidance, harvesting and preparation, when performed
INCLUDES Radiologic guidance (76942, 77002, 77012, 77021)
EXCLUDES *Blood collection (36415, 36592)*
Bone marrow procedures (38220-38222, 38230)
Injection platelet rich plasma (0232T)
Injections to tendon, ligament, or fascia (20550-20551)
Joint aspiration or injection (20600-20611)
Other tissue grafts ([15769], 15771-15774)
Pooling platelets (86965)
0.00 0.00 **FUD** 000 Q1
AMA: 2019,Oct,5

0483T-0484T

INCLUDES Access and closure
Angiography
Balloon valvuloplasty
Contrast injections
Fluoroscopy
Radiological supervision and interpretation
Valve deployment and repositioning
Ventriculography

EXCLUDES *Diagnostic heart catheterization (93451-93453, 93456-93461, 93530-93533)*
Transcatheter mitral valve annulus reconstruction (0544T)
Transcatheter mitral valve repair through coronary sinus (0345T)
Transcatheter mitral valve repair with transseptal puncture, when performed (33418-33419)
Transcatheter tricuspid valve annulus reconstruction (0545T)

Code also cardiopulmonary bypass when provided (33367-33369)
Code also diagnostic cardiac catheterization procedures when no previous study available and append modifier 59 when:
Patient condition has changed
Previous study inadequate

0483T Transcatheter mitral valve implantation/replacement (TMVI) with prosthetic valve; percutaneous approach, including transseptal puncture, when performed
0.00 0.00 **FUD** 000 C 80

0484T transthoracic exposure (eg, thoracotomy, transapical)
0.00 0.00 **FUD** 000 C 80

0485T-0486T

0485T Optical coherence tomography (OCT) of middle ear, with interpretation and report; unilateral
0.00 0.00 **FUD** XXX Q1 50

0486T bilateral
0.00 0.00 **FUD** XXX Q1

0487T-0488T [0488T]

0487T Biomechanical mapping, transvaginal, with report
0.00 0.00 **FUD** XXX Q1 N1

0488T **Resequenced code. See code following 0403T.**

0489T-0490T

EXCLUDES *Joint injection/aspiration (20600, 20604)*
Liposuction procedures (15876-15879)
Tissue grafts ([15769], 15771-15774)

Code also for complete procedure report both codes (0489T-0490T)

0489T Autologous adipose-derived regenerative cell therapy for scleroderma in the hands; adipose tissue harvesting, isolation and preparation of harvested cells including incubation with cell dissociation enzymes, removal of non-viable cells and debris, determination of concentration and dilution of regenerative cells
0.00 0.00 **FUD** 000 E
AMA: 2019,Oct,5; 2018,Sep,12

0490T multiple injections in one or both hands
EXCLUDES *Single injections*
0.00 0.00 **FUD** 000 E
AMA: 2019,Oct,5; 2018,Sep,12

0491T-0493T

0491T Ablative laser treatment, non-contact, full field and fractional ablation, open wound, per day, total treatment surface area; first 20 sq cm or less
0.00 0.00 **FUD** 000 T G2

+ **0492T each additional 20 sq cm, or part thereof (List separately in addition to code for primary procedure)**
EXCLUDES *Laser fenestration scars (0479T-0480T)*
Code first (0491T)
0.00 0.00 **FUD** ZZZ N N1

0493T Near-infrared spectroscopy studies of lower extremity wounds (eg, for oxyhemoglobin measurement)
0.00 0.00 **FUD** XXX N N1

0494T-0496T

0494T Surgical preparation and cannulation of marginal (extended) cadaver donor lung(s) to ex vivo organ perfusion system, including decannulation, separation from the perfusion system, and cold preservation of the allograft prior to implantation, when performed
0.00 0.00 **FUD** XXX C 80

0495T Initiation and monitoring marginal (extended) cadaver donor lung(s) organ perfusion system by physician or qualified health care professional, including physiological and laboratory assessment (eg, pulmonary artery flow, pulmonary artery pressure, left atrial pressure, pulmonary vascular resistance, mean/peak and plateau airway pressure, dynamic compliance and perfusate gas analysis), including bronchoscopy and X ray when performed; first two hours in sterile field
0.00 0.00 **FUD** XXX C

+ **0496T each additional hour (List separately in addition to code for primary procedure)**
Code first (0495T)
0.00 0.00 **FUD** ZZZ C

0497T-0498T

EXCLUDES *ECG event monitoring (93268, 93271-93272)*
ECG rhythm strips (93040-93042)
Remote telemetry (93228-93229)

0497T External patient-activated, physician- or other qualified health care professional-prescribed, electrocardiographic rhythm derived event recorder without 24 hour attended monitoring; in-office connection
0.00 0.00 **FUD** XXX Q1 TC

0498T review and interpretation by a physician or other qualified health care professional per 30 days with at least one patient-generated triggered event
0.00 0.00 **FUD** XXX M 26

0499T-0500T

0499T **Cystourethroscopy, with mechanical dilation and urethral therapeutic drug delivery for urethral stricture or stenosis, including fluoroscopy, when performed**

EXCLUDES *Cystourethroscopy for stricture (52281, 52283)*

0.00 0.00 FUD 000 E

0500T **Infectious agent detection by nucleic acid (DNA or RNA), human papillomavirus (HPV) for five or more separately reported high-risk HPV types (eg, 16, 18, 31, 33, 35, 39, 45, 51, 52, 56, 58, 59, 68) (ie, genotyping)**

EXCLUDES *Less than five high-risk HPV types ([87624, 87625])*

0.00 0.00 FUD XXX A

0501T-0523T [0523T, 0623T, 0624T, 0625T, 0626T]

EXCLUDES *Reporting code more than one time for each CT angiogram*

0501T **Noninvasive estimated coronary fractional flow reserve (FFR) derived from coronary computed tomography angiography data using computation fluid dynamics physiologic simulation software analysis of functional data to assess the severity of coronary artery disease; data preparation and transmission, analysis of fluid dynamics and simulated maximal coronary hyperemia, generation of estimated FFR model, with anatomical data review in comparison with estimated FFR model to reconcile discordant data, interpretation and report**

INCLUDES All complete test components (0501T-0504T)

EXCLUDES *Automated coronary plaque characterization/quantification using coronary CT angiography data ([0623T, 0624T, 0625T, 0626T])*

0.00 0.00 FUD XXX M

AMA: 2018,Sep,10

0502T **data preparation and transmission**

EXCLUDES *Automated coronary plaque characterization/quantification using coronary CT angiography data ([0623T, 0624T, 0625T, 0626T])*

0.00 0.00 FUD XXX N N1 TC

AMA: 2018,Sep,10

0503T **analysis of fluid dynamics and simulated maximal coronary hyperemia, and generation of estimated FFR model**

EXCLUDES *Automated coronary plaque characterization/quantification using coronary CT angiography data ([0623T, 0624T, 0625T, 0626T])*

0.00 0.00 FUD XXX S N1 TC

AMA: 2018,Sep,10

0504T **anatomical data review in comparison with estimated FFR model to reconcile discordant data, interpretation and report**

EXCLUDES *Automated coronary plaque characterization/quantification using coronary CT angiography data ([0623T, 0624T, 0625T, 0626T])*

0.00 0.00 FUD XXX M 26

AMA: 2018,Sep,10

● # **0623T** **Automated quantification and characterization of coronary atherosclerotic plaque to assess severity of coronary disease, using data from coronary computed tomographic angiography; data preparation and transmission, computerized analysis of data, with review of computerized analysis output to reconcile discordant data, interpretation and report**

INCLUDES All complete test components ([0623T, 0624T, 0625T, 0626T])

EXCLUDES *3D rendering (76376-76377)*

Noninvasive estimated coronary fractional flow reserve (FFR) (0501T-0504T)

0.00 0.00 FUD 000

● # **0624T** **data preparation and transmission**

EXCLUDES *3D rendering (76376-76377)*

Noninvasive estimated coronary fractional flow reserve (FFR) (0501T-0504T)

0.00 0.00 FUD 000

● # **0625T** **computerized analysis of data from coronary computed tomographic angiography**

EXCLUDES *3D rendering (76376-76377)*

Noninvasive estimated coronary fractional flow reserve (FFR) (0501T-0504T)

0.00 0.00 FUD 000

● # **0626T** **review of computerized analysis output to reconcile discordant data, interpretation and report**

EXCLUDES *3D rendering (76376-76377)*

Noninvasive estimated coronary fractional flow reserve (FFR) (0501T-0504T)

0.00 0.00 FUD 000

+ # **0523T** **Intraprocedural coronary fractional flow reserve (FFR) with 3D functional mapping of color-coded FFR values for the coronary tree, derived from coronary angiogram data, for real-time review and interpretation of possible atherosclerotic stenosis(es) intervention (List separately in addition to code for primary procedure)**

EXCLUDES *3D rendering (76376-76377)*

Coronary artery doppler studies (93571-93572)

Noninvasive estimated coronary fractional flow reserve (FFR) (0501T-0504T)

Procedure reported more than one time each session

Code first (93454-93461)

0.00 0.00 FUD ZZZ N1 80

0505T-0514T [0510T, 0511T, 0512T, 0513T, 0620T]

0505T **Endovenous femoral-popliteal arterial revascularization, with transcatheter placement of intravascular stent graft(s) and closure by any method, including percutaneous or open vascular access, ultrasound guidance for vascular access when performed, all catheterization(s) and intraprocedural roadmapping and imaging guidance necessary to complete the intervention, all associated radiological supervision and interpretation, when performed, with crossing of the occlusive lesion in an extraluminal fashion**

INCLUDES All procedures performed on same side:

- Catheterization (arterial and venous)
- Diagnostic imaging for arteriography
- Radiologic supervision and interpretation

Ultrasound guidance (76937)

EXCLUDES *Balloon angioplasty arteries other than dialysis circuit ([37248, 37249])*

Revascularization femoral or popliteal artery (37224-37227)

Venous stenting (37238-37239)

0.00 0.00 FUD YYY 80

● # **0620T** **Endovascular venous arterialization, tibial or peroneal vein, with transcatheter placement of intravascular stent graft(s) and closure by any method, including percutaneous or open vascular access, ultrasound guidance for vascular access when performed, all catheterization(s) and intraprocedural roadmapping and imaging guidance necessary to complete the intervention, all associated radiological supervision and interpretation, when performed**

INCLUDES All procedures performed on same side:

- Catheterization (arterial and venous)
- Diagnostic imaging for arteriography
- Radiologic supervision and interpretation

EXCLUDES *When performed within tibial-peroneal segment:*

- *Endovascular revascularization procedures (37228-37231)*
- *Transcatheter intravascular stent placement (37238-37239)*
- *Transluminal balloon angioplasty ([37248, 37249])*

0.00 0.00 FUD 000

0506T Macular pigment optical density measurement by heterochromatic flicker photometry, unilateral or bilateral, with interpretation and report
    🚑 0.00   ⚕ 0.00   **FUD** XXX   [80] 🔲
    AMA: 2018,Dec,6; 2018,Dec,6

0507T Near-infrared dual imaging (ie, simultaneous reflective and trans-illuminated light) of meibomian glands, unilateral or bilateral, with interpretation and report
    EXCLUDES   *External ocular photography (92285)*
        Tear film imaging (0330T)
    🚑 0.00   ⚕ 0.00   **FUD** XXX   [80] 🔲

0508T Pulse-echo ultrasound bone density measurement resulting in indicator of axial bone mineral density, tibia
    🚑 0.00   ⚕ 0.00   **FUD** XXX   [Z2][80] 🔲

0509T Electroretinography (ERG) with interpretation and report, pattern (PERG)
    EXCLUDES   *Full field ERG (92273)*
        Multifocal ERG (92274)
    🚑 2.24   ⚕ 2.24   **FUD** XXX   [80] 🔲
    AMA: 2019,Jan,12

0510T   **Resequenced code. See code following 0335T.**

0511T   **Resequenced code. See code following 0335T.**

0512T   **Resequenced code. See code following 0102T.**

0513T   **Resequenced code. See code following 0102T.**

+ **0514T** Intraoperative visual axis identification using patient fixation (List separately in addition to code for primary procedure)
    Code first (66982, 66984)
    🚑 0.00   ⚕ 0.00   **FUD** ZZZ   [N1] 🔲
    AMA: 2018,Dec,6; 2018,Dec,6

0515T-0523T [0523T]

INCLUDES   Complete system with two components
    Pulse generator including battery and transmitter
    Wireless endocardial left ventricular electrode

0515T Insertion of wireless cardiac stimulator for left ventricular pacing, including device interrogation and programming, and imaging supervision and interpretation, when performed; complete system (includes electrode and generator [transmitter and battery])
    INCLUDES   Catheterization (93452-93453, 93458-93461, 93531-93533)
        Creation pockets
        Electrode insertion
        Imaging guidance (76000, 76998, 93303-93355)
        Insertion complete wireless cardiac stimulator system
        Interrogation device (0521T)
        Programming device (0522T)
        Pulse generator (battery and transmitter) (0517T)
        Revision and repositioning
    EXCLUDES   *Insertion electrode as separate procedure (0516T)*
        Removal/replacement device or components (0518T-0520T)
    🚑 0.00   ⚕ 0.00   **FUD** YYY   🔲

0516T electrode only
    INCLUDES   Catheterization (93452-93453, 93458-93461, 93531-93533)
        Imaging guidance (76000, 76998, 93303-93355)
        Interrogation device (0521T)
        Programming device (0522T)
    EXCLUDES   *Removal/replacement device or components (0518T-0520T)*
    🚑 0.00   ⚕ 0.00   **FUD** YYY   🔲

0517T pulse generator component(s) (battery and/or transmitter) only
    INCLUDES   Catheterization (93452-93453, 93458-93461, 93531-93533)
        Imaging guidance (76000, 76998, 93303-93355)
        Interrogation device (0521T)
        Programming device (0522T)
    EXCLUDES   *Removal/replacement device or components (0518T-0520T)*
    🚑 0.00   ⚕ 0.00   **FUD** YYY   🔲

0518T Removal of only pulse generator component(s) (battery and/or transmitter) of wireless cardiac stimulator for left ventricular pacing
    INCLUDES   Catheterization (93452-93453, 93458-93461, 93531-93533)
        Imaging guidance (76000, 76998, 93303-93355)
        Interrogation device (0521T)
        Programming device (0522T)
        Pulse generator (battery and transmitter) (0517T)
    EXCLUDES   *Complete procedure (0515T)*
        Insertion electrode only (0516T)
        Removal/replacement device or components (0519T-0520T)
    🚑 0.00   ⚕ 0.00   **FUD** YYY   🔲

0519T Removal and replacement of wireless cardiac stimulator for left ventricular pacing; pulse generator component(s) (battery and/or transmitter)
    INCLUDES   Catheterization (93452-93453, 93458-93461, 93531-93533)
        Imaging guidance (76000, 76998, 93303-93355)
        Interrogation device (0521T)
        Programming device (0522T)
        Pulse generator (battery and transmitter) (0517T)
    EXCLUDES   *Complete procedure (0515T)*
        Insertion electrode only (0516T)
        Removal/replacement device or components (0518T)
    🚑 0.00   ⚕ 0.00   **FUD** YYY   🔲

0520T pulse generator component(s) (battery and/or transmitter), including placement of a new electrode
    INCLUDES   Catheterization (93452-93453, 93458-93461, 93531-93533)
        Imaging guidance (76000, 76998, 93303-93355)
        Interrogation device (0521T)
        Programming device (0522T)
        Pulse generator (battery and transmitter) (0517T)
    EXCLUDES   *Complete procedure (0515T)*
        Insertion electrode only (0516T)
        Removal only device or components (0518T)
    🚑 0.00   ⚕ 0.00   **FUD** YYY   🔲

0521T Interrogation device evaluation (in person) with analysis, review and report, includes connection, recording, and disconnection per patient encounter, wireless cardiac stimulator for left ventricular pacing
    INCLUDES   Programming device (0522T)
        Pulse generator (battery and transmitter) (0517T)
    EXCLUDES   *Complete procedure (0515T)*
        Insertion electrode only (0516T)
        Removal/replacement device or components (0518T-0520T)
    🚑 0.00   ⚕ 0.00   **FUD** XXX   🔲

0522T **Programming device evaluation (in person) with iterative adjustment of the implantable device to test the function of the device and select optimal permanent programmed values with analysis, including review and report, wireless cardiac stimulator for left ventricular pacing**

INCLUDES Interrogation device (0521T)
Pulse generator (battery and transmitter) (0517T)

EXCLUDES *Complete procedure (0515T)*
Insertion electrode only (0516T)
Removal/replacement device or components (0518T-0520T)

0.00 0.00 FUD XXX

0523T **Resequenced code. See code before 0505T.**

0524T

0524T **Endovenous catheter directed chemical ablation with balloon isolation of incompetent extremity vein, open or percutaneous, including all vascular access, catheter manipulation, diagnostic imaging, imaging guidance and monitoring**

0.00 0.00 FUD YYY G2 50

0525T-0532T

0525T **Insertion or replacement of intracardiac ischemia monitoring system, including testing of the lead and monitor, initial system programming, and imaging supervision and interpretation; complete system (electrode and implantable monitor)**

INCLUDES Electrocardiography (93000, 93005, 93010)
Interrogation device (0529T)
Programming device (0528T)

EXCLUDES *Removal intracardiac ischemia monitor or components (0530T-0532T)*

0.00 0.00 FUD YYY J8

0526T **electrode only**

INCLUDES Electrocardiography (93000, 93005, 93010)
Interrogation device (0529T)
Programming device (0528T)

EXCLUDES *Removal intracardiac ischemia monitor or components (0530T-0532T)*

0.00 0.00 FUD YYY J8

0527T **implantable monitor only**

INCLUDES Electrocardiography (93000, 93005, 93010)
Interrogation device (0529T)
Programming device (0528T)

EXCLUDES *Removal intracardiac ischemia monitor or components (0530T-0532T)*

0.00 0.00 FUD YYY J8

0528T **Programming device evaluation (in person) of intracardiac ischemia monitoring system with iterative adjustment of programmed values, with analysis, review, and report**

INCLUDES Electrocardiography (93000, 93005, 93010)

EXCLUDES *Insertion/replacement intracardiac ischemia monitor or components (0525T-0527T)*
Interrogation device (0529T)
Removal intracardiac ischemia monitor or components (0530T-0532T)

0.00 0.00 FUD XXX

0529T **Interrogation device evaluation (in person) of intracardiac ischemia monitoring system with analysis, review, and report**

INCLUDES Electrocardiography (93000, 93005, 93010)

EXCLUDES *Insertion/replacement electrode only (0526T)*
Insertion/replacement intracardiac ischemia monitor or components (0525T-0527T)
Programming device (0528T)
Removal intracardiac ischemia monitor or components (0530T-0532T)

0.00 0.00 FUD XXX

0530T **Removal of intracardiac ischemia monitoring system, including all imaging supervision and interpretation; complete system (electrode and implantable monitor)**

EXCLUDES *Interrogation device (0529T)*
Programming device (0528T)

0.00 0.00 FUD YYY G2

0531T **electrode only**

EXCLUDES *Interrogation device (0529T)*
Programming device (0528T)

0.00 0.00 FUD YYY G2

0532T **implantable monitor only**

EXCLUDES *Interrogation device (0529T)*
Programming device (0528T)

0.00 0.00 FUD YYY G2

0533T-0536T

0533T **Continuous recording of movement disorder symptoms, including bradykinesia, dyskinesia, and tremor for 6 days up to 10 days; includes set-up, patient training, configuration of monitor, data upload, analysis and initial report configuration, download review, interpretation and report**

0.00 0.00 FUD XXX

0534T **set-up, patient training, configuration of monitor**

0.00 0.00 FUD XXX

0535T **data upload, analysis and initial report configuration**

0.00 0.00 FUD XXX

0536T **download review, interpretation and report**

0.00 0.00 FUD XXX

0537T-0540T

INCLUDES Administration genetically modified cells for treatment serious diseases (e.g., cancer)
Evaluation prior to, during, and after CAR-T cell administration
Infusion fluids and supportive medications provided with administration
Management clinical staff
Management untoward events (e.g., nausea)
Physician certification, processing cells
Physician presence during cell administration

Code also care provided not directly related to CAR-T cell administration (e.g., other medical problems) may be reported separately using appropriate E/M code and modifier 25

0537T **Chimeric antigen receptor T-cell (CAR-T) therapy; harvesting of blood-derived T lymphocytes for development of genetically modified autologous CAR-T cells, per day**

EXCLUDES *Reporting more than one time per day despite times cells are collected*

0.00 0.00 FUD XXX

AMA: 2019,Jun,5

0538T **preparation of blood-derived T lymphocytes for transportation (eg, cryopreservation, storage)**

0.00 0.00 FUD XXX

AMA: 2019,Jun,5

0539T **receipt and preparation of CAR-T cells for administration**

0.00 0.00 FUD XXX

AMA: 2019,Jun,5

0540T **CAR-T cell administration, autologous**

EXCLUDES *Reporting more than one time per day despite units administered*

0.00 0.00 FUD YYY

AMA: 2019,Jun,5

0541T-0542T

0541T **Myocardial imaging by magnetocardiography (MCG) for detection of cardiac ischemia, by signal acquisition using minimum 36 channel grid, generation of magnetic-field time-series images, quantitative analysis of magnetic dipoles, machine learning-derived clinical scoring, and automated report generation, single study;**

0.00 0.00 FUD XXX TC

0542T **interpretation and report**
0.00 0.00 **FUD** XXX 26

0543T

EXCLUDES *Transesophageal echocardiography (93355)*

0543T **Transapical mitral valve repair, including transthoracic echocardiography, when performed, with placement of artificial chordae tendineae**
0.00 0.00 **FUD** YYY 80

0544T-0545T

INCLUDES Adjustment/deployment reconstruction device
Catheterization
Insertion temporary pacemaker
Vascular access and closure

EXCLUDES *Fluoroscopic guidance (76000)*
Percutaneous mitral valve repair

Code also diagnostic angiography or catheterization and append modifier 59, when:
Prior study available but inadequate or patient's condition has changed
Prior study not available and full diagnostic study performed
Code also transcatheter implantation/replacement mitral valve (0483T)
Code also when performed:
Balloon pump insertion (33967, 33970, 33973)
Central bypass (33369)
Peripheral bypass (33367-33368)
Ventricular assist device (33990-33993)

0544T **Transcatheter mitral valve annulus reconstruction, with implantation of adjustable annulus reconstruction device, percutaneous approach including transseptal puncture**
EXCLUDES *Transcatheter mitral valve repair (33418-33419)*
Transcatheter mitral valve repair via coronary sinus (0345T)
0.00 0.00 **FUD** YYY 80

0545T **Transcatheter tricuspid valve annulus reconstruction with implantation of adjustable annulus reconstruction device, percutaneous approach**
EXCLUDES *Repositioning/plication tricuspid valve (33468)*
0.00 0.00 **FUD** YYY 80

0546T

EXCLUDES *Reporting code for re-excision of site*
Reporting code more than one time per partial mastectomy site

0546T **Radiofrequency spectroscopy, real time, intraoperative margin assessment, at the time of partial mastectomy, with report**
0.00 0.00 **FUD** YYY 80
AMA: 2020,May,9

0547T

0547T **Bone-material quality testing by microindentation(s) of the tibia(s), with results reported as a score**
0.00 0.00 **FUD** XXX 80

0548T-0551T

0548T **Transperineal periurethral balloon continence device; bilateral placement, including cystoscopy and fluoroscopy**
0.00 0.00 **FUD** YYY J8 80
AMA: 2020,Aug,6

0549T **unilateral placement, including cystoscopy and fluoroscopy**
0.00 0.00 **FUD** YYY J8 80
AMA: 2020,Aug,6

0550T **removal, each balloon**
0.00 0.00 **FUD** YYY G2 80
AMA: 2020,Aug,6

0551T **adjustment of balloon(s) fluid volume**
EXCLUDES *Insertion or removal periurethral balloon continence device (0548T-0550T)*
0.00 0.00 **FUD** YYY R2 80
AMA: 2020,Aug,6

0552T

0552T **Low-level laser therapy, dynamic photonic and dynamic thermokinetic energies, provided by a physician or other qualified health care professional**
0.00 0.00 **FUD** YYY 80

0553T

EXCLUDES *Angiography extremity (75710)*
Endovascular revascularization (37220-37221, 37224, 37226, 37238)
Injection for venography (36005)
Insertion catheter/needle, upper or lower extremity artery (36140)
Selective catheter placement (36011-36012, 36245-36246)
Transluminal balloon angioplasty ([37248])
Venography (75820)

0553T **Percutaneous transcatheter placement of iliac arteriovenous anastomosis implant, inclusive of all radiological supervision and interpretation, intraprocedural roadmapping, and imaging guidance necessary to complete the intervention**
0.00 0.00 **FUD** YYY 80

0554T-0557T

0554T **Bone strength and fracture risk using finite element analysis of functional data, and bone-mineral density, utilizing data from a computed tomography scan; retrieval and transmission of the scan data, assessment of bone strength and fracture risk and bone mineral density, interpretation and report**
INCLUDES Assessment, interpretation and report, and retrieval and transmission of data (0555T-0557T)
0.00 0.00 **FUD** XXX 80
AMA: 2020,Sep,11

0555T **retrieval and transmission of the scan data**
0.00 0.00 **FUD** XXX 80
AMA: 2020,Sep,11

0556T **assessment of bone strength and fracture risk and bone mineral density**
0.00 0.00 **FUD** XXX 80
AMA: 2020,Sep,11

0557T **interpretation and report**
0.00 0.00 **FUD** XXX 80
AMA: 2020,Sep,11

0558T

EXCLUDES *Computed tomography:*
abdominal aorta (75635)
abdomen/pelvis (72191-72194, 74150-74178)
chest/thorax (71250-71270, 71275)
colonography (74261-74263)
heart (75571-75574)
spine (72125-72133)
whole body (78816)

0558T **Computed tomography scan taken for the purpose of biomechanical computed tomography analysis**
0.00 0.00 **FUD** XXX Z2 80
AMA: 2020,Sep,11

0559T-0562T

EXCLUDES *3D rendering (76376-76377)*

0559T **Anatomic model 3D-printed from image data set(s); first individually prepared and processed component of an anatomic structure**
INCLUDES 3D printed anatomical model production
0.00 0.00 **FUD** XXX 80

\+ 0560T **each additional individually prepared and processed component of an anatomic structure (List separately in addition to code for primary procedure)**
INCLUDES 3D printed anatomical model production
Code first (0559T)
0.00 0.00 **FUD** ZZZ 80

0561T **Anatomic guide 3D-printed and designed from image data set(s); first anatomic guide**

INCLUDES 3D printed cutting or drilling guides for use during surgery

0.00 0.00 FUD XXX 80

\+ **0562T** **each additional anatomic guide (List separately in addition to code for primary procedure)**

INCLUDES 3D printed cutting or drilling guides for use during surgery

Code first (0561T)

0.00 0.00 FUD ZZZ 80

0563T-0564T [0563T]

0563T **Resequenced code. See code before code 0208T.**

0564T **Oncology, chemotherapeutic drug cytotoxicity assay of cancer stem cells (CSCs), from cultured CSCs and primary tumor cells, categorical drug response reported based on percent of cytotoxicity observed, a minimum of 14 drugs or drug combinations**

0.00 0.00 FUD YYY 80

0565T-0566T

0565T **Autologous cellular implant derived from adipose tissue for the treatment of osteoarthritis of the knees; tissue harvesting and cellular implant creation**

EXCLUDES *Other tissue grafts ([15769], 15771-15774)*

0.00 0.00 FUD YYY 80

0566T **injection of cellular implant into knee joint including ultrasound guidance, unilateral**

INCLUDES Guidance for needle placement:
- Fluoroscopy (77002)
- Ultrasound (76942)

EXCLUDES *Arthrocentesis, with or without imaging guidance (20610-20611)*

0.00 0.00 FUD YYY R2 80

0567T-0568T

0567T **Permanent fallopian tube occlusion with degradable biopolymer implant, transcervical approach, including transvaginal ultrasound** ♀

INCLUDES Transvaginal ultrasound (76830)

EXCLUDES *Catheter insertion and introduction saline/contrast for sonohysterography or hysterosalpingography (58340)*
Hysterosalpingography (74740)
Nonobstetric pelvic ultrasound (76856-76857)
Surgical hysteroscopy with bilateral occlusion fallopian tube (58565)
Transcervical catheterization fallopian tube (74742)

0.00 0.00 FUD YYY 80

0568T **Introduction of mixture of saline and air for sonosalpingography to confirm occlusion of fallopian tubes, transcervical approach, including transvaginal ultrasound and pelvic ultrasound** ♀

INCLUDES Transvaginal ultrasound (76830)

EXCLUDES *Catheter insertion and introduction saline/contrast for sonohysterography or hysterosalpingography (58340)*
Hysterosalpingography (74740)
Nonobstetric pelvic ultrasound (76856-76857)
Sonohysterography (SIS) (76831)
Surgical hysteroscopy with bilateral occlusion fallopian tube (58565)
Transcervical catheterization fallopian tube (74742)

0.00 0.00 FUD YYY 80

0569T-0570T

INCLUDES Adjustment/deployment prosthetic device
Catheterization
Fluoroscopic guidance (76000)
Intracardiac echocardiography (93662)
Vascular access and closure

EXCLUDES *Open tricuspid valve procedures (33460, 33463-33465, 33468)*

Code also diagnostic angiography or catheterization and append modifier 59, when:
- Prior study available but inadequate or patient's condition has changed
- Prior study not available and full diagnostic study performed

Code also when performed:
- Balloon pump insertion (33967, 33970, 33973)
- Central bypass (33369)
- Peripheral bypass (33367-33368)
- Ventricular assist device (33990-33993)
- TEE, when done by different operator (93355)

0569T **Transcatheter tricuspid valve repair, percutaneous approach; initial prosthesis**

EXCLUDES *Reporting code more than once per session*

0.00 0.00 FUD YYY 80

\+ **0570T** **each additional prosthesis during same session (List separately in addition to code for primary procedure)**

Code first (0569T)

0.00 0.00 FUD ZZZ 80

0571T-0614T [0614T]

EXCLUDES *Defibrillator or pacemaker device evaluations (93279-93284, 93285-93289, 93290-93298)*
Implantable defibrillator procedures (33215-33220, 33223-33226, 33240-33249 [33230, 33231, 33262, 33263, 33264])
Pacemaker procedures (33202-33220 [33221], 33222-33226, 33233-33238 [33227, 33228, 33229])
Subcutaneous implantable defibrillator system procedures:
- *Electrophysiological evaluation (93644)*
- *Insertion electrode ([33271])*
- *Insertion/replacement entire system ([33270])*
- *Interrogation ([93261])*
- *Programming ([93260])*
- *Removal electrode ([33272])*
- *Repositioning electrode ([33273])*

Transcatheter permanent leadless pacemaker procedures:
- *Insertion or replacement ([33274])*

0571T **Insertion or replacement of implantable cardioverter-defibrillator system with substernal electrode(s), including all imaging guidance and electrophysiological evaluation (includes defibrillation threshold evaluation, induction of arrhythmia, evaluation of sensing for arrhythmia termination, and programming or reprogramming of sensing or therapeutic parameters), when performed**

INCLUDES Imaging guidance
Programming, interrogation, and electrophysiological evaluations (0575T-0577T)

EXCLUDES *Substernal electrode insertion only (0572T)*

Code also removal implantable cardioverter-defibrillator generator and substernal electrode(s), when total system replaced:
- Electrode(s) (0573T)
- Generator (0580T)

0.00 0.00 FUD YYY 80

0572T **Insertion of substernal implantable defibrillator electrode**

INCLUDES Imaging guidance

EXCLUDES *Insertion generator and electrode (0571T)*
Programming, interrogation, and electrophysiological evaluations (0575T-0577T)
Removal generator only (0580T)

0.00 0.00 FUD YYY 80

0573T Removal of substernal implantable defibrillator electrode

INCLUDES Imaging guidance

EXCLUDES *Programming, interrogation, and electrophysiological evaluations (0575T-0577T)*

Code also removal implantable cardioverter-defibrillator generator and insertion new generator/electrode, when total system replaced:
Insertion new system (0571T)
Removal generator (0580T)
Code also removal generator when system not replaced (0580T)

0.00 0.00 FUD YYY 80

0574T Repositioning of previously implanted substernal implantable defibrillator-pacing electrode

INCLUDES Imaging guidance

EXCLUDES *Programming, interrogation, and electrophysiological evaluations (0575T-0577T)*
Substernal electrode insertion only (0572T)

0.00 0.00 FUD YYY 80

0575T Programming device evaluation (in person) of implantable cardioverter-defibrillator system with substernal electrode, with iterative adjustment of the implantable device to test the function of the device and select optimal permanent programmed values with analysis, review and report by a physician or other qualified health care professional

EXCLUDES *Interrogation and programming device (93260 [93260], 93282, 93287, 0576T)*
Programming during:
Electrode insertion (0572T)
Electrode removal (0573T)
Electrode repositioning (0574T)
Generator removal (0580T)
Insertion/replacement entire system (0571T)
Removal and replacement generator ([0614T])

0.00 0.00 FUD YYY 80

0576T Interrogation device evaluation (in person) of implantable cardioverter-defibrillator system with substernal electrode, with analysis, review and report by a physician or other qualified health care professional, includes connection, recording and disconnection per patient encounter

EXCLUDES *Interrogation and programming device (93261 [93261], 93289, 0575T)*
Interrogation during:
Electrode insertion (0572T)
Electrode removal (0573T)
Electrode repositioning (0574T)
Generator removal (0580T)
Insertion/replacement entire system (0571T)
Removal and replacement generator ([0614T])

0.00 0.00 FUD YYY 80

0577T Electrophysiologic evaluation of implantable cardioverter-defibrillator system with substernal electrode (includes defibrillation threshold evaluation, induction of arrhythmia, evaluation of sensing for arrhythmia termination, and programming or reprogramming of sensing or therapeutic parameters)

EXCLUDES *Electrophysiologic evaluation during:*
Electrode insertion (0572T)
Electrode removal (0573T)
Electrode repositioning (0574T)
Generator removal (0580T)
Insertion/replacement entire system (0571T)
Removal and replacement generator ([0614T])
Electrophysiologic evaluation of subcutaneous implantable defibrillator (93644)

0.00 0.00 FUD YYY 80

0578T Interrogation device evaluation(s) (remote), up to 90 days, substernal lead implantable cardioverter-defibrillator system with interim analysis, review(s) and report(s) by a physician or other qualified health care professional

EXCLUDES *In person device interrogation (0576T)*
Reporting code more than once per 90 days

0.00 0.00 FUD YYY 80

0579T Interrogation device evaluation(s) (remote), up to 90 days, substernal lead implantable cardioverter-defibrillator system, remote data acquisition(s), receipt of transmissions and technician review, technical support and distribution of results

EXCLUDES *In person device interrogation (0576T)*
Reporting code more than once per 90 days

0.00 0.00 FUD YYY 80

0580T Removal of substernal implantable defibrillator pulse generator only

INCLUDES Removal generator when system not replaced

EXCLUDES *Programming, interrogation, and electrophysiological evaluations (0575T-0577T)*
Removal and replacement generator ([33262])

Code also removal substernal electrode and insertion new generator/electrode, when total system replaced:
Insertion new system (0571T)

0.00 0.00 FUD YYY 80

● # **0614T Removal and replacement of substernal implantable defibrillator pulse generator**

EXCLUDES *Electrode insertion (0572T)*
Insertion/replacement entire system (0571T)
Programming, interrogation, and electrophysiological evaluations (0575T-0577T)
Removal generator only (0580T)
Removal/replacement single lead system ([33262])

0.00 0.00 FUD YYY J8 80

0581T-0582T

0581T Ablation, malignant breast tumor(s), percutaneous, cryotherapy, including imaging guidance when performed, unilateral

INCLUDES Ultrasound for:
Breast imaging (76641-76642)
Monitoring tissue ablation (76940)
Needle placement (76942)

EXCLUDES *Cryoablation for breast fibroadenoma(s) (19105)*
Reporting code more than once per treated breast

0.00 0.00 FUD YYY 80

0582T Transurethral ablation of malignant prostate tissue by high-energy water vapor thermotherapy, including intraoperative imaging and needle guidance ♂

INCLUDES 3D rendering (76376-76377)
Cystourethroscopy (52000)
MRI pelvis (72195-72197)
Radiologic guidance for:
Needle placement (76942, 77021)
Tissue ablation monitoring (76940, 77022)
Transrectal ultrasound (76872)

EXCLUDES *Destruction by radiofrequency-generated water vapor thermotherapy for benign prostatic hypertrophy (BPH) (53854)*

0.00 0.00 FUD YYY 80

0583T

0583T Tympanostomy (requiring insertion of ventilating tube), using an automated tube delivery system, iontophoresis local anesthesia

INCLUDES Binocular microscopy (92504)
Iontophoresis (97033)
Operating microscope (69990)

EXCLUDES *Myringotomy (69420-69421)*
Removal impacted cerumen (69209-69210)
Tympanostomy without automated delivery system (69433, 69436)

0.00 0.00 FUD YYY 80

0584T-0586T

0584T Islet cell transplant, includes portal vein catheterization and infusion, including all imaging, including guidance, and radiological supervision and interpretation, when performed; percutaneous

0.00 0.00 FUD YYY 80

0585T laparoscopic

0.00 0.00 FUD YYY 80

0586T open

0.00 0.00 FUD YYY 80

0587T-0590T

0587T Percutaneous implantation or replacement of integrated single device neurostimulation system including electrode array and receiver or pulse generator, including analysis, programming, and imaging guidance when performed, posterior tibial nerve

INCLUDES Electronic analysis (95970-95972, 0589T-0590T)

EXCLUDES *Insertion other neurostimulator devices (64555, 64566, 64575, 64590)*
Revision or removal integrated neurostimulation system (0588T)

0.00 0.00 FUD YYY J8 80

0588T Revision or removal of integrated single device neurostimulation system including electrode array and receiver or pulse generator, including analysis, programming, and imaging guidance when performed, posterior tibial nerve

INCLUDES Electronic analysis (95970-95972, 0589T-0590T)

EXCLUDES *Initial insertion or replacement integrated neurostimulation system (0587T)*
Insertion other neurostimulator devices (64555, 64566, 64575, 64590)

0.00 0.00 FUD YYY R2 80

0589T Electronic analysis with simple programming of implanted integrated neurostimulation system (eg, electrode array and receiver), including contact group(s), amplitude, pulse width, frequency (Hz), on/off cycling, burst, dose lockout, patient-selectable parameters, responsive neurostimulation, detection algorithms, closed-loop parameters, and passive parameters, when performed by physician or other qualified health care professional, posterior tibial nerve, 1-3 parameters

EXCLUDES *Electronic analysis other implanted neurostimulators (95970-95977, [95983, 95984])*
Electronic analysis with complex programming (0590T)
Reporting code during insertion, replacement, revision, or removal integrated neurostimulation system (0587T-0588T)
Reporting code during insertion, replacement, revision, or removal other neurostimulator device (generator and/or electrode) (43647-43648, 43881-43882, 61850-61888, 63650, 63655, 63661-63688, 64553-64595)

0.00 0.00 FUD YYY 80

0590T Electronic analysis with complex programming of implanted integrated neurostimulation system (eg, electrode array and receiver), including contact group(s), amplitude, pulse width, frequency (Hz), on/off cycling, burst, dose lockout, patient-selectable parameters, responsive neurostimulation, detection algorithms, closed-loop parameters, and passive parameters, when performed by physician or other qualified health care professional, posterior tibial nerve, 4 or more parameters

EXCLUDES *Electronic analysis other implanted neurostimulators (95970-95977, [95983, 95984])*
Electronic analysis with simple programming (0589T)
Reporting code during insertion, replacement, revision, or removal integrated neurostimulation system (0587T-0588T)
Reporting code during insertion, replacement, revision, or removal other neurostimulator device (generator and/or electrode) (43647-43648, 43881-43882, 61850-61888, 63650, 63655, 63661-63688, 64553-64595)

0.00 0.00 FUD YYY 80

0591T-0593T

INCLUDES Nonphysician health care professional coach trained to assist patients in obtaining improved health and well-being goals through:
Accountability
Active learning processes
Self-discovery

0591T Health and well-being coaching face-to-face; individual, initial assessment

EXCLUDES *Health and well-being coaching, follow-up session (0592T)*
Health and well-being coaching, group session (0593T)

0.00 0.00 FUD YYY 80

AMA: 2020,Jul,7

0592T individual, follow-up session, at least 30 minutes

EXCLUDES *Diabetic preventative behavior change program ([0488T])*
Education/training for self-management (98960)
Health and well-being coaching, group session (0593T)
Health and well-being coaching, initial session (0591T)
Health behavior assessment/intervention (96156-96159)
Medical nutrition therapy (97802-97804)

0.00 0.00 FUD YYY 80

AMA: 2020,Jul,7

0593T group (2 or more individuals), at least 30 minutes

EXCLUDES *Diabetic preventative behavior change program (0403T)*
Education/training for self-management (98961-98962)
Group therapy procedure (97150)
Health and well-being coaching, individual (0591T-0592T)
Health behavior assessment/intervention ([96164, 96165])

0.00 0.00 FUD YYY 80

AMA: 2020,Jul,7

0594T

● **0594T Osteotomy, humerus, with insertion of an externally controlled intramedullary lengthening device, including intraoperative imaging, initial and subsequent alignment assessments, computations of adjustment schedules, and management of the intramedullary lengthening device**

EXCLUDES *Application multiplane external fixation device (20696)*
Osteoplasty, humerus (24420)
Osteotomy, humerus (24400-24410)
Revision externally controlled intramedullary lengthening device (24999)
Treatment humeral shaft fracture (24516)

0.00 0.00 FUD YYY J8 80

0596T-0597T

EXCLUDES Bladder irrigation (51700)
Change cystostomy tube (51705)
Injection retrograde urethrocystography (51610)
Insertion bladder catheter (51701-51703)

● 0596T **Temporary female intraurethral valve-pump (ie, voiding prosthesis); initial insertion, including urethral measurement** ♀
0.00 0.00 FUD YYY P2 80

● 0597T **replacement** ♀
0.00 0.00 FUD YYY P2 80

0598T-0599T

● 0598T **Noncontact real-time fluorescence wound imaging, for bacterial presence, location, and load, per session; first anatomic site (eg, lower extremity)**
0.00 0.00 FUD YYY Z2 80

● + 0599T **each additional anatomic site (eg, upper extremity) (List separately in addition to code for primary procedure)**
Code first (0598T)
0.00 0.00 FUD YYY N1 80

0600T-0601T

● 0600T **Ablation, irreversible electroporation; 1 or more tumors per organ, including imaging guidance, when performed, percutaneous**
INCLUDES Radiological guidance (76940, 77002, 77013, 77022)
0.00 0.00 FUD YYY J8 80

● 0601T **1 or more tumors, including fluoroscopic and ultrasound guidance, when performed, open**
INCLUDES Fluoroscopic guidance (76940)
Ultrasound guidance (77002)
0.00 0.00 FUD YYY J8 80

0602T-0603T

● 0602T **Glomerular filtration rate (GFR) measurement(s), transdermal, including sensor placement and administration of a single dose of fluorescent pyrazine agent**
EXCLUDES Glomerular filtration rate (GFR) monitoring (0603T)
0.00 0.00 FUD YYY 80

● 0603T **Glomerular filtration rate (GFR) monitoring, transdermal, including sensor placement and administration of more than one dose of fluorescent pyrazine agent, each 24 hours**
EXCLUDES Glomerular filtration rate (GFR) measurement(s) (0602T)
0.00 0.00 FUD YYY 80

0604T-0606T

EXCLUDES Remote physiologic monitoring treament management services ([99457], [99458])

● 0604T **Optical coherence tomography (OCT) of retina, remote, patient-initiated image capture and transmission to a remote surveillance center unilateral or bilateral; initial device provision, set-up and patient education on use of equipment**
0.00 0.00 FUD YYY 80

● 0605T **remote surveillance center technical support, data analyses and reports, with a minimum of 8 daily recordings, each 30 days**
0.00 0.00 FUD YYY 80

● 0606T **review, interpretation and report by the prescribing physician or other qualified health care professional of remote surveillance center data analyses, each 30 days**
0.00 0.00 FUD YYY 80

0607T-0608T

EXCLUDES During same monitoring period:
Cardiac event monitor (93268-93272)
External mobile cardiovascular telemetry (93228-93229)
Holter monitor procedures (93224-93227)
Interrogation cardiovasular physiologic monitoring system (93297)
Remote monitoring pulmonary artery pressure sensor ([93264])

● 0607T **Remote monitoring of an external continuous pulmonary fluid monitoring system, including measurement of radiofrequency-derived pulmonary fluid levels, heart rate, respiration rate, activity, posture, and cardiovascular rhythm (eg, ECG data), transmitted to a remote 24-hour attended surveillance center; set-up and patient education on use of equipment**
EXCLUDES Remote monitoring physiologic parameters, initial during same monitoring period ([99453])
0.00 0.00 FUD YYY 80

● 0608T **analysis of data received and transmission of reports to the physician or other qualified health care professional**
EXCLUDES Remote monitoring physiologic parameters, each 30 days, during same monitoring period ([99454])
Reporting more than once per 30 days
0.00 0.00 FUD YYY 80

0609T-0612T

EXCLUDES Magnetic resonance angiography, spine (72159)
Magnetic resonance imaging, spine (72141-72158)
Other magnetic spectroscopy (76390)

● 0609T **Magnetic resonance spectroscopy, determination and localization of discogenic pain (cervical, thoracic, or lumbar); acquisition of single voxel data, per disc, on biomarkers (ie, lactic acid, carbohydrate, alanine, laal, propionic acid, proteoglycan, and collagen) in at least 3 discs**
0.00 0.00 FUD YYY 80

● 0610T **transmission of biomarker data for software analysis**
0.00 0.00 FUD YYY 80

● 0611T **postprocessing for algorithmic analysis of biomarker data for determination of relative chemical differences between discs**
0.00 0.00 FUD YYY 80

● 0612T **interpretation and report**
0.00 0.00 FUD YYY 80

0613T

EXCLUDES Heart catheterization (93451-93453, 93456-93462)
Heart catheterization for congenital defect(s) (93530-93533)
Intracardiac echocardiography (93662)
Transcatheter/transvenous procedures atrial septectomy/septostomy (33741-33746)
Transesophageal echocardiography procedures (93313-93314, 93318, 93355)
Ultrasound guidance (76937)

● 0613T **Percutaneous transcatheter implantation of interatrial septal shunt device, including right and left heart catheterization, intracardiac echocardiography, and imaging guidance by the proceduralist, when performed**
0.00 0.00 FUD YYY 80

0614T-0615T [0614T]

0614T **Resequenced code. See code following code 0580T.**

● 0615T **Eye-movement analysis without spatial calibration, with interpretation and report**
EXCLUDES Vestibular function tests (92540-92542, 92544-92547)
0.00 0.00 FUD YYY 80

0616T-0618T

EXCLUDES *Iridectomy (66600)*
Repair/suture iris (66680, 66682)

● **0616T Insertion of iris prosthesis, including suture fixation and repair or removal of iris, when performed; without removal of crystalline lens or intraocular lens, without insertion of intraocular lens**
0.00 0.00 FUD YYY J8 80

● **0617T with removal of crystalline lens and insertion of intraocular lens**
EXCLUDES *Cataract extraction/removal:*
Extracapsular (66982, 66984)
Intracapsular (66983)
0.00 0.00 FUD YYY J8 80

● **0618T with secondary intraocular lens placement or intraocular lens exchange**
EXCLUDES *Intraocular lens:*
Exchange (66986)
Insertion, secondary implant (66985)
0.00 0.00 FUD YYY J8 80

0619T

INCLUDES Cystourethroscopy (separate procedure) (52000)
EXCLUDES *Cystourethroscopy:*
with insertion transprostatic implant (52441-52442)
with mechanical dilation/drug delivery (0499T)
Laser:
Coagulation (52647)
Enucleation (52649)
Vaporization (52648)
Prostate, transurethral:
Destruction (53850-53854)
Incision (52450)
Resection (52500, 52601, 52630, 52640)
Transrectal ultrasound (76872)

● **0619T Cystourethroscopy with transurethral anterior prostate commissurotomy and drug delivery, including transrectal ultrasound and fluoroscopy, when performed** ♂
0.00 0.00 FUD YYY J8 80

0620T-0622T [0620T]

0620T **Resequenced code. See code following 0505T.**

● **0621T Trabeculostomy ab interno by laser**
EXCLUDES *Gonioscopy (92020)*

● **0622T with use of ophthalmic endoscope**
EXCLUDES *Gonioscopy (92020)*

0623T-0626T [0623T, 0624T, 0625T, 0626T]

0623T **Resequenced code. See code following 0504T.**
0624T **Resequenced code. See code following 0504T.**
0625T **Resequenced code. See code following 0504T.**
0626T **Resequenced code. See code following 0504T.**

0627T-0630T

● **0627T Percutaneous injection of allogeneic cellular and/or tissue-based product, intervertebral disc, unilateral or bilateral injection, with fluoroscopic guidance, lumbar; first level**
INCLUDES Fluoroscopic guidance (77003)

● + **0628T each additional level (List separately in addition to code for primary procedure)**
EXCLUDES *Fluoroscopic guidance (77003)*
Code first (0627T)
0.00 0.00 FUD 000

● **0629T Percutaneous injection of allogeneic cellular and/or tissue-based product, intervertebral disc, unilateral or bilateral injection, with CT guidance, lumbar; first level**
INCLUDES CT guidance (77012)

● + **0630T each additional level (List separately in addition to code for primary procedure)**
INCLUDES CT guidance (77012)
Code first (0629T)
0.00 0.00 FUD 000

0631T

EXCLUDES *Pulse oximetry (94760-94762)*
Transcutaneous biomarker measurement (0061U)

● **0631T Transcutaneous visible light hyperspectral imaging measurement of oxyhemoglobin, deoxyhemoglobin, and tissue oxygenation, with interpretation and report, per extremity**

0632T

● **0632T Percutaneous transcatheter ultrasound ablation of nerves innervating the pulmonary arteries, including right heart catheterization, pulmonary artery angiography, and all imaging guidance**
INCLUDES Heart catheterization (93451, 93453, 93456, 93460)
Pulmonary artery angiography/injection (75741, 75743, 75746, 93568)
Pulmonary artery catheterization (36013-36015)
Swan-Ganz catheter insertion (93503)
EXCLUDES *Endomyocardial biopsy (93505)*

0633T-0638T

INCLUDES 3D rendering (76376-76377)
EXCLUDES *Diagnostic/interventional CT (76497)*
Limited/localized follow-up CT (76380)

● **0633T Computed tomography, breast, including 3D rendering, when performed, unilateral; without contrast material**
● **0634T with contrast material(s)**
● **0635T without contrast, followed by contrast material(s)**
● **0636T Computed tomography, breast, including 3D rendering, when performed, bilateral; without contrast material(s)**
● **0637T with contrast material(s)**
● **0638T without contrast, followed by contrast material(s)**

0639T

EXCLUDES *Ultrasound guidance (76998-76999)*

● **0639T Wireless skin sensor thermal anisotropy measurement(s) and assessment of flow in cerebrospinal fluid shunt, including ultrasound guidance, when performed**

Appendix A — Modifiers

CPT Modifiers

A modifier is a two-position alpha or numeric code appended to a CPT® code to clarify the services being billed. Modifiers provide a means by which a service can be altered without changing the procedure code. They add more information, such as the anatomical site, to the code. In addition, they help to eliminate the appearance of duplicate billing and unbundling. Modifiers are used to increase accuracy in reimbursement, coding consistency, editing, and to capture payment data.

22 **Increased Procedural Services:** When the work required to provide a service is substantially greater than typically required, it may be identified by adding modifier 22 to the usual procedure code. Documentation must support the substantial additional work and the reason for the additional work (ie, increased intensity, time, technical difficulty of procedure, severity of patient's condition, physical and mental effort required).
Note: This modifier should not be appended to an E/M service.

23 **Unusual Anesthesia:** Occasionally, a procedure, which usually requires either no anesthesia or local anesthesia, because of unusual circumstances must be done under general anesthesia. This circumstance may be reported by adding modifier 23 to the procedure code of the basic service.

24 **Unrelated Evaluation and Management Service by the Same Physician or Other Qualified Health Care Professional During a Postoperative Period:** The physician or other qualified health care professional may need to indicate that an evaluation and management service was performed during a postoperative period for a reason(s) unrelated to the original procedure. This circumstance may be reported by adding modifier 24 to the appropriate level of E/M service.

25 **Significant, Separately Identifiable Evaluation and Management Service by the Same Physician or Other Qualified Health Care Professional on the Same Day of the Procedure or Other Service:** It may be necessary to indicate that on the day a procedure or service identified by a CPT code was performed, the patient's condition required a significant, separately identifiable E/M service above and beyond the other service provided or beyond the usual preoperative and postoperative care associated with the procedure that was performed. A significant, separately identifiable E/M service is defined or substantiated by documentation that satisfies the relevant criteria for the respective E/M service to be reported (see Evaluation and Management Services Guidelines for instructions on determining level of E/M service). The E/M service may be prompted by the symptom or condition for which the procedure and/or service was provided. As such, different diagnoses are not required for reporting of the E/M services on the same date. This circumstance may be reported by adding modifier 25 to the appropriate level of E/M service.
Note: This modifier is not used to report an E/M service that resulted in a decision to perform surgery. See modifier 57. For significant, separately identifiable non-E/M services, see modifier 59.

26 **Professional Component:** Certain procedures are a combination of a physician or other qualified health care professional component and a technical component. When the physician or other qualified health care professional component is reported separately, the service may be identified by adding modifier 26 to the usual procedure number.

32 **Mandated Services:** Services related to *mandated* consultation and/or related services (eg, third party payer, governmental, legislative or regulatory requirement) may be identified by adding modifier 32 to the basic procedure.

33 **Preventive Services:** When the primary purpose of the service is the delivery of an evidence based service in accordance with a US Preventive Services Task Force A or B rating in effect and other preventive services identified in preventive services mandates (legislative or regulatory), the service may be identified by adding 33 to the procedure. For separately reported services specifically identified as preventive, the modifier should not be used.

47 **Anesthesia by Surgeon:** Regional or general anesthesia provided by the surgeon may be reported by adding modifier 47 to the basic service. (This does not include local anesthesia.)
Note: Modifier 47 would not be used as a modifier for the anesthesia procedures.

50 **Bilateral Procedure:** Unless otherwise identified in the listings, bilateral procedures that are performed at the same session should be identified by adding modifier 50 to the appropriate 5 digit code.
Note: This modifier should not be appended to designated "add-on" codes (see Appendix F).

51 **Multiple Procedures:** When multiple procedures, other than E/M services, Physical Medicine and Rehabilitation services or provision of supplies (eg, vaccines), are performed at the same session by the same individual, the primary procedure or service may be reported as listed. The additional procedure(s) or service(s) may be identified by appending modifier 51 to the additional procedure or service code(s).
Note: This modifier should not be appended to designated "add-on" codes (see Appendix F).

52 **Reduced Services:** Under certain circumstances a service or procedure is partially reduced or eliminated at the discretion of the physician or other qualified health care professional. Under these circumstances the service provided can be identified by its usual procedure number and the addition of modifier 52, signifying that the service is reduced. This provides a means of reporting reduced services without disturbing the identification of the basic service.
Note: For hospital outpatient reporting of a previously scheduled procedure/service that is partially reduced or cancelled as a result of extenuating circumstances or those that threaten the well-being of the patient prior to or after administration of anesthesia, see modifiers 73 and 74 (see modifiers approved for ASC hospital outpatient use).

53 **Discontinued Procedure:** Under certain circumstances, the physician or other qualified health care professional may elect to terminate a surgical or diagnostic procedure. Due to extenuating circumstances or those that threaten the well being of the patient, it may be necessary to indicate that a surgical or diagnostic procedure was started but discontinued. This circumstance may be reported by adding modifier 53 to the code reported by the physician for the discontinued procedure.
Note: This modifier is not used to report the elective cancellation of a procedure prior to the patient's anesthesia induction and/or surgical preparation in the operating suite. For outpatient hospital/ambulatory surgery center (ASC) reporting of a previously scheduled procedure/service that is partially reduced or cancelled as a result of extenuating circumstances or those that threaten the well being of the patient prior to or after administration of anesthesia, see modifiers 73 and 74 (see modifiers approved for ASC hospital outpatient use).

54 **Surgical Care Only:** When 1 physician or other qualified health care professional performs a surgical procedure and another provides preoperative and/or postoperative management, surgical services may be identified by adding modifier 54 to the usual procedure number.

55 **Postoperative Management Only:** When 1 physician or other qualified health care professional performed the postoperative management and another performed the surgical procedure, the postoperative component may be identified by adding modifier 55 to the usual procedure number.

56 **Preoperative Management Only:** When 1 physician or other qualified health care professional performed the preoperative care and evaluation and another performed the surgical procedure, the preoperative component may be identified by adding modifier 56 to the usual procedure number.

57 **Decision for Surgery:** An evaluation and management service that resulted in the initial decision to perform the surgery may be identified by adding modifier 57 to the appropriate level of E/M service.

58 Staged or Related Procedure or Service by the Same Physician or Other Qualified Health Care Professional During the Postoperative Period: It may be necessary to indicate that the performance of a procedure or service during the postoperative period was (a) planned or anticipated (staged); (b) more extensive than the original procedure; or (c) for therapy following a surgical procedure. This circumstance may be reported by adding modifier 58 to the staged or related procedure.
Note: For treatment of a problem that requires a return to the operating/procedure room (eg, unanticipated clinical condition), see modifier 78.

59 Distinct Procedural Service: Under certain circumstances, it may be necessary to indicate that a procedure or service was distinct or independent from other non-E/M services performed on the same day. Modifier 59 is used to identify procedures/services, other than E/M services, that are not normally reported together but are appropriate under the circumstances. Documentation must support a different session, different procedure or surgery, different site or organ system, separate incision/excision, separate lesion, or separate injury (or area of injury in extensive injuries) not ordinarily encountered or performed on the same day by the same individual. However, when another already established modifier is appropriate it should be used rather than modifier 59. Only if no more descriptive modifier is available, and the use of modifier 59 best explains the circumstances, should modifier 59 be used.
Note: Modifier 59 should not be appended to an E/M service. To report a separate and distinct E/M service with a non-E/M service performed on the same date, see modifier 25.

62 Two Surgeons: When 2 surgeons work together as primary surgeons performing distinct part(s) of a procedure, each surgeon should report his/her distinct operative work by adding modifier 62 to the procedure code and any associated add-on code(s) for that procedure as long as both surgeons continue to work together as primary surgeons. Each surgeon should report the co-surgery once using the same procedure code. If additional procedure(s) (including add-on procedure[s]) are performed during the same surgical session, separate code(s) may also be reported with modifier 62 added.
Note: If a co-surgeon acts as an assistant in the performance of additional procedure(s), other than those reported with the modifier 62, during the same surgical session, those services may be reported using separate procedure code(s) with modifier 80 or modifier 82 added, as appropriate.

63 Procedure Performed on Infants less than 4 kg: Procedures performed on neonates and infants up to a present body weight of 4 kg may involve significantly increased complexity and physician or other qualified health care professional work commonly associated with these patients. This circumstance may be reported by adding modifier 63 to the procedure number.
Note: Unless otherwise designated, this modifier may only be appended to procedures/services listed in the 20100-69990 code series and 92920, 92928, 92953, 92960, 92986, 92987, 92990, 92997, 92998, 93312, 93313, 93314, 93315, 93316, 93317, 93318, 93452, 93505, 93530, 93531, 93532, 93533, 93561, 93562, 93563, 93564, 93568, 93580, 93582, 93590, 93591, 93592, 93615, 93616 from the Medicine/Cardiovascular section.

Modifier 63 should not be appended to any CPT codes listed in the Evaluation and Management Services, Anesthesia, Radiology, Pathology/Laboratory, or Medicine sections (other than those identified above from the Medicine/Cardiovascular section).

66 Surgical Team: Under some circumstances, highly complex procedures (requiring the concomitant services of several physicians or other qualified health care professionals, often of different specialties, plus other highly skilled, specially trained personnel, various types of complex equipment) are carried out under the "surgical team" concept. Such circumstances may be identified by each participating individual with the addition of modifier 66 to the basic procedure number used for reporting services.

76 Repeat Procedure or Service by Same Physician or Other Qualified Health Care Professional: It may be necessary to indicate that a procedure or service was repeated by the same physician or other qualified health care professional subsequent to the original procedure or service. This circumstance may be reported by adding modifier 76 to the repeated procedure or service.
Note: This modifier should not be appended to an E/M service.

77 Repeat Procedure by Another Physician or Other Qualified Health Care Professional: It may be necessary to indicate that a basic procedure or service was repeated by another physician or other qualified health care professional subsequent to the original procedure or service. This circumstance may be reported by adding modifier 77 to the repeated procedure or service.
Note: This modifier should not be appended to an E/M service.

78 Unplanned Return to the Operating/Procedure Room by the Same Physician or Other Qualified Health Care Professional Following Initial Procedure for a Related Procedure During the Postoperative Period: It may be necessary to indicate that another procedure was performed during the postoperative period of the initial procedure (unplanned procedure following initial procedure). When this procedure is related to the first, and requires the use of an operating/procedure room, it may be reported by adding modifier 78 to the related procedure. (For repeat procedures, see modifier 76.)

79 Unrelated Procedure or Service by the Same Physician or Other Qualified Health Care Professional During the Postoperative Period: The individual may need to indicate that the performance of a procedure or service during the postoperative period was unrelated to the original procedure. This circumstance may be reported by using modifier 79. (For repeat procedures on the same day, see modifier 76.)

80 Assistant Surgeon: Surgical assistant services may be identified by adding modifier 80 to the usual procedure number(s).

81 Minimum Assistant Surgeon: Minimum surgical assistant services are identified by adding modifier 81 to the usual procedure number.

82 Assistant Surgeon (when qualified resident surgeon not available): The unavailability of a qualified resident surgeon is a prerequisite for use of modifier 82 appended to the usual procedure code number(s).

90 Reference (Outside) Laboratory: When laboratory procedures are performed by a party other than the treating or reporting physician or other qualified health care professional, the procedure may be identified by adding modifier 90 to the usual procedure number.

91 Repeat Clinical Diagnostic Laboratory Test: In the course of treatment of the patient, it may be necessary to repeat the same laboratory test on the same day to obtain subsequent (multiple) test results. Under these circumstances, the laboratory test performed can be identified by its usual procedure number and the addition of modifier 91.
Note: This modifier may not be used when tests are rerun to confirm initial results; due to testing problems with specimens or equipment; or for any other reason when a normal, one-time, reportable result is all that is required. This modifier may not be used when other code(s) describe a series of test results (eg, glucose tolerance tests, evocative/suppression testing). This modifier may only be used for laboratory test(s) performed more than once on the same day on the same patient.

92 Alternative Laboratory Platform Testing: When laboratory testing is being performed using a kit or transportable instrument that wholly or in part consists of a single use, disposable analytical chamber, the service may be identified by adding modifier 92 to the usual laboratory procedure code (HIV testing 86701-86703, and 87389). The test does not require permanent dedicated space, hence by its design may be hand carried or transported to the vicinity of the patient for immediate testing at that site, although location of the testing is not in itself determinative of the use of this modifier.

95 **Synchronous Telemedicine Service Rendered Via a Real-Time Interactive Audio and Video Telecommunications System:** Synchronous telemedicine service is defined as a **real-time** interaction between a physician or other qualified health care professional and a patient who is located at a distant site from the physician or other qualified health care professional. The totality of the communication of information exchanged between the physician or other qualified health care professional and patient during the course of the synchronous telemedicine service must be of an amount and nature that would be sufficient to meet the key components and/or requirements of the same service when rendered via a face-to-face interaction. Modifier 95 may only be appended to the services listed in Appendix F. Appendix F is the list of CPT codes for services that are typically performed face-to-face, but may be rendered via real-time (synchronous) interactive audio and video telecommunications system.

96 **Habilitative Services:** When a service or procedure that may be either habilitative or rehabilitative in nature is provided for habilitative purposes, the physician or other qualified health care professional may add modifier 96 to the service or procedure code to indicate that the service or procedure provided was a habilitative service. Habilitative services help an individual learn skills and functioning for daily living that the individual has not yet developed, and then keep and/or improve those learned skills. Habilitative services also help an individual keep, learn, or improve skills and functioning for daily living.

97 **Rehabilitative Services:** When a service or procedure that may be either habilitative or rehabilitative in nature is provided for rehabilitative purposes, the physician or other qualified health care professional may add modifier 97 to the service or procedure code to indicate that the service or procedure provided was a rehabilitative service. Rehabilitative services help an individual keep, get back, or improve skills and functioning for daily living that have been lost or impaired because the individual was sick, hurt, or disabled.

99 **Multiple Modifiers:** Under certain circumstances 2 or more modifiers may be necessary to completely delineate a service. In such situations modifier 99 should be added to the basic procedure, and other applicable modifiers may be listed as part of the description of the service.

Anesthesia Physical Status Modifiers

All anesthesia services are reported by use of the five-digit anesthesia procedure code with the appropriate physical status modifier appended.

Under certain circumstances, when other modifier(s) are appropriate, they should be reported in addition to the physical status modifier.

P1 A normal healthy patient

P2 A patient with mild systemic disease

P3 A patient with severe systemic disease

P4 A patient with severe systemic disease that is a constant threat to life

P5 A moribund patient who is not expected to survive without the operation

P6 A declared brain-dead patient whose organs are being removed for donor purposes

Modifiers Approved for Ambulatory Surgery Center (ASC) Hospital Outpatient Use

CPT Level I Modifiers

25 **Significant, Separately Identifiable Evaluation and Management Service by the Same Physician or Other Qualified Health Care Professional on the Same Day of the Procedure or Other Service:** It may be necessary to indicate that on the day a procedure or service identified by a CPT code was performed, the patient's condition required a significant, separately identifiable E/M service above and beyond the other service provided or beyond the usual preoperative and postoperative care associated with the procedure that was performed. A significant, separately identifiable E/M service is defined or substantiated by documentation that satisfies the relevant criteria for the respective E/M service to be reported (see Evaluation and Management Services Guidelines for instructions on determining level of E/M service). The E/M service may be prompted by the symptom or condition for which the procedure and/or service was provided. As such, different diagnoses are not required for reporting of the E/M services on the same date. This circumstance may be reported by adding modifier 25 to the appropriate level of E/M service.
Note: This modifier is not used to report an E/M service that resulted in a decision to perform surgery. See modifier 57. For significant, separately identifiable non-E/M services, see modifier 59.

27 **Multiple Outpatient Hospital E/M Encounters on the Same Date:** For hospital outpatient reporting purposes, utilization of hospital resources related to separate and distinct E/M encounters performed in multiple outpatient hospital settings on the same date may be reported by adding modifier 27 to each appropriate level outpatient and/or emergency department E/M code(s). This modifier provides a means of reporting circumstances involving evaluation and management services provided by a physician(s) in more than one (multiple) outpatient hospital setting(s) (eg, hospital emergency department, clinic).
Note: This modifier is not to be used for physician reporting of multiple E/M services performed by the same physician on the same date. For physician reporting of all outpatient evaluation and management services provided by the same physician on the same date and performed in multiple outpatient settings (eg, hospital emergency department, clinic), see Evaluation and Management, Emergency Department, or Preventive Medicine Services codes.

33 **Preventive Services:** When the primary purpose of the service is the delivery of an evidence based service in accordance with a US Preventive Services Task Force A or B rating in effect and other preventive services identified in preventive services mandates (legislative or regulatory), the service may be identified by adding 33 to the procedure. For separately reported services specifically identified as preventive, the modifier should not be used.

50 **Bilateral Procedure:** Unless otherwise identified in the listings, bilateral procedures that are performed at the same session should be identified by adding modifier 50 to the appropriate 5 digit code.
Note: This modifier should not be appended to designated "add-on" codes (see appendix F).

52 **Reduced Services:** Under certain circumstances a service or procedure is partially reduced or eliminated at the discretion of the physician or other qualified health care professional. Under these circumstances the service provided can be identified by its usual procedure number and the addition of modifier 52, signifying that the service is reduced. This provides a means of reporting reduced services without disturbing the identification of the basic service.
Note: For hospital outpatient reporting of a previously scheduled procedure/service that is partially reduced or cancelled as a result of extenuating circumstances or those that threaten the well-being of the patient prior to or after administration of anesthesia, see modifiers 73 and 74 (see modifiers approved for ASC hospital outpatient use).

58 **Staged or Related Procedure or Service by the Same Physician or Other Qualified Health Care Professional During the Postoperative Period:** It may be necessary to indicate that the performance of a procedure or service during the postoperative period was (a) planned or anticipated (staged); (b) more extensive than the original procedure; or (c) for therapy following a surgical procedure. This circumstance may be reported by adding modifier 58 to the staged or related procedure.
Note: For treatment of a problem that requires a return to the operating or procedure room (eg, unanticipated clinical condition), see modifier 78.

59 **Distinct Procedural Service:** Under certain circumstances, it may be necessary to indicate that a procedure or service was distinct or independent from other non-E/M services performed on the same day. Modifier 59 is used to identify procedures/services, other than E/M services, that are not normally reported together but are appropriate under the circumstances. Documentation must support a different session, different procedure or surgery,

different site or organ system, separate incision/excision, separate lesion, or separate injury (or area of injury in extensive injuries) not ordinarily encountered or performed on the same day by the same individual. However, when another already established modifier is appropriate it should be used rather than modifier 59. Only if no more descriptive modifier is available, and the use of modifier 59 best explains the circumstances, should modifier 59 be used.
Note: Modifier 59 should not be appended to an E/M service. To report a separate and distinct E/M service with a non-E/M service performed on the same date, see modifier 25.

73 Discontinued Out-Patient Hospital/Ambulatory Surgery Center (ASC) Procedure Prior to the Administration of Anesthesia: Due to extenuating circumstances or those that threaten the well being of the patient, the physician may cancel a surgical or diagnostic procedure subsequent to the patient's surgical preparation (including sedation when provided, and being taken to the room where the procedure is to be performed), but prior to the administration of anesthesia (local, regional block(s) or general). Under these circumstances, the intended service that is prepared for but cancelled can be reported by its usual procedure number and the addition of modifier 73.
Note: The elective cancellation of a service prior to the administration of anesthesia and/or surgical preparation of the patient should not be reported. For physician reporting of a discontinued procedure, see modifier 53.

74 Discontinued Out-Patient Hospital/Ambulatory Surgery Center (ASC) Procedure After Administration of Anesthesia: Due to extenuating circumstances or those that threaten the well being of the patient, the physician may terminate a surgical or diagnostic procedure after the administration of anesthesia (local, regional block(s), general) or after the procedure was started (incision made, intubation started, scope inserted, etc.). Under these circumstances, the procedure started but terminated can be reported by its usual procedure number and the addition of modifier 74.
Note: The elective cancellation of a service prior to the administration of anesthesia and/or surgical preparation of the patient should not be reported. For physician reporting of a discontinued procedure, see modifier 53.

76 Repeat Procedure or Service by Same Physician or Other Qualified Health Care Professional: It may be necessary to indicate that a procedure or service was repeated by the same physician or other qualified health care professional subsequent to the original procedure or service. This circumstance may be reported by adding modifier 76 to the repeated procedure or service.
Note: This modifier should not be appended to an E/M service.

77 Repeat Procedure by Another Physician or Other Qualified Health Care Professional: It may be necessary to indicate that a basic procedure or service was repeated by another physician or other qualified health care professional subsequent to the original procedure or service. This circumstance may be reported by adding modifier 77 to the repeated procedure or service.
Note: This modifier should not be appended to an E/M service.

78 Unplanned Return to the Operating/Procedure Room by the Same Physician or Other Qualified Health Care Professional Following Initial Procedure for a Related Procedure During the Postoperative Period: It may be necessary to indicate that another procedure was performed during the postoperative period of the initial procedure (unplanned procedure following initial procedure). When this procedure is related to the first, and requires the use of an operating/procedure room, it may be reported by adding modifier 78 to the related procedure. (For repeat procedures, see modifier 76.)

79 Unrelated Procedure or Service by the Same Physician During the Postoperative Period: The individual may need to indicate that the performance of a procedure or service during the postoperative period was unrelated to the original procedure. This circumstance may be reported by using modifier 79. (For repeat procedures on the same day, see modifier 76.)

91 Repeat Clinical Diagnostic Laboratory Test: In the course of treatment of the patient, it may be necessary to repeat the same laboratory test on the same day to obtain subsequent (multiple) test results. Under these circumstances, the laboratory test performed can be identified by its usual procedure number and the addition of modifier 91.
Note: This modifier may not be used when tests are rerun to confirm initial results; due to testing problems with specimens or equipment; or for any other reason when a normal, one-time, reportable result is all that is required. This modifier may not be used when other code(s) describe a series of test results (eg, glucose tolerance tests, evocative/suppression testing). This modifier may only be used for laboratory test(s) performed more than once on the same day on the same patient.

Level II (HCPCS/National) Modifiers

The HCPCS Level II modifiers included here are those most commonly used when coding procedures. See your 2021 HCPCS Level II book for a complete listing.

Anatomical Modifiers

E1 Upper left, eyelid
E2 Lower left, eyelid
E3 Upper right, eyelid
E4 Lower right, eyelid
FA Left hand, thumb
F1 Left hand, second digit
F2 Left hand, third digit
F3 Left hand, fourth digit
F4 Left hand, fifth digit
F5 Right hand, thumb
F6 Right hand, second digit
F7 Right hand, third digit
F8 Right hand, fourth digit
F9 Right hand, fifth digit
LT Left side (used to identify procedures performed on the left side of the body)
RT Right side (used to identify procedures performed on the right side of the body)
TA Left foot, great toe
T1 Left foot, second digit
T2 Left foot, third digit
T3 Left foot, fourth digit
T4 Left foot, fifth digit
T5 Right foot, great toe
T6 Right foot, second digit
T7 Right foot, third digit
T8 Right foot, fourth digit
T9 Right foot, fifth digit

Anesthesia Modifiers

AA Anesthesia services performed personally by anesthesiologist
AD Medical supervision by a physician: more than four concurrent anesthesia procedures
G8 Monitored anesthesia care (MAC) for deep complex, complicated, or markedly invasive surgical procedure
G9 Monitored anesthesia care for patient who has history of severe cardiopulmonary condition
QK Medical direction of two, three, or four concurrent anesthesia procedures involving qualified individuals
QS Monitored anesthesiology care service
QX CRNA service: with medical direction by a physician
QY Medical direction of one certified registered nurse anesthetist (CRNA) by an anesthesiologist
QZ CRNA service: without medical direction by a physician

Coronary Artery Modifiers

LC Left circumflex coronary artery

LD Left anterior descending coronary artery

LM Left main coronary artery

RC Right coronary artery

RI Ramus intermedius coronary artery

Other Modifiers

CT Computed tomography services furnished using equipment that does not meet each of the attributes of the national electrical manufacturers association (NEMA) XR-29-2013 standard

EA Erythropoetic stimulating agent (ESA) administered to treat anemia due to anticancer chemotherapy

EB Erythropoetic stimulating agent (ESA) administered to treat anemia due to anticancer radiotherapy

EC Erythropoetic stimulating agent (ESA) administered to treat anemia not due to anticancer radiotherapy or anticancer chemotherapy

FP Service provided as part of family planning program

FX X-ray taken using film

G7 Pregnancy resulted from rape or incest or pregnancy certified by physician as life threatening

GA Waiver of liability statement issued as required by payer policy, individual case

GG Performance and payment of a screening mammogram and diagnostic mammogram on the same patient, same day

GH Diagnostic mammogram converted from screening mammogram on same day

GQ Via asynchronous telecommunications system

GT Via interactive audio and video telecommunication systems

GU Waiver of liability statement issued as required by payer policy, routine notice

GX Notice of liability issued, voluntary under payer policy

GY Item or service statutorily excluded, does not meet the definition of any Medicare benefit or, for non-Medicare insurers, is not a contract benefit

GZ Item or service expected to be denied as not reasonable and necessary

PI Positron emission tomography (PET) or PET/computed tomography (CT) to inform the initial treatment strategy of tumors that are biopsy proven or strongly suspected of being cancerous based on other diagnostic testing

PS Positron emission tomography (PET) or PET/computed tomography (CT) to inform the subsequent treatment strategy of cancerous tumors when the beneficiary's treating physician determines that the PET study is needed to inform subsequent antitumor strategy

PT Colorectal cancer screening test; converted to diagnostic test or other procedure

Q7 One Class A finding

Q8 Two Class B findings

Q9 One Class B and two Class C findings

QC Single channel monitoring

QM Ambulance service provided under arrangement by a provider of services

QN Ambulance service furnished directly by a provider of services

QW CLIA waived test

TC Technical component; under certain circumstances, a charge may be made for the technical component alone; under those circumstances the technical component charge is identified by adding modifier TC to the usual procedure number; technical component charges are institutional charges and not billed separately by physicians; however, portable x-ray suppliers only bill for technical component and should utilize modifier TC; the charge data from portable x-ray suppliers will then be used to build customary and prevailing profiles

* **XE** Separate encounter, a service that is distinct because it occurred during a separate encounter

* **XP** Separate practitioner, a service that is distinct because it was performed by a different practitioner

* **XS** Separate structure, a service that is distinct because it was performed on a separate organ/structure

* **XU** Unusual nonoverlapping service, the use of a service that is distinct because it does not overlap usual components of the main service

* CMS instituted additional HCPCS modifiers to define explicit subsets of modifier 59 Distinct Procedural Service.

Category II Modifiers

1P Performance Measure Exclusion Modifier due to Medical Reasons

Reasons include:

- Not indicated (absence of organ/limb, already received/performed, other)
- Contraindicated (patient allergic history, potential adverse drug interaction, other)
- Other medical reasons

2P Performance Measure Exclusion Modifier due to Patient Reasons

Reasons include:

- Patient declined
- Economic, social, or religious reasons
- Other patient reasons

3P Performance Measure Exclusion Modifier due to System Reasons

Reasons include:

- Resources to perform the services not available
- Insurance coverage/payor-related limitations
- Other reasons attributable to health care delivery system

Modifier 8P is intended to be used as a "reporting modifier" to allow the reporting of circumstances when an action described in a measure's numerator is not performed and the reason is not otherwise specified.

8P Performance measure reporting modifier-action not performed, reason not otherwise specified

Appendix B — New, Revised, and Deleted Codes

New Codes

30468 Repair of nasal valve collapse with subcutaneous/submucosal lateral wall implant(s)

32408 Core needle biopsy, lung or mediastinum, percutaneous, including imaging guidance, when performed

33741 Transcatheter atrial septostomy (TAS) for congenital cardiac anomalies to create effective atrial flow, including all imaging guidance by the proceduralist, when performed, any method (eg, Rashkind, Sang-Park, balloon, cutting balloon, blade)

33745 Transcatheter intracardiac shunt (TIS) creation by stent placement for congenital cardiac anomalies to establish effective intracardiac flow, including all imaging guidance by the proceduralist, when performed, left and right heart diagnostic cardiac catherization for congenital cardiac anomalies, and target zone angioplasty, when performed (eg, atrial septum, Fontan fenestration, right ventricular outflow tract, Mustard/Senning/Warden baffles); initial intracardiac shunt

33746 each additional intracardiac shunt location (List separately in addition to code for primary procedure)

33995 Insertion of ventricular assist device, percutaneous, including radiological supervision and interpretation; right heart, venous access only

33997 Removal of percutaneous right heart ventricular assist device, venous cannula, at separate and distinct session from insertion

55880 Ablation of malignant prostate tissue, transrectal, with high intensity-focused ultrasound (HIFU), including ultrasound guidance

57465 Computer-aided mapping of cervix uteri during colposcopy, including optical dynamic spectral imaging and algorithmic quantification of the acetowhitening effect (List separately in addition to code for primary procedure)

69705 Nasopharyngoscopy, surgical, with dilation of eustachian tube (ie, balloon dilation); unilateral

69706 bilateral

71271 Computed tomography, thorax, low dose for lung cancer screening, without contrast material(s)

76145 Medical physics dose evaluation for radiation exposure that exceeds institutional review threshold, including report

80143 Acetaminophen

80151 Amiodarone

80161 -10,11-epoxide

80167 Felbamate

80179 Salicylate

80181 Flecainide

80189 Itraconazole

80193 Leflunomide

80204 Methotrexate

80210 Rufinamide

81168 CCND1/IGH (t(11;14)) (eg, mantle cell lymphoma) translocation analysis, major breakpoint, qualitative and quantitative, if performed

81191 NTRK1 (neurotrophic receptor tyrosine kinase 1) (eg, solid tumors) translocation analysis

81192 NTRK2 (neurotrophic receptor tyrosine kinase 2) (eg, solid tumors) translocation analysis

81193 NTRK3 (neurotrophic receptor tyrosine kinase 3) (eg, solid tumors) translocation analysis

81194 NTRK (neurotrophic-tropomyosin receptor tyrosine kinase 1, 2, and 3) (eg, solid tumors) translocation analysis

81278 IGH@/BCL2 (t(14;18)) (eg, follicular lymphoma) translocation analysis, major breakpoint region (MBR) and minor cluster region (mcr) breakpoints, qualitative or quantitative

81279 JAK2 (Janus kinase 2) (eg, myeloproliferative disorder) targeted sequence analysis (eg, exons 12 and 13)

81338 MPL (MPL proto-oncogene, thrombopoietin receptor) (eg, myeloproliferative disorder) gene analysis; common variants (eg, W515A, W515K, W515L, W515R)

81339 sequence analysis, exon 10

81347 SF3B1 (splicing factor [3b] subunit B1) (eg, myelodysplastic syndrome/acute myeloid leukemia) gene analysis, common variants (eg, A672T, E622D, L833F, R625C, R625L)

81348 SRSF2 (serine and arginine-rich splicing factor 2) (eg, myelodysplastic syndrome, acute myeloid leukemia) gene analysis, common variants (eg, P95H, P95L)

81351 TP53 (tumor protein 53) (eg, Li-Fraumeni syndrome) gene analysis; full gene sequence

81352 targeted sequence analysis (eg, 4 oncology)

81353 known familial variant

81357 U2AF1 (U2 small nuclear RNA auxiliary factor 1) (eg, myelodysplastic syndrome, acute myeloid leukemia) gene analysis, common variants (eg, S34F, S34Y, Q157R, Q157P)

81360 ZRSR2 (zinc finger CCCH-type, RNA binding motif and serine/arginine-rich 2) (eg, myelodysplastic syndrome, acute myeloid leukemia) gene analysis, common variant(s) (eg, E65fs, E122fs, R448fs)

81419 Epilepsy genomic sequence analysis panel, must include analyses for ALDH7A1, CACNA1A, CDKL5, CHD2, GABRG2, GRIN2A, KCNQ2, MECP2, PCDH19, POLG, PRRT2, SCN1A, SCN1B, SCN2A, SCN8A, SLC2A1, SLC9A6, STXBP1, SYNGAP1, TCF4, TPP1, TSC1, TSC2, and ZEB2

81513 Infectious disease, bacterial vaginosis, quantitative real-time amplification of RNA markers for Atopobium vaginae, Gardnerella vaginalis, and Lactobacillus species, utilizing vaginal-fluid specimens, algorithm reported as a positive or negative result for bacterial vaginosis

81514 Infectious disease, bacterial vaginosis and vaginitis, quantitative real-time amplification of DNA markers for Gardnerella vaginalis, Atopobium vaginae, Megasphaera type 1, Bacterial Vaginosis Associated Bacteria-2 (BVAB-2), and Lactobacillus species (L. crispatus and L. jensenii), utilizing vaginal-fluid specimens, algorithm reported as a positive or negative for high likelihood of bacterial vaginosis, includes separate detection of Trichomonas vaginalis and/or Candida species (C. albicans, C. tropicalis, C. parapsilosis, C. dubliniensis), Candida glabrata, Candida krusei, when reported

81529 Oncology (cutaneous melanoma), mRNA, gene expression profiling by real-time RT-PCR of 31 genes (28 content and 3 housekeeping), utilizing formalin-fixed paraffin-embedded tissue, algorithm reported as recurrence risk, including likelihood of sentinel lymph node metastasis

81546 Oncology (thyroid), mRNA, gene expression analysis of 10,196 genes, utilizing fine needle aspirate, algorithm reported as a categorical result (eg, benign or suspicious)

81554 Pulmonary disease (idiopathic pulmonary fibrosis [IPF]), mRNA, gene expression analysis of 190 genes, utilizing transbronchial biopsies, diagnostic algorithm reported as categorical result (eg, positive or negative for high probability of usual interstitial pneumonia [UIP])

82077 Alcohol (ethanol); any specimen except urine and breath, immunoassay (eg, IA, EIA, ELISA, RIA, EMIT, FPIA) and enzymatic methods (eg, alcohol dehydrogenase)

82681 Estradiol; free, direct measurement (eg, equilibrium dialysis)

86328 Immunoassay for infectious agent antibody(ies), qualitative or semiquantitative, single-step method (eg, reagent strip); severe acute respiratory syndrome coronavirus 2 (SARS-CoV-2) (Coronavirus disease [COVID-19])

86769 Antibody; severe acute respiratory syndrome coronavirus 2 (SARS-CoV-2) (Coronavirus disease [COVID-19])

87635 Infectious agent detection by nucleic acid (DNA or RNA); severe acute respiratory syndrome coronavirus 2 (SARS-CoV-2) (Coronavirus disease [COVID-19]), amplified probe technique

90377 Rabies immune globulin, heat- and solvent/detergent-treated (RIg-HT S/D), human, for intramuscular and/or subcutaneous use

92229 Imaging of retina for detection or monitoring of disease; point-of-care automated analysis and report, unilateral or bilateral

92517 Vestibular evoked myogenic potential (VEMP) testing, with interpretation and report; cervical (cVEMP)

92518 ocular (oVEMP)

92519 cervical (cVEMP) and ocular (oVEMP)

92650 Auditory evoked potentials; screening of auditory potential with broadband stimuli, automated analysis

92651 for hearing status determination, broadband stimuli, with interpretation and report

92652 for threshold estimation at multiple frequencies, with interpretation and report

92653 neurodiagnostic, with interpretation and report

93241 External electrocardiographic recording for more than 48 hours up to 7 days by continuous rhythm recording and storage; includes recording, scanning analysis with report, review and interpretation

93242 recording (includes connection and initial recording)

93243 scanning analysis with report

93244 review and interpretation

93245 External electrocardiographic recording for more than 7 days up to 15 days by continuous rhythm recording and storage; includes recording, scanning analysis with report, review and interpretation

93246 recording (includes connection and initial recording)

93247 scanning analysis with report

93248 review and interpretation

94619 Exercise test for bronchospasm, including pre- and post-spirometry and pulse oximetry; without electrocardiographic recording(s)

99417 Prolonged office or other outpatient evaluation and management service(s) beyond the minimum required time of the primary procedure which has been selected using total time, requiring total time with or without direct patient contact beyond the usual service, on the date of the primary service, each 15 minutes of total time (List separately in addition to codes 99205, 99215 for office or other outpatient Evaluation and Management services)

99439 Chronic care management services with the following required elements: multiple (two or more) chronic conditions expected to last at least 12 months, or until the death of the patient, chronic conditions place the patient at significant risk of death, acute exacerbation/decompensation, or functional decline, comprehensive care plan established, implemented, revised, or monitored; each additional 20 minutes of clinical staff time directed by a physician or other qualified health care professional, per calendar month (List separately in addition to code for primary procedure)

0139U Neurology (autism spectrum disorder [ASD]), quantitative measurements of 6 central carbon metabolites (ie, α-ketoglutarate, alanine, lactate, phenylalanine, pyruvate, and succinate), LC-MS/MS, plasma, algorithmic analysis with result reported as negative or positive (with metabolic subtypes of ASD)

0140U Infectious disease (fungi), fungal pathogen identification, DNA (15 fungal targets), blood culture, amplified probe technique, each target reported as detected or not detected

0141U Infectious disease (bacteria and fungi), gram-positive organism identification and drug resistance element detection, DNA (20 gram-positive bacterial targets, 4 resistance genes, 1 pan gram-negative bacterial target, 1 pan Candida target), blood culture, amplified probe technique, each target reported as detected or not detected

0142U Infectious disease (bacteria and fungi), gram-negative bacterial identification and drug resistance element detection, DNA (21 gram-negative bacterial targets, 6 resistance genes, 1 pan gram-positive bacterial target, 1 pan Candida target), amplified probe technique, each target reported as detected or not detected

0143U Drug assay, definitive, 120 or more drugs or metabolites, urine, quantitative liquid chromatography with tandem mass spectrometry (LC-MS/MS) using multiple reaction monitoring (MRM), with drug or metabolite description, comments including sample validation, per date of service

0144U Drug assay, definitive, 160 or more drugs or metabolites, urine, quantitative liquid chromatography with tandem mass spectrometry (LC-MS/MS) using multiple reaction monitoring (MRM), with drug or metabolite description, comments including sample validation, per date of service

0145U Drug assay, definitive, 65 or more drugs or metabolites, urine, quantitative liquid chromatography with tandem mass spectrometry (LC-MS/MS) using multiple reaction monitoring (MRM), with drug or metabolite description, comments including sample validation, per date of service

0146U Drug assay, definitive, 80 or more drugs or metabolites, urine, by quantitative liquid chromatography with tandem mass spectrometry (LC-MS/MS) using multiple reaction monitoring (MRM), with drug or metabolite description, comments including sample validation, per date of service

0147U Drug assay, definitive, 85 or more drugs or metabolites, urine, quantitative liquid chromatography with tandem mass spectrometry (LC-MS/MS) using multiple reaction monitoring (MRM), with drug or metabolite description, comments including sample validation, per date of service

0148U Drug assay, definitive, 100 or more drugs or metabolites, urine, quantitative liquid chromatography with tandem mass spectrometry (LC-MS/MS) using multiple reaction monitoring (MRM), with drug or metabolite description, comments including sample validation, per date of service

0149U Drug assay, definitive, 60 or more drugs or metabolites, urine, quantitative liquid chromatography with tandem mass spectrometry (LC-MS/MS) using multiple reaction monitoring (MRM), with drug or metabolite description, comments including sample validation, per date of service

0150U Drug assay, definitive, 120 or more drugs or metabolites, urine, quantitative liquid chromatography with tandem mass spectrometry (LC-MS/MS) using multiple reaction monitoring (MRM), with drug or metabolite description, comments including sample validation, per date of service

0151U Infectious disease (bacterial or viral respiratory tract infection), pathogen specific nucleic acid (DNA or RNA), 33 targets, real-time semi-quantitative PCR, bronchoalveolar lavage, sputum, or endotracheal aspirate, detection of 33 organismal and antibiotic resistance genes with limited semi-quantitative results

0153U Oncology (breast), mRNA, gene expression profiling by next-generation sequencing of 101 genes, utilizing formalin-fixed paraffin-embedded tissue, algorithm reported as a triple negative breast cancer clinical subtype(s) with information on immune cell involvement

0156U Copy number (eg, intellectual disability, dysmorphology), sequence analysis

0157U APC (APC regulator of WNT signaling pathway) (eg, familial adenomatosis polyposis [FAP]) mRNA sequence analysis (List separately in addition to code for primary procedure)

0158U MLH1 (mutL homolog 1) (eg, hereditary non-polyposis colorectal cancer, Lynch syndrome) mRNA sequence analysis (List separately in addition to code for primary procedure)

0159U MSH2 (mutS homolog 2) (eg, hereditary colon cancer, Lynch syndrome) mRNA sequence analysis (List separately in addition to code for primary procedure)

0160U MSH6 (mutS homolog 6) (eg, hereditary colon cancer, Lynch syndrome) mRNA sequence analysis (List separately in addition to code for primary procedure)

0161U PMS2 (PMS1 homolog 2, mismatch repair system component) (eg, hereditary non-polyposis colorectal cancer, Lynch syndrome) mRNA sequence analysis (List separately in addition to code for primary procedure)

0162U Hereditary colon cancer (Lynch syndrome), targeted mRNA sequence analysis panel (MLH1, MSH2, MSH6, PMS2) (List separately in addition to code for primary procedure)

0163U Oncology (colorectal) screening, biochemical enzyme-linked immunosorbent assay (ELISA) of 3 plasma or serum proteins (teratocarcinoma derived growth factor-1 [TDGF-1, Cripto-1], carcinoembryonic antigen [CEA], extracellular matrix protein [ECM]), with demographic data (age, gender, CRC-screening compliance) using a proprietary algorithm and reported as likelihood of CRC or advanced adenomas

0164U Gastroenterology (irritable bowel syndrome [IBS]), immunoassay for anti-CdtB and anti-vinculin antibodies, utilizing plasma, algorithm for elevated or not elevated qualitative results

0166U Liver disease, 10 biochemical assays (α2-macroglobulin, haptoglobin, apolipoprotein A1, bilirubin, GGT, ALT, AST, triglycerides, cholesterol, fasting glucose) and biometric and demographic data, utilizing serum, algorithm reported as scores for fibrosis, necroinflammatory activity, and steatosis with a summary interpretation

0167U Gonadotropin, chorionic (hCG), immunoassay with direct optical observation, blood

0168U Fetal aneuploidy (trisomy 21, 18, and 13) DNA sequence analysis of selected regions using maternal plasma without fetal fraction cutoff, algorithm reported as a risk score for each trisomy

0169U NUDT15 (nudix hydrolase 15) and TPMT (thiopurine S-methyltransferase) (eg, drug metabolism) gene analysis, common variants

0170U Neurology (autism spectrum disorder [ASD]), RNA, next-generation sequencing, saliva, algorithmic analysis, and results reported as predictive probability of ASD diagnosis

0171U Targeted genomic sequence analysis panel, acute myeloid leukemia, myelodysplastic syndrome, and myeloproliferative neoplasms, DNA analysis, 23 genes, interrogation for sequence variants, rearrangements and minimal residual disease, reported as presence/absence

0172U Oncology (solid tumor as indicated by the label), somatic mutation analysis of BRCA1 (BRCA1, DNA repair associated), BRCA2 (BRCA2, DNA repair associated) and analysis of homologous recombination deficiency pathways, DNA, formalin-fixed paraffin-embedded tissue, algorithm quantifying tumor genomic instability score

0173U Psychiatry (ie, depression, anxiety), genomic analysis panel, includes variant analysis of 14 genes

0174U Oncology (solid tumor), mass spectrometric 30 protein targets, formalin-fixed paraffin-embedded tissue, prognostic and predictive algorithm reported as likely, unlikely, or uncertain benefit of 39 chemotherapy and targeted therapeutic oncology agents

0175U Psychiatry (eg, depression, anxiety), genomic analysis panel, variant analysis of 15 genes

0176U Cytolethal distending toxin B (CdtB) and vinculin IgG antibodies by immunoassay (ie, ELISA)

0177U Oncology (breast cancer), DNA, PIK3CA (phosphatidylinositol-4,5-bisphosphate 3-kinase catalytic subunit alpha) gene analysis of 11 gene variants utilizing plasma, reported as PIK3CA gene mutation status

0178U Peanut allergen-specific quantitative assessment of multiple epitopes using enzyme-linked immunosorbent assay (ELISA), blood, report of minimum eliciting exposure for a clinical reaction

0179U Oncology (non-small cell lung cancer), cell-free DNA, targeted sequence analysis of 23 genes (single nucleotide variations, insertions and deletions, fusions without prior knowledge of partner/breakpoint, copy number variations), with report of significant mutation(s)

0180U Red cell antigen (ABO blood group) genotyping (ABO), gene analysis Sanger/chain termination/conventional sequencing, ABO (ABO, alpha 1-3-N-acetylgalactosaminyltransferase and alpha 1-3-galactosyltransferase) gene, including subtyping, 7 exons

0181U Red cell antigen (Colton blood group) genotyping (CO), gene analysis, AQP1 (aquaporin 1 [Colton blood group]) exon 1

0182U Red cell antigen (Cromer blood group) genotyping (CROM), gene analysis, CD55 (CD55 molecule [Cromer blood group]) exons 1-10

0183U Red cell antigen (Diego blood group) genotyping (DI), gene analysis, SLC4A1 (solute carrier family 4 member 1 [Diego blood group]) exon 19

0184U Red cell antigen (Dombrock blood group) genotyping (DO), gene analysis, ART4 (ADP-ribosyltransferase 4 [Dombrock blood group]) exon 2

0185U Red cell antigen (H blood group) genotyping (FUT1), gene analysis, FUT1 (fucosyltransferase 1 [H blood group]) exon 4

0186U Red cell antigen (H blood group) genotyping (FUT2), gene analysis, FUT2 (fucosyltransferase 2) exon 2

0187U Red cell antigen (Duffy blood group) genotyping (FY), gene analysis, ACKR1 (atypical chemokine receptor 1 [Duffy blood group]) exons 1-2

0188U Red cell antigen (Gerbich blood group) genotyping (GE), gene analysis, GYPC (glycophorin C [Gerbich blood group]) exons 1-4

0189U Red cell antigen (MNS blood group) genotyping (GYPA), gene analysis, GYPA (glycophorin A [MNS blood group]) introns 1, 5, exon 2

0190U Red cell antigen (MNS blood group) genotyping (GYPB), gene analysis, GYPB (glycophorin B [MNS blood group]) introns 1, 5, pseudoexon 3

0191U Red cell antigen (Indian blood group) genotyping (IN), gene analysis, CD44 (CD44 molecule [Indian blood group]) exons 2, 3, 6

0192U Red cell antigen (Kidd blood group) genotyping (JK), gene analysis, SLC14A1 (solute carrier family 14 member 1 [Kidd blood group]) gene promoter, exon 9

0193U Red cell antigen (JR blood group) genotyping (JR), gene analysis, ABCG2 (ATP binding cassette subfamily G member 2 [Junior blood group]) exons 2-26

0194U Red cell antigen (Kell blood group) genotyping (KEL), gene analysis, KEL (Kell metallo-endopeptidase [Kell blood group]) exon 8

0195U KLF1 (Kruppel-like factor 1), targeted sequencing (ie, exon 13)

0196U Red cell antigen (Lutheran blood group) genotyping (LU), gene analysis, BCAM (basal cell adhesion molecule [Lutheran blood group]) exon 3

0197U Red cell antigen (Landsteiner-Wiener blood group) genotyping (LW), gene analysis, ICAM4 (intercellular adhesion molecule 4 [Landsteiner-Wiener blood group]) exon 1

0198U Red cell antigen (RH blood group) genotyping (RHD and RHCE), gene analysis Sanger/chain termination/conventional sequencing, RHD (Rh blood group D antigen) exons 1-10 and RHCE (Rh blood group CcEe antigens) exon 5

0199U Red cell antigen (Scianna blood group) genotyping (SC), gene analysis, ERMAP (erythroblast membrane associated protein [Scianna blood group]) exons 4, 12

0200U Red cell antigen (Kx blood group) genotyping (XK), gene analysis, XK (X-linked Kx blood group) exons 1-3

0201U Red cell antigen (Yt blood group) genotyping (YT), gene analysis, ACHE (acetylcholinesterase [Cartwright blood group]) exon 2

0202U Infectious disease (bacterial or viral respiratory tract infection), pathogen-specific nucleic acid (DNA or RNA), 22 targets including severe acute respiratory syndrome coronavirus 2 (SARS-CoV-2), qualitative RT-PCR, nasopharyngeal swab, each pathogen reported as detected or not detected

0203U Autoimmune (inflammatory bowel disease), mRNA, gene expression profiling by quantitative RT-PCR, 17 genes (15 target and 2 reference genes), whole blood, reported as a continuous risk score and classification of inflammatory bowel disease aggressiveness

0204U Oncology (thyroid), mRNA, gene expression analysis of 593 genes (including BRAF, RAS, RET, PAX8, and NTRK) for sequence variants and rearrangements, utilizing fine needle aspirate, reported as detected or not detected

0205U Ophthalmology (age-related macular degeneration), analysis of 3 gene variants (2 CFH gene, 1 ARMS2 gene), using PCR and MALDI-TOF, buccal swab, reported as positive or negative for neovascular age-related macular-degeneration risk associated with zinc supplements

0206U Neurology (Alzheimer disease); cell aggregation using morphometric imaging and protein kinase C-epsilon (PKCe) concentration in response to amylospheroid treatment by ELISA, cultured skin fibroblasts, each reported as positive or negative for Alzheimer disease

0207U quantitative imaging of phosphorylated ERK1 and ERK2 in response to bradykinin treatment by in situ immunofluorescence, using cultured skin fibroblasts, reported as a probability index for Alzheimer disease (List separately in addition to code for primary procedure)

0208U Oncology (medullary thyroid carcinoma), mRNA, gene expression analysis of 108 genes, utilizing fine needle aspirate, algorithm reported as positive or negative for medullary thyroid carcinoma

0209U Cytogenomic constitutional (genome-wide) analysis, interrogation of genomic regions for copy number, structural changes and areas of homozygosity for chromosomal abnormalities

0210U Syphilis test, non-treponemal antibody, immunoassay, quantitative (RPR)

0211U Oncology (pan-tumor), DNA and RNA by next-generation sequencing, utilizing formalin-fixed paraffin-embedded tissue, interpretative report for single nucleotide variants, copy number alterations, tumor mutational burden, and microsatellite instability, with therapy association

0212U Rare diseases (constitutional/heritable disorders), whole genome and mitochondrial DNA sequence analysis, including small sequence changes, deletions, duplications, short tandem repeat gene expansions, and variants in non-uniquely mappable regions, blood or saliva, identification and categorization of genetic variants, proband

0213U Rare diseases (constitutional/heritable disorders), whole genome and mitochondrial DNA sequence analysis, including small sequence changes, deletions, duplications, short tandem repeat gene expansions, and variants in non-uniquely mappable regions, blood or saliva, identification and categorization of genetic variants, each comparator genome (eg, parent, sibling)

0214U Rare diseases (constitutional/heritable disorders), whole exome and mitochondrial DNA sequence analysis, including small sequence changes, deletions, duplications, short tandem repeat gene expansions, and variants in non-uniquely mappable regions, blood or saliva, identification and categorization of genetic variants, proband

0215U Rare diseases (constitutional/heritable disorders), whole exome and mitochondrial DNA sequence analysis, including small sequence changes, deletions, duplications, short tandem repeat gene expansions, and variants in non-uniquely mappable regions, blood or saliva, identification and categorization of genetic variants, each comparator exome (eg, parent, sibling)

0216U Neurology (inherited ataxias), genomic DNA sequence analysis of 12 common genes including small sequence changes, deletions, duplications, short tandem repeat gene expansions, and variants in non-uniquely mappable regions, blood or saliva, identification and categorization of genetic variants

0217U Neurology (inherited ataxias), genomic DNA sequence analysis of 51 genes including small sequence changes, deletions, duplications, short tandem repeat gene expansions, and variants in non-uniquely mappable regions, blood or saliva, identification and categorization of genetic variants

0218U Neurology (muscular dystrophy), DMD gene sequence analysis, including small sequence changes, deletions, duplications, and variants in non-uniquely mappable regions, blood or saliva, identification and characterization of genetic variants

0219U Infectious agent (human immunodeficiency virus), targeted viral next-generation sequence analysis (ie, protease [PR], reverse transcriptase [RT], integrase [INT]) algorithm reported as prediction of antiviral drug susceptibility

0220U Oncology (breast cancer), image analysis with artificial intelligence assessment of 12 histologic and immunohistochemical features, reported as a recurrence score

0221U Red cell antigen (ABO blood group) genotyping (ABO), gene analysis, next-generation sequencing, ABO (ABO, alpha 1-3-N-acetylgalactosaminyltransferase and alpha 1-3-galactosyltransferase) gene

0222U Red cell antigen (RH blood group) genotyping (RHD and RHCE), gene analysis, next-generation sequencing, RH proximal promoter, exons 1-10, portions of introns 2-3

0594T Osteotomy, humerus, with insertion of an externally controlled intramedullary lengthening device, including intraoperative imaging, initial and subsequent alignment assessments, computations of adjustment schedules, and management of the intramedullary lengthening device

0596T Temporary female intraurethral valve-pump (ie, voiding prosthesis); initial insertion, including urethral measurement

0597T replacement

0598T Noncontact real-time fluorescence wound imaging, for bacterial presence, location, and load, per session; first anatomic site (eg, lower extremity)

0599T each additional anatomic site (eg, upper extremity) (List separately in addition to code for primary procedure)

0600T Ablation, irreversible electroporation; 1 or more tumors per organ, including imaging guidance, when performed, percutaneous

0601T 1 or more tumors per organ, including fluoroscopic and ultrasound guidance, when performed, open

0602T Glomerular filtration rate (GFR) measurement(s), transdermal, including sensor placement and administration of a single dose of fluorescent pyrazine agent

0603T Glomerular filtration rate (GFR) monitoring, transdermal, including sensor placement and administration of more than one dose of fluorescent pyrazine agent, each 24 hours

0604T Optical coherence tomography (OCT) of retina, remote, patient-initiated image capture and transmission to a remote surveillance center, unilateral or bilateral; initial device provision, set-up and patient education on use of equipment

0605T remote surveillance center technical support, data analyses and reports, with a minimum of 8 daily recordings, each 30 days

0606T review, interpretation and report by the prescribing physician or other qualified health care professional of remote surveillance center data analyses, each 30 days

0607T Remote monitoring of an external continuous pulmonary fluid monitoring system, including measurement of radiofrequency-derived pulmonary fluid levels, heart rate, respiration rate, activity, posture, and cardiovascular rhythm (eg, ECG data), transmitted to a remote 24-hour attended surveillance center; set-up and patient education on use of equipment

0608T analysis of data received and transmission of reports to the physician or other qualified health care professional

0609T Magnetic resonance spectroscopy, determination and localization of discogenic pain (cervical, thoracic, or lumbar); acquisition of single voxel data, per disc, on biomarkers (ie, lactic acid, carbohydrate, alanine, laal, propionic acid, proteoglycan, and collagen) in at least 3 discs

0610T transmission of biomarker data for software analysis

0611T postprocessing for algorithmic analysis of biomarker data for determination of relative chemical differences between discs

0612T interpretation and report

0613T Percutaneous transcatheter implantation of interatrial septal shunt device, including right and left heart catheterization, intracardiac echocardiography, and imaging guidance by the proceduralist, when performed

0614T Removal and replacement of substernal implantable defibrillator pulse generator

0615T Eye-movement analysis without spatial calibration, with interpretation and report

0616T Insertion of iris prosthesis, including suture fixation and repair or removal of iris, when performed; without removal of crystalline lens or intraocular lens, without insertion of intraocular lens

0617T with removal of crystalline lens and insertion of intraocular lens

0618T with secondary intraocular lens placement or intraocular lens exchange

0619T Cystourethroscopy with transurethral anterior prostate commissurotomy and drug delivery, including transrectal ultrasound and fluoroscopy, when performed

0620T Endovascular venous arterialization, tibial or peroneal vein, with transcatheter placement of intravascular stent graft(s) and closure by any method, including percutaneous or open vascular access, ultrasound guidance for vascular access when performed, all catheterization(s) and intraprocedural roadmapping and imaging guidance necessary to complete the intervention, all associated radiological supervision and interpretation, when performed

0621T Trabeculostomy ab interno by laser;

0622T with use of ophthalmic endoscope

0623T Automated quantification and characterization of coronary atherosclerotic plaque to assess severity of coronary disease, using data from coronary computed tomographic angiography; data preparation and transmission, computerized analysis of data, with review of computerized analysis output to reconcile discordant data, interpretation and report

0624T data preparation and transmission

0625T computerized analysis of data from coronary computed tomographic angiography

0626T review of computerized analysis output to reconcile discordant data, interpretation and report

0627T Percutaneous injection of allogeneic cellular and/or tissue-based product, intervertebral disc, unilateral or bilateral injection, with fluoroscopic guidance, lumbar; first level

0628T each additional level (List separately in addition to code for primary procedure)

0629T Percutaneous injection of allogeneic cellular and/or tissue-based product, intervertebral disc, unilateral or bilateral injection, with CT guidance, lumbar; first level

0630T each additional level (List separately in addition to code for primary procedure)

0631T Transcutaneous visible light hyperspectral imaging measurement of oxyhemoglobin, deoxyhemoglobin, and tissue oxygenation, with interpretation and report, per extremity

0632T Percutaneous transcatheter ultrasound ablation of nerves innervating the pulmonary arteries, including right heart catheterization, pulmonary artery angiography, and all imaging guidance

0633T Computed tomography, breast, including 3D rendering, when performed, unilateral; without contrast material

0634T with contrast material(s)

0635T without contrast, followed by contrast material(s)

0636T Computed tomography, breast, including 3D rendering, when performed, bilateral; without contrast material(s)

0637T with contrast material(s)

0638T without contrast, followed by contrast material(s)

0639T Wireless skin sensor thermal anisotropy measurement(s) and assessment of flow in cerebrospinal fluid shunt, including ultrasound guidance, when performed

0014M Liver disease, analysis of 3 biomarkers (hyaluronic acid [HA], procollagen III amino terminal peptide [PIIINP], tissue inhibitor of metalloproteinase 1 [TIMP-1]), using immunoassays, utilizing serum, prognostic algorithm reported as a risk score and risk of liver fibrosis and liver-related clinical events within 5 years

0015M Adrenal cortical tumor, biochemical assay of 25 steroid markers, utilizing 24-hour urine specimen and clinical parameters, prognostic algorithm reported as a clinical risk and integrated clinical steroid risk for adrenal cortical carcinoma, adenoma, or other adrenal malignancy

0016M Oncology (bladder), mRNA, microarray gene expression profiling of 209 genes, utilizing formalin-fixed paraffin-embedded tissue, algorithm reported as molecular subtype (luminal, luminal infiltrated, basal, basal claudin-low, neuroendocrine-like)

Revised Codes

11970 Replacement of tissue expander with permanent ~~prosthesis~~ implant

11971 Removal of tissue expander~~(s)~~ without insertion of ~~prosthesis~~ implant

19318 Breast ~~R~~ reduction ~~mammaplasty~~

19325 ~~Mammaplasty, augmentation~~ Breast augmentation with implant~~;~~ ~~with prosthetic implant~~

19328 Removal of intact ~~mammary~~ breast implant

19330 Removal of ~~mammary~~ ruptured breast implant ~~material,~~ including implant contents (eg, saline, silicone gel)

19340 ~~Immediate i~~Insertion of breast implant ~~prosthesis following mastopexy, mastectomy or in reconstruction~~ on same day of mastectomy (ie, immediate)

19342 ~~Delayed i~~Insertion or replacement of breast ~~prosthesis following mastopexy, mastectomy or in reconstruction~~ implant on separate day from mastectomy

19357 ~~Breast reconstruction, immediate or delayed, with tissue expander~~ Tissue expander placement in breast reconstruction, including subsequent expansion(s)

19361 Breast reconstruction; with latissimus dorsi flap~~, without prosthetic implant~~

19364 ~~Breast reconstruction~~ with free flap (eg, fTRAM, DIEP, SIEA, GAP flap)

19367 ~~Breast reconstruction~~ with single-pedicled transverse rectus abdominis myocutaneous (TRAM) flap ~~(TRAM), single pedicle, including closure of donor site;~~

19368 with single-pedicled transverse rectus abdominis myocutaneous (TRAM) flap, requiring separate microvascular anastomosis (supercharging)

19369 with bipedicled transverse rectus abdominis myocutaneous (TRAM) flap ~~Breast reconstruction with transverse rectus abdominis myocutaneous flap (TRAM), double pedicle, including closure of donor site~~

19370 ~~Open periprosthetic~~ Revision of peri-implant capsule, breast, including capsulotomy, capsulorrhaphy, ~~breast~~ and/or partial capsulectomy

19371 Peri~~prosthetic~~-implant capsulectomy, breast, complete, including removal of all intracapsular contents

19380 Revision of reconstructed breast (eg, significant removal of tissue, re-advancement and/or re-inset of flaps in autologous reconstruction or significant capsular revision combined with soft tissue excision in implant-based reconstruction)

29822 Arthroscopy, shoulder, surgical; debridement, limited, 1 or 2 discrete structures (eg, humeral bone, humeral articular cartilage, glenoid bone, glenoid articular cartilage, biceps tendon, biceps anchor complex, labrum, articular capsule, articular side of the rotator cuff, bursal side of the rotator cuff, subacromial bursa, foreign body[ies])

29823 debridement, extensive, 3 or more discrete structures (eg, humeral bone, humeral articular cartilage, glenoid bone, glenoid articular cartilage, biceps tendon, biceps anchor complex, labrum, articular capsule, articular side of the rotator cuff, bursal side of the rotator cuff, subacromial bursa, foreign body[ies])

33990 Insertion of ventricular assist device, percutaneous, including radiological supervision and interpretation; left heart, arterial access only

33991 left heart, both arterial and venous access, with transseptal puncture

Appendix B — New, Revised, and Deleted Codes

33992 Removal of percutaneous left heart ventricular assist device, arterial or arterial and venous cannula(s), at separate and distinct session from insertion

33993 Repositioning of percutaneous right or left heart ventricular assist device with imaging guidance at separate and distinct session from insertion

64455 Injection(s), anesthetic agent(s) and/or steroid; plantar common digital nerve(s) (eg, Morton's neuroma)

64479 transforaminal epidural, with imaging guidance (fluoroscopy or CT), cervical or thoracic, single level

64480 transforaminal epidural, with imaging guidance (fluoroscopy or CT), cervical or thoracic, each additional level (List separately in addition to code for primary procedure)

64483 transforaminal epidural, with imaging guidance (fluoroscopy or CT), lumbar or sacral, single level

64484 transforaminal epidural, with imaging guidance (fluoroscopy or CT), lumbar or sacral, each additional level (List separately in addition to code for primary procedure)

71250 Computed tomography, thorax, diagnostic; without contrast material

71260 with contrast material(s)

71270 without contrast material, followed by contrast material(s) and further sections

74425 Urography, antegrade ~~(pyelostogram, nephrostogram, loopogram)~~, radiological supervision and interpretation

76513 [Ophthalmic ultrasound, diagnostic;] anterior segment ultrasound, immersion (water bath) B-scan or high resolution biomicroscopy, unilateral or bilateral

78130 Red cell survival study~~;~~

80415 estradiol response

81401 Molecular pathology procedure, Level 2 (eg, 2-10 SNPs, 1 methylated variant, or 1 somatic variant [typically using nonsequencing target variant analysis], or detection of a dynamic mutation disorder/triplet repeat) ~~CCND1/IGH (BCL1/IgH, t(11;14)) (eg, mantle cell lymphoma) translocation analysis, major breakpoint, qualitative, and quantitative, if performed ETV6/NTRK3 (t(12;15)) (eg, congenital/infantile fibrosarcoma), translocation analysis, qualitative, and quantitative, if performed~~

81402 Molecular pathology procedure, Level 3 (eg, >10 SNPs, 2-10 methylated variants, or 2-10 somatic variants [typically using non-sequencing target variant analysis], immunoglobulin and T-cell receptor gene rearrangements, duplication/deletion variants of 1 exon, loss of heterozygosity [LOH], uniparental disomy [UPD]) ~~IGH@/BCL2 (t(14;18)) (eg, follicular lymphoma), translocation analysis; major breakpoint region (MBR) and minor cluster region (mcr) breakpoints, qualitative or quantitative MPL (myeloproliferative leukemia virus oncogene, thrombopoietin receptor, TPOR) (eg, myeloproliferative disorder), common variants (eg, W515A, W515K, W515L, W515R)~~

81403 Molecular pathology procedure, Level 4 (eg, analysis of single exon by DNA sequence analysis, analysis of >10 amplicons using multiplex PCR in 2 or more independent reactions, mutation scanning or duplication/deletion variants of 2-5 exons) ~~JAK2 (Janus kinase 2) (eg, myeloproliferative disorder), exon 12 sequence and exon 13 sequence, if performed MPL (myeloproliferative leukemia virus oncogene, thrombopoietin receptor, TPOR) (eg, myeloproliferative disorder), exon 10 sequence~~

81404 Molecular pathology procedure, Level 5 (eg, analysis of 2-5 exons by DNA sequence analysis, mutation scanning or duplication/deletion variants of 6-10 exons, or characterization of a dynamic mutation disorder/triplet repeat by Southern blot analysis) ~~TP53 (tumor protein 53) (eg, tumor samples), targeted sequence analysis of 2-5 exons~~

81405 Molecular pathology procedure, Level 6 (eg, analysis of 6-10 exons by DNA sequence analysis, mutation scanning or duplication/deletion variants of 11-25 exons, regionally targeted cytogenomic array analysis) ~~TP53 (tumor protein 53) (eg, Li-Fraumeni syndrome, tumor samples), full gene sequence or targeted sequence analysis of >5 exons~~

82075 Alcohol (ethanol)~~, breath;~~ breath

82670 Estradiol; total

86318 Immunoassay for infectious agent antibody(ies), qualitative or semiquantitative, single-step method (eg, reagent strip);

0154U Oncology (urothelial cancer), RNA, analysis by real-time RT-PCR of the FGFR3 (fibroblast growth factor receptor 3) gene analysis (ie, p.R248C [c.742C>T], p.S249C [c.746C>G], p.G370C [c.1108G>T], p.Y373C [c.1118A>G], FGFR3-TACC3v1, and FGFR3-TACC3v3), utilizing formalin-fixed paraffin-embedded urothelial cancer tumor tissue, reported as FGFR gene alteration status

0155U Oncology (breast cancer), DNA, *PIK3CA (phosphatidylinositol-4,5-bisphosphate 3-kinase, catalytic subunit alpha)* (eg, breast cancer) gene analysis (ie, p.C420R, p.E542K, p.E545A, p.E545D [g.1635G>T only], p.E545G, p.E545K, p.Q546E, p.Q546R, p.H1047L, p.H1047R, p.H1047Y[UL]), utilizing formalin-fixed paraffin-embedded breast tumor tissue, reported as PIK3CA gene mutation status

0165U Peanut allergen-specific ~~IgE and~~ quantitative assessment of 64 multiple epitopes using enzyme-linked immunosorbent assay (ELISA), blood, individual epitope results and ~~interpretation~~ probability of peanut allergy

92227 ~~Remote imaging~~ Imaging of retina for detection or monitoring of ~~retinal~~ disease ~~(eg, retinopathy in a patient with diabetes) with analysis and report under physician supervision, unilateral or bilateral~~ ; with remote clinical staff review and report, unilateral or bilateral

92228 ~~Remote imaging for monitoring and management of active retinal disease (eg, diabetic retinopathy)~~ with remote physician ~~review~~ or other qualified health care professional interpretation and report, unilateral or bilateral

94617 Exercise test for bronchospasm, including pre- and post-spirometry~~, electrocardiographic recording(s),~~ and pulse oximetry; with electrocardiographic recording(s)

95070 Inhalation bronchial challenge testing (not including necessary pulmonary function tests)~~;~~ , with histamine, methacholine, or similar compounds

99202 Office or other outpatient visit for the evaluation and management of a new patient, which requires ~~these 3 key components:~~ a medically appropriate history and/or examination and straightforward medical decision making. ~~An expanded problem focused history; An expanded problem focused examination; Straightforward medical decision making. Counseling and/or coordination of care with other physicians, other qualified health care professionals~~ When using time for code selection, ~~or agencies are provided consistent with the nature~~ 15-29 minutes of ~~the problem(s) and the patient's and/or family's needs~~ total time is spent on the date of the encounter. ~~Usually, the presenting problem(s) are of low to moderate severity. Typically, 20 minutes are spent face-to-face with the patient and/or family.~~

99203 Office or other outpatient visit for the evaluation and management of a new patient, which requires ~~these 3 key components:~~ a medically appropriate history and/or examination and low level of medical decision making. ~~A detailed history; A detailed examination; Medical decision making of low complexity. Counseling and/or coordination of care with other physicians, other qualified health care professionals~~ When using time for code selection, ~~or agencies are provided consistent with the nature~~ 30-44 minutes of ~~the problem(s) and the patient's and/or family's needs~~ total time is spent on the date of the encounter. ~~Usually, the presenting problem(s) are of moderate severity. Typically, 30 minutes are spent face-to-face with the patient and/or family.~~

99204 Office or other outpatient visit for the evaluation and management of a new patient, which requires ~~these 3 key components:~~ a medically appropriate history and/or examination and moderate level of medical decision making. ~~A comprehensive history; A comprehensive examination; Medical decision making of moderate complexity. Counseling and/or coordination of care with other physicians, other qualified health care professionals~~ When using time for code selection, ~~or agencies are provided consistent with the nature~~ 45-59 minutes of ~~the problem(s) and the patient's~~

~~and/or family's needs~~ total time is spent on the date of the encounter. ~~Usually, the presenting problem(s) are of moderate to high severity. Typically, 45 minutes are spent face-to-face with the patient and/or family.~~

99205 Office or other outpatient visit for the evaluation and management of a new patient, which requires ~~these 3 key components:~~ a medically appropriate history and/or examination and high level of medical decision making. ~~A comprehensive history; A comprehensive examination; Medical decision making of high complexity. Counseling and/or coordination of care with other physicians, other qualified health care professionals~~ When using time for code selection, ~~or agencies are provided consistent with the nature~~ 60-74 minutes of ~~the problem(s) and the patient's and/or family's needs~~ total time is spent on the date of the encounter. ~~Usually, the presenting problem(s) are of moderate to high severity. Typically, 60 minutes are spent face-to-face with the patient and/or family~~

99211 Office or other outpatient visit for the evaluation and management of an established patient, that may not require the presence of a physician or other qualified health care professional. Usually, the presenting problem(s) are minimal.~~ Typically, 5 minutes are spent performing or supervising these services~~

99212 Office or other outpatient visit for the evaluation and management of an established patient, which requires a~~t least 2 of these 3 key components:~~ medically appropriate history and/or examination and straightforward medical decision making. ~~A problem focused history; A problem focused examination; Straightforward medical decision making. Counseling and/or coordination of care with other physicians, other qualified health care professionals~~ When using time for code selection, ~~or agencies are provided consistent with the nature~~ 10-19 minutes of ~~the problem(s) and the patient's and/or family's needs~~ total time is spent on the date of the encounter. ~~Usually, the presenting problem(s) are self limited or minor. Typically, 10 minutes are spent face-to-face with the patient and/or family.~~

99213 Office or other outpatient visit for the evaluation and management of an established patient, which requires a~~t least 2 of these 3 key components:~~ medically appropriate history and/or examination and low level of medical decision making. ~~An expanded problem focused history; An expanded problem focused examination; Medical decision making of low complexity. Counseling and coordination of care with other physicians, other qualified health care professionals~~ When using time for code selection, ~~or agencies are provided consistent with the nature~~ 20-29 minutes of ~~the problem(s) and the patient's and/or family's needs~~ total time is spent on the date of the encounter. ~~Usually, the presenting problem(s) are of low to moderate severity. Typically, 15 minutes are spent face-to-face with the patient and/or family.~~

99214 Office or other outpatient visit for the evaluation and management of an established patient, which requires a~~t least 2 of these 3 key components:~~ medically appropriate history and/or examination and moderate level of medical decision making. ~~A detailed history; A detailed examination; Medical decision making of moderate complexity. Counseling and/or coordination of care with other physicians, other qualified health care professionals~~ When using time for code selection, ~~or agencies are provided consistent with the nature~~ 30-39 minutes of ~~the problem(s) and the patient's and/or family's needs~~ total time is spent on the date of the encounter. ~~Usually, the presenting problem(s) are of moderate to high severity. Typically, 25 minutes are spent face-to-face with the patient and/or family.~~

99215 Office or other outpatient visit for the evaluation and management of an established patient, which requires a~~t least 2 of these 3 key components:~~ medically appropriate history and/or examination and high level of medical decision making. ~~A comprehensive history; A comprehensive examination; Medical decision making of high complexity. Counseling and/or coordination of care with other physicians, other qualified health care professionals~~ When using time for code selection, ~~or agencies are provided consistent with the nature~~ 40-54 minutes of ~~the problem(s) and the patient's and/or family's needs~~ total time is spent on the date of the encounter. ~~Usually, the presenting problem(s) are of moderate to high severity. Typically, 40 minutes are spent face-to-face with the patient and/or family.~~

99354 Prolonged ~~evaluation and management or psychotherapy~~ service(s) ~~(beyond the typical service time of the primary procedure)~~ in the ~~office or other~~ outpatient setting requiring direct patient contact beyond the time of the usual service; first hour (List separately in addition to code for ~~office or other~~ outpatient Evaluation and Management or psychotherapy service, except with office or other outpatient services [99202, 99203, 99204, 99205, 99212, 99213, 99214, 99215])

99355 each additional 30 minutes (List separately in addition to code for prolonged service)

99356 Prolonged service in the inpatient or observation setting, requiring unit/floor time beyond the usual service; first hour (List separately in addition to code for inpatient or observation Evaluation and Management service)

99415 Prolonged clinical staff service (the service beyond the highest time in the range of total ~~typical service~~ time of the service) during an evaluation and management service in the office or outpatient setting, direct patient contact with physician supervision; first hour (List separately in addition to code for outpatient Evaluation and Management service)

99416 each additional 30 minutes (List separately in addition to code for prolonged service)

99487 Complex chronic care management services, with the following required elements: multiple (two or more) chronic conditions expected to last at least 12 months, or until the death of the patient, chronic conditions place the patient at significant risk of death, acute exacerbation/decompensation, or functional decline, ~~establishment or substantial revision of a comprehensive care plan~~comprehensive care plan established, implemented, revised, or monitored, moderate or high complexity medical decision making; ~~60 minutes of clinical staff time directed by a physician or other qualified health care professional, per calendar month.~~ first 60 minutes of clinical staff time directed by a physician or other qualified health care professional, per calendar month.

99489 each additional 30 minutes of clinical staff time directed by a physician or other qualified health care professional, per calendar month (List separately in addition to code for primary procedure)

99490 Chronic care management services, ~~at least 20 minutes of clinical staff time directed by a physician or other qualified health care professional, per calendar month,~~ with the following required elements: multiple (two or more) chronic conditions expected to last at least 12 months, or until the death of the patient,~~;~~ chronic conditions place the patient at significant risk of death, acute exacerbation/decompensation, or functional decline,~~;~~ comprehensive care plan established, implemented, revised, or monitored; first 20 minutes of clinical staff time directed by a physician or other qualified health care professional, per calendar month.

3170F ~~Flow~~ Baseline flow cytometry studies performed at time of diagnosis or prior to initiating treatment (HEM)[1]

0577T Electrophysiologic~~al~~ evaluation of implantable cardioverter-defibrillator system with substernal electrode (includes defibrillation threshold evaluation, induction of arrhythmia, evaluation of sensing for arrhythmia termination, and programming or reprogramming of sensing or therapeutic parameters)

Deleted Codes

0006U	0124U	0125U	0126U	0127U	0128U	0058T
0085T	0111T	0126T	0228T	0229T	0230T	0231T
0295T	0296T	0297T	0298T	0381T	0382T	0383T
0384T	0385T	0386T	0396T	0400T	0401T	0405T
0595T	19324	19366	32405	49220	57112	58293
61870	62163	63180	63182	69605	76970	78135
81545	92585	92586	92992	92993	94250	94400
94750	94770	95071	99201			

Resequenced Icon Added

33995	33997	80161	80167	80176	80179	80181
80189	80193	80204	80210	81168	81191	81192

81193	81194	81278	81279	81338	81339	81347
81348	81351	81352	81353	81357	81419	81546
81595	81500	81503	81504	81540	81595	81596
82681	86328	87811	92517	92518	92519	92650
92651	92652	92653	93241	93242	93243	93244
93245	93246	93247	93248	94619	99417	99439
0614T	0620T	0623T	0624T	0625T	0626T	

Web Release New and Revised Codes

Codes indicated as "Web Release" codes indicate CPT codes that are in *Current Procedural Coding Expert* for the current year, but will not be in the AMA CPT book until the following year. This can also include those codes designated by the AMA as new or revised for 2021 but that actually appeared in the 2020 Optum360 book. These codes will have the appropriate new or revised icon appended to match the CPT code book, however. See the complete list that follows:

New codes, deleted codes, and revisions to codes in the 2021 *Current Procedural Coding Expert* that will not appear in the CPT code book until 2022

These codes are indicated with the following icons: ● ▲ These icons will be green in the body of the book.

New Codes

86408 Neutralizing antibody, severe acute respiratory syndrome coronavirus 2 (SARS-CoV-2) (Coronavirus disease [COVID-19]); screen

86409 titer

86413 Severe acute respiratory syndrome coronavirus 2 (SARS-CoV-2) (Coronavirus disease [COVID-19]) antibody, quantitative

87636 Infectious agent detection by nucleic acid (DNA or RNA); severe acute respiratory syndrome coronavirus 2 (SARS-CoV-2) (Coronavirus disease [COVID-19]) and influenza virus types A and B, multiplex amplified probe technique

87637 severe acute respiratory syndrome coronavirus 2 (SARS-CoV-2) (Coronavirus disease [COVID-19]), influenza virus types A and B, and respiratory syncytial virus, multiplex amplified probe technique

87811 Infectious agent antigen detection by immunoassay with direct optical (ie, visual) observation; severe acute respiratory syndrome coronavirus 2 (SARS-CoV-2) (Coronavirus disease [COVID-19])

99072 Additional supplies, materials, and clinical staff time over and above those usually included in an office visit or other nonfacility service(s), when performed during a Public Health Emergency, as defined by law, due to respiratory-transmitted infectious disease

0223U Infectious disease (bacterial or viral respiratory tract infection), pathogen-specific nucleic acid (DNA or RNA), 22 targets including severe acute respiratory syndrome coronavirus 2 (SARS-CoV-2), qualitative RT-PCR, nasopharyngeal swab, each pathogen reported as detected or not detected

0224U Antibody, severe acute respiratory syndrome coronavirus 2 (SARS-CoV-2) (Coronavirus disease [COVID-19]), includes titer(s), when performed

0225U Infectious disease (bacterial or viral respiratory tract infection) pathogen-specific DNA and RNA, 21 targets, including severe acute respiratory syndrome coronavirus 2 (SARS-CoV-2), amplified probe technique, including multiplex reverse transcription for RNA targets, each analyte reported as detected or not detected

0226U Surrogate viral neutralization test (sVNT), severe acute respiratory syndrome coronavirus 2 (SARS-CoV-2) (Coronavirus disease [COVID-19]), ELISA, plasma, serum

0227U Drug assay, presumptive, 30 or more drugs or metabolites, urine, liquid chromatography with tandem mass spectrometry (LC-MS/MS) using multiple reaction monitoring (MRM), with drug or metabolite description, includes sample validation

0228U Oncology (prostate), multianalyte molecular profile by photometric detection of macromolecules adsorbed on nanosponge array slides with machine learning, utilizing first morning voided urine, algorithm reported as likelihood of prostate cancer

0229U *BCAT1 (Branched chain amino acid transaminase 1)* or *IKZF1 (IKAROS family zinc finger 1)* (eg, colorectal cancer) promoter methylation analysis

0230U *AR (androgen receptor)* (eg, spinal and bulbar muscular atrophy, Kennedy disease, X chromosome inactivation), full sequence analysis, including small sequence changes in exonic and intronic regions, deletions, duplications, short tandem repeat (STR) expansions, mobile element insertions, and variants in non-uniquely mappable regions

0231U *CACNA1A (calcium voltage-gated channel subunit alpha 1A)* (eg, spinocerebellar ataxia), full gene analysis, including small sequence changes in exonic and intronic regions, deletions, duplications, short tandem repeat (STR) gene expansions, mobile element insertions, and variants in non-uniquely mappable regions

0232U *CSTB (cystatin B)* (eg, progressive myoclonic epilepsy type 1A, Unverricht-Lundborg disease), full gene analysis, including small sequence changes in exonic and intronic regions, deletions, duplications, short tandem repeat (STR) expansions, mobile element insertions, and variants in non-uniquely mappable regions

0233U *FXN (frataxin)* (eg, Friedreich ataxia), gene analysis, including small sequence changes in exonic and intronic regions, deletions, duplications, short tandem repeat (STR) expansions, mobile element insertions, and variants in non-uniquely mappable regions

0234U *MECP2 (methyl CpG binding protein 2)* (eg, Rett syndrome), full gene analysis, including small sequence changes in exonic and intronic regions, deletions, duplications, mobile element insertions, and variants in non-uniquely mappable regions

0235U *PTEN (phosphatase and tensin homolog)* (eg, Cowden syndrome, PTEN hamartoma tumor syndrome), full gene analysis, including small sequence changes in exonic and intronic regions, deletions, duplications, mobile element insertions, and variants in non-uniquely mappable regions

0236U *SMN1 (survival of motor neuron 1, telomeric)* and *SMN2 (survival of motor neuron 2, centromeric)* (eg, spinal muscular atrophy) full gene analysis, including small sequence changes in exonic and intronic regions, duplications and deletions, and mobile element insertions

0237U Cardiac ion channelopathies (eg, Brugada syndrome, long QT syndrome, short QT syndrome, catecholaminergic polymorphic ventricular tachycardia), genomic sequence analysis panel including *ANK2, CASQ2, CAV3, KCNE1, KCNE2, KCNH2, KCNJ2, KCNQ1, RYR2,* and *SCN5A,* including small sequence changes in exonic and intronic regions, deletions, duplications, mobile element insertions, and variants in non-uniquely mappable regions

0238U Oncology (Lynch syndrome), genomic DNA sequence analysis of *MLH1, MSH2, MSH6, PMS2,* and *EPCAM,* including small sequence changes in exonic and intronic regions, deletions, duplications, mobile element insertions, and variants in non-uniquely mappable regions

0239U Targeted genomic sequence analysis panel, solid organ neoplasm, cell-free DNA, analysis of 311 or more genes, interrogation for sequence variants, including substitutions, insertions, deletions, select rearrangements, and copy number variations

0240U Infectious disease (viral respiratory tract infection), pathogen-specific RNA, 3 targets (severe acute respiratory syndrome coronavirus 2 [SARS-CoV-2], influenza A, influenza B), upper respiratory specimen, each pathogen reported as detected or not detected

0241U Infectious disease (viral respiratory tract infection), pathogen-specific RNA, 4 targets (severe acute respiratory syndrome coronavirus 2 [SARS-CoV-2], influenza A, influenza B, respiratory syncytial virus [RSV]), upper respiratory specimen, each pathogen reported as detected or not detected

Revised Codes

87301 Infectious agent antigen detection by immunoassay technique, (eg, enzyme immunoassay [EIA], enzyme-linked immunosorbent assay [ELISA], fluorescence immunoassay [FIA], immunochemiluminometric assay [IMCA]) qualitative or semiquantitative, ~~multiple-step method~~; adenovirus enteric types 40/41

87305 Aspergillus

87320 Chlamydia trachomatis

87324 Clostridium difficile toxin(s)

87327 Cryptococcus neoformans

87328 cryptosporidium

87329 giardia

87332 cytomegalovirus

87335 Escherichia coli 0157

87336 Entamoeba histolytica dispar group

87337 Entamoeba histolytica group

87338 Helicobacter pylori, stool

87339 Helicobacter pylori

87340 hepatitis B surface antigen (HBsAg)

87341 hepatitis B surface antigen (HBsAg) neutralization

87350 hepatitis Be antigen (HBeAg)

87380 hepatitis, delta agent

87385 Histoplasma capsulatum

87389 HIV-1 antigen(s), with HIV-1 and HIV-2 antibodies, single result

87390 HIV-1

87391 HIV-2

87400 Influenza, A or B, each

87420 respiratory syncytial virus

87425 rotavirus

87426 severe acute respiratory syndrome coronavirus (eg, SARS-CoV, SARS-CoV-2 [COVID-19])

87427 Shiga-like toxin

87430 Streptococcus, group A

87449 not otherwise specified, each organism

87451 polyvalent for multiple organisms, each polyvalent antiserum

87802 Infectious agent antigen detection by immunoassay with direct optical (ie, visual) observation; Streptococcus, group B

87803 Clostridium difficile toxin A

87806 HIV-1 antigen(s), with HIV-1 and HIV-2 antibodies

87804 Influenza

87807 respiratory syncytial virus

87808 Trichomonas vaginalis

87809 adenovirus

87810 Chlamydia trachomatis

87850 Neisseria gonorrhoeae

87880 Streptococcus, group A

87899 not otherwise specified

0152U Infectious disease (bacteria, fungi, parasites, and DNA viruses), microbial cell-free DNA, ~~PCR and~~ plasma, untargeted next-generation sequencing, ~~plasma, detection of >1,000 potential microbial organisms for~~ report for significant positive pathogens

Deleted Codes

87450 Infectious agent antigen detection by immunoassay technique, (eg, enzyme immunoassay [EIA], enzyme-linked immunosorbent assay [ELISA], immunochemiluminometric assay [IMCA]), qualitative or semiquantitative; single step method, not otherwise specified, each organism

Appendix C — Evaluation and Management Extended Guidelines

This appendix provides an overview of evaluation and management (E/M) services, tables that identify the documentation elements associated with each code, the 2021 changes to some E/M services, and the federal documentation guidelines with emphasis on the 1997 exam guidelines. The new 2021 guidelines affect codes 99202–99215 only. The 1997 version identifies both general multi-system physical examinations and single-system examinations, but providers may also use the original 1995 version of the E/M guidelines; both are currently supported by the Centers for Medicare and Medicaid Services (CMS) for audit purposes when reporting 99217–99499.

The levels of E/M services define the wide variations in skill, effort, and time and are required for preventing and/or diagnosing and treating illness or injury, and promoting optimal health. These codes are intended to represent physician work, and because much of this work involves the amount of training, experience, expertise, and knowledge that a provider may employ when treating a given patient, the true indications of the level of this work may be difficult to recognize without some explanation.

Providers

The AMA advises coders that while a particular service or procedure may be assigned to a specific section, the service or procedure itself is not limited to use only by that specialty group (see paragraphs 2 and 3 under "Instructions for Use of the CPT® Codebook" on page xiv of the AMA CPT Book). Additionally, the procedures and services listed throughout the book are for use by any qualified physician or other qualified health care professional or entity (e.g., hospitals, laboratories, or home health agencies).

The use of the phrase "physician or other qualified health care professional" (OQHCP) was adopted to identify a health care provider other than a physician. This type of provider is further described in CPT as an individual "qualified by education, training, licensure/regulation (when applicable), and facility privileging (when applicable)." State licensure guidelines determine the scope of practice and an OQHCP must practice within these guidelines, even if more restrictive than the CPT guidelines. The OQHCP may report services independently or under incident-to guidelines. The professionals within this definition are separate from "clinical staff" and are able to practice independently. CPT defines clinical staff as "a person who works under the supervision of a physician or OQHCP and who is allowed, by law, regulation, and facility policy to perform or assist in the performance of a specified professional service, but who does not individually report that professional service." Keep in mind that there may be other policies or guidance that can affect who may report a specific service.

Types of E/M Services

When approaching E/M, the first choice that a provider must make is what type of code to use. The following tables outline the E/M codes for different levels of care for:

- Office or other outpatient services—new patient
- Office or other outpatient services—established patient
- Hospital observation services—initial care, subsequent, and discharge
- Hospital inpatient services—initial care, subsequent, and discharge
- Observation or inpatient care (including admission and discharge services)
- Consultations—office or other outpatient
- Consultations—inpatient
- Emergency department services
- Critical care
- Nursing facility—initial services
- Nursing facility—subsequent services
- Nursing facility—discharge and annual assessment
- Domiciliary, rest home, or custodial care—new patient
- Domiciliary, rest home, or custodial care—established patient
- Home services—new patient
- Home services—established patient
- Newborn care services
- Neonatal and pediatric interfacility transport
- Neonatal and pediatric critical care—inpatient
- Neonate and infant intensive care services—initial and continuing

The specifics of the code components that determine code selection are listed in the table and discussed in the next section. Before a level of service is decided upon, the correct type of service is identified.

A new patient is a patient who has not received any face-to-face professional services from the physician or OQHCP within the past three years. An established patient is a patient who has received face-to-face professional services from the physician or OQHCP within the past three years. In the case of group practices, if a physician or OQHCP of the exact same specialty or subspecialty has seen the patient within three years, the patient is considered established.

If a physician or OQHCP is on call or covering for another physician or OQHCP, the patient's encounter is classified as it would have been by the physician or OQHCP who is not available. Thus, a locum tenens physician or OQHCP who sees a patient on behalf of the patient's attending physician or OQHCP may not bill a new patient code unless the attending physician or OQHCP has not seen the patient for any problem within three years.

Office or other outpatient services are E/M services provided in the physician or OQHCP office, the outpatient area, or other ambulatory facility. Until the patient is admitted to a health care facility, he/she is considered to be an outpatient. Hospital observation services are E/M services provided to patients who are designated or admitted as "observation status" in a hospital.

Codes 99218-99220 are used to indicate initial observation care. These codes include the initiation of the observation status, supervision of patient care including writing orders, and the performance of periodic reassessments. These codes are used only by the provider "admitting" the patient for observation.

Codes 99234-99236 are used to indicate evaluation and management services to a patient who is admitted to and discharged from observation status or hospital inpatient on the same day. If the patient is admitted as an inpatient from observation on the same day, use the appropriate level of Initial Hospital Care (99221-99223).

Code 99217 indicates discharge from observation status. It includes the final physical examination of the patient, instructions, and preparation of the discharge records. It should not be used when admission and discharge are on the same date of service. As mentioned above, report codes 99234-99236 to appropriately describe same day observation services.

If a patient is in observation longer than one day, subsequent observation care codes 99224-99226 should be reported. If the patient is discharged on the second day, observation discharge code 99217 should be reported. If the patient status is changed to inpatient on a subsequent date, the appropriate inpatient code, 99221-99233, should be reported.

Initial hospital care is defined as E/M services provided during the first hospital inpatient encounter with the patient by the admitting provider. (If a physician other than the admitting physician performs the initial inpatient encounter, refer to consultations or subsequent hospital care in the CPT book.) Subsequent hospital care includes all follow-up encounters with the patient by all physicians or OQHCP. As there may only be one admitting physician, HCPCS Level II modifier AI Principal physician of record, should be appended to the initial hospital care code by the attending physician or OQHCP.

A consultation is the provision of a physician or OQHCP's opinion or advice about a patient for a specific problem at the request of another physician or other appropriate source. CPT also states that a consultation may be performed when a physician or OQHCP is determining whether to accept the transfer of patient care at the request of another physician or appropriate source. An office or other outpatient consultation is a consultation provided in the consultant's office, in the emergency department, or in an outpatient or other ambulatory facility including hospital observation services, home services, domiciliary, rest home, or custodial care. An inpatient consultation is a consultation provided in the hospital or partial hospital nursing facility setting. Report only one inpatient consultation by a consultant for each admission to the hospital or nursing facility.

If a consultant participates in the patient's management after the opinion or advice is provided, use codes for subsequent hospital or observation care or for office or other outpatient services (established patient), as appropriate.

Under CMS guidelines, the inpatient and office/outpatient consultation codes contained in the CPT manual are not covered services.

All outpatient consultation services will be reported for Medicare using the appropriate new or established evaluation and management (E/M) codes. Inpatient consultation services for the initial encounter should be reported by the physician providing the service using initial hospital care codes 99221–99223, and subsequent inpatient care codes 99231–99233.

Codes 99439, 99487, 99489, 99490, and 99491 are used to report evaluation and management services for chronic care management. These codes represent management and support services provided by clinical staff, under the direction of a physician or OQHCP, to patients residing at home or in a domiciliary, rest home, or assisted living facility. The qualified provider oversees the management and/or coordination of services for all medical conditions, psychosocial needs, and activities of daily living. These codes are reported only once per calendar month and have specific time-based thresholds.

Codes 99497-99498 are used to report the discussion and explanation of advanced directives by a physician or OQHCP. These codes represent a face-to-face service between the provider and a patient, family member, or surrogate. These codes are time-based codes and, since no active management of the problem(s) is undertaken during this time, may be reported on the same day as another E/M service.

Certain codes that CPT considers appropriate telehealth services are identified with the ★ icon and reported with modifier 95 Synchronous telemedicine service rendered via a real-time interactive audio and video telecommunications system. Medicare recognizes certain CPT and HCPCS Level II G codes as telehealth services reported with modifier GT. Check with individual payers for telehealth modifier guidance.

Revised E/M Services—Codes 99202 OCG: I.C.1.g.1.b; I.C.1.d
99215

These revised codes are used to report office or other outpatient services for a new (99202–99205) or established (99212–99215) patient.

A medically appropriate history and physical examination, as determined by the treating provider, should be documented. The level of history and physical examination are no longer used when determining the level of service. Codes should be selected based upon the CPT 2021 Medical Decision Making (MDM) table or time as documented in the patient record.

The 2021 Medical Decision Making table requires two of three levels of the three elements be met or exceeded to determine the level of code reported. The three elements are

- Number and complexity of problems addressed at the encounter
- Amount and/or complexity of data to be reviewed and analyzed
- Risk of complications and/or morbidity or mortality of patient management

Instructions and examples of each element are given in the table to enable accurate selection of the level of MDM and E/M service from 99202–99215 to be reported.

Alternatively time alone may be used to select the appropriate level of service. Total time for reporting these services includes face-to-face and non-face-to-face time personally spent by the physician or other qualified health care professional on the date of the encounter. The revised E/M codes 99202–99205 and 99212–99215 include specific time ranges used to select the appropriate code. Report new code 99417 for prolonged services when the time for code 99205 or 99215 is exceeded. Report 99417 for each minimum of 15 minutes additional prolonged services.

Code 99211 was revised but is still used to report the E/M service that does not require the presence of the physician or other qualified health care professional. The time element has also been removed from the code description.

The Centers for Medicare and Medicaid Services (CMS) recognizes these changes and will adopt the code description changes and use of time or the MDM table for codes 99202–99215 beginning January 1, 2021.

E/M Code	History	Exam	Medical Decision Making	Time Spent Face-to-Face (avg.)
99202	Medically appropriate	Medically appropriate	Straightforward	15–29 min.
99203	Medically appropriate	Medically appropriate	Low	30–44 min.
99204	Medically appropriate	Medically appropriate	Moderate	45–59 min.
99205	Medically appropriate	Medically appropriate	High	60–74 min.

Office or Other Outpatient Services—Established Patient[1]

E/M Code	History	Exam	Medical Decision Making	Time Spent Face-to-Face (avg.)
99211	—	—	Physician supervision, but presence not required	—
99212	Medically appropriate	Medically appropriate	Straightforward	10–19 min.
99213	Medically appropriate	Medically appropriate	Low	20–29 min.
99214	Medically appropriate	Medically appropriate	Moderate	30–39 min.
99215	Medically appropriate	Medically appropriate	High	40–54 min.

1 Includes follow-up, periodic reevaluation, and evaluation and management of new problems.

Hospital Observation Services

E/M Code	History[1]	Exam[1]	Medical Decision Making[1]	Problem Severity	Coordination of Care; Counseling	Time Spent Bedside and on Unit/Floor (avg.)
99217	Observation care discharge day management					
99218	Detailed or comprehensive	Detailed or comprehensive	Straightforward or low complexity	Low	Consistent with problem(s) and patient's needs	30 min.
99219	Comprehensive	Comprehensive	Moderate complexity	Moderate	Consistent with problem(s) and patient's needs	50 min.
99220	Comprehensive	Comprehensive	High complexity	High	Consistent with problem(s) and patient's needs	70 min.

1 Key component. All three components (history, exam, and medical decision making) are crucial for selecting the correct code.

Subsequent Hospital Observation Services[1]

E/M Code[2]	History[3]	Exam[3]	Medical Decision Making[3]	Problem Severity	Coordination of Care; Counseling	Time Spent Bedside and on Unit/Floor (avg.)
99224	Problem-focused interval	Problem-focused	Straightforward or low complexity	Stable, recovering, or improving	Consistent with problem(s) and patient's needs	15 min.
99225	Expanded problem-focused interval	Expanded problem-focused	Moderate complexity	Inadequate response to treatment; minor complications	Consistent with problem(s) and patient's needs	25 min.
99226	Detailed interval	Detailed	High complexity	Unstable; significant new problem or significant complication	Consistent with problem(s) and patient's needs	35 min.

1 All subsequent levels of service include reviewing the medical record, diagnostic studies, and changes in the patient's status, such as history, physical condition, and response to treatment since the last assessment.
2 These codes are resequenced in CPT and are printed following codes 99217-99220.
3 Key component. For subsequent care, at least two of the three components (history, exam, and medical decision making) are needed to select the correct code.

Hospital Inpatient Services—Initial Care[1]

E/M Code	History[2]	Exam[2]	Medical Decision Making[2]	Problem Severity	Coordination of Care; Counseling	Time Spent Bedside and on Unit/Floor (avg.)
99221	Detailed or comprehensive	Detailed or comprehensive	Straightforward or low complexity	Low	Consistent with problem(s) and patient's needs	30 min.
99222	Comprehensive	Comprehensive	Moderate complexity	Moderate	Consistent with problem(s) and patient's needs	50 min.
99223	Comprehensive	Comprehensive	High complexity	High	Consistent with problem(s) and patient's needs	70 min.

1 The admitting physician should append modifier AI, Principal physician of record, for Medicare patients

2 Key component. For initial care, all three components (history, exam, and medical decision making) are crucial for selecting the correct code.

Hospital Inpatient Services—Subsequent Care[1]

E/M Code	History[2]	Exam[2]	Medical Decision Making[2]	Problem Severity	Coordination of Care; Counseling	Time Spent Bedside and on Unit/Floor (avg.)
99231	Problem-focused interval	Problem-focused	Straightforward or low complexity	Stable, recovering or Improving	Consistent with problem(s) and patient's needs	15 min.
99232	Expanded problem-focused interval	Expanded problem-focused	Moderate complexity	Inadequate response to treatment; minor complications	Consistent with problem(s) and patient's needs	25 min.
99233	Detailed interval	Detailed	High complexity	Unstable; significant new problem or significant complication	Consistent with problem(s) and patient's needs	35 min.
99238	Hospital discharge day management					30 min. or less
99239	Hospital discharge day management					> 30 min.

1 All subsequent levels of service include reviewing the medical record, diagnostic studies, and changes in the patient's status, such as history, physical condition, and response to treatment since the last assessment.

2 Key component. For subsequent care, at least two of the three components (history, exam, and medical decision making) are needed to select the correct code.

Observation or Inpatient Care Services (Including Admission and Discharge Services)

E/M Code	History[1]	Exam[1]	Medical Decision Making[1]	Problem Severity	Coordination of Care; Counseling	Time
99234	Detailed or comprehensive	Detailed or comprehensive	Straightforward or low complexity	Low	Consistent with problem(s) and patient's needs	40 min.
99235	Comprehensive	Comprehensive	Moderate	Moderate	Consistent with problem(s) and patient's needs	50 min.
99236	Comprehensive	Comprehensive	High	High	Consistent with problem(s) and patient's needs	55 min.

1 Key component. All three components (history, exam, and medical decision making) are crucial for selecting the correct code.

Consultations—Office or Other Outpatient

E/M Code	History[1]	Exam[1]	Medical Decision Making[1]	Problem Severity	Coordination of Care; Counseling	Time Spent Face-to-Face (avg.)
99241	Problem-focused	Problem-focused	Straightforward	Minor or self-limited	Consistent with problem(s) and patient's needs	15 min.
99242	Expanded problem-focused	Expanded problem-focused	Straightforward	Low	Consistent with problem(s) and patient's needs	30 min.
99243	Detailed	Detailed	Low complexity	Moderate	Consistent with problem(s) and patient's needs	40 min.
99244	Comprehensive	Comprehensive	Moderate complexity	Moderate to high	Consistent with problem(s) and patient's needs	60 min.
99245	Comprehensive	Comprehensive	High complexity	Moderate to high	Consistent with problem(s) and patient's needs	80 min.

1 Key component. For office or other outpatient consultations, all three components (history, exam, and medical decision making) are crucial for selecting the correct code.

Consultations—Inpatient[1]

E/M Code	History[2]	Exam[2]	Medical Decision Making[2]	Problem Severity	Coordination of Care; Counseling	Time Spent Bedside and on Unit/Floor (avg.)
99251	Problem-focused	Problem-focused	Straightforward	Minor or self-limited	Consistent with problem(s) and patient's needs	20 min.
99252	Expanded problem-focused	Expanded problem-focused	Straightforward	Low	Consistent with problem(s) and patient's needs	40 min.
99253	Detailed	Detailed	Low complexity	Moderate	Consistent with problem(s) and patient's needs	55 min.
99254	Comprehensive	Comprehensive	Moderate complexity	Moderate to high	Consistent with problem(s) and patient's needs	80 min.
99255	Comprehensive	Comprehensive	High complexity	Moderate to high	Consistent with problem(s) and patient's needs	110 min.

1 These codes are used for hospital inpatients, residents of nursing facilities or patients in a partial hospital setting.
2 Key component. For initial inpatient consultations, all three components (history, exam, and medical decision making) are crucial for selecting the correct code.

Emergency Department Services, New or Established Patient

E/M Code	History[1]	Exam[1]	Medical Decision Making[1]	Problem Severity[3]	Coordination of Care; Counseling	Time Spent[2] Face-to-Face (avg.)
99281	Problem-focused	Problem-focused	Straightforward	Minor or self-limited	Consistent with problem(s) and patient's needs	N/A
99282	Expanded problem-focused	Expanded problem-focused	Low complexity	Low to moderate	Consistent with problem(s) and patient's needs	N/A
99283	Expanded problem-focused	Expanded problem-focused	Moderate complexity	Moderate	Consistent with problem(s) and patient's needs	N/A
99284	Detailed	Detailed	Moderate complexity	High; requires urgent evaluation	Consistent with problem(s) and patient's needs	N/A
99285	Comprehensive	Comprehensive	High complexity	High; poses immediate/significant threat to life or physiologic function	Consistent with problem(s) and patient's needs	N/A
99288[4]			High complexity			N/A

1 Key component. For emergency department services, all three components (history, exam, and medical decision making) are crucial for selecting the correct code and must be adequately documented in the medical record to substantiate the level of service reported.
2 Typical times have not been established for this category of services.
3 NOTE: The severity of the patient's problem, while taken into consideration when evaluating and treating the patient, does not automatically determine the level of E/M service unless the medical record documentation reflects the severity of the patient's illness, injury, or condition in the details of the history, physical examination, and medical decision making process. Federal auditors will "downcode" the level of E/M service despite the nature of the patient's problem when the documentation does not support the E/M code reported.
4 Code 99288 is used to report two-way communication with emergency medical services personnel in the field.

Critical Care

E/M Code	Patient Status	Physician Attendance	Time[1]
99291	Critically ill or critically injured	Constant	First 30–74 minutes
99292	Critically ill or critically injured	Constant	Each additional 30 minutes beyond the first 74 minutes

1 Per the guidelines for time in *CPT 2016 page xv*, "A unit of time is attained when the mid-point is passed. For example, an hour is attained when 31 minutes have elapsed (more than midway between zero and 60 minutes)."

Nursing Facility Services—Initial Nursing Facility Care[1]

E/M Code	History[1]	Exam[1]	Medical Decision Making[1]	Problem Severity	Coordination of Care; Counseling
99304	Detailed or comprehensive	Detailed or comprehensive	Straightforward or low complexity	Low	25 min.
99305	Comprehensive	Comprehensive	Moderate complexity	Moderate	35 min.
99306	Comprehensive	Comprehensive	High complexity	High	45 min.

1 These services must be performed by the physician. See CPT Corrections Document – CPT 2013 page 3 or guidelines CPT 2016 page 26.
2 Key component. For new patients, all three components (history, exam, and medical decision making) are crucial for selecting the correct code.

Nursing Facility Services—Subsequent Nursing Facility Care

E/M Code	History[1]	Exam[1]	Medical Decision Making[2]	Problem Severity	Coordination of Care; Counseling
99307	Problem-focused interval	Problem-focused	Straightforward	Stable, recovering or improving	10 min.
99308	Expanded problem-focused interval	Expanded problem-focused	Low complexity	Responding inadequately or has developed a minor complication	15 min.
99309	Detailed interval	Detailed	Moderate complexity	Significant complication or a significant new problem	25 min.
99310	Comprehensive interval	Comprehensive	High complexity	Developed a significant new problem requiring immediate attention	35 min.

1 Key component. For established patients, at least two of the three components (history, exam, and medical decision making) are needed for selecting the correct code.

Nursing Facility Discharge and Annual Assessment

E/M Code	History[1]	Exam[1]	Medical Decision Making[1]	Problem Severity	Time Spent Bedside and on Unit/Floor (avg.)
99315	Nursing facility discharge day management				30 min. or less
99316	Nursing facility discharge day management				more than 30 min.
99318	Detailed interval	Comprehensive	Low to moderate complexity	Stable, recovering or improving	30 min.

1 Key component. For annual nursing facility assessment, all three components (history, exam, and medical decision making) are crucial for selecting the correct code.

Domiciliary, Rest Home (e.g., Boarding Home) or Custodial Care Services—New Patient

E/M Code	History[1]	Exam[1]	Medical Decision Making[1]	Problem Severity	Coordination of Care; Counseling	Time Spent Face-to-Face (avg.)
99324	Problem-focused	Problem focused	Straightforward	Low	Consistent with problem(s) and patient's needs	20 min.
99325	Expanded problem-focused	Expanded problem-focused	Low complexity	Moderate	Consistent with problem(s) and patient's needs	30 min.
99326	Detailed	Detailed	Moderate complexity	Moderate to high	Consistent with problem(s) and patient's needs	45 min.
99327	Comprehensive	Comprehensive	Moderate complexity	High	Consistent with problem(s) and patient's needs	60 min.
99328	Comprehensive	Comprehensive	High complexity	Unstable or developed a new problem requiring immediate physician attention	Consistent with problem(s) and patient's needs	75 min.

1 Key component. For new patients, all three components (history, exam, and medical decision making) are crucial for selecting the correct code and must be adequately documented in the medical record to substantiate the level of service reported.

Domiciliary, Rest Home (e.g., Boarding Home) or Custodial Care Services— Established Patient

E/M Code	History[1]	Exam[1]	Medical Decision Making[1]	Problem Severity	Coordination of Care; Counseling	Time Spent Face-to-Face (avg.)
99334	Problem-focused interval	Problem-focused	Straightforward	Minor or self-limited	Consistent with problem(s) and patient's needs	15 min.
99335	Expanded problem-focused interval	Expanded problem-focused	Low complexity	Low to moderate	Consistent with problem(s) and patient's needs	25 min.
99336	Detailed interval	Detailed	Moderate complexity	Moderate to high	Consistent with problem(s) and patient's needs	40 min.
99337	Comprehensive interval	Comprehensive	Moderate to high complexity	Moderate to high	Consistent with problem(s) and patient's needs	60 min.

1 Key component. For established patients, at least two of the three components (history, exam, and medical decision making) are needed for selecting the correct code.

Domiciliary, Rest Home (e.g., Assisted Living Facility), or Home Care Plan Oversight Services

E/M Code	Intent of Service	Presence of Patient	Time
99339	Individual physician supervision of a patient (patient not present) in home, domiciliary or rest home (e.g., assisted living facility) requiring complex and multidisciplinary care modalities involving regular physician development and/or revision of care plans, review of subsequent reports of patient status, review of related laboratory and other studies, communication (including telephone calls) for purposes of assessment or care decisions with health care professional(s), family member(s), surrogate decision maker(s) (e.g., legal guardian) and/or key caregiver(s) involved in patient's care, integration of new information into the medical treatment plan and/or adjustment of medical therapy, within a calendar month	Patient not present	15–29 min.
99340	Same as 99339	Patient not present	30 min. or more

Home Services—New Patient

E/M Code	History[1]	Exam[1]	Medical Decision Making[1]	Problem Severity	Coordination of Care; Counseling	Time Spent Face-to-Face (avg.)
99341	Problem-focused	Problem-focused	Straightforward complexity	Low	Consistent with problem(s) and patient's needs	20 min.
99342	Expanded problem-focused	Expanded problem-focused	Low complexity	Moderate	Consistent with problem(s) and patient's needs	30 min.
99343	Detailed	Detailed	Moderate complexity	Moderate to high	Consistent with problem(s) and patient's needs	45 min.
99344	Comprehensive	Comprehensive	Moderate complexity	High	Consistent with problem(s) and patient's needs	60 min.
99345	Comprehensive	Comprehensive	High complexity	Usually the patient has developed a significant new problem requiring immediate physician attention	Consistent with problem(s) and patient's needs	75 min.

1 Key component. For new patients, all three components (history, exam, and medical decision making) are crucial for selecting the correct code and must be adequately documented in the medical record to substantiate the level of service reported.

Home Services—Established Patient

E/M Code	History[1]	Exam[1]	Medical Decision Making[1]	Problem Severity	Coordination of Care; Counseling	Time Spent Face-to-Face (avg.)
99347	Problem-focused interval	Problem-focused	Straightforward	Minor or self-limited	Consistent with problem(s) and patient's needs	15 min.
99348	Expanded problem-focused interval	Expanded problem-focused	Low complexity	Low to moderate	Consistent with problem(s) and patient's needs	25 min.
99349	Detailed interval	Detailed	Moderate complexity	Moderate to high	Consistent with problem(s) and patient's needs	40 min.
99350	Comprehensive interval	Comprehensive	Moderate to high complexity	Moderate to high Usually the patient has developed a significant new problem requiring immediate physician attention	Consistent with problem(s) and patient's needs	60 min.

1 Key component. For established patients, at least two of the three components (history, exam, and medical decision making) are needed for selecting the correct code.

Newborn Care Services

E/M Code	Patient Status	Type of Visit
99460	Normal newborn	Inpatient initial inpatient hospital or birthing center per day
99461	Normal newborn	Inpatient initial treatment not in hospital or birthing center per day
99462	Normal newborn	Inpatient subsequent per day
99463	Normal newborn	Inpatient initial inpatient and discharge in hospital or birthing center per day
99464	Unstable newborn	Attendance at delivery
99465	High-risk newborn at delivery	Resuscitation, ventilation, and cardiac treatment

Neonatal and Pediatric Interfacility Transportation

E/M Code	Patient Status	Type of Visit
99466	Critically ill or injured infant or young child, to 24 months	Face-to-face transportation from one facility to another, initial 30-74 minutes
99467	Critically ill or injured infant or young child, to 24 months	Face-to-face transportation from one facility to another, each additional 30 minutes
99485[1]	Critically ill or injured infant or young child, to 24 months	Supervision of patient transport from one facility to another, initial 30 minutes
99486[1]	Critically ill or injured infant or young child, to 24 months	Supervision of patient transport from one facility to another, each additional 30 minutes

1 These codes are resequenced in CPT and are printed following codes 99466-99467.

Inpatient Neonatal and Pediatric Critical Care

E/M Code	Patient Status	Type of Visit
99468[1]	Critically ill neonate, aged 28 days or less	Inpatient initial per day
99469[2]	Critically ill neonate, aged 28 days or less	Inpatient subsequent per day
99471	Critically ill infant or young child, aged 29 days to 24 months	Inpatient initial per day
99472	Critically ill infant or young child, aged 29 days to 24 months	Inpatient subsequent per day
99475	Critically ill infant or young child, 2 to 5 years[3]	Inpatient initial per day
99476	Critically ill infant or young child, 2 to 5 years	Inpatient subsequent per day

1 Codes 99468, 99471, and 99475 may be reported only once per admission.
2 Codes 99469, 99472, and 99476 may be reported only once per day and by only one provider.
3 See 99291-99292 for patients 6 years of age and older.

Neonate and Infant Initial and Continuing Intensive Care Services

E/M Code	Patient Status	Type of Visit
99477	Neonate, aged 28 days or less	Inpatient initial per day
99478	Infant with present body weight of less than 1500 grams, no longer critically ill	Inpatient subsequent per day
99479	Infant with present body weight of 1500-2500 grams, no longer critically ill	Inpatient subsequent per day
99480	Infant with present body weight of 2501-5000 grams, no longer critically ill	Inpatient subsequent per day

Levels of E/M Services Codes 99217–99499

Confusion may be experienced when first approaching E/M codes 99217–99499 due to the way that each description of a code component or element seems to have another layer of description beneath. The three key components—history, exam, and decision making—are each comprised of elements that combine to create varying levels of that component.

For example, an expanded problem-focused history includes the chief complaint, a brief history of the present illness, and a system review focusing on the patient's problems. The level of exam is not made up of different elements but rather distinguished by the extent of exam across body areas or organ systems.

The single largest source of confusion are the "labels" or names applied to the varying degrees of history, exam, and decision-making. Terms such as expanded problem-focused, detailed, and comprehensive are somewhat meaningless unless they are defined. The lack of definition in CPT guidelines relative to these terms is precisely what caused the first set of federal guidelines to be developed in 1995 and again in 1997.

Documentation Guidelines for Evaluation and Management Services

Both versions of the federal guidelines go well beyond CPT guidelines in defining specific code requirements. The current version of the CPT guidelines does not explain the number of history of present illness (HPI) elements or the specific number of organ systems or body areas to be examined as they are in the federal guidelines. Adherence to some version of the guidelines is required when billing E/M to federal payers, but at this time, the CPT guidelines do not incorporate this level of detail into the code definitions. Although that could be interpreted to mean that non-governmental payers have a lesser documentation standard, it is best to adopt one set of the federal versions for all payer types for both consistency and ease of use.

The 1997 guidelines supply a great amount of detail relative to history and exam and will give the provider clear direction to follow when documenting elements. With that stated, the 1995 guidelines are equally valid and place a lesser documentation burden on the provider in regard to the physical exam.

The 1995 guidelines ask only for a notation of "normal" on systems with normal findings. The only narrative required is for abnormal findings. The 1997 version calls for much greater detail, or an "elemental" or "bullet-point" approach to organ systems, although a notation of normal is sufficient when addressing the elements within a system. The 1997 version works well in a template or electronic health record (EHR) format for recording E/M services.

The 1997 version did produce the single system specialty exam guidelines. When reviewing the complete guidelines listed below, note the differences between exam requirements in the 1995 and 1997 versions.

A Comparison of 1995 and 1997 Exam Guidelines

There are four types of exams indicated in the levels of E/M codes. Although the descriptors or labels are the same under 1995 and 1997 guidelines, the degree of detail required is different. The remaining content on this topic references the 1997 general multi-system specialty examination, at the end of this chapter.

The levels under each set of guidelines are:

1995 Exam Guidelines:

Problem focused:	One body area or system
Expanded problem focused:	Two to seven body areas or organ systems
Detailed:	Two to seven body areas or organ systems
Comprehensive:	Eight or more organ systems or a complete single-system examination

1997 Exam Guidelines:

Problem-focused:	Perform and document examination of one to five bullet point elements in one or more organ systems/body areas from the general multi-system examination
OR	
	Perform or document examination of one to five bullet point elements from one of the 10 single-organ-system examinations, shaded or unshaded boxes
Expanded problem-focused:	Perform and document examination of at least six bullet point elements in one or more organ systems from the general multi-system examination
OR	
	Perform and document examination of at least six bullet point elements from one of the 10 single-organ-system examinations, shaded or unshaded boxes
Detailed:	Perform and document examination of at least six organ systems or body areas, including at least two bullet point elements for each organ system or body area from the general multi-system examination
OR	
	Perform and document examination of at least 12 bullet point elements in two or more organ systems or body areas from the general multisystem examination
OR	
	Perform and document examination of at least 12 bullet elements from one of the single-organ-system examinations, shaded or unshaded boxes
Comprehensive:	Perform and document examination of at least nine organ systems or body areas, with all bullet elements for each organ system or body area (unless specific instructions are expected to limit examination content with at least two bullet elements for each organ system or body area) from the general multi-system examination
OR	
	Perform and document examination of all bullet point elements from one of the 10 single-organ system examinations with documentation of every element in shaded boxes and at least one element in each unshaded box from the single-organ-system examination.

The Documentation Guidelines

The following guidelines were developed jointly by the American Medical Association (AMA) and the Centers for Medicare and Medicaid Services (CMS). Their mutual goal was to provide physicians and claims reviewers with advice about preparing or reviewing documentation for Evaluation and Management (E/M) services.

I. Introduction

What is Documentation and Why Is It Important?

Medical record documentation is required to record pertinent facts, findings, and observations about an individual's health history, including past and present illnesses, examinations, tests, treatments, and outcomes. The medical record chronologically documents the care of the patient and is an important element contributing to high quality care. The medical record facilitates:

- The ability of the physician and other health care professionals to evaluate and plan the patient's immediate treatment and to monitor his/her health care over time
- Communication and continuity of care among physicians and other health care professionals involved in the patient's care
- Accurate and timely claims review and payment
- Appropriate utilization review and quality of care evaluations
- Collection of data that may be useful for research and education

An appropriately documented medical record can reduce many of the problems associated with claims processing and may serve as a legal document to verify the care provided, if necessary.

What Do Payers Want and Why?

Because payers have a contractual obligation to enrollees, they may require reasonable documentation that services are consistent with the insurance coverage provided. They may request information to validate:

- The site of service
- The medical necessity and appropriateness of the diagnostic and/or therapeutic services provided
- Services provided have been accurately reported

II. General Principles of Medical Record Documentation

The principles of documentation listed below are applicable to all types of medical and surgical services in all settings. For Evaluation and Management (E/M) services, the nature and amount of physician work and documentation varies by type of service, place of service, and the patient's status. The general principles listed below may be modified to account for these variable circumstances in providing E/M services.

- The medical record should be complete and legible
- The documentation of each patient encounter should include:
  - A reason for the encounter and relevant history, physical examination findings, and prior diagnostic test results
  - Assessment, clinical impression, or diagnosis
  - Plan for care
  - Date and legible identity of the practitioner
- If not documented, the rationale for ordering diagnostic and other ancillary services should be easily inferred
- Past and present diagnoses should be accessible to the treating and/or consulting physician
- Appropriate health risk factors should be identified
- The patient's progress, response to, and changes in treatment and revision of diagnosis should be documented
- The CPT and ICD-9-CM codes reported on the health insurance claim form or billing statement should be supported by the documentation in the medical record

III. Documentation of E/M Services 1995 and 1997

The following information provides definitions and documentation guidelines for the three key components of E/M services and for visits that consist predominately of counseling or coordination of care. The three key components—history, examination, and medical decision making—appear in the descriptors for office and other outpatient services, hospital observation services, hospital inpatient services, consultations, emergency department services, nursing facility services, domiciliary care services, and home services. While some of the text of the CPT guidelines has been repeated in this document, the reader should refer to CMS or CPT for the complete descriptors for E/M services and instructions for selecting a level of service. Documentation guidelines are identified by the symbol DG.

The descriptors for the levels of E/M services recognize seven components that are used in defining the levels of E/M services. These components are:

- History
- Examination
- Medical decision making
- Counseling
- Coordination of care
- Nature of presenting problem
- Time

The first three of these components (i.e., history, examination, and medical decision making) are the key components in selecting the level of E/M services. In the case of visits that consist predominately of counseling or coordination of care, time is the key or controlling factor to qualify for a particular level of E/M service.

Because the level of E/M service is dependent on two or three key components, performance and documentation of one component (e.g., examination) at the highest level does not necessarily mean that the encounter in its entirety qualifies for the highest level of E/M service.

These Documentation Guidelines for E/M services reflect the needs of the typical adult population. For certain groups of patients, the recorded information may vary slightly from that described here. Specifically, the medical records of infants, children, adolescents, and pregnant women may have additional or modified information, as appropriate, recorded in each history and examination area.

As an example, newborn records may include under history of the present illness (HPI) the details of the mother's pregnancy and the infant's status at birth; social history will focus on family structure; and family history will focus on congenital anomalies and hereditary disorders in the family. In addition, the content of a pediatric examination will vary with the age and development of the child. Although not specifically defined in these documentation guidelines, these patient group variations on history and examination are appropriate.

A. Documentation of History

The levels of E/M services are based on four types of history (Problem Focused, Expanded Problem Focused, Detailed, and Comprehensive). Each type of history includes some or all of the following elements:

- Chief complaint (CC)
- History of present illness (HPI)
- Review of systems (ROS)
- Past, family, and/or social history (PFSH)

The extent of history of present illness, review of systems, and past, family, and/or social history that is obtained and documented is dependent upon clinical judgment and the nature of the presenting problem.

The chart below shows the progression of the elements required for each type of history. To qualify for a given type of history all three elements in the table must be met. (A chief complaint is indicated at all levels.)

- DG: The CC, ROS, and PFSH may be listed as separate elements of history or they may be included in the description of the history of present illness

- DG: A ROS and/or a PFSH obtained during an earlier encounter does not need to be re-recorded if there is evidence that the physician reviewed and updated the previous information. This may occur when a physician updates his/her own record or in an institutional setting or group practice where many physicians use a common record. The review and update may be documented by:

  - Describing any new ROS and/or PFSH information or noting there has been no change in the information

  - Noting the date and location of the earlier ROS and/or PFSH

- DG: The ROS and/or PFSH may be recorded by ancillary staff or on a form completed by the patient. To document that the physician reviewed the information, there must be a notation supplementing or confirming the information recorded by others

- DG: If the physician is unable to obtain a history from the patient or other source, the record should describe the patient's condition or other circumstance that precludes obtaining a history

Definitions and specific documentation guidelines for each of the elements of history are listed below.

Chief Complaint (CC)

The CC is a concise statement describing the symptom, problem, condition, diagnosis, physician recommended return, or other factor that is the reason for the encounter, usually stated in the patient's words.

- DG: The medical record should clearly reflect the chief complaint

History of Present Illness (HPI)

The HPI is a chronological description of the development of the patient's present illness from the first sign and/or symptom or from the previous encounter to the present. It includes the following elements:

- Location
- Quality
- Severity
- Duration
- Timing
- Context
- Modifying factors
- Associated signs and symptoms

Brief and extended HPIs are distinguished by the amount of detail needed to accurately characterize the clinical problem.

A brief HPI consists of one to three elements of the HPI.

- DG: The medical record should describe one to three elements of the present illness (HPI)

An extended HPI consists of at least four elements of the HPI or the status of at least three chronic or inactive conditions.

- DG: The medical record should describe at least four elements of the present illness (HPI) or the status of at least three chronic or inactive conditions

Beginning with services performed on or after September 10, 2013, CMS has stated that physicians and OQHCP will be able to use the 1997 guidelines for an extended history of present illness (HPI) in combination with other elements from the 1995 documentation guidelines to document a particular level of evaluation and management service.

History of Present Illness	Review of systems (ROS)	PFSH	Type of History
Brief	N/A	N/A	Problem-focused
Brief	Problem Pertinent	N/A	Expanded Problem-Focused
Extended	Extended	Pertinent	Detailed
Extended	Complete	Complete	Comprehensive

Review of Systems (ROS)

A ROS is an inventory of body systems obtained through a series of questions seeking to identify signs and/or symptoms that the patient may be experiencing or has experienced. For purposes of ROS, the following systems are recognized:

- Constitutional symptoms (e.g., fever, weight loss)
- Eyes
- Ears, nose, mouth, throat
- Cardiovascular
- Respiratory
- Gastrointestinal
- Genitourinary
- Musculoskeletal
- Integumentary (skin and/or breast)
- Neurological
- Psychiatric
- Endocrine
- Hematologic/lymphatic
- Allergic/immunologic

A problem pertinent ROS inquires about the system directly related to the problem identified in the HPI.

- DG: The patient's positive responses and pertinent negatives for the system related to the problem should be documented

An extended ROS inquires about the system directly related to the problem identified in the HPI and a limited number of additional systems.

- DG: The patient's positive responses and pertinent negatives for two to nine systems should be documented

A complete ROS inquires about the system directly related to the problem identified in the HPI plus all additional body systems.

- DG: At least 10 organ systems must be reviewed. Those systems with positive or pertinent negative responses must be individually documented. For the remaining systems, a notation indicating all other systems are negative is permissible. In the absence of such a notation, at least 10 systems must be individually documented

Past, Family, and/or Social History (PFSH)

The PFSH consists of a review of three areas:

- Past history (the patient's past experiences with illnesses, operations, injuries, and treatment)
- Family history (a review of medical events in the patient's family, including diseases that may be hereditary or place the patient at risk)
- Social history (an age appropriate review of past and current activities)

For certain categories of E/M services that include only an interval history, it is not necessary to record information about the PFSH. Those categories are subsequent hospital care, follow-up inpatient consultations, and subsequent nursing facility care.

A pertinent PFSH is a review of the history area directly related to the problem identified in the HPI.

- DG: At least one specific item from any of the three history areas must be documented for a pertinent PFSH

A complete PFSH is a review of two or all three of the PFSH history areas, depending on the category of the E/M service. A review of all three history areas is required for services that by their nature include a comprehensive assessment or reassessment of the patient. A review of two of the three history areas is sufficient for other services.

- DG: A least one specific item from two of the three history areas must be documented for a complete PFSH for the following categories of E/M services: office or other outpatient services, established patient; emergency department; domiciliary care, established patient; and home care, established patient

- DG: At least one specific item from each of the three history areas must be documented for a complete PFSH for the following categories of E/M services: office or other outpatient services, new patient; hospital observation services; hospital inpatient services, initial care; consultations; comprehensive nursing facility assessments; domiciliary care, new patient; and home care, new patient

B. *Documentation of Examination 1997 Guidelines*

The levels of E/M services are based on four types of examination:

- Problem Focused: A limited examination of the affected body area or organ system
- Expanded Problem Focused: A limited examination of the affected body area or organ system and any other symptomatic or related body area or organ system
- Detailed: An extended examination of the affected body area or organ system and any other symptomatic or related body area or organ system
- Comprehensive: A general multi-system examination or complete examination of a single organ system and other symptomatic or related body area or organ system

These types of examinations have been defined for general multi-system and the following single organ systems:

- Cardiovascular
- Ears, nose, mouth, and throat
- Eyes
- Genitourinary (Female)
- Genitourinary (Male)
- Hematologic/lymphatic/immunologic
- Musculoskeletal
- Neurological
- Psychiatric
- Respiratory
- Skin

Any physician regardless of specialty may perform a general multi-system examination or any of the single organ system examinations. The type (general multi-system or single organ system) and content of examination are selected by the examining physician and are based upon clinical judgment, the patient's history, and the nature of the presenting problem.

The content and documentation requirements for each type and level of examination are summarized below and described in detail in a table found later on in this document. In the table, organ systems and body areas recognized by CPT for purposes of describing examinations are shown in the left column. The content, or individual elements, of the examination pertaining to that body area or organ system are identified by bullets (•) in the right column.

Parenthetical examples "(e.g., ...)," have been used for clarification and to provide guidance regarding documentation. Documentation for each element must satisfy any numeric requirements (such as "Measurement of any three of the following seven...") included in the description of the element. Elements with multiple components but with no specific numeric requirement (such as "Examination of liver and spleen") require documentation of at least one component. It is possible for a given examination to be expanded beyond what is defined here. When that occurs, findings related to the additional systems and/or areas should be documented.

- DG: Specific abnormal and relevant negative findings from the examination of the affected or symptomatic body area or organ system should be documented. A notation of "abnormal" without elaboration is insufficient

- DG: Abnormal or unexpected findings from the examination of any asymptomatic body area or organ system should be described

- DG: A brief statement or notation indicating "negative" or "normal" is sufficient to document normal findings related to an unaffected areas or asymptomatic organ system

General Multi-System Examinations

General multi-system examinations are described in detail later in this document. To qualify for a given level of multi-system examination, the following content and documentation requirements should be met:

- Problem Focused Examination: It should include performance and documentation of one to five elements identified by a bullet (•) in one or more organ systems or body areas
- Expanded Problem Focused Examination: It should include performance and documentation of at least six elements identified by a bullet (•) in one or more organ systems or body areas
- Detailed Examination: It should include at least six organ systems or body areas. For each system/area selected, performance and documentation of at least two elements identified by a bullet (•) is expected. Alternatively, a detailed examination may include performance and documentation of at least 12 elements identified by a bullet (•) in two or more organ systems or body areas
- Comprehensive Examination: It should include at least nine organ systems or body areas. For each system/area selected, all elements of the examination identified by a bullet (•) should be performed, unless specific directions limit the content of the examination. For each area/system, documentation of at least two elements identified by a bullet (•) is expected

Single Organ System Examinations

The single organ system examinations recognized by CMS include eyes; ears, nose, mouth, and throat; cardiovascular; respiratory; genitourinary (male and female); musculoskeletal; neurologic; hematologic, lymphatic, and immunologic; skin; and psychiatric. Note that for each specific single organ examination type, the performance and documentation of the stated number of elements, identified by a bullet (•) should be included, whether in a box with a shaded or unshaded border. The following content and documentation requirements must be met to qualify for a given level:

- Problem Focused Examination: one to five elements
- Expanded Problem Focused Examination: at least six elements
- Detailed Examination: at least 12 elements (other than eye and psychiatric examinations)
- Comprehensive Examination: all elements (Documentation of every element in a box with a shaded border and at least one element in a box with an unshaded border is expected)

Content and Documentation Requirements

General Multisystem Examination 1997

System/Body Area	Elements of Examination
Constitutional	• Measurement of any three of the following seven vital signs: 1) sitting or standing blood pressure, 2) supine blood pressure, 3) pulse rate and regularity, 4) respiration, 5) temperature, 6) height, 7) weight (May be measured and recorded by ancillary staff). • General appearance of patient (e.g., development, nutrition, body habitus, deformities attention to grooming)
Eyes	• Inspection of conjunctivae and lids • Examination of pupils and irises (e.g., reaction to light and accommodation, size and symmetry) • Ophthalmoscopic examination of optic discs (e.g., size, C/D ratio, appearance) and posterior segments (e.g., vessel changes, exudates, hemorrhages)
Ears, nose, mouth, and throat	• External inspection of ears and nose (e.g., overall appearance, scars, lesions, masses) • Otoscopic examination of external auditory canals and tympanic membranes • Assessment of hearing (e.g., whispered voice, finger rub, tuning fork) • Inspection of nasal mucosa, septum and turbinates • Inspection of lips, teeth and gums • Examination of oropharynx: oral mucosa, salivary glands, hard and soft palates, tongue, tonsils and posterior pharynx
Neck	• Examination of neck (e.g., masses, overall appearance, symmetry, tracheal position, crepitus) • Examination of thyroid (e.g., enlargement, tenderness, mass)
Respiratory	• Assessment of respiratory effort (e.g., intercostal retractions, use of accessory muscles, diaphragmatic movement) • Percussion of chest (e.g., dullness, flatness, hyperresonance) • Palpation of chest (e.g., tactile fremitus) • Auscultation of lungs (e.g., breath sounds, adventitious sounds, rubs)
Cardiovascular	• Palpation of heart (e.g., location, size, thrills) • Auscultation of heart with notation of abnormal sounds and murmurs • Examination of: — carotid arteries (e.g., pulse amplitude, bruits) — abdominal aorta (e.g., size, bruits) — femoral arteries (e.g., pulse amplitude, bruits) — pedal pulses (e.g., pulse amplitude) — extremities for edema and/or varicosities
Chest (Breasts)	• Inspection of breasts (e.g., symmetry, nipple discharge) • Palpation of breasts and axillae (e.g., masses or lumps, tenderness)
Gastrointestinal (Abdomen)	• Examination of abdomen with notation of presence of masses or tenderness • Examination of liver and spleen • Examination for presence or absence of hernia • Examination (when indicated) of anus, perineum and rectum, including sphincter tone, presence of hemorrhoids, rectal masses • Obtain stool sample for occult blood test when indicated

System/Body Area	Elements of Examination
Genitourinary	**Male:** • Examination of the scrotal contents (e.g., hydrocele, spermatocele, tenderness of cord, testicular mass) • Examination of the penis • Digital rectal examination of prostate gland (e.g., size, symmetry, nodularity tenderness) **Female**: • Pelvic examination (with or without specimen collection for smears and cultures), including: — examination of external genitalia (e.g., general appearance, hair distribution, lesions) and vagina (e.g., general appearance, estrogen effect, discharge, lesions, pelvic support, cystocele, rectocele) — examination of urethra (e.g., masses, tenderness, scarring) — examination of bladder (e.g., fullness, masses, tenderness) • Cervix (e.g., general appearance, lesions, discharge) • Uterus (e.g., size, contour, position, mobility, tenderness, consistency, descent or support) • Adnexa/parametria (e.g., masses, tenderness)
Lymphatic	Palpation of lymph nodes in **two or more** areas: • Neck • Groin • Axillae • Other
Musculoskeletal	• Examination of gait and station *(if circled, add to total at bottom of column to the left) • Inspection and/or palpation of digits and nails (e.g., clubbing, cyanosis, inflammatory conditions, petechiae, ischemia, infections, nodes) *(if circled, add to total at bottom of column to the left) Examination of joints, bones and muscles of **one or more of the following six** areas: 1) head and neck; 2) spine, ribs, and pelvis; 3) right upper extremity; 4) left upper extremity; 5) right lower extremity; and 6) left lower extremity. The examination of a given area includes: • Inspection and/or palpation with notation of presence of any misalignment, asymmetry, crepitation, defects, tenderness, masses, effusions • Assessment of range of motion with notation of any pain, crepitation or contracture • Assessment of stability with notation of any dislocation (luxation), subluxation, or laxity • Assessment of muscle strength and tone (e.g., flaccid, cog wheel, spastic) with notation of any atrophy or abnormal movements
Skin	• Inspection of skin and subcutaneous tissue (e.g., rashes, lesions, ulcers) • Palpation of skin and subcutaneous tissue (e.g., induration, subcutaneous nodules, tightening)
Neurologic	• Test cranial nerves with notation of any deficits • Examination of deep tendon reflexes with notation of pathological reflexes (e.g., Babinski) • Examination of sensation (e.g., by touch, pin, vibration, proprioception)
Psychiatric	• Description of patient's judgment and insight • Brief assessment of mental status including: — Orientation to time, place and person — Recent and remote memory — Mood and affect (e.g., depression, anxiety, agitation)

Content and Documentation Requirements

Level of exam	Perform and document
Problem focused	**One to five** elements identified by a bullet
Expanded problem focused	**At least six** elements identified by a bullet
Detailed	**At least 12** elements identified by a bullet, whether in a box with a shaded or unshaded border
Comprehensive	Performance of **all** elements identified by a bullet; whether in a box or with a shaded or unshaded box. Documentation of every element in each with a shaded border and at least one element in a box with an unshaded border is expected

Number of Diagnoses or Management Options	Amount and/or Complexity of Data to be Reviewed	Risk of Complications and/or Morbidity or Mortality	Type of Decision Making
Minimal	Minimal or None	Minimal	Straightforward
Limited	Limited	Low	Low Complexity
Multiple	Moderate	Moderate	Moderate Complexity
Extensive	Extensive	High	High Complexity

C. *Documentation of the Complexity of Medical Decision Making 1995 and 1997*

The levels of E/M services recognize four types of medical decision-making (straightforward, low complexity, moderate complexity, and high complexity). Medical decision-making refers to the complexity of establishing a diagnosis and/or selecting a management option as measured by:

- The number of possible diagnoses and/or the number of management options that must be considered
- The amount and/or complexity of medical records, diagnostic tests, and/or other information that must be obtained, reviewed, and analyzed
- The risk of significant complications, morbidity, and/or mortality, as well as comorbidities, associated with the patient's presenting problem, the diagnostic procedure, and/or the possible management options

The following chart shows the progression of the elements required for each level of medical decision-making. To qualify for a given type of decision-making, two of the three elements in the table must be either met or exceeded.

Each of the elements of medical decision-making is described below.

Number of Diagnoses or Management Options

The number of possible diagnoses and/or the number of management options that must be considered is based on the number and types of problems addressed during the encounter, the complexity of establishing a diagnosis, and the management decisions that are made by the physician.

Generally, decision making with respect to a diagnosed problem is easier than that for an identified but undiagnosed problem. The number and type of diagnostic tests employed may be an indicator of the number of possible diagnoses. Problems that are improving or resolving are less complex than those that are worsening or failing to change as expected. The need to seek advice from others is another indicator of complexity of diagnostic or management problems.

- DG: For each encounter, an assessment, clinical impression, or diagnosis should be documented. It may be explicitly stated or implied in documented decisions regarding management plans and/or further evaluation
    - For a presenting problem with an established diagnosis, the record should reflect whether the problem is: a) improved, well controlled, resolving, or resolved; or b) inadequately controlled, worsening, or failing to change as expected
    - For a presenting problem without an established diagnosis, the assessment or clinical impression may be stated in the form of a differential diagnosis or as a "possible," "probable," or "rule-out" (R/O) diagnosis
- DG: The initiation of, or changes in, treatment should be documented. Treatment includes a wide range of management options including patient instructions, nursing instructions, therapies, and medications
- DG: If referrals are made, consultations requested, or advice sought, the record should indicate to whom or where the referral or consultation is made or from whom the advice is requested

Amount and/or Complexity of Data to be Reviewed

The amount and complexity of data to be reviewed is based on the types of diagnostic testing ordered or reviewed. A decision to obtain and review old medical records and/or obtain history from sources other than the patient increases the amount and complexity of data to be reviewed.

Discussion of contradictory or unexpected test results with the physician who performed or interpreted the test is an indication of the complexity of data being reviewed. On occasion, the physician who ordered a test may personally review the image, tracing, or specimen to supplement information from the physician who prepared the test report or interpretation; this is another indication of the complexity of data being reviewed.

- DG: If a diagnostic service (test or procedure) is ordered, planned, scheduled, or performed at the time of the E/M encounter, the type of service (e.g., lab or x-ray) should be documented
- DG: The review of lab, radiology, and/or other diagnostic tests should be documented. A simple notation such as WBC elevated" or "chest x-ray unremarkable" is acceptable. Alternatively, the review may be documented by initialing and dating the report containing the test results
- DG: A decision to obtain old records or a decision to obtain additional history from the family, caretaker, or other source to supplement that obtained from the patient should be documented
- DG: Relevant findings from the review of old records and/or the receipt of additional history from the family, caretaker, or other source to supplement that obtained from the patient should be documented. If there is no relevant information beyond that already obtained, that fact should be documented. A notation of "old records reviewed" or "additional history obtained from family" without elaboration is insufficient
- DG: The results of discussion of laboratory, radiology, or other diagnostic tests with the physician who performed or interpreted the study should be documented
- DG: The direct visualization and independent interpretation of an image, tracing, or specimen previously or subsequently interpreted by another physician should be documented

Risk of Significant Complications, Morbidity, and/or Mortality

The risk of significant complications, morbidity, and/or mortality is based on the risks associated with the presenting problem, the diagnostic procedure, and the possible management options.

- DG: Comorbidities/underlying disease or other factors that increase the complexity of medical decision making by increasing the risk of complications, morbidity, and/or mortality should be documented
- DG: If a surgical or invasive diagnostic procedure is ordered, planned, or scheduled at the time of the E/M encounter, the type of procedure (e.g., laparoscopy) should be documented
- DG: If a surgical or invasive diagnostic procedure is performed at the time of the E/M encounter, the specific procedure should be documented
- DG: The referral for or decision to perform a surgical or invasive diagnostic procedure on an urgent basis should be documented or implied

The following Table of Risk may be used to help determine whether the risk of significant complications, morbidity, and/or mortality is minimal, low, moderate, or high. Because the determination of risk is complex and not readily quantifiable, the table includes common clinical examples rather than absolute measures of risk. The assessment of risk of the presenting problem is based on the risk related to the disease process anticipated between the present encounter and the next one. The assessment of risk of selecting diagnostic procedures and management options is based on the risk during and immediately following any procedures or treatment. The highest level of risk in any one category (presenting problem, diagnostic procedure, or management options) determines the overall risk.

Table of Risk

Level of Risk	Presenting Problem(s)	Diagnostic Procedure(s) Ordered	Management Options Selected
Minimal	One self-limited or minor problem (e.g., cold, insect bite, tinea corporis)	Laboratory test requiring venipuncture Chest x-rays EKG/EEG Urinalysis Ultrasound (e.g., echocardiography) KOH prep	Rest Gargles Elastic bandages Superficial dressings
Low	Two or more self-limited or minor problems One stable chronic illness (e.g., well controlled hypertension, non-insulin dependent diabetes, cataract, BPH) Acute, uncomplicated illness or injury (e.g., cystitis, allergic rhinitis, simple sprain)	Physiologic tests not under stress (e.g., pulmonary function tests) Non-cardiovascular imaging studies with contrast (e.g., barium enema) Superficial needle biopsies Clinical laboratory tests requiring arterial puncture Skin biopsies	Over-the-counter drugs Minor surgery with no identified risk factors Physical therapy Occupational therapy IV fluids without additives
Moderate	One or more chronic illnesses with mild exacerbation, progression or side effects of treatment Two or more stable chronic illnesses Undiagnosed new problem with uncertain prognosis (e.g., lump in breast) Acute illness with systemic symptoms (e.g., pyelonephritis, pneumonitis, colitis) Acute complicated injury (e.g., head injury with brief loss of consciousness)	Physiologic tests not under stress (e.g., cardiac stress test, fetal contraction stress test) Diagnostic endoscopies with no identified risk factors Deep needle or incisional biopsy Cardiovascular imaging studies with contrast and no identified risk factors (e.g., arteriogram, cardiac catheterization) Obtain fluid from body cavity (e.g., lumbar puncture, thoracentesis, culdocentesis)	Minor surgery with identified risk factors Effective major surgery (open, percutaneous or endoscopic) with no identified risk factors Prescription drug management Therapeutic nuclear medicine IV fluids with additives Closed treatment of fracture or dislocation without manipulation
High	One or more chronic illnesses with severe exacerbation, progression or side effects of treatment Acute/chronic illnesses that may pose a threat to life or bodily function (e.g., multiple trauma, acute MI, pulmonary embolus, severe respiratory distress, progressive severe rheumatoid arthritis, psychiatric illness with potential threat to self or others, peritonitis, acute renal failure An abrupt change in neurologic status (e.g., seizure, TIA, weakness or sensory loss)	Cardiovascular imaging studies with contrast with identified risk factors Cardiac electrophysiological tests Diagnostic endoscopies with identified risk factors Discography	Elective major surgery (open, percutaneous or endoscopic) with identified risk factors Emergency major surgery (open, percutaneous or endoscopic) Parenteral controlled substances Drug therapy requiring intensive monitoring for toxicity Decision not to resuscitate or to de-escalate care because of poor prognosis

D. Documentation of an Encounter Dominated by Counseling or Coordination of Care

In the case where counseling and/or coordination of care dominates (more than 50 percent) the physician/patient and/or family encounter (face-to-face time in the office or other outpatient setting or floor-unit time in the hospital or nursing facility), time is considered the key or controlling factor to qualify for a particular level of E/M service.

- DG: If the physician elects to report the level of service based on counseling and/or coordination of care, the total length of time of the encounter (face-to-face or floor time, as appropriate) should be documented and the record should describe the counseling and/or activities to coordinate care

Appendix D — Crosswalk of Deleted Codes

The deleted code crosswalk is meant to be used as a reference tool to find active codes that could be used in place of the deleted code. This will not always be an exact match. Please review the code descriptions and guidelines before selecting a code.

Code	Cross reference
0058T	To report, see 89398
0085T	To report, see 84999
0111T	To report, see 82726
0126T	To report, see 93998
0228T	To report, see 64999
0229T	To report, see 64999
0230T	To report, see 64999
0231T	To report, see 64999
0295T	To report, see [93241, 93242, 93243, 93244, 93245, 93246, 93247, 93248]
0296T	To report, see [93241, 93242, 93243, 93244, 93245, 93246, 93247, 93248]
0297T	To report, see [93241, 93242, 93243, 93244, 93245, 93246, 93247, 93248]
0298T	To report, see [93241, 93242, 93243, 93244, 93245, 93246, 93247, 93248]
0381T	To report, see 95999
0382T	To report, see 95999
0383T	To report, see 95999
0384T	To report, see 95999
0385T	To report, see 95999
0386T	To report, see 95999
0396T	To report, see 27599
0400T	To report, see 96999
0401T	To report, see 96999
0405T	To report, see 99499
19324	To report, see 15771-15772
32405	To report, see 32408
87450	To report, see 87301-87451, 87802-87899 [87806, 87811]
92585	To report, see 92652-92653
92586	To report, see 92650-92651
99201	To report, see 99202

Appendix E — Resequenced Codes

This appendix contains a list of codes that are not in numeric order in the book. AMA resequenced some code numbers to relocate codes in the same category but not in numeric sequence. In addition to the list of resequenced codes, the page number where the code may be found is provided for ease of use.

Code	Page	Reference
10004	13	See code following 10021.
10005	13	See code following 10021.
10006	13	See code following 10021.
10007	13	See code following 10021.
10008	13	See code following 10021.
10009	13	See code following 10021.
10010	13	See code following 10021.
10011	13	See code following 10021.
10012	13	See code following 10021.
11045	15	See code following 11042.
11046	15	See code following 11043.
15769	28	See code following 15770.
20560	40	See code following 20553.
20561	40	See code before 20555.
21552	51	See code following 21555.
21554	51	See code following 21556.
22858	61	See code following 22856.
22859	60	See code following 22854.
23071	63	See code following 23075.
23073	63	See code following 23076.
24071	66	See code following 24075.
24073	66	See code following 24076.
25071	70	See code following 25075.
25073	70	See code following 25076.
26111	76	See code following 26115.
26113	76	See code following 26116.
27043	82	See code following 27047.
27045	82	See code following 27048.
27059	83	See code following 27049.
27329	88	See code following 27360.
27337	87	See code following 27327.
27339	87	See code before 27330.
27632	93	See code following 27618.
27634	93	See code following 27619.
28039	97	See code following 28043.
28041	97	See code following 28045.
28295	100	See code following 28296.
29914	107	See code following 29863.
29915	107	See code following 29863.
29916	107	See code before 29866.
31253	112	See code following 31255.
31257	112	See code following 31255.
31259	112	See code following 31255.
31551	116	See code following 31580.
31552	116	See code following 31580.
31553	116	See code following 31580.
31554	116	See code following 31580.
31572	116	See code following 31578.
31573	116	See code following 31578.
31574	116	See code following 31578.
31651	118	See code following 31647.
32994	124	See code following 32998.
33221	127	See code following 33213.
33227	128	See code following 33233.
33228	128	See code following 33233.
33229	128	See code before 33234.
33230	129	See code following 33240.
33231	129	See code before 33241.
33262	129	See code following 33241.
33263	130	See code following 33241.
33264	130	See code before 33243.
33270	130	See code following 33249.
33271	130	See code following 33249.
33272	130	See code following 33249.
33273	131	See code following 33249.
33274	131	See code following 33249.
33275	131	See code following 33249.
33440	134	See code following 33410.
33962	145	See code following 33959.
33963	146	See code following 33959.
33964	146	See code following 33959.
33965	146	See code following 33959.
33966	146	See code following 33959.
33969	146	See code following 33959.
33984	146	See code following 33959.
33985	146	See code following 33959.
33986	146	See code following 33959.
33987	146	See code following 33959.
33988	146	See code following 33959.
33989	146	See code following 33959.
33995	148	See code following 33983.
33997	148	See code following 33992.
34717	150	See code following 34708.
34718	151	See code following 34709.
34812	151	See code following 34713.
34820	151	See code following 34714.
34833	152	See code following 34714.
34834	152	See code following 34714.
36465	164	See code following 36471.
36466	164	See code following 36471.
36482	165	See code following 36479.
36483	165	See code following 36479.
36572	167	See code following 36569.
36573	167	See code following 36569.
37246	174	See code following 37235.
37247	175	See code following 37235.
37248	175	See code following 37235.
37249	175	See code following 37235.
38243	179	See code following 38241.
43210	195	See code following 43259.
43211	192	See code following 43217.
43212	192	See code following 43217.
43213	192	See code following 43220.
43214	192	See code following 43220.
43233	195	See code following 43249.
43266	195	See code following 43255.
43270	195	See code following 43257.
43274	197	See code following numeric code 43270.
43275	197	See code following numeric code 43270.
43276	197	See code following numeric code 43270.
43277	197	See code following numeric code 43270.
43278	197	See code following numeric code 43270.
44381	208	See code following 44382.
44401	208	See code following 44392.
45346	212	See code following 45338.
45388	213	See code following 45382.
45390	214	See code following 45392.
45398	214	See code following 45393.
45399	215	See code before 45990.
46220	216	See code before 46230.
46320	216	See code following 46230.
46945	215	See code following 46221.
46946	216	See code following resequenced code 46945.
46947	218	See code following 46761.
46948	216	See code before resequenced code 46220.
50430	235	See code following 50396.
50431	236	See code following 50396.
50432	236	See code following 50396.
50433	236	See code following 50396.
50434	236	See code following 50396.
50435	236	See code following 50396.
50436	235	See code following 50391.
50437	235	See code following 50391.
51797	242	See code following 51729.
52356	246	See code following 52353.
58674	264	See code before 58541.
62328	289	See code following 62270.
62329	289	See code following 62272.
64461	300	See code following 64484.

Code	Page	Reference
64462	300	See code following 64484.
64463	300	See code following 64484.
64624	302	See code following 64610.
64625	302	See code before 64611.
64633	303	See code following 64620.
64634	303	See code following 64620.
64635	303	See code following 64620.
64636	303	See code before 64630.
66987	314	See code following 66982.
66988	314	See code following 66984.
67810	319	See code following 67715.
77085	352	See code following 77081.
77086	352	See code before 77084.
77295	353	See code before 77300.
77385	364	See code following 77417.
77386	354	See code following 77417.
77387	354	See code following 77417.
77424	354	See code following 77417.
77425	354	See code following 77417.
78429	359	See code following 78459.
78430	359	See code following 78491.
78431	359	See code following 78492.
78432	359	See code following 78492.
78433	359	See code following 78492.
78434	359	See code following 78492.
78804	361	See code following 78802.
78830	361	See code following numeric code 78804.
78831	361	See code following numeric code 78804.
78832	361	See code following numeric code 78804.
78835	361	See code following numeric code 78804.
80081	363	See code following 80055.
80161	366	See code following 80157.
80164	367	See code following 80201.
80165	367	See code following 80201.
80167	366	See code following 80169.
80171	366	See code before 80170.
80176	366	See code following 80177.
80179	367	See code before 80195.
80181	366	See code following resequenced code 80167.
80189	366	See code following resequenced code 80230.
80193	366	See code before 80177.
80204	367	See code following 80178.
80210	367	See code following 80194.
80230	366	See code following 80173.
80235	366	See code before 80175.
80280	367	See code following 80202.
80285	367	See code before 80203.
80305	364	See code before 80143.
80306	364	See code before 80143.
80307	364	See code before 80143.

Code	Page	Reference
80320	364	See code before 80143.
80321	364	See code before 80143.
80322	364	See code before 80143.
80323	364	See code before 80143.
80324	364	See code before 80143.
80325	364	See code before 80143.
80326	364	See code before 80143.
80327	364	See code before 80143.
80328	364	See code before 80143.
80329	364	See code before 80143.
80330	364	See code before 80143.
80331	364	See code before 80143.
80332	364	See code before 80143.
80333	365	See code before 80143.
80334	365	See code before 80143.
80335	365	See code before 80143.
80336	365	See code before 80143.
80337	365	See code before 80143.
80338	365	See code before 80143.
80339	365	See code before 80143.
80340	365	See code before 80145.
80341	365	See code before 80143.
80342	365	See code before 80143.
80343	365	See code before 80143.
80344	365	See code before 80143.
80345	365	See code before 80143.
80346	365	See code before 80143.
80347	365	See code before 80143.
80348	365	See code before 80143.
80349	365	See code before 80143.
80350	365	See code before 80143.
80351	365	See code before 80143.
80352	365	See code before 80143.
80353	365	See code before 80143.
80354	365	See code before 80143.
80355	365	See code before 80143.
80356	365	See code before 80143.
80357	365	See code before 80143.
80358	365	See code before 80143.
80359	365	See code before 80143.
80360	365	See code before 80143.
80361	365	See code before 80143.
80362	365	See code before 80143.
80363	365	See code before 80143.
80364	365	See code before 80143.
80365	365	See code before 80143.
80366	365	See code before 80143.
80367	365	See code before 80143.
80368	365	See code before 80143.
80369	365	See code before 80143.
80370	365	See code before 80143.
80371	366	See code before 80143.
80372	366	See code before 80143.
80373	366	See code before 80143.

Code	Page	Reference
80374	366	See code before 80143.
80375	366	See code before 80143.
80376	366	See code before 80143.
80377	366	See code before 80143.
81105	375	See code before 81260.
81106	375	See code before 81260.
81107	375	See code before 81260.
81108	375	See code before 81260.
81109	375	See code before 81260.
81110	375	See code before 81260.
81111	375	See code before 81260.
81112	375	See code before 81260.
81120	375	See code before 81260.
81121	375	See code before 81260.
81161	373	See code following numeric code 81231.
81162	371	See code following resequenced code 81210.
81163	371	See code following resequenced code 81210.
81164	371	See code before 81212.
81165	372	See code following 81212.
81166	372	See code following 81212.
81167	372	See code following 81216.
81168	372	See code before 81218.
81173	370	See code following resequenced code 81204.
81174	370	See code following resequenced code 81204.
81184	372	See code following resequenced code 81233.
81185	372	See code following resequenced code 81233.
81186	372	See code following resequenced code 81233.
81187	372	See code following resequenced code 81268.
81188	373	See code following resequenced code 81266.
81189	373	See code following resequenced code 81266.
81190	373	See code following resequenced code 81266.
81191	377	See code following numeric code 81312.
81192	377	See code following numeric code 81312.
81193	377	See code following numeric code 81312.
81194	377	See code following numeric code 81312.
81200	370	See code before 81175.
81201	370	See code following numeric code 81174.
81202	370	See code following numeric code 81174.
81203	370	See code following numeric code 81174.

Code	Page	Reference
81204	370	See code following numeric code 81174.
81205	371	See code following numeric code 81210.
81206	371	See code following numeric code 81210.
81207	371	See code following numeric code 81210.
81208	371	See code following numeric code 81210.
81209	371	See code following numeric code 81210.
81210	371	See code following numeric code 81210.
81219	372	See code before 81218.
81227	373	See code before 81225.
81230	373	See code following numeric code 81227.
81231	373	See code following numeric code 81227.
81233	372	See code following 81217.
81234	373	See code following numeric code 81231.
81238	373	See code following 81241.
81239	373	See code before 81232.
81245	374	See code following 81242.
81246	374	See code following 81242.
81250	374	See code before 81247.
81257	374	See code following 81254.
81258	374	See code following 81254.
81259	374	See code following 81254.
81261	375	See code before 81260.
81262	375	See code before 81260.
81263	375	See code before 81260.
81264	375	See code before 81260.
81265	372	See code following resequenced code 81187.
81266	372	See code following resequenced code 81187.
81267	372	See code following 81224.
81268	372	See code following 81224.
81269	374	See code following resequenced code 81259.
81271	375	See code following numeric code 81259.
81274	375	See code following resequenced code 81271.
81277	373	See code following 81229.
81278	375	See code following resequenced code 81263.
81279	375	See code following 81270.
81283	375	See code following resequenced code 81121.
81284	374	See code following numeric code 81246.
81285	374	See code following numeric code 81246.
81286	374	See code following numeric code 81246.

Code	Page	Reference
81287	376	See code following resequenced code 81304.
81288	376	See code following resequenced code 81292.
81289	374	See code following numeric code 81246.
81291	377	See code before 81305.
81292	376	See code before numeric code 81291.
81293	376	See code before numeric code 81291.
81294	376	See code before numeric code 81291.
81295	376	See code before numeric code 81291.
81301	376	See code following resequenced code 81287.
81302	376	See code following 81290.
81303	376	See code following 81290.
81304	376	See code following 81290.
81306	377	See code following resequenced code 81194.
81307	377	See code before 81313.
81308	377	See code before 81313.
81309	377	See code following 81314.
81312	377	See code before resequenced code 81307.
81320	377	See code before 81315.
81324	377	See code following 81316.
81325	377	See code following 81316.
81326	377	See code following 81316.
81332	378	See code following 81327.
81334	378	See code following numeric code 81326.
81336	378	See code following 81329.
81337	378	See code following 81329.
81338	376	See code following resequenced code 81294.
81339	376	See code before resequenced code 81295.
81343	377	See code following numeric code 81320.
81344	378	See code following numeric code 81332.
81345	378	See code following numeric code 81332.
81347	378	See code before 81328.
81348	378	See code following numeric code 81312.
81351	378	See code before 81335.
81352	378	See code before 81335.
81353	378	See code before 81335.
81357	379	See code before 81350.
81361	374	See code following 81254.
81362	374	See code following 81254.
81363	374	See code following 81254.
81364	374	See code following 81254.
81419	391	See code following 81414.

Code	Page	Reference
81443	391	See code following 81422.
81448	392	See code following 81438.
81479	391	See code following 81408.
81500	394	See code following 81538.
81503	394	See code before 81539.
81504	395	See code following resequenced code 81546.
81522	394	See code following 81518.
81540	395	See code before 81552.
81546	395	See code following 81551.
81595	393	See code following 81490.
81596	394	See code following 81514.
82042	396	See code following 82045.
82652	397	See code following 82306.
82681	400	See code following 82670.
83992	365	See code following resequenced code 80365.
86152	415	See code following 86147.
86153	415	See code before 86148.
86328	416	See code following 86318.
86408	417	See code following 86382.
86409	417	See code following 86382.
86413	417	See code following resequenced code 86409.
87623	428	See code following 87539.
87624	428	See code following 87539.
87625	428	See code before 87540.
87806	430	See code following 87803.
87811	430	See code following 87807.
87906	430	See code following 87901.
87910	430	See code following 87900.
87912	430	See code before 87902.
88177	432	See code following 88173.
88341	436	See code following 88342.
88350	436	See code following 88346.
88364	437	See code following 88365.
88373	437	See code following 88367.
88374	437	See code following 88367.
88377	437	See code following 88369.
90619	457	See code following 90734.
90620	457	See code following 90734.
90621	457	See code following 90734.
90625	457	See code following 90723.
90630	455	See code following 90654.
90644	457	See code following 90732.
90672	455	See code following 90660.
90673	455	See code before 90662.
90674	455	See code following 90661.
90694	456	See code following 90689.
90750	458	See code following 90736.
90756	455	See code following 90661.
92517	470	See code following 92549.
92518	470	See code following 92549.
92519	470	See code following 92549.
92558	471	See code before 92587.

Code	Page	Reference
92597	472	See code following 92604.
92618	472	See code following 92605.
92650	471	See code following 92584.
92651	471	See code following 92584.
92652	471	See code following 92584.
92653	471	See code following 92584.
92920	475	See code following 92998.
92921	475	See code following 92998.
92924	475	See code following 92998.
92925	475	See code following 92998.
92928	475	See code following 92998.
92929	475	See code following 92998.
92933	475	See code following 92998.
92934	476	See code following 92998.
92937	476	See code following 92998.
92938	476	See code following 92998.
92941	476	See code following 92998.
92943	476	See code following 92998.
92944	476	See code following 92998.
92973	476	See code following 92998.
92974	476	See code following 92998.
92975	476	See code following 92998.
92977	476	See code following 92998.
92978	476	See code following 92998.
92979	476	See code following 92998.
93241	478	See code following 93227.
93242	478	See code following 93227.
93243	478	See code following 93227.
93244	478	See code following 93227.
93245	478	See code following 93227.
93246	478	See code following 93227.
93247	478	See code following 93227.
93248	478	See code following 93227.
93260	480	See code following 93284.
93261	480	See code following 93289.
93264	479	See code before 93279.
93356	483	See code following 93351.
94619	496	See code following 94617.
95249	499	See code following 95250.
95700	508	See code following 95967.
95705	508	See code following 95967.
95706	508	See code following 95967.
95707	508	See code following 95967.
95708	508	See code following 95967.
95709	508	See code following 95967.
95710	508	See code following 95967.
95711	508	See code following 95967.
95712	508	See code following 95967.
95713	508	See code following 95967.
95714	508	See code following 95967.
95715	508	See code following 95967.
95716	508	See code following 95967.
95717	508	See code following 95967.
95718	508	See code following 95967.

Code	Page	Reference
95719	508	See code following 95967.
95720	509	See code following 95967.
95721	509	See code following 95967.
95722	509	See code following 95967.
95723	509	See code following 95967.
95724	509	See code following 95967.
95725	509	See code following 95967.
95726	509	See code following 95967.
95782	501	See code following 95811.
95783	501	See code following 95811.
95800	501	See code following 95806.
95801	501	See code following 95806.
95829	502	See code following 95830.
95836	503	See code following 95830.
95885	504	See code following 95872.
95886	504	See code following 95872.
95887	504	See code before 95873.
95938	506	See code following 95926.
95939	506	See code following 95929.
95940	505	See code following 95913.
95941	505	See code following 95913.
95943	506	See code following 95924.
95983	510	See code following 95977.
95984	510	See code following 95977.
96125	513	See code following 96105.
96127	513	See code following 96113.
96164	514	See code following 96159.
96165	514	See code following 96159.
96167	514	See code following 96159.
96168	514	See code following 96159.
96170	514	See code following 96159.
96171	514	See code following 96159.
97151	511	See code following 96040.
97152	511	See code following 96040.
97153	512	See code following 96040.
97154	512	See code following 96040.
97155	512	See code following 96040.
97156	512	See code following 96040.
97157	512	See code following 96040.
97158	512	See code following 96040.
97161	521	See code before 97010.
97162	522	See code before 97010.
97163	522	See code before 97010.
97164	522	See code before 97010.
97165	522	See code before 97010.
97166	522	See code before 97010.
97167	523	See code before 97010.
97168	523	See code before 97010.
97169	523	See code before 97010.
97170	523	See code before 97010.
97171	523	See code before 97010.
97172	523	See code before 97010.
99091	557	See code following resequenced code 99454.

Code	Page	Reference
99177	531	See code following 99174.
99224	544	See code following 99220.
99225	544	See code following 99220.
99226	544	See code following 99220.
99415	553	See code following 99359.
99416	554	See code following 99359.
99417	554	See code following resequenced code 99416.
99421	556	See code following 99443.
99422	556	See code following 99443.
99423	556	See code following 99443.
99439	561	See code following resequenced code 99490.
99451	557	See code following 99449.
99452	557	See code following 99449.
99453	557	See code following 99449.
99454	557	See code following 99449.
99457	558	See code before 99450.
99458	558	See code before 99450.
99473	558	See code before 99450.
99474	558	See code before 99450.
99484	563	See code following 99498.
99485	559	See code following 99467.
99486	559	See code following 99467.
99490	561	See code before 99487.
99491	561	See code before 99487.
2033F	569	See code following 2026F.
3051F	570	See code following 3044F.
3052F	570	See code before 3046F.
0253T	582	See code before 0198T.
0376T	582	See code following 0191T.
0464T	585	See code following 0333T.
0488T	587	See code following 0403T.
0510T	585	See code following 0335T.
0511T	585	See code following 0335T.
0512T	581	See code following 0102T.
0513T	581	See code following 0102T.
0523T	593	See code before 0505T.
0563T	583	See code following 0207T.
0614T	598	See code following 0580T.
0620T	593	See code following 0505T.
0623T	593	See code following 0504T.
0624T	596	See code following 0504T.
0625T	593	See code following 0504T.
0626T	593	See code following 0504T.

Appendix F — Add-on Codes, Optum Modifier 50 Exempt, Modifier 51 Exempt, Optum Modifier 51 Exempt, Modifier 63 Exempt, and Modifier 95 Telemedicine Services

Codes specified as add-on, exempt from modifiers 50, 51 and 63, and modifier 95 (telemedicine services) are listed. The lists are designed to be read left to right rather than vertically.

Add-on Codes

0054T	0055T	0076T	0095T	0098T	0163T	0164T
0165T	0174T	0214T	0215T	0217T	0218T	0222T
0290T	0376T	0397T	0437T	0439T	0443T	0450T
0466T	0471T	0480T	0492T	0496T	0513T	0514T
0523T	0560T	0562T	0570T	0599T	0628T	0630T
0071U	0072U	0073U	0074U	0075U	0076U	0130U
0131U	0132U	0133U	0134U	0135U	0136U	0137U
0138U	0157U	0158U	0159U	0160U	0161U	0162U
0207U	01953	01968	01969	10004	10006	10008
10010	10012	10036	11001	11008	11045	11046
11047	11103	11105	11107	11201	11732	11922
13102	13122	13133	13153	14302	15003	15005
15101	15111	15116	15121	15131	15136	15151
15152	15156	15157	15201	15221	15241	15261
15272	15274	15276	15278	15772	15774	15777
15787	15847	16036	17003	17312	17314	17315
19001	19082	19084	19086	19126	19282	19284
19286	19288	19294	19297	20700	20701	20702
20703	20704	20705	20930	20931	20932	20933
20934	20936	20937	20938	20939	20985	22103
22116	22208	22216	22226	22328	22512	22515
22527	22534	22552	22585	22614	22632	22634
22840	22841	22842	22843	22844	22845	22846
22847	22848	22853	22854	22858	22859	22868
22870	26125	26861	26863	27358	27692	29826
31627	31632	31633	31637	31649	31651	31654
32501	32506	32507	32667	32668	32674	33141
33225	33257	33258	33259	33367	33368	33369
33419	33508	33517	33518	33519	33521	33522
33523	33530	33572	33746	33768	33866	33884
33924	33929	33987	34709	34711	34713	34714
34715	34716	34717	34808	34812	34813	34820
34833	34834	35306	35390	35400	35500	35572
35600	35681	35682	35683	35685	35686	35697
35700	36218	36227	36228	36248	36474	36476
36479	36483	36907	36908	36909	37185	37186
37222	37223	37232	37233	37234	37235	37237
37239	37247	37249	37252	37253	38102	38746
38747	38900	43273	43283	43338	43635	44015
44121	44128	44139	44203	44213	44701	44955
47001	47542	47543	47544	47550	48400	49326
49327	49412	49435	49568	49905	50606	50705
50706	51797	52442	56606	57267	57465	58110
58611	59525	60512	61316	61517	61611	61641
61642	61651	61781	61782	61783	61797	61799
61800	61864	61868	62148	62160	63035	63043
63044	63048	63057	63066	63076	63078	63082
63086	63088	63091	63103	63295	63308	63621
64421	64462	64480	64484	64491	64492	64494
64495	64634	64636	64643	64645	64727	64778
64783	64787	64832	64837	64859	64872	64874
64876	64901	64902	64913	65757	66990	67225
67320	67331	67332	67334	67335	67340	69990
74248	74301	74713	75565	75774	76125	76802
76810	76812	76814	76937	76979	76983	77001
77002	77003	77063	77293	78020	78434	78496
78730	78835	81266	81416	81426	81536	82952
86826	87187	87503	87904	88155	88177	88185
88311	88314	88332	88334	88341	88350	88364
88369	88373	88388	90461	90472	90474	90785
90833	90836	90838	90840	90863	90913	91013
92547	92608	92618	92621	92627	92921	92925
92929	92934	92938	92944	92973	92974	92978
92979	92998	93320	93321	93325	93352	93356
93462	93463	93464	93563	93564	93565	93566
93567	93568	93571	93572	93592	93609	93613
93621	93622	93623	93655	93657	93662	94645
94729	94781	95079	95873	95874	95885	95886
95887	95940	95941	95962	95967	95984	96113
96121	96131	96133	96137	96139	96159	96165
96168	96171	96361	96366	96367	96368	96370
96371	96375	96376	96411	96415	96417	96423
96570	96571	96934	96935	96936	97130	97546
97598	97811	97814	99100	99116	99135	99140
99153	99157	99292	99354	99355	99356	99357
99359	99415	99416	99417	99439	99458	99467
99486	99489	99494	99498	99602	99607	

Optum Modifier 50 Exempt Codes

0214T	0215T	0217T	0218T	15777	20939	34713
34714	34715	34716	34717	34812	34820	34833
34834	35572	36227	36228	49568	63035	63043
63044	64421	64462	64480	64484	64491	64492
64494	64495	64634	64636			

AMA Modifier 51 Exempt Codes

20697	20974	20975	44500	61107	93600	93602
93603	93610	93612	93615	93616	93618	94610
95905	99151	99152				

Optum Modifier 51 Exempt Codes

22585	22614	22632	69990	90281	90283	90284
90287	90288	90291	90296	90371	90375	90376
90377	90378	90384	90385	90386	90389	90393
90396	90399	90476	90477	90581	90585	90586
90587	90619	90620	90621	90625	90630	90632
90633	90634	90636	90644	90647	90648	90649
90650	90651	90653	90654	90655	90656	90657
90658	90660	90661	90662	90664	90666	90667
90668	90670	90672	90673	90674	90675	90676
90680	90681	90682	90685	90686	90687	90688
90689	90690	90691	90694	90696	90697	90698
90700	90702	90707	90710	90713	90714	90715
90716	90717	90723	90732	90733	90734	90736
90738	90739	90740	90743	90744	90746	90747
90748	90749	90750	90756	97010	97012	97014
97016	97018	97022	97024	97026	97028	97032
97033	97034	97035	97036	97110	97112	97113
97116	97124	97129	97130	97140	97150	97161
97162	97163	97164	97165	97166	97167	97168
97169	97170	97171	97172	97530	97533	97535
97537	97542	97545	97546	97597	97598	97602
97605	97606	97607	97608	97610	97750	97755
97760	97761	97763	99050	99051	99053	99056
99058	99060					

Modifier 63 Exempt Codes

30540	30545	31520	33470	33502	33503	33505
33506	33610	33611	33619	33647	33670	33690
33694	33730	33732	33735	33736	33750	33755
33762	33778	33786	33922	33946	33947	33948
33949	36415	36420	36450	36456	36460	36510
36660	39503	43313	43314	43520	43831	44055
44126	44127	44128	46070	46705	46715	46716

46730	46735	46740	46742	46744	47700	47701
49215	49491	49492	49495	49496	49600	49605
49606	49610	49611	53025	54000	54150	54160
63700	63702	63704	63706	65820		

Telemedicine Services Codes

The codes on the following list may be used to report telemedicine services when modifier 95 Synchronous Telemedicine Service Rendered via a Real-Time Interactive Audio and Visual Telecommunications System, is appended.

90791	90792	90832	90833	90834	90836	90837
90838	90845	90846	90847	90863	90951	90952
90954	90955	90957	90958	90960	90961	92227
92228	93228	93229	93268	93270	93271	93272
96040	96116	97802	97803	97804	98960	98961
98962	99202	99203	99204	99205	99212	99213
99214	99215	99231	99232	99233	*99241	*99242
*99243	*99244	*99245	*99251	*99252	*99253	*99254
*99255	99307	99308	99309	99310	99354	99355
99406	99407	99408	99409	99417	99495	99496

* Consultations are noncovered by Medicare

Appendix G — Medicare Internet-only Manuals (IOMs)

The Centers for Medicare and Medicaid Services restructured its paper-based manual system as a web-based system on October 1, 2003. Called the online CMS manual system, it combines all of the various program instructions into internet-only manuals (IOMs), which are used by all CMS programs and contractors. In many instances, the references from the online manuals in appendix G contain a mention of the old paper manuals from which the current information was obtained when the manuals were converted. This information is shown in the header of the text, in the following format, when applicable, as A3-3101, HO-210, and B3-2049.

Effective with implementation of the IOMs, the former method of publishing program memoranda (PMs) to communicate program instructions was replaced by the following four templates:

- One-time notification
- Manual revisions
- Business requirements
- Confidential requirements

The web-based system has been organized by functional area (e.g., eligibility, entitlement, claims processing, benefit policy, program integrity) in an effort to eliminate redundancy within the manuals, simplify updating, and make CMS program instructions available more quickly. The web-based system contains the functional areas included below:

Pub. 100	Introduction
Pub. 100-01	Medicare General Information, Eligibility and Entitlement Manual
Pub. 100-02	Medicare Benefit Policy Manual
Pub. 100-03	Medicare National Coverage Determinations (NCD) Manual
Pub. 100-04	Medicare Claims Processing Manual
Pub. 100-05	Medicare Secondary Payer Manual
Pub. 100-06	Medicare Financial Management Manual
Pub. 100-07	State Operations Manual
Pub. 100-08	Medicare Program Integrity Manual
Pub. 100-09	Medicare Contractor Beneficiary and Provider Communications Manual
Pub. 100-10	Quality Improvement Organization Manual
Pub. 100-11	Programs of All-Inclusive Care for the Elderly (PACE) Manual
Pub. 100-12	State Medicaid Manual (under development)
Pub. 100-13	Medicaid State Children's Health Insurance Program (under development)
Pub. 100-14	Medicare ESRD Network Organizations Manual
Pub. 100-15	Medicaid Integrity Program (MIP)
Pub. 100-16	Medicare Managed Care Manual
Pub. 100-17	CMS/Business Partners Systems Security Manual
Pub. 100-18	Medicare Prescription Drug Benefit Manual
Pub. 100-19	Demonstrations
Pub. 100-20	One-Time Notification
Pub. 100-21	Reserved
Pub. 100-22	Medicare Quality Reporting Incentive Programs Manual
Pub. 100-24	State Buy-In Manual
Pub. 100-25	Information Security Acceptable Risk Safeguards Manual

A brief description of the Medicare manuals primarily used for *CPC Expert* follows:

The ***National Coverage Determinations Manual*** (NCD), is organized according to categories such as diagnostic services, supplies, and medical procedures. The table of contents lists each category and subject within that category. Revision transmittals identify any new or background material, recap the changes, and provide an effective date for the change. The manual contains four sections and is organized in accordance with CPT category sequence and contains a list of HCPCS codes related to coverage determinations, where appropriate.

The ***Medicare Benefit Policy Manual*** contains Medicare general coverage instructions that are not national coverage determinations. As a general rule, in the past these instructions have been found in chapter II of the ***Medicare Carriers Manual,*** the ***Medicare Intermediary Manual***, other provider manuals, and program memoranda.

The ***Medicare Claims Processing Manual*** contains instructions for processing claims for contractors and providers.

The ***Medicare Program Integrity Manual*** communicates the priorities and standards for the Medicare integrity programs.

Medicare IOM References

A printed version of the Medicare IOM references will no longer be published in Optum360's *Current Procedural Coding* product. Complete versions of all the manuals can be found online at https://www.cms.gov/Regulations-and-Guidance/Guidance/Manuals/Internet-Only-Manuals-IOMs.

Appendix H — Quality Payment Program

In 2015, Congress passed the Medicare Access and CHIP Reauthorization Act (MACRA), which included sweeping changes for practitioners who provide services reimbursed under the Medicare physician fee schedule (MPFS). The act focused on repealing the faulty Medicare sustainable growth rate, focusing on quality of patient outcomes, and controlling Medicare spending.

A MACRA final rule in October 2016 established the Quality Payment Program (QPP) that was effective January 1, 2017.

The QPP has two tracks:

- The merit-based incentive payment system (MIPS)
- Alternative payment models (APMs)

MIPS uses the existing quality and value reporting, Medicare meaningful use (MU), and value-based modifier (VBM) programs to define certain performance categories that determine an overall score. Eligible clinicians (ECs) can obtain a composite performance score (CPS) of up to 100 points from these weighted performance categories. This performance score then defines the payment adjustments in the second calendar year after the year the score is obtained. For instance, the score obtained for the 2019 performance year is linked to payment for Medicare Part B services in 2021.

The performance categories, along with the weights used to determine the overall score, are:

- Quality
- Advancing care information (previously called meaningful use)
- Clinical practice improvement activities (CPIA)
- Resource use

ECs may also choose to participate in APMs. These payment models, created in conjunction with the clinician community, provide additional incentives to those clinicians in the APM who provide high-quality care as cost-efficiently as possible. APMs can be created around specific clinical conditions, a care episode, or a patient population type. An APM can also be described as a new way of paying the healthcare provider for the care rendered to Medicare patients.

Advanced APMs are a subset of APMs; practices participating in an advanced APM can earn even more incentives because the ECs take on risk related to their patients' outcomes. For calendar years 2019 through 2024, clinicians participating in advanced APMs have the potential to earn an additional 5 percent incentive payment; furthermore, they are exempt from having to participate in MIPS as long as they have sufficiently participated in the advanced APM.

Eligible clinicians have flexible options for submitting data to the MIPS and an option to join advanced APMs. Under the QPP, providers can receive increased payment by providing high-quality care and by controlling costs. ECs who successfully report determined criteria—defined by the pathway chosen—receive a larger payment depending on how successful they are at meeting performance thresholds. Those who do not participate or who do not fulfill the defined requirements receive a negative penalty; failure to participate in a track in 2021 results in 9 percent payment reduction in 2022.

ECs can receive incentives under the QPP. Once the performance threshold is established, ALL ECs who score above that threshold are eligible to receive a positive payment adjustment. Keep in mind that the key requirement is that an EC **submit data** to avoid the negative payment adjustment and receive the incentives. CMS has redesigned the scoring so that clinicians are able to know how well they are doing in the program, as benchmarks are known in advance of participating.

Proposed 2021 Changes

A number of revisions have been proposed for 2021. As noted earlier, in 2021, the maximum negative payment for payment adjustment is negative 9 percent. The positive payment, not including additional positive payments adjustments for exceptional performance, is also up to a 9 percent adjustment. CMS is proposing additions, revisions, and deletions to many of the current reporting measures. Other proposals affecting the MIPS program for 2021 include:

- In the MIPS performance category, CMS proposes to reduce the Quality performance category weight from 45 percent to 40 percent and to increase the Cost performance category weight from 15 percent to 20 percent. This is in accordance with CMS's effort to equalize weighting between the Quality and Cost performance categories by 2022 as indicated in MACRA.
- New specialty sets would be added for Speech Language Pathology, Audiology, Clinical Social Work, Chiropractic Medicine, Pulmonology, Nutrition/Dietician, and Endocrinology.
- CMS proposes adding telehealth services to existing total per capital cost (TPCC) and episode-based cost measures.
- In the Improvement Activities performance category, CMS recommends modification of two existing activities. Additional criteria for nomination of new improvement activity includes linking to existing and related MIPS quality and cost measures.

Within the advanced alternative payment models (APMs), CMS has proposed MIPS quality reporting options for APM participants. Previously, CMS has tried to streamline APM participation in MIPS; however, the agency feels that allowing MIPS quality measures to be reported by the APMs would offer flexibility and improve meaningful measurement.

Appendix I — Medically Unlikely Edits (MUEs)

The Centers for Medicare & Medicaid Services (CMS) began to publish many of the edits used in the medically unlikely edits (MUE) program for the first time effective October 2008. What follows below is a list of the published CPT codes that have MUEs assigned to them and the number of units allowed with each code. CMS publishes the updates on a quarterly basis. Not all MUEs will be published, however. MUEs intended to detect and discourage any questionable payments will not be published as the agency feels the efficacy of these edits would be compromised. CMS added another component to the MUEs—the MUE Adjudication Indicator (MAI). The appropriate MAI can be found in parentheses following the MUE in this table and specify the maximum units of service (UOS) for a CPT/HCPCS code for the service. The MAI designates whether the UOS edit is applied to the line or claim.

The three MAIs are defined as follows:

MAI 1 (Line Edit) This MAI will continué to be adjudicated as the line edit on the claim and is auto-adjudicated by the contractor.

MAI 2 (Date of Service Edit, Policy) This MAI is considered to be the "absolute date of service edit" and is based on policy. The total unit of services (UOS) for that CPT code and that date of service (DOS) are combined for this edit. Medicare contractors are required to review all claims for the same patient, same date of service, and same provider.

MAI 3 (Date of Service Edit: Clinical) This MAI is also a date-of-service edit but is based upon clinical standards. The review takes current and previously submitted claims for the same patient, same date of service, and same provider into account. When medical necessity is clearly documented, the edit may be bypassed or the claim resubmitted.

The quarterly updates are published on the CMS website at https://www.cms.gov/Medicare/Coding/NationalCorrectCodInitEd/MUE. The following was updated on 10/01/2020.

Professional

CPT	*MUE*
0001U	1(2)
0002M	1(3)
0002U	1(2)
0003M	1(3)
0003U	1(2)
0004M	1(2)
0005U	1(2)
0006M	1(2)
0007M	1(2)
0007U	1(2)
0008U	1(3)
0009U	2(3)
0010U	2(3)
0011M	1(2)
0011U	1(2)
0012M	1(2)
0012U	1(2)
0013M	1(2)
0013U	1(3)
0014M	1(2)
0014U	1(3)
0016U	1(3)
0017U	1(3)
0018U	1(1)
0019U	1(3)
0021U	1(2)
0022U	2(3)
0023U	1(2)
0024U	1(2)
0025U	1(2)
0026U	1(3)
0027U	1(2)
0029U	1(2)
0030U	1(2)
0031U	1(2)
0032U	1(2)
0033U	1(2)
0034U	1(2)
0035U	1(2)
0036U	1(3)
0037U	1(3)
0038U	1(2)
0039U	1(2)

CPT	*MUE*
0040U	1(2)
0041U	1(2)
0042T	1(3)
0042U	1(2)
0043U	1(2)
0044U	1(2)
0045U	1(3)
0046U	1(3)
0047U	1(3)
0048U	1(3)
0049U	1(3)
0050U	1(3)
0051U	1(2)
0052U	1(2)
0053U	1(3)
0054T	1(3)
0054U	1(2)
0055T	1(3)
0055U	1(2)
0056U	1(3)
0058T	1(2)
0058U	1(2)
0059U	1(2)
0060U	1(2)
0061U	2(3)
0062U	1(2)
0063U	1(2)
0064U	2(3)
0065U	2(3)
0066U	1(3)
0067U	2(3)
0068U	1(3)
0069U	1(3)
0070U	1(2)
0071T	1(2)
0071U	1(2)
0072T	1(2)
0072U	1(2)
0073U	1(2)
0074U	1(2)
0075T	1(2)
0075U	1(2)
0076T	1(2)
0076U	1(2)

CPT	*MUE*
0077U	2(2)
0078U	1(2)
0079U	0(3)
0080U	1(2)
0082U	1(2)
0083U	1(3)
0084U	1(2)
0085T	0(3)
0086U	1(3)
0087U	1(2)
0088U	1(2)
0089U	1(2)
0090U	1(2)
0091U	1(2)
0092U	1(2)
0093U	1(2)
0094U	1(2)
0095T	1(3)
0095U	1(2)
0096U	1(2)
0097U	1(2)
0098T	2(3)
0098U	1(2)
0099U	1(2)
0100T	1(2)
0100U	1(2)
0101T	1(3)
0101U	1(2)
0102T	2(2)
0102U	1(2)
0103U	1(2)
0105U	1(2)
0106T	4(2)
0106U	1(2)
0107T	4(2)
0107U	1(3)
0108T	4(2)
0108U	1(2)
0109T	4(2)
0109U	1(3)
0110T	4(2)
0110U	1(2)
0111T	1(3)
0111U	1(2)

CPT	*MUE*
0112U	1(3)
0113U	1(2)
0114U	1(2)
0115U	1(3)
0116U	1(2)
0117U	1(2)
0118U	1(2)
0119U	1(2)
0120U	1(2)
0121U	1(2)
0122U	1(2)
0123U	1(2)
0126T	1(3)
0129U	1(2)
0130U	1(2)
0131U	1(2)
0132U	1(2)
0133U	1(2)
0134U	1(2)
0135U	1(2)
0136U	1(2)
0137U	1(2)
0138U	1(2)
0139U	1(2)
0140U	1(2)
0141U	1(2)
0142U	1(2)
0143U	1(2)
0144U	1(2)
0145U	1(2)
0146U	1(2)
0147U	1(2)
0148U	1(2)
0149U	1(2)
0150U	1(2)
0151U	1(2)
0152U	1(2)
0153U	1(2)
0154U	1(2)
0155U	1(2)
0156U	1(2)
0157U	1(2)
0158U	1(2)
0159U	1(2)

CPT	*MUE*
0160U	1(2)
0161U	1(2)
0162U	1(2)
0163T	1(3)
0163U	0(3)
0164T	4(2)
0164U	1(2)
0165T	4(2)
0165U	1(2)
0166U	1(2)
0167U	1(2)
0168U	1(2)
0169U	1(2)
0170U	1(2)
0171U	1(2)
0172U	1(2)
0173U	1(2)
0174T	1(3)
0174U	1(2)
0175T	1(3)
0175U	1(2)
0176U	1(3)
0177U	1(2)
0178U	1(2)
0179U	1(2)
0184T	1(3)
0191T	2(2)
0198T	2(2)
01996	1(2)
0200T	1(2)
0201T	1(2)
0202T	1(3)
0202U	1(3)
0207T	2(2)
0208T	1(3)
0209T	1(3)
0210T	1(3)
0211T	1(3)
0212T	1(3)
0213T	1(2)
0214T	1(2)
0215T	1(2)
0216T	1(2)
0217T	1(2)

CPT	*MUE*
0218T	1(2)
0219T	1(2)
0220T	1(2)
0221T	1(2)
0222T	1(3)
0223U	1(3)
0224U	3(3)
0228T	1(2)
0229T	2(3)
0230T	1(2)
0231T	2(3)
0232T	1(3)
0234T	2(2)
0235T	2(3)
0236T	1(2)
0237T	2(3)
0238T	2(3)
0253T	1(3)
0263T	1(3)
0264T	1(3)
0265T	1(3)
0266T	1(2)
0267T	1(3)
0268T	1(3)
0269T	1(2)
0270T	1(3)
0271T	1(3)
0272T	1(3)
0273T	1(3)
0274T	1(2)
0275T	1(2)
0278T	1(3)
0290T	1(3)
0295T	1(2)
0296T	1(2)
0297T	1(2)
0298T	1(2)
0308T	1(3)
0312T	1(3)
0313T	1(3)
0314T	1(3)
0315T	1(3)
0316T	1(3)
0317T	1(3)

CPT	*MUE*
0329T	1(2)
0330T	1(2)
0331T	1(3)
0332T	1(3)
0333T	1(2)
0335T	2(2)
0338T	1(2)
0339T	1(2)
0342T	1(3)
0345T	1(2)
0347T	1(3)
0348T	1(3)
0349T	1(3)
0350T	1(3)
0351T	5(3)
0352T	5(3)
0353T	2(3)
0354T	2(3)
0355T	1(2)
0356T	4(2)
0358T	1(2)
0362T	8(3)
0373T	24(3)
0376T	2(3)
0378T	1(2)
0379T	1(2)
0381T	1(2)
0382T	1(2)
0383T	1(2)
0384T	1(2)
0385T	1(2)
0386T	1(2)
0394T	2(3)
0395T	2(3)
0396T	2(2)
0397T	1(3)
0398T	1(3)
0400T	1(2)
0401T	1(2)
0402T	2(2)
0403T	1(2)
0404T	1(2)
0405T	1(2)
0408T	1(3)

CPT	*MUE*
0409T	1(3)
0410T	1(3)
0411T	1(3)
0412T	1(2)
0413T	1(3)
0414T	1(2)
0415T	1(3)
0416T	1(3)
0417T	1(3)
0418T	1(3)
0419T	1(2)
0420T	1(2)
0421T	1(2)
0422T	1(3)
0423T	1(3)
0424T	1(3)
0425T	1(3)
0426T	1(3)
0427T	1(3)
0428T	1(2)
0429T	1(2)
0430T	1(2)
0431T	1(2)
0432T	1(3)
0433T	1(3)
0434T	1(3)
0435T	1(3)
0436T	1(3)
0437T	1(3)
0439T	1(3)
0440T	3(3)
0441T	3(3)
0442T	3(3)
0443T	1(2)
0444T	1(2)
0445T	1(2)
0446T	1(3)
0447T	1(3)
0448T	1(3)
0449T	1(2)
0450T	1(3)
0451T	1(3)
0452T	1(3)
0453T	1(3)

CPT	MUE
0454T	3(3)
0455T	1(3)
0456T	1(3)
0457T	1(3)
0458T	3(3)
0459T	1(3)
0460T	3(3)
0461T	1(3)
0462T	1(2)
0463T	1(2)
0464T	1(2)
0465T	1(3)
0466T	1(3)
0467T	1(3)
0468T	1(3)
0469T	1(2)
0470T	1(2)
0471T	2(1)
0472T	1(2)
0473T	1(2)
0474T	2(2)
0475T	1(3)
0476T	1(3)
0477T	1(3)
0478T	1(3)
0479T	1(2)
0480T	4(1)
0481T	1(3)
0483T	1(2)
0484T	1(2)
0485T	1(2)
0486T	1(2)
0487T	1(3)
0488T	1(2)
0489T	1(2)
0490T	1(2)
0491T	1(2)
0492T	4(3)
0493T	1(3)
0494T	1(2)
0495T	1(2)
0496T	4(3)
0497T	1(3)
0498T	1(2)
0499T	1(2)
0500T	1(3)
0501T	1(2)
0502T	1(2)
0503T	1(2)
0504T	1(2)
0505T	1(3)
0506T	1(2)
0507T	1(2)
0508T	1(3)
0509T	1(2)
0510T	1(2)
0511T	1(2)
0512T	1(2)
0513T	2(3)
0514T	2(2)
0515T	1(3)
0516T	1(3)
0517T	1(3)
0518T	1(3)
0519T	1(3)

CPT	MUE
0520T	1(3)
0521T	1(3)
0522T	1(3)
0523T	1(3)
0524T	3(3)
0525T	1(3)
0526T	1(3)
0527T	1(3)
0528T	1(3)
0529T	1(3)
0530T	1(3)
0531T	1(3)
0532T	1(3)
0533T	1(2)
0534T	1(2)
0535T	1(2)
0536T	1(2)
0537T	1(2)
0538T	1(3)
0539T	1(3)
0540T	1(3)
0541T	1(3)
0542T	1(3)
0543T	1(2)
0544T	1(2)
0545T	1(2)
0546T	2(2)
0547T	1(2)
0548T	1(2)
0549T	1(2)
0550T	2(3)
0551T	1(2)
0552T	1(3)
0553T	2(2)
0554T	1(2)
0555T	1(2)
0556T	1(2)
0557T	1(2)
0558T	1(2)
0559T	1(2)
0560T	1(3)
0561T	1(2)
0562T	1(3)
0563T	1(2)
0564T	1(2)
0565T	1(2)
0566T	1(2)
0567T	1(2)
0568T	1(2)
0569T	1(2)
0570T	1(3)
0571T	1(2)
0572T	1(2)
0573T	1(2)
0574T	1(2)
0575T	1(2)
0576T	1(2)
0577T	1(2)
0578T	1(2)
0579T	1(2)
0580T	1(2)
0581T	0(3)
0582T	0(3)
0583T	2(2)
0584T	1(2)

CPT	MUE
0585T	1(2)
0586T	1(2)
0587T	1(2)
0588T	1(2)
0589T	1(2)
0590T	1(2)
0591T	1(2)
0592T	1(2)
0593T	1(2)
10004	3(3)
10005	1(2)
10006	3(3)
10007	1(2)
10008	2(3)
10009	1(2)
10010	3(3)
10011	1(2)
10012	3(3)
10021	1(2)
10030	2(3)
10035	1(2)
10036	2(3)
10040	1(2)
10060	1(2)
10061	1(2)
10080	1(3)
10081	1(3)
10120	3(3)
10121	2(3)
10140	2(3)
10160	3(3)
10180	2(3)
11000	1(2)
11001	1(3)
11004	1(2)
11005	1(2)
11006	1(2)
11008	1(2)
11010	2(3)
11011	2(3)
11012	2(3)
11042	1(2)
11043	1(2)
11044	1(2)
11045	12(3)
11046	10(3)
11047	10(3)
11055	1(2)
11056	1(2)
11057	1(2)
11102	1(2)
11103	6(3)
11104	1(2)
11105	3(3)
11106	1(2)
11107	2(3)
11200	1(2)
11201	1(3)
11300	5(3)
11301	6(3)
11302	4(3)
11303	3(3)
11305	4(3)
11306	4(3)
11307	3(3)

CPT	MUE
11308	2(3)
11310	4(3)
11311	4(3)
11312	3(3)
11313	3(3)
11400	3(3)
11401	3(3)
11402	3(3)
11403	2(3)
11404	2(3)
11406	2(3)
11420	3(3)
11421	3(3)
11422	3(3)
11423	2(3)
11424	2(3)
11426	2(3)
11440	4(3)
11441	3(3)
11442	3(3)
11443	2(3)
11444	2(3)
11446	2(3)
11450	1(2)
11451	1(2)
11462	1(2)
11463	1(2)
11470	3(2)
11471	2(3)
11600	2(3)
11601	2(3)
11602	3(3)
11603	2(3)
11604	2(3)
11606	2(3)
11620	2(3)
11621	2(3)
11622	2(3)
11623	2(3)
11624	2(3)
11626	2(3)
11640	2(3)
11641	2(3)
11642	3(3)
11643	2(3)
11644	2(3)
11646	2(3)
11719	1(2)
11720	1(2)
11721	1(2)
11730	1(2)
11732	4(3)
11740	2(3)
11750	6(3)
11755	2(3)
11760	4(3)
11762	2(3)
11765	4(3)
11770	1(3)
11771	1(3)
11772	1(3)
11900	1(2)
11901	1(2)
11920	1(2)
11921	1(2)

CPT	MUE
11922	1(3)
11950	1(2)
11951	1(2)
11952	1(2)
11954	1(3)
11960	2(3)
11970	2(3)
11971	2(3)
11976	1(2)
11980	1(2)
11981	1(3)
11982	1(3)
11983	1(3)
12001	1(2)
12002	1(2)
12004	1(2)
12005	1(2)
12006	1(2)
12007	1(2)
12011	1(2)
12013	1(2)
12014	1(2)
12015	1(2)
12016	1(2)
12017	1(2)
12018	1(2)
12020	2(3)
12021	3(3)
12031	1(2)
12032	1(2)
12034	1(2)
12035	1(2)
12036	1(2)
12037	1(2)
12041	1(2)
12042	1(2)
12044	1(2)
12045	1(2)
12046	1(2)
12047	1(2)
12051	1(2)
12052	1(2)
12053	1(2)
12054	1(2)
12055	1(2)
12056	1(2)
12057	1(2)
13100	1(2)
13101	1(2)
13102	9(3)
13120	1(2)
13121	1(2)
13122	9(3)
13131	1(2)
13132	1(2)
13133	7(3)
13151	1(2)
13152	1(2)
13153	2(3)
13160	2(3)
14000	2(3)
14001	2(3)
14020	2(3)
14021	2(3)
14040	2(3)

CPT	MUE
14041	3(3)
14060	2(3)
14061	2(3)
14301	2(3)
14302	8(3)
14350	2(3)
15002	1(2)
15003	60(3)
15004	1(2)
15005	19(3)
15040	1(2)
15050	1(3)
15100	1(2)
15101	40(3)
15110	1(2)
15111	5(3)
15115	1(2)
15116	2(3)
15120	1(2)
15121	8(3)
15130	1(2)
15131	2(3)
15135	1(2)
15136	1(3)
15150	1(2)
15151	1(2)
15152	5(3)
15155	1(2)
15156	1(2)
15157	1(3)
15200	1(2)
15201	7(3)
15220	1(2)
15221	9(3)
15240	1(2)
15241	9(3)
15260	1(2)
15261	6(3)
15271	1(2)
15272	3(3)
15273	1(2)
15274	60(3)
15275	1(2)
15276	3(2)
15277	1(2)
15278	15(3)
15570	2(3)
15572	2(3)
15574	2(3)
15576	2(3)
15600	2(3)
15610	2(3)
15620	2(3)
15630	2(3)
15650	1(3)
15730	1(3)
15731	1(3)
15733	2(3)
15734	4(3)
15736	2(3)
15738	3(3)
15740	2(3)
15750	2(3)
15756	2(3)
15757	2(3)

CPT	MUE
15758	2(3)
15760	2(3)
15769	1(3)
15770	2(3)
15771	1(2)
15772	9(3)
15773	1(2)
15774	3(3)
15775	1(2)
15776	1(2)
15777	1(3)
15780	1(2)
15781	1(3)
15782	1(3)
15783	1(3)
15786	1(2)
15787	2(3)
15788	1(2)
15789	1(2)
15792	1(3)
15793	1(3)
15819	1(2)
15820	1(2)
15821	1(2)
15822	1(2)
15823	1(2)
15824	1(2)
15825	1(2)
15826	1(2)
15828	1(2)
15829	1(2)
15830	1(2)
15832	1(2)
15833	1(2)
15834	1(2)
15835	1(3)
15836	1(2)
15837	2(3)
15838	1(2)
15839	2(3)
15840	1(3)
15841	2(3)
15842	2(3)
15845	2(3)
15847	1(2)
15850	0(3)
15851	1(2)
15852	1(3)
15860	1(3)
15876	1(2)
15877	1(2)
15878	1(2)
15879	1(2)
15920	1(3)
15922	1(3)
15931	1(3)
15933	1(3)
15934	1(3)
15935	1(3)
15936	1(3)
15937	1(3)
15940	2(3)
15941	2(3)
15944	2(3)
15945	2(3)

CPT	MUE
15946	2(3)
15950	2(3)
15951	2(3)
15952	2(3)
15953	2(3)
15956	2(3)
15958	2(3)
15999	1(3)
16000	1(2)
16020	1(3)
16025	1(3)
16030	1(3)
16035	1(2)
16036	8(3)
17000	1(2)
17003	13(2)
17004	1(2)
17106	1(2)
17107	1(2)
17108	1(2)
17110	1(2)
17111	1(2)
17250	4(3)
17260	7(3)
17261	7(3)
17262	6(3)
17263	3(3)
17264	3(3)
17266	2(3)
17270	6(3)
17271	4(3)
17272	5(3)
17273	4(3)
17274	2(3)
17276	2(3)
17280	6(3)
17281	5(3)
17282	4(3)
17283	4(3)
17284	2(3)
17286	2(3)
17311	4(3)
17312	6(3)
17313	3(3)
17314	4(3)
17315	15(3)
17340	1(2)
17360	1(2)
17380	1(3)
17999	1(3)
19000	2(3)
19001	5(3)
19020	2(3)
19030	1(2)
19081	1(2)
19082	2(3)
19083	1(2)
19084	2(3)
19085	1(2)
19086	2(3)
19100	4(3)
19101	3(3)
19105	2(3)
19110	1(3)
19112	2(3)

CPT	MUE
19120	1(2)
19125	1(2)
19126	3(3)
19281	1(2)
19282	2(3)
19283	1(2)
19284	2(3)
19285	1(2)
19286	2(3)
19287	1(2)
19288	2(3)
19294	2(3)
19296	1(3)
19297	2(3)
19298	1(2)
19300	1(2)
19301	1(2)
19302	1(2)
19303	1(2)
19305	1(2)
19306	1(2)
19307	1(2)
19316	1(2)
19318	1(2)
19324	1(2)
19325	1(2)
19328	1(2)
19330	1(2)
19340	1(2)
19342	1(2)
19350	1(2)
19355	1(2)
19357	1(2)
19361	1(2)
19364	1(2)
19366	1(2)
19367	1(2)
19368	1(2)
19369	1(2)
19370	1(2)
19371	1(2)
19380	1(2)
19396	1(2)
19499	1(3)
20100	2(3)
20101	2(3)
20102	3(3)
20103	3(3)
20150	2(3)
20200	2(3)
20205	3(3)
20206	3(3)
20220	3(3)
20225	2(3)
20240	4(3)
20245	3(3)
20250	1(3)
20251	2(3)
20500	2(3)
20501	2(3)
20520	2(3)
20525	4(3)
20526	1(2)
20527	2(3)
20550	5(3)

CPT	MUE
20551	5(3)
20552	1(2)
20553	1(2)
20555	1(3)
20560	1(2)
20561	1(2)
20600	6(3)
20604	4(3)
20605	2(3)
20606	2(3)
20610	2(3)
20611	2(3)
20612	2(3)
20615	1(3)
20650	4(3)
20660	1(2)
20661	1(2)
20662	1(2)
20663	1(2)
20664	1(2)
20665	1(2)
20670	3(3)
20680	3(3)
20690	2(3)
20692	2(3)
20693	2(3)
20694	2(3)
20696	2(3)
20697	4(3)
20700	1(3)
20701	1(3)
20702	1(3)
20703	1(3)
20704	1(3)
20705	1(3)
20802	1(2)
20805	1(2)
20808	1(2)
20816	3(3)
20822	3(3)
20824	1(2)
20827	1(2)
20838	1(2)
20900	2(3)
20902	2(3)
20910	1(3)
20912	1(3)
20920	1(3)
20922	1(3)
20924	2(3)
20930	0(3)
20931	1(2)
20932	1(3)
20933	1(3)
20934	1(3)
20936	0(3)
20937	1(2)
20938	1(2)
20939	1(3)
20950	2(3)
20955	1(3)
20956	1(3)
20957	1(3)
20962	1(3)
20969	2(3)

CPT	MUE
20970	1(3)
20972	2(3)
20973	1(2)
20974	1(3)
20975	1(3)
20979	1(3)
20982	1(2)
20983	1(2)
20985	2(3)
20999	1(3)
21010	1(2)
21011	4(3)
21012	3(3)
21013	2(3)
21014	2(3)
21015	1(3)
21016	2(3)
21025	2(3)
21026	2(3)
21029	1(3)
21030	1(3)
21031	2(3)
21032	1(3)
21034	1(3)
21040	2(3)
21044	1(3)
21045	1(3)
21046	2(3)
21047	2(3)
21048	2(3)
21049	1(3)
21050	1(2)
21060	1(2)
21070	1(2)
21073	1(2)
21076	1(2)
21077	1(2)
21079	1(2)
21080	1(2)
21081	1(2)
21082	1(2)
21083	1(2)
21084	1(2)
21085	1(3)
21086	1(2)
21087	1(2)
21088	1(2)
21089	1(3)
21100	1(2)
21110	2(3)
21116	1(2)
21120	1(2)
21121	1(2)
21122	1(2)
21123	1(2)
21125	2(2)
21127	2(3)
21137	1(2)
21138	1(2)
21139	1(2)
21141	1(2)
21142	1(2)
21143	1(2)
21145	1(2)
21146	1(2)

CPT	MUE
21147	1(2)
21150	1(2)
21151	1(2)
21154	1(2)
21155	1(2)
21159	1(2)
21160	1(2)
21172	1(3)
21175	1(2)
21179	1(2)
21180	1(2)
21181	1(3)
21182	1(2)
21183	1(2)
21184	1(2)
21188	1(2)
21193	1(2)
21194	1(2)
21195	1(2)
21196	1(2)
21198	1(3)
21199	1(2)
21206	1(3)
21208	1(3)
21209	1(3)
21210	2(3)
21215	2(3)
21230	2(3)
21235	2(3)
21240	1(2)
21242	1(2)
21243	1(2)
21244	1(2)
21245	2(2)
21246	2(2)
21247	1(2)
21248	2(3)
21249	2(3)
21255	1(2)
21256	1(2)
21260	1(2)
21261	1(2)
21263	1(2)
21267	1(2)
21268	1(2)
21270	1(2)
21275	1(2)
21280	1(2)
21282	1(2)
21295	1(2)
21296	1(2)
21299	1(3)
21310	1(2)
21315	1(2)
21320	1(2)
21325	1(2)
21330	1(2)
21335	1(2)
21336	1(2)
21337	1(2)
21338	1(2)
21339	1(2)
21340	1(2)
21343	1(2)
21344	1(2)

CPT	MUE
21345	1(2)
21346	1(2)
21347	1(2)
21348	1(2)
21355	1(2)
21356	1(2)
21360	1(2)
21365	1(2)
21366	1(2)
21385	1(2)
21386	1(2)
21387	1(2)
21390	1(2)
21395	1(2)
21400	1(2)
21401	1(2)
21406	1(2)
21407	1(2)
21408	1(2)
21421	1(2)
21422	1(2)
21423	1(2)
21431	1(2)
21432	1(2)
21433	1(2)
21435	1(2)
21436	1(2)
21440	2(2)
21445	2(2)
21450	1(2)
21451	1(2)
21452	1(2)
21453	1(2)
21454	1(2)
21461	1(2)
21462	1(2)
21465	1(2)
21470	1(2)
21480	1(2)
21485	1(2)
21490	1(2)
21497	1(2)
21499	1(3)
21501	3(3)
21502	1(3)
21510	1(3)
21550	2(3)
21552	2(3)
21554	2(3)
21555	2(3)
21556	2(3)
21557	1(3)
21558	1(3)
21600	5(3)
21601	2(3)
21602	1(3)
21603	1(3)
21610	1(3)
21615	1(2)
21616	1(2)
21620	1(2)
21627	1(2)
21630	1(2)
21632	1(2)
21685	1(2)

CPT	MUE
21700	1(2)
21705	1(2)
21720	1(3)
21725	1(3)
21740	1(2)
21742	1(2)
21743	1(2)
21750	1(2)
21811	1(2)
21812	1(2)
21813	1(2)
21820	1(2)
21825	1(2)
21899	1(3)
21920	2(3)
21925	2(3)
21930	5(3)
21931	3(3)
21932	2(3)
21933	2(3)
21935	1(3)
21936	1(3)
22010	2(3)
22015	2(3)
22100	1(2)
22101	1(2)
22102	1(2)
22103	3(3)
22110	1(2)
22112	1(2)
22114	1(2)
22116	3(3)
22206	1(2)
22207	1(2)
22208	5(3)
22210	1(2)
22212	1(2)
22214	1(2)
22216	6(3)
22220	1(2)
22222	1(2)
22224	1(2)
22226	4(3)
22310	1(2)
22315	1(2)
22318	1(2)
22319	1(2)
22325	1(2)
22326	1(2)
22327	1(2)
22328	6(3)
22505	1(2)
22510	1(2)
22511	1(2)
22512	3(3)
22513	1(2)
22514	1(2)
22515	4(3)
22526	0(3)
22527	0(3)
22532	1(2)
22533	1(2)
22534	3(3)
22548	1(2)
22551	1(2)

CPT	MUE
22552	5(3)
22554	1(2)
22556	1(2)
22558	1(2)
22585	5(3)
22586	1(2)
22590	1(2)
22595	1(2)
22600	1(2)
22610	1(2)
22612	1(2)
22614	13(3)
22630	1(2)
22632	4(2)
22633	1(2)
22634	4(2)
22800	1(2)
22802	1(2)
22804	1(2)
22808	1(2)
22810	1(2)
22812	1(2)
22818	1(2)
22819	1(2)
22830	1(2)
22840	1(3)
22841	0(3)
22842	1(3)
22843	1(3)
22844	1(3)
22845	1(3)
22846	1(3)
22847	1(3)
22848	1(2)
22849	1(2)
22850	1(2)
22852	1(2)
22853	4(3)
22854	4(3)
22855	1(2)
22856	1(2)
22857	1(2)
22858	1(2)
22859	4(3)
22861	1(2)
22862	1(2)
22864	1(2)
22865	1(2)
22867	1(2)
22868	1(2)
22869	1(2)
22870	1(2)
22899	1(3)
22900	3(3)
22901	2(3)
22902	4(3)
22903	3(3)
22904	1(3)
22905	1(3)
22999	1(3)
23000	1(2)
23020	1(2)
23030	2(3)
23031	1(3)
23035	1(3)

CPT	MUE
23040	1(2)
23044	1(3)
23065	2(3)
23066	2(3)
23071	2(3)
23073	2(3)
23075	2(3)
23076	2(3)
23077	1(3)
23078	1(3)
23100	1(2)
23101	1(3)
23105	1(2)
23106	1(2)
23107	1(2)
23120	1(2)
23125	1(2)
23130	1(2)
23140	1(3)
23145	1(3)
23146	1(3)
23150	1(3)
23155	1(3)
23156	1(3)
23170	1(3)
23172	1(3)
23174	1(3)
23180	1(3)
23182	1(3)
23184	1(3)
23190	1(3)
23195	1(2)
23200	1(3)
23210	1(3)
23220	1(3)
23330	2(3)
23333	1(3)
23334	1(2)
23335	1(2)
23350	1(2)
23395	1(2)
23397	1(3)
23400	1(2)
23405	2(3)
23406	1(3)
23410	1(2)
23412	1(2)
23415	1(2)
23420	1(2)
23430	1(2)
23440	1(2)
23450	1(2)
23455	1(2)
23460	1(2)
23462	1(2)
23465	1(2)
23466	1(2)
23470	1(2)
23472	1(2)
23473	1(2)
23474	1(2)
23480	1(2)
23485	1(2)
23490	1(2)
23491	1(2)

CPT	MUE
23500	1(2)
23505	1(2)
23515	1(2)
23520	1(2)
23525	1(2)
23530	1(2)
23532	1(2)
23540	1(2)
23545	1(2)
23550	1(2)
23552	1(2)
23570	1(2)
23575	1(2)
23585	1(2)
23600	1(2)
23605	1(2)
23615	1(2)
23616	1(2)
23620	1(2)
23625	1(2)
23630	1(2)
23650	1(2)
23655	1(2)
23660	1(2)
23665	1(2)
23670	1(2)
23675	1(2)
23680	1(2)
23700	1(2)
23800	1(2)
23802	1(2)
23900	1(2)
23920	1(2)
23921	1(2)
23929	1(3)
23930	2(3)
23931	2(3)
23935	2(3)
24000	1(2)
24006	1(2)
24065	2(3)
24066	2(3)
24071	2(3)
24073	2(3)
24075	5(3)
24076	4(3)
24077	1(3)
24079	1(3)
24100	1(2)
24101	1(2)
24102	1(2)
24105	1(2)
24110	1(3)
24115	1(3)
24116	1(3)
24120	1(3)
24125	1(3)
24126	1(3)
24130	1(2)
24134	1(3)
24136	1(3)
24138	1(3)
24140	1(3)
24145	1(3)
24147	1(2)

CPT	MUE
24149	1(2)
24150	1(3)
24152	1(3)
24155	1(2)
24160	1(2)
24164	1(2)
24200	3(3)
24201	3(3)
24220	1(2)
24300	1(2)
24301	2(3)
24305	4(3)
24310	2(3)
24320	2(3)
24330	1(3)
24331	1(3)
24332	1(2)
24340	1(2)
24341	2(3)
24342	2(3)
24343	1(2)
24344	1(2)
24345	1(2)
24346	1(2)
24357	1(3)
24358	1(3)
24359	2(3)
24360	1(2)
24361	1(2)
24362	1(2)
24363	1(2)
24365	1(2)
24366	1(2)
24370	1(2)
24371	1(2)
24400	1(3)
24410	1(2)
24420	1(2)
24430	1(3)
24435	1(3)
24470	1(2)
24495	1(2)
24498	1(2)
24500	1(2)
24505	1(2)
24515	1(2)
24516	1(2)
24530	1(2)
24535	1(2)
24538	1(2)
24545	1(2)
24546	1(2)
24560	1(3)
24565	1(3)
24566	1(3)
24575	1(3)
24576	1(3)
24577	1(3)
24579	1(3)
24582	1(3)
24586	1(3)
24587	1(2)
24600	1(2)
24605	1(2)
24615	1(2)

CPT	MUE
24620	1(2)
24635	1(2)
24640	1(2)
24650	1(2)
24655	1(2)
24665	1(2)
24666	1(2)
24670	1(2)
24675	1(2)
24685	1(2)
24800	1(2)
24802	1(2)
24900	1(2)
24920	1(2)
24925	1(2)
24930	1(2)
24931	1(2)
24935	1(2)
24940	1(2)
24999	1(3)
25000	2(3)
25001	1(3)
25020	1(2)
25023	1(2)
25024	1(2)
25025	1(2)
25028	4(3)
25031	2(3)
25035	2(3)
25040	1(3)
25065	2(3)
25066	2(3)
25071	3(3)
25073	2(3)
25075	6(3)
25076	3(3)
25077	1(3)
25078	1(3)
25085	1(2)
25100	1(2)
25101	1(2)
25105	1(2)
25107	1(2)
25109	4(3)
25110	2(3)
25111	1(3)
25112	1(3)
25115	1(3)
25116	1(3)
25118	5(3)
25119	1(2)
25120	1(3)
25125	1(3)
25126	1(3)
25130	1(3)
25135	1(3)
25136	1(3)
25145	1(3)
25150	1(3)
25151	1(3)
25170	1(3)
25210	2(3)
25215	1(2)
25230	1(2)
25240	1(2)

CPT	MUE
25246	1(2)
25248	3(3)
25250	1(2)
25251	1(2)
25259	1(2)
25260	9(3)
25263	4(3)
25265	4(3)
25270	8(3)
25272	4(3)
25274	4(3)
25275	2(3)
25280	9(3)
25290	10(3)
25295	9(3)
25300	1(2)
25301	1(2)
25310	5(3)
25312	4(3)
25315	1(3)
25316	1(3)
25320	1(2)
25332	1(2)
25335	1(2)
25337	1(2)
25350	1(3)
25355	1(3)
25360	1(3)
25365	1(3)
25370	1(2)
25375	1(2)
25390	1(2)
25391	1(2)
25392	1(2)
25393	1(2)
25394	1(3)
25400	1(2)
25405	1(2)
25415	1(2)
25420	1(2)
25425	1(2)
25426	1(2)
25430	1(3)
25431	1(3)
25440	1(2)
25441	1(2)
25442	1(2)
25443	1(2)
25444	1(2)
25445	1(2)
25446	1(2)
25447	4(3)
25449	1(2)
25450	1(2)
25455	1(2)
25490	1(2)
25491	1(2)
25492	1(2)
25500	1(2)
25505	1(2)
25515	1(2)
25520	1(2)
25525	1(2)
25526	1(2)
25530	1(2)

CPT	MUE
25535	1(2)
25545	1(2)
25560	1(2)
25565	1(2)
25574	1(2)
25575	1(2)
25600	1(2)
25605	1(2)
25606	1(2)
25607	1(2)
25608	1(2)
25609	1(2)
25622	1(2)
25624	1(2)
25628	1(2)
25630	1(3)
25635	1(3)
25645	1(3)
25650	1(2)
25651	1(2)
25652	1(2)
25660	1(2)
25670	1(2)
25671	1(2)
25675	1(2)
25676	1(2)
25680	1(2)
25685	1(2)
25690	1(2)
25695	1(2)
25800	1(2)
25805	1(2)
25810	1(2)
25820	1(2)
25825	1(2)
25830	1(2)
25900	1(2)
25905	1(2)
25907	1(2)
25909	1(2)
25915	1(2)
25920	1(2)
25922	1(2)
25924	1(2)
25927	1(2)
25929	1(2)
25931	1(2)
25999	1(3)
26010	2(3)
26011	3(3)
26020	4(3)
26025	1(2)
26030	1(2)
26034	2(3)
26035	1(3)
26037	1(3)
26040	1(2)
26045	1(2)
26055	5(3)
26060	5(3)
26070	2(3)
26075	3(3)
26080	3(3)
26100	1(3)
26105	2(3)

CPT	MUE
26110	2(3)
26111	4(3)
26113	3(3)
26115	4(3)
26116	2(3)
26117	2(3)
26118	1(3)
26121	1(2)
26123	1(2)
26125	4(3)
26130	1(3)
26135	4(3)
26140	2(3)
26145	6(3)
26160	4(3)
26170	4(3)
26180	4(3)
26185	1(3)
26200	2(3)
26205	1(3)
26210	2(3)
26215	2(3)
26230	2(3)
26235	2(3)
26236	2(3)
26250	2(3)
26260	1(3)
26262	1(3)
26320	4(3)
26340	4(3)
26341	2(3)
26350	6(3)
26352	2(3)
26356	4(3)
26357	2(3)
26358	2(3)
26370	3(3)
26372	1(3)
26373	2(3)
26390	2(3)
26392	2(3)
26410	4(3)
26412	3(3)
26415	2(3)
26416	2(3)
26418	4(3)
26420	3(3)
26426	4(3)
26428	2(3)
26432	2(3)
26433	2(3)
26434	2(3)
26437	4(3)
26440	6(3)
26442	5(3)
26445	5(3)
26449	5(3)
26450	6(3)
26455	6(3)
26460	4(3)
26471	4(3)
26474	4(3)
26476	4(3)
26477	2(3)
26478	6(3)

CPT	MUE
26479	4(3)
26480	4(3)
26483	4(3)
26485	4(3)
26489	2(3)
26490	3(3)
26492	2(3)
26494	1(3)
26496	1(3)
26497	2(3)
26498	1(3)
26499	2(3)
26500	3(3)
26502	2(3)
26508	1(2)
26510	4(3)
26516	1(2)
26517	1(2)
26518	1(2)
26520	4(3)
26525	4(3)
26530	4(3)
26531	4(3)
26535	3(3)
26536	4(3)
26540	4(3)
26541	4(3)
26542	4(3)
26545	4(3)
26546	2(3)
26548	3(3)
26550	1(2)
26551	1(2)
26553	1(3)
26554	1(3)
26555	2(3)
26556	2(3)
26560	2(3)
26561	2(3)
26562	2(3)
26565	2(3)
26567	3(3)
26568	2(3)
26580	1(2)
26587	2(3)
26590	2(3)
26591	4(3)
26593	8(3)
26596	1(3)
26600	2(3)
26605	3(3)
26607	2(3)
26608	4(3)
26615	3(3)
26641	1(2)
26645	1(2)
26650	1(2)
26665	1(2)
26670	2(3)
26675	1(3)
26676	2(3)
26685	3(3)
26686	3(3)
26700	2(3)
26705	3(3)

CPT	MUE
26706	2(3)
26715	3(3)
26720	4(3)
26725	3(3)
26727	3(3)
26735	4(3)
26740	3(3)
26742	3(3)
26746	3(3)
26750	3(3)
26755	2(3)
26756	2(3)
26765	3(3)
26770	3(3)
26775	2(3)
26776	4(3)
26785	3(3)
26820	1(2)
26841	1(2)
26842	1(2)
26843	2(3)
26844	2(3)
26850	5(3)
26852	2(3)
26860	1(2)
26861	4(3)
26862	1(2)
26863	2(3)
26910	4(3)
26951	8(3)
26952	4(3)
26989	1(3)
26990	2(3)
26991	1(3)
26992	2(3)
27000	1(3)
27001	1(3)
27003	1(2)
27005	1(2)
27006	1(2)
27025	1(3)
27027	1(2)
27030	1(2)
27033	1(2)
27035	1(2)
27036	1(2)
27040	2(3)
27041	3(3)
27043	2(3)
27045	3(3)
27047	2(3)
27048	2(3)
27049	1(3)
27050	1(2)
27052	1(2)
27054	1(2)
27057	1(2)
27059	1(3)
27060	1(2)
27062	1(2)
27065	1(3)
27066	1(3)
27067	1(3)
27070	1(3)
27071	1(3)

CPT	MUE
27075	1(3)
27076	1(2)
27077	1(2)
27078	1(2)
27080	1(2)
27086	1(3)
27087	1(3)
27090	1(2)
27091	1(2)
27093	1(2)
27095	1(2)
27096	1(2)
27097	1(3)
27098	1(2)
27100	1(2)
27105	1(3)
27110	1(2)
27111	1(2)
27120	1(2)
27122	1(2)
27125	1(2)
27130	1(2)
27132	1(2)
27134	1(2)
27137	1(2)
27138	1(2)
27140	1(2)
27146	1(3)
27147	1(3)
27151	1(3)
27156	1(2)
27158	1(2)
27161	1(2)
27165	1(2)
27170	1(2)
27175	1(2)
27176	1(2)
27177	1(2)
27178	1(2)
27179	1(2)
27181	1(2)
27185	1(2)
27187	1(2)
27197	1(2)
27198	1(2)
27200	1(2)
27202	1(2)
27215	0(3)
27216	0(3)
27217	0(3)
27218	0(3)
27220	1(2)
27222	1(2)
27226	1(2)
27227	1(2)
27228	1(2)
27230	1(2)
27232	1(2)
27235	1(2)
27236	1(2)
27238	1(2)
27240	1(2)
27244	1(2)
27245	1(2)
27246	1(2)

CPT	MUE
27248	1(2)
27250	1(2)
27252	1(2)
27253	1(2)
27254	1(2)
27256	1(2)
27257	1(2)
27258	1(2)
27259	1(2)
27265	1(2)
27266	1(2)
27267	1(2)
27268	1(2)
27269	1(2)
27275	2(2)
27279	1(2)
27280	1(2)
27282	1(2)
27284	1(2)
27286	1(2)
27290	1(2)
27295	1(2)
27299	1(3)
27301	3(3)
27303	2(3)
27305	1(2)
27306	1(2)
27307	1(2)
27310	1(2)
27323	2(3)
27324	3(3)
27325	1(2)
27326	1(2)
27327	5(3)
27328	3(3)
27329	1(3)
27330	1(2)
27331	1(2)
27332	1(2)
27333	1(2)
27334	1(2)
27335	1(2)
27337	3(3)
27339	4(3)
27340	1(2)
27345	1(2)
27347	1(2)
27350	1(2)
27355	1(3)
27356	1(3)
27357	1(3)
27358	1(3)
27360	2(3)
27364	1(3)
27365	1(3)
27369	1(2)
27372	2(3)
27380	1(2)
27381	1(2)
27385	2(3)
27386	2(3)
27390	1(2)
27391	1(2)
27392	1(2)
27393	1(2)

CPT	MUE
27394	1(2)
27395	1(2)
27396	1(2)
27397	1(2)
27400	1(2)
27403	1(3)
27405	2(2)
27407	2(2)
27409	1(2)
27412	1(2)
27415	1(2)
27416	1(2)
27418	1(2)
27420	1(2)
27422	1(2)
27424	1(2)
27425	1(2)
27427	1(2)
27428	1(2)
27429	1(2)
27430	1(2)
27435	1(2)
27437	1(2)
27438	1(2)
27440	1(2)
27441	1(2)
27442	1(2)
27443	1(2)
27445	1(2)
27446	1(2)
27447	1(2)
27448	1(3)
27450	1(3)
27454	1(2)
27455	1(3)
27457	1(3)
27465	1(2)
27466	1(2)
27468	1(2)
27470	1(2)
27472	1(2)
27475	1(2)
27477	1(2)
27479	1(2)
27485	1(2)
27486	1(2)
27487	1(2)
27488	1(2)
27495	1(2)
27496	1(2)
27497	1(2)
27498	1(2)
27499	1(2)
27500	1(2)
27501	1(2)
27502	1(2)
27503	1(2)
27506	1(2)
27507	1(2)
27508	1(2)
27509	1(2)
27510	1(2)
27511	1(2)
27513	1(2)
27514	1(2)

CPT	MUE
27516	1(2)
27517	1(2)
27519	1(2)
27520	1(2)
27524	1(2)
27530	1(2)
27532	1(2)
27535	1(2)
27536	1(2)
27538	1(2)
27540	1(2)
27550	1(2)
27552	1(2)
27556	1(2)
27557	1(2)
27558	1(2)
27560	1(2)
27562	1(2)
27566	1(2)
27570	1(2)
27580	1(2)
27590	1(2)
27591	1(2)
27592	1(2)
27594	1(2)
27596	1(2)
27598	1(2)
27599	1(3)
27600	1(2)
27601	1(2)
27602	1(2)
27603	2(3)
27604	2(3)
27605	1(2)
27606	1(2)
27607	2(3)
27610	1(2)
27612	1(2)
27613	3(3)
27614	3(3)
27615	1(3)
27616	1(3)
27618	3(3)
27619	2(3)
27620	1(2)
27625	1(2)
27626	1(2)
27630	2(3)
27632	3(3)
27634	2(3)
27635	1(3)
27637	1(3)
27638	1(3)
27640	1(3)
27641	1(3)
27645	1(3)
27646	1(3)
27647	1(3)
27648	1(2)
27650	1(2)
27652	1(2)
27654	1(2)
27656	1(3)
27658	2(3)
27659	2(3)

CPT	MUE
27664	2(3)
27665	2(3)
27675	1(2)
27676	1(2)
27680	2(3)
27681	1(2)
27685	2(3)
27686	3(3)
27687	1(2)
27690	2(3)
27691	2(3)
27692	4(3)
27695	1(2)
27696	1(2)
27698	2(2)
27700	1(2)
27702	1(2)
27703	1(2)
27704	1(2)
27705	1(3)
27707	1(3)
27709	1(3)
27712	1(2)
27715	1(2)
27720	1(2)
27722	1(2)
27724	1(2)
27725	1(2)
27726	1(2)
27727	1(2)
27730	1(2)
27732	1(2)
27734	1(2)
27740	1(2)
27742	1(2)
27745	1(2)
27750	1(2)
27752	1(2)
27756	1(2)
27758	1(2)
27759	1(2)
27760	1(2)
27762	1(2)
27766	1(2)
27767	1(2)
27768	1(2)
27769	1(2)
27780	1(2)
27781	1(2)
27784	1(2)
27786	1(2)
27788	1(2)
27792	1(2)
27808	1(2)
27810	1(2)
27814	1(2)
27816	1(2)
27818	1(2)
27822	1(2)
27823	1(2)
27824	1(2)
27825	1(2)
27826	1(2)
27827	1(2)
27828	1(2)

CPT	MUE
27829	1(2)
27830	1(2)
27831	1(2)
27832	1(2)
27840	1(2)
27842	1(2)
27846	1(2)
27848	1(2)
27860	1(2)
27870	1(2)
27871	1(3)
27880	1(2)
27881	1(2)
27882	1(2)
27884	1(2)
27886	1(2)
27888	1(2)
27889	1(2)
27892	1(2)
27893	1(2)
27894	1(2)
27899	1(3)
28001	2(3)
28002	3(3)
28003	2(3)
28005	3(3)
28008	2(3)
28010	4(3)
28011	4(3)
28020	2(3)
28022	3(3)
28024	4(3)
28035	1(2)
28039	2(3)
28041	2(3)
28043	4(3)
28045	4(3)
28046	1(3)
28047	1(3)
28050	2(3)
28052	2(3)
28054	2(3)
28055	1(3)
28060	1(2)
28062	1(2)
28070	2(3)
28072	4(3)
28080	3(3)
28086	2(3)
28088	2(3)
28090	2(3)
28092	2(3)
28100	1(3)
28102	1(3)
28103	1(3)
28104	2(3)
28106	1(3)
28107	1(3)
28108	2(3)
28110	1(2)
28111	1(2)
28112	4(3)
28113	1(2)
28114	1(2)
28116	1(2)

CPT	MUE
28118	1(2)
28119	1(2)
28120	2(3)
28122	4(3)
28124	4(3)
28126	4(3)
28130	1(2)
28140	3(3)
28150	4(3)
28153	4(3)
28160	5(3)
28171	1(3)
28173	2(3)
28175	2(3)
28190	3(3)
28192	2(3)
28193	2(3)
28200	4(3)
28202	2(3)
28208	4(3)
28210	2(3)
28220	1(2)
28222	1(2)
28225	1(2)
28226	1(2)
28230	1(2)
28232	6(3)
28234	6(3)
28238	1(2)
28240	1(2)
28250	1(2)
28260	1(2)
28261	1(3)
28262	1(2)
28264	1(2)
28270	6(3)
28272	6(3)
28280	1(2)
28285	4(3)
28286	1(2)
28288	4(3)
28289	1(2)
28291	1(2)
28292	1(2)
28295	1(2)
28296	1(2)
28297	1(2)
28298	1(2)
28299	1(2)
28300	1(2)
28302	1(2)
28304	1(3)
28305	1(3)
28306	1(2)
28307	1(2)
28308	4(3)
28309	1(2)
28310	1(2)
28312	4(3)
28313	4(3)
28315	1(2)
28320	1(2)
28322	2(3)
28340	2(3)
28341	2(3)

CPT	MUE
28344	1(2)
28345	2(3)
28360	1(2)
28400	1(2)
28405	1(2)
28406	1(2)
28415	1(2)
28420	1(2)
28430	1(2)
28435	1(2)
28436	1(2)
28445	1(2)
28446	1(2)
28450	2(3)
28455	3(3)
28456	2(3)
28465	3(3)
28470	2(3)
28475	5(3)
28476	4(3)
28485	5(3)
28490	1(2)
28495	1(2)
28496	1(2)
28505	1(2)
28510	4(3)
28515	4(3)
28525	4(3)
28530	1(2)
28531	1(2)
28540	1(3)
28545	1(3)
28546	1(3)
28555	1(3)
28570	1(2)
28575	1(2)
28576	1(2)
28585	1(3)
28600	2(3)
28605	2(3)
28606	3(3)
28615	5(3)
28630	2(3)
28635	2(3)
28636	4(3)
28645	4(3)
28660	4(3)
28665	3(3)
28666	4(3)
28675	3(3)
28705	1(2)
28715	1(2)
28725	1(2)
28730	1(2)
28735	1(2)
28737	1(2)
28740	1(2)
28750	1(2)
28755	1(2)
28760	1(2)
28800	1(2)
28805	1(2)
28810	5(3)
28820	6(3)
28825	8(2)

CPT	MUE
28890	1(2)
28899	1(3)
29000	1(3)
29010	1(3)
29015	1(3)
29035	1(3)
29040	1(3)
29044	1(3)
29046	1(3)
29049	1(3)
29055	1(3)
29058	1(3)
29065	1(3)
29075	1(3)
29085	1(3)
29086	2(3)
29105	1(2)
29125	1(2)
29126	1(2)
29130	3(3)
29131	2(3)
29200	1(2)
29240	1(2)
29260	1(3)
29280	2(3)
29305	1(3)
29325	1(3)
29345	1(3)
29355	1(3)
29358	1(3)
29365	1(3)
29405	1(3)
29425	1(3)
29435	1(3)
29440	1(2)
29445	1(3)
29450	1(3)
29505	1(2)
29515	1(2)
29520	1(2)
29530	1(2)
29540	1(2)
29550	1(2)
29580	1(2)
29581	1(2)
29584	1(2)
29700	2(3)
29705	1(3)
29710	1(2)
29720	1(2)
29730	1(3)
29740	1(3)
29750	1(3)
29799	1(3)
29800	1(2)
29804	1(2)
29805	1(2)
29806	1(2)
29807	1(2)
29819	1(2)
29820	1(2)
29821	1(2)
29822	1(2)
29823	1(2)
29824	1(2)

CPT	MUE
29825	1(2)
29826	1(2)
29827	1(2)
29828	1(2)
29830	1(2)
29834	1(2)
29835	1(2)
29836	1(2)
29837	1(2)
29838	1(2)
29840	1(2)
29843	1(2)
29844	1(2)
29845	1(2)
29846	1(2)
29847	1(2)
29848	1(2)
29850	1(2)
29851	1(2)
29855	1(2)
29856	1(2)
29860	1(2)
29861	1(2)
29862	1(2)
29863	1(2)
29866	1(2)
29867	1(2)
29868	1(3)
29870	1(2)
29871	1(2)
29873	1(2)
29874	1(2)
29875	1(2)
29876	1(2)
29877	1(2)
29879	1(2)
29880	1(2)
29881	1(2)
29882	1(2)
29883	1(2)
29884	1(2)
29885	1(2)
29886	1(2)
29887	1(2)
29888	1(2)
29889	1(2)
29891	1(2)
29892	1(2)
29893	1(2)
29894	1(2)
29895	1(2)
29897	1(2)
29898	1(2)
29899	1(2)
29900	2(3)
29901	2(3)
29902	2(3)
29904	1(2)
29905	1(2)
29906	1(2)
29907	1(2)
29914	1(2)
29915	1(2)
29916	1(2)
29999	1(3)

CPT	MUE
30000	1(3)
30020	1(3)
30100	2(3)
30110	1(2)
30115	1(2)
30117	2(3)
30118	1(3)
30120	1(2)
30124	2(3)
30125	1(3)
30130	1(2)
30140	1(2)
30150	1(2)
30160	1(2)
30200	1(2)
30210	1(3)
30220	1(2)
30300	1(3)
30310	1(3)
30320	1(3)
30400	1(2)
30410	1(2)
30420	1(2)
30430	1(2)
30435	1(2)
30450	1(2)
30460	1(2)
30462	1(2)
30465	1(2)
30520	1(2)
30540	1(2)
30545	1(2)
30560	1(2)
30580	2(3)
30600	1(3)
30620	1(2)
30630	1(2)
30801	1(2)
30802	1(2)
30901	1(3)
30903	1(3)
30905	1(2)
30906	1(3)
30915	1(3)
30920	1(3)
30930	1(2)
30999	1(3)
31000	1(2)
31002	1(2)
31020	1(2)
31030	1(2)
31032	1(2)
31040	1(2)
31050	1(2)
31051	1(2)
31070	1(2)
31075	1(2)
31080	1(2)
31081	1(2)
31084	1(2)
31085	1(2)
31086	1(2)
31087	1(2)
31090	1(2)
31200	1(2)

CPT	MUE
31201	1(2)
31205	1(2)
31225	1(2)
31230	1(2)
31231	1(2)
31233	1(2)
31235	1(2)
31237	1(2)
31238	1(3)
31239	1(2)
31240	1(2)
31241	1(2)
31253	1(2)
31254	1(2)
31255	1(2)
31256	1(2)
31257	1(2)
31259	1(2)
31267	1(2)
31276	1(2)
31287	1(2)
31288	1(2)
31290	1(2)
31291	1(2)
31292	1(2)
31293	1(2)
31294	1(2)
31295	1(2)
31296	1(2)
31297	1(2)
31298	1(2)
31299	1(3)
31300	1(2)
31360	1(2)
31365	1(2)
31367	1(2)
31368	1(2)
31370	1(2)
31375	1(2)
31380	1(2)
31382	1(2)
31390	1(2)
31395	1(2)
31400	1(3)
31420	1(2)
31500	2(3)
31502	1(3)
31505	1(3)
31510	1(2)
31511	1(3)
31512	1(3)
31513	1(3)
31515	1(3)
31520	1(3)
31525	1(3)
31526	1(3)
31527	1(2)
31528	1(2)
31529	1(3)
31530	1(3)
31531	1(3)
31535	1(3)
31536	1(3)
31540	1(3)
31541	1(3)

CPT	MUE
31545	1(2)
31546	1(2)
31551	1(2)
31552	1(2)
31553	1(2)
31554	1(2)
31560	1(2)
31561	1(2)
31570	1(2)
31571	1(2)
31572	1(2)
31573	1(2)
31574	1(2)
31575	1(3)
31576	1(3)
31577	1(3)
31578	1(3)
31579	1(2)
31580	1(2)
31584	1(2)
31587	1(2)
31590	1(2)
31591	1(2)
31592	1(2)
31599	1(3)
31600	1(2)
31601	1(2)
31603	1(2)
31605	1(2)
31610	1(2)
31611	1(2)
31612	1(3)
31613	1(2)
31614	1(2)
31615	1(3)
31622	1(3)
31623	1(3)
31624	1(3)
31625	1(2)
31626	1(2)
31627	1(3)
31628	1(2)
31629	1(2)
31630	1(3)
31631	1(2)
31632	2(3)
31633	2(3)
31634	1(3)
31635	1(3)
31636	1(2)
31637	2(3)
31638	1(3)
31640	1(3)
31641	1(3)
31643	1(2)
31645	1(2)
31646	2(3)
31647	1(2)
31648	1(2)
31649	2(3)
31651	3(3)
31652	1(2)
31653	1(2)
31654	1(3)
31660	1(2)

CPT	MUE
31661	1(2)
31717	1(3)
31720	1(3)
31725	1(3)
31730	1(3)
31750	1(2)
31755	1(2)
31760	1(2)
31766	1(2)
31770	2(3)
31775	1(3)
31780	1(2)
31781	1(2)
31785	1(3)
31786	1(3)
31800	1(3)
31805	1(3)
31820	1(2)
31825	1(2)
31830	1(2)
31899	1(3)
32035	1(2)
32036	1(3)
32096	1(3)
32097	1(3)
32098	1(2)
32100	1(3)
32110	1(3)
32120	1(3)
32124	1(3)
32140	1(3)
32141	1(3)
32150	1(3)
32151	1(3)
32160	1(3)
32200	2(3)
32215	1(2)
32220	1(2)
32225	1(2)
32310	1(3)
32320	1(3)
32400	2(3)
32405	2(3)
32440	1(2)
32442	1(2)
32445	1(2)
32480	1(2)
32482	1(2)
32484	2(3)
32486	1(3)
32488	1(2)
32491	1(2)
32501	1(3)
32503	1(2)
32504	1(2)
32505	1(2)
32506	3(3)
32507	2(3)
32540	1(3)
32550	2(3)
32551	2(3)
32552	2(2)
32553	1(2)
32554	2(3)
32555	2(3)

CPT	MUE
32556	2(3)
32557	2(3)
32560	1(3)
32561	1(2)
32562	1(2)
32601	1(3)
32604	1(3)
32606	1(3)
32607	1(3)
32608	1(3)
32609	1(3)
32650	1(2)
32651	1(2)
32652	1(2)
32653	1(3)
32654	1(3)
32655	1(3)
32656	1(2)
32658	1(3)
32659	1(2)
32661	1(3)
32662	1(3)
32663	1(3)
32664	1(2)
32665	1(2)
32666	1(3)
32667	3(3)
32668	2(3)
32669	2(3)
32670	1(2)
32671	1(2)
32672	1(3)
32673	1(2)
32674	1(2)
32701	1(2)
32800	1(3)
32810	1(3)
32815	1(3)
32820	1(2)
32850	1(2)
32851	1(2)
32852	1(2)
32853	1(2)
32854	1(2)
32855	1(2)
32856	1(2)
32900	1(2)
32905	1(2)
32906	1(2)
32940	1(3)
32960	1(2)
32994	1(2)
32997	1(2)
32998	1(2)
32999	1(3)
33016	1(3)
33017	1(3)
33018	1(3)
33019	1(3)
33020	1(3)
33025	1(2)
33030	1(2)
33031	1(2)
33050	1(2)
33120	1(3)

CPT	MUE
33130	1(3)
33140	1(2)
33141	1(2)
33202	1(2)
33203	1(2)
33206	1(3)
33207	1(3)
33208	1(3)
33210	1(3)
33211	1(3)
33212	1(3)
33213	1(3)
33214	1(3)
33215	2(3)
33216	1(3)
33217	1(3)
33218	1(3)
33220	1(3)
33221	1(3)
33222	1(3)
33223	1(3)
33224	1(3)
33225	1(3)
33226	1(3)
33227	1(3)
33228	1(3)
33229	1(3)
33230	1(3)
33231	1(3)
33233	1(2)
33234	1(2)
33235	1(2)
33236	1(2)
33237	1(2)
33238	1(2)
33240	1(3)
33241	1(2)
33243	1(2)
33244	1(2)
33249	1(3)
33250	1(2)
33251	1(2)
33254	1(2)
33255	1(2)
33256	1(2)
33257	1(2)
33258	1(2)
33259	1(2)
33261	1(2)
33262	1(3)
33263	1(3)
33264	1(3)
33265	1(2)
33266	1(2)
33270	1(3)
33271	1(3)
33272	1(3)
33273	1(3)
33274	1(3)
33275	1(3)
33285	1(3)
33286	1(3)
33289	1(3)
33300	1(3)
33305	1(3)

CPT	MUE	CPT	MUE	CPT	MUE	CPT	MUE	CPT	MUE	CPT	MUE	CPT	MUE	CPT	MUE
33310	1(2)	33514	1(2)	33771	1(2)	33953	1(3)	34710	1(2)	35236	2(3)	35600	2(3)	36100	2(3)
33315	1(2)	33516	1(2)	33774	1(2)	33954	1(3)	34711	2(3)	35241	2(3)	35601	1(3)	36140	3(3)
33320	1(3)	33517	1(2)	33775	1(2)	33955	1(3)	34712	1(2)	35246	2(3)	35606	1(3)	36160	2(3)
33321	1(3)	33518	1(2)	33776	1(2)	33956	1(3)	34713	1(2)	35251	2(3)	35612	1(3)	36200	2(3)
33322	1(3)	33519	1(2)	33777	1(2)	33957	1(3)	34714	1(2)	35256	2(3)	35616	1(3)	36215	6(3)
33330	1(3)	33521	1(2)	33778	1(2)	33958	1(3)	34715	1(2)	35261	1(3)	35621	1(3)	36216	4(3)
33335	1(3)	33522	1(2)	33779	1(2)	33959	1(3)	34716	1(2)	35266	2(3)	35623	1(3)	36217	2(3)
33340	1(2)	33523	1(2)	33780	1(2)	33962	1(3)	34717	2(2)	35271	2(3)	35626	3(3)	36218	6(3)
33361	1(2)	33530	1(2)	33781	1(2)	33963	1(3)	34718	2(2)	35276	2(3)	35631	4(3)	36221	1(3)
33362	1(2)	33533	1(2)	33782	1(2)	33964	1(3)	34808	1(3)	35281	2(3)	35632	1(3)	36222	1(3)
33363	1(2)	33534	1(2)	33783	1(2)	33965	1(3)	34812	1(2)	35286	2(3)	35633	1(3)	36223	1(3)
33364	1(2)	33535	1(2)	33786	1(2)	33966	1(3)	34813	1(2)	35301	2(3)	35634	1(3)	36224	1(3)
33365	1(2)	33536	1(2)	33788	1(2)	33967	1(3)	34820	1(2)	35302	1(2)	35636	1(3)	36225	1(3)
33366	1(3)	33542	1(2)	33800	1(2)	33968	1(3)	34830	1(2)	35303	1(2)	35637	1(3)	36226	1(3)
33367	1(2)	33545	1(2)	33802	1(3)	33969	1(3)	34831	1(2)	35304	1(2)	35638	1(3)	36227	2(2)
33368	1(2)	33548	1(2)	33803	1(3)	33970	1(3)	34832	1(2)	35305	1(2)	35642	1(3)	36228	4(3)
33369	1(2)	33572	3(2)	33813	1(2)	33971	1(3)	34833	1(2)	35306	2(3)	35645	1(3)	36245	6(3)
33390	1(2)	33600	1(3)	33814	1(2)	33973	1(3)	34834	1(2)	35311	1(2)	35646	1(3)	36246	4(3)
33391	1(2)	33602	1(3)	33820	1(2)	33974	1(3)	34839	1(2)	35321	1(2)	35647	1(3)	36247	3(3)
33404	1(2)	33606	1(2)	33822	1(2)	33975	1(3)	34841	1(2)	35331	1(2)	35650	1(3)	36248	6(3)
33405	1(2)	33608	1(2)	33824	1(2)	33976	1(3)	34842	1(2)	35341	3(3)	35654	1(3)	36251	1(3)
33406	1(2)	33610	1(2)	33840	1(2)	33977	1(3)	34843	1(2)	35351	1(3)	35656	1(3)	36252	1(3)
33410	1(2)	33611	1(2)	33845	1(2)	33978	1(3)	34844	1(2)	35355	1(2)	35661	1(3)	36253	1(3)
33411	1(2)	33612	1(2)	33851	1(2)	33979	1(3)	34845	1(2)	35361	1(2)	35663	1(3)	36254	1(3)
33412	1(2)	33615	1(2)	33852	1(2)	33980	1(3)	34846	1(2)	35363	1(2)	35665	1(3)	36260	1(2)
33413	1(2)	33617	1(2)	33853	1(2)	33981	1(3)	34847	1(2)	35371	1(2)	35666	2(3)	36261	1(2)
33414	1(2)	33619	1(2)	33858	1(2)	33982	1(3)	34848	1(2)	35372	1(2)	35671	2(3)	36262	1(2)
33415	1(2)	33620	1(2)	33859	1(2)	33983	1(3)	35001	1(2)	35390	1(3)	35681	1(3)	36299	1(3)
33416	1(2)	33621	1(3)	33863	1(2)	33984	1(3)	35002	1(2)	35400	1(3)	35682	1(2)	36400	1(3)
33417	1(2)	33622	1(2)	33864	1(2)	33985	1(3)	35005	1(2)	35500	2(3)	35683	1(2)	36405	1(3)
33418	1(3)	33641	1(2)	33866	1(2)	33986	1(3)	35011	1(2)	35501	1(3)	35685	2(3)	36406	1(3)
33419	1(2)	33645	1(2)	33871	1(2)	33987	1(3)	35013	1(2)	35506	1(3)	35686	1(3)	36410	3(3)
33420	1(2)	33647	1(2)	33875	1(2)	33988	1(3)	35021	1(2)	35508	1(3)	35691	1(3)	36415	2(3)
33422	1(2)	33660	1(2)	33877	1(2)	33989	1(3)	35022	1(2)	35509	1(3)	35693	1(3)	36416	0(3)
33425	1(2)	33665	1(2)	33880	1(2)	33990	1(3)	35045	1(3)	35510	1(3)	35694	1(3)	36420	2(3)
33426	1(2)	33670	1(2)	33881	1(2)	33991	1(3)	35081	1(2)	35511	1(3)	35695	1(3)	36425	2(3)
33427	1(2)	33675	1(2)	33883	1(2)	33992	1(2)	35082	1(2)	35512	1(3)	35697	2(3)	36430	1(2)
33430	1(2)	33676	1(2)	33884	2(3)	33993	1(3)	35091	1(2)	35515	1(3)	35700	2(3)	36440	1(3)
33440	1(2)	33677	1(2)	33886	1(2)	33999	1(3)	35092	1(2)	35516	1(3)	35701	1(2)	36450	1(3)
33460	1(2)	33681	1(2)	33889	1(2)	34001	1(3)	35102	1(2)	35518	1(3)	35702	2(2)	36455	1(3)
33463	1(2)	33684	1(2)	33891	1(2)	34051	1(3)	35103	1(2)	35521	1(3)	35703	2(2)	36456	1(3)
33464	1(2)	33688	1(2)	33910	1(3)	34101	1(3)	35111	1(2)	35522	1(3)	35800	2(3)	36460	2(3)
33465	1(2)	33690	1(2)	33915	1(3)	34111	2(3)	35112	1(2)	35523	1(3)	35820	2(3)	36465	1(2)
33468	1(2)	33692	1(2)	33916	1(3)	34151	1(3)	35121	1(3)	35525	1(3)	35840	2(3)	36466	1(2)
33470	1(2)	33694	1(2)	33917	1(2)	34201	1(3)	35122	1(3)	35526	1(3)	35860	2(3)	36468	2(3)
33471	1(2)	33697	1(2)	33920	1(2)	34203	1(2)	35131	1(2)	35531	1(3)	35870	1(3)	36470	1(2)
33474	1(2)	33702	1(2)	33922	1(2)	34401	1(3)	35132	1(2)	35533	1(3)	35875	2(3)	36471	1(2)
33475	1(2)	33710	1(2)	33924	1(2)	34421	1(3)	35141	1(2)	35535	1(3)	35876	2(3)	36473	1(3)
33476	1(2)	33720	1(2)	33925	1(2)	34451	1(3)	35142	1(2)	35536	1(3)	35879	2(3)	36474	1(3)
33477	1(2)	33722	1(3)	33926	1(2)	34471	1(2)	35151	1(2)	35537	1(3)	35881	1(3)	36475	1(3)
33478	1(2)	33724	1(2)	33927	1(3)	34490	1(2)	35152	1(2)	35538	1(3)	35883	1(3)	36476	2(3)
33496	1(3)	33726	1(2)	33928	1(3)	34501	1(2)	35180	2(3)	35539	1(3)	35884	1(3)	36478	1(3)
33500	1(3)	33730	1(2)	33929	1(3)	34502	1(2)	35182	2(3)	35540	1(3)	35901	1(3)	36479	2(3)
33501	1(3)	33732	1(2)	33930	1(2)	34510	2(3)	35184	2(3)	35556	1(3)	35903	2(3)	36481	1(3)
33502	1(3)	33735	1(2)	33933	1(2)	34520	1(3)	35188	2(3)	35558	1(3)	35905	1(3)	36482	1(3)
33503	1(3)	33736	1(2)	33935	1(2)	34530	1(2)	35189	1(3)	35560	1(3)	35907	1(3)	36483	2(3)
33504	1(3)	33737	1(2)	33940	1(2)	34701	1(2)	35190	2(3)	35563	1(3)	36000	4(3)	36500	4(3)
33505	1(3)	33750	1(3)	33944	1(2)	34702	1(2)	35201	2(3)	35565	1(3)	36002	2(3)	36510	1(3)
33506	1(3)	33755	1(2)	33945	1(2)	34703	1(2)	35206	2(3)	35566	1(3)	36005	2(3)	36511	1(3)
33507	1(3)	33762	1(2)	33946	1(2)	34704	1(2)	35207	3(3)	35570	1(3)	36010	2(3)	36512	1(3)
33508	1(2)	33764	1(3)	33947	1(2)	34705	1(2)	35211	3(3)	35571	1(3)	36011	4(3)	36513	1(3)
33510	1(2)	33766	1(2)	33948	1(2)	34706	1(2)	35216	2(3)	35572	2(3)	36012	4(3)	36514	1(3)
33511	1(2)	33767	1(2)	33949	1(2)	34707	1(2)	35221	3(3)	35583	1(2)	36013	2(3)	36516	1(3)
33512	1(2)	33768	1(2)	33951	1(3)	34708	1(2)	35226	3(3)	35585	2(3)	36014	2(3)	36522	1(3)
33513	1(2)	33770	1(2)	33952	1(3)	34709	3(3)	35231	2(3)	35587	1(3)	36015	4(3)	36555	2(3)

CPT	MUE
36556	2(3)
36557	2(3)
36558	2(3)
36560	2(3)
36561	2(3)
36563	1(3)
36565	1(3)
36566	1(3)
36568	2(3)
36569	2(3)
36570	2(3)
36571	2(3)
36572	1(3)
36573	1(3)
36575	2(3)
36576	2(3)
36578	2(3)
36580	2(3)
36581	2(3)
36582	2(3)
36583	2(3)
36584	2(3)
36585	2(3)
36589	2(3)
36590	2(3)
36591	2(3)
36592	1(3)
36593	2(3)
36595	2(3)
36596	2(3)
36597	2(3)
36598	2(3)
36600	4(3)
36620	3(3)
36625	2(3)
36640	1(3)
36660	1(3)
36680	1(3)
36800	1(3)
36810	1(3)
36815	1(3)
36818	1(3)
36819	1(3)
36820	1(3)
36821	2(3)
36823	1(3)
36825	1(3)
36830	2(3)
36831	1(3)
36832	2(3)
36833	1(3)
36835	1(3)
36838	1(3)
36860	2(3)
36861	2(3)
36901	1(3)
36902	1(3)
36903	1(3)
36904	1(3)
36905	1(3)
36906	1(3)
36907	1(3)
36908	1(3)
36909	1(3)
37140	1(2)

CPT	MUE
37145	1(3)
37160	1(3)
37180	1(2)
37181	1(2)
37182	1(2)
37183	1(2)
37184	1(2)
37185	2(3)
37186	2(3)
37187	1(3)
37188	1(3)
37191	1(3)
37192	1(3)
37193	1(3)
37195	1(3)
37197	2(3)
37200	2(3)
37211	1(2)
37212	1(2)
37213	1(2)
37214	1(2)
37215	1(2)
37216	0(3)
37217	1(2)
37218	1(2)
37220	1(2)
37221	1(2)
37222	2(2)
37223	2(2)
37224	1(2)
37225	1(2)
37226	1(2)
37227	1(2)
37228	1(2)
37229	1(2)
37230	1(2)
37231	1(2)
37232	2(3)
37233	2(3)
37234	2(3)
37235	2(3)
37236	1(2)
37237	2(3)
37238	1(2)
37239	2(3)
37241	2(3)
37242	2(3)
37243	1(3)
37244	2(3)
37246	1(2)
37247	2(3)
37248	1(2)
37249	3(3)
37252	1(2)
37253	5(3)
37500	1(3)
37501	1(3)
37565	1(2)
37600	1(3)
37605	1(3)
37606	1(3)
37607	1(3)
37609	1(2)
37615	2(3)
37616	1(3)

CPT	MUE
37617	3(3)
37618	2(3)
37619	1(2)
37650	1(2)
37660	1(2)
37700	1(2)
37718	1(2)
37722	1(2)
37735	1(2)
37760	1(2)
37761	1(2)
37765	1(2)
37766	1(2)
37780	1(2)
37785	1(2)
37788	1(2)
37790	1(2)
37799	1(3)
38100	1(2)
38101	1(3)
38102	1(2)
38115	1(3)
38120	1(2)
38129	1(3)
38200	1(3)
38204	0(3)
38205	1(3)
38206	1(3)
38207	0(3)
38208	0(3)
38209	0(3)
38210	0(3)
38211	0(3)
38212	0(3)
38213	0(3)
38214	0(3)
38215	0(3)
38220	1(3)
38221	1(3)
38222	1(2)
38230	1(2)
38232	1(2)
38240	1(3)
38241	1(2)
38242	1(2)
38243	1(3)
38300	1(3)
38305	1(3)
38308	1(3)
38380	1(2)
38381	1(2)
38382	1(2)
38500	2(3)
38505	2(3)
38510	1(2)
38520	1(2)
38525	1(2)
38530	1(2)
38531	1(2)
38542	1(2)
38550	1(3)
38555	1(3)
38562	1(2)
38564	1(2)
38570	1(2)

CPT	MUE
38571	1(2)
38572	1(2)
38573	1(2)
38589	1(3)
38700	1(2)
38720	1(2)
38724	1(2)
38740	1(2)
38745	1(2)
38746	1(2)
38747	1(2)
38760	1(2)
38765	1(2)
38770	1(2)
38780	1(2)
38790	1(2)
38792	1(3)
38794	1(2)
38900	1(3)
38999	1(3)
39000	1(2)
39010	1(2)
39200	1(2)
39220	1(2)
39401	1(3)
39402	1(3)
39499	1(3)
39501	1(3)
39503	1(2)
39540	1(2)
39541	1(2)
39545	1(2)
39560	1(3)
39561	1(3)
39599	1(3)
40490	2(3)
40500	2(3)
40510	2(3)
40520	2(3)
40525	2(3)
40527	2(3)
40530	2(3)
40650	2(3)
40652	2(3)
40654	2(3)
40700	1(2)
40701	1(2)
40702	1(2)
40720	1(2)
40761	1(2)
40799	1(3)
40800	2(3)
40801	2(3)
40804	1(3)
40805	2(3)
40806	2(2)
40808	2(3)
40810	2(3)
40812	2(3)
40814	4(3)
40816	2(3)
40818	2(3)
40819	2(2)
40820	2(3)
40830	2(3)

CPT	MUE
40831	2(3)
40840	1(2)
40842	1(2)
40843	1(2)
40844	1(2)
40845	1(3)
40899	1(3)
41000	1(3)
41005	1(3)
41006	2(3)
41007	2(3)
41008	2(3)
41009	2(3)
41010	1(2)
41015	2(3)
41016	1(3)
41017	2(3)
41018	2(3)
41019	1(2)
41100	2(3)
41105	2(3)
41108	2(3)
41110	2(3)
41112	2(3)
41113	2(3)
41114	2(3)
41115	1(2)
41116	2(3)
41120	1(2)
41130	1(2)
41135	1(2)
41140	1(2)
41145	1(2)
41150	1(2)
41153	1(2)
41155	1(2)
41250	2(3)
41251	2(3)
41252	2(3)
41510	1(2)
41512	1(2)
41520	1(3)
41530	1(3)
41599	1(3)
41800	2(3)
41805	1(3)
41806	1(3)
41820	4(2)
41821	2(3)
41822	1(2)
41823	1(2)
41825	2(3)
41826	2(3)
41827	2(3)
41828	4(2)
41830	2(3)
41850	2(3)
41870	2(3)
41872	4(2)
41874	4(2)
41899	1(3)
42000	1(3)
42100	2(3)
42104	2(3)
42106	2(3)

CPT	MUE
42107	2(3)
42120	1(2)
42140	1(2)
42145	1(2)
42160	1(3)
42180	1(3)
42182	1(3)
42200	1(2)
42205	1(2)
42210	1(2)
42215	1(2)
42220	1(2)
42225	1(2)
42226	1(2)
42227	1(2)
42235	1(2)
42260	1(3)
42280	1(2)
42281	1(2)
42299	1(3)
42300	2(3)
42305	2(3)
42310	2(3)
42320	2(3)
42330	1(3)
42335	2(2)
42340	1(2)
42400	2(3)
42405	2(3)
42408	1(3)
42409	1(3)
42410	1(2)
42415	1(2)
42420	1(2)
42425	1(2)
42426	1(2)
42440	1(2)
42450	1(3)
42500	2(3)
42505	2(3)
42507	1(2)
42509	1(2)
42510	1(2)
42550	2(3)
42600	1(3)
42650	2(3)
42660	2(3)
42665	2(3)
42699	1(3)
42700	2(3)
42720	1(3)
42725	1(3)
42800	3(3)
42804	1(3)
42806	1(3)
42808	2(3)
42809	1(3)
42810	1(3)
42815	1(3)
42820	1(2)
42821	1(2)
42825	1(2)
42826	1(2)
42830	1(2)
42831	1(2)

CPT	MUE
42835	1(2)
42836	1(2)
42842	1(3)
42844	1(3)
42845	1(3)
42860	1(3)
42870	1(3)
42890	1(2)
42892	1(3)
42894	1(3)
42900	1(3)
42950	1(2)
42953	1(3)
42955	1(2)
42960	1(3)
42961	1(3)
42962	1(3)
42970	1(3)
42971	1(3)
42972	1(3)
42999	1(3)
43020	1(2)
43030	1(2)
43045	1(2)
43100	1(3)
43101	1(3)
43107	1(2)
43108	1(2)
43112	1(2)
43113	1(2)
43116	1(2)
43117	1(2)
43118	1(2)
43121	1(2)
43122	1(2)
43123	1(2)
43124	1(2)
43130	1(3)
43135	1(3)
43180	1(2)
43191	1(3)
43192	1(3)
43193	1(3)
43194	1(3)
43195	1(3)
43196	1(3)
43197	1(3)
43198	1(3)
43200	1(3)
43201	1(2)
43202	1(2)
43204	1(2)
43205	1(2)
43206	1(2)
43210	1(2)
43211	1(3)
43212	1(3)
43213	1(2)
43214	1(3)
43215	1(3)
43216	1(2)
43217	1(2)
43220	1(3)
43226	1(3)
43227	1(3)

CPT	MUE
43229	1(3)
43231	1(2)
43232	1(2)
43233	1(3)
43235	1(3)
43236	1(2)
43237	1(2)
43238	1(2)
43239	1(2)
43240	1(2)
43241	1(3)
43242	1(2)
43243	1(2)
43244	1(2)
43245	1(2)
43246	1(2)
43247	1(2)
43248	1(3)
43249	1(3)
43250	1(2)
43251	1(2)
43252	1(2)
43253	1(3)
43254	1(3)
43255	2(3)
43257	1(2)
43259	1(2)
43260	1(3)
43261	1(2)
43262	2(2)
43263	1(2)
43264	1(2)
43265	1(2)
43266	1(3)
43270	1(3)
43273	1(2)
43274	2(3)
43275	1(3)
43276	2(3)
43277	3(3)
43278	1(3)
43279	1(2)
43280	1(2)
43281	1(2)
43282	1(2)
43283	1(2)
43284	1(2)
43285	1(2)
43286	1(2)
43287	1(2)
43288	1(2)
43289	1(3)
43300	1(2)
43305	1(2)
43310	1(2)
43312	1(2)
43313	1(2)
43314	1(2)
43320	1(2)
43325	1(2)
43327	1(2)
43328	1(2)
43330	1(2)
43331	1(2)
43332	1(2)

CPT	MUE
43333	1(2)
43334	1(2)
43335	1(2)
43336	1(2)
43337	1(2)
43338	1(2)
43340	1(2)
43341	1(2)
43351	1(2)
43352	1(2)
43360	1(2)
43361	1(2)
43400	1(2)
43405	1(2)
43410	1(3)
43415	1(3)
43420	1(3)
43425	1(3)
43450	1(3)
43453	1(3)
43460	1(3)
43496	1(3)
43499	1(3)
43500	1(2)
43501	1(3)
43502	1(2)
43510	1(2)
43520	1(2)
43605	1(2)
43610	2(3)
43611	2(3)
43620	1(2)
43621	1(2)
43622	1(2)
43631	1(2)
43632	1(2)
43633	1(2)
43634	1(2)
43635	1(2)
43640	1(2)
43641	1(2)
43644	1(2)
43645	1(2)
43647	1(2)
43648	1(2)
43651	1(2)
43652	1(2)
43653	1(2)
43659	1(3)
43752	2(3)
43753	1(3)
43754	1(3)
43755	1(3)
43756	1(2)
43757	1(2)
43761	2(3)
43762	2(3)
43763	2(3)
43770	1(2)
43771	1(2)
43772	1(2)
43773	1(2)
43774	1(2)
43775	1(2)
43800	1(2)

CPT	MUE
43810	1(2)
43820	1(2)
43825	1(2)
43830	1(2)
43831	1(2)
43832	1(2)
43840	2(3)
43842	0(3)
43843	1(2)
43845	1(2)
43846	1(2)
43847	1(2)
43848	1(2)
43850	1(2)
43855	1(2)
43860	1(2)
43865	1(2)
43870	1(2)
43880	1(3)
43881	1(3)
43882	1(3)
43886	1(2)
43887	1(2)
43888	1(2)
43999	1(3)
44005	1(2)
44010	1(2)
44015	1(2)
44020	2(3)
44021	1(3)
44025	1(3)
44050	1(2)
44055	1(2)
44100	1(2)
44110	1(2)
44111	1(2)
44120	1(2)
44121	2(3)
44125	1(2)
44126	1(2)
44127	1(2)
44128	2(3)
44130	2(3)
44132	1(2)
44133	1(2)
44135	1(2)
44136	1(2)
44137	1(2)
44139	1(2)
44140	2(3)
44141	1(3)
44143	1(2)
44144	1(3)
44145	1(2)
44146	1(2)
44147	1(3)
44150	1(2)
44151	1(2)
44155	1(2)
44156	1(2)
44157	1(2)
44158	1(2)
44160	1(2)
44180	1(2)
44186	1(2)

CPT	MUE
44187	1(3)
44188	1(3)
44202	1(2)
44203	2(3)
44204	2(3)
44205	1(2)
44206	1(2)
44207	1(2)
44208	1(2)
44210	1(2)
44211	1(2)
44212	1(2)
44213	1(2)
44227	1(3)
44238	1(3)
44300	1(3)
44310	2(3)
44312	1(2)
44314	1(2)
44316	1(2)
44320	1(2)
44322	1(2)
44340	1(2)
44345	1(2)
44346	1(2)
44360	1(3)
44361	1(2)
44363	1(3)
44364	1(2)
44365	1(2)
44366	1(3)
44369	1(2)
44370	1(2)
44372	1(2)
44373	1(2)
44376	1(3)
44377	1(2)
44378	1(3)
44379	1(2)
44380	1(3)
44381	1(3)
44382	1(2)
44384	1(3)
44385	1(3)
44386	1(2)
44388	1(3)
44389	1(2)
44390	1(3)
44391	1(3)
44392	1(2)
44394	1(2)
44401	1(2)
44402	1(3)
44403	1(3)
44404	1(3)
44405	1(3)
44406	1(3)
44407	1(2)
44408	1(3)
44500	1(3)
44602	1(2)
44603	1(2)
44604	1(2)
44605	1(2)
44615	3(3)

CPT	MUE
44620	2(3)
44625	1(3)
44626	1(3)
44640	2(3)
44650	2(3)
44660	1(3)
44661	1(3)
44680	1(3)
44700	1(2)
44701	1(2)
44705	1(3)
44715	1(2)
44720	2(3)
44721	2(3)
44799	1(3)
44800	1(3)
44820	1(3)
44850	1(3)
44899	1(3)
44900	1(2)
44950	1(2)
44955	1(2)
44960	1(2)
44970	1(2)
44979	1(3)
45000	1(3)
45005	1(3)
45020	1(3)
45100	2(3)
45108	1(2)
45110	1(2)
45111	1(2)
45112	1(2)
45113	1(2)
45114	1(2)
45116	1(2)
45119	1(2)
45120	1(2)
45121	1(2)
45123	1(2)
45126	1(2)
45130	1(2)
45135	1(2)
45136	1(2)
45150	1(2)
45160	1(3)
45171	2(3)
45172	2(3)
45190	1(3)
45300	1(3)
45303	1(3)
45305	1(2)
45307	1(3)
45308	1(2)
45309	1(2)
45315	1(2)
45317	1(3)
45320	1(2)
45321	1(2)
45327	1(2)
45330	1(3)
45331	1(2)
45332	1(3)
45333	1(2)
45334	1(3)

CPT	MUE
45335	1(2)
45337	1(2)
45338	1(2)
45340	1(2)
45341	1(2)
45342	1(2)
45346	1(2)
45347	1(3)
45349	1(3)
45350	1(2)
45378	1(3)
45379	1(3)
45380	1(2)
45381	1(2)
45382	1(3)
45384	1(2)
45385	1(2)
45386	1(2)
45388	1(2)
45389	1(3)
45390	1(3)
45391	1(2)
45392	1(2)
45393	1(3)
45395	1(2)
45397	1(2)
45398	1(2)
45399	1(3)
45400	1(2)
45402	1(2)
45499	1(3)
45500	1(2)
45505	1(2)
45520	1(2)
45540	1(2)
45541	1(2)
45550	1(2)
45560	1(2)
45562	1(2)
45563	1(2)
45800	1(3)
45805	1(3)
45820	1(3)
45825	1(3)
45900	1(2)
45905	1(2)
45910	1(2)
45915	1(2)
45990	1(2)
45999	1(3)
46020	2(3)
46030	1(3)
46040	2(3)
46045	2(3)
46050	2(3)
46060	2(3)
46070	1(2)
46080	1(2)
46083	2(3)
46200	1(3)
46220	1(2)
46221	1(2)
46230	1(2)
46250	1(2)
46255	1(2)

CPT	MUE
46257	1(2)
46258	1(2)
46260	1(2)
46261	1(2)
46262	1(2)
46270	1(3)
46275	1(3)
46280	1(2)
46285	1(3)
46288	1(3)
46320	2(3)
46500	1(2)
46505	1(2)
46600	1(3)
46601	1(3)
46604	1(2)
46606	1(2)
46607	1(2)
46608	1(3)
46610	1(2)
46611	1(2)
46612	1(2)
46614	1(3)
46615	1(2)
46700	1(2)
46705	1(2)
46706	1(3)
46707	1(3)
46710	1(3)
46712	1(3)
46715	1(2)
46716	1(2)
46730	1(2)
46735	1(2)
46740	1(2)
46742	1(2)
46744	1(2)
46746	1(2)
46748	1(2)
46750	1(2)
46751	1(2)
46753	1(2)
46754	1(3)
46760	1(2)
46761	1(2)
46900	1(2)
46910	1(2)
46916	1(2)
46917	1(2)
46922	1(2)
46924	1(2)
46930	1(2)
46940	1(2)
46942	1(3)
46945	1(2)
46946	1(2)
46947	1(2)
46948	1(2)
46999	1(3)
47000	3(3)
47001	3(3)
47010	1(3)
47015	1(2)
47100	3(3)
47120	2(3)

CPT	MUE
47122	1(2)
47125	1(2)
47130	1(2)
47133	1(2)
47135	1(2)
47140	1(2)
47141	1(2)
47142	1(2)
47143	1(2)
47144	1(2)
47145	1(2)
47146	2(3)
47147	1(3)
47300	2(3)
47350	1(3)
47360	1(3)
47361	1(3)
47362	1(3)
47370	1(2)
47371	1(2)
47379	1(3)
47380	1(2)
47381	1(2)
47382	1(2)
47383	1(2)
47399	1(3)
47400	1(3)
47420	1(2)
47425	1(2)
47460	1(2)
47480	1(2)
47490	1(2)
47531	2(3)
47532	1(3)
47533	1(3)
47534	2(3)
47535	1(3)
47536	2(3)
47537	1(3)
47538	2(3)
47539	2(3)
47540	2(3)
47541	1(3)
47542	2(3)
47543	1(3)
47544	1(3)
47550	1(3)
47552	1(3)
47553	1(2)
47554	1(3)
47555	1(2)
47556	1(2)
47562	1(2)
47563	1(2)
47564	1(2)
47570	1(2)
47579	1(3)
47600	1(2)
47605	1(2)
47610	1(2)
47612	1(2)
47620	1(2)
47700	1(2)
47701	1(2)
47711	1(2)

CPT	MUE
47712	1(2)
47715	1(2)
47720	1(2)
47721	1(2)
47740	1(2)
47741	1(2)
47760	1(2)
47765	1(2)
47780	1(2)
47785	1(2)
47800	1(2)
47801	1(3)
47802	1(2)
47900	1(2)
47999	1(3)
48000	1(2)
48001	1(2)
48020	1(3)
48100	1(3)
48102	1(3)
48105	1(2)
48120	1(3)
48140	1(2)
48145	1(2)
48146	1(2)
48148	1(2)
48150	1(2)
48152	1(2)
48153	1(2)
48154	1(2)
48155	1(2)
48160	0(3)
48400	1(3)
48500	1(3)
48510	1(3)
48520	1(3)
48540	1(3)
48545	1(3)
48547	1(2)
48548	1(2)
48550	1(2)
48551	1(2)
48552	2(3)
48554	1(2)
48556	1(2)
48999	1(3)
49000	1(2)
49002	1(3)
49010	1(3)
49013	1(2)
49014	1(3)
49020	2(3)
49040	2(3)
49060	2(3)
49062	1(3)
49082	1(3)
49083	2(3)
49084	1(3)
49180	2(3)
49185	2(3)
49203	1(2)
49204	1(2)
49205	1(2)
49215	1(2)
49220	1(2)

CPT	MUE
49250	1(2)
49255	1(2)
49320	1(3)
49321	1(2)
49322	1(2)
49323	1(2)
49324	1(2)
49325	1(2)
49326	1(2)
49327	1(2)
49329	1(3)
49400	1(3)
49402	1(3)
49405	2(3)
49406	2(3)
49407	1(3)
49411	1(2)
49412	1(2)
49418	1(3)
49419	1(2)
49421	1(2)
49422	1(2)
49423	2(3)
49424	3(3)
49425	1(2)
49426	1(3)
49427	1(3)
49428	1(2)
49429	1(2)
49435	1(2)
49436	1(2)
49440	1(3)
49441	1(3)
49442	1(3)
49446	1(2)
49450	1(3)
49451	1(3)
49452	1(3)
49460	1(3)
49465	1(3)
49491	1(2)
49492	1(2)
49495	1(2)
49496	1(2)
49500	1(2)
49501	1(2)
49505	1(2)
49507	1(2)
49520	1(2)
49521	1(2)
49525	1(2)
49540	1(2)
49550	1(2)
49553	1(2)
49555	1(2)
49557	1(2)
49560	2(3)
49561	1(3)
49565	2(3)
49566	2(3)
49568	2(3)
49570	1(3)
49572	1(3)
49580	1(2)
49582	1(2)

CPT	MUE
49585	1(2)
49587	1(2)
49590	1(2)
49600	1(2)
49605	1(2)
49606	1(2)
49610	1(2)
49611	1(2)
49650	1(2)
49651	1(2)
49652	2(3)
49653	2(3)
49654	1(3)
49655	1(3)
49656	1(3)
49657	1(3)
49659	1(3)
49900	1(3)
49904	1(3)
49905	1(3)
49906	1(3)
49999	1(3)
50010	1(2)
50020	1(3)
50040	1(2)
50045	1(2)
50060	1(2)
50065	1(2)
50070	1(2)
50075	1(2)
50080	1(2)
50081	1(2)
50100	1(2)
50120	1(2)
50125	1(2)
50130	1(2)
50135	1(2)
50200	1(3)
50205	1(3)
50220	1(2)
50225	1(2)
50230	1(2)
50234	1(2)
50236	1(2)
50240	1(2)
50250	1(3)
50280	1(2)
50290	1(3)
50300	1(2)
50320	1(2)
50323	1(2)
50325	1(2)
50327	2(3)
50328	1(3)
50329	1(3)
50340	1(2)
50360	1(2)
50365	1(2)
50370	1(2)
50380	1(2)
50382	1(3)
50384	1(3)
50385	1(3)
50386	1(3)
50387	1(3)

CPT	MUE
50389	1(3)
50390	2(3)
50391	1(3)
50396	1(3)
50400	1(2)
50405	1(2)
50430	2(3)
50431	2(3)
50432	2(3)
50433	2(3)
50434	2(3)
50435	2(3)
50436	1(3)
50437	1(3)
50500	1(3)
50520	1(3)
50525	1(3)
50526	1(3)
50540	1(2)
50541	1(2)
50542	1(2)
50543	1(2)
50544	1(2)
50545	1(2)
50546	1(2)
50547	1(2)
50548	1(2)
50549	1(3)
50551	1(3)
50553	1(3)
50555	1(2)
50557	1(2)
50561	1(2)
50562	1(3)
50570	1(3)
50572	1(3)
50574	1(2)
50575	1(2)
50576	1(2)
50580	1(2)
50590	1(2)
50592	1(2)
50593	1(2)
50600	1(3)
50605	1(3)
50606	1(3)
50610	1(2)
50620	1(2)
50630	1(2)
50650	1(2)
50660	1(3)
50684	1(3)
50686	2(3)
50688	2(3)
50690	2(3)
50693	2(3)
50694	2(3)
50695	2(3)
50700	1(2)
50705	2(3)
50706	2(3)
50715	1(2)
50722	1(2)
50725	1(3)
50727	1(3)

CPT	MUE
50728	1(3)
50740	1(2)
50750	1(2)
50760	1(2)
50770	1(2)
50780	1(2)
50782	1(2)
50783	1(2)
50785	1(2)
50800	1(2)
50810	1(3)
50815	1(2)
50820	1(2)
50825	1(3)
50830	1(3)
50840	1(2)
50845	1(2)
50860	1(2)
50900	1(3)
50920	2(3)
50930	2(3)
50940	1(2)
50945	1(2)
50947	1(2)
50948	1(2)
50949	1(3)
50951	1(3)
50953	1(3)
50955	1(2)
50957	1(2)
50961	1(2)
50970	1(3)
50972	1(3)
50974	1(2)
50976	1(2)
50980	1(2)
51020	1(2)
51030	1(2)
51040	1(3)
51045	2(3)
51050	1(3)
51060	1(3)
51065	1(3)
51080	1(3)
51100	1(3)
51101	1(3)
51102	1(3)
51500	1(2)
51520	1(2)
51525	1(2)
51530	1(2)
51535	1(2)
51550	1(2)
51555	1(2)
51565	1(2)
51570	1(2)
51575	1(2)
51580	1(2)
51585	1(2)
51590	1(2)
51595	1(2)
51596	1(2)
51597	1(2)
51600	1(3)
51605	1(3)

CPT	MUE
51610	1(3)
51700	1(3)
51701	2(3)
51702	2(3)
51703	2(3)
51705	1(3)
51710	1(3)
51715	1(2)
51720	1(3)
51725	1(3)
51726	1(3)
51727	1(3)
51728	1(3)
51729	1(3)
51736	1(3)
51741	1(3)
51784	1(3)
51785	1(3)
51792	1(3)
51797	1(3)
51798	1(3)
51800	1(2)
51820	1(2)
51840	1(2)
51841	1(2)
51845	1(2)
51860	1(3)
51865	1(3)
51880	1(2)
51900	1(3)
51920	1(3)
51925	1(2)
51940	1(2)
51960	1(2)
51980	1(2)
51990	1(2)
51992	1(2)
51999	1(3)
52000	1(3)
52001	1(3)
52005	2(3)
52007	1(2)
52010	1(2)
52204	1(2)
52214	1(2)
52224	1(2)
52234	1(2)
52235	1(2)
52240	1(2)
52250	1(2)
52260	1(2)
52265	1(2)
52270	1(2)
52275	1(2)
52276	1(2)
52277	1(2)
52281	1(2)
52282	1(2)
52283	1(2)
52285	1(2)
52287	1(2)
52290	1(2)
52300	1(2)
52301	1(2)
52305	1(2)

CPT	MUE
52310	1(3)
52315	2(3)
52317	1(3)
52318	1(3)
52320	1(2)
52325	1(3)
52327	1(2)
52330	1(2)
52332	1(2)
52334	1(2)
52341	1(2)
52342	1(2)
52343	1(2)
52344	1(2)
52345	1(2)
52346	1(2)
52351	1(3)
52352	1(2)
52353	1(2)
52354	1(3)
52355	1(3)
52356	1(2)
52400	1(2)
52402	1(2)
52441	1(2)
52442	6(3)
52450	1(2)
52500	1(2)
52601	1(2)
52630	1(2)
52640	1(2)
52647	1(2)
52648	1(2)
52649	1(2)
52700	1(3)
53000	1(2)
53010	1(2)
53020	1(2)
53025	1(2)
53040	1(3)
53060	1(3)
53080	1(3)
53085	1(3)
53200	1(3)
53210	1(2)
53215	1(2)
53220	1(3)
53230	1(3)
53235	1(3)
53240	1(3)
53250	1(3)
53260	1(2)
53265	1(3)
53270	1(2)
53275	1(2)
53400	1(2)
53405	1(2)
53410	1(2)
53415	1(2)
53420	1(2)
53425	1(2)
53430	1(2)
53431	1(2)
53440	1(2)
53442	1(2)

CPT	MUE
53444	1(3)
53445	1(2)
53446	1(2)
53447	1(2)
53448	1(2)
53449	1(2)
53450	1(2)
53460	1(2)
53500	1(2)
53502	1(3)
53505	1(3)
53510	1(3)
53515	1(3)
53520	1(3)
53600	1(3)
53601	1(3)
53605	1(3)
53620	1(2)
53621	1(3)
53660	1(2)
53661	1(3)
53665	1(3)
53850	1(2)
53852	1(2)
53854	1(2)
53855	1(2)
53860	1(2)
53899	1(3)
54000	1(2)
54001	1(2)
54015	1(3)
54050	1(2)
54055	1(2)
54056	1(2)
54057	1(2)
54060	1(2)
54065	1(2)
54100	2(3)
54105	2(3)
54110	1(2)
54111	1(2)
54112	1(3)
54115	1(3)
54120	1(2)
54125	1(2)
54130	1(2)
54135	1(2)
54150	1(2)
54160	1(2)
54161	1(2)
54162	1(2)
54163	1(2)
54164	1(2)
54200	1(2)
54205	1(2)
54220	1(3)
54230	1(3)
54231	1(3)
54235	1(3)
54240	1(2)
54250	1(2)
54300	1(2)
54304	1(2)
54308	1(2)
54312	1(2)

CPT	MUE
54316	1(2)
54318	1(2)
54322	1(2)
54324	1(2)
54326	1(2)
54328	1(2)
54332	1(2)
54336	1(2)
54340	1(2)
54344	1(2)
54348	1(2)
54352	1(2)
54360	1(2)
54380	1(2)
54385	1(2)
54390	1(2)
54400	1(2)
54401	1(2)
54405	1(2)
54406	1(2)
54408	1(2)
54410	1(2)
54411	1(2)
54415	1(2)
54416	1(2)
54417	1(2)
54420	1(2)
54430	1(2)
54435	1(2)
54437	1(2)
54438	1(2)
54440	1(2)
54450	1(2)
54500	1(3)
54505	1(3)
54512	1(3)
54520	1(2)
54522	1(2)
54530	1(2)
54535	1(2)
54550	1(2)
54560	1(2)
54600	1(2)
54620	1(2)
54640	1(2)
54650	1(2)
54660	1(2)
54670	1(3)
54680	1(2)
54690	1(2)
54692	1(2)
54699	1(3)
54700	1(3)
54800	1(2)
54830	1(2)
54840	1(2)
54860	1(2)
54861	1(2)
54865	1(3)
54900	1(2)
54901	1(2)
55000	1(3)
55040	1(2)
55041	1(2)
55060	1(2)

CPT	MUE
55100	2(3)
55110	1(2)
55120	1(3)
55150	1(2)
55175	1(2)
55180	1(2)
55200	1(2)
55250	1(2)
55300	1(2)
55400	1(2)
55500	1(2)
55520	1(2)
55530	1(2)
55535	1(2)
55540	1(2)
55550	1(2)
55559	1(3)
55600	1(2)
55605	1(2)
55650	1(2)
55680	1(3)
55700	1(2)
55705	1(2)
55706	1(2)
55720	1(3)
55725	1(3)
55801	1(2)
55810	1(2)
55812	1(2)
55815	1(2)
55821	1(2)
55831	1(2)
55840	1(2)
55842	1(2)
55845	1(2)
55860	1(2)
55862	1(2)
55865	1(2)
55866	1(2)
55870	1(2)
55873	1(2)
55874	1(2)
55875	1(2)
55876	1(2)
55899	1(3)
55920	1(2)
55970	1(2)
55980	1(2)
56405	2(3)
56420	1(3)
56440	1(3)
56441	1(2)
56442	1(2)
56501	1(2)
56515	1(2)
56605	1(2)
56606	6(3)
56620	1(2)
56625	1(2)
56630	1(2)
56631	1(2)
56632	1(2)
56633	1(2)
56634	1(2)
56637	1(2)

CPT	MUE
56640	1(2)
56700	1(2)
56740	1(3)
56800	1(2)
56805	1(2)
56810	1(2)
56820	1(2)
56821	1(2)
57000	1(3)
57010	1(3)
57020	1(3)
57022	1(3)
57023	1(3)
57061	1(2)
57065	1(2)
57100	2(3)
57105	2(3)
57106	1(2)
57107	1(2)
57109	1(2)
57110	1(2)
57111	1(2)
57112	1(2)
57120	1(2)
57130	1(2)
57135	2(3)
57150	1(3)
57155	1(3)
57156	1(3)
57160	1(2)
57170	1(2)
57180	1(3)
57200	1(3)
57210	1(3)
57220	1(2)
57230	1(2)
57240	1(2)
57250	1(2)
57260	1(2)
57265	1(2)
57267	2(3)
57268	1(2)
57270	1(2)
57280	1(2)
57282	1(2)
57283	1(2)
57284	1(2)
57285	1(2)
57287	1(2)
57288	1(2)
57289	1(2)
57291	1(2)
57292	1(2)
57295	1(2)
57296	1(2)
57300	1(3)
57305	1(3)
57307	1(3)
57308	1(3)
57310	1(3)
57311	1(3)
57320	1(3)
57330	1(3)
57335	1(2)
57400	1(2)

CPT	MUE
57410	1(2)
57415	1(3)
57420	1(3)
57421	1(3)
57423	1(2)
57425	1(2)
57426	1(2)
57452	1(3)
57454	1(3)
57455	1(3)
57456	1(3)
57460	1(3)
57461	1(3)
57500	1(3)
57505	1(3)
57510	1(3)
57511	1(3)
57513	1(3)
57520	1(3)
57522	1(3)
57530	1(3)
57531	1(2)
57540	1(2)
57545	1(3)
57550	1(3)
57555	1(2)
57556	1(2)
57558	1(3)
57700	1(3)
57720	1(3)
57800	1(3)
58100	1(3)
58110	1(3)
58120	1(3)
58140	1(3)
58145	1(3)
58146	1(3)
58150	1(3)
58152	1(2)
58180	1(3)
58200	1(2)
58210	1(2)
58240	1(2)
58260	1(3)
58262	1(3)
58263	1(2)
58267	1(2)
58270	1(2)
58275	1(2)
58280	1(2)
58285	1(3)
58290	1(3)
58291	1(2)
58292	1(2)
58293	1(2)
58294	1(2)
58300	0(3)
58301	1(3)
58321	1(2)
58322	1(2)
58323	1(3)
58340	1(3)
58345	1(3)
58346	1(2)
58350	1(2)

CPT	MUE
58353	1(3)
58356	1(3)
58400	1(3)
58410	1(2)
58520	1(2)
58540	1(3)
58541	1(3)
58542	1(2)
58543	1(3)
58544	1(2)
58545	1(2)
58546	1(2)
58548	1(2)
58550	1(3)
58552	1(3)
58553	1(3)
58554	1(2)
58555	1(3)
58558	1(3)
58559	1(3)
58560	1(3)
58561	1(3)
58562	1(3)
58563	1(3)
58565	1(2)
58570	1(3)
58571	1(2)
58572	1(3)
58573	1(2)
58575	1(2)
58578	1(3)
58579	1(3)
58600	1(2)
58605	1(2)
58611	1(2)
58615	1(2)
58660	1(2)
58661	1(2)
58662	1(2)
58670	1(2)
58671	1(2)
58672	1(2)
58673	1(2)
58674	1(2)
58679	1(3)
58700	1(2)
58720	1(2)
58740	1(2)
58750	1(2)
58752	1(2)
58760	1(2)
58770	1(2)
58800	1(2)
58805	1(2)
58820	1(3)
58822	1(3)
58825	1(2)
58900	1(2)
58920	1(2)
58925	1(3)
58940	1(2)
58943	1(2)
58950	1(2)
58951	1(2)
58952	1(2)

CPT	MUE
58953	1(2)
58954	1(2)
58956	1(2)
58957	1(2)
58958	1(2)
58960	1(2)
58970	1(3)
58974	1(3)
58976	2(3)
58999	1(3)
59000	2(3)
59001	2(3)
59012	2(3)
59015	2(3)
59020	2(3)
59025	2(3)
59030	2(3)
59050	2(3)
59051	2(3)
59070	2(3)
59072	2(3)
59074	2(3)
59076	2(3)
59100	1(2)
59120	1(3)
59121	1(3)
59130	1(3)
59135	1(3)
59136	1(3)
59140	1(2)
59150	1(3)
59151	1(3)
59160	1(2)
59200	1(3)
59300	1(2)
59320	1(2)
59325	1(2)
59350	1(2)
59400	1(2)
59409	2(3)
59410	1(2)
59412	1(3)
59414	1(3)
59425	1(2)
59426	1(2)
59430	1(2)
59510	1(2)
59514	1(3)
59515	1(2)
59525	1(2)
59610	1(2)
59612	2(3)
59614	1(2)
59618	1(2)
59620	1(2)
59622	1(2)
59812	1(2)
59820	1(2)
59821	1(2)
59830	1(2)
59840	1(2)
59841	1(2)
59850	1(2)
59851	1(2)
59852	1(2)

CPT	MUE
59855	1(2)
59856	1(2)
59857	1(2)
59866	1(2)
59870	1(2)
59871	1(2)
59897	1(3)
59898	1(3)
59899	1(3)
60000	1(3)
60100	3(3)
60200	2(3)
60210	1(2)
60212	1(2)
60220	1(3)
60225	1(2)
60240	1(2)
60252	1(2)
60254	1(2)
60260	1(2)
60270	1(2)
60271	1(2)
60280	1(3)
60281	1(3)
60300	2(3)
60500	1(2)
60502	1(3)
60505	1(3)
60512	1(3)
60520	1(2)
60521	1(2)
60522	1(2)
60540	1(2)
60545	1(2)
60600	1(3)
60605	1(3)
60650	1(2)
60659	1(3)
60699	1(3)
61000	1(2)
61001	1(2)
61020	2(3)
61026	2(3)
61050	1(3)
61055	1(3)
61070	2(3)
61105	1(3)
61107	1(3)
61108	1(3)
61120	1(3)
61140	1(3)
61150	1(3)
61151	1(3)
61154	1(3)
61156	1(3)
61210	1(3)
61215	1(3)
61250	1(3)
61253	1(3)
61304	1(3)
61305	1(3)
61312	2(3)
61313	2(3)
61314	2(3)
61315	1(3)

CPT	MUE
61316	1(3)
61320	2(3)
61321	1(3)
61322	1(3)
61323	1(3)
61330	1(2)
61333	1(2)
61340	1(2)
61343	1(2)
61345	1(3)
61450	1(3)
61458	1(2)
61460	1(2)
61500	1(3)
61501	1(3)
61510	1(3)
61512	1(3)
61514	2(3)
61516	1(3)
61517	1(3)
61518	1(3)
61519	1(3)
61520	1(3)
61521	1(3)
61522	1(3)
61524	2(3)
61526	1(3)
61530	1(3)
61531	1(2)
61533	2(3)
61534	1(3)
61535	2(3)
61536	1(3)
61537	1(3)
61538	1(2)
61539	1(3)
61540	1(3)
61541	1(2)
61543	1(2)
61544	1(3)
61545	1(2)
61546	1(2)
61548	1(2)
61550	1(2)
61552	1(2)
61556	1(3)
61557	1(2)
61558	1(3)
61559	1(3)
61563	2(3)
61564	1(2)
61566	1(3)
61567	1(2)
61570	1(3)
61571	1(3)
61575	1(2)
61576	1(2)
61580	1(2)
61581	1(2)
61582	1(2)
61583	1(2)
61584	1(2)
61585	1(2)
61586	1(3)
61590	1(2)

CPT	MUE
61591	1(2)
61592	1(2)
61595	1(2)
61596	1(2)
61597	1(2)
61598	1(3)
61600	1(3)
61601	1(3)
61605	1(3)
61606	1(3)
61607	1(3)
61608	1(3)
61611	1(3)
61613	1(3)
61615	1(3)
61616	1(3)
61618	2(3)
61619	2(3)
61623	2(3)
61624	2(3)
61626	2(3)
61630	1(3)
61635	2(3)
61640	0(3)
61641	0(3)
61642	0(3)
61645	1(3)
61650	1(2)
61651	2(2)
61680	1(3)
61682	1(3)
61684	1(3)
61686	1(3)
61690	1(3)
61692	1(3)
61697	2(3)
61698	1(3)
61700	2(3)
61702	1(3)
61703	1(3)
61705	1(3)
61708	1(3)
61710	1(3)
61711	1(3)
61720	1(3)
61735	1(3)
61750	2(3)
61751	2(3)
61760	1(2)
61770	1(2)
61781	1(3)
61782	1(3)
61783	1(3)
61790	1(2)
61791	1(2)
61796	1(2)
61797	4(3)
61798	1(2)
61799	4(3)
61800	1(2)
61850	1(3)
61860	1(3)
61863	1(2)
61864	1(3)
61867	1(2)

CPT	MUE
61868	2(3)
61870	1(3)
61880	1(2)
61885	1(3)
61886	1(3)
61888	1(3)
62000	1(3)
62005	1(3)
62010	1(3)
62100	1(3)
62115	1(2)
62117	1(2)
62120	1(2)
62121	1(2)
62140	1(3)
62141	1(3)
62142	2(3)
62143	2(3)
62145	2(3)
62146	2(3)
62147	1(3)
62148	1(3)
62160	1(3)
62161	1(3)
62162	1(3)
62163	1(3)
62164	1(3)
62165	1(2)
62180	1(3)
62190	1(3)
62192	1(3)
62194	1(3)
62200	1(2)
62201	1(2)
62220	1(3)
62223	1(3)
62225	2(3)
62230	2(3)
62252	2(3)
62256	1(3)
62258	1(3)
62263	1(2)
62264	1(2)
62267	2(3)
62268	1(3)
62269	2(3)
62270	2(3)
62272	1(3)
62273	2(3)
62280	1(3)
62281	1(3)
62282	1(3)
62284	1(3)
62287	1(2)
62290	5(2)
62291	4(3)
62292	1(2)
62294	1(3)
62302	1(3)
62303	1(3)
62304	1(3)
62305	1(3)
62320	1(3)
62321	1(3)
62322	1(3)

CPT	MUE
62323	1(3)
62324	1(3)
62325	1(3)
62326	1(3)
62327	1(3)
62328	2(3)
62329	1(3)
62350	1(3)
62351	1(3)
62355	1(3)
62360	1(2)
62361	1(2)
62362	1(2)
62365	1(2)
62367	1(3)
62368	1(3)
62369	1(3)
62370	1(3)
62380	2(3)
63001	1(2)
63003	1(2)
63005	1(2)
63011	1(2)
63012	1(2)
63015	1(2)
63016	1(2)
63017	1(2)
63020	1(2)
63030	1(2)
63035	4(3)
63040	1(2)
63042	1(2)
63043	4(3)
63044	4(2)
63045	1(2)
63046	1(2)
63047	1(2)
63048	5(3)
63050	1(2)
63051	1(2)
63055	1(2)
63056	1(2)
63057	3(3)
63064	1(2)
63066	1(3)
63075	1(2)
63076	3(3)
63077	1(2)
63078	3(3)
63081	1(2)
63082	6(2)
63085	1(2)
63086	2(3)
63087	1(2)
63088	3(3)
63090	1(2)
63091	3(3)
63101	1(2)
63102	1(2)
63103	3(3)
63170	1(3)
63172	1(3)
63173	1(3)
63180	1(2)
63182	1(2)

CPT	MUE
63185	1(2)
63190	1(2)
63191	1(2)
63194	1(2)
63195	1(2)
63196	1(2)
63197	1(2)
63198	1(2)
63199	1(2)
63200	1(2)
63250	1(3)
63251	1(3)
63252	1(3)
63265	1(3)
63266	1(3)
63267	1(3)
63268	1(3)
63270	1(3)
63271	1(3)
63272	1(3)
63273	1(3)
63275	1(3)
63276	1(3)
63277	1(3)
63278	1(3)
63280	1(3)
63281	1(3)
63282	1(3)
63283	1(3)
63285	1(3)
63286	1(3)
63287	1(3)
63290	1(3)
63295	1(2)
63300	1(2)
63301	1(2)
63302	1(2)
63303	1(2)
63304	1(2)
63305	1(2)
63306	1(2)
63307	1(2)
63308	3(3)
63600	2(3)
63610	1(3)
63620	1(2)
63621	2(2)
63650	2(3)
63655	1(3)
63661	1(2)
63662	1(2)
63663	1(3)
63664	1(3)
63685	1(3)
63688	1(3)
63700	1(3)
63702	1(3)
63704	1(3)
63706	1(3)
63707	1(3)
63709	1(3)
63710	1(3)
63740	1(3)
63741	1(3)
63744	1(3)

CPT	MUE
63746	1(2)
64400	4(3)
64405	1(3)
64408	1(3)
64415	1(3)
64416	1(2)
64417	1(3)
64418	1(3)
64420	2(2)
64421	3(3)
64425	1(3)
64430	1(3)
64435	1(3)
64445	1(3)
64446	1(2)
64447	1(3)
64448	1(2)
64449	1(2)
64450	10(3)
64451	2(2)
64454	2(2)
64455	1(2)
64461	1(2)
64462	1(2)
64463	1(3)
64479	1(2)
64480	4(3)
64483	1(2)
64484	4(3)
64486	1(3)
64487	1(2)
64488	1(3)
64489	1(2)
64490	1(2)
64491	1(2)
64492	1(2)
64493	1(2)
64494	1(2)
64495	1(2)
64505	1(3)
64510	1(3)
64517	1(3)
64520	1(3)
64530	1(3)
64553	1(3)
64555	2(3)
64561	1(3)
64566	1(3)
64568	1(3)
64569	1(3)
64570	1(3)
64575	2(3)
64580	2(3)
64581	2(3)
64585	2(3)
64590	1(3)
64595	1(3)
64600	2(3)
64605	1(2)
64610	1(2)
64611	1(2)
64612	1(2)
64615	1(2)
64616	1(2)
64617	1(2)

CPT	MUE
64620	5(3)
64624	2(2)
64625	2(2)
64630	1(3)
64632	1(2)
64633	1(2)
64634	4(3)
64635	1(2)
64636	4(2)
64640	5(3)
64642	1(2)
64643	3(2)
64644	1(2)
64645	3(2)
64646	1(2)
64647	1(2)
64650	1(2)
64653	1(2)
64680	1(2)
64681	1(2)
64702	2(3)
64704	4(3)
64708	3(3)
64712	1(2)
64713	1(2)
64714	1(2)
64716	2(3)
64718	1(2)
64719	1(2)
64721	1(2)
64722	4(3)
64726	2(3)
64727	2(3)
64732	1(2)
64734	1(2)
64736	1(2)
64738	1(2)
64740	1(2)
64742	1(2)
64744	1(2)
64746	1(2)
64755	1(2)
64760	1(2)
64763	1(2)
64766	1(2)
64771	2(3)
64772	2(3)
64774	2(3)
64776	1(2)
64778	1(3)
64782	2(2)
64783	2(3)
64784	3(3)
64786	1(3)
64787	4(3)
64788	5(3)
64790	1(3)
64792	2(3)
64795	2(3)
64802	1(2)
64804	1(2)
64809	1(2)
64818	1(2)
64820	4(3)
64821	1(2)

CPT	MUE
64822	1(2)
64823	1(2)
64831	1(2)
64832	3(3)
64834	1(2)
64835	1(2)
64836	1(2)
64837	2(3)
64840	1(2)
64856	2(3)
64857	2(3)
64858	1(2)
64859	2(3)
64861	1(2)
64862	1(2)
64864	2(3)
64865	1(3)
64866	1(3)
64868	1(3)
64872	1(3)
64874	1(3)
64876	1(3)
64885	1(3)
64886	1(3)
64890	2(3)
64891	2(3)
64892	2(3)
64893	2(3)
64895	2(3)
64896	2(3)
64897	2(3)
64898	2(3)
64901	2(3)
64902	1(3)
64905	1(3)
64907	1(3)
64910	3(3)
64911	2(3)
64912	3(3)
64913	3(3)
64999	1(3)
65091	1(2)
65093	1(2)
65101	1(2)
65103	1(2)
65105	1(2)
65110	1(2)
65112	1(2)
65114	1(2)
65125	1(2)
65130	1(2)
65135	1(2)
65140	1(2)
65150	1(2)
65155	1(2)
65175	1(2)
65205	1(3)
65210	1(3)
65220	1(3)
65222	1(3)
65235	1(3)
65260	1(3)
65265	1(3)
65270	1(3)
65272	1(3)

CPT	MUE
65273	1(3)
65275	1(3)
65280	1(3)
65285	1(3)
65286	1(3)
65290	1(3)
65400	1(3)
65410	1(3)
65420	1(2)
65426	1(2)
65430	1(2)
65435	1(2)
65436	1(2)
65450	1(3)
65600	1(2)
65710	1(2)
65730	1(2)
65750	1(2)
65755	1(2)
65756	1(2)
65757	1(3)
65760	0(3)
65765	0(3)
65767	0(3)
65770	1(2)
65771	0(3)
65772	1(2)
65775	1(2)
65778	1(2)
65779	1(2)
65780	1(2)
65781	1(2)
65782	1(2)
65785	1(2)
65800	1(2)
65810	1(2)
65815	1(3)
65820	1(2)
65850	1(2)
65855	1(2)
65860	1(2)
65865	1(2)
65870	1(2)
65875	1(2)
65880	1(2)
65900	1(3)
65920	1(2)
65930	1(3)
66020	1(3)
66030	1(3)
66130	1(3)
66150	1(2)
66155	1(2)
66160	1(2)
66170	1(2)
66172	1(2)
66174	1(2)
66175	1(2)
66179	1(2)
66180	1(2)
66183	1(3)
66184	1(2)
66185	1(2)
66225	1(2)
66250	1(2)

CPT	MUE
66500	1(2)
66505	1(2)
66600	1(2)
66605	1(2)
66625	1(2)
66630	1(2)
66635	1(2)
66680	1(2)
66682	1(2)
66700	1(2)
66710	1(2)
66711	1(2)
66720	1(2)
66740	1(2)
66761	1(2)
66762	1(2)
66770	1(3)
66820	1(2)
66821	1(2)
66825	1(2)
66830	1(2)
66840	1(2)
66850	1(2)
66852	1(2)
66920	1(2)
66930	1(2)
66940	1(2)
66982	1(2)
66983	1(2)
66984	1(2)
66985	1(2)
66986	1(2)
66987	2(2)
66988	2(2)
66990	1(3)
66999	1(3)
67005	1(2)
67010	1(2)
67015	1(2)
67025	1(2)
67027	1(2)
67028	1(3)
67030	1(2)
67031	1(2)
67036	1(2)
67039	1(2)
67040	1(2)
67041	1(2)
67042	1(2)
67043	1(2)
67101	1(2)
67105	1(2)
67107	1(2)
67108	1(2)
67110	1(2)
67113	1(2)
67115	1(2)
67120	1(2)
67121	1(2)
67141	1(2)
67145	1(2)
67208	1(2)
67210	1(2)
67218	1(2)
67220	1(2)

CPT	MUE
67221	1(2)
67225	1(2)
67227	1(2)
67228	1(2)
67229	1(2)
67250	1(2)
67255	1(2)
67299	1(3)
67311	1(2)
67312	1(2)
67314	1(2)
67316	1(2)
67318	1(2)
67320	2(3)
67331	1(2)
67332	1(2)
67334	1(2)
67335	1(2)
67340	2(2)
67343	1(2)
67345	1(3)
67346	1(3)
67399	1(3)
67400	1(2)
67405	1(2)
67412	1(2)
67413	1(2)
67414	1(2)
67415	1(3)
67420	1(2)
67430	1(2)
67440	1(2)
67445	1(2)
67450	1(2)
67500	1(3)
67505	1(3)
67515	1(3)
67550	1(2)
67560	1(2)
67570	1(2)
67599	1(3)
67700	2(3)
67710	1(2)
67715	1(3)
67800	1(2)
67801	1(2)
67805	1(2)
67808	1(2)
67810	2(3)
67820	1(2)
67825	1(2)
67830	1(2)
67835	1(2)
67840	3(3)
67850	3(3)
67875	1(2)
67880	1(2)
67882	1(2)
67900	1(2)
67901	1(2)
67902	1(2)
67903	1(2)
67904	1(2)
67906	1(2)
67908	1(2)

CPT	MUE
67909	1(2)
67911	2(3)
67912	1(2)
67914	2(3)
67915	2(3)
67916	2(3)
67917	2(3)
67921	2(3)
67922	2(3)
67923	2(3)
67924	2(3)
67930	2(3)
67935	2(3)
67938	2(3)
67950	2(2)
67961	2(3)
67966	2(3)
67971	1(2)
67973	1(2)
67974	1(2)
67975	1(2)
67999	1(3)
68020	1(3)
68040	1(2)
68100	1(3)
68110	1(3)
68115	1(3)
68130	1(3)
68135	1(3)
68200	1(3)
68320	1(2)
68325	1(2)
68326	1(2)
68328	1(2)
68330	1(3)
68335	1(3)
68340	1(3)
68360	1(3)
68362	1(3)
68371	1(3)
68399	1(3)
68400	1(2)
68420	1(2)
68440	2(3)
68500	1(2)
68505	1(2)
68510	1(2)
68520	1(2)
68525	1(2)
68530	1(2)
68540	1(2)
68550	1(2)
68700	1(2)
68705	2(3)
68720	1(2)
68745	1(2)
68750	1(2)
68760	4(2)
68761	4(2)
68770	1(3)
68801	4(2)
68810	1(2)
68811	1(2)
68815	1(2)
68816	1(2)

CPT	MUE
68840	1(2)
68850	1(3)
68899	1(3)
69000	1(3)
69005	1(3)
69020	1(3)
69090	0(3)
69100	3(3)
69105	1(3)
69110	1(2)
69120	1(3)
69140	1(2)
69145	1(3)
69150	1(3)
69155	1(3)
69200	1(2)
69205	1(3)
69209	1(2)
69210	1(2)
69220	1(2)
69222	1(2)
69300	1(2)
69310	1(2)
69320	1(2)
69399	1(3)
69420	1(2)
69421	1(2)
69424	1(2)
69433	1(2)
69436	1(2)
69440	1(2)
69450	1(2)
69501	1(3)
69502	1(2)
69505	1(2)
69511	1(2)
69530	1(2)
69535	1(2)
69540	1(3)
69550	1(3)
69552	1(2)
69554	1(2)
69601	1(2)
69602	1(2)
69603	1(2)
69604	1(2)
69605	1(2)
69610	1(2)
69620	1(2)
69631	1(2)
69632	1(3)
69633	1(2)
69635	1(3)
69636	1(3)
69637	1(3)
69641	1(2)
69642	1(2)
69643	1(2)
69644	1(2)
69645	1(2)
69646	1(2)
69650	1(2)
69660	1(2)
69661	1(2)
69662	1(2)

CPT	MUE
69666	1(2)
69667	1(2)
69670	1(2)
69676	1(2)
69700	1(3)
69710	0(3)
69711	1(2)
69714	1(2)
69715	1(3)
69717	1(2)
69718	1(2)
69720	1(2)
69725	1(2)
69740	1(2)
69745	1(2)
69799	1(3)
69801	1(3)
69805	1(3)
69806	1(3)
69905	1(2)
69910	1(2)
69915	1(3)
69930	1(2)
69949	1(3)
69950	1(2)
69955	1(2)
69960	1(2)
69970	1(3)
69979	1(3)
69990	1(3)
70010	1(3)
70015	1(3)
70030	2(2)
70100	2(3)
70110	2(3)
70120	1(3)
70130	1(3)
70134	1(3)
70140	2(3)
70150	1(3)
70160	1(3)
70170	2(2)
70190	1(2)
70200	2(3)
70210	1(3)
70220	1(3)
70240	1(2)
70250	2(3)
70260	1(3)
70300	1(3)
70310	1(3)
70320	1(3)
70328	1(3)
70330	1(3)
70332	2(3)
70336	1(3)
70350	1(3)
70355	1(3)
70360	2(3)
70370	1(3)
70371	1(2)
70380	2(3)
70390	2(3)
70450	3(3)
70460	1(3)

CPT	MUE
70470	2(3)
70480	1(3)
70481	1(3)
70482	1(3)
70486	1(3)
70487	1(3)
70488	1(3)
70490	1(3)
70491	1(3)
70492	1(3)
70496	2(3)
70498	2(3)
70540	1(3)
70542	1(3)
70543	1(3)
70544	2(3)
70545	1(3)
70546	1(3)
70547	1(3)
70548	1(3)
70549	1(3)
70551	2(3)
70552	2(3)
70553	2(3)
70554	1(3)
70555	1(3)
70557	1(3)
70558	1(3)
70559	1(3)
71045	4(3)
71046	2(3)
71047	1(3)
71048	1(3)
71100	2(3)
71101	2(3)
71110	1(3)
71111	1(3)
71120	1(3)
71130	1(3)
71250	2(3)
71260	2(3)
71270	1(3)
71275	1(3)
71550	1(3)
71551	1(3)
71552	1(3)
71555	1(3)
72020	4(3)
72040	3(3)
72050	1(3)
72052	1(3)
72070	1(3)
72072	1(3)
72074	1(3)
72080	1(3)
72081	1(3)
72082	1(3)
72083	1(3)
72084	1(3)
72100	2(3)
72110	1(3)
72114	1(3)
72120	1(3)
72125	1(3)
72126	1(3)

CPT	MUE
72127	1(3)
72128	1(3)
72129	1(3)
72130	1(3)
72131	1(3)
72132	1(3)
72133	1(3)
72141	1(3)
72142	1(3)
72146	1(3)
72147	1(3)
72148	1(3)
72149	1(3)
72156	1(3)
72157	1(3)
72158	1(3)
72159	1(3)
72170	2(3)
72190	1(3)
72191	1(3)
72192	1(3)
72193	1(3)
72194	1(3)
72195	1(3)
72196	1(3)
72197	1(3)
72198	1(3)
72200	2(3)
72202	1(3)
72220	1(3)
72240	1(2)
72255	1(2)
72265	1(2)
72270	1(2)
72275	1(3)
72285	4(3)
72295	5(3)
73000	2(3)
73010	2(3)
73020	2(3)
73030	4(3)
73040	2(2)
73050	1(3)
73060	2(3)
73070	2(3)
73080	2(3)
73085	2(2)
73090	2(3)
73092	2(3)
73100	2(3)
73110	3(3)
73115	2(2)
73120	2(3)
73130	3(3)
73140	3(3)
73200	2(3)
73201	2(3)
73202	2(3)
73206	2(3)
73218	2(3)
73219	2(3)
73220	2(3)
73221	2(3)
73222	2(3)
73223	2(3)

CPT	MUE
73225	2(3)
73501	2(3)
73502	2(3)
73503	2(3)
73521	2(3)
73522	2(3)
73523	2(3)
73525	2(2)
73551	2(3)
73552	2(3)
73560	4(3)
73562	3(3)
73564	4(3)
73565	1(3)
73580	2(2)
73590	3(3)
73592	2(3)
73600	2(3)
73610	3(3)
73615	2(2)
73620	2(3)
73630	3(3)
73650	2(3)
73660	2(3)
73700	2(3)
73701	2(3)
73702	2(3)
73706	2(3)
73718	2(3)
73719	2(3)
73720	2(3)
73721	3(3)
73722	2(3)
73723	2(3)
73725	2(3)
74018	3(3)
74019	2(3)
74021	2(3)
74022	2(3)
74150	1(3)
74160	1(3)
74170	1(3)
74174	1(3)
74175	1(3)
74176	2(3)
74177	2(3)
74178	1(3)
74181	1(3)
74182	1(3)
74183	1(3)
74185	1(3)
74190	1(3)
74210	1(3)
74220	1(3)
74221	1(3)
74230	1(3)
74235	1(3)
74240	2(3)
74246	1(3)
74248	1(2)
74250	1(3)
74251	1(3)
74261	1(2)
74262	1(2)
74263	0(3)

CPT	MUE
74270	1(3)
74280	1(3)
74283	1(3)
74290	1(3)
74300	1(3)
74301	1(3)
74328	1(3)
74329	1(3)
74330	1(3)
74340	1(3)
74355	1(3)
74360	1(3)
74363	2(3)
74400	1(3)
74410	1(3)
74415	1(3)
74420	2(3)
74425	2(3)
74430	1(3)
74440	1(2)
74445	1(2)
74450	1(3)
74455	1(3)
74470	2(2)
74485	2(3)
74710	1(3)
74712	1(3)
74713	2(3)
74740	1(3)
74742	2(2)
74775	1(2)
75557	1(3)
75559	1(3)
75561	1(3)
75563	1(3)
75565	1(3)
75571	1(3)
75572	1(3)
75573	1(3)
75574	1(3)
75600	1(3)
75605	1(3)
75625	1(3)
75630	1(3)
75635	1(3)
75705	20(3)
75710	2(3)
75716	1(3)
75726	3(3)
75731	1(3)
75733	1(3)
75736	2(3)
75741	1(3)
75743	1(3)
75746	1(3)
75756	2(3)
75774	7(3)
75801	1(3)
75803	1(3)
75805	1(2)
75807	1(2)
75809	1(3)
75810	1(3)
75820	2(3)
75822	1(3)

CPT	MUE	CPT	MUE	CPT	MUE	CPT	MUE	CPT	MUE	CPT	MUE	CPT	MUE	CPT	MUE
75825	1(3)	76801	1(2)	77061	1(2)	77520	1(3)	78268	1(2)	78709	1(2)	80185	2(3)	80362	1(3)
75827	1(3)	76802	2(3)	77062	1(2)	77522	1(3)	78278	2(3)	78725	1(3)	80186	2(3)	80363	1(3)
75831	1(3)	76805	1(2)	77063	1(2)	77523	1(3)	78282	1(2)	78730	1(2)	80187	1(3)	80364	1(3)
75833	1(3)	76810	2(3)	77065	1(2)	77525	1(3)	78290	1(3)	78740	1(2)	80188	2(3)	80365	1(3)
75840	1(3)	76811	1(2)	77066	1(2)	77600	1(3)	78291	1(3)	78761	1(2)	80190	2(3)	80366	1(3)
75842	1(3)	76812	2(3)	77067	1(2)	77605	1(3)	78299	1(3)	78799	1(3)	80192	2(3)	80367	1(3)
75860	2(3)	76813	1(2)	77071	1(3)	77610	1(3)	78300	1(2)	78800	1(2)	80194	2(3)	80368	1(3)
75870	1(3)	76814	2(3)	77072	1(2)	77615	1(3)	78305	1(2)	78801	1(2)	80195	2(3)	80369	1(3)
75872	1(3)	76815	1(2)	77073	1(2)	77620	1(3)	78306	1(2)	78802	1(2)	80197	2(3)	80370	1(3)
75880	1(3)	76816	2(3)	77074	1(2)	77750	1(3)	78315	1(2)	78803	1(2)	80198	2(3)	80371	1(3)
75885	1(3)	76817	1(3)	77075	1(2)	77761	1(3)	78350	0(3)	78804	1(2)	80199	1(3)	80372	1(3)
75887	1(3)	76818	2(3)	77076	1(2)	77762	1(3)	78351	0(3)	78808	1(2)	80200	2(3)	80373	1(3)
75889	1(3)	76819	2(3)	77077	1(2)	77763	1(3)	78399	1(3)	78811	1(2)	80201	2(3)	80374	1(3)
75891	1(3)	76820	3(3)	77078	1(2)	77767	2(3)	78414	1(2)	78812	1(2)	80202	2(3)	80375	1(3)
75893	2(3)	76821	2(3)	77080	1(2)	77768	2(3)	78428	1(3)	78813	1(2)	80203	1(3)	80376	1(3)
75894	2(3)	76825	2(3)	77081	1(2)	77770	2(3)	78429	1(2)	78814	1(2)	80230	1(3)	80377	1(3)
75898	2(3)	76826	2(3)	77084	1(2)	77771	2(3)	78430	1(2)	78815	1(2)	80235	1(3)	80400	1(3)
75901	1(3)	76827	2(3)	77085	1(2)	77772	2(3)	78431	1(2)	78816	1(2)	80280	1(3)	80402	1(3)
75902	2(3)	76828	2(3)	77086	1(2)	77778	1(3)	78432	1(2)	78830	1(2)	80285	1(3)	80406	1(3)
75956	1(2)	76830	1(3)	77261	1(3)	77789	2(3)	78433	1(2)	78831	1(2)	80299	3(3)	80408	1(3)
75957	1(2)	76831	1(3)	77262	1(3)	77790	1(3)	78434	1(2)	78832	1(2)	80305	1(2)	80410	1(3)
75958	2(3)	76856	1(3)	77263	1(3)	77799	1(3)	78445	1(3)	78835	4(3)	80306	1(2)	80412	1(3)
75959	1(2)	76857	1(3)	77280	2(3)	78012	1(3)	78451	1(2)	78999	1(3)	80307	1(2)	80414	1(3)
75970	1(3)	76870	1(2)	77285	1(3)	78013	1(3)	78452	1(2)	79005	1(3)	80320	1(3)	80415	1(3)
75984	2(3)	76872	1(3)	77290	1(3)	78014	1(2)	78453	1(2)	79101	1(3)	80321	1(3)	80416	1(3)
75989	2(3)	76873	1(2)	77293	1(3)	78015	1(3)	78454	1(2)	79200	1(3)	80322	1(3)	80417	1(3)
76000	3(3)	76881	2(3)	77295	1(3)	78016	1(3)	78456	1(3)	79300	1(3)	80323	1(3)	80418	1(3)
76010	2(3)	76882	2(3)	77299	1(3)	78018	1(2)	78457	1(2)	79403	1(3)	80324	1(3)	80420	1(2)
76080	3(3)	76885	1(2)	77300	10(3)	78020	1(3)	78458	1(2)	79440	1(3)	80325	1(3)	80422	1(3)
76098	3(3)	76886	1(2)	77301	1(3)	78070	1(2)	78459	1(3)	79445	1(3)	80326	1(3)	80424	1(3)
76100	2(3)	76932	1(2)	77306	1(3)	78071	1(3)	78466	1(3)	79999	1(3)	80327	1(3)	80426	1(3)
76101	1(3)	76936	1(3)	77307	1(3)	78072	1(3)	78468	1(3)	80047	2(3)	80328	1(3)	80428	1(3)
76102	1(3)	76937	2(3)	77316	1(3)	78075	1(2)	78469	1(3)	80048	2(3)	80329	1(3)	80430	1(3)
76120	1(3)	76940	1(3)	77317	1(3)	78099	1(3)	78472	1(2)	80050	0(3)	80330	1(3)	80432	1(3)
76125	1(3)	76941	3(3)	77318	1(3)	78102	1(2)	78473	1(2)	80051	2(3)	80331	1(3)	80434	1(3)
76140	0(3)	76942	1(3)	77321	1(2)	78103	1(2)	78481	1(2)	80053	1(3)	80332	1(3)	80435	1(3)
76376	2(3)	76945	1(3)	77331	3(3)	78104	1(2)	78483	1(2)	80055	1(3)	80333	1(3)	80436	1(3)
76377	2(3)	76946	1(3)	77332	4(3)	78110	1(2)	78491	1(3)	80061	1(3)	80334	1(3)	80438	1(3)
76380	2(3)	76948	1(2)	77333	2(3)	78111	1(2)	78492	1(2)	80069	1(3)	80335	1(3)	80439	1(3)
76390	0(3)	76965	2(3)	77334	10(3)	78120	1(2)	78494	1(3)	80074	1(2)	80336	1(3)	80500	1(3)
76391	1(3)	76970	2(3)	77336	1(2)	78121	1(2)	78496	1(3)	80076	1(3)	80337	1(3)	80502	1(3)
76496	1(3)	76975	1(3)	77338	1(3)	78122	1(2)	78499	1(3)	80081	1(2)	80338	1(3)	81000	2(3)
76497	1(3)	76977	1(2)	77370	1(3)	78130	1(2)	78579	1(3)	80145	1(3)	80339	1(3)	81001	2(3)
76498	1(3)	76978	1(2)	77371	1(2)	78135	1(3)	78580	1(3)	80150	2(3)	80340	1(3)	81002	2(3)
76499	1(3)	76979	3(3)	77372	1(2)	78140	1(3)	78582	1(3)	80155	1(3)	80341	1(3)	81003	2(3)
76506	1(2)	76981	1(3)	77373	1(3)	78185	1(2)	78597	1(3)	80156	2(3)	80342	1(3)	81005	2(3)
76510	2(2)	76982	1(2)	77385	1(3)	78191	1(2)	78598	1(3)	80157	2(3)	80343	1(3)	81007	1(3)
76511	2(2)	76983	2(3)	77386	1(3)	78195	1(2)	78599	1(3)	80158	1(3)	80344	1(3)	81015	2(3)
76512	2(2)	76998	1(3)	77387	1(3)	78199	1(3)	78600	1(3)	80159	2(3)	80345	1(3)	81020	1(3)
76513	2(2)	76999	1(3)	77399	1(3)	78201	1(3)	78601	1(3)	80162	2(3)	80346	1(3)	81025	1(3)
76514	1(2)	77001	2(3)	77401	1(2)	78202	1(3)	78605	1(3)	80163	1(3)	80347	1(3)	81050	2(3)
76516	1(2)	77002	1(3)	77402	2(3)	78215	1(3)	78606	1(3)	80164	2(3)	80348	1(3)	81099	1(3)
76519	2(2)	77003	1(3)	77407	2(3)	78216	1(3)	78608	1(3)	80165	1(3)	80349	1(3)	81105	1(2)
76529	2(2)	77011	1(3)	77412	2(3)	78226	1(3)	78609	0(3)	80168	2(3)	80350	1(3)	81106	1(2)
76536	1(3)	77012	1(3)	77417	1(2)	78227	1(3)	78610	1(3)	80169	1(3)	80351	1(3)	81107	1(2)
76604	1(3)	77013	1(3)	77423	1(3)	78230	1(3)	78630	1(3)	80170	2(3)	80352	1(3)	81108	1(2)
76641	2(2)	77014	2(3)	77424	1(2)	78231	1(3)	78635	1(3)	80171	1(3)	80353	1(3)	81109	1(2)
76642	2(2)	77021	1(3)	77425	1(3)	78232	1(3)	78645	1(3)	80173	2(3)	80354	1(3)	81110	1(2)
76700	1(3)	77022	1(3)	77427	1(2)	78258	1(2)	78650	1(3)	80175	1(3)	80355	1(3)	81111	1(2)
76705	2(3)	77046	1(2)	77431	1(2)	78261	1(2)	78660	1(2)	80176	1(3)	80356	1(3)	81112	1(2)
76706	1(2)	77047	1(2)	77432	1(2)	78262	1(2)	78699	1(3)	80177	1(3)	80357	1(3)	81120	1(3)
76770	1(3)	77048	1(2)	77435	1(2)	78264	1(2)	78700	1(3)	80178	2(3)	80358	1(3)	81121	1(3)
76775	2(3)	77049	1(2)	77469	1(2)	78265	1(2)	78701	1(3)	80180	1(3)	80359	1(3)	81161	1(3)
76776	2(3)	77053	2(2)	77470	1(2)	78266	1(2)	78707	1(2)	80183	1(3)	80360	1(3)	81162	1(2)
76800	1(3)	77054	2(2)	77499	1(3)	78267	1(2)	78708	1(2)	80184	2(3)	80361	1(3)	81163	1(2)

CPT	MUE	CPT	MUE	CPT	MUE	CPT	MUE	CPT	MUE	CPT	MUE	CPT	MUE	CPT	MUE
81164	1(2)	81243	1(3)	81313	1(3)	81414	1(2)	82013	1(3)	82378	1(3)	82728	1(3)	83080	2(3)
81165	1(2)	81244	1(3)	81314	1(3)	81415	1(2)	82016	1(3)	82379	1(3)	82731	1(3)	83088	1(3)
81166	1(2)	81245	1(3)	81315	1(3)	81416	2(3)	82017	1(3)	82380	1(3)	82735	1(3)	83090	2(3)
81167	1(2)	81246	1(3)	81316	1(2)	81417	1(3)	82024	4(3)	82382	1(2)	82746	1(2)	83150	1(3)
81170	1(2)	81247	1(2)	81317	1(2)	81420	1(2)	82030	1(3)	82383	1(3)	82747	1(2)	83491	1(3)
81171	1(2)	81248	1(2)	81318	1(3)	81422	1(2)	82040	1(3)	82384	2(3)	82757	1(2)	83497	1(3)
81172	1(2)	81249	1(2)	81319	1(2)	81425	1(2)	82042	2(3)	82387	1(3)	82759	1(3)	83498	2(3)
81173	1(2)	81250	1(3)	81320	1(3)	81426	2(3)	82043	1(3)	82390	1(2)	82760	1(3)	83500	1(3)
81174	1(2)	81251	1(3)	81321	1(3)	81427	1(3)	82044	1(3)	82397	3(3)	82775	1(3)	83505	1(3)
81175	1(3)	81252	1(3)	81322	1(3)	81430	1(2)	82045	1(3)	82415	1(3)	82776	1(2)	83516	4(3)
81176	1(3)	81253	1(3)	81323	1(3)	81431	1(2)	82075	2(3)	82435	1(3)	82777	1(3)	83518	1(3)
81177	1(2)	81254	1(3)	81324	1(3)	81432	1(2)	82085	1(3)	82436	1(3)	82784	6(3)	83519	5(3)
81178	1(2)	81255	1(3)	81325	1(3)	81433	1(2)	82088	2(3)	82438	1(3)	82785	1(3)	83520	9(3)
81179	1(2)	81256	1(2)	81326	1(3)	81434	1(2)	82103	1(3)	82441	1(2)	82787	4(3)	83525	4(3)
81180	1(2)	81257	1(2)	81327	1(2)	81435	1(2)	82104	1(2)	82465	1(3)	82800	1(3)	83527	1(3)
81181	1(2)	81258	1(2)	81328	1(2)	81436	1(2)	82105	1(3)	82480	2(3)	82803	2(3)	83528	1(3)
81182	1(2)	81259	1(2)	81329	1(2)	81437	1(2)	82106	2(3)	82482	1(3)	82805	2(3)	83540	2(3)
81183	1(2)	81260	1(3)	81330	1(3)	81438	1(2)	82107	1(3)	82485	1(3)	82810	2(3)	83550	1(3)
81184	1(2)	81261	1(3)	81331	1(3)	81439	1(2)	82108	1(3)	82495	1(2)	82820	1(3)	83570	1(3)
81185	1(2)	81262	1(3)	81332	1(3)	81440	1(2)	82120	1(3)	82507	1(3)	82930	1(3)	83582	1(3)
81186	1(2)	81263	1(3)	81333	1(2)	81442	1(2)	82127	1(3)	82523	1(3)	82938	1(3)	83586	1(3)
81187	1(2)	81264	1(3)	81334	1(3)	81443	1(2)	82128	2(3)	82525	2(3)	82941	1(3)	83593	1(3)
81188	1(2)	81265	1(3)	81335	1(2)	81445	1(2)	82131	2(3)	82528	1(3)	82943	1(3)	83605	1(3)
81189	1(2)	81266	2(3)	81336	1(2)	81448	1(2)	82135	1(3)	82530	4(3)	82945	4(3)	83615	2(3)
81190	1(2)	81267	1(3)	81337	1(2)	81450	1(2)	82136	2(3)	82533	5(3)	82946	1(2)	83625	1(3)
81200	1(2)	81268	4(3)	81340	1(3)	81455	1(2)	82139	2(3)	82540	1(3)	82947	5(3)	83630	1(3)
81201	1(2)	81269	1(2)	81341	1(3)	81460	1(2)	82140	2(3)	82542	6(3)	82948	2(3)	83631	1(3)
81202	1(3)	81270	1(2)	81342	1(3)	81465	1(2)	82143	2(3)	82550	3(3)	82950	3(3)	83632	1(3)
81203	1(3)	81271	1(2)	81343	1(2)	81470	1(2)	82150	2(3)	82552	3(3)	82951	1(2)	83633	1(3)
81204	1(2)	81272	1(3)	81344	1(2)	81471	1(2)	82154	1(3)	82553	3(3)	82952	3(3)	83655	2(3)
81205	1(3)	81273	1(3)	81345	1(3)	81479	3(3)	82157	1(3)	82554	1(3)	82955	1(2)	83661	3(3)
81206	1(3)	81274	1(2)	81346	1(2)	81490	1(2)	82160	1(3)	82565	2(3)	82960	1(2)	83662	4(3)
81207	1(3)	81275	1(3)	81350	1(3)	81493	1(2)	82163	1(3)	82570	3(3)	82962	2(3)	83663	3(3)
81208	1(3)	81276	1(3)	81355	1(3)	81500	1(2)	82164	1(3)	82575	1(3)	82963	1(3)	83664	3(3)
81209	1(3)	81277	1(2)	81361	1(2)	81503	1(2)	82172	2(3)	82585	1(2)	82965	1(3)	83670	1(3)
81210	1(3)	81283	1(2)	81362	1(2)	81504	1(2)	82175	2(3)	82595	1(3)	82977	1(3)	83690	2(3)
81212	1(2)	81284	1(2)	81363	1(2)	81506	1(2)	82180	1(2)	82600	1(3)	82978	1(3)	83695	1(3)
81215	1(2)	81285	1(2)	81364	1(2)	81507	1(2)	82190	2(3)	82607	1(2)	82979	1(3)	83698	1(3)
81216	1(2)	81286	1(2)	81370	1(2)	81508	1(2)	82232	2(3)	82608	1(2)	82985	1(3)	83700	1(2)
81217	1(2)	81287	1(3)	81371	1(2)	81509	1(2)	82239	1(3)	82610	1(3)	83001	1(3)	83701	1(3)
81218	1(3)	81288	1(3)	81372	1(2)	81510	1(2)	82240	1(3)	82615	1(3)	83002	1(3)	83704	1(3)
81219	1(3)	81289	1(2)	81373	2(2)	81511	1(2)	82247	2(3)	82626	1(3)	83003	5(3)	83718	1(3)
81220	1(3)	81290	1(3)	81374	1(3)	81512	1(2)	82248	2(3)	82627	1(3)	83006	1(2)	83719	1(3)
81221	1(3)	81291	1(3)	81375	1(2)	81518	1(2)	82252	1(3)	82633	1(3)	83009	1(3)	83721	1(3)
81222	1(3)	81292	1(2)	81376	5(3)	81519	1(2)	82261	1(3)	82634	1(3)	83010	1(3)	83722	1(2)
81223	1(2)	81293	1(3)	81377	2(3)	81520	1(2)	82270	1(3)	82638	1(3)	83012	1(2)	83727	1(3)
81224	1(3)	81294	1(3)	81378	1(2)	81521	1(2)	82271	1(3)	82642	1(2)	83013	1(3)	83735	4(3)
81225	1(3)	81295	1(2)	81379	1(2)	81522	1(2)	82272	1(3)	82652	1(2)	83014	1(2)	83775	1(3)
81226	1(3)	81296	1(3)	81380	2(2)	81525	1(2)	82274	1(3)	82656	1(3)	83015	1(2)	83785	1(3)
81227	1(3)	81297	1(3)	81381	3(3)	81528	1(2)	82286	1(3)	82657	2(3)	83018	4(3)	83789	4(3)
81228	1(3)	81298	1(2)	81382	6(3)	81535	1(2)	82300	1(3)	82658	2(3)	83020	2(3)	83825	2(3)
81229	1(3)	81299	1(3)	81383	2(3)	81536	11(3)	82306	1(2)	82664	2(3)	83021	2(3)	83835	2(3)
81230	1(2)	81300	1(3)	81400	2(3)	81538	1(2)	82308	1(3)	82668	1(3)	83026	1(3)	83857	1(3)
81231	1(2)	81301	1(3)	81401	2(3)	81539	1(2)	82310	2(3)	82670	2(3)	83030	1(3)	83861	2(2)
81232	1(2)	81302	1(3)	81402	1(3)	81540	1(2)	82330	2(3)	82671	1(3)	83033	1(3)	83864	1(2)
81233	1(3)	81303	1(3)	81403	4(3)	81541	1(2)	82331	1(3)	82672	1(3)	83036	1(2)	83872	2(3)
81234	1(2)	81304	1(3)	81404	5(3)	81542	1(2)	82340	1(3)	82677	1(3)	83037	1(2)	83873	1(3)
81235	1(3)	81305	1(3)	81405	2(3)	81545	1(2)	82355	2(3)	82679	1(3)	83045	1(3)	83874	2(3)
81236	1(3)	81306	1(2)	81406	2(3)	81551	1(2)	82360	2(3)	82693	2(3)	83050	1(3)	83876	1(3)
81237	1(3)	81307	1(2)	81407	1(3)	81552	1(2)	82365	2(3)	82696	1(3)	83051	1(3)	83880	1(3)
81238	1(2)	81308	1(2)	81408	2(3)	81595	1(2)	82370	2(3)	82705	1(3)	83060	1(3)	83883	4(3)
81239	1(2)	81309	1(2)	81410	1(2)	81596	1(2)	82373	1(3)	82710	1(3)	83065	1(2)	83885	2(3)
81240	1(2)	81310	1(3)	81411	1(2)	81599	1(3)	82374	1(3)	82715	3(3)	83068	1(2)	83915	1(3)
81241	1(2)	81311	1(3)	81412	1(2)	82009	1(3)	82375	1(3)	82725	1(3)	83069	1(3)	83916	2(3)
81242	1(3)	81312	1(2)	81413	1(2)	82010	1(3)	82376	1(3)	82726	1(3)	83070	1(2)	83918	2(3)

CPT	MUE
83919	1(3)
83921	2(3)
83930	2(3)
83935	2(3)
83937	1(3)
83945	2(3)
83950	1(2)
83951	1(2)
83970	2(3)
83986	2(3)
83987	1(3)
83992	2(3)
83993	1(3)
84030	1(2)
84035	1(2)
84060	1(3)
84066	1(3)
84075	2(3)
84078	1(2)
84080	1(3)
84081	1(3)
84085	1(2)
84087	1(3)
84100	2(3)
84105	1(3)
84106	1(2)
84110	1(3)
84112	1(3)
84119	1(2)
84120	1(3)
84126	1(3)
84132	2(3)
84133	2(3)
84134	1(3)
84135	1(3)
84138	1(3)
84140	1(3)
84143	2(3)
84144	1(3)
84145	1(3)
84146	3(3)
84150	2(3)
84152	1(2)
84153	1(2)
84154	1(2)
84155	1(3)
84156	1(3)
84157	2(3)
84160	2(3)
84163	1(3)
84165	1(2)
84166	2(3)
84181	3(3)
84182	6(3)
84202	1(2)
84203	1(2)
84206	1(2)
84207	1(2)
84210	1(3)
84220	1(3)
84228	1(3)
84233	1(3)
84234	1(3)
84235	1(3)
84238	3(3)

CPT	MUE
84244	2(3)
84252	1(2)
84255	2(3)
84260	1(3)
84270	1(3)
84275	1(3)
84285	1(3)
84295	1(3)
84300	2(3)
84302	1(3)
84305	1(3)
84307	1(3)
84311	2(3)
84315	1(3)
84375	1(3)
84376	1(3)
84377	1(3)
84378	2(3)
84379	1(3)
84392	1(3)
84402	1(3)
84403	2(3)
84410	1(2)
84425	1(2)
84430	1(3)
84431	1(3)
84432	1(2)
84436	1(2)
84437	1(2)
84439	1(2)
84442	1(2)
84443	4(2)
84445	1(2)
84446	1(2)
84449	1(3)
84450	1(3)
84460	1(3)
84466	1(3)
84478	1(3)
84479	1(2)
84480	1(2)
84481	1(2)
84482	1(2)
84484	2(3)
84485	1(3)
84488	1(3)
84490	1(2)
84510	1(3)
84512	1(3)
84520	1(3)
84525	1(3)
84540	2(3)
84545	1(3)
84550	1(3)
84560	2(3)
84577	1(3)
84578	1(3)
84580	1(3)
84583	1(3)
84585	1(2)
84586	1(2)
84588	1(3)
84590	1(2)
84591	1(3)
84597	1(3)

CPT	MUE
84600	2(3)
84620	1(2)
84630	2(3)
84681	1(3)
84702	2(3)
84703	1(3)
84704	1(3)
84830	1(2)
84999	1(3)
85002	1(3)
85004	1(3)
85007	1(3)
85008	1(3)
85009	1(3)
85013	1(3)
85014	2(3)
85018	2(3)
85025	2(3)
85027	2(3)
85032	1(3)
85041	1(3)
85044	1(2)
85045	1(2)
85046	1(2)
85048	2(3)
85049	2(3)
85055	1(3)
85060	1(3)
85097	2(3)
85130	1(3)
85170	1(3)
85175	1(3)
85210	2(3)
85220	2(3)
85230	2(3)
85240	2(3)
85244	1(3)
85245	2(3)
85246	2(3)
85247	2(3)
85250	2(3)
85260	2(3)
85270	2(3)
85280	2(3)
85290	2(3)
85291	1(3)
85292	1(3)
85293	1(3)
85300	2(3)
85301	1(3)
85302	1(3)
85303	2(3)
85305	2(3)
85306	2(3)
85307	2(3)
85335	2(3)
85337	1(3)
85345	1(3)
85347	3(3)
85348	1(3)
85360	1(3)
85362	2(3)
85366	1(3)
85370	1(3)
85378	1(3)

CPT	MUE
85379	2(3)
85380	1(3)
85384	2(3)
85385	1(3)
85390	3(3)
85396	1(2)
85397	2(3)
85400	1(3)
85410	1(3)
85415	2(3)
85420	2(3)
85421	1(3)
85441	1(2)
85445	1(2)
85460	1(3)
85461	1(2)
85475	1(3)
85520	1(3)
85525	2(3)
85530	1(3)
85536	1(2)
85540	1(2)
85547	1(2)
85549	1(3)
85555	1(2)
85557	1(2)
85576	7(3)
85597	1(3)
85598	1(3)
85610	4(3)
85611	2(3)
85612	1(3)
85613	3(3)
85635	1(3)
85651	1(2)
85652	1(2)
85660	2(3)
85670	2(3)
85675	1(3)
85705	1(3)
85730	4(3)
85732	4(3)
85810	2(3)
85999	1(3)
86000	6(3)
86001	20(3)
86005	2(3)
86008	20(3)
86021	1(2)
86022	1(2)
86023	3(3)
86038	1(3)
86039	1(3)
86060	1(3)
86063	1(3)
86077	1(2)
86078	1(3)
86079	1(3)
86140	1(2)
86141	1(2)
86146	3(3)
86147	4(3)
86148	3(3)
86152	1(3)
86153	1(3)

CPT	MUE
86155	1(3)
86156	1(2)
86157	1(2)
86160	4(3)
86161	2(3)
86162	1(2)
86171	2(3)
86200	1(3)
86215	1(3)
86225	1(3)
86226	1(3)
86235	10(3)
86255	5(3)
86256	9(3)
86277	1(3)
86280	1(3)
86294	1(3)
86300	2(3)
86301	1(2)
86304	1(2)
86305	1(2)
86308	1(2)
86309	1(2)
86310	1(2)
86316	2(3)
86317	6(3)
86318	2(3)
86320	1(2)
86325	2(3)
86327	1(3)
86328	3(3)
86329	3(3)
86331	12(3)
86332	1(3)
86334	2(2)
86335	2(3)
86336	1(3)
86337	1(2)
86340	1(2)
86341	1(3)
86343	1(3)
86344	1(2)
86352	1(3)
86353	7(3)
86355	1(2)
86356	7(3)
86357	1(2)
86359	1(2)
86360	1(2)
86361	1(2)
86367	1(3)
86376	2(3)
86382	3(3)
86384	1(3)
86386	1(2)
86403	2(3)
86406	2(3)
86430	2(3)
86431	2(3)
86480	1(3)
86481	1(3)
86485	1(2)
86486	2(3)
86490	1(2)
86510	1(2)

CPT	MUE
86580	1(2)
86590	1(3)
86592	2(3)
86593	2(3)
86602	3(3)
86603	2(3)
86609	14(3)
86611	4(3)
86612	2(3)
86615	6(3)
86617	2(3)
86618	2(3)
86619	2(3)
86622	2(3)
86625	1(3)
86628	3(3)
86631	6(3)
86632	3(3)
86635	4(3)
86638	6(3)
86641	2(3)
86644	2(3)
86645	1(3)
86648	2(3)
86651	2(3)
86652	2(3)
86653	2(3)
86654	2(3)
86658	12(3)
86663	2(3)
86664	2(3)
86665	2(3)
86666	4(3)
86668	2(3)
86671	3(3)
86674	3(3)
86677	3(3)
86682	2(3)
86684	2(3)
86687	1(3)
86688	1(3)
86689	2(3)
86692	2(3)
86694	2(3)
86695	2(3)
86696	2(3)
86698	3(3)
86701	1(3)
86702	2(3)
86703	1(2)
86704	1(2)
86705	1(2)
86706	2(3)
86707	1(3)
86708	1(2)
86709	1(2)
86710	4(3)
86711	2(3)
86713	3(3)
86717	8(3)
86720	2(3)
86723	2(3)
86727	2(3)
86732	2(3)
86735	2(3)

CPT	MUE
86738	2(3)
86741	2(3)
86744	2(3)
86747	2(3)
86750	4(3)
86753	3(3)
86756	2(3)
86757	6(3)
86759	2(3)
86762	2(3)
86765	2(3)
86768	5(3)
86769	3(3)
86771	2(3)
86774	2(3)
86777	2(3)
86778	2(3)
86780	2(3)
86784	1(3)
86787	2(3)
86788	2(3)
86789	2(3)
86790	4(3)
86793	2(3)
86794	1(3)
86800	1(3)
86803	1(3)
86804	1(2)
86805	2(3)
86806	2(3)
86807	2(3)
86808	1(3)
86812	1(2)
86813	1(2)
86816	1(2)
86817	1(2)
86821	1(3)
86825	1(3)
86826	2(3)
86828	1(3)
86829	1(3)
86830	2(3)
86831	2(3)
86832	2(3)
86833	1(3)
86834	1(3)
86835	1(3)
86849	1(3)
86850	3(3)
86860	2(3)
86870	2(3)
86880	4(3)
86885	2(3)
86886	3(3)
86890	1(3)
86891	1(3)
86900	1(3)
86901	1(3)
86902	6(3)
86904	2(3)
86905	8(3)
86906	1(2)
86910	0(3)
86911	0(3)
86920	9(3)

CPT	MUE
86921	2(3)
86922	5(3)
86923	10(3)
86927	2(3)
86930	0(3)
86931	1(3)
86932	1(3)
86940	1(3)
86941	1(3)
86945	2(3)
86950	1(3)
86960	1(3)
86965	1(3)
86970	1(3)
86971	1(3)
86972	1(3)
86975	1(3)
86976	1(3)
86977	1(3)
86978	1(3)
86985	1(3)
86999	1(3)
87003	1(3)
87015	3(3)
87040	2(3)
87045	3(3)
87046	6(3)
87070	3(3)
87071	2(3)
87073	2(3)
87075	6(3)
87076	2(3)
87077	4(3)
87081	2(3)
87084	1(3)
87086	3(3)
87088	3(3)
87101	2(3)
87102	4(3)
87103	2(3)
87106	3(3)
87107	4(3)
87109	2(3)
87110	2(3)
87116	2(3)
87118	3(3)
87140	3(3)
87143	2(3)
87149	4(3)
87150	12(3)
87152	1(3)
87153	3(3)
87158	1(3)
87164	2(3)
87166	2(3)
87168	2(3)
87169	2(3)
87172	1(3)
87176	2(3)
87177	3(3)
87181	12(3)
87184	8(3)
87185	4(3)
87186	12(3)
87187	3(3)

CPT	MUE
87188	6(3)
87190	9(3)
87197	1(3)
87205	3(3)
87206	6(3)
87207	3(3)
87209	4(3)
87210	4(3)
87220	3(3)
87230	2(3)
87250	1(3)
87252	2(3)
87253	2(3)
87254	7(3)
87255	2(3)
87260	1(3)
87265	1(3)
87267	1(3)
87269	1(3)
87270	1(3)
87271	1(3)
87272	1(3)
87273	1(3)
87274	1(3)
87275	1(3)
87276	1(3)
87278	1(3)
87279	1(3)
87280	1(3)
87281	1(3)
87283	1(3)
87285	1(3)
87290	1(3)
87299	1(3)
87300	2(3)
87301	1(3)
87305	1(3)
87320	1(3)
87324	2(3)
87327	1(3)
87328	2(3)
87329	2(3)
87332	1(3)
87335	1(3)
87336	1(3)
87337	1(3)
87338	1(3)
87339	1(3)
87340	1(2)
87341	1(2)
87350	1(2)
87380	1(2)
87385	2(3)
87389	1(3)
87390	1(3)
87391	1(3)
87400	2(3)
87420	1(3)
87425	1(3)
87426	3(3)
87427	2(3)
87430	1(3)
87449	3(3)
87450	2(3)
87451	2(3)

CPT	MUE
87471	1(3)
87472	1(3)
87475	1(3)
87476	1(3)
87480	1(3)
87481	5(3)
87482	1(3)
87483	1(2)
87485	1(3)
87486	1(3)
87487	1(3)
87490	1(3)
87491	3(3)
87492	1(3)
87493	2(3)
87495	1(3)
87496	1(3)
87497	2(3)
87498	1(3)
87500	1(3)
87501	1(3)
87502	1(3)
87503	1(3)
87505	1(2)
87506	1(2)
87507	1(2)
87510	1(3)
87511	1(3)
87512	1(3)
87516	1(3)
87517	1(3)
87520	1(3)
87521	1(3)
87522	1(3)
87525	1(3)
87526	1(3)
87527	1(3)
87528	1(3)
87529	2(3)
87530	2(3)
87531	1(3)
87532	1(3)
87533	1(3)
87534	1(3)
87535	1(3)
87536	1(3)
87537	1(3)
87538	1(3)
87539	1(3)
87540	1(3)
87541	1(3)
87542	1(3)
87550	1(3)
87551	2(3)
87552	1(3)
87555	1(3)
87556	1(3)
87557	1(3)
87560	1(3)
87561	1(3)
87562	1(3)
87563	3(3)
87580	1(3)
87581	1(3)
87582	1(3)

CPT	MUE
87590	1(3)
87591	3(3)
87592	1(3)
87623	1(2)
87624	1(3)
87625	1(3)
87631	1(3)
87632	1(3)
87633	1(3)
87634	1(3)
87635	2(3)
87640	1(3)
87641	1(3)
87650	1(3)
87651	1(3)
87652	1(3)
87653	1(3)
87660	1(3)
87661	1(3)
87662	2(3)
87797	3(3)
87798	13(3)
87799	3(3)
87800	2(3)
87801	3(3)
87802	2(3)
87803	3(3)
87804	3(3)
87806	1(2)
87807	2(3)
87808	1(3)
87809	2(3)
87810	2(3)
87850	1(3)
87880	2(3)
87899	4(3)
87900	1(2)
87901	1(2)
87902	1(2)
87903	1(2)
87904	14(3)
87905	2(3)
87906	2(3)
87910	1(3)
87912	1(3)
87999	1(3)
88000	0(3)
88005	0(3)
88007	0(3)
88012	0(3)
88014	0(3)
88016	0(3)
88020	0(3)
88025	0(3)
88027	0(3)
88028	0(3)
88029	0(3)
88036	0(3)
88037	0(3)
88040	0(3)
88045	0(3)
88099	0(3)
88104	5(3)
88106	5(3)
88108	6(3)

CPT	MUE
88112	6(3)
88120	2(3)
88121	2(3)
88125	1(3)
88130	1(2)
88140	1(2)
88141	1(3)
88142	1(3)
88143	1(3)
88147	1(3)
88148	1(3)
88150	1(3)
88152	1(3)
88153	1(3)
88155	1(3)
88160	4(3)
88161	4(3)
88162	3(3)
88164	1(3)
88165	1(3)
88166	1(3)
88167	1(3)
88172	5(3)
88173	5(3)
88174	1(3)
88175	1(3)
88177	6(3)
88182	2(3)
88184	2(3)
88185	35(3)
88187	2(3)
88188	2(3)
88189	2(3)
88199	1(3)
88230	2(3)
88233	2(3)
88235	2(3)
88237	4(3)
88239	3(3)
88240	1(3)
88241	3(3)
88245	1(2)
88248	1(2)
88249	1(2)
88261	2(3)
88262	2(3)
88263	1(3)
88264	1(3)
88267	2(3)
88269	2(3)
88271	16(3)
88272	12(3)
88273	3(3)
88274	5(3)
88275	12(3)
88280	1(3)
88283	5(3)
88285	10(3)
88289	1(3)
88291	1(3)
88299	1(3)
88300	4(3)
88302	4(3)
88304	5(3)
88305	16(3)

CPT	MUE
88307	8(3)
88309	3(3)
88311	4(3)
88312	9(3)
88313	8(3)
88314	6(3)
88319	11(3)
88321	1(2)
88323	1(2)
88325	1(2)
88329	2(3)
88331	11(3)
88332	13(3)
88333	4(3)
88334	5(3)
88341	13(3)
88342	4(3)
88344	6(3)
88346	2(3)
88348	1(3)
88350	8(3)
88355	1(3)
88356	3(3)
88358	2(3)
88360	6(3)
88361	6(3)
88362	1(3)
88363	2(3)
88364	3(3)
88365	4(3)
88366	2(3)
88367	3(3)
88368	3(3)
88369	3(3)
88371	1(3)
88372	1(3)
88373	3(3)
88374	5(3)
88375	1(3)
88377	5(3)
88380	1(3)
88381	1(3)
88387	2(3)
88388	1(3)
88399	1(3)
88720	1(3)
88738	1(3)
88740	1(2)
88741	1(2)
88749	1(3)
89049	1(3)
89050	2(3)
89051	2(3)
89055	2(3)
89060	2(3)
89125	2(3)
89160	1(3)
89190	1(3)
89220	2(3)
89230	1(2)
89240	1(3)
89250	1(2)
89251	1(2)
89253	1(3)
89254	1(3)

CPT	MUE
89255	1(3)
89257	1(3)
89258	1(2)
89259	1(2)
89260	1(2)
89261	1(2)
89264	1(3)
89268	1(2)
89272	1(2)
89280	1(2)
89281	1(2)
89290	1(2)
89291	1(2)
89300	1(2)
89310	1(2)
89320	1(2)
89321	1(2)
89322	1(2)
89325	1(2)
89329	1(2)
89330	1(2)
89331	1(2)
89335	1(3)
89337	1(2)
89342	1(2)
89343	1(2)
89344	1(2)
89346	1(2)
89352	1(2)
89353	1(3)
89354	1(3)
89356	2(3)
89398	1(3)
90281	0(3)
90283	0(3)
90284	0(3)
90287	0(3)
90288	0(3)
90291	0(3)
90296	1(2)
90371	10(3)
90375	20(3)
90376	20(3)
90378	4(3)
90384	0(3)
90385	1(2)
90386	0(3)
90389	0(3)
90393	1(2)
90396	1(2)
90399	0(3)
90460	9(3)
90461	8(3)
90471	1(2)
90472	8(3)
90473	1(2)
90474	1(3)
90476	1(2)
90477	1(2)
90581	1(2)
90585	1(2)
90586	1(2)
90587	1(2)
90619	1(2)
90620	1(2)

CPT	MUE
90621	1(2)
90625	1(2)
90630	1(2)
90632	1(2)
90633	1(2)
90634	1(2)
90636	1(2)
90644	1(2)
90647	1(2)
90648	1(2)
90649	1(2)
90650	1(2)
90651	1(2)
90653	1(2)
90654	1(2)
90655	1(2)
90656	1(2)
90657	1(2)
90658	1(2)
90660	1(2)
90661	1(2)
90662	1(2)
90664	1(2)
90666	1(2)
90667	1(2)
90668	1(2)
90670	1(2)
90672	1(2)
90673	1(2)
90674	1(2)
90675	1(2)
90676	1(2)
90680	1(2)
90681	1(2)
90682	1(2)
90685	1(2)
90686	1(2)
90687	1(2)
90688	1(2)
90689	1(2)
90690	1(2)
90691	1(2)
90694	1(2)
90696	1(2)
90697	1(2)
90698	1(2)
90700	1(2)
90702	1(2)
90707	1(2)
90710	1(2)
90713	1(2)
90714	1(2)
90715	1(2)
90716	1(2)
90717	1(2)
90723	0(3)
90732	1(2)
90733	1(2)
90734	1(2)
90736	1(2)
90738	1(2)
90739	1(2)
90740	1(2)
90743	1(2)
90744	1(2)

CPT	MUE
90746	1(2)
90747	1(2)
90748	0(3)
90749	1(3)
90750	1(2)
90756	1(2)
90785	3(3)
90791	1(3)
90792	1(3)
90832	2(3)
90833	2(3)
90834	2(3)
90836	2(3)
90837	2(3)
90838	2(3)
90839	1(2)
90840	3(3)
90845	1(2)
90846	1(3)
90847	1(3)
90849	1(3)
90853	1(3)
90863	1(3)
90865	1(3)
90867	1(2)
90868	1(3)
90869	1(3)
90870	2(3)
90875	1(3)
90876	0(3)
90880	1(3)
90882	0(3)
90885	0(3)
90887	0(3)
90889	0(3)
90899	1(3)
90901	1(3)
90912	1(2)
90913	3(3)
90935	1(3)
90937	1(3)
90940	1(3)
90945	1(3)
90947	1(3)
90951	1(2)
90952	1(2)
90953	1(2)
90954	1(2)
90955	1(2)
90956	1(2)
90957	1(2)
90958	1(2)
90959	1(2)
90960	1(2)
90961	1(2)
90962	1(2)
90963	1(2)
90964	1(2)
90965	1(2)
90966	1(2)
90967	1(2)
90968	1(2)
90969	1(2)
90970	1(2)
90989	1(2)

CPT	MUE
90993	1(3)
90997	1(3)
90999	1(3)
91010	1(2)
91013	1(3)
91020	1(2)
91022	1(2)
91030	1(2)
91034	1(2)
91035	1(2)
91037	1(2)
91038	1(2)
91040	1(2)
91065	2(2)
91110	1(2)
91111	1(2)
91112	1(3)
91117	1(2)
91120	1(2)
91122	1(2)
91132	1(3)
91133	1(3)
91200	1(2)
91299	1(3)
92002	1(2)
92004	1(2)
92012	1(3)
92014	1(3)
92015	0(3)
92018	1(2)
92019	1(2)
92020	1(2)
92025	1(2)
92060	1(2)
92065	1(2)
92071	2(2)
92072	1(2)
92081	1(2)
92082	1(2)
92083	1(2)
92100	1(2)
92132	1(2)
92133	1(2)
92134	1(2)
92136	2(2)
92145	1(2)
92201	1(2)
92202	1(2)
92227	1(2)
92228	1(2)
92230	2(2)
92235	1(2)
92240	1(2)
92242	1(2)
92250	1(2)
92260	1(2)
92265	1(2)
92270	1(2)
92273	1(2)
92274	1(2)
92283	1(2)
92284	1(2)
92285	1(2)
92286	1(2)
92287	1(2)

CPT	MUE
92310	0(3)
92311	1(2)
92312	1(2)
92313	1(3)
92314	0(3)
92315	1(2)
92316	1(2)
92317	1(3)
92325	1(3)
92326	2(2)
92340	0(3)
92341	0(3)
92342	0(3)
92352	0(3)
92353	0(3)
92354	0(3)
92355	0(3)
92358	0(3)
92370	0(3)
92371	0(3)
92499	1(3)
92502	1(3)
92504	1(3)
92507	1(3)
92508	1(3)
92511	1(3)
92512	1(2)
92516	1(3)
92520	1(2)
92521	1(2)
92522	1(2)
92523	1(2)
92524	1(2)
92526	1(2)
92531	0(3)
92532	0(3)
92533	0(3)
92534	0(3)
92537	1(2)
92538	1(2)
92540	1(3)
92541	1(3)
92542	1(3)
92544	1(3)
92545	1(3)
92546	1(3)
92547	1(3)
92548	1(3)
92549	1(3)
92550	1(2)
92551	0(3)
92552	1(2)
92553	1(2)
92555	1(2)
92556	1(2)
92557	1(2)
92558	0(3)
92559	0(3)
92560	0(3)
92561	1(2)
92562	1(2)
92563	1(2)
92564	1(2)
92565	1(2)
92567	1(2)

CPT	MUE
92568	1(2)
92570	1(2)
92571	1(2)
92572	1(2)
92575	1(2)
92576	1(2)
92577	1(2)
92579	1(2)
92582	1(2)
92583	1(2)
92584	1(2)
92585	1(2)
92586	1(2)
92587	1(2)
92588	1(2)
92590	0(3)
92591	0(3)
92592	0(3)
92593	0(3)
92594	0(3)
92595	0(3)
92596	1(2)
92597	1(3)
92601	1(3)
92602	1(3)
92603	1(3)
92604	1(3)
92605	0(3)
92606	0(3)
92607	1(3)
92608	4(3)
92609	1(3)
92610	1(2)
92611	1(3)
92612	1(3)
92613	1(2)
92614	1(3)
92615	1(2)
92616	1(3)
92617	1(2)
92618	1(3)
92620	1(2)
92621	2(3)
92625	1(2)
92626	1(2)
92627	6(3)
92630	0(3)
92633	0(3)
92640	1(3)
92700	1(3)
92920	3(3)
92921	6(2)
92924	2(3)
92925	6(2)
92928	3(3)
92929	6(2)
92933	2(3)
92934	6(2)
92937	2(3)
92938	6(3)
92941	1(3)
92943	2(3)
92944	3(3)
92950	2(3)
92953	2(3)

CPT	MUE
92960	2(3)
92961	1(3)
92970	1(3)
92971	1(3)
92973	2(3)
92974	1(3)
92975	1(3)
92977	1(3)
92978	1(3)
92979	2(3)
92986	1(2)
92987	1(2)
92990	1(2)
92992	1(2)
92993	1(2)
92997	1(2)
92998	2(3)
93000	3(3)
93005	3(3)
93010	5(3)
93015	1(3)
93016	1(3)
93017	1(3)
93018	1(3)
93024	1(3)
93025	1(2)
93040	3(3)
93041	2(3)
93042	3(3)
93050	1(3)
93224	1(2)
93225	1(2)
93226	1(2)
93227	1(2)
93228	1(2)
93229	1(2)
93260	1(2)
93261	1(3)
93264	1(2)
93268	1(2)
93270	1(2)
93271	1(2)
93272	1(2)
93278	1(3)
93279	1(3)
93280	1(3)
93281	1(3)
93282	1(3)
93283	1(3)
93284	1(3)
93285	1(3)
93286	2(3)
93287	2(3)
93288	1(3)
93289	1(3)
93290	1(3)
93291	1(3)
93292	1(3)
93293	1(2)
93294	1(2)
93295	1(2)
93296	1(2)
93297	1(2)
93298	1(2)
93303	1(3)

CPT	MUE
93304	1(3)
93306	1(3)
93307	1(3)
93308	1(3)
93312	1(3)
93313	1(3)
93314	1(3)
93315	1(3)
93316	1(3)
93317	1(3)
93318	1(3)
93320	2(3)
93321	1(3)
93325	2(3)
93350	1(2)
93351	1(2)
93352	1(3)
93355	1(3)
93356	1(3)
93451	1(3)
93452	1(3)
93453	1(3)
93454	1(3)
93455	1(3)
93456	1(3)
93457	1(3)
93458	1(3)
93459	1(3)
93460	1(3)
93461	1(3)
93462	1(3)
93463	1(3)
93464	1(3)
93503	2(3)
93505	1(2)
93530	1(3)
93531	1(3)
93532	1(3)
93533	1(3)
93561	1(3)
93562	1(3)
93563	1(3)
93564	1(3)
93565	1(3)
93566	1(3)
93567	1(3)
93568	1(3)
93571	1(3)
93572	2(3)
93580	1(3)
93581	1(3)
93582	1(2)
93583	1(2)
93590	1(2)
93591	1(2)
93592	2(3)
93600	1(3)
93602	1(3)
93603	1(3)
93609	1(3)
93610	1(3)
93612	1(3)
93613	1(3)
93615	1(3)
93616	1(3)

CPT	MUE
93618	1(3)
93619	1(3)
93620	1(3)
93621	1(3)
93622	1(3)
93623	1(3)
93624	1(3)
93631	1(3)
93640	1(3)
93641	1(2)
93642	1(3)
93644	1(3)
93650	1(2)
93653	1(3)
93654	1(3)
93655	2(3)
93656	1(3)
93657	2(3)
93660	1(3)
93662	1(3)
93668	1(3)
93701	1(2)
93702	1(2)
93724	1(3)
93740	0(3)
93745	1(2)
93750	4(3)
93770	0(3)
93784	1(2)
93786	1(2)
93788	1(2)
93790	1(2)
93792	1(2)
93793	1(2)
93797	2(2)
93798	2(2)
93799	1(3)
93880	1(3)
93882	1(3)
93886	1(3)
93888	1(3)
93890	1(3)
93892	1(3)
93893	1(3)
93895	1(3)
93922	2(2)
93923	2(2)
93924	1(2)
93925	1(3)
93926	1(3)
93930	1(3)
93931	1(3)
93970	1(3)
93971	1(3)
93975	1(3)
93976	1(3)
93978	1(3)
93979	1(3)
93980	1(3)
93981	1(3)
93985	1(3)
93986	1(3)
93990	2(3)
93998	1(3)
94002	1(2)

CPT	MUE
94003	1(2)
94004	1(2)
94005	1(3)
94010	1(3)
94011	1(3)
94012	1(3)
94013	1(3)
94014	1(2)
94015	1(2)
94016	1(2)
94060	1(3)
94070	1(2)
94150	0(3)
94200	1(3)
94250	1(3)
94375	1(3)
94400	1(3)
94450	1(3)
94452	1(2)
94453	1(2)
94610	2(3)
94617	1(3)
94618	1(3)
94621	1(3)
94640	4(3)
94642	1(3)
94644	1(2)
94645	2(3)
94660	1(2)
94662	1(2)
94664	1(3)
94667	1(2)
94668	2(3)
94669	2(3)
94680	1(3)
94681	1(3)
94690	1(3)
94726	1(3)
94727	1(3)
94728	1(3)
94729	1(3)
94750	1(3)
94760	1(3)
94761	1(2)
94762	1(2)
94770	1(3)
94772	1(2)
94774	1(2)
94775	1(2)
94776	1(2)
94777	1(2)
94780	1(2)
94781	2(3)
94799	1(3)
95004	80(3)
95012	2(3)
95017	27(3)
95018	19(3)
95024	40(3)
95027	90(3)
95028	30(3)
95044	80(3)
95052	20(3)
95056	1(2)
95060	1(2)

CPT	MUE
95065	1(3)
95070	1(3)
95071	1(2)
95076	1(2)
95079	2(3)
95115	1(2)
95117	1(2)
95120	0(3)
95125	0(3)
95130	0(3)
95131	0(3)
95132	0(3)
95133	0(3)
95134	0(3)
95144	30(3)
95145	10(3)
95146	10(3)
95147	10(3)
95148	10(3)
95149	10(3)
95165	30(3)
95170	10(3)
95180	6(3)
95199	1(3)
95249	1(2)
95250	1(2)
95251	1(2)
95700	1(2)
95705	1(2)
95706	1(2)
95707	1(2)
95708	4(3)
95709	4(3)
95710	4(3)
95711	1(2)
95712	1(2)
95713	1(2)
95714	4(3)
95715	4(3)
95716	4(3)
95717	1(2)
95718	1(2)
95719	1(2)
95720	1(2)
95721	1(2)
95722	1(2)
95723	1(2)
95724	1(2)
95725	1(2)
95726	1(2)
95782	1(2)
95783	1(2)
95800	1(2)
95801	1(2)
95803	1(2)
95805	1(2)
95806	1(2)
95807	1(2)
95808	1(2)
95810	1(2)
95811	1(2)
95812	1(3)
95813	1(3)
95816	1(3)
95819	1(3)

CPT	MUE
95822	1(3)
95824	1(3)
95829	1(3)
95830	1(3)
95836	1(2)
95851	3(3)
95852	1(3)
95857	1(2)
95860	1(3)
95861	1(3)
95863	1(3)
95864	1(3)
95865	1(3)
95866	1(3)
95867	1(3)
95868	1(3)
95869	1(3)
95870	4(3)
95872	4(3)
95873	1(2)
95874	1(2)
95875	2(3)
95885	4(2)
95886	4(2)
95887	1(2)
95905	2(3)
95907	1(2)
95908	1(2)
95909	1(2)
95910	1(2)
95911	1(2)
95912	1(2)
95913	1(2)
95921	1(3)
95922	1(3)
95923	1(3)
95924	1(3)
95925	1(3)
95926	1(3)
95927	1(3)
95928	1(3)
95929	1(3)
95930	1(3)
95933	1(3)
95937	4(3)
95938	1(3)
95939	1(3)
95940	32(3)
95941	0(3)
95943	1(3)
95954	1(3)
95955	1(3)
95957	1(3)
95958	1(3)
95961	1(2)
95962	5(3)
95965	1(3)
95966	1(3)
95967	3(3)
95970	1(3)
95971	1(3)
95972	1(3)
95976	1(3)
95977	1(3)
95980	1(3)

CPT	MUE
95981	1(3)
95982	1(3)
95983	1(2)
95984	11(3)
95990	1(3)
95991	1(3)
95992	1(2)
95999	1(3)
96000	1(2)
96001	1(2)
96002	1(3)
96003	1(3)
96004	1(2)
96020	1(2)
96040	4(3)
96105	3(3)
96110	3(3)
96112	1(2)
96113	6(3)
96116	1(2)
96121	3(3)
96125	2(3)
96127	2(3)
96130	1(2)
96131	7(3)
96132	1(2)
96133	7(3)
96136	1(2)
96137	11(3)
96138	1(2)
96139	11(3)
96146	1(2)
96156	1(3)
96158	1(2)
96159	4(3)
96160	3(3)
96161	1(3)
96164	1(2)
96165	6(3)
96167	1(2)
96168	6(3)
96170	1(3)
96171	1(3)
96360	1(3)
96361	8(3)
96365	1(3)
96366	8(3)
96367	4(3)
96368	1(2)
96369	1(2)
96370	3(3)
96371	1(3)
96372	4(3)
96373	2(3)
96374	1(3)
96375	6(3)
96376	0(3)
96377	1(3)
96379	1(3)
96401	3(3)
96402	2(3)
96405	1(2)
96406	1(2)
96409	1(3)
96411	3(3)

CPT	MUE
96413	1(3)
96415	8(3)
96416	1(3)
96417	3(3)
96420	1(3)
96422	2(3)
96423	1(3)
96425	1(3)
96440	1(3)
96446	1(3)
96450	1(3)
96521	2(3)
96522	1(3)
96523	1(3)
96542	1(3)
96549	1(3)
96567	1(3)
96570	1(2)
96571	2(3)
96573	1(2)
96574	1(2)
96900	1(3)
96902	0(3)
96904	1(2)
96910	1(3)
96912	1(3)
96913	1(3)
96920	1(2)
96921	1(2)
96922	1(2)
96931	1(2)
96932	1(2)
96933	1(2)
96934	2(3)
96935	2(3)
96936	2(3)
96999	1(3)
97010	0(3)
97012	1(3)
97014	0(3)
97016	1(3)
97018	1(3)
97022	1(3)
97024	1(3)
97026	1(3)
97028	1(3)
97032	4(3)
97033	4(3)
97034	2(3)
97035	2(3)
97036	3(3)
97039	1(3)
97110	6(3)
97112	4(3)
97113	6(3)
97116	4(3)
97124	4(3)
97129	1(2)
97130	7(3)
97139	1(3)
97140	6(3)
97150	1(3)
97151	8(3)
97152	8(3)
97153	32(3)

CPT	MUE
97154	12(3)
97155	24(3)
97156	16(3)
97157	16(3)
97158	16(3)
97161	1(2)
97162	1(2)
97163	1(2)
97164	1(2)
97165	1(2)
97166	1(2)
97167	1(2)
97168	1(2)
97169	0(3)
97170	0(3)
97171	0(3)
97172	0(3)
97530	6(3)
97533	4(3)
97535	8(3)
97537	6(3)
97542	8(3)
97545	1(2)
97546	2(3)
97597	1(3)
97598	8(3)
97602	0(3)
97605	1(3)
97606	1(3)
97607	1(3)
97608	1(3)
97610	1(2)
97750	8(3)
97755	8(3)
97760	6(3)
97761	6(3)
97763	6(3)
97799	1(3)
97802	8(3)
97803	8(3)
97804	6(3)
97810	1(2)
97811	2(3)
97813	1(2)
97814	2(3)
98925	1(2)
98926	1(2)
98927	1(2)
98928	1(2)
98929	1(2)
98940	1(2)
98941	1(2)
98942	1(2)
98943	0(3)
98960	0(3)
98961	0(3)
98962	0(3)
98966	1(2)
98967	1(2)
98968	1(2)
98970	1(2)
98971	1(2)
98972	1(2)
99000	0(3)
99001	0(3)

CPT	MUE
99002	0(3)
99024	1(3)
99026	0(3)
99027	0(3)
99050	0(3)
99051	0(3)
99053	0(3)
99056	0(3)
99058	0(3)
99060	0(3)
99070	0(3)
99071	0(3)
99075	0(3)
99078	0(3)
99080	0(3)
99082	1(3)
99091	1(2)
99100	1(3)
99116	0(3)
99135	0(3)
99140	0(3)
99151	1(3)
99152	2(3)
99153	9(3)
99155	1(3)
99156	1(3)
99157	6(3)
99170	1(3)
99172	0(3)
99173	0(3)
99174	0(3)
99175	1(3)
99177	1(2)
99183	1(3)
99184	1(2)
99188	1(2)
99190	1(3)
99191	1(3)
99192	1(3)
99195	2(3)
99199	1(3)
99201	1(2)
99202	1(2)
99203	1(2)
99204	1(2)
99205	1(2)
99211	1(3)
99212	2(3)
99213	2(3)
99214	2(3)
99215	1(3)
99217	1(2)
99218	1(2)
99219	1(2)
99220	1(2)
99221	1(3)
99222	1(3)
99223	1(3)
99224	1(2)
99225	1(2)
99226	1(2)
99231	1(3)
99232	1(3)
99233	1(3)
99234	1(3)

CPT	MUE
99235	1(3)
99236	1(3)
99238	1(3)
99239	1(3)
99241	0(3)
99242	0(3)
99243	0(3)
99244	0(3)
99245	0(3)
99251	0(3)
99252	0(3)
99253	0(3)
99254	0(3)
99255	0(3)
99281	1(3)
99282	1(3)
99283	1(3)
99284	1(3)
99285	1(3)
99288	0(3)
99291	1(2)
99292	8(3)
99304	1(2)
99305	1(2)
99306	1(2)
99307	1(2)
99308	1(2)
99309	1(2)
99310	1(2)
99315	1(2)
99316	1(2)
99318	1(2)
99324	1(2)
99325	1(2)
99326	1(2)
99327	1(2)
99328	1(2)
99334	1(3)
99335	1(3)
99336	1(3)
99337	1(3)
99339	0(3)
99340	0(3)
99341	1(2)
99342	1(2)
99343	1(2)
99344	1(2)
99345	1(2)
99347	1(3)
99348	1(3)
99349	1(3)
99350	1(3)
99354	1(2)
99355	4(3)
99356	1(2)
99357	4(3)
99358	1(2)
99359	2(3)
99360	1(3)
99366	0(3)
99367	0(3)
99368	0(3)
99374	0(3)
99375	0(3)
99377	0(3)

CPT	MUE
99378	0(3)
99379	0(3)
99380	0(3)
99381	0(3)
99382	0(3)
99383	0(3)
99384	0(3)
99385	0(3)
99386	0(3)
99387	0(3)
99391	0(3)
99392	0(3)
99393	0(3)
99394	0(3)
99395	0(3)
99396	0(3)
99397	0(3)
99401	0(3)
99402	0(3)
99403	0(3)
99404	0(3)
99406	1(2)
99407	1(2)
99408	0(3)
99409	0(3)
99411	0(3)
99412	0(3)
99415	1(2)
99416	3(3)
99421	1(2)
99422	1(2)
99423	1(2)
99429	0(3)
99441	1(2)
99442	1(2)
99443	1(2)
99446	1(2)
99447	1(2)
99448	1(2)
99449	1(2)
99450	0(3)
99451	1(2)
99452	1(2)
99453	1(2)
99454	1(2)
99455	1(3)
99456	1(3)
99457	1(2)
99458	3(3)
99460	1(2)
99461	1(2)
99462	1(2)
99463	1(2)
99464	1(2)
99465	1(2)
99466	1(2)
99467	4(3)
99468	1(2)
99469	1(2)
99471	1(2)
99472	1(2)
99473	1(2)
99474	1(2)
99475	1(2)
99476	1(2)

CPT	MUE
99477	1(2)
99478	1(2)
99479	1(2)
99480	1(2)
99483	1(2)
99484	1(2)
99485	1(3)
99486	4(1)
99487	1(2)
99489	10(3)
99490	1(2)
99491	1(2)
99492	1(2)
99493	1(2)
99494	2(3)
99495	1(2)
99496	1(2)
99497	1(2)
99498	3(3)
99499	1(3)
99500	0(3)
99501	0(3)
99502	0(3)
99503	0(3)
99504	0(3)
99505	0(3)
99506	0(3)
99507	0(3)
99509	0(3)
99510	0(3)
99511	0(3)
99512	0(3)
99600	0(3)
99601	0(3)
99602	0(3)
99605	0(2)
99606	0(3)
99607	0(3)
A0021	0(3)
A0080	0(3)
A0090	0(3)
A0100	0(3)
A0110	0(3)
A0120	0(3)
A0130	0(3)
A0140	0(3)
A0160	0(3)
A0170	0(3)
A0180	0(3)
A0190	0(3)
A0200	0(3)
A0210	0(3)
A0225	0(3)
A0380	0(3)
A0382	0(3)
A0384	0(3)
A0390	0(3)
A0392	0(3)
A0394	0(3)
A0396	0(3)
A0398	0(3)
A0420	0(3)
A0422	0(3)
A0424	0(3)
A0425	250(1)

CPT	MUE
A0426	2(3)
A0427	2(3)
A0428	2(3)
A0429	2(3)
A0430	1(3)
A0431	1(3)
A0432	1(3)
A0433	1(3)
A0434	2(3)
A0435	999(3)
A0436	300(3)
A0888	0(3)
A0998	0(3)
A0999	1(3)
A4206	0(3)
A4207	0(3)
A4208	0(3)
A4209	0(3)
A4210	0(3)
A4211	0(3)
A4212	0(3)
A4213	0(3)
A4215	0(3)
A4216	0(3)
A4217	0(3)
A4218	0(3)
A4220	1(3)
A4221	0(3)
A4222	0(3)
A4223	0(3)
A4224	0(3)
A4225	0(3)
A4226	0(3)
A4230	0(3)
A4231	0(3)
A4232	0(3)
A4233	0(3)
A4234	0(3)
A4235	0(3)
A4236	0(3)
A4244	0(3)
A4245	0(3)
A4246	0(3)
A4247	0(3)
A4248	0(3)
A4250	0(3)
A4252	0(3)
A4253	0(3)
A4255	0(3)
A4256	0(3)
A4257	0(3)
A4258	0(3)
A4259	0(3)
A4261	0(3)
A4262	0(3)
A4263	0(3)
A4264	0(3)
A4265	0(3)
A4266	0(3)
A4267	0(3)
A4268	0(3)
A4269	0(3)
A4270	0(3)
A4280	0(3)
A4281	0(3)
A4282	0(3)
A4283	0(3)
A4284	0(3)
A4285	0(3)
A4286	0(3)
A4290	2(3)
A4300	0(3)
A4301	1(2)
A4305	0(3)
A4306	0(3)
A4310	0(3)
A4311	0(3)
A4312	0(3)
A4313	0(3)
A4314	0(3)
A4315	0(3)
A4316	0(3)
A4320	0(3)
A4321	1(3)
A4322	0(3)
A4326	0(3)
A4327	0(3)
A4328	0(3)
A4330	0(3)
A4331	1(3)
A4332	2(3)
A4333	1(3)
A4334	1(3)
A4335	0(3)
A4336	1(3)
A4337	0(3)
A4338	0(3)
A4340	0(3)
A4344	0(3)
A4346	0(3)
A4349	1(3)
A4351	0(3)
A4352	0(3)
A4353	1(3)
A4354	0(3)
A4355	0(3)
A4356	0(3)
A4357	0(3)
A4358	0(3)
A4360	1(3)
A4361	0(3)
A4362	0(3)
A4363	1(3)
A4364	0(3)
A4366	1(3)
A4367	0(3)
A4368	1(3)
A4369	1(3)
A4371	1(3)
A4372	1(3)
A4373	1(3)
A4375	2(3)
A4376	2(3)
A4377	2(3)
A4378	2(3)
A4379	2(3)
A4380	2(3)
A4381	2(3)
A4382	2(3)
A4383	2(3)
A4384	2(3)
A4385	2(3)
A4387	1(3)
A4388	1(3)
A4389	2(3)
A4390	1(3)
A4391	1(3)
A4392	2(3)
A4393	1(3)
A4394	1(3)
A4395	3(3)
A4396	2(3)
A4397	0(3)
A4398	0(3)
A4399	0(3)
A4400	0(3)
A4402	0(3)
A4404	0(3)
A4405	1(3)
A4406	1(3)
A4407	2(3)
A4408	1(3)
A4409	1(3)
A4410	2(3)
A4411	1(3)
A4412	1(3)
A4413	2(3)
A4414	1(3)
A4415	1(3)
A4416	2(3)
A4417	2(3)
A4418	2(3)
A4419	2(3)
A4420	1(3)
A4422	7(3)
A4423	2(3)
A4424	1(3)
A4425	1(3)
A4426	2(3)
A4427	1(3)
A4428	1(3)
A4429	2(3)
A4430	1(3)
A4431	1(3)
A4432	2(3)
A4433	1(3)
A4434	1(3)
A4435	2(3)
A4450	0(3)
A4452	0(3)
A4455	0(3)
A4458	0(3)
A4459	0(3)
A4461	2(3)
A4463	0(3)
A4465	0(3)
A4467	0(3)
A4470	0(3)
A4480	0(3)
A4481	0(3)
A4483	0(3)
A4490	0(3)
A4495	0(3)
A4500	0(3)
A4510	0(3)
A4520	0(3)
A4550	0(3)
A4553	0(3)
A4554	0(3)
A4555	0(3)
A4556	0(3)
A4557	0(3)
A4558	0(3)
A4559	0(3)
A4561	1(3)
A4562	1(3)
A4563	1(2)
A4565	2(3)
A4566	0(3)
A4570	0(3)
A4575	0(3)
A4580	0(3)
A4590	0(3)
A4595	0(3)
A4600	0(3)
A4601	0(3)
A4602	0(3)
A4604	0(3)
A4605	0(3)
A4606	0(3)
A4608	0(3)
A4611	0(3)
A4612	0(3)
A4613	0(3)
A4614	0(3)
A4615	0(3)
A4616	0(3)
A4617	0(3)
A4618	1(3)
A4619	0(3)
A4620	0(3)
A4623	0(3)
A4624	0(3)
A4625	30(3)
A4626	0(3)
A4627	0(3)
A4628	0(3)
A4629	0(3)
A4630	0(3)
A4633	0(3)
A4634	0(3)
A4635	0(3)
A4636	0(3)
A4637	0(3)
A4638	0(3)
A4639	0(3)
A4640	0(3)
A4642	1(3)
A4648	5(3)
A4649	1(3)
A4650	3(3)
A4651	0(3)
A4652	0(3)
A4653	0(3)
A4657	0(3)
A4660	0(3)
A4663	0(3)
A4670	0(3)
A4671	0(3)
A4672	0(3)
A4673	0(3)
A4674	0(3)
A4680	0(3)
A4690	0(3)
A4706	0(3)
A4707	0(3)
A4708	0(3)
A4709	0(3)
A4714	0(3)
A4719	0(3)
A4720	0(3)
A4721	0(3)
A4722	0(3)
A4723	0(3)
A4724	0(3)
A4725	0(3)
A4726	0(3)
A4728	0(3)
A4730	0(3)
A4736	0(3)
A4737	0(3)
A4740	0(3)
A4750	0(3)
A4755	0(3)
A4760	0(3)
A4765	0(3)
A4766	0(3)
A4770	0(3)
A4771	0(3)
A4772	0(3)
A4773	0(3)
A4774	0(3)
A4802	0(3)
A4860	0(3)
A4870	0(3)
A4890	0(3)
A4911	0(3)
A4913	0(3)
A4918	0(3)
A4927	0(3)
A4928	0(3)
A4929	0(3)
A4930	0(3)
A4931	0(3)
A4932	0(3)
A5051	0(3)
A5052	0(3)
A5053	0(3)
A5054	0(3)
A5055	0(3)
A5056	90(3)
A5057	90(3)
A5061	0(3)
A5062	0(3)
A5063	0(3)
A5071	0(3)
A5072	0(3)
A5073	0(3)
A5081	0(3)
A5082	0(3)
A5083	5(3)
A5093	0(3)
A5102	0(3)
A5105	0(3)
A5112	0(3)
A5113	0(3)
A5114	0(3)
A5120	150(3)
A5121	0(3)
A5122	0(3)
A5126	0(3)
A5131	0(3)
A5200	2(3)
A5500	0(3)
A5501	0(3)
A5503	0(3)
A5504	0(3)
A5505	0(3)
A5506	0(3)
A5507	0(3)
A5508	0(3)
A5510	0(3)
A5512	0(3)
A5513	0(3)
A5514	0(3)
A6000	0(3)
A6010	0(3)
A6011	0(3)
A6021	0(3)
A6022	0(3)
A6023	0(3)
A6024	0(3)
A6025	0(3)
A6154	0(3)
A6196	0(3)
A6197	0(3)
A6198	0(3)
A6199	0(3)
A6203	0(3)
A6204	0(3)
A6205	0(3)
A6206	0(3)
A6207	0(3)
A6208	0(3)
A6209	0(3)
A6210	0(3)
A6211	0(3)
A6212	0(3)
A6213	0(3)
A6214	0(3)
A6215	0(3)
A6216	0(3)
A6217	0(3)
A6218	0(3)
A6219	0(3)
A6220	0(3)
A6221	0(3)
A6222	0(3)
A6223	0(3)
A6224	0(3)
A6228	0(3)
A6229	0(3)
A6230	0(3)
A6231	0(3)
A6232	0(3)
A6233	0(3)
A6234	0(3)
A6235	0(3)
A6236	0(3)
A6237	0(3)
A6238	0(3)
A6239	0(3)
A6240	0(3)
A6241	0(3)
A6242	0(3)
A6243	0(3)
A6244	0(3)
A6245	0(3)
A6246	0(3)
A6247	0(3)
A6248	0(3)
A6250	0(3)
A6251	0(3)
A6252	0(3)
A6253	0(3)
A6254	0(3)
A6255	0(3)
A6256	0(3)
A6257	0(3)
A6258	0(3)
A6259	0(3)
A6260	0(3)
A6261	0(3)
A6262	0(3)
A6266	0(3)
A6402	0(3)
A6403	0(3)
A6404	0(3)
A6407	0(3)
A6410	2(3)
A6411	0(3)
A6412	0(3)
A6413	0(3)
A6441	0(3)
A6442	0(3)
A6443	0(3)
A6444	0(3)
A6445	0(3)
A6446	0(3)
A6447	0(3)
A6448	0(3)
A6449	0(3)
A6450	0(3)
A6451	0(3)
A6452	0(3)
A6453	0(3)
A6454	0(3)
A6455	0(3)
A6456	0(3)
A6457	0(3)
A6460	1(1)
A6461	1(1)
A6501	0(3)
A6502	0(3)
A6503	0(3)
A6504	0(3)
A6505	0(3)
A6506	0(3)
A6507	0(3)
A6508	0(3)
A6509	0(3)
A6510	0(3)
A6511	0(3)
A6513	0(3)
A6530	0(3)
A6531	0(3)
A6532	0(3)
A6533	0(3)
A6534	0(3)
A6535	0(3)
A6536	0(3)
A6537	0(3)
A6538	0(3)
A6539	0(3)
A6540	0(3)
A6541	0(3)
A6544	0(3)
A6545	0(3)
A6549	0(3)
A6550	0(3)
A7000	0(3)
A7001	0(3)
A7002	0(3)
A7003	0(3)
A7004	0(3)
A7005	0(3)
A7006	0(3)
A7007	0(3)
A7008	0(3)
A7009	0(3)
A7010	0(3)
A7012	0(3)
A7013	0(3)
A7014	0(3)
A7015	0(3)
A7016	0(3)
A7017	0(3)
A7018	0(3)
A7020	0(3)
A7025	0(3)
A7026	0(3)
A7027	0(3)
A7028	0(3)
A7029	0(3)
A7030	0(3)
A7031	0(3)
A7032	0(3)
A7033	0(3)
A7034	0(3)
A7035	0(3)
A7036	0(3)
A7037	0(3)
A7038	0(3)
A7039	0(3)
A7040	2(3)
A7041	2(3)
A7044	0(3)
A7045	0(3)
A7046	0(3)
A7047	0(3)
A7048	2(3)
A7501	0(3)
A7502	0(3)
A7503	0(3)
A7504	0(3)
A7505	0(3)
A7506	0(3)
A7507	0(3)
A7508	0(3)
A7509	0(3)

CPT	MUE
A7520	0(3)
A7521	0(3)
A7522	0(3)
A7523	0(3)
A7524	0(3)
A7525	0(3)
A7526	0(3)
A7527	0(3)
A8000	0(3)
A8001	0(3)
A8002	0(3)
A8003	0(3)
A8004	0(3)
A9152	0(3)
A9153	0(3)
A9155	1(3)
A9180	0(3)
A9270	0(3)
A9272	0(3)
A9273	0(3)
A9274	0(3)
A9275	0(3)
A9276	0(3)
A9277	0(3)
A9278	0(3)
A9279	0(3)
A9280	0(3)
A9281	0(3)
A9282	0(3)
A9283	0(3)
A9284	0(3)
A9285	0(3)
A9286	0(3)
A9300	0(3)
A9500	3(3)
A9501	1(3)
A9502	3(3)
A9503	1(3)
A9504	1(3)
A9505	4(3)
A9507	1(3)
A9508	2(3)
A9509	5(3)
A9510	1(3)
A9512	30(3)
A9513	200(3)
A9515	1(3)
A9516	4(3)
A9517	200(3)
A9520	1(3)
A9521	2(3)
A9524	10(3)
A9526	2(3)
A9527	195(3)
A9528	10(3)
A9529	10(3)
A9530	200(3)
A9531	100(3)
A9532	10(3)
A9536	1(3)
A9537	1(3)
A9538	1(3)
A9539	2(3)
A9540	2(3)
A9541	1(3)

CPT	MUE
A9542	1(3)
A9543	1(3)
A9546	1(3)
A9547	2(3)
A9548	2(3)
A9550	1(3)
A9551	1(3)
A9552	1(3)
A9553	1(3)
A9554	1(3)
A9555	2(3)
A9556	10(3)
A9557	2(3)
A9558	7(3)
A9559	1(3)
A9560	2(3)
A9561	1(3)
A9562	2(3)
A9563	10(3)
A9564	20(3)
A9566	1(3)
A9567	2(3)
A9568	0(3)
A9569	1(3)
A9570	1(3)
A9571	1(3)
A9572	1(3)
A9575	300(3)
A9576	40(3)
A9577	50(3)
A9578	50(3)
A9579	100(3)
A9580	1(3)
A9581	20(3)
A9582	1(3)
A9583	18(3)
A9584	1(3)
A9585	300(3)
A9586	1(3)
A9587	54(3)
A9588	10(3)
A9589	1(3)
A9590	675(3)
A9600	7(3)
A9604	1(3)
A9606	224(3)
A9698	2(3)
A9700	2(3)
A9900	1(3)
A9901	0(3)
A9999	1(3)
B4034	0(3)
B4035	0(3)
B4036	0(3)
B4081	0(3)
B4082	0(3)
B4083	0(3)
B4087	0(3)
B4088	0(3)
B4100	0(3)
B4102	0(3)
B4103	0(3)
B4104	0(3)
B4149	0(3)
B4150	0(3)

CPT	MUE
B4152	0(3)
B4153	0(3)
B4154	0(3)
B4155	0(3)
B4157	0(3)
B4158	0(3)
B4159	0(3)
B4160	0(3)
B4161	0(3)
B4162	0(3)
B4164	0(3)
B4168	0(3)
B4172	0(3)
B4176	0(3)
B4178	0(3)
B4180	0(3)
B4185	0(3)
B4189	0(3)
B4193	0(3)
B4197	0(3)
B4199	0(3)
B4216	0(3)
B4220	0(3)
B4222	0(3)
B4224	0(3)
B5000	0(3)
B5100	0(3)
B5200	0(3)
B9002	0(3)
B9004	0(3)
B9006	0(3)
B9998	0(3)
B9999	0(3)
C1713	20(3)
C1714	4(3)
C1715	45(3)
C1716	4(3)
C1717	10(3)
C1719	99(3)
C1721	1(3)
C1722	1(3)
C1724	5(3)
C1725	9(3)
C1726	5(3)
C1727	4(3)
C1728	5(3)
C1729	6(3)
C1730	4(3)
C1731	2(3)
C1732	3(3)
C1733	3(3)
C1734	2(3)
C1749	1(3)
C1750	2(3)
C1751	3(3)
C1752	2(3)
C1753	2(3)
C1754	2(3)
C1755	2(3)
C1756	2(3)
C1757	6(3)
C1758	2(3)
C1759	2(3)
C1760	4(3)
C1762	4(3)

CPT	MUE
C1763	4(3)
C1764	1(3)
C1765	4(3)
C1766	4(3)
C1767	2(3)
C1768	3(3)
C1769	9(3)
C1770	3(3)
C1771	1(3)
C1772	1(3)
C1773	3(3)
C1776	10(3)
C1777	2(3)
C1778	4(3)
C1779	2(3)
C1780	2(3)
C1781	4(3)
C1782	1(3)
C1783	2(3)
C1784	2(3)
C1785	1(3)
C1786	1(3)
C1787	2(3)
C1788	2(3)
C1789	2(3)
C1813	1(3)
C1814	2(3)
C1815	1(3)
C1816	2(3)
C1817	1(3)
C1818	2(3)
C1819	4(3)
C1820	2(3)
C1821	4(3)
C1822	1(3)
C1823	1(3)
C1824	1(2)
C1830	2(3)
C1839	2(2)
C1840	1(3)
C1841	1(2)
C1842	1(2)
C1874	5(3)
C1875	4(3)
C1876	5(3)
C1877	5(3)
C1878	2(3)
C1880	2(3)
C1881	2(3)
C1882	1(3)
C1883	4(3)
C1884	4(3)
C1885	2(3)
C1886	1(3)
C1887	7(3)
C1888	2(3)
C1889	1(3)
C1890	1(3)
C1891	1(3)
C1892	6(3)
C1893	6(3)
C1894	6(3)
C1895	2(3)
C1896	2(3)
C1897	2(3)

CPT	MUE
C1898	2(3)
C1899	2(3)
C1900	1(3)
C1982	1(3)
C2596	1(3)
C2613	2(3)
C2614	3(3)
C2615	2(3)
C2616	1(3)
C2617	4(3)
C2618	4(3)
C2619	1(3)
C2620	1(3)
C2621	1(3)
C2622	1(3)
C2623	2(3)
C2624	1(3)
C2625	4(3)
C2626	1(3)
C2627	2(3)
C2628	4(3)
C2629	4(3)
C2630	3(3)
C2631	1(3)
C2634	24(3)
C2635	124(3)
C2636	690(3)
C2637	0(3)
C2638	150(3)
C2639	150(3)
C2640	150(3)
C2641	150(3)
C2642	120(3)
C2643	120(3)
C2644	500(1)
C2645	4608(3)
C5271	1(2)
C5272	3(2)
C5273	1(2)
C5274	35(3)
C5275	1(2)
C5276	3(2)
C5277	1(2)
C5278	15(3)
C8900	1(3)
C8901	1(3)
C8902	1(3)
C8903	1(3)
C8905	1(3)
C8906	1(3)
C8908	1(3)
C8909	1(3)
C8910	1(3)
C8911	1(3)
C8912	1(3)
C8913	1(3)
C8914	1(3)
C8918	1(3)
C8919	1(3)
C8920	1(3)
C8921	1(3)
C8922	1(3)
C8923	1(3)
C8924	1(3)
C8925	1(3)

CPT	MUE
C8926	1(3)
C8927	1(3)
C8928	1(2)
C8929	1(3)
C8930	1(2)
C8931	1(3)
C8932	1(3)
C8933	1(3)
C8934	2(3)
C8935	2(3)
C8936	2(3)
C8937	2(2)
C8957	2(3)
C9046	160(3)
C9047	22(3)
C9055	400(3)
C9113	10(3)
C9132	5500(3)
C9248	25(3)
C9250	1(3)
C9254	400(3)
C9257	5(3)
C9285	2(3)
C9290	266(3)
C9293	700(3)
C9352	3(3)
C9353	4(3)
C9354	300(3)
C9355	3(3)
C9356	125(3)
C9358	800(3)
C9359	30(3)
C9360	300(3)
C9361	10(3)
C9362	60(3)
C9363	500(3)
C9364	600(3)
C9460	1(3)
C9462	600(3)
C9482	150(3)
C9488	20(3)
C9600	3(3)
C9601	2(3)
C9602	2(3)
C9603	2(3)
C9604	2(3)
C9605	2(3)
C9606	1(3)
C9607	1(2)
C9608	2(3)
C9725	1(3)
C9726	2(3)
C9727	1(2)
C9728	1(2)
C9733	1(3)
C9734	1(3)
C9738	1(3)
C9739	1(2)
C9740	1(2)
C9745	2(2)
C9747	1(2)
C9749	1(2)
C9751	1(3)
C9752	1(2)
C9753	3(3)

CPT	MUE
C9756	1(3)
C9757	2(2)
C9758	1(2)
C9803	2(3)
D0150	1(3)
D0240	1(3)
D0250	2(3)
D0270	1(3)
D0272	1(3)
D0274	1(3)
D0277	1(3)
D0412	0(3)
D0416	1(3)
D0431	1(3)
D0460	1(2)
D0484	1(2)
D0485	1(2)
D0601	1(2)
D0602	1(2)
D0603	1(2)
D1510	2(2)
D1516	1(2)
D1517	1(2)
D1520	2(2)
D1526	1(2)
D1527	1(2)
D1551	1(2)
D1552	1(2)
D1553	2(2)
D1575	4(2)
D4260	4(2)
D4263	4(2)
D4264	3(3)
D4270	4(3)
D4273	1(2)
D4277	1(2)
D4278	3(3)
D4355	1(2)
D4381	12(3)
D5282	0(3)
D5283	0(3)
D5876	0(3)
D5911	1(3)
D5912	1(2)
D5983	1(3)
D5984	1(3)
D5985	1(3)
D7111	20(3)
D7140	32(2)
D7210	32(2)
D7220	6(3)
D7230	6(3)
D7240	6(3)
D7241	6(3)
D7250	32(2)
D7260	1(3)
D7261	1(3)
D7283	4(3)
D7288	2(3)
D7321	4(2)
D9110	1(3)
D9130	0(3)
D9230	1(3)
D9248	1(3)
D9613	0(3)

CPT	MUE
D9930	1(2)
D9944	0(3)
D9945	0(3)
D9946	0(3)
D9950	1(3)
D9951	1(3)
D9952	1(3)
D9961	0(3)
D9990	0(3)
E0100	0(3)
E0105	0(3)
E0110	0(3)
E0111	0(3)
E0112	0(3)
E0113	0(3)
E0114	0(3)
E0116	0(3)
E0117	0(3)
E0118	0(3)
E0130	0(3)
E0135	0(3)
E0140	0(3)
E0141	0(3)
E0143	0(3)
E0144	0(3)
E0147	0(3)
E0148	0(3)
E0149	0(3)
E0153	0(3)
E0154	0(3)
E0155	0(3)
E0156	0(3)
E0157	0(3)
E0158	0(3)
E0159	2(2)
E0160	0(3)
E0161	0(3)
E0162	0(3)
E0163	0(3)
E0165	0(3)
E0167	0(3)
E0168	0(3)
E0170	0(3)
E0171	0(3)
E0172	0(3)
E0175	0(3)
E0181	0(3)
E0182	0(3)
E0184	0(3)
E0185	0(3)
E0186	0(3)
E0187	0(3)
E0188	0(3)
E0189	0(3)
E0190	0(3)
E0191	0(3)
E0193	0(3)
E0194	0(3)
E0196	0(3)
E0197	0(3)
E0198	0(3)
E0199	0(3)
E0200	0(3)
E0202	0(3)
E0203	0(3)

CPT	MUE
E0205	0(3)
E0210	0(3)
E0215	0(3)
E0217	0(3)
E0218	0(3)
E0221	0(3)
E0225	0(3)
E0231	0(3)
E0232	0(3)
E0235	0(3)
E0236	0(3)
E0239	0(3)
E0240	0(3)
E0241	0(3)
E0242	0(3)
E0243	0(3)
E0244	0(3)
E0245	0(3)
E0246	0(3)
E0247	0(3)
E0248	0(3)
E0249	0(3)
E0250	0(3)
E0251	0(3)
E0255	0(3)
E0256	0(3)
E0260	0(3)
E0261	0(3)
E0265	0(3)
E0266	0(3)
E0270	0(3)
E0271	0(3)
E0272	0(3)
E0273	0(3)
E0274	0(3)
E0275	0(3)
E0276	0(3)
E0277	0(3)
E0280	0(3)
E0290	0(3)
E0291	0(3)
E0292	0(3)
E0293	0(3)
E0294	0(3)
E0295	0(3)
E0296	0(3)
E0297	0(3)
E0300	0(3)
E0301	0(3)
E0302	0(3)
E0303	0(3)
E0304	0(3)
E0305	0(3)
E0310	0(3)
E0315	0(3)
E0316	0(3)
E0325	0(3)
E0326	0(3)
E0328	0(3)
E0329	0(3)
E0350	0(3)
E0352	0(3)
E0370	0(3)
E0371	0(3)
E0372	0(3)

CPT	MUE
E0373	0(3)
E0424	0(3)
E0425	0(3)
E0430	0(3)
E0431	0(3)
E0433	0(3)
E0434	0(3)
E0435	0(3)
E0439	0(3)
E0440	0(3)
E0441	0(3)
E0442	0(3)
E0443	0(3)
E0444	0(3)
E0445	0(3)
E0446	0(3)
E0447	0(3)
E0455	0(3)
E0457	0(3)
E0459	0(3)
E0462	0(3)
E0465	0(3)
E0466	0(3)
E0467	0(3)
E0470	0(3)
E0471	0(3)
E0472	0(3)
E0480	0(3)
E0481	0(3)
E0482	0(3)
E0483	0(3)
E0484	0(3)
E0485	0(3)
E0486	0(3)
E0487	0(3)
E0500	0(3)
E0550	0(3)
E0555	0(3)
E0560	0(3)
E0561	0(3)
E0562	0(3)
E0565	0(3)
E0570	0(3)
E0572	0(3)
E0574	0(3)
E0575	0(3)
E0580	0(3)
E0585	0(3)
E0600	0(3)
E0601	0(3)
E0602	0(3)
E0603	0(3)
E0604	0(3)
E0605	0(3)
E0606	0(3)
E0607	0(3)
E0610	0(3)
E0615	0(3)
E0616	1(2)
E0617	0(3)
E0618	0(3)
E0619	0(3)
E0620	0(3)
E0621	0(3)
E0625	0(3)

CPT	MUE
E0627	0(3)
E0629	0(3)
E0630	0(3)
E0635	0(3)
E0636	0(3)
E0637	0(3)
E0638	0(3)
E0639	0(3)
E0640	0(3)
E0641	0(3)
E0642	0(3)
E0650	0(3)
E0651	0(3)
E0652	0(3)
E0655	0(3)
E0656	0(3)
E0657	0(3)
E0660	0(3)
E0665	0(3)
E0666	0(3)
E0667	0(3)
E0668	0(3)
E0669	0(3)
E0670	0(3)
E0671	0(3)
E0672	0(3)
E0673	0(3)
E0675	0(3)
E0676	1(3)
E0691	0(3)
E0692	0(3)
E0693	0(3)
E0694	0(3)
E0700	0(3)
E0705	0(3)
E0710	0(3)
E0720	0(3)
E0730	0(3)
E0731	0(3)
E0740	0(3)
E0744	0(3)
E0745	0(3)
E0746	1(3)
E0747	0(3)
E0748	0(3)
E0749	1(3)
E0755	0(3)
E0760	0(3)
E0761	0(3)
E0762	0(3)
E0764	0(3)
E0765	0(3)
E0766	0(3)
E0769	0(3)
E0770	1(3)
E0776	0(3)
E0779	0(3)
E0780	0(3)
E0781	1(2)
E0782	1(2)
E0783	1(2)
E0784	0(3)
E0785	1(2)
E0786	1(2)
E0787	0(3)

CPT	MUE
E0791	0(3)
E0830	0(3)
E0840	0(3)
E0849	0(3)
E0850	0(3)
E0855	0(3)
E0856	0(3)
E0860	0(3)
E0870	0(3)
E0880	0(3)
E0890	0(3)
E0900	0(3)
E0910	0(3)
E0911	0(3)
E0912	0(3)
E0920	0(3)
E0930	0(3)
E0935	0(3)
E0936	0(3)
E0940	0(3)
E0941	0(3)
E0942	0(3)
E0944	0(3)
E0945	0(3)
E0946	0(3)
E0947	0(3)
E0948	0(3)
E0950	0(3)
E0951	0(3)
E0952	0(3)
E0953	0(3)
E0954	0(3)
E0955	0(3)
E0956	0(3)
E0957	0(3)
E0958	0(3)
E0959	0(3)
E0960	0(3)
E0961	0(3)
E0966	0(3)
E0967	0(3)
E0968	0(3)
E0969	0(3)
E0970	0(3)
E0971	0(3)
E0973	0(3)
E0974	0(3)
E0978	0(3)
E0980	0(3)
E0981	0(3)
E0982	0(3)
E0983	0(3)
E0984	0(3)
E0985	0(3)
E0986	0(3)
E0988	0(3)
E0990	0(3)
E0992	0(3)
E0994	0(3)
E0995	0(3)
E1002	0(3)
E1003	0(3)
E1004	0(3)
E1005	0(3)
E1006	0(3)

CPT	MUE
E1007	0(3)
E1008	0(3)
E1009	0(3)
E1010	0(3)
E1011	0(3)
E1012	0(3)
E1014	0(3)
E1015	0(3)
E1016	0(3)
E1017	0(3)
E1018	0(3)
E1020	0(3)
E1028	0(3)
E1029	0(3)
E1030	0(3)
E1031	0(3)
E1035	0(3)
E1036	0(3)
E1037	0(3)
E1038	0(3)
E1039	0(3)
E1050	0(3)
E1060	0(3)
E1070	0(3)
E1083	0(3)
E1084	0(3)
E1085	0(3)
E1086	0(3)
E1087	0(3)
E1088	0(3)
E1089	0(3)
E1090	0(3)
E1092	0(3)
E1093	0(3)
E1100	0(3)
E1110	0(3)
E1130	0(3)
E1140	0(3)
E1150	0(3)
E1160	0(3)
E1161	0(3)
E1170	0(3)
E1171	0(3)
E1172	0(3)
E1180	0(3)
E1190	0(3)
E1195	0(3)
E1200	0(3)
E1220	0(3)
E1221	0(3)
E1222	0(3)
E1223	0(3)
E1224	0(3)
E1225	0(3)
E1226	0(3)
E1227	0(3)
E1228	0(3)
E1229	0(3)
E1230	0(3)
E1231	0(3)
E1232	0(3)
E1233	0(3)
E1234	0(3)
E1235	0(3)
E1236	0(3)

CPT	MUE
E1237	0(3)
E1238	0(3)
E1239	0(3)
E1240	0(3)
E1250	0(3)
E1260	0(3)
E1270	0(3)
E1280	0(3)
E1285	0(3)
E1290	0(3)
E1295	0(3)
E1296	0(3)
E1297	0(3)
E1298	0(3)
E1300	0(3)
E1310	0(3)
E1352	0(3)
E1353	0(3)
E1354	0(3)
E1355	0(3)
E1356	0(3)
E1357	0(3)
E1358	0(3)
E1372	0(3)
E1390	0(3)
E1391	0(3)
E1392	0(3)
E1399	1(3)
E1405	0(3)
E1406	0(3)
E1500	0(3)
E1510	0(3)
E1520	0(3)
E1530	0(3)
E1540	0(3)
E1550	0(3)
E1560	0(3)
E1570	0(3)
E1575	0(3)
E1580	0(3)
E1590	0(3)
E1592	0(3)
E1594	0(3)
E1600	0(3)
E1610	0(3)
E1615	0(3)
E1620	0(3)
E1625	0(3)
E1630	0(3)
E1632	0(3)
E1634	0(3)
E1635	0(3)
E1636	0(3)
E1637	0(3)
E1639	0(3)
E1699	0(3)
E1700	0(3)
E1701	0(3)
E1702	0(3)
E1800	0(3)
E1801	0(3)
E1802	0(3)
E1805	0(3)
E1806	0(3)
E1810	0(3)

CPT	MUE
E1811	0(3)
E1812	0(3)
E1815	0(3)
E1816	0(3)
E1818	0(3)
E1820	0(3)
E1821	0(3)
E1825	0(3)
E1830	0(3)
E1831	0(3)
E1840	0(3)
E1841	0(3)
E1902	0(3)
E2000	0(3)
E2100	0(3)
E2101	0(3)
E2120	0(3)
E2201	0(3)
E2202	0(3)
E2203	0(3)
E2204	0(3)
E2205	0(3)
E2206	0(3)
E2207	0(3)
E2208	0(3)
E2209	0(3)
E2210	0(3)
E2211	0(3)
E2212	0(3)
E2213	0(3)
E2214	0(3)
E2215	0(3)
E2216	0(3)
E2217	0(3)
E2218	0(3)
E2219	0(3)
E2220	0(3)
E2221	0(3)
E2222	0(3)
E2224	0(3)
E2225	0(3)
E2226	0(3)
E2227	0(3)
E2228	0(3)
E2230	0(3)
E2231	0(3)
E2291	1(2)
E2292	1(2)
E2293	1(2)
E2294	1(2)
E2295	0(3)
E2300	0(3)
E2301	0(3)
E2310	0(3)
E2311	0(3)
E2312	0(3)
E2313	0(3)
E2321	0(3)
E2322	0(3)
E2323	0(3)
E2324	0(3)
E2325	0(3)
E2326	0(3)
E2327	0(3)
E2328	0(3)

CPT	MUE
E2329	0(3)
E2330	0(3)
E2331	0(3)
E2340	0(3)
E2341	0(3)
E2342	0(3)
E2343	0(3)
E2351	0(3)
E2358	0(3)
E2359	0(3)
E2360	0(3)
E2361	0(3)
E2362	0(3)
E2363	0(3)
E2364	0(3)
E2365	0(3)
E2366	0(3)
E2367	0(3)
E2368	0(3)
E2369	0(3)
E2370	0(3)
E2371	0(3)
E2372	0(3)
E2373	0(3)
E2374	0(3)
E2375	0(3)
E2376	0(3)
E2377	0(3)
E2378	0(3)
E2381	0(3)
E2382	0(3)
E2383	0(3)
E2384	0(3)
E2385	0(3)
E2386	0(3)
E2387	0(3)
E2388	0(3)
E2389	0(3)
E2390	0(3)
E2391	0(3)
E2392	0(3)
E2394	0(3)
E2395	0(3)
E2396	0(3)
E2397	0(3)
E2398	0(3)
E2402	0(3)
E2500	0(3)
E2502	0(3)
E2504	0(3)
E2506	0(3)
E2508	0(3)
E2510	0(3)
E2511	0(3)
E2512	0(3)
E2599	0(3)
E2601	0(3)
E2602	0(3)
E2603	0(3)
E2604	0(3)
E2605	0(3)
E2606	0(3)
E2607	0(3)
E2608	0(3)
E2609	0(3)

CPT	MUE
E2610	0(3)
E2611	0(3)
E2612	0(3)
E2613	0(3)
E2614	0(3)
E2615	0(3)
E2616	0(3)
E2617	0(3)
E2619	0(3)
E2620	0(3)
E2621	0(3)
E2622	0(3)
E2623	0(3)
E2624	0(3)
E2625	0(3)
E2626	0(3)
E2627	0(3)
E2628	0(3)
E2629	0(3)
E2630	0(3)
E2631	0(3)
E2632	0(3)
E2633	0(3)
E8000	0(3)
E8001	0(3)
E8002	0(3)
G0008	1(2)
G0009	1(2)
G0010	1(3)
G0027	1(2)
G0068	16(3)
G0069	16(3)
G0070	16(3)
G0071	1(3)
G0076	1(3)
G0077	1(3)
G0078	1(3)
G0079	1(3)
G0080	1(3)
G0081	1(3)
G0082	1(3)
G0083	1(3)
G0084	1(3)
G0085	1(3)
G0086	1(3)
G0087	1(3)
G0101	1(2)
G0102	1(2)
G0103	1(2)
G0104	1(2)
G0105	1(2)
G0106	1(2)
G0108	6(3)
G0109	12(3)
G0117	1(2)
G0118	1(2)
G0120	1(2)
G0121	1(2)
G0122	0(3)
G0123	1(3)
G0124	1(3)
G0127	1(2)
G0128	1(3)
G0130	1(2)
G0141	1(3)

CPT	MUE
G0143	1(3)
G0144	1(3)
G0145	1(3)
G0147	1(3)
G0148	1(3)
G0166	2(3)
G0168	2(3)
G0175	1(3)
G0177	0(3)
G0179	1(2)
G0180	1(2)
G0181	1(2)
G0182	1(2)
G0186	1(2)
G0219	0(3)
G0235	1(3)
G0237	8(3)
G0238	8(3)
G0239	1(3)
G0245	1(2)
G0246	1(2)
G0247	1(2)
G0248	1(2)
G0249	3(3)
G0250	1(2)
G0252	0(3)
G0255	0(3)
G0257	0(3)
G0259	2(3)
G0260	2(3)
G0268	1(2)
G0269	0(3)
G0270	8(3)
G0271	4(3)
G0276	1(3)
G0277	5(3)
G0278	1(2)
G0279	1(2)
G0281	1(3)
G0282	0(3)
G0283	1(3)
G0288	1(2)
G0289	1(2)
G0293	1(2)
G0294	1(2)
G0295	0(3)
G0296	1(2)
G0297	1(2)
G0302	1(2)
G0303	1(2)
G0304	1(2)
G0305	1(2)
G0306	1(3)
G0307	1(3)
G0328	1(2)
G0329	1(3)
G0333	0(3)
G0337	1(2)
G0339	1(2)
G0340	1(3)
G0341	1(2)
G0342	1(2)
G0343	1(2)
G0372	1(2)
G0378	0(3)

CPT	MUE
G0379	0(3)
G0380	0(3)
G0381	0(3)
G0382	0(3)
G0383	0(3)
G0384	0(3)
G0390	0(3)
G0396	1(2)
G0397	1(2)
G0398	1(2)
G0399	1(2)
G0400	1(2)
G0402	1(2)
G0403	1(2)
G0404	1(2)
G0405	1(2)
G0406	1(3)
G0407	1(3)
G0408	1(3)
G0410	4(3)
G0411	4(3)
G0412	1(2)
G0413	1(2)
G0414	1(2)
G0415	1(2)
G0416	1(2)
G0420	2(3)
G0421	2(3)
G0422	6(2)
G0423	6(2)
G0424	2(2)
G0425	1(3)
G0426	1(3)
G0427	1(3)
G0428	0(3)
G0429	1(2)
G0432	1(2)
G0433	1(2)
G0435	1(2)
G0438	1(2)
G0439	1(2)
G0442	1(2)
G0443	1(2)
G0444	1(2)
G0445	1(2)
G0446	1(3)
G0447	4(3)
G0448	1(3)
G0451	1(3)
G0452	6(3)
G0453	40(3)
G0454	1(2)
G0455	1(2)
G0458	1(3)
G0459	1(3)
G0460	1(3)
G0463	0(3)
G0466	1(2)
G0467	1(3)
G0468	1(2)
G0469	1(2)
G0470	1(3)
G0471	2(3)
G0472	1(2)
G0473	1(3)

CPT	MUE
G0475	1(2)
G0476	1(2)
G0480	1(2)
G0481	1(2)
G0482	1(2)
G0483	1(2)
G0490	1(3)
G0491	1(3)
G0492	1(3)
G0493	1(3)
G0494	1(3)
G0495	1(3)
G0496	1(3)
G0498	1(2)
G0499	1(2)
G0500	1(3)
G0501	0(3)
G0506	1(2)
G0508	1(2)
G0509	1(2)
G0511	1(2)
G0512	1(2)
G0513	1(2)
G0514	1(1)
G0516	1(2)
G0517	1(2)
G0518	1(2)
G0659	1(2)
G2000	1(3)
G2001	1(3)
G2002	1(3)
G2003	1(3)
G2004	1(3)
G2005	1(3)
G2006	1(3)
G2007	1(3)
G2008	1(3)
G2009	1(3)
G2010	1(3)
G2011	1(2)
G2012	1(3)
G2013	1(3)
G2014	1(3)
G2015	1(3)
G2023	2(3)
G2024	2(3)
G2058	2(3)
G2061	1(2)
G2062	1(2)
G2063	1(2)
G2064	1(2)
G2065	1(2)
G2066	1(2)
G2067	1(2)
G2068	1(2)
G2069	1(2)
G2070	1(2)
G2071	1(2)
G2072	1(2)
G2073	1(2)
G2074	1(2)
G2075	1(2)
G2076	1(2)
G2078	3(3)
G2079	3(3)

CPT	MUE
G2081	1(2)
G2082	1(2)
G2083	1(2)
G2086	1(3)
G2087	2(3)
G6001	2(3)
G6002	2(3)
G6003	2(3)
G6004	2(3)
G6005	2(3)
G6006	2(3)
G6007	2(3)
G6008	2(3)
G6009	2(3)
G6010	2(3)
G6011	2(3)
G6012	2(3)
G6013	2(3)
G6014	2(3)
G6015	2(3)
G6016	2(3)
G6017	2(3)
G9143	1(2)
G9147	0(3)
G9148	1(3)
G9149	1(3)
G9150	1(3)
G9151	1(3)
G9152	1(3)
G9153	1(3)
G9156	1(2)
G9157	1(2)
G9187	1(3)
G9480	1(3)
G9481	1(3)
G9482	1(3)
G9483	1(3)
G9484	1(3)
G9485	1(3)
G9486	1(3)
G9487	1(3)
G9488	1(3)
G9489	1(3)
G9490	1(3)
G9678	1(2)
G9685	1(3)
G9978	1(3)
G9979	1(3)
G9980	1(3)
G9981	1(3)
G9982	1(3)
G9983	1(3)
G9984	1(3)
G9985	1(3)
G9986	1(3)
G9987	1(3)
J0120	1(3)
J0121	200(3)
J0122	300(3)
J0129	100(3)
J0130	4(3)
J0131	400(3)
J0132	12(3)
J0133	1200(3)
J0135	8(3)

CPT	MUE
J0153	180(3)
J0171	20(3)
J0178	4(2)
J0179	12(2)
J0180	140(3)
J0185	130(3)
J0190	0(3)
J0200	0(3)
J0202	12(3)
J0205	0(3)
J0207	4(3)
J0210	4(3)
J0215	30(3)
J0220	1(3)
J0221	250(3)
J0222	300(3)
J0223	756(3)
J0256	1600(3)
J0257	1400(3)
J0270	32(3)
J0275	1(3)
J0278	15(3)
J0280	7(3)
J0282	5(3)
J0285	5(3)
J0287	50(3)
J0288	0(3)
J0289	50(3)
J0290	24(3)
J0291	500(3)
J0295	12(3)
J0300	8(3)
J0330	10(3)
J0348	200(3)
J0350	0(3)
J0360	2(3)
J0364	6(3)
J0365	0(3)
J0380	1(3)
J0390	0(3)
J0395	0(3)
J0400	39(3)
J0401	400(3)
J0456	4(3)
J0461	200(3)
J0470	2(3)
J0475	8(3)
J0476	2(3)
J0480	1(3)
J0485	1500(3)
J0490	160(3)
J0500	4(3)
J0515	3(3)
J0517	30(3)
J0520	0(3)
J0558	24(3)
J0561	24(3)
J0565	200(3)
J0567	300(3)
J0570	4(3)
J0571	0(3)
J0572	0(3)
J0573	0(3)
J0574	0(3)
J0575	0(3)

CPT	MUE
J0583	250(3)
J0584	90(3)
J0585	600(3)
J0586	300(3)
J0587	300(3)
J0588	600(3)
J0592	6(3)
J0593	300(3)
J0594	320(3)
J0595	8(3)
J0596	840(3)
J0597	250(3)
J0598	100(3)
J0599	900(3)
J0600	3(3)
J0606	150(3)
J0610	15(3)
J0620	1(3)
J0630	1(3)
J0636	100(3)
J0637	20(3)
J0638	300(3)
J0640	24(3)
J0641	600(3)
J0642	600(3)
J0670	10(3)
J0690	12(3)
J0691	300(3)
J0692	12(3)
J0694	8(3)
J0695	60(3)
J0696	16(3)
J0697	4(3)
J0698	10(3)
J0702	18(3)
J0706	1(3)
J0710	0(3)
J0712	120(3)
J0713	12(3)
J0714	4(3)
J0715	0(3)
J0716	4(3)
J0717	400(3)
J0720	15(3)
J0725	10(3)
J0735	50(3)
J0740	2(3)
J0743	16(3)
J0744	6(3)
J0745	2(3)
J0770	5(3)
J0775	180(3)
J0780	4(3)
J0795	100(3)
J0800	3(3)
J0834	3(3)
J0840	6(3)
J0841	20(3)
J0850	9(3)
J0875	300(3)
J0878	1500(3)
J0881	500(3)
J0882	300(3)
J0883	1125(3)
J0884	1125(3)

CPT	MUE
J0885	60(3)
J0887	360(3)
J0888	360(3)
J0890	0(3)
J0894	100(3)
J0895	12(3)
J0897	120(3)
J0945	4(3)
J1000	1(3)
J1020	8(3)
J1030	8(3)
J1040	4(3)
J1050	1000(3)
J1071	400(3)
J1094	0(3)
J1095	1034(2)
J1096	4(3)
J1097	4(3)
J1100	120(3)
J1110	3(3)
J1120	2(3)
J1130	300(3)
J1160	2(3)
J1162	1(3)
J1165	50(3)
J1170	350(3)
J1180	0(3)
J1190	8(3)
J1200	8(3)
J1205	4(3)
J1212	1(3)
J1230	3(3)
J1240	6(3)
J1245	6(3)
J1250	2(3)
J1260	2(3)
J1265	20(3)
J1267	150(3)
J1270	8(3)
J1290	30(3)
J1300	120(3)
J1301	60(3)
J1303	360(3)
J1320	0(3)
J1322	150(3)
J1324	108(3)
J1325	1(3)
J1327	1(3)
J1330	1(3)
J1335	2(3)
J1364	2(3)
J1380	4(3)
J1410	4(3)
J1428	450(3)
J1430	10(3)
J1435	1(3)
J1436	0(3)
J1438	2(3)
J1439	750(3)
J1442	1500(3)
J1443	272(3)
J1444	272(3)
J1447	960(3)
J1450	4(3)
J1451	1(3)

CPT	MUE
J1452	0(3)
J1453	150(3)
J1454	1(3)
J1455	18(3)
J1457	0(3)
J1458	100(3)
J1459	300(3)
J1460	10(2)
J1555	480(3)
J1556	300(3)
J1557	300(3)
J1559	300(3)
J1560	1(2)
J1561	300(3)
J1562	0(3)
J1566	300(3)
J1568	300(3)
J1569	300(3)
J1570	4(3)
J1571	20(3)
J1572	300(3)
J1573	130(3)
J1575	650(3)
J1580	9(3)
J1595	1(3)
J1599	300(3)
J1600	2(3)
J1602	300(3)
J1610	2(3)
J1620	0(3)
J1626	30(3)
J1627	100(3)
J1628	100(3)
J1630	5(3)
J1631	9(3)
J1640	672(3)
J1642	100(3)
J1644	40(3)
J1645	10(3)
J1650	30(3)
J1652	20(3)
J1655	0(3)
J1670	1(3)
J1675	0(3)
J1700	0(3)
J1710	0(3)
J1720	10(3)
J1726	28(3)
J1729	25(3)
J1730	0(3)
J1740	3(3)
J1741	8(3)
J1742	2(3)
J1743	66(3)
J1744	30(3)
J1745	150(3)
J1746	200(3)
J1750	45(3)
J1756	500(3)
J1786	680(3)
J1790	2(3)
J1800	6(3)
J1810	0(3)
J1815	8(3)
J1817	0(3)

CPT	MUE
J1826	1(3)
J1830	1(3)
J1833	372(3)
J1835	0(3)
J1840	3(3)
J1850	4(3)
J1885	8(3)
J1890	0(3)
J1930	120(3)
J1931	377(3)
J1940	6(3)
J1943	675(3)
J1944	1064(3)
J1945	0(3)
J1950	12(3)
J1953	300(3)
J1955	11(3)
J1956	4(3)
J1960	0(3)
J1980	2(3)
J1990	0(3)
J2001	60(3)
J2010	10(3)
J2020	6(3)
J2060	4(3)
J2062	10(3)
J2150	8(3)
J2170	8(3)
J2175	4(3)
J2180	0(3)
J2182	300(3)
J2185	30(3)
J2186	600(3)
J2210	1(3)
J2212	240(3)
J2248	150(3)
J2250	22(3)
J2260	4(3)
J2265	400(3)
J2270	9(3)
J2274	250(3)
J2278	1000(3)
J2280	4(3)
J2300	4(3)
J2310	4(3)
J2315	380(3)
J2320	4(3)
J2323	300(3)
J2325	0(3)
J2326	120(3)
J2350	600(3)
J2353	60(3)
J2354	60(3)
J2355	2(3)
J2357	90(3)
J2358	405(3)
J2360	2(3)
J2370	2(3)
J2400	4(3)
J2405	64(3)
J2407	120(3)
J2410	2(3)
J2425	125(3)
J2426	819(3)
J2430	3(3)

CPT	MUE
J2440	4(3)
J2460	0(3)
J2469	10(3)
J2501	2(3)
J2502	60(3)
J2503	2(3)
J2504	15(3)
J2505	1(3)
J2507	8(3)
J2510	4(3)
J2513	1(3)
J2515	1(3)
J2540	75(3)
J2543	16(3)
J2545	1(3)
J2547	600(3)
J2550	3(3)
J2560	1(3)
J2562	48(3)
J2590	3(3)
J2597	45(3)
J2650	0(3)
J2670	0(3)
J2675	1(3)
J2680	4(3)
J2690	4(3)
J2700	48(3)
J2704	80(3)
J2710	2(3)
J2720	5(3)
J2724	3500(3)
J2725	0(3)
J2730	2(3)
J2760	2(3)
J2765	10(3)
J2770	6(3)
J2778	10(2)
J2780	16(3)
J2783	60(3)
J2785	4(3)
J2786	500(3)
J2787	2(3)
J2788	1(3)
J2790	1(3)
J2791	15(3)
J2792	450(3)
J2793	320(3)
J2794	100(3)
J2795	200(3)
J2796	150(3)
J2797	333(3)
J2798	240(3)
J2800	3(3)
J2805	3(3)
J2810	5(3)
J2820	15(3)
J2840	160(3)
J2850	16(3)
J2860	170(3)
J2910	0(3)
J2916	20(3)
J2920	25(3)
J2930	25(3)
J2940	0(3)
J2941	8(3)

CPT	MUE
J2950	0(3)
J2993	2(3)
J2995	0(3)
J2997	8(3)
J3000	2(3)
J3010	100(3)
J3030	1(3)
J3031	675(3)
J3060	760(3)
J3070	3(3)
J3090	200(3)
J3095	150(3)
J3101	50(3)
J3105	2(3)
J3110	2(3)
J3111	210(3)
J3121	400(3)
J3145	750(3)
J3230	2(3)
J3240	1(3)
J3243	150(3)
J3245	100(3)
J3246	1(3)
J3250	2(3)
J3260	8(3)
J3262	800(3)
J3265	0(3)
J3280	0(3)
J3285	1(3)
J3300	160(3)
J3301	16(3)
J3302	0(3)
J3303	24(3)
J3304	64(2)
J3305	0(3)
J3310	0(3)
J3315	6(3)
J3316	6(3)
J3320	0(3)
J3350	0(3)
J3355	1(3)
J3357	90(3)
J3358	520(3)
J3360	6(3)
J3364	0(3)
J3365	0(3)
J3370	12(3)
J3380	300(3)
J3385	80(3)
J3396	150(3)
J3397	600(3)
J3398	150(2)
J3400	0(3)
J3410	8(3)
J3411	4(3)
J3415	6(3)
J3420	1(3)
J3430	25(3)
J3465	40(3)
J3470	3(3)
J3471	999(2)
J3472	2(3)
J3473	450(3)
J3475	20(3)
J3480	40(3)

CPT	MUE
J3485	160(3)
J3486	4(3)
J3489	5(3)
J3520	0(3)
J3530	0(3)
J3535	0(3)
J3570	0(3)
J7030	5(3)
J7040	6(3)
J7042	6(3)
J7050	10(3)
J7060	10(3)
J7070	4(3)
J7100	2(3)
J7110	2(3)
J7120	4(3)
J7121	4(3)
J7131	500(3)
J7169	180(3)
J7170	1800(3)
J7175	9000(1)
J7177	10500(3)
J7178	7700(1)
J7179	7500(1)
J7180	6000(1)
J7181	3850(1)
J7182	22000(1)
J7183	7500(1)
J7185	22000(1)
J7186	7500(1)
J7187	7500(1)
J7188	22000(1)
J7189	13000(1)
J7190	22000(1)
J7191	0(3)
J7192	22000(1)
J7193	4000(1)
J7194	9000(1)
J7195	6000(1)
J7196	175(3)
J7197	6300(1)
J7198	6000(1)
J7200	20000(1)
J7201	9000(1)
J7202	11550(1)
J7203	12000(1)
J7205	9750(1)
J7207	22500(1)
J7208	12000(1)
J7209	7500(1)
J7210	22000(1)
J7211	22000(1)
J7296	0(3)
J7297	0(3)
J7298	0(3)
J7300	0(3)
J7301	0(3)
J7303	0(3)
J7304	0(3)
J7306	0(3)
J7307	0(3)
J7308	3(3)
J7309	1(3)
J7310	0(3)
J7311	118(2)

CPT	MUE
J7312	14(2)
J7313	38(2)
J7314	36(2)
J7315	2(3)
J7316	3(3)
J7318	120(3)
J7320	50(3)
J7321	2(2)
J7322	48(3)
J7323	2(2)
J7324	2(2)
J7325	96(3)
J7326	2(2)
J7327	2(2)
J7328	336(3)
J7329	50(2)
J7330	1(3)
J7331	40(3)
J7332	40(3)
J7336	1120(3)
J7340	1(3)
J7342	10(3)
J7345	200(3)
J7401	270(2)
J7500	0(3)
J7501	1(3)
J7502	0(3)
J7503	0(3)
J7504	15(3)
J7505	1(3)
J7507	0(3)
J7508	0(3)
J7509	0(3)
J7510	0(3)
J7511	9(3)
J7512	0(3)
J7513	0(3)
J7515	0(3)
J7516	1(3)
J7517	0(3)
J7518	0(3)
J7520	0(3)
J7525	2(3)
J7527	0(3)
J7599	1(3)
J7604	0(3)
J7605	2(3)
J7606	2(3)
J7607	0(3)
J7608	3(3)
J7609	0(3)
J7610	0(3)
J7611	10(3)
J7612	10(3)
J7613	10(3)
J7614	10(3)
J7615	0(3)
J7620	6(3)
J7622	0(3)
J7624	0(3)
J7626	2(3)
J7627	0(3)
J7628	0(3)
J7629	0(3)
J7631	4(3)

CPT	MUE
J7632	0(3)
J7633	0(3)
J7634	0(3)
J7635	0(3)
J7636	0(3)
J7637	0(3)
J7638	0(3)
J7639	3(3)
J7640	0(3)
J7641	0(3)
J7642	0(3)
J7643	0(3)
J7644	3(3)
J7645	0(3)
J7647	0(3)
J7648	0(3)
J7649	0(3)
J7650	0(3)
J7657	0(3)
J7658	0(3)
J7659	0(3)
J7660	0(3)
J7665	0(3)
J7667	0(3)
J7668	0(3)
J7669	0(3)
J7670	0(3)
J7674	100(3)
J7676	0(3)
J7677	175(3)
J7680	0(3)
J7681	0(3)
J7682	2(3)
J7683	0(3)
J7684	0(3)
J7685	0(3)
J7686	1(3)
J7699	1(3)
J7799	2(3)
J7999	2(3)
J8498	0(3)
J8499	0(3)
J8501	0(3)
J8510	0(3)
J8515	0(3)
J8520	0(3)
J8521	0(3)
J8530	0(3)
J8540	0(3)
J8560	0(3)
J8562	0(3)
J8565	0(3)
J8597	0(3)
J8600	0(3)
J8610	0(3)
J8650	0(3)
J8655	1(3)
J8670	0(3)
J8700	0(3)
J8705	0(3)
J8999	0(3)
J9000	20(3)
J9015	1(3)
J9017	30(3)
J9019	60(3)

CPT	MUE
J9020	0(3)
J9022	168(3)
J9023	140(3)
J9025	300(3)
J9027	100(3)
J9030	50(3)
J9032	300(3)
J9033	300(3)
J9034	360(3)
J9035	170(3)
J9036	360(3)
J9039	210(3)
J9040	4(3)
J9041	35(3)
J9042	200(3)
J9043	60(3)
J9044	35(3)
J9045	22(3)
J9047	160(3)
J9050	6(3)
J9055	120(3)
J9057	60(3)
J9060	24(3)
J9065	100(3)
J9070	55(3)
J9098	5(3)
J9100	120(3)
J9118	750(3)
J9119	350(3)
J9120	5(3)
J9130	24(3)
J9145	240(3)
J9150	12(3)
J9151	12(3)
J9153	132(3)
J9155	240(3)
J9160	7(3)
J9165	0(3)
J9171	240(3)
J9173	150(3)
J9175	10(3)
J9176	3000(3)
J9178	150(3)
J9179	50(3)
J9181	100(3)
J9185	2(3)
J9190	20(3)
J9200	5(3)
J9201	20(3)
J9202	3(3)
J9203	180(3)
J9204	160(3)
J9205	215(3)
J9206	42(3)
J9207	90(3)
J9208	15(3)
J9209	55(3)
J9210	1500(3)
J9211	6(3)
J9212	0(3)
J9213	12(3)
J9214	100(3)
J9215	0(3)
J9216	2(3)
J9217	6(3)

CPT	MUE
J9218	1(3)
J9219	1(3)
J9225	1(3)
J9226	1(3)
J9228	1100(3)
J9229	27(3)
J9230	5(3)
J9245	9(3)
J9250	25(3)
J9260	20(3)
J9261	80(3)
J9262	700(3)
J9263	700(3)
J9264	600(3)
J9266	2(3)
J9267	750(3)
J9268	1(3)
J9270	0(3)
J9271	400(3)
J9280	12(3)
J9285	200(3)
J9293	8(3)
J9295	800(3)
J9299	480(3)
J9301	100(3)
J9302	200(3)
J9303	90(3)
J9305	150(3)
J9306	840(3)
J9307	60(3)
J9308	280(3)
J9309	280(3)
J9311	160(3)
J9312	150(3)
J9313	600(3)
J9315	40(3)
J9320	4(3)
J9325	400(3)
J9328	400(3)
J9330	50(3)
J9340	4(3)
J9351	120(3)
J9352	40(3)
J9354	600(3)
J9355	105(3)
J9356	60(3)
J9357	4(3)
J9360	40(3)
J9370	4(3)
J9371	5(3)
J9390	36(3)
J9395	20(3)
J9400	500(3)
J9600	4(3)
K0001	0(3)
K0002	0(3)
K0003	0(3)
K0004	0(3)
K0005	0(3)
K0006	0(3)
K0007	0(3)
K0008	0(3)
K0009	0(3)
K0010	0(3)
K0011	0(3)

CPT	MUE
K0012	0(3)
K0013	0(3)
K0014	0(3)
K0015	0(3)
K0017	0(3)
K0018	0(3)
K0019	0(3)
K0020	0(3)
K0037	0(3)
K0038	0(3)
K0039	0(3)
K0040	0(3)
K0041	0(3)
K0042	0(3)
K0043	0(3)
K0044	0(3)
K0045	0(3)
K0046	0(3)
K0047	0(3)
K0050	0(3)
K0051	0(3)
K0052	0(3)
K0053	0(3)
K0056	0(3)
K0065	0(3)
K0069	0(3)
K0070	0(3)
K0071	0(3)
K0072	0(3)
K0073	0(3)
K0077	0(3)
K0098	0(3)
K0105	0(3)
K0108	0(3)
K0195	0(3)
K0455	0(3)
K0462	0(3)
K0553	0(3)
K0554	0(3)
K0602	0(3)
K0604	0(3)
K0605	0(3)
K0606	0(3)
K0607	0(3)
K0608	0(3)
K0609	0(3)
K0669	0(3)
K0672	0(3)
K0730	0(3)
K0733	0(3)
K0738	0(3)
K0740	0(3)
K0743	0(3)
K0744	0(3)
K0745	0(3)
K0746	0(3)
K0800	0(3)
K0801	0(3)
K0802	0(3)
K0806	0(3)
K0807	0(3)
K0808	0(3)
K0812	0(3)
K0813	0(3)
K0814	0(3)

CPT	MUE
K0815	0(3)
K0816	0(3)
K0820	0(3)
K0821	0(3)
K0822	0(3)
K0823	0(3)
K0824	0(3)
K0825	0(3)
K0826	0(3)
K0827	0(3)
K0828	0(3)
K0829	0(3)
K0830	0(3)
K0831	0(3)
K0835	0(3)
K0836	0(3)
K0837	0(3)
K0838	0(3)
K0839	0(3)
K0840	0(3)
K0841	0(3)
K0842	0(3)
K0843	0(3)
K0848	0(3)
K0849	0(3)
K0850	0(3)
K0851	0(3)
K0852	0(3)
K0853	0(3)
K0854	0(3)
K0855	0(3)
K0856	0(3)
K0857	0(3)
K0858	0(3)
K0859	0(3)
K0860	0(3)
K0861	0(3)
K0862	0(3)
K0863	0(3)
K0864	0(3)
K0868	0(3)
K0869	0(3)
K0870	0(3)
K0871	0(3)
K0877	0(3)
K0878	0(3)
K0879	0(3)
K0880	0(3)
K0884	0(3)
K0885	0(3)
K0886	0(3)
K0890	0(3)
K0891	0(3)
K0898	1(2)
K0899	0(3)
K0900	0(3)
K1001	0(3)
K1002	0(3)
K1003	0(3)
K1004	0(3)
K1005	0(3)
L0112	0(3)
L0113	0(3)
L0120	0(3)
L0130	0(3)

CPT	MUE
L0140	0(3)
L0150	0(3)
L0160	0(3)
L0170	0(3)
L0172	0(3)
L0174	0(3)
L0180	0(3)
L0190	0(3)
L0200	0(3)
L0220	0(3)
L0450	0(3)
L0452	0(3)
L0454	0(3)
L0455	0(3)
L0456	0(3)
L0457	0(3)
L0458	0(3)
L0460	0(3)
L0462	0(3)
L0464	0(3)
L0466	0(3)
L0467	0(3)
L0468	0(3)
L0469	0(3)
L0470	0(3)
L0472	0(3)
L0480	0(3)
L0482	0(3)
L0484	0(3)
L0486	0(3)
L0488	0(3)
L0490	0(3)
L0491	0(3)
L0492	0(3)
L0621	0(3)
L0622	0(3)
L0623	0(3)
L0624	0(3)
L0625	0(3)
L0626	0(3)
L0627	0(3)
L0628	0(3)
L0629	0(3)
L0630	0(3)
L0631	0(3)
L0632	0(3)
L0633	0(3)
L0634	0(3)
L0635	0(3)
L0636	0(3)
L0637	0(3)
L0638	0(3)
L0639	0(3)
L0640	0(3)
L0641	0(3)
L0642	0(3)
L0643	0(3)
L0648	0(3)
L0649	0(3)
L0650	0(3)
L0651	0(3)
L0700	0(3)
L0710	0(3)
L0810	0(3)
L0820	0(3)

CPT	MUE
L0830	0(3)
L0859	0(3)
L0861	0(3)
L0970	0(3)
L0972	0(3)
L0974	0(3)
L0976	0(3)
L0978	0(3)
L0980	0(3)
L0982	0(3)
L0984	0(3)
L0999	0(3)
L1000	0(3)
L1001	0(3)
L1005	0(3)
L1010	0(3)
L1020	0(3)
L1025	0(3)
L1030	0(3)
L1040	0(3)
L1050	0(3)
L1060	0(3)
L1070	0(3)
L1080	0(3)
L1085	0(3)
L1090	0(3)
L1100	0(3)
L1110	0(3)
L1120	0(3)
L1200	0(3)
L1210	0(3)
L1220	0(3)
L1230	0(3)
L1240	0(3)
L1250	0(3)
L1260	0(3)
L1270	0(3)
L1280	0(3)
L1290	0(3)
L1300	0(3)
L1310	0(3)
L1499	1(3)
L1600	0(3)
L1610	0(3)
L1620	0(3)
L1630	0(3)
L1640	0(3)
L1650	0(3)
L1652	0(3)
L1660	0(3)
L1680	0(3)
L1685	0(3)
L1686	0(3)
L1690	0(3)
L1700	0(3)
L1710	0(3)
L1720	0(3)
L1730	0(3)
L1755	0(3)
L1810	0(3)
L1812	0(3)
L1820	0(3)
L1830	0(3)
L1831	0(3)
L1832	0(3)

CPT	MUE
L1833	0(3)
L1834	0(3)
L1836	0(3)
L1840	0(3)
L1843	0(3)
L1844	0(3)
L1845	0(3)
L1846	0(3)
L1847	0(3)
L1848	0(3)
L1850	0(3)
L1851	0(3)
L1852	0(3)
L1860	0(3)
L1900	0(3)
L1902	0(3)
L1904	0(3)
L1906	0(3)
L1907	0(3)
L1910	0(3)
L1920	0(3)
L1930	0(3)
L1932	0(3)
L1940	0(3)
L1945	0(3)
L1950	0(3)
L1951	0(3)
L1960	0(3)
L1970	0(3)
L1971	0(3)
L1980	0(3)
L1990	0(3)
L2000	0(3)
L2005	0(3)
L2006	0(3)
L2010	0(3)
L2020	0(3)
L2030	0(3)
L2034	0(3)
L2035	0(3)
L2036	0(3)
L2037	0(3)
L2038	0(3)
L2040	0(3)
L2050	0(3)
L2060	0(3)
L2070	0(3)
L2080	0(3)
L2090	0(3)
L2106	0(3)
L2108	0(3)
L2112	0(3)
L2114	0(3)
L2116	0(3)
L2126	0(3)
L2128	0(3)
L2132	0(3)
L2134	0(3)
L2136	0(3)
L2180	0(3)
L2182	0(3)
L2184	0(3)
L2186	0(3)
L2188	0(3)
L2190	0(3)

CPT	MUE
L2192	0(3)
L2200	0(3)
L2210	0(3)
L2220	0(3)
L2230	0(3)
L2232	0(3)
L2240	0(3)
L2250	0(3)
L2260	0(3)
L2265	0(3)
L2270	0(3)
L2275	0(3)
L2280	0(3)
L2300	0(3)
L2310	0(3)
L2320	0(3)
L2330	0(3)
L2335	0(3)
L2340	0(3)
L2350	0(3)
L2360	0(3)
L2370	0(3)
L2375	0(3)
L2380	0(3)
L2385	0(3)
L2387	0(3)
L2390	0(3)
L2395	0(3)
L2397	0(3)
L2405	0(3)
L2415	0(3)
L2425	0(3)
L2430	0(3)
L2492	0(3)
L2500	0(3)
L2510	0(3)
L2520	0(3)
L2525	0(3)
L2526	0(3)
L2530	0(3)
L2540	0(3)
L2550	0(3)
L2570	0(3)
L2580	0(3)
L2600	0(3)
L2610	0(3)
L2620	0(3)
L2622	0(3)
L2624	0(3)
L2627	0(3)
L2628	0(3)
L2630	0(3)
L2640	0(3)
L2650	0(3)
L2660	0(3)
L2670	0(3)
L2680	0(3)
L2750	0(3)
L2755	0(3)
L2760	0(3)
L2768	0(3)
L2780	0(3)
L2785	0(3)
L2795	0(3)
L2800	0(3)

CPT	MUE
L2810	0(3)
L2820	0(3)
L2830	0(3)
L2840	0(3)
L2850	0(3)
L2861	0(3)
L2999	0(3)
L3000	0(3)
L3001	0(3)
L3002	0(3)
L3003	0(3)
L3010	0(3)
L3020	0(3)
L3030	0(3)
L3031	0(3)
L3040	0(3)
L3050	0(3)
L3060	0(3)
L3070	0(3)
L3080	0(3)
L3090	0(3)
L3100	0(3)
L3140	0(3)
L3150	0(3)
L3160	0(3)
L3170	0(3)
L3201	0(3)
L3202	0(3)
L3203	0(3)
L3204	0(3)
L3206	0(3)
L3207	0(3)
L3208	0(3)
L3209	0(3)
L3211	0(3)
L3212	0(3)
L3213	0(3)
L3214	0(3)
L3215	0(3)
L3216	0(3)
L3217	0(3)
L3219	0(3)
L3221	0(3)
L3222	0(3)
L3224	0(3)
L3225	0(3)
L3230	0(3)
L3250	0(3)
L3251	0(3)
L3252	0(3)
L3253	0(3)
L3254	0(3)
L3255	0(3)
L3257	0(3)
L3260	0(3)
L3265	0(3)
L3300	0(3)
L3310	0(3)
L3320	0(3)
L3330	0(3)
L3332	0(3)
L3334	0(3)
L3340	0(3)
L3350	0(3)
L3360	0(3)

CPT	MUE	CPT	MUE	CPT	MUE	CPT	MUE	CPT	MUE	CPT	MUE	CPT	MUE	CPT	MUE
L3370	0(3)	L3915	0(3)	L5050	0(3)	L5647	0(3)	L5812	0(3)	L6320	0(3)	L6694	0(3)	L7402	0(3)
L3380	0(3)	L3916	0(3)	L5060	0(3)	L5648	0(3)	L5814	0(3)	L6350	0(3)	L6695	0(3)	L7403	0(3)
L3390	0(3)	L3917	0(3)	L5100	0(3)	L5649	0(3)	L5816	0(3)	L6360	0(3)	L6696	0(3)	L7404	0(3)
L3400	0(3)	L3918	0(3)	L5105	0(3)	L5650	0(3)	L5818	0(3)	L6370	0(3)	L6697	0(3)	L7405	0(3)
L3410	0(3)	L3919	0(3)	L5150	0(3)	L5651	0(3)	L5822	0(3)	L6380	0(3)	L6698	0(3)	L7499	0(3)
L3420	0(3)	L3921	0(3)	L5160	0(3)	L5652	0(3)	L5824	0(3)	L6382	0(3)	L6703	0(3)	L7510	4(3)
L3430	0(3)	L3923	0(3)	L5200	0(3)	L5653	0(3)	L5826	0(3)	L6384	0(3)	L6704	0(3)	L7600	0(3)
L3440	0(3)	L3924	0(3)	L5210	0(3)	L5654	0(3)	L5828	0(3)	L6386	0(3)	L6706	0(3)	L7700	0(3)
L3450	0(3)	L3925	0(3)	L5220	0(3)	L5655	0(3)	L5830	0(3)	L6388	0(3)	L6707	0(3)	L7900	0(3)
L3455	0(3)	L3927	0(3)	L5230	0(3)	L5656	0(3)	L5840	0(3)	L6400	0(3)	L6708	0(3)	L7902	0(3)
L3460	0(3)	L3929	0(3)	L5250	0(3)	L5658	0(3)	L5845	0(3)	L6450	0(3)	L6709	0(3)	L8000	0(3)
L3465	0(3)	L3930	0(3)	L5270	0(3)	L5661	0(3)	L5848	0(3)	L6500	0(3)	L6711	0(3)	L8001	0(3)
L3470	0(3)	L3931	0(3)	L5280	0(3)	L5665	0(3)	L5850	0(3)	L6550	0(3)	L6712	0(3)	L8002	0(3)
L3480	0(3)	L3933	0(3)	L5301	0(3)	L5666	0(3)	L5855	0(3)	L6570	0(3)	L6713	0(3)	L8010	0(3)
L3485	0(3)	L3935	0(3)	L5312	0(3)	L5668	0(3)	L5856	0(3)	L6580	0(3)	L6714	0(3)	L8015	0(3)
L3500	0(3)	L3956	0(3)	L5321	0(3)	L5670	0(3)	L5857	0(3)	L6582	0(3)	L6715	0(3)	L8020	0(3)
L3510	0(3)	L3960	0(3)	L5331	0(3)	L5671	0(3)	L5858	0(3)	L6584	0(3)	L6721	0(3)	L8030	0(3)
L3520	0(3)	L3961	0(3)	L5341	0(3)	L5672	0(3)	L5859	0(3)	L6586	0(3)	L6722	0(3)	L8031	0(3)
L3530	0(3)	L3962	0(3)	L5400	0(3)	L5673	0(3)	L5910	0(3)	L6588	0(3)	L6805	0(3)	L8032	0(3)
L3540	0(3)	L3967	0(3)	L5410	0(3)	L5676	0(3)	L5920	0(3)	L6590	0(3)	L6810	0(3)	L8033	0(3)
L3550	0(3)	L3971	0(3)	L5420	0(3)	L5677	0(3)	L5925	0(3)	L6600	0(3)	L6880	0(3)	L8035	0(3)
L3560	0(3)	L3973	0(3)	L5430	0(3)	L5678	0(3)	L5930	0(3)	L6605	0(3)	L6881	0(3)	L8039	0(3)
L3570	0(3)	L3975	0(3)	L5450	0(3)	L5679	0(3)	L5940	0(3)	L6610	0(3)	L6882	0(3)	L8040	0(3)
L3580	0(3)	L3976	0(3)	L5460	0(3)	L5680	0(3)	L5950	0(3)	L6611	0(3)	L6883	0(3)	L8041	0(3)
L3590	0(3)	L3977	0(3)	L5500	0(3)	L5681	0(3)	L5960	0(3)	L6615	0(3)	L6884	0(3)	L8042	0(3)
L3595	0(3)	L3978	0(3)	L5505	0(3)	L5682	0(3)	L5961	0(3)	L6616	0(3)	L6885	0(3)	L8043	0(3)
L3600	0(3)	L3980	0(3)	L5510	0(3)	L5683	0(3)	L5962	0(3)	L6620	0(3)	L6890	0(3)	L8044	0(3)
L3610	0(3)	L3981	0(3)	L5520	0(3)	L5684	0(3)	L5964	0(3)	L6621	0(3)	L6895	0(3)	L8045	0(3)
L3620	0(3)	L3982	0(3)	L5530	0(3)	L5685	0(3)	L5966	0(3)	L6623	0(3)	L6900	0(3)	L8046	0(3)
L3630	0(3)	L3984	0(3)	L5535	0(3)	L5686	0(3)	L5968	0(3)	L6624	0(3)	L6905	0(3)	L8047	0(3)
L3640	0(3)	L3995	0(3)	L5540	0(3)	L5688	0(3)	L5969	0(3)	L6625	0(3)	L6910	0(3)	L8048	1(3)
L3649	0(3)	L3999	0(3)	L5560	0(3)	L5690	0(3)	L5970	0(3)	L6628	0(3)	L6915	0(3)	L8049	0(3)
L3650	0(3)	L4000	0(3)	L5570	0(3)	L5692	0(3)	L5971	0(3)	L6629	0(3)	L6920	0(3)	L8300	0(3)
L3660	0(3)	L4002	0(3)	L5580	0(3)	L5694	0(3)	L5972	0(3)	L6630	0(3)	L6925	0(3)	L8310	0(3)
L3670	0(3)	L4010	0(3)	L5585	0(3)	L5695	0(3)	L5973	0(3)	L6632	0(3)	L6930	0(3)	L8320	0(3)
L3671	0(3)	L4020	0(3)	L5590	0(3)	L5696	0(3)	L5974	0(3)	L6635	0(3)	L6935	0(3)	L8330	0(3)
L3674	0(3)	L4030	0(3)	L5595	0(3)	L5697	0(3)	L5975	0(3)	L6637	0(3)	L6940	0(3)	L8400	0(3)
L3675	0(3)	L4040	0(3)	L5600	0(3)	L5698	0(3)	L5976	0(3)	L6638	0(3)	L6945	0(3)	L8410	0(3)
L3677	0(3)	L4045	0(3)	L5610	0(3)	L5699	0(3)	L5978	0(3)	L6640	0(3)	L6950	0(3)	L8415	0(3)
L3678	0(3)	L4050	0(3)	L5611	0(3)	L5700	0(3)	L5979	0(3)	L6641	0(3)	L6955	0(3)	L8417	0(3)
L3702	0(3)	L4055	0(3)	L5613	0(3)	L5701	0(3)	L5980	0(3)	L6642	0(3)	L6960	0(3)	L8420	0(3)
L3710	0(3)	L4060	0(3)	L5614	0(3)	L5702	0(3)	L5981	0(3)	L6645	0(3)	L6965	0(3)	L8430	0(3)
L3720	0(3)	L4070	0(3)	L5616	0(3)	L5703	0(3)	L5982	0(3)	L6646	0(3)	L6970	0(3)	L8435	0(3)
L3730	0(3)	L4080	0(3)	L5617	0(3)	L5704	0(3)	L5984	0(3)	L6647	0(3)	L6975	0(3)	L8440	0(3)
L3740	0(3)	L4090	0(3)	L5618	0(3)	L5705	0(3)	L5985	0(3)	L6648	0(3)	L7007	0(3)	L8460	0(3)
L3760	0(3)	L4100	0(3)	L5620	0(3)	L5706	0(3)	L5986	0(3)	L6650	0(3)	L7008	0(3)	L8465	0(3)
L3761	0(3)	L4110	0(3)	L5622	0(3)	L5707	0(3)	L5987	0(3)	L6655	0(3)	L7009	0(3)	L8470	0(3)
L3762	0(3)	L4130	0(3)	L5624	0(3)	L5710	0(3)	L5988	0(3)	L6660	0(3)	L7040	0(3)	L8480	0(3)
L3763	0(3)	L4205	0(3)	L5626	0(3)	L5711	0(3)	L5990	0(3)	L6665	0(3)	L7045	0(3)	L8485	0(3)
L3764	0(3)	L4210	0(3)	L5628	0(3)	L5712	0(3)	L5999	0(3)	L6670	0(3)	L7170	0(3)	L8499	1(3)
L3765	0(3)	L4350	0(3)	L5629	0(3)	L5714	0(3)	L6000	0(3)	L6672	0(3)	L7180	0(3)	L8500	0(3)
L3766	0(3)	L4360	0(3)	L5630	0(3)	L5716	0(3)	L6010	0(3)	L6675	0(3)	L7181	0(3)	L8501	0(3)
L3806	0(3)	L4361	0(3)	L5631	0(3)	L5718	0(3)	L6020	0(3)	L6676	0(3)	L7185	0(3)	L8505	0(3)
L3807	0(3)	L4370	0(3)	L5632	0(3)	L5722	0(3)	L6026	0(3)	L6677	0(3)	L7186	0(3)	L8507	0(3)
L3808	0(3)	L4386	0(3)	L5634	0(3)	L5724	0(3)	L6050	0(3)	L6680	0(3)	L7190	0(3)	L8509	1(3)
L3809	0(3)	L4387	0(3)	L5636	0(3)	L5726	0(3)	L6055	0(3)	L6682	0(3)	L7191	0(3)	L8510	0(3)
L3891	0(3)	L4392	0(3)	L5637	0(3)	L5728	0(3)	L6100	0(3)	L6684	0(3)	L7259	0(3)	L8511	1(3)
L3900	0(3)	L4394	0(3)	L5638	0(3)	L5780	0(3)	L6110	0(3)	L6686	0(3)	L7360	0(3)	L8512	1(3)
L3901	0(3)	L4396	0(3)	L5639	0(3)	L5781	0(3)	L6120	0(3)	L6687	0(3)	L7362	0(3)	L8513	1(3)
L3904	0(3)	L4397	0(3)	L5640	0(3)	L5782	0(3)	L6130	0(3)	L6688	0(3)	L7364	0(3)	L8514	1(3)
L3905	0(3)	L4398	0(3)	L5642	0(3)	L5785	0(3)	L6200	0(3)	L6689	0(3)	L7366	0(3)	L8515	1(3)
L3906	0(3)	L4631	0(3)	L5643	0(3)	L5790	0(3)	L6205	0(3)	L6690	0(3)	L7367	0(3)	L8600	2(3)
L3908	0(3)	L5000	0(3)	L5644	0(3)	L5795	0(3)	L6250	0(3)	L6691	0(3)	L7368	0(3)	L8603	4(3)
L3912	0(3)	L5010	0(3)	L5645	0(3)	L5810	0(3)	L6300	0(3)	L6692	0(3)	L7400	0(3)	L8604	3(3)
L3913	0(3)	L5020	0(3)	L5646	0(3)	L5811	0(3)	L6310	0(3)	L6693	0(3)	L7401	0(3)	L8605	4(3)

CPT	MUE
L8606	5(3)
L8607	20(3)
L8609	1(3)
L8610	1(3)
L8612	1(3)
L8613	1(3)
L8614	1(3)
L8615	2(3)
L8616	2(3)
L8617	2(3)
L8618	2(3)
L8619	2(3)
L8621	360(3)
L8622	2(3)
L8625	1(3)
L8627	2(2)
L8628	2(2)
L8629	2(2)
L8631	1(3)
L8641	4(3)
L8642	2(3)
L8658	2(3)
L8659	2(3)
L8670	2(3)
L8679	1(3)
L8681	1(3)
L8682	2(3)
L8683	1(3)
L8684	1(3)
L8685	1(3)
L8686	2(3)
L8687	1(3)
L8688	1(3)
L8689	1(3)
L8690	2(2)
L8691	1(3)
L8692	0(3)
L8693	1(3)
L8694	1(3)
L8695	1(3)
L8696	1(3)
L8701	0(3)
L8702	0(3)
M0075	0(3)
M0076	0(3)
M0100	0(3)
M0300	0(3)
M0301	0(3)
P2028	1(2)
P2029	1(2)
P2031	0(3)
P2033	1(2)
P2038	1(2)
P3000	1(3)
P3001	1(3)
P7001	0(3)
P9010	2(3)
P9011	2(3)

CPT	MUE
P9012	8(3)
P9016	3(3)
P9017	2(3)
P9019	2(3)
P9020	2(3)
P9021	3(3)
P9022	2(3)
P9023	2(3)
P9031	12(3)
P9032	12(3)
P9033	12(3)
P9034	2(3)
P9035	2(3)
P9036	2(3)
P9037	2(3)
P9038	2(3)
P9039	2(3)
P9040	3(3)
P9041	5(3)
P9043	5(3)
P9044	10(3)
P9045	20(3)
P9046	25(3)
P9047	20(3)
P9048	1(3)
P9050	1(3)
P9051	2(3)
P9052	2(3)
P9053	2(3)
P9054	2(3)
P9055	2(3)
P9056	2(3)
P9057	2(3)
P9058	2(3)
P9059	2(3)
P9060	2(3)
P9070	2(3)
P9071	2(3)
P9073	2(3)
P9099	1(3)
P9100	2(3)
P9603	300(3)
P9604	2(3)
P9612	1(3)
P9615	1(3)
Q0035	1(3)
Q0081	1(3)
Q0083	1(3)
Q0084	1(3)
Q0085	1(3)
Q0091	1(3)
Q0111	2(3)
Q0112	3(3)
Q0113	1(3)
Q0114	1(3)
Q0115	1(3)
Q0138	510(3)
Q0139	510(3)

CPT	MUE
Q0144	0(3)
Q0161	0(3)
Q0162	0(3)
Q0163	0(3)
Q0164	0(3)
Q0166	0(3)
Q0167	0(3)
Q0169	0(3)
Q0173	0(3)
Q0174	0(3)
Q0175	0(3)
Q0177	0(3)
Q0180	0(3)
Q0181	0(3)
Q0477	1(1)
Q0478	1(3)
Q0479	1(3)
Q0480	1(3)
Q0481	1(2)
Q0482	1(3)
Q0483	1(3)
Q0484	1(3)
Q0485	1(3)
Q0486	1(3)
Q0487	1(3)
Q0488	1(3)
Q0489	1(3)
Q0490	1(3)
Q0491	1(3)
Q0492	1(3)
Q0493	1(3)
Q0494	1(3)
Q0495	1(3)
Q0496	1(3)
Q0497	2(3)
Q0498	1(3)
Q0499	1(3)
Q0501	1(3)
Q0502	1(3)
Q0503	3(3)
Q0504	1(3)
Q0506	8(3)
Q0507	1(3)
Q0508	4(3)
Q0509	2(3)
Q0510	0(3)
Q0511	0(3)
Q0512	0(3)
Q0513	0(3)
Q0514	0(3)
Q0515	0(3)
Q1004	2(2)
Q1005	2(2)
Q2004	1(3)
Q2009	100(3)
Q2017	12(3)
Q2026	30(3)
Q2028	1470(3)

CPT	MUE
Q2034	1(2)
Q2035	1(2)
Q2036	1(2)
Q2037	1(2)
Q2038	1(2)
Q2039	1(2)
Q2043	1(2)
Q2049	10(3)
Q2050	14(3)
Q2052	1(3)
Q3014	1(3)
Q3027	30(3)
Q3028	0(3)
Q3031	1(3)
Q4001	1(3)
Q4002	1(3)
Q4003	2(3)
Q4004	2(3)
Q4012	2(3)
Q4013	2(3)
Q4014	2(3)
Q4018	2(3)
Q4021	2(3)
Q4025	1(3)
Q4026	1(3)
Q4027	1(3)
Q4028	1(3)
Q4030	2(3)
Q4037	2(3)
Q4042	2(3)
Q4046	2(3)
Q4050	2(3)
Q4051	2(3)
Q4074	3(3)
Q4081	100(3)
Q5101	1500(3)
Q5103	150(3)
Q5104	150(3)
Q5105	100(3)
Q5106	60(3)
Q5107	170(3)
Q5108	12(3)
Q5109	150(3)
Q5110	1500(3)
Q5111	12(3)
Q5112	120(3)
Q5113	120(3)
Q5114	120(3)
Q5115	120(3)
Q5116	120(3)
Q5117	120(3)
Q5118	230(3)
Q9950	5(3)
Q9951	0(3)
Q9953	10(3)
Q9954	18(3)
Q9955	0(3)
Q9956	9(3)

CPT	MUE
Q9957	3(3)
Q9958	300(3)
Q9959	0(3)
Q9960	250(3)
Q9961	200(3)
Q9962	150(3)
Q9963	240(3)
Q9964	0(3)
Q9966	250(3)
Q9967	300(3)
Q9969	3(3)
Q9982	1(3)
Q9983	1(3)
Q9991	1(2)
Q9992	1(2)
R0070	2(3)
R0075	2(3)
R0076	1(3)
U0001	2(3)
U0002	2(3)
U0003	2(3)
U0004	2(3)
V2020	0(3)
V2025	0(3)
V2100	0(3)
V2101	0(3)
V2102	0(3)
V2103	0(3)
V2104	0(3)
V2105	0(3)
V2106	0(3)
V2107	0(3)
V2108	0(3)
V2109	0(3)
V2110	0(3)
V2111	0(3)
V2112	0(3)
V2113	0(3)
V2114	0(3)
V2115	0(3)
V2118	0(3)
V2121	0(3)
V2199	2(3)
V2200	0(3)
V2201	0(3)
V2202	0(3)
V2203	0(3)
V2204	0(3)
V2205	0(3)
V2206	0(3)
V2207	0(3)
V2208	0(3)
V2209	0(3)
V2210	0(3)
V2211	0(3)
V2212	0(3)
V2213	0(3)
V2214	0(3)

CPT	MUE
V2215	0(3)
V2218	0(3)
V2219	0(3)
V2220	0(3)
V2221	0(3)
V2299	0(3)
V2300	0(3)
V2301	0(3)
V2302	0(3)
V2303	0(3)
V2304	0(3)
V2305	0(3)
V2306	0(3)
V2307	0(3)
V2308	0(3)
V2309	0(3)
V2310	0(3)
V2311	0(3)
V2312	0(3)
V2313	0(3)
V2314	0(3)
V2315	0(3)
V2318	0(3)
V2319	0(3)
V2320	0(3)
V2321	0(3)
V2399	0(3)
V2410	0(3)
V2430	0(3)
V2499	2(3)
V2500	0(3)
V2501	0(3)
V2502	0(3)
V2503	0(3)
V2510	0(3)
V2511	0(3)
V2512	0(3)
V2513	0(3)
V2520	2(3)
V2521	2(3)
V2522	2(3)
V2523	2(3)
V2530	0(3)
V2531	0(3)
V2599	2(3)
V2600	0(2)
V2610	0(2)
V2615	0(2)
V2623	0(3)
V2624	0(3)
V2625	0(3)
V2626	0(3)
V2627	0(3)
V2628	0(3)
V2629	0(3)
V2630	2(2)
V2631	2(2)
V2632	2(2)

CPT	MUE
V2700	0(3)
V2702	0(3)
V2710	0(3)
V2715	0(3)
V2718	0(3)
V2730	0(3)
V2744	0(3)
V2745	0(3)
V2750	0(3)
V2755	0(3)
V2756	0(3)
V2760	0(3)
V2761	0(2)
V2762	0(3)
V2770	0(3)
V2780	0(3)
V2781	0(2)
V2782	0(3)
V2783	0(3)
V2784	0(3)
V2785	2(2)
V2786	0(3)
V2787	0(3)
V2788	0(3)
V2790	1(3)
V2797	0(3)
V5008	0(3)
V5010	0(3)
V5011	0(3)
V5014	0(3)
V5020	0(3)
V5030	0(3)
V5040	0(3)
V5050	0(3)
V5060	0(3)
V5070	0(3)
V5080	0(3)
V5090	0(3)
V5095	0(3)
V5100	0(3)
V5110	0(3)
V5120	0(3)
V5130	0(3)
V5140	0(3)
V5150	0(3)
V5160	0(3)
V5171	0(3)
V5172	0(3)
V5181	0(3)
V5190	0(3)
V5200	0(3)
V5211	0(3)
V5212	0(3)
V5213	0(3)
V5214	0(3)
V5215	0(3)
V5221	0(3)
V5230	0(3)

CPT	MUE
V5240	0(3)
V5241	0(3)
V5242	0(3)
V5243	0(3)
V5244	0(3)
V5245	0(3)
V5246	0(3)
V5247	0(3)
V5248	0(3)
V5249	0(3)
V5250	0(3)
V5251	0(3)
V5252	0(3)
V5253	0(3)
V5254	0(3)
V5255	0(3)
V5256	0(3)
V5257	0(3)
V5258	0(3)
V5259	0(3)
V5260	0(3)
V5261	0(3)
V5262	0(3)
V5263	0(3)
V5264	0(3)
V5265	0(3)
V5266	0(3)
V5267	0(3)
V5268	0(3)
V5269	0(3)
V5270	0(3)
V5271	0(3)
V5272	0(3)
V5273	0(3)
V5274	0(3)
V5275	0(3)
V5281	0(3)
V5282	0(3)
V5283	0(3)
V5284	0(3)
V5285	0(3)
V5286	0(3)
V5287	0(3)
V5288	0(3)
V5289	0(3)
V5290	0(3)
V5298	0(3)
V5299	1(3)
V5336	0(3)
V5362	0(3)
V5363	0(3)
V5364	0(3)

OPPS

CPT	MUE
0001U	1(2)
0002M	1(3)
0002U	1(2)
0003M	1(3)
0003U	1(2)
0004M	1(2)
0005U	1(2)
0006M	1(2)
0007M	1(2)
0007U	1(2)
0008U	1(3)
0009U	2(3)
0010U	2(3)
0011M	1(2)
0011U	1(2)
0012M	1(2)
0012U	1(2)
0013M	1(2)
0013U	1(3)
0014M	1(2)
0014U	1(3)
0016U	1(3)
0017U	1(3)
0018U	1(1)
0019U	1(3)
0021U	1(2)
0022U	2(3)
0023U	1(2)
0024U	1(2)
0025U	1(2)
0026U	1(3)
0027U	1(2)
0029U	1(2)
0030U	1(2)
0031U	1(2)
0032U	1(2)
0033U	1(2)
0034U	1(2)
0035U	1(2)
0036U	1(3)
0037U	1(3)
0038U	1(2)
0039U	1(2)
0040U	1(2)
0041U	1(2)
0042T	1(3)
0042U	1(2)
0043U	1(2)
0044U	1(2)
0045U	1(3)
0046U	1(3)
0047U	1(3)
0048U	1(3)
0049U	1(3)
0050U	1(3)
0051U	1(2)
0052U	1(2)
0053U	1(3)
0054T	1(3)
0054U	1(2)
0055T	1(3)
0055U	1(2)
0056U	1(3)
0058T	1(2)

CPT	MUE
0058U	1(2)
0059U	1(2)
0060U	1(2)
0061U	2(3)
0062U	1(2)
0063U	1(2)
0064U	2(3)
0065U	2(3)
0066U	1(3)
0067U	2(3)
0068U	1(3)
0069U	1(3)
0070U	1(2)
0071T	1(2)
0071U	1(2)
0072T	1(2)
0072U	1(2)
0073U	1(2)
0074U	1(2)
0075T	1(2)
0075U	1(2)
0076T	1(2)
0076U	1(2)
0077U	2(2)
0078U	1(2)
0079U	0(3)
0080U	1(2)
0082U	1(2)
0083U	1(3)
0084U	1(2)
0085T	0(3)
0086U	1(3)
0087U	1(2)
0088U	1(2)
0089U	1(2)
0090U	1(2)
0091U	1(2)
0092U	1(2)
0093U	1(2)
0094U	1(2)
0095T	1(3)
0095U	1(2)
0096U	1(2)
0097U	1(2)
0098T	2(3)
0098U	1(2)
0099U	1(2)
0100T	1(2)
0100U	1(2)
0101T	1(3)
0101U	1(2)
0102T	2(2)
0102U	1(2)
0103U	1(2)
0105U	1(2)
0106T	4(2)
0106U	1(2)
0107T	4(2)
0107U	1(3)
0108T	4(2)
0108U	1(2)
0109T	4(2)
0109U	1(3)
0110T	4(2)

CPT	MUE
0110U	1(2)
0111T	1(3)
0111U	1(2)
0112U	1(3)
0113U	1(2)
0114U	1(2)
0115U	1(3)
0116U	1(2)
0117U	1(2)
0118U	1(2)
0119U	1(2)
0120U	1(2)
0121U	1(2)
0122U	1(2)
0123U	1(2)
0126T	1(3)
0129U	1(2)
0130U	1(2)
0131U	1(2)
0132U	1(2)
0133U	1(2)
0134U	1(2)
0135U	1(2)
0136U	1(2)
0137U	1(2)
0138U	1(2)
0139U	1(2)
0140U	1(2)
0141U	1(2)
0142U	1(2)
0143U	1(2)
0144U	1(2)
0145U	1(2)
0146U	1(2)
0147U	1(2)
0148U	1(2)
0149U	1(2)
0150U	1(2)
0151U	1(2)
0152U	1(2)
0153U	1(2)
0154U	1(2)
0155U	1(2)
0156U	1(2)
0157U	1(2)
0158U	1(2)
0159U	1(2)
0160U	1(2)
0161U	1(2)
0162U	1(2)
0163T	1(3)
0163U	0(3)
0164T	4(2)
0164U	1(2)
0165T	4(2)
0165U	1(2)
0166U	1(2)
0167U	1(2)
0168U	1(2)
0169U	1(2)
0170U	1(2)
0171U	1(2)
0172U	1(2)
0173U	1(2)

CPT	MUE
0174T	1(3)
0174U	1(2)
0175T	1(3)
0175U	1(2)
0176U	1(3)
0177U	1(2)
0178U	1(2)
0179U	1(2)
0184T	1(3)
0191T	2(2)
0198T	2(2)
01996	1(2)
0200T	1(2)
0201T	1(2)
0202T	1(3)
0202U	1(3)
0207T	2(2)
0208T	1(3)
0209T	1(3)
0210T	1(3)
0211T	1(3)
0212T	1(3)
0213T	1(2)
0214T	1(2)
0215T	1(2)
0216T	1(2)
0217T	1(2)
0218T	1(2)
0219T	1(2)
0220T	1(2)
0221T	1(2)
0222T	1(3)
0223U	1(3)
0224U	3(3)
0228T	1(2)
0229T	2(3)
0230T	1(2)
0231T	2(3)
0232T	1(3)
0234T	2(2)
0235T	2(3)
0236T	1(2)
0237T	2(3)
0238T	2(3)
0253T	1(3)
0263T	1(3)
0264T	1(3)
0265T	1(3)
0266T	1(2)
0267T	1(3)
0268T	1(3)
0269T	1(2)
0270T	1(3)
0271T	1(3)
0272T	1(3)
0273T	1(3)
0274T	1(2)
0275T	1(2)
0278T	1(3)
0290T	1(3)
0295T	1(2)
0296T	1(2)
0297T	1(2)
0298T	1(2)

CPT	MUE
0308T	1(3)
0312T	1(3)
0313T	1(3)
0314T	1(3)
0315T	1(3)
0316T	1(3)
0317T	1(3)
0329T	0(3)
0330T	1(2)
0331T	1(3)
0332T	1(3)
0333T	0(3)
0335T	2(2)
0338T	1(2)
0339T	1(2)
0342T	1(3)
0345T	1(2)
0347T	1(3)
0348T	1(3)
0349T	1(3)
0350T	1(3)
0351T	5(3)
0352T	5(3)
0353T	2(3)
0354T	2(3)
0355T	1(2)
0356T	4(2)
0358T	1(2)
0362T	8(3)
0373T	24(3)
0376T	2(3)
0378T	1(2)
0379T	1(2)
0381T	1(2)
0382T	1(2)
0383T	1(2)
0384T	1(2)
0385T	1(2)
0386T	1(2)
0394T	2(3)
0395T	2(3)
0396T	2(2)
0397T	1(3)
0398T	1(3)
0400T	1(2)
0401T	1(2)
0402T	2(2)
0403T	0(3)
0404T	1(2)
0405T	1(2)
0408T	1(3)
0409T	1(3)
0410T	1(3)
0411T	1(3)
0412T	1(2)
0413T	1(3)
0414T	1(2)
0415T	1(3)
0416T	1(3)
0417T	1(3)
0418T	1(3)
0419T	1(2)
0420T	1(2)
0421T	1(2)

CPT	MUE
0422T	1(3)
0423T	1(3)
0424T	1(3)
0425T	1(3)
0426T	1(3)
0427T	1(3)
0428T	1(2)
0429T	1(2)
0430T	1(2)
0431T	1(2)
0432T	1(3)
0433T	1(3)
0434T	1(3)
0435T	1(3)
0436T	1(3)
0437T	1(3)
0439T	1(3)
0440T	3(3)
0441T	3(3)
0442T	3(3)
0443T	1(2)
0444T	1(2)
0445T	1(2)
0446T	1(3)
0447T	1(3)
0448T	1(3)
0449T	1(2)
0450T	1(3)
0451T	1(3)
0452T	1(3)
0453T	1(3)
0454T	3(3)
0455T	1(3)
0456T	1(3)
0457T	1(3)
0458T	3(3)
0459T	1(3)
0460T	3(3)
0461T	1(3)
0462T	1(2)
0463T	1(2)
0464T	1(2)
0465T	1(3)
0466T	1(3)
0467T	1(3)
0468T	1(3)
0469T	1(2)
0470T	1(2)
0471T	2(1)
0472T	1(2)
0473T	1(2)
0474T	0(3)
0475T	1(3)
0476T	1(3)
0477T	1(3)
0478T	1(3)
0479T	1(2)
0480T	4(1)
0481T	1(3)
0483T	1(2)
0484T	1(2)
0485T	1(2)
0486T	1(2)
0487T	1(3)

CPT	MUE
0488T	1(2)
0489T	1(2)
0490T	1(2)
0491T	1(2)
0492T	4(3)
0493T	1(3)
0494T	1(2)
0495T	1(2)
0496T	4(3)
0497T	1(3)
0498T	1(2)
0499T	1(2)
0500T	1(3)
0501T	1(2)
0502T	1(2)
0503T	1(2)
0504T	1(2)
0505T	1(3)
0506T	1(2)
0507T	1(2)
0508T	1(3)
0509T	1(2)
0510T	1(2)
0511T	1(2)
0512T	1(2)
0513T	2(3)
0514T	2(2)
0515T	1(3)
0516T	1(3)
0517T	1(3)
0518T	1(3)
0519T	1(3)
0520T	1(3)
0521T	1(3)
0522T	1(3)
0523T	1(3)
0524T	3(3)
0525T	1(3)
0526T	1(3)
0527T	1(3)
0528T	1(3)
0529T	1(3)
0530T	1(3)
0531T	1(3)
0532T	1(3)
0533T	1(2)
0534T	1(2)
0535T	1(2)
0536T	1(2)
0537T	1(2)
0538T	1(3)
0539T	1(3)
0540T	1(3)
0541T	1(3)
0542T	1(3)
0543T	1(2)
0544T	1(2)
0545T	1(2)
0546T	2(2)
0547T	1(2)
0548T	1(2)
0549T	1(2)
0550T	2(3)
0551T	1(2)

CPT	MUE
0552T	0(3)
0553T	0(3)
0554T	0(3)
0555T	1(2)
0556T	1(2)
0557T	0(3)
0558T	1(2)
0559T	1(2)
0560T	1(3)
0561T	1(2)
0562T	1(3)
0563T	1(2)
0564T	1(2)
0565T	1(2)
0566T	1(2)
0567T	1(2)
0568T	1(2)
0569T	1(2)
0570T	1(3)
0571T	1(2)
0572T	1(2)
0573T	1(2)
0574T	1(2)
0575T	1(2)
0576T	1(2)
0577T	1(2)
0578T	1(2)
0579T	1(2)
0580T	1(2)
0581T	0(3)
0582T	0(3)
0583T	2(2)
0584T	1(2)
0585T	1(2)
0586T	1(2)
0587T	1(2)
0588T	1(2)
0589T	1(2)
0590T	1(2)
0591T	1(2)
0592T	1(2)
0593T	1(2)
10004	3(3)
10005	1(2)
10006	3(3)
10007	1(2)
10008	2(3)
10009	1(2)
10010	3(3)
10011	1(2)
10012	3(3)
10021	1(2)
10030	2(3)
10035	1(2)
10036	3(3)
10040	1(2)
10060	1(2)
10061	1(2)
10080	1(3)
10081	1(3)
10120	3(3)
10121	2(3)
10140	2(3)
10160	3(3)

CPT	MUE
10180	2(3)
11000	1(2)
11001	1(3)
11004	1(2)
11005	1(2)
11006	1(2)
11008	1(2)
11010	2(3)
11011	2(3)
11012	2(3)
11042	1(2)
11043	1(2)
11044	1(2)
11045	12(3)
11046	4(3)
11047	4(3)
11055	1(2)
11056	1(2)
11057	1(2)
11102	1(2)
11103	6(3)
11104	1(2)
11105	3(3)
11106	1(2)
11107	2(3)
11200	1(2)
11201	1(3)
11300	5(3)
11301	6(3)
11302	4(3)
11303	3(3)
11305	4(3)
11306	4(3)
11307	3(3)
11308	2(3)
11310	4(3)
11311	4(3)
11312	3(3)
11313	3(3)
11400	3(3)
11401	3(3)
11402	3(3)
11403	2(3)
11404	2(3)
11406	2(3)
11420	3(3)
11421	3(3)
11422	3(3)
11423	2(3)
11424	2(3)
11426	2(3)
11440	4(3)
11441	3(3)
11442	3(3)
11443	2(3)
11444	2(3)
11446	2(3)
11450	1(2)
11451	1(2)
11462	1(2)
11463	1(2)
11470	3(2)
11471	2(3)
11600	2(3)
11601	2(3)

CPT	MUE
11602	3(3)
11603	2(3)
11604	2(3)
11606	2(3)
11620	2(3)
11621	2(3)
11622	2(3)
11623	2(3)
11624	2(3)
11626	2(3)
11640	2(3)
11641	2(3)
11642	3(3)
11643	2(3)
11644	2(3)
11646	2(3)
11719	1(2)
11720	1(2)
11721	1(2)
11730	1(2)
11732	4(3)
11740	2(3)
11750	6(3)
11755	2(3)
11760	4(3)
11762	2(3)
11765	4(3)
11770	1(3)
11771	1(3)
11772	1(3)
11900	1(2)
11901	1(2)
11920	1(2)
11921	1(2)
11922	1(3)
11950	1(2)
11951	1(2)
11952	1(2)
11954	1(3)
11960	2(3)
11970	2(3)
11971	2(3)
11976	1(2)
11980	1(2)
11981	1(3)
11982	1(3)
11983	1(3)
12001	1(2)
12002	1(2)
12004	1(2)
12005	1(2)
12006	1(2)
12007	1(2)
12011	1(2)
12013	1(2)
12014	1(2)
12015	1(2)
12016	1(2)
12017	1(2)
12018	1(2)
12020	2(3)
12021	3(3)
12031	1(2)
12032	1(2)
12034	1(2)

CPT	MUE
12035	1(2)
12036	1(2)
12037	1(2)
12041	1(2)
12042	1(2)
12044	1(2)
12045	1(2)
12046	1(2)
12047	1(2)
12051	1(2)
12052	1(2)
12053	1(2)
12054	1(2)
12055	1(2)
12056	1(2)
12057	1(2)
13100	1(2)
13101	1(2)
13102	9(3)
13120	1(2)
13121	1(2)
13122	9(3)
13131	1(2)
13132	1(2)
13133	7(3)
13151	1(2)
13152	1(2)
13153	2(3)
13160	2(3)
14000	2(3)
14001	2(3)
14020	2(3)
14021	2(3)
14040	2(3)
14041	3(3)
14060	2(3)
14061	2(3)
14301	2(3)
14302	8(3)
14350	2(3)
15002	1(2)
15003	9(3)
15004	1(2)
15005	2(3)
15040	1(2)
15050	1(3)
15100	1(2)
15101	9(3)
15110	1(2)
15111	2(3)
15115	1(2)
15116	2(3)
15120	1(2)
15121	5(3)
15130	1(2)
15131	2(3)
15135	1(2)
15136	1(3)
15150	1(2)
15151	1(2)
15152	2(3)
15155	1(2)
15156	1(2)
15157	1(3)
15200	1(2)

CPT	MUE
15201	7(3)
15220	1(2)
15221	9(3)
15240	1(2)
15241	9(3)
15260	1(2)
15261	6(3)
15271	1(2)
15272	3(3)
15273	1(2)
15274	6(3)
15275	1(2)
15276	3(2)
15277	1(2)
15278	3(3)
15570	2(3)
15572	2(3)
15574	2(3)
15576	2(3)
15600	2(3)
15610	2(3)
15620	2(3)
15630	2(3)
15650	1(3)
15730	1(3)
15731	1(3)
15733	2(3)
15734	4(3)
15736	2(3)
15738	3(3)
15740	2(3)
15750	2(3)
15756	2(3)
15757	2(3)
15758	2(3)
15760	2(3)
15769	1(3)
15770	2(3)
15771	1(2)
15772	9(3)
15773	1(2)
15774	3(3)
15775	1(2)
15776	1(2)
15777	1(3)
15780	1(2)
15781	1(3)
15782	1(3)
15783	1(3)
15786	1(2)
15787	2(3)
15788	1(2)
15789	1(2)
15792	1(3)
15793	1(3)
15819	1(2)
15820	1(2)
15821	1(2)
15822	1(2)
15823	1(2)
15824	1(2)
15825	1(2)
15826	1(2)
15828	1(2)
15829	1(2)

CPT	MUE
15830	1(2)
15832	1(2)
15833	1(2)
15834	1(2)
15835	1(3)
15836	1(2)
15837	2(3)
15838	1(2)
15839	2(3)
15840	1(3)
15841	2(3)
15842	2(3)
15845	2(3)
15847	1(2)
15850	1(2)
15851	1(2)
15852	1(3)
15860	1(3)
15876	1(2)
15877	1(2)
15878	1(2)
15879	1(2)
15920	1(3)
15922	1(3)
15931	1(3)
15933	1(3)
15934	1(3)
15935	1(3)
15936	1(3)
15937	1(3)
15940	2(3)
15941	2(3)
15944	2(3)
15945	2(3)
15946	2(3)
15950	2(3)
15951	2(3)
15952	2(3)
15953	2(3)
15956	2(3)
15958	2(3)
15999	1(3)
16000	1(2)
16020	1(3)
16025	1(3)
16030	1(3)
16035	1(2)
16036	2(3)
17000	1(2)
17003	13(2)
17004	1(2)
17106	1(2)
17107	1(2)
17108	1(2)
17110	1(2)
17111	1(2)
17250	4(3)
17260	7(3)
17261	7(3)
17262	6(3)
17263	3(3)
17264	3(3)
17266	2(3)
17270	6(3)
17271	4(3)

CPT	MUE
17272	5(3)
17273	4(3)
17274	2(3)
17276	2(3)
17280	6(3)
17281	5(3)
17282	4(3)
17283	4(3)
17284	2(3)
17286	2(3)
17311	4(3)
17312	6(3)
17313	3(3)
17314	4(3)
17315	15(3)
17340	1(2)
17360	1(2)
17380	1(3)
17999	1(3)
19000	2(3)
19001	5(3)
19020	2(3)
19030	1(2)
19081	1(2)
19082	2(3)
19083	1(2)
19084	2(3)
19085	1(2)
19086	2(3)
19100	4(3)
19101	3(3)
19105	2(3)
19110	1(3)
19112	2(3)
19120	1(2)
19125	1(2)
19126	3(3)
19281	1(2)
19282	2(3)
19283	1(2)
19284	2(3)
19285	1(2)
19286	2(3)
19287	1(2)
19288	2(3)
19294	2(3)
19296	1(3)
19297	2(3)
19298	1(2)
19300	1(2)
19301	1(2)
19302	1(2)
19303	1(2)
19305	1(2)
19306	1(2)
19307	1(2)
19316	1(2)
19318	1(2)
19324	1(2)
19325	1(2)
19328	1(2)
19330	1(2)
19340	1(2)
19342	1(2)
19350	1(2)

CPT	MUE
19355	1(2)
19357	1(2)
19361	1(2)
19364	1(2)
19366	1(2)
19367	1(2)
19368	1(2)
19369	1(2)
19370	1(2)
19371	1(2)
19380	1(2)
19396	1(2)
19499	1(3)
20100	2(3)
20101	2(3)
20102	3(3)
20103	3(3)
20150	2(3)
20200	2(3)
20205	3(3)
20206	3(3)
20220	3(3)
20225	2(3)
20240	4(3)
20245	3(3)
20250	1(3)
20251	2(3)
20500	2(3)
20501	2(3)
20520	2(3)
20525	4(3)
20526	1(2)
20527	2(3)
20550	5(3)
20551	5(3)
20552	1(2)
20553	1(2)
20555	1(3)
20560	1(2)
20561	1(2)
20600	6(3)
20604	4(3)
20605	2(3)
20606	2(3)
20610	2(3)
20611	2(3)
20612	2(3)
20615	1(3)
20650	4(3)
20660	1(2)
20661	1(2)
20662	1(2)
20663	1(2)
20664	1(2)
20665	1(2)
20670	3(3)
20680	3(3)
20690	2(3)
20692	2(3)
20693	2(3)
20694	2(3)
20696	2(3)
20697	4(3)
20700	1(3)
20701	1(3)

CPT	MUE
20702	1(3)
20703	1(3)
20704	1(3)
20705	1(3)
20802	1(2)
20805	1(2)
20808	1(2)
20816	3(3)
20822	3(3)
20824	1(2)
20827	1(2)
20838	1(2)
20900	2(3)
20902	2(3)
20910	1(3)
20912	1(3)
20920	1(3)
20922	1(3)
20924	2(3)
20930	1(3)
20931	1(2)
20932	1(3)
20933	1(3)
20934	1(3)
20936	1(3)
20937	1(2)
20938	1(2)
20939	1(3)
20950	2(3)
20955	1(3)
20956	1(3)
20957	1(3)
20962	1(3)
20969	2(3)
20970	1(3)
20972	2(3)
20973	1(2)
20974	1(3)
20975	1(3)
20979	1(3)
20982	1(2)
20983	1(2)
20985	2(3)
20999	1(3)
21010	1(2)
21011	4(3)
21012	3(3)
21013	2(3)
21014	2(3)
21015	1(3)
21016	2(3)
21025	2(3)
21026	2(3)
21029	1(3)
21030	1(3)
21031	2(3)
21032	1(3)
21034	1(3)
21040	2(3)
21044	1(3)
21045	1(3)
21046	2(3)
21047	2(3)
21048	2(3)
21049	1(3)

CPT	MUE
21050	1(2)
21060	1(2)
21070	1(2)
21073	1(2)
21076	1(2)
21077	1(2)
21079	1(2)
21080	1(2)
21081	1(2)
21082	1(2)
21083	1(2)
21084	1(2)
21085	1(3)
21086	1(2)
21087	1(2)
21088	1(2)
21089	1(3)
21100	1(2)
21110	2(3)
21116	1(2)
21120	1(2)
21121	1(2)
21122	1(2)
21123	1(2)
21125	2(2)
21127	2(3)
21137	1(2)
21138	1(2)
21139	1(2)
21141	1(2)
21142	1(2)
21143	1(2)
21145	1(2)
21146	1(2)
21147	1(2)
21150	1(2)
21151	1(2)
21154	1(2)
21155	1(2)
21159	1(2)
21160	1(2)
21172	1(3)
21175	1(2)
21179	1(2)
21180	1(2)
21181	1(3)
21182	1(2)
21183	1(2)
21184	1(2)
21188	1(2)
21193	1(2)
21194	1(2)
21195	1(2)
21196	1(2)
21198	1(3)
21199	1(2)
21206	1(3)
21208	1(3)
21209	1(3)
21210	2(3)
21215	2(3)
21230	2(3)
21235	2(3)
21240	1(2)
21242	1(2)

CPT	MUE
21243	1(2)
21244	1(2)
21245	2(2)
21246	2(2)
21247	1(2)
21248	2(3)
21249	2(3)
21255	1(2)
21256	1(2)
21260	1(2)
21261	1(2)
21263	1(2)
21267	1(2)
21268	1(2)
21270	1(2)
21275	1(2)
21280	1(2)
21282	1(2)
21295	1(2)
21296	1(2)
21299	1(3)
21310	1(2)
21315	1(2)
21320	1(2)
21325	1(2)
21330	1(2)
21335	1(2)
21336	1(2)
21337	1(2)
21338	1(2)
21339	1(2)
21340	1(2)
21343	1(2)
21344	1(2)
21345	1(2)
21346	1(2)
21347	1(2)
21348	1(2)
21355	1(2)
21356	1(2)
21360	1(2)
21365	1(2)
21366	1(2)
21385	1(2)
21386	1(2)
21387	1(2)
21390	1(2)
21395	1(2)
21400	1(2)
21401	1(2)
21406	1(2)
21407	1(2)
21408	1(2)
21421	1(2)
21422	1(2)
21423	1(2)
21431	1(2)
21432	1(2)
21433	1(2)
21435	1(2)
21436	1(2)
21440	2(2)
21445	2(2)
21450	1(2)
21451	1(2)

CPT	MUE
21452	1(2)
21453	1(2)
21454	1(2)
21461	1(2)
21462	1(2)
21465	1(2)
21470	1(2)
21480	1(2)
21485	1(2)
21490	1(2)
21497	1(2)
21499	1(3)
21501	3(3)
21502	1(3)
21510	1(3)
21550	2(3)
21552	2(3)
21554	2(3)
21555	2(3)
21556	2(3)
21557	1(3)
21558	1(3)
21600	5(3)
21601	2(3)
21602	1(3)
21603	1(3)
21610	1(3)
21615	1(2)
21616	1(2)
21620	1(2)
21627	1(2)
21630	1(2)
21632	1(2)
21685	1(2)
21700	1(2)
21705	1(2)
21720	1(3)
21725	1(3)
21740	1(2)
21742	1(2)
21743	1(2)
21750	1(2)
21811	1(2)
21812	1(2)
21813	1(2)
21820	1(2)
21825	1(2)
21899	1(3)
21920	2(3)
21925	2(3)
21930	5(3)
21931	3(3)
21932	2(3)
21933	2(3)
21935	1(3)
21936	1(3)
22010	2(3)
22015	2(3)
22100	1(2)
22101	1(2)
22102	1(2)
22103	3(3)
22110	1(2)
22112	1(2)
22114	1(2)

CPT	MUE
22116	3(3)
22206	1(2)
22207	1(2)
22208	5(3)
22210	1(2)
22212	1(2)
22214	1(2)
22216	6(3)
22220	1(2)
22222	1(2)
22224	1(2)
22226	4(3)
22310	1(2)
22315	1(2)
22318	1(2)
22319	1(2)
22325	1(2)
22326	1(2)
22327	1(2)
22328	6(3)
22505	1(2)
22510	1(2)
22511	1(2)
22512	3(3)
22513	1(2)
22514	1(2)
22515	4(3)
22526	0(3)
22527	0(3)
22532	1(2)
22533	1(2)
22534	3(3)
22548	1(2)
22551	1(2)
22552	5(3)
22554	1(2)
22556	1(2)
22558	1(2)
22585	5(3)
22586	1(2)
22590	1(2)
22595	1(2)
22600	1(2)
22610	1(2)
22612	1(2)
22614	13(3)
22630	1(2)
22632	4(2)
22633	1(2)
22634	4(2)
22800	1(2)
22802	1(2)
22804	1(2)
22808	1(2)
22810	1(2)
22812	1(2)
22818	1(2)
22819	1(2)
22830	1(2)
22840	1(3)
22841	0(3)
22842	1(3)
22843	1(3)
22844	1(3)
22845	1(3)

CPT	MUE
22846	1(3)
22847	1(3)
22848	1(2)
22849	1(2)
22850	1(2)
22852	1(2)
22853	4(3)
22854	4(3)
22855	1(2)
22856	1(2)
22857	1(2)
22858	1(2)
22859	4(3)
22861	1(2)
22862	1(2)
22864	1(2)
22865	1(2)
22867	1(2)
22868	1(2)
22869	1(2)
22870	1(2)
22899	1(3)
22900	3(3)
22901	2(3)
22902	4(3)
22903	3(3)
22904	1(3)
22905	1(3)
22999	1(3)
23000	1(2)
23020	1(2)
23030	2(3)
23031	1(3)
23035	1(3)
23040	1(2)
23044	1(3)
23065	2(3)
23066	2(3)
23071	2(3)
23073	2(3)
23075	2(3)
23076	2(3)
23077	1(3)
23078	1(3)
23100	1(2)
23101	1(3)
23105	1(2)
23106	1(2)
23107	1(2)
23120	1(2)
23125	1(2)
23130	1(2)
23140	1(3)
23145	1(3)
23146	1(3)
23150	1(3)
23155	1(3)
23156	1(3)
23170	1(3)
23172	1(3)
23174	1(3)
23180	1(3)
23182	1(3)
23184	1(3)
23190	1(3)

CPT	MUE
23195	1(2)
23200	1(3)
23210	1(3)
23220	1(3)
23330	2(3)
23333	1(3)
23334	1(2)
23335	1(2)
23350	1(2)
23395	1(2)
23397	1(3)
23400	1(2)
23405	2(3)
23406	1(3)
23410	1(2)
23412	1(2)
23415	1(2)
23420	1(2)
23430	1(2)
23440	1(2)
23450	1(2)
23455	1(2)
23460	1(2)
23462	1(2)
23465	1(2)
23466	1(2)
23470	1(2)
23472	1(2)
23473	1(2)
23474	1(2)
23480	1(2)
23485	1(2)
23490	1(2)
23491	1(2)
23500	1(2)
23505	1(2)
23515	1(2)
23520	1(2)
23525	1(2)
23530	1(2)
23532	1(2)
23540	1(2)
23545	1(2)
23550	1(2)
23552	1(2)
23570	1(2)
23575	1(2)
23585	1(2)
23600	1(2)
23605	1(2)
23615	1(2)
23616	1(2)
23620	1(2)
23625	1(2)
23630	1(2)
23650	1(2)
23655	1(2)
23660	1(2)
23665	1(2)
23670	1(2)
23675	1(2)
23680	1(2)
23700	1(2)
23800	1(2)
23802	1(2)

CPT	MUE
23900	1(2)
23920	1(2)
23921	1(2)
23929	1(3)
23930	2(3)
23931	2(3)
23935	2(3)
24000	1(2)
24006	1(2)
24065	2(3)
24066	2(3)
24071	2(3)
24073	2(3)
24075	5(3)
24076	4(3)
24077	1(3)
24079	1(3)
24100	1(2)
24101	1(2)
24102	1(2)
24105	1(2)
24110	1(3)
24115	1(3)
24116	1(3)
24120	1(3)
24125	1(3)
24126	1(3)
24130	1(2)
24134	1(3)
24136	1(3)
24138	1(3)
24140	1(3)
24145	1(3)
24147	1(2)
24149	1(2)
24150	1(3)
24152	1(3)
24155	1(2)
24160	1(2)
24164	1(2)
24200	3(3)
24201	3(3)
24220	1(2)
24300	1(2)
24301	2(3)
24305	4(3)
24310	2(3)
24320	2(3)
24330	1(3)
24331	1(3)
24332	1(2)
24340	1(2)
24341	2(3)
24342	2(3)
24343	1(2)
24344	1(2)
24345	1(2)
24346	1(2)
24357	1(3)
24358	1(3)
24359	2(3)
24360	1(2)
24361	1(2)
24362	1(2)
24363	1(2)

CPT	MUE
24365	1(2)
24366	1(2)
24370	1(2)
24371	1(2)
24400	1(3)
24410	1(2)
24420	1(2)
24430	1(3)
24435	1(3)
24470	1(2)
24495	1(2)
24498	1(2)
24500	1(2)
24505	1(2)
24515	1(2)
24516	1(2)
24530	1(2)
24535	1(2)
24538	1(2)
24545	1(2)
24546	1(2)
24560	1(3)
24565	1(3)
24566	1(3)
24575	1(3)
24576	1(3)
24577	1(3)
24579	1(3)
24582	1(3)
24586	1(3)
24587	1(2)
24600	1(2)
24605	1(2)
24615	1(2)
24620	1(2)
24635	1(2)
24640	1(2)
24650	1(2)
24655	1(2)
24665	1(2)
24666	1(2)
24670	1(2)
24675	1(2)
24685	1(2)
24800	1(2)
24802	1(2)
24900	1(2)
24920	1(2)
24925	1(2)
24930	1(2)
24931	1(2)
24935	1(2)
24940	1(2)
24999	1(3)
25000	2(3)
25001	1(3)
25020	1(2)
25023	1(2)
25024	1(2)
25025	1(2)
25028	4(3)
25031	2(3)
25035	2(3)
25040	1(3)
25065	2(3)

CPT	MUE
25066	2(3)
25071	3(3)
25073	2(3)
25075	6(3)
25076	3(3)
25077	1(3)
25078	1(3)
25085	1(2)
25100	1(2)
25101	1(2)
25105	1(2)
25107	1(2)
25109	4(3)
25110	2(3)
25111	1(3)
25112	1(3)
25115	1(3)
25116	1(3)
25118	5(3)
25119	1(2)
25120	1(3)
25125	1(3)
25126	1(3)
25130	1(3)
25135	1(3)
25136	1(3)
25145	1(3)
25150	1(3)
25151	1(3)
25170	1(3)
25210	2(3)
25215	1(2)
25230	1(2)
25240	1(2)
25246	1(2)
25248	3(3)
25250	1(2)
25251	1(2)
25259	1(2)
25260	7(3)
25263	4(3)
25265	4(3)
25270	8(3)
25272	4(3)
25274	4(3)
25275	2(3)
25280	9(3)
25290	10(3)
25295	9(3)
25300	1(2)
25301	1(2)
25310	5(3)
25312	4(3)
25315	1(3)
25316	1(3)
25320	1(2)
25332	1(2)
25335	1(2)
25337	1(2)
25350	1(3)
25355	1(3)
25360	1(3)
25365	1(3)
25370	1(2)
25375	1(2)

CPT	MUE
25390	1(2)
25391	1(2)
25392	1(2)
25393	1(2)
25394	1(3)
25400	1(2)
25405	1(2)
25415	1(2)
25420	1(2)
25425	1(2)
25426	1(2)
25430	1(3)
25431	1(3)
25440	1(2)
25441	1(2)
25442	1(2)
25443	1(2)
25444	1(2)
25445	1(2)
25446	1(2)
25447	4(3)
25449	1(2)
25450	1(2)
25455	1(2)
25490	1(2)
25491	1(2)
25492	1(2)
25500	1(2)
25505	1(2)
25515	1(2)
25520	1(2)
25525	1(2)
25526	1(2)
25530	1(2)
25535	1(2)
25545	1(2)
25560	1(2)
25565	1(2)
25574	1(2)
25575	1(2)
25600	1(2)
25605	1(2)
25606	1(2)
25607	1(2)
25608	1(2)
25609	1(2)
25622	1(2)
25624	1(2)
25628	1(2)
25630	1(3)
25635	1(3)
25645	1(3)
25650	1(2)
25651	1(2)
25652	1(2)
25660	1(2)
25670	1(2)
25671	1(2)
25675	1(2)
25676	1(2)
25680	1(2)
25685	1(2)
25690	1(2)
25695	1(2)
25800	1(2)

CPT	MUE
25805	1(2)
25810	1(2)
25820	1(2)
25825	1(2)
25830	1(2)
25900	1(2)
25905	1(2)
25907	1(2)
25909	1(2)
25915	1(2)
25920	1(2)
25922	1(2)
25924	1(2)
25927	1(2)
25929	1(2)
25931	1(2)
25999	1(3)
26010	2(3)
26011	3(3)
26020	4(3)
26025	1(2)
26030	1(2)
26034	2(3)
26035	1(3)
26037	1(3)
26040	1(2)
26045	1(2)
26055	5(3)
26060	5(3)
26070	2(3)
26075	3(3)
26080	3(3)
26100	1(3)
26105	2(3)
26110	2(3)
26111	4(3)
26113	3(3)
26115	4(3)
26116	2(3)
26117	2(3)
26118	1(3)
26121	1(2)
26123	1(2)
26125	4(3)
26130	1(3)
26135	4(3)
26140	2(3)
26145	6(3)
26160	4(3)
26170	4(3)
26180	4(3)
26185	1(3)
26200	2(3)
26205	1(3)
26210	2(3)
26215	2(3)
26230	2(3)
26235	2(3)
26236	2(3)
26250	2(3)
26260	1(3)
26262	1(3)
26320	4(3)
26340	4(3)
26341	2(3)

CPT	MUE
26350	6(3)
26352	2(3)
26356	4(3)
26357	2(3)
26358	2(3)
26370	3(3)
26372	1(3)
26373	2(3)
26390	2(3)
26392	2(3)
26410	4(3)
26412	3(3)
26415	2(3)
26416	2(3)
26418	4(3)
26420	3(3)
26426	4(3)
26428	2(3)
26432	2(3)
26433	2(3)
26434	2(3)
26437	4(3)
26440	6(3)
26442	5(3)
26445	5(3)
26449	5(3)
26450	6(3)
26455	6(3)
26460	4(3)
26471	4(3)
26474	4(3)
26476	4(3)
26477	2(3)
26478	6(3)
26479	4(3)
26480	4(3)
26483	4(3)
26485	4(3)
26489	2(3)
26490	3(3)
26492	2(3)
26494	1(3)
26496	1(3)
26497	2(3)
26498	1(3)
26499	2(3)
26500	3(3)
26502	2(3)
26508	1(2)
26510	4(3)
26516	1(2)
26517	1(2)
26518	1(2)
26520	4(3)
26525	4(3)
26530	4(3)
26531	4(3)
26535	3(3)
26536	4(3)
26540	4(3)
26541	4(3)
26542	4(3)
26545	4(3)
26546	2(3)
26548	3(3)

CPT	MUE
26550	1(2)
26551	1(2)
26553	1(3)
26554	1(3)
26555	2(3)
26556	2(3)
26560	2(3)
26561	2(3)
26562	2(3)
26565	2(3)
26567	3(3)
26568	2(3)
26580	1(2)
26587	2(3)
26590	2(3)
26591	4(3)
26593	8(3)
26596	1(3)
26600	2(3)
26605	3(3)
26607	2(3)
26608	4(3)
26615	3(3)
26641	1(2)
26645	1(2)
26650	1(2)
26665	1(2)
26670	2(3)
26675	1(3)
26676	2(3)
26685	3(3)
26686	3(3)
26700	2(3)
26705	3(3)
26706	2(3)
26715	3(3)
26720	4(3)
26725	3(3)
26727	3(3)
26735	4(3)
26740	3(3)
26742	3(3)
26746	3(3)
26750	3(3)
26755	2(3)
26756	2(3)
26765	3(3)
26770	3(3)
26775	2(3)
26776	4(3)
26785	3(3)
26820	1(2)
26841	1(2)
26842	1(2)
26843	2(3)
26844	2(3)
26850	5(3)
26852	2(3)
26860	1(2)
26861	4(3)
26862	1(2)
26863	2(3)
26910	4(3)
26951	8(3)
26952	4(3)

CPT	MUE
26989	1(3)
26990	2(3)
26991	1(3)
26992	2(3)
27000	1(3)
27001	1(3)
27003	1(2)
27005	1(2)
27006	1(2)
27025	1(3)
27027	1(2)
27030	1(2)
27033	1(2)
27035	1(2)
27036	1(2)
27040	2(3)
27041	3(3)
27043	2(3)
27045	3(3)
27047	2(3)
27048	2(3)
27049	1(3)
27050	1(2)
27052	1(2)
27054	1(2)
27057	1(2)
27059	1(3)
27060	1(2)
27062	1(2)
27065	1(3)
27066	1(3)
27067	1(3)
27070	1(3)
27071	1(3)
27075	1(3)
27076	1(2)
27077	1(2)
27078	1(2)
27080	1(2)
27086	1(3)
27087	1(3)
27090	1(2)
27091	1(2)
27093	1(2)
27095	1(2)
27096	1(2)
27097	1(3)
27098	1(2)
27100	1(2)
27105	1(3)
27110	1(2)
27111	1(2)
27120	1(2)
27122	1(2)
27125	1(2)
27130	1(2)
27132	1(2)
27134	1(2)
27137	1(2)
27138	1(2)
27140	1(2)
27146	1(3)
27147	1(3)
27151	1(3)
27156	1(2)

CPT	MUE
27158	1(2)
27161	1(2)
27165	1(2)
27170	1(2)
27175	1(2)
27176	1(2)
27177	1(2)
27178	1(2)
27179	1(2)
27181	1(2)
27185	1(2)
27187	1(2)
27197	1(2)
27198	1(2)
27200	1(2)
27202	1(2)
27215	0(3)
27216	0(3)
27217	0(3)
27218	0(3)
27220	1(2)
27222	1(2)
27226	1(2)
27227	1(2)
27228	1(2)
27230	1(2)
27232	1(2)
27235	1(2)
27236	1(2)
27238	1(2)
27240	1(2)
27244	1(2)
27245	1(2)
27246	1(2)
27248	1(2)
27250	1(2)
27252	1(2)
27253	1(2)
27254	1(2)
27256	1(2)
27257	1(2)
27258	1(2)
27259	1(2)
27265	1(2)
27266	1(2)
27267	1(2)
27268	1(2)
27269	1(2)
27275	2(2)
27279	1(2)
27280	1(2)
27282	1(2)
27284	1(2)
27286	1(2)
27290	1(2)
27295	1(2)
27299	1(3)
27301	3(3)
27303	2(3)
27305	1(2)
27306	1(2)
27307	1(2)
27310	1(2)
27323	2(3)
27324	3(3)

CPT	MUE
27325	1(2)
27326	1(2)
27327	5(3)
27328	3(3)
27329	1(3)
27330	1(2)
27331	1(2)
27332	1(2)
27333	1(2)
27334	1(2)
27335	1(2)
27337	3(3)
27339	4(3)
27340	1(2)
27345	1(2)
27347	1(2)
27350	1(2)
27355	1(3)
27356	1(3)
27357	1(3)
27358	1(3)
27360	2(3)
27364	1(3)
27365	1(3)
27369	1(2)
27372	2(3)
27380	1(2)
27381	1(2)
27385	2(3)
27386	2(3)
27390	1(2)
27391	1(2)
27392	1(2)
27393	1(2)
27394	1(2)
27395	1(2)
27396	1(2)
27397	1(2)
27400	1(2)
27403	1(3)
27405	2(2)
27407	2(2)
27409	1(2)
27412	1(2)
27415	1(2)
27416	1(2)
27418	1(2)
27420	1(2)
27422	1(2)
27424	1(2)
27425	1(2)
27427	1(2)
27428	1(2)
27429	1(2)
27430	1(2)
27435	1(2)
27437	1(2)
27438	1(2)
27440	1(2)
27441	1(2)
27442	1(2)
27443	1(2)
27445	1(2)
27446	1(2)
27447	1(2)

CPT	MUE
27448	1(3)
27450	1(3)
27454	1(2)
27455	1(3)
27457	1(3)
27465	1(2)
27466	1(2)
27468	1(2)
27470	1(2)
27472	1(2)
27475	1(2)
27477	1(2)
27479	1(2)
27485	1(2)
27486	1(2)
27487	1(2)
27488	1(2)
27495	1(2)
27496	1(2)
27497	1(2)
27498	1(2)
27499	1(2)
27500	1(2)
27501	1(2)
27502	1(2)
27503	1(2)
27506	1(2)
27507	1(2)
27508	1(2)
27509	1(2)
27510	1(2)
27511	1(2)
27513	1(2)
27514	1(2)
27516	1(2)
27517	1(2)
27519	1(2)
27520	1(2)
27524	1(2)
27530	1(2)
27532	1(2)
27535	1(2)
27536	1(2)
27538	1(2)
27540	1(2)
27550	1(2)
27552	1(2)
27556	1(2)
27557	1(2)
27558	1(2)
27560	1(2)
27562	1(2)
27566	1(2)
27570	1(2)
27580	1(2)
27590	1(2)
27591	1(2)
27592	1(2)
27594	1(2)
27596	1(2)
27598	1(2)
27599	1(3)
27600	1(2)
27601	1(2)
27602	1(2)

CPT	MUE
27603	2(3)
27604	2(3)
27605	1(2)
27606	1(2)
27607	2(3)
27610	1(2)
27612	1(2)
27613	3(3)
27614	3(3)
27615	1(3)
27616	1(3)
27618	3(3)
27619	2(3)
27620	1(2)
27625	1(2)
27626	1(2)
27630	2(3)
27632	3(3)
27634	2(3)
27635	1(3)
27637	1(3)
27638	1(3)
27640	1(3)
27641	1(3)
27645	1(3)
27646	1(3)
27647	1(3)
27648	1(2)
27650	1(2)
27652	1(2)
27654	1(2)
27656	1(3)
27658	2(3)
27659	2(3)
27664	2(3)
27665	2(3)
27675	1(2)
27676	1(2)
27680	2(3)
27681	1(2)
27685	2(3)
27686	3(3)
27687	1(2)
27690	2(3)
27691	2(3)
27692	4(3)
27695	1(2)
27696	1(2)
27698	2(2)
27700	1(2)
27702	1(2)
27703	1(2)
27704	1(2)
27705	1(3)
27707	1(3)
27709	1(3)
27712	1(2)
27715	1(2)
27720	1(2)
27722	1(2)
27724	1(2)
27725	1(2)
27726	1(2)
27727	1(2)
27730	1(2)

CPT	MUE
27732	1(2)
27734	1(2)
27740	1(2)
27742	1(2)
27745	1(2)
27750	1(2)
27752	1(2)
27756	1(2)
27758	1(2)
27759	1(2)
27760	1(2)
27762	1(2)
27766	1(2)
27767	1(2)
27768	1(2)
27769	1(2)
27780	1(2)
27781	1(2)
27784	1(2)
27786	1(2)
27788	1(2)
27792	1(2)
27808	1(2)
27810	1(2)
27814	1(2)
27816	1(2)
27818	1(2)
27822	1(2)
27823	1(2)
27824	1(2)
27825	1(2)
27826	1(2)
27827	1(2)
27828	1(2)
27829	1(2)
27830	1(2)
27831	1(2)
27832	1(2)
27840	1(2)
27842	1(2)
27846	1(2)
27848	1(2)
27860	1(2)
27870	1(2)
27871	1(3)
27880	1(2)
27881	1(2)
27882	1(2)
27884	1(2)
27886	1(2)
27888	1(2)
27889	1(2)
27892	1(2)
27893	1(2)
27894	1(2)
27899	1(3)
28001	2(3)
28002	3(3)
28003	2(3)
28005	3(3)
28008	2(3)
28010	4(3)
28011	4(3)
28020	2(3)
28022	3(3)

CPT	MUE
28024	4(3)
28035	1(2)
28039	2(3)
28041	2(3)
28043	4(3)
28045	4(3)
28046	1(3)
28047	1(3)
28050	2(3)
28052	2(3)
28054	2(3)
28055	1(3)
28060	1(2)
28062	1(2)
28070	2(3)
28072	4(3)
28080	3(3)
28086	2(3)
28088	2(3)
28090	2(3)
28092	2(3)
28100	1(3)
28102	1(3)
28103	1(3)
28104	2(3)
28106	1(3)
28107	1(3)
28108	2(3)
28110	1(2)
28111	1(2)
28112	4(3)
28113	1(2)
28114	1(2)
28116	1(2)
28118	1(2)
28119	1(2)
28120	2(3)
28122	4(3)
28124	4(3)
28126	4(3)
28130	1(2)
28140	3(3)
28150	4(3)
28153	4(3)
28160	5(3)
28171	1(3)
28173	2(3)
28175	2(3)
28190	3(3)
28192	2(3)
28193	2(3)
28200	4(3)
28202	2(3)
28208	4(3)
28210	2(3)
28220	1(2)
28222	1(2)
28225	1(2)
28226	1(2)
28230	1(2)
28232	6(3)
28234	6(3)
28238	1(2)
28240	1(2)
28250	1(2)

CPT	MUE
28260	1(2)
28261	1(3)
28262	1(2)
28264	1(2)
28270	6(3)
28272	6(3)
28280	1(2)
28285	4(3)
28286	1(2)
28288	4(3)
28289	1(2)
28291	1(2)
28292	1(2)
28295	1(2)
28296	1(2)
28297	1(2)
28298	1(2)
28299	1(2)
28300	1(2)
28302	1(2)
28304	1(3)
28305	1(3)
28306	1(2)
28307	1(2)
28308	4(3)
28309	1(2)
28310	1(2)
28312	4(3)
28313	4(3)
28315	1(2)
28320	1(2)
28322	2(3)
28340	2(3)
28341	2(3)
28344	1(2)
28345	2(3)
28360	1(2)
28400	1(2)
28405	1(2)
28406	1(2)
28415	1(2)
28420	1(2)
28430	1(2)
28435	1(2)
28436	1(2)
28445	1(2)
28446	1(2)
28450	2(3)
28455	3(3)
28456	2(3)
28465	3(3)
28470	2(3)
28475	5(3)
28476	4(3)
28485	5(3)
28490	1(2)
28495	1(2)
28496	1(2)
28505	1(2)
28510	4(3)
28515	4(3)
28525	4(3)
28530	1(2)
28531	1(2)
28540	1(3)

CPT	MUE
28545	1(3)
28546	1(3)
28555	1(3)
28570	1(2)
28575	1(2)
28576	1(2)
28585	1(3)
28600	2(3)
28605	2(3)
28606	3(3)
28615	5(3)
28630	2(3)
28635	2(3)
28636	4(3)
28645	4(3)
28660	4(3)
28665	3(3)
28666	4(3)
28675	3(3)
28705	1(2)
28715	1(2)
28725	1(2)
28730	1(2)
28735	1(2)
28737	1(2)
28740	1(2)
28750	1(2)
28755	1(2)
28760	1(2)
28800	1(2)
28805	1(2)
28810	5(3)
28820	6(3)
28825	8(2)
28890	1(2)
28899	1(3)
29000	1(3)
29010	1(3)
29015	1(3)
29035	1(3)
29040	1(3)
29044	1(3)
29046	1(3)
29049	1(3)
29055	1(3)
29058	1(3)
29065	1(3)
29075	1(3)
29085	1(3)
29086	2(3)
29105	1(2)
29125	1(2)
29126	1(2)
29130	3(3)
29131	2(3)
29200	1(2)
29240	1(2)
29260	1(3)
29280	2(3)
29305	1(3)
29325	1(3)
29345	1(3)
29355	1(3)
29358	1(3)
29365	1(3)

CPT	MUE
29405	1(3)
29425	1(3)
29435	1(3)
29440	1(2)
29445	1(3)
29450	1(3)
29505	1(2)
29515	1(2)
29520	1(2)
29530	1(2)
29540	1(2)
29550	1(2)
29580	1(2)
29581	1(2)
29584	1(2)
29700	2(3)
29705	1(3)
29710	1(2)
29720	1(2)
29730	1(3)
29740	1(3)
29750	1(3)
29799	1(3)
29800	1(2)
29804	1(2)
29805	1(2)
29806	1(2)
29807	1(2)
29819	1(2)
29820	1(2)
29821	1(2)
29822	1(2)
29823	1(2)
29824	1(2)
29825	1(2)
29826	1(2)
29827	1(2)
29828	1(2)
29830	1(2)
29834	1(2)
29835	1(2)
29836	1(2)
29837	1(2)
29838	1(2)
29840	1(2)
29843	1(2)
29844	1(2)
29845	1(2)
29846	1(2)
29847	1(2)
29848	1(2)
29850	1(2)
29851	1(2)
29855	1(2)
29856	1(2)
29860	1(2)
29861	1(2)
29862	1(2)
29863	1(2)
29866	1(2)
29867	1(2)
29868	1(3)
29870	1(2)
29871	1(2)
29873	1(2)

CPT	MUE
29874	1(2)
29875	1(2)
29876	1(2)
29877	1(2)
29879	1(2)
29880	1(2)
29881	1(2)
29882	1(2)
29883	1(2)
29884	1(2)
29885	1(2)
29886	1(2)
29887	1(2)
29888	1(2)
29889	1(2)
29891	1(2)
29892	1(2)
29893	1(2)
29894	1(2)
29895	1(2)
29897	1(2)
29898	1(2)
29899	1(2)
29900	2(3)
29901	2(3)
29902	2(3)
29904	1(2)
29905	1(2)
29906	1(2)
29907	1(2)
29914	1(2)
29915	1(2)
29916	1(2)
29999	1(3)
30000	1(3)
30020	1(3)
30100	2(3)
30110	1(2)
30115	1(2)
30117	2(3)
30118	1(3)
30120	1(2)
30124	2(3)
30125	1(3)
30130	1(2)
30140	1(2)
30150	1(2)
30160	1(2)
30200	1(2)
30210	1(3)
30220	1(2)
30300	1(3)
30310	1(3)
30320	1(3)
30400	1(2)
30410	1(2)
30420	1(2)
30430	1(2)
30435	1(2)
30450	1(2)
30460	1(2)
30462	1(2)
30465	1(2)
30520	1(2)
30540	1(2)

CPT	MUE
30545	1(2)
30560	1(2)
30580	2(3)
30600	1(3)
30620	1(2)
30630	1(2)
30801	1(2)
30802	1(2)
30901	1(3)
30903	1(3)
30905	1(2)
30906	1(3)
30915	1(3)
30920	1(3)
30930	1(2)
30999	1(3)
31000	1(2)
31002	1(2)
31020	1(2)
31030	1(2)
31032	1(2)
31040	1(2)
31050	1(2)
31051	1(2)
31070	1(2)
31075	1(2)
31080	1(2)
31081	1(2)
31084	1(2)
31085	1(2)
31086	1(2)
31087	1(2)
31090	1(2)
31200	1(2)
31201	1(2)
31205	1(2)
31225	1(2)
31230	1(2)
31231	1(2)
31233	1(2)
31235	1(2)
31237	1(2)
31238	1(3)
31239	1(2)
31240	1(2)
31241	1(2)
31253	1(2)
31254	1(2)
31255	1(2)
31256	1(2)
31257	1(2)
31259	1(2)
31267	1(2)
31276	1(2)
31287	1(2)
31288	1(2)
31290	1(2)
31291	1(2)
31292	1(2)
31293	1(2)
31294	1(2)
31295	1(2)
31296	1(2)
31297	1(2)
31298	1(2)

CPT	MUE
31299	1(3)
31300	1(2)
31360	1(2)
31365	1(2)
31367	1(2)
31368	1(2)
31370	1(2)
31375	1(2)
31380	1(2)
31382	1(2)
31390	1(2)
31395	1(2)
31400	1(3)
31420	1(2)
31500	2(3)
31502	1(3)
31505	1(3)
31510	1(2)
31511	1(3)
31512	1(3)
31513	1(3)
31515	1(3)
31520	1(3)
31525	1(3)
31526	1(3)
31527	1(2)
31528	1(2)
31529	1(3)
31530	1(3)
31531	1(3)
31535	1(3)
31536	1(3)
31540	1(3)
31541	1(3)
31545	1(2)
31546	1(2)
31551	1(2)
31552	1(2)
31553	1(2)
31554	1(2)
31560	1(2)
31561	1(2)
31570	1(2)
31571	1(2)
31572	1(2)
31573	1(2)
31574	1(2)
31575	1(3)
31576	1(3)
31577	1(3)
31578	1(3)
31579	1(2)
31580	1(2)
31584	1(2)
31587	1(2)
31590	1(2)
31591	1(2)
31592	1(2)
31599	1(3)
31600	1(2)
31601	1(2)
31603	1(2)
31605	1(2)
31610	1(2)
31611	1(2)

CPT	MUE
31612	1(3)
31613	1(2)
31614	1(2)
31615	1(3)
31622	1(3)
31623	1(3)
31624	1(3)
31625	1(2)
31626	1(2)
31627	1(3)
31628	1(2)
31629	1(2)
31630	1(3)
31631	1(2)
31632	2(3)
31633	2(3)
31634	1(3)
31635	1(3)
31636	1(2)
31637	2(3)
31638	1(3)
31640	1(3)
31641	1(3)
31643	1(2)
31645	1(2)
31646	2(3)
31647	1(2)
31648	1(2)
31649	2(3)
31651	3(3)
31652	1(2)
31653	1(2)
31654	1(3)
31660	1(2)
31661	1(2)
31717	1(3)
31720	3(3)
31725	1(3)
31730	1(3)
31750	1(2)
31755	1(2)
31760	1(2)
31766	1(2)
31770	2(3)
31775	1(3)
31780	1(2)
31781	1(2)
31785	1(3)
31786	1(3)
31800	1(3)
31805	1(3)
31820	1(2)
31825	1(2)
31830	1(2)
31899	1(3)
32035	1(2)
32036	1(3)
32096	1(3)
32097	1(3)
32098	1(2)
32100	1(3)
32110	1(3)
32120	1(3)
32124	1(3)
32140	1(3)

CPT	MUE
32141	1(3)
32150	1(3)
32151	1(3)
32160	1(3)
32200	2(3)
32215	1(2)
32220	1(2)
32225	1(2)
32310	1(3)
32320	1(3)
32400	2(3)
32405	2(3)
32440	1(2)
32442	1(2)
32445	1(2)
32480	1(2)
32482	1(2)
32484	2(3)
32486	1(3)
32488	1(2)
32491	1(2)
32501	1(3)
32503	1(2)
32504	1(2)
32505	1(2)
32506	3(3)
32507	2(3)
32540	1(3)
32550	2(3)
32551	2(3)
32552	2(2)
32553	1(2)
32554	2(3)
32555	2(3)
32556	2(3)
32557	2(3)
32560	1(3)
32561	1(2)
32562	1(2)
32601	1(3)
32604	1(3)
32606	1(3)
32607	1(3)
32608	1(3)
32609	1(3)
32650	1(2)
32651	1(2)
32652	1(2)
32653	1(3)
32654	1(3)
32655	1(3)
32656	1(2)
32658	1(3)
32659	1(2)
32661	1(3)
32662	1(3)
32663	1(3)
32664	1(2)
32665	1(2)
32666	1(3)
32667	3(3)
32668	2(3)
32669	2(3)
32670	1(2)
32671	1(2)

CPT	MUE
32672	1(3)
32673	1(2)
32674	1(2)
32701	1(2)
32800	1(3)
32810	1(3)
32815	1(3)
32820	1(2)
32850	1(2)
32851	1(2)
32852	1(2)
32853	1(2)
32854	1(2)
32855	1(2)
32856	1(2)
32900	1(2)
32905	1(2)
32906	1(2)
32940	1(3)
32960	1(2)
32994	1(2)
32997	1(2)
32998	1(2)
32999	1(3)
33016	1(3)
33017	1(3)
33018	1(3)
33019	1(3)
33020	1(3)
33025	1(2)
33030	1(2)
33031	1(2)
33050	1(2)
33120	1(3)
33130	1(3)
33140	1(2)
33141	1(2)
33202	1(2)
33203	1(2)
33206	1(3)
33207	1(3)
33208	1(3)
33210	1(3)
33211	1(3)
33212	1(3)
33213	1(3)
33214	1(3)
33215	2(3)
33216	1(3)
33217	1(3)
33218	1(3)
33220	1(3)
33221	1(3)
33222	1(3)
33223	1(3)
33224	1(3)
33225	1(3)
33226	1(3)
33227	1(3)
33228	1(3)
33229	1(3)
33230	1(3)
33231	1(3)
33233	1(2)
33234	1(2)

CPT	MUE
33235	1(2)
33236	1(2)
33237	1(2)
33238	1(2)
33240	1(3)
33241	1(2)
33243	1(2)
33244	1(2)
33249	1(3)
33250	1(2)
33251	1(2)
33254	1(2)
33255	1(2)
33256	1(2)
33257	1(2)
33258	1(2)
33259	1(2)
33261	1(2)
33262	1(3)
33263	1(3)
33264	1(3)
33265	1(2)
33266	1(2)
33270	1(3)
33271	1(3)
33272	1(3)
33273	1(3)
33274	1(3)
33275	1(3)
33285	1(3)
33286	1(3)
33289	1(3)
33300	1(3)
33305	1(3)
33310	1(2)
33315	1(2)
33320	1(3)
33321	1(3)
33322	1(3)
33330	1(3)
33335	1(3)
33340	1(2)
33361	1(2)
33362	1(2)
33363	1(2)
33364	1(2)
33365	1(2)
33366	1(3)
33367	1(2)
33368	1(2)
33369	1(2)
33390	1(2)
33391	1(2)
33404	1(2)
33405	1(2)
33406	1(2)
33410	1(2)
33411	1(2)
33412	1(2)
33413	1(2)
33414	1(2)
33415	1(2)
33416	1(2)
33417	1(2)
33418	1(3)

CPT	MUE
33419	1(2)
33420	1(2)
33422	1(2)
33425	1(2)
33426	1(2)
33427	1(2)
33430	1(2)
33440	1(2)
33460	1(2)
33463	1(2)
33464	1(2)
33465	1(2)
33468	1(2)
33470	1(2)
33471	1(2)
33474	1(2)
33475	1(2)
33476	1(2)
33477	1(2)
33478	1(2)
33496	1(3)
33500	1(3)
33501	1(3)
33502	1(3)
33503	1(3)
33504	1(3)
33505	1(3)
33506	1(3)
33507	1(3)
33508	1(2)
33510	1(2)
33511	1(2)
33512	1(2)
33513	1(2)
33514	1(2)
33516	1(2)
33517	1(2)
33518	1(2)
33519	1(2)
33521	1(2)
33522	1(2)
33523	1(2)
33530	1(2)
33533	1(2)
33534	1(2)
33535	1(2)
33536	1(2)
33542	1(2)
33545	1(2)
33548	1(2)
33572	3(2)
33600	1(3)
33602	1(3)
33606	1(2)
33608	1(2)
33610	1(2)
33611	1(2)
33612	1(2)
33615	1(2)
33617	1(2)
33619	1(2)
33620	1(2)
33621	1(3)
33622	1(2)
33641	1(2)

CPT	MUE
33645	1(2)
33647	1(2)
33660	1(2)
33665	1(2)
33670	1(2)
33675	1(2)
33676	1(2)
33677	1(2)
33681	1(2)
33684	1(2)
33688	1(2)
33690	1(2)
33692	1(2)
33694	1(2)
33697	1(2)
33702	1(2)
33710	1(2)
33720	1(2)
33722	1(3)
33724	1(2)
33726	1(2)
33730	1(2)
33732	1(2)
33735	1(2)
33736	1(2)
33737	1(2)
33750	1(3)
33755	1(2)
33762	1(2)
33764	1(3)
33766	1(2)
33767	1(2)
33768	1(2)
33770	1(2)
33771	1(2)
33774	1(2)
33775	1(2)
33776	1(2)
33777	1(2)
33778	1(2)
33779	1(2)
33780	1(2)
33781	1(2)
33782	1(2)
33783	1(2)
33786	1(2)
33788	1(2)
33800	1(2)
33802	1(3)
33803	1(3)
33813	1(2)
33814	1(2)
33820	1(2)
33822	1(2)
33824	1(2)
33840	1(2)
33845	1(2)
33851	1(2)
33852	1(2)
33853	1(2)
33858	1(2)
33859	1(2)
33863	1(2)
33864	1(2)
33866	1(2)

CPT	MUE
33871	1(2)
33875	1(2)
33877	1(2)
33880	1(2)
33881	1(2)
33883	1(2)
33884	2(3)
33886	1(2)
33889	1(2)
33891	1(2)
33910	1(3)
33915	1(3)
33916	1(3)
33917	1(2)
33920	1(2)
33922	1(2)
33924	1(2)
33925	1(2)
33926	1(2)
33927	1(3)
33928	1(3)
33929	1(3)
33930	1(2)
33933	1(2)
33935	1(2)
33940	1(2)
33944	1(2)
33945	1(2)
33946	1(2)
33947	1(2)
33948	1(2)
33949	1(2)
33951	1(3)
33952	1(3)
33953	1(3)
33954	1(3)
33955	1(3)
33956	1(3)
33957	1(3)
33958	1(3)
33959	1(3)
33962	1(3)
33963	1(3)
33964	1(3)
33965	1(3)
33966	1(3)
33967	1(3)
33968	1(3)
33969	1(3)
33970	1(3)
33971	1(3)
33973	1(3)
33974	1(3)
33975	1(3)
33976	1(3)
33977	1(3)
33978	1(3)
33979	1(3)
33980	1(3)
33981	1(3)
33982	1(3)
33983	1(3)
33984	1(3)
33985	1(3)
33986	1(3)

CPT	MUE
33987	1(3)
33988	1(3)
33989	1(3)
33990	1(3)
33991	1(3)
33992	1(2)
33993	1(3)
33999	1(3)
34001	1(3)
34051	1(3)
34101	1(3)
34111	2(3)
34151	1(3)
34201	1(3)
34203	1(2)
34401	1(3)
34421	1(3)
34451	1(3)
34471	1(2)
34490	1(2)
34501	1(2)
34502	1(2)
34510	2(3)
34520	1(3)
34530	1(2)
34701	1(2)
34702	1(2)
34703	1(2)
34704	1(2)
34705	1(2)
34706	1(2)
34707	1(2)
34708	1(2)
34709	3(3)
34710	1(2)
34711	2(3)
34712	1(2)
34713	1(2)
34714	1(2)
34715	1(2)
34716	1(2)
34717	2(2)
34718	2(2)
34808	1(3)
34812	1(2)
34813	1(2)
34820	1(2)
34830	1(2)
34831	1(2)
34832	1(2)
34833	1(2)
34834	1(2)
34839	1(2)
34841	1(2)
34842	1(2)
34843	1(2)
34844	1(2)
34845	1(2)
34846	1(2)
34847	1(2)
34848	1(2)
35001	1(2)
35002	1(2)
35005	1(2)
35011	1(2)

CPT	MUE
35013	1(2)
35021	1(2)
35022	1(2)
35045	1(3)
35081	1(2)
35082	1(2)
35091	1(2)
35092	1(2)
35102	1(2)
35103	1(2)
35111	1(2)
35112	1(2)
35121	1(3)
35122	1(3)
35131	1(2)
35132	1(2)
35141	1(2)
35142	1(2)
35151	1(2)
35152	1(2)
35180	2(3)
35182	2(3)
35184	2(3)
35188	2(3)
35189	1(3)
35190	2(3)
35201	2(3)
35206	2(3)
35207	3(3)
35211	3(3)
35216	2(3)
35221	3(3)
35226	3(3)
35231	2(3)
35236	2(3)
35241	2(3)
35246	2(3)
35251	2(3)
35256	2(3)
35261	1(3)
35266	2(3)
35271	2(3)
35276	2(3)
35281	2(3)
35286	2(3)
35301	2(3)
35302	1(2)
35303	1(2)
35304	1(2)
35305	1(2)
35306	2(3)
35311	1(2)
35321	1(2)
35331	1(2)
35341	3(3)
35351	1(3)
35355	1(2)
35361	1(2)
35363	1(2)
35371	1(2)
35372	1(2)
35390	1(3)
35400	1(3)
35500	2(3)
35501	1(3)

CPT	MUE
35506	1(3)
35508	1(3)
35509	1(3)
35510	1(3)
35511	1(3)
35512	1(3)
35515	1(3)
35516	1(3)
35518	1(3)
35521	1(3)
35522	1(3)
35523	1(3)
35525	1(3)
35526	1(3)
35531	1(3)
35533	1(3)
35535	1(3)
35536	1(3)
35537	1(3)
35538	1(3)
35539	1(3)
35540	1(3)
35556	1(3)
35558	1(3)
35560	1(3)
35563	1(3)
35565	1(3)
35566	1(3)
35570	1(3)
35571	1(3)
35572	2(3)
35583	1(2)
35585	2(3)
35587	1(3)
35600	2(3)
35601	1(3)
35606	1(3)
35612	1(3)
35616	1(3)
35621	1(3)
35623	1(3)
35626	3(3)
35631	4(3)
35632	1(3)
35633	1(3)
35634	1(3)
35636	1(3)
35637	1(3)
35638	1(3)
35642	1(3)
35645	1(3)
35646	1(3)
35647	1(3)
35650	1(3)
35654	1(3)
35656	1(3)
35661	1(3)
35663	1(3)
35665	1(3)
35666	2(3)
35671	2(3)
35681	1(3)
35682	1(2)
35683	1(2)
35685	2(3)

CPT	MUE
35686	1(3)
35691	1(3)
35693	1(3)
35694	1(3)
35695	1(3)
35697	2(3)
35700	2(3)
35701	1(2)
35702	2(2)
35703	2(2)
35800	2(3)
35820	2(3)
35840	2(3)
35860	2(3)
35870	1(3)
35875	2(3)
35876	2(3)
35879	2(3)
35881	1(3)
35883	1(3)
35884	1(3)
35901	1(3)
35903	2(3)
35905	1(3)
35907	1(3)
36000	4(3)
36002	2(3)
36005	2(3)
36010	2(3)
36011	4(3)
36012	4(3)
36013	2(3)
36014	2(3)
36015	4(3)
36100	2(3)
36140	3(3)
36160	2(3)
36200	2(3)
36215	2(3)
36216	2(3)
36217	2(3)
36218	2(3)
36221	1(3)
36222	1(3)
36223	1(3)
36224	1(3)
36225	1(3)
36226	1(3)
36227	2(2)
36228	2(3)
36245	3(3)
36246	4(3)
36247	2(3)
36248	2(3)
36251	1(3)
36252	1(3)
36253	1(3)
36254	1(3)
36260	1(2)
36261	1(2)
36262	1(2)
36299	1(3)
36400	1(3)
36405	1(3)
36406	1(3)

CPT	MUE
36410	3(3)
36415	2(3)
36416	6(3)
36420	2(3)
36425	2(3)
36430	1(2)
36440	1(3)
36450	1(3)
36455	1(3)
36456	1(3)
36460	2(3)
36465	1(2)
36466	1(2)
36468	2(3)
36470	1(2)
36471	1(2)
36473	1(3)
36474	1(3)
36475	1(3)
36476	2(3)
36478	1(3)
36479	2(3)
36481	1(3)
36482	1(3)
36483	2(3)
36500	4(3)
36510	1(3)
36511	1(3)
36512	1(3)
36513	1(3)
36514	1(3)
36516	1(3)
36522	1(3)
36555	2(3)
36556	2(3)
36557	2(3)
36558	2(3)
36560	2(3)
36561	2(3)
36563	1(3)
36565	1(3)
36566	1(3)
36568	2(3)
36569	2(3)
36570	2(3)
36571	2(3)
36572	1(3)
36573	1(3)
36575	2(3)
36576	2(3)
36578	2(3)
36580	2(3)
36581	2(3)
36582	2(3)
36583	2(3)
36584	2(3)
36585	2(3)
36589	2(3)
36590	2(3)
36591	2(3)
36592	1(3)
36593	2(3)
36595	2(3)
36596	2(3)
36597	2(3)

CPT	MUE
36598	2(3)
36600	4(3)
36620	3(3)
36625	2(3)
36640	1(3)
36660	1(3)
36680	1(3)
36800	1(3)
36810	1(3)
36815	1(3)
36818	1(3)
36819	1(3)
36820	1(3)
36821	2(3)
36823	1(3)
36825	1(3)
36830	2(3)
36831	1(3)
36832	2(3)
36833	1(3)
36835	1(3)
36838	1(3)
36860	2(3)
36861	2(3)
36901	1(3)
36902	1(3)
36903	1(3)
36904	1(3)
36905	1(3)
36906	1(3)
36907	1(3)
36908	1(3)
36909	1(3)
37140	1(2)
37145	1(3)
37160	1(3)
37180	1(2)
37181	1(2)
37182	1(2)
37183	1(2)
37184	1(2)
37185	2(3)
37186	2(3)
37187	1(3)
37188	1(3)
37191	1(3)
37192	1(3)
37193	1(3)
37195	1(3)
37197	2(3)
37200	2(3)
37211	1(2)
37212	1(2)
37213	1(2)
37214	1(2)
37215	1(2)
37216	0(3)
37217	1(2)
37218	1(2)
37220	1(2)
37221	1(2)
37222	2(2)
37223	2(2)
37224	1(2)
37225	1(2)

CPT	MUE
37226	1(2)
37227	1(2)
37228	1(2)
37229	1(2)
37230	1(2)
37231	1(2)
37232	2(3)
37233	2(3)
37234	2(3)
37235	2(3)
37236	1(2)
37237	2(3)
37238	1(2)
37239	2(3)
37241	2(3)
37242	2(3)
37243	1(3)
37244	2(3)
37246	1(2)
37247	2(3)
37248	1(2)
37249	3(3)
37252	1(2)
37253	5(3)
37500	1(3)
37501	1(3)
37565	1(2)
37600	1(3)
37605	1(3)
37606	1(3)
37607	1(3)
37609	1(2)
37615	2(3)
37616	1(3)
37617	3(3)
37618	2(3)
37619	1(2)
37650	1(2)
37660	1(2)
37700	1(2)
37718	1(2)
37722	1(2)
37735	1(2)
37760	1(2)
37761	1(2)
37765	1(2)
37766	1(2)
37780	1(2)
37785	1(2)
37788	1(2)
37790	1(2)
37799	1(3)
38100	1(2)
38101	1(3)
38102	1(2)
38115	1(3)
38120	1(2)
38129	1(3)
38200	1(3)
38204	1(2)
38205	1(3)
38206	1(3)
38207	1(3)
38208	1(3)
38209	1(3)

CPT	MUE	CPT	MUE	CPT	MUE	CPT	MUE	CPT	MUE	CPT	MUE	CPT	MUE	CPT	MUE
38210	1(3)	39545	1(2)	41140	1(2)	42410	1(2)	43117	1(2)	43264	1(2)	43620	1(2)	44050	1(2)
38211	1(3)	39560	1(3)	41145	1(2)	42415	1(2)	43118	1(2)	43265	1(2)	43621	1(2)	44055	1(2)
38212	1(3)	39561	1(3)	41150	1(2)	42420	1(2)	43121	1(2)	43266	1(3)	43622	1(2)	44100	1(2)
38213	1(3)	39599	1(3)	41153	1(2)	42425	1(2)	43122	1(2)	43270	1(3)	43631	1(2)	44110	1(2)
38214	1(3)	40490	2(3)	41155	1(2)	42426	1(2)	43123	1(2)	43273	1(2)	43632	1(2)	44111	1(2)
38215	1(3)	40500	2(3)	41250	2(3)	42440	1(2)	43124	1(2)	43274	2(3)	43633	1(2)	44120	1(2)
38220	1(3)	40510	2(3)	41251	2(3)	42450	1(3)	43130	1(3)	43275	1(3)	43634	1(2)	44121	2(3)
38221	1(3)	40520	2(3)	41252	2(3)	42500	2(3)	43135	1(3)	43276	2(3)	43635	1(2)	44125	1(2)
38222	1(2)	40525	2(3)	41510	1(2)	42505	2(3)	43180	1(2)	43277	3(3)	43640	1(2)	44126	1(2)
38230	1(2)	40527	2(3)	41512	1(2)	42507	1(2)	43191	1(3)	43278	1(3)	43641	1(2)	44127	1(2)
38232	1(2)	40530	2(3)	41520	1(3)	42509	1(2)	43192	1(3)	43279	1(2)	43644	1(2)	44128	2(3)
38240	1(3)	40650	2(3)	41530	1(3)	42510	1(2)	43193	1(3)	43280	1(2)	43645	1(2)	44130	2(3)
38241	1(2)	40652	2(3)	41599	1(3)	42550	2(3)	43194	1(3)	43281	1(2)	43647	1(2)	44132	1(2)
38242	1(2)	40654	2(3)	41800	2(3)	42600	1(3)	43195	1(3)	43282	1(2)	43648	1(2)	44133	1(2)
38243	1(3)	40700	1(2)	41805	1(3)	42650	2(3)	43196	1(3)	43283	1(2)	43651	1(2)	44135	1(2)
38300	1(3)	40701	1(2)	41806	1(3)	42660	2(3)	43197	1(3)	43284	1(2)	43652	1(2)	44136	1(2)
38305	1(3)	40702	1(2)	41820	4(2)	42665	2(3)	43198	1(3)	43285	1(2)	43653	1(2)	44137	1(2)
38308	1(3)	40720	1(2)	41821	2(3)	42699	1(3)	43200	1(3)	43286	1(2)	43659	1(3)	44139	1(2)
38380	1(2)	40761	1(2)	41822	1(2)	42700	2(3)	43201	1(2)	43287	1(2)	43752	2(3)	44140	2(3)
38381	1(2)	40799	1(3)	41823	1(2)	42720	1(3)	43202	1(2)	43288	1(2)	43753	1(3)	44141	1(3)
38382	1(2)	40800	2(3)	41825	2(3)	42725	1(3)	43204	1(2)	43289	1(3)	43754	1(3)	44143	1(2)
38500	2(3)	40801	2(3)	41826	2(3)	42800	3(3)	43205	1(2)	43300	1(2)	43755	1(3)	44144	1(3)
38505	2(3)	40804	1(3)	41827	2(3)	42804	1(3)	43206	1(2)	43305	1(2)	43756	1(2)	44145	1(2)
38510	1(2)	40805	2(3)	41828	4(2)	42806	1(3)	43210	1(2)	43310	1(2)	43757	1(2)	44146	1(2)
38520	1(2)	40806	2(2)	41830	2(3)	42808	2(3)	43211	1(3)	43312	1(2)	43761	2(3)	44147	1(3)
38525	1(2)	40808	2(3)	41850	2(3)	42809	1(3)	43212	1(3)	43313	1(2)	43762	2(3)	44150	1(2)
38530	1(2)	40810	2(3)	41870	2(3)	42810	1(3)	43213	1(2)	43314	1(2)	43763	2(3)	44151	1(2)
38531	1(2)	40812	2(3)	41872	4(2)	42815	1(3)	43214	1(3)	43320	1(2)	43770	1(2)	44155	1(2)
38542	1(2)	40814	4(3)	41874	4(2)	42820	1(2)	43215	1(3)	43325	1(2)	43771	1(2)	44156	1(2)
38550	1(3)	40816	2(3)	41899	1(3)	42821	1(2)	43216	1(2)	43327	1(2)	43772	1(2)	44157	1(2)
38555	1(3)	40818	2(3)	42000	1(3)	42825	1(2)	43217	1(2)	43328	1(2)	43773	1(2)	44158	1(2)
38562	1(2)	40819	2(2)	42100	2(3)	42826	1(2)	43220	1(3)	43330	1(2)	43774	1(2)	44160	1(2)
38564	1(2)	40820	2(3)	42104	2(3)	42830	1(2)	43226	1(3)	43331	1(2)	43775	1(2)	44180	1(2)
38570	1(2)	40830	2(3)	42106	2(3)	42831	1(2)	43227	1(3)	43332	1(2)	43800	1(2)	44186	1(2)
38571	1(2)	40831	2(3)	42107	2(3)	42835	1(2)	43229	1(3)	43333	1(2)	43810	1(2)	44187	1(3)
38572	1(2)	40840	1(2)	42120	1(2)	42836	1(2)	43231	1(2)	43334	1(2)	43820	1(2)	44188	1(3)
38573	1(2)	40842	1(2)	42140	1(2)	42842	1(3)	43232	1(2)	43335	1(2)	43825	1(2)	44202	1(2)
38589	1(3)	40843	1(2)	42145	1(2)	42844	1(3)	43233	1(3)	43336	1(2)	43830	1(2)	44203	2(3)
38700	1(2)	40844	1(2)	42160	1(3)	42845	1(3)	43235	1(3)	43337	1(2)	43831	1(2)	44204	2(3)
38720	1(2)	40845	1(3)	42180	1(3)	42860	1(3)	43236	1(2)	43338	1(2)	43832	1(2)	44205	1(2)
38724	1(2)	40899	1(3)	42182	1(3)	42870	1(3)	43237	1(2)	43340	1(2)	43840	2(3)	44206	1(2)
38740	1(2)	41000	1(3)	42200	1(2)	42890	1(2)	43238	1(2)	43341	1(2)	43842	0(3)	44207	1(2)
38745	1(2)	41005	1(3)	42205	1(2)	42892	1(3)	43239	1(2)	43351	1(2)	43843	1(2)	44208	1(2)
38746	1(2)	41006	2(3)	42210	1(2)	42894	1(3)	43240	1(2)	43352	1(2)	43845	1(2)	44210	1(2)
38747	1(2)	41007	2(3)	42215	1(2)	42900	1(3)	43241	1(3)	43360	1(2)	43846	1(2)	44211	1(2)
38760	1(2)	41008	2(3)	42220	1(2)	42950	1(2)	43242	1(2)	43361	1(2)	43847	1(2)	44212	1(2)
38765	1(2)	41009	2(3)	42225	1(2)	42953	1(3)	43243	1(2)	43400	1(2)	43848	1(2)	44213	1(2)
38770	1(2)	41010	1(2)	42226	1(2)	42955	1(2)	43244	1(2)	43405	1(2)	43850	1(2)	44227	1(3)
38780	1(2)	41015	2(3)	42227	1(2)	42960	1(3)	43245	1(2)	43410	1(3)	43855	1(2)	44238	1(3)
38790	1(2)	41016	1(3)	42235	1(2)	42961	1(3)	43246	1(2)	43415	1(3)	43860	1(2)	44300	1(3)
38792	1(3)	41017	2(3)	42260	1(3)	42962	1(3)	43247	1(2)	43420	1(3)	43865	1(2)	44310	2(3)
38794	1(2)	41018	2(3)	42280	1(2)	42970	1(3)	43248	1(3)	43425	1(3)	43870	1(2)	44312	1(2)
38900	1(3)	41019	1(2)	42281	1(2)	42971	1(3)	43249	1(3)	43450	1(3)	43880	1(3)	44314	1(2)
38999	1(3)	41100	2(3)	42299	1(3)	42972	1(3)	43250	1(2)	43453	1(3)	43881	1(3)	44316	1(2)
39000	1(2)	41105	2(3)	42300	2(3)	42999	1(3)	43251	1(2)	43460	1(3)	43882	1(3)	44320	1(2)
39010	1(2)	41108	2(3)	42305	2(3)	43020	1(2)	43252	1(2)	43496	1(3)	43886	1(2)	44322	1(2)
39200	1(2)	41110	2(3)	42310	2(3)	43030	1(2)	43253	1(3)	43499	1(3)	43887	1(2)	44340	1(2)
39220	1(2)	41112	2(3)	42320	2(3)	43045	1(2)	43254	1(3)	43500	1(2)	43888	1(2)	44345	1(2)
39401	1(3)	41113	2(3)	42330	1(3)	43100	1(3)	43255	2(3)	43501	1(3)	43999	1(3)	44346	1(2)
39402	1(3)	41114	2(3)	42335	2(2)	43101	1(3)	43257	1(2)	43502	1(2)	44005	1(2)	44360	1(3)
39499	1(3)	41115	1(2)	42340	1(2)	43107	1(2)	43259	1(2)	43510	1(2)	44010	1(2)	44361	1(2)
39501	1(3)	41116	2(3)	42400	2(3)	43108	1(2)	43260	1(3)	43520	1(2)	44015	1(2)	44363	1(3)
39503	1(2)	41120	1(2)	42405	2(3)	43112	1(2)	43261	1(2)	43605	1(2)	44020	2(3)	44364	1(2)
39540	1(2)	41130	1(2)	42408	1(3)	43113	1(2)	43262	2(2)	43610	2(3)	44021	1(3)	44365	1(2)
39541	1(2)	41135	1(2)	42409	1(3)	43116	1(2)	43263	1(2)	43611	2(3)	44025	1(3)	44366	1(3)

CPT	MUE
44369	1(2)
44370	1(2)
44372	1(2)
44373	1(2)
44376	1(3)
44377	1(2)
44378	1(3)
44379	1(2)
44380	1(3)
44381	1(3)
44382	1(2)
44384	1(3)
44385	1(3)
44386	1(2)
44388	1(3)
44389	1(2)
44390	1(3)
44391	1(3)
44392	1(2)
44394	1(2)
44401	1(2)
44402	1(3)
44403	1(3)
44404	1(3)
44405	1(3)
44406	1(3)
44407	1(2)
44408	1(3)
44500	1(3)
44602	1(2)
44603	1(2)
44604	1(2)
44605	1(2)
44615	3(3)
44620	2(3)
44625	1(3)
44626	1(3)
44640	2(3)
44650	2(3)
44660	1(3)
44661	1(3)
44680	1(3)
44700	1(2)
44701	1(2)
44705	1(3)
44715	1(2)
44720	2(3)
44721	2(3)
44799	1(3)
44800	1(3)
44820	1(3)
44850	1(3)
44899	1(3)
44900	1(2)
44950	1(2)
44955	1(2)
44960	1(2)
44970	1(2)
44979	1(3)
45000	1(3)
45005	1(3)
45020	1(3)
45100	2(3)
45108	1(2)
45110	1(2)

CPT	MUE
45111	1(2)
45112	1(2)
45113	1(2)
45114	1(2)
45116	1(2)
45119	1(2)
45120	1(2)
45121	1(2)
45123	1(2)
45126	1(2)
45130	1(2)
45135	1(2)
45136	1(2)
45150	1(2)
45160	1(3)
45171	2(3)
45172	2(3)
45190	1(3)
45300	1(3)
45303	1(3)
45305	1(2)
45307	1(3)
45308	1(2)
45309	1(2)
45315	1(2)
45317	1(3)
45320	1(2)
45321	1(2)
45327	1(2)
45330	1(3)
45331	1(2)
45332	1(3)
45333	1(2)
45334	1(3)
45335	1(2)
45337	1(2)
45338	1(2)
45340	1(2)
45341	1(2)
45342	1(2)
45346	1(2)
45347	1(3)
45349	1(3)
45350	1(2)
45378	1(3)
45379	1(3)
45380	1(2)
45381	1(2)
45382	1(3)
45384	1(2)
45385	1(2)
45386	1(2)
45388	1(2)
45389	1(3)
45390	1(3)
45391	1(2)
45392	1(2)
45393	1(3)
45395	1(2)
45397	1(2)
45398	1(2)
45399	1(3)
45400	1(2)
45402	1(2)
45499	1(3)

CPT	MUE
45500	1(2)
45505	1(2)
45520	1(2)
45540	1(2)
45541	1(2)
45550	1(2)
45560	1(2)
45562	1(2)
45563	1(2)
45800	1(3)
45805	1(3)
45820	1(3)
45825	1(3)
45900	1(2)
45905	1(2)
45910	1(2)
45915	1(2)
45990	1(2)
45999	1(3)
46020	2(3)
46030	1(3)
46040	2(3)
46045	2(3)
46050	2(3)
46060	2(3)
46070	1(2)
46080	1(2)
46083	2(3)
46200	1(3)
46220	1(2)
46221	1(2)
46230	1(2)
46250	1(2)
46255	1(2)
46257	1(2)
46258	1(2)
46260	1(2)
46261	1(2)
46262	1(2)
46270	1(3)
46275	1(3)
46280	1(2)
46285	1(3)
46288	1(3)
46320	2(3)
46500	1(2)
46505	1(2)
46600	1(3)
46601	1(3)
46604	1(2)
46606	1(2)
46607	1(2)
46608	1(3)
46610	1(2)
46611	1(2)
46612	1(2)
46614	1(3)
46615	1(2)
46700	1(2)
46705	1(2)
46706	1(3)
46707	1(3)
46710	1(3)
46712	1(3)
46715	1(2)

CPT	MUE
46716	1(2)
46730	1(2)
46735	1(2)
46740	1(2)
46742	1(2)
46744	1(2)
46746	1(2)
46748	1(2)
46750	1(2)
46751	1(2)
46753	1(2)
46754	1(3)
46760	1(2)
46761	1(2)
46900	1(2)
46910	1(2)
46916	1(2)
46917	1(2)
46922	1(2)
46924	1(2)
46930	1(2)
46940	1(2)
46942	1(3)
46945	1(2)
46946	1(2)
46947	1(2)
46948	1(2)
46999	1(3)
47000	3(3)
47001	3(3)
47010	1(3)
47015	1(2)
47100	3(3)
47120	2(3)
47122	1(2)
47125	1(2)
47130	1(2)
47133	1(2)
47135	1(2)
47140	1(2)
47141	1(2)
47142	1(2)
47143	1(2)
47144	1(2)
47145	1(2)
47146	2(3)
47147	1(3)
47300	2(3)
47350	1(3)
47360	1(3)
47361	1(3)
47362	1(3)
47370	1(2)
47371	1(2)
47379	1(3)
47380	1(2)
47381	1(2)
47382	1(2)
47383	1(2)
47399	1(3)
47400	1(3)
47420	1(2)
47425	1(2)
47460	1(2)
47480	1(2)

CPT	MUE
47490	1(2)
47531	2(3)
47532	1(3)
47533	1(3)
47534	2(3)
47535	1(3)
47536	2(3)
47537	1(3)
47538	2(3)
47539	2(3)
47540	2(3)
47541	1(3)
47542	2(3)
47543	1(3)
47544	1(3)
47550	1(3)
47552	1(3)
47553	1(2)
47554	1(3)
47555	1(2)
47556	1(2)
47562	1(2)
47563	1(2)
47564	1(2)
47570	1(2)
47579	1(3)
47600	1(2)
47605	1(2)
47610	1(2)
47612	1(2)
47620	1(2)
47700	1(2)
47701	1(2)
47711	1(2)
47712	1(2)
47715	1(2)
47720	1(2)
47721	1(2)
47740	1(2)
47741	1(2)
47760	1(2)
47765	1(2)
47780	1(2)
47785	1(2)
47800	1(2)
47801	1(3)
47802	1(2)
47900	1(2)
47999	1(3)
48000	1(2)
48001	1(2)
48020	1(3)
48100	1(3)
48102	1(3)
48105	1(2)
48120	1(3)
48140	1(2)
48145	1(2)
48146	1(2)
48148	1(2)
48150	1(2)
48152	1(2)
48153	1(2)
48154	1(2)
48155	1(2)

CPT	MUE
48160	0(3)
48400	1(3)
48500	1(3)
48510	1(3)
48520	1(3)
48540	1(3)
48545	1(3)
48547	1(2)
48548	1(2)
48550	1(2)
48551	1(2)
48552	2(3)
48554	1(2)
48556	1(2)
48999	1(3)
49000	1(2)
49002	1(3)
49010	1(3)
49013	1(2)
49014	1(3)
49020	2(3)
49040	2(3)
49060	2(3)
49062	1(3)
49082	1(3)
49083	2(3)
49084	1(3)
49180	2(3)
49185	2(3)
49203	1(2)
49204	1(2)
49205	1(2)
49215	1(2)
49220	1(2)
49250	1(2)
49255	1(2)
49320	1(3)
49321	1(2)
49322	1(2)
49323	1(2)
49324	1(2)
49325	1(2)
49326	1(2)
49327	1(2)
49329	1(3)
49400	1(3)
49402	1(3)
49405	2(3)
49406	2(3)
49407	1(3)
49411	1(2)
49412	1(2)
49418	1(3)
49419	1(2)
49421	1(2)
49422	1(2)
49423	2(3)
49424	3(3)
49425	1(2)
49426	1(3)
49427	1(3)
49428	1(2)
49429	1(2)
49435	1(2)
49436	1(2)

CPT	MUE
49440	1(3)
49441	1(3)
49442	1(3)
49446	1(2)
49450	1(3)
49451	1(3)
49452	1(3)
49460	1(3)
49465	1(3)
49491	1(2)
49492	1(2)
49495	1(2)
49496	1(2)
49500	1(2)
49501	1(2)
49505	1(2)
49507	1(2)
49520	1(2)
49521	1(2)
49525	1(2)
49540	1(2)
49550	1(2)
49553	1(2)
49555	1(2)
49557	1(2)
49560	2(3)
49561	1(3)
49565	2(3)
49566	2(3)
49568	2(3)
49570	1(3)
49572	1(3)
49580	1(2)
49582	1(2)
49585	1(2)
49587	1(2)
49590	1(2)
49600	1(2)
49605	1(2)
49606	1(2)
49610	1(2)
49611	1(2)
49650	1(2)
49651	1(2)
49652	2(3)
49653	2(3)
49654	1(3)
49655	1(3)
49656	1(3)
49657	1(3)
49659	1(3)
49900	1(3)
49904	1(3)
49905	1(3)
49906	1(3)
49999	1(3)
50010	1(2)
50020	1(3)
50040	1(2)
50045	1(2)
50060	1(2)
50065	1(2)
50070	1(2)
50075	1(2)
50080	1(2)

CPT	MUE
50081	1(2)
50100	1(2)
50120	1(2)
50125	1(2)
50130	1(2)
50135	1(2)
50200	1(3)
50205	1(3)
50220	1(2)
50225	1(2)
50230	1(2)
50234	1(2)
50236	1(2)
50240	1(2)
50250	1(3)
50280	1(2)
50290	1(3)
50300	1(2)
50320	1(2)
50323	1(2)
50325	1(2)
50327	2(3)
50328	1(3)
50329	1(3)
50340	1(2)
50360	1(2)
50365	1(2)
50370	1(2)
50380	1(2)
50382	1(3)
50384	1(3)
50385	1(3)
50386	1(3)
50387	1(3)
50389	1(3)
50390	2(3)
50391	1(3)
50396	1(3)
50400	1(2)
50405	1(2)
50430	2(3)
50431	2(3)
50432	2(3)
50433	2(3)
50434	2(3)
50435	2(3)
50436	1(3)
50437	1(3)
50500	1(3)
50520	1(3)
50525	1(3)
50526	1(3)
50540	1(2)
50541	1(2)
50542	1(2)
50543	1(2)
50544	1(2)
50545	1(2)
50546	1(2)
50547	1(2)
50548	1(2)
50549	1(3)
50551	1(3)
50553	1(3)
50555	1(2)

CPT	MUE
50557	1(2)
50561	1(2)
50562	1(3)
50570	1(3)
50572	1(3)
50574	1(2)
50575	1(2)
50576	1(2)
50580	1(2)
50590	1(2)
50592	1(2)
50593	1(2)
50600	1(3)
50605	1(3)
50606	1(3)
50610	1(2)
50620	1(2)
50630	1(2)
50650	1(2)
50660	1(3)
50684	1(3)
50686	2(3)
50688	2(3)
50690	2(3)
50693	2(3)
50694	2(3)
50695	2(3)
50700	1(2)
50705	2(3)
50706	2(3)
50715	1(2)
50722	1(2)
50725	1(3)
50727	1(3)
50728	1(3)
50740	1(2)
50750	1(2)
50760	1(2)
50770	1(2)
50780	1(2)
50782	1(2)
50783	1(2)
50785	1(2)
50800	1(2)
50810	1(3)
50815	1(2)
50820	1(2)
50825	1(3)
50830	1(3)
50840	1(2)
50845	1(2)
50860	1(2)
50900	1(3)
50920	2(3)
50930	2(3)
50940	1(2)
50945	1(2)
50947	1(2)
50948	1(2)
50949	1(3)
50951	1(3)
50953	1(3)
50955	1(2)
50957	1(2)
50961	1(2)

CPT	MUE
50970	1(3)
50972	1(3)
50974	1(2)
50976	1(2)
50980	1(2)
51020	1(2)
51030	1(2)
51040	1(3)
51045	2(3)
51050	1(3)
51060	1(3)
51065	1(3)
51080	1(3)
51100	1(3)
51101	1(3)
51102	1(3)
51500	1(2)
51520	1(2)
51525	1(2)
51530	1(2)
51535	1(2)
51550	1(2)
51555	1(2)
51565	1(2)
51570	1(2)
51575	1(2)
51580	1(2)
51585	1(2)
51590	1(2)
51595	1(2)
51596	1(2)
51597	1(2)
51600	1(3)
51605	1(3)
51610	1(3)
51700	1(3)
51701	2(3)
51702	2(3)
51703	2(3)
51705	2(3)
51710	1(3)
51715	1(2)
51720	1(3)
51725	1(3)
51726	1(3)
51727	1(3)
51728	1(3)
51729	1(3)
51736	1(3)
51741	1(3)
51784	1(3)
51785	1(3)
51792	1(3)
51797	1(3)
51798	1(3)
51800	1(2)
51820	1(2)
51840	1(2)
51841	1(2)
51845	1(2)
51860	1(3)
51865	1(3)
51880	1(2)
51900	1(3)
51920	1(3)

CPT	MUE
51925	1(2)
51940	1(2)
51960	1(2)
51980	1(2)
51990	1(2)
51992	1(2)
51999	1(3)
52000	1(3)
52001	1(3)
52005	2(3)
52007	1(2)
52010	1(2)
52204	1(2)
52214	1(2)
52224	1(2)
52234	1(2)
52235	1(2)
52240	1(2)
52250	1(2)
52260	1(2)
52265	1(2)
52270	1(2)
52275	1(2)
52276	1(2)
52277	1(2)
52281	1(2)
52282	1(2)
52283	1(2)
52285	1(2)
52287	1(2)
52290	1(2)
52300	1(2)
52301	1(2)
52305	1(2)
52310	1(3)
52315	2(3)
52317	1(3)
52318	1(3)
52320	1(2)
52325	1(3)
52327	1(2)
52330	1(2)
52332	1(2)
52334	1(2)
52341	1(2)
52342	1(2)
52343	1(2)
52344	1(2)
52345	1(2)
52346	1(2)
52351	1(3)
52352	1(2)
52353	1(2)
52354	1(3)
52355	1(3)
52356	1(2)
52400	1(2)
52402	1(2)
52441	1(2)
52442	6(3)
52450	1(2)
52500	1(2)
52601	1(2)
52630	1(2)
52640	1(2)

CPT	MUE
52647	1(2)
52648	1(2)
52649	1(2)
52700	1(3)
53000	1(2)
53010	1(2)
53020	1(2)
53025	1(2)
53040	1(3)
53060	1(3)
53080	1(3)
53085	1(3)
53200	1(3)
53210	1(2)
53215	1(2)
53220	1(3)
53230	1(3)
53235	1(3)
53240	1(3)
53250	1(3)
53260	1(2)
53265	1(3)
53270	1(2)
53275	1(2)
53400	1(2)
53405	1(2)
53410	1(2)
53415	1(2)
53420	1(2)
53425	1(2)
53430	1(2)
53431	1(2)
53440	1(2)
53442	1(2)
53444	1(3)
53445	1(2)
53446	1(2)
53447	1(2)
53448	1(2)
53449	1(2)
53450	1(2)
53460	1(2)
53500	1(2)
53502	1(3)
53505	1(3)
53510	1(3)
53515	1(3)
53520	1(3)
53600	1(3)
53601	1(3)
53605	1(3)
53620	1(2)
53621	1(3)
53660	1(2)
53661	1(3)
53665	1(3)
53850	1(2)
53852	1(2)
53854	1(2)
53855	1(2)
53860	1(2)
53899	1(3)
54000	1(2)
54001	1(2)
54015	1(3)

CPT	MUE
54050	1(2)
54055	1(2)
54056	1(2)
54057	1(2)
54060	1(2)
54065	1(2)
54100	2(3)
54105	2(3)
54110	1(2)
54111	1(2)
54112	1(3)
54115	1(3)
54120	1(2)
54125	1(2)
54130	1(2)
54135	1(2)
54150	1(2)
54160	1(2)
54161	1(2)
54162	1(2)
54163	1(2)
54164	1(2)
54200	1(2)
54205	1(2)
54220	1(3)
54230	1(3)
54231	1(3)
54235	1(3)
54240	1(2)
54250	1(2)
54300	1(2)
54304	1(2)
54308	1(2)
54312	1(2)
54316	1(2)
54318	1(2)
54322	1(2)
54324	1(2)
54326	1(2)
54328	1(2)
54332	1(2)
54336	1(2)
54340	1(2)
54344	1(2)
54348	1(2)
54352	1(2)
54360	1(2)
54380	1(2)
54385	1(2)
54390	1(2)
54400	1(2)
54401	1(2)
54405	1(2)
54406	1(2)
54408	1(2)
54410	1(2)
54411	1(2)
54415	1(2)
54416	1(2)
54417	1(2)
54420	1(2)
54430	1(2)
54435	1(2)
54437	1(2)
54438	1(2)

CPT	MUE
54440	1(2)
54450	1(2)
54500	1(3)
54505	1(3)
54512	1(3)
54520	1(2)
54522	1(2)
54530	1(2)
54535	1(2)
54550	1(2)
54560	1(2)
54600	1(2)
54620	1(2)
54640	1(2)
54650	1(2)
54660	1(2)
54670	1(3)
54680	1(2)
54690	1(2)
54692	1(2)
54699	1(3)
54700	1(3)
54800	1(2)
54830	1(2)
54840	1(2)
54860	1(2)
54861	1(2)
54865	1(3)
54900	1(2)
54901	1(2)
55000	1(3)
55040	1(2)
55041	1(2)
55060	1(2)
55100	2(3)
55110	1(2)
55120	1(3)
55150	1(2)
55175	1(2)
55180	1(2)
55200	1(2)
55250	1(2)
55300	1(2)
55400	1(2)
55500	1(2)
55520	1(2)
55530	1(2)
55535	1(2)
55540	1(2)
55550	1(2)
55559	1(3)
55600	1(2)
55605	1(2)
55650	1(2)
55680	1(3)
55700	1(2)
55705	1(2)
55706	1(2)
55720	1(3)
55725	1(3)
55801	1(2)
55810	1(2)
55812	1(2)
55815	1(2)
55821	1(2)

CPT	MUE
55831	1(2)
55840	1(2)
55842	1(2)
55845	1(2)
55860	1(2)
55862	1(2)
55865	1(2)
55866	1(2)
55870	1(2)
55873	1(2)
55874	1(2)
55875	1(2)
55876	1(2)
55899	1(3)
55920	1(2)
55970	1(2)
55980	1(2)
56405	2(3)
56420	1(3)
56440	1(3)
56441	1(2)
56442	1(2)
56501	1(2)
56515	1(2)
56605	1(2)
56606	6(3)
56620	1(2)
56625	1(2)
56630	1(2)
56631	1(2)
56632	1(2)
56633	1(2)
56634	1(2)
56637	1(2)
56640	1(2)
56700	1(2)
56740	1(3)
56800	1(2)
56805	1(2)
56810	1(2)
56820	1(2)
56821	1(2)
57000	1(3)
57010	1(3)
57020	1(3)
57022	1(3)
57023	1(3)
57061	1(2)
57065	1(2)
57100	2(3)
57105	2(3)
57106	1(2)
57107	1(2)
57109	1(2)
57110	1(2)
57111	1(2)
57112	1(2)
57120	1(2)
57130	1(2)
57135	2(3)
57150	1(3)
57155	1(3)
57156	1(3)
57160	1(2)
57170	1(2)

CPT	MUE
57180	1(3)
57200	1(3)
57210	1(3)
57220	1(2)
57230	1(2)
57240	1(2)
57250	1(2)
57260	1(2)
57265	1(2)
57267	2(3)
57268	1(2)
57270	1(2)
57280	1(2)
57282	1(2)
57283	1(2)
57284	1(2)
57285	1(2)
57287	1(2)
57288	1(2)
57289	1(2)
57291	1(2)
57292	1(2)
57295	1(2)
57296	1(2)
57300	1(3)
57305	1(3)
57307	1(3)
57308	1(3)
57310	1(3)
57311	1(3)
57320	1(3)
57330	1(3)
57335	1(2)
57400	1(2)
57410	1(2)
57415	1(3)
57420	1(3)
57421	1(3)
57423	1(2)
57425	1(2)
57426	1(2)
57452	1(3)
57454	1(3)
57455	1(3)
57456	1(3)
57460	1(3)
57461	1(3)
57500	1(3)
57505	1(3)
57510	1(3)
57511	1(3)
57513	1(3)
57520	1(3)
57522	1(3)
57530	1(3)
57531	1(2)
57540	1(2)
57545	1(3)
57550	1(3)
57555	1(2)
57556	1(2)
57558	1(3)
57700	1(3)
57720	1(3)
57800	1(3)

CPT	MUE
58100	1(3)
58110	1(3)
58120	1(3)
58140	1(3)
58145	1(3)
58146	1(3)
58150	1(3)
58152	1(2)
58180	1(3)
58200	1(2)
58210	1(2)
58240	1(2)
58260	1(3)
58262	1(3)
58263	1(2)
58267	1(2)
58270	1(2)
58275	1(2)
58280	1(2)
58285	1(3)
58290	1(3)
58291	1(2)
58292	1(2)
58293	1(2)
58294	1(2)
58300	0(3)
58301	1(3)
58321	1(2)
58322	1(2)
58323	1(3)
58340	1(3)
58345	1(3)
58346	1(2)
58350	1(2)
58353	1(3)
58356	1(3)
58400	1(3)
58410	1(2)
58520	1(2)
58540	1(3)
58541	1(3)
58542	1(2)
58543	1(3)
58544	1(2)
58545	1(2)
58546	1(2)
58548	1(2)
58550	1(3)
58552	1(3)
58553	1(3)
58554	1(2)
58555	1(3)
58558	1(3)
58559	1(3)
58560	1(3)
58561	1(3)
58562	1(3)
58563	1(3)
58565	1(2)
58570	1(3)
58571	1(2)
58572	1(3)
58573	1(2)
58575	1(2)
58578	1(3)
58579	1(3)
58600	1(2)
58605	1(2)
58611	1(2)
58615	1(2)
58660	1(2)
58661	1(2)
58662	1(2)
58670	1(2)
58671	1(2)
58672	1(2)
58673	1(2)
58674	1(2)
58679	1(3)
58700	1(2)
58720	1(2)
58740	1(2)
58750	1(2)
58752	1(2)
58760	1(2)
58770	1(2)
58800	1(2)
58805	1(2)
58820	1(3)
58822	1(3)
58825	1(2)
58900	1(2)
58920	1(2)
58925	1(3)
58940	1(2)
58943	1(2)
58950	1(2)
58951	1(2)
58952	1(2)
58953	1(2)
58954	1(2)
58956	1(2)
58957	1(2)
58958	1(2)
58960	1(2)
58970	1(3)
58974	1(3)
58976	2(3)
58999	1(3)
59000	2(3)
59001	2(3)
59012	2(3)
59015	2(3)
59020	2(3)
59025	2(3)
59030	2(3)
59050	2(3)
59051	2(3)
59070	2(3)
59072	2(3)
59074	2(3)
59076	2(3)
59100	1(2)
59120	1(3)
59121	1(3)
59130	1(3)
59135	1(3)
59136	1(3)
59140	1(2)
59150	1(3)
59151	1(3)
59160	1(2)
59200	1(3)
59300	1(2)
59320	1(2)
59325	1(2)
59350	1(2)
59400	1(2)
59409	2(3)
59410	1(2)
59412	1(3)
59414	1(3)
59425	1(2)
59426	1(2)
59430	1(2)
59510	1(2)
59514	1(3)
59515	1(2)
59525	1(2)
59610	1(2)
59612	2(3)
59614	1(2)
59618	1(2)
59620	1(2)
59622	1(2)
59812	1(2)
59820	1(2)
59821	1(2)
59830	1(2)
59840	1(2)
59841	1(2)
59850	1(2)
59851	1(2)
59852	1(2)
59855	1(2)
59856	1(2)
59857	1(2)
59866	1(2)
59870	1(2)
59871	1(2)
59897	1(3)
59898	1(3)
59899	1(3)
60000	1(3)
60100	3(3)
60200	2(3)
60210	1(2)
60212	1(2)
60220	1(3)
60225	1(2)
60240	1(2)
60252	1(2)
60254	1(2)
60260	1(2)
60270	1(2)
60271	1(2)
60280	1(3)
60281	1(3)
60300	2(3)
60500	1(2)
60502	1(3)
60505	1(3)
60512	1(3)
60520	1(2)
60521	1(2)
60522	1(2)
60540	1(2)
60545	1(2)
60600	1(3)
60605	1(3)
60650	1(2)
60659	1(3)
60699	1(3)
61000	1(2)
61001	1(2)
61020	2(3)
61026	2(3)
61050	1(3)
61055	1(3)
61070	2(3)
61105	1(3)
61107	1(3)
61108	1(3)
61120	1(3)
61140	1(3)
61150	1(3)
61151	1(3)
61154	1(3)
61156	1(3)
61210	1(3)
61215	1(3)
61250	1(3)
61253	1(3)
61304	1(3)
61305	1(3)
61312	2(3)
61313	2(3)
61314	2(3)
61315	1(3)
61316	1(3)
61320	2(3)
61321	1(3)
61322	1(3)
61323	1(3)
61330	1(2)
61333	1(2)
61340	1(2)
61343	1(2)
61345	1(3)
61450	1(3)
61458	1(2)
61460	1(2)
61500	1(3)
61501	1(3)
61510	1(3)
61512	1(3)
61514	2(3)
61516	1(3)
61517	1(3)
61518	1(3)
61519	1(3)
61520	1(3)
61521	1(3)
61522	1(3)
61524	2(3)
61526	1(3)
61530	1(3)
61531	1(2)
61533	2(3)
61534	1(3)
61535	2(3)
61536	1(3)
61537	1(3)
61538	1(2)
61539	1(3)
61540	1(3)
61541	1(2)
61543	1(2)
61544	1(3)
61545	1(2)
61546	1(2)
61548	1(2)
61550	1(2)
61552	1(2)
61556	1(3)
61557	1(2)
61558	1(3)
61559	1(3)
61563	2(3)
61564	1(2)
61566	1(3)
61567	1(2)
61570	1(3)
61571	1(3)
61575	1(2)
61576	1(2)
61580	1(2)
61581	1(2)
61582	1(2)
61583	1(2)
61584	1(2)
61585	1(2)
61586	1(3)
61590	1(2)
61591	1(2)
61592	1(2)
61595	1(2)
61596	1(2)
61597	1(2)
61598	1(3)
61600	1(3)
61601	1(3)
61605	1(3)
61606	1(3)
61607	1(3)
61608	1(3)
61611	1(3)
61613	1(3)
61615	1(3)
61616	1(3)
61618	2(3)
61619	2(3)
61623	2(3)
61624	2(3)
61626	2(3)
61630	1(3)
61635	2(3)
61640	0(3)
61641	0(3)
61642	0(3)
61645	1(3)
61650	1(2)
61651	2(2)
61680	1(3)
61682	1(3)
61684	1(3)
61686	1(3)
61690	1(3)
61692	1(3)
61697	2(3)
61698	1(3)
61700	2(3)
61702	1(3)
61703	1(3)
61705	1(3)
61708	1(3)
61710	1(3)
61711	1(3)
61720	1(3)
61735	1(3)
61750	2(3)
61751	2(3)
61760	1(2)
61770	1(2)
61781	1(3)
61782	1(3)
61783	1(3)
61790	1(2)
61791	1(2)
61796	1(2)
61797	4(3)
61798	1(2)
61799	4(3)
61800	1(2)
61850	1(3)
61860	1(3)
61863	1(2)
61864	1(3)
61867	1(2)
61868	2(3)
61870	1(3)
61880	1(2)
61885	1(3)
61886	1(3)
61888	1(3)
62000	1(3)
62005	1(3)
62010	1(3)
62100	1(3)
62115	1(2)
62117	1(2)
62120	1(2)
62121	1(2)
62140	1(3)
62141	1(3)
62142	2(3)
62143	2(3)
62145	2(3)
62146	2(3)
62147	1(3)
62148	1(3)
62160	1(3)
62161	1(3)
62162	1(3)
62163	1(3)
62164	1(3)
62165	1(2)
62180	1(3)
62190	1(3)
62192	1(3)
62194	1(3)
62200	1(2)
62201	1(2)
62220	1(3)
62223	1(3)
62225	2(3)
62230	2(3)
62252	2(3)
62256	1(3)
62258	1(3)
62263	1(2)
62264	1(2)
62267	2(3)
62268	1(3)
62269	2(3)
62270	2(3)
62272	2(3)
62273	2(3)
62280	1(3)
62281	1(3)
62282	1(3)
62284	1(3)
62287	1(2)
62290	5(2)
62291	4(3)
62292	1(2)
62294	1(3)
62302	1(3)
62303	1(3)
62304	1(3)
62305	1(3)
62320	1(3)
62321	1(3)
62322	1(3)
62323	1(3)
62324	1(3)
62325	1(3)
62326	1(3)
62327	1(3)
62328	2(3)
62329	1(3)
62350	1(3)
62351	1(3)
62355	1(3)
62360	1(2)
62361	1(2)
62362	1(2)
62365	1(2)
62367	1(3)
62368	1(3)
62369	1(3)
62370	1(3)
62380	2(3)
63001	1(2)
63003	1(2)
63005	1(2)
63011	1(2)
63012	1(2)
63015	1(2)
63016	1(2)
63017	1(2)
63020	1(2)
63030	1(2)
63035	4(3)
63040	1(2)
63042	1(2)
63043	4(3)
63044	4(2)
63045	1(2)
63046	1(2)
63047	1(2)
63048	5(3)
63050	1(2)
63051	1(2)
63055	1(2)
63056	1(2)
63057	3(3)
63064	1(2)
63066	1(3)
63075	1(2)
63076	3(3)
63077	1(2)
63078	3(3)
63081	1(2)
63082	6(2)
63085	1(2)
63086	2(3)
63087	1(2)
63088	3(3)
63090	1(2)
63091	3(3)
63101	1(2)
63102	1(2)
63103	3(3)
63170	1(3)
63172	1(3)
63173	1(3)
63180	1(2)
63182	1(2)
63185	1(2)
63190	1(2)
63191	1(2)
63194	1(2)
63195	1(2)
63196	1(2)
63197	1(2)
63198	1(2)
63199	1(2)
63200	1(2)
63250	1(3)
63251	1(3)
63252	1(3)
63265	1(3)
63266	1(3)
63267	1(3)
63268	1(3)
63270	1(3)
63271	1(3)
63272	1(3)
63273	1(3)
63275	1(3)
63276	1(3)
63277	1(3)
63278	1(3)
63280	1(3)
63281	1(3)
63282	1(3)
63283	1(3)
63285	1(3)
63286	1(3)

CPT	MUE
63287	1(3)
63290	1(3)
63295	1(2)
63300	1(2)
63301	1(2)
63302	1(2)
63303	1(2)
63304	1(2)
63305	1(2)
63306	1(2)
63307	1(2)
63308	3(3)
63600	2(3)
63610	1(3)
63620	1(2)
63621	2(2)
63650	2(3)
63655	1(3)
63661	1(2)
63662	1(2)
63663	1(3)
63664	1(3)
63685	1(3)
63688	1(3)
63700	1(3)
63702	1(3)
63704	1(3)
63706	1(3)
63707	1(3)
63709	1(3)
63710	1(3)
63740	1(3)
63741	1(3)
63744	1(3)
63746	1(2)
64400	4(3)
64405	1(3)
64408	1(3)
64415	1(3)
64416	1(2)
64417	1(3)
64418	1(3)
64420	2(2)
64421	3(3)
64425	1(3)
64430	1(3)
64435	1(3)
64445	1(3)
64446	1(2)
64447	1(3)
64448	1(2)
64449	1(2)
64450	10(3)
64451	2(2)
64454	2(2)
64455	1(2)
64461	1(2)
64462	1(2)
64463	1(3)
64479	1(2)
64480	4(3)
64483	1(2)
64484	4(3)
64486	1(3)
64487	1(2)

CPT	MUE
64488	1(3)
64489	1(2)
64490	1(2)
64491	1(2)
64492	1(2)
64493	1(2)
64494	1(2)
64495	1(2)
64505	1(3)
64510	1(3)
64517	1(3)
64520	1(3)
64530	1(3)
64553	1(3)
64555	2(3)
64561	1(3)
64566	1(3)
64568	1(3)
64569	1(3)
64570	1(3)
64575	2(3)
64580	2(3)
64581	2(3)
64585	2(3)
64590	1(3)
64595	1(3)
64600	2(3)
64605	1(2)
64610	1(2)
64611	1(2)
64612	1(2)
64615	1(2)
64616	1(2)
64617	1(2)
64620	5(3)
64624	2(2)
64625	2(2)
64630	1(3)
64632	1(2)
64633	1(2)
64634	4(3)
64635	1(2)
64636	4(2)
64640	5(3)
64642	1(2)
64643	3(2)
64644	1(2)
64645	3(2)
64646	1(2)
64647	1(2)
64650	1(2)
64653	1(2)
64680	1(2)
64681	1(2)
64702	2(3)
64704	4(3)
64708	3(3)
64712	1(2)
64713	1(2)
64714	1(2)
64716	2(3)
64718	1(2)
64719	1(2)
64721	1(2)
64722	4(3)

CPT	MUE
64726	2(3)
64727	2(3)
64732	1(2)
64734	1(2)
64736	1(2)
64738	1(2)
64740	1(2)
64742	1(2)
64744	1(2)
64746	1(2)
64755	1(2)
64760	1(2)
64763	1(2)
64766	1(2)
64771	2(3)
64772	2(3)
64774	2(3)
64776	1(2)
64778	1(3)
64782	2(2)
64783	2(3)
64784	3(3)
64786	1(3)
64787	4(3)
64788	5(3)
64790	1(3)
64792	2(3)
64795	2(3)
64802	1(2)
64804	1(2)
64809	1(2)
64818	1(2)
64820	4(3)
64821	1(2)
64822	1(2)
64823	1(2)
64831	1(2)
64832	3(3)
64834	1(2)
64835	1(2)
64836	1(2)
64837	2(3)
64840	1(2)
64856	2(3)
64857	2(3)
64858	1(2)
64859	2(3)
64861	1(2)
64862	1(2)
64864	2(3)
64865	1(3)
64866	1(3)
64868	1(3)
64872	1(3)
64874	1(3)
64876	1(3)
64885	1(3)
64886	1(3)
64890	2(3)
64891	2(3)
64892	2(3)
64893	2(3)
64895	2(3)
64896	2(3)
64897	2(3)

CPT	MUE
64898	2(3)
64901	2(3)
64902	1(3)
64905	1(3)
64907	1(3)
64910	3(3)
64911	2(3)
64912	3(3)
64913	3(3)
64999	1(3)
65091	1(2)
65093	1(2)
65101	1(2)
65103	1(2)
65105	1(2)
65110	1(2)
65112	1(2)
65114	1(2)
65125	1(2)
65130	1(2)
65135	1(2)
65140	1(2)
65150	1(2)
65155	1(2)
65175	1(2)
65205	1(3)
65210	1(3)
65220	1(3)
65222	1(3)
65235	1(3)
65260	1(3)
65265	1(3)
65270	1(3)
65272	1(3)
65273	1(3)
65275	1(3)
65280	1(3)
65285	1(3)
65286	1(3)
65290	1(3)
65400	1(3)
65410	1(3)
65420	1(2)
65426	1(2)
65430	1(2)
65435	1(2)
65436	1(2)
65450	1(3)
65600	1(2)
65710	1(2)
65730	1(2)
65750	1(2)
65755	1(2)
65756	1(2)
65757	1(3)
65760	0(3)
65765	0(3)
65767	0(3)
65770	1(2)
65771	0(3)
65772	1(2)
65775	1(2)
65778	1(2)
65779	1(2)
65780	1(2)

CPT	MUE
65781	1(2)
65782	1(2)
65785	1(2)
65800	1(2)
65810	1(2)
65815	1(3)
65820	1(2)
65850	1(2)
65855	1(2)
65860	1(2)
65865	1(2)
65870	1(2)
65875	1(2)
65880	1(2)
65900	1(3)
65920	1(2)
65930	1(3)
66020	1(3)
66030	1(3)
66130	1(3)
66150	1(2)
66155	1(2)
66160	1(2)
66170	1(2)
66172	1(2)
66174	1(2)
66175	1(2)
66179	1(2)
66180	1(2)
66183	1(3)
66184	1(2)
66185	1(2)
66225	1(2)
66250	1(2)
66500	1(2)
66505	1(2)
66600	1(2)
66605	1(2)
66625	1(2)
66630	1(2)
66635	1(2)
66680	1(2)
66682	1(2)
66700	1(2)
66710	1(2)
66711	1(2)
66720	1(2)
66740	1(2)
66761	1(2)
66762	1(2)
66770	1(3)
66820	1(2)
66821	1(2)
66825	1(2)
66830	1(2)
66840	1(2)
66850	1(2)
66852	1(2)
66920	1(2)
66930	1(2)
66940	1(2)
66982	1(2)
66983	1(2)
66984	1(2)
66985	1(2)

CPT	MUE
66986	1(2)
66987	2(2)
66988	2(2)
66990	1(3)
66999	1(3)
67005	1(2)
67010	1(2)
67015	1(2)
67025	1(2)
67027	1(2)
67028	1(3)
67030	1(2)
67031	1(2)
67036	1(2)
67039	1(2)
67040	1(2)
67041	1(2)
67042	1(2)
67043	1(2)
67101	1(2)
67105	1(2)
67107	1(2)
67108	1(2)
67110	1(2)
67113	1(2)
67115	1(2)
67120	1(2)
67121	1(2)
67141	1(2)
67145	1(2)
67208	1(2)
67210	1(2)
67218	1(2)
67220	1(2)
67221	1(2)
67225	1(2)
67227	1(2)
67228	1(2)
67229	1(2)
67250	1(2)
67255	1(2)
67299	1(3)
67311	1(2)
67312	1(2)
67314	1(2)
67316	1(2)
67318	1(2)
67320	2(3)
67331	1(2)
67332	1(2)
67334	1(2)
67335	1(2)
67340	2(2)
67343	1(2)
67345	1(3)
67346	1(3)
67399	1(3)
67400	1(2)
67405	1(2)
67412	1(2)
67413	1(2)
67414	1(2)
67415	1(3)
67420	1(2)
67430	1(2)

CPT	MUE
67440	1(2)
67445	1(2)
67450	1(2)
67500	1(3)
67505	1(3)
67515	1(3)
67550	1(2)
67560	1(2)
67570	1(2)
67599	1(3)
67700	2(3)
67710	1(2)
67715	1(3)
67800	1(2)
67801	1(2)
67805	1(2)
67808	1(2)
67810	2(3)
67820	1(2)
67825	1(2)
67830	1(2)
67835	1(2)
67840	3(3)
67850	3(3)
67875	1(2)
67880	1(2)
67882	1(2)
67900	1(2)
67901	1(2)
67902	1(2)
67903	1(2)
67904	1(2)
67906	1(2)
67908	1(2)
67909	1(2)
67911	2(3)
67912	1(2)
67914	2(3)
67915	2(3)
67916	2(3)
67917	2(3)
67921	2(3)
67922	2(3)
67923	2(3)
67924	2(3)
67930	2(3)
67935	2(3)
67938	2(3)
67950	2(2)
67961	2(3)
67966	2(3)
67971	1(2)
67973	1(2)
67974	1(2)
67975	1(2)
67999	1(3)
68020	1(3)
68040	1(2)
68100	1(3)
68110	1(3)
68115	1(3)
68130	1(3)
68135	1(3)
68200	1(3)
68320	1(2)

CPT	MUE
68325	1(2)
68326	1(2)
68328	1(2)
68330	1(3)
68335	1(3)
68340	1(3)
68360	1(3)
68362	1(3)
68371	1(3)
68399	1(3)
68400	1(2)
68420	1(2)
68440	2(3)
68500	1(2)
68505	1(2)
68510	1(2)
68520	1(2)
68525	1(2)
68530	1(2)
68540	1(2)
68550	1(2)
68700	1(2)
68705	2(3)
68720	1(2)
68745	1(2)
68750	1(2)
68760	4(2)
68761	4(2)
68770	1(3)
68801	4(2)
68810	1(2)
68811	1(2)
68815	1(2)
68816	1(2)
68840	1(2)
68850	1(3)
68899	1(3)
69000	1(3)
69005	1(3)
69020	1(3)
69090	0(3)
69100	3(3)
69105	1(3)
69110	1(2)
69120	1(3)
69140	1(2)
69145	1(3)
69150	1(3)
69155	1(3)
69200	1(2)
69205	1(3)
69209	1(2)
69210	1(2)
69220	1(2)
69222	1(2)
69300	1(2)
69310	1(2)
69320	1(2)
69399	1(3)
69420	1(2)
69421	1(2)
69424	1(2)
69433	1(2)
69436	1(2)
69440	1(2)

CPT	MUE
69450	1(2)
69501	1(3)
69502	1(2)
69505	1(2)
69511	1(2)
69530	1(2)
69535	1(2)
69540	1(3)
69550	1(3)
69552	1(2)
69554	1(2)
69601	1(2)
69602	1(2)
69603	1(2)
69604	1(2)
69605	1(2)
69610	1(2)
69620	1(2)
69631	1(2)
69632	1(3)
69633	1(2)
69635	1(3)
69636	1(3)
69637	1(3)
69641	1(2)
69642	1(2)
69643	1(2)
69644	1(2)
69645	1(2)
69646	1(2)
69650	1(2)
69660	1(2)
69661	1(2)
69662	1(2)
69666	1(2)
69667	1(2)
69670	1(2)
69676	1(2)
69700	1(3)
69710	0(3)
69711	1(2)
69714	1(2)
69715	1(3)
69717	1(2)
69718	1(2)
69720	1(2)
69725	1(2)
69740	1(2)
69745	1(2)
69799	1(3)
69801	1(3)
69805	1(3)
69806	1(3)
69905	1(2)
69910	1(2)
69915	1(3)
69930	1(2)
69949	1(3)
69950	1(2)
69955	1(2)
69960	1(2)
69970	1(3)
69979	1(3)
69990	1(3)
70010	1(3)

CPT	MUE
70015	1(3)
70030	2(2)
70100	2(3)
70110	2(3)
70120	1(3)
70130	1(3)
70134	1(3)
70140	2(3)
70150	1(3)
70160	1(3)
70170	2(2)
70190	1(2)
70200	2(3)
70210	1(3)
70220	1(3)
70240	1(2)
70250	2(3)
70260	1(3)
70300	1(3)
70310	1(3)
70320	1(3)
70328	1(3)
70330	1(3)
70332	2(3)
70336	1(3)
70350	1(3)
70355	1(3)
70360	2(3)
70370	1(3)
70371	1(2)
70380	2(3)
70390	2(3)
70450	3(3)
70460	1(3)
70470	2(3)
70480	1(3)
70481	1(3)
70482	1(3)
70486	1(3)
70487	1(3)
70488	1(3)
70490	1(3)
70491	1(3)
70492	1(3)
70496	2(3)
70498	2(3)
70540	1(3)
70542	1(3)
70543	1(3)
70544	2(3)
70545	1(3)
70546	1(3)
70547	1(3)
70548	1(3)
70549	1(3)
70551	2(3)
70552	2(3)
70553	2(3)
70554	1(3)
70555	1(3)
70557	1(3)
70558	1(3)
70559	1(3)
71045	4(3)
71046	3(3)

CPT	MUE
71047	2(3)
71048	1(3)
71100	2(3)
71101	2(3)
71110	1(3)
71111	1(3)
71120	1(3)
71130	1(3)
71250	2(3)
71260	2(3)
71270	1(3)
71275	1(3)
71550	1(3)
71551	1(3)
71552	1(3)
71555	1(3)
72020	4(3)
72040	3(3)
72050	1(3)
72052	1(3)
72070	1(3)
72072	1(3)
72074	1(3)
72080	1(3)
72081	1(3)
72082	1(3)
72083	1(3)
72084	1(3)
72100	2(3)
72110	1(3)
72114	1(3)
72120	1(3)
72125	1(3)
72126	1(3)
72127	1(3)
72128	1(3)
72129	1(3)
72130	1(3)
72131	1(3)
72132	1(3)
72133	1(3)
72141	1(3)
72142	1(3)
72146	1(3)
72147	1(3)
72148	1(3)
72149	1(3)
72156	1(3)
72157	1(3)
72158	1(3)
72159	1(3)
72170	2(3)
72190	1(3)
72191	1(3)
72192	1(3)
72193	1(3)
72194	1(3)
72195	1(3)
72196	1(3)
72197	1(3)
72198	1(3)
72200	2(3)
72202	1(3)
72220	1(3)
72240	1(2)

CPT	MUE
72255	1(2)
72265	1(2)
72270	1(2)
72275	1(3)
72285	4(3)
72295	5(3)
73000	2(3)
73010	2(3)
73020	2(3)
73030	4(3)
73040	2(2)
73050	1(3)
73060	2(3)
73070	2(3)
73080	2(3)
73085	2(2)
73090	2(3)
73092	2(3)
73100	2(3)
73110	3(3)
73115	2(2)
73120	2(3)
73130	3(3)
73140	3(3)
73200	2(3)
73201	2(3)
73202	2(3)
73206	2(3)
73218	2(3)
73219	2(3)
73220	2(3)
73221	2(3)
73222	2(3)
73223	2(3)
73225	2(3)
73501	2(3)
73502	2(3)
73503	2(3)
73521	2(3)
73522	2(3)
73523	2(3)
73525	2(2)
73551	2(3)
73552	2(3)
73560	4(3)
73562	3(3)
73564	4(3)
73565	1(3)
73580	2(2)
73590	3(3)
73592	2(3)
73600	2(3)
73610	3(3)
73615	2(2)
73620	2(3)
73630	3(3)
73650	2(3)
73660	2(3)
73700	2(3)
73701	2(3)
73702	2(3)
73706	2(3)
73718	2(3)
73719	2(3)
73720	2(3)

CPT	MUE
73721	3(3)
73722	2(3)
73723	2(3)
73725	2(3)
74018	3(3)
74019	2(3)
74021	2(3)
74022	2(3)
74150	1(3)
74160	1(3)
74170	1(3)
74174	1(3)
74175	1(3)
74176	2(3)
74177	2(3)
74178	1(3)
74181	1(3)
74182	1(3)
74183	1(3)
74185	1(3)
74190	1(3)
74210	1(3)
74220	1(3)
74221	1(3)
74230	1(3)
74235	1(3)
74240	2(3)
74246	1(3)
74248	1(2)
74250	1(3)
74251	1(3)
74261	1(2)
74262	1(2)
74263	0(3)
74270	1(3)
74280	1(3)
74283	1(3)
74290	1(3)
74300	1(3)
74301	1(3)
74328	1(3)
74329	1(3)
74330	1(3)
74340	1(3)
74355	1(3)
74360	1(3)
74363	2(3)
74400	1(3)
74410	1(3)
74415	1(3)
74420	2(3)
74425	2(3)
74430	1(3)
74440	1(2)
74445	1(2)
74450	1(3)
74455	1(3)
74470	2(2)
74485	2(3)
74710	1(3)
74712	1(3)
74713	2(3)
74740	1(3)
74742	2(2)
74775	1(2)

CPT	MUE
75557	1(3)
75559	1(3)
75561	1(3)
75563	1(3)
75565	1(3)
75571	1(3)
75572	1(3)
75573	1(3)
75574	1(3)
75600	1(3)
75605	1(3)
75625	1(3)
75630	1(3)
75635	1(3)
75705	20(3)
75710	2(3)
75716	1(3)
75726	3(3)
75731	1(3)
75733	1(3)
75736	2(3)
75741	1(3)
75743	1(3)
75746	1(3)
75756	2(3)
75774	7(3)
75801	1(3)
75803	1(3)
75805	1(2)
75807	1(2)
75809	1(3)
75810	1(3)
75820	2(3)
75822	1(3)
75825	1(3)
75827	1(3)
75831	1(3)
75833	1(3)
75840	1(3)
75842	1(3)
75860	2(3)
75870	1(3)
75872	1(3)
75880	1(3)
75885	1(3)
75887	1(3)
75889	1(3)
75891	1(3)
75893	2(3)
75894	2(3)
75898	2(3)
75901	1(3)
75902	2(3)
75956	1(2)
75957	1(2)
75958	2(3)
75959	1(2)
75970	1(3)
75984	2(3)
75989	2(3)
76000	3(3)
76010	2(3)
76080	3(3)
76098	3(3)
76100	2(3)

CPT	MUE
76101	1(3)
76102	1(3)
76120	1(3)
76125	1(3)
76140	0(3)
76376	2(3)
76377	2(3)
76380	2(3)
76390	0(3)
76391	1(3)
76496	1(3)
76497	1(3)
76498	1(3)
76499	1(3)
76506	1(2)
76510	2(2)
76511	2(2)
76512	2(2)
76513	2(2)
76514	1(2)
76516	1(2)
76519	1(3)
76529	2(2)
76536	1(3)
76604	1(3)
76641	2(2)
76642	2(2)
76700	1(3)
76705	2(3)
76706	1(2)
76770	1(3)
76775	2(3)
76776	2(3)
76800	1(3)
76801	1(2)
76802	2(3)
76805	1(2)
76810	2(3)
76811	1(2)
76812	2(3)
76813	1(2)
76814	2(3)
76815	1(2)
76816	2(3)
76817	1(3)
76818	2(3)
76819	2(3)
76820	3(3)
76821	2(3)
76825	2(3)
76826	2(3)
76827	2(3)
76828	2(3)
76830	1(3)
76831	1(3)
76856	1(3)
76857	1(3)
76870	1(2)
76872	1(3)
76873	1(2)
76881	2(3)
76882	2(3)
76885	1(2)
76886	1(2)
76932	1(2)

CPT	MUE
76936	1(3)
76937	2(3)
76940	1(3)
76941	3(3)
76942	1(3)
76945	1(3)
76946	1(3)
76948	1(2)
76965	2(3)
76970	2(3)
76975	1(3)
76977	1(2)
76978	1(2)
76979	3(3)
76981	1(3)
76982	1(2)
76983	2(3)
76998	1(3)
76999	1(3)
77001	2(3)
77002	1(3)
77003	1(3)
77011	1(3)
77012	1(3)
77013	1(3)
77014	2(3)
77021	1(3)
77022	1(3)
77046	1(2)
77047	1(2)
77048	1(2)
77049	1(2)
77053	2(2)
77054	2(2)
77061	1(2)
77062	1(2)
77063	1(2)
77065	1(2)
77066	1(2)
77067	1(2)
77071	1(3)
77072	1(2)
77073	1(2)
77074	1(2)
77075	1(2)
77076	1(2)
77077	1(2)
77078	1(2)
77080	1(2)
77081	1(2)
77084	1(2)
77085	1(2)
77086	1(2)
77261	1(3)
77262	1(3)
77263	1(3)
77280	2(3)
77285	1(3)
77290	1(3)
77293	1(3)
77295	1(3)
77299	1(3)
77300	10(3)
77301	1(3)
77306	1(3)

CPT	MUE
77307	1(3)
77316	1(3)
77317	1(3)
77318	1(3)
77321	1(2)
77331	3(3)
77332	4(3)
77333	2(3)
77334	10(3)
77336	1(2)
77338	1(3)
77370	1(3)
77371	1(2)
77372	1(2)
77373	1(3)
77385	2(3)
77386	2(3)
77387	2(3)
77399	1(3)
77401	1(2)
77402	2(3)
77407	2(3)
77412	2(3)
77417	1(2)
77423	1(3)
77424	1(2)
77425	1(3)
77427	1(2)
77431	1(2)
77432	1(2)
77435	1(2)
77469	1(2)
77470	1(2)
77499	1(3)
77520	2(3)
77522	2(3)
77523	2(3)
77525	2(3)
77600	1(3)
77605	1(3)
77610	1(3)
77615	1(3)
77620	1(3)
77750	1(3)
77761	1(3)
77762	1(3)
77763	1(3)
77767	2(3)
77768	2(3)
77770	2(3)
77771	2(3)
77772	2(3)
77778	1(3)
77789	2(3)
77790	1(3)
77799	1(3)
78012	1(3)
78013	1(3)
78014	1(2)
78015	1(3)
78016	1(3)
78018	1(2)
78020	1(3)
78070	1(2)
78071	1(3)

CPT	MUE
78072	1(3)
78075	1(2)
78099	1(3)
78102	1(2)
78103	1(2)
78104	1(2)
78110	1(2)
78111	1(2)
78120	1(2)
78121	1(2)
78122	1(2)
78130	1(2)
78135	1(3)
78140	1(3)
78185	1(2)
78191	1(2)
78195	1(2)
78199	1(3)
78201	1(3)
78202	1(3)
78215	1(3)
78216	1(3)
78226	1(3)
78227	1(3)
78230	1(3)
78231	1(3)
78232	1(3)
78258	1(2)
78261	1(2)
78262	1(2)
78264	1(2)
78265	1(2)
78266	1(2)
78267	1(2)
78268	1(2)
78278	2(3)
78282	1(2)
78290	1(3)
78291	1(3)
78299	1(3)
78300	1(2)
78305	1(2)
78306	1(2)
78315	1(2)
78350	0(3)
78351	0(3)
78399	1(3)
78414	1(2)
78428	1(3)
78429	1(2)
78430	1(2)
78431	1(2)
78432	1(2)
78433	1(2)
78434	1(2)
78445	1(3)
78451	1(2)
78452	1(2)
78453	1(2)
78454	1(2)
78456	1(3)
78457	1(2)
78458	1(2)
78459	1(3)
78466	1(3)

CPT	MUE
78468	1(3)
78469	1(3)
78472	1(2)
78473	1(2)
78481	1(2)
78483	1(2)
78491	1(3)
78492	1(2)
78494	1(3)
78496	1(3)
78499	1(3)
78579	1(3)
78580	1(3)
78582	1(3)
78597	1(3)
78598	1(3)
78599	1(3)
78600	1(3)
78601	1(3)
78605	1(3)
78606	1(3)
78608	1(3)
78609	0(3)
78610	1(3)
78630	1(3)
78635	1(3)
78645	1(3)
78650	1(3)
78660	1(2)
78699	1(3)
78700	1(3)
78701	1(3)
78707	1(2)
78708	1(2)
78709	1(2)
78725	1(3)
78730	1(2)
78740	1(2)
78761	1(2)
78799	1(3)
78800	1(2)
78801	1(2)
78802	1(2)
78803	1(2)
78804	1(2)
78808	1(2)
78811	1(2)
78812	1(2)
78813	1(2)
78814	1(2)
78815	1(2)
78816	1(2)
78830	1(2)
78831	1(2)
78832	1(2)
78835	4(3)
78999	1(3)
79005	1(3)
79101	1(3)
79200	1(3)
79300	1(3)
79403	1(3)
79440	1(3)
79445	1(3)
79999	1(3)

CPT	MUE
80047	2(3)
80048	2(3)
80050	0(3)
80051	4(3)
80053	1(3)
80055	1(3)
80061	1(3)
80069	1(3)
80074	1(2)
80076	1(3)
80081	1(2)
80145	1(3)
80150	2(3)
80155	1(3)
80156	2(3)
80157	2(3)
80158	2(3)
80159	2(3)
80162	2(3)
80163	1(3)
80164	2(3)
80165	1(3)
80168	2(3)
80169	2(3)
80170	2(3)
80171	1(3)
80173	2(3)
80175	1(3)
80176	1(3)
80177	1(3)
80178	2(3)
80180	1(3)
80183	1(3)
80184	2(3)
80185	2(3)
80186	2(3)
80187	1(3)
80188	2(3)
80190	2(3)
80192	2(3)
80194	2(3)
80195	2(3)
80197	2(3)
80198	2(3)
80199	1(3)
80200	2(3)
80201	2(3)
80202	2(3)
80203	1(3)
80230	1(3)
80235	1(3)
80280	1(3)
80285	1(3)
80299	3(3)
80305	1(2)
80306	1(2)
80307	1(2)
80320	2(3)
80321	1(3)
80322	1(3)
80323	1(3)
80324	1(3)
80325	1(3)
80326	1(3)
80327	1(3)

CPT	MUE
80328	1(3)
80329	2(3)
80330	1(3)
80331	1(3)
80332	1(3)
80333	1(3)
80334	1(3)
80335	1(3)
80336	1(3)
80337	1(3)
80338	1(3)
80339	2(3)
80340	1(3)
80341	1(3)
80342	1(3)
80343	1(3)
80344	1(3)
80345	2(3)
80346	1(3)
80347	1(3)
80348	1(3)
80349	1(3)
80350	1(3)
80351	1(3)
80352	1(3)
80353	1(3)
80354	1(3)
80355	1(3)
80356	1(3)
80357	1(3)
80358	1(3)
80359	1(3)
80360	1(3)
80361	2(3)
80362	1(3)
80363	1(3)
80364	1(3)
80365	2(3)
80366	1(3)
80367	1(3)
80368	1(3)
80369	1(3)
80370	1(3)
80371	1(3)
80372	1(3)
80373	1(3)
80374	1(3)
80375	1(3)
80376	1(3)
80377	1(3)
80400	1(3)
80402	1(3)
80406	1(3)
80408	1(3)
80410	1(3)
80412	1(3)
80414	1(3)
80415	1(3)
80416	1(3)
80417	1(3)
80418	1(3)
80420	1(2)
80422	1(3)
80424	1(3)
80426	1(3)

CPT	MUE
80428	1(3)
80430	1(3)
80432	1(3)
80434	1(3)
80435	1(3)
80436	1(3)
80438	1(3)
80439	1(3)
80500	1(3)
80502	1(3)
81000	2(3)
81001	2(3)
81002	2(3)
81003	2(3)
81005	2(3)
81007	1(3)
81015	2(3)
81020	1(3)
81025	1(3)
81050	2(3)
81099	1(3)
81105	1(2)
81106	1(2)
81107	1(2)
81108	1(2)
81109	1(2)
81110	1(2)
81111	1(2)
81112	1(2)
81120	1(3)
81121	1(3)
81161	1(3)
81162	1(2)
81163	1(2)
81164	1(2)
81165	1(2)
81166	1(2)
81167	1(2)
81170	1(2)
81171	1(2)
81172	1(2)
81173	1(2)
81174	1(2)
81175	1(3)
81176	1(3)
81177	1(2)
81178	1(2)
81179	1(2)
81180	1(2)
81181	1(2)
81182	1(2)
81183	1(2)
81184	1(2)
81185	1(2)
81186	1(2)
81187	1(2)
81188	1(2)
81189	1(2)
81190	1(2)
81200	1(2)
81201	1(2)
81202	1(3)
81203	1(3)
81204	1(2)
81205	1(3)

CPT	MUE
81206	1(3)
81207	1(3)
81208	1(3)
81209	1(3)
81210	1(3)
81212	1(2)
81215	1(2)
81216	1(2)
81217	1(2)
81218	1(3)
81219	1(3)
81220	1(3)
81221	1(3)
81222	1(3)
81223	1(2)
81224	1(3)
81225	1(3)
81226	1(3)
81227	1(3)
81228	1(3)
81229	1(3)
81230	1(2)
81231	1(2)
81232	1(2)
81233	1(3)
81234	1(2)
81235	1(3)
81236	1(3)
81237	1(3)
81238	1(2)
81239	1(2)
81240	1(2)
81241	1(2)
81242	1(3)
81243	1(3)
81244	1(3)
81245	1(3)
81246	1(3)
81247	1(2)
81248	1(2)
81249	1(2)
81250	1(3)
81251	1(3)
81252	1(3)
81253	1(3)
81254	1(3)
81255	1(3)
81256	1(2)
81257	1(2)
81258	1(2)
81259	1(2)
81260	1(3)
81261	1(3)
81262	1(3)
81263	1(3)
81264	1(3)
81265	1(3)
81266	2(3)
81267	1(3)
81268	4(3)
81269	1(2)
81270	1(2)
81271	1(2)
81272	1(3)
81273	1(3)

CPT	MUE
81274	1(2)
81275	1(3)
81276	1(3)
81277	1(2)
81283	1(2)
81284	1(2)
81285	1(2)
81286	1(2)
81287	1(3)
81288	1(3)
81289	1(2)
81290	1(3)
81291	1(3)
81292	1(2)
81293	1(3)
81294	1(3)
81295	1(2)
81296	1(3)
81297	1(3)
81298	1(2)
81299	1(3)
81300	1(3)
81301	1(3)
81302	1(3)
81303	1(3)
81304	1(3)
81305	1(3)
81306	1(2)
81307	1(2)
81308	1(2)
81309	1(2)
81310	1(3)
81311	1(3)
81312	1(2)
81313	1(3)
81314	1(3)
81315	1(3)
81316	1(2)
81317	1(2)
81318	1(3)
81319	1(2)
81320	1(3)
81321	1(3)
81322	1(3)
81323	1(3)
81324	1(3)
81325	1(3)
81326	1(3)
81327	1(2)
81328	1(2)
81329	1(2)
81330	1(3)
81331	1(3)
81332	1(3)
81333	1(2)
81334	1(3)
81335	1(2)
81336	1(2)
81337	1(2)
81340	1(3)
81341	1(3)
81342	1(3)
81343	1(2)
81344	1(2)
81345	1(3)

CPT	MUE
81346	1(2)
81350	1(3)
81355	1(3)
81361	1(2)
81362	1(2)
81363	1(2)
81364	1(2)
81370	1(2)
81371	1(2)
81372	1(2)
81373	2(2)
81374	1(3)
81375	1(2)
81376	5(3)
81377	2(3)
81378	1(2)
81379	1(2)
81380	2(2)
81381	3(3)
81382	6(3)
81383	2(3)
81400	2(3)
81401	3(3)
81402	1(3)
81403	3(3)
81404	3(3)
81405	2(3)
81406	3(3)
81407	1(3)
81408	1(3)
81410	1(2)
81411	1(2)
81412	1(2)
81413	1(2)
81414	1(2)
81415	1(2)
81416	2(3)
81417	1(3)
81420	1(2)
81422	1(2)
81425	1(2)
81426	2(3)
81427	1(3)
81430	1(2)
81431	1(2)
81432	1(2)
81433	1(2)
81434	1(2)
81435	1(2)
81436	1(2)
81437	1(2)
81438	1(2)
81439	1(2)
81440	1(2)
81442	1(2)
81443	1(2)
81445	1(2)
81448	1(2)
81450	1(2)
81455	1(2)
81460	1(2)
81465	1(2)
81470	1(2)
81471	1(2)
81479	3(3)

CPT	MUE
81490	1(2)
81493	1(2)
81500	1(2)
81503	1(2)
81504	1(2)
81506	1(2)
81507	1(2)
81508	1(2)
81509	1(2)
81510	1(2)
81511	1(2)
81512	1(2)
81518	1(2)
81519	1(2)
81520	1(2)
81521	1(2)
81522	1(2)
81525	1(2)
81528	1(2)
81535	1(2)
81536	11(3)
81538	1(2)
81539	1(2)
81540	1(2)
81541	1(2)
81542	1(2)
81545	1(2)
81551	1(2)
81552	1(2)
81595	1(2)
81596	1(2)
81599	1(3)
82009	3(3)
82010	3(3)
82013	1(3)
82016	1(3)
82017	1(3)
82024	4(3)
82030	1(3)
82040	1(3)
82042	2(3)
82043	1(3)
82044	1(3)
82045	1(3)
82075	2(3)
82085	1(3)
82088	2(3)
82103	1(3)
82104	1(2)
82105	1(3)
82106	2(3)
82107	1(3)
82108	1(3)
82120	1(3)
82127	1(3)
82128	2(3)
82131	2(3)
82135	1(3)
82136	2(3)
82139	2(3)
82140	2(3)
82143	2(3)
82150	4(3)
82154	1(3)
82157	1(3)

CPT	MUE
82160	1(3)
82163	1(3)
82164	1(3)
82172	2(3)
82175	2(3)
82180	1(2)
82190	2(3)
82232	2(3)
82239	1(3)
82240	1(3)
82247	2(3)
82248	2(3)
82252	1(3)
82261	1(3)
82270	1(3)
82271	3(3)
82272	1(3)
82274	1(3)
82286	1(3)
82300	1(3)
82306	1(2)
82308	1(3)
82310	4(3)
82330	4(3)
82331	1(3)
82340	1(3)
82355	2(3)
82360	2(3)
82365	2(3)
82370	2(3)
82373	1(3)
82374	2(3)
82375	4(3)
82376	2(3)
82378	1(3)
82379	1(3)
82380	1(3)
82382	1(2)
82383	1(3)
82384	2(3)
82387	1(3)
82390	1(2)
82397	4(3)
82415	1(3)
82435	2(3)
82436	1(3)
82438	1(3)
82441	1(2)
82465	1(3)
82480	2(3)
82482	1(3)
82485	1(3)
82495	1(2)
82507	1(3)
82523	1(3)
82525	2(3)
82528	1(3)
82530	4(3)
82533	5(3)
82540	1(3)
82542	6(3)
82550	3(3)
82552	3(3)
82553	3(3)
82554	2(3)

CPT	MUE
82565	2(3)
82570	3(3)
82575	1(3)
82585	1(2)
82595	1(3)
82600	1(3)
82607	1(2)
82608	1(2)
82610	1(3)
82615	1(3)
82626	1(3)
82627	1(3)
82633	1(3)
82634	1(3)
82638	1(3)
82642	1(2)
82652	1(2)
82656	1(3)
82657	2(3)
82658	2(3)
82664	2(3)
82668	1(3)
82670	2(3)
82671	1(3)
82672	1(3)
82677	1(3)
82679	1(3)
82693	2(3)
82696	1(3)
82705	1(3)
82710	1(3)
82715	3(3)
82725	1(3)
82726	1(3)
82728	1(3)
82731	1(3)
82735	1(3)
82746	1(2)
82747	1(2)
82757	1(2)
82759	1(3)
82760	1(3)
82775	1(3)
82776	1(2)
82777	1(3)
82784	6(3)
82785	1(3)
82787	4(3)
82800	2(3)
82805	3(3)
82810	4(3)
82820	1(3)
82930	1(3)
82938	1(3)
82941	1(3)
82943	1(3)
82945	4(3)
82946	1(2)
82947	5(3)
82950	3(3)
82951	1(2)
82952	3(3)
82955	1(2)
82960	1(2)
82963	1(3)

CPT	MUE
82965	1(3)
82977	1(3)
82978	1(3)
82979	1(3)
82985	1(3)
83001	1(3)
83002	1(3)
83003	5(3)
83006	1(2)
83009	1(3)
83010	1(3)
83012	1(2)
83013	1(3)
83014	1(2)
83015	1(2)
83018	4(3)
83020	2(3)
83021	2(3)
83026	1(3)
83030	1(3)
83033	1(3)
83036	1(2)
83037	1(2)
83045	1(3)
83050	2(3)
83051	1(3)
83060	1(3)
83065	1(2)
83068	1(2)
83069	1(3)
83070	1(2)
83080	2(3)
83088	1(3)
83090	2(3)
83150	1(3)
83491	1(3)
83497	1(3)
83498	2(3)
83500	1(3)
83505	1(3)
83516	5(3)
83518	1(3)
83519	5(3)
83520	9(3)
83525	4(3)
83527	1(3)
83528	1(3)
83540	2(3)
83550	1(3)
83570	1(3)
83582	1(3)
83586	1(3)
83593	1(3)
83605	2(3)
83615	3(3)
83625	1(3)
83630	1(3)
83631	1(3)
83632	1(3)
83633	1(3)
83655	2(3)
83661	3(3)
83662	4(3)
83663	3(3)
83664	3(3)

CPT	MUE
83670	1(3)
83690	2(3)
83695	1(3)
83698	1(3)
83700	1(2)
83701	1(3)
83704	1(3)
83718	1(3)
83719	1(3)
83721	1(3)
83722	1(2)
83727	1(3)
83735	4(3)
83775	1(3)
83785	1(3)
83789	4(3)
83825	2(3)
83835	2(3)
83857	1(3)
83861	2(2)
83864	1(2)
83872	2(3)
83873	1(3)
83874	4(3)
83876	1(3)
83880	1(3)
83883	4(3)
83885	2(3)
83915	1(3)
83916	2(3)
83918	2(3)
83919	1(3)
83921	2(3)
83930	2(3)
83935	2(3)
83937	1(3)
83945	2(3)
83950	1(2)
83951	1(2)
83970	4(3)
83986	2(3)
83987	1(3)
83992	2(3)
83993	1(3)
84030	1(2)
84035	1(2)
84060	1(3)
84066	1(3)
84075	2(3)
84078	1(2)
84080	1(3)
84081	1(3)
84085	1(2)
84087	1(3)
84100	2(3)
84105	1(3)
84106	1(2)
84110	1(3)
84112	1(3)
84119	1(2)
84120	1(3)
84126	1(3)
84132	3(3)
84133	2(3)
84134	1(3)

CPT	MUE
84135	1(3)
84138	1(3)
84140	1(3)
84143	2(3)
84144	1(3)
84145	1(3)
84146	3(3)
84150	2(3)
84152	1(2)
84153	1(2)
84154	1(2)
84155	1(3)
84156	1(3)
84157	2(3)
84160	2(3)
84163	1(3)
84165	1(2)
84166	2(3)
84181	3(3)
84182	6(3)
84202	1(2)
84203	1(2)
84206	1(2)
84207	1(2)
84210	1(3)
84220	1(3)
84228	1(3)
84233	1(3)
84234	1(3)
84235	1(3)
84238	3(3)
84244	2(3)
84252	1(2)
84255	2(3)
84260	1(3)
84270	1(3)
84275	1(3)
84285	1(3)
84295	2(3)
84300	2(3)
84302	1(3)
84305	1(3)
84307	1(3)
84311	2(3)
84315	1(3)
84375	1(3)
84376	1(3)
84377	1(3)
84378	2(3)
84379	1(3)
84392	1(3)
84402	1(3)
84403	2(3)
84410	1(2)
84425	1(2)
84430	1(3)
84431	1(3)
84432	1(2)
84436	1(2)
84437	1(2)
84439	1(2)
84442	1(2)
84443	4(2)
84445	1(2)
84446	1(2)

CPT	MUE
84449	1(3)
84450	1(3)
84460	1(3)
84466	1(3)
84478	1(3)
84479	1(2)
84480	1(2)
84481	1(2)
84482	1(2)
84484	4(3)
84485	1(3)
84488	1(3)
84490	1(2)
84510	1(3)
84512	3(3)
84520	2(3)
84525	1(3)
84540	2(3)
84545	1(3)
84550	1(3)
84560	2(3)
84577	1(3)
84578	1(3)
84580	1(3)
84583	1(3)
84585	1(2)
84586	1(2)
84588	1(3)
84590	1(2)
84591	1(3)
84597	1(3)
84600	2(3)
84620	1(2)
84630	2(3)
84681	1(3)
84702	2(3)
84703	1(3)
84704	1(3)
84830	1(2)
84999	1(3)
85002	1(3)
85004	2(3)
85007	1(3)
85008	1(3)
85009	1(3)
85013	1(3)
85014	4(3)
85018	4(3)
85025	4(3)
85027	4(3)
85032	2(3)
85041	1(3)
85044	1(2)
85045	1(2)
85046	1(2)
85048	2(3)
85049	2(3)
85055	1(3)
85060	1(3)
85097	2(3)
85130	1(3)
85170	1(3)
85175	1(3)
85210	2(3)
85220	2(3)

CPT	MUE
85230	2(3)
85240	2(3)
85244	1(3)
85245	2(3)
85246	2(3)
85247	2(3)
85250	2(3)
85260	2(3)
85270	2(3)
85280	2(3)
85290	2(3)
85291	1(3)
85292	1(3)
85293	1(3)
85300	2(3)
85301	1(3)
85302	1(3)
85303	2(3)
85305	2(3)
85306	2(3)
85307	2(3)
85335	2(3)
85337	1(3)
85345	1(3)
85347	9(3)
85348	4(3)
85360	1(3)
85362	2(3)
85366	1(3)
85370	1(3)
85378	2(3)
85379	2(3)
85380	2(3)
85384	2(3)
85385	1(3)
85390	3(3)
85396	1(2)
85397	2(3)
85400	1(3)
85410	1(3)
85415	2(3)
85420	2(3)
85421	1(3)
85441	1(2)
85445	1(2)
85460	1(3)
85461	1(2)
85475	1(3)
85520	3(3)
85525	2(3)
85530	1(3)
85536	1(2)
85540	1(2)
85547	1(2)
85549	1(3)
85555	1(2)
85557	1(2)
85576	7(3)
85597	1(3)
85598	1(3)
85610	4(3)
85611	2(3)
85612	1(3)
85613	3(3)
85635	1(3)

CPT	MUE
85651	1(2)
85652	1(2)
85660	2(3)
85670	2(3)
85675	1(3)
85705	1(3)
85730	4(3)
85732	4(3)
85810	2(3)
85999	1(3)
86000	6(3)
86001	20(3)
86005	6(3)
86008	20(3)
86021	1(2)
86022	1(2)
86023	3(3)
86038	1(3)
86039	1(3)
86060	1(3)
86063	1(3)
86077	1(2)
86078	1(3)
86079	1(3)
86140	1(2)
86141	1(2)
86146	3(3)
86147	4(3)
86148	3(3)
86152	1(3)
86153	1(3)
86155	1(3)
86156	1(2)
86157	1(2)
86160	4(3)
86161	2(3)
86162	1(2)
86171	2(3)
86200	1(3)
86215	1(3)
86225	1(3)
86226	1(3)
86235	10(3)
86255	5(3)
86256	9(3)
86277	1(3)
86280	1(3)
86294	1(3)
86300	2(3)
86301	1(2)
86304	1(2)
86305	1(2)
86308	1(2)
86309	1(2)
86310	1(2)
86316	2(3)
86317	6(3)
86318	2(3)
86320	1(2)
86325	2(3)
86327	1(3)
86328	3(3)
86329	3(3)
86331	12(3)
86332	1(3)

CPT	MUE
86334	2(2)
86335	2(3)
86336	1(3)
86337	1(2)
86340	1(2)
86341	1(3)
86343	1(3)
86344	1(2)
86352	1(3)
86353	7(3)
86355	1(2)
86356	7(3)
86357	1(2)
86359	1(2)
86360	1(2)
86361	1(2)
86367	2(3)
86376	2(3)
86382	3(3)
86384	1(3)
86386	1(2)
86403	3(3)
86406	2(3)
86430	2(3)
86431	2(3)
86480	1(3)
86481	1(3)
86485	1(2)
86486	2(3)
86490	1(2)
86510	1(2)
86580	1(2)
86590	1(3)
86592	2(3)
86593	2(3)
86602	3(3)
86603	2(3)
86609	14(3)
86611	4(3)
86612	2(3)
86615	6(3)
86617	2(3)
86618	2(3)
86619	2(3)
86622	2(3)
86625	1(3)
86628	3(3)
86631	6(3)
86632	3(3)
86635	4(3)
86638	6(3)
86641	2(3)
86644	2(3)
86645	1(3)
86648	2(3)
86651	2(3)
86652	2(3)
86653	2(3)
86654	2(3)
86658	12(3)
86663	2(3)
86664	2(3)
86665	2(3)
86666	4(3)
86668	2(3)

CPT	MUE
86671	3(3)
86674	3(3)
86677	3(3)
86682	2(3)
86684	2(3)
86687	1(3)
86688	1(3)
86689	2(3)
86692	2(3)
86694	2(3)
86695	2(3)
86696	2(3)
86698	3(3)
86701	1(3)
86702	2(3)
86703	1(2)
86704	1(2)
86705	1(2)
86706	2(3)
86707	1(3)
86708	1(2)
86709	1(2)
86710	4(3)
86711	2(3)
86713	3(3)
86717	8(3)
86720	2(3)
86723	2(3)
86727	2(3)
86732	2(3)
86735	2(3)
86738	2(3)
86741	2(3)
86744	2(3)
86747	2(3)
86750	4(3)
86753	3(3)
86756	2(3)
86757	6(3)
86759	2(3)
86762	2(3)
86765	2(3)
86768	5(3)
86769	3(3)
86771	2(3)
86774	2(3)
86777	2(3)
86778	2(3)
86780	2(3)
86784	1(3)
86787	2(3)
86788	2(3)
86789	2(3)
86790	4(3)
86793	2(3)
86794	1(3)
86800	1(3)
86803	1(3)
86804	1(2)
86805	12(3)
86806	2(3)
86807	2(3)
86808	1(3)
86812	1(2)
86813	1(2)

CPT	MUE
86816	1(2)
86817	1(2)
86821	1(3)
86825	1(3)
86826	8(3)
86828	2(3)
86829	2(3)
86830	2(3)
86831	2(3)
86832	2(3)
86833	1(3)
86834	1(3)
86835	1(3)
86849	1(3)
86850	3(3)
86860	2(3)
86870	6(3)
86880	4(3)
86885	3(3)
86886	3(3)
86890	2(3)
86891	2(3)
86900	3(3)
86901	3(3)
86902	40(3)
86905	28(3)
86906	1(2)
86910	0(3)
86911	0(3)
86920	19(3)
86922	10(3)
86923	10(3)
86930	3(3)
86931	4(3)
86940	3(3)
86941	3(3)
86945	5(3)
86950	1(3)
86960	3(3)
86965	4(3)
86971	6(3)
86972	2(3)
86975	2(3)
86976	2(3)
86977	2(3)
86999	1(3)
87003	1(3)
87015	3(3)
87045	3(3)
87046	6(3)
87071	2(3)
87073	2(3)
87075	6(3)
87076	4(3)
87077	6(3)
87081	4(3)
87084	1(3)
87086	3(3)
87088	3(3)
87101	3(3)
87102	4(3)
87103	2(3)
87106	4(3)
87107	4(3)
87109	2(3)

CPT	MUE
87110	2(3)
87118	3(3)
87140	3(3)
87143	2(3)
87149	11(3)
87150	12(3)
87152	1(3)
87153	3(3)
87164	2(3)
87166	2(3)
87168	2(3)
87169	2(3)
87172	1(3)
87176	3(3)
87177	3(3)
87181	12(3)
87184	8(3)
87185	4(3)
87186	12(3)
87187	3(3)
87188	14(3)
87190	10(3)
87197	1(3)
87206	6(3)
87207	3(3)
87209	4(3)
87210	4(3)
87220	3(3)
87230	2(3)
87250	1(3)
87252	4(3)
87253	3(3)
87254	10(3)
87255	2(3)
87260	1(3)
87265	1(3)
87267	1(3)
87269	1(3)
87270	1(3)
87271	1(3)
87272	1(3)
87273	1(3)
87274	1(3)
87275	1(3)
87276	1(3)
87278	1(3)
87279	1(3)
87280	1(3)
87281	1(3)
87283	1(3)
87285	1(3)
87290	1(3)
87299	1(3)
87300	2(3)
87301	1(3)
87305	1(3)
87320	1(3)
87324	2(3)
87327	1(3)
87328	2(3)
87329	2(3)
87332	1(3)
87335	1(3)
87336	1(3)
87337	1(3)

CPT	MUE
87338	1(3)
87339	1(3)
87340	1(2)
87341	1(2)
87350	1(2)
87380	1(2)
87385	2(3)
87389	1(3)
87390	1(3)
87391	1(3)
87400	2(3)
87420	1(3)
87425	1(3)
87426	3(3)
87427	2(3)
87430	1(3)
87449	3(3)
87450	2(3)
87451	2(3)
87471	1(3)
87472	1(3)
87475	1(3)
87476	1(3)
87480	1(3)
87481	6(3)
87482	1(3)
87483	1(2)
87485	1(3)
87486	1(3)
87487	1(3)
87490	1(3)
87491	3(3)
87492	1(3)
87493	2(3)
87495	1(3)
87496	1(3)
87497	2(3)
87498	1(3)
87500	1(3)
87501	1(3)
87502	1(3)
87503	1(3)
87505	1(2)
87506	1(2)
87507	1(2)
87510	1(3)
87511	1(3)
87512	1(3)
87516	1(3)
87517	1(3)
87520	1(3)
87521	1(3)
87522	1(3)
87525	1(3)
87526	1(3)
87527	1(3)
87528	1(3)
87529	2(3)
87530	2(3)
87531	1(3)
87532	1(3)
87533	1(3)
87534	1(3)
87535	1(3)
87536	1(3)

CPT	MUE
87537	1(3)
87538	1(3)
87539	1(3)
87540	1(3)
87541	1(3)
87542	1(3)
87550	1(3)
87551	2(3)
87552	1(3)
87555	1(3)
87556	1(3)
87557	1(3)
87560	1(3)
87561	1(3)
87562	1(3)
87563	3(3)
87580	1(3)
87581	1(3)
87582	1(3)
87590	1(3)
87591	3(3)
87592	1(3)
87623	1(2)
87624	1(3)
87625	1(3)
87631	1(3)
87632	1(3)
87633	1(3)
87634	1(3)
87635	2(3)
87640	1(3)
87641	1(3)
87650	1(3)
87651	1(3)
87652	1(3)
87653	1(3)
87660	1(3)
87661	1(3)
87662	2(3)
87797	3(3)
87798	21(3)
87799	3(3)
87800	2(3)
87801	3(3)
87802	2(3)
87803	3(3)
87804	3(3)
87806	1(2)
87807	2(3)
87808	1(3)
87809	2(3)
87810	2(3)
87850	1(3)
87880	2(3)
87899	6(3)
87900	1(2)
87901	1(2)
87902	1(2)
87903	1(2)
87904	14(3)
87905	2(3)
87906	2(3)
87910	1(3)
87912	1(3)
87999	1(3)

CPT	MUE	CPT	MUE	CPT	MUE	CPT	MUE	CPT	MUE	CPT	MUE	CPT	MUE	CPT	MUE
88000	0(3)	88263	1(3)	88738	1(3)	90386	0(3)	90700	1(2)	90953	1(2)	92201	1(2)	92547	1(3)
88005	0(3)	88264	1(3)	88740	1(2)	90389	0(3)	90702	1(2)	90954	1(2)	92202	1(2)	92548	1(3)
88007	0(3)	88267	2(3)	88741	1(2)	90393	1(2)	90707	1(2)	90955	1(2)	92227	1(2)	92549	1(3)
88012	0(3)	88269	2(3)	88749	1(3)	90396	1(2)	90710	1(2)	90956	1(2)	92228	1(2)	92550	1(2)
88014	0(3)	88271	16(3)	89049	1(3)	90399	0(3)	90713	1(2)	90957	1(2)	92230	2(2)	92551	0(3)
88016	0(3)	88272	12(3)	89050	2(3)	90460	9(3)	90714	1(2)	90958	1(2)	92235	1(2)	92552	1(2)
88020	0(3)	88273	3(3)	89051	2(3)	90461	8(3)	90715	1(2)	90959	1(2)	92240	1(2)	92553	1(2)
88025	0(3)	88274	5(3)	89055	2(3)	90471	1(2)	90716	1(2)	90960	1(2)	92242	1(2)	92555	1(2)
88027	0(3)	88275	12(3)	89060	2(3)	90472	8(3)	90717	1(2)	90961	1(2)	92250	1(2)	92556	1(2)
88028	0(3)	88280	1(3)	89125	2(3)	90473	1(2)	90723	0(3)	90962	1(2)	92260	1(2)	92557	1(2)
88029	0(3)	88283	5(3)	89160	1(3)	90474	1(3)	90732	1(2)	90963	1(2)	92265	1(2)	92558	0(3)
88036	0(3)	88285	10(3)	89190	1(3)	90476	1(2)	90733	1(2)	90964	1(2)	92270	1(2)	92559	0(3)
88037	0(3)	88289	1(3)	89220	2(3)	90477	1(2)	90734	1(2)	90965	1(2)	92273	1(2)	92560	0(3)
88040	0(3)	88291	0(3)	89230	1(2)	90581	1(2)	90736	1(2)	90966	1(2)	92274	1(2)	92561	1(2)
88045	0(3)	88299	1(3)	89240	1(3)	90585	1(2)	90738	1(2)	90967	1(2)	92283	1(2)	92562	1(2)
88099	0(3)	88300	4(3)	89250	1(2)	90586	1(2)	90739	1(2)	90968	1(2)	92284	1(2)	92563	1(2)
88104	5(3)	88302	4(3)	89251	1(2)	90587	1(2)	90740	1(2)	90969	1(2)	92285	1(2)	92564	1(2)
88106	5(3)	88304	5(3)	89253	1(3)	90619	1(2)	90743	1(2)	90970	1(2)	92286	1(2)	92565	1(2)
88108	6(3)	88305	16(3)	89254	1(3)	90620	1(2)	90744	1(2)	90989	1(2)	92287	1(2)	92567	1(2)
88112	6(3)	88307	8(3)	89255	1(3)	90621	1(2)	90746	1(2)	90993	1(3)	92310	0(3)	92568	1(2)
88120	2(3)	88309	3(3)	89257	1(3)	90625	1(2)	90747	1(2)	90997	1(3)	92311	1(2)	92570	1(2)
88121	2(3)	88311	4(3)	89258	1(2)	90630	1(2)	90748	0(3)	90999	1(3)	92312	1(2)	92571	1(2)
88125	1(3)	88312	9(3)	89259	1(2)	90632	1(2)	90749	1(3)	91010	1(2)	92313	1(3)	92572	1(2)
88130	1(2)	88313	8(3)	89260	1(2)	90633	1(2)	90750	1(2)	91013	1(3)	92314	0(3)	92575	1(2)
88140	1(2)	88314	6(3)	89261	1(2)	90634	1(2)	90756	1(2)	91020	1(2)	92315	1(2)	92576	1(2)
88141	1(3)	88319	11(3)	89264	1(3)	90636	1(2)	90785	3(3)	91022	1(2)	92316	1(2)	92577	1(2)
88142	1(3)	88321	1(2)	89268	1(2)	90644	1(2)	90791	1(3)	91030	1(2)	92317	1(3)	92579	1(2)
88143	1(3)	88323	1(2)	89272	1(2)	90647	1(2)	90792	2(3)	91034	1(2)	92325	1(3)	92582	1(2)
88147	1(3)	88325	1(2)	89280	1(2)	90648	1(2)	90832	3(3)	91035	1(2)	92326	2(2)	92583	1(2)
88148	1(3)	88329	2(3)	89281	1(2)	90649	1(2)	90833	3(3)	91037	1(2)	92340	0(3)	92584	1(2)
88150	1(3)	88331	11(3)	89290	1(2)	90650	1(2)	90834	3(3)	91038	1(2)	92341	0(3)	92585	1(2)
88152	1(3)	88332	13(3)	89291	1(2)	90651	1(2)	90836	3(3)	91040	1(2)	92342	0(3)	92586	1(2)
88153	1(3)	88333	4(3)	89300	1(2)	90653	1(2)	90837	3(3)	91065	2(2)	92352	1(3)	92587	1(2)
88155	1(3)	88334	5(3)	89310	1(2)	90654	1(2)	90838	3(3)	91110	1(2)	92353	1(3)	92588	1(2)
88160	4(3)	88341	13(3)	89320	1(2)	90655	1(2)	90839	1(2)	91111	1(2)	92354	1(3)	92590	0(3)
88161	4(3)	88342	4(3)	89321	1(2)	90656	1(2)	90840	4(3)	91112	1(3)	92355	1(3)	92591	0(3)
88162	3(3)	88344	6(3)	89322	1(2)	90657	1(2)	90845	1(2)	91117	1(2)	92358	1(3)	92592	0(3)
88164	1(3)	88346	2(3)	89325	1(2)	90658	1(2)	90846	2(3)	91120	1(2)	92370	0(3)	92593	0(3)
88165	1(3)	88348	1(3)	89329	1(2)	90660	1(2)	90847	2(3)	91122	1(2)	92371	1(3)	92594	0(3)
88166	1(3)	88350	8(3)	89330	1(2)	90661	1(2)	90849	2(3)	91132	1(3)	92499	1(3)	92595	0(3)
88167	1(3)	88355	1(3)	89331	1(2)	90662	1(2)	90853	4(3)	91133	1(3)	92502	1(3)	92596	1(2)
88172	7(3)	88356	3(3)	89335	1(3)	90664	1(2)	90863	1(3)	91200	1(2)	92504	1(3)	92597	1(3)
88173	7(3)	88358	2(3)	89337	1(2)	90666	1(2)	90865	1(3)	91299	1(3)	92507	1(3)	92601	1(3)
88174	1(3)	88360	6(3)	89342	1(2)	90667	1(2)	90867	1(2)	92002	1(2)	92508	1(3)	92602	1(3)
88175	1(3)	88361	6(3)	89343	1(2)	90668	1(2)	90868	1(3)	92004	1(2)	92511	1(3)	92603	1(3)
88177	6(3)	88362	1(3)	89344	1(2)	90670	1(2)	90869	1(3)	92012	1(3)	92512	1(2)	92604	1(3)
88182	2(3)	88363	2(3)	89346	1(2)	90672	1(2)	90870	2(3)	92014	1(3)	92516	1(3)	92605	1(2)
88184	2(3)	88364	3(3)	89352	1(2)	90673	1(2)	90875	1(3)	92015	0(3)	92520	1(2)	92606	1(2)
88185	35(3)	88365	4(3)	89353	1(3)	90674	1(2)	90876	0(3)	92018	1(2)	92521	1(2)	92607	1(3)
88187	2(3)	88366	2(3)	89354	1(3)	90675	1(2)	90880	1(3)	92019	1(2)	92522	1(2)	92608	4(3)
88188	2(3)	88367	3(3)	89356	2(3)	90676	1(2)	90882	0(3)	92020	1(2)	92523	1(2)	92609	1(3)
88189	2(3)	88368	3(3)	89398	1(3)	90680	1(2)	90885	1(3)	92025	1(2)	92524	1(2)	92610	1(2)
88199	1(3)	88369	3(3)	90281	0(3)	90681	1(2)	90887	1(3)	92060	1(2)	92526	1(2)	92611	1(3)
88230	2(3)	88371	1(3)	90283	0(3)	90682	1(2)	90889	1(3)	92065	1(2)	92531	1(3)	92612	1(3)
88233	2(3)	88372	1(3)	90284	0(3)	90685	1(2)	90899	1(3)	92071	2(2)	92532	1(3)	92613	1(2)
88235	2(3)	88373	3(3)	90287	0(3)	90686	1(2)	90901	1(3)	92072	1(2)	92533	4(2)	92614	1(3)
88237	4(3)	88374	5(3)	90288	0(3)	90687	1(2)	90912	1(2)	92081	1(2)	92534	1(3)	92615	1(2)
88239	3(3)	88375	1(3)	90291	0(3)	90688	1(2)	90913	3(3)	92082	1(2)	92537	1(2)	92616	1(3)
88240	3(3)	88377	5(3)	90296	1(2)	90689	1(2)	90935	1(3)	92083	1(2)	92538	1(2)	92617	1(2)
88241	3(3)	88380	1(3)	90371	10(3)	90690	1(2)	90937	1(3)	92100	1(2)	92540	1(3)	92618	1(3)
88245	1(2)	88381	1(3)	90375	20(3)	90691	1(2)	90940	1(3)	92132	1(2)	92541	1(3)	92620	1(2)
88248	1(2)	88387	2(3)	90376	20(3)	90694	1(2)	90945	1(3)	92133	1(2)	92542	1(3)	92621	4(3)
88249	1(2)	88388	1(3)	90378	4(3)	90696	1(2)	90947	1(3)	92134	1(2)	92544	1(3)	92625	1(2)
88261	2(3)	88399	1(3)	90384	0(3)	90697	1(2)	90951	1(2)	92136	1(3)	92545	1(3)	92626	1(2)
88262	2(3)	88720	1(3)	90385	1(2)	90698	1(2)	90952	1(2)	92145	1(2)	92546	1(3)	92627	6(3)

CPT	MUE
92630	0(3)
92633	0(3)
92640	1(3)
92700	1(3)
92920	3(3)
92921	6(2)
92924	2(3)
92925	6(2)
92928	3(3)
92929	6(2)
92933	2(3)
92934	6(2)
92937	2(3)
92938	6(3)
92941	1(3)
92943	2(3)
92944	3(3)
92950	2(3)
92953	2(3)
92960	2(3)
92961	1(3)
92970	1(3)
92971	1(3)
92973	2(3)
92974	1(3)
92975	1(3)
92977	1(3)
92978	1(3)
92979	2(3)
92986	1(2)
92987	1(2)
92990	1(2)
92992	1(2)
92993	1(2)
92997	1(2)
92998	2(3)
93000	3(3)
93005	5(3)
93010	5(3)
93015	1(3)
93016	1(3)
93017	1(3)
93018	1(3)
93024	1(3)
93025	1(2)
93040	3(3)
93041	3(3)
93042	3(3)
93050	1(3)
93224	1(2)
93225	1(2)
93226	1(2)
93227	1(2)
93228	1(2)
93229	1(2)
93260	1(2)
93261	1(3)
93264	1(2)
93268	1(2)
93270	1(2)
93271	1(2)
93272	1(2)
93278	1(3)
93279	1(3)
93280	1(3)

CPT	MUE
93281	1(3)
93282	1(3)
93283	1(3)
93284	1(3)
93285	1(3)
93286	2(3)
93287	2(3)
93288	1(3)
93289	1(3)
93290	1(3)
93291	1(3)
93292	1(3)
93293	1(2)
93294	1(2)
93295	1(2)
93296	1(2)
93297	1(2)
93298	1(2)
93303	1(3)
93304	1(3)
93306	1(3)
93307	1(3)
93308	1(3)
93312	1(3)
93313	1(3)
93314	1(3)
93315	1(3)
93316	1(3)
93317	1(3)
93318	1(3)
93320	2(3)
93321	1(3)
93325	2(3)
93350	1(2)
93351	1(2)
93352	1(3)
93355	1(3)
93356	1(3)
93451	1(3)
93452	1(3)
93453	1(3)
93454	1(3)
93455	1(3)
93456	1(3)
93457	1(3)
93458	1(3)
93459	1(3)
93460	1(3)
93461	1(3)
93462	1(3)
93463	1(3)
93464	1(3)
93503	2(3)
93505	1(2)
93530	1(3)
93531	1(3)
93532	1(3)
93533	1(3)
93561	1(3)
93562	1(3)
93563	1(3)
93564	1(3)
93565	1(3)
93566	1(3)
93567	1(3)

CPT	MUE
93568	1(3)
93571	1(3)
93572	2(3)
93580	1(3)
93581	1(3)
93582	1(2)
93583	1(2)
93590	1(2)
93591	1(2)
93592	2(3)
93600	1(3)
93602	1(3)
93603	1(3)
93609	1(3)
93610	1(3)
93612	1(3)
93613	1(3)
93615	1(3)
93616	1(3)
93618	1(3)
93619	1(3)
93620	1(3)
93621	1(3)
93622	1(3)
93623	1(3)
93624	1(3)
93631	1(3)
93640	1(3)
93641	1(2)
93642	1(3)
93644	1(3)
93650	1(2)
93653	1(3)
93654	1(3)
93655	2(3)
93656	1(3)
93657	2(3)
93660	1(3)
93662	1(3)
93668	1(3)
93701	1(2)
93702	1(2)
93724	1(3)
93740	1(3)
93745	1(2)
93750	1(3)
93770	1(3)
93784	1(2)
93786	1(2)
93788	1(2)
93790	1(2)
93792	1(2)
93793	1(2)
93797	2(2)
93798	2(2)
93799	1(3)
93880	1(3)
93882	1(3)
93886	1(3)
93888	1(3)
93890	1(3)
93892	1(3)
93893	1(3)
93895	1(3)
93922	2(2)

CPT	MUE
93923	2(2)
93924	1(2)
93925	1(3)
93926	1(3)
93930	1(3)
93931	1(3)
93970	1(3)
93971	1(3)
93975	1(3)
93976	1(3)
93978	1(3)
93979	1(3)
93980	1(3)
93981	1(3)
93985	1(3)
93986	1(3)
93990	2(3)
93998	1(3)
94002	1(2)
94003	1(2)
94004	1(2)
94005	1(3)
94010	1(3)
94011	1(3)
94012	1(3)
94013	1(3)
94014	1(2)
94015	1(2)
94016	1(2)
94060	1(3)
94070	1(2)
94150	2(3)
94200	1(3)
94250	1(3)
94375	1(3)
94400	1(3)
94450	1(3)
94452	1(2)
94453	1(2)
94610	2(3)
94617	1(3)
94618	1(3)
94621	1(3)
94640	1(3)
94642	1(3)
94644	1(2)
94645	4(3)
94660	1(2)
94662	1(2)
94664	1(3)
94667	1(2)
94668	5(3)
94669	4(3)
94680	1(3)
94681	1(3)
94690	1(3)
94726	1(3)
94727	1(3)
94728	1(3)
94729	1(3)
94750	1(3)
94760	1(3)
94761	1(2)
94762	1(2)
94770	1(3)

CPT	MUE
94772	1(2)
94774	1(2)
94775	1(2)
94776	1(2)
94777	1(2)
94780	1(2)
94781	2(3)
94799	1(3)
95004	80(3)
95012	2(3)
95017	27(3)
95018	19(3)
95024	40(3)
95027	90(3)
95028	30(3)
95044	80(3)
95052	20(3)
95056	1(2)
95060	1(2)
95065	1(3)
95070	1(3)
95071	1(2)
95076	1(2)
95079	2(3)
95115	1(2)
95117	1(2)
95120	0(3)
95125	0(3)
95130	0(3)
95131	0(3)
95132	0(3)
95133	0(3)
95134	0(3)
95144	30(3)
95145	10(3)
95146	10(3)
95147	10(3)
95148	10(3)
95149	10(3)
95165	30(3)
95170	10(3)
95180	8(3)
95199	1(3)
95249	1(2)
95250	1(2)
95251	1(2)
95700	1(2)
95705	1(2)
95706	1(2)
95707	1(2)
95708	4(3)
95709	4(3)
95710	4(3)
95711	1(2)
95712	1(2)
95713	1(2)
95714	4(3)
95715	4(3)
95716	4(3)
95717	1(2)
95718	1(2)
95719	1(2)
95720	1(2)
95721	1(2)
95722	1(2)

CPT	MUE
95723	1(2)
95724	1(2)
95725	1(2)
95726	1(2)
95782	1(2)
95783	1(2)
95800	1(2)
95801	1(2)
95803	1(2)
95805	1(2)
95806	1(2)
95807	1(2)
95808	1(2)
95810	1(2)
95811	1(2)
95812	1(3)
95813	1(3)
95816	1(3)
95819	1(3)
95822	1(3)
95824	1(3)
95829	1(3)
95830	1(3)
95836	1(2)
95851	3(3)
95852	1(3)
95857	1(2)
95860	1(3)
95861	1(3)
95863	1(3)
95864	1(3)
95865	1(3)
95866	1(3)
95867	1(3)
95868	1(3)
95869	1(3)
95870	4(3)
95872	4(3)
95873	1(2)
95874	1(2)
95875	2(3)
95885	4(2)
95886	4(2)
95887	1(2)
95905	2(3)
95907	1(2)
95908	1(2)
95909	1(2)
95910	1(2)
95911	1(2)
95912	1(2)
95913	1(2)
95921	1(3)
95922	1(3)
95923	1(3)
95924	1(3)
95925	1(3)
95926	1(3)
95927	1(3)
95928	1(3)
95929	1(3)
95930	1(3)
95933	1(3)
95937	4(3)
95938	1(3)

CPT	MUE
95939	1(3)
95940	20(3)
95941	8(3)
95943	1(3)
95954	1(3)
95955	1(3)
95957	1(3)
95958	1(3)
95961	1(2)
95962	3(3)
95965	1(3)
95966	1(3)
95967	3(3)
95970	1(3)
95971	1(3)
95972	1(3)
95976	1(3)
95977	1(3)
95980	1(3)
95981	1(3)
95982	1(3)
95983	1(2)
95984	11(3)
95990	1(3)
95991	1(3)
95992	1(2)
95999	1(3)
96000	1(2)
96001	1(2)
96002	1(3)
96003	1(3)
96004	1(2)
96020	1(2)
96040	4(3)
96105	3(3)
96110	3(3)
96112	1(2)
96113	6(3)
96116	1(2)
96121	3(3)
96125	2(3)
96127	2(3)
96130	1(2)
96131	7(3)
96132	1(2)
96133	7(3)
96136	1(2)
96137	11(3)
96138	1(2)
96139	11(3)
96146	1(2)
96156	1(3)
96158	1(2)
96159	4(3)
96160	3(3)
96161	1(3)
96164	1(2)
96165	6(3)
96167	1(2)
96168	6(3)
96170	1(3)
96171	1(3)
96360	2(3)
96361	24(3)
96365	2(3)

CPT	MUE
96366	24(3)
96367	4(3)
96368	1(2)
96369	1(2)
96370	3(3)
96371	1(3)
96372	5(3)
96373	3(3)
96374	1(3)
96375	6(3)
96376	10(3)
96377	1(3)
96379	2(3)
96401	4(3)
96402	2(3)
96405	1(2)
96406	1(2)
96409	1(3)
96411	3(3)
96413	1(3)
96415	8(3)
96416	1(3)
96417	3(3)
96420	2(3)
96422	2(3)
96423	2(3)
96425	1(3)
96440	1(3)
96446	1(3)
96450	1(3)
96521	2(3)
96522	1(3)
96523	2(3)
96542	1(3)
96549	1(3)
96567	1(3)
96570	1(2)
96571	2(3)
96573	1(2)
96574	1(2)
96900	1(3)
96902	1(3)
96904	1(2)
96910	1(3)
96912	1(3)
96913	1(3)
96920	1(2)
96921	1(2)
96922	1(2)
96931	1(2)
96932	1(2)
96933	1(2)
96934	2(3)
96935	2(3)
96936	2(3)
96999	1(3)
97010	1(3)
97012	1(3)
97014	0(3)
97016	1(3)
97018	1(3)
97022	1(3)
97024	1(3)
97026	1(3)
97028	1(3)

CPT	MUE
97032	4(3)
97033	4(3)
97034	2(3)
97035	2(3)
97036	3(3)
97039	1(3)
97110	8(3)
97112	6(3)
97113	6(3)
97116	4(3)
97124	4(3)
97129	1(2)
97130	7(3)
97139	1(3)
97140	6(3)
97150	2(3)
97151	8(3)
97152	8(3)
97153	32(3)
97154	12(3)
97155	24(3)
97156	16(3)
97157	16(3)
97158	16(3)
97161	1(2)
97162	1(2)
97163	1(2)
97164	1(2)
97165	1(2)
97166	1(2)
97167	1(2)
97168	1(2)
97169	0(3)
97170	0(3)
97171	0(3)
97172	0(3)
97530	6(3)
97533	4(3)
97535	8(3)
97537	8(3)
97542	8(3)
97545	1(2)
97546	2(3)
97597	1(3)
97598	8(3)
97602	1(3)
97605	1(3)
97606	1(3)
97607	1(3)
97608	1(3)
97610	1(2)
97750	8(3)
97755	8(3)
97760	6(3)
97761	6(3)
97763	6(3)
97799	1(3)
97802	8(3)
97803	8(3)
97804	6(3)
97810	1(2)
97811	2(3)
97813	1(2)
97814	2(3)
98925	1(2)

CPT	MUE
98926	1(2)
98927	1(2)
98928	1(2)
98929	1(2)
98940	1(2)
98941	1(2)
98942	1(2)
98943	0(3)
98960	0(3)
98961	0(3)
98962	0(3)
98966	1(2)
98967	1(2)
98968	1(2)
98970	1(2)
98971	1(2)
98972	1(2)
99000	0(3)
99001	0(3)
99002	1(3)
99024	1(3)
99026	0(3)
99027	0(3)
99050	1(3)
99051	1(3)
99053	1(3)
99056	1(3)
99058	1(3)
99060	1(3)
99070	1(3)
99071	1(3)
99075	0(3)
99078	3(3)
99080	1(3)
99082	1(3)
99091	1(2)
99100	1(3)
99116	1(3)
99135	1(3)
99140	2(3)
99151	1(3)
99152	2(3)
99153	12(3)
99155	1(3)
99156	1(3)
99157	6(3)
99170	1(3)
99172	0(3)
99173	0(3)
99174	0(3)
99175	1(3)
99177	1(2)
99183	1(3)
99184	1(2)
99188	1(2)
99190	1(3)
99191	1(3)
99192	1(3)
99195	2(3)
99199	1(3)
99201	1(2)
99202	1(2)
99203	1(2)
99204	1(2)
99205	1(2)

CPT	MUE
99211	2(3)
99212	2(3)
99213	2(3)
99214	2(3)
99215	2(3)
99217	1(2)
99218	1(2)
99219	1(2)
99220	1(2)
99221	0(3)
99222	0(3)
99223	0(3)
99224	1(2)
99225	1(2)
99226	1(2)
99231	0(3)
99232	0(3)
99233	0(3)
99234	1(3)
99235	1(3)
99236	1(3)
99238	0(3)
99239	0(3)
99241	0(3)
99242	0(3)
99243	0(3)
99244	0(3)
99245	0(3)
99251	0(3)
99252	0(3)
99253	0(3)
99254	0(3)
99255	0(3)
99281	2(3)
99282	2(3)
99283	2(3)
99284	2(3)
99285	2(3)
99288	1(3)
99291	1(2)
99292	8(3)
99304	1(2)
99305	1(2)
99306	1(2)
99307	1(2)
99308	1(2)
99309	1(2)
99310	1(2)
99315	1(2)
99316	1(2)
99318	1(2)
99324	1(2)
99325	1(2)
99326	1(2)
99327	1(2)
99328	1(2)
99334	1(3)
99335	1(3)
99336	1(3)
99337	1(3)
99339	1(2)
99340	1(2)
99341	1(2)
99342	1(2)
99343	1(2)

CPT	MUE
99344	1(2)
99345	1(2)
99347	1(3)
99348	1(3)
99349	1(3)
99350	1(3)
99354	1(2)
99355	4(3)
99356	1(2)
99357	1(3)
99358	1(2)
99359	1(3)
99360	1(3)
99366	2(3)
99367	1(3)
99368	2(3)
99374	1(2)
99375	0(3)
99377	1(2)
99378	0(3)
99379	1(2)
99380	1(2)
99381	0(3)
99382	0(3)
99383	0(3)
99384	0(3)
99385	0(3)
99386	0(3)
99387	0(3)
99391	0(3)
99392	0(3)
99393	0(3)
99394	0(3)
99395	0(3)
99396	0(3)
99397	0(3)
99401	0(3)
99402	0(3)
99403	0(3)
99404	0(3)
99406	1(2)
99407	1(2)
99408	0(3)
99409	0(3)
99411	0(3)
99412	0(3)
99415	1(2)
99416	3(3)
99421	1(2)
99422	1(2)
99423	1(2)
99429	0(3)
99441	1(2)
99442	1(2)
99443	1(2)
99446	1(2)
99447	1(2)
99448	1(2)
99449	1(2)
99450	0(3)
99451	1(2)
99452	1(2)
99453	1(2)
99454	1(2)
99455	1(3)

CPT	MUE
99456	1(3)
99457	1(2)
99458	3(3)
99460	1(2)
99461	1(2)
99462	1(2)
99463	1(2)
99464	1(2)
99465	1(2)
99466	1(2)
99467	4(3)
99468	1(2)
99469	1(2)
99471	1(2)
99472	1(2)
99473	1(2)
99474	1(2)
99475	1(2)
99476	1(2)
99477	1(2)
99478	1(2)
99479	1(2)
99480	1(2)
99483	1(2)
99484	1(2)
99485	1(3)
99486	4(1)
99487	1(2)
99489	4(3)
99490	1(2)
99491	1(2)
99492	1(2)
99493	1(2)
99494	2(3)
99495	1(2)
99496	1(2)
99497	1(2)
99498	3(3)
99499	1(3)
99500	0(3)
99501	0(3)
99502	0(3)
99503	0(3)
99504	0(3)
99505	0(3)
99506	0(3)
99507	0(3)
99509	0(3)
99510	0(3)
99511	0(3)
99512	0(3)
99600	0(3)
99601	0(3)
99602	0(3)
99605	0(2)
99606	0(3)
99607	0(3)
A0021	0(3)
A0080	0(3)
A0090	0(3)
A0100	0(3)
A0110	0(3)
A0120	0(3)
A0130	0(3)
A0140	0(3)

CPT	MUE
A0160	0(3)
A0170	0(3)
A0180	0(3)
A0190	0(3)
A0200	0(3)
A0210	0(3)
A0225	0(3)
A0380	0(3)
A0382	0(3)
A0384	0(3)
A0390	0(3)
A0392	0(3)
A0394	0(3)
A0396	0(3)
A0398	0(3)
A0420	0(3)
A0422	0(3)
A0424	0(3)
A0425	250(1)
A0426	2(3)
A0427	2(3)
A0428	2(3)
A0429	2(3)
A0430	1(3)
A0431	1(3)
A0432	1(3)
A0433	1(3)
A0434	2(3)
A0435	999(3)
A0436	300(3)
A0888	0(3)
A0998	0(3)
A0999	1(3)
A4206	1(3)
A4207	1(3)
A4208	4(3)
A4209	6(3)
A4210	0(3)
A4211	1(3)
A4212	2(3)
A4213	5(3)
A4215	9(3)
A4216	25(3)
A4217	4(3)
A4218	20(3)
A4220	1(3)
A4221	1(3)
A4222	2(3)
A4223	1(3)
A4224	1(2)
A4225	1(3)
A4226	0(3)
A4230	1(3)
A4231	1(3)
A4232	0(3)
A4233	0(3)
A4234	0(3)
A4235	1(3)
A4236	0(3)
A4244	1(3)
A4245	1(3)
A4246	1(3)
A4247	1(3)
A4248	10(3)
A4250	0(3)

CPT	MUE
A4252	0(3)
A4253	0(3)
A4255	0(3)
A4256	1(3)
A4257	0(3)
A4258	0(3)
A4259	0(3)
A4261	0(3)
A4262	4(2)
A4263	4(2)
A4264	0(3)
A4265	1(3)
A4266	0(3)
A4267	0(3)
A4268	0(3)
A4269	0(3)
A4270	3(3)
A4280	1(3)
A4281	0(3)
A4282	0(3)
A4283	0(3)
A4284	0(3)
A4285	0(3)
A4286	0(3)
A4290	2(3)
A4300	4(3)
A4301	1(2)
A4305	2(3)
A4306	2(3)
A4310	2(3)
A4311	2(3)
A4312	1(3)
A4313	1(3)
A4314	2(3)
A4315	2(3)
A4316	1(3)
A4320	2(3)
A4321	1(3)
A4322	2(3)
A4326	1(3)
A4327	2(3)
A4328	1(3)
A4330	1(3)
A4331	3(3)
A4332	2(3)
A4335	1(3)
A4336	1(3)
A4337	2(3)
A4338	3(3)
A4340	2(3)
A4344	2(3)
A4346	2(3)
A4351	2(3)
A4352	2(3)
A4353	3(3)
A4354	2(3)
A4355	2(3)
A4356	2(3)
A4357	2(3)
A4360	1(3)
A4361	1(3)
A4362	2(3)
A4363	0(3)
A4364	2(3)
A4366	1(3)

CPT	MUE
A4367	1(3)
A4368	1(3)
A4369	1(3)
A4371	1(3)
A4372	1(3)
A4373	1(3)
A4375	2(3)
A4376	2(3)
A4377	2(3)
A4378	2(3)
A4379	2(3)
A4380	2(3)
A4381	2(3)
A4382	2(3)
A4383	2(3)
A4384	2(3)
A4385	2(3)
A4387	1(3)
A4388	1(3)
A4389	2(3)
A4390	1(3)
A4391	1(3)
A4392	2(3)
A4393	1(3)
A4394	1(3)
A4395	3(3)
A4396	2(3)
A4397	1(3)
A4398	2(3)
A4399	1(3)
A4400	1(3)
A4402	1(3)
A4404	1(3)
A4405	1(3)
A4406	1(3)
A4407	2(3)
A4408	1(3)
A4409	1(3)
A4410	2(3)
A4411	1(3)
A4412	1(3)
A4413	2(3)
A4414	1(3)
A4415	1(3)
A4416	2(3)
A4417	2(3)
A4418	2(3)
A4419	2(3)
A4420	1(3)
A4423	2(3)
A4424	1(3)
A4425	1(3)
A4426	2(3)
A4427	1(3)
A4428	1(3)
A4429	2(3)
A4430	1(3)
A4431	1(3)
A4432	2(3)
A4433	1(3)
A4434	1(3)
A4435	2(3)
A4450	20(3)
A4452	4(3)
A4455	1(3)

CPT	MUE
A4458	1(3)
A4459	1(3)
A4461	2(3)
A4463	2(3)
A4465	1(3)
A4467	0(3)
A4470	1(3)
A4480	1(3)
A4481	2(3)
A4483	1(3)
A4490	0(3)
A4495	0(3)
A4500	0(3)
A4510	0(3)
A4520	0(3)
A4550	3(3)
A4553	0(3)
A4554	0(3)
A4555	0(3)
A4556	2(3)
A4557	2(3)
A4558	1(3)
A4559	1(3)
A4561	1(3)
A4562	1(3)
A4563	1(2)
A4565	2(3)
A4566	0(3)
A4570	0(3)
A4575	0(3)
A4580	0(3)
A4590	0(3)
A4595	2(3)
A4600	0(3)
A4601	0(3)
A4602	1(3)
A4604	1(3)
A4605	1(3)
A4606	1(3)
A4608	1(3)
A4611	0(3)
A4612	0(3)
A4613	0(3)
A4614	1(2)
A4615	2(3)
A4616	1(3)
A4617	1(3)
A4618	1(3)
A4619	1(3)
A4620	1(3)
A4623	10(3)
A4624	2(3)
A4625	30(3)
A4626	1(3)
A4627	0(3)
A4628	1(3)
A4629	1(3)
A4630	0(3)
A4633	0(3)
A4634	1(3)
A4635	0(3)
A4636	0(3)
A4637	0(3)
A4638	0(3)
A4639	0(3)

CPT	MUE
A4640	0(3)
A4642	1(3)
A4648	3(3)
A4650	3(3)
A4651	2(3)
A4652	2(3)
A4653	0(3)
A4657	0(3)
A4660	0(3)
A4663	0(3)
A4670	0(3)
A4671	0(3)
A4672	0(3)
A4673	0(3)
A4674	0(3)
A4680	0(3)
A4690	0(3)
A4706	0(3)
A4707	0(3)
A4708	0(3)
A4709	0(3)
A4714	0(3)
A4719	0(3)
A4720	0(3)
A4721	0(3)
A4722	0(3)
A4723	0(3)
A4724	0(3)
A4725	0(3)
A4726	0(3)
A4728	0(3)
A4730	0(3)
A4736	0(3)
A4737	0(3)
A4740	0(3)
A4750	0(3)
A4755	0(3)
A4760	0(3)
A4765	0(3)
A4766	0(3)
A4770	0(3)
A4771	0(3)
A4772	0(3)
A4773	0(3)
A4774	0(3)
A4802	0(3)
A4860	0(3)
A4870	0(3)
A4890	0(3)
A4911	0(3)
A4913	0(3)
A4918	0(3)
A4927	0(3)
A4928	0(3)
A4929	0(3)
A4930	0(3)
A4931	0(3)
A4932	0(3)
A5051	1(3)
A5052	1(3)
A5053	2(3)
A5054	1(3)
A5055	1(3)
A5056	90(3)
A5057	90(3)

CPT	MUE
A5061	2(3)
A5062	1(3)
A5063	1(3)
A5071	2(3)
A5072	1(3)
A5073	1(3)
A5081	2(3)
A5082	1(3)
A5083	5(3)
A5093	2(3)
A5102	1(3)
A5105	1(3)
A5112	2(3)
A5113	0(3)
A5114	0(3)
A5120	150(3)
A5121	1(3)
A5122	1(3)
A5126	2(3)
A5131	1(3)
A5200	2(3)
A5500	0(3)
A5501	0(3)
A5503	0(3)
A5504	0(3)
A5505	0(3)
A5506	0(3)
A5507	0(3)
A5508	0(3)
A5510	0(3)
A5512	0(3)
A5513	0(3)
A5514	0(3)
A6000	0(3)
A6010	3(3)
A6011	20(3)
A6024	1(3)
A6025	4(3)
A6154	1(3)
A6205	1(3)
A6221	9(3)
A6228	2(3)
A6230	1(3)
A6236	1(3)
A6238	3(3)
A6239	1(3)
A6240	2(3)
A6241	1(3)
A6244	1(3)
A6246	3(3)
A6247	2(3)
A6250	1(3)
A6256	3(3)
A6259	3(3)
A6261	3(3)
A6262	3(3)
A6404	2(3)
A6407	4(3)
A6410	2(3)
A6411	2(3)
A6412	2(3)
A6413	0(3)
A6441	8(3)
A6442	8(3)
A6443	8(3)

CPT	MUE
A6444	4(3)
A6445	8(3)
A6446	14(3)
A6447	6(3)
A6448	24(3)
A6449	12(3)
A6450	8(3)
A6451	8(3)
A6452	22(3)
A6453	6(3)
A6454	25(3)
A6455	4(3)
A6456	20(3)
A6457	12(3)
A6460	1(1)
A6461	1(1)
A6501	1(3)
A6502	1(3)
A6503	1(3)
A6504	2(3)
A6505	2(3)
A6506	2(3)
A6507	2(3)
A6508	2(3)
A6509	1(3)
A6510	1(3)
A6511	1(3)
A6513	1(3)
A6530	0(3)
A6531	2(3)
A6532	2(3)
A6533	0(3)
A6534	0(3)
A6535	0(3)
A6536	0(3)
A6537	0(3)
A6538	0(3)
A6539	0(3)
A6540	0(3)
A6541	0(3)
A6544	0(3)
A6545	2(3)
A6549	0(3)
A6550	1(3)
A7000	0(3)
A7001	0(3)
A7002	0(3)
A7003	0(3)
A7004	0(3)
A7005	0(3)
A7006	0(3)
A7007	0(3)
A7008	0(3)
A7009	0(3)
A7010	0(3)
A7012	0(3)
A7013	0(3)
A7014	0(3)
A7015	0(3)
A7016	0(3)
A7017	0(3)
A7018	0(3)
A7020	0(3)
A7025	0(3)
A7026	0(3)

CPT	MUE
A7027	0(3)
A7028	0(3)
A7029	0(3)
A7030	0(3)
A7031	0(3)
A7032	0(3)
A7033	0(3)
A7034	0(3)
A7035	0(3)
A7036	0(3)
A7037	0(3)
A7038	0(3)
A7039	0(3)
A7040	2(3)
A7041	2(3)
A7044	0(3)
A7045	0(3)
A7046	0(3)
A7047	1(3)
A7048	2(3)
A7501	1(3)
A7502	1(3)
A7503	1(3)
A7504	180(3)
A7505	1(3)
A7506	0(3)
A7507	200(3)
A7508	0(3)
A7509	0(3)
A7520	1(3)
A7521	1(3)
A7522	0(3)
A7523	0(3)
A7524	1(3)
A7525	0(3)
A7526	0(3)
A7527	1(3)
A8000	0(3)
A8001	0(3)
A8002	0(3)
A8003	0(3)
A8004	0(3)
A9152	0(3)
A9153	0(3)
A9155	1(3)
A9180	0(3)
A9270	0(3)
A9272	0(3)
A9273	0(3)
A9274	0(3)
A9275	0(3)
A9276	0(3)
A9277	0(3)
A9278	0(3)
A9279	0(3)
A9280	0(3)
A9281	0(3)
A9282	0(3)
A9283	0(3)
A9284	0(3)
A9285	0(3)
A9286	0(3)
A9300	0(3)
A9500	3(3)
A9501	1(3)

CPT	MUE
A9502	3(3)
A9503	1(3)
A9504	1(3)
A9505	4(3)
A9507	1(3)
A9508	2(3)
A9509	5(3)
A9510	1(3)
A9512	30(3)
A9513	200(3)
A9515	1(3)
A9516	4(3)
A9517	200(3)
A9520	1(3)
A9521	2(3)
A9524	10(3)
A9526	2(3)
A9527	195(3)
A9528	10(3)
A9529	10(3)
A9530	200(3)
A9531	100(3)
A9532	10(3)
A9536	1(3)
A9537	1(3)
A9538	1(3)
A9539	2(3)
A9540	2(3)
A9541	1(3)
A9542	1(3)
A9543	1(3)
A9546	1(3)
A9547	2(3)
A9548	2(3)
A9550	1(3)
A9551	1(3)
A9552	1(3)
A9553	1(3)
A9554	1(3)
A9555	2(3)
A9556	10(3)
A9557	2(3)
A9558	7(3)
A9559	1(3)
A9560	2(3)
A9561	1(3)
A9562	2(3)
A9563	10(3)
A9564	0(3)
A9566	1(3)
A9567	2(3)
A9568	0(3)
A9569	1(3)
A9570	1(3)
A9571	1(3)
A9572	1(3)
A9575	300(3)
A9576	100(3)
A9577	50(3)
A9578	50(3)
A9579	100(3)
A9580	1(3)
A9581	20(3)
A9582	1(3)
A9583	18(3)

CPT	MUE
A9584	1(3)
A9585	300(3)
A9586	1(3)
A9587	54(3)
A9588	10(3)
A9589	1(3)
A9590	675(3)
A9600	7(3)
A9604	1(3)
A9606	224(3)
A9698	3(3)
A9700	2(3)
A9900	0(3)
A9901	0(3)
A9999	0(3)
B4034	0(3)
B4035	0(3)
B4036	0(3)
B4081	0(3)
B4082	0(3)
B4083	0(3)
B4087	0(3)
B4088	0(3)
B4100	0(3)
B4102	0(3)
B4103	0(3)
B4104	0(3)
B4149	0(3)
B4150	0(3)
B4152	0(3)
B4153	0(3)
B4154	0(3)
B4155	0(3)
B4157	0(3)
B4158	0(3)
B4159	0(3)
B4160	0(3)
B4161	0(3)
B4162	0(3)
B4164	0(3)
B4168	0(3)
B4172	0(3)
B4176	0(3)
B4178	0(3)
B4180	0(3)
B4185	0(3)
B4189	0(3)
B4193	0(3)
B4197	0(3)
B4199	0(3)
B4216	0(3)
B4220	0(3)
B4222	0(3)
B4224	0(3)
B5000	0(3)
B5100	0(3)
B5200	0(3)
B9002	0(3)
B9004	0(3)
B9006	0(3)
B9998	0(3)
B9999	0(3)
C1713	20(3)
C1714	4(3)
C1715	45(3)

CPT	MUE
C1716	4(3)
C1717	10(3)
C1719	99(3)
C1721	1(3)
C1722	1(3)
C1724	5(3)
C1725	9(3)
C1726	5(3)
C1727	4(3)
C1728	5(3)
C1729	6(3)
C1730	4(3)
C1731	2(3)
C1732	3(3)
C1733	3(3)
C1734	2(3)
C1749	1(3)
C1750	2(3)
C1751	3(3)
C1752	2(3)
C1753	2(3)
C1754	2(3)
C1755	2(3)
C1756	2(3)
C1757	6(3)
C1758	2(3)
C1759	2(3)
C1760	4(3)
C1762	4(3)
C1763	4(3)
C1764	1(3)
C1765	4(3)
C1766	4(3)
C1767	2(3)
C1768	3(3)
C1769	9(3)
C1770	3(3)
C1771	1(3)
C1772	1(3)
C1773	3(3)
C1776	10(3)
C1777	2(3)
C1778	4(3)
C1779	2(3)
C1780	2(3)
C1781	4(3)
C1782	1(3)
C1783	2(3)
C1784	2(3)
C1785	1(3)
C1786	1(3)
C1787	2(3)
C1788	2(3)
C1789	2(3)
C1813	1(3)
C1814	2(3)
C1815	1(3)
C1816	2(3)
C1817	1(3)
C1818	2(3)
C1819	4(3)
C1820	2(3)
C1821	4(3)
C1822	1(3)
C1823	1(3)

CPT	MUE
C1824	1(2)
C1830	2(3)
C1839	2(2)
C1840	1(3)
C1841	1(2)
C1842	0(3)
C1874	5(3)
C1875	4(3)
C1876	5(3)
C1877	5(3)
C1878	2(3)
C1880	2(3)
C1881	2(3)
C1882	1(3)
C1883	4(3)
C1884	4(3)
C1885	2(3)
C1886	1(3)
C1887	7(3)
C1888	2(3)
C1889	2(3)
C1890	1(3)
C1891	1(3)
C1892	6(3)
C1893	6(3)
C1894	6(3)
C1895	2(3)
C1896	2(3)
C1897	2(3)
C1898	2(3)
C1899	2(3)
C1900	1(3)
C1982	1(3)
C2596	1(3)
C2613	2(3)
C2614	3(3)
C2615	2(3)
C2616	1(3)
C2617	4(3)
C2618	4(3)
C2619	1(3)
C2620	1(3)
C2621	1(3)
C2622	1(3)
C2623	4(3)
C2624	1(3)
C2625	4(3)
C2626	1(3)
C2627	2(3)
C2628	4(3)
C2629	4(3)
C2630	3(3)
C2631	1(3)
C2634	24(3)
C2635	124(3)
C2636	690(3)
C2637	0(3)
C2638	150(3)
C2639	150(3)
C2640	150(3)
C2641	150(3)
C2642	120(3)
C2643	120(3)
C2644	0(3)
C2645	4608(3)

CPT	MUE
C5271	1(2)
C5272	3(2)
C5273	1(2)
C5274	35(3)
C5275	1(2)
C5276	3(2)
C5277	1(2)
C5278	15(3)
C8900	1(3)
C8901	1(3)
C8902	1(3)
C8903	1(3)
C8905	1(3)
C8906	1(3)
C8908	1(3)
C8909	1(3)
C8910	1(3)
C8911	1(3)
C8912	1(3)
C8913	1(3)
C8914	1(3)
C8918	1(3)
C8919	1(3)
C8920	1(3)
C8921	1(3)
C8922	1(3)
C8923	1(3)
C8924	1(3)
C8925	1(3)
C8926	1(3)
C8927	1(3)
C8928	1(2)
C8929	1(3)
C8930	1(2)
C8931	1(3)
C8932	1(3)
C8933	1(3)
C8934	2(3)
C8935	2(3)
C8936	2(3)
C8937	2(2)
C8957	2(3)
C9046	160(3)
C9047	22(3)
C9055	400(3)
C9113	10(3)
C9132	5500(3)
C9248	25(3)
C9250	5(3)
C9254	400(3)
C9257	8000(3)
C9285	2(3)
C9290	266(3)
C9293	700(3)
C9352	3(3)
C9353	4(3)
C9354	300(3)
C9355	3(3)
C9356	125(3)
C9358	800(3)
C9359	30(3)
C9360	300(3)
C9361	10(3)
C9362	60(3)
C9363	500(3)

CPT	MUE
C9364	600(3)
C9460	100(3)
C9462	600(3)
C9482	300(3)
C9488	40(3)
C9600	3(3)
C9601	2(3)
C9602	2(3)
C9603	2(3)
C9604	2(3)
C9605	2(3)
C9606	1(3)
C9607	1(2)
C9608	2(3)
C9725	1(3)
C9726	2(3)
C9727	1(2)
C9728	1(2)
C9733	1(3)
C9734	1(3)
C9738	1(3)
C9739	1(2)
C9740	1(2)
C9745	1(2)
C9747	1(2)
C9749	1(2)
C9751	1(3)
C9752	1(2)
C9753	3(3)
C9756	1(3)
C9757	2(2)
C9758	1(2)
C9803	2(3)
C9898	1(3)
D0150	1(3)
D0240	1(3)
D0250	2(3)
D0270	1(3)
D0272	1(3)
D0274	1(3)
D0277	1(3)
D0412	0(3)
D0416	1(3)
D0431	1(3)
D0460	1(2)
D0484	1(2)
D0485	1(2)
D0601	0(3)
D0602	0(3)
D0603	0(3)
D1510	2(2)
D1516	1(2)
D1517	1(2)
D1520	2(2)
D1526	1(2)
D1527	1(2)
D1551	1(2)
D1552	1(2)
D1553	2(2)
D1575	4(2)
D1999	0(3)
D4260	4(2)
D4263	4(2)
D4264	3(3)
D4270	4(3)

CPT	MUE
D4273	1(2)
D4277	0(3)
D4278	0(3)
D4355	1(2)
D4381	12(3)
D5282	0(3)
D5283	0(3)
D5876	0(3)
D5911	1(3)
D5912	1(2)
D5951	0(3)
D5983	1(3)
D5984	1(3)
D5985	1(3)
D6052	0(3)
D7111	20(3)
D7140	32(2)
D7210	32(2)
D7220	6(3)
D7230	6(3)
D7240	6(3)
D7241	6(3)
D7250	32(2)
D7260	1(3)
D7261	1(3)
D7283	4(3)
D7288	2(3)
D7321	4(2)
D9110	1(3)
D9130	0(3)
D9230	1(3)
D9248	1(3)
D9613	0(3)
D9930	1(2)
D9944	2(2)
D9945	2(2)
D9946	2(2)
D9950	1(3)
D9951	1(3)
D9952	1(3)
D9961	0(3)
D9990	0(3)
E0100	0(3)
E0105	0(3)
E0110	0(3)
E0111	0(3)
E0112	0(3)
E0113	0(3)
E0114	0(3)
E0116	0(3)
E0117	0(3)
E0118	0(3)
E0130	0(3)
E0135	0(3)
E0140	0(3)
E0141	0(3)
E0143	0(3)
E0144	0(3)
E0147	0(3)
E0148	0(3)
E0149	0(3)
E0153	0(3)
E0154	0(3)
E0155	0(3)
E0156	0(3)

CPT	MUE
E0157	0(3)
E0158	0(3)
E0159	0(3)
E0160	0(3)
E0161	0(3)
E0162	0(3)
E0163	0(3)
E0165	0(3)
E0167	0(3)
E0168	0(3)
E0170	0(3)
E0171	0(3)
E0172	0(3)
E0175	0(3)
E0181	0(3)
E0182	0(3)
E0184	0(3)
E0185	0(3)
E0186	0(3)
E0187	0(3)
E0188	0(3)
E0189	0(3)
E0190	0(3)
E0191	0(3)
E0193	0(3)
E0194	0(3)
E0196	0(3)
E0197	0(3)
E0198	0(3)
E0199	0(3)
E0200	0(3)
E0202	0(3)
E0203	0(3)
E0205	0(3)
E0210	0(3)
E0215	0(3)
E0217	0(3)
E0218	0(3)
E0221	0(3)
E0225	0(3)
E0231	0(3)
E0232	0(3)
E0235	0(3)
E0236	0(3)
E0239	0(3)
E0240	0(3)
E0241	0(3)
E0242	0(3)
E0243	0(3)
E0244	0(3)
E0245	0(3)
E0246	0(3)
E0247	0(3)
E0248	0(3)
E0249	0(3)
E0250	0(3)
E0251	0(3)
E0255	0(3)
E0256	0(3)
E0260	0(3)
E0261	0(3)
E0265	0(3)
E0266	0(3)
E0270	0(3)
E0271	0(3)

CPT	MUE
E0272	0(3)
E0273	0(3)
E0274	0(3)
E0275	0(3)
E0276	0(3)
E0277	0(3)
E0280	0(3)
E0290	0(3)
E0291	0(3)
E0292	0(3)
E0293	0(3)
E0294	0(3)
E0295	0(3)
E0296	0(3)
E0297	0(3)
E0300	0(3)
E0301	0(3)
E0302	0(3)
E0303	0(3)
E0304	0(3)
E0305	0(3)
E0310	0(3)
E0315	0(3)
E0316	0(3)
E0325	0(3)
E0326	0(3)
E0328	0(3)
E0329	0(3)
E0350	0(3)
E0352	0(3)
E0370	0(3)
E0371	0(3)
E0372	0(3)
E0373	0(3)
E0424	0(3)
E0425	0(3)
E0430	0(3)
E0431	0(3)
E0433	0(3)
E0434	0(3)
E0435	0(3)
E0439	0(3)
E0440	0(3)
E0441	0(3)
E0442	0(3)
E0443	0(3)
E0444	0(3)
E0445	0(3)
E0446	0(3)
E0447	0(3)
E0455	0(3)
E0457	0(3)
E0459	0(3)
E0462	0(3)
E0465	0(3)
E0466	0(3)
E0467	0(3)
E0470	0(3)
E0471	0(3)
E0472	0(3)
E0480	0(3)
E0481	0(3)
E0482	0(3)
E0483	0(3)
E0484	0(3)

CPT	MUE
E0485	0(3)
E0486	0(3)
E0487	0(3)
E0500	0(3)
E0550	0(3)
E0555	0(3)
E0560	0(3)
E0561	0(3)
E0562	0(3)
E0565	0(3)
E0570	0(3)
E0572	0(3)
E0574	0(3)
E0575	0(3)
E0580	0(3)
E0585	0(3)
E0600	0(3)
E0601	0(3)
E0602	0(3)
E0603	0(3)
E0604	0(3)
E0605	0(3)
E0606	0(3)
E0607	0(3)
E0610	0(3)
E0615	0(3)
E0616	1(2)
E0617	0(3)
E0618	0(3)
E0619	0(3)
E0620	0(3)
E0621	0(3)
E0625	0(3)
E0627	0(3)
E0629	0(3)
E0630	0(3)
E0635	0(3)
E0636	0(3)
E0637	0(3)
E0638	0(3)
E0639	0(3)
E0640	0(3)
E0641	0(3)
E0642	0(3)
E0650	0(3)
E0651	0(3)
E0652	0(3)
E0655	0(3)
E0656	0(3)
E0657	0(3)
E0660	0(3)
E0665	0(3)
E0666	0(3)
E0667	0(3)
E0668	0(3)
E0669	0(3)
E0670	0(3)
E0671	0(3)
E0672	0(3)
E0673	0(3)
E0675	0(3)
E0676	1(3)
E0691	0(3)
E0692	0(3)
E0693	0(3)

CPT	MUE
E0694	0(3)
E0700	0(3)
E0705	1(2)
E0710	0(3)
E0720	0(3)
E0730	0(3)
E0731	0(3)
E0740	0(3)
E0744	0(3)
E0745	0(3)
E0746	1(3)
E0747	0(3)
E0748	0(3)
E0749	1(3)
E0755	0(3)
E0760	0(3)
E0761	0(3)
E0762	1(3)
E0764	0(3)
E0765	0(3)
E0766	0(3)
E0769	0(3)
E0770	1(3)
E0776	0(3)
E0779	0(3)
E0780	0(3)
E0781	0(3)
E0782	1(2)
E0783	1(2)
E0784	0(3)
E0785	1(2)
E0786	1(2)
E0787	0(3)
E0791	0(3)
E0830	0(3)
E0840	0(3)
E0849	0(3)
E0850	0(3)
E0855	0(3)
E0856	0(3)
E0860	0(3)
E0870	0(3)
E0880	0(3)
E0890	0(3)
E0900	0(3)
E0910	0(3)
E0911	0(3)
E0912	0(3)
E0920	0(3)
E0930	0(3)
E0935	0(3)
E0936	0(3)
E0940	0(3)
E0941	0(3)
E0942	0(3)
E0944	0(3)
E0945	0(3)
E0946	0(3)
E0947	0(3)
E0948	0(3)
E0950	0(3)
E0951	0(3)
E0952	0(3)
E0953	0(3)
E0954	0(3)

CPT	MUE	CPT	MUE	CPT	MUE	CPT	MUE	CPT	MUE	CPT	MUE	CPT	MUE	CPT	MUE
E0955	0(3)	E1092	0(3)	E1520	0(3)	E2216	0(3)	E2384	0(3)	G0070	16(3)	G0268	1(2)	G0425	1(3)
E0956	0(3)	E1093	0(3)	E1530	0(3)	E2217	0(3)	E2385	0(3)	G0071	1(3)	G0269	2(3)	G0426	1(3)
E0957	0(3)	E1100	0(3)	E1540	0(3)	E2218	0(3)	E2386	0(3)	G0076	1(3)	G0270	8(3)	G0427	1(3)
E0958	0(3)	E1110	0(3)	E1550	0(3)	E2219	0(3)	E2387	0(3)	G0077	1(3)	G0271	4(3)	G0428	0(3)
E0959	2(2)	E1130	0(3)	E1560	0(3)	E2220	0(3)	E2388	0(3)	G0078	1(3)	G0276	1(3)	G0429	1(2)
E0960	0(3)	E1140	0(3)	E1570	0(3)	E2221	0(3)	E2389	0(3)	G0079	1(3)	G0277	5(3)	G0432	1(2)
E0961	2(2)	E1150	0(3)	E1575	0(3)	E2222	0(3)	E2390	0(3)	G0080	1(3)	G0278	1(2)	G0433	1(2)
E0966	1(2)	E1160	0(3)	E1580	0(3)	E2224	0(3)	E2391	0(3)	G0081	1(3)	G0279	1(2)	G0435	1(2)
E0967	0(3)	E1161	0(3)	E1590	0(3)	E2225	0(3)	E2392	0(3)	G0082	1(3)	G0281	1(3)	G0438	1(2)
E0968	0(3)	E1170	0(3)	E1592	0(3)	E2226	0(3)	E2394	0(3)	G0083	1(3)	G0282	0(3)	G0439	1(2)
E0969	0(3)	E1171	0(3)	E1594	0(3)	E2227	0(3)	E2395	0(3)	G0084	1(3)	G0283	1(3)	G0442	1(2)
E0970	0(3)	E1172	0(3)	E1600	0(3)	E2228	0(3)	E2396	0(3)	G0085	1(3)	G0288	1(2)	G0443	1(2)
E0971	2(3)	E1180	0(3)	E1610	0(3)	E2230	0(3)	E2397	0(3)	G0086	1(3)	G0289	1(2)	G0444	1(2)
E0973	2(2)	E1190	0(3)	E1615	0(3)	E2231	0(3)	E2398	0(3)	G0087	1(3)	G0293	1(2)	G0445	1(2)
E0974	2(2)	E1195	0(3)	E1620	0(3)	E2291	1(2)	E2402	0(3)	G0101	1(2)	G0294	1(2)	G0446	1(3)
E0978	1(3)	E1200	0(3)	E1625	0(3)	E2292	1(2)	E2500	0(3)	G0102	1(2)	G0295	0(3)	G0447	4(3)
E0980	0(3)	E1220	0(3)	E1630	0(3)	E2293	1(2)	E2502	0(3)	G0103	1(2)	G0296	1(2)	G0448	1(3)
E0981	0(3)	E1221	0(3)	E1632	0(3)	E2294	1(2)	E2504	0(3)	G0104	1(2)	G0297	1(2)	G0451	1(3)
E0982	0(3)	E1222	0(3)	E1634	0(3)	E2295	0(3)	E2506	0(3)	G0105	1(2)	G0302	1(2)	G0452	1(3)
E0983	0(3)	E1223	0(3)	E1635	0(3)	E2300	0(3)	E2508	0(3)	G0106	1(2)	G0303	1(2)	G0453	10(3)
E0984	0(3)	E1224	0(3)	E1636	0(3)	E2301	0(3)	E2510	0(3)	G0108	8(3)	G0304	1(2)	G0454	1(2)
E0985	0(3)	E1225	0(3)	E1637	0(3)	E2310	0(3)	E2511	0(3)	G0109	12(3)	G0305	1(2)	G0455	1(2)
E0986	0(3)	E1226	1(2)	E1639	0(3)	E2311	0(3)	E2512	0(3)	G0117	1(2)	G0306	4(3)	G0458	1(3)
E0988	0(3)	E1227	0(3)	E1699	1(3)	E2312	0(3)	E2599	0(3)	G0118	1(2)	G0307	4(3)	G0459	1(3)
E0990	2(2)	E1228	0(3)	E1700	0(3)	E2313	0(3)	E2601	0(3)	G0120	1(2)	G0328	1(2)	G0460	1(3)
E0992	1(2)	E1229	0(3)	E1701	0(3)	E2321	0(3)	E2602	0(3)	G0121	1(2)	G0329	1(3)	G0463	4(3)
E0994	0(3)	E1230	0(3)	E1702	0(3)	E2322	0(3)	E2603	0(3)	G0122	0(3)	G0333	0(3)	G0466	1(2)
E0995	2(2)	E1231	0(3)	E1800	0(3)	E2323	0(3)	E2604	0(3)	G0123	1(3)	G0337	1(2)	G0467	1(3)
E1002	0(3)	E1232	0(3)	E1801	0(3)	E2324	0(3)	E2605	0(3)	G0124	1(3)	G0339	1(2)	G0468	1(2)
E1003	0(3)	E1233	0(3)	E1802	0(3)	E2325	0(3)	E2606	0(3)	G0127	1(2)	G0340	1(3)	G0469	1(2)
E1004	0(3)	E1234	0(3)	E1805	0(3)	E2326	0(3)	E2607	0(3)	G0128	1(3)	G0341	1(2)	G0470	1(3)
E1005	0(3)	E1235	0(3)	E1806	0(3)	E2327	0(3)	E2608	0(3)	G0129	6(3)	G0342	1(2)	G0471	2(3)
E1006	0(3)	E1236	0(3)	E1810	0(3)	E2328	0(3)	E2609	0(3)	G0130	1(2)	G0343	1(2)	G0472	1(2)
E1007	0(3)	E1237	0(3)	E1811	0(3)	E2329	0(3)	E2610	1(3)	G0141	1(3)	G0372	1(2)	G0473	1(3)
E1008	0(3)	E1238	0(3)	E1812	0(3)	E2330	0(3)	E2611	0(3)	G0143	1(3)	G0379	1(2)	G0475	1(2)
E1009	0(3)	E1239	0(3)	E1815	0(3)	E2331	0(3)	E2612	0(3)	G0144	1(3)	G0380	2(3)	G0476	1(2)
E1010	0(3)	E1240	0(3)	E1816	0(3)	E2340	0(3)	E2613	0(3)	G0145	1(3)	G0381	2(3)	G0480	1(2)
E1011	0(3)	E1250	0(3)	E1818	0(3)	E2341	0(3)	E2614	0(3)	G0147	1(3)	G0382	2(3)	G0481	1(2)
E1012	0(3)	E1260	0(3)	E1820	0(3)	E2342	0(3)	E2615	0(3)	G0148	1(3)	G0383	2(3)	G0482	1(2)
E1014	0(3)	E1270	0(3)	E1821	0(3)	E2343	0(3)	E2616	0(3)	G0166	2(3)	G0384	2(3)	G0483	1(2)
E1015	0(3)	E1280	0(3)	E1825	0(3)	E2351	0(3)	E2617	0(3)	G0168	2(3)	G0390	1(2)	G0490	1(3)
E1016	0(3)	E1285	0(3)	E1830	0(3)	E2358	0(3)	E2619	0(3)	G0175	1(3)	G0396	1(2)	G0491	1(3)
E1017	0(3)	E1290	0(3)	E1831	0(3)	E2359	0(3)	E2620	0(3)	G0176	5(3)	G0397	1(2)	G0492	1(3)
E1018	0(3)	E1295	0(3)	E1840	0(3)	E2360	0(3)	E2621	0(3)	G0177	5(3)	G0398	1(2)	G0493	1(3)
E1020	0(3)	E1296	0(3)	E1841	0(3)	E2361	0(3)	E2622	0(3)	G0179	1(2)	G0399	1(2)	G0494	1(3)
E1028	0(3)	E1297	0(3)	E1902	0(3)	E2362	0(3)	E2623	0(3)	G0180	1(2)	G0400	1(2)	G0495	1(3)
E1029	0(3)	E1298	0(3)	E2000	0(3)	E2363	0(3)	E2624	0(3)	G0181	1(2)	G0402	1(2)	G0496	1(3)
E1030	0(3)	E1300	0(3)	E2100	0(3)	E2364	0(3)	E2625	0(3)	G0182	1(2)	G0403	1(2)	G0498	1(2)
E1031	0(3)	E1310	0(3)	E2101	0(3)	E2365	0(3)	E2626	0(3)	G0186	1(2)	G0404	1(2)	G0499	1(2)
E1035	0(3)	E1352	0(3)	E2120	0(3)	E2366	0(3)	E2627	0(3)	G0219	0(3)	G0405	1(2)	G0500	1(3)
E1036	0(3)	E1353	0(3)	E2201	0(3)	E2367	0(3)	E2628	0(3)	G0235	1(3)	G0406	1(3)	G0501	1(3)
E1037	0(3)	E1354	0(3)	E2202	0(3)	E2368	0(3)	E2629	0(3)	G0237	8(3)	G0407	1(3)	G0506	1(2)
E1038	0(3)	E1355	0(3)	E2203	0(3)	E2369	0(3)	E2630	0(3)	G0238	8(3)	G0408	1(3)	G0508	1(2)
E1039	0(3)	E1356	0(3)	E2204	0(3)	E2370	0(3)	E2631	0(3)	G0239	2(3)	G0410	6(3)	G0509	1(2)
E1050	0(3)	E1357	0(3)	E2205	0(3)	E2371	0(3)	E2632	0(3)	G0245	1(2)	G0411	6(3)	G0511	1(2)
E1060	0(3)	E1358	0(3)	E2206	0(3)	E2372	0(3)	E2633	0(3)	G0246	1(2)	G0412	1(2)	G0512	1(2)
E1070	0(3)	E1372	0(3)	E2207	0(3)	E2373	0(3)	E8000	0(3)	G0247	1(2)	G0413	1(2)	G0513	1(2)
E1083	0(3)	E1390	0(3)	E2208	0(3)	E2374	0(3)	E8001	0(3)	G0248	1(2)	G0414	1(2)	G0514	1(1)
E1084	0(3)	E1391	0(3)	E2209	0(3)	E2375	0(3)	E8002	0(3)	G0249	3(3)	G0415	1(2)	G0516	1(2)
E1085	0(3)	E1392	0(3)	E2210	0(3)	E2376	0(3)	G0008	1(2)	G0250	1(2)	G0416	1(2)	G0517	1(2)
E1086	0(3)	E1399	0(3)	E2211	0(3)	E2377	0(3)	G0009	1(2)	G0252	0(3)	G0420	2(3)	G0518	1(2)
E1087	0(3)	E1405	0(3)	E2212	0(3)	E2378	0(3)	G0010	1(3)	G0255	0(3)	G0421	2(3)	G0659	1(2)
E1088	0(3)	E1406	0(3)	E2213	0(3)	E2381	0(3)	G0027	1(2)	G0257	1(3)	G0422	6(2)	G2000	1(3)
E1089	0(3)	E1500	0(3)	E2214	0(3)	E2382	0(3)	G0068	16(3)	G0259	2(3)	G0423	6(2)	G2001	1(3)
E1090	0(3)	E1510	0(3)	E2215	0(3)	E2383	0(3)	G0069	16(3)	G0260	2(3)	G0424	2(2)	G2002	1(3)

CPT	MUE	CPT	MUE	CPT	MUE	CPT	MUE	CPT	MUE	CPT	MUE	CPT	MUE	CPT	MUE
G2003	1(3)	G9157	1(2)	J0300	8(3)	J0696	16(3)	J1230	5(3)	J1627	100(3)	J2185	60(3)	J2725	0(3)
G2004	1(3)	G9187	0(3)	J0330	50(3)	J0697	12(3)	J1240	6(3)	J1628	100(3)	J2186	600(3)	J2730	2(3)
G2005	1(3)	G9480	1(3)	J0348	200(3)	J0698	12(3)	J1245	6(3)	J1630	7(3)	J2210	5(3)	J2760	2(3)
G2006	1(3)	G9481	2(3)	J0350	0(3)	J0702	20(3)	J1250	4(3)	J1631	9(3)	J2212	240(3)	J2765	18(3)
G2007	1(3)	G9482	2(3)	J0360	6(3)	J0706	16(3)	J1260	2(3)	J1640	672(3)	J2248	300(3)	J2770	7(3)
G2008	1(3)	G9483	2(3)	J0364	6(3)	J0710	0(3)	J1265	100(3)	J1642	150(3)	J2250	30(3)	J2778	10(2)
G2009	1(3)	G9484	2(3)	J0365	0(3)	J0712	180(3)	J1267	150(3)	J1644	50(3)	J2260	16(3)	J2780	16(3)
G2010	1(3)	G9485	2(3)	J0380	1(3)	J0713	12(3)	J1270	16(3)	J1645	10(3)	J2265	400(3)	J2783	60(3)
G2011	1(2)	G9486	2(3)	J0390	0(3)	J0714	12(3)	J1290	60(3)	J1650	30(3)	J2270	15(3)	J2785	4(3)
G2012	1(3)	G9487	2(3)	J0395	0(3)	J0715	0(3)	J1300	120(3)	J1652	20(3)	J2274	100(3)	J2786	500(3)
G2013	1(3)	G9488	2(3)	J0400	120(3)	J0716	4(1)	J1301	60(3)	J1655	0(3)	J2278	1000(3)	J2787	2(3)
G2014	1(3)	G9489	2(3)	J0401	400(3)	J0717	400(3)	J1303	360(3)	J1670	2(3)	J2280	8(3)	J2788	1(3)
G2015	1(3)	G9490	2(3)	J0456	4(3)	J0720	15(3)	J1320	0(3)	J1675	0(3)	J2300	10(3)	J2790	3(3)
G2023	2(3)	G9678	1(2)	J0461	800(3)	J0725	10(3)	J1322	150(3)	J1700	0(3)	J2310	10(3)	J2791	15(3)
G2024	2(3)	G9685	1(3)	J0470	2(3)	J0735	50(3)	J1324	0(3)	J1710	0(3)	J2315	380(3)	J2792	450(3)
G2058	2(3)	G9978	2(3)	J0475	8(3)	J0740	2(3)	J1325	18(3)	J1720	10(3)	J2320	4(3)	J2793	320(3)
G2061	1(2)	G9979	2(3)	J0476	2(3)	J0743	16(3)	J1327	99(3)	J1726	28(3)	J2323	300(3)	J2794	100(3)
G2062	1(2)	G9980	2(3)	J0480	1(3)	J0744	8(3)	J1330	0(3)	J1729	25(3)	J2325	34(3)	J2795	2400(3)
G2063	1(2)	G9981	2(3)	J0485	1500(3)	J0745	8(3)	J1335	2(3)	J1730	0(3)	J2326	120(3)	J2796	150(3)
G2064	1(2)	G9982	2(3)	J0490	160(3)	J0770	5(3)	J1364	8(3)	J1740	3(3)	J2350	600(3)	J2797	333(3)
G2065	1(2)	G9983	2(3)	J0500	4(3)	J0775	180(3)	J1380	4(3)	J1741	32(3)	J2353	60(3)	J2798	240(3)
G2066	1(2)	G9984	2(3)	J0515	6(3)	J0780	10(3)	J1410	4(3)	J1742	4(3)	J2354	60(3)	J2800	3(3)
G2067	1(2)	G9985	2(3)	J0517	30(3)	J0795	100(3)	J1428	450(3)	J1743	66(3)	J2355	2(3)	J2805	3(3)
G2068	1(2)	G9986	2(3)	J0520	0(3)	J0800	3(3)	J1430	10(3)	J1744	90(3)	J2357	90(3)	J2810	20(3)
G2069	1(2)	G9987	2(3)	J0558	24(3)	J0834	3(3)	J1435	0(3)	J1745	150(3)	J2358	405(3)	J2820	10(3)
G2070	1(2)	J0120	1(3)	J0561	24(3)	J0840	18(3)	J1436	0(3)	J1746	200(3)	J2360	3(3)	J2840	160(3)
G2071	1(2)	J0121	200(3)	J0565	200(3)	J0841	24(3)	J1438	2(3)	J1750	45(3)	J2370	30(3)	J2850	48(3)
G2072	1(2)	J0122	300(3)	J0567	300(3)	J0850	9(3)	J1439	750(3)	J1756	500(3)	J2400	4(3)	J2860	170(3)
G2073	1(2)	J0129	100(3)	J0570	4(3)	J0875	300(3)	J1442	1500(3)	J1786	680(3)	J2405	64(3)	J2910	0(3)
G2074	1(2)	J0130	6(3)	J0571	0(3)	J0878	1500(3)	J1443	0(3)	J1790	2(3)	J2407	120(3)	J2916	20(3)
G2075	1(2)	J0131	400(3)	J0572	0(3)	J0881	500(3)	J1444	272(3)	J1800	12(3)	J2410	2(3)	J2920	25(3)
G2076	1(2)	J0132	300(3)	J0573	0(3)	J0882	300(3)	J1447	960(3)	J1810	0(3)	J2425	125(3)	J2930	25(3)
G2078	3(3)	J0133	1200(3)	J0574	0(3)	J0883	1250(3)	J1450	4(3)	J1815	200(3)	J2426	819(3)	J2940	0(3)
G2079	3(3)	J0135	8(3)	J0575	0(3)	J0884	1250(3)	J1451	200(3)	J1817	0(3)	J2430	3(3)	J2941	8(3)
G2081	1(2)	J0153	180(3)	J0583	1250(3)	J0885	60(3)	J1452	0(3)	J1826	1(3)	J2440	4(3)	J2950	0(3)
G2082	1(2)	J0171	120(3)	J0584	90(3)	J0887	360(3)	J1453	150(3)	J1830	1(3)	J2460	0(3)	J2993	2(3)
G2083	1(2)	J0178	4(2)	J0585	600(3)	J0888	360(3)	J1454	1(3)	J1833	1116(3)	J2469	10(3)	J2995	0(3)
G2086	1(3)	J0179	12(2)	J0586	300(3)	J0890	0(3)	J1455	18(3)	J1835	0(3)	J2501	25(3)	J2997	100(3)
G2087	2(3)	J0180	140(3)	J0587	300(3)	J0894	100(3)	J1457	0(3)	J1840	3(3)	J2502	60(3)	J3000	2(3)
G6001	2(3)	J0185	130(3)	J0588	600(3)	J0895	12(3)	J1458	100(3)	J1850	14(3)	J2503	2(3)	J3010	100(3)
G6002	2(3)	J0190	0(3)	J0592	12(3)	J0897	120(3)	J1459	300(3)	J1885	8(3)	J2504	15(3)	J3030	2(3)
G6003	2(3)	J0200	0(3)	J0593	300(3)	J0945	4(3)	J1460	10(2)	J1890	0(3)	J2505	1(3)	J3031	675(3)
G6004	2(3)	J0202	12(3)	J0594	320(3)	J1000	1(3)	J1555	480(3)	J1930	120(3)	J2507	8(3)	J3060	760(3)
G6005	2(3)	J0205	0(3)	J0595	12(3)	J1020	8(3)	J1556	300(3)	J1931	609(3)	J2510	4(3)	J3070	3(3)
G6006	2(3)	J0207	4(3)	J0596	840(3)	J1030	8(3)	J1557	300(3)	J1940	10(3)	J2513	1(3)	J3090	200(3)
G6007	2(3)	J0210	16(3)	J0597	250(3)	J1040	4(3)	J1559	300(3)	J1943	675(3)	J2515	8(3)	J3095	150(3)
G6008	2(3)	J0215	0(3)	J0598	100(3)	J1050	1000(3)	J1560	1(2)	J1944	1064(3)	J2540	75(3)	J3101	50(3)
G6009	2(3)	J0220	20(3)	J0599	900(3)	J1071	400(3)	J1561	300(3)	J1945	0(3)	J2543	20(3)	J3105	4(3)
G6010	2(3)	J0221	300(3)	J0600	3(3)	J1094	0(3)	J1562	0(3)	J1950	12(3)	J2545	1(3)	J3110	2(3)
G6011	2(3)	J0222	300(3)	J0606	150(3)	J1095	1034(2)	J1566	300(3)	J1953	300(3)	J2547	600(3)	J3111	210(3)
G6012	2(3)	J0223	756(3)	J0610	15(3)	J1096	4(3)	J1568	300(3)	J1955	11(3)	J2550	3(3)	J3121	400(3)
G6013	2(3)	J0256	1600(3)	J0620	1(3)	J1097	4(3)	J1569	300(3)	J1956	4(3)	J2560	16(3)	J3145	750(3)
G6014	2(3)	J0257	1400(3)	J0630	8(3)	J1100	120(3)	J1570	4(3)	J1960	0(3)	J2562	48(3)	J3230	6(3)
G6015	2(3)	J0270	32(3)	J0636	100(3)	J1110	3(3)	J1571	20(3)	J1980	8(3)	J2590	15(3)	J3240	1(3)
G6016	2(3)	J0275	1(3)	J0637	20(3)	J1120	2(3)	J1572	300(3)	J1990	0(3)	J2597	45(3)	J3243	200(3)
G6017	2(3)	J0278	15(3)	J0638	300(3)	J1130	300(3)	J1573	130(3)	J2001	400(3)	J2650	0(3)	J3245	100(3)
G9143	1(2)	J0280	10(3)	J0640	24(3)	J1160	3(3)	J1575	650(3)	J2010	10(3)	J2670	0(3)	J3246	100(3)
G9147	0(3)	J0282	70(3)	J0641	1200(3)	J1162	10(3)	J1580	9(3)	J2020	6(3)	J2675	1(3)	J3250	4(3)
G9148	0(3)	J0285	5(3)	J0642	1200(3)	J1165	50(3)	J1595	2(3)	J2060	10(3)	J2680	4(3)	J3260	12(3)
G9149	0(3)	J0287	60(3)	J0670	10(3)	J1170	50(3)	J1599	300(3)	J2062	10(3)	J2690	4(3)	J3262	800(3)
G9150	0(3)	J0288	0(3)	J0690	16(3)	J1180	0(3)	J1600	0(3)	J2150	8(3)	J2700	48(3)	J3265	0(3)
G9151	0(3)	J0289	115(3)	J0691	300(3)	J1190	8(3)	J1602	300(3)	J2170	8(3)	J2704	400(3)	J3280	0(3)
G9152	0(3)	J0290	24(3)	J0692	12(3)	J1200	8(3)	J1610	3(3)	J2175	6(3)	J2710	10(3)	J3285	9(3)
G9153	0(3)	J0291	500(3)	J0694	12(3)	J1205	4(3)	J1620	0(3)	J2180	0(3)	J2720	10(3)	J3300	160(3)
G9156	1(2)	J0295	12(3)	J0695	60(3)	J1212	1(3)	J1626	30(3)	J2182	300(3)	J2724	3500(3)	J3301	16(3)

CPT	MUE
J3302	0(3)
J3303	24(3)
J3304	64(2)
J3305	0(3)
J3310	0(3)
J3315	6(3)
J3316	6(3)
J3320	0(3)
J3350	0(3)
J3355	0(3)
J3357	90(3)
J3358	520(3)
J3360	6(3)
J3364	0(3)
J3365	0(3)
J3370	12(3)
J3380	300(3)
J3385	80(3)
J3396	150(3)
J3397	600(3)
J3398	150(2)
J3400	0(3)
J3410	16(3)
J3411	8(3)
J3415	6(3)
J3420	1(3)
J3430	50(3)
J3465	120(3)
J3470	3(3)
J3471	999(2)
J3472	2(3)
J3473	450(3)
J3475	80(3)
J3480	200(3)
J3485	160(3)
J3486	4(3)
J3489	5(3)
J3520	0(3)
J3530	0(3)
J3535	0(3)
J3570	0(3)
J7030	20(3)
J7040	12(3)
J7042	12(3)
J7050	20(3)
J7060	10(3)
J7070	7(3)
J7100	2(3)
J7110	3(3)
J7120	20(3)
J7121	5(3)
J7131	500(3)
J7169	180(3)
J7170	1800(3)
J7175	9000(1)
J7177	10500(3)
J7178	7700(1)
J7179	9600(1)
J7180	6000(1)
J7181	3850(1)
J7182	22000(1)
J7183	9600(1)
J7185	22000(1)
J7186	9600(1)
J7187	9600(1)

CPT	MUE
J7188	22000(1)
J7189	26000(1)
J7190	22000(1)
J7191	0(3)
J7192	22000(1)
J7193	20000(1)
J7194	9000(1)
J7195	20000(1)
J7196	175(3)
J7197	6300(1)
J7198	30000(1)
J7200	20000(1)
J7201	9000(1)
J7202	11550(1)
J7203	12000(1)
J7205	9750(1)
J7207	22500(1)
J7208	18000(1)
J7209	7500(1)
J7210	22000(1)
J7211	22000(1)
J7296	0(3)
J7297	0(3)
J7298	0(3)
J7300	0(3)
J7301	0(3)
J7303	0(3)
J7304	0(3)
J7306	0(3)
J7307	0(3)
J7308	3(3)
J7309	0(3)
J7310	0(3)
J7311	118(2)
J7312	14(2)
J7313	38(2)
J7314	36(2)
J7315	2(3)
J7316	3(3)
J7318	120(3)
J7320	50(3)
J7321	2(2)
J7322	48(3)
J7323	2(2)
J7324	2(2)
J7325	96(3)
J7326	2(2)
J7327	2(2)
J7328	336(3)
J7329	0(3)
J7330	1(3)
J7331	40(3)
J7332	40(3)
J7336	1120(3)
J7340	1(3)
J7342	10(3)
J7345	200(3)
J7401	270(2)
J7500	15(3)
J7501	8(3)
J7502	60(3)
J7503	120(3)
J7504	15(3)
J7505	1(3)
J7507	40(3)

CPT	MUE
J7508	300(3)
J7509	60(3)
J7510	60(3)
J7511	9(3)
J7512	300(3)
J7513	0(3)
J7515	90(3)
J7516	4(3)
J7517	16(3)
J7518	12(3)
J7520	40(3)
J7525	2(3)
J7527	20(3)
J7599	1(3)
J7604	0(3)
J7605	0(3)
J7606	0(3)
J7607	0(3)
J7608	0(3)
J7609	0(3)
J7610	0(3)
J7611	0(3)
J7612	0(3)
J7613	0(3)
J7614	0(3)
J7615	0(3)
J7620	0(3)
J7622	0(3)
J7624	0(3)
J7626	0(3)
J7627	0(3)
J7628	0(3)
J7629	0(3)
J7631	0(3)
J7632	0(3)
J7633	0(3)
J7634	0(3)
J7635	0(3)
J7636	0(3)
J7637	0(3)
J7638	0(3)
J7639	0(3)
J7640	0(3)
J7641	0(3)
J7642	0(3)
J7643	0(3)
J7644	0(3)
J7645	0(3)
J7647	0(3)
J7648	0(3)
J7649	0(3)
J7650	0(3)
J7657	0(3)
J7658	0(3)
J7659	0(3)
J7660	0(3)
J7665	0(3)
J7667	0(3)
J7668	0(3)
J7669	0(3)
J7670	0(3)
J7674	100(3)
J7676	0(3)
J7677	175(3)
J7680	0(3)

CPT	MUE
J7681	0(3)
J7682	0(3)
J7683	0(3)
J7684	0(3)
J7685	0(3)
J7686	0(3)
J7699	0(3)
J7799	2(3)
J7999	6(3)
J8498	1(3)
J8499	0(3)
J8501	57(3)
J8510	5(3)
J8515	0(3)
J8520	50(3)
J8521	15(3)
J8530	60(3)
J8540	48(3)
J8560	6(3)
J8562	12(3)
J8565	0(3)
J8597	4(3)
J8600	40(3)
J8610	20(3)
J8650	0(3)
J8655	1(3)
J8670	180(3)
J8700	120(3)
J8705	22(3)
J8999	2(3)
J9000	20(3)
J9015	1(3)
J9017	30(3)
J9019	60(3)
J9020	0(3)
J9022	168(3)
J9023	140(3)
J9025	300(3)
J9027	100(3)
J9030	50(3)
J9032	300(3)
J9033	300(3)
J9034	360(3)
J9035	170(3)
J9036	360(3)
J9039	210(3)
J9040	4(3)
J9041	35(3)
J9042	200(3)
J9043	60(3)
J9044	35(3)
J9045	22(3)
J9047	160(3)
J9050	6(3)
J9055	120(3)
J9057	60(3)
J9060	24(3)
J9065	100(3)
J9070	55(3)
J9098	5(3)
J9100	120(3)
J9118	750(3)
J9119	350(3)
J9120	5(3)
J9130	24(3)

CPT	MUE
J9145	240(3)
J9150	12(3)
J9151	12(3)
J9153	132(3)
J9155	240(3)
J9160	0(3)
J9165	0(3)
J9171	240(3)
J9173	150(3)
J9175	10(3)
J9176	3000(3)
J9178	150(3)
J9179	50(3)
J9181	100(3)
J9185	2(3)
J9190	20(3)
J9200	20(3)
J9201	20(3)
J9202	3(3)
J9203	180(3)
J9204	160(3)
J9205	215(3)
J9206	42(3)
J9207	90(3)
J9208	15(3)
J9209	55(3)
J9210	1500(3)
J9211	6(3)
J9212	0(3)
J9213	12(3)
J9214	100(3)
J9215	0(3)
J9216	0(3)
J9217	6(3)
J9218	1(3)
J9219	0(3)
J9225	1(3)
J9226	1(3)
J9228	1100(3)
J9229	27(3)
J9230	5(3)
J9245	11(3)
J9250	50(3)
J9260	20(3)
J9261	80(3)
J9262	700(3)
J9263	700(3)
J9264	600(3)
J9266	2(3)
J9267	750(3)
J9268	1(3)
J9270	0(3)
J9271	400(3)
J9280	12(3)
J9285	200(3)
J9293	8(3)
J9295	800(3)
J9299	480(3)
J9301	100(3)
J9302	200(3)
J9303	90(3)
J9305	150(3)
J9306	840(3)
J9307	80(3)
J9308	280(3)

CPT	MUE
J9309	280(3)
J9311	160(3)
J9312	150(3)
J9313	600(3)
J9315	40(3)
J9320	4(3)
J9325	400(3)
J9328	400(3)
J9330	50(3)
J9340	4(3)
J9351	120(3)
J9352	40(3)
J9354	600(3)
J9355	105(3)
J9356	60(3)
J9357	4(3)
J9360	40(3)
J9370	4(3)
J9371	5(3)
J9390	36(3)
J9395	20(3)
J9400	500(3)
J9600	4(3)
K0001	0(3)
K0002	0(3)
K0003	0(3)
K0004	0(3)
K0005	0(3)
K0006	0(3)
K0007	0(3)
K0008	0(3)
K0009	0(3)
K0010	0(3)
K0011	0(3)
K0012	0(3)
K0013	0(3)
K0014	0(3)
K0015	0(3)
K0017	0(3)
K0018	0(3)
K0019	0(3)
K0020	0(3)
K0037	0(3)
K0038	0(3)
K0039	0(3)
K0040	0(3)
K0041	0(3)
K0042	0(3)
K0043	0(3)
K0044	0(3)
K0045	0(3)
K0046	0(3)
K0047	0(3)
K0050	0(3)
K0051	0(3)
K0052	0(3)
K0053	0(3)
K0056	0(3)
K0065	0(3)
K0069	0(3)
K0070	0(3)
K0071	0(3)
K0072	0(3)
K0073	0(3)
K0077	0(3)

CPT	MUE
K0098	0(3)
K0105	0(3)
K0108	0(3)
K0195	0(3)
K0455	0(3)
K0462	0(3)
K0552	0(3)
K0553	0(3)
K0554	0(3)
K0601	0(3)
K0602	0(3)
K0603	0(3)
K0604	0(3)
K0605	0(3)
K0606	0(3)
K0607	0(3)
K0608	0(3)
K0609	0(3)
K0669	0(3)
K0672	4(3)
K0730	0(3)
K0733	0(3)
K0738	0(3)
K0740	0(3)
K0743	0(3)
K0800	0(3)
K0801	0(3)
K0802	0(3)
K0806	0(3)
K0807	0(3)
K0808	0(3)
K0812	0(3)
K0813	0(3)
K0814	0(3)
K0815	0(3)
K0816	0(3)
K0820	0(3)
K0821	0(3)
K0822	0(3)
K0823	0(3)
K0824	0(3)
K0825	0(3)
K0826	0(3)
K0827	0(3)
K0828	0(3)
K0829	0(3)
K0830	0(3)
K0831	0(3)
K0835	0(3)
K0836	0(3)
K0837	0(3)
K0838	0(3)
K0839	0(3)
K0840	0(3)
K0841	0(3)
K0842	0(3)
K0843	0(3)
K0848	0(3)
K0849	0(3)
K0850	0(3)
K0851	0(3)
K0852	0(3)
K0853	0(3)
K0854	0(3)
K0855	0(3)

CPT	MUE
K0856	0(3)
K0857	0(3)
K0858	0(3)
K0859	0(3)
K0860	0(3)
K0861	0(3)
K0862	0(3)
K0863	0(3)
K0864	0(3)
K0868	0(3)
K0869	0(3)
K0870	0(3)
K0871	0(3)
K0877	0(3)
K0878	0(3)
K0879	0(3)
K0880	0(3)
K0884	0(3)
K0885	0(3)
K0886	0(3)
K0890	0(3)
K0891	0(3)
K0898	1(2)
K0899	0(3)
K0900	0(3)
K1001	0(3)
K1002	0(3)
K1003	0(3)
K1004	0(3)
K1005	0(3)
L0112	1(2)
L0113	1(2)
L0120	1(2)
L0130	1(2)
L0140	1(2)
L0150	1(2)
L0160	1(2)
L0170	1(2)
L0172	1(2)
L0174	1(2)
L0180	1(2)
L0190	1(2)
L0200	1(2)
L0220	1(3)
L0450	1(2)
L0452	1(2)
L0454	1(2)
L0455	1(2)
L0456	1(2)
L0457	1(2)
L0458	1(2)
L0460	1(2)
L0462	1(2)
L0464	1(2)
L0466	1(2)
L0467	1(2)
L0468	1(2)
L0469	1(2)
L0470	1(2)
L0472	1(2)
L0480	1(2)
L0482	1(2)
L0484	1(2)
L0486	1(2)
L0488	1(2)

CPT	MUE	CPT	MUE	CPT	MUE	CPT	MUE	CPT	MUE	CPT	MUE	CPT	MUE	CPT	MUE
L0490	1(2)	L1220	1(3)	L1990	2(2)	L2425	4(2)	L3209	1(3)	L3670	1(3)	L4020	2(2)	L5590	2(2)
L0491	1(2)	L1230	1(2)	L2000	2(2)	L2430	4(2)	L3211	1(3)	L3671	1(3)	L4030	2(2)	L5595	2(2)
L0492	1(2)	L1240	1(3)	L2005	2(2)	L2492	4(2)	L3212	1(3)	L3674	1(3)	L4040	2(2)	L5600	2(2)
L0621	1(2)	L1250	2(3)	L2006	0(3)	L2500	2(2)	L3213	1(3)	L3675	1(2)	L4045	2(2)	L5610	2(2)
L0622	1(2)	L1260	1(3)	L2010	2(2)	L2510	2(2)	L3214	1(3)	L3677	1(2)	L4050	2(2)	L5611	2(2)
L0623	1(2)	L1270	3(3)	L2020	2(2)	L2520	2(2)	L3215	0(3)	L3678	1(2)	L4055	2(2)	L5613	2(2)
L0624	1(2)	L1280	2(3)	L2030	2(2)	L2525	2(2)	L3216	0(3)	L3702	2(2)	L4060	2(2)	L5614	2(2)
L0625	1(2)	L1290	2(3)	L2034	2(2)	L2526	2(2)	L3217	0(3)	L3710	2(2)	L4070	2(3)	L5616	2(2)
L0626	1(2)	L1300	1(2)	L2035	2(2)	L2530	2(2)	L3219	0(3)	L3720	2(2)	L4080	2(2)	L5617	2(3)
L0627	1(2)	L1310	1(2)	L2036	2(2)	L2540	2(2)	L3221	0(3)	L3730	2(2)	L4090	4(2)	L5618	4(3)
L0628	1(2)	L1499	1(3)	L2037	2(2)	L2550	2(2)	L3222	0(3)	L3740	2(2)	L4100	2(2)	L5620	4(3)
L0629	1(2)	L1600	1(2)	L2038	2(2)	L2570	2(2)	L3224	2(2)	L3760	2(2)	L4110	4(2)	L5622	4(3)
L0630	1(2)	L1610	1(2)	L2040	1(2)	L2580	2(2)	L3225	2(2)	L3761	2(2)	L4130	2(2)	L5624	4(3)
L0631	1(2)	L1620	1(2)	L2050	1(2)	L2600	2(2)	L3230	2(2)	L3762	2(2)	L4205	8(3)	L5626	4(3)
L0632	1(2)	L1630	1(2)	L2060	1(2)	L2610	2(2)	L3250	2(2)	L3763	2(2)	L4210	4(3)	L5628	2(3)
L0633	1(2)	L1640	1(2)	L2070	1(2)	L2620	2(2)	L3251	2(2)	L3764	2(2)	L4350	2(2)	L5629	2(2)
L0634	1(2)	L1650	1(2)	L2080	1(2)	L2622	2(2)	L3252	2(2)	L3765	2(2)	L4360	2(2)	L5630	2(2)
L0635	1(2)	L1652	1(2)	L2090	1(2)	L2624	2(2)	L3253	2(2)	L3766	2(2)	L4361	2(2)	L5631	2(2)
L0636	1(2)	L1660	1(2)	L2106	2(2)	L2627	1(3)	L3254	1(3)	L3806	2(2)	L4370	2(2)	L5632	2(2)
L0637	1(2)	L1680	1(2)	L2108	2(2)	L2628	1(3)	L3255	1(3)	L3807	2(2)	L4386	2(2)	L5634	2(2)
L0638	1(2)	L1685	1(2)	L2112	2(2)	L2630	1(2)	L3257	1(3)	L3808	2(2)	L4387	2(2)	L5636	2(2)
L0639	1(2)	L1686	1(3)	L2114	2(2)	L2640	1(2)	L3260	0(3)	L3809	2(2)	L4392	2(3)	L5637	2(2)
L0640	1(2)	L1690	1(2)	L2116	2(2)	L2650	2(3)	L3265	1(3)	L3891	0(3)	L4394	2(3)	L5638	2(2)
L0641	1(2)	L1700	1(2)	L2126	2(2)	L2660	1(3)	L3300	4(3)	L3900	2(2)	L4396	2(2)	L5639	2(2)
L0642	1(2)	L1710	1(2)	L2128	2(2)	L2670	2(3)	L3310	4(3)	L3901	2(2)	L4397	2(2)	L5640	2(2)
L0643	1(2)	L1720	2(2)	L2132	2(2)	L2680	2(3)	L3330	2(2)	L3904	2(2)	L4398	2(2)	L5642	2(2)
L0648	1(2)	L1730	1(2)	L2134	2(2)	L2750	8(3)	L3332	2(2)	L3905	2(2)	L4631	2(2)	L5643	2(2)
L0649	1(2)	L1755	2(2)	L2136	2(2)	L2755	8(3)	L3334	4(3)	L3906	2(2)	L5000	2(3)	L5644	2(2)
L0650	1(2)	L1810	2(2)	L2180	2(2)	L2760	8(2)	L3340	2(2)	L3908	2(2)	L5010	2(2)	L5645	2(2)
L0651	1(2)	L1812	2(2)	L2182	4(2)	L2768	4(2)	L3350	2(2)	L3912	2(3)	L5020	2(2)	L5646	2(2)
L0700	1(2)	L1820	2(2)	L2184	4(2)	L2780	8(3)	L3360	2(2)	L3913	2(2)	L5050	2(2)	L5647	2(2)
L0710	1(2)	L1830	2(2)	L2186	4(2)	L2785	4(2)	L3370	2(2)	L3915	2(2)	L5060	2(2)	L5648	2(2)
L0810	1(2)	L1831	2(2)	L2188	2(2)	L2795	2(2)	L3380	2(2)	L3916	2(3)	L5100	2(2)	L5649	2(2)
L0820	1(2)	L1832	2(2)	L2190	2(2)	L2800	2(2)	L3390	2(2)	L3917	2(2)	L5105	2(2)	L5650	2(2)
L0830	1(2)	L1833	2(2)	L2192	2(2)	L2810	4(2)	L3400	2(2)	L3918	2(2)	L5150	2(2)	L5651	2(2)
L0859	1(2)	L1834	2(2)	L2200	4(2)	L2820	2(3)	L3410	2(2)	L3919	2(2)	L5160	2(2)	L5652	2(2)
L0861	1(2)	L1836	2(2)	L2210	4(2)	L2830	2(3)	L3420	2(2)	L3921	2(2)	L5200	2(2)	L5653	2(2)
L0970	1(2)	L1840	2(2)	L2220	4(2)	L2861	0(3)	L3430	2(2)	L3923	2(2)	L5210	2(2)	L5654	2(2)
L0972	1(2)	L1843	2(2)	L2230	2(2)	L2999	2(3)	L3440	2(2)	L3924	2(2)	L5220	2(2)	L5655	2(2)
L0974	1(2)	L1844	2(2)	L2232	2(2)	L3000	2(3)	L3450	2(2)	L3925	4(3)	L5230	2(2)	L5656	2(2)
L0976	1(2)	L1845	2(2)	L2240	2(2)	L3001	2(3)	L3455	2(2)	L3927	4(3)	L5250	2(2)	L5658	2(2)
L0978	2(3)	L1846	2(2)	L2250	2(2)	L3002	2(3)	L3460	2(2)	L3929	2(2)	L5270	2(2)	L5661	2(2)
L0980	1(2)	L1847	2(2)	L2260	2(2)	L3003	2(3)	L3465	2(2)	L3930	2(2)	L5280	2(2)	L5665	2(2)
L0982	1(3)	L1848	2(2)	L2265	2(2)	L3010	2(3)	L3470	2(2)	L3931	2(2)	L5301	2(2)	L5666	2(2)
L0984	3(3)	L1850	2(2)	L2270	2(3)	L3020	2(3)	L3480	2(2)	L3933	3(3)	L5312	2(2)	L5668	2(2)
L0999	1(3)	L1851	2(2)	L2275	2(3)	L3030	2(3)	L3485	2(2)	L3935	3(3)	L5321	2(2)	L5670	2(2)
L1000	1(2)	L1852	2(2)	L2280	2(2)	L3031	2(3)	L3500	2(2)	L3956	4(3)	L5331	2(2)	L5671	2(2)
L1001	1(2)	L1860	2(2)	L2300	1(2)	L3040	2(3)	L3510	2(2)	L3960	1(3)	L5341	2(2)	L5672	2(2)
L1005	1(2)	L1900	2(2)	L2310	1(2)	L3050	2(3)	L3520	2(2)	L3961	1(3)	L5400	2(2)	L5673	4(3)
L1010	2(2)	L1902	2(2)	L2320	2(3)	L3060	2(3)	L3530	2(2)	L3962	1(3)	L5410	2(2)	L5676	2(2)
L1020	2(3)	L1904	2(2)	L2330	2(3)	L3070	2(3)	L3540	2(2)	L3967	1(3)	L5420	2(2)	L5677	2(2)
L1025	1(3)	L1906	2(2)	L2335	2(2)	L3080	2(3)	L3550	2(2)	L3971	1(3)	L5430	2(2)	L5678	2(2)
L1030	1(3)	L1907	2(2)	L2340	2(2)	L3090	2(3)	L3560	2(2)	L3973	1(3)	L5450	2(2)	L5679	4(3)
L1040	1(3)	L1910	2(2)	L2350	2(2)	L3100	2(2)	L3570	2(2)	L3975	1(3)	L5460	2(2)	L5680	2(2)
L1050	1(3)	L1920	2(2)	L2360	2(2)	L3140	1(2)	L3580	2(2)	L3976	1(3)	L5500	2(2)	L5681	2(2)
L1060	1(3)	L1930	2(2)	L2370	2(2)	L3150	1(2)	L3590	2(2)	L3977	1(3)	L5505	2(2)	L5682	2(2)
L1070	2(2)	L1932	2(2)	L2375	2(2)	L3160	2(2)	L3595	2(2)	L3978	1(3)	L5510	2(2)	L5683	2(2)
L1080	2(2)	L1940	2(2)	L2380	2(3)	L3170	2(2)	L3600	2(2)	L3980	2(2)	L5520	2(2)	L5684	2(3)
L1085	1(2)	L1945	2(2)	L2385	4(2)	L3201	1(3)	L3610	2(2)	L3981	2(2)	L5530	2(2)	L5685	4(3)
L1090	1(3)	L1950	2(2)	L2387	4(2)	L3202	1(3)	L3620	2(2)	L3982	2(2)	L5535	2(2)	L5686	2(2)
L1100	2(2)	L1951	2(2)	L2390	4(2)	L3203	1(3)	L3630	2(2)	L3984	2(2)	L5540	2(2)	L5688	2(3)
L1110	2(2)	L1960	2(2)	L2395	4(2)	L3204	1(3)	L3640	1(2)	L3999	2(3)	L5560	2(2)	L5690	2(3)
L1120	3(3)	L1970	2(2)	L2397	4(3)	L3206	1(3)	L3649	2(3)	L4000	1(2)	L5570	2(2)	L5692	2(2)
L1200	1(2)	L1971	2(2)	L2405	4(2)	L3207	1(3)	L3650	1(2)	L4002	4(3)	L5580	2(2)	L5694	2(2)
L1210	2(3)	L1980	2(2)	L2415	4(2)	L3208	1(3)	L3660	1(2)	L4010	2(2)	L5585	2(2)	L5695	2(3)

CPT	MUE
L5696	2(2)
L5697	2(2)
L5698	2(2)
L5699	2(3)
L5700	2(2)
L5701	2(2)
L5702	2(2)
L5703	2(2)
L5704	2(2)
L5705	2(2)
L5706	2(2)
L5707	2(2)
L5710	2(2)
L5711	2(2)
L5712	2(2)
L5714	2(2)
L5716	2(2)
L5718	2(2)
L5722	2(2)
L5724	2(2)
L5726	2(2)
L5728	2(2)
L5780	2(2)
L5781	2(2)
L5782	2(2)
L5785	2(2)
L5790	2(2)
L5795	2(2)
L5810	2(2)
L5811	2(2)
L5812	2(2)
L5814	2(2)
L5816	2(2)
L5818	2(2)
L5822	2(2)
L5824	2(2)
L5826	2(2)
L5828	2(2)
L5830	2(2)
L5840	2(2)
L5845	2(2)
L5848	2(2)
L5850	2(2)
L5855	2(2)
L5856	2(2)
L5857	2(2)
L5858	2(2)
L5859	2(2)
L5910	2(2)
L5920	2(2)
L5925	2(3)
L5930	2(2)
L5940	2(2)
L5950	2(2)
L5960	2(2)
L5961	1(3)
L5962	2(2)
L5964	2(2)
L5966	2(2)
L5968	2(2)
L5969	0(3)
L5970	2(2)
L5971	2(2)
L5972	2(2)
L5973	2(3)

CPT	MUE
L5974	2(2)
L5975	2(2)
L5976	2(2)
L5978	2(2)
L5979	2(2)
L5980	2(2)
L5981	2(2)
L5982	2(2)
L5984	2(2)
L5985	2(2)
L5986	2(2)
L5987	2(2)
L5988	2(2)
L5990	2(2)
L5999	2(3)
L6000	2(2)
L6010	2(2)
L6020	2(2)
L6026	2(2)
L6050	2(2)
L6055	2(2)
L6100	2(2)
L6110	2(2)
L6120	2(2)
L6130	2(2)
L6200	2(2)
L6205	2(2)
L6250	2(2)
L6300	2(2)
L6310	2(2)
L6320	2(2)
L6350	2(2)
L6360	2(2)
L6370	2(2)
L6380	2(2)
L6382	2(2)
L6384	2(2)
L6386	2(2)
L6388	2(2)
L6400	2(2)
L6450	2(2)
L6500	2(2)
L6550	2(2)
L6570	2(2)
L6580	2(2)
L6582	2(2)
L6584	2(2)
L6586	2(2)
L6588	2(2)
L6590	2(2)
L6600	2(2)
L6605	2(2)
L6610	2(2)
L6611	2(3)
L6615	2(2)
L6616	2(2)
L6620	2(2)
L6621	2(2)
L6623	2(2)
L6624	2(2)
L6625	2(2)
L6628	2(2)
L6629	2(2)
L6630	2(2)
L6632	4(3)

CPT	MUE
L6635	2(2)
L6637	2(2)
L6638	2(2)
L6640	2(2)
L6641	2(3)
L6642	2(3)
L6645	2(2)
L6646	2(2)
L6647	2(2)
L6648	2(2)
L6650	2(2)
L6655	4(3)
L6660	4(3)
L6665	4(3)
L6670	2(2)
L6672	2(2)
L6675	2(2)
L6676	2(2)
L6677	2(2)
L6680	4(3)
L6682	4(3)
L6684	4(3)
L6686	2(2)
L6687	2(2)
L6688	2(2)
L6689	2(2)
L6690	2(2)
L6691	2(3)
L6692	2(3)
L6693	2(2)
L6694	2(3)
L6695	2(3)
L6696	2(2)
L6697	2(2)
L6698	2(2)
L6703	2(2)
L6704	2(2)
L6706	2(2)
L6707	2(2)
L6708	2(2)
L6709	2(2)
L6711	2(2)
L6712	2(2)
L6713	2(2)
L6714	2(2)
L6715	5(3)
L6721	2(2)
L6722	2(2)
L6805	2(2)
L6810	2(3)
L6880	2(2)
L6881	2(2)
L6882	2(2)
L6883	2(2)
L6884	2(2)
L6885	2(2)
L6890	2(3)
L6895	2(3)
L6900	2(2)
L6905	2(2)
L6910	2(2)
L6915	2(2)
L6920	2(2)
L6925	2(2)
L6930	2(2)

CPT	MUE
L6935	2(2)
L6940	2(2)
L6945	2(2)
L6950	2(2)
L6955	2(2)
L6960	2(2)
L6965	2(2)
L6970	2(2)
L6975	2(2)
L7007	2(2)
L7008	2(2)
L7009	2(2)
L7040	2(2)
L7045	2(2)
L7170	2(2)
L7180	2(2)
L7181	2(2)
L7185	2(2)
L7186	2(2)
L7190	2(2)
L7191	2(2)
L7259	2(2)
L7360	1(3)
L7362	1(2)
L7364	1(3)
L7366	1(2)
L7367	2(3)
L7368	1(2)
L7400	2(2)
L7401	2(2)
L7402	2(2)
L7403	2(2)
L7404	2(2)
L7405	2(2)
L7499	2(3)
L7510	4(3)
L7600	0(3)
L7700	2(1)
L7900	0(3)
L7902	0(3)
L8000	6(3)
L8001	4(3)
L8002	4(3)
L8010	4(3)
L8015	4(3)
L8020	4(3)
L8030	2(3)
L8031	2(3)
L8032	2(2)
L8033	0(3)
L8035	2(3)
L8039	2(3)
L8040	1(2)
L8041	1(2)
L8042	2(2)
L8043	1(2)
L8044	1(2)
L8045	2(2)
L8046	1(3)
L8047	1(2)
L8048	1(3)
L8049	6(3)
L8300	1(3)
L8310	1(3)
L8320	2(3)

CPT	MUE
L8330	2(3)
L8400	12(3)
L8410	12(3)
L8415	6(3)
L8417	12(3)
L8420	14(3)
L8430	12(3)
L8435	12(3)
L8440	4(3)
L8460	4(3)
L8465	4(3)
L8470	14(3)
L8480	12(3)
L8485	12(3)
L8499	1(3)
L8500	1(2)
L8501	2(3)
L8507	3(3)
L8509	1(3)
L8510	1(2)
L8511	1(3)
L8512	1(3)
L8513	1(3)
L8514	1(3)
L8515	1(3)
L8600	2(3)
L8603	4(3)
L8604	3(3)
L8605	4(3)
L8606	5(3)
L8607	20(3)
L8609	1(3)
L8610	2(3)
L8612	1(3)
L8613	2(3)
L8614	2(3)
L8615	2(3)
L8616	2(3)
L8617	2(3)
L8618	2(3)
L8619	2(3)
L8621	360(3)
L8622	2(3)
L8625	1(3)
L8627	2(2)
L8628	2(2)
L8629	2(2)
L8631	2(3)
L8641	4(3)
L8642	2(3)
L8658	3(3)
L8659	4(3)
L8670	3(3)
L8679	3(3)
L8680	0(3)
L8681	1(3)
L8682	2(3)
L8683	1(3)
L8684	1(3)
L8685	0(3)
L8686	0(3)
L8687	0(3)
L8688	0(3)
L8689	1(3)
L8690	2(2)

CPT	MUE
L8691	1(3)
L8692	0(3)
L8693	1(3)
L8694	1(3)
L8695	1(3)
L8696	1(3)
L8701	1(3)
L8702	1(3)
M0075	0(3)
M0076	0(3)
M0100	0(3)
M0300	0(3)
M0301	0(3)
P2028	1(2)
P2029	1(2)
P2031	0(3)
P2033	1(2)
P2038	1(2)
P3000	1(3)
P3001	1(3)
P7001	0(3)
P9010	4(3)
P9011	4(3)
P9012	12(3)
P9016	12(3)
P9017	24(3)
P9019	12(3)
P9020	5(3)
P9021	8(3)
P9022	12(3)
P9023	15(3)
P9031	12(3)
P9032	12(3)
P9033	12(3)
P9034	4(3)
P9035	4(3)
P9036	4(3)
P9037	4(3)
P9038	4(3)
P9039	2(3)
P9040	8(3)
P9041	100(3)
P9043	10(3)
P9044	20(3)
P9045	20(3)
P9046	40(3)
P9047	20(3)
P9048	2(3)
P9050	1(3)
P9051	4(3)
P9052	3(3)
P9053	3(3)
P9054	2(3)
P9055	2(3)
P9056	3(3)
P9057	4(3)
P9058	4(3)
P9059	15(3)
P9060	4(3)
P9070	15(3)
P9071	15(3)
P9073	4(3)
P9099	1(3)
P9100	12(3)
P9603	100(3)

CPT	MUE
P9604	2(3)
P9612	1(3)
P9615	1(3)
Q0035	1(3)
Q0081	2(3)
Q0083	2(3)
Q0084	2(3)
Q0085	2(3)
Q0091	1(3)
Q0092	2(3)
Q0111	2(3)
Q0112	3(3)
Q0113	1(3)
Q0114	1(3)
Q0115	1(3)
Q0138	510(3)
Q0139	510(3)
Q0144	0(3)
Q0161	66(3)
Q0162	24(3)
Q0163	6(3)
Q0164	8(3)
Q0166	2(3)
Q0167	108(3)
Q0169	12(3)
Q0173	5(3)
Q0174	0(3)
Q0175	6(3)
Q0177	16(3)
Q0180	1(3)
Q0181	2(3)
Q0477	1(1)
Q0478	1(3)
Q0479	1(3)
Q0480	1(3)
Q0481	1(2)
Q0482	1(3)
Q0483	1(3)
Q0484	1(3)
Q0485	1(3)
Q0486	1(3)
Q0487	1(3)
Q0488	1(3)
Q0489	1(3)
Q0490	1(3)
Q0491	1(3)
Q0492	1(3)
Q0493	1(3)
Q0494	1(3)
Q0495	1(3)
Q0497	2(3)
Q0498	1(3)
Q0499	1(3)
Q0501	1(3)
Q0502	1(3)
Q0503	3(3)
Q0504	1(3)
Q0506	8(3)
Q0507	1(3)
Q0508	24(3)
Q0509	2(3)
Q0510	1(2)
Q0511	1(2)
Q0512	4(3)
Q0513	1(2)

CPT	MUE
Q0514	1(2)
Q0515	0(3)
Q1004	0(3)
Q1005	0(3)
Q2004	1(3)
Q2009	100(3)
Q2017	12(3)
Q2026	30(3)
Q2028	1470(3)
Q2034	1(2)
Q2035	1(2)
Q2036	1(2)
Q2037	1(2)
Q2038	1(2)
Q2039	1(2)
Q2043	1(2)
Q2049	10(3)
Q2050	20(3)
Q2052	0(3)
Q3014	2(3)
Q3027	30(3)
Q3028	0(3)
Q3031	1(3)
Q4001	1(3)
Q4002	1(3)
Q4003	2(3)
Q4004	2(3)
Q4012	2(3)
Q4013	2(3)
Q4014	2(3)
Q4018	2(3)
Q4021	2(3)
Q4025	1(3)
Q4026	1(3)
Q4027	1(3)
Q4028	1(3)
Q4030	2(3)
Q4037	2(3)
Q4042	2(3)
Q4046	2(3)
Q4050	2(3)
Q4051	2(3)
Q4074	0(3)
Q4081	400(3)
Q5101	1500(3)
Q5103	150(3)
Q5104	150(3)
Q5105	400(3)
Q5106	60(3)
Q5107	170(3)
Q5108	12(3)
Q5109	150(3)
Q5110	1500(3)
Q5111	12(3)
Q5112	120(3)
Q5113	120(3)
Q5114	120(3)
Q5115	120(3)
Q5116	120(3)
Q5117	120(3)
Q5118	230(3)
Q9950	5(3)
Q9951	0(3)
Q9953	10(3)
Q9954	18(3)

CPT	MUE
Q9955	0(3)
Q9956	9(3)
Q9957	3(3)
Q9958	600(3)
Q9959	0(3)
Q9960	250(3)
Q9961	200(3)
Q9962	200(3)
Q9963	240(3)
Q9964	0(3)
Q9966	250(3)
Q9967	300(3)
Q9969	3(3)
Q9982	1(3)
Q9983	1(3)
Q9991	1(2)
Q9992	1(2)
R0070	2(3)
R0075	2(3)
R0076	1(3)
U0001	2(3)
U0002	2(3)
U0003	2(3)
U0004	2(3)
V2020	1(3)
V2025	0(3)
V2100	2(3)
V2101	2(3)
V2102	2(3)

CPT	MUE
V2103	2(3)
V2104	2(3)
V2105	2(3)
V2106	2(3)
V2107	2(3)
V2108	2(3)
V2109	2(3)
V2110	2(3)
V2111	2(3)
V2112	2(3)
V2113	2(3)
V2114	2(3)
V2115	2(3)
V2118	2(3)
V2121	2(3)
V2199	2(3)
V2200	2(3)
V2201	2(3)
V2202	2(3)
V2203	2(3)
V2204	2(3)
V2205	2(3)
V2206	2(3)
V2207	2(3)
V2208	2(3)
V2209	2(3)
V2210	2(3)
V2211	2(3)
V2212	2(3)

CPT	MUE
V2213	2(3)
V2214	2(3)
V2215	2(3)
V2218	2(3)
V2219	2(3)
V2220	2(3)
V2221	2(3)
V2299	2(3)
V2300	2(3)
V2301	2(3)
V2302	2(3)
V2303	2(3)
V2304	2(3)
V2305	2(3)
V2306	2(3)
V2307	2(3)
V2308	2(3)
V2309	2(3)
V2310	2(3)
V2311	2(3)
V2312	2(3)
V2313	2(3)
V2314	2(3)
V2315	2(3)
V2318	2(3)
V2319	2(3)
V2320	2(3)
V2321	2(3)
V2399	2(3)

CPT	MUE
V2410	2(3)
V2430	2(3)
V2499	2(3)
V2500	2(3)
V2501	2(3)
V2502	2(3)
V2503	2(3)
V2510	2(3)
V2511	2(3)
V2512	2(3)
V2513	2(3)
V2520	2(3)
V2521	2(3)
V2522	2(3)
V2523	2(3)
V2530	2(3)
V2531	2(3)
V2599	2(3)
V2600	0(2)
V2610	0(2)
V2615	0(2)
V2623	2(2)
V2624	2(2)
V2625	2(2)
V2626	2(2)
V2627	2(2)
V2628	2(3)
V2629	2(2)
V2630	2(2)

CPT	MUE
V2631	2(2)
V2632	2(2)
V2700	2(3)
V2702	0(3)
V2710	2(3)
V2715	4(3)
V2718	2(3)
V2730	2(3)
V2744	2(3)
V2745	2(3)
V2750	2(3)
V2755	2(3)
V2756	0(3)
V2760	0(3)
V2761	0(2)
V2762	0(3)
V2770	2(3)
V2780	2(3)
V2781	0(2)
V2782	2(3)
V2783	2(3)
V2784	2(3)
V2785	2(2)
V2786	0(3)
V2787	0(3)
V2788	0(3)
V2790	1(3)
V2797	0(3)
V5008	0(3)

CPT	MUE
V5010	0(3)
V5011	0(3)
V5014	0(3)
V5020	0(3)
V5030	0(3)
V5040	0(3)
V5050	0(3)
V5060	0(3)
V5070	0(3)
V5080	0(3)
V5090	0(3)
V5095	0(3)
V5100	0(3)
V5110	0(3)
V5120	0(3)
V5130	0(3)
V5140	0(3)
V5150	0(3)
V5160	0(3)
V5171	0(3)
V5172	0(3)
V5181	0(3)
V5190	0(3)
V5200	0(3)
V5211	0(3)
V5212	0(3)
V5213	0(3)
V5214	0(3)
V5215	0(3)

CPT	MUE
V5221	0(3)
V5230	0(3)
V5240	0(3)
V5241	0(3)
V5242	0(3)
V5243	0(3)
V5244	0(3)
V5245	0(3)
V5246	0(3)
V5247	0(3)
V5248	0(3)
V5249	0(3)
V5250	0(3)
V5251	0(3)
V5252	0(3)
V5253	0(3)
V5254	0(3)
V5255	0(3)
V5256	0(3)
V5257	0(3)
V5258	0(3)
V5259	0(3)
V5260	0(3)
V5261	0(3)
V5262	0(3)
V5263	0(3)
V5264	0(3)
V5265	0(3)
V5266	0(3)

CPT	MUE
V5267	0(3)
V5268	0(3)
V5269	0(3)
V5270	0(3)
V5271	0(3)
V5272	0(3)
V5273	0(3)
V5274	0(3)
V5275	0(3)
V5281	0(3)
V5282	0(3)
V5283	0(3)
V5284	0(3)
V5285	0(3)
V5286	0(3)
V5287	0(3)
V5288	0(3)
V5289	0(3)
V5290	0(3)
V5298	0(3)
V5299	1(3)
V5336	0(3)
V5362	0(3)
V5363	0(3)
V5364	0(3)

Appendix J — Inpatient-Only Procedures

Inpatient Only Procedures—This appendix identifies services with the status indicator C. Medicare will not pay an OPPS hospital or ASC when they are performed on a Medicare patient as an outpatient. Physicians should refer to this list when scheduling Medicare patients for surgical procedures. CMS updates this list quarterly. The following was updated 10/01/2020.

00176 Anesth pharyngeal surgery
00192 Anesth facial bone surgery
00211 Anesth cran surg hematoma
00214 Anesth skull drainage
00215 Anesth skull repair/fract
00474 Anesth surgery of rib
00524 Anesth chest drainage
00540 Anesth chest surgery
00542 Anesthesia removal pleura
00546 Anesth lung chest wall surg
00560 Anesth heart surg w/o pump
00561 Anesth heart surg <1 yr
00562 Anesth hrt surg w/pmp age 1+
00567 Anesth CABG w/pump
00580 Anesth heart/lung transplnt
00604 Anesth sitting procedure
00632 Anesth removal of nerves
0075T Perq stent/chest vert art
0076T S&i stent/chest vert art
00792 Anesth hemorr/excise liver
00794 Anesth pancreas removal
00796 Anesth for liver transplant
00844 Anesth pelvis surgery
00846 Anesth hysterectomy
00848 Anesth pelvic organ surg
00864 Anesth removal of bladder
00866 Anesth removal of adrenal
00868 Anesth kidney transplant
00882 Anesth major vein ligation
00904 Anesth perineal surgery
00908 Anesth removal of prostate
00932 Anesth amputation of penis
00934 Anesth penis nodes removal
00936 Anesth penis nodes removal
0095T Rmvl artific disc addl crvcl
0098T Rev artific disc addl
01140 Anesth amputation at pelvis
01150 Anesth pelvic tumor surgery
01212 Anesth hip disarticulation
01232 Anesth amputation of femur
01234 Anesth radical femur surg
01272 Anesth femoral artery surg
01274 Anesth femoral embolectomy
01404 Anesth amputation at knee
01442 Anesth knee artery surg
01444 Anesth knee artery repair
01486 Anesth ankle replacement
01502 Anesth lwr leg embolectomy
01634 Anesth shoulder joint amput
01636 Anesth forequarter amput
01638 Anesth shoulder replacement
0163T Lumb artif diskectomy addl
0164T Remove lumb artif disc addl
01652 Anesth shoulder vessel surg
01654 Anesth shoulder vessel surg
01656 Anesth arm-leg vessel surg
0165T Revise lumb artif disc addl
01756 Anesth radical humerus surg
01990 Support for organ donor
0202T Post vert arthrplst 1 lumbar
0219T Plmt post facet implt cerv
0220T Plmt post facet implt thor
0235T Trluml perip athrc visceral
0345T Transcath mtral vlve repair
0451T Insj/rplcmt aortic ventr sys
0452T Insj/rplcmt dev vasc seal
0455T Remvl aortic ventr cmpl sys
0456T Remvl aortic dev vasc seal
0459T Relocaj rplcmt aortic ventr
0461T Repos aortic contrpulsj dev
0483T Tmvi percutaneous approach
0484T Tmvi transthoracic exposure
0494T Prep & cannulj cdvr don lung
0495T Mntr cdvr don lng 1st 2 hrs
0496T Mntr cdvr don lng ea addl hr
0543T Ta mv rpr w/artif chord tend
0544T Tcat mv annulus rcnstj
0545T Tcat tv annulus rcnstj
0569T Ttvr perq appr 1st prosth
0570T Ttvr perq ea addl prosth
0584T Perq islet cell transplant
0585T Laps islet cell transplant
0586T Open islet cell transplant
11004 Debride genitalia & perineum
11005 Debride abdom wall
11006 Debride genit/per/abdom wall
11008 Remove mesh from abd wall
15756 Free myo/skin flap microvasc
15757 Free skin flap microvasc
15758 Free fascial flap microvasc
16036 Escharotomy addl incision
19305 Mast radical
19306 Mast rad urban type
19361 Breast reconstr w/lat flap
19364 Breast reconstruction
19367 Breast reconstruction
19368 Breast reconstruction
19369 Breast reconstruction
20661 Application of head brace
20664 Application of halo
20802 Replantation arm complete
20805 Replant forearm complete
20808 Replantation hand complete
20816 Replantation digit complete
20824 Replantation thumb complete
20827 Replantation thumb complete
20838 Replantation foot complete
20955 Fibula bone graft microvasc
20956 Iliac bone graft microvasc
20957 Mt bone graft microvasc
20962 Other bone graft microvasc
20969 Bone/skin graft microvasc
20970 Bone/skin graft iliac crest
21045 Extensive jaw surgery
21141 Lefort i-1 piece w/o graft
21142 Lefort i-2 piece w/o graft
21143 Lefort i-3/> piece w/o graft
21145 Lefort i-1 piece w/ graft
21146 Lefort i-2 piece w/ graft
21147 Lefort i-3/> piece w/ graft
21151 Lefort ii w/bone grafts
21154 Lefort iii w/o lefort i
21155 Lefort iii w/ lefort i
21159 Lefort iii w/fhdw/o lefort i
21160 Lefort iii w/fhd w/ lefort i
21179 Reconstruct entire forehead
21180 Reconstruct entire forehead
21182 Reconstruct cranial bone
21183 Reconstruct cranial bone
21184 Reconstruct cranial bone
21188 Reconstruction of midface
21194 Reconst lwr jaw w/graft
21196 Reconst lwr jaw w/fixation
21247 Reconstruct lower jaw bone
21255 Reconstruct lower jaw bone
21268 Revise eye sockets
21343 Open tx dprsd front sinus fx
21344 Open tx compl front sinus fx
21347 Opn tx nasomax fx multple
21348 Opn tx nasomax fx w/graft
21366 Opn tx complx malar w/grft
21422 Treat mouth roof fracture
21423 Treat mouth roof fracture
21431 Treat craniofacial fracture
21432 Treat craniofacial fracture
21433 Treat craniofacial fracture
21435 Treat craniofacial fracture
21436 Treat craniofacial fracture
21510 Drainage of bone lesion
21602 Exc ch wal tum w/o lymphadec
21603 Exc ch wal tum w/lymphadec
21615 Removal of rib
21616 Removal of rib and nerves
21620 Partial removal of sternum
21627 Sternal debridement
21630 Extensive sternum surgery
21632 Extensive sternum surgery
21705 Revision of neck muscle/rib
21740 Reconstruction of sternum

21750 Repair of sternum separation
21825 Treat sternum fracture
22010 I&d p-spine c/t/cerv-thor
22015 I&d abscess p-spine l/s/ls
22110 Remove part of neck vertebra
22112 Remove part thorax vertebra
22114 Remove part lumbar vertebra
22116 Remove extra spine segment
22206 Incis spine 3 column thorac
22207 Incis spine 3 column lumbar
22208 Incis spine 3 column adl seg
22210 Incis 1 vertebral seg cerv
22212 Incis 1 vertebral seg thorac
22214 Incis 1 vertebral seg lumbar
22216 Incis addl spine segment
22220 Incis w/discectomy cervical
22222 Incis w/discectomy thoracic
22224 Incis w/discectomy lumbar
22226 Revise extra spine segment
22318 Treat odontoid fx w/o graft
22319 Treat odontoid fx w/graft
22325 Treat spine fracture
22326 Treat neck spine fracture
22327 Treat thorax spine fracture
22328 Treat each add spine fx
22532 Lat thorax spine fusion
22533 Lat lumbar spine fusion
22534 Lat thor/lumb addl seg
22548 Neck spine fusion
22556 Thorax spine fusion
22558 Lumbar spine fusion
22586 Prescrl fuse w/ instr l5-s1
22590 Spine & skull spinal fusion
22595 Neck spinal fusion
22600 Neck spine fusion
22610 Thorax spine fusion
22630 Lumbar spine fusion
22632 Spine fusion extra segment
22800 Post fusion </6 vert seg
22802 Post fusion 7-12 vert seg
22804 Post fusion 13/> vert seg
22808 Ant fusion 2-3 vert seg
22810 Ant fusion 4-7 vert seg
22812 Ant fusion 8/> vert seg
22818 Kyphectomy 1-2 segments
22819 Kyphectomy 3 or more
22830 Exploration of spinal fusion
22841 Insert spine fixation device
22843 Insert spine fixation device
22844 Insert spine fixation device
22846 Insert spine fixation device
22847 Insert spine fixation device
22848 Insert pelv fixation device
22849 Reinsert spinal fixation
22850 Remove spine fixation device
22852 Remove spine fixation device
22855 Remove spine fixation device
22857 Lumbar artif diskectomy
22861 Revise cerv artific disc
22862 Revise lumbar artif disc
22864 Remove cerv artif disc
22865 Remove lumb artif disc
23200 Resect clavicle tumor
23210 Resect scapula tumor
23220 Resect prox humerus tumor
23335 Shoulder prosthesis removal
23472 Reconstruct shoulder joint
23474 Revis reconst shoulder joint
23900 Amputation of arm & girdle
23920 Amputation at shoulder joint
24900 Amputation of upper arm
24920 Amputation of upper arm
24930 Amputation follow-up surgery
24931 Amputate upper arm & implant
24940 Revision of upper arm
25900 Amputation of forearm
25905 Amputation of forearm
25915 Amputation of forearm
25920 Amputate hand at wrist
25924 Amputation follow-up surgery
25927 Amputation of hand
26551 Great toe-hand transfer
26553 Single transfer toe-hand
26554 Double transfer toe-hand
26556 Toe joint transfer
26992 Drainage of bone lesion
27005 Incision of hip tendon
27025 Incision of hip/thigh fascia
27030 Drainage of hip joint
27036 Excision of hip joint/muscle
27054 Removal of hip joint lining
27070 Part remove hip bone super
27071 Part removal hip bone deep
27075 Resect hip tumor
27076 Resect hip tum incl acetabul
27077 Resect hip tum w/innom bone
27078 Rsect hip tum incl femur
27090 Removal of hip prosthesis
27091 Removal of hip prosthesis
27120 Reconstruction of hip socket
27122 Reconstruction of hip socket
27125 Partial hip replacement
27132 Total hip arthroplasty
27134 Revise hip joint replacement
27137 Revise hip joint replacement
27138 Revise hip joint replacement
27140 Transplant femur ridge
27146 Incision of hip bone
27147 Revision of hip bone
27151 Incision of hip bones
27156 Revision of hip bones
27158 Revision of pelvis
27161 Incision of neck of femur
27165 Incision/fixation of femur
27170 Repair/graft femur head/neck
27175 Treat slipped epiphysis
27176 Treat slipped epiphysis
27177 Treat slipped epiphysis
27178 Treat slipped epiphysis
27181 Treat slipped epiphysis
27185 Revision of femur epiphysis
27187 Reinforce hip bones
27222 Treat hip socket fracture
27226 Treat hip wall fracture
27227 Treat hip fracture(s)
27228 Treat hip fracture(s)
27232 Treat thigh fracture
27236 Treat thigh fracture
27240 Treat thigh fracture
27244 Treat thigh fracture
27245 Treat thigh fracture
27248 Treat thigh fracture
27253 Treat hip dislocation
27254 Treat hip dislocation
27258 Treat hip dislocation
27259 Treat hip dislocation
27268 Cltx thigh fx w/mnpj
27269 Optx thigh fx
27280 Fusion of sacroiliac joint
27282 Fusion of pubic bones
27284 Fusion of hip joint
27286 Fusion of hip joint
27290 Amputation of leg at hip
27295 Amputation of leg at hip
27303 Drainage of bone lesion
27365 Resect femur/knee tumor
27445 Revision of knee joint
27448 Incision of thigh
27450 Incision of thigh
27454 Realignment of thigh bone
27455 Realignment of knee
27457 Realignment of knee
27465 Shortening of thigh bone
27466 Lengthening of thigh bone
27468 Shorten/lengthen thighs
27470 Repair of thigh
27472 Repair/graft of thigh
27486 Revise/replace knee joint
27487 Revise/replace knee joint
27488 Removal of knee prosthesis
27495 Reinforce thigh
27506 Treatment of thigh fracture
27507 Treatment of thigh fracture
27511 Treatment of thigh fracture
27513 Treatment of thigh fracture
27514 Treatment of thigh fracture
27519 Treat thigh fx growth plate
27535 Treat knee fracture
27536 Treat knee fracture
27540 Treat knee fracture
27556 Treat knee dislocation
27557 Treat knee dislocation
27558 Treat knee dislocation
27580 Fusion of knee
27590 Amputate leg at thigh
27591 Amputate leg at thigh
27592 Amputate leg at thigh

27596 Amputation follow-up surgery
27598 Amputate lower leg at knee
27645 Resect tibia tumor
27646 Resect fibula tumor
27702 Reconstruct ankle joint
27703 Reconstruction ankle joint
27712 Realignment of lower leg
27715 Revision of lower leg
27724 Repair/graft of tibia
27725 Repair of lower leg
27727 Repair of lower leg
27880 Amputation of lower leg
27881 Amputation of lower leg
27882 Amputation of lower leg
27886 Amputation follow-up surgery
27888 Amputation of foot at ankle
28800 Amputation of midfoot
31225 Removal of upper jaw
31230 Removal of upper jaw
31290 Nasal/sinus endoscopy surg
31291 Nasal/sinus endoscopy surg
31360 Removal of larynx
31365 Removal of larynx
31367 Partial removal of larynx
31368 Partial removal of larynx
31370 Partial removal of larynx
31375 Partial removal of larynx
31380 Partial removal of larynx
31382 Partial removal of larynx
31390 Removal of larynx & pharynx
31395 Reconstruct larynx & pharynx
31725 Clearance of airways
31760 Repair of windpipe
31766 Reconstruction of windpipe
31770 Repair/graft of bronchus
31775 Reconstruct bronchus
31780 Reconstruct windpipe
31781 Reconstruct windpipe
31786 Remove windpipe lesion
31800 Repair of windpipe injury
31805 Repair of windpipe injury
32035 Thoracostomy w/rib resection
32036 Thoracostomy w/flap drainage
32096 Open wedge/bx lung infiltr
32097 Open wedge/bx lung nodule
32098 Open biopsy of lung pleura
32100 Exploration of chest
32110 Explore/repair chest
32120 Re-exploration of chest
32124 Explore chest free adhesions
32140 Removal of lung lesion(s)
32141 Remove/treat lung lesions
32150 Removal of lung lesion(s)
32151 Remove lung foreign body
32160 Open chest heart massage
32200 Drain open lung lesion
32215 Treat chest lining
32220 Release of lung
32225 Partial release of lung
32310 Removal of chest lining
32320 Free/remove chest lining
32440 Remove lung pneumonectomy
32442 Sleeve pneumonectomy
32445 Removal of lung extrapleural
32480 Partial removal of lung
32482 Bilobectomy
32484 Segmentectomy
32486 Sleeve lobectomy
32488 Completion pneumonectomy
32491 Lung volume reduction
32501 Repair bronchus add-on
32503 Resect apical lung tumor
32504 Resect apical lung tum/chest
32505 Wedge resect of lung initial
32506 Wedge resect of lung add-on
32507 Wedge resect of lung diag
32540 Removal of lung lesion
32650 Thoracoscopy w/pleurodesis
32651 Thoracoscopy remove cortex
32652 Thoracoscopy rem totl cortex
32653 Thoracoscopy remov fb/fibrin
32654 Thoracoscopy contrl bleeding
32655 Thoracoscopy resect bullae
32656 Thoracoscopy w/pleurectomy
32658 Thoracoscopy w/sac fb remove
32659 Thoracoscopy w/sac drainage
32661 Thoracoscopy w/pericard exc
32662 Thoracoscopy w/mediast exc
32663 Thoracoscopy w/lobectomy
32664 Thoracoscopy w/ th nrv exc
32665 Thoracoscop w/esoph musc exc
32666 Thoracoscopy w/wedge resect
32667 Thoracoscopy w/w resect addl
32668 Thoracoscopy w/w resect diag
32669 Thoracoscopy remove segment
32670 Thoracoscopy bilobectomy
32671 Thoracoscopy pneumonectomy
32672 Thoracoscopy for lvrs
32673 Thoracoscopy w/thymus resect
32674 Thoracoscopy lymph node exc
32800 Repair lung hernia
32810 Close chest after drainage
32815 Close bronchial fistula
32820 Reconstruct injured chest
32850 Donor pneumonectomy
32851 Lung transplant single
32852 Lung transplant with bypass
32853 Lung transplant double
32854 Lung transplant with bypass
32855 Prepare donor lung single
32856 Prepare donor lung double
32900 Removal of rib(s)
32905 Revise & repair chest wall
32906 Revise & repair chest wall
32940 Revision of lung
32997 Total lung lavage
33017 Prcrd drg 6yr+ w/o cgen car
33018 Prcrd drg 0-5yr or w/anomly
33019 Perq prcrd drg insj cath ct
33020 Incision of heart sac
33025 Incision of heart sac
33030 Partial removal of heart sac
33031 Partial removal of heart sac
33050 Resect heart sac lesion
33120 Removal of heart lesion
33130 Removal of heart lesion
33140 Heart revascularize (tmr)
33141 Heart tmr w/other procedure
33202 Insert epicard eltrd open
33203 Insert epicard eltrd endo
33236 Remove electrode/thoracotomy
33237 Remove electrode/thoracotomy
33238 Remove electrode/thoracotomy
33243 Remove eltrd/thoracotomy
33250 Ablate heart dysrhythm focus
33251 Ablate heart dysrhythm focus
33254 Ablate atria lmtd
33255 Ablate atria w/o bypass ext
33256 Ablate atria w/bypass exten
33257 Ablate atria lmtd add-on
33258 Ablate atria x10sv add-on
33259 Ablate atria w/bypass add-on
33261 Ablate heart dysrhythm focus
33265 Ablate atria lmtd endo
33266 Ablate atria x10sv endo
33300 Repair of heart wound
33305 Repair of heart wound
33310 Exploratory heart surgery
33315 Exploratory heart surgery
33320 Repair major blood vessel(s)
33321 Repair major vessel
33322 Repair major blood vessel(s)
33330 Insert major vessel graft
33335 Insert major vessel graft
33340 Perq clsr tcat l atr apndge
33361 Replace aortic valve perq
33362 Replace aortic valve open
33363 Replace aortic valve open
33364 Replace aortic valve open
33365 Replace aortic valve open
33366 Trcath replace aortic valve
33367 Replace aortic valve w/byp
33368 Replace aortic valve w/byp
33369 Replace aortic valve w/byp
33390 Valvuloplasty aortic valve
33391 Valvuloplasty aortic valve
33404 Prepare heart-aorta conduit
33405 Replacement of aortic valve
33406 Replacement of aortic valve
33410 Replacement of aortic valve
33411 Replacement of aortic valve
33412 Replacement of aortic valve
33413 Replacement of aortic valve
33414 Repair of aortic valve
33415 Revision subvalvular tissue
33416 Revise ventricle muscle
33417 Repair of aortic valve

33418 Repair tcat mitral valve
33420 Revision of mitral valve
33422 Revision of mitral valve
33425 Repair of mitral valve
33426 Repair of mitral valve
33427 Repair of mitral valve
33430 Replacement of mitral valve
33440 Rplcmt a-valve tlcj autol pv
33460 Revision of tricuspid valve
33463 Valvuloplasty tricuspid
33464 Valvuloplasty tricuspid
33465 Replace tricuspid valve
33468 Revision of tricuspid valve
33470 Revision of pulmonary valve
33471 Valvotomy pulmonary valve
33474 Revision of pulmonary valve
33475 Replacement pulmonary valve
33476 Revision of heart chamber
33477 Implant tcat pulm vlv perq
33478 Revision of heart chamber
33496 Repair prosth valve clot
33500 Repair heart vessel fistula
33501 Repair heart vessel fistula
33502 Coronary artery correction
33503 Coronary artery graft
33504 Coronary artery graft
33505 Repair artery w/tunnel
33506 Repair artery translocation
33507 Repair art intramural
33510 Cabg vein single
33511 Cabg vein two
33512 Cabg vein three
33513 Cabg vein four
33514 Cabg vein five
33516 Cabg vein six or more
33517 Cabg artery-vein single
33518 Cabg artery-vein two
33519 Cabg artery-vein three
33521 Cabg artery-vein four
33522 Cabg artery-vein five
33523 Cabg art-vein six or more
33530 Coronary artery bypass/reop
33533 Cabg arterial single
33534 Cabg arterial two
33535 Cabg arterial three
33536 Cabg arterial four or more
33542 Removal of heart lesion
33545 Repair of heart damage
33548 Restore/remodel ventricle
33572 Open coronary endarterectomy
33600 Closure of valve
33602 Closure of valve
33606 Anastomosis/artery-aorta
33608 Repair anomaly w/conduit
33610 Repair by enlargement
33611 Repair double ventricle
33612 Repair double ventricle
33615 Repair modified fontan
33617 Repair single ventricle
33619 Repair single ventricle
33620 Apply r&l pulm art bands
33621 Transthor cath for stent
33622 Redo compl cardiac anomaly
33641 Repair heart septum defect
33645 Revision of heart veins
33647 Repair heart septum defects
33660 Repair of heart defects
33665 Repair of heart defects
33670 Repair of heart chambers
33675 Close mult vsd
33676 Close mult vsd w/resection
33677 Cl mult vsd w/rem pul band
33681 Repair heart septum defect
33684 Repair heart septum defect
33688 Repair heart septum defect
33690 Reinforce pulmonary artery
33692 Repair of heart defects
33694 Repair of heart defects
33697 Repair of heart defects
33702 Repair of heart defects
33710 Repair of heart defects
33720 Repair of heart defect
33722 Repair of heart defect
33724 Repair venous anomaly
33726 Repair pul venous stenosis
33730 Repair heart-vein defect(s)
33732 Repair heart-vein defect
33735 Revision of heart chamber
33736 Revision of heart chamber
33737 Revision of heart chamber
33750 Major vessel shunt
33755 Major vessel shunt
33762 Major vessel shunt
33764 Major vessel shunt & graft
33766 Major vessel shunt
33767 Major vessel shunt
33768 Cavopulmonary shunting
33770 Repair great vessels defect
33771 Repair great vessels defect
33774 Repair great vessels defect
33775 Repair great vessels defect
33776 Repair great vessels defect
33777 Repair great vessels defect
33778 Repair great vessels defect
33779 Repair great vessels defect
33780 Repair great vessels defect
33781 Repair great vessels defect
33782 Nikaidoh proc
33783 Nikaidoh proc w/ostia implt
33786 Repair arterial trunk
33788 Revision of pulmonary artery
33800 Aortic suspension
33802 Repair vessel defect
33803 Repair vessel defect
33813 Repair septal defect
33814 Repair septal defect
33820 Revise major vessel
33822 Revise major vessel
33824 Revise major vessel
33840 Remove aorta constriction
33845 Remove aorta constriction
33851 Remove aorta constriction
33852 Repair septal defect
33853 Repair septal defect
33858 As-aort grf f/aortic dsj
33859 As-aort grf f/ds oth/thn dsj
33863 Ascending aortic graft
33864 Ascending aortic graft
33871 Transvrs a-arch grf hypthrm
33875 Thoracic aortic graft
33877 Thoracoabdominal graft
33880 Endovasc taa repr incl subcl
33881 Endovasc taa repr w/o subcl
33883 Insert endovasc prosth taa
33884 Endovasc prosth taa add-on
33886 Endovasc prosth delayed
33889 Artery transpose/endovas taa
33891 Car-car bp grft/endovas taa
33910 Remove lung artery emboli
33915 Remove lung artery emboli
33916 Surgery of great vessel
33917 Repair pulmonary artery
33920 Repair pulmonary atresia
33922 Transect pulmonary artery
33924 Remove pulmonary shunt
33925 Rpr pul art unifocal w/o cpb
33926 Repr pul art unifocal w/cpb
33927 Impltj tot rplcmt hrt sys
33928 Rmvl & rplcmt tot hrt sys
33929 Rmvl rplcmt hrt sys f/trnspl
33930 Removal of donor heart/lung
33933 Prepare donor heart/lung
33935 Transplantation heart/lung
33940 Removal of donor heart
33944 Prepare donor heart
33945 Transplantation of heart
33946 Ecmo/ecls initiation venous
33947 Ecmo/ecls initiation artery
33948 Ecmo/ecls daily mgmt-venous
33949 Ecmo/ecls daily mgmt artery
33951 Ecmo/ecls insj prph cannula
33952 Ecmo/ecls insj prph cannula
33953 Ecmo/ecls insj prph cannula
33954 Ecmo/ecls insj prph cannula
33955 Ecmo/ecls insj ctr cannula
33956 Ecmo/ecls insj ctr cannula
33957 Ecmo/ecls repos perph cnula
33958 Ecmo/ecls repos perph cnula
33959 Ecmo/ecls repos perph cnula
33962 Ecmo/ecls repos perph cnula
33963 Ecmo/ecls repos perph cnula
33964 Ecmo/ecls repos perph cnula
33965 Ecmo/ecls rmvl perph cannula
33966 Ecmo/ecls rmvl prph cannula
33967 Insert i-aort percut device
33968 Remove aortic assist device
33969 Ecmo/ecls rmvl perph cannula

33970	Aortic circulation assist
33971	Aortic circulation assist
33973	Insert balloon device
33974	Remove intra-aortic balloon
33975	Implant ventricular device
33976	Implant ventricular device
33977	Remove ventricular device
33978	Remove ventricular device
33979	Insert intracorporeal device
33980	Remove intracorporeal device
33981	Replace vad pump ext
33982	Replace vad intra w/o bp
33983	Replace vad intra w/bp
33984	Ecmo/ecls rmvl prph cannula
33985	Ecmo/ecls rmvl ctr cannula
33986	Ecmo/ecls rmvl ctr cannula
33987	Artery expos/graft artery
33988	Insertion of left heart vent
33989	Removal of left heart vent
33990	Insert vad artery access
33991	Insert vad art&vein access
33992	Remove vad different session
33993	Reposition vad diff session
34001	Removal of artery clot
34051	Removal of artery clot
34151	Removal of artery clot
34401	Removal of vein clot
34451	Removal of vein clot
34502	Reconstruct vena cava
34701	Evasc rpr a-ao ndgft
34702	Evasc rpr a-ao ndgft rpt
34703	Evasc rpr a-unilac ndgft
34704	Evasc rpr a-unilac ndgft rpt
34705	Evac rpr a-biiliac ndgft
34706	Evasc rpr a-biiliac rpt
34707	Evasc rpr ilio-iliac ndgft
34708	Evasc rpr ilio-iliac rpt
34709	Plmt xtn prosth evasc rpr
34710	Dlyd plmt xtn prosth 1st vsl
34711	Dlyd plmt xtn prosth ea addl
34712	Tcat dlvr enhncd fixj dev
34717	Evasc rpr a-iliac ndgft
34718	Evasc rpr n/a a-iliac ndgft
34808	Endovas iliac a device addon
34812	Xpose for endoprosth femorl
34813	Femoral endovas graft add-on
34820	Xpose for endoprosth iliac
34830	Open aortic tube prosth repr
34831	Open aortoiliac prosth repr
34832	Open aortofemor prosth repr
34833	Xpose for endoprosth iliac
34834	Xpose endoprosth brachial
34841	Endovasc visc aorta 1 graft
34842	Endovasc visc aorta 2 graft
34843	Endovasc visc aorta 3 graft
34844	Endovasc visc aorta 4 graft
34845	Visc & infraren abd 1 prosth
34846	Visc & infraren abd 2 prosth
34847	Visc & infraren abd 3 prosth
34848	Visc & infraren abd 4+ prost
35001	Repair defect of artery
35002	Repair artery rupture neck
35005	Repair defect of artery
35013	Repair artery rupture arm
35021	Repair defect of artery
35022	Repair artery rupture chest
35081	Repair defect of artery
35082	Repair artery rupture aorta
35091	Repair defect of artery
35092	Repair artery rupture aorta
35102	Repair defect of artery
35103	Repair artery rupture aorta
35111	Repair defect of artery
35112	Repair artery rupture spleen
35121	Repair defect of artery
35122	Repair artery rupture belly
35131	Repair defect of artery
35132	Repair artery rupture groin
35141	Repair defect of artery
35142	Repair artery rupture thigh
35151	Repair defect of artery
35152	Repair ruptd popliteal art
35182	Repair blood vessel lesion
35189	Repair blood vessel lesion
35211	Repair blood vessel lesion
35216	Repair blood vessel lesion
35221	Repair blood vessel lesion
35241	Repair blood vessel lesion
35246	Repair blood vessel lesion
35251	Repair blood vessel lesion
35271	Repair blood vessel lesion
35276	Repair blood vessel lesion
35281	Repair blood vessel lesion
35301	Rechanneling of artery
35302	Rechanneling of artery
35303	Rechanneling of artery
35304	Rechanneling of artery
35305	Rechanneling of artery
35306	Rechanneling of artery
35311	Rechanneling of artery
35331	Rechanneling of artery
35341	Rechanneling of artery
35351	Rechanneling of artery
35355	Rechanneling of artery
35361	Rechanneling of artery
35363	Rechanneling of artery
35371	Rechanneling of artery
35372	Rechanneling of artery
35390	Reoperation carotid add-on
35400	Angioscopy
35501	Art byp grft ipsilat carotid
35506	Art byp grft subclav-carotid
35508	Art byp grft carotid-vertbrl
35509	Art byp grft contral carotid
35510	Art byp grft carotid-brchial
35511	Art byp grft subclav-subclav
35512	Art byp grft subclav-brchial
35515	Art byp grft subclav-vertbrl
35516	Art byp grft subclav-axilary
35518	Art byp grft axillary-axilry
35521	Art byp grft axill-femoral
35522	Art byp grft axill-brachial
35523	Art byp grft brchl-ulnr-rdl
35525	Art byp grft brachial-brchl
35526	Art byp grft aor/carot/innom
35531	Art byp grft aorcel/aormesen
35533	Art byp grft axill/fem/fem
35535	Art byp grft hepatorenal
35536	Art byp grft splenorenal
35537	Art byp grft aortoiliac
35538	Art byp grft aortobi-iliac
35539	Art byp grft aortofemoral
35540	Art byp grft aortbifemoral
35556	Art byp grft fem-popliteal
35558	Art byp grft fem-femoral
35560	Art byp grft aortorenal
35563	Art byp grft ilioiliac
35565	Art byp grft iliofemoral
35566	Art byp fem-ant-post tib/prl
35570	Art byp tibial-tib/peroneal
35571	Art byp pop-tibl-prl-other
35583	Vein byp grft fem-popliteal
35585	Vein byp fem-tibial peroneal
35587	Vein byp pop-tibl peroneal
35600	Harvest art for cabg add-on
35601	Art byp common ipsi carotid
35606	Art byp carotid-subclavian
35612	Art byp subclav-subclavian
35616	Art byp subclav-axillary
35621	Art byp axillary-femoral
35623	Art byp axillary-pop-tibial
35626	Art byp aorsubcl/carot/innom
35631	Art byp aor-celiac-msn-renal
35632	Art byp ilio-celiac
35633	Art byp ilio-mesenteric
35634	Art byp iliorenal
35636	Art byp spenorenal
35637	Art byp aortoiliac
35638	Art byp aortobi-iliac
35642	Art byp carotid-vertebral
35645	Art byp subclav-vertebrl
35646	Art byp aortobifemoral
35647	Art byp aortofemoral
35650	Art byp axillary-axillary
35654	Art byp axill-fem-femoral
35656	Art byp femoral-popliteal
35661	Art byp femoral-femoral
35663	Art byp ilioiliac
35665	Art byp iliofemoral
35666	Art byp fem-ant-post tib/prl
35671	Art byp pop-tibl-prl-other
35681	Composite byp grft pros&vein
35682	Composite byp grft 2 veins
35683	Composite byp grft 3/> segmt
35691	Art trnsposj vertbrl carotid
35693	Art trnsposj subclavian
35694	Art trnsposj subclav carotid

35695 Art trnsposj carotid subclav
35697 Reimplant artery each
35700 Reoperation bypass graft
35701 Exploration carotid artery
35702 Expl n/flwd surg uxtr art
35703 Expl n/flwd surg lxtr art
35721 Exploration femoral artery
35800 Explore neck vessels
35820 Explore chest vessels
35840 Explore abdominal vessels
35870 Repair vessel graft defect
35901 Excision graft neck
35905 Excision graft thorax
35907 Excision graft abdomen
36660 Insertion catheter artery
36823 Insertion of cannula(s)
37140 Revision of circulation
37145 Revision of circulation
37160 Revision of circulation
37180 Revision of circulation
37181 Splice spleen/kidney veins
37182 Insert hepatic shunt (tips)
37215 Transcath stent cca w/eps
37217 Stent placemt retro carotid
37218 Stent placemt ante carotid
37616 Ligation of chest artery
37617 Ligation of abdomen artery
37618 Ligation of extremity artery
37660 Revision of major vein
37788 Revascularization penis
38100 Removal of spleen total
38101 Removal of spleen partial
38102 Removal of spleen total
38115 Repair of ruptured spleen
38380 Thoracic duct procedure
38381 Thoracic duct procedure
38382 Thoracic duct procedure
38562 Removal pelvic lymph nodes
38564 Removal abdomen lymph nodes
38724 Removal of lymph nodes neck
38746 Remove thoracic lymph nodes
38747 Remove abdominal lymph nodes
38765 Remove groin lymph nodes
38770 Remove pelvis lymph nodes
38780 Remove abdomen lymph nodes
39000 Exploration of chest
39010 Exploration of chest
39200 Resect mediastinal cyst
39220 Resect mediastinal tumor
39499 Chest procedure
39501 Repair diaphragm laceration
39503 Repair of diaphragm hernia
39540 Repair of diaphragm hernia
39541 Repair of diaphragm hernia
39545 Revision of diaphragm
39560 Resect diaphragm simple
39561 Resect diaphragm complex
39599 Diaphragm surgery procedure
41130 Partial removal of tongue
41135 Tongue and neck surgery
41140 Removal of tongue
41145 Tongue removal neck surgery
41150 Tongue mouth jaw surgery
41153 Tongue mouth neck surgery
41155 Tongue jaw & neck surgery
42426 Excise parotid gland/lesion
42845 Extensive surgery of throat
42894 Revision of pharyngeal walls
42953 Repair throat esophagus
42961 Control throat bleeding
42971 Control nose/throat bleeding
43045 Incision of esophagus
43100 Excision of esophagus lesion
43101 Excision of esophagus lesion
43107 Removal of esophagus
43108 Removal of esophagus
43112 Removal of esophagus
43113 Removal of esophagus
43116 Partial removal of esophagus
43117 Partial removal of esophagus
43118 Partial removal of esophagus
43121 Partial removal of esophagus
43122 Partial removal of esophagus
43123 Partial removal of esophagus
43124 Removal of esophagus
43135 Removal of esophagus pouch
43279 Lap myotomy heller
43283 Lap esoph lengthening
43286 Esphg tot w/laps moblj
43287 Esphg dstl 2/3 w/laps moblj
43288 Esphg thrsc moblj
43300 Repair of esophagus
43305 Repair esophagus and fistula
43310 Repair of esophagus
43312 Repair esophagus and fistula
43313 Esophagoplasty congenital
43314 Tracheo-esophagoplasty cong
43320 Fuse esophagus & stomach
43325 Revise esophagus & stomach
43327 Esoph fundoplasty lap
43328 Esoph fundoplasty thor
43330 Esophagomyotomy abdominal
43331 Esophagomyotomy thoracic
43332 Transab esoph hiat hern rpr
43333 Transab esoph hiat hern rpr
43334 Transthor diaphrag hern rpr
43335 Transthor diaphrag hern rpr
43336 Thorabd diaphr hern repair
43337 Thorabd diaphr hern repair
43338 Esoph lengthening
43340 Fuse esophagus & intestine
43341 Fuse esophagus & intestine
43351 Surgical opening esophagus
43352 Surgical opening esophagus
43360 Gastrointestinal repair
43361 Gastrointestinal repair
43400 Ligate esophagus veins
43405 Ligate/staple esophagus
43410 Repair esophagus wound
43415 Repair esophagus wound
43425 Repair esophagus opening
43460 Pressure treatment esophagus
43496 Free jejunum flap microvasc
43500 Surgical opening of stomach
43501 Surgical repair of stomach
43502 Surgical repair of stomach
43520 Incision of pyloric muscle
43605 Biopsy of stomach
43610 Excision of stomach lesion
43611 Excision of stomach lesion
43620 Removal of stomach
43621 Removal of stomach
43622 Removal of stomach
43631 Removal of stomach partial
43632 Removal of stomach partial
43633 Removal of stomach partial
43634 Removal of stomach partial
43635 Removal of stomach partial
43640 Vagotomy & pylorus repair
43641 Vagotomy & pylorus repair
43644 Lap gastric bypass/roux-en-y
43645 Lap gastr bypass incl smll i
43771 Lap revise gastr adj device
43775 Lap sleeve gastrectomy
43800 Reconstruction of pylorus
43810 Fusion of stomach and bowel
43820 Fusion of stomach and bowel
43825 Fusion of stomach and bowel
43832 Place gastrostomy tube
43840 Repair of stomach lesion
43843 Gastroplasty w/o v-band
43845 Gastroplasty duodenal switch
43846 Gastric bypass for obesity
43847 Gastric bypass incl small i
43848 Revision gastroplasty
43850 Revise stomach-bowel fusion
43855 Revise stomach-bowel fusion
43860 Revise stomach-bowel fusion
43865 Revise stomach-bowel fusion
43880 Repair stomach-bowel fistula
43881 Impl/redo electrd antrum
43882 Revise/remove electrd antrum
44005 Freeing of bowel adhesion
44010 Incision of small bowel
44015 Insert needle cath bowel
44020 Explore small intestine
44021 Decompress small bowel
44025 Incision of large bowel
44050 Reduce bowel obstruction
44055 Correct malrotation of bowel
44110 Excise intestine lesion(s)
44111 Excision of bowel lesion(s)
44120 Removal of small intestine
44121 Removal of small intestine
44125 Removal of small intestine
44126 Enterectomy w/o taper cong
44127 Enterectomy w/taper cong

44128	Enterectomy cong add-on
44130	Bowel to bowel fusion
44132	Enterectomy cadaver donor
44133	Enterectomy live donor
44135	Intestine transplnt cadaver
44136	Intestine transplant live
44137	Remove intestinal allograft
44139	Mobilization of colon
44140	Partial removal of colon
44141	Partial removal of colon
44143	Partial removal of colon
44144	Partial removal of colon
44145	Partial removal of colon
44146	Partial removal of colon
44147	Partial removal of colon
44150	Removal of colon
44151	Removal of colon/ileostomy
44155	Removal of colon/ileostomy
44156	Removal of colon/ileostomy
44157	Colectomy w/ileoanal anast
44158	Colectomy w/neo-rectum pouch
44160	Removal of colon
44187	Lap ileo/jejuno-stomy
44188	Lap colostomy
44202	Lap enterectomy
44203	Lap resect s/intestine addl
44204	Laparo partial colectomy
44205	Lap colectomy part w/ileum
44206	Lap part colectomy w/stoma
44207	L colectomy/coloproctostomy
44208	L colectomy/coloproctostomy
44210	Laparo total proctocolectomy
44211	Lap colectomy w/proctectomy
44212	Laparo total proctocolectomy
44213	Lap mobil splenic fl add-on
44227	Lap close enterostomy
44300	Open bowel to skin
44310	Ileostomy/jejunostomy
44314	Revision of ileostomy
44316	Devise bowel pouch
44320	Colostomy
44322	Colostomy with biopsies
44345	Revision of colostomy
44346	Revision of colostomy
44602	Suture small intestine
44603	Suture small intestine
44604	Suture large intestine
44605	Repair of bowel lesion
44615	Intestinal strictureplasty
44620	Repair bowel opening
44625	Repair bowel opening
44626	Repair bowel opening
44640	Repair bowel-skin fistula
44650	Repair bowel fistula
44660	Repair bowel-bladder fistula
44661	Repair bowel-bladder fistula
44680	Surgical revision intestine
44700	Suspend bowel w/prosthesis
44715	Prepare donor intestine
44720	Prep donor intestine/venous
44721	Prep donor intestine/artery
44800	Excision of bowel pouch
44820	Excision of mesentery lesion
44850	Repair of mesentery
44899	Bowel surgery procedure
44900	Drain appendix abscess open
44960	Appendectomy
45110	Removal of rectum
45111	Partial removal of rectum
45112	Removal of rectum
45113	Partial proctectomy
45114	Partial removal of rectum
45116	Partial removal of rectum
45119	Remove rectum w/reservoir
45120	Removal of rectum
45121	Removal of rectum and colon
45123	Partial proctectomy
45126	Pelvic exenteration
45130	Excision of rectal prolapse
45135	Excision of rectal prolapse
45136	Excise ileoanal reservior
45395	Lap removal of rectum
45397	Lap remove rectum w/pouch
45400	Laparoscopic proc
45402	Lap proctopexy w/sig resect
45540	Correct rectal prolapse
45550	Repair rectum/remove sigmoid
45562	Exploration/repair of rectum
45563	Exploration/repair of rectum
45800	Repair rect/bladder fistula
45805	Repair fistula w/colostomy
45820	Repair rectourethral fistula
45825	Repair fistula w/colostomy
46705	Repair of anal stricture
46710	Repr per/vag pouch sngl proc
46712	Repr per/vag pouch dbl proc
46715	Rep perf anoper fistu
46716	Rep perf anoper/vestib fistu
46730	Construction of absent anus
46735	Construction of absent anus
46740	Construction of absent anus
46742	Repair of imperforated anus
46744	Repair of cloacal anomaly
46746	Repair of cloacal anomaly
46748	Repair of cloacal anomaly
46751	Repair of anal sphincter
47010	Open drainage liver lesion
47015	Inject/aspirate liver cyst
47100	Wedge biopsy of liver
47120	Partial removal of liver
47122	Extensive removal of liver
47125	Partial removal of liver
47130	Partial removal of liver
47133	Removal of donor liver
47135	Transplantation of liver
47140	Partial removal donor liver
47141	Partial removal donor liver
47142	Partial removal donor liver
47143	Prep donor liver whole
47144	Prep donor liver 3-segment
47145	Prep donor liver lobe split
47146	Prep donor liver/venous
47147	Prep donor liver/arterial
47300	Surgery for liver lesion
47350	Repair liver wound
47360	Repair liver wound
47361	Repair liver wound
47362	Repair liver wound
47380	Open ablate liver tumor rf
47381	Open ablate liver tumor cryo
47400	Incision of liver duct
47420	Incision of bile duct
47425	Incision of bile duct
47460	Incise bile duct sphincter
47480	Incision of gallbladder
47550	Bile duct endoscopy add-on
47570	Laparo cholecystoenterostomy
47600	Removal of gallbladder
47605	Removal of gallbladder
47610	Removal of gallbladder
47612	Removal of gallbladder
47620	Removal of gallbladder
47700	Exploration of bile ducts
47701	Bile duct revision
47711	Excision of bile duct tumor
47712	Excision of bile duct tumor
47715	Excision of bile duct cyst
47720	Fuse gallbladder & bowel
47721	Fuse upper gi structures
47740	Fuse gallbladder & bowel
47741	Fuse gallbladder & bowel
47760	Fuse bile ducts and bowel
47765	Fuse liver ducts & bowel
47780	Fuse bile ducts and bowel
47785	Fuse bile ducts and bowel
47800	Reconstruction of bile ducts
47801	Placement bile duct support
47802	Fuse liver duct & intestine
47900	Suture bile duct injury
48000	Drainage of abdomen
48001	Placement of drain pancreas
48020	Removal of pancreatic stone
48100	Biopsy of pancreas open
48105	Resect/debride pancreas
48120	Removal of pancreas lesion
48140	Partial removal of pancreas
48145	Partial removal of pancreas
48146	Pancreatectomy
48148	Removal of pancreatic duct
48150	Partial removal of pancreas
48152	Pancreatectomy
48153	Pancreatectomy
48154	Pancreatectomy
48155	Removal of pancreas
48400	Injection intraop add-on
48500	Surgery of pancreatic cyst
48510	Drain pancreatic pseudocyst

48520 Fuse pancreas cyst and bowel
48540 Fuse pancreas cyst and bowel
48545 Pancreatorrhaphy
48547 Duodenal exclusion
48548 Fuse pancreas and bowel
48551 Prep donor pancreas
48552 Prep donor pancreas/venous
48554 Transpl allograft pancreas
48556 Removal allograft pancreas
49000 Exploration of abdomen
49002 Reopening of abdomen
49010 Exploration behind abdomen
49013 Prpertl pel pack hemrrg trma
49014 Reexploration pelvic wound
49020 Drainage abdom abscess open
49040 Drain open abdom abscess
49060 Drain open retroperi abscess
49062 Drain to peritoneal cavity
49203 Exc abd tum 5 cm or less
49204 Exc abd tum over 5 cm
49205 Exc abd tum over 10 cm
49215 Excise sacral spine tumor
49220 Multiple surgery abdomen
49255 Removal of omentum
49412 Ins device for rt guide open
49425 Insert abdomen-venous drain
49428 Ligation of shunt
49605 Repair umbilical lesion
49606 Repair umbilical lesion
49610 Repair umbilical lesion
49611 Repair umbilical lesion
49900 Repair of abdominal wall
49904 Omental flap extra-abdom
49905 Omental flap intra-abdom
49906 Free omental flap microvasc
50010 Exploration of kidney
50040 Drainage of kidney
50045 Exploration of kidney
50060 Removal of kidney stone
50065 Incision of kidney
50070 Incision of kidney
50075 Removal of kidney stone
50100 Revise kidney blood vessels
50120 Exploration of kidney
50125 Explore and drain kidney
50130 Removal of kidney stone
50135 Exploration of kidney
50205 Renal biopsy open
50220 Remove kidney open
50225 Removal kidney open complex
50230 Removal kidney open radical
50234 Removal of kidney & ureter
50236 Removal of kidney & ureter
50240 Partial removal of kidney
50250 Cryoablate renal mass open
50280 Removal of kidney lesion
50290 Removal of kidney lesion
50300 Remove cadaver donor kidney
50320 Remove kidney living donor
50323 Prep cadaver renal allograft
50325 Prep donor renal graft
50327 Prep renal graft/venous
50328 Prep renal graft/arterial
50329 Prep renal graft/ureteral
50340 Removal of kidney
50360 Transplantation of kidney
50365 Transplantation of kidney
50370 Remove transplanted kidney
50380 Reimplantation of kidney
50400 Revision of kidney/ureter
50405 Revision of kidney/ureter
50500 Repair of kidney wound
50520 Close kidney-skin fistula
50525 Close nephrovisceral fistula
50526 Close nephrovisceral fistula
50540 Revision of horseshoe kidney
50545 Laparo radical nephrectomy
50546 Laparoscopic nephrectomy
50547 Laparo removal donor kidney
50548 Laparo remove w/ureter
50600 Exploration of ureter
50605 Insert ureteral support
50610 Removal of ureter stone
50620 Removal of ureter stone
50630 Removal of ureter stone
50650 Removal of ureter
50660 Removal of ureter
50700 Revision of ureter
50715 Release of ureter
50722 Release of ureter
50725 Release/revise ureter
50728 Revise ureter
50740 Fusion of ureter & kidney
50750 Fusion of ureter & kidney
50760 Fusion of ureters
50770 Splicing of ureters
50780 Reimplant ureter in bladder
50782 Reimplant ureter in bladder
50783 Reimplant ureter in bladder
50785 Reimplant ureter in bladder
50800 Implant ureter in bowel
50810 Fusion of ureter & bowel
50815 Urine shunt to intestine
50820 Construct bowel bladder
50825 Construct bowel bladder
50830 Revise urine flow
50840 Replace ureter by bowel
50845 Appendico-vesicostomy
50860 Transplant ureter to skin
50900 Repair of ureter
50920 Closure ureter/skin fistula
50930 Closure ureter/bowel fistula
50940 Release of ureter
51525 Removal of bladder lesion
51530 Removal of bladder lesion
51550 Partial removal of bladder
51555 Partial removal of bladder
51565 Revise bladder & ureter(s)
51570 Removal of bladder
51575 Removal of bladder & nodes
51580 Remove bladder/revise tract
51585 Removal of bladder & nodes
51590 Remove bladder/revise tract
51595 Remove bladder/revise tract
51596 Remove bladder/create pouch
51597 Removal of pelvic structures
51800 Revision of bladder/urethra
51820 Revision of urinary tract
51840 Attach bladder/urethra
51841 Attach bladder/urethra
51865 Repair of bladder wound
51900 Repair bladder/vagina lesion
51920 Close bladder-uterus fistula
51925 Hysterectomy/bladder repair
51940 Correction of bladder defect
51960 Revision of bladder & bowel
51980 Construct bladder opening
53415 Reconstruction of urethra
53448 Remov/replc ur sphinctr comp
54125 Removal of penis
54130 Remove penis & nodes
54135 Remove penis & nodes
54390 Repair penis and bladder
54430 Revision of penis
54438 Replantation of penis
55605 Incise sperm duct pouch
55650 Remove sperm duct pouch
55801 Removal of prostate
55810 Extensive prostate surgery
55812 Extensive prostate surgery
55815 Extensive prostate surgery
55821 Removal of prostate
55831 Removal of prostate
55840 Extensive prostate surgery
55842 Extensive prostate surgery
55845 Extensive prostate surgery
55862 Extensive prostate surgery
55865 Extensive prostate surgery
56630 Extensive vulva surgery
56631 Extensive vulva surgery
56632 Extensive vulva surgery
56633 Extensive vulva surgery
56634 Extensive vulva surgery
56637 Extensive vulva surgery
56640 Extensive vulva surgery
57110 Remove vagina wall complete
57111 Remove vagina tissue compl
57112 Vaginectomy w/nodes compl
57270 Repair of bowel pouch
57280 Suspension of vagina
57296 Revise vag graft open abd
57305 Repair rectum-vagina fistula
57307 Fistula repair & colostomy
57308 Fistula repair transperine
57311 Repair urethrovaginal lesion
57531 Removal of cervix radical
57540 Removal of residual cervix

57545 Remove cervix/repair pelvis
58140 Myomectomy abdom method
58146 Myomectomy abdom complex
58150 Total hysterectomy
58152 Total hysterectomy
58180 Partial hysterectomy
58200 Extensive hysterectomy
58210 Extensive hysterectomy
58240 Removal of pelvis contents
58267 Vag hyst w/urinary repair
58275 Hysterectomy/revise vagina
58280 Hysterectomy/revise vagina
58285 Extensive hysterectomy
58293 Vag hyst w/uro repair compl
58400 Suspension of uterus
58410 Suspension of uterus
58520 Repair of ruptured uterus
58540 Revision of uterus
58548 Lap radical hyst
58575 Laps tot hyst resj mal
58605 Division of fallopian tube
58611 Ligate oviduct(s) add-on
58700 Removal of fallopian tube
58720 Removal of ovary/tube(s)
58740 Adhesiolysis tube ovary
58750 Repair oviduct
58752 Revise ovarian tube(s)
58760 Fimbrioplasty
58822 Drain ovary abscess percut
58825 Transposition ovary(s)
58940 Removal of ovary(s)
58943 Removal of ovary(s)
58950 Resect ovarian malignancy
58951 Resect ovarian malignancy
58952 Resect ovarian malignancy
58953 Tah rad dissect for debulk
58954 Tah rad debulk/lymph remove
58956 Bso omentectomy w/tah
58957 Resect recurrent gyn mal
58958 Resect recur gyn mal w/lym
58960 Exploration of abdomen
59120 Treat ectopic pregnancy
59121 Treat ectopic pregnancy
59130 Treat ectopic pregnancy
59135 Treat ectopic pregnancy
59136 Treat ectopic pregnancy
59140 Treat ectopic pregnancy
59325 Revision of cervix
59350 Repair of uterus
59514 Cesarean delivery only
59525 Remove uterus after cesarean
59620 Attempted vbac delivery only
59830 Treat uterus infection
59850 Abortion
59851 Abortion
59852 Abortion
59855 Abortion
59856 Abortion
59857 Abortion

60254 Extensive thyroid surgery
60270 Removal of thyroid
60505 Explore parathyroid glands
60521 Removal of thymus gland
60522 Removal of thymus gland
60540 Explore adrenal gland
60545 Explore adrenal gland
60600 Remove carotid body lesion
60605 Remove carotid body lesion
60650 Laparoscopy adrenalectomy
61105 Twist drill hole
61107 Drill skull for implantation
61108 Drill skull for drainage
61120 Burr hole for puncture
61140 Pierce skull for biopsy
61150 Pierce skull for drainage
61151 Pierce skull for drainage
61154 Pierce skull & remove clot
61156 Pierce skull for drainage
61210 Pierce skull implant device
61250 Pierce skull & explore
61253 Pierce skull & explore
61304 Open skull for exploration
61305 Open skull for exploration
61312 Open skull for drainage
61313 Open skull for drainage
61314 Open skull for drainage
61315 Open skull for drainage
61316 Implt cran bone flap to abdo
61320 Open skull for drainage
61321 Open skull for drainage
61322 Decompressive craniotomy
61323 Decompressive lobectomy
61333 Explore orbit/remove lesion
61340 Subtemporal decompression
61343 Incise skull (press relief)
61345 Relieve cranial pressure
61450 Incise skull for surgery
61458 Incise skull for brain wound
61460 Incise skull for surgery
61500 Removal of skull lesion
61501 Remove infected skull bone
61510 Removal of brain lesion
61512 Remove brain lining lesion
61514 Removal of brain abscess
61516 Removal of brain lesion
61517 Implt brain chemotx add-on
61518 Removal of brain lesion
61519 Remove brain lining lesion
61520 Removal of brain lesion
61521 Removal of brain lesion
61522 Removal of brain abscess
61524 Removal of brain lesion
61526 Removal of brain lesion
61530 Removal of brain lesion
61531 Implant brain electrodes
61533 Implant brain electrodes
61534 Removal of brain lesion
61535 Remove brain electrodes

61536 Removal of brain lesion
61537 Removal of brain tissue
61538 Removal of brain tissue
61539 Removal of brain tissue
61540 Removal of brain tissue
61541 Incision of brain tissue
61543 Removal of brain tissue
61544 Remove & treat brain lesion
61545 Excision of brain tumor
61546 Removal of pituitary gland
61548 Removal of pituitary gland
61550 Release of skull seams
61552 Release of skull seams
61556 Incise skull/sutures
61557 Incise skull/sutures
61558 Excision of skull/sutures
61559 Excision of skull/sutures
61563 Excision of skull tumor
61564 Excision of skull tumor
61566 Removal of brain tissue
61567 Incision of brain tissue
61570 Remove foreign body brain
61571 Incise skull for brain wound
61575 Skull base/brainstem surgery
61576 Skull base/brainstem surgery
61580 Craniofacial approach skull
61581 Craniofacial approach skull
61582 Craniofacial approach skull
61583 Craniofacial approach skull
61584 Orbitocranial approach/skull
61585 Orbitocranial approach/skull
61586 Resect nasopharynx skull
61590 Infratemporal approach/skull
61591 Infratemporal approach/skull
61592 Orbitocranial approach/skull
61595 Transtemporal approach/skull
61596 Transcochlear approach/skull
61597 Transcondylar approach/skull
61598 Transpetrosal approach/skull
61600 Resect/excise cranial lesion
61601 Resect/excise cranial lesion
61605 Resect/excise cranial lesion
61606 Resect/excise cranial lesion
61607 Resect/excise cranial lesion
61608 Resect/excise cranial lesion
61611 Transect artery sinus
61613 Remove aneurysm sinus
61615 Resect/excise lesion skull
61616 Resect/excise lesion skull
61618 Repair dura
61619 Repair dura
61624 Transcath occlusion cns
61630 Intracranial angioplasty
61635 Intracran angioplsty w/stent
61645 Perq art m-thrombect &/nfs
61650 Evasc prlng admn rx agnt 1st
61651 Evasc prlng admn rx agnt add
61680 Intracranial vessel surgery
61682 Intracranial vessel surgery

61684 Intracranial vessel surgery
61686 Intracranial vessel surgery
61690 Intracranial vessel surgery
61692 Intracranial vessel surgery
61697 Brain aneurysm repr complx
61698 Brain aneurysm repr complx
61700 Brain aneurysm repr simple
61702 Inner skull vessel surgery
61703 Clamp neck artery
61705 Revise circulation to head
61708 Revise circulation to head
61710 Revise circulation to head
61711 Fusion of skull arteries
61735 Incise skull/brain surgery
61750 Incise skull/brain biopsy
61751 Brain biopsy w/ct/mr guide
61760 Implant brain electrodes
61850 Implant neuroelectrodes
61860 Implant neuroelectrodes
61863 Implant neuroelectrode
61864 Implant neuroelectrde addl
61867 Implant neuroelectrode
61868 Implant neuroelectrde addl
61870 Implant neuroelectrodes
62005 Treat skull fracture
62010 Treatment of head injury
62100 Repair brain fluid leakage
62115 Reduction of skull defect
62117 Reduction of skull defect
62120 Repair skull cavity lesion
62121 Incise skull repair
62140 Repair of skull defect
62141 Repair of skull defect
62142 Remove skull plate/flap
62143 Replace skull plate/flap
62145 Repair of skull & brain
62146 Repair of skull with graft
62147 Repair of skull with graft
62148 Retr bone flap to fix skull
62161 Dissect brain w/scope
62162 Remove colloid cyst w/scope
62163 Zneuroendoscopy w/fb removal
62164 Remove brain tumor w/scope
62165 Remove pituit tumor w/scope
62180 Establish brain cavity shunt
62190 Establish brain cavity shunt
62192 Establish brain cavity shunt
62200 Establish brain cavity shunt
62201 Brain cavity shunt w/scope
62220 Establish brain cavity shunt
62223 Establish brain cavity shunt
62256 Remove brain cavity shunt
62258 Replace brain cavity shunt
63050 Cervical laminoplsty 2/> seg
63051 C-laminoplasty w/graft/plate
63077 Spine disk surgery thorax
63078 Spine disk surgery thorax
63081 Remove vert body dcmprn crvl
63082 Remove vertebral body add-on
63085 Remove vert body dcmprn thrc
63086 Remove vertebral body add-on
63087 Remov vertbr dcmprn thrclmbr
63088 Remove vertebral body add-on
63090 Remove vert body dcmprn lmbr
63091 Remove vertebral body add-on
63101 Remove vert body dcmprn thrc
63102 Remove vert body dcmprn lmbr
63103 Remove vertebral body add-on
63170 Incise spinal cord tract(s)
63172 Drainage of spinal cyst
63173 Drainage of spinal cyst
63180 Revise spinal cord ligaments
63182 Revise spinal cord ligaments
63185 Incise spine nrv half segmnt
63190 Incise spine nrv >2 segmnts
63191 Incise spine accessory nerve
63194 Incise spine & cord cervical
63195 Incise spine & cord thoracic
63196 Incise spine&cord 2 trx crvl
63197 Incise spine&cord 2 trx thrc
63198 Incise spin&cord 2 stgs crvl
63199 Incise spin&cord 2 stgs thrc
63200 Release spinal cord lumbar
63250 Revise spinal cord vsls crvl
63251 Revise spinal cord vsls thrc
63252 Revise spine cord vsl thrlmb
63270 Excise intrspinl lesion crvl
63271 Excise intrspinl lesion thrc
63272 Excise intrspinl lesion lmbr
63273 Excise intrspinl lesion scrl
63275 Bx/exc xdrl spine lesn crvl
63276 Bx/exc xdrl spine lesn thrc
63277 Bx/exc xdrl spine lesn lmbr
63278 Bx/exc xdrl spine lesn scrl
63280 Bx/exc idrl spine lesn crvl
63281 Bx/exc idrl spine lesn thrc
63282 Bx/exc idrl spine lesn lmbr
63283 Bx/exc idrl spine lesn scrl
63285 Bx/exc idrl imed lesn cervl
63286 Bx/exc idrl imed lesn thrc
63287 Bx/exc idrl imed lesn thrlmb
63290 Bx/exc xdrl/idrl lsn any lvl
63295 Repair laminectomy defect
63300 Remove vert xdrl body crvcl
63301 Remove vert xdrl body thrc
63302 Remove vert xdrl body thrlmb
63303 Remov vert xdrl bdy lmbr/sac
63304 Remove vert idrl body crvcl
63305 Remove vert idrl body thrc
63306 Remov vert idrl bdy thrclmbr
63307 Remov vert idrl bdy lmbr/sac
63308 Remove vertebral body add-on
63700 Repair of spinal herniation
63702 Repair of spinal herniation
63704 Repair of spinal herniation
63706 Repair of spinal herniation
63707 Repair spinal fluid leakage
63709 Repair spinal fluid leakage
63710 Graft repair of spine defect
63740 Install spinal shunt
64755 Incision of stomach nerves
64760 Incision of vagus nerve
64809 Remove sympathetic nerves
64818 Remove sympathetic nerves
64866 Fusion of facial/other nerve
64868 Fusion of facial/other nerve
65273 Repair of eye wound
69155 Extensive ear/neck surgery
69535 Remove part of temporal bone
69554 Remove ear lesion
69950 Incise inner ear nerve
75956 Xray endovasc thor ao repr
75957 Xray endovasc thor ao repr
75958 Xray place prox ext thor ao
75959 Xray place dist ext thor ao
92941 Prq card revasc mi 1 vsl
92970 Cardioassist internal
92971 Cardioassist external
92975 Dissolve clot heart vessel
92992 Revision of heart chamber
92993 Revision of heart chamber
93583 Perq transcath septal reduxn
99184 Hypothermia ill neonate
99190 Special pump services
99191 Special pump services
99192 Special pump services
99356 Prolonged service inpatient
99357 Prolonged service inpatient
99462 Sbsq nb em per day hosp
99468 Neonate crit care initial
99469 Neonate crit care subsq
99471 Ped critical care initial
99472 Ped critical care subsq
99475 Ped crit care age 2-5 init
99476 Ped crit care age 2-5 subsq
99477 Init day hosp neonate care
99478 Ic lbw inf < 1500 gm subsq
99479 Ic lbw inf 1500-2500 g subsq
99480 Ic inf pbw 2501-5000 g subsq
C9606 PC H rev ac tot/subtot occl 1 ves
G0341 Percutaneous islet celltrans
G0342 Laparoscopy islet cell trans
G0343 Laparotomy islet cell transp
G0412 Open tx iliac spine uni/bil
G0414 Pelvic ring fx treat int fix
G0415 Open tx post pelvic fxcture

Appendix K — Place of Service and Type of Service

Place-of-Service Codes for Professional Claims

Listed below are place of service codes and descriptions. These codes should be used on professional claims to specify the entity where service(s) were rendered. Check with individual payers (e.g., Medicare, Medicaid, other private insurance) for reimbursement policies regarding these codes. To comment on a code(s) or description(s), please send your request to posinfo@cms.gov.

01	Pharmacy	A facility or location where drugs and other medically related items and services are sold, dispensed, or otherwise provided directly to patients.
02	Telehealth	The location where health services and health related services are provided or received through telecommunication technology.
03	School	A facility whose primary purpose is education.
04	Homeless shelter	A facility or location whose primary purpose is to provide temporary housing to homeless individuals (e.g., emergency shelters, individual or family shelters).
05	Indian Health Service freestanding facility	A facility or location, owned and operated by the Indian Health Service, which provides diagnostic, therapeutic (surgical and non-surgical), and rehabilitation services to American Indians and Alaska natives who do not require hospitalization.
06	Indian Health Service provider-based facility	A facility or location, owned and operated by the Indian Health Service, which provides diagnostic, therapeutic (surgical and nonsurgical), and rehabilitation services rendered by, or under the supervision of, physicians to American Indians and Alaska natives admitted as inpatients or outpatients.
07	Tribal 638 freestanding facility	A facility or location owned and operated by a federally recognized American Indian or Alaska native tribe or tribal organization under a 638 agreement, which provides diagnostic, therapeutic (surgical and nonsurgical), and rehabilitation services to tribal members who do not require hospitalization.
08	Tribal 638 provider-based Facility	A facility or location owned and operated by a federally recognized American Indian or Alaska native tribe or tribal organization under a 638 agreement, which provides diagnostic, therapeutic (surgical and nonsurgical), and rehabilitation services to tribal members admitted as inpatients or outpatients.
09	Prison/correctional facility	A prison, jail, reformatory, work farm, detention center, or any other similar facility maintained by either federal, state or local authorities for the purpose of confinement or rehabilitation of adult or juvenile criminal offenders.
10	Unassigned	N/A
11	Office	Location, other than a hospital, skilled nursing facility (SNF), military treatment facility, community health center, State or local public health clinic, or intermediate care facility (ICF), where the health professional routinely provides health examinations, diagnosis, and treatment of illness or injury on an ambulatory basis.
12	Home	Location, other than a hospital or other facility, where the patient receives care in a private residence.
13	Assisted living facility	Congregate residential facility with self-contained living units providing assessment of each resident's needs and on-site support 24 hours a day, 7 days a week, with the capacity to deliver or arrange for services including some health care and other services.
14	Group home	A residence, with shared living areas, where clients receive supervision and other services such as social and/or behavioral services, custodial service, and minimal services (e.g., medication administration).
15	Mobile unit	A facility/unit that moves from place-to-place equipped to provide preventive, screening, diagnostic, and/or treatment services.
16	Temporary lodging	A short-term accommodation such as a hotel, campground, hostel, cruise ship or resort where the patient receives care, and which is not identified by any other POS code.
17	Walk-in retail health clinic	A walk-in health clinic, other than an office, urgent care facility, pharmacy, or independent clinic and not described by any other place of service code, that is located within a retail operation and provides preventive and primary care services on an ambulatory basis.
18	Place of employment/ worksite	A location, not described by any other POS code, owned or operated by a public or private entity where the patient is employed, and where a health professional provides on-going or episodic occupational medical, therapeutic or rehabilitative services to the individual.
19	Off campus-outpatient hospital	A portion of an off-campus hospital provider based department which provides diagnostic, therapeutic (both surgical and nonsurgical), and rehabilitation services to sick or injured persons who do not require hospitalization or institutionalization.
20	Urgent care facility	Location, distinct from a hospital emergency room, an office, or a clinic, whose purpose is to diagnose and treat illness or injury for unscheduled, ambulatory patients seeking immediate medical attention.

21	Inpatient hospital	A facility, other than psychiatric, which primarily provides diagnostic, therapeutic (both surgical and nonsurgical), and rehabilitation services by, or under, the supervision of physicians to patients admitted for a variety of medical conditions.
22	On campus-outpatient hospital	A portion of a hospital's main campus which provides diagnostic, therapeutic (both surgical and nonsurgical), and rehabilitation services to sick or injured persons who do not require hospitalization or institutionalization.
23	Emergency room—hospital	A portion of a hospital where emergency diagnosis and treatment of illness or injury is provided.
24	Ambulatory surgical center	A freestanding facility, other than a physician's office, where surgical and diagnostic services are provided on an ambulatory basis.
25	Birthing center	A facility, other than a hospital's maternity facilities or a physician's office, which provides a setting for labor, delivery, and immediate post-partum care as well as immediate care of new born infants.
26	Military treatment facility	A medical facility operated by one or more of the uniformed services. Military treatment facility (MTF) also refers to certain former U.S. Public Health Service (USPHS) facilities now designated as uniformed service treatment facilities (USTF).
27-30	Unassigned	N/A
31	Skilled nursing facility	A facility which primarily provides inpatient skilled nursing care and related services to patients who require medical, nursing, or rehabilitative services but does not provide the level of care or treatment available in a hospital.
32	Nursing facility	A facility which primarily provides to residents skilled nursing care and related services for the rehabilitation of injured, disabled, or sick persons, or, on a regular basis, health-related care services above the level of custodial care to individuals other than those with intellectual disabilities.
33	Custodial care facility	A facility which provides room, board, and other personal assistance services, generally on a long-term basis, and which does not include a medical component.
34	Hospice	A facility, other than a patient's home, in which palliative and supportive care for terminally ill patients and their families is provided.
35-40	Unassigned	N/A
41	Ambulance—land	A land vehicle specifically designed, equipped and staffed for lifesaving and transporting the sick or injured.
42	Ambulance—air or water	An air or water vehicle specifically designed, equipped and staffed for lifesaving and transporting the sick or injured.
43-48	Unassigned	N/A
49	Independent clinic	A location, not part of a hospital and not described by any other place-of-service code, that is organized and operated to provide preventive, diagnostic, therapeutic, rehabilitative, or palliative services to outpatients only.
50	Federally qualified health center	A facility located in a medically underserved area that provides Medicare beneficiaries with preventive primary medical care under the general direction of a physician.
51	Inpatient psychiatric facility	A facility that provides inpatient psychiatric services for the diagnosis and treatment of mental illness on a 24-hour basis, by or under the supervision of a physician.
52	Psychiatric facility-partial hospitalization	A facility for the diagnosis and treatment of mental illness that provides a planned therapeutic program for patients who do not require full time hospitalization, but who need broader programs than are possible from outpatient visits to a hospital-based or hospital-affiliated facility.
53	Community mental health center	A facility that provides the following services: outpatient services, including specialized outpatient services for children, the elderly, individuals who are chronically ill, and residents of the CMHC's mental health services area who have been discharged from inpatient treatment at a mental health facility; 24 hour a day emergency care services; day treatment, other partial hospitalization services, or psychosocial rehabilitation services; screening for patients being considered for admission to state mental health facilities to determine the appropriateness of such admission; and consultation and education services.
54	Intermediate care facility/individuals with intellectual disabilities	A facility which primarily provides health-related care and services above the level of custodial care to individuals with Intellectual Disabilities but does not provide the level of care or treatment available in a hospital or SNF.
55	Residential substance abuse treatment facility	A facility which provides treatment for substance (alcohol and drug) abuse to live-in residents who do not require acute medical care. Services include individual and group therapy and counseling, family counseling, laboratory tests, drugs and supplies, psychological testing, and room and board.
56	Psychiatric residential treatment center	A facility or distinct part of a facility for psychiatric care which provides a total 24-hour therapeutically planned and professionally staffed group living and learning environment.
57	Non-residential substance abuse treatment facility	A location which provides treatment for substance (alcohol and drug) abuse on an ambulatory basis. Services include individual and group therapy and counseling, family counseling, laboratory tests, drugs and supplies, and psychological testing.

58	Non-residential opioid treatment facility	A location that provides treatment for opioid use disorder on an ambulatory basis. Services include methadone and other forms of medication assisted treatment (MAT).
59	Unassigned	N/A
60	Mass immunization center	A location where providers administer pneumococcal pneumonia and influenza virus vaccinations and submit these services as electronic media claims, paper claims, or using the roster billing method. This generally takes place in a mass immunization setting, such as, a public health center, pharmacy, or mall but may include a physician office setting.
61	Comprehensive inpatient rehabilitation facility	A facility that provides comprehensive rehabilitation services under the supervision of a physician to inpatients with physical disabilities. Services include physical therapy, occupational therapy, speech pathology, social or psychological services, and orthotics and prosthetics services.
62	Comprehensive outpatient rehabilitation facility	A facility that provides comprehensive rehabilitation services under the supervision of a physician to outpatients with physical disabilities. Services include physical therapy, occupational therapy, and speech pathology services.
63-64	Unassigned	N/A
65	End-stage renal disease treatment facility	A facility other than a hospital, which provides dialysis treatment, maintenance, and/or training to patients or caregivers on an ambulatory or home-care basis.
66-70	Unassigned	N/A
71	Public health clinic	A facility maintained by either state or local health departments that provides ambulatory primary medical care under the general direction of a physician.
72	Rural health clinic	A certified facility which is located in a rural medically underserved area that provides ambulatory primary medical care under the general direction of a physician.
73-80	Unassigned	N/A
81	Independent laboratory	A laboratory certified to perform diagnostic and/or clinical tests independent of an institution or a physician's office.
82-98	Unassigned	N/A
99	Other place of service	Other place of service not identified above.

Type of Service

Common Working File Type of Service (TOS) Indicators

For submitting a claim to the Common Working File (CWF), use the following table to assign the proper TOS. Some procedures may have more than one applicable TOS. CWF will reject codes with incorrect TOS designations. CWF will produce alerts on codes with incorrect TOS designations.

The only exceptions to this annual update are:

- Surgical services billed for dates of service through December 31, 2007, containing the ASC facility service modifier SG must be reported as TOS F. Effective for services on or after January 1, 2008, the SG modifier is no longer applicable for Medicare services. ASC providers should discontinue applying the SG modifier on ASC facility claims. The indicator F does not appear in the TOS table because its use depends upon claims submitted with POS 24 (ASC facility) from an ASC (specialty 49). This became effective for dates of service January 1, 2008, or after.
- Surgical services billed with an assistant-at-surgery modifier (80-82, AS) must be reported with TOS 8. The 8 indicator does not appear on the TOS table because its use is dependent upon the use of the appropriate modifier. (See Pub. 100-4 *Medicare Claims Processing Manual,* chapter 12, "Physician/Practitioner Billing," for instructions on when assistant-at-surgery is allowable.)
- TOS H appears in the list of descriptors. However, it does not appear in the table. In CWF, "H" is used only as an indicator for hospice. The contractor should not submit TOS H to CWF at this time.
- For outpatient services, when a transfusion medicine code appears on a claim that also contains a blood product, the service is paid under reasonable charge at 80 percent; coinsurance and deductible apply. When transfusion medicine codes are paid under the clinical laboratory fee schedule they are paid at 100 percent; coinsurance and deductible do not apply.

Note: For injection codes with more than one possible TOS designation, use the following guidelines when assigning the TOS:

When the choice is L or 1:

- Use TOS L when the drug is used related to ESRD; or
- Use TOS 1 when the drug is not related to ESRD and is administered in the office.

When the choice is G or 1:

- Use TOS G when the drug is an immunosuppressive drug; or
- Use TOS 1 when the drug is used for other than immunosuppression.

When the choice is P or 1:

- Use TOS P if the drug is administered through durable medical equipment (DME); or
- Use TOS 1 if the drug is administered in the office.

The place of service or diagnosis may be considered when determining the appropriate TOS. The descriptors for each of the TOS codes listed in the annual HCPCS update are:

0	Whole blood
1	Medical care
2	Surgery
3	Consultation
4	Diagnostic radiology
5	Diagnostic laboratory
6	Therapeutic radiology
7	Anesthesia
8	Assistant at surgery
9	Other medical items or services
A	Used DME
B	High risk screening mammography
C	Low risk screening mammography
D	Ambulance
E	Enteral/parenteral nutrients/supplies
F	Ambulatory surgical center (facility usage for surgical services)
G	Immunosuppressive drugs
H	Hospice
J	Diabetic shoes
K	Hearing items and services
L	ESRD supplies
M	Monthly capitation payment for dialysis
N	Kidney donor
P	Lump sum purchase of DME, prosthetics, orthotics
Q	Vision items or services

R	Rental of DME
S	Surgical dressings or other medical supplies
U	Occupational therapy
V	Pneumococcal/flu vaccine
W	Physical therapy

Appendix L — Multianalyte Assays with Algorithmic Analyses

The following tables contain the Administrative Codes for Multianalyte Assays with Algorithmic Analyses (MAAA), category I codes for MAAA and the most current list of Proprietary Laboratory Analysis (PLA) codes.

The following is a list of MAAA procedures that are usually exclusive to one single clinical laboratory or manufacturer. These tests use the results from several different assays, including molecular pathology assays, fluorescent in situ hybridization assays, and nonnucleic acid-based assays (e.g., proteins, polypeptides, lipids, and carbohydrates) to perform an algorithmic analysis that is reported as a numeric score or probability. Although the laboratory report may list results of individual component tests of the MAAAs, these assays are not separately reportable.

The following list includes the proprietary name and clinical laboratory/manufacturer, an alphanumeric code, and the code descriptor.

The format for the code descriptor usually includes:

- Type of disease (e.g., oncology, autoimmune, tissue rejection)
- Chemical(s) analyzed (e.g., DNA, RNA, protein, antibody)
- Number of markers (e.g., number of genes, number of proteins)
- Methodology(s) (e.g., microarray, real-time [RT]-PCR, in situ hybridization [ISH], enzyme linked immunosorbent assays [ELISA])
- Number of functional domains (when indicated)
- Type of specimen (e.g., blood, fresh tissue, formalin-fixed paraffin embedded)
- Type of algorithm result (e.g., prognostic, diagnostic)
- Report (e.g., probability index, risk score)

MAAA procedures with a Category I code are noted on the following list and can also be found in code range 81500–81599 in the pathology and laboratory chapter. If a specific MAAA test does not have a Category I code, it is denoted with a four-digit number and the letter M. Use code 81599 if an MAAA test is not included on the following list or in the Category I codes. The codes on the list are exclusive to the assays identified by proprietary name. Report code 81599 also when an analysis is performed that may possibly fall within a specific descriptor but the proprietary name is not included in the list. The list does not contain all MAAA procedures.

Proprietary Name/Clinical Laboratory/Manufacturer	Code	Descriptor
Administrative Codes for Multianalyte Assays with Algorithmic Analyses (MAAA)		
	0001M (0001M has been deleted. To report, see 81596.)	
ASH FibroSURE™, BioPredictive S.A.S	0002M	Liver disease, ten biochemical assays (ALT, A2-macroglobulin, apolipoprotein A-1, total bilirubin, GGT, haptoglobin, AST, glucose, total cholesterol and triglycerides) utilizing serum, prognostic algorithm reported as quantitative scores for fibrosis, steatosis and alcoholic steatohepatitis (ASH)
NASH FibroSURE™, BioPredictive S.A.S	0003M	Liver disease, ten biochemical assays (ALT, A2-macroglobulin, apolipoprotein A-1, total bilirubin, GGT, haptoglobin, AST, glucose, total cholesterol and triglycerides) utilizing serum, prognostic algorithm reported as quantitative scores for fibrosis, steatosis and nonalcoholic steatohepatitis (NASH)
ScoliScore™ Transgenomic	0004M	Scoliosis, DNA analysis of 53 single nucleotide polymorphisms (SNPs), using saliva, prognostic algorithm reported as a risk score
HeproDX™, GoPath Laboratories, LLC	0006M	Oncology (hepatic), mRNA expression levels of 161 genes, utilizing fresh hepatocellular carcinoma tumor tissue, with alpha-fetoprotein level, algorithm reported as a risk classifier
NETest (Wren Laboratories, LLC)	0007M	Oncology (gastrointestinal neuroendocrine tumors), real-time PCR expression analysis of 51 genes, utilizing whole peripheral blood, algorithm reported as a nomogram of tumor disease index
	(0009M has been deleted)	
NeoLAB™ Prostate Liquid Biopsy, NeoGenomics Laboratories	0011M	Oncology, prostate cancer, mRNA expression assay of 12 genes (10 content and 2 housekeeping), RT-PCR test utilizing blood plasma and urine, algorithms to predict high-grade prostate cancer risk
Cxbladder™ Detect, Pacific Edge Diagnostics USA, Ltd.	0012M	Oncology (urothelial), mRNA, gene expression profiling by real-time quantitative PCR of five genes (*MDK, HOXA13, CDC2 [CDK1], IGFBP5*, and *CXCR2*), utilizing urine, algorithm reported as a risk score for having urothelial carcinoma
Cxbladder™ Monitor, Pacific Edge Diagnostics USA, Ltd.	0013M	Oncology (urothelial), mRNA, gene expression profiling by real-time quantitative PCR of five genes (*MDK, HOXA13, CDC2 [CDK1], IGFBP5*, and *CXCR2*), utilizing urine, algorithm reported as a risk score for having recurrent urothelial carcinoma
Enhanced Liver Fibrosis™ (ELF™) Test, Siemens Healthcare Diagnostics Inc/Siemens Healthcare Laboratory LLC	● 0014M	Liver disease, analysis of 3 biomarkers (hyaluronic acid [HA], procollagen III amino terminal peptide [PIIINP], tissue inhibitor of metalloproteinase 1 [TIMP-1]), using immunoassays, utilizing serum, prognostic algorithm reported as a risk score and risk of liver fibrosis and liver-related clinical events within 5 years
Adrenal Mass Panel, 24 Hour, Urine, Mayo Clinic Laboratories (MCL), Mayo Clinic	● 0015M	Adrenal cortical tumor, biochemical assay of 25 steroid markers, utilizing 24-hour urine specimen and clinical parameters, prognostic algorithm reported as a clinical risk and integrated clinical steroid risk for adrenal cortical carcinoma, adenoma, or other adrenal malignancy

Proprietary Name/Clinical Laboratory/Manufacturer	Code	Descriptor
Decipher Bladder TURBT®, Decipher Biosciences, Inc	● 0016M	Oncology (bladder), mRNA, microarray gene expression profiling of 209 genes, utilizing formalin fixed paraffin-embedded tissue, algorithm reported as molecular subtype (luminal, luminal infiltrated, basal, basal claudin-low, neuroendocrine-like)
Category I Codes for Multianalyte Assays with Algorithmic Analyses (MAAA)		
Vectra® DA, Crescendo Bioscience, Inc	81490	Autoimmune (rheumatoid arthritis), analysis of 12 biomarkers using immunoassays, utilizing serum, prognostic algorithm reported as a disease activity score (Do not report 81490 with 86140)
AlloMap®, CareDx, Inc	# 81595	Cardiology (heart transplant), mRNA, gene expression profiling by real-time quantitative PCR of 20 genes (11 content and 9 housekeeping), utilizing subfraction of peripheral blood, algorithm reported as a rejection risk score
Corus® CAD, CardioDx, Inc	81493	Coronary artery disease, mRNA, gene expression profiling by real-time RT-PCR of 23 genes, utilizing whole peripheral blood, algorithm reported as a risk score
PreDx Diabetes Risk Score™, Tethys Clinical Laboratory	81506	Endocrinology (type 2 diabetes), biochemical assays of seven analytes (glucose, HbA1c, insulin, hs-CRP, adiponectin, ferritin, interleukin 2-receptor alpha), utilizing serum or plasma, algorithm reporting a risk score
Harmony™ Prenatal Test, Ariosa Diagnostics	81507	Fetal aneuploidy (trisomy 21, 18, and 13) DNA sequence analysis of selected regions using maternal plasma, algorithm reported as a risk score for each trisomy
No proprietary name and clinical laboratory or manufacturer. Maternal serum screening procedures are performed by many labs and are not exclusive to a single facility.	81508	Fetal congenital abnormalities, biochemical assays of two proteins (PAPP-A, hCG [any form]), utilizing maternal serum, algorithm reported as a risk score
	81509	Fetal congenital abnormalities, biochemical assays of three proteins (PAPP-A, hCG [any form], DIA), utilizing maternal serum, algorithm reported as a risk score
	81510	Fetal congenital abnormalities, biochemical assays of three analytes (AFP, uE3, hCG [any form]), utilizing maternal serum, algorithm reported as a risk score
	81511	Fetal congenital abnormalities, biochemical assays of four analytes (AFP, uE3, hCG [any form], DIA) utilizing maternal serum, algorithm reported as a risk score (may include additional results from previous biochemical testing)
	81512	Fetal congenital abnormalities, biochemical assays of five analytes (AFP, uE3, total hCG, hyperglycosylated hCG, DIA) utilizing maternal serum, algorithm reported as a risk score
Aptima® BV Assay, Hologic, Inc	● 81513	Infectious disease, bacterial vaginosis, quantitative real-time amplification of RNA markers for Atopobium vaginae, Gardnerella vaginalis, and Lactobacillus species, utilizing vaginal-fluid specimens, algorithm reported as a positive or negative result for bacterial vaginosis
BD MAX™ Vaginal Panel, Becton Dickson and Company	● 81514	Infectious disease, bacterial vaginosis and vaginitis, quantitative real-time amplification of DNA markers for Gardnerella vaginalis, Atopobium vaginae, Megasphaera type 1, Bacterial Vaginosis Associated Bacteria-2 (BVAB-2), and Lactobacillus species (L. crispatus and L. jensenii), utilizing vaginal-fluid specimens, algorithm reported as a positive or negative for high likelihood of bacterial vaginosis, includes separate detection of Trichomonas vaginalis and/or Candida species (C. albicans, C. tropicalis, C. parapsilosis, C. dubliniensis), Candida glabrata, Candida krusei, when reported
HCV FibroSURE™, FibroTest™, BioPredictive S.A.S.	# 81596	Infectious disease, chronic hepatitis C virus (HCV) infection, six biochemical assays (ALT, A2-macroglobulin, apolipoprotein A-1, total bilirubin, GGT, and haptoglobin) utilizing serum, prognostic algorithm reported as scores for fibrosis and necroinflammatory activity in liver
Breast Cancer Index, Biotheranostics, Inc	81518	Oncology (breast), mRNA, gene expression profiling by real-time RT-PCR of 11 genes (7 content and 4 housekeeping), utilizing formalin-fixed paraffin-embedded tissue, algorithms reported as percentage risk for metastatic recurrence and likelihood of benefit from extended endocrine therapy
EndoPredict®, Myriad Genetic Laboratories, Inc	# 81522	Oncology (breast), mRNA, gene expression profiling by RT-PCR of 12 genes (8 content and 4 housekeeping), utilizing formalin-fixed paraffin-embedded tissue, algorithm reported as recurrence risk score
Oncotype DX® Genomic Health	81519	Oncology (breast), mRNA, gene expression profiling by real-time RT-PCR of 21 genes, utilizing formalin-fixed paraffin embedded tissue, algorithm reported as recurrence score
Prosigna® Breast Cancer Assay, NanoString Technologies, Inc	81520	Oncology (breast), mRNA gene expression profiling by hybrid capture of 58 genes (50 content and 8 housekeeping), utilizing formalin-fixed paraffin-embedded tissue, algorithm reported as a recurrence risk score
MammaPrint®, Agendia, Inc	81521	Oncology (breast), mRNA, microarray gene expression profiling of 70 content genes and 465 housekeeping genes, utilizing fresh frozen or formalin-fixed paraffin-embedded tissue, algorithm reported as index related to risk of distant metastasis
Oncotype DX® Colon Cancer Assay, Genomic Health	81525	Oncology (colon), mRNA, gene expression profiling by real-time RT-PCR of 12 genes (7 content and 5 housekeeping), utilizing formalin-fixed paraffin-embedded tissue, algorithm reported as a recurrence score

Proprietary Name/Clinical Laboratory/Manufacturer	Code	Descriptor
Cologuard™, Exact Sciences, Inc	81528	Oncology (colorectal) screening, quantitative real-time target and signal amplification of 10 DNA markers (*KRAS* mutations, promoter methylation of *NDRG4* and *BMP3*) and fecal hemoglobin, utilizing stool, algorithm reported as a positive or negative result
Decision Dx® Melanoma, Castle Biosciences, Inc	● 81529	Oncology (cutaneous melanoma), mRNA, gene expression profiling by real-time RT-PCR of 31 genes (28 content and 3 housekeeping), utilizing formalin-fixed paraffin-embedded tissue, algorithm reported as recurrence risk, including likelihood of sentinel lymph node metastasis
ChemoFX®, Helomics, Corp.	81535	Oncology (gynecologic), live tumor cell culture and chemotherapeutic response by DAPI stain and morphology, predictive algorithm reported as a drug response score; first single drug or drug combination
ChemoFX®, Helomics, Corp.	+ 81536	Oncology (gynecologic), live tumor cell culture and chemotherapeutic response by DAPI stain and morphology, predictive algorithm reported as a drug response score; each additional single drug or drug combination (List separately in addition to code for primary procedure)
VeriStrat, Biodesix, Inc	81538	Oncology (lung), mass spectrometric 8-protein signature, including amyloid A, utilizing serum, prognostic and predictive algorithm reported as good versus poor overall survival
Risk of Ovarian Malignancy Algorithm (ROMA)™, Fujirebio Diagnostics	# 81500	Oncology (ovarian), biochemical assays of two proteins (CA-125 and HE4), utilizing serum, with menopausal status, algorithm reported as a risk score
OVA1™, Vermillion, Inc	# 81503	Oncology (ovarian), biochemical assays of five proteins (CA-125, apolipoprotein A1, beta-2 microglobulin, transferrin, and pre-albumin), utilizing serum, algorithm reported as a risk score
4Kscore test, OPKO Health Inc	81539	Oncology (high-grade prostate cancer), biochemical assay of four proteins (Total PSA, Free PSA, Intact PSA, and human kallikrein-2 [hK2]), utilizing plasma or serum, prognostic algorithm reported as a probability score
Prolaris®, Myriad Genetic Laboratories, Inc	81541	Oncology (prostate), mRNA gene expression profiling by real-time RT-PCR of 46 genes (31 content and 15 housekeeping), utilizing formalin-fixed paraffin-embedded tissue, algorithm reported as a disease-specific mortality risk score
Decipher® Prostate, Decipher® Biosciences	81542	Oncology (prostate), mRNA, microarray gene expression profiling of 22 content genes, utilizing formalin-fixed paraffin-embedded tissue, algorithm reported as metastasis risk score
	(81545 has been deleted)	
ConfirmMDx® for Prostate Cancer, MDxHealth, Inc	81551	Oncology (prostate), promoter methylation profiling by real-time PCR of 3 genes (*GSTP1, APC, RASSF1*), utilizing formalin-fixed paraffin-embedded tissue, algorithm reported as a likelihood of prostate cancer detection on repeat biopsy
Afirma® Genomic Sequencing Classifier, Veracyte, Inc	# ● 81546	Oncology (thyroid), mRNA, gene expression analysis of 10,196 genes, utilizing fine needle aspirate, algorithm reported as a categorical result (eg, benign or suspicious)
Tissue of Origin Test, Kit-FFPE, Cancer Genetics, Inc	# 81504	Oncology (tissue of origin), microarray gene expression profiling of >2000 genes, utilizing formalin-fixed paraffin-embedded tissue, algorithm reported as tissue similarity scores
CancerTYPE ID, bioTheranostics, Inc	# 81540	Oncology (tumor of unknown origin), mRNA, gene expression profiling by real-time RT-PCR of 92 genes (87 content and 5 housekeeping) to classify tumor into main cancer type and subtype, utilizing formalin-fixed paraffin-embedded tissue, algorithm reported as a probability of a predicted main cancer type and subtype
DecisionDx®-UM test, Castle Biosciences, Inc	81552	Oncology (uveal melanoma), mRNA, gene expression profiling by real-time RT-PCR of 15 genes (12 content and 3 housekeeping), utilizing fine needle aspirate or formalin-fixed paraffin-embedded tissue, algorithm reported as risk of metastasis
Envisia® Genomic Classifier, Veracyte, Inc	● 81554	Pulmonary disease (idiopathic pulmonary fibrosis [IPF]), mRNA, gene expression analysis of 190 genes, utilizing transbronchial biopsies, diagnostic algorithm reported as categorical result (eg, positive or negative for high probability of usual interstitial pneumonia [UIP])
Proprietary Laboratory Analyses (PLA)		
PreciseType® HEA Test, Immucor, Inc	0001U	Red blood cell antigen typing, DNA, human erythrocyte antigen gene analysis of 35 antigens from 11 blood groups, utilizing whole blood, common RBC alleles reported
PolypDX™, Atlantic Diagnostic Laboratories, LLC, Metabolomic Technologies, Inc	0002U	Oncology (colorectal), quantitative assessment of three urine metabolites (ascorbic acid, succinic acid and carnitine) by liquid chromatography with tandem mass spectrometry (LC-MS/MS) using multiple reaction monitoring acquisition, algorithm reported as likelihood of adenomatous polyps
Overa (OVA1 Next Generation), Aspira Labs, Inc, Vermillion, Inc	0003U	Oncology (ovarian) biochemical assays of five proteins (apolipoprotein A-1, CA 125 II, follicle stimulating hormone, human epididymis protein 4, transferrin), utilizing serum, algorithm reported as a likelihood score
	(0004U has been deleted)	

Proprietary Name/Clinical Laboratory/Manufacturer	Code	Descriptor
ExosomeDx®, Prostate (IntelliScore), Exosome Diagnostics, Inc, Exosome Diagnostics, Inc	0005U	Oncology (prostate) gene expression profile by real-time RT-PCR of 3 genes *ERG, PCA3,* and *SPDEF),* urine, algorithm reported as risk score
	(0006U has been deleted)	
ToxProtect, Genotox Laboratories Ltd	0007U	Drug test(s), presumptive, with definitive confirmation of positive results, any number of drug classes, urine, includes specimen verification including DNA authentication in comparison to buccal DNA, per date of service.
AmHPR® H. pylori Antibiotic Resistance Panel, American Molecular Laboratories, Inc	0008U	Helicobacter pylori detection and antibiotic resistance, DNA, 16S and 23S rRNA, gyrA, pbp1,rdxA and rpoB, next generation sequencing, formalin-fixed paraffin-embedded or fresh tissue or fecal sample, predictive, reported as positive or negative for resistance to clarithromycin, fluoroquinolones, metronidazole, amoxicillin, tetracycline, and rifabutin
DEPArray™HER2, PacificDx	0009U	Oncology (breast cancer), *ERBB2* (HER2) copy number by FISH, tumor cells from formalin-fixed paraffin-embedded tissue isolated using image-based dielectrophoresis (DEP) sorting, reported as *ERBB2* gene amplified or non-amplified
Bacterial Typing by Whole Genome Sequencing, Mayo Clinic	0010U	Infectious disease (bacterial), strain typing by whole genome sequencing, phylogenetic-based report of strain relatedness, per submitted isolate
Cordant CORE™, Cordant Health Solutions	0011U	Prescription drug monitoring, evaluation of drugs present by LC-MS/MS, using oral fluid, reported as a comparison to an estimated steady-state range, per date of service including all drug compounds and metabolites
MatePair Targeted Rearrangements, Congenital, Mayo Clinic	0012U	Germline disorders, gene rearrangement detection by whole genome next-generation sequencing, DNA, whole blood, report of specific gene rearrangement(s)
MatePair Targeted Rearrangements, Oncology, Mayo Clinic	0013U	Oncology (solid organ neoplasia), gene rearrangement detection by whole genome next-generation sequencing, DNA, fresh or frozen tissue or cells, report of specific gene rearrangement(s)
MatePair Targeted Rearrangements, Hematologic, Mayo Clinic	0014U	Hematology (hematolymphoid neoplasia), gene rearrangement detection by whole genome next-generation sequencing, DNA, whole blood or bone marrow, report of specific gene rearrangement(s)
	(0015U has been deleted)	
BCR-ABL1 major and minor breakpoint fusion transcripts, University of Iowa, Department of Pathology, Asuragen	0016U	Oncology (hematolymphoid neoplasia), RNA, *BCR/ABL1* major and minor breakpoint fusion transcripts, quantitative PCR amplification, blood or bone marrow, report of fusion not detected or detected with quantitation
JAK2 Mutation, University of Iowa, Department of Pathology	0017U	Oncology (hematolymphoid neoplasia), *JAK2* mutation, DNA, PCR amplification of exons 12-14 and sequence analysis, blood or bone marrow, report of JAK2 mutation not detected or detected
ThyraMIR™, Interpace Diagnostics	0018U	Oncology (thyroid), microRNA profiling by RT-PCR of 10 microRNA sequences, utilizing fine needle aspirate, algorithm reported as a positive or negative result for moderate to high risk of malignancy
OncoTarget/OncoTreat, Columbia University Department of Pathology and Cell Biology, Darwin Health	0019U	Oncology, RNA, gene expression by whole transcriptome sequencing, formalin-fixed paraffin embedded tissue or fresh frozen tissue, predictive algorithm reported as potential targets for therapeutic agents
	(0020U has been deleted)	
Apifiny®, Armune BioScience, Inc	0021U	Oncology (prostate), detection of 8 autoantibodies (ARF 6, NKX3-1, 5'-UTR-BMI1, CEP 164, 3'-UTR-Ropporin, Desmocollin, AURKAIP-1, CSNK2A2), multiplexed immunoassay and flow cytometry serum, algorithm reported as risk score
Oncomine™ Dx Target Test, Thermo Fisher Scientific	0022U	Targeted genomic sequence analysis panel, non-small cell lung neoplasia, DNA and RNA analysis, 23 genes, interrogation for sequence variants and rearrangements, reported as presence/absence of variants and associated therapy(ies) to consider
LeukoStrat® CDx *FLT3* Mutation Assay, LabPMM LLC, an Invivoscribe Technologies, Inc Company, Invivoscribe Technologies, Inc	0023U	Oncology (acute myelogenous leukemia), DNA, genotyping of internal tandem duplication, p.D835, p.I836, using mononuclear cells, reported as detection or non-detection of *FLT3* mutation and indication for or against the use of midostaurin
GlycA, Laboratory Corporation of America, Laboratory Corporation of America	0024U	Glycosylated acute phase proteins (GlycA), nuclear magnetic resonance spectroscopy, quantitative
UrSure Tenofovir Quantification Test, Synergy Medical Laboratories, UrSure Inc	0025U	Tenofovir, by liquid chromatography with tandem mass spectrometry (LC-MS/MS), urine, quantitative
Thyroseq Genomic Classifier, CBLPath, Inc, University of Pittsburgh Medical Center	0026U	Oncology (thyroid), DNA and mRNA of 112 genes, next-generation sequencing, fine needle aspirate of thyroid nodule, algorithmic analysis reported as a categorical result ("Positive, high probability of malignancy" or "Negative, low probability of malignancy")
JAK2 Exons 12 to 15 Sequencing, Mayo Clinic, Mayo Clinic	0027U	*JAK2 (Janus kinase 2)* (eg, myeloproliferative disorder) gene analysis, targeted sequence analysis exons 12-15
	(0028U has been deleted)	
Focused Pharmacogenomics Panel, Mayo Clinic, Mayo Clinic	0029U	Drug metabolism (adverse drug reactions and drug response), targeted sequence analysis (ie, *CYP1A2, CYP2C19, CYP2C9, CYP2D6, CYP3A4, CYP3A5, CYP4F2, SLCO1B1, VKORC1* and rs12777823)

Proprietary Name/Clinical Laboratory/Manufacturer	Code	Descriptor
Warfarin Response Genotype, Mayo Clinic, Mayo Clinic	0030U	Drug metabolism (warfarin drug response), targeted sequence analysis (i.e., *CYP2C9, CYP4F2, VKORC1*, rs12777823)
Cytochrome P450 1A2 Genotype, Mayo Clinic, Mayo Clinic	0031U	*CYP1A2 (cytochrome P450 family 1, subfamily A, member 2)* (eg, drug metabolism) gene analysis, common variants (ie, *1F, *1K, *6, *7)
Catechol-O- Methyltransferase *(COMT)* Genotype, Mayo Clinic, Mayo Clinic	0032U	*COMT (catechol-O-methyltransferase)* (eg, drug metabolism) gene analysis, c.472G>A (rs4680) variant
Serotonin Receptor Genotype *(HTR2A* and *HTR2C)*, Mayo Clinic, Mayo Clinic	0033U	*HTR2A (5-hydroxytryptamine receptor 2A), HTR2C (5-hydroxytryptamine receptor 2C) (eg, citalopram metabolism) gene analysis, common variants* (i.e., *HTR2A* rs7997012 [c.614-2211T>C], *HTR2C* rs3813929 [c.- 759C>T] and rs1414334 [c.551-3008C>G])
Thiopurine Methyltransferase *(TPMT)* and Nudix Hydrolase *(NUDT15)* Genotyping, Mayo Clinic, Mayo Clinic	0034U	*TPMT (thiopurine S-methyltransferase), NUDT15 (nudix hydroxylase 15)* (eg, thiopurine metabolism) gene analysis, common variants (i.e., *TPMT* *2, *3A, *3B, *3C, *4, *5, *6, *8, *12; *NUDT15* *3, *4, *5)
Real-time quaking induced conversion for prion detection (RT QuIC), National Prion Disease Pathology Surveillance Center	0035U	Neurology (prion disease), cerebrospinal fluid, detection of prion protein by quaking induced conformational conversion, qualitative
EXaCT-1 Whole Exome Testing, Lab of Oncology-Molecular Detection, Weill Cornell Medicine-Clinical Genomics Laboratory	0036U	Exome (ie, somatic mutations), paired formalin-fixed paraffin-embedded tumor tissue and normal specimen, sequence analyses
FoundationOne CDx™ (F1CDx), Foundation Medicine, Inc, Foundation Medicine, Inc	0037U	Targeted genomic sequence analysis, solid organ neoplasm, DNA analysis of 324 genes, interrogation for sequence variants, gene copy number amplifications, gene rearrangements, microsatellite instability and tumor mutational burden
Sensieva ™ Droplet 25OH Vitamin D2/D3 Microvolume LC/MS Assay, InSource Diagnostics, InSource Diagnostics	0038U	Vitamin D, 25 hydroxy D2 and D3, by LC- MS/MS, serum microsample, quantitative
Anti-dsDNA, High Salt/Avidity, University of Washington, Department of Laboratory Medicine, Bio-Rad	0039U	Deoxyribonucleic acid (DNA) antibody, double stranded, high avidity
MRDx BCR-ABL Test, MolecularMD, MolecularMD	0040U	*BCR/ABL1 (t(9;22))* (eg, chronic myelogenous leukemia) translocation analysis, major breakpoint, quantitative
Lyme ImmunoBlot IgM, IGeneX Inc, ID-FISH Technology Inc (ASR) (Lyme ImmunoBlot IgM Strips Only)	0041U	Borrelia burgdorferi, antibody detection of 5 recombinant protein groups, by immunoblot, IgM
Lyme ImmunoBlot IgG, IGeneX Inc, ID-FISH Technology Inc (ASR) (Lyme ImmunoBlot IgG Strips Only)	0042U	Borrelia burgdorferi, antibody detection of 12 recombinant protein groups, by immunoblot, IgG
Tick-Borne Relapsing Fever (TBRF) Borrelia ImmunoBlots IgM Test, IGeneX Inc, ID-FISH Technology Inc (Provides TBRF ImmunoBlot IgM Strips)	0043U	Tick-borne relapsing fever Borrelia group, antibody detection to 4 recombinant protein groups, by immunoblot, IgM
Tick-Borne Relapsing Fever (TBRF) Borrelia ImmunoBlots IgG Test, IGeneX Inc, ID-FISH Technology Inc (Provides TBRF ImmunoBlot IgG Strips)	0044U	Tick-borne relapsing fever Borrelia group, antibody detection to 4 recombinant protein groups, by immunoblot, IgG
The Oncotype DX® Breast DCIS Score™ Test, Genomic Health, Inc, Genomic Health, Inc	0045U	Oncology (breast ductal carcinoma in situ), mRNA, gene expression profiling by real- time RT-PCR of 12 genes (7 content and 5 housekeeping), utilizing formalin-fixed paraffin-embedded tissue, algorithm reported as recurrence score
FLT3 ITD MRD by NGS, LabPMM LLC, an Invivoscribe Technologies, Inc Company	0046U	*FLT3 (fms-related tyrosine kinase 3)* (eg, acute myeloid leukemia) internal tandem duplication (ITD) variants, quantitative
Oncotype DX Genomic Prostate Score, Genomic Health, Inc, Genomic Health, Inc	0047U	Oncology (prostate), mRNA, gene expression profiling by real-time RT-PCR of 17 genes (12 content and 5 housekeeping), utilizing formalin-fixed paraffin-embedded tissue, algorithm reported as a risk score
MSK-IMPACT (Integrated Mutation Profiling of Actionable Cancer Targets), Memorial Sloan Kettering Cancer Center	0048U	Oncology (solid organ neoplasia), DNA, targeted sequencing of protein-coding exons of 468 cancer-associated genes, including interrogation for somatic mutations and microsatellite instability, matched with normal specimens, utilizing formalin-fixed paraffin-embedded tumor tissue, report of clinically significant mutation(s)
NPM1 MRD by NGS, LabPMM LLC, an Invivoscribe Technologies, Inc Company	0049U	*NPM1 (nucleophosmin)* (eg, acute myeloid leukemia) gene analysis, quantitative
MyAML NGS Panel, LabPMM LLC, an Invivoscribe Technologies, Inc Company	0050U	Targeted genomic sequence analysis panel, acute myelogenous leukemia, DNA analysis, 194 genes, interrogation for sequence variants, copy number variants or rearrangements
UCompliDx, Elite Medical Laboratory Solutions, LLC, Elite Medical Laboratory Solutions, LLC (LDT)	0051U	Prescription drug monitoring, evaluation of drugs present by LC-MS/MS, urine, 31 drug panel, reported as quantitative results, detected or not detected, per date of service
VAP Cholesterol Test, VAP Diagnostics Laboratory, Inc, VAP Diagnostics Laboratory, Inc	0052U	Lipoprotein, blood, high resolution fractionation and quantitation of lipoproteins, including all five major lipoprotein classes and subclasses of HDL, LDL, and VLDL by vertical auto profile ultracentrifugation

Proprietary Name/Clinical Laboratory/Manufacturer	Code	Descriptor
Prostate Cancer Risk Panel, Mayo Clinic, Laboratory Developed Test	0053U	Oncology (prostate cancer), FISH analysis of 4 genes (*ASAP1, HDAC9, CHD1 and PTEN*), needle biopsy specimen, algorithm reported as probability of higher tumor grade
AssuranceRx Micro Serum, Firstox Laboratories, LLC, Firstox Laboratories, LLC	0054U	Prescription drug monitoring, 14 or more classes of drugs and substances, definitive tandem mass spectrometry with chromatography, capillary blood, quantitative report with therapeutic and toxic ranges, including steady-state range for the prescribed dose when detected, per date of service
myTAIHEART, TAI Diagnostics, Inc, TAI Diagnostics, Inc	0055U	Cardiology (heart transplant), cell-free DNA, PCR assay of 96 DNA target sequences (94 single nucleotide polymorphism targets and two control targets), plasma
MatePair Acute Myeloid Leukemia Panel, Mayo Clinic, Laboratory Developed Test	0056U	Hematology (acute myelogenous leukemia), DNA, whole genome next-generation sequencing to detect gene rearrangement(s), blood or bone marrow, report of specific gene rearrangement(s)
	(0057U has been deleted)	
Merkel SmT Oncoprotein Antibody Titer, University of Washington, Department of Laboratory Medicine	0058U	Oncology (Merkel cell carcinoma), detection of antibodies to the Merkel cell polyoma virus oncoprotein (small T antigen), serum, quantitative
Merkel Virus VP1 Capsid Antibody, University of Washington, Department of Laboratory Medicine	0059U	Oncology (Merkel cell carcinoma), detection of antibodies to the Merkel cell polyoma virus capsid protein (VP1), serum, reported as positive or negative
Twins Zygosity PLA, Natera, Inc, Natera, Inc	0060U	Twin zygosity, genomic-targeted sequence analysis of chromosome 2, using circulating cell-free fetal DNA in maternal blood
Transcutaneous multispectral measurement of tissue oxygenation and hemoglobin using spatial frequency domain imaging (SFDI), Modulated Imaging, Inc, Modulated Imaging, Inc	0061U	Transcutaneous measurement of five biomarkers (tissue oxygenation [StO2], oxyhemoglobin [ctHbO2], deoxyhemoglobin [ctHbR], papillary and reticular dermal hemoglobin concentrations [ctHb1 and ctHb2]), using spatial frequency domain imaging (SFDI) and multi-spectral analysis
SLE-key® Rule Out, Veracis Inc, Veracis Inc	0062U	Autoimmune (systemic lupus erythematosus), IgG and IgM analysis of 80 biomarkers, utilizing serum, algorithm reported with a risk score
NPDX ASD ADM Panel I, Stemina Biomarker Discovery, Inc, Stemina Biomarker Discovery, Inc d/b/a NeuroPointDX	0063U	Neurology (autism), 32 amines by LC-MS/MS, using plasma, algorithm reported as metabolic signature associated with autism spectrum disorder
BioPlex 2200 Syphilis Total & RPR Assay, Bio-Rad Laboratories, Bio-Rad Laboratories	0064U	Antibody, Treponema pallidum, total and rapid plasma reagin (RPR), immunoassay, qualitative
BioPlex 2200 RPR Assay, Bio-Rad Laboratories, Bio-Rad Laboratories	0065U	Syphilis test, non-treponemal antibody, immunoassay, qualitative (RPR)
PartoSure™ Test, Parsagen Diagnostics, Inc, Parsagen Diagnostics, Inc, a QIAGEN Company	0066U	Placental alpha-micro globulin-1 (PAMG-1), immunoassay with direct optical observation, cervico-vaginal fluid, each specimen
BBDRisk Dx™, Silbiotech, Inc, Silbiotech, Inc	0067U	Oncology (breast), immunohistochemistry, protein expression profiling of 4 biomarkers (matrix metalloproteinase-1 [MMP-1], carcinoembryonic antigen-related cell adhesion molecule 6 [CEACAM6], hyaluronoglucosaminidase [HYAL1], highly expressed in cancer protein [HEC1]), formalin-fixed paraffin-embedded precancerous breast tissue, algorithm reported as carcinoma risk score
MYCODART Dual Amplification Real Time PCR Panel for 6 Candida species, RealTime Laboratories, Inc/MycoDART, Inc, RealTime Laboratories, Inc	0068U	Candida species panel (*C. albicans, C. glabrata, C. parapsilosis, C. kruseii, C tropicalis, and C. auris*), amplified probe technique with qualitative report of the presence or absence of each species
miR-31*now*™, GoPath Laboratories, GoPath Laboratories	0069U	Oncology (colorectal), microRNA, RT-PCR expression profiling of miR-31-3p, formalin-fixed paraffin-embedded tissue, algorithm reported as an expression score
CYP2D6 Common Variants and Copy Number, Mayo Clinic, Laboratory Developed Test	0070U	*CYP2D6 (cytochrome P450, family 2, subfamily D, polypeptide 6)* (eg, drug metabolism) gene analysis, common and select rare variants (ie, *2, *3, *4, *4N, *5, *6, *7, *8, *9, *10, *11, *12, *13, *14A, *14B, *15, *17, *29, *35, *36, *41, *57, *61, *63, *68, *83, *xN)
CYP2D6 Full Gene Sequencing, Mayo Clinic, Laboratory Developed Test	+ 0071U	*CYP2D6 (cytochrome P450, family 2, subfamily D, polypeptide 6)* (eg, drug metabolism) gene analysis, full gene sequence (List separately in addition to code for primary procedure)
CYP2D6-2D7 Hybrid Gene Targeted Sequence Analysis, Mayo Clinic, Laboratory Developed Test	+ 0072U	*CYP2D6 (cytochrome P450, family 2, subfamily D, polypeptide 6)* (eg, drug metabolism) gene analysis, targeted sequence analysis (ie, CYP2D6-2D7 hybrid gene) (List separately in addition to code for primary procedure)
CYP2D7-2D6 Hybrid Gene Targeted Sequence Analysis, Mayo Clinic, Laboratory Developed Test	+ 0073U	*CYP2D6 (cytochrome P450, family 2, subfamily D, polypeptide 6)* (eg, drug metabolism) gene analysis, targeted sequence analysis (ie, CYP2D7-2D6 hybrid gene) (List separately in addition to code for primary procedure)
CYP2D6 trans-duplication/multiplication non-duplicated gene targeted sequence analysis, Mayo Clinic, Laboratory Developed Test	+ 0074U	*CYP2D6 (cytochrome P450, family 2, subfamily D, polypeptide 6)* (eg, drug metabolism) gene analysis, targeted sequence analysis (ie, non-duplicated gene when duplication/multiplication is trans) (List separately in addition to code for primary procedure)
CYP2D6 5′ gene duplication/multiplication targeted sequence analysis, Mayo Clinic, Laboratory Developed Test	+ 0075U	*CYP2D6 (cytochrome P450, family 2, subfamily D, polypeptide 6)* (eg, drug metabolism) gene analysis, targeted sequence analysis (ie, 5′ gene duplication/multiplication) (List separately in addition to code for primary procedure)

Proprietary Name/Clinical Laboratory/Manufacturer	Code	Descriptor
CYP2D6 3' gene duplication/multiplication targeted sequence analysis, Mayo Clinic, Laboratory Developed Test	+ 0076U	*CYP2D6 (cytochrome P450, family 2, subfamily D, polypeptide 6)* (eg, drug metabolism) gene analysis, targeted sequence analysis (ie, 3' gene duplication/multiplication) (List separately in addition to code for primary procedure)
M-Protein Detection and Isotyping by MALDI-TOF Mass Spectrometry, Mayo Clinic, Laboratory Developed Test	0077U	Immunoglobulin paraprotein (M-protein), qualitative, immunoprecipitation and mass spectrometry, blood or urine, including isotype
INFINITI® Neural Response Panel, PersonalizeDx Labs, AutoGenomics Inc	0078U	Pain management (opioid-use disorder) genotyping panel, 16 common variants (ie, *ABCB1, COMT, DAT1, DBH, DOR, DRD1, DRD2, DRD4, GABA, GAL, HTR2A, HTTLPR, MTHFR, MUOR, OPRK1, OPRM1*), buccal swab or other germline tissue sample, algorithm reported as positive or negative risk of opioid-use disorder
ToxLok™, InSource Diagnostics, InSource Diagnostics	0079U	Comparative DNA analysis using multiple selected single-nucleotide polymorphisms (SNPs), urine and buccal DNA, for specimen identity verification
BDX-XL2, Biodesix®, Inc, Biodesix®, Inc	0080U	Oncology (lung), mass spectrometric analysis of galectin-3-binding protein and scavenger receptor cysteine-rich type 1 protein M130, with five clinical risk factors (age, smoking status, nodule diameter, nodule-spiculation status and nodule location), utilizing plasma, algorithm reported as a categorical probability of malignancy
	(0081U has been deleted. To report, use 81552)	
NextGen Precision™ Testing, Precision Diagnostics, Precision Diagnostics LBN Precision Toxicology, LLC	0082U	Drug test(s), definitive, 90 or more drugs or substances, definitive chromatography with mass spectrometry, and presumptive, any number of drug classes, by instrument chemistry analyzer (utilizing immunoassay), urine, report of presence or absence of each drug, drug metabolite or substance with description and severity of significant interactions per date of service
Onco4D™, Animated Dynamics, Inc, Animated Dynamics, Inc	0083U	Oncology, response to chemotherapy drugs using motility contrast tomography, fresh or frozen tissue, reported as likelihood of sensitivity or resistance to drugs or drug combinations
BLOODchip®, ID CORE XT™, Grifols Diagnostic Solutions Inc	0084U	Red blood cell antigen typing, DNA, genotyping of 10 blood groups with phenotype prediction of 37 red blood cell antigens
	(0085U has been deleted)	
Accelerate PhenoTest™ BC kit, Accelerate Diagnostics, Inc	0086U	Infectious disease (bacterial and fungal), organism identification, blood culture, using rRNA FISH, 6 or more organism targets, reported as positive or negative with phenotypic minimum inhibitory concentration (MIC)-based antimicrobial susceptibility
Molecular Microscope® MMDx—Heart, Kashi Clinical Laboratories	0087U	Cardiology (heart transplant), mRNA gene expression profiling by microarray of 1283 genes, transplant biopsy tissue, allograft rejection and injury algorithm reported as a probability score
Molecular Microscope® MMDx—Kidney, Kashi Clinical Laboratories	0088U	Transplantation medicine (kidney allograft rejection), microarray gene expression profiling of 1494 genes, utilizing transplant biopsy tissue, algorithm reported as a probability score for rejection
Pigmented Lesion Assay (PLA), DermTech	0089U	Oncology (melanoma), gene expression profiling by RTqPCR, *PRAME* and *LINC00518*, superficial collection using adhesive patch(es)
myPath® Melanoma, Myriad Genetic Laboratories	0090U	Oncology (cutaneous melanoma), mRNA gene expression profiling by RT-PCR of 23 genes (14 content and 9 housekeeping), utilizing formalin-fixed paraffin-embedded tissue, algorithm reported as a categorical result (ie, benign, indeterminate, malignant)
FirstSight[CRC], CellMax Life	0091U	Oncology (colorectal) screening, cell enumeration of circulating tumor cells, utilizing whole blood, algorithm, for the presence of adenoma or cancer, reported as a positive or negative result
REVEAL Lung Nodule Characterization, MagArray, Inc	0092U	Oncology (lung), three protein biomarkers, immunoassay using magnetic nanosensor technology, plasma, algorithm reported as risk score for likelihood of malignancy
ComplyRX, Claro Labs	0093U	Prescription drug monitoring, evaluation of 65 common drugs by LC-MS/MS, urine, each drug reported detected or not detected
RCIGM Rapid Whole Genome Sequencing, Rady Children's Institute for Genomic Medicine (RCIGM)	0094U	Genome (eg, unexplained constitutional or heritable disorder or syndrome), rapid sequence analysis
Esophageal String Test™ (EST), Cambridge Biomedical, Inc	0095U	Inflammation (eosinophilic esophagitis), ELISA analysis of eotaxin-3 *(CCL26 [C-C motif chemokine ligand 26])* and major basic protein *(PRG2 [proteoglycan 2, pro eosinophil major basic protein])*, specimen obtained by swallowed nylon string, algorithm reported as predictive probability index for active eosinophilic esophagitis
HPV, High-Risk, Male Urine, Molecular Testing Labs	0096U	Human papillomavirus (HPV), high-risk types (ie, 16, 18, 31, 33, 35, 39, 45, 51, 52, 56, 58, 59, 66, 68), male urine

Proprietary Name/Clinical Laboratory/Manufacturer	Code	Descriptor
BioFire® FilmArray® Gastrointestinal (GI) Panel, BioFire® Diagnostics	0097U	Gastrointestinal pathogen, multiplex reverse transcription and multiplex amplified probe technique, multiple types or subtypes, 22 targets (Campylobacter [C. jejuni/C. coli/C. upsaliensis], Clostridium difficile [C. difficile] toxin A/B, Plesiomonas shigelloides, Salmonella, Vibrio [V. parahaemolyticus/V. vulnificus/V. cholerae], including specific identification of Vibrio cholerae, Yersinia enterocolitica, Enteroaggregative Escherichia coli [EAEC], Enteropathogenic Escherichia coli [EPEC], Enterotoxigenic Escherichia coli [ETEC] lt/st, Shiga-like toxin-producing Escherichia coli [STEC] stx1/stx2 [including specific identification of the E. coli O157 serogroup within STEC], Shigella/Enteroinvasive Escherichia coli [EIEC], Cryptosporidium, Cyclospora cayetanensis, Entamoeba histolytica, Giardia lamblia [also known as G. intestinalis and G. duodenalis], adenovirus F 40/41, astrovirus, norovirus GI/GII, rotavirus A, sapovirus [Genogroups I, II, IV, and V])
BioFire® FilmArray® Respiratory Panel (RP) EZ, BioFire® Diagnostics	0098U	Respiratory pathogen, multiplex reverse transcription and multiplex amplified probe technique, multiple types or subtypes, 14 targets (adenovirus, coronavirus, human metapneumovirus, influenza A, influenza A subtype H1, influenza A subtype H3, influenza A subtype H1-2009, influenza B, parainfluenza virus, human rhinovirus/enterovirus, respiratory syncytial virus, Bordetella pertussis, Chlamydophila pneumoniae, Mycoplasma pneumoniae)
BioFire® FilmArray® Respiratory Panel (RP), BioFire® Diagnostics	0099U	Respiratory pathogen, multiplex reverse transcription and multiplex amplified probe technique, multiple types or subtypes, 20 targets (adenovirus, coronavirus 229E, coronavirus HKU1, coronavirus, coronavirus OC43, human metapneumovirus, influenza A, influenza A subtype, influenza A subtype H3, influenza A subtype H1-2009, influenza, parainfluenza virus, parainfluenza virus 2, parainfluenza virus 3, parainfluenza virus 4, human rhinovirus/enterovirus, respiratory syncytial virus, Bordetella pertussis, Chlamydophila pneumonia, Mycoplasma pneumoniae)
BioFire® FilmArray® Respiratory Panel 2 (RP2), BioFire® Diagnostics	0100U	Respiratory pathogen, multiplex reverse transcription and multiplex amplified probe technique, multiple types or subtypes, 21 targets (adenovirus, coronavirus 229E, coronavirus HKU1, coronavirus NL63, coronavirus OC43, human metapneumovirus, human rhinovirus/enterovirus, influenza A, including subtypes H1, H1-2009, and H3, influenza B, parainfluenza virus 1, parainfluenza virus 2, parainfluenza virus 3, parainfluenza virus 4, respiratory syncytial virus, Bordetella parapertussis [IS1001], Bordetella pertussis [ptxP], Chlamydia pneumoniae, Mycoplasma pneumoniae)
ColoNext®, Ambry Genetics®, Ambry Genetics®	0101U	Hereditary colon cancer disorders (eg, Lynch syndrome, *PTEN* hamartoma syndrome, Cowden syndrome, familial adenomatosis polyposis), genomic sequence analysis panel utilizing a combination of NGS, Sanger, MLPA, and array CGH, with MRNA analytics to resolve variants of unknown significance when indicated (15 genes [sequencing and deletion/duplication], *EPCAM* and *GREM1* [deletion/duplication only])
BreastNext®, Ambry Genetics®, Ambry Genetics®	0102U	Hereditary breast cancer-related disorders (eg, hereditary breast cancer, hereditary ovarian cancer, hereditary endometrial cancer), genomic sequence analysis panel utilizing a combination of NGS, Sanger, MLPA, and array CGH, with MRNA analytics to resolve variants of unknown significance when indicated (17 genes [sequencing and deletion/duplication])
OvaNext®, Ambry Genetics®, Ambry Genetics®	0103U	Hereditary ovarian cancer (eg, hereditary ovarian cancer, hereditary endometrial cancer), genomic sequence analysis panel utilizing a combination of NGS, Sanger, MLPA, and array CGH, with MRNA analytics to resolve variants of unknown significance when indicated (24 genes [sequencing and deletion/duplication], *EPCAM* [deletion/duplication only])
	(0104U has been deleted)	
KidneyIntelXT™, RenalytixAI, RenalytixAI	0105U	Nephrology (chronic kidney disease), multiplex electrochemiluminescent immunoassay (ECLIA) of tumor necrosis factor receptor 1A, receptor superfamily 2 *(TNFR1, TNFR2)*, and kidney injury molecule-1 (KIM-1) combined with longitudinal clinical data, including *APOL1* genotype if available, and plasma (isolated fresh or frozen), algorithm reported as probability score for rapid kidney function decline (RKFD)
13C-Spirulina Gastric Emptying Breath Test (GEBT), Cairn Diagnostics d/b/a Advanced Breath Diagnostics, LLC, Cairn Diagnostics d/b/a Advanced Breath Diagnostics, LLC	0106U	Gastric emptying, serial collection of 7 timed breath specimens, non-radioisotope carbon-13(^{13}C) spirulina substrate, analysis of each specimen by gas isotope ratio mass spectrometry, reported as rate of $^{13}CO_2$ excretion
Singulex Clarity C.diff toxins A/B Assay, Singulex	0107U	Clostridium difficile toxin(s) antigen detection by immunoassay technique, stool, qualitative, multiple-step method
TissueCypher® Barrett's Esophagus Assay, Cernostics, Cernostics	0108U	Gastroenterology (Barrett's esophagus), whole slide-digital imaging, including morphometric analysis, computer-assisted quantitative immunolabeling of 9 protein biomarkers (p16, AMACR, p53, CD68, COX-2, CD45RO, HIF1a, HER-2, K20) and morphology, formalin-fixed paraffin-embedded tissue, algorithm reported as risk of progression to high-grade dysplasia or cancer
MYCODART Dual Amplification Real Time PCR Panel for 4 Aspergillus species, RealTime Laboratories, Inc/MycoDART, Inc	0109U	Infectious disease (Aspergillus species), real-time PCR for detection of DNA from 4 species *(A. fumigatus, A. terreus, A. niger,* and *A. flavus)*, blood, lavage fluid, or tissue, qualitative reporting of presence or absence of each species

Proprietary Name/Clinical Laboratory/Manufacturer	Code	Descriptor
Oral OncolyticAssuranceRX, Firstox Laboratories, LLC, Firstox Laboratories, LLC	0110U	Prescription drug monitoring, one or more oral oncology drug(s) and substances, definitive tandem mass spectrometry with chromatography, serum or plasma from capillary blood or venous blood, quantitative report with steady-state range for the prescribed drug(s) when detected
Praxis(™) Extended RAS Panel, Illumina, Illumina	0111U	Oncology (colon cancer), targeted *KRAS* (codons 12, 13, and 61) and *NRAS* (codons 12, 13, and 61) gene analysis utilizing formalin-fixed paraffin-embedded tissue
MicroGenDX qPCR & NGS For Infection, MicroGenDX, MicroGenDX	0112U	Infectious agent detection and identification, targeted sequence analysis (16S and 18S rRNA genes) with drug-resistance gene
MiPS (Mi-Prostate Score), MLabs, MLabs	0113U	Oncology (prostate), measurement of *PCA3* and *TMPRSS2-ERG* in urine and PSA in serum following prostatic massage, by RNA amplification and fluorescence-based detection, algorithm reported as risk score
EsoGuard™, Lucid Diagnostics, Lucid Diagnostics	0114U	Gastroenterology (Barrett's esophagus), *VIM* and *CCNA1* methylation analysis, esophageal cells, algorithm reported as likelihood for Barrett's esophagus
ePlex Respiratory Pathogen (RP) Panel, GenMark Diagnostics, Inc, GenMark Diagnostics, Inc	0115U	Respiratory infectious agent detection by nucleic acid (DNA and RNA), 18 viral types and subtypes and 2 bacterial targets, amplified probe technique, including multiplex reverse transcription for RNA targets, each analyte reported as detected or not detected
Snapshot Oral Fluid Compliance, Ethos Laboratories	0116U	Prescription drug monitoring, enzyme immunoassay of 35 or more drugs confirmed with LC-MS/MS, oral fluid, algorithm results reported as a patient-compliance measurement with risk of drug to drug interactions for prescribed medications
Foundation PI℠, Ethos Laboratories	0117U	Pain management, analysis of 11 endogenous analytes (methylmalonic acid, xanthurenic acid, homocysteine, pyroglutamic acid, vanilmandelate, 5-hydroxyindoleacetic acid, hydroxymethylglutarate, ethylmalonate, 3-hydroxypropyl mercapturic acid (3-HPMA), quinolinic acid, kynurenic acid), LC-MS/MS, urine, algorithm reported as a pain-index score with likelihood of atypical biochemical function associated with pain
Viracor TRAC™ dd-cfDNA, Viracor Eurofins, Viracor Eurofins	0118U	Transplantation medicine, quantification of donor-derived cell-free DNA using whole genome next-generation sequencing, plasma, reported as percentage of donor-derived cell-free DNA in the total cell-free DNA
MI-HEART Ceramides, Plasma, Mayo Clinic, Laboratory Developed Test	0119U	Cardiology, ceramides by liquid chromatography-tandem mass spectrometry, plasma, quantitative report with risk score for major cardiovascular events
Lymph3Cx Lymphoma Molecular Subtyping Assay, Mayo Clinic, Laboratory Developed Test	0120U	Oncology (B-cell lymphoma classification), mRNA, gene expression profiling by fluorescent probe hybridization of 58 genes (45 content and 13 housekeeping genes), formalin-fixed paraffin-embedded tissue, algorithm reported as likelihood for primary mediastinal B-cell lymphoma (PMBCL) and diffuse large B-cell lymphoma (DLBCL) with cell of origin subtyping in the latter
Flow Adhesion of Whole Blood on VCAM-1 (FAB-V), Functional Fluidics, Functional Fluidics	0121U	Sickle cell disease, microfluidic flow adhesion (VCAM-1), whole blood
Flow Adhesion of Whole Blood to P-SELECTIN (WB-PSEL), Functional Fluidics, Functional Fluidics	0122U	Sickle cell disease, microfluidic flow adhesion (P-Selectin), whole blood
Mechanical Fragility, RBC by shear stress profiling and spectral analysis, Functional Fluidics, Functional Fluidics	0123U	Mechanical fragility, RBC, shear stress and spectral analysis profiling
	(0124U has been deleted)	
	(0125U has been deleted)	
	(0126U has been deleted)	
	(0127U has been deleted)	
	(0128U has been deleted)	
BRCAplus, Ambry Genetics	0129U	Hereditary breast cancer-related disorders (eg, hereditary breast cancer, hereditary ovarian cancer, hereditary endometrial cancer), genomic sequence analysis and deletion/duplication analysis panel *(ATM, BRCA1, BRCA2, CDH1, CHEK2, PALB2, PTEN,* and *TP53)*
+RNAinsight™ for ColoNext®, Ambry Genetics	+ 0130U	Hereditary colon cancer disorders (eg, Lynch syndrome, PTEN hamartoma syndrome, Cowden syndrome, familial adenomatosis polyposis), targeted mRNA sequence analysis panel *(APC, CDH1, CHEK2, MLH1, MSH2, MSH6, MUTYH, PMS2, PTEN,* and *TP53)* (List separately in addition to code for primary procedure)
+RNAinsight™ for BreastNext®, Ambry Genetics	+ 0131U	Hereditary breast cancer-related disorders (eg, hereditary breast cancer, hereditary ovarian cancer, hereditary endometrial cancer), targeted mRNA sequence analysis panel (13 genes) (List separately in addition to code for primary procedure)
+RNAinsight™ for OvaNext®, Ambry Genetics	+ 0132U	Hereditary ovarian cancer-related disorders (eg, hereditary breast cancer, hereditary ovarian cancer, hereditary endometrial cancer), targeted mRNA sequence analysis panel (17 genes) (List separately in addition to code for primary procedure)
+RNAinsight™ for ProstateNext®, Ambry Genetics	+ 0133U	Hereditary prostate cancer-related disorders, targeted mRNA sequence analysis panel (11 genes) (List separately in addition to code for primary procedure)

Proprietary Name/Clinical Laboratory/Manufacturer	Code	Descriptor
+RNAinsight™ for CancerNext®, Ambry Genetics	+ 0134U	Hereditary pan cancer (eg, hereditary breast and ovarian cancer, hereditary endometrial cancer, hereditary colorectal cancer), targeted mRNA sequence analysis panel (18 genes) (List separately in addition to code for primary procedure)
+RNAinsight™ for GYNPlus®, Ambry Genetics	+ 0135U	Hereditary gynecological cancer (eg, hereditary breast and ovarian cancer, hereditary endometrial cancer, hereditary colorectal cancer), targeted mRNA sequence analysis panel (12 genes) (List separately in addition to code for primary procedure)
+RNAinsight™ for *ATM*, Ambry Genetics	+ 0136U	*ATM (ataxia telangiectasia mutated)* (eg, ataxia telangiectasia) mRNA sequence analysis (List separately in addition to code for primary procedure)
+RNAinsight™ for *PALB2*, Ambry Genetics	+ 0137U	*PALB2 (partner and localizer of BRCA2)* (eg, breast and pancreatic cancer) mRNA sequence analysis (List separately in addition to code for primary procedure)
+RNAinsight™ for *BRCA1/2*, Ambry Genetics	+ 0138U	*BRCA1 (BRCA1, DNA repair associated), BRCA2 (BRCA2, DNA repair associated)* (eg, hereditary breast and ovarian cancer) mRNA sequence analysis (List separately in addition to code for primary procedure)
NPDX ASD Energy Metabolism, Stemina Biomarker Discovery, Inc, Stemina Biomarker Discovery, Inc	● 0139U	Neurology (autism spectrum disorder [ASD]), quantitative measurements of 6 central carbon metabolites (ie, α-ketoglutarate, alanine, lactate, phenylalanine, pyruvate, and succinate), LC-MS/MS, plasma, algorithmic analysis with result reported as negative or positive (with metabolic subtypes of ASD)
ePlex® BCID Fungal Pathogens Panel, GenMark Diagnostics, Inc, GenMark Diagnostics, Inc	● 0140U	Infectious disease (fungi), fungal pathogen identification, DNA (15 fungal targets), blood culture, amplified probe technique, each target reported as detected or not detected
ePlex® BCID Gram-Positive Panel, GenMark Diagnostics, Inc, GenMark Diagnostics, Inc	● 0141U	Infectious disease (bacteria and fungi), gram-positive organism identification and drug resistance element detection, DNA (20 gram-positive bacterial targets, 4 resistance genes, 1 pan gram-negative bacterial target, 1 pan Candida target), blood culture, amplified probe technique, each target reported as detected or not detected
ePlex® BCID Gram-Negative Panel, GenMark Diagnostics, Inc, GenMark Diagnostics, Inc	● 0142U	Infectious disease (bacteria and fungi), gram-negative bacterial identification and drug resistance element detection, DNA (21 gram-negative bacterial targets, 6 resistance genes, 1 pan gram-positive bacterial target, 1 pan Candida target), amplified probe technique, each target reported as detected or not detected
CareViewRx, Newstar Medical Laboratories, LLC, Newstar Medical Laboratories, LLC PsychViewRx Plus analysis by Newstar Medical Laboratories, LLC. To report, see (~0150U)	● 0143U	Drug assay, definitive, 120 or more drugs or metabolites, urine, quantitative liquid chromatography with tandem mass spectrometry (LC-MS/MS) using multiple reaction monitoring (MRM), with drug or metabolite description, comments including sample validation, per date of service
CareViewRx Plus, Newstar Medical Laboratories, LLC, Newstar Medical Laboratories, LLC	● 0144U	Drug assay, definitive, 160 or more drugs or metabolites, urine, quantitative liquid chromatography with tandem mass spectrometry (LC-MS/MS) using multiple reaction monitoring (MRM), with drug or metabolite description, comments including sample validation, per date of service
PainViewRx, Newstar Medical Laboratories, LLC, Newstar Medical Laboratories, LLC	● 0145U	Drug assay, definitive, 65 or more drugs or metabolites, urine, quantitative liquid chromatography with tandem mass spectrometry (LC-MS/MS) using multiple reaction monitoring (MRM), with drug or metabolite description, comments including sample validation, per date of service
PainViewRx Plus, Newstar Medical Laboratories, LLC, Newstar Medical Laboratories, LLC	● 0146U	Drug assay, definitive, 80 or more drugs or metabolites, urine, by quantitative liquid chromatography with tandem mass spectrometry (LC-MS/MS) using multiple reaction monitoring (MRM), with drug or metabolite description, comments including sample validation, per date of service
RiskViewRx, Newstar Medical Laboratories, LLC, Newstar Medical Laboratories, LLC	● 0147U	Drug assay, definitive, 85 or more drugs or metabolites, urine, quantitative liquid chromatography with tandem mass spectrometry (LC-MS/MS) using multiple reaction monitoring (MRM), with drug or metabolite description, comments including sample validation, per date of service
RiskViewRx Plus, Newstar Medical Laboratories, LLC, Newstar Medical Laboratories, LLC	● 0148U	Drug assay, definitive, 100 or more drugs or metabolites, urine, quantitative liquid chromatography with tandem mass spectrometry (LC-MS/MS) using multiple reaction monitoring (MRM), with drug or metabolite description, comments including sample validation, per date of service
PsychViewRx, Newstar Medical Laboratories, LLC, Newstar Medical Laboratories, LLC	● 0149U	Drug assay, definitive, 60 or more drugs or metabolites, urine, quantitative liquid chromatography with tandem mass spectrometry (LC-MS/MS) using multiple reaction monitoring (MRM), with drug or metabolite description, comments including sample validation, per date of service
PsychViewRx Plus, Newstar Medical Laboratories, LLC, Newstar Medical Laboratories, LLC CareViewRx analysis by Newstar Medical Laboratories, LLC. To report, see (~0143U)	● 0150U	Drug assay, definitive, 120 or more drugs or metabolites, urine, quantitative liquid chromatography with tandem mass spectrometry (LC-MS/MS) using multiple reaction monitoring (MRM), with drug or metabolite description, comments including sample validation, per date of service
BioFire® FilmArray® Pneumonia Panel, BioFire® Diagnostics, BioFire® Diagnostics	● 0151U	Infectious disease (bacterial or viral respiratory tract infection), pathogen specific nucleic acid (DNA or RNA), 33 targets, real-time semi-quantitative PCR, bronchoalveolar lavage, sputum, or endotracheal aspirate, detection of 33 organismal and antibiotic resistance genes with limited semi-quantitative results

Proprietary Name/Clinical Laboratory/Manufacturer	Code	Descriptor
Karius® Test, Karius Inc, Karius Inc	● 0152U	Infectious disease (bacteria, fungi, parasites, and DNA viruses), microbial cell-free DNA, plasma, untargeted next-generation sequencing, report for significant positive pathogens
Insight TNBCtype™, Insight Molecular Labs	● 0153U	Oncology (breast), mRNA, gene expression profiling by next-generation sequencing of 101 genes, utilizing formalin-fixed paraffin-embedded tissue, algorithm reported as a triple negative breast cancer clinical subtype(s) with information on immune cell involvement
therascreen® *FGFR* RGQ RT-PCR Kit, QIAGEN, QIAGEN GmbH	● 0154U	Oncology (urothelial cancer), RNA, analysis by real-time RT-PCR of the *FGFR3 (fibroblast growth factor receptor3)* gene analysis (ie, p.R248C [c.742C>T], p.S249C [c.746C>G], p.G370C [c.1108G>T], p.Y373C [c.1118A>G], FGFR3-TACC3v1, and FGFR3-TACC3v3) utilizing formalin-fixed paraffin-embedded urothelial cancer tumor tissue, reported as *FGFR* gene alteration status
therascreen *PIK3CA* RGQ PCR Kit, QIAGEN, QIAGEN GmbH	● 0155U	Oncology (breast cancer), DNA, *PIK3CA (phosphatidylinositol-4,5-bisphosphate 3 kinase, catalytic subunit alpha)* (eg, breast cancer) gene analysis (ie, p.C420R, p.E542K, p.E545A, p.E545D [g.1635G>T only], p.E545G, p.E545K, p.Q546E, p.Q546R, p.H1047L, p.H1047R, p.H1047Y), utilizing formalin-fixed paraffin-embedded breast tumor tissue, reported as *PIK3CA* gene mutation status
SMASH™, New York Genome Center, Marvel Genomics™	● 0156U	Copy number (eg, intellectual disability, dysmorphology), sequence analysis
CustomNext + RNA: *APC*, Ambry Genetics®, Ambry Genetics®	+● 0157U	*APC (APC regulator of WNT signaling pathway)* (eg, familial adenomatosis polyposis [FAP]) mRNA sequence analysis (List separately in addition to code for primary procedure)
CustomNext + RNA: *MLH1*, Ambry Genetics®, Ambry Genetics®	+● 0158U	*MLH1 (mutL homolog 1)* (eg, hereditary non-polyposis colorectal cancer, Lynch syndrome) mRNA sequence analysis (List separately in addition to code for primary procedure)
CustomNext + RNA: *MSH2*, Ambry Genetics®, Ambry Genetics®	+● 0159U	*MSH2 (mutS homolog 2)* (eg, hereditary colon cancer, Lynch syndrome) mRNA sequence analysis (List separately in addition to code for primary procedure)
CustomNext + RNA: *MSH6*, Ambry Genetics®, Ambry Genetics®	+● 0160U	*MSH6 (mutS homolog 6)* (eg, hereditary colon cancer, Lynch syndrome) mRNA sequence analysis (List separately in addition to code for primary procedure)
CustomNext + RNA: *PMS2*, Ambry Genetics®, Ambry Genetics®	+● 0161U	*PMS2 (PMS1 homolog 2, mismatch repair system component)* (eg, hereditary non-polyposis colorectal cancer, Lynch syndrome) mRNA sequence analysis (List separately in addition to code for primary procedure)
CustomNext + RNA: Lynch *(MLH1, MSH2, MSH6, PMS2)*, Ambry Genetics®, Ambry Genetics®	+● 0162U	Hereditary colon cancer (Lynch syndrome), targeted mRNA sequence analysis panel *(MLH1, MSH2, MSH6, PMS2)* (List separately in addition to code for primary procedure)
BeScreened™-CRC, Beacon Biomedical Inc, Beacon Biomedical Inc	● 0163U	Oncology (colorectal) screening, biochemical enzyme-linked immunosorbent assay (ELISA) of 3 plasma or serum proteins (teratocarcinoma derived growth factor-1 [TDGF-1, Cripto-1], carcinoembryonic antigen [CEA], extracellular matrix protein [ECM]), with demographic data (age, gender, CRC-screening compliance) using a proprietary algorithm and reported as likelihood of CRC or advanced adenomas
ibs-smart™, Gemelli Biotech, Gemelli Biotech	● 0164U	Gastroenterology (irritable bowel syndrome [IBS]), immunoassay for anti-CdtB and anti-vinculin antibodies, utilizing plasma, algorithm for elevated or not elevated qualitative results
VeriMAP™ Peanut Dx—Bead-based Epitope Assay, AllerGenis™ Clinical Laboratory, AllerGenis™ LLC	▲ 0165U	Peanut allergen-specific quantitative assessment of multiple epitopes using enzyme-linked immunosorbent assay (ELISA), blood, individual epitope results and interpretation probability of peanut allergy
LiverFASt™, Fibronostics, Fibronostics	● 0166U	Liver disease, 10 biochemical assays (a2-macroglobulin, haptoglobin, apolipoprotein A1, bilirubin, GGT, ALT, AST, triglycerides, cholesterol, fasting glucose) and biometric and demographic data, utilizing serum, algorithm reported as scores for fibrosis, necroinflammatory activity, and steatosis with a summary interpretation
ADEXUSDx hCG Test, NOWDiagnostics, NOWDiagnostics	● 0167U	Gonadotropin, chorionic (hCG), immunoassay with direct optical observation, blood
Vanadis® NIPT, PerkinElmer, Inc, PerkinElmer Genomics	● 0168U	Fetal aneuploidy (trisomy 21, 18, and 13) DNA sequence analysis of selected regions using maternal plasma without fetal fraction cutoff, algorithm reported as a risk score for each trisomy
NT *(NUDT15* and *TPMT)* genotyping panel, RPRD Diagnostics	● 0169U	*NUDT15 (nudix hydrolase 15)* and *TPMT (thiopurine S-methyltransferase)* (eg, drug metabolism) gene analysis, common variants
Clarifi™, Quadrant Biosciences, Inc, Quadrant Biosciences, Inc	● 0170U	Neurology (autism spectrum disorder [ASD]), RNA, next-generation sequencing, saliva, algorithmic analysis, and results reported as predictive probability of ASD diagnosis
MyMRD® NGS Panel, Laboratory for Personalized Molecular Medicine, Laboratory for Personalized Molecular Medicine	● 0171U	Targeted genomic sequence analysis panel, acute myeloid leukemia, myelodysplastic syndrome, and myeloproliferative neoplasms, DNA analysis, 23 genes, interrogation for sequence variants, rearrangements and minimal residual disease, reported as presence/absence

Proprietary Name/Clinical Laboratory/Manufacturer	Code	Descriptor
myChoice® CDx, Myriad Genetics Laboratories, Inc, Myriad Genetics Laboratories, Inc	● 0172U	Oncology (solid tumor as indicated by the label), somatic mutation analysis of *BRCA1 (BRCA1, DNA repair associated), BRCA2 (BRCA2, DNA repair associated)* and analysis of homologous recombination deficiency pathways, DNA, formalin-fixed paraffin-embedded tissue, algorithm quantifying tumor genomic instability score
Psych HealthPGx Panel, RPRD Diagnostics, RPRD Diagnostics	● 0173U	Psychiatry (ie, depression, anxiety), genomic analysis panel, includes variant analysis of 14 genes
LC-MS/MS Targeted Proteomic Assay, OncoOmicDx Laboratory, LDT	● 0174U	Oncology (solid tumor), mass spectrometric 30 protein targets, formalin-fixed paraffin-embedded tissue, prognostic and predictive algorithm reported as likely, unlikely, or uncertain benefit of 39 chemotherapy and targeted therapeutic oncology agents
Genomind® Professional PGx Express™ CORE, Genomind, Inc, Genomind, Inc	● 0175U	Psychiatry (eg, depression, anxiety), genomic analysis panel, variant analysis of 15 genes
IB*Schek*®, Commonwealth Diagnostics International, Inc, Commonwealth Diagnostics International, Inc	● 0176U	Cytolethal distending toxin B (CdtB) and vinculin IgG antibodies by immunoassay (ie, ELISA)
therascreen® *PIK3CA* RGQ PCR Kit, QIAGEN, QIAGEN GmbH	● 0177U	Oncology (breast cancer), DNA, *PIK3CA (phosphatidylinositol-4,5-bisphosphate 3-kinase catalytic subunit alpha)* gene analysis of 11 gene variants utilizing plasma, reported as PIK3CA gene mutation status
VeriMAP™ Peanut Sensitivity - Bead Based Epitope Assay, AllerGenis™ Clinical Laboratory, AllerGenis™ LLC	● 0178U	Peanut allergen-specific quantitative assessment of multiple epitopes using enzyme-linked immunosorbent assay (ELISA), blood, report of minimum eliciting exposure for a clinical reaction
Resolution ctDx Lung™, Resolution Bioscience, Resolution Bioscience, Inc	● 0179U	Oncology (non-small cell lung cancer), cell-free DNA, targeted sequence analysis of 23 genes (single nucleotide variations, insertions and deletions, fusions without prior knowledge of partner/breakpoint, copy number variations), with report of significant mutation(s)
Navigator ABO Sequencing, Grifols Immunohematology Center, Grifols Immunohematology Center	● 0180U	Red cell antigen (ABO blood group) genotyping *(ABO), gene analysis Sanger/chain termination/conventional sequencing, ABO (ABO, alpha 1-3-N-acetylgalactosaminyltransferase and alpha 1-3-galactosyltransferase)* gene, including subtyping, 7 exons
Navigator CO Sequencing, Grifols Immunohematology Center, Grifols Immunohematology Center	● 0181U	Red cell antigen (Colton blood group) genotyping (CO), gene analysis, *AQP1 (aquaporin 1 [Colton blood group])* exon 1
Navigator CROM Sequencing, Grifols Immunohematology Center, Grifols Immunohematology Center	● 0182U	Red cell antigen (Cromer blood group) genotyping (CROM), gene analysis, *CD55 (CD55 molecule [Cromer blood group])* exons 1-10
Navigator DI Sequencing, Grifols Immunohematology Center, Grifols Immunohematology Center	● 0183U	Red cell antigen (Diego blood group) genotyping (DI), gene analysis, *SLC4A1 (solute carrier family 4 member 1 [Diego blood group])* exon 19
Navigator DO Sequencing, Grifols Immunohematology Center, Grifols Immunohematology Center	● 0184U	Red cell antigen (Dombrock blood group) genotyping (DO), gene analysis, *ART4 (ADP-ribosyltransferase 4 [Dombrock blood group])* exon 2
Navigator FUT1 Sequencing, Grifols Immunohematology Center, Grifols Immunohematology Center	● 0185U	Red cell antigen (H blood group) genotyping (FUT1), gene analysis, *FUT1 (fucosyltransferase 1 [H blood group])* exon 4
Navigator FUT2 Sequencing, Grifols Immunohematology Center, Grifols Immunohematology Center	● 0186U	Red cell antigen (H blood group) genotyping (FUT2), gene analysis, *FUT2 (fucosyltransferase 2)* exon 2
Navigator FY Sequencing, Grifols Immunohematology Center, Grifols Immunohematology Center	● 0187U	Red cell antigen (Duffy blood group) genotyping (FY), gene analysis, *ACKR1 (atypical chemokine receptor 1 [Duffy blood group])* exons 1-2
Navigator GE Sequencing, Grifols Immunohematology Center, Grifols Immunohematology Center	● 0188U	Red cell antigen (Gerbich blood group) genotyping (GE), gene analysis, *GYPC (glycophorin C [Gerbich blood group])* exons 1-4
Navigator GYPA Sequencing, Grifols Immunohematology Center, Grifols Immunohematology Center	● 0189U	Red cell antigen (MNS blood group) genotyping (GYPA), gene analysis, *GYPA (glycophorin A [MNS blood group])* introns 1, 5, exon 2
Navigator GYPB Sequencing, Grifols Immunohematology Center, Grifols Immunohematology Center	● 0190U	Red cell antigen (MNS blood group) genotyping (GYPB), gene analysis, *GYPB (glycophorin B [MNS blood group])* introns 1, 5, pseudoexon 3
Navigator IN Sequencing, Grifols Immunohematology Center, Grifols Immunohematology Center	● 0191U	Red cell antigen (Indian blood group) genotyping (IN), gene analysis, *CD44 (CD44 molecule [Indian blood group])* exons 2, 3, 6
Navigator JK Sequencing, Grifols Immunohematology Center, Grifols Immunohematology Center	● 0192U	Red cell antigen (Kidd blood group) genotyping (JK), gene analysis, *SLC14A1 (solute carrier family 14 member 1 [Kidd blood group])* gene promoter, exon 9
Navigator JR Sequencing, Grifols Immunohematology Center, Grifols Immunohematology Center	● 0193U	Red cell antigen (JR blood group) genotyping (JR), gene analysis, *ABCG2 (ATP binding cassette subfamily G member 2 [Junior blood group])* exons 2-26
Navigator KEL Sequencing, Grifols Immunohematology Center, Grifols Immunohematology Center	● 0194U	Red cell antigen (Kell blood group) genotyping (KEL), gene analysis, *KEL (Kell metallo-endopeptidase [Kell blood group])* exon 8
Navigator KLF1 Sequencing, Grifols Immunohematology Center, Grifols Immunohematology Center	● 0195U	*KLF1 (Kruppel-like factor 1)*, targeted sequencing (ie, exon 13)
Navigator LU Sequencing, Grifols Immunohematology Center, Grifols Immunohematology Center	● 0196U	Red cell antigen (Lutheran blood group) genotyping (LU), gene analysis, *BCAM (basal cell adhesion molecule [Lutheran blood group])* exon 3
Navigator LW Sequencing, Grifols Immunohematology Center, Grifols Immunohematology Center	● 0197U	Red cell antigen (Landsteiner-Wiener blood group) genotyping (LW), gene analysis, *ICAM4 (intercellular adhesion molecule 4 [Landsteiner-Wiener blood group])* exon 1

Proprietary Name/Clinical Laboratory/Manufacturer	Code	Descriptor
Navigator RHD/CE Sequencing, Grifols Immunohematology Center, Grifols Immunohematology Center	● 0198U	Red cell antigen (RH blood group) genotyping (RHD and RHCE), gene analysis Sanger/chain termination/conventional sequencing, *RHD (Rh blood group D antigen)* exons 1-10 and *RHCE (Rh blood group CcEe antigens)* exon 5
Navigator SC Sequencing, Grifols Immunohematology Center, Grifols Immunohematology Center	● 0199U	Red cell antigen (Scianna blood group) genotyping (SC), gene analysis, *ERMAP (erythroblast membrane associated protein [Scianna blood group])* exons 4, 12
Navigator XK Sequencing, Grifols Immunohematology Center, Grifols Immunohematology Center	● 0200U	Red cell antigen (Kx blood group) genotyping (XK), gene analysis, *XK (X-linked Kx blood group)* exons 1-3
Navigator YT Sequencing, Grifols Immunohematology Center, Grifols Immunohematology Center	● 0201U	Red cell antigen (Yt blood group) genotyping (YT), gene analysis, *ACHE (acetylcholinesterase [Cartwright blood group])* exon 2
BioFire® Respiratory Panel 2.1 (RP2.1), BioFire® Diagnostics, BioFire® Diagnostics, LLC QIAstat-Dx Respiratory SARS CoV-2 Panel, QIAGEN Sciences, QIAGEN GmbH. To report, see (~0223U)	● 0202U	Infectious disease (bacterial or viral respiratory tract infection), pathogen-specific nucleic acid (DNA or RNA), 22 targets including severe acute respiratory syndrome coronavirus 2 (SARS-CoV-2), qualitative RT-PCR, nasopharyngeal swab, each pathogen reported as detected or not detected
PredictSURE IBD™ Test, KSL Diagnostics, PredictImmune Ltd	● 0203U	Autoimmune (inflammatory bowel disease), mRNA, gene expression profiling by quantitative RT-PCR, 17 genes (15 target and 2 reference genes), whole blood, reported as a continuous risk score and classification of inflammatory bowel disease aggressiveness
Afirma Xpression Atlas, Veracyte, Inc, Veracyte, Inc	● 0204U	Oncology (thyroid), mRNA, gene expression analysis of 593 genes (including *BRAF, RAS, RET, PAX8,* and *NTRK*) for sequence variants and rearrangements, utilizing fine needle aspirate, reported as detected or not detected
Vita Risk®, Arctic Medical Laboratories, Arctic Medical Laboratories	● 0205U	Ophthalmology (age-related macular degeneration), analysis of 3 gene variants (2 *CFH* gene, 1 *ARMS2* gene), using PCR and MALDI-TOF, buccal swab, reported as positive or negative for neovascular age-related macular-degeneration risk associated with zinc supplements
DISCERN™, NeuroDiagnostics, NeuroDiagnostics	● 0206U	Neurology (Alzheimer disease); cell aggregation using morphometric imaging and protein kinase C-epsilon (PKCe) concentration in response to amylospheroid treatment by ELISA, cultured skin fibroblasts, each reported as positive or negative for Alzheimer disease
DISCERN™, NeuroDiagnostics, NeuroDiagnostics	+● 0207U	Neurology (Alzheimer disease); quantitative imaging of phosphorylated *ERK1* and *ERK2* in response to bradykinin treatment by in situ immunofluorescence, using cultured skin fibroblasts, reported as a probability index for Alzheimer disease (List separately in addition to code for primary procedure)
Afirma Medullary Thyroid Carcinoma (MTC) Classifier, Veracyte, Inc, Veracyte, Inc	● 0208U	Oncology (medullary thyroid carcinoma), mRNA, gene expression analysis of 108 genes, utilizing fine needle aspirate, algorithm reported as positive or negative for medullary thyroid carcinoma
CNGnome™, PerkinElmer Genomics, PerkinElmer Genomics	● 0209U	Cytogenomic constitutional (genome-wide) analysis, interrogation of genomic regions for copy number, structural changes and areas of homozygosity for chromosomal abnormalities
BioPlex 2200 RPR Assay - Quantitative, Bio-Rad Laboratories, Bio-Rad Laboratories	● 0210U	Syphilis test, non-treponemal antibody, immunoassay, quantitative (RPR)
MI Cancer Seek™ - NGS Analysis, Caris MPI d/b/a Caris Life Sciences, Caris MPI d/b/a Caris Life Sciences	● 0211U	Oncology (pan-tumor), DNA and RNA by next-generation sequencing, utilizing formalin-fixed paraffin-embedded tissue, interpretative report for single nucleotide variants, copy number alterations, tumor mutational burden, and microsatellite instability, with therapy association
Genomic Unity® Whole Genome Analysis—Proband, Variantyx Inc, Variantyx Inc	● 0212U	Rare diseases (constitutional/heritable disorders), whole genome and mitochondrial DNA sequence analysis, including small sequence changes, deletions, duplications, short tandem repeat gene expansions, and variants in non-uniquely mappable regions, blood or saliva, identification and categorization of genetic variants, proband
Genomic Unity® Whole Genome Analysis - Comparator, Variantyx Inc, Variantyx Inc	● 0213U	Rare diseases (constitutional/heritable disorders), whole genome and mitochondrial DNA sequence analysis, including small sequence changes, deletions, duplications, short tandem repeat gene expansions, and variants in non-uniquely mappable regions, blood or saliva, identification and categorization of genetic variants, each comparator genome (eg, parent, sibling)
Genomic Unity® Exome Plus Analysis - Proband, Variantyx Inc, Variantyx Inc	● 0214U	Rare diseases (constitutional/heritable disorders), whole exome and mitochondrial DNA sequence analysis, including small sequence changes, deletions, duplications, short tandem repeat gene expansions, and variants in non-uniquely mappable regions, blood or saliva, identification and categorization of genetic variants, proband
Genomic Unity® Exome Plus Analysis - Comparator, Variantyx Inc, Variantyx Inc	● 0215U	Rare diseases (constitutional/heritable disorders), whole exome and mitochondrial DNA sequence analysis, including small sequence changes, deletions, duplications, short tandem repeat gene expansions, and variants in non-uniquely mappable regions, blood or saliva, identification and categorization of genetic variants, each comparator exome (eg, parent, sibling)
Genomic Unity® Ataxia Repeat Expansion and Sequence Analysis, Variantyx Inc, Variantyx Inc	● 0216U	Neurology (inherited ataxias), genomic DNA sequence analysis of 12 common genes including small sequence changes, deletions, duplications, short tandem repeat gene expansions, and variants in non-uniquely mappable regions, blood or saliva, identification and categorization of genetic variants

Proprietary Name/Clinical Laboratory/Manufacturer	Code	Descriptor
Genomic Unity® Comprehensive Ataxia Repeat Expansion and Sequence Analysis, Variantyx Inc, Variantyx Inc	● 0217U	Neurology (inherited ataxias), genomic DNA sequence analysis of 51 genes including small sequence changes, deletions, duplications, short tandem repeat gene expansions, and variants in non-uniquely mappable regions, blood or saliva, identification and categorization of genetic variants
Genomic Unity® DMD Analysis, Variantyx Inc, Variantyx Inc	● 0218U	Neurology (muscular dystrophy), *DMD* gene sequence analysis, including small sequence changes, deletions, duplications, and variants in non-uniquely mappable regions, blood or saliva, identification and characterization of genetic variants
Sentosa® SQ HIV-1 Genotyping Assay, Vela Diagnostics USA, Inc, Vela Operations Singapore Pte Ltd	● 0219U	Infectious agent (human immunodeficiency virus), targeted viral next-generation sequence analysis (ie, protease [PR], reverse transcriptase [RT], integrase [INT]), algorithm reported as prediction of antiviral drug susceptibility
PreciseDx™ Breast Cancer Test, PreciseDx, PreciseDx	● 0220U	Oncology (breast cancer), image analysis with artificial intelligence assessment of 12 histologic and immunohistochemical features, reported as a recurrence score
Navigator ABO Blood Group NGS, Grifols Immunohematology Center, Grifols Immunohematology Center	● 0221U	Red cell antigen (ABO blood group) genotyping (ABO), gene analysis, next-generation sequencing, *ABO (ABO, alpha 1-3-N-acetylgalactosaminyltransferase and alpha 1-3-galactosyltransferase)* gene
Navigator Rh Blood Group NGS, Grifols Immunohematology Center, Grifols Immunohematology Center	● 0222U	Red cell antigen (RH blood group) genotyping (RHD and RHCE), gene analysis, next-generation sequencing, RH proximal promoter, exons 1-10, portions of introns 2-3
QIAstat-Dx Respiratory SARS CoV-2 Panel, QIAGEN Sciences, QIAGEN GmbH BioFire® Respiratory Panel 2.1 (RP2.1), BioFire® Diagnostics, BioFire® Diagnostics, LLC. To report, see (~0202U)	● 0223U	Infectious disease (bacterial or viral respiratory tract infection), pathogen-specific nucleic acid (DNA or RNA), 22 targets including severe acute respiratory syndrome coronavirus 2 (SARS-CoV-2), qualitative RT-PCR, nasopharyngeal swab, each pathogen reported as detected or not detected
COVID-19 Antibody Test, Mt Sinai, Mount Sinai Laboratory	● 0224U	Antibody, severe acute respiratory syndrome coronavirus 2 (SARS-CoV-2) (Coronavirus disease [COVID-19]), includes titer(s), when performed
ePlex® Respiratory Pathogen Panel 2, GenMark Dx, GenMark Diagnostics, Inc	● 0225U	Infectious disease (bacterial or viral respiratory tract infection) pathogen-specific DNA and RNA, 21 targets, including severe acute respiratory syndrome coronavirus 2 (SARS-CoV-2), amplified probe technique, including multiplex reverse transcription for RNA targets, each analyte reported as detected or not detected
Tru-Immune™, Ethos Laboratories, GenScript® USA Inc	● 0226U	Surrogate viral neutralization test (sVNT), severe acute respiratory syndrome coronavirus 2 (SARS-CoV-2) (Coronavirus disease [COVID-19]), ELISA, plasma, serum
Comprehensive Screen, Aspenti Health	● 0227U	Drug assay, presumptive, 30 or more drugs or metabolites, urine, liquid chromatography with tandem mass spectrometry (LC-MS/MS) using multiple reaction monitoring (MRM), with drug or metabolite description, includes sample validation
PanGIA Prostate, Genetics Institute of America, Entopsis, LLC	● 0228U	Oncology (prostate), multianalyte molecular profile by photometric detection of macromolecules adsorbed on nanosponge array slides with machine learning, utilizing first morning voided urine, algorithm reported as likelihood of prostate cancer
Colvera®, Clinical Genomic Pathology Inc	● 0229U	*BCAT1 (Branched chain amino acid transaminase 1) or IKZF1 (IKAROS family zinc finger 1)* (eg, colorectal cancer) promoter methylation analysis
Genomic Unity® AR Analysis, Variantyx Inc, Variantyx Inc	● 0230U	*AR (androgen receptor)* (eg, spinal and bulbar muscular atrophy, Kennedy disease, X chromosome inactivation), full sequence analysis, including small sequence changes in exonic and intronic regions, deletions, duplications, short tandem repeat (STR) expansions, mobile element insertions, and variants in non-uniquely mappable regions
Genomic Unity® CACNA1A Analysis, Variantyx Inc, Variantyx Inc	● 0231U	*CACNA1A (calcium voltage-gated channel subunit alpha 1A)* (eg, spinocerebellar ataxia), full gene analysis, including small sequence changes in exonic and intronic regions, deletions, duplications, short tandem repeat (STR) gene expansions, mobile element insertions, and variants in non-uniquely mappable regions
Genomic Unity® CSTB Analysis, Variantyx Inc, Variantyx Inc	● 0232U	*CSTB (cystatin B)* (eg, progressive myoclonic epilepsy type 1A, Unverricht-Lundborg disease), full gene analysis, including small sequence changes in exonic and intronic regions, deletions, duplications, short tandem repeat (STR) expansions, mobile element insertions, and variants in non-uniquely mappable regions
Genomic Unity® FXN Analysis, Variantyx Inc, Variantyx Inc	● 0233U	*FXN (frataxin)* (eg, Friedreich ataxia), gene analysis, including small sequence changes in exonic and intronic regions, deletions, duplications, short tandem repeat (STR) expansions, mobile element insertions, and variants in non-uniquely mappable regions
Genomic Unity® MECP2 Analysis, Variantyx Inc, Variantyx Inc	● 0234U	*MECP2 (methyl CpG binding protein 2)* (eg, Rett syndrome), full gene analysis, including small sequence changes in exonic and intronic regions, deletions, duplications, mobile element insertions, and variants in non-uniquely mappable regions

Proprietary Name/Clinical Laboratory/Manufacturer	Code	Descriptor
Genomic Unity® PTEN Analysis, Variantyx Inc, Variantyx Inc	0235U	*PTEN (phosphatase and tensin homolog)* (eg, Cowden syndrome, PTEN hamartoma tumor syndrome), full gene analysis, including small sequence changes in exonic and intronic regions, deletions, duplications, mobile element insertions, and variants in non-uniquely mappable regions
Genomic Unity® SMN1/2 Analysis, Variantyx Inc, Variantyx Inc	0236U	*SMN1 (survival of motor neuron 1, telomeric)* and *SMN2 (survival of motor neuron 2, centromeric)* (eg, spinal muscular atrophy) full gene analysis, including small sequence changes in exonic and intronic regions, duplications and deletions, and mobile element insertions
Genomic Unity® Cardiac Ion Channelopathies Analysis, Variantyx Inc, Variantyx Inc	0237U	Cardiac ion channelopathies (eg, Brugada syndrome, long QT syndrome, short QT syndrome, catecholaminergic polymorphic ventricular tachycardia), genomic sequence analysis panel including *ANK2, CASQ2, CAV3, KCNE1, KCNE2, KCNH2, KCNJ2, KCNQ1, RYR2,* and *SCN5A,* including small sequence changes in exonic and intronic regions, deletions, duplications, mobile element insertions, and variants in non-uniquely mappable regions
Genomic Unity® Lynch Syndrome Analysis, Variantyx Inc, Variantyx Inc	0238U	Oncology (Lynch syndrome), genomic DNA sequence analysis of *MLH1, MSH2, MSH6, PMS2,* and *EPCAM,* including small sequence changes in exonic and intronic regions, deletions, duplications, mobile element insertions, and variants in non-uniquely mappable regions
FoundationOne® Liquid CDx, FOUNDATION MEDICINE, INC, FOUNDATION MEDICINE, INC	0239U	Targeted genomic sequence analysis panel, solid organ neoplasm, cell-free DNA, analysis of 311 or more genes, interrogation for sequence variants, including substitutions, insertions, deletions, select rearrangements, and copy number variations
Xpert® Xpress SARS-CoV-2/Flu/RSV (SARS-CoV-2 & Flu targets only), Cepheid	0240U	Infectious disease (viral respiratory tract infection), pathogen-specific RNA, 3 targets (severe acute respiratory syndrome coronavirus 2 [SARS-CoV-2], influenza A, influenza B), upper respiratory specimen, each pathogen reported as detected or not detected
Xpert® Xpress SARS-CoV-2/Flu/RSV (all targets), Cepheid	0241U	Infectious disease (viral respiratory tract infection), pathogen-specific RNA, 4 targets (severe acute respiratory syndrome coronavirus 2 [SARS-CoV-2], influenza A, influenza B, respiratory syncytial virus [RSV]), upper respiratory specimen, each pathogen reported as detected or not detected

Appendix M — Glossary

-centesis. Puncture, as with a needle, trocar, or aspirator; often done for withdrawing fluid from a cavity.

-ectomy. Excision, removal.

-orrhaphy. Suturing.

-ostomy. Indicates a surgically created artificial opening.

-otomy. Making an incision or opening.

-plasty. Indicates surgically formed or molded.

abdominal lymphadenectomy. Surgical removal of the abdominal lymph nodes grouping, with or without para-aortic and vena cava nodes.

ablation. Removal or destruction of a body part or tissue or its function. Ablation may be performed by surgical means, hormones, drugs, radiofrequency, heat, chemical application, or other methods.

abnormal alleles. Form of gene that includes disease-related variations.

absorbable sutures. Strands prepared from collagen or a synthetic polymer and capable of being absorbed by tissue over time. Examples include surgical gut and collagen sutures; or synthetics like polydioxanone (PDS), polyglactin 910 (Vicryl), poliglecaprone 25 (Monocryl), polyglyconate (Maxon), and polyglycolic acid (Dexon).

acetabuloplasty. Surgical repair or reconstruction of the large cup-shaped socket in the hipbone (acetabulum) with which the head of the femur articulates.

Achilles tendon. Tendon attached to the back of the heel bone (calcaneus) that flexes the foot downward.

acromioclavicular joint. Junction between the clavicle and the scapula. The acromion is the projection from the back of the scapula that forms the highest point of the shoulder and connects with the clavicle. Trauma or injury to the acromioclavicular joint is often referred to as a dislocation of the shoulder. This is not correct, however, as a dislocation of the shoulder is a disruption of the glenohumeral joint.

acromionectomy. Surgical treatment for acromioclavicular arthritis in which the distal portion of the acromion process is removed.

acromioplasty. Repair of the part of the shoulder blade that connects to the deltoid muscles and clavicle.

actigraphy. Science of monitoring activity levels, particularly during sleep. In most cases, the patient wears a wristband that records motion while sleeping. The data are recorded, analyzed, and interpreted to study sleep/wake patterns and circadian rhythms.

air conduction. Transportation of sound from the air, through the external auditory canal, to the tympanic membrane and ossicular chain. Air conduction hearing is tested by presenting an acoustic stimulus through earphones or a loudspeaker to the ear.

air puff device. Instrument that measures intraocular pressure by evaluating the force of a reflected amount of air blown against the cornea.

alleles. Form of gene usually arising from a mutation responsible for a hereditary variation.

allogeneic collection. Collection of blood or blood components from one person for the use of another. Allogeneic collection was formerly termed homologous collection.

allograft. Graft from one individual to another of the same species.

amniocentesis. Surgical puncture through the abdominal wall, with a specialized needle and under ultrasonic guidance, into the interior of the pregnant uterus and directly into the amniotic sac to collect fluid for diagnostic analysis or therapeutic reduction of fluid levels.

anastomosis. Surgically created connection between ducts, blood vessels, or bowel segments to allow flow from one to the other.

anesthesia time. Time period factored into anesthesia procedures beginning with the anesthesiologist preparing the patient for surgery and ending when the patient is turned over to the recovery department.

Angelman syndrome. Early childhood emergence of a pattern of interrupted development, stiff, jerky gait, absence or impairment of speech, excessive laughter, and seizures.

angioplasty. Reconstruction or repair of a diseased or damaged blood vessel.

annuloplasty. Surgical plication of weakened tissue of the heart, to improve its muscular function. Annuli are thick, fibrous rings and one is found surrounding each of the cardiac chambers. The atrial and ventricular muscle fibers attach to the annuli. In annuloplasty, weakened annuli may be surgically plicated, or tucked, to improve muscular functions.

anorectal anometry. Measurement of pressure generated by anal sphincter to diagnose incontinence.

anterior chamber lenses. Lenses inserted into the anterior chamber following intracapsular cataract extraction.

applanation tonometer. Instrument that measures intraocular pressure by recording the force required to flatten an area of the cornea.

appropriateness of care. Proper setting of medical care that best meets the patient's care or diagnosis, as defined by a health care plan or other legal entity.

aqueous humor. Fluid within the anterior and posterior chambers of the eye that is continually replenished as it diffuses out into the blood. When the flow of aqueous is blocked, a build-up of fluid in the eye causes increased intraocular pressure and leads to glaucoma and blindness.

arteriogram. Radiograph of arteries.

arteriovenous fistula. Connecting passage between an artery and a vein.

arteriovenous malformation. Connecting passage between an artery and a vein.

arthrotomy. Surgical incision into a joint that may include exploration, drainage, or removal of a foreign body.

ASA. 1) Acetylsalicylic acid. Synonym(s): aspirin. 2) American Society of Anesthesiologists. National organization for anesthesiology that maintains and publishes the guidelines and relative values for anesthesia coding.

aspirate. To withdraw fluid or air from a body cavity by suction.

assay. Chemical analysis of a substance to establish the presence and strength of its components. A therapeutic drug assay is used to determine if a drug is within the expected therapeutic range for a patient.

atrial septal defect. Cardiac anomaly consisting of a patent opening in the atrial septum due to a fusion failure, classified as ostium secundum type, ostium primum defect, or endocardial cushion defect.

attended surveillance. Ability of a technician at a remote surveillance center or location to respond immediately to patient transmissions regarding rhythm or device alerts as they are produced and received at the remote location. These transmissions may originate from wearable or implanted therapy or monitoring devices.

auricle. External ear, which is a single elastic cartilage covered in skin and normal adnexal features (hair follicles, sweat glands, and sebaceous glands), shaped to channel sound waves into the acoustic meatus.

autogenous transplant. Tissue, such as bone, that is harvested from the patient and used for transplantation back into the same patient.

autograft. Any tissue harvested from one anatomical site of a person and grafted to another anatomical site of the same person. Most commonly, blood vessels, skin, tendons, fascia, and bone are used as autografts.

autologous. Tissue, cells, or structure obtained from the same individual.

AVF. Arteriovenous fistula.

AVM. Arteriovenous malformation. Clusters of abnormal blood vessels that grow in the brain comprised of a blood vessel "nidus" or nest through which arteries and veins connect directly without going through the capillaries. As time passes, the nidus may enlarge resulting in the formation of a mass that may bleed. AVMs are more prone to bleeding in patients ages 10 to 55. Once older than age 55, the possibility of bleeding is reduced dramatically.

backbench preparation. Procedures performed on a donor organ following procurement to prepare the organ for transplant into the recipient. Excess fat and other tissue may be removed, the organ may be perfused, and vital arteries may be sized, repaired, or modified to fit the patient. These procedures are done on a back table in the operating room before transplantation can begin.

Bartholin's gland. Mucous-producing gland found in the vestibular bulbs on either side of the vaginal orifice and connected to the mucosal membrane at the opening by a duct.

Bartholin's gland abscess. Pocket of pus and surrounding cellulitis caused by infection of the Bartholin's gland and causing localized swelling and pain in the posterior labia majora that may extend into the lower vagina.

basic value. Relative weighted value based upon the usual anesthesia services and the relative work or cost of the specific anesthesia service assigned to each anesthesia-specific procedure code.

Berman locator. Small, sensitive tool used to detect the location of a metallic foreign body in the eye.

bifurcated. Having two branches or divisions, such as the left pulmonary veins that split off from the left atrium to carry oxygenated blood away from the heart.

Billroth's operation. Anastomosis of the stomach to the duodenum or jejunum.

bioprosthetic heart valve. Replacement cardiac valve made of biological tissue. Allograft, xenograft or engineered tissue.

biopsy. Tissue or fluid removed for diagnostic purposes through analysis of the cells in the biopsy material.

Blalock-Hanlon procedure. Atrial septectomy procedure to allow free mixing of the blood from the right and left atria.

Blalock-Taussig procedure. Anastomosis of the left subclavian artery to the left pulmonary artery or the right subclavian artery to the right pulmonary artery in order to shunt some of the blood flow from the systemic to the pulmonary circulation.

blepharochalasis. Loss of elasticity and relaxation of skin of the eyelid, thickened or indurated skin on the eyelid associated with recurrent episodes of edema, and intracellular atrophy.

blepharoplasty. Plastic surgery of the eyelids to remove excess fat and redundant skin weighting down the lid. The eyelid is pulled tight and sutured to support sagging muscles.

blepharoptosis. Droop or displacement of the upper eyelid, caused by paralysis, muscle problems, or outside mechanical forces.

blepharorrhaphy. Suture of a portion or all of the opposing eyelids to shorten the palpebral fissure or close it entirely.

bone conduction. Transportation of sound through the bones of the skull to the inner ear.

bone mass measurement. Radiologic or radioisotopic procedure or other procedure approved by the FDA for identifying bone mass, detecting bone loss, or determining bone quality. The procedure includes a physician's interpretation of the results. Qualifying individuals must be an estrogen-deficient woman at clinical risk for osteoporosis with vertebral abnormalities

brachytherapy. Form of radiation therapy in which radioactive pellets or seeds are implanted directly into the tissue being treated to deliver their dose of radiation in a more directed fashion. Brachytherapy provides radiation to the prescribed body area while minimizing exposure to normal tissue.

breakpoint. Point at which a chromosome breaks.

Bristow procedure. Anterior capsulorrhaphy prevents chronic separation of the shoulder. In this procedure, the bone block is affixed to the anterior glenoid rim with a screw.

buccal mucosa. Tissue from the mucous membrane on the inside of the cheek.

bundle of His. Bundle of modified cardiac fibers that begins at the atrioventricular node and passes through the right atrioventricular fibrous ring to the interventricular septum, where it divides into two branches. Bundle of His recordings are taken for intracardiac electrograms.

Caldwell-Luc operation. Intraoral antrostomy approach into the maxillary sinus for the removal of tooth roots or tissue, or for packing the sinus to reduce zygomatic fractures by creating a window above the teeth in the canine fossa area.

canthorrhaphy. Suturing of the palpebral fissure, the juncture between the eyelids, at either end of the eye.

canthotomy. Horizontal incision at the canthus (junction of upper and lower eyelids) to divide the outer canthus and enlarge lid margin separation.

cardio-. Relating to the heart.

cardiopulmonary bypass. Venous blood is diverted to a heart-lung machine, which mechanically pumps and oxygenates the blood temporarily so the heart can be bypassed while an open procedure on the heart or coronary arteries is performed. During bypass, the lungs are deflated and immobile.

cardioverter-defibrillator. Device that uses both low energy cardioversion or defibrillating shocks and antitachycardia pacing to treat ventricular tachycardia or ventricular fibrillation.

care plan oversight services. Physician's ongoing review and revision of a patient's care plan involving complex or multidisciplinary care modalities.

case management services. Physician case management is a process of involving direct patient care as well as coordinating and controlling access to the patient or initiating and/or supervising other necessary health care services.

cataract extraction. Surgical removal of the cataract or cloudy lens. Anterior chamber lenses are inserted in conjunction with intracapsular cataract extraction and posterior chamber lenses are inserted in conjunction with extracapsular cataract extraction.

catheter. Flexible tube inserted into an area of the body for introducing or withdrawing fluid.

Centers for Medicare and Medicaid Services. Federal agency that oversees the administration of the public health programs such as Medicare, Medicaid, and State Children's Insurance Program.

certified nurse midwife. Registered nurse who has successfully completed a program of study and clinical experience or has been certified by a recognized organization for the care of pregnant or delivering patients.

CFR. Code of Federal Regulations.

CGMS. Continuous glucose monitoring system.

CHAMPUS. Civilian Health and Medical Program of the Uniformed Services. See Tricare.

CHAMPVA. Civilian Health and Medical Program of the Department of Veterans Affairs.

chemodenervation. Chemical destruction of nerves. A substance, for example, Botox, is used to temporarily inhibit the transfer of chemicals at the presynaptic membrane, blocking the neuromuscular junctions.

chemoembolization. Administration of chemotherapeutic agents directly to a tumor in combination with the percutaneous administration of an occlusive substance into a vessel to deprive the tumor of its blood supply. This ensures a prolonged level of therapy directed at the tumor. Chemoembolization is primarily being used for cancers of the liver and endocrine system.

chemosurgery. Application of chemical agents to destroy tissue, originally referring to the in situ chemical fixation of premalignant or malignant lesions to facilitate surgical excision.

Chiari osteotomy. Top of the femur is altered to correct a dislocated hip caused by congenital conditions or cerebral palsy. Plate and screws are often used.

chimera. Organ or anatomic structure consisting of tissues of diverse genetic constitution.

choanal atresia. Congenital, membranous, or bony closure of one or both posterior nostrils due to failure of the embryonic bucconasal membrane to rupture and open up the nasal passageway.

chondromalacia. Condition in which the articular cartilage softens, seen in various body sites but most often in the patella, and may be congenital or acquired.

chorionic villus sampling. Aspiration of a placental sample through a catheter, under ultrasonic guidance. The specialized needle is placed transvaginally through the cervix or transabdominally into the uterine cavity.

chronic pain management services. Distinct services frequently performed by anesthesiologists who have additional training in pain management procedures. Pain management services include initial and subsequent evaluation and management (E/M) services, trigger point injections, spine and spinal cord injections, and nerve blocks.

cineplastic amputation. Amputation in which muscles and tendons of the remaining portion of the extremity are arranged so that they may be utilized for motor functions. Following this type of amputation, a specially constructed prosthetic device allows the individual to execute more complex movements because the muscles and tendons are able to communicate independent movements to the device.

circadian. Relating to a cyclic, 24-hour period.

CLIA. Clinical Laboratory Improvement Amendments. Requirements set in 1988, CLIA imposes varying levels of federal regulations on clinical procedures. Few laboratories, including those in physician offices, are exempt. Adopted by Medicare and Medicaid, CLIA regulations redefine laboratory testing in regard to laboratory certification and accreditation, proficiency testing, quality assurance, personnel standards, and program administration.

clinical social worker. Individual who possesses a master's or doctor's degree in social work and, after obtaining the degree, has performed at least two years of supervised clinical social work. A clinical social worker must be licensed by the state or, in the case of states without licensure, must completed at least two years or 3,000 hours of post-master's degree supervised clinical social work practice under the supervision of a master's level social worker.

clinical staff. Someone who works for, or under, the direction of a physician or qualified health care professional and does not bill services separately. The person may be licensed or regulated to help the physician perform specific duties.

clonal. Originating from one cell.

CMS. Centers for Medicare and Medicaid Services. Federal agency that administers the public health programs.

CO_2 laser. Carbon dioxide laser that emits an invisible beam and vaporizes water-rich tissue. The vapor is suctioned from the site.

codons. Series of three adjoining bases in one polynucleotide chain of a DNA or RNA molecule that provides the codes for a specific amino acid.

cognitive. Being aware by drawing from knowledge, such as judgment, reason, perception, and memory.

colostomy. Artificial surgical opening anywhere along the length of the colon to the skin surface for the diversion of feces.

commissurotomy. Surgical division or disruption of any two parts that are joined to form a commissure in order to increase the opening. The procedure most often refers to opening the adherent leaflet bands of fibrous tissue in a stenosed mitral valve.

common variants. Nucleotide sequence differences associated with abnormal gene function. Tests are usually performed in a single series of laboratory testing (in a single, typically multiplex, assay arrangement or using more than one assay to include all variants to be examined). Variants are representative of a mutation that mainly causes a single disease, such as cystic fibrosis. Other uncommon variants could provide additional information. Tests may be performed based on society recommendations and guidelines.

community mental health center. Facility providing outpatient mental health day treatment, assessments, and education as appropriate to community members.

component code. In the National Correct Coding Initiative (NCCI), the column II code that cannot be charged to Medicare when the column I code is reported.

comprehensive code. In the National Correct Coding Initiative (NCCI), the column I code that is reported to Medicare and precludes reporting column II codes.

computerized corneal topography. Digital imaging and analysis by computer of the shape of the corneal.

conjunctiva. Mucous membrane lining of the eyelids and covering of the exposed, anterior sclera.

conjunctivodacryocystostomy. Surgical connection of the lacrimal sac directly to the conjunctival sac.

conjunctivorhinostomy. Correction of an obstruction of the lacrimal canal achieved by suturing the posterior flaps and removing any lacrimal obstruction, preserving the conjunctiva.

constitutional. Cells containing genetic code that may be passed down to future generations. May also be referred to as germline.

consultation. Advice or opinion regarding diagnosis and treatment or determination to accept transfer of care of a patient rendered by a medical professional at the request of the primary care provider.

continuous positive airway pressure device. Pressurized device used to maintain the patient's airway for spontaneous or mechanically aided breathing. Often used for patients with mild to moderate sleep apnea.

core needle biopsy. Large-bore biopsy needle inserted into a mass and a core of tissue is removed for diagnostic study.

corpectomy. Removal of the body of a bone, such as a vertebra.

costochondral. Pertaining to the ribs and the scapula.

COTD. Cardiac output thermodilution. Cardiac output measured by thermodilution method that requires heart catheterization and then injection of a thermal indicator, usually iced saline. A computer calculates the cardiac output using an equation that incorporates body temperature, injectate volume and temperature, time, and other calculated ratios over a denominator of the integral of the change in blood temperature during the cold injection, reflected by the area of the inscribed curve.

CPT. 1) Chest physical therapy. 2) Cold pressor test. 3) Current Procedural Terminology.

craniosynostosis. Congenital condition in which one or more of the cranial sutures fuse prematurely, creating a deformed or aberrant head shape.

craterization. Excision of a portion of bone creating a crater-like depression to facilitate drainage from infected areas of bone.

cricoid. Circular cartilage around the trachea.

CRNA. Certified registered nurse anesthetist. Nurse trained and specializing in the administration of anesthesia.

cryolathe. Tool used for reshaping a button of corneal tissue.

cryosurgery. Application of intense cold, usually produced using liquid nitrogen, to locally freeze diseased or unwanted tissue and induce tissue necrosis without causing harm to adjacent tissue.

CT. Computed tomography.

cutdown. Small, incised opening in the skin to expose a blood vessel, especially over a vein (venous cutdown) to allow venipuncture and permit a needle or cannula to be inserted for the withdrawal of blood or administration of fluids.

cyclophotocoagulation. Procedure done to prevent vision loss from glaucoma in which a neodymium: YAG laser is used to burn and destroy a portion of the ciliary body in order to decrease the amount of aqueous humor being produced in the eye. This procedure is only done when creating a drain for aqueous humor to reduce intraocular pressure would not be successful. Destroying portions of the ciliary body reduces the amount of fluid present in the eye.

cytogenetic studies. Procedures in CPT that are related to the branch of genetics that studies cellular (cyto) structure and function as it relates to heredity (genetics). White blood cells, specifically T-lymphocytes, are the most commonly used specimen for chromosome analysis.

cytogenomic. Chromosomic evaluation using molecular methods.

dacryocystotome. Instrument used for incising the lacrimal duct strictures.

DBS. Deep brain stimulation. Treatment for disabling neurological symptoms associated with diseases including Parkinson's. DBS requires three components: the implanted electrode, extension, and neurostimulator. Electrical impulses are sent from the neurostimulator to the implant to block tremors.

debride. To remove all foreign objects and devitalized or infected tissue from a burn or wound to prevent infection and promote healing.

definitive drug testing. Drug tests used to further analyze or confirm the presence or absence of specific drugs or classes of drugs used by the patient. These tests are able to provide more conclusive information regarding the concentration of the drug and their metabolites. May be used for medical, workplace, or legal purposes.

definitive identification. Identification of microorganisms using additional tests to specify the genus or species (e.g., slide cultures or biochemical panels).

dentoalveolar structure. Area of alveolar bone surrounding the teeth and adjacent tissue.

Department of Health and Human Services. Cabinet department that oversees the operating divisions of the federal government responsible for health and welfare. HHS oversees the Centers for Medicare and Medicaid Services, Food and Drug Administration, Public Health Service, and other such entities.

Department of Justice. Attorneys from the DOJ and the United States Attorney's Office have, under the memorandum of understanding, the same direct access to contractor data and records as the OIG and the Federal Bureau of Investigation (FBI). DOJ is responsible for prosecution of fraud and civil or criminal cases presented.

dermis. Skin layer found under the epidermis that contains a papillary upper layer and the deep reticular layer of collagen, vascular bed, and nerves.

dermis graft. Skin graft that has been separated from the epidermal tissue and the underlying subcutaneous fat, used primarily as a substitute for fascia grafts in plastic surgery.

desensitization. 1) Administration of extracts of allergens periodically to build immunity in the patient. 2) Application of medication to decrease the symptoms, usually pain, associated with a dental condition or disease.

destruction. Ablation or eradication of a structure or tissue.

diabetes outpatient self-management training services. Educational and training services furnished by a certified provider in an outpatient setting. The physician managing the individual's diabetic condition must certify that the services are needed under a comprehensive plan of care and provide the patient with the skills and knowledge necessary for therapeutic program compliance (including skills related to the self-administration of injectable drugs). The provider must meet applicable standards established by the National Diabetes Advisory or be recognized by an organization that represents individuals with diabetes as meeting standards for furnishing the services.

diagnostic procedures. Procedure performed on a patient to obtain information to assess the medical condition of the patient or to identify a disease and to determine the nature and severity of an illness or injury.

dialysis. Artificial filtering of the blood to remove contaminating waste elements and restore normal balance.

diaphragm. 1) Muscular wall separating the thorax and its structures from the abdomen. 2) Flexible disk inserted into the vagina and against the cervix as a method of birth control.

diaphysectomy. Surgical removal of a portion of the shaft of a long bone, often done to facilitate drainage from infected bone.

diathermy. Applying heat to body tissues by various methods for therapeutic treatment or surgical purposes to coagulate and seal tissue.

dilation. Artificial increase in the diameter of an opening or lumen made by medication or by instrumentation.

dissect. Cut apart or separate tissue for surgical purposes or for visual or microscopic study.

DNA. Deoxyribonucleic acid. Chemical containing the genetic information necessary to produce and propagate living organisms. Molecules are comprised of two twisting paired strands, called a double helix.

DNA marker. Specific gene sequence within a chromosome indicating the inheritance of a certain trait.

dorsal. Pertaining to the back or posterior aspect.

drugs and biologicals. Drugs and biologicals included - or approved for inclusion - in the United States Pharmacopoeia, the National Formulary, the United States Homeopathic Pharmacopoeia, in New Drugs or Accepted Dental Remedies, or approved by the pharmacy and drug therapeutics committee of the medical staff of the hospital. Also included are medically accepted and FDA approved drugs used in an anticancer chemotherapeutic regimen. The carrier determines medical acceptance based on supportive clinical evidence.

dual-lead device. Implantable cardiac device (pacemaker or implantable cardioverter-defibrillator [ICD]) in which pacing and sensing components are placed in only two chambers of the heart.

duplex scan. Noninvasive vascular diagnostic technique that uses ultrasonic scanning to identify the pattern and direction of blood flow within arteries or veins displayed in real time images. Duplex scanning combines B-mode two-dimensional pictures of the vessel structure with spectra and/or color flow Doppler mapping or imaging of the blood as it moves through the vessels.

duplication/deletion (DUP/DEL). Term used in molecular testing which examines genomic regions to determine if there are extra chromosomes (duplication) or missing chromosomes (deletions). Normal gene dosage is two copies per cell except for the sex chromosomes which have one per cell.

DuToit staple capsulorrhaphy. Reattachment of the capsule of the shoulder and glenoid labrum to the glenoid lip using staples to anchor the avulsed capsule and glenoid labrum.

Dx. Diagnosis.

DXA. Dual energy x-ray absorptiometry. Radiological technique for bone density measurement using a two-dimensional projection system in which two x-ray beams with different levels of energy are pulsed alternately and the results are given in two scores, reported as standard deviations from peak bone mass density.

dynamic mutation. Unstable or changing polynucleotides resulting in repeats related to genes that can undergo disease-producing increases or decreases in the repeats that differ within tissues or over generations.

ECMO. Extracorporeal membrane oxygenation.

ectropion. Drooping of the lower eyelid away from the eye or outward turning or eversion of the edge of the eyelid, exposing the palpebral conjunctiva and causing irritation.

Eden-Hybinette procedure. Anterior shoulder repair using an anterior bone block to augment the bony anterior glenoid lip.

EDTA. Drug used to inhibit damage to the cornea by collagenase. EDTA is especially effective in alkali burns as it neutralizes soluble alkali, including lye.

effusion. Escape of fluid from within a body cavity.

electrocardiographic rhythm derived. Analysis of data obtained from readings of the heart's electrical activation, including heart rate and rhythm, variability of heart rate, ST analysis, and T-wave alternans. Other data may also be assessed when warranted.

electrocautery. Division or cutting of tissue using high-frequency electrical current to produce heat, which destroys cells.

electrode array. Electronic device containing more than one contact whose function can be adjusted during programming services. Electrodes are specialized for a particular electrochemical reaction that acts as a medium between a body surface and another instrument.

electromyography. Test that measures muscle response to nerve stimulation determining if muscle weakness is present and if it is related to the muscles themselves or a problem with the nerves that supply the muscles.

electrooculogram (EOG). Record of electrical activity associated with eye movements.

electrophysiologic studies. Electrical stimulation and monitoring to diagnose heart conduction abnormalities that predispose patients to bradyarrhythmias and to determine a patient's chance for developing ventricular and supraventricular tachyarrhythmias.

embolization. Placement of a clotting agent, such as a coil, plastic particles, gel, foam, etc., into an area of hemorrhage to stop the bleeding or to block blood flow to a problem area, such as an aneurysm or a tumor.

emergency. Serious medical condition or symptom (including severe pain) resulting from injury, sickness, or mental illness that arises suddenly and requires immediate care and treatment, generally received within 24 hours of onset, to avoid jeopardy to the life, limb, or health of a covered person.

empyema. Accumulation of pus within the respiratory, or pleural, cavity.

EMTALA. Emergency Medical Treatment and Active Labor Act.

end-stage renal disease. Chronic, advanced kidney disease requiring renal dialysis or a kidney transplant to prevent imminent death.

endarterectomy. Removal of the thickened, endothelial lining of a diseased or damaged artery.

endomicroscopy. Diagnostic technology that allows for the examination of tissue at the cellular level during endoscopy. The technology decreases the need for biopsy with histological examination for some types of lesions.

endovascular embolization. Procedure whereby vessels are occluded by a variety of therapeutic substances for the treatment of abnormal blood vessels by inhibiting the flow of blood to a tumor, arteriovenous malformations, lymphatic malformation, and to prevent or stop hemorrhage.

entropion. Inversion of the eyelid, turning the edge in toward the eyeball and causing irritation from contact of the lashes with the surface of the eye.

enucleation. Removal of a growth or organ cleanly so as to extract it in one piece.

epidermis. Outermost, nonvascular layer of skin that contains four to five differentiated layers depending on its body location: stratum corneum, lucidum, granulosum, spinosum, and basale.

epiphysiodesis. Surgical fusion of an epiphysis performed to prematurely stop further bone growth.

escharotomy. Surgical incision into the scab or crust resulting from a severe burn in order to relieve constriction and allow blood flow to the distal unburned tissue.

established patient. 1) Patient who has received professional services in a face-to-face setting within the last three years from the same physician/qualified health care professional or another physician/qualified health care professional of the exact same specialty and subspecialty who belongs to the same group practice. 2) For OPPS hospitals, patient who has been registered as an inpatient or outpatient in a hospital's provider-based clinic or emergency department within the past three years.

evacuation. Removal or purging of waste material.

evaluation and management codes. Assessment and management of a patient's health care.

evaluation and management service components. Key components of history, examination, and medical decision making that are key to selecting the correct E/M codes. Other non-key components include counseling, coordination of care, nature of presenting problem, and time.

event recorder. Portable, ambulatory heart monitor worn by the patient that makes electrocardiographic recordings of the length and frequency of aberrant cardiac rhythm to help diagnose heart conditions and to assess pacemaker functioning or programming.

exenteration. Surgical removal of the entire contents of a body cavity, such as the pelvis or orbit.

exon. One of multiple nucleic acid sequences used to encode information for a gene polypeptide or protein. Exons are separated from other exons by non-protein-coding sequences known as introns.

extended care services. Items and services provided to an inpatient of a skilled nursing facility, including nursing care, physical or occupational therapy, speech pathology, drugs and supplies, and medical social services.

external electrical capacitor device. External electrical stimulation device designed to promote bone healing. This device may also promote neural regeneration, revascularization, epiphyseal growth, and ligament maturation.

external pulsating electromagnetic field. External stimulation device designed to promote bone healing. This device may also promote neural regeneration, revascularization, epiphyseal growth, and ligament maturation.

extracorporeal. Located or taking place outside the body.

Eyre-Brook capsulorrhaphy. Reattachment of the capsule of the shoulder and glenoid labrum to the glenoid lip.

False Claims Act. Governs civil actions for filing false claims. Liability under this act pertains to any person who knowingly presents or causes to be presented a false or fraudulent claim to the government for payment or approval.

fascia. Fibrous sheet or band of tissue that envelops organs, muscles, and groupings of muscles.

fasciectomy. Excision of fascia or strips of fascial tissue.

fasciotomy. Incision or transection of fascial tissue.

fat graft. Graft composed of fatty tissue completely freed from surrounding tissue that is used primarily to fill in depressions.

FDA. Food and Drug Administration. Federal agency responsible for protecting public health by substantiating the safety, efficacy, and security of human and veterinary drugs, biological products, medical devices, national food supply, cosmetics, and items that give off radiation.

filtered speech test. Test most commonly used to identify central auditory dysfunction in which the patient is presented monosyllabic words that are low pass filtered, allowing only the parts of each word below a certain pitch to be presented. A score is given on the number of correct responses. This may be a subset of a standard battery of tests provided during a single encounter.

fissure. Deep furrow, groove, or cleft in tissue structures.

fistulization. Creation of a communication between two structures that were not previously connected.

flexor digitorum profundus tendon. Tendon originating in the proximal forearm and extending to the index finger and wrist. A thickened FDP sheath, usually caused by age, illness, or injury, can fill the carpal canal and lead to impingement of the median nerve.

fluoroscopy. Radiology technique that allows visual examination of part of the body or a function of an organ using a device that projects an x-ray image on a fluorescent screen.

focal length. Distance between the object in focus and the lens.

focused medical review. Process of targeting and directing medical review efforts on Medicare claims where the greatest risk of inappropriate program payment exists. The goal is to reduce the number of noncovered claims or unnecessary services. CMS analyzes national data such as internal billing, utilization, and payment data and provides its findings to the FI. Local medical review policies are developed identifying aberrances, abuse, and overutilized services. Providers are responsible for knowing national Medicare coverage and billing guidelines and local medical review policies, and for determining whether the services provided to Medicare beneficiaries are covered by Medicare.

fragile X syndrome. Intellectual disabilities, enlarged testes, big jaw, high forehead, and long ears in males. In females, fragile X presents with mild intellectual disabilities and heterozygous sexual structures. In some families, males have shown no symptoms but carry the gene.

free flap. Tissue that is completely detached from the donor site and transplanted to the recipient site, receiving its blood supply from capillary ingrowth at the recipient site.

free microvascular flap. Tissue that is completely detached from the donor site following careful dissection and preservation of the blood vessels, then attached to the recipient site with the transferred blood vessels anastomosed to the vessels in the recipient bed.

fulguration. Destruction of living tissue by using sparks from a high-frequency electric current.

gas tamponade. Absorbable gas may be injected to force the retina against the choroid. Common gases include room air, short-acting sulfahexafluoride, intermediate-acting perfluoroethane, or long-acting perfluorooctane.

Gaucher disease. Genetic metabolic disorder in which fat deposits may accumulate in the spleen, liver, lungs, bone marrow, and brain.

gene. Basic unit of heredity that contains nucleic acid. Genes are arranged in different and unique sequences or strings that determine the gene's function. Human genes usually include multiple protein coding regions such as exons separated by introns which are nonprotein coding sections.

genome. Complete set of DNA of an organism. Each cell in the human body is comprised of a complete copy of the approximately three billion DNA base pairs that constitute the human genome.

habilitative services. Procedures or services provided to assist a patient in learning, keeping, and improving new skills needed to perform daily living activities. Habilitative services assist patients in acquiring a skill for the first time.

HCPCS. Healthcare Common Procedure Coding System.

HCPCS Level I. Healthcare Common Procedure Coding System Level I. Numeric coding system used by physicians, facility outpatient departments, and ambulatory surgery centers (ASC) to code ambulatory, laboratory, radiology, and other diagnostic services for Medicare billing. This coding system contains only the American Medical Association's Physicians' Current Procedural Terminology (CPT) codes. The AMA updates codes annually.

HCPCS Level II. Healthcare Common Procedure Coding System Level II. National coding system, developed by CMS, that contains alphanumeric codes for physician and nonphysician services not included in the CPT coding system. HCPCS Level II covers such things as ambulance services, durable medical equipment, and orthotic and prosthetic devices.

HCPCS modifiers. Two-character code (AA-ZZ) that identifies circumstances that alter or enhance the description of a service or supply. They are recognized by carriers nationally and are updated annually by CMS.

Hct. Hematocrit.

health care provider. Entity that administers diagnostic and therapeutic services.

hemilaminectomy. Excision of a portion of the vertebral lamina.

hemodialysis. Cleansing of wastes and contaminating elements from the blood by virtue of different diffusion rates through a semipermeable membrane, which separates blood from a filtration solution that diffuses other elements out of the blood. The blood is slowly filtered extracorporeally through special dialysis equipment and returned to the body. Synonym(s): renal dialysis.

hemodialysis. Cleansing of wastes and contaminating elements from the blood by virtue of different diffusion rates through a semipermeable membrane, which separates blood from a filtration solution that diffuses other elements out of the blood.

hemoperitoneum. Effusion of blood into the peritoneal cavity, the space between the continuous membrane lining the abdominopelvic walls and encasing the visceral organs.

heterograft. Surgical graft of tissue from one animal species to a different animal species. A common type of heterograft is porcine (pig) tissue, used for temporary wound closure.

heterotopic transplant. Tissue transplanted from a different anatomical site for usage as is natural for that tissue, for example, buccal mucosa to a conjunctival site.

HGNC. HUGO gene nomenclature committee.

HGVS. Human genome variation society.

Hickman catheter. Central venous catheter used for long-term delivery of medications, such as antibiotics, nutritional substances, or chemotherapeutic agents.

HLA. Human leukocyte antigen.

home health services. Services furnished to patients in their homes under the care of physicians. These services include part-time or intermittent skilled nursing care, physical therapy, medical social services, medical supplies, and some rehabilitation equipment. Home health supplies and services must be prescribed by a physician, and the beneficiary must be confined at home in order for Medicare to pay the benefits in full.

homograft. Graft from one individual to another of the same species.

hospice care. Items and services provided to a terminally ill individual by a hospice program under a written plan established and periodically reviewed by the individual's attending physician and by the medical director: Nursing care provided by or under the supervision of a registered professional nurse; Physical or occupational therapy or speech-language pathology services; Medical social services under the direction of a physician; Services of a home health aide who has successfully completed a training program; Medical supplies (including drugs and biologicals) and the use of medical appliances; Physicians' services; Short-term inpatient care (including both respite care and procedures necessary for pain control and acute and chronic symptom management) in an inpatient facility on an intermittent basis and not consecutively over longer than five days; Counseling (including dietary counseling) with respect to care of the terminally ill individual and adjustment to his death; Any item or service which is specified in the plan and for which payment may be made.

hospital. Institution that provides, under the supervision of physicians, diagnostic, therapeutic, and rehabilitation services for medical diagnosis, treatment, and care of patients. Hospitals receiving federal funds must maintain clinical records on all patients, provide 24-hour nursing services, and have a discharge planning process in place. The term "hospital" also includes religious nonmedical health care institutions and facilities of 50 beds or less located in rural areas.

HUGO. Human genome organization

IA. Intra-arterial.

ICD. Implantable cardioverter defibrillator.

ICD-10-CM. International Classification of Diseases, 10th Revision, Clinical Modification. Clinical modification of the alphanumeric classification of diseases used by the World Health Organization, already in use in much of the world, and used for mortality reporting in the United States. The implementation date for ICD-10-CM diagnostic coding system to replace ICD-9-CM in the United States was October 1, 2015.

ICD-10-PCS. International Classification of Diseases, 10th Revision, Procedure Coding System. Beginning October 1, 2015, inpatient hospital services and surgical procedures must be coded using ICD-10-PCS codes, replacing ICD-9-CM, Volume 3 for procedures.

ICM. Implantable cardiovascular monitor.

ileostomy. Artificial surgical opening that brings the end of the ileum out through the abdominal wall to the skin surface for the diversion of feces through a stoma.

iliopsoas tendon. Fibrous tissue that connects muscle to bone in the pelvic region, common to the iliacus and psoas major.

ILR. Implantable loop recorder.

IM. 1) Infectious mononucleosis. 2) Internal medicine. 3) Intramuscular.

immunotherapy. Therapeutic use of serum or gamma globulin.

implant. Material or device inserted or placed within the body for therapeutic, reconstructive, or diagnostic purposes.

implantable cardiovascular monitor. Implantable electronic device that stores cardiovascular physiologic data such as intracardiac pressure waveforms collected from internal sensors or data such as weight and blood pressure collected from external sensors. The information stored in these devices is used as an aid in managing patients with heart failure and other cardiac conditions that are non-rhythm related. The data may be transmitted via local telemetry or remotely to a surveillance technician or an internet-based file server.

implantable cardioverter-defibrillator. Implantable electronic cardiac device used to control rhythm abnormalities such as tachycardia, fibrillation, or bradycardia by producing high- or low-energy stimulation and pacemaker functions. It may also have the capability to provide the functions of an implantable loop recorder or implantable cardiovascular monitor.

implantable loop recorder. Implantable electronic cardiac device that constantly monitors and records electrocardiographic rhythm. It may be triggered by the patient when a symptomatic episode occurs or activated automatically by rapid or slow heart rates. This may be the sole purpose of the device or it may be a component of another cardiac device, such as a pacemaker or implantable cardioverter-defibrillator. The data can be transmitted via local telemetry or remotely to a surveillance technician or an internet-based file server.

implantable venous access device. Catheter implanted for continuous access to the venous system for long-term parenteral feeding or for the administration of fluids or medications.

IMRT. Intensity modulated radiation therapy. External beam radiation therapy delivery using computer planning to specify the target dose and to modulate the radiation intensity, usually as a treatment for a malignancy. The delivery system approaches the patient from multiple angles, minimizing damage to normal tissue.

in situ. Located in the natural position or contained within the origin site, not spread into neighboring tissue.

incontinence. Inability to control urination or defecation.

infundibulectomy. Excision of the anterosuperior portion of the right ventricle of the heart.

internal direct current stimulator. Electrostimulation device placed directly into the surgical site designed to promote bone regeneration by encouraging cellular healing response in bone and ligaments.

interrogation device evaluation. Assessment of an implantable cardiac device (pacemaker, cardioverter-defibrillator, cardiovascular monitor, or loop recorder) in which collected data about the patient's heart rate and rhythm, battery and pulse generator function, and any leads or sensors present, are retrieved and evaluated. Determinations regarding device programming and appropriate treatment settings are made based on the findings. CPT provides required components for evaluation of the various types of devices.

intramedullary implants. Nail, rod, or pin placed into the intramedullary canal at the fracture site. Intramedullary implants not only provide a method of aligning the fracture, they also act as a splint and may reduce fracture pain. Implants may be rigid or flexible. Rigid implants are preferred for prophylactic treatment of diseased bone, while flexible implants are preferred for traumatic injuries.

intraocular lens. Artificial lens implanted into the eye to replace a damaged natural lens or cataract.

intravenous. Within a vein or veins.

introducer. Instrument, such as a catheter, needle, or tube, through which another instrument or device is introduced into the body.

intron. Nonprotein section of a gene that separates exons in human genes. Contains vital sequences that allow splicing of exons to produce a functional protein from a gene. Sometimes referred to as intervening sequences (IVS).

IP. 1) Interphalangeal. 2) Intraperitoneal.

irrigation. To wash out or cleanse a body cavity, wound, or tissue with water or other fluid.

Kayser-Fleischer ring. Condition found in Wilson's disease in which deposits of copper cause a pigmented ring around the cornea's outer border in the deep epithelial layers.

keratoprosthesis. Surgical procedure in which the physician creates a new anterior chamber with a plastic optical implant to replace a severely damaged cornea that cannot be repaired.

keratotomy. Surgical incision of the cornea.

krypton laser. Laser light energy that uses ionized krypton by electric current as the active source, has a radiation beam between the visible yellow-red spectrum, and is effective in photocoagulation of retinal bleeding, macular lesions, and vessel aberrations of the choroid.

lacrimal. Tear-producing gland or ducts that provides lubrication and flushing of the eyes and nasal cavities.

lacrimal punctum. Opening of the lacrimal papilla of the eyelid through which tears flow to the canaliculi to the lacrimal sac.

lacrimotome. Knife for cutting the lacrimal sac or duct.

lacrimotomy. Incision of the lacrimal sac or duct.

laparotomy. Incision through the flank or abdomen for therapeutic or diagnostic purposes.

laryngoscopy. Examination of the hypopharynx, larynx, and tongue base with an endoscope.

larynx. Musculocartilaginous structure between the trachea and the pharynx that functions as the valve preventing food and other particles from entering the respiratory tract, as well as the voice mechanism. Also called the voicebox, the larynx is composed of three single cartilages: cricoid, epiglottis, and thyroid; and three paired cartilages: arytenoid, corniculate, and cuneiform.

laser surgery. Use of concentrated, sharply defined light beams to cut, cauterize, coagulate, seal, or vaporize tissue.

LEEP. Loop electrode excision procedure. Biopsy specimen or cone shaped wedge of cervical tissue is removed using a hot cautery wire loop with an electrical current running through it.

levonorgestrel. Drug inhibiting ovulation and preventing sperm from penetrating cervical mucus. It is delivered subcutaneously in polysiloxone capsules. The capsules can be effective for up to five years, and provide a cumulative pregnancy rate of less than 2 percent. The capsules are not biodegradable, and therefore must be removed. Removal is more difficult than insertion of levonorgestrel capsules because fibrosis develops around the capsules. Normal hormonal activity and a return to fertility begins immediately upon removal.

ligament. Band or sheet of fibrous tissue that connects the articular surfaces of bones or supports visceral organs.

ligation. Tying off a blood vessel or duct with a suture or a soft, thin wire.

lymphadenectomy. Dissection of lymph nodes free from the vessels and removal for examination by frozen section in a separate procedure to detect early-stage metastases.

lysis. Destruction, breakdown, dissolution, or decomposition of cells or substances by a specific catalyzing agent.

Magnuson-Stack procedure. Treatment for recurrent anterior dislocation of the shoulder that involves tightening and realigning the subscapularis tendon.

maintenance of wakefulness test. Attended study determining the patient's ability to stay awake.

Manchester operation. Preservation of the uterus following prolapse by amputating the vaginal portion of the cervix, shortening the cardinal ligaments, and performing a colpoperineorrhaphy posteriorly.

mapping. Multidimensional depiction of a tachycardia that identifies its site of origin and its electrical conduction pathway after tachycardia has been induced. The recording is made from multiple catheter sites within the heart, obtaining electrograms simultaneously or sequentially.

marsupialization. Creation of a pouch in surgical treatment of a cyst in which one wall is resected and the remaining cut edges are sutured to adjacent tissue creating an open pouch of the previously enclosed cyst.

mastectomy. Surgical removal of one or both breasts.

McDonald procedure. Polyester tape is placed around the cervix with a running stitch to assist in the prevention of pre-term delivery. Tape is removed at term for vaginal delivery.

MCP. Metacarpophalangeal.

medial. Middle or midline.

mediastinotomy. Incision into the mediastinum for purposes of exploration, foreign body removal, drainage, or biopsy.

medical review. Review by a Medicare administrative contractor, carrier, and/or quality improvement organization (QIO) of services and items provided by physicians, other health care practitioners, and providers of health care services under Medicare. The review determines if the items and services are reasonable and necessary and meet Medicare coverage requirements, whether the quality meets professionally recognized standards of health care, and whether the services are medically appropriate in an inpatient, outpatient, or other setting as supported by documentation.

Medicare contractor. Medicare Part A fiscal intermediary, Medicare Part B carrier, Medicare administrative contractor (MAC), or a durable medical equipment Medicare administrative contractor (DME MAC).

Medicare physician fee schedule. List of payments Medicare allows by procedure or service. Payments may vary through geographic adjustments. The MPFS is based on the resource-based relative value scale (RBRVS). A national total relative value unit (RVU) is given to each procedure (HCPCS Level I CPT, Level II national codes). Each total RVU has three components: physician work, practice expense, and malpractice insurance.

meibomian gland. Sebaceous gland located in the tarsal plates along the eyelid margins that produces the lipid components found in tears.

metabolite. Chemical compound resulting from the natural process of metabolism. In drug testing, the metabolite of the drug may endure in a higher concentration or for a longer duration than the initial "parent" drug.

methylation. Mechanism used to regulate genes and protect DNA from some types of cleavage.

microarray. Small surface onto which multiple specific nucleic acid sequences can be attached to be used for analysis. Microarray may also be known as a gene chip or DNA chip. Tests can be run on the sequences for any variants that may be present.

mitral valve. Valve with two cusps that is between the left atrium and left ventricle of the heart.

moderate sedation. Medically controlled state of depressed consciousness, with or without analgesia, while maintaining the patient's airway, protective reflexes, and ability to respond to stimulation or verbal commands.

Mohs micrographic surgery. Special technique used to treat complex or ill-defined skin cancer and requires a single physician to provide two distinct services. The first service is surgical and involves the destruction of the lesion by a combination of chemosurgery and excision. The second service is that of a pathologist and includes mapping, color coding of specimens, microscopic examination of specimens, and complete histopathologic preparation.

monitored anesthesia care. Sedation, with or without analgesia, used to achieve a medically controlled state of depressed consciousness while maintaining the patient's airway, protective reflexes, and ability to respond to stimulation or verbal commands. In dental conscious sedation, the patient is rendered free of fear, apprehension, and anxiety through the use of pharmacological agents.

monoclonal. Relating to a single clone of cells.

mosaicplasty. Multiple, small grafts composed of bone and cartilage placed to treat osteochondral defects of the knee. The grafts are cylindrical in shape and are placed in corresponding size holes made to the desired depth to fill the defect and allow for a more naturally shaped reconstruction.

multiple sleep latency test (MSLT). Attended study to determine the tendency of the patient to fall asleep.

multiple-lead device. Implantable cardiac device (pacemaker or implantable cardioverter-defibrillator [ICD]) in which pacing and sensing components are placed in at least three chambers of the heart.

Mustard procedure. Corrective measure for transposition of great vessels involves an intra-atrial baffle made of pericardial tissue or synthetic material. The baffle is secured between pulmonary veins and mitral valve and between mitral and tricuspid valves. The baffle directs systemic venous flow into the left ventricle and lungs and pulmonary venous flow into the right ventricle and aorta.

mutation. Alteration in gene function that results in changes to a gene or chromosome. Can cause deficits or disease that can be inherited, can have beneficial effects, or result in no noticeable change.

mutation scanning. Process normally used on multiple polymerase chain reaction (PCR) amplicons to determine DNA sequence variants by differences in characteristics compared to normal. Specific DNA variants can then be studied further.

myotomy. Surgical cutting of a muscle to gain access to underlying tissues or for therapeutic reasons.

myringotomy. Incision in the eardrum done to prevent spontaneous rupture precipitated by fluid pressure build-up behind the tympanic membrane and to prevent stagnant infection and erosion of the ossicles.

nasal polyp. Fleshy outgrowth projecting from the mucous membrane of the nose or nasal sinus cavity that may obstruct ventilation or affect the sense of smell.

nasal sinus. Air-filled cavities in the cranial bones lined with mucous membrane and continuous with the nasal cavity, draining fluids through the nose.

nasogastric tube. Long, hollow, cylindrical catheter made of soft rubber or plastic that is inserted through the nose down into the stomach, and is used for feeding, instilling medication, or withdrawing gastric contents.

nasolacrimal punctum. Opening of the lacrimal duct near the nose.

nasopharynx. Membranous passage above the level of the soft palate.

Nd:YAG laser. Laser light energy that uses an yttrium, aluminum, and garnet crystal doped with neodymium ions as the active source, has a radiation beam nearing the infrared spectrum, and is effective in photocoagulation, photoablation, cataract extraction, and lysis of vitreous strands.

nebulizer. Latin for mist, a device that converts liquid into a fine spray and is commonly used to deliver medicine to the upper respiratory, bronchial, and lung areas.

nerve conduction study. Diagnostic test performed to assess muscle or nerve damage. Nerves are stimulated with electric shocks along the course of the muscle. Sensors are utilized to measure and record nerve functions, including conduction and velocity.

neurectomy. Excision of all or a portion of a nerve.

neuromuscular junction. Nerve synapse at the meeting point between the terminal end of a nerve (motor neuron) and a muscle fiber.

neuropsychological testing. Evaluation of a patient's behavioral abilities wherein a physician or other health care professional administers a series of tests in thinking, reasoning, and judgment.

new patient. Patient who is receiving face-to-face care from a provider/qualified health care professional or another physician/qualified health care professional of the exact same specialty and subspecialty who belongs to the same group practice for the first time in three years. For OPPS hospitals, a patient who has not been registered as an inpatient or outpatient, including off-campus provider based clinic or emergency department, within the past three years.

Niemann-Pick syndrome. Accumulation of phospholipid in histiocytes in the bone marrow, liver, lymph nodes, and spleen, cerebral involvement, and red macular spots similar to Tay-Sachs disease. Most commonly found in Jewish infants.

Nissen fundoplasty. Surgical repair technique that involves the fundus of the stomach being wrapped around the lower end of the esophagus to treat reflux esophagitis.

nonabsorbable sutures. Strands of natural or synthetic material that resist absorption into living tissue and are removed once healing is under way. Nonabsorbable sutures are commonly used to close skin wounds and repair tendons or collagenous tissue.

obturator. Prosthesis used to close an acquired or congenital opening in the palate that aids in speech and chewing.

obturator nerve. Lumbar plexus nerve with anterior and posterior divisions that innervate the adductor muscles (e.g., adductor longus, adductor brevis) of the leg and the skin over the medial area of the thigh or a sacral plexus nerve with anterior and posterior divisions that innervate the superior gemellus muscles.

occult blood test. Chemical or microscopic test to determine the presence of blood in a specimen.

ocular implant. Implant inside muscular cone.

oophorectomy. Surgical removal of all or part of one or both ovaries, either as open procedure or laparoscopically. Menstruation and childbearing ability continues when one ovary is removed.

orthosis. Derived from a Greek word meaning "to make straight," it is an artificial appliance that supports, aligns, or corrects an anatomical deformity or improves the use of a moveable body part. Unlike a prosthesis, an orthotic device is always functional in nature.

osteo-. Having to do with bone.

osteogenesis stimulator. Device used to stimulate the growth of bone by electrical impulses or ultrasound.

osteotomy. Surgical cutting of a bone

ostomy. Artificial (surgical) opening in the body used for drainage or for delivery of medications or nutrients.

pacemaker. Implantable cardiac device that controls the heart's rhythm and maintains regular beats by artificial electric discharges. This device consists of the pulse generator with a battery and the electrodes, or leads, which are placed in single or dual chambers of the heart, usually transvenously.

palmaris longus tendon. Tendon located in the hand that flexes the wrist joint.

paracentesis. Surgical puncture of a body cavity with a specialized needle or hollow tubing to aspirate fluid for diagnostic or therapeutic reasons.

paratenon graft. Graft composed of the fatty tissue found between a tendon and its sheath.

passive mobilization. Pressure, movement, or pulling of a limb or body part utilizing an apparatus or device.

pedicle flap. Full-thickness skin and subcutaneous tissue for grafting that remains partially attached to the donor site by a pedicle or stem in which the blood vessels supplying the flap remain intact.

Pemberton osteotomy. Osteotomy is performed to position triradiate cartilage as a hinge for rotating the acetabular roof in cases of dysplasia of the hip in children.

penetrance. Being formed by, or pertaining to, a single clone.

percutaneous intradiscal electrothermal annuloplasty. Procedure corrects tears in the vertebral annulus by applying heat to the collagen disc walls percutaneously through a catheter. The heat contracts and thickens the wall, which may contract and close any annular tears.

percutaneous skeletal fixation. Treatment that is neither open nor closed and the injury site is not directly visualized. Fixation devices (pins, screws) are placed through the skin to stabilize the dislocation using x-ray guidance.

pericardium. Thin and slippery case in which the heart lies that is lined with fluid so that the heart is free to pulse and move as it beats.

peripheral arterial tonometry (PAT). Pulsatile volume changes in a digit are measured to determine activity in the sympathetic nervous system for respiratory analysis.

peritoneal. Space between the lining of the abdominal wall, or parietal peritoneum, and the surface layer of the abdominal organs, or visceral peritoneum. It contains a thin, watery fluid that keeps the peritoneal surfaces moist.

peritoneal dialysis. Dialysis that filters waste from blood inside the body using the peritoneum, the natural lining of the abdomen, as the semipermeable membrane across which ultrafiltration is accomplished. A special catheter is inserted into the abdomen and a dialysis solution is drained into the abdomen. This solution extracts fluids and wastes, which are then discarded when the fluid is drained. Various forms of peritoneal dialysis include CAPD, CCPD, and NIDP.

peritoneal effusion. Persistent escape of fluid within the peritoneal cavity.

pessary. Device placed in the vagina to support and reposition a prolapsing or retropositioned uterus, rectum, or vagina.

phacoemulsification. Cataract extraction in which the lens is fragmented by ultrasonic vibrations and simultaneously irrigated and aspirated.

phenotype. Physical expression of a trait or characteristic as determined by an individual's genetic makeup or genotype.

photocoagulation. Application of an intense laser beam of light to disrupt tissue and condense protein material to a residual mass, used especially for treating ocular conditions.

physical status modifiers. Alphanumeric modifier used to identify the patient's health status as it affects the work related to providing the anesthesia service.

physical therapy modality. Therapeutic agent or regimen applied or used to provide appropriate treatment of the musculoskeletal system.

physician. Legally authorized practitioners including a doctor of medicine or osteopathy, a doctor of dental surgery or of dental medicine, a doctor of podiatric medicine, a doctor of optometry, and a chiropractor only with respect to treatment by means of manual manipulation of the spine (to correct a subluxation).

PICC. Peripherally inserted central catheter. PICC is inserted into one of the large veins of the arm and threaded through the vein until the tip sits in a large vein just above the heart.

PKR. Photorefractive therapy. Procedure involving the removal of the surface layer of the cornea (epithelium) by gentle scraping and use of a computer-controlled excimer laser to reshape the stroma.

pleurodesis. Injection of a sclerosing agent into the pleural space for creating adhesions between the parietal and the visceral pleura to treat a collapsed lung caused by air trapped in the pleural cavity, or severe cases of pleural effusion.

plication. Surgical technique involving folding, tucking, or pleating to reduce the size of a hollow structure or organ.

polyclonal. Containing one or more cells.

polymorphism. Genetic variation in the same species that does not harm the gene function or create disease.

polypeptide. Chain of amino acids held together by covalent bonds. Proteins are made up of amino acids.

polysomnography. Test involving monitoring of respiratory, cardiac, muscle, brain, and ocular function during sleep.

Potts-Smith-Gibson procedure. Side-to-side anastomosis of the aorta and left pulmonary artery creating a shunt that enlarges as the child grows.

Prader-Willi syndrome. Rounded face, almond-shaped eyes, strabismus, low forehead, hypogonadism, hypotonia, intellectual disabilities, and an insatiable appetite.

presumptive drug testing. Drug screening tests to identify the presence or absence of drugs in a patient's system. Tests are usually able to identify low concentrations of the drug. These tests may be used for medical, workplace, or legal purposes.

presumptive identification. Identification of microorganisms using media growth, colony morphology, gram stains, or up to three specific tests (e.g., catalase, indole, oxidase, urease).

professional component. Portion of a charge for health care services that represents the physician's (or other practitioner's) work in providing the service, including interpretation and report of the procedure. This component of the service usually is charged for and billed separately from the inpatient hospital charges.

profunda. Denotes a part of a structure that is deeper from the surface of the body than the rest of the structure.

prolonged physician services. Extended pre- or post-service care provided to a patient whose condition requires services beyond the usual.

prostate. Male gland surrounding the bladder neck and urethra that secretes a substance into the seminal fluid.

prosthetic. Device that replaces all or part of an internal body organ or body part, or that replaces part of the function of a permanently inoperable or malfunctioning internal body organ or body part.

provider of services. Institution, individual, or organization that provides health care.

proximal. Located closest to a specified reference point, usually the midline or trunk.

psychiatric hospital. Specialized institution that provides, under the supervision of physicians, services for the diagnosis and treatment of mentally ill persons.

pterygium. Benign, wedge-shaped, conjunctival thickening that advances from the inner corner of the eye toward the cornea.

pterygomaxillary fossa. Wide depression on the external surface of the maxilla above and to the side of the canine tooth socket.

pulmonary artery banding. Surgical constriction of the pulmonary artery to prevent irreversible pulmonary vascular obstructive changes and overflow into the left ventricle.

Putti-Platt procedure. Realignment of the subscapularis tendon to treat recurrent anterior dislocation, thereby partially eliminating external rotation. The anterior capsule is also tightened and reinforced.

pyloroplasty. Enlargement and reconstruction of the lower portion of the stomach opening into the duodenum performed after vagotomy to speed gastric emptying and treat duodenal ulcers.

qualified health care professional. Educated, licensed or certified, and regulated professional operating under a specified scope of practice to provide patient services that are separate and distinct from other clinical staff. Services may be billed independently or under the facility's services.

RAC. Recovery audit contractor. National program using CMS-affiliated contractors to review claims prior to payment as well as for payments on claims already processed, including overpayments and underpayments.

radiation therapy simulation. Radiation therapy simulation. Procedure by which the specific body area to be treated with radiation is defined and marked. A CT scan is performed to define the body contours and these images are used to create a plan customized treatment for the patient, targeting the area to be treated while sparing adjacent tissue. The center of the area to be treated is marked and an immobilization device (e.g., cradle, mold) is created to make sure the patient is in the same position each time for treatment. Complexity of treatment depends on the number of treatment areas and the use of tools to isolate the area of treatment.

radioactive substances. Materials used in the diagnosis and treatment of disease that emit high-speed particles and energy-containing rays.

radiology services. Services that include diagnostic and therapeutic radiology, nuclear medicine, CT scan procedures, magnetic resonance imaging services, ultrasound, and other imaging procedures.

radiotherapy afterloading. Part of the radiation therapy process in which the chemotherapy agent is actually instilled into the tumor area subsequent to surgery and placement of an expandable catheter into the void remaining after tumor excision. The specialized catheter remains in place and the patient may come in for multiple treatments with radioisotope placed to treat the margin of tissue surrounding the excision. After the radiotherapy is completed, the patient returns to have the catheter emptied and removed. This is a new therapy in breast cancer treatment.

Rashkind procedure. Transvenous balloon atrial septectomy or septostomy performed by cardiac catheterization. A balloon catheter is inserted into the heart either to create or enlarge an opening in the interatrial septal wall.

rehabilitation services. Therapy services provided primarily for assisting in a rehabilitation program of evaluation and service including cardiac rehabilitation, medical social services, occupational therapy, physical therapy, respiratory therapy, skilled nursing, speech therapy, psychiatric rehabilitation, and alcohol and substance abuse rehabilitation.

respiratory airflow (ventilation). Assessment of air movement during inhalation and exhalation as measured by nasal pressure sensors and thermistor.

respiratory analysis. Assessment of components of respiration obtained by other methods such as airflow or peripheral arterial tone.

respiratory effort. Measurement of diaphragm and/or intercostal muscle for airflow using transducers to estimate thoracic and abdominal motion.

respiratory movement. Measurement of chest and abdomen movement during respiration.

ribbons. In oncology, small plastic tubes containing radioactive sources for interstitial placement that may be cut into specific lengths tailored to the size of the area receiving ionizing radiation treatment.

Ridell sinusotomy. Frontal sinus tissue is destroyed to eliminate tumors.

RNA. Ribonucleic acid.

rural health clinic. Clinic in an area where there is a shortage of health services staffed by a nurse practitioner, physician assistant, or certified nurse midwife under physician direction that provides routine diagnostic services, including clinical laboratory services, drugs, and biologicals and that has prompt access to additional diagnostic services from facilities meeting federal requirements.

Salter osteotomy. Innominate bone of the hip is cut, removed, and repositioned to repair a congenital dislocation, subluxation, or deformity.

saucerization. Creation of a shallow, saucer-like depression in the bone to facilitate drainage of infected areas.

Schiotz tonometer. Instrument that measures intraocular pressure by recording the depth of an indentation on the cornea by a plunger of known weight.

screening mammography. Radiologic images taken of the female breast for the early detection of breast cancer.

screening pap smear. Diagnostic laboratory test consisting of a routine exfoliative cytology test (Papanicolaou test) provided to a woman for the early detection of cervical or vaginal cancer. The exam includes a clinical breast examination and a physician's interpretation of the results.

seeds. Small (1 mm or less) sources of radioactive material that are permanently placed directly into tumors.

Senning procedure. Flaps of intra-atrial septum and right atrial wall are used to create two interatrial channels to divert the systemic and pulmonary venous circulation.

sensitivity tests. Number of methods of applying selective suspected allergens to the skin or mucous.

sensorineural conduction. Transportation of sound from the cochlea to the acoustic nerve and central auditory pathway to the brain.

sentinel lymph node. First node to which lymph drainage and metastasis from a cancer can occur.

separate procedures. Services commonly carried out as a fundamental part of a total service and, as such, do not usually warrant separate identification. These services are identified in CPT with the parenthetical phrase (separate procedure) at the end of the description and are payable only when performed alone.

septectomy. 1) Surgical removal of all or part of the nasal septum. 2) Submucosal resection of the nasal septum.

Shirodkar procedure. Treatment of an incompetent cervical os by placing nonabsorbent suture material in purse-string sutures as a cerclage to support the cervix.

short tandem repeat (STR). Short sequences of a DNA pattern that are repeated. Can be used as genetic markers for human identity testing.

sialodochoplasty. Surgical repair of a salivary gland duct.

single-lead device. Implantable cardiac device (pacemaker or implantable cardioverter-defibrillator [ICD]) in which pacing and sensing components are placed in only one chamber of the heart.

single-nucleotide polymorphism (SNP). Single nucleotide (A, T, C, or G that is different in a DNA sequence. This difference occurs at a significant frequency in the population.

sinus of Valsalva. Any of three sinuses corresponding to the individual cusps of the aortic valve, located in the most proximal part of the aorta just above the cusps. These structures are contained within the pericardium and appear as distinct but subtle outpouchings or dilations of the aortic wall between each of the semilunar cusps of the valve.

sleep apnea. Intermittent cessation of breathing during sleep that may cause hypoxemia and pulmonary arterial hypertension.

sleep latency. Time period between lying down in bed and the onset of sleep.

sleep staging. Determination of the separate levels of sleep according to physiological measurements.

somatic. 1) Pertaining to the body or trunk. 2) In genetics acquired or occurring after birth.

SPECT. Single photon emission computerized tomography. SPECT images are taken after the injection of a radionuclide using a special camera containing a detector crystal, usually sodium iodide. Images are captured as the gamma radiation from the radionuclide scintillates or gives off its energy in a flash of light when coming in contact with the crystal. This type of imaging is reported for the anatomical area and purpose such as detecting liver function or myocardial perfusion after an ischemic event.

speculoscopy. Viewing the cervix utilizing a magnifier and a special wavelength of light, allowing detection of abnormalities that may not be discovered on a routine Pap smear.

speech-language pathology services. Speech, language, and related function assessment and rehabilitation service furnished by a qualified speech-language pathologist. Audiology services include hearing and balance assessment services furnished by a qualified audiologist. A qualified speech pathologist and audiologist must have a master's or doctoral degree in their respective fields and be licensed to serve in the state. Speech pathologists and audiologists practicing in states without licensure must complete 350 hours of supervised clinical work and perform at least nine months of supervised full-time service after earning their degrees.

sphincteroplasty. Surgical repair done to correct, augment, or improve the muscular function of a sphincter, such as the anus or intestines.

spirometry. Measurement of the lungs' breathing capacity.

splint. Brace or support. 1) dynamic splint: brace that permits movement of an anatomical structure such as a hand, wrist, foot, or other part of the body after surgery or injury. 2) static splint: brace that prevents movement and maintains support and position for an anatomical structure after surgery or injury.

stent. Tube to provide support in a body cavity or lumen.

stereotactic radiosurgery. Delivery of externally-generated ionizing radiation to specific targets for destruction or inactivation. Most often utilized in the treatment of brain or spinal tumors, high-resolution stereotactic imaging is used to identify the target and then deliver the treatment. Computer-assisted planning may also be employed. Simple and complex cranial lesions and spinal lesions are typically treated in a single planning and treatment session, although a maximum of five sessions may be required. No incision is made for stereotactic radiosurgery procedures.

stereotaxis. Three-dimensional method for precisely locating structures.

Stoffel rhizotomy. Nerve roots are sectioned to relieve pain or spastic paralysis.

strabismus. Misalignment of the eyes due to an imbalance in extraocular muscles.

surgical package. Normal, uncomplicated performance of specific surgical services, with the assumption that, on average, all surgical procedures of a given type are similar with respect to skill level, duration, and length of normal follow-up care.

symblepharopterygium. Adhesion in which the eyelid is adhered to the eyeball by a band that resembles a pterygium.

sympathectomy. Surgical interruption or transection of a sympathetic nervous system pathway.

tarso-. 1) Relating to the foot. 2) Relating to the margin of the eyelid.

tarsocheiloplasty. Plastic operation upon the edge of the eyelid for the treatment of trichiasis.

tarsorrhaphy. Suture of a portion or all of the opposing eyelids together for the purpose of shortening the palpebral fissure or closing it entirely.

technical component. Portion of a health care service that identifies the provision of the equipment, supplies, technical personnel, and costs attendant to the performance of the procedure other than the professional services.

tendon. Fibrous tissue that connects muscle to bone, consisting primarily of collagen and containing little vasculature.

tendon allograft. Allografts are tissues obtained from another individual of the same species. Tendon allografts are usually obtained from cadavers and frozen or freeze dried for later use in soft tissue repairs where the physician elects not to obtain an autogenous graft (a graft obtained from the individual on whom the surgery is being performed).

tendon suture material. Tendons are composed of fibrous tissue consisting primarily of collagen and containing few cells or blood vessels. This tissue heals more slowly than tissues with more vascularization. Because of this, tendons are usually repaired with nonabsorbable suture material. Examples include surgical silk, surgical cotton, linen, stainless steel, surgical nylon, polyester fiber, polybutester (Novafil), polyethylene (Dermalene), and polypropylene (Prolene, Surilene).

tendon transplant. Replacement of a tendon with another tendon.

tenon's capsule. Connective tissue that forms the capsule enclosing the posterior eyeball, extending from the conjunctival fornix and continuous with the muscular fascia of the eye.

tenonectomy. Excision of a portion of a tendon to make it shorter.

tenotomy. Cutting into a tendon.

TENS. Transcutaneous electrical nerve stimulator. TENS is applied by placing electrode pads over the area to be stimulated and connecting the electrodes to a transmitter box, which sends a current through the skin to sensory nerve fibers to help decrease pain in that nerve distribution.

tensilon. Edrophonium chloride. Agent used for evaluation and treatment of myasthenia gravis.

terminally ill. Individual whose medical prognosis for life expectancy is six months or less.

tetralogy of Fallot. Specific combination of congenital cardiac defects: obstruction of the right ventricular outflow tract with pulmonary stenosis, interventricular septal defect, malposition of the aorta, overriding the interventricular septum and receiving blood from both the venous and arterial systems, and enlargement of the right ventricle.

therapeutic services. Services performed for treatment of a specific diagnosis. These services include performance of the procedure, various incidental elements, and normal, related follow-up care.

thoracentesis. Surgical puncture of the chest cavity with a specialized needle or hollow tubing to aspirate fluid from within the pleural space for diagnostic or therapeutic reasons.

thoracic lymphadenectomy. Procedure to cut out the lymph nodes near the lungs, around the heart, and behind the trachea.

thoracostomy. Creation of an opening in the chest wall for drainage.

thyroglossal duct. Embryonic duct at the front of the neck, which becomes the pyramidal lobe of the thyroid gland with obliteration of the remaining duct, but may form a cyst or sinus in adulthood if it persists.

total disc arthroplasty with artificial disc. Removal of an intravertebral disc and its replacement with an implant. The implant is an artificial disc consisting of two metal plates with a weight-bearing surface of polyethylene between the plates. The plates are anchored to the vertebral immediately above and below the affected disc.

total shoulder replacement. Prosthetic replacement of the entire shoulder joint, including the humeral head and the glenoid fossa.

trabeculae carneae cordis. Bands of muscular tissue that line the walls of the ventricles in the heart.

trabeculectomy. Surgical incision between the anterior portion of the eye and the canal of Schlemm to drain the aqueous humor.

tracheostomy. Formation of a tracheal opening on the neck surface with tube insertion to allow for respiration in cases of obstruction or decreased patency. A tracheostomy may be planned or performed on an emergency basis for temporary or long-term use.

tracheotomy. Formation of a tracheal opening on the neck surface with tube insertion to allow for respiration in cases of obstruction or decreased patency. A tracheotomy may be planned or performed on an emergency basis for temporary or long-term use.

traction. Drawing out or holding tension on an area by applying a direct therapeutic pulling force.

transcranial magnetic stimulation. Application of electromagnetic energy to the brain through a coil placed on the scalp. The procedure stimulates cortical neurons and is intended to activate and normalize their processes.

transcription. Process by which messenger RNA is synthesized from a DNA template resulting in the transfer of genetic information from the DNA molecule to the messenger RNA.

translocation. Disconnection of all or part of a chromosome that reattaches to another position in the DNA sequence of the same or another chromosome. Often results in a reciprocal exchange of DNA sequences between two differently numbered chromosomes. May or may not result in a clinically significant loss of DNA.

trephine. 1) Specialized round saw for cutting circular holes in bone, especially the skull. 2) Instrument that removes small disc-shaped buttons of corneal tissue for transplanting.

tricuspid atresia. Congenital absence of the valve that may occur with other defects, such as atrial septal defect, pulmonary atresia, and transposition of great vessels.

turbinates. Scroll or shell-shaped elevations from the wall of the nasal cavity, the inferior turbinate being a separate bone, while the superior and middle turbinates are of the ethmoid bone.

tympanic membrane. Thin, sensitive membrane across the entrance to the middle ear that vibrates in response to sound waves, allowing the waves to be transmitted via the ossicular chain to the internal ear.

tympanoplasty. Surgical repair of the structures of the middle ear, including the eardrum and the three small bones, or ossicles.

unlisted procedure. Procedural descriptions used when the overall procedure and outcome of the procedure are not adequately described by an existing procedure code. Such codes are used as a last resort and only when there is not a more appropriate procedure code.

ureterorrhaphy. Surgical repair using sutures to close an open wound or injury of the ureter.

vagotomy. Division of the vagus nerves, interrupting impulses resulting in lower gastric acid production and hastening gastric emptying. Used in the treatment of chronic gastric, pyloric, and duodenal ulcers that can cause severe pain and difficulties in eating and sleeping.

variant. Nucleotide deviation from the normal sequence of a region. Variations are usually either substitutions or deletions. Substitution variations are the result of one nucleotide taking the place of another. A deletion occurs when one or more nucleotides are left out. In some cases, several in a reasonably close proximity on the same chromosome in a DNA strand. These variations result in amino acid changes in the protein made by the gene. However, the term variant does not itself imply a functional change. Intron variations are usually described in one of two ways: 1) the changed nucleotide is defined by a plus or a minus sign indicating the position relative to the first or last nucleotide to the intron, or 2) the second variant description is indicated relative to the last nucleotide of the preceding exon or first nucleotide of the following exon.

vascular family. Group of vessels (family) that branch from the aorta or vena cava. At each branching, the vascular order increases by one. The first order vessel is the primary branch off the aorta or vena cava. The second order vessel branches from the first order, the third order branches from the second order, and any further branching is beyond the third order. For example, for the inferior vena cava, the common iliac artery is a first order vessel. The internal and external iliac arteries are second order vessels, as they each originate from the first order common iliac artery. The external iliac artery extends directly from the common iliac artery and the internal iliac artery bifurcates from the common iliac artery. A third order vessel from the external iliac artery is the inferior epigastric artery and a third order vessel from the internal iliac artery is the obturator artery. Note orders are not always identical bilaterally (e.g., the left common carotid artery is a first order and the right common carotid is a second order. Synonym(s): vascular origins and distributions.

vasectomy. Surgical procedure involving the removal of all or part of the vas deferens, usually performed for sterilization or in conjunction with a prostatectomy.

vena cava interruption. Procedure that places a filter device, called an umbrella or sieve, within the large vein returning deoxygenated blood to the heart to prevent pulmonary embolism caused by clots.

ventricular assist device. Temporary measure used to support the heart by substituting for left and/or right heart function. The device replaces the work of the left and/or right ventricle when a patient has a damaged or weakened heart. A left ventricular assist device (VAD) helps the heart pump blood through the rest of the body. A right VAD helps the heart pump blood to the lungs to become oxygenated again. Catheters are inserted to circulate the blood through external tubing to a pump machine located outside of the body and back to the correct artery.

ventricular septal defect. Congenital cardiac anomaly resulting in a continual opening in the septum between the ventricles that, in severe cases, causes oxygenated blood to flow back into the lungs, resulting in pulmonary hypertension.

vertebral interspace. Non-bony space between two adjacent vertebral bodies that contains the cushioning intervertebral disk.

volar. Palm of the hand (palmar) or sole of the foot (plantar).

Waterston procedure. Type of aortopulmonary shunting done to increase pulmonary blood flow. The ascending aorta is anastomosed to the right pulmonary artery.

Wharton's ducts. Salivary ducts below the mandible.

wick catheter. Device used to monitor interstitial fluid pressure, and sometimes used intraoperatively during fasciotomy procedures to evaluate the effectiveness of the decompression.

wound closure. Closure or repair of a wound created surgically or due to trauma (e.g., laceration). The closure technique depends on the type, site, and depth of the defect. Consideration is also given to cosmetic and functional outcome. A single layer closure involves approximation of the edges of the wound. The second type of closure involves closing the one or more deeper layers of tissue prior to skin closure. The most complex type of closure may include techniques such as debridement or undermining, which involves manipulation of tissue around the wound to allow the skin to cover the wound. The AMA CPT® book defines these as Simple, Intermediate and Complex repair.

xenograft. Tissue that is nonhuman and harvested from one species and grafted to another. Pigskin is the most common xenograft for human skin and is applied to a wound as a temporary closure until a permanent option is performed.

z-plasty. Plastic surgery technique used primarily to release tension or elongate contractured scar tissue in which a Z-shaped incision is made with the middle line of the Z crossing the area of greatest tension. The triangular flaps are then rotated so that they cross the incision line in the opposite direction, creating a reversed Z.

ZPIC. Zone Program Integrity Contractor. CMS contractor that replaced the existing Program Safeguard Contractors (PSC). Contractors are responsible for ensuring the integrity of all Medicare-related claims under Parts A and B (hospital, skilled nursing, home health, provider, and durable medical equipment claims), Part C (Medicare Advantage health plans), Part D (prescription drug plans), and coordination of Medicare-Medicaid data matches (Medi-Medi).

Appendix N — Listing of Sensory, Motor, and Mixed Nerves

This list contains the sensory, motor, and mixed nerves assigned to each nerve conduction study to improve coding accuracy. Each nerve makes up one single unit of service.

Motor Nerves Assigned to Codes 95907-95913

I. Upper extremity, cervical plexus, and brachial plexus motor nerves
   - A. Axillary motor nerve to the deltoid
   - B. Long thoracic motor nerve to the serratus anterior
   - C. Median nerve
     1. Median motor nerve to the abductor pollicis brevis
     2. Median motor nerve, anterior interosseous branch, to the flexor pollicis longus
     3. Median motor nerve, anterior interosseous branch, to the pronator quadratus
     4. Median motor nerve to the first lumbrical
     5. Median motor nerve to the second lumbrical
   - D. Musculocutaneous motor nerve to the biceps brachii
   - E. Radial nerve
     1. Radial motor nerve to the extensor carpi ulnaris
     2. Radial motor nerve to the extensor digitorum communis
     3. Radial motor nerve to the extensor indicis proprius
     4. Radial motor nerve to the brachioradialis
   - F. Suprascapular nerve
     1. Suprascapular motor nerve to the supraspinatus
     2. Suprascapular motor nerve to the infraspinatus
   - G. Thoracodorsal motor nerve to the latissimus dorsi
   - H. Ulnar nerve
     1. Ulnar motor nerve to the abductor digiti minimi
     2. Ulnar motor nerve to the palmar interosseous
     3. Ulnar motor nerve to the first dorsal interosseous
     4. Ulnar motor nerve to the flexor carpi ulnaris
   - I. Other

II. Lower extremity motor nerves
   - A. Femoral motor nerve to the quadriceps
     1. Femoral motor nerve to vastus medialis
     2. Femoral motor nerve to vastus lateralis
     3. Femoral motor nerve to vastus intermedius
     4. Femoral motor nerve to rectus femoris
   - B. Ilioinguinal motor nerve
   - C. Peroneal (fibular) nerve
     1. Peroneal motor nerve to the extensor digitorum brevis
     2. Peroneal motor nerve to the peroneus brevis
     3. Peroneal motor nerve to the peroneus longus
     4. Peroneal motor nerve to the tibialis anterior
   - D. Plantar motor nerve
   - E. Sciatic nerve
   - F. Tibial nerve
     1. Tibial motor nerve, inferior calcaneal branch, to the abductor digiti minimi
     2. Tibial motor nerve, medial plantar branch, to the abductor hallucis
     3. Tibial motor nerve, lateral plantar branch, to the flexor digiti minimi brevis
   - G. Other

III. Cranial nerves and trunk
   - A. Cranial nerve VII (facial motor nerve)
     1. Facial nerve to the frontalis
     2. Facial nerve to the nasalis
     3. Facial nerve to the orbicularis oculi
     4. Facial nerve to the orbicularis oris
   - B. Cranial nerve XI (spinal accessory motor nerve)
   - C. Cranial nerve XII (hypoglossal motor nerve)
   - D. Intercostal motor nerve
   - E. Phrenic motor nerve to the diaphragm
   - F. Recurrent laryngeal nerve
   - G. Other

IV. Nerve Roots
   - A. Cervical nerve root stimulation
     1. Cervical level 5 (C5)
     2. Cervical level 6 (C6)
     3. Cervical level 7 (C7)
     4. Cervical level 8 (C8)
   - B. Thoracic nerve root stimulation
     1. Thoracic level 1 (T1)
     2. Thoracic level 2 (T2)
     3. Thoracic level 3 (T3)
     4. Thoracic level 4 (T4)
     5. Thoracic level 5 (T5)
     6. Thoracic level 6 (T6)
     7. Thoracic level 7 (T7)
     8. Thoracic level 8 (T8)
     9. Thoracic level 9 (T9)
     10. Thoracic level 10 (T10)
     11. Thoracic level 11 (T11)
     12. Thoracic level 12 (T12)
   - C. Lumbar nerve root stimulation
     1. Lumbar level 1 (L1)
     2. Lumbar level 2 (L2)
     3. Lumbar level 3 (L3)
     4. Lumbar level 4 (L4)
     5. Lumbar level 5 (L5)
   - D. Sacral nerve root stimulation
     1. Sacral level 1 (S1)
     2. Sacral level 2 (S2)
     3. Sacral level 3 (S3)
     4. Sacral level 4 (S4)

Sensory and Mixed Nerves Assigned to Codes 95907–95913

I. Upper extremity sensory and mixed nerves
  A. Lateral antebrachial cutaneous sensory nerve
  B. Medial antebrachial cutaneous sensory nerve
  C. Medial brachial cutaneous sensory nerve
  D. Median nerve
    1. Median sensory nerve to the first digit
    2. Median sensory nerve to the second digit
    3. Median sensory nerve to the third digit
    4. Median sensory nerve to the fourth digit
    5. Median palmar cutaneous sensory nerve
    6. Median palmar mixed nerve
  E. Posterior antebrachial cutaneous sensory nerve
  F. Radial sensory nerve
    1. Radial sensory nerve to the base of the thumb
    2. Radial sensory nerve to digit 1
  G. Ulnar nerve
    1. Ulnar dorsal cutaneous sensory nerve
    2. Ulnar sensory nerve to the fourth digit
    3. Ulnar sensory nerve to the fifth digit
    4. Ulnar palmar mixed nerve
  H. Intercostal sensory nerve
  I. Other

II. Lower extremity sensory and mixed nerves
  A. Lateral femoral cutaneous sensory nerve
  B. Medical calcaneal sensory nerve
  C. Medial femoral cutaneous sensory nerve
  D. Peroneal nerve
    1. Deep peroneal sensory nerve
    2. Superficial peroneal sensory nerve, medial dorsal cutaneous branch
    3. Superficial peroneal sensory nerve, intermediate dorsal cutaneous branch
  E. Posterior femoral cutaneous sensory nerve
  F. Saphenous nerve
    1. Saphenous sensory nerve (distal technique)
    2. Saphenous sensory nerve (proximal technique)
  G. Sural nerve
    1. Sural sensory nerve, lateral dorsal cutaneous branch
    2. Sural sensory nerve
  H. Tibial sensory nerve (digital nerve to toe 1)
  I. Tibial sensory nerve (medial plantar nerve)
  J. Tibial sensory nerve (lateral plantar nerve)
  K. Other

III. Head and trunk sensory nerves
  A. Dorsal nerve of the penis
  B. Greater auricular nerve
  C. Ophthalmic branch of the trigeminal nerve
  D. Pudendal sensory nerve
  E. Suprascapular sensory nerves
  F. Other

In the following table, the reasonable maximum number of studies per diagnostic category is listed that allows for a physician or other qualified health care professional to obtain a diagnosis for 90 percent of patients with that same final diagnosis. The numbers denote the suggested number of studies, although the decision is up to the provider.

Type of Study/Maximum Number of Studies

Indication	Limbs Studied by Needle EMG (95860–95864, 95867–95870, 95885–95887)	Nerve Conduction Studies (Total nerves studied, 95907-95913)	Neuromuscular Junction Testing (Repetitive Stimulation 95937)
Carpal Tunnel (Unilateral)	1	7	—
Carpal Tunnel (Bilateral)	2	10	—
Radiculopathy	2	7	—
Mononeuropathy	1	8	—
Polyneuropathy/Mononeuropathy Multiplex	3	10	—
Myopathy	2	4	2
Motor Neuronopathy (e.g., ALS)	4	6	2
Plexopathy	2	12	—
Neuromuscular Junction	2	4	3
Tarsal Tunnel Syndrome (Unilateral)	1	8	—
Tarsal Tunnel Syndrome (Bilateral)	2	11	—
Weakness, Fatigue, Cramps, or Twitching (Focal)	2	7	2
Weakness, Fatigue, Cramps, or Twitching (General)	4	8	2
Pain, Numbness, or Tingling (Unilateral)	1	9	—
Pain, Numbness, or Tingling (Bilateral)	2	12	—

Notes

Notes